**LifeExtension®**

# Disease
# Prevention
# and
# Treatment

## Fifth Edition

130 Evidence-Based Protocols to
Combat the Diseases of Aging

*Based on Thousands of Scientific Articles
and the Clinical Experience of Physicians
from Around the World*

**LifeExtension®**

**Editorial Staff**
*Chief Editor*: Blake Gossard
*Managing Editor*: Lori Feldman RD, LD, CCRC

**Scientific Staff**
*Scientific Director*: Kira Schmid, ND
*Vice President of Product Innovation & Scientific Development*: Luke Huber, ND, MBA

**Page Design and Production**
Graphic World, Inc.

**Cover Design**
Carlos Macedo

This information (and any accompanying printed material) is not intended to replace the attention or advice of a physician or other qualified health care professional. Anyone who wishes to embark on any dietary, drug, exercise, or other lifestyle change intended to prevent or treat a specific disease or condition should first consult with and seek clearance from a physician or other qualified health care professional. Pregnant women in particular should seek the advice of a physician before using any protocol listed in this book. The protocols described in this book are for adults only, unless otherwise specified. Product labels may contain important safety information and the most recent product information provided by the product manufacturers should be carefully reviewed prior to use to verify the dose, administration, and contraindications. National, state, and local laws may vary regarding the use and application of many of the treatments discussed. The reader assumes the risk of any injuries. The authors and publishers, their affiliates and assigns are not liable for any injury and/or damage to persons arising from this publication and expressly disclaim responsibility for any adverse effects resulting from the use of the information in this book.

The information published in the protocols is only as current as the day the manuscript was sent to the printer. The protocols raise many issues that are subject to change as new data emerge. None of our suggested protocol regimens can guarantee a cure. The publisher has not performed independent verification of the data contained herein, and expressly disclaims responsibility for any error in the literature, transcription, or typography. The most current protocols are available at **www.lef.org**.

1-800-544-4440

FIFTH EDITION

ISBN 978-0-9658777-8-7

# TABLE OF CONTENTS

# OPENING REMARKS FROM THE FOUNDERS OF LIFE EXTENSION FOUNDATION...

## *Why There Are Not <u>More</u> Cures!*

Once you or a loved one is stricken with a serious illness, all other issues become largely irrelevant. Your only concern is whether a nontoxic *cure* is available.

Unlike rapid advances occurring in other technologies, *medical progress* is brutally hindered by excessive bureaucracy.

The American public does not yet comprehend the lethal consequences of today's regulatory barriers. This oversight turns into harsh reality when one is diagnosed with an illness for which there is no effective treatment.

We at Life Extension® are involved in a relentless campaign to alert policymakers and the public about the urgent need to *accelerate* the introduction of new therapies.

This book is dedicated to enlightening readers about documented methods of protecting against disease that are *overlooked* by the medical establishment.

In this process, we also seek to convey a message in this book about the vast number of life-saving techniques that are being repressed by physician *apathy* and governmental *overregulation*.

Failure to meaningfully *reform* the way health care is approached will result in *catastrophic losses* of human life. This is no longer just the opinion of health freedom activists, but also the current and former *commissioners of the Food and Drug Administration (FDA)*!

## FDA ASSAILED BY ITS OWN LEADERS

Since *1980*, we at *Life Extension* have been harshly critical of the FDA's drug approval process, arguing that medical innovation has been suffocated by *high costs* and *bureaucratic uncertainties*.

An increasing number of respected individuals are agreeing that delaying lifesaving therapies can no longer be tolerated, including former *FDA Commissioner Andrew von Eschenbach*.

Dr. von Eschenbach is a former director of the National Cancer Institute and served as FDA Commissioner from 2005 to 2009.[1] He authored an editorial published in *The Wall Street Journal* that was critical of the FDA's ability to evaluate and approve new life-saving therapies.[2]

The editorial opened by Dr. von Eschenbach stating:

> **We stand on the cusp of a revolution in health care. Advances in molecular medicine will allow us to develop powerful new treatments that can cure or even prevent diseases like Alzheimer's and cancer.**[2]

"What's missing," according to Dr. von Eschenbach, "is a modernized Food and Drug Administration that can rapidly and efficiently bring new discoveries to patients."[2]

Dr. von Eschenbach cited *current* FDA Commissioner Margaret Hamburg's concession before Congress that, "The FDA is relying on 20th-century regulatory science to evaluate 21st century medical products."[3]

The most compelling arguments Dr. von Eschenbach made for meaningful reform were:

> The FDA should approve drugs based on safety and leave efficacy testing for post-market studies. Congress can ensure that the FDA serves as a bridge—not a barrier—to cutting-edge technologies.[2]

Said differently, once a potentially effective therapy has been cleared for safety, it should be made *immediately* available to human beings who will otherwise suffer and die.

Brain tumor patients, for example, don't have years to wait for FDA-mandated efficacy studies. They need rapid access to new therapies that offer some hope of saving their lives.

## BRIDGING THE FDA'S "DEATH VALLEY"

Newly diagnosed cancer patients are usually given several treatment choices, all laden with guaranteed side effects with no promise of a cure or even a significant remission.

For most types of cancer, progress has been excruciatingly slow, even though there are more scientific studies being published about cancer now than at any time in human history. The term "death valley" is increasingly being used to describe the gap that separates what is discovered in the scientific setting from what actually makes it into patients' bodies.

The sad fact is there are so many bureaucratic roadblocks that potentially effective therapies aren't making it out of the laboratory setting. The high costs of conducting human efficacy trials deny smaller companies equal opportunity to bring what may be superior medications to market.

Dr. von Eschenbach's proposal to allow new therapies on the market as soon as *safety* is established would liberate many promising therapies currently trapped in the FDA's oppressive quagmire.

## WHAT TO DO *BEFORE* MEANINGFUL REFORM OCCURS

A surprising number of effective therapies are already available to better treat the diseases of aging.

In the treatment of many *cancers*, for instance, the proper use of the drugs *metformin*, *aspirin*, and *cimetidine* markedly improves clinical outcomes. (See Appendix A at the back of this book.)

None of these drugs, however, are *approved* by the FDA to treat cancer, despite hundreds of studies published in the world's most prestigious scientific journals documenting their safety and efficacy. Oncologists read about the off-label use of these drugs in their own journals, yet almost universally fail to prescribe them.

*Disease Prevention and Treatment* breaks down these bureaucratic barriers to enlighten readers about proven methods to mitigate serious disease and enhance the odds of achieving a meaningful response or outright cure.

The cost of researching, analyzing, compiling, and writing this book totals many *millions of dollars*. We know of no other organization that has come close to expending these kinds of resources to spare human beings needless suffering and death.

*Disease Prevention and Treatment* was not produced to generate a financial profit. The objective is to communicate in user-friendly form, data from peer-reviewed scientific publications that is not effectively being used to save human lives.

June 2013

William Faloon

Saul Kent

*Founders of the Life Extension Foundation (1980)*

# DON'T BLAME THE DOCTORS
## *Preamble*

There was a time when medical doctors were respected with resolute trust. This physician esteem was well deserved, since those who contracted illness often had nowhere else to turn.

In conventional medicine's bygone golden era, doctors routinely delivered state-of-the-art care. One reason yesteryear's physicians kept abreast of new developments was that medical progress back then was very slow. In other words, it was not particularly difficult to prescribe the best standard treatment, since medical advancements occurred at such a sluggish pace.

Times have changed.

For any given disease, there are more new scientific studies published in a *month* than previously came out in a *year*. It has become *impossible* for practicing physicians to stay current with what has become an avalanche of new research findings.

In today's world, scientific information is plentiful. This creates an unsettling predicament for those suffering from a serious illness. The dilemma is that a significant amount of time and expertise is required to review complex medical literature and then translate that data into a practical treatment plan.

Gathering information that pertains to any given disease often entails spending hundreds of hours poring over thousands of scientific reports. While the reliability of these reports varies, the undeniable fact is that the proper utilization of these data could mean the difference between life and death for those with severe disease.

The difficulty is that even with advanced electronic communications and data mining, doctors lack the time to analyze every new study published in the world's medical journals. The quandary faced by patients is that their very lives may be at stake, yet up until now, they have had nowhere to turn to uncover novel therapies that could result in a significant improvement in their health and wellbeing.

Since 1980, the Life Extension Foundation® has identified enormous amounts of evidence indicating that effective, but overlooked approaches already exist to mitigate many of today's lethal diseases. This abundance of new scientific findings has created the need to publish an updated edition of our *Disease Prevention and Treatment* reference book.

The purpose of publishing this fifth edition of *Disease Prevention and Treatment* is to break down the barriers of ignorance that result in unnecessary suffering and death. Life Extension has spent tens of thousands of hours reviewing the scientific literature in order to develop the novel approaches to disease prevention and treatment you are about to read.

# DEADLY HEALTH CARE
## *Foreword*

For decades, those involved in alternative medicine have criticized mainstream doctors for failing to integrate natural approaches into conventional treatment regimens.

A stark example of this neglect can be seen with the millions of prescriptions written each year for cholesterol-lowering statin drugs. It was long ago established that the very mechanism by which statin drugs inhibit cholesterol production also interferes with the natural synthesis of *coenzyme Q10* in the body.

For those who don't know, *coenzyme Q10* is required by virtually every cell to support vital life functions. A deficiency of coenzyme Q10 predisposes aging people to a host of degenerative disorders, including heart failure, which happens to be one of the diseases that statins are prescribed for.[4,5]

Despite a huge body of scientific literature documenting the critical importance of coenzyme Q10, few doctors recommend it to their patients when prescribing statin drugs. The result is an epidemic deficiency of coenzyme Q10, especially in aging individuals taking statin drugs.

Few doctors understand the critical importance of coenzyme Q10 in maintaining cardiac, renal, immunologic, and neurologic health. Intriguing studies indicate that coenzyme Q10 may also be of benefit in cancer prevention and treatment.[4,5]

So in America, we have an aging population that is increasingly being prescribed statin drugs, but not coenzyme Q10. Is it any wonder that despite record amounts of money being spent on health care, life expectancy rates are not proportionally climbing?

## CONVENTIONAL CARE IS UNIFORMLY MEDIOCRE

While the failure of mainstream doctors to incorporate proven natural therapies into their practice has long been known, still more disturbing are reports that even accepted conventional treatments are often not properly administered to those in need.

According to a report published in the *New England Journal of Medicine*, medical care in the United States is uniformly *mediocre*. This report was based on one of the largest studies ever conducted of health care quality in the United States.[6]

The findings from this study revealed that all Americans—rich, poor, black, white—get roughly equal medical treatment and it is consistently *mediocre* for all groups. Even by today's pathetic conventional standards, which don't incorporate the novel findings revealed in this book, patients were found to receive proper care only 55% of the time.[6]

This *New England Journal of Medicine* study brought to light a well-founded fear that no one is safe from poor quality medical care. The study used conventionally accepted criteria to evaluate the care received for 30 common disorders, including high blood pressure, diabetes, and heart disease.[6] The researchers found that it is almost a coin flip as to whether patients get what conventional medicine recommends as proper health care, even though these standard treatments are widely known.

If you suffer from any one of the 130 health concerns covered in this book, you will learn much of what conventional medicine is supposed to be doing, plus a whole lot more that is documented in the scientific literature, but remains largely ignored by mainstream practitioners.

## UNITED STATES LEADS IN MEDICAL ERRORS

It is bad enough that today's medical system provides only 55% of patients with proper care.[6] What has patients even more concerned are the well-publicized risks of medical error when any procedure is performed.

According to a survey, the United States leads six first-world countries in medical errors. Findings from this study showed a startling 34% of Americans reported at least one medical error occurring in the previous 2 years.[7] These included receiving a wrong drug, incorrect treatment, incorrect test results, and delayed test results.

The report stated that while Americans spent *more* for health care than countries such as Germany, England, Australia, Canada, and New Zealand, *"the United States often ranks last or tied for last for safety, efficiency, and access."*[7]

Another study found that if the health care system in the United States performed as efficiently as that of countries such as France, Japan, and Australia, *101 000 preventable* deaths could be avoided each year.[8] A 2012 analysis revealed the rate of preventable deaths is falling twice as fast in the United Kingdom as in the United States, largely due to failure of the U.S. health care system to efficiently treat cardiovascular diseases.[9]

## EXPOSING THESE MEDICAL ATROCITIES

The medical establishment's admission of its own ineptitudes is a frightening revelation for those who depend on mainstream physicians to keep them alive. Yet a report published by the Life Extension Foundation reveals a far more pervasive epidemic of harm inflicted by conventional medicine.

For the past four decades, Life Extension Foundation has cited a myriad of statistics to show how many Americans needlessly suffer and die at the hands of the medical establishment. No one, however, had ever analyzed and combined *all* of the published literature dealing with injuries and deaths caused by government-protected medicine.

That changed when a group of researchers meticulously reviewed the published statistical evidence and compiled a startling fully referenced report. According to the data compiled by these researchers, the number of people having adverse reactions to prescribed drugs in the hospital is 2.2 million per year. The number of unnecessary antibiotics prescribed annually for viral infections is 20 million per year. The number of unnecessary medical and surgical procedures performed annually is 7.5 million per year. The number of people exposed to unnecessary hospitalization annually is 8.9 million per year.[10–17]

The most stunning statistic, however, is the total number of deaths caused by conventional medicine. According to the statistics compiled by these researchers, an astounding *783 936* Americans die each year as a result of the medical care they receive. It is now evident that today's medical system is the *leading cause of death and injury* in the United States.[10–17] By contrast, 577 190 deaths due to cancer and about 600 000 due to heart disease have been estimated for 2012.[18,19]

Despite the overwhelming size of this comprehensive exposé of conventional medicine, it was published in its entirety in *Life Extension* magazine.[17] By revealing these shocking statistics in painstaking detail, a basis is provided for competent and compassionate medical professionals to recognize the inadequacies of today's system and at least attempt to institute meaningful reforms.

In recognition of the deadly dangers posed by conventional medicine, the Life Extension Foundation has published this fifth edition of *Disease Prevention and Treatment*. It is our sincere belief that the information contained in this book will protect tens of thousands of human beings against the adverse consequences posed by today's deadly health care system.

# WHY DID WE PUBLISH THIS BOOK?
## *Introduction*

At any given time, hundreds of different health books are offered to the American public. Most of these books provide some good information, but none adequately addresses the archaic state of medical practice that patients with serious disease are confronted with.

As the underlying mechanisms of diseases are better identified, more books are authored that provide the lay reader with partial solutions to incurable diseases. The problem is that to success-fully overcome a serious disorder, a comprehensive approach is required that must address *all* of the causative factors involved in the disease process.

While superficial treatments might provide some relief, they almost always fail to provide long-term remission or cure. One example of this is *cancer* treatment. In most cases, there is only *one* opportunity to completely eradicate a tumor from one's body. If the initial treatment protocol fails, the residual cancer cells often develop survival characteristics that make them resistant to even the most aggressive therapies.

Despite having the knowledge that cancer cells should be attacked using multimodal therapies to increase the odds of a complete eradication, most oncologists fail to implement a comprehensive individualized treatment protocol. They instead rely on "one-size-fits-all" recipes that were long ago shown to have a high failure rate.

Another illustration of the inadequacy of both conventional and alternative medicine can be seen in the treatment of *atherosclerosis*, a major cause of *heart attack* and *stroke*. Atherosclerosis has more than 17 readily identifiable causes, yet most cardiologists fail to test their patient's blood for all of these proven risk factors, let alone take aggressive steps to correct them. Those who suffer ministrokes or angina are often left to fend for themselves, while proven ways to reduce risks of future occurrences are ignored.

From the quality-of-life-robbing effects of depression, to the DNA damage inflicted by viral infections, to the degenerative suffering endured by those with age-related disease, proven rem-edies are available, but egregiously underutilized. *Disease Prevention and Treatment* was written to provide innovative solutions to *130* common health concerns that have not been adequately addressed by mainstream physicians.

## WHY DOCTORS NEED THIS BOOK

We live in a world where medical discoveries seem to be routine events. The sheer volume of new findings, however, has inundated practicing physicians. While the media superficially re-ports on a few discoveries, the vast majority of medical breakthroughs remain buried in the mil-lions of pages of scientific journals that are published each year.

When medical discoveries are not delivered to patients, the result is less-than-optimal care. For patients suffering from a non life-threatening condition, this absence of applied knowledge means their agony may not subside. If they suffer from a serious disorder, the result of the physician not taking advantage of current treatment findings can result in premature death.

In order to help bridge the gap between scientific research findings and conventional medical practice, *Disease Prevention and Treatment* was written not only for the lay reader, but also for physicians who seek to provide more comprehensive care to their patients.

We express our sincerest gratitude to the numerous physicians who have used the information published in previous editions of this book to alleviate human suffering.

## THE 33-YEAR HISTORY OF THIS BOOK

Starting in the 1970s, the founders of a nonprofit group called The Life Extension Foundation began to uncover information that could be used to improve patient outcomes and, in many cases, prevent people from dying prematurely. Conveying these data to those with health problems often resulted in significant improvements in their condition.

As Life Extension's founders delved deeper into the scientific literature, it became clear that many people were dying from medical ignorance. This startling revelation did not go totally unnoticed. A growing number of individuals began asking the Life Extension founders for help when confronted with difficult-to-treat disorders. As more cases were presented, it became blatantly apparent that a lethal communication gap exists between scientists making discoveries in the laboratory and physicians in the clinical setting.

While intriguing discoveries are published in prestigious medical journals today, little of this information is utilized to actually save human lives. It's as if a brick wall separates newly discovered scientific solutions from those in critical need of this knowledge. The mission of *Disease Prevention and Treatment* is to tear down the walls of ignorance and apathy that have become the underlying reasons why human beings needlessly suffer and die today.

A classic historical example of scientific advance being overruled by bureaucracy occurred when a young Hungarian doctor named *Ignaz Semmelweis* discovered that a contagious disease was being transmitted to hospital patients because medical personnel failed to wash their hands.

In the 19th century, tens of thousands of women died every year from puerperal sepsis (childbed fever). The reason for this epidemic was that doctors were performing autopsies and then conducting vaginal exams with their hands covered with decomposing necrotic tissue. Dr. Semmelweis observed that women who used midwives instead of doctors had low rates of childbed fever.

To test these observations, Semmelweis implemented a policy in his department that required doctors to wash their hands with disinfectant prior to attending to patients. Mortality rates from childbed fever immediately declined from about *18%* to about *1–2%*.[20]

When Semmelweis published his meticulous findings about the importance of hand washing, the medical community reacted with hostility or dismissal. The prevailing belief at the time was that childbed fever was caused by bad air. After strident attempts to persuade skeptics, Semmelweis was committed to an insane asylum where he died at age 47.

It is regrettable that even today hospitals are still failing to follow proper sanitary and sterile techniques. The result is that too many hospitalized patients needlessly contract infectious diseases, some of which are lethal.

## WHAT TO DO IF YOU ARE HOSPITALIZED

Hospital confinement exposes one to increased risk of contracting bacterial infections that are sometimes antibiotic-resistant. What few people understand is that the infectious bacterium does not always emanate from the hospital. It is often a bacterium that is in you already, but is kept in check by your healthy immune system.

In many cases, a *Staphylococcus* (staph) bacterium called S. *aureus* inhabits your nasal passages, and if the hospital swabs this area with an antimicrobial product called *mupirocin* upon admitting you, your risks of developing infection arising from nasal colonization with S. *aureus* are markedly reduced.

A *2010* report published in the *New England Journal of Medicine* referenced three studies (published in 1959, 2001, and 2004) that showed 80% of staph infections acquired in the hospital are endogenous, which means that these infections were caused by the patient's own bacterial contamination. This study showed that if a patient's nasal passages were decolonized with *mupirocin* applied twice daily for 5 days, combined with a *chlorhexidine* body wash, the risk of staph infection was reduced by nearly 60%.[21]

Despite these solid data showing dramatic reductions in hospital-acquired infections, too many hospitals *fail* to swab their patient's nasal passages twice daily with mupirocin combined with chlorhexidine body wash. If you are ever hospitalized, insist on it!

We at Life Extension strongly believe that the lethal combination of *insufficient vitamin D* (due to no sunlight exposure and no supplements given), *lack of sleep* (due to chronic hospital staff disturbance), and *nutrition deficit* (due to micronutrient-depleted food and stress-inducing commotion) conspire to rob hospitalized patients of immune function required to suppress bacteria carried in their own bodies.

It does not matter how many sanitary procedures an institution performs if the patient's *immune function* is being compromised by standard hospital practices. Anyone hospitalized for an extended period should take assertive measures to maintain immune function as most hospitals fail to pay attention to it. At a minimum, every hospitalized patient should immediately be given enough *vitamin D* to achieve optimal blood levels of over 50 ng/mL of *25-hydroxyvitamin D*.

A number of studies confirm the potent *antimicrobial* effects of *vitamin D*, making it essential for hospital-confined patients.[22,23]

## CRITERIA FOR INCLUSION IN THIS BOOK

Every day, many new studies are published in peer-reviewed journals that reveal better ways of preventing and treating disease. The Life Extension Foundation evaluates many of these studies for their value in health care and medicine. When sufficient evidence accumulates to validate a new approach, it is then considered for inclusion in Life Extension's ever-evolving disease prevention and treatment protocols.

Many of the therapies discussed in *Disease Prevention and Treatment* have not yet been accepted by mainstream medicine. This book was not published, however, to maintain the status quo of medical mediocrity.

This updated edition of *Disease Prevention and Treatment* has been published to highlight scientific findings that can be incorporated into treatment protocols that will save the lives of individuals who may otherwise perish as a result of indifference and unawareness.

## WHY THIS BOOK MAY BE MORE IMPORTANT THAN EVER...

### Not Enough Doctors!

The first edition of *Disease Prevention and Treatment* was published in 1996. A problem facing our health care system today makes it even more important that people empower themselves with knowledge to protect against disease.

As the population ages, demand for medical services is sharply escalating. Little has been done, however, to provide a corresponding increase in supply of health care providers. Increased demand without additional supply equals *shortages*.

When it comes to *shortages of medical services*, the tragic result is needless suffering and death.

As this book is being finalized, the Affordable Care Act is coming into force. This law is supposed to provide virtually every American with medical coverage. No one, however, knows where the *physicians* will come from to treat these "newly insured" individuals.[24]

In many parts of the country, hoards of the newly insured, along with people who are merely growing old, are creating *severe* physician shortages.[25]

### Doctor Shortages Not a New Problem

People exposed to conventional health care are aware that most doctors lack the time to provide optimal care. This is evidenced by delays in getting appointments, jammed waiting rooms, and long hold-ups in exam rooms.

Some physicians are not taking new patients, while others crowd whoever calls into a clogged schedule that does not allow sufficient time to treat each patient.

You can drive your car in for a "10-minute oil change," but you are unlikely to get that much time with most physicians, even though your life may be on the line.

As more scientific advances occur in the medical arena, the inability of physicians to devote enough time to their patients will result in greater numbers of tragic outcomes.

Warnings of *physician shortages* are no longer confined to Life Extension's publications. These dire predictions are now coming from the medical establishment itself!

## The Frightening Numbers

The *Association of American Medical Colleges* estimates that within 2 years the United States will have 62 900 *fewer* doctors than needed. By 2025, the shortfall of doctors will exceed *100 000*.[26]

Mainstream experts, including many who supported the Affordable Care Act, say there is little that anyone can do to close the gap as the law will extend coverage to about *30 million* Americans.

It typically takes a decade to train a doctor. Even if medical schools significantly increased enrollment, they would not come close to generating enough physicians to treat the newly insured *and* the rapidly aging population.

High tuition costs, stringent academic requirements, and brutal internships create barriers that limit the supply of new doctors. The Harvard School of Medicine, for example, accepts only 165 new admissions each year, and not all these students graduate into medical practice.

Some in the mainstream describe a *doctor shortage* as an "invisible problem." Patients still get care, they say, but the process is often slow and difficult. It can force patients to drive long distances, languish on waiting lists, overuse emergency rooms, and even forgo care. Those who delay treatment place an even greater future burden on what is already a broken sick-care system.

Even more ominous for many of the "newly insured" is that since *2008*, more than *50%* of *primary care* doctors have stopped accepting new Medicaid patients.[27-29] The consequence will be that certain patients entitled to free health care may not find a willing physician.

To avoid this looming catastrophe of *doctor shortages*, radical changes must be made in the way sick-care is dispensed in the United States.

In the meantime, patients must empower themselves with more *knowledge* about medical problems that affect them. *Disease Prevention and Treatment* was written to provide individuals with practical information they can use to better protect against the onslaught of aging-related disease.

## Nearly Half of Doctors Already Suffering Burn Out

A national survey of physicians finds the prevalence of burnout is already "*alarming*."

The report describes the looming physician shortage as millions of "newly insured" crowd waiting rooms, but the report stated that *45.8%* of physicians already suffer from one or more symptoms of burnout.[30]

One doctor describes that being asked to see more patients, while not having enough time to devote to them makes one feel like "*being on a hamster wheel*."

Experts were surprised at the high rate of burnout in frontline physicians and stated that this will adversely affect patient outcomes and ultimately drive up costs, as sick people aren't being efficiently cured.[31]

When you develop a medical problem, you don't want your life to depend on a "burned-out" doctor. If adults acquire knowledge to better treat relatively simple problems such as elevated LDL, hypertension, and obesity, then the quality of care can increase as the patient load decreases.

## Penalties of Failing to Face Reality

The looming shortage of physicians will affect most everyone reading this book. It is just one symptom of a sick-care system plagued by *regulatory inefficiency*.

The best way of avoiding becoming a victim is to take aggressive care of your precious health every single day. *Comprehensive blood tests* performed annually and an at-home *blood pressure monitor* are two simple steps aging Americans can use to become "empowered patients," thereby not being 100% reliant on hurried physicians.

As you will read in the 130 chapters contained in this book, there is a lot you can do in cooperation with your physician to improve the quality of your health care, and thus reduce your odds of being victimized by the pending shortage of physicians.

# ACKNOWLEDGMENT

It is impossible to thank all the dedicated physicians, scientists, writers, editors, and Life Extension members who contributed to this work. Any attempt at a complete list of names would leave out many who informed us of research findings that represent essential elements of these protocols.

A common attribute of the people who contributed to this book is a passion for knowledge relating to biological mechanisms. It is this curiosity that motivates them to discover new methods of preventing and treating disease.

History describes medical pioneers who share common traits with those who contributed to this book. One such pioneer was *Antony van Leeuwenhoek*, a tradesman with no university degrees. This would normally have excluded him from the scientific community. Yet with skill, diligence, curiosity, and an open mind, Leeuwenhoek made some of the most important discoveries in the history of biology. Leeuwenhoek discovered bacteria, sperm cells, blood cells, microscopic nematodes and rotifers, and much more. His research findings were widely circulated and opened up an entire world of microscopic life to scientists.

What distinguished Leeuwenhoek was his desire to observe anything that could be placed under his lenses along with his ability to describe what he saw. Although Leeuwenhoek could not draw well, he hired an illustrator to prepare drawings of the things he saw to accompany his written descriptions.

In 1673, Leeuwenhoek began writing letters to the Royal Society of London, describing what he had seen with his microscopes. For the next 50 years he corresponded with the Royal Society. Leeuwenhoek's letters were eagerly awaited by scientists fascinated by the microscopic world.

Despite Leeuwenhoek's documenting the existence of microorganisms, it took several more centuries before physicians discerned that what Leeuwenhoek first observed under his microscope were the culprits behind the leading causes of death in those days, that is, bacterial infections.

Seven years before his death, Leeuwenhoek wrote the following to explain why he had devoted his life to making discoveries and disseminating his findings to the world:

> [M]y work, which I've done for a long time, was not pursued in order to gain the praise I now enjoy, but chiefly from a craving after knowledge, which I notice resides in me more than in most other men. And therewithal, whenever I found out anything remarkable, I have thought it my duty to put down my discovery on paper, so that all ingenious people might be informed thereof.
>
> Antony van Leeuwenhoek
> Letter of June 12, 1716

Other physicians and scientists throughout the ages have made groundbreaking discoveries that have propelled medical science forward.

Some of the most innovative minds in the history of medicine include Andreas Vesalius, a Flemish scientist who is considered the founder of modern human anatomy. Using dissection as his primary tool of investigation, Vesalius disproved numerous widely held but incorrect principles of anatomy that had been established by leading thinkers such as Galen and Aristotle. Vesalius showed that the heart had four chambers, the liver had two lobes, and that the blood vessels originated in the heart, not the liver, as was the current paradigm. In 1543, Vesalius published *On the Fabric of the Human Body*, a groundbreaking seven-volume work on human anatomy.

In the early 17th century, Dr. William Harvey described the detailed functions of the heart and circulatory system in his book, *On the Motion of the Heart*. While the prevailing theory of the time held that blood flow was caused by a sucking action of the heart and liver, William Harvey proposed that the heart acted like a pump to move blood throughout the body. Furthermore, he noted that blood flowed through the heart in two separate closed loops, with one connecting the circulatory system to the lungs, and the second causing blood flow to the body's organs and tissues. While his theories were initially attacked, Harvey's ideas were eventually accepted during his lifetime. William Harvey's elucidation of the functioning of the circulatory system has been dubbed the *"greatest medical achievement of all time."*

Some of the greatest scientists have reaped tremendous discoveries based on fortunate accidents. After noticing that he felt no pain from an injury when he was under the influence of ether at a party, Dr. Crawford Long developed the idea for surgical anesthesia in 1842. At that time, surgeries were traumatic for both patients and doctors, since patients were not sedated and often experienced unbearable pain. While doctors tried to relax their patients before surgery with alcohol or hypnotism, these methods did little to alleviate patients' agony. Crawford Long's discovery led the way for doctors to prevent their patients from feeling pain by using anesthesia during surgical procedures.

In the early 1900s, Ross Harrison developed a method for growing living cells outside of the body. This breakthrough led the way for the study of living organisms at the cellular and molecular levels and the development of vaccines, as well as investigations into the causes of maladies such as cancer and AIDS. Thanks to Ross Harrison's pioneering work in tissue culture, scientists have learned more about the mechanisms of disease in the last 50 years than in the previous 5000 years.

In the early 1950s, Maurice Williams isolated and studied a single fiber of DNA. His work paved the way for scientists James Watson and Frances Crick, who developed the double helix model of DNA. The elucidation of the structure of DNA has opened the door to the field of genetic research. The three scientists shared the Nobel Prize for their discoveries about the structure of DNA.

While many contributors to this book are highly credentialed physicians and scientists, they share with Leeuwenhoek and these other medical pioneers the craving for knowledge and desire to pass on their findings to others.

The innovative methods in *Disease Prevention and Treatment* stem from the desire of the Life Extension Foundation to inform the world about life-saving medical discoveries. Life Extension's objective is to do everything rational to keep you alive and healthy for as long as possible.

# A BIT OF MEDICAL HISTORY

**Louis Pasteur's theory of germs is ridiculous fiction.**

**Pierre Pachet, professor of physiology at Toulouse, 1872**

Acursory reading of medical history reveals startling examples of scientific discoveries that were suppressed by whatever "establishment" ruled the day. Rejecting new ideas has long been a common medical ideology, and those who became ill suffered horrendous deaths as a result.

One example of a scientific breakthrough ignored by the medical mainstream was the development of the smallpox vaccine. Smallpox was humankind's worst scourge, killing a larger percentage of populations than any other disease.

In 1789, a British doctor named Edward Jenner performed an experiment that laid the foundation for the eradication of smallpox. Jenner tested this hypothesis by inoculating his own son with material obtained from a cowpox lesion. Six weeks later, his son proved resistant when challenged with material from a smallpox lesion. The principle of immunization was thus established. This is an epic story when you realize that Edward Jenner's young son would likely have died if Jenner was wrong.

Putting his son's life on the line was only the first challenge Jenner faced in convincing the world to accept his new idea. An article sent to the Royal Medical Society in 1796 describing 13 successfully vaccinated persons was rejected. Jenner was forced to pay the costs of publishing his own treatise in 1798, but it was not well received. Jenner's work was subjected to fierce criticism by the medical profession. Some physicians were opposed to any new ideas, while others had financial interests in less effective forms of smallpox treatment. Jenner endured severe abuse from the press, religious groups, and the medical establishment. In today's regulated legal environment, Jenner almost certainly would have been jailed for practicing "unapproved" medicine.

Millions died of smallpox while medical authorities suppressed Jenner's life-saving discovery. Regrettably, the same situation exists currently vis-à-vis today's lethal diseases. Doctors routinely overlook novel therapies that have shown efficacy in published scientific studies. The result is that people die while potentially effective therapies wait to be accepted by the medical establishment or the FDA.

## THE DELAY IN RECOGNIZING PENICILLIN

There are people alive today who remember the carnage inflicted by bacterial infections such as tuberculosis, diphtheria, rheumatic fever, cholera, syphilis, pneumonia, and so on. Before the advent of antibiotics, agonizing deaths from bacterial infections were commonplace, especially in children.

In 1928, Dr. Alexander Fleming discovered penicillin. His work was published the very next year in the *British Journal of Experimental Pathology*. Nevertheless, the medical profession did not begin treating humans with this life-saving therapy until 1941, and the general population did not gain access to penicillin until 1946.

Millions of people suffered and died from bacterial/infectious diseases when a cure (penicillin) had already been discovered and published in a respected medical journal. For 18 years, millions of people could only watch helplessly as their loved ones suffered and died from diseases that penicillin could have cured.

Dr. Fleming and two other scientists who assisted in making sufficient quantities of penicillin to save human lives were awarded a Nobel Prize in 1945.

## THE COVER-UP OF THE DANGERS OF RADIOACTIVE FALLOUT

A U.S. government study released in the year 2002 says that radioactive fallout from nuclear weapons testing has caused at least 15 000 cancer deaths in the United States. This report was prepared as a joint effort by the *National Cancer Institute* and *Centers for Disease Control and Prevention*. Here is a chilling revelation from this report based on above-ground tests that took place between 1951 and 1962:

**Any person living in the contiguous United States since 1951 has been exposed to radioactive fallout, and all organs and tissues of the body have received some radiation exposure.**

For decades, the federal government contended that radioactive fallout from nuclear testing was harmless. Government propaganda films in the 1950s even showed American children playing in fresh radioactive ash to demonstrate that it was as "safe as snow."

Linus Pauling knew in the 1950s that radioactive fallout would cause cancer and other diseases in humans. Pauling joined with Albert Einstein and five others to form the Emergency Committee of Atomic Scientists. Their mission was to inform the public about the dangerous consequences that nuclear weapons and nuclear testing held for civilization.

In 1957, Pauling wrote a scientific appeal petition calling for a nuclear test ban treaty and distributed it throughout the scientific community. He soon gathered over 9000 signatures from 49 countries including 2000 American scientists. In 1958, Pauling presented the petition to the Secretary General of the United Nations, announcing that it represented the general consensus of the world's scientists and their plea for a ban on future nuclear testing.

Pauling gave hundreds of lectures against nuclear weapons testing and war. Unfortunately, he toured during a time of heightened Cold War suspicions and was marked a Communist supporter. The federal government refused to give Pauling a passport, thus denying him the opportunity to attend international scientific conventions. Pauling was twice subpoenaed to appear before congressional committees investigating anti-American activities to declare that he was not a Communist. On October 11, 1960, Pauling was threatened to be held in contempt of Congress because he refused to reveal the names of those who helped circulate his petition to ban nuclear testing.

Despite unrelenting government oppression, Pauling remained undaunted and continued his crusade by writing a draft resolution for a nuclear test ban treaty. He sent letters and copies of his resolution to both President Kennedy and Premier Khrushchev. The two superpowers agreed on a limited test ban treaty, one that was strikingly similar to Pauling's. The treaty went into effect on October 10, 1963, the very day it was announced that Pauling was to receive his second Nobel Prize.

By disseminating his knowledge about the lethal dangers of radioactive fallout, Pauling became a target of government harassment, persecution in the press, and charges of working for the enemy. He could have been jailed for refusing to provide Congress with the names of those involved in gathering more than 9000 signatures for the scientific petition to ban above-ground nuclear testing.

We now know that the government knew about the effects of above-ground nuclear testing, but covered it up. In the 1950s, for example, government officials notified suppliers of photographic film of expected fallout patterns so they could protect their film, but did not share the information with milk producers. Many children drank this radioactive contaminated milk.

Almost sixty years ago, Dr. Linus Pauling formulated a public health response to eradicate the problem caused by above-ground nuclear testing, but the federal government chose instead to persecute this brilliant scientist so that the practice of raining radioactive fallout throughout the United States could continue.

As has so often been the case when the government makes a criminal accusation against a political dissident (in this case, Linus Pauling), history later shows that it was the government itself who was involved in the sinister activities. What could be more anti-American than inflicting cancer on 15000 innocent people?

## WE CANNOT FORGET THE PAST, OR WE MAY HAVE TO RELIVE IT

Those with new ideas often face fierce attack by the establishment and the federal government. An example was the announcement that human embryonic stem cells had been produced and that there was an opportunity to cure many of today's lethal diseases.

You would think that the scientist who made this remarkable discovery, Dr. Mike West, would be proclaimed a hero. Instead, government leaders immediately vowed to pass new laws to make it a crime to create embryonic stem cells for therapeutic purposes.

The concern of the Life Extension Foundation is that only a precious few brilliant minds like Edward Jenner, Alexander Fleming, and Linus Pauling are ever born. When Linus Pauling stated that radioactive fallout caused cancer in humans, he was ridiculed, persecuted, and almost incarcerated. Pauling has now been proven right. This vindication does nothing for the 15000 Americans who have perished from radioactive fallout-induced cancer.

Today, there are pockets of exceptional intelligence that are stifled by bureaucratic red tape. In order to create the scientific renaissance needed to radically extend the healthy human life span, the barriers that suppress implementation of new ideas must be broken down.

This book is dedicated to eradicating the ignorance that is causing humans to suffer and die from diseases that may already have cures, or at least palliative therapies. Almost every therapy discussed in this book has been documented extensively by peer-reviewed, published studies from medical journals around the world. Despite this scientific evidence, the medical establishment largely ignores many of these therapies.

**Each progressive spirit is opposed by a thousand mediocre minds appointed to guard the past.**

**Maurice Maeterlinck**

**References** available at: www.lef.org/dpt5/fm

# SCIENTIFIC ADVISORY BOARD

**Aubrey de Grey, PhD**, is a biomedical gerontologist and Editor-in-Chief of Rejuvenation Research, the world's highest-impact peer-reviewed journal focused on intervention in aging. He received his BA and PhD from the University of Cambridge in 1985 and 2000, respectively. Dr. de Grey is a fellow of both the Gerontological Society of America and the American Aging Association, and sits on the editorial and scientific advisory boards of numerous journals and organizations.

**Örn Adalsteinsson, PhD**, holds a master's and doctorate from the Massachusetts Institute of Technology (MIT). He has specialized in human therapeutics including vaccines, monoclonal antibodies, product development, nutraceuticals, formulations, artificial intelligence, hormones, and nutritional supplementation. He has also authored articles and contributed to peer-reviewed publications, and served as an editor for the *Journal of Medicinal Food*.

**John Boik, PhD**, is the author of two books on cancer therapy, *Cancer and Natural Medicine* (1996) and *Natural Compounds in Cancer Therapy* (2001). He obtained his doctorate at the University of Texas Graduate School of Biomedical Sciences with research at the MD Anderson Cancer Center, focusing on screening models to identify promising new anticancer drugs. He conducted his postdoctoral training at Stanford University Department of Statistics. He is currently president of New Earth BioMed, a nonprofit cancer research corporation that studies mixtures of natural products.

**Frank Eichorn, MD**, is a urologist who has specialized in prostate cancer for the past 10 years. He has a private practice in Bad Reichenhall, Germany, and is prostate cancer consultant at the Urologische Klinik Castringius, Planegg, Munich. In his integrative approach to prostate cancer he is working with an international network of experts to improve treatment outcomes for prostate cancer patients with a special focus on natural and translational medicine.

**Deborah F. Harding, MD**, is founder of the Harding Anti-Aging Center. She is triple board certified in internal medicine, sleep disorder medicine, and anti-aging medicine. She also earned the Cenegenics certification in age management medicine. She is a faculty member of the new University of Central Florida Medical School.

**Steven B. Harris, MD**, is president and director of research at Critical Care Research, a company that grew out of 21st-century medicine in Rancho Cucamonga, CA. Dr. Harris participates in groundbreaking hypothermia, cryothermia, and ischemia research. His research interests include antioxidant and dietary-restriction effects in animals and humans.

**Stanley W. Jacob, MD**, is Gerlinger Distinguished Professor, Department of Surgery, Oregon Health and Science University. He has authored 175 scientific articles and 15 books, and holds three patents, including the initial patent on the therapeutic implications of dimethyl sulfoxide (DMSO).

**Richard Kratz, MD, DSci**, is clinical professor of ophthalmology at the University of California, Irvine, and the University of Southern California (Los Angeles). Dr. Kratz pioneered the cataract-removal technique called phacoemulsification and developed intraocular lenses to replace the crystalline lens. He is currently involved in projects relating to glaucoma, cataract extraction, and facilitating eyesight for the totally blind.

**Peter H. Langsjoen, MD, FACC**, is a cardiologist specializing in congestive heart failure, primary and statin-induced diastolic dysfunction, and other heart diseases. A leading authority on coenzyme Q10, Dr. Langsjoen has been involved with its clinical application since 1983. He is a founding member of the Executive Committee of the International Coenzyme Q10 Association, a fellow of the American College of Cardiology, and a member of numerous other medical associations.

**Ralph W. Moss, PhD**, is the author of books such as *Antioxidants against Cancer*, *Cancer Therapy*, *Questioning Chemotherapy*, and *The Cancer Industry*, as well as the award-winning PBS documentary, "The Cancer War." Dr. Moss has independently evaluated the claims of various cancer treatments, and currently directs The Moss Reports, an updated library of detailed reports on more than 200 varieties of cancer diagnoses.

**Michael D. Ozner, MD, FACC, FAHA**, is a board-certified cardiologist who specializes in cardiovascular disease prevention. He serves as medical director for the Cardiovascular Prevention Institute of South Florida, and is a noted national speaker on heart disease prevention. Dr. Ozner is also author of *The Great American Heart Hoax* (2010, BenBella Books) and *The Miami Mediterranean Diet* (2008, BenBella Books). For more information, visit www.drozner.com.

**Robert Pastore, PhD, CNS**, is a clinical nutritionist practicing in New York City. Due to his thorough nature and focus on organic chemistry and biochemistry, his colleagues have termed his practice forensic nutrition. He is a member of Harvard Medical School Postgraduate Association, the American College of Nutrition, New York Academy of Sciences, and the American Association of Pharmaceutical Scientists.

**Jonathan V. Wright, MD**, is medical director of the Tahoma Clinic in Renton, WA. He received his MD from the University of Michigan and has taught natural biochemical medical treatments since 1983. Dr. Wright pioneered the use of bioidentical estrogens and DHEA in daily medical practice. He has authored 11 books and publishes *Nutrition and Healing*, a monthly newsletter with a worldwide circulation of more than 100 000.

# AN IMPECCABLE SCIENTIFIC TRACK RECORD

Since 1980, the Life Extension Foundation has been reporting and funding research to fight the diseases of aging.

This short overview will give you just a brief glimpse of what we've worked to accomplish. Its purpose is to demonstrate our consistent, ongoing commitment to health care innovation. Our goal is and always has been to help you live a longer, healthier life.

## THE 1980s: DHEA, ASPIRIN, CoQ10

1981: Life Extension recommended B-complex vitamins to lower homocysteine blood levels. High homocysteine levels are now a recognized risk factor for heart disease and stroke. Foundation members have been keeping their homocysteine levels low by taking folic acid, vitamin B12, trimethylglycine (TMG), and vitamin B6.

1983: The Foundation was the first organization in the world to recommend the Japanese cardiac drug coenzyme Q10 (CoQ10) as an antiaging nutrient. The use of high-dose CoQ10 in the United States is enabling people with congestive heart failure to resume normal lives because this nutrient significantly boosts cardiac energy output. High-dose CoQ10 also has been shown to significantly slow the progression of Parkinson's disease—something that drugs cannot yet do. A breakthrough in the field of antiaging medicine occurred in 2006 with the publication of a study showing that CoQ10 (ubiquinol) slowed aging in middle-aged, senescent-accelerated mice by 40%. This ubiquinol form of CoQ10 is what most Life Extension members now supplement with.

1983: Life Extension recommended the use of low-dose aspirin on a daily basis to prevent vascular disease. The majority of cardiologists in the United States now prescribe low-dose aspirin to protect against a heart attack in cardiac patients and studies now show that daily low-dose aspirin also reduces cancer risk.

1985: The Foundation published an article suggesting that the progression of AIDS could be slowed by vitamin supplementation. The U.S. FDA raided Life Extension's premises in 1987 because the agency at that time did not believe that nutrition had anything to do with HIV progression. In the April 1995 issue of *FDA Consumer*, the FDA recommended vitamin supplements to slow the progression of AIDS— and a federal judge eventually forced the FDA to return everything it seized from Life Extension in 1987. Since we published the article in 1985, hundreds of published studies have shown that the proper nutrient supplementation can dramatically slow the progression of the immune system decline that leads to AIDS.

1985: The Foundation recommended the drug cimetidine (Tagamet®) as an adjuvant cancer therapy. Since then, published studies reveal that this drug (most commonly associated with heartburn relief) can reduce the recurrence of certain cancers by as much as 69%.

1986: The Foundation recommended the drug ribavirin to treat lethal viral infections. It took 12 years for the FDA to approve ribavirin as a treatment for hepatitis C. Hundreds of thousands of Americans died because the FDA denied Americans access to this broad-spectrum anti-viral medication.

# THE 1990s: ALZHEIMER'S, CANCER, AND HEART DISEASE

1991: The Foundation sued the U.S. FDA because the FDA failed to approve tacrine (THA) to treat Alzheimer's disease. While the lawsuit was dismissed on technical grounds, it forced the FDA to finally approve THA several years after it was shown in a *New England Journal of Medicine* report to improve cognitive symptoms in Alzheimer's patients.

1994: The Foundation warned that the commonly prescribed estrogen and synthetic progestin drugs could increase breast and ovarian cancer risk. Findings published years later confirmed these dangers.

1994: Congress passed the Dietary Supplement Health and Education Act (DSHEA) by an overwhelming majority and it was signed into law. The Life Extension Foundation spearheaded this legislation beginning in 1989 at a time when no one believed that Congress would ever pass such a sweeping bill that took away FDA's draconian powers to deny Americans access to truthful nonmisleading information about dietary supplements.

1997: The Foundation recommended that certain patients temporarily take a combination of statin and COX-2–inhibiting drugs to inhibit cancer cell growth. Since then, several studies have confirmed the anticancer effects of these drugs that are not commonly associated with cancer therapy.

1997: The Foundation warned of taking only the "alpha tocopherol" form of vitamin E. Since then, a number of published studies confirmed that aging people would benefit by also taking the "gamma tocopherol" form of vitamin E that Life Extension has long advocated.

1998: The Foundation introduced to the United States a natural herbal supplement called *Urtica dioica* that has been used for more than 10 years in Europe to relieve the symptoms of benign prostatic hypertrophy.

1998: The Foundation introduced Americans to a Japanese drug called methylcobalamin, a form of vitamin B12 that was particularly effective in protecting the brain against damaging excitotoxicity and also reversing the course of certain neurologic disorders.

1999: The Foundation showed how vitamin C may prevent nitroglycerin drug intolerance in patients with coronary artery disease.

1999: The Foundation showed how certain FDA-approved estrogen drugs may not protect against heart disease. A few years later, these very drugs were shown to increase cardiovascular disease in women.

# 2000 TO 2003: ANTIOXIDANTS, PARKINSON'S, AND METFORMIN

2000: The Foundation revealed how COX-2 inhibiting drugs could increase proinflammatory factors in the body, potentially leading to permanent joint damage and vascular disease. In 2004, two of these drugs were taken off the market because of increased risks of heart attack in those who took them. For the COX-2–inhibiting drugs like Celebrex® that remained on the market, black-box warnings are now placed on their label cautioning about increased heart attack risk when using these drugs. (Note that the proper use of Celebrex still plays a role in the treatment of certain cancers.)

2000:  The Foundation conducted original research using carotid ultrasound tests to show that people taking high doses of antioxidants over an extended period of time may be protected against atherosclerosis.

2001:  The Foundation funded research to identify genes linked to aging versus those that act to extend life. This research has led to the discovery of agents that mimic the longevity-promoting effects of calorie restriction.

2001:  The Foundation recommended a drug to treat Alzheimer's disease and Parkinson's disease called memantine that had been used in Germany since 1991 but was not approved by the FDA. (The FDA approved memantine 2.5 years later.)

2002:  The Foundation introduced methylselenocysteine, the form of selenium found naturally in garlic and broccoli that protects against mammary tumor development.

2003:  The Foundation advised members to stock up on an antiviral drug called Tamiflu® in case they were exposed to the common flu virus. Two years later, the world became so frightened about a potential SARS virus pandemic that Tamiflu disappeared from pharmacy shelves worldwide. Foundation members who heeded Life Extension's early warning already had their personal supply of Tamiflu in their medicine cabinet.

2003:  The Foundation introduced the first therapeutic program to slow the progression of Parkinson's disease.

2003:  The Foundation revealed an effective strategy for reducing the frequency and intensity of debilitating migraine headaches by restoring hormone balance.

2003:  The Foundation discovered that the drug metformin could mimic many of the beneficial effects of calorie restriction. The findings from Life Extension's study were published in the *Proceedings of the National Academy of Sciences*.

2003:  Life Extension introduced a plant extract to protect against DNA mutations and neutralize carcinogens.

## 2004 TO 2006: OSTEOPOROSIS, PROSTATE CANCER, STEM CELLS

2004:  The Foundation warned of the hidden dangers of osteoporosis in men.

2004:  Life Extension reported that optimal glucose levels should be lower than current guidelines to reduce heart attack risk by 40%. (Soon thereafter, national standards for the upper-scale limit of blood glucose were lowered but still not to the lower levels recommended by Life Extension.)

2005:  The Foundation conducted a clinical study showing that sesame lignans significantly enhance the antioxidant and anti-inflammatory effects of gamma tocopherol. Furthermore, Life Extension reported that standardized sesame seed lignans increase vitamin E activity and enhance the benefits of borage and fish oil supplements.

2005:  Life Extension announced the startling finding that PSA (prostate-specific antigen) itself could promote prostate cancer and provided novel methods to lower PSA levels in aging men.

2005:  Life Extension conducted a clinical study showing that an orally ingested agent could naturally increase superoxide dismutase (SOD) and catalase in the body.

SOD and catalase are naturally produced antioxidants that are more potent than orally ingested antioxidants.

2005: The National Academy of Sciences released a report confirming what the Life Extension Foundation has argued for years—that x-rays at any dose pose health risks to humans.

2005: The Foundation alerted the public to the disease-causing toxins present in fish and provided a strategy for safely capturing the health-promoting benefits of fish oil.

2005: The Foundation revealed data showing that blueberry extract can help reverse the memory and motor impairments associated with aging.

2005: The Foundation revealed an effective strategy for reducing the frequency and intensity of debilitating migraine headaches using an herbal extract from Europe, and for restoring youthful hormone balance.

2006: The Foundation revealed why vegetarians do not live that much longer than meat-eaters and how easy it is to correct this problem by supplementing with one critical nutrient (carnosine).

2006: The Foundation exposed how drug companies are seeking to shut down compounding pharmacies that offer Americans access to safer and less expensive drugs.

2006: The Foundation showed a novel form of vitamin K could guard against arterial calcification and osteoporosis.

2006: The Foundation presented a summary of cumulative findings showing how the proper intake of a plant extract could reverse atherosclerosis and slow the progression of prostate cancer.

2006: The Foundation identified how one missing plant extract was responsible for the epidemic of macular degeneration afflicting aging humans.

2006: The Foundation introduced a form of coenzyme Q10 (ubiquinol) that is vastly superior to commercial CoQ10 supplements in absorbing into the human bloodstream, reducing fatigue and slowing age-related markers.

2006: The Foundation uncovered findings to show that new stem cell formation can be promoted in the body by ingesting commonly available nutrients.

2006: The Foundation exposed how the FDA was attempting to censor truthful information about the health benefits of fruits and vegetables.

## 2007–2009: VITAMIN D, HORMONES, AND OBESITY

2007: The Foundation revealed how the ubiquinol form of CoQ10 reversed congestive heart failure in cases where conventional CoQ10 was shown to be ineffective.

2007: The Foundation ascertained what dose of green tea was required to protect against certain cancers and vascular diseases, and why drinking only a few cups of green tea a day may not be enough.

2007: The Foundation showed how cancer cells lurk in the prostate glands of many aging men, and how to inhibit an enzyme (5-lipoxygenase) that enables these isolated malignant cells to develop into full-blown prostate cancer.

2007: The Foundation showed that those drinking bottled water were at significant risk of suffering a lethal magnesium deficiency.

2007: The Foundation revealed one overlooked reason why humans contract the flu (vitamin D deficiency) much more frequently in winter months and what could be done to guard against this.

2007: The Foundation revealed published findings about how people with higher blood levels of vitamin E slashed their risk of dying over a 19-year period and showed that it was not possible to attain adequate vitamin E levels through diet alone.

2007: The Foundation unveiled a comprehensive program to sharply reduce the high cost of prescription drugs while also protecting consumers against dangerous side effects.

2007: The Foundation showed for the first time how Coumadin® (warfarin) drug users could safely benefit from low-dose vitamin K. Most doctors still tell their Coumadin patients to avoid even foods that contain vitamin K, whereas Life Extension showed that most Coumadin users can benefit from consistent low-dose vitamin K, which can help stabilize coagulation markers in the blood while protecting against arterial calcification and bone density loss—two common side effects associated with this drug.

2007: The Foundation showed that low blood levels of the omega-3 fatty acids EPA and DHA are independent risk factors for heart attack and angina.

2007: The Foundation exposed how pharmaceutical special interests were seeking to ban over-the-counter sales of DHEA so they could sell this safe, antiaging hormone as a prescription drug. Life Extension members inundated Congress with protests and prevented DHEA from being removed from the supplement marketplace.

2007: The Foundation uncovered five anticancer drugs that the FDA was not approving, despite human clinical studies documenting both safety and efficacy. Life Extension organized patient advocate groups to contact their members of Congress to protest the unjust denial of these medications to terminally ill cancer patients. One of these drugs (Provenge®) was approved in 2010.

2007: The Foundation compiled data showing that supplementing with higher-dose vitamin D could significantly reduce the risk of the most common age-related disorders, including cancer, chronic inflammation, and heart disease. The Foundation wrote the president of the United States urging that a national emergency be declared to urge every adult to consume at least 1000 IU a day of vitamin D. The Foundation also offered to donate 50000 one-year-supply bottles of vitamin D to the federal government to give to those who could not afford this low-cost supplement.

2007: The Foundation showed how mainstream oncologists are failing to optimally prescribe FDA-approved therapies and offered a practical solution for cancer patients to consider.

2007: The Foundation unveiled its multipronged scientific research program to more efficiently develop new cancer drugs.

2008: The Foundation revealed how the consumption of specific plant lignans can slash prostate cancer risk.

2008: The Foundation published data showing why more Americans are depressed, overweight, and suffer sleep disturbances than ever before. The Foundation then revealed a novel method to enable tryptophan supplements to safely increase brain serotonin to improve mood, decrease carbohydrate craving, and facilitate restful sleep.

2008: The Foundation issued a meticulous rebuttal to the FDA's attack against bioidentical hormones and provided a scientific rationale for using natural testosterone and estrogen to reverse certain manifestations of aging.

2008:   The Foundation launched a political campaign to radically overhaul the FDA. The Foundation's position paper revealed how the FDA is the major impediment to life-saving advances in medicine.

2008:   The Foundation uncovered an orally ingested supplement that protects the skin from solar radiation.

2008:   The Foundation announced a startling breakthrough whereby the clinical course of Alzheimer's disease was reversed. The Foundation then announced it was funding an expanded research program to further validate the remarkable cognitive improvements observed in Alzheimer's patients receiving this novel drug therapy.

2009:   Obese Americans were shown for the first time to outnumber those who are merely overweight. Life Extension published overlooked research findings indicating substantial fat-loss effects in response to the proper use of bioidentical hormones, certain prescription drugs and nutrients, along with lifestyle changes. The reason these proven weight-loss strategies have still not caught on, the Foundation asserted, is that when used in isolation, they often fail to meet the expectations of corpulent individuals. In an eye-opening report, Life Extension revealed how to interpret blood test results to utilize an armada of medications, natural hormones, and lifestyle alterations that can safely induce substantial weight loss.

2009:   The Foundation introduced the American public to a noninvasive diagnostic procedure available in Europe to detect the presence of small, and otherwise undetectable, lymph node lesions in patients with cancer.

2009:   The Foundation cut through the heated debate on statin drugs and revealed why the Vytorin® trial failed to live up to conventional medicine's expectations. In this rare instance, Life Extension found itself defending the interest of a pharmaceutical company that appeared to be too overwhelmed by negative media coverage to put this study in proper scientific context.

2009:   The Foundation analyzed 13 892 blood tests measuring 25-hydroxyvitamin D levels in a group of dedicated supplement users and discovered that 85.7% had insufficient vitamin D status. A startling 38% of them were deficient in vitamin D according to conventional reference ranges. This unprecedented analysis of achieved vitamin D serum levels in a large group of high-dose supplement users reveals that most aging people require a dose of 5000 IU or higher of this critical disease-preventing nutrient.

## 2010 AND THE FUTURE...

2010:   A landmark study of caloric restriction in primates demonstrating a three-fold reduction in mortality, confirmed what Life Extension published 30 years prior.

2010:   To counter the abnormally high blood sugar and dangerous prediabetic state suffered by an estimated 60 million Americans, Life Extension uncovered a novel group of enzyme-inhibitors shown to control glucose levels, improve blood markers of health, and regain glycemic balance.

2010:   Life Extension announced a revolutionary new test, currently available in Europe that measures the characteristics of circulating tumor cells and allows for specific conventional and natural treatments to be tailored to cancer patients.

2010: Life Extension reminded male Life Extension members about the critical need to maintain estrogen blood levels between 20–30 pg/mL. This longstanding recommendation was confirmed the year before when the Journal of the American Medical Association published a study that showed men with unbalanced estrogen levels were up to 317% more likely to die from heart failure.

2010: Life Extension reported on a strawberry extract called fisetin that has been shown to enhance the calorie restriction mimetic action of resveratrol.

2010: A groundbreaking scientific study, partially funded by the Life Extension Foundation and published in the journal Regenerative Medicine, demonstrated that the aging of human cells can be reversed in vitro.

2010: Life Extension unveiled a multi-modal weight loss program that for the first time combines the use of natural hormones, certain drugs, and novel nutrients that attack the underlying causes of age-related weight gain.

2010: The federal government admitted that radiation from CT scans contributes to 29 000 cases of cancer in one year and 15 000 needless deaths. Since its inception, Life Extension warned its members to avoid any kind of medical x-ray unless absolutely necessary because of increased cancer risks.

2010: The FDA finally approved Provenge® to treat prostate cancer. Life Extension had battled the FDA to have Provenge approved for nearly a decade. The FDA's delay of this immune-boosting therapy is calculated to have caused 82 000 lost life years.

2010: Life Extension introduced a novel compound called PQQ (Pyrroloquinoline quinone), that has been shown to rejuvenate aging cells by promoting the growth of new mitochondria.

2010: Life Extension reported that the berry extract C3G (cyanidin-3-glucoside) has demonstrated the ability to enhance visual acuity in low-light conditions.

2010: Life Extension reported on a safer, better, and clinically proven form of chromium that has been shown to improve glucose control and insulin sensitivity in a study of diabetics taking one of three common oral hypoglycemic medications.

2010: Formulated first soups that provide a full spectrum of cruciferous and other vegetables with no rice, pasta, potatoes, corn, or sugar found in commercial soups that can spike blood glucose levels.

2011: Life Extension reports a landmark aging-reversal study published in the November 28, 2010, online edition of the scientific journal Nature, which showed that prematurely aged mice whose telomeres were lengthened experienced a rapid reversal of degenerative pathologies. In response to this unprecedented finding, Life Extension funded $2 million for a new aging-reversal study that will include telomere lengthening.

2011: Life Extension introduced a better form of magnesium to enhance memory and cognitive function.

2011: Life Extension exposed how the FDA's failure to allow widespread use of low-dose aspirin resulted in 3 million needless cancer deaths in the United States. In an eye-opening report published by Oxford University in The Lancet in 2010, long-term, low-dose aspirin therapy (75 mg per day) reduced the overall risk of cancer death by 20%. These findings demonstrate that low-dose aspirin therapy could have saved millions from cancer and vascular diseases since Life Extension first recommended daily aspirin use in 1983.

2011: Life Extension introduces a complex of bioactive milk peptides, widely used in Europe to promote sustained and restful sleep patterns and a healthy response to stress.

2011: Life Extension published a book (Pharmocracy) that exposed how inefficient and corrupt government practices stifle medical innovation and cause health care prices to spiral out of control. Pharmocracy advocates the repeal of draconian laws that have granted a virtual monopoly to the entrenched medical establishment and warns the nation's solvency is at stake unless free market reforms are implemented.

2011: Life Extension identified more therapies being irrationally suppressed by the FDA that could save the lives of cancer victims.

2011: Life Extension revealed the lethal dangers of even one omission. In this instance, it appears that legendary health guru Jack LaLanne died too early from a disorder that could have been prevented.

2011: Life Extension introduced the novel ingredient Green Coffee Bean Extract, standardized to 50% chlorogenic acid, a potent polyphenol shown to induce weight loss by inhibiting absorption of calories from starches and sugars while lowering lipids and inhibiting after-meal blood glucose spikes.

2011: At the French-American BioTech Symposium, Dr. Michael West presented data on the restoration of cell life span using transcriptional reprogramming technology. This was funded in part with millions of dollars contributed by the Life Extension Foundation.

2012: In an effort to combat the increasing incidence of nonalcoholic fatty liver disease, Life Extension introduced a phyto-supplement containing extracts from the adaptogenic vine Schisandra chinensis and from muskmelon. This formulation helps to detoxify the liver and restore its antioxidant function to youthful levels.

2012: To help support healthy blood pressure, Life Extension formulated a product featuring oleuropein, a compound found in high concentration in the olive leaf, which has been shown to favorably modulate arterial resistance or stiffness.

2012: Life Extension published findings on a nontoxic experimental treatment it funded that resulted in 80% survival of women with stage IV breast cancer.

To view Life Extension's entire track record, visit our website at www.LifeExtension.com/track.

Membership in the nonprofit Life Extension Foundation is at an all-time high. Life Extension is growing because people are becoming aware that recommendations published by the Foundation in the early 1980s are now scientifically validated, and many are even accepted by the medical establishment.

Membership is low cost, and this minimal expense is quickly offset because members save substantially on blood tests, compounded prescription drugs, state-of-the-art nutritional supplements, and free telephone access to knowledgeable health advisors.

# CONTRIBUTORS

Adam Cloe, PhD

Kevin M. Connolly, PhD

Aaron Csicseri, PharmD

Leah DiPlacido, PhD

Cindy Embleton, MS

Michael Gertner, MS

Grace P. Ibay, MHS

Curtis James

Tina Kaczor, ND, FABNO

William Lagakos, PhD

Eileen M. Lynch, PhD

Elaine A. Richman, PhD

Yusuf (J.P.) Saleeby, MD

Paula Simpson, B.Sc., RNCP

Benjamin S. Weeks, PhD

Eric Yarnell, ND, RH(AHG)

# STAFF ACKNOWLEDGMENTS

Life Extension wishes to thank the many employees who contributed to this book. We would like to recognize the following individuals who contributed to the research and editorial development of this edition.

Alex Benitez, BS

Tatiana Enriquez, CpHt

Scott Fogle, ND

Justin Henry, MPH, MHE

Crystal Moore, MS, CNS

Steven Nemeroff, ND

Erica Neyland, MS

Marie Parks, BS

April Roberts, BS

Maylin Paez, RN, BS

Richard A. Stein, MD, PhD

Heidi Yanoti, DC

Peter Zhang, MD, PhD

# DISCLAIMER AND SAFETY INFORMATION

This information (and any accompanying printed material) is not intended to replace the attention or advice of a physician or other qualified health care professional. Anyone who wishes to embark on any dietary, drug, exercise, or other lifestyle change intended to prevent or treat a specific disease or condition should first consult with and seek clearance from a physician or other qualified health care professional. Pregnant women in particular should seek the advice of a physician before using any protocol listed in this book. The protocols described in this book are for adults only, unless otherwise specified. Product labels may contain important safety information and the most recent product information provided by the product manufacturers should be carefully reviewed prior to use to verify the dose, administration, and contraindications. National, state, and local laws may vary regarding the use and application of many of the treatments discussed. The reader assumes the risk of any injuries. The authors and publishers, and their affiliates and assigns are not liable for any injury and/or damage to persons arising from this publication and expressly disclaim responsibility for any adverse effects resulting from the use of the information in this book.

The information published in the protocols is only as current as the day the manuscript was sent to the printer. The protocols raise many issues that are subject to change as new data emerge. None of our suggested protocol regimens can guarantee a cure. The publisher has not performed independent verification of the data contained herein, and expressly disclaims responsibility for any error in the literature, transcription, or typography. The most current protocols are available at *www.lef.org*.

# 1

# Acetaminophen and NSAID Toxicity

Nonsteroidal anti-inflammatory drugs (NSAIDs) are a diverse group of drugs with analgesic, anti-inflammatory, and antipyretic (fever-reducing) properties. NSAIDs are typically used to relieve mild to moderate pain related to a variety of conditions.[1–3]

Acetaminophen, also called paracetamol, is not an NSAID, but a distinct analgesic and fever-reducing drug with a similarly broad usage.[4,5]

Acetaminophen overdose is the leading cause of acute liver failure in the developed world,[6,7] accounting for more than 56 000 emergency room visits, 26 000 hospitalizations, and 450 deaths per year in the United States.[4] Acetaminophen can also contribute to kidney toxicity.[8]

Although the "safe" dose of acetaminophen is up to 4 g daily, chronic daily ingestion of this dose has been shown to cause elevations of liver enzymes, even in healthy people.[9] Since alcohol, especially when consumed chronically, augments the toxic potential of acetaminophen, many people unknowingly put themselves at risk of significant liver damage by consuming acetaminophen and alcohol together.[10,11]

Aspirin and NSAID usage has been associated with gastrointestinal toxicity including bleeding ulcer.[12,13] Certain NSAIDs (eg, selective COX-2 inhibitors) have been linked to an increased risk of cardiovascular events, and in particular heart attack. In addition, chronic use of some types of NSAIDs has been associated with kidney damage that may persist even after drug withdrawal in some cases.[14–17]

This protocol discusses the mechanisms of acetaminophen and NSAID function and toxicity, and outlines dietary and lifestyle approaches for minimizing their toxic potential.

## ACETAMINOPHEN AND NSAIDs: BACKGROUND AND OVERVIEW

Acetaminophen has been available as an over-the-counter analgesic and antipyretic for over 50 years. More than 100 million people use acetaminophen each year in the United States alone, with up to 50 million Americans using acetaminophen-containing products in a given week.[4] While generally considered a safe therapy when taken below the recommended maximum daily dose of 4 g, acetaminophen overdoses are not uncommon.[4,18]

Although most patients recover spontaneously from an acetaminophen overdose, the drug can cause life-threatening liver injury. Acetaminophen accounts for up to 50% of all adult cases of acute liver failure in the United States.[4,7] Even in the absence of overt overdose symptoms, therapeutic acetaminophen dosages can still increase the blood concentrations of liver enzymes (markers of liver damage).[9] Other potential negative consequences of acetaminophen include increased fracture risk,[19] inhibition of testosterone production,[20,21] and kidney toxicity.[8]

NSAIDs are among the most widely used of all drugs, with 20–30 billion tablets sold each year in the United States alone.[22,23] The prototypical member, aspirin, is one of the oldest analgesics, in use as an anti-inflammatory therapy long before the molecular mechanics of inflammation had been discovered. Low-dose aspirin (eg, 75–100 mg) is often used to reduce the risk of cardiovascular events in high-risk patient populations.[24] Regular use of aspirin has also been associated with a significantly reduced risk of several cancers.[25]

The anti-inflammatory properties of NSAIDs are due to their inhibition of the cyclooxygenase (COX) enzymes, which catalyze the synthesis of localized proinflammatory signaling molecules called prostaglandins.[26]

The two COX enzymes with well-defined roles in humans are COX-1 and COX-2. COX-2 is normally inactive, but can be turned on during inflammation to produce proinflammatory prostaglandins. In contrast, COX-1 is normally active in many tissues, where it has roles unrelated to inflammation (eg, clotting function in blood platelets and mucus production from cells lining the GI tract).[1,26] The inhibition of prostaglandins in the central nervous system also raises the pain threshold and acts on the hypothalamus to reduce body temperature.[4]

Nonselective NSAIDs (aspirin, naproxen [eg, Aleve®], ibuprofen [eg, Advil®], diclofenac [eg, Cambia®], and indomethacin [Indocin®]) inhibit the activity of both COX enzymes.[1] COX-2 selective NSAIDs (ie, COX-2 inhibitors or coxibs) inhibit COX-2 more strongly than COX-1, resulting in less gastrointestinal side effects, but potential cardiovascular complications, most notably an increase in the risk of heart attack due to increased blood clotting propensity.[1]

# MECHANISMS OF ACETAMINOPHEN AND NSAID TOXICITY

Despite similarities in activity, the potential toxicities of acetaminophen and NSAIDs arise from different mechanisms.

## Acetaminophen Toxicity

Acetaminophen is toxic to the liver and kidneys primarily through its ability to overwhelm the liver's innate detoxification systems (see Life Extension's "Metabolic Detoxification" protocol for a review of this system).[8,27]

The liver uses multiple enzyme systems to metabolize acetaminophen; at low doses, these systems are able to remove excess acetaminophen from the body. However, if the acetaminophen dosage is increased, some of these enzyme systems may become overwhelmed.

The majority of acetaminophen is first converted into the toxic metabolite *N-acetyl-p-benzoquinoneimine* (*NAPQI*) by phase I CYP (cytochrome P450) enzymes, and then conjugated with glutathione using the phase II enzyme glutathione-S-transferase (GST). As acetaminophen detoxification proceeds in this fashion, glutathione, a ubiquitous cellular antioxidant, eventually becomes depleted,[27] and NAPQI can no longer be sufficiently detoxified.[28] Rising levels of NAPQI in the liver cause widespread damage, including lipid peroxidation, inactivation of cellular proteins, and disruption of DNA metabolism.[8] Furthermore, the loss of cellular glutathione leads to increased oxidative damage, the inability of mitochondria to produce cellular energy (ATP), and eventual cell death.[29] The outcome of excessive acetaminophen is liver toxicity, which, if left untreated, can lead to liver failure.[30] Similarly, toxicity can be observed in the kidneys and may lead to acute renal failure.[8,31]

## NSAID Toxicity

In contrast to the liver toxicity of acetaminophen, NSAIDs exhibit varying degrees of gastrointestinal, cardiovascular, and kidney toxicity.

### NSAID COX-1 AND COX-2 SELECTIVITY

It should be noted that even nonselective NSAIDs have different degrees of selectivity toward COX-1 and COX-2 enzymes.[32] For example, diclofenac, while considered a nonselective NSAID, may inhibit COX-2 significantly more than COX-1; naproxen inhibits COX-1 more readily than COX-2.[32] These differences may partially explain why various NSAIDs carry different cardiovascular and gastrointestinal risk profiles.

**NSAIDs–COX-1 inhibition and gastrointestinal toxicity.** Cyclooxygenases and the prostaglandins they form also have roles beyond inflammation. In the gastrointestinal tract, COX-1-derived prostaglandins function to increase production of the thick mucus/bicarbonate layer that coats gastric surfaces and buffers them against stomach acid.[13] Inhibition of COX-1 activity by nonselective NSAIDs (such as aspirin or ibuprofen) results in degradation of the protective mucus layer.[13] Damage to the lining of the stomach and small intestine results in symptoms that range from relatively minor heartburn, nausea, and abdominal pain (affecting 15–40% of NSAID users) to life-threatening ulceration, perforation, and bleeding (affecting 1–2% of chronic NSAID users).[13]

**NSAIDs–COX-2 inhibition and cardiovascular toxicity.** While inhibition of COX-1 can have serious gastrointestinal consequences, selective inhibition of COX-2 carries cardiovascular risks. Blood platelets express a blood clotting, vessel-constricting compound called thromboxane A2 or TXA2, which is synthesized by COX-1. Blood vessels produce an anticlotting compound called prostaglandin I2 or PGI2. During blood vessel injury, the relative ratios of TXA2 and PGI2 are controlled by COX enzymes to balance the opposing actions of clotting and blood flow. COX-2 specific inhibitors (eg, coxibs) preferentially reduce amounts of PGI2, tipping the balance toward thrombosis.[13] The increased risk of thrombosis and heart attack observed in some studies of COX-2 inhibitors may result from this mechanism.[1] Increases in blood vessel constriction by COX-2 inhibition can also lead to the hypertension and renal failure seen in some studies of nonselective and COX-2 selective NSAIDs.[1] COX-2 inhibitors may also impair the removal of excess cholesterol from blood vessel walls, a process known as reverse cholesterol transport.[33] Moreover, COX-2 inhibitors can cause metabolic imbalances that result in overproduction of two toxic cytokines—tumor necrosis factor alpha (TNF-$\alpha$) and interleukin 1 beta (IL-1$\beta$).[34,35]

**NSAIDs—kidney toxicity.** An underappreciated side effect of NSAID use is kidney toxicity. Long-term use of NSAIDs can lead to impaired glomerular filtration, renal tubular necrosis, and ultimately chronic renal failure by disrupting prostaglandin synthesis, which can impair renal blood flow.[36] This is because prostaglandins, which are blocked by COX inhibition, are important for proper blood vessel function within the kidneys.[17]

In a study involving more than 10000 elderly individuals, long-term, high-dose NSAID therapy was associated with a significantly increased risk of progression of chronic kidney disease.[37] Even in NSAID users with healthy kidneys, subclinical irregularities in kidney function are sometimes observed.[17] Other consequences of kidney toxicity related to NSAID use include high blood pressure, salt and water retention, and electrolyte imbalances.[17]

**NSAIDs—mitochondrial dysfunction and oxidative stress.** An underappreciated side effect of NSAIDs is their contribution to mitochondrial dysfunction, thereby causing the formation of highly reactive free radicals. Free radicals cause tissue damage and may contribute to toxicity associated with NSAIDs.[38,39]

Mitochondria generate energy for cells in the form of adenosine triphosphate (ATP). A byproduct of this metabolically intensive process is creation of free radicals. When mitochondria are functioning normally, they generate minimal oxidative products and the body's antioxidant defense systems keep them in check. However, when toxins, in this case NSAIDs and/or their metabolites, interfere with the efficiency of this process, the amount of free-radical products generated can increase considerably.[40,41] This mechanism has been associated with NSAID-related gastrointestinal[41] and liver toxicity.[42,43] NSAIDs have also been shown to cause oxidative stress via a mitochondria-independent mechanism in vascular tissue.[44]

---

### DAILY LOW-DOSE (75–100 MG) ASPIRIN: LIFE-SAVING BENEFITS WITH MANAGEABLE RISK

Life Extension originally began recommending low-dose aspirin for the prevention of cardiovascular events in the early 1980s. This was based on evidence for reduction in the risk of certain cardiovascular events such as heart attack and ischemic stroke.

Today, the role of daily low-dose aspirin therapy in reducing the risk of cardiovascular events is well known.[45]

However, there is another emerging benefit of this low-cost drug—*cancer prevention*.

In a landmark study published in early 2011 in *The Lancet*, Oxford University researchers found that daily low-dose aspirin therapy reduces overall risk of cancer death by 20% and colorectal cancer death risk by nearly 40%, proving especially effective in populations *55 and older*.[46] Subsequently, additional evidence corroborated these findings.[24]

Aspirin, like other NSAIDs, inhibits COX-2, which is one way it combats cancer. However, aspirin has several other anticancer mechanisms. It inhibits signaling through the nuclear factor kappa B (NF-κB) pathway, which is involved in inflammation and carcinogenesis.[47] Other anticancer mechanisms of aspirin include COX-1 inhibition, inhibition of platelet aggregation, and induction of apoptosis.[48–50]

Many important decisions in medicine are based on careful consideration of the potential risk versus potential benefit of using or not using a drug or therapy. Aspirin is associated with peptic ulcer and, less commonly, hemorrhagic stroke. For these reasons, individuals should discuss the risks and benefits of low-dose aspirin with their health care practitioners prior to initiating an aspirin regimen.[51–54] In addition, those using daily low-dose aspirin are encouraged to consider the suggestions in this protocol for protecting against gastrointestinal damage related to COX-1 inhibition.

---

## CAUSES AND RISK FACTORS FOR ACETAMINOPHEN AND NSAID TOXICITY

### Acetaminophen

Liver necrosis, the primary outcome of acetaminophen toxicity in humans, is predominantly a function of overdose.[29] For an adult, the maximum recommended single dose is 1 g and the maximum dose in a 24-hour period is 4 g.[18] Acetaminophen overdose has occurred over a wide range of daily intakes. Acute toxicity studies in animals, if extrapolated to humans, implicate a single dose of 10–15 g as necessary to produce significant liver toxicity, although several human case reports have shown toxicity at doses less than 4 g per day (likely due to having one or more risk factors for sensitivity to toxicity).[4] Accidental overdose (taking an over-the-counter acetaminophen-containing product concurrently with a prescription acetaminophen-containing therapy) represents a significant number of acetaminophen toxicities.

Factors that can lower the threshold for overdose or increase the likelihood of liver failure include the following:

**Delays in treatment.** Delays in treatment following overdose are associated with increased mortality. The conventional antidote for acetaminophen toxicity, N-acetyl cysteine (NAC), begins to lose efficacy if administered more than 8–10 hours following overdose.[30,55]

**Alcohol use.** Chronic alcohol use lowers the threshold for acetaminophen toxicity by induction of CYP enzymes and depletion of glutathione stores.[4]

**Medications.** Anticonvulsants, antibiotics, antivirals, antigout, and anti-GERD treatments can increase the toxicity of an acetaminophen dose by induction of CYP enzymes, depletion of glutathione stores, or saturation of other liver detoxification systems.[4]

**Starvation and malnutrition.** Starvation can increase the toxicity of an acetaminophen dose. It may also be responsible for toxicity and liver failure seen at lower doses.[4] Starvation may deplete liver glutathione stores, as well as precursors for other acetaminophen detoxification pathways. Malnourishment, eating disorders, and cachexia (muscle wasting) can also increase the risk of liver injury following overdose.[18] Animal models have demonstrated a protective effect of caloric restriction with optimal nutrition against experimentally induced acetaminophen toxicity.[56,57] Low dietary protein (a source of sulfur-containing amino acids used in glutathione synthesis) has been associated with increased sensitivity to acetaminophen toxicity in animals.[58]

**Age and gender.** Acetaminophen toxicity, more common in women than men, is most common in people aged 30–40 years. Note that these observations are based on case reports, and do not necessarily reflect susceptibility of these demographics to toxicity.[4]

**Genetics.** Several mutations have been identified in the phase I and II detoxification genes required for acetaminophen metabolism, which may affect the rate of acetaminophen clearance or production of the toxic metabolite NAPQI.[59]

## NSAIDs

NSAID use is associated with significant adverse effects such as gastrointestinal bleeding, peptic ulcer disease, high blood pressure, edema (ie, swelling), and kidney disease.[60]

There are several factors that influence risk of toxicity due to NSAID use[13,61]:

**Age.** Individuals over 60 are 5–6 times more likely to develop NSAID-related ulcers. Because older people generally have greater cardiovascular risk than younger people, their risk of NSAID-related cardiovascular events may also be elevated.

**Medical conditions.** Prior history of ulcer or other gastrointestinal complications increase risk of NSAID ulcers 4- to 5-fold. Cardiovascular or respiratory disease, renal or hepatic impairment, diabetes, *Helicobacter pylori* infection, rheumatoid arthritis, and hypertension are also associated with increased risk. Individuals with cardiovascular risk factors such as hypertension, high cholesterol, or history of heart attack or bypass surgery are at increased risk of having an NSAID-related cardiovascular event.[1]

**Dose and duration of treatment.** Use of high-dose or multiple NSAIDs increases the risk of gastrointestinal complications up to 10-fold. Cardiovascular risk appears to increase in tandem with duration of NSAID use.[1]

**Medications.** Simultaneous use of NSAIDs with corticosteroids, anticoagulants, aspirin, platelet inhibitors, and serotonin reuptake inhibitors can increase gastrointestinal toxicity up to 15-fold.

**NSAID selection.** As mentioned above, different NSAIDs carry different risks of either gastrointestinal or cardiovascular toxicity. While COX-2 selective inhibitors and diclofenac are associated with greater cardiovascular but lower gastrointestinal risks than nonselective NSAIDs, nonselective NSAIDs demonstrate the opposite effect. NSAIDs with longer half-lives, such as piroxicam (Feldene®), are associated with greater risk of gastrointestinal bleeding than those metabolized more quickly.[62] For people with high cardiovascular risk, the NSAID naproxen is typically recommended because it has been associated with fewer cardiovascular events compared with other NSAIDs in several studies.[1]

## AVOIDING UNINTENTIONAL TOXIC OVERDOSE

Most cases of unintentional acetaminophen overdose result from either failure to follow dosing instructions, or inadvertently combining multiple acetaminophen-containing products (such as "cold medicines" with analgesics). In one study, nearly one quarter of adults surveyed reported that they were likely to take more than the maximum 4 g of acetaminophen in a 24-hour period, while just over 5% (in error) were likely to take more than 6 g in the same period.[63] Therefore, *strict attention to dosing instructions* for all medications is imperative.

Avoiding the potential gastrointestinal and cardiovascular risk(s) of sustained NSAID usage necessitates the recognition of risk factors for each, as well as choosing an appropriate treatment strategy (eg, reduced dosage or pairing with a gastroprotective agent).[13]

## DIAGNOSIS AND TREATMENT OF ACETAMINOPHEN/NSAID TOXICITY

### Acetaminophen Overdose

Within a few hours of acetaminophen overdose, typical symptoms include nausea and vomiting. Tenderness and pain in the upper right abdomen may be present. Initial signs of liver failure (eg, jaundice, impaired consciousness, and hemorrhage) can begin within 24 hours of ingestion, but may be delayed for 2–3 days. Very large doses can result in lactic acidosis (a drop in pH of the blood) and coma.[18,29]

Several additional tests can support a diagnosis of acetaminophen overdose. Elevated levels of liver enzymes gamma-glutamyl transpeptidase (GGT), alanine aminotransferase (ALT), and aspartate aminotransferase (AST) can indicate liver damage, as can elevated serum bilirubin (a breakdown product of the red blood cell component hemoglobin normally cleared by a healthy liver). Increased prothrombin time (determined by a PTT test) also indicates liver dysfunction. Recovery from acetaminophen overdose is less favorable if these tests are abnormal by the time medical treatment is initiated. Blood levels of acetaminophen are also determined to guide treatment.[18,29]

A mainstay of conventional treatment for acetaminophen overdose is N-acetyl cysteine (NAC). NAC, a therapeutic form of the conditionally essential amino acid cysteine, is the rate-limiting reagent for the production of glutathione.[8] Health care practitioners prescribe NAC either orally (1330 mg/kg of body weight, given over 72 hours) or intravenously (300 mg/kg of body weight, given over 20 hours).[4] At these doses, the most common side effects of NAC are nausea and vomiting, although severe allergic reactions can occur in susceptible individuals.[18] NAC should be given relatively quickly after an overdose, as its efficacy begins to decline 8–10 hours following intoxication.[30,55] If administered within this window, however, NAC is very effective at mitigating toxicity. In a study of cancer patients taking high-dose acetaminophen (an average dose of 400 mg/kg/day, up to a maximum of 1 g/kg/day), a rescue dose of NAC within 8 hours of acetaminophen dosing prevented severe liver toxicity.[64]

If taken within 2 hours of acetaminophen overdose, activated charcoal may absorb excess drug.[30] Once acute liver failure has occurred or seems likely, however, the course of action is intensive supportive therapy or liver transplantation.[18]

### NSAID Toxicity

Gastrointestinal NSAID toxicity is managed by minimizing NSAID exposure, or pairing the NSAIDs with drugs that protect the integrity of the gastrointestinal tract. The American College of Rheumatology has recommended acetaminophen as first-line analgesic therapy for arthritis pain; if other NSAIDs are used, then the lowest effective dose for the shortest possible duration is recommended.[22] For individuals at moderate risk of gastrointestinal complications, combined therapy of NSAIDs with a gastroprotective agent should be considered.

Conventional gastroprotective drugs commonly prescribed to minimize NSAID toxicity or heal NSAID-induced ulcers include H2-receptor antagonists (cimetidine, ranitidine, famotidine), proton pump inhibitors (omeprazole, lansoprazole, esomeprazole), and misoprostol (a synthetic prostaglandin analog).[13]

## NOVEL AND EMERGING THERAPIES

One approach to avoiding gastrointestinal toxicity of NSAIDs is to pair them with fixed doses of gastroprotective agents in single-tablet formulations. For example, Arthrotec®, a combination product of diclofenac and misoprostol, is approved for use in osteoarthritis or rheumatoid arthritis patients at high risk of gastrointestinal disorders. A single-tablet combination of naproxen and esomeprazole is available by prescription under the brand name Vimovo®, and HZT-501 (a combination product of ibuprofen and famotidine) is being developed under the brand name Duexa®.[1,65] In two multicenter studies of over 1500 patients requiring NSAID therapy, HZT-501 demonstrated a ~55% reduction in the risk of ulcer (determined by endoscopy) compared to ibuprofen alone over 24 weeks.[65] Single-tablet preparations may also help overcome poor compliance to prescription NSAID/gastroprotectant regimens (reported at only 68% in one survey).[66]

*Topical NSAIDs*, unlike oral NSAIDs, deliver the drug directly to the target tissue, resulting in significantly lower systemic concentrations (<10% of an equivalent oral dose) and reduced gastrointestinal symptoms. Therefore, topical NSAIDs may have advantages over oral NSAIDs in some cases (eg, osteoarthritis). In the United States, only topical diclofenac (solution and gel) has been approved by the Food and Drug Administration (FDA) for use in osteoarthritis patients; its efficacy is comparable to oral diclofenac.[62]

## AVOIDING ACETAMINOPHEN/ NSAID TOXICITY

The most effective approach to minimizing acetaminophen and NSAID toxicity would be avoiding their usage altogether and choosing alternative means for treatment of inflammation and pain. (For more information, see Life Extension's Inflammation [Chronic] and Pain [Chronic] protocols.) However, because of their efficacy at reducing fever, treating inflammation, and minimizing thrombotic and cancer risk,[24] a complete cessation of NSAIDs, aspirin, or acetaminophen usage may not be suitable for everyone.

Whenever acetaminophen is taken, at least 600 mg of N-acetyl cysteine should be taken along with it to help protect against liver toxicity.

Chronic users of acetaminophen or NSAIDs should have regular blood tests to monitor the health of their liver and kidneys. A simple *chemistry panel* can help assess both liver and kidney function, and a *cystatin-C* blood test helps evaluate kidney health.

*If an acetaminophen overdose is suspected, call 911 or the National Poison Control Center (1-800-222-1222) immediately.*[67]

# NUTRITIONAL SUPPORT

People who take acetaminophen and NSAIDs regularly should be aware that these drugs can cause liver and kidney toxicity. When taking these medications, it is a good idea to provide antioxidant support to protect these organs.

Much of the data below are derived from animal models in which nutritional interventions garnered protection against acetaminophen and NSAID toxicity. The specific dosages studied in many of these animal models are very high when extrapolated to human equivalent doses; but lower dosages, such as those available in nutritional products, may offer antioxidant protection when used regularly in conjunction with typical doses of acetaminophen and NSAIDs in humans.[68,69]

## Sulfur-Containing Amino Acids

Sulfur-containing amino acids support liver health following exposure to acetaminophen. For those on a regimen of chronic acetaminophen or NSAID use, supplementing daily with sulfur-containing amino acids and other compounds to support glutathione levels may protect against drug-induced toxicity.

**N-acetyl cysteine (NAC).** High-dose NAC is a conventional treatment for acetaminophen overdose. It is an effective treatment for acute liver failure due to nonacetaminophen drug toxicity as well.[70] Any time acetaminophen is taken, at least 600 mg of N-acetyl cysteine should be taken along with it to help protect against liver toxicity.

**Methionine.** Methionine is the essential amino acid precursor to several sulfur-containing antioxidants (including cysteine and glutathione), and sufficient dietary methionine is necessary for maintaining glutathione levels. Methionine is used as an alternate conventional antidote for acetaminophen overdose, although a lack of comparative controlled trials makes it difficult to determine its relative efficacy to NAC in humans.[30] In some parts of the world, methionine (10%) is included

in acetaminophen products to protect against accidental intoxication. A study in rats of a single-tablet combination demonstrated that including methionine could minimize liver toxicity (measured by serum ALT and AST) at therapeutic (100 mg/kg) and highly toxic (1000 mg/kg) acetaminophen doses.[71]

**S-adenosylmethionine (SAMe).** SAMe, a methionine derivative, is critical for the synthesis of nucleic acids, proteins, and phospholipids (compounds necessary for recovery after an acetaminophen overdose). Acetaminophen decreases SAMe levels in the nuclei and mitochondria of liver cells.[72] In one study, the efficacy (as an antidote) of SAMe and NAC were comparable when given to mice within 1 hour of acetaminophen overdose.[73]

## Selenium

Selenium is a cofactor for enzymes that synthesize glutathione and detoxify acetaminophen. In an experimental mouse model, selenium deficiency significantly reduced the size of a lethal acetaminophen dose.[74] Injecting rats with selenium 24 hours prior to acetaminophen overdose provided significant protection against hepatotoxicity, lowered levels of ALT and AST (markers of liver damage), and increased liver glutathione levels.[75] Oral selenium (0.5 mg/kg body weight) combined with NAC (500 mg/kg body weight) demonstrated a greater protective effect than NAC alone when administered to rats within 1 hour of acetaminophen overdose.[76]

## Carotenoids

Several carotenoids have been examined for protection against acetaminophen overdose in rat models. *Lutein* (50–250 mg/kg/day) administered 7 days before overdose preserved glutathione levels and reduced elevations of ALT and AST in response to acetaminophen.[77] *Lycopene*-rich tomato extract (5 mg/kg/day) given for 7 consecutive days after overdose had a similar protective effect.[78] Single doses of *beta-carotene* (30 mg/kg) or *mesozeaxanthin* (50–250 mg/kg) given concurrently with a toxic acetaminophen dose reduced serum liver enzymes and in the case of mesozeaxanthin, microscopic evidence of liver tissue damage.[68,79]

## Silymarin

Silymarin, a mixture of several related polyphenolic compounds from *milk thistle*,[80] promotes detoxification by several complementary mechanisms. The antioxidant capacity of silymarin can lower oxidative stress (in the liver) associated with acetaminophen metabolism in rats, which has the effect of conserving cellular glutathione levels.[81] Like NAC, silymarin can protect against acetaminophen toxicity. Furthermore, an animal study suggests that it may be more effective than NAC for acetaminophen toxicity if the treatment is delayed. In a mouse model, it was effective when administered up to 24 hours after overdose.[82]

## Curcumin

When administered to rats within 30 minutes of experimental acetaminophen intoxication, 200 mg/kg of curcumin prevented the microscopic appearance of kidney damage, prevented elevations in renal lipid peroxidation, and maintained glutathione levels compared to control rats.[83] Oral preconditioning of rats with 50 or 100 mg/kg/day for 7 days significantly reduced markers of liver damage (ALT, AST, and lipid peroxidation) following experimental acetaminophen overdose.[84] Curcumin may also increase the efficacy of NAC as an acetaminophen antidote; the addition of 25 mg/kg curcumin to 200 mg/kg NAC protected rat liver and kidney from acetaminophen toxicity with an efficacy equivalent to 800mg/kg of NAC.[85]

## Polyphenols

Polyphenolic antioxidants have been tested for their ability to mitigate liver damage in mouse models of acetaminophen overdose. Pretreatment of mice with either *grape seed extract* (100 mg/kg/day for 7 days) or *green tea extract* (0.25–1% of diet for 5 days) protected livers from acetaminophen-mediated damage, as determined by serum levels of ALT and microscopic examination.[86–89] *Resveratrol* (75 mg/kg) injected into mice 1 or 6 hours after acetaminophen intoxication significantly reduced ALT levels compared to control animals.[90] In addition, an injection of resveratrol (30 mg/kg) following acetaminophen-induced intoxication in mice resulted in reduced markers of hepatotoxicity.[91]

## Coenzyme Q10 (CoQ10)

Treating rats by injection with CoQ10 either before or after acetaminophen overdose conferred protection from liver damage. Pretreatment with intravenous CoQ10 (5 mg/kg) reduced serum ALT and markers of oxidative stress, but had no effect on liver glutathione levels.[92] Two injections of CoQ10 (10 mg/kg each) given 1 and 12 hours after acetaminophen intoxication significantly reduced levels of ALT, AST, and inflammatory cytokines, suppressed lipid peroxidation, preserved glutathione, and reduced tissue death.[93]

## Vitamin C

High doses of ascorbyl palmitate (equivalent to 600 mg/kg of free vitamin C) given concurrently with acetaminophen prevented the elevation of serum liver enzymes in mice and reduced acetaminophen-mediated mortality.[94] Free vitamin C (ascorbic acid) did not protect against liver or kidney damage in mouse models.[94,95]

## Botanicals

Several botanicals have been examined for protection against acetaminophen overdose in animal models. Rats pretreated with the traditional liver tonics *Andrographis paniculata* (100–200 mg/kg/day) and *Picrorhiza kurroa* (50–100 mg/kg/day) had lower markers of liver damage (ALT, AST, lipid peroxidation) after acetaminophen intoxication.[84,96] When given at 6 mg/kg, *andrographolides*, the principle bioactive compounds from andrographis, demonstrated nearly 100% survival of liver cells following acetaminophen overdose.[97] A rescue injection of *Gingko biloba* following acetaminophen overdose reversed the increases in serum liver enzymes, lipid oxidation, and inflammatory cytokines due to acetaminophen intoxication.[98] Several compounds from *garlic*, including ajoene,[99] diallyl disulfide,[100] S-allylmercaptocysteine,[101] and fresh garlic homogenates[102] have been shown to preserve liver glutathione levels as well as reduce serum markers of liver damage, liver tissue death, and animal mortality in rodent models of acetaminophen overdose when supplied in sufficient quantities (up to 5 g/kg for fresh garlic homogenates).

## Melatonin

Treatment of mice with oral melatonin (50 or 100 mg/kg) 4 or 8 hours before acetaminophen overdose suppressed the increase in serum ALT and AST activities in a dose- and a time-dependent manner, but had no effect on liver glutathione levels. When given 4 hours before overdose, marked inhibition of liver necrosis was observed.[103] Melatonin injections (10 mg/kg) prior to acetaminophen overdose may be more effective than "rescue" doses for reducing liver toxicity,[104] although rescue treatments at this same dose have been shown to effectively protect kidney tissue from cell death.[105]

## Gastrointestinal Support

Some gastrointestinal side effects of NSAIDs may be addressed using gastroprotective nutrients. (For more information, see Life Extension's Gastroesophageal Reflux Disease protocol.) Gastroprotective nutrients include the following:

**Zinc-carnosine.** Zinc-carnosine (ie, the carnosine chelate of zinc) is a gastroprotective agent that can reduce NSAID-induced gastrointestinal epithelial cell death, possibly by quenching reactive oxygen species.[106] Zinc-carnosine is a prescription antiulcer drug in Japan, where it has been studied for over a decade.[107,108] Using tracer compounds to monitor the course of the preparation in animal stomachs, researchers observed the combination adhering to the stomach wall more efficiently than either zinc or carnosine alone, allowing the beneficial effects of both components to be delivered to the site where protection is needed.[109] A protective effect was observed in a 2007 human trial; 10 healthy volunteers taking zinc-carnosine (37.5 mg twice daily) were protected against the 3-fold increase in gastrointestinal permeability caused by indomethacin treatment.[110]

**Licorice.** Licorice has been used historically in Europe as a gastroprotective/ulcer-healing agent.[111,112] The over-the-counter ulcer treatment carbenoxolone is a derivative of a naturally occurring compound in licorice. A licorice decoction (given at 2.5 g/kg of body weight) healed aspirin-induced ulcers in the stomachs of rats. The healing effect was similar to two prescription treatments (the proton-pump inhibitor omeprazole and synthetic prostaglandin misoprostol), but was not effective prophylactically (before ulceration had occurred).[113] In another animal study, deglycyrrhizinated licorice (DGL) in combination with the reflux drug cimetidine provided greater protection against aspirin-induced mucosal damage than either substance alone.[114] Unlike whole licorice, DGL extracts provide gastroprotective effects without glycyrrhizin (a component of whole licorice that has been shown to cause side effects such as high blood pressure).[114,115]

**Boswellia serrata.** Boswellic acids, extracted from *Boswellia serrata*, are anti-inflammatory compounds in their own right; they inhibit the activity of the proinflammatory enzyme 5-lipoxygenase and have demonstrated improvements in animal and human models of inflammatory diseases (including asthma, osteoarthritis, and Crohn's disease).[116] Boswellic acids may also protect against NSAID-induced gastric ulceration; in one study, rats pretreated with oral boswellia extract (250 mg/kg) demonstrated significantly less aspirin- or indomethacin-induced gastric ulceration (as determined by qualitative determination) than control animals.[117]

## ANTIOXIDANTS: TARGETING MITOCHONDRIAL HEALTH AND OXIDATIVE STRESS TO REDUCE NSAID TOXICITY

NSAIDs are known to damage the gastric mucosa and contribute to conditions such as ulcers. When examining the mechanisms driving this and other NSAID-related toxicities, much of the scientific community focuses on factors closely related to COX-1 and COX-2 inhibition. However, mitochondrial dysfunction function and oxidative stress appears to be important aspects of this equation as well (see above).

Several studies have shown that nutrients with antioxidant capacity may be able to mitigate NSAID toxicity. For example, *melatonin*, *quercetin*, and *curcumin* have been shown to ease gastric toxicity of NSAIDs by ameliorating oxidative stress.[38,118,119]

In addition, nutrients that support mitochondrial function such as *coenzyme Q10* and *pyrroloquinoline quinone (PQQ)* may be able to blunt some of the mitochondrial toxicity caused by NSAIDs, although this hypothesis has yet to be confirmed in clinical trials.

## Life Extension Suggestions

*If an acetaminophen overdose is suspected, call 911 or the National Poison Control Center (1-800-222-1222) immediately.*[67]

By supporting antioxidant defenses and bodily detoxification systems, the following nutrients may help combat acetaminophen and NSAID-related toxicity.

- **N-acetyl-cysteine** (NAC): 600–1800 mg daily
- **L-methionine:** 1000 mg daily
- **S-adenosylmethionine** (SAMe): 200–1200 mg daily
- **Selenium:** 200–400 mcg daily
- **Lutein:** 10–20 mg daily
- **Lycopene extract:** 15 mg daily
- **Beta-carotene:** 4500 IU daily
- **Zeaxanthin and meso-zeaxanthin blend:** 3.75 mg daily
- **Milk thistle,** standardized extract: 750 mg daily
- **Curcumin,** as highly absorbed BCM-95®: 400–800 mg daily
- **Grape seed extract:** 100 mg daily
- **Green tea extract** (standardized to 98% polyphenols): 725–1450 mg daily
- **Trans-resveratrol:** 250 mg daily

- **Coenzyme Q10,** as ubiquinol: 100–300 mg daily
- **Ascorbyl palmitate:** 500 mg daily
- **Andrographis paniculata extract:** 150–300 mg daily
- **Picrorhiza kurroa extract:** 4 mg daily
- **Ginkgo biloba** (standardized extract): 120 mg daily
- **Garlic extract,** standardized to 10 000 ppm allicin potential (12 mg): 1200–4800 mg daily
- **Melatonin:** 0.3–5 mg before bed (sometimes up to 10 mg)
- **Quercetin,** as quercetin dihydrate, glycoside derivatives, and free quercetin: 250–500 mg daily
- **Pyrroloquinoline quinone** (PQQ): 10–20 mg daily

The following nutrients may support the health of the gastric mucosa:

- **Zinc-L-carnosine:** 50 mg daily
- **Deglycyrrhizinated licorice extract:** 500 mg daily
- **Boswellia serrata extract,** standardized to 20% AKBA: 100 mg daily

In addition, the following blood tests may provide helpful information:

- Chemistry Panel and Complete Blood Count (CBC)
- Cystatin-C

## REFERENCES

References available at: www.lef.org/dpt5/ch1

# 2

# Acne

Acne (acne vulgaris) is a dermatologic condition characterized by lesions that most often appear on the face and neck, but also develop on the chest, back, shoulders, and upper arms. Approximately 80–95% of adolescents develop some degree of acne, but its prevalence declines over subsequent years until middle age, when it still affects about 12% of women and 3% of men.[1,2] Acne can be a significant source of misery, and it is difficult to treat. Many over-the-counter (OTC) medications and washes are sold and marketed for acne (many with harmful chemicals), along with strong prescription medications.

Acne is characterized by pimples, cysts, and abscesses. It occurs when the pores in the skin are blocked, trapping oil, dead skin, and bacteria in the hair follicles. Under normal circumstances, glands (called sebaceous glands) attached to hair follicles secrete an oily substance known as sebum. This sebum typically travels up the hair follicle and onto the skin. However, if the hair follicle is blocked, the sebum can not get out, sometimes causing the formation of a blackhead. This is the result of the blocked oil oxidizing, causing inflammation and an influx of white blood cells. Meanwhile, normally present bacteria (*Propionibacterium acnes*) begin to break down the trapped sebum within the hair follicle. This results in further inflammation, as white blood cells attack the bacteria. Pus forms as the lesion enters the whitehead stage. In more severe stages, an abscess—a pus-filled pocket within the skin—may form. Although most pimples won't leave lasting scars, anything that damages the dermis (the layer of skin just underneath the epidermis) can leave a permanent scar.

## TYPES OF ACNE LESIONS

- Open comedones (blackheads): These are dilated hair follicles that are filled with sebum, dead cells and bacteria, and which have central, dark, solid plugs. The follicles are not completely blocked; the black appearance is caused by oxidation, not dirt.
- Closed comedones (whiteheads): These form when skin cells and oil completely block the opening of a hair follicle, usually after a blackhead has formed.
- Nodules: These are solid, dome- or irregular-shaped, inflamed lesions that extend deep into the skin, sometimes causing tissue damage and scarring if not treated. Nodular acne, which can be painful, is the most severe form of the disease.
- Papules: This type of whitehead (≤5 mm) is one that has become swollen, red and inflamed.
- Cysts: These sac-like lesions contain white blood cells, bacteria, and dead cells in a liquid or semiliquid state. They can result in scarring, and may be very painful and severely inflamed. Cysts and nodules often appear together to form nodulocystic acne, also very severe.
- Pustules: This whitehead is pus-filled and inflamed. Once they rupture into the skin, they form pustular heads.

## CAUSES

Acne can be caused by environmental and genetic factors, but genetics seems to predominate. In one large twin study, for example, 81% of disease variance—that is, the difference from what would normally be expected—was attributed to genetic effects, and the remaining 19% to environmental factors. The study also showed that having a family history of acne is significantly associated with increased personal risk.[3]

The role of hormones in the development of acne is apparent at puberty, when there is a surge in the production of male hormones (which are present in both males and females), enlarging the sebaceous glands in the skin. This results in increased sebum production, which leads to the aforementioned plug formation, creating as well a fertile environment in which bacteria can multiply. Unlike male hormones (androgens), female hormones (estrogens) have a beneficial effect on acne, which is why some doctors recommend birth control pills for women who have acne. But when a woman's estrogen levels decline, as they do just before the beginning of a menstrual cycle, acne may worsen.[4]

Acne or acne-like lesions can develop in response to various substances, including corticosteroids, lithium,[5] and some psychotropic drugs. Other causes include exposure to tobacco smoke, coal tar derivatives, industrial oils, and chlorinated hydrocarbons. Further, oils in aerosol sprays, as well as excessive washing or scrubbing of the skin, can exacerbate acne because these cause increased skin-oil production. Use of many types of cosmetics, oil-based hair products, and suntan lotions can block oil glands and worsen acne; hypoallergenic, oil-free, water-based products that do not clog pores are better choices.[4] Despite popular opinion, the conventional medical view is that acne is not caused by poor hygiene or consuming specific foods, such as chocolate, pizza, and soda (although the evidence is mixed—see "The Role of Diet in Acne" below).

# CONVENTIONAL TREATMENT OPTIONS

Many people who have mild-to-moderate cases of acne choose to treat themselves, using topical and/or systemic (oral) products that are available over the counter (OTC). More severe acne requires a professional approach designed by a physician (usually a dermatologist), and typically includes topical and/or systemic prescription medications.

## Topical Treatment

When choosing a topical product, the type of vehicle— the cream, gel, lotion, or solution that contains the active ingredient—may be as important as the medicinal agent. For example, creams are appropriate for sensitive or dry skin, and gels and solutions can be helpful for oily skin. Lotions can be used with any skin type and are easily spread over hairy skin surfaces. Most topical treatments dry the skin to some degree and cause minor peeling that loosens oil-gland plugs. This peeling smoothes facial skin and helps resolve old and new lesions. On the downside, topical medications can cause minor irritation. For mild acne, self-treatment with OTC topical products may be sufficient, while more severe or resistant cases may respond to prescription products.

The active ingredients found in commonly used OTC and prescription topical preparations include benzoyl peroxide (which kills bacteria), salicylic acid (encourages shedding of cells), alphahydroxy acid, sulfur (which breaks down blackheads and whiteheads), azelaic acid (an antibacterial agent), retinoids (suppressing skin oil production), antioxidants, and antibiotics. Combination therapy is used for people who have comedones (clogged pores) and inflammatory acne. Once topical treatment begins, it often takes 4–6 weeks for any significant improvement to become evident, and treatment should continue until no new lesions appear. As with most medical treatment, it is very important that medication be used consistently. This can be especially challenging when the patient is an adolescent.

**Topical retinoids.** Topical retinoids (eg, Retin-A®, or tretinoin) are available as creams, gels, and solutions. Retinoids are naturally occurring or synthetic compounds that are chemically similar to vitamin A (retinol), which is necessary for skin growth, differentiation, and maintenance. Mild acne responds well to tretinoin, which acts on oil glands and reduces clogged

pores. Further, long-term use of tretinoin increases collagen synthesis and the shedding of dead skin, and can produce a more even skin tone. Side effects include burning, stinging, itching, peeling, scaling, dryness, tightness, and reddened skin—all are sensations most noticeable with solutions and least with gels. Topical retinoids are sometimes used with antibiotics; combination therapy is faster acting and less irritating than single therapies.[6]

The retinoid Tazorac® (tazarotene) is available in gel and cream and often used along with a topical antibiotic. It is more effective than tretinoin and Accutane® (isotretinoin).[7] Yet another topical medication is adapalene, a "designer" topical retinoid agent that acts rapidly, but has been found to be less effective than tazarotene in a comparison study.[8]

## Systemic Treatment

Oral medications are usually reserved for severe cases of acne, and may include antibiotics, oral retinoids, and antiandrogens. Antibiotics may be used to prevent formation of new blemishes by killing bacteria present in the skin.[9] Accutane®, a chemical look-alike of retinoic acid, inhibits sebaceous gland function and keratinization (accumulation of dead skin cells). Another oral retinoid, acitretin, is also used for severe acne. However, caution is necessary: Oral retinoids are associated with liver damage and a high risk of fetal deformity if taken during pregnancy. They are absolutely contraindicated in women who might become pregnant.

Antiandrogens block the action of androgens, which cause increased sebum secretion by stimulating the sebaceous gland. In women, birth control pills are often prescribed.[10] Women who have more resistant acne and excess androgens may be prescribed 5-alpha-reductase inhibitors (eg, finasteride or Avodart®), which block the metabolism of testosterone to dihydrotestosterone (DHT), or flutamide, which blocks testosterone receptor sites on cell membranes.[11] Two other drugs that may have antiandrogen action are isotretinoin.[12] and the anti-acne antibiotic roxithromycin[13]

**New drugs.** Several new drugs are being studied. They include steroid sulfatase inhibitors, which block production of sex steroids,[14] glycylglycine antibiotics (tigecycline),[15] and lipoxygenase inhibitors for inflammation.[16]

# THE ROLE OF DIET IN ACNE

Diet has long been suspected as a contributor to acne. Many people strongly believe that such foods as greasy pizza, chocolate, and refined sugars cause acne. Meanwhile, the conventional dermatological community is adamant that diet does not contribute to acne, dismissing most dietary concerns as myths.

According to the few well-designed scientific studies, the truth is probably somewhere between these 2 extremes. There is some very preliminary evidence that a diet with a high glycemic index—that is, one contributing to glucose in the blood—may contribute to acne. In one small study, researchers noted that, by avoiding glycemia-inducing foods, "some results appeared promising," but that the sample size (11 young men aged 15–20) was not large enough to draw significant conclusions.[17] Another study conducted at the Harvard School of Public Health, Department of Nutrition, examined the role of dairy consumption in acne. Researchers studied questionnaires submitted by more than 47000 high-school-age women, and found a "positive association" between acne and total milk and skim milk consumption. They speculated that the association may be due to hormones and bioactive molecules found in dairy milk.[18] Other studies have confirmed that the Western diet in general, which is high in fats, refined carbohydrates, and sugar, is conducive to acne. In one survey, researchers did not find a single case of acne among sample natives on the Pacific island of Kitava, Papua New Guinea, or Ache hunter-gatherers in Paraguay, in contrast to the 79–95% of American adolescents who are afflicted with acne.[1] Researchers concluded that these remarkable differences could not be attributed to genetics alone.

Although more research is needed to fully understand the interaction between diet and acne, Life Extension recommends that people who suffer from acne should strive for the "cleanest" diet possible, concentrating on fresh, organic fruits and vegetables, and reducing intake of saturated fat and processed sugar. Patients with acne should also drink organic, hormone-free dairy products, which may reduce the presence of hormones that cause acne. Finally, acne patients should drink plenty of clean, filtered water.

# NUTRITIONAL AND ALTERNATIVE THERAPIES

Nutritional and alternative therapies for acne can help reduce inflammation, and infection, and may be used alone or to complement conventional medical treatment, especially in cases of severe or difficult-to-treat acne.

## Vitamins A and E

The benefits of vitamins A and E in acne were highlighted in a study in which investigators identified plasma vitamin A and E concentrations in 100 untreated patients with acne, compared with 100 healthy controls. Plasma concentrations of both vitamins in patients with acne were significantly lower than those of the controls, and a strong relationship between a decline in vitamin A and E levels and an increase in the severity of acne was noted.[19]

This study supports previous work in which researchers found that supplementation with vitamin A is beneficial in inflammatory conditions, including acne, and conversely that vitamin A deficiency induces inflammation and aggravates existing inflammatory conditions.[20] In fact, vitamin A in retinoid form has long been an important treatment for acne.

## Lipoic Acid

Research into the efficacy of lipoic acid in the treatment of acne goes back several decades. Reportedly, lipoic acid activates a factor in the body known as AP-1, which produces enzymes that digest damaged collagen and helps erase scars, including acne scars.[21] Lipoic acid is an ingredient in several topical acne remedies, but it can be taken as an oral supplement as well.

## Zinc

This mineral appears to perform a threefold role in the treatment of acne. It helps reduce inflammation, kills *Propionibacterium acnes*, the main bacteria associated with the disease, and produces changes in the skin environment that make it more hostile to this bacterium for a longer time. A 2-month study of the efficacy of zinc gluconate (30 mg once daily) in 30 patients with inflammatory acne showed a reduction in the number of inflammatory lesions after the treatment period, and improved effectiveness of the antibiotic erythromycin among patients with antibiotic-resistant organisms.[22] In a double-blind study, a combination of 1.2% zinc and 4% erythromycin in a topical lotion was used by 14 individuals with acne. The combination significantly reduced secretion of sebum after 6 weeks of treatment.[23] Further, a topical preparation of zinc acetate was found to prolong the duration of erythromycin on skin, potentially overcoming some mechanisms of erythromycin resistance.[24]

In addition, clinical trials of zinc preparations have demonstrated their equivalence to antibiotics, with the added benefit of more convenient dosing schedules. A study that compared a cream containing chloroxylenol and zinc oxide showed no difference in efficacy compared with 5% benzoyl peroxide, but it did find significantly less skin drying and irritation with the zinc-containing cream.[25] Finally, a 2005 study demonstrated that a gel containing clindamycin plus zinc, applied once or twice daily, achieved the same benefit obtained by clindamycin lotion alone used twice daily.[26]

## Niacinamide (nicotinamide)

One of the 2 principal forms of niacin, niacinamide is effective when applied topically to acne. In a State University of New York study, a 4% nicotinamide gel was compared to a 1% clindamycin gel for the treatment of moderate inflammatory acne in 76 patients. Treatment was applied twice daily for 8 weeks. At the end of treatment, 82% of the nicotinamide patients and 68% of the clindamycin patients were improved. The fact that the use of topical clindamycin is also associated with the development of resistant microorganisms makes niacinamide even more preferred.[27] Nicotinamide cream has also been shown to reduce the amount of sebum present on the skin.[28]

## Essential Fatty Acids

The omega-3 fatty acids eicosapentaenoic acid (EPA) and docosahexaenoic acid (DHA) are well-known anti-inflammatories that have been shown in dozens of studies to reduce inflammation. Although they have not been extensively studied in acne or skin inflammation, their ability to reduce inflammation in general suggests a role in the treatment of acne. Several studies have found that omega-3 fatty acids are absorbed through the skin and can reduce inflammation in a particular area.[29,30]

## Herbal Therapy

Herbal therapy is often suggested for acne, but few controlled scientific studies have been conducted to verify any claims. In a double-blind, placebo-controlled clinical trial of Ayurvedic (ancient Hindu) herbal preparations, researchers randomly assigned either placebo or 1 of 4 Ayurvedic formulas to 82 people with moderate acne. One formulation, Sunder Vati, significantly reduced the number of inflammatory and noninflammatory acne lesions. Sunder Vati consists of ginger (*Zingiber officinale*), *Holarrhena antidysenterica*, and *Embelia ribes*.[31]

Several other herbs have anti-inflammatory properties that may be helpful in the treatment of skin conditions, although no scientific studies have been performed with acne. The herbs include calendula (*Calendula officinalis*), German chamomile (*Matricaria recutita*), witch hazel (*Hamamelis virginiana*), and licorice root (*Glycyrrhiza glabra*).[32] These are found in some natural skin-care products, and may be effective on an individual basis.

## Light-based Therapies

Numerous studies have shown that laser and other light-based therapies are safe and effective in the treatment of acne. In a study in which 45 patients with mild-to-moderate acne were treated with high-intensity pure blue light (two 20-minute treatments per week for 4–8 weeks), 50% were highly satisfied with the treatment, 20% had complete clearing at 8 weeks, and no side effects were reported.[33] Similarly, researchers in Japan reported a 64.7% improvement in acne lesions among 28 adults who were treated with a total of 8 biweekly 15-minute treatments,[34] while in yet another study investigators reported that 85% of acne had cleared 2 months after 8 pulsed-light and heat-energy treatments.[35]

In addition, a combination of topical medication and light therapy has also proved effective. Santos and colleagues found that topical 5-aminolevulinic acid, along with intense pulsed light, is superior to light treatment alone in the treatment of acne, and may be used with other acne treatment methods.[36]

## NATURAL TOPICAL PRODUCTS

A wide range of natural products, from facial scrubs and moisturizers to antiseptics and facial masks, are available for acne and skin care. Note that many of these products contain ingredients with claims that are supported by anecdotal reports but not scientific research. Results may vary based on individual skin sensitivities and severity of acne.

- **Skin healing.** Gels that contain some of the following: lipoic acid, carnosine, dimethylaminoethanol (DMAE), collagen, protein, and vitamins A, C, and E. These ingredients reportedly repair damaged tissue and mitigate free-radical damage.
- **Inflammation and redness.** Creams that contain chamomile, cat's claw, and geranium extract help to reduce inflammation from infection or irritating topical medications.
- **Cleansers.** Facial washes contain fruit and vegetable extracts such as lemon, apricot, and cucumber, and herbal extracts such as ginseng, green tea, and ginkgo for deep pore cleansing. Remember that excessive scrubbing or washing with any product increases sebum production and can aggravate acne.
- **Antibacterial/antifungal.** Tea tree oil contains chemicals known as terpenoids, which kill bacteria, including some bacteria that are resistant to antibiotics. In a double-blind study in which 5% tea tree oil was compared with 5% benzoyl peroxide in the treatment of acne, the oil was more effective overall and had far fewer side effects,

although it was slower in action than the benzoyl peroxide.[37] In a subsequent study, researchers determined that the major components of tea tree oil are active against *Propionibacterium acnes*, lending further support to its use in the treatment of acne.[38] Echinacea and white willow bark contain antiseptics that kill microbes. Calendula and marigold possess antibacterial activity.

- **Astringents.** Witch hazel, herbal extracts, citrus seed extracts, and calendula remove excess facial oil.
- **Facial masks.** Formulations that combine the following minerals, extracts, and antioxidants can provide a multi-modal system in lessening the severity of acne and improve the skin's appearance.
  - **Seaweed extract.** Stimulates, revitalizes, and nourishes skin due to its content of iodine and sulfur, which also give it soothing, anti-inflammatory, and disinfectant abilities.[39]
  - **Bentonite clay** (a combination of montmorillonite and volcanic ash). Pulls oils and toxins from the skin.
  - **Sulfur.** When applied topically, interacts with the cysteine present in the outermost layer of the epidermis to form hydrogen sulfide. This hydrogen sulfide effectively breaks down the tough, keratin-containing dead skin cells that comprise this outer layer and gently removes them. In addition to this exfoliating action, sulfur also has an inhibitory effect on the growth of bacteria involved in acne, possibly from its ability to inactivate bacterial enzyme systems. Sulfur is an excellent anti-inflammatory that also effectively downregulates the production of histamines by macrophage cells that cause infected skin to become red, swollen, and painful.[40]
  - **Antioxidant tea blend.** Helps reduce the production of inflammatory agents that promote new acne infections.[41]

## Life Extension Suggestions

### Lifestyle Modifications
- Avoid the sun. Overexposure to the sun can worsen acne.
- Use cosmetics sparingly. Use only hypoallergenic, oil-free cosmetics.
- Wash face gently with unscented, oil-free cleansers and keep skin clean. Remember: Acne is not caused by dirt. Scrubbing inflamed skin makes acne worse.
- Resist the urge to squeeze, scratch, or pick at acne lesions. Let them drain when they are ready.
- Try products that contain benzoyl peroxide for mild-to-moderate acne.
- Young men with moderate-to-severe acne should use a new razor blade every time they shave to lessen risk of infection.
- Avoid alcohol-based aftershaves. Instead, use herbal alternatives that include essential oils of lavender, chamomile, or tea tree oil.

- Eliminate foods high in fat, hormones, and iodine.
- Eat a range of whole, natural foods, especially raw foods. Avoid processed foods with additives and trans-fatty acids.
- Drink adequate liquids, especially pure water and green tea.

In addition, the following nutrients may be considered:

- **Vitamin A:** 5000–10000 international units (IU) daily
- **Vitamin E:** 400 IU, with 200 mg gamma tocopherols daily
- **R-lipoic acid:** 150–300 mg daily
- **Zinc:** 50 mg daily
- **EPA/DHA:** 1400 mg EPA and 1000 mg DHA daily
- **Niacinamide:** As a topical gel
- **Tea tree oil:** Topical oil, as needed
- **Sulfur and antioxidant blend facial mask:** Per label instructions
- **Seaweed extract:** Found in certain formulated creams, lotions, and gels

For people who cannot find relief with the above recommendations, prescription medications may be warranted. Consult a medical professional if acne does not respond to self-treatment. Your physician may consider several drug therapies, including Retin-A®, Accutane®, antibiotics, or antiandrogens.

Oral and topical antibiotics help prevent new blemishes by killing bacteria and breaking down sebum into free fatty acids. Prescription-strength antibiotics must be obtained from a physician. However, some lesser-strength antibiotics are available as OTC preparations. For women who do not respond to other therapies, birth control pills may be prescribed.

In addition, the following blood testing resources may be helpful:

- **Female Comprehensive Hormone Panel**
- **Male Comprehensive Hormone Panel**

## REFERENCES

References available at: www.lef.org/dpt5/ch2

# 3

---

# Adrenal Disorders (Addison's Disease and Cushing's Syndrome)

---

The adrenal glands are a pair of triangular-shaped, hormone-producing glands; one is located on top of each kidney. They regulate several fundamental aspects of human physiology via secretion of specific hormones including *glucocorticoids* (eg, cortisol), *mineralocorticoids* (eg, aldosterone), *catecholamines* (eg, epinephrine), and *adrenal androgens* (eg, dehydroepiandrosterone [DHEA]).[1-6]

- *Glucocorticoids* help regulate blood sugar, blood pressure, fat and protein metabolism, and immunity.[7]
- *Mineralocorticoids* help regulate kidney and cardiovascular function (via maintenance of salt and water balance within the body).[8]
- *Catecholamines* help regulate the *fight or flight* response to stress.[3,9]
- *Adrenal androgens* are precursors to sex hormones such as testosterone and estrogen.[6]

Disordered adrenal function can lead to a barrage of significant complications, including diabetes, high blood pressure, prolonged fatigue, and depression.[10,11] *Addison's disease* and *Cushing's syndrome* are two major adrenal gland disorders, and they can be *deadly* if left untreated.[10,12,13]

Typical conventional treatment strategies for Addison's and Cushing's comprise side-effect-laden drugs that may require regular clinical monitoring, or invasive surgical procedures.[14,15] However, emergent treatment strategies such as stimulation of *adrenal stem cells* for Addison's disease and the novel drug *pasireotide* for Cushing's syndrome represent the potential next generation of minimally invasive treatment strategies for these debilitating conditions.[16,17]

This protocol will provide an overview of adrenal function and examine the development and consequences of the two primary adrenal disorders: Addison's disease and Cushing's syndrome. Conventional strategies for managing adrenal disorders will be discussed, as well as emerging medical approaches and scientifically studied natural therapies.

## ADRENAL GLAND FUNCTION

Each adrenal gland has an outer region, called the *cortex*, and an inner region, called the *medulla*. Each of these regions contains highly specialized cells that secrete distinct hormones to carry out different physiologic functions.[3]

The *adrenal cortex* secretes three types of hormones: *glucocorticoids*, *mineralocorticoids*, and *androgens*.

- *Glucocorticoids* (eg, *cortisol*) control inflammation and regulate the body's response to infections and stress. They also play a role in maintaining blood pressure, blood sugar, and cardiovascular function.[7]
- *Mineralocorticoids* (eg, *aldosterone*) regulate sodium and potassium levels in the body and thereby help maintain blood pressure and water balance, mainly via the kidneys.[8]
- *Adrenal androgens* (eg, *dehydroepiandrosterone [DHEA]*) are precursors of the sex hormones testosterone and estrogen.[6] In addition, the adrenal glands also produce a small amount of testosterone.[3]

The *adrenal medulla* produces the *catecholamine hormones*, which comprise epinephrine (also known as adrenaline), norepinephrine (noradrenaline), and dopamine.[3] Norepinephrine and epinephrine are primarily responsible for the "fight or flight" response to stress or fear.[9]

The "fight or flight" response manifests as increased heart rate and blood pressure, rapid breathing, and greater blood flow to muscles.[18,19] These physiologic responses arise via activation of the *sympathetic nervous system*. The sympathetic nervous system is a part of the involuntary nervous system, which controls processes such as breathing, heart rate, and metabolism.[19,20]

A precisely regulated relationship exists between the adrenal hormones and hormones secreted by the *hypothalamus* (a small region located at the center of the brain) and the pituitary gland (a pea-shaped structure located at the base of the brain). These 3 structures influence one another and collectively comprise the *hypothalamic-pituitary-adrenal (HPA) axis*.[18,21] The HPA axis is crucial to the regulation of a variety of physiologic functions including the body's response to stress. For example, one of the actions of the hypothalamus is to direct the pituitary gland to release *adrenocorticotropic hormone (ACTH)*, which regulates the production and secretion of hormones from the adrenal cortex.

Under normal healthy conditions, the secretion of hypothalamic, pituitary, and adrenal cortex hormones is finely controlled by each of the other glands.[18] For instance, increasing cortisol levels signal the pituitary to reduce ACTH secretion, which in turn decreases cortisol secretion.[18,21] Under chronic stress or disease conditions, however, this feedback system can become imbalanced.[22,23]

## Impaired Adrenal Function

Impaired function of the adrenal glands may lead to either increased or decreased production of adrenal hormones. Cushing's syndrome and Addison's disease are conditions characterized by abnormal adrenal function.

**Cushing's syndrome.** In Cushing's syndrome, blood levels of cortisol remain high over an extended period of time and cause characteristic changes in the body.[13,24] People with Cushing's typically have a rounded "moon" face, gain weight around the trunk, and have slender arms and legs. Their skin is often thin and can have a bruised appearance with stretch marks. Other features include muscle weakness, susceptibility to infection, elevated blood sugar levels (hyperglycemia), and weak bones (osteoporosis). These changes are often accompanied by mood disorders such as anxiety and depression. In children, excess cortisol can lead to stunted growth. Furthermore, men can exhibit reduced fertility and libido, while women can exhibit hirsutism (abnormal hair growth on face, neck, thighs, and chest) and menstrual disorders.[11,25] Excess secretion of adrenal androgens may also lead to virilization (presence of external male characteristics in females or in boys before puberty).[25]

**Addison's disease.** Addison's disease is an uncommon, debilitating disease that is rarely identified in its early stages. In Addison's disease, the function of the adrenal cortex progressively declines over time, resulting in glucocorticoid and mineralocorticoid deficiency, as well as reduced levels of DHEA and androgens.[10,26–28] The typical early symptoms of Addison's disease are weakness, low blood pressure upon standing, and fatigue. People with Addison's disease gradually develop an often heavy pigmentation of the skin (especially around bony prominences, skin folds, and on the back of arms and legs) and a bluish discoloration of the mucous membrane lining the mouth.[10] Cortisol and aldosterone deficiency together cause changes in blood levels of sodium and potassium and a decrease in plasma volume, which can lead to extreme dehydration and shock.[29] Trauma, surgery, and infections in people with reduced adrenal function may result in *adrenal crisis*, a life-threatening condition that can lead to extreme weakness, severe body pain, low blood pressure, and fever.[30,31]

## ADRENAL FATIGUE

Although not a diagnosis recognized by the conventional medical establishment, some innovative doctors characterize "adrenal fatigue" as a condition that shares some symptoms with Addison's disease, such as tiredness, depression, muscle pain, poor concentration, low blood sugar, craving for stimulants, and difficulty sleeping. However, in adrenal fatigue it is thought that the adrenal glands are unable to perform normally due to exposure to chronic stress. More information is available in Life Extension's Stress Management protocol.[32]

## CAUSES AND RISK FACTORS

### Addison's Disease

Adrenal insufficiency, or decreased production of adrenal hormones, can occur for several reasons. *Autoimmune Addison's disease*, in which the body's own immune system attacks the adrenal glands, is the most common cause. In other cases, diseases such as tuberculosis, cancer, or adrenal hemorrhage can damage the adrenal glands, leading to reduced function or complete loss of function.[10,33] Sometimes, mutations in certain genes at birth or an inherent inability of the adrenal glands to respond to *adrenocorticotropic hormone* (ACTH) can lead to the stunted growth of the glands, thereby causing them to secrete abnormally low levels of adrenal hormones. In some severe cases, people with gene mutations can be deficient in all 3 types of adrenal cortex hormones—glucocorticoids, mineralocorticoids, and androgens.[10] Drugs that inhibit the synthesis of steroids in the adrenal cortex (eg, the antifungal drug ketoconazole) can also impair adrenal hormone production.[34–37] Finally, since adrenal gland function is controlled by the hypothalamus and pituitary gland, decreased adrenal function can arise from conditions or events that affect these brain regions, such as pituitary or hypothalamic tumors, pituitary surgery or radiation treatment, or head trauma.[33]

> **Note:** *ACTH is secreted from the pituitary gland and regulates the production and secretion of hormones from the adrenal cortex.*

### Cushing's Syndrome

ACTH signals the adrenal glands to produce cortisol, thus excess secretion of ACTH results in excessive elevation of cortisol levels. A common cause of elevated cortisol is the presence of a pituitary gland tumor that continually secretes ACTH.[24,38] This is referred to as Cushing's *disease* and is considered distinct from Cushing's *syndrome*. In Cushing's syndrome, increased cortisol levels manifest after ACTH secretion from ectopic tumors (tumors in other organs, such as the lung).[24] Since increased cortisol levels in these two conditions are a result of excess ACTH secretion, they are considered to be "ACTH-dependent." Cushing's syndrome can also occur due to the direct over-secretion of cortisol from adrenal gland tumors. This type of cortisol elevation is considered to be "ACTH-independent".[25] Over-treatment with glucocorticoid medications is considered to be the most common cause of Cushing's syndrome.[15]

# DIAGNOSIS AND BIOMARKERS OF ADRENAL GLAND DYSFUNCTION

## Addison's Disease

Addison's disease is typically diagnosed based on assessment of the clinical signs and symptoms described earlier. Laboratory tests are performed to assess electrolyte levels in the blood as well as serum levels of cortisol and ACTH; computed tomography (CT) scans of the adrenal or pituitary glands are sometimes performed as well.[33] Low serum cortisol with increased serum ACTH levels is indicative of Addison's disease.[39] Cortisol levels vary according to the time of the day (diurnal variation), with levels normally peaking no later than 8 a.m.[40] Therefore, an 8 a.m. cortisol test is performed to check for cortisol levels in the blood, which are decreased (<3 μg/dL) in Addison's disease.[33,40,41] Further, individuals with Addison's disease do not show an increase in serum cortisol level when given an injection of cosyntropin (a synthetic form of ACTH); this procedure is referred to as an ACTH stimulation test.[33,42]

On the other hand, people with Addison's disease specifically due to hypothalamic or pituitary disorders will show low levels of both ACTH *and* cortisol.[42] Upon fasting, these individuals often develop very low glucose levels in the blood (hypoglycemia), as their body is unable to produce glucose from stored fat and proteins.[33] Abnormally low blood levels of levels of DHEA-sulfate (DHEA-S) along with decreased cortisol and aldosterone levels are indicative of *adrenal insufficiency*, warranting further testing of HPA axis function.[39]

## Cushing's Syndrome

The typical physical characteristics of Cushing's syndrome are diagnostic and are further confirmed by laboratory test results. People with Cushing's syndrome generally have grossly increased levels of free cortisol in their urine and, although cortisol levels normally show diurnal variation, this variation is not observed in Cushing's syndrome.[43] Measurement of ACTH levels can also help to distinguish between the 2 variants of Cushing's syndrome (ACTH-dependent and ACTH-independent).[15,44] Magnetic resonance imaging (MRI) and CT scans are useful for the diagnosis of pituitary and adrenal tumors.[15,45]

# CONVENTIONAL TREATMENTS

## Addison's Disease

**Hydrocortisone.** The standard therapy for treating Addison's disease consists of replacing the deficient hormones.[10] Hydrocortisone, which is a synthetic glucocorticoid, is one of the most common cortisol replacement therapies.[46] In acute illnesses, such as adrenal crisis, immediate administration of intravenous hydrocortisone and saline is needed to prevent potentially life-threatening complications.[47]

Although effective, there are many challenges associated with using hydrocortisone. Since cortisol levels follow a diurnal variation, it is difficult to choose an optimal drug dosing regimen to simulate this natural *circadian rhythm*.[10,48] Furthermore, it is difficult to regulate levels of ACTH after administering hydrocortisone; ACTH levels can become very high because the hydrocortisone is released into the blood several hours after the morning dose.[10] Persistently high ACTH levels can lead to an increase in the size of the pituitary gland or even, in rare cases, to the development of a pituitary tumor.[49,50] Since the optimum glucocorticoid dose is difficult to determine, there is significant risk of overtreatment. Signs of overtreatment include dark pigmentation of the skin, weight gain, high blood pressure, high blood glucose, easy bruising, osteoporosis, and osteonecrosis (death of bone tissue).[10,51]

**Fludrocortisone.** With regard to the replacement of aldosterone, fludrocortisone (also known as 9α-fluorohydrocortisone, a synthetic compound chemically similar to aldosterone with glucocorticoid and mineralocorticoid activity) can be orally administered. However, care needs to be taken to deliver an optimal dose because overtreatment can lead to hypertension.[10]

## Cushing's Syndrome

**Surgery.** Cushing's disease resulting from a pituitary tumor is treated by surgically removing the tumor.[11,52] However, only about 50% of people with large tumors benefit from surgery because the complete removal of the tumor is challenging. The tumors are also known to recur in up to 45% of people.[11,15,52] Moreover, repeat surgeries to the pituitary or adrenal gland are required in almost 25% of the people with a recurrence of Cushing's syndrome.[53,54]

In Cushing's syndrome where the cause is an ectopic tumor, removal of the tumor is required.[15,52] However, this is not always possible since: 1) identifying and locating the primary ACTH-secreting ectopic tumor may be difficult; 2) the tumor may have spread to different organs via the blood stream (metastasis); or 3) the tumor may be located at a site where surgery is difficult, such as in the pancreas.[11,15,52]

**Pharmaceutical treatment.** Pharmacologic treatment of Cushing's syndrome includes the administration of drugs that prevent steroid production or that suppress the release of ACTH from pituitary or ectopic tumors.[15] With the exception of mifepristone, which was approved by the Food and Drug Administration (FDA) in 2012 for the treatment of high blood sugar in people with Cushing's syndrome who are either not surgical candidates or who had failed surgery, none of the other medications are FDA-approved for use in Cushing's syndrome as of the time of this writing.[15] There are also limitations of these pharmacologic treatments. For instance, blocking steroid production has its own challenges—people on these medicines require frequent hospital visits and laboratory tests to ensure that the treatment does not result in adrenal insufficiency or adrenal crisis.[15,37] If adrenal insufficiency is detected, glucocorticoids can be started; however, great care must be taken to ensure that this preventive measure does not worsen Cushing's syndrome.[15]

The antifungal drug *ketoconazole* inhibits several steps in steroid synthesis within the adrenal cortex. It is also likely that ketoconazole directly inhibits ACTH secretion from the pituitary gland. It is one of the most widely used and effective medications for Cushing's syndrome.[15] However, prolonged treatment with ketoconazole has been shown to cause adrenal crisis.[36,37] Other side effects associated with ketoconazole are erectile dysfunction in men, low libido, and an increase in certain liver enzymes.[15] This increase in liver enzymes occurs through injury to liver cells.[55] Moreover, ketoconazole is known to interact with and possibly interfere with actions of several other medications through the inhibition of the cytochrome P450 enzymes, which are critical for the metabolism of several drugs.[15,35]

*Mitotane* (Lysodren™) is used to treat people with tumors of the adrenal cortex. It prevents the production of steroids by interfering with enzymes involved in the conversion of cholesterol to various other steroid hormones. Although effective, mitotane has a late onset of action—it can take up to 2 weeks before showing beneficial effects. Mitotane

has teratogenic effects (potential to cause birth defects) and can cause nervous system and gastrointestinal side effects.[15]

# NOVEL AND EMERGING THERAPIES

Given the side effects of currently available medications and the burden of repeated laboratory testing necessary to monitor hormone levels, scientists are trying to find novel treatment approaches for adrenal disorders that may be more effective and have an acceptable range of side effects.[11]

## Stem Cells

It is believed that the adrenal cortex contains dormant adrenal stem cells, which are specialized cells that can multiply and differentiate to replenish all cell types that make up the adrenal gland.[56] Further in-depth studies are needed to provide insights into the biology of these stem cells and to characterize their role in adrenal diseases before they can be utilized as a treatment option.[57]

Since cells of the adrenal cortex are sensitive to ACTH levels in the blood, investigators explored the possibility of stimulating adrenal cortex stem cells with ACTH, to push them to differentiate into steroid-producing cells. The assessment of serum cortisol levels after an ACTH stimulation test was the main criterion to check if functioning adrenal cortical cells have been generated or not.[17] This trial could open the doors to a new treatment option for conditions, such as autoimmune Addison's disease, in which the adrenal glands do not secrete adequate amount of hormones but have not lost their ability to respond to ACTH stimulation.

## Pasireotide (Signifor®)

A new drug called pasireotide has shown promising results in reducing cortisol levels in Cushing's disease. This drug is similar in structure and function to the naturally-occurring hormone somatostatin, which has been suggested as a therapeutic target for pituitary-dependent Cushing's disease, following a study revealing that adrenal cortex tumor cells have sites to which somatostatins can bind to prevent the release of ACTH.[58] Results of a clinical trial examining the use of pasireotide in Cushing's disease were published in the New England Journal of Medicine in March 2012. The drug was administered for 12 months to 162 people with Cushing's disease who were divided into 2 groups receiving either 600 or 900 mcg of the drug by subcutaneous injection twice daily. In both groups, the levels of free cortisol in the urine decreased by approximately 50% by the second month of treatment and remained stable. The levels of cortisol in the serum and saliva also decreased. In addition, the overall symptoms of Cushing's disease diminished.[16]

# DIETARY AND LIFESTYLE MANAGEMENT STRATEGIES

The following dietary and lifestyle considerations may support healthy adrenal function.[59]

## Avoiding Simple Carbohydrates

Cortisol increases the levels of glucose in the blood and low glucose levels signal the adrenals to produce more cortisol.[60] Low levels of glucose can occur when meals are skipped or taken at irregular intervals, or by eating foods rich in simple carbohydrates, since simple carbohydrates are metabolized and absorbed faster by the body. This quick absorption triggers a quick spike in blood glucose levels, which subsequently declines quickly as insulin levels rise. This can trigger the stress response mechanism and increase cortisol levels.[60,61] Hence, eating meals at regular intervals and consuming foods rich in fiber, which slows carbohydrate absorption, may prevent the increase in cortisol levels caused by quickly absorbed carbohydrates.

Proper glucose control is paramount not only for mitigating sugar-induced spikes in stress hormone levels, but for controlling and preventing a myriad of age-related diseases. Life Extension recommends a comprehensive approach to glucose control and weight management that takes several important, but often overlooked factors into account. A comprehensive, strategically developed approach to glucose and weight management is outlined in the *Life Extension magazine* article titled *The Nine Pillars of Successful Weight Loss*, and in the Life Extension protocol titled Obesity and Weight Loss.

## Dieting Properly

Chronic stress is associated with increased cortisol levels, which promote overeating and increases in abdominal fat.[62] Studies indicate that the brain limits weight gain above a set point, which is ultimately regulated by the levels of *leptin*, a hormone that regulates energy intake and expenditure. When one exceeds their set point, high leptin levels tell the hypothalamus that energy storage (ie, weight) is adequate and appetite is suppressed. However, when dieting, the blood levels of leptin are decreased, which notifies the brain as to the presence of the decreased energy

storage. The brain then reacts by increasing appetite and decreasing metabolism. Consequently, "yo-yo dieting" (an endless cycle of losing and gaining weight due to poor control of calorie intake) can disrupt the hormonal feedback to the brain and improperly disrupt appetite and metabolism.[62] On the other hand, well-planned diets that supply the body with all its essential nutrients can be useful for controlling weight, reducing stress, and improving performance. A clinical study evaluating the effect of calorie restriction for 1 month in otherwise healthy overweight women aged 20–36 found that, along with an average weight loss of almost 13 lbs, there was a significant decrease in blood pressure, heart rate, and cortisol concentration, improved hand–eye coordination, and no evidence of increased physiologic or psychological stress.[63]

## Limiting Stimulants

Consumption of stimulants, such as energy drinks, has been linked to the perception of stress.[64] Caffeine is known to exacerbate the stress response and to increase cortisol production. Therefore, caffeine should be consumed in moderation or avoided by people exposed to chronic stress or with impaired adrenal function.[60] Nicotine exposure in habitual smokers also increases serum cortisol levels.[65]

## Exercising

Exercise stimulates the production of cortisol and other glucocorticoids from the adrenals.[60] As such, people who exercise regularly, such as athletes undergoing endurance training, are continuously exposed to high levels of glucocorticoids. However, studies have shown that regular exercise can modulate the HPA axis whereby people undergoing regular exercise are less sensitive to the effects of elevated glucocorticoid secretion.[60,66] In fact, a clinical study showed that physical conditioning, as performed by moderately- and highly-trained runners, was linked to a reduction in adrenal-pituitary activation.[67] Interestingly, another study evaluating the effect of exercise intensity on the HPA axis in moderately-trained men showed that low-intensity exercise resulted in a reduction of circulating cortisol levels.[68] These studies suggest that low- to moderate-intensity exercise could be beneficial in Cushing's syndrome.

## Maintaining a Positive Outlook and Good Self Esteem

Low self-esteem and loneliness are known to increase cortisol levels, while maintaining a positive outlook on life and a good social support system is associated with lower stress hormone levels.[69]

## Sleep

Along with chronic stress, sleep deprivation is a common cause of high cortisol levels.[70] Disturbed sleep, overactivity of the HPA axis, and metabolic disturbances are often observed in people with Cushing's syndrome, insomnia, and depression.[71] High glucocorticoid concentrations in Cushing's syndrome have a deleterious effect on sleep.[71] Sleep deprivation can have a direct effect on the HPA axis and may be an important risk factor leading to stress-related disorders. Some studies have shown that lack of sleep in healthy people can lead to mild increases in cortisol levels, and that restful sleep can slightly decrease the cortisol levels.[72] Thus, changing one's lifestyle to get adequate sleep at regular intervals may help prevent HPA axis disturbances and stress-related disorders.

# TARGETED NUTRITIONAL INTERVENTIONS

Given the crucial role of the adrenal glands in maintaining normal body function and the extended (often life-long) treatment needed for adrenal disorders, there is a pressing need for alternative strategies that can help people cope with the debilitating effects of Cushing's syndrome, Addison's disease, and related conditions. Research has shown that several natural compounds have an impact on adrenal physiology.[60] In this section, several nutritional interventions that may play a supportive role in the treatment of adrenal disorders will be reviewed. Additional discussion about natural compounds that may support adrenal health (eg, in "adrenal fatigue") is available in the Stress Management protocol.

## Nutritional Interventions in Cushing's Syndrome

**Melatonin.** Melatonin is a hormone secreted by the pineal gland in the brain during the night. It plays a role in inducing sleep and regulating the circadian rhythm.[73,74] Cushing's syndrome has been associated with low melatonin levels and disruption of its circadian secretion.[75,76] A study assessing the effects of melatonin on adrenal hormone production in healthy men found that melatonin reduced cortisol secretion in response to an ACTH stimulation test, but did not affect the levels of other steroid hormones. This suggests that melatonin may have a direct action on the adrenal glands.[77]

**Vitamin D and calcium.** Vitamin D supports calcium absorption and its deficiency can contribute to osteoporosis. In Cushing's syndrome, high cortisol levels lead to osteoporosis.[15] Similarly, long-term glucocorticoid treatment can also result in osteoporosis. Vitamin D supplementation is considered to be an important step for preventing osteoporosis due to glucocorticoid treatment.[78] A group of researchers analyzed studies conducted over 33 years and concluded that vitamin D and calcium supplements should be given to people receiving long-term corticosteroids.[79] A second analysis of studies conducted between 1970 and 2011 showed that adults who received glucocorticoid treatment had less than optimal levels of vitamin D, which were inadequate for the prevention of osteoporosis.[78] Thus, vitamin D supplements may be useful in people with Cushing's syndrome who have high cortisol levels, as well as in Addison's disease where long-term hormone replacement is necessary.

**Potassium.** Potassium levels are known to be low in individuals with Cushing's syndrome, and low potassium levels are a significant determinant of cardiovascular complications in this population.[80,81] Hence, potassium supplements could be useful in people with Cushing's syndrome. However, people on ketoconazole treatment for Cushing's syndrome should avoid potassium supplements since ketoconazole treatment can also increase potassium levels.[82]

**Additional support for Cushing's disease.** The following interventions may provide support for Cushing's disease, though more studies are needed to confirm their efficacy in humans.

- **Vitamin A.** Laboratory and animal studies have shown that retinoic acid (a form of vitamin A) decreases ACTH synthesis and decreases proliferation (or multiplication) and survival of pituitary tumor cells.[11,83] It also decreased proliferation and corticosterone production in adrenal cortex cells.[84] In one study, animals with Cushing's disease were given either ketoconazole or retinoic acid. After 90 and 180 days of treatment there was a significant decrease in ACTH levels in the retinoic acid treated animals compared to no change in the ketoconazole group. The retinoic acid treated animals also showed improvements in clinical signs and survival time, and a significant reduction in pituitary tumor size.[85]

- **Curcumin.** Curcumin, one of the active constituents of *Curcuma longa* (a spice commonly used in South Asian cooking), has been widely studied for its therapeutic properties. ACTH-secreting pituitary tumors are one of the most common causes of Cushing's disease.[38] Using pituitary tumor cells from mice, a laboratory study showed that curcumin suppresses ACTH secretion, stops tumor cell growth and proliferation, and induces the death of tumor cells.[86]

## Nutritional Interventions in Addison's Disease

**Licorice.** Licorice (*Glycyrrhiza glabra*) has been used for hundreds, if not thousands of years in both Eastern and Western cultures to treat myriad illnesses and to increase physical endurance.[87] Licorice may also protect against DNA damage induced by carcinogens (cancer-causing compounds) and induce the death of cancer cells.[88] It was used for the treatment of stomach and duodenal ulcers until the advent of modern anti-ulcer medicines. It was in the context of its use as an antiulcer compound that the mineralocorticoid-like actions of licorice were noticed. People taking licorice extracts for extended periods of time showed sodium and water retention and increased excretion of potassium.[87] This effect was also observed in animal experiments.[89] Further research showed that licorice appeared to be successful in reversing the effects of Addison's disease. With advances in scientific research in the 1980s, it was found that a chemical compound, called glycyrrhetinic acid, present in licorice causes changes in adrenal steroid metabolism, resulting in increased levels of corticosterone in animals and cortisol in humans.[87]

Licorice is also known to regulate the HPA axis. Healthy male and female volunteers who consumed a licorice-containing confectionary showed increased levels of DHEA and testosterone in the saliva.[90] Thus, licorice may also be useful for androgen deficiency in adrenal disorders. In one study, people with Addison's disease on cortisone replacement therapy who were given licorice were found to have increased cortisol tissue levels.[91]

**Dehydroepiandrosterone.** Individuals with Addison's disease, in addition to cortisol insufficiency, have been reported in some studies to have low dehydroepiandrosterone (DHEA) levels, which researchers speculate may contribute to decreased quality of life. A small clinical study of DHEA supplementation among Addison's patients revealed an immunomodulatory role for the hormone in this population, whereby supplementation appeared to improve regulation of inflammation and immune response.[92] In another clinical trial, men and women aged 25–69 with Addison's disease were given DHEA daily for 12 weeks. Their DHEA levels increased from below normal to a normal range for healthy young people.[93] In a year-long study, 106 people with Addison's disease were given 50 mg of DHEA daily or no supplement. The group receiving DHEA showed increased levels of circulating DHEA-S and androstenedione, a reversal of bone density loss at the neck of the femur (thigh bone), and improved emotional health.[6] DHEA

supplementation may also counter some consequences of adrenal insufficiency that arise secondarily to impaired pituitary gland function.[94]

There are several variables that can influence DHEA levels among individuals with adrenal dysfunction, whether due to Addison's or Cushing's, and DHEA supplementation may not be ideal for everyone with impaired adrenal function. Therefore, a diligent approach entails testing blood levels of DHEA-S, a major metabolite of DHEA, to determine if DHEA concentrations are outside the optimal range and initiating supplementation if an insufficiency or deficiency is observed. Life Extension suggests an optimal DHEA-S level of 350–490 µg/dL in men and 274–400 µg/dL in women.

**Pantothenic acid.** Pantothenic acid (vitamin B5) plays a role in the synthesis and maintenance of coenzyme A (CoA), a crucial cofactor for many biological enzymatic reactions and a primary component of lipid and carbohydrate metabolism.[95] Pantothenic acid is thought to be needed to maintain normal adrenal structure and function, as the administration of pantothenic acid to deficient animals improves adrenal function.[96] Adrenal gland cells from rodents treated with pantothenic acid produced higher levels of corticosterone and progesterone than adrenal cells from rats that did not receive treatment.[97]

Prolonged stress from physical, mental, or environmental causes has deleterious effects on the body, including increased levels of cortisol, reduced immune function, and a disruption of the gastrointestinal microflora (beneficial bacteria).[96] Pantothenic acid administered to human subjects with various diseases better controlled the increase in cortisol metabolites in the urine following ACTH stimulation. This suggests pantothenic acid can modulate cortisol secretion in response to stress.[96]

**Coenzyme Q10 (CoQ10).** Coenzyme Q10, in the form of ubiquinone or ubiquinol, is essential for cellular energy production. It has antioxidant properties and protects cell membranes from damage. It is also commonly taken as an antiaging supplement and to increase endurance in athletes.[98,99] When coenzyme Q10 is utilized as an antioxidant within the body, its availability for energy production may decrease.[98] This is the rationale behind the dietary replenishment of coenzyme Q10 in many disease conditions. Preliminary data suggest that adrenal hormone secretion is related to coenzyme Q10 levels. Analysis of coenzyme Q10 levels in people with irregular pituitary-adrenal axis function showed that coenzyme Q10 levels are considerably lower in people with isolated decreases in adrenal function compared to people with adrenal hyperplasia or multiple pituitary deficiencies.[100] The ubiquinol form of coenzyme Q10 has been shown to absorb better into the bloodstream than ubiquinone.

## Life Extension Suggestions

The following interventions may be supportive in conditions involving *excessive adrenal function*:

- **Melatonin:** 0.3–10 mg daily at bedtime
- **Vitamin D3:** 2000–5000 IU daily
- **Calcium:** 1000–1200 mg daily (along with magnesium and boron to further support bone health)
- **Potassium:** 99 mg daily as needed in accordance with blood test results
- **Vitamin A:** 2500 IU daily
- **Curcumin,** as highly absorbed BCM-95®: 400–800 mg daily

The following interventions may be supportive in conditions involving *low adrenal function*:

- **Licorice tea or capsules (not DGL):** per label instructions
- **DHEA:** 50 mg daily, based on appropriate laboratory tests (see DHEA Restoration Therapy protocol for more information)

- **Pantothenic acid (vitamin B5):** 500 mg daily
- **Coenzyme Q10,** as ubiquinol: 100–200 mg daily

Additional suggestions of natural compounds that support adrenal health are available in the Stress Management protocol.

In addition, the following *blood tests* may provide helpful information:

- Chemistry panel (includes potassium levels)
- Aldosterone
- Adrenocorticotropic hormone (ACTH)
- Dehydroepiandrosterone sulfate (DHEA-S)
- Coenzyme Q10
- Cortisol or 24-hour urine cortisol

## REFERENCES

References available at: www.lef.org/dpt5/ch3

*4*

# Age-Related Cognitive Decline

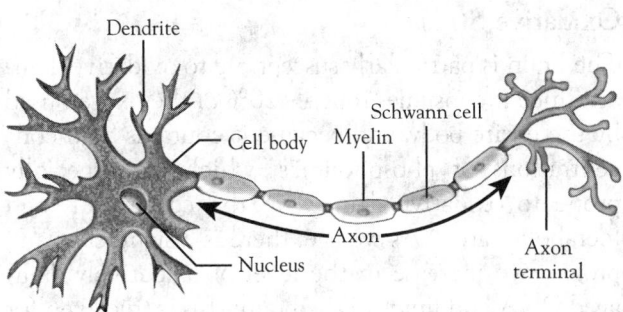

**Anatomy of a neuron**

All aging humans will develop some degree of decline in cognitive capacity as time progresses. Data indicate that deterioration of the biological framework that underlies the ability to think and reason begins as early as the mid-twenties and includes a drop in regional brain volume[1-5]; loss of myelin integrity[6,7]; cortical thinning[8,9]; impaired serotonin, acetylcholine, and dopamine receptor binding and signaling[10-13]; accumulation of neurofibrillary tangles[14]; and altered concentrations of various brain metabolites.[15] Cumulatively, these changes give rise to a variety of symptoms associated with aging, such as forgetfulness, decreased ability to maintain focus, and decreased problem-solving capability. If left unchecked, symptoms often progress into more serious conditions, such as dementia and depression, or even Alzheimer's disease.

Cognitive decline does not affect all individuals equally; clear associations exist between the rate and severity of cognitive decline and a variety of factors, including oxidative stress and free radical damage,[16-18] chronic low-level inflammation,[19] declining hormone levels,[20] endothelial dysfunction,[21] excess body weight,[22] suboptimal nutrition,[23] lifestyle,[24] social network,[25] other medical conditions,[26] and various biomarkers.[27] Fortunately, many of these factors are modifiable to a significant extent, and proactive lifestyle changes, cognitive training, and nutritional interventions have been shown to decrease the rate of intellectual decay and potentially reverse age-related cognitive decline.

## THE AGING BRAIN

The aging process profoundly impacts the brain in ways that can be observed on multiple levels, ranging from subcellularly to macrostructurally. On a diminutive scale, aging causes deterioration of neuronal and mitochondrial membranes, which leads to the loss of cellular integrity and impaired neuronal function.[28-30] Steep age-related declines in neurotransmitter synthesis and signaling,[31-33] coupled with reductions in synaptic density and plasticity (adaptability),[34] and loss of as much as 50% of the length of myelinated axons[35] make the brain increasingly less efficient as we age.

In a broader sense, the physical structure of the brain as a whole also deteriorates with age. Shrinkage and death of neurons, and reductions in the number of synaptic spines and functional synapses contribute to annual reductions of as much as 0.5–1.0% in cortical thickness (the cortex is the outermost layer of the brain) and subcortical volume in some regions of the brain.[36] Specifically, even in healthy individuals, aging accounts for volume variances of 37% in the thalamus, which is involved in sight, hearing, and the sleep–wake cycle; 36% in the nucleus accumbens, which plays a major role in mood regulation (eg, pleasure, fear, reward); and 33% in the hippocampus, a critical site for consolidation of short-term to long-term memory.[36] Taken together, age-related neuroanatomic changes account for an estimated 25 to 100% of the variance in cognitive ability between young and aged individuals.[36] In other words, age-related cognitive decline occurs in tandem with the physical degradation of brain structure. Thus, conserving cognitive vigilance into late life requires early and aggressive intervention to preserve the brain in its youthful physical and functional state.

## BIOLOGICAL RISK FACTORS CONTRIBUTING TO COGNITIVE DECLINE

Various biological systems work in conjunction to maintain optimal brain function and cognitive ability. Perturbations in the harmony of these systems caused by such age-associated insults as chronic inflammation,[37] oxidative stress,[38] insulin resistance,[39] declining hormone levels,[40] and endothelial dysfunction,[41] result in physical deterioration of the brain and subsequent cognitive decline.

## Oxidative Stress

The brain is particularly susceptible to oxidative damage since it consumes roughly 20% of the oxygen used by the entire body, and because it contains high concentrations of phospholipids, which are especially prone to oxidative damage in the context of high metabolic rate.[16] As we age, there is a significant and progressive increase in the level of oxidatively damaged DNA and lipids in the brain; this is true even for healthy individuals.[42] Over time, this free radical damage leads to the death of neurons.

Numerous studies have implicated oxidative stress in the pathology of mild cognitive impairment and Alzheimer's disease alike.[16–18]

In a study of 338 individuals, researchers analyzed blood samples from patients with various neurodegenerative diseases and found that the antioxidant capacity of their blood was reduced by as much as 28%, relative to healthy controls. Subjects with a neurodegenerative condition also exhibited significantly increased levels of thiobarbituric acid reactive substances, a marker of free radical damage.[43]

A separate study, in which researchers examined the plasma of 34 subjects with mild cognitive impairment, 45 with Alzheimer's disease, and 28 age-matched healthy controls, revealed that patients with mild cognitive impairment or Alzheimer's disease displayed markedly increased oxidative damage. Subjects with mild cognitive impairment or Alzheimer's disease exhibited increased protein oxidation (protein carbonyls) and decreased levels of glutathione, a powerful endogenous antioxidant.[44]

In aged rodents exhibiting signs of cognitive deterioration, increased oxidation of key proteins involved in neuronal metabolism and energy production has been observed.[45] Old animals also display dramatically reduced ability to combat oxidative stress, as assessed by a loss of efficiency of thiol-reducing systems.[45]

## Inflammation

The inflammatory process in the brain is unique in that the blood–brain barrier (BBB) (tight layer of endothelial cells that separates the brain from regular systemic circulation), during healthy conditions, prevents the infiltration of inflammatory agents and allows only select nutrients and small molecules into the central nervous system (CNS).[46] However, chronic systemic inflammation induced by stimuli such as cigarette smoking, obesity, disrupted sleep patterns, and poor dietary habits compromises the integrity of the BBB, allowing irritants to enter the brain and stimulate the production of inflammatory cytokines, such as IL-1β, IL-6, and IL-18.[47] Inside the CNS, these cytokines impair *neurogenesis*, the process by which new neurons are generated.[48–51] Aside from inhibiting neurogenesis, some inflammatory cytokines, such as IL-1β, IL-6, and TNF-α, damage and destroy existing neurons.[52,53]

Several studies have linked biomarkers of inflammation with cognitive impairment.

A prospective study of 779 healthy, high-functioning men and women found that subjects in the highest tertile (one-third) for blood levels of IL-6 were significantly more likely to score below the median when assessed for cognitive function at baseline. During follow-up 7 years later, those same individuals more frequently exhibited declines in cognition compared to their counterparts with lower baseline IL-6 levels.[54]

In a study of 97 women between 60 and 70 years of age, elevated baseline high-sensitivity C-reactive protein (hs-CRP) levels were correlated with worsening of memory at the 12-year follow-up. These data led the authors to conclude that *"hs-CRP may be a useful biomarker to identify individuals at an increased risk for cognitive decline."*[55] Likewise, in a study assessing over 4000 subjects, higher levels of CRP *and* IL-6 were found to be associated with decreased cognition and executive function. IL-6 was also associated with steeper declines in memory performance during follow-up at up to 5 years.[19]

Another study found that, even in healthy individuals, baseline CRP levels were inversely correlated with the results of a learning and recall test at follow-up 6 years later. The investigators concluded that *"relatively high concentrations of … CRP may be indicative for impaired cognitive performance."*[37] In a similar study, biological markers were measured in the blood of 93 healthy individuals aged 57 years (mean). At 6 years follow-up time, those individuals with the highest baseline CRP levels scored lower on a word learning test. In this study it was concluded that *"concentrations of serum markers related to inflammation … are not only associated with Alzheimer's disease, but also with cognitive functioning in the cognitively healthy aging population."*[56]

The deleterious effects of inflammation on cognitive function are observable in real time as well. Researchers administered a typhoid vaccination, which is known to induce an inflammatory response, or a placebo injection to 16 healthy men aged 18 to 35. Study subjects then completed a series of tests designed to assess cognitive vigilance. Participants who received the typhoid vaccination exhibited significantly slower reaction times than their counterparts who received the placebo, and the degree of delay in reaction time correlated with the intensity of inflammation, as measured by circulating IL-6 levels.[57]

## Hormonal Imbalance

Distributed throughout the brain are steroid hormone receptors that function to regulate the transcription of a vast array of genes involved in cognition and behavior.[58] Adequate steroid hormone-receptor activation in the brain is a fundamental determinant in many aspects of our lives that we take for granted. When hormonal imbalances or deficiencies disrupt receptor activation, cognitive deficits and emotional turmoil are the result.

### Estrogen

Animal models indicate that experimentally-induced alterations in the levels of steroid hormones, particularly estradiol, in the brain cause significant behavioral changes observable within minutes, leading some researchers to conclude that steroid hormones actually have the capacity to function directly as neurotransmitters in the central nervous system.[59] In humans, suboptimal (low) levels of estradiol are associated with decreased scores on standardized assessments of cognition in both men and women.[20] Postmenopausal women with higher levels of endogenous estradiol also have better semantic memory than do those deficient in the estrogen.[40] Accordingly, postmenopausal women treated with estradiol displayed improvements in executive function compared to those taking a placebo.[60]

### Testosterone

Maintaining optimal levels of testosterone can help preserve cognitive ability as well. In a study involving over 500 aging men and women, higher levels of testosterone were linked with better performance on the Mini-Mental State Examination (MMSE) at baseline. Men with the lowest levels of testosterone at the beginning of the study period were more likely to exhibit a sharp decline in cognitive ability over the following 2-year period as well.[61] Several other studies also conclude that testosterone levels are positively associated with multiple aspects of cognitive function.[62, 63]

Aging men given testosterone replacement therapy display improved cognitive function. In one study healthy men between the ages of 50 and 85 years responded to supplemental testosterone restoration treatment with significantly improved spatial and verbal memory, and spatial ability.[64] Likewise, men with mild cognitive impairment or Alzheimer's disease responded to testosterone therapy with enhanced spatial and verbal memory, and constructional abilities.[65]

Experimental studies indicate that the connection between testosterone and cognitive function is due in part to the dependence of the hippocampus on androgens to maintain synaptic density. Intriguing data show that male nonhuman primates devoid of androgens have a dramatically reduced number of synapses in the hippocampus, which is of paramount importance for consolidation of short-term and long-term memory, as well as learning.[66] Additional experimental data show that hippocampal synaptic maintenance is androgen dependent.[67]

### Dehydroepiandrosterone (DHEA)

Age-associated decline in levels of the adrenal hormone dehydroepiandrosterone (DHEA), which is very active in the central nervous system,[68] is also tied to worsening cognitive performance.[69] In a study involving over 750 aging subjects, MMSE scores were significantly associated with levels of DHEA-S, the sulfated metabolic derivative of DHEA, which is more highly concentrated in humans. Moreover, those individuals with the lowest levels of DHEA-S at baseline displayed greater cognitive decline over time than those with higher initial levels.[70] In a separate community-based study involving nearly 300 healthy women, levels of DHEA-S correlated positively with superior executive function, concentration, and working memory.[71] Accordingly, in a double-blind, placebo controlled clinical trial, 6 months of supplementation with 25 mg of DHEA daily improved measures of cognitive function, especially verbal fluency, in aging women.[72]

### Pregnenolone

Another neurosteroid, pregnenolone, is also involved with a number of cognition-related functions within the brain. For example, experimental studies indicate that pregnenolone modulates neurotransmitter signaling through interaction with select receptor sites, which translates to improvements in long-term memory in rodents.[73,74] In human clinical trials, supplementation with pregnenolone improved cognition in subjects with neurologic disorders.[75] Additionally, levels of pregnenolone metabolites are reduced significantly in the prefrontal cortex—an area involved with higher-order processing—in Alzheimer's disease patients, leading some researchers to speculate that pregnenolone levels may be relevant in the pathology of the disease.[76]

Research indicates that DHEA, pregnenolone, and metabolites thereof exert numerous activities in the central nervous system through activation of the *Sigma-1 receptor*. This effect may confer benefits including protecting neurons against ischemia (ie, stroke),[77] and enhancement of long-term potentiation (memory formation).[78]

### Thyroid hormones

During the developmental period, thyroid hormones play a critical role in ensuring proper growth and maturation of the brain.[79] Thyroid hormone levels may also be related to cognitive function in adults, though the evidence in this area is inconsistent. However, limited associations with both hypo- (low) and hyper- (high) thyroid function and cognitive impairment exist in the peer-reviewed literature; thus maintaining levels of TSH, T3, and T4 within normal ranges is suggested.[80]

## Cerebrovascular Health

The brain depends on the carotid arteries to obtain the oxygen and nutrient-rich blood that it needs to sustain its high rate of metabolic activity. The carotid arteries emerge from the aorta and carry blood through the neck into the brain where they branch and diverge into many smaller capillaries, which facilitate circulation across the various brain regions. Like other blood vessels, the carotid arteries and their subsidiaries (smaller branches) are susceptible to endothelial dysfunction, dysregulation, and damage to the delicate cells that line blood vessels. Endothelial dysfunction is a critical step in both the initiation, and progression, of atherosclerosis.

If the integrity of the blood vessels that supply the brain is compromised, cognition suffers as a result. Multiple correlates between measures of vascular health and cognitive function are identified in the peer-reviewed literature.

### HDL levels

HDL serves to shuttle cholesterol from the blood vessel walls back to the liver for excretion, and thus insufficient levels of HDL are associated with increased endothelial dysfunction and arterial plaque deposition. Studies have linked low HDL levels with declining brain health and function.

Researchers examined the brains of 183 subjects, mean age 58 years, using magnetic resonance imaging (MRI). Tests revealed that HDL levels were positively associated with brain gray matter volume. Not surprisingly, then, subjects with higher HDL levels also scored significantly higher on a visuo-spatial memory test than their counterparts with lower HDL levels. These findings led the investigators to conclude that "adults with decreased levels of HDL cholesterol may be experiencing cognitive changes and grey matter reductions in regions associated with neurodegenerative disease and therefore, may be at greater risk for future cognitive decline."[81]

In a study of 139 very elderly subjects, plasma HDL levels were strongly associated with cognitive acuity. Subjects with higher HDL levels performed much better on the MMSE than those with lower HDL levels. In fact, "each decrease in plasma HDL tertile (74.9 ± 2.1, 50.6 ± 0.5, and 36.8 ± 1.0 mg/dl) was associated with a significant decrease in MMSE [score]."[82]

### Homocysteine

Homocysteine is an endogenous amino acid derivative that damages the endothelial cells which line the inside of blood vessels and contributes to the pathogenesis of atherosclerosis and vascular dysfunction.[83] Elevated homocysteine has been linked with reduced blood flow to the brain,[84] memory impairment,[85] poorer global cognitive function,[86] smaller overall brain volume,[87] and increased silent brain infarcts (subclinical stroke-like blood vessel occlusions in the brain).[87]

In a randomized, placebo-controlled clinical trial, which included over 5500 subjects with known cardiovascular disease, treatment with the homocysteine-lowering B vitamins folic acid (2.5 mg), B6 (50 mg), and B12 (1000 mcg) was shown to significantly reduce the risk of stroke versus placebo, highlighting the link between cerebrovascular health and homocysteine levels.[88]

Similarly, lowering homocysteine in individuals over 70 years of age through supplementation with 800 mcg folic acid, 500 mcg B12, and 20 mg B6 daily for a period of 24 months was shown to reduce the rate of brain atrophy by 53% versus placebo control in a randomized, double-blind trial. Subjects receiving the homocysteine lowering B-vitamins also scored much better on their final cognitive tests at the end of the study period.[89]

### Hypertension

Small, delicate capillaries, like those that perpetuate the flow of blood throughout the brain, are particularly susceptible to damage caused by elevated blood pressure. Chronic hypertension leads to the breakdown of cerebrocapillaries, a condition associated with the development of neurodegenerative diseases and cognitive impairment.[90]

A case–control study of over 700 patients found a statistically significant correlation between blood pressure and rate of cognitive decline over a 6-month period for subjects younger than 65 years.[91] Accordingly, an observational study of more than 1800 people revealed that individuals taking an antihypertensive medication were less likely to have dementia at the study onset, and were also less likely to develop dementia over the following 3-year period. Significantly, subjects who *did* have dementia at baseline and were *not* taking blood pressure medication exhibited a two-fold faster rate of cognitive decline than demented individuals with medication-controlled hypertension.[92]

In a study that followed 717 individuals for 38 years starting from age 45, researchers found that subjects with systolic blood pressure ≥140 mmHg throughout the study period "*performed consistently less well than the normal systolic blood pressure subgroups on a composite measure of verbal learning and memory.*"[93]

Evidence suggests that blood pressure of 115/75 mmHg significantly reduces the risk for cardiovascular disease,[94] and thus may be an ideal target for those who wish to maintain optimal cognitive performance as well.

## Diabetes and Insulin Resistance

Due to the high metabolic demand for energy in the brain, even small perturbations in glucose metabolism can noticeably impact cognitive performance. Diabetes (hyperglycemia) has been linked with lower levels of neuronal growth factors,[95] decreased brain volume,[96] and higher incidence of all types of dementia.[97]

Cerebral glucose metabolism was measured by flu-deoxyglucose–positron emission tomography (FDG-PET) in 23 adults aged 74 years (mean), who met criteria for diabetes or prediabetes. The results were compared to those of six 74-year-old (mean) adults without diabetes or prediabetes. Subjects were asked to memorize and recall a list of 20 random words they heard through a pair of headphones. FDG-PET scans revealed markedly different patterns of glucose utilization and brain activity between diabetic/prediabetic subjects and healthy controls during the memorization task. Subjects with healthy glucose metabolism remembered more words upon recall attempt. Interestingly, FDG-PET scans of those with prediabetes/diabetes resembled brain scans of Alzheimer's patients.[98]

Researchers in another study compared MRI-assessed manifestations of cerebral degeneration in 89 nondemented subjects with type-2 diabetes to 438 age-matched healthy controls over a 3-year period. Individuals with diabetes displayed increased progression of brain atrophy, and performed less well on tests of cognitive performance and learning. The investigators concluded the following: "*[O]ur data show that elderly patients with [type-2 diabetes] without dementia have accelerated progression of brain atrophy with significant consequences in cognition compared to subjects without [type-2 diabetes]. Our findings add further evidence to the hypothesis that diabetes exerts deleterious effects on neuronal integrity.*"[99]

In over 1300 aging men, researchers observed an inverse correlation between fasting insulin levels and cognitive function in nondiabetics. Baseline insulin levels were assessed and followed by a battery of cognitive testing an average 3.3 years later. Subjects with *higher* initial insulin levels scored more *poorly* on all four tests administered. These results indicate that "*higher fasting insulin and greater insulin secretion in older men may be related to overall cognitive decline, even in the absence of diabetes.*"[39]

## Obesity

Adipose tissue secretes molecules that directly influence multiple functions within the brain. There is a clearly established reciprocal relationship between adiposity (amount of body fat) and overall brain volume and cognitive function. In other words, as body weight *increases*, brain volume drops and cognitive function *worsens*.[100–103]

In a study utilizing MRI brain imaging technology to explore the link between obesity and brain volume, researchers discovered that visceral abdominal obesity in particular was associated with deteriorating brain structure. This was true even in individuals without pre-existing cognitive deficits. The findings were statistically significant and independent of vascular risk factors and overall body mass index (BMI).[22]

Similar findings were reported by another group, but this time in 700 patients with a prior diagnosis of Alzheimer's disease or cognitive impairment. Investigators identified a strong correlation between higher BMI and brain volume deficits in the frontal, temporal, parietal, and occipital lobes. It was concluded that "*cardiovascular risk factors, especially obesity, should be considered as influencing brain structure in those already afflicted by cognitive impairment and dementia.*"[104]

In 90 healthy middle-aged and older adults (ages 54–81) who performed tests of manual dexterity, motor speed, and executive function, greater central obesity as manifested by higher waist circumference was associated with poorer performance. Not surprisingly, high blood pressure exacerbated the correlation between increasing waist circumference and declining cognition: "*in healthy older adults, there are similar, negative relations of central and total obesity to cognitive function that are potentiated by higher [blood pressure] levels.*"[105]

Mid-life obesity was strongly linked to later-life dementia in over 1000 participants in a longitudinal study carried out over a 36-year period. Subjects with the greatest waist diameters at baseline were nearly three-fold more likely to develop dementia over the following three decades. The investigators in this study concluded that "*central obesity in midlife increases risk of dementia independent of diabetes and cardiovascular comorbidities.*"[106]

# PSYCHOLOGICAL RISK FACTORS CONTRIBUTING TO COGNITIVE DECLINE

There is a tendency to focus on the biological aspects of a disease state because they are perceived as tangible, measurable, and modifiable. However, more loosely defined facets of life related to psychological condition contribute to mental fluency as well. The ways in which the brain is utilized and stimulated impact its functional state at all ages.

Psychoanalytical tests have found that cognitive impairment is closely correlated with traits such as boredom-proneness, loneliness,[107] small social network,[108] and high stress.[109]

## Anxiety and Stress

Research in patients with anxiety has shown that, compared to nonanxious control subjects, those with high-anxiety levels must exert greater effort (dedicate more brain resources) to maintain the same level of performance on cognitive tests.[110] More severe anxiety is also predicative of earlier conversion from mild cognitive impairment to Alzheimer's disease.[111] In men, even subclinical (low-level) anxiety is tied to cognitive impairment.[112]

Excessive stress leads to cognitive dysfunction as well. In a study involving 36 women between the ages of 25 and 53, those with the highest work-related stress levels displayed decreased attention and visuo-spatial memory.[113] Likewise, in a cohort of 811 aging men, subjects reporting higher stress levels scored lower on the MMSE than their low-stress counterparts. This indicates that "*psychological stress had an independent inverse association with cognition.*"[109]

Posttraumatic stress disorder (PTSD) is a condition characterized by chronic, lingering anxiety and stress related to a traumatic event in the past. A comprehensive review of eight studies highlighted a strong association between PTSD and smaller brain size (total brain volume).[114] The duration of PTSD influences the extent to which the brain deteriorates; developing effective coping strategies as soon as possible may help to limit PTSD-induced decreases in brain volume.[115]

Meditation is an effective method for relieving stress. With the connection between stress and cognitive dysfunction in mind, researchers studied the effects of an 8-week audio-guided meditation program on cerebral blood flow and cognition in 14 subjects with memory problems. Tests revealed that meditation significantly increased cerebral blood flow in several major brain regions. Improvements in tests of verbal fluency and logical memory were attributed to meditation as well.[116]

## Depression

An intimate relationship exists between depression and cognitive dysfunction. Many studies have closely examined this link and allude to the intertwinement of these two conditions, rather than a causal effect of one on the other. Interestingly, depression seems to worsen cognitive dysfunction, but poorer cognitive health predisposes aging individuals to depression as well.[117]

In fact, studies designed specifically to assess age-related cognitive performance in depression show an interrelationship between the two conditions. A group of aging subjects diagnosed with depression completed various cognitive tests, and their results were compared to those of age- and sex-matched, nondepressed control subjects. More than half of the depressed subjects scored below the 10th percentile of the control group on the battery of tests that they completed. The conclusion drawn from this evidence was that "*late-life depression is characterized by slowed information processing, which affects all realms of cognition.*"[118]

Continuing research has led to the delineation of "*depression-associated reversible dementia,*" which is cognitive impairment associated with depression that subsides upon improvement of depression. Nonetheless, in a study of 57 elderly subjects with major depression, those who displayed depression-associated reversible dementia were nearly *five times more* likely to develop true dementia over a roughly 3-year period.[119]

Several cognitive and neuropsychological deficits accompany depression, including impairments in executive function, attention, episodic memory, visuo-spatial skills, and information processing.[120] Other research indicates that deterioration in structural integrity of specific brain regions involved in emotional processing is observed in depressed patients.[121]

## Social Network and Personal Relationships

Several studies have suggested that maintaining a large network of friends and other personal relationships, and regularly engaging in social and productive activities is associated with a decreased risk of cognitive decline.[122,123] Conversely, social *disengagement*, defined as having very few or no social relationships, is a strong risk factor for cognitive decline.[124]

Among 2249 women aged 78 or older, those with smaller social networks at baseline had a significantly greater chance of having developed dementia within 1 year than women with larger social networks. The investigators stated the following: "[O]ur *findings suggest that larger social networks have a protective influence on cognitive function among elderly women.*"[123] In another study, researchers assessed work history data for nearly 1000 subjects, who were then followed for up to 6 years. Participants in the study whose careers involved regularly working closely with people on complex tasks were much less likely to develop dementia over time than subjects who did not regularly work closely with other people.[125]

Sixteen behavioral measures were correlated with MMSE scores for 1437 elderly subjects in an Austrian study. Among other measures, living alone and perceiving life as being generally stressful were independently associated with lower MMSE scores.[126] These findings are supported by a separate study that identified being unmarried as an independent risk factor for cognitive impairment in over 7000 Italian subjects.[25]

Social integration, defined by marital status, volunteer activity, and frequency of contact with children, parents, and neighbors, conveys a memory-preserving effect in elderly adults. Over a 6-year period, memory among those with the lowest level of social integration declined at twice the rate of subjects with the higher levels of social integration.[127]

Maintaining close ties with friends and loved ones, and being involved in various group-oriented activities, especially outdoors, is an effective method for stimulating and maintaining your brain as you age.

# MENTAL AND PHYSICAL ACTIVITY

The brain consists of a vast network of approximately 90 billion neurons interconnected by 1000 trillion synaptic junctions.[128] Each mental and physical task that we perform stimulates this massive network in a unique way. Regular stimulation of diverse synaptic pathways by engaging in a wide range of mentally and physically challenging activities directly influences our ability to learn by enhancing synaptic plasticity, and initiating the process of neurogenesis in critical areas of the brain.[129,130] In fact, it is now clear that neural plasticity allows the structure and function of the adult human brain to change significantly as a result of new experiences.[131]

## Physical Activity and Brain-Derived Neurotrophic Factor

A critical driving force behind neural plasticity (and therefore overall cognitive function) is a protein called brain-derived neurotrophic factor (BDNF). BDNF acts on areas of the brain involved in learning, memory, and higher-order thinking to stimulate genesis of new neurons, survival of existing neurons, and synaptic adaptation.[132–134] Low levels of BDNF are observed in a variety of brain disorders, including cognitive decline, depression, dementia, and Alzheimer's disease.[135,136]

Physical exercise is known to enhance cognitive function in humans and other animals, and many researchers now believe that an increase in levels of BDNF induced by exercise mediates this improvement.[137–139] Several studies have demonstrated that moderate- to high-intensity aerobic or anaerobic exercise induces sharp (intensity-dependent) increases in BDNF levels in humans.[140,141]

Gold et al noted a marked increase in serum BDNF levels induced by a 30-minute bout of moderate intensity cycling; this was observed in both healthy subjects and in patients with multiple sclerosis.[142] These findings are supported by Tang *et al* who found that only 15 minutes of a high-intensity, stair-climbing exercise significantly bolstered serum BDNF levels in healthy men.[143] At the highest intensity level, exercise induces sharp increases in serum BDNF levels in as little as 3 minutes, as reported by Winter et al, who documented the effects of very-high intensity sprinting exercises in healthy young men.[144] In this last study, the postexercise spike in BDNF levels corresponded with a 20% improvement in short-term memory.[144]

Animal models allow scientists to more closely study the dynamic effect of physical activity on the brain. Work conducted by researchers in Taiwan indicates that, while both leisurely (voluntary) physical activity (ie, briskly walking in the park) and targeted physical exercise (ie, going to the gym) boost levels of BDNF and enhance plasticity in animals, they do so in different regions of the brain.[138] These findings highlight the importance of not only engaging in exercise routines, but leading a generally active lifestyle as well in order to promote overall brain health.

The beneficial effects of exercise on brain health appear to be limited only by the duration of exercise. Studies conducted in rats reveal a direct correlation between the amount of time spent exercising (wheel running) and the genetic expression of BDNF. In other words, the longer the rats exercised, the more robust the increase in BDNF gene expression.[145]

The protective effects of regular exercise on cognitive health were documented in a comprehensive analysis of 15 studies including over 33 000 subjects who were followed for up to 12 years. Individuals with the highest levels of physical activity were a striking 38% less likely to show signs of cognitive decline over time compared to those with very-low activity levels. Amazingly, even low to moderate levels of physical activity conveyed a robust 35% reduction in risk for cognitive decline. The importance of physical activity for brain health was reflected in the authors' concluding statements: "[T]he present results suggest a significant and consistent protection for all levels of physical activity against the occurrence of cognitive decline."[146]

## Mental Activity, Brain Plasticity, and Cognitive Reserve

Neural plasticity, the dynamic ability of the brain to adapt and respond to novel stimuli in a unique and reinforceable way, is a pivotal aspect of cognition. Plasticity serves as a key medium for the effects of practicing a physical activity—ie, getting better at a physical task over time. As we practice an activity repetitively, signals are transmitted through the brain in a specific pattern over and over again. This redundant signaling ultimately strengthens the connections between neurons in the signaling pathway required to execute the task, leading to greater efficiency and accuracy of signal transmission.

An important limitation of *physical* practice, though, is that improvements in ability are generally confined to the task being practiced. In other words, practicing tennis does not increase proficiency in bowling. Repetitive *mental* stimulation, on the other hand, exerts domain-wide improvements that impact other tasks as well. To elaborate, practicing a mentally challenging activity that requires utilization of higher-order cognitive processes, such as playing chess, can improve fluency in other activities that require similar cognitive processes, like driving a vehicle.[147,148]

Brain plasticity also serves as a prerequisite for a more global effect known as cognitive reserve. This phenomenon arises from, and is dependent on, synaptogenesis—the formation of new synapses, the hallmark physical effect of mental training.

The introduction of novel cognitive stimuli encourages the brain to establish new neural networks through synaptogenesis, which can then be used to bypass breakdowns in other neural networks arising from age-related or pathologic deterioration in brain circuitry.

Cognitive reserve is measurable as a function of life experiences, and studies have shown that cognitive reserve scores correlate with overall cognitive function in an aging population.[149] In subjects with Alzheimer's disease or mild cognitive impairment, higher cognitive reserve mitigates the loss of function typical with these conditions.[150] The same study found that individuals with higher cognitive reserve scores performed better on assessments of visuo-spatial ability than those with lower scores, despite presenting with equal pathologic progression of Alzheimer's disease or mild cognitive impairment as assessed by brain imaging.

Just as the desire to maintain a fit and functional body into late life necessitates regular physical exercise, ensuring cognitive dexterity with advancing age requires constantly pushing the brain to new limits in order to evoke plastic changes that strengthen existing, and encourage new, synaptic connections. This becomes clear when considering that individuals with mentally demanding careers appear to be at significantly decreased risk of developing Alzheimer's dementia in later life, compared to those whose careers centered on physical labor.[151]

Plasticity is an intrinsic property of the brain maintained throughout life; and so cognitive stimulation and training enhance cognitive reserve and convey protection against loss of brain function regardless of age.[152] In a study including nearly 500 individuals with clinical cognitive impairment, computerized cognitive training significantly improved several measures of cognitive function.[153] Improvement was still evident up to 3 months post training in some cognitive assessments. Moreover, as little as 2 hours of cognitive training initiates structural changes in the brain suggesting that those who chose to challenge their intellectual capacity reap the benefits instantaneously.[154]

A 2005 case study of a chess player reveals the true compensatory ability of the brain given regular cognitive stimulation. The chess player, an aging gentleman whom heretofore displayed excellent cognitive function, presented with complaints of slight memory loss, which over the next 2 years progressed into mild cognitive impairment. The man then fell ill with an unrelated illness and passed 7 months later. The autopsy revealed that he had been living with advanced Alzheimer's pathology in his brain, which would normally cause severe deterioration of cognitive ability. Remarkably, the man displayed only mild cognitive impairment until his death.[155] Regularly playing chess had imbued him with a great deal of cognitive reserve, allowing for relatively normal neural efficiency despite stark deterioration of the structural integrity of the brain.

Speaking more than one language is also a strong inducer of plasticity and cognitive reserve. Learning a second language requires the brain to constantly categorize information in ways that are unnecessary when only a single language is spoken; this establishes numerous new neuronal communication streams. In a study of more than 200 individuals clinically likely to have Alzheimer's disease, being bilingual was found to delay that onset of symptoms by over 5 years, and delay diagnosis by nearly 4.5 years relative to monolingual speakers.[156]

Cognitive stimulation and training also benefit the brain by enhancing cerebral blood flow. Mozolic et al have shown that an 8-week attention and distractibility cognitive training program significantly increased blood flow to the prefrontal cortex, a brain region involved in personality expression and decision making. The control group in this study, who were exposed to education material, but not intensive cognitive training, displayed no increase in cerebral perfusion.[157]

A lifestyle incorporating frequent physical exercise, continual learning, and regular cognitive stimulation is likely to be the most effective means for preserving, and possibly enhancing, cognitive function at any age.

## MEDICAL APPROACHES TO COMBATING COGNITIVE DECLINE

While various pharmacologic therapeutics have been studied in hopes of identifying an effective intervention for preserving cognition with aging, and preventing diseases of the brain such as Alzheimer's disease, evidence in support of medical therapies are equivocal at best.[158] However, preliminary data suggest that some drugs may provide limited benefits for brain health, and thus may adjunctively synergize with increased mental and physical activity levels, dietary changes, and nutraceutical options to optimize brain function with advancing age.

### Piracetam

Piracetam has been studied in a wide range of patient populations, and has demonstrated small benefits in a variety of models of neurologic disorders. Multiple mechanisms for the observable effects of piracetam on brain function have been proposed, although a precise description of its mechanism(s) of action has yet to be elucidated. Preliminary studies suggest that piracetam may modulate the signaling of multiple neurotransmitter receptors,[159] and improve neuronal membrane fluidity.[160]

A comprehensive review which assessed the efficacy of piracetam in older subjects suggests that the drug may provide appreciable benefits for cognitive dysfunction. The reviewers concluded that *"the results of this analysis provide compelling evidence for the global efficacy of piracetam in a diverse group of older subjects with cognitive impairment."*[161]

### Hydergine

Like piracetam, hydergine has been proposed to affect the brain in multiple ways. The drug, which largely fell out of clinical use decades ago after it was shown to be largely ineffective for Alzheimer's disease, is still incorporated by some integrative physicians into regimens for brain support. Proposed mechanisms include enhancing brain glucose utilization,[162] increasing acetylcholine signaling,[163] and preserving hippocampal structure with advancing age,[164] among others.

Collectively, data indicate that hydergine may be slightly more effective than placebo for treating dementia; however, a review concluded that *"the efficacy of [h]ydergine remains inadequately defined."*[165]

### Deprenyl

Deprenyl in low doses is a selective MAO-B inhibitor, and thus slows the breakdown of various neurotransmitters in the central nervous system, especially dopamine, so it may enhance mood and energy.[166] The drug has been shown to preserve some regions of the rodent brain with increasing age,[167] and to ameliorate HIV-related cognitive impairment in a double-blind, placebo-controlled human trial.[168]

### Centrophenoxine

Centrophenoxine is structurally related to dimethylethanolamine (DMAE), a metabolic precursor to acetylcholine. It has been shown that centrophenoxine increases acetylcholinergic synaptic signaling,[169] and improves memory and mental alertness in healthy elderly subjects.[170] Other proposed mechanisms by which centrophenoxine may benefit brain function are improving neuronal hydration through enhanced membrane fluidity[171] and the ability to reduce neuronal oxidative stress.[172]

## DIETARY CONSIDERATIONS FOR A HEALTHY BRAIN

The exceptionally high rate of metabolism in the brain makes it particularly responsive to the nutritional content of the diet. A Western dietary pattern, typified by excess consumption of simple carbohydrates and dietary fat (in particular, saturated fat and omega-6 polyunsaturated fatty acids), is a detrimental, yet alterable, modulator of cognitive function. Numerous studies have identified high intakes of simple sugars and saturated fats as being especially deleterious for brain health.[173–175] Transitioning to a slightly calorie-restricted Mediterranean diet high in mono- and poly-unsaturated omega-3 fats, fiber, and polyphenols will provide the brain with nutrition to function at high capacity and efficiency.

Some dietary considerations that may be easily overlooked provide substantial brain benefits as well.

## Calorie Restriction

Calorie restriction is the restriction of caloric intake to a level modestly below normal, typically 20% to 30% less, but the diet should be dense with micronutrients to maintain optimal nutrition. Caloric restriction is well-known for its ability to induce favorable changes in peripheral insulin sensitivity, which enhances insulin signaling in the central nervous system. The brain relies heavily on proper insulin signaling for a variety of functions that impact cognition, and so it is not surprising that caloric restriction has been shown to benefit cognitive function in many animal and human studies.[176,177]

A study conducted in 124 hypertensive individuals who led generally sedentary lifestyles found that 4 months of caloric restriction in conjunction with a diet designed to help control blood pressure produced several neurocognitive improvements in domains including executive learning and psychomotor speed.[178]

Caloric restriction also boosts levels of several neurotrophic factors, including BDNF, and thus creates an ideal environment for plastic adaptation of the brain in response to mental stimulation.[179]

## Mediterranean Diet

A great deal of scientific literature validates the Mediterranean diet as a staple for those concerned with cardiovascular health, cognitive health, and longevity. The diet centers on "good" fats—mono- and poly-unsaturated fats, especially omega-3's and olive oil, multicolored fruits and vegetables, and moderate red wine consumption.[180] Adherence to the Mediterranean diet has been linked with improved insulin sensitivity,[181] lipid metabolism,[182] blood pressure,[183] and reduced risk of developing cancer[184] or metabolic syndrome,[185] as well as an overall decrease in mortality.[186,187]

The brain also benefits greatly from the health-promoting lipids and antioxidants that are ample in the Mediterranean diet.[188] An abundance of scientific literature concedes that adherence to the Mediterranean diet is associated with better cognitive performance in a variety of populations.[189]

In 1393 individuals participating in a prospective study with follow-up of 4.5 years, greater Mediterranean diet adherence was shown to decrease the risk of developing mild cognitive impairment by 28% compared to lesser adherence. Additionally, in those who consistently consumed a Mediterranean diet, but *did* develop mild cognitive impairment, risk of converting to Alzheimer's disease was cut by 48% relative to subjects whose diet deviated from the Mediterranean style.[23] Several additional studies have similar conclusions.[190–192]

## Moderate Alcohol Consumption

While there is no question that heavy alcohol consumption is deleterious to nearly all aspects of health, including cognition, moderate alcohol consumption, characterized as two drinks daily, seems to convey protection against cognitive decline with aging. Fifteen studies were summarized in a comprehensive review that included data for over 36 000 subjects; those classified as "moderate" drinkers were roughly 25–30% less likely to develop Alzheimer's disease, vascular dementia, or any type of dementia, than nondrinkers or heavy drinkers.[193]

Light to moderate alcohol consumption during midlife appears to convey protection against cognitive decline in late life. A study following over 1400 individuals for nearly 23 years found that mid-life moderate drinkers were less likely to display signs of cognitive impairment later in life than their teetotaling and heavy-drinking peers.[194]

Evidence suggests that red wine may be the alcoholic beverage of choice for maintaining cognitive health, as it contains many phenolic antioxidant compounds that are suspected to impede the pathologic progress of Alzheimer's disease,[195] and limit the neurologic consequences of high cholesterol.[196] Indeed, a 7-year longitudinal study including over 5000 healthy subjects found that those who regularly drank a moderate amount of red wine scored better on every test of cognitive performance that the investigators administered than nondrinkers.[197] Other studies have produced similar findings.[198]

Many of the benefits of moderate drinking are likely attributable to alcohol's profound positive impact on levels of HDL ("good") cholesterol and enhancement of cholesterol efflux.[199–201] Alcohol consumption protects against cardiovascular and neurologic disease and degeneration via mechanisms that may be thought of as hormetic (stress adaptive) in nature. The concluding statements of a review on this topic suggest that "*to a certain extent, moderate alcohol exposure appears to trigger analogous mild stress-associated, anti-inflammatory mechanisms in the heart, vasculature, and brain that tend to promote cellular survival pathways.*"[202]

## Moderate Caffeinated Coffee Consumption

Coffee, like red wine, is an excellent source of antioxidant and neuroprotective compounds.[203–206] However, it has been suggested that the antioxidant compounds in coffee may synergize with caffeine to enhance the protective effect against brain pathology, and that decaffeinated coffee does not provide the same level of neuroprotection observed with caffeinated coffee.[207] Accordingly, a study that followed nearly 700 elderly men for a 10-year period revealed that coffee consumption, roughly equivalent to 3 cups daily, was associated with a 4.3-fold slower rate of cognitive decline when compared to subjects who did not drink coffee.[208]

A team of Scottish researchers found that coffee consumption was tied to superior reading ability and higher scores on some other cognitive assessments in a cohort of over 900 healthy adults.[209]

Moreover, a level of evidence that is strongly suggestive has accumulated indicating that caffeine itself exerts a variety of protective and augmentative effects in various cognitive domains.[210–213] Animal models have identified several mechanisms by which caffeine protects the aging brain, including preservation of blood–brain barrier integrity and suppression of brain and plasma amyloid-beta levels.[214–216]

In addition to preserving cognition, coffee consumption may also protect against type 2 diabetes and some cancers.[217,218] Black coffee or espresso appear to be superior choices when selecting a coffee beverage for health benefits, since adding sugar or non-dairy creamer has been shown to blunt the ability of coffee to increase the levels of antioxidants in circulation.[219]

## Nutraceuticals to Support Brain Health

Healthy dietary habits ensure that food is an excellent source of nutrients that serve to support the brain both structurally and functionally. However, optimal neuroprotection and cognitive preservation often require micronutrient intakes in excess of those obtainable in a typical Western diet, or intake of specialized nutrients not common in most foods.

Many nutrients known to modulate physiologic processes important for brain health have been shown to slow cognitive deterioration or enhance mental performance.

### Fish Oil

Phospholipids are an integral component of all cells in the body, without which the integrity of cell membranes would fail, as would cellular function. In the brain omega-3 fatty acids are incorporated liberally into cellular phospholipid bilayers; DHA alone accounts for 40% of the phospholipid content of neuronal membranes.[220] Along with EPA, DHA plays a central role in neurotransmitter signaling and synthesis, and together the omega-3 fatty acids modulate numerous aspects of cognition and behavior.[221–223]

Evidence suggests that the typical Western diet is severely deficient in beneficial omega-3's, and supplies omega-6's in excess, which creates a fatty acid milieu that promotes inflammation and contributes to several age-related degenerative diseases.[224] Numerous studies have concluded accordingly, indicating that supplementation with omega-3 fatty acids optimizes cognitive health.

Slightly less than 2 g of fish oil daily over a 24-week period was shown to significantly improve scores on a standardized assessment of cognitive function in subjects with mild cognitive impairment. Increases in red blood cell EPA confirmed that supplemental fish oil was biologically available and responsible for the improvement in cognition.[225] A similar but longer-term study involving nearly 1500 subjects found that daily omega-3 supplementation was independently associated with a dramatic reduction in cognitive decline over a 1.5-year period in an aging study population, compared to those not taking omega-3 supplements. Importantly, this study also found that dietary fish consumption was *not* associated with cognition, while omega-3 supplements were, highlighting the superiority of supplementing with omega-3's for supporting brain health.[226]

In addition to the numerous studies that have associated increased dietary omega-3 intake with better cognitive performance,[227,228] a more detailed study confirms the principal role the role of DHA in mediating this improvement. Researchers assessed serum phospholipid levels in 280 middle-aged (35–54) healthy study volunteers, which were then correlated to cognitive function. It was found that subjects with the highest serum levels of DHA performed significantly better in multiple domains of cognition than their cohorts with lower DHA levels. This association remained significant even after adjustment for various other confounding factors.[229]

### Polyphenols and Anthocyanins

The disproportionately large metabolic demand of the brain compared to other parts of the body gives rise to an environment in the CNS primed for generation of cell-damaging oxygen free radicals. Polyphenolic antioxidants, such as resveratrol from grapes, catechins from green tea, and anthocyanins from blueberries are among the strongest naturally occurring free radical neutralizers, and several laboratory in vitro studies have confirmed the neuroprotective properties of these antioxidants. In the past, some scientists questioned the utility of these compounds in protecting neural health *in vivo* due to concerns over oral bioavailability. However, data clearly indicate that these protective compounds are not only adequately bioavailable ingested orally, but accumulate in the brain after oral ingestion, indicating blood–brain barrier permeability as well.[230–235]

**Blueberries.** Multiple animal studies have provided mechanistic insights into the well-documented brain health benefits of blueberry constituents. In addition to strongly attenuating neural oxidative stress, blueberry components also inhibit *acetylcholinesterase* (AChE), an enzyme responsible for catabolizing the important neurotransmitter acetylcholine, thus preserving acetylcholine-related memory and learning.[235] Blueberry supplementation also stimulates neurogenesis and enhances neuronal plasticity (adaptability) in the hippocampus, the region of the brain chiefly affected by Alzheimer's disease.[236] Other research has revealed that blueberry compounds may optimize cognitive performance through modulation of genetic expression within the brain.[237]

These biochemical actions translate into observable improvements in learning, memory, and overall cognitive performance resulting from blueberry supplementation or dietary fortification in both animal and human studies.[238–240]

Other beneficial effects of blueberry consumption include enhanced insulin sensitivity in obese subjects,[241] and improved vascular smooth muscle contractility after prolonged supplementation.[242]

**Tea polyphenols.** Interest in studying components of tea in the context of brain health was generated by publication of epidemiologic evidence that linked increased tea consumption with superior cognitive function in aged populations.[243,244] Investigations were fruitful in that they led to the elucidation of powerful tea constituents, including *epigallocatechin-3-gallate* (EGCG) and other phenolic antioxidants, and findings that these compounds possess tremendous disease-modifying potential in Alzheimer's disease and the ability to preserve cognition in healthy aging individuals and animals.[245–247]

In a double-blind, placebo-controlled trial, co-ingestion of green tea polyphenols and L-theanine, an amino acid found in tea, was shown to improve memory and attention in subjects with mild cognitive impairment. Those subjects who consumed the supplement also displayed significantly increased theta brain wave activity as measured by electroencephalography (EEG); theta waves are associated with learning and memory.[248–250] Similar results were observed in animal models of cognitive impairment, in which some of the benefits were attributed to the free radical scavenging ability of green tea polyphenols.[251,252] Other research has shown that daily green tea supplementation attenuates age-related cognitive dysfunction in mice, even when treatment is initiated well into adulthood. These results suggest that green tea might protect neurons and preserve cognition regardless of age.[247]

Tea polyphenols and theanine may also ameliorate the damaging effects of amyloid-beta proteins, which accumulate in the brain as the hallmark pathology of Alzheimer's disease causing severe oxidative stress and neuronal death. Several animal studies have found that EGCG and related catechins suppress amyloid-beta–induced cognitive dysfunction and neurotoxicity.[253–255]

Green tea supplementation has also been shown to optimize insulin signaling[256] and endothelial function,[257] which may provide additional neuroprotective benefits. Additional clinical trials have established that daily green tea supplementation favorably modulates multiple other metabolic parameters related to brain health, including body weight and lipid peroxidation.[258]

**Resveratrol.** Many researchers believe that at least some of the health benefits of red wine consumption may be due to its modest content of the well-known phenolic antioxidant molecule resveratrol. In addition to a multitude of evidence suggesting that resveratrol extends lifespan in experimental settings, likely by mimicking the genetic effects of calorie restriction,[259] numerous publications also highlight various roles for resveratrol in optimizing brain function.

Resveratrol may benefit the brain via mechanisms including increased synthesis of the growth factors IGF-1[260] and BDNF[261] in the hippocampus, suppressing formation of inflammatory metabolic products within the brain,[262,263] reinforcing the integrity of the blood–brain barrier,[264] and optimizing overall brain metabolism.[265] Other studies have shown that resveratrol supplementation preserves cerebrovascular integrity with aging,[266] and protects the brain after traumatic brain injury as well.[267]

In a double-blind, randomized, placebo-controlled human clinical trial, doses of resveratrol ranging from 250–500 mg were shown to dose-dependently enhance cerebral circulation and brain oxygenation. In a trial involving non-human primates resveratrol supplementation was shown to increase physical activity levels and enhance both working and spatial memory. The investigators concluded that *"these results suggest that resveratrol could be a good candidate to mimic long-term CR effects and support the growing evidences that nutritional interventions can have beneficial effects on brain functions even in adults."*[268]

### B-vitamins

Inside the central nervous system B-vitamin–dependent reactions are responsible for ensuring the proper function of a vast array of neurochemical processes. When levels of B vitamins, especially B6, B12, and folic acid, are insufficient to optimally support these reactions, consequences such as impaired neurotransmitter synthesis and neurocapillary-damaging hyperhomocysteinemia can result.[269]

Multiple human studies have associated low plasma levels of B vitamins, and even subclinical deficiencies, with cognitive decline and dementia.[270–272] Scott et al have shown that in elderly patients, levels of folate correlate positively with the volume of the hippocampus and amygdala, and inversely with white matter hyperintensities, a marker of neuropathology observable upon MRI brain imaging.[273]

The brain may be the first organ affected by insufficient intake of various other B-vitamins as well, including pantothenic acid, riboflavin, and nicotinamide, since these nutrients are important intermediaries in the mitochondrial oxidative phosphorylation (OXPHOS) process, a series of reactions by which chemical energy in the form of adenosine triphosphate (ATP) is produced. The brain produces more energy per unit mass than any other organ in the body, thus reflecting the sheer number of OXPHOS reactions taking place therein.[274–276]

### Coenzyme Q10

A critical component of the OXPHOS reaction pathway, CoQ10 serves to shuttle electrons between two "stations" along the mitochondrial inner membrane on the pathway to ATP formation. Without adequate CoQ10 supply, electron transport may slow, resulting in fewer ATP molecules being produced, and ultimately less available cellular energy.

CoQ10 supplementation has been shown to improve outcomes in several neurodegenerative disorders involving loss of mitochondrial function, such as Parkinson's disease, Huntington's disease, and amyotrophic lateral sclerosis.[277,278] Some animal data provide evidence for CoQ10's potential for preserving cognitive function in conditions such as experimental Alzheimer's disease.[279]

Inhibition of HMG-CoA by the widely prescribed cholesterol-lowering statin drugs is known to deplete levels of CoQ10 in the body. Indeed, studies have shown that coadministration of CoQ10 with statins may ameliorate some of the side effects of the drugs, and individuals with memory complaints who are also taking statin drugs may benefit from supplementation.[280–282]

### Acetyl-L-Carnitine

The amino acids lysine and methionine are biochemically conjoined in vivo to form the compound carnitine. Carnitine is essential for ensuring that fatty acids are transported into the mitochondrial matrix where they fuel aspects of OXPHOS, but under certain conditions, including age-related cognitive decline, endogenous synthesis may be insufficient to support optimal fatty acid transport. Subsequent to delineation of the role of carnitine in energy production, many researchers began to study the effects of supplementation with carnitine and its more brain-permeable derivative acetyl-L-carnitine on various energy-demanding systems and reactions in the body.[283]

Supplementation with carnitine and acetyl-L-carnitine has been well-documented to ameliorate consequences of disease states with widespread implications for health, including type 2 diabetes and stroke.[284,285] However, more impressive is the efficacy of acetyl-L-carnitine in supporting brain health and cognition during normal age related cognitive decline and Alzheimer's disease. Acetyl-L-carnitine optimizes cognition by acting upon multiple facets of neuronal function, including enhancing efficiency of cholinergic neurotransmission,[286] stabilization of neuronal mitochondrial membranes,[287] increasing neural antioxidant defenses,[288] and enhancing neuron growth through sensitization to neurotrophic factors.[289,290]

A meta-analysis (comprehensive systematic review) of randomized, controlled human clinical trials involving data from 21 studies and data for over 1200 subjects with mild cognitive impairment or mild to moderate Alzheimer's disease provides unequivocal evidence that supplementation with acetyl-L-carnitine ameliorates cognitive deficits observed during aging and during pathological brain deterioration.[291] The reviewers found that daily doses of acetyl-L-carnitine ranging from 1.5–3.0 g consistently provided a statistically significant benefit over placebo for preserving cognition as assessed by multiple standardized tests. Moreover, there was a clear trend for a cumulative effect of acetyl-L-carnitine supplementation over time, suggesting that long-term use of acetyl-L-carnitine may provide the greatest benefit.

### Phosphatidylserine

Like the omega-3's EPA and DHA, phosphatidylserine is an especially important component of cellular membranes. In the brain phosphatidylserine conjugates with DHA and helps maintain the proper electrical gradient along neuronal membranes, thus facilitating proper neural communication.[292] Human clinical trials have found that orally administered phosphatidylserine in doses ranging from 200 mg to 600 mg daily improves cognitive function in aging subjects with cognitive impairment.[293–295]

### Ginkgo Biloba

The leaves of the ginkgo biloba tree have been highly regarded throughout human history and used as a food additive and as a traditional medicine. Although widely regarded a nootropic, or cognitive enhancer, human clinical data as a whole suggest that supplementation with ginkgo biloba extract alone, not in combination with other cognitive support ingredients, is minimally effective for improving cognitive function in those with Alzheimer's disease or cognitive impairment.[296] Nonetheless, because studies have shown that supplementation with ginkgo improves cerebral blood flow,[297] and other cerebrovascular-related aspects of cognition,[297] its use in combination with other brain-supporting nutrients may provide synergistic benefits for cognition. Indeed, results in both animals and humans suggest that, when ginkgo is combined with nutrients such as phosphatidylerine, B vitamins, or vitamin E, the combination of ingredients confer cognitive benefits.[298,299] In fact, in one study comparing the effects of supplementation with ginkgo biloba extract alone, to ginkgo biloba extract together with phosphatidylserine, the combination of the two ingredients resulted in improvements in at least two aspects of memory performance, while ginkgo alone did not.[299]

### Bacopa Monnieri

In India, where the Bacopa monnieri herb grows, the leaves are held in high regard, and have long been believed in Ayurvedic medical tradition to promote cognitive health. More recently, modern scientific inquiry into the origins of these Ayurvedic tenets has revealed that the herb supports brain function through various mechanisms.

Bacopa is rich in free-radical–scavenging compounds including polyphenols and sulfur-based molecules, and so may ameliorate the oxidative stress generated by the brains' intense metabolic rate.[300] It also contains

various phytochemicals with known anti-inflammatory properties, such as luteolin and apigenin.[301,302] Several human clinical trials have revealed cognitive-enhancing and memory-improving effects of supplementation with Bacopa extract.

In one double-blind, placebo-controlled trial, daily doses of 300 mg of Bacopa extract significantly improved visual information–processing speed, memory consolidation, and lessened anxiety in healthy individuals after 12 weeks of supplementation.[303] Another double-blind, placebo-controlled study of the same duration, using the same dose of Bacopa extract, found that the benefits extend to elderly subjects as well. In this study, the group receiving Bacopa fared better on an auditory verbal learning test, and scored lower on anxiety and depression scales than those taking placebo.[304] Additional promising results were achieved in a similar study in which healthy adults received either 300 mg of Bacopa extract daily, or a placebo, for 90 days. Improvements in working memory were noted in the Bacopa group, but not in the placebo group.[305]

### Huperzine A

A compound derived from the plant Huperzia serrata, commonly known as clubmoss or firmoss, huperzine A is a well-established inhibitor of the *acetylcholinesterase* enzyme, a mechanism that it shares with many commonly prescribed pharmaceutical treatments for Alzheimer's disease.[306,307] Inhibition of acetylcholinesterase preserves levels of the neurotransmitter acetylcholine, which is critical for cognition and memory.

Huperzine A has been shown to enhance memory in healthy young humans, and in a comprehensive literature review, it was found that high doses of huperzine A significantly improved scores on standardized cognitive tests achieved by patients with Alzheimer's disease in a time-dependent manner.[308]

### Glyceryl Phosphoryl Choline

Glyceryl phosphoryl choline (GPC) is a form of choline that is naturally present in all the body's cells. Among aging adults, the rationale for GPC therapy goes back to the hypothesis, developed more than 30 years ago, that declining levels of acetylcholine—and a concurrent decrease in the number of neurons that are its intended target—are responsible for a range of cognitive deficits.[309] Acetylcholine is an essential neurotransmitter involved in muscle control, sleep, and cognition. Research has shown that GPC is a precursor of acetylcholine that is safe and well tolerated.[310] A review of 13 published studies, involving more than 4000 participants, found that patients taking GPC exhibited neurological improvement and relief of clinical symptoms of chronic cerebral deterioration that was clearly superior to placebo and "*superior or equivalent*" to that obtained with prescription drugs. The same authors found that GPC was superior to choline and lecithin and that it deserved wider study as a therapy for stroke patients seeking to regain full cognitive function.[311]

### Vinpocetine

A semisynthetic derivative of the lesser periwinkle plant (*Vinca minor*), vinpocetine has been shown to exert a variety of biological effects that may benefit brain health. It is known to regulate the action of sodium in neurons, lessening the damaging effects of hypoxia as seen in stroke, as well as mitigating oxidative stress.[312] Vinpocetine also blunts the activity of an enzyme called *phosphodiesterase type 1*, an effect that may increase neuronal energy by upregulating the energy "throttle" *cyclic AMP*.[313] Also, vinpocetine itself has demonstrated the ability to neutralize particularly damaging hydroxyl radicals.[314] Moreover, vinpocetine supports healthy blood flow by enhancing vasodilation and blunting platelet aggregation, effects that may enhance cerebral circulation.[315,316] Indeed, human clinical trials show that large doses of IV vinpocetine, followed by 3 months of oral supplementation with 30 mg vinpocetine, eases blood flow in patients with chronic cardiovascular disease.[317]

### Multivitamin

Even the healthiest diets may not provide the optimal levels of micronutrients, vitamins, and minerals needed to support healthy brain function. A comprehensive multivitamin supplement may help to fill these nutritional gaps and ameliorate some consequences of insufficient dietary nutrition. In a double-blind, controlled clinical trial involving over 200 healthy middle-aged individuals subjects were given either a multivitamin or placebo for more than 2 months, and both groups were then assessed for cognitive function. It was shown that those taking the multivitamin displayed less fatigue during extended cognitive challenges, and were also more accurate. Also, those taking multivitamins were able to more quickly complete mathematical processing tests than subjects receiving placebo.[318]

## Life Extension Suggestions

- **Fish oil:** 2–6 g daily (minimum of 1400 mg EPA and 1000 mg of DHA)
- **Glyceryl phosphoryl choline:** 600 mg daily
- **Phosphatidylserine:** 100–200 mg daily
- **DHEA:** 15–50 mg daily (depending on blood test results)
- **Vinpocetine:** 15–30 mg daily
- **Acetyl-L-carnitine:** 1500–3000 mg daily
- **Trans-resveratrol:** 250–500 mg daily
- **Blueberry**, standardized extract: 500–1000 mg daily
- **Green tea**, standardized extract: 725–1450 mg daily
- **Huperzine A:** 50–100 mcg daily
- **B-vitamin complex:** per label instructions
- **Complete multivitamin:** per label instructions
- **CoQ10** (as ubiquinol): 100–300 mg daily
- **Bacopa**, standardized extract: 450–900 mg daily
- **Ginkgo biloba**, standardized extract: 120 mg daily
- **Pregnenolone:** 50–100 mg daily

In addition, the following *blood testing* resources may be helpful:

- Male and Female Panel
- Omega Score®
- CoQ10 (Coenzyme Q10)
- C-Reactive Protein (CRP)

## REFERENCES

References available at: www.lef.org/dpt5/ch4

# 5

# Age-Related Macular Degeneration

The macula or macula *lutea* (from Latin *macula*, "spot" + *lutea*, "yellow") is a highly pigmented yellow spot near the center of the retina of the human eye, providing the clearest, most distinct vision needed in reading, driving, seeing fine detail, and recognizing facial features.

Age-related macular degeneration (AMD) is a devastating condition characterized by the deterioration of the macula in which central vision becomes severely impaired. There are two forms of macular degeneration: atrophic (dry) and neovascular (wet). Both forms of the disease may affect both eyes simultaneously.

Age-related declines in the retinal carotenoid pigment content, coupled with photo damage induced by harmful ultraviolet (UV) rays, give rise to this debilitating condition. The progression and severity of macular degeneration, as with all age-related diseases, are exacerbated by factors such as oxidative stress, inflammation, high blood sugar, and poor vascular health.

Scientifically studied natural compounds that help restore waning carotenoid levels within the macula, boost the antioxidant defenses of the eye, and support healthy circulation offer an effective adjunct to conventional treatment, which may greatly improve the outlook for those with AMD.

This protocol explores the pathology, weighs the risks and benefits of conventional treatment, and reveals exciting new scientific findings on innovative natural approaches for ameliorating the effects of AMD.

## PREVALENCE

AMD is the leading cause of irreversible visual impairment and blindness among North Americans and Europeans aged 60. According to the National Institute of Health, more Americans are affected by AMD than cataracts and glaucoma combined. The eye-health organization Macular Degeneration Partnership estimates that as many as 15 million Americans currently exhibit evidence of macular degeneration.[1]

Approximately 85–90% of AMD cases are the dry form. Wet AMD, which represents only 10–15% of AMD cases, is responsible for more than 80% of blindness. AMD is equally common in men and women, and has a heritable nature.[2,3] A positive development is that the estimated prevalence of AMD in Americans aged 40 has decreased from 9.4% in 1988–1994 to 6.5% in 2005–2008.[2]

## PATHOLOGY OF AMD

The retina, the innermost layer of the eye, contains nerves that communicate sight. Behind the retina is the choroid, which supplies the blood to the macula and retina. In the atrophic (dry) form of AMD, cellular debris called *drusen* accumulates between the retina and the choroid. The macular degeneration progresses slowly as vision is lost painlessly. In the wet form of AMD, blood vessels below the retina undergo abnormal growth into the retina beneath the macula. These newly formed blood vessels frequently bleed, causing the macula to bulge or form a mound, often surrounded by small hemorrhages and tissue scarring. The results are a distortion in central vision and the appearance of dark spots. Whereas the progression of atrophic AMD may take place

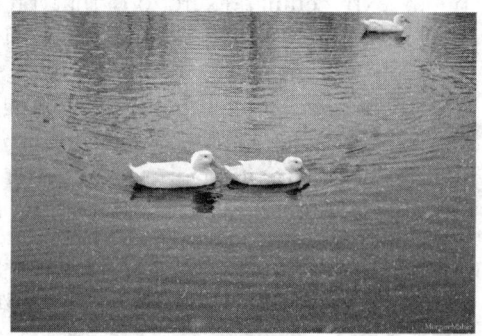

Normal Vision

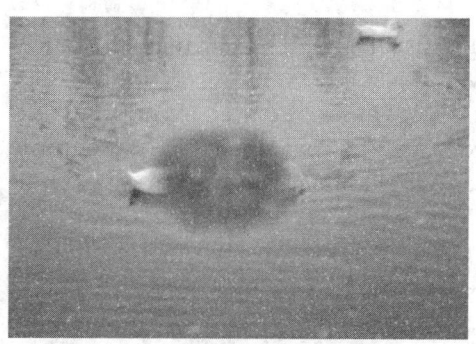

The same scene as viewed by a person with age-related macular degeneration

**How vision is affected in macular degeneration**

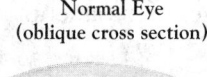

Normal Eye
(oblique cross section)

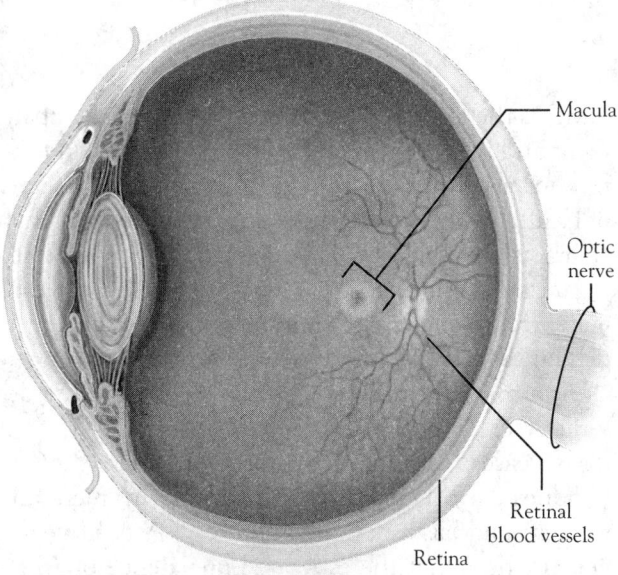

Macula

Optic
nerve

Retinal
blood vessels

Retina

Age-related Macular Degeneration

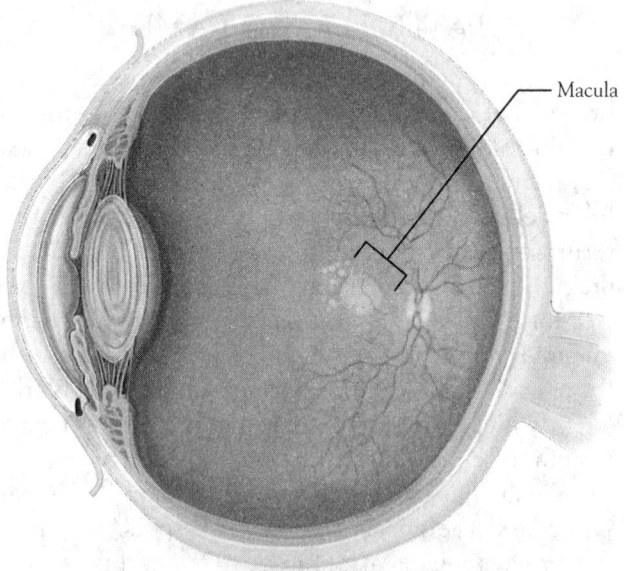

Macula

Macular Degeneration

over years, neovascular AMD can progress in mere months or even weeks.[4]

While the exact causes of AMD are not fully understood, recent scientific evidence points to chronic vascular disease, including cardiovascular disease, as a potential cause. Scientists believe that slow degradation of the blood vessels in the choroid, which provides blood to the retina, may lead to macular degeneration.

A complementary theory suggests an alteration in the dynamics of the choroidal blood circulation as an important pathophysiologic mechanism. Blockages within the choroidal blood vessels, possibly due to vascular disease, lead to increased ocular rigidity and decreased efficiency in the choroidal blood circulation system. Specifically, the increased capillary resistance (due to blockages) causes elevated pressure, resulting in the extracellular release of proteins and lipids that form drusen deposits.[5]

Cholesterol exists in the drusen. Researchers suggest that the formation of AMD lesions and their aftermath may be a pathologic response to the retention of a subendothelial apolipoprotein B, similar to a widely accepted model of atherosclerotic coronary artery disease.[6] As such, researchers have now found that biomarkers predictive of cardiovascular risk (eg, elevated homocysteine and C-reactive protein [CRP] levels) are risk factors for AMD.[7]

Small drusen are extremely common, with approximately 80% of the general population over 30 manifesting at least one. The depositing of large drusen (63 μm) are characteristic of atrophic AMD, in which this drusen causes thinning of macular tissue, experienced as blurry or distorted vision with possible blank spots in central vision. Drusen continue to accumulate and aggregate with advancing age; people over 75 are 16 times more likely to develop aggregated large drusen compared to 43–54 year-olds.[8]

Along with drusen formation, there may be deterioration in the elastin and collagen in Bruch's membrane—the barrier between the retina and the choroids—causing calcification and fragmentation. This, coupled with an increase in a protein called vascular endothelial growth factor (VEGF), allows capillaries (or very small blood vessels) to grow up from the choroid into the retina, ultimately leading to blood and protein leakage below the macula (wet-form AMD).[9,10]

Other theories postulate that abnormalities in the enzymatic activity of aged retinal pigment epithelium (RPE) cells lead to the accumulation of metabolic byproducts. When the RPE cells become engorged, their normal cellular metabolism is obstructed, resulting in extracellular excretions that produce drusen and lead to neovascularization.

People who have a close relative with AMD have a 50% higher risk of eventually developing it compared to 12% for other people. Scientists believe a newly discovered genetic association will better help predict those at risk and ultimately lead to better treatments.[11]

## RISK FACTORS OF AMD

**Cigarette Smoking.** Increased incidence of neovascular and atrophic AMD has been consistently demonstrated among smokers.[12,13]

The macular pigment (MP) optical density in 34 cigarette smokers was compared against the MP optical density in 34 nonsmokers matched for age, sex, and dietary patterns. It was found that tobacco users had significantly less MP than control subjects. Further, smoking frequency (cigarettes per day) was inversely related to MP density.[14]

In a study investigating the relationship between smoking and the risk of developing AMD in Caucasians, 435 cases with end-stage AMD were compared to 280 controls. The authors demonstrated a strong association between the risk of both dry- and wet-form AMD and the amount of cigarette smoking. More specifically, for subjects with 40 pack years (number of pack years = packs smoked per day × years as a smoker), the odds ratio (probability of the condition occurring) was 2.75 compared with nonsmokers. Both types of AMD showed a similar relation; smoking more than 40 pack years of cigarettes was associated with an odds ratio of 3.43 for dry AMD and 2.49 for wet AMD. Stopping smoking was associated with reduced odds of AMD. Also, the risk in those who had not smoked for over 20 years was comparable to nonsmokers. The risk profile was similar for males and females. Passive smoking exposure was also associated with an increased risk of AMD in nonsmokers.[15]

**Oxidative Stress.** The retina is particularly susceptible to oxidative stress because of its high consumption of oxygen, high proportion of polyunsaturated fatty acids, and exposure to visible light. In vitro studies have consistently shown that photochemical retinal injury is attributable to oxidative stress. Furthermore, there is strong evidence suggesting that lipofuscin (a photoreactive substance) is derived, at least in part, from oxidatively damaged photoreceptor outer segments.[16] While naturally occurring antioxidants typically manage this, environmental factors and stress can decrease circulating antioxidants. For example, levels of the endogenous antioxidant glutathione decrease as people age, making the lens nucleus and retina susceptible to oxidative stress.[17]

Vitamin C, normally highly concentrated in the aqueous humor and corneal epithelium, helps absorb damaging ultraviolet radiation, protect the basal layer of the epithelium, and prevent AMD.[18] L-carnosine and vitamin E also mitigate oxidative stress and free-radical damage.[17]

**Inflammation.** Injury and inflammation to the pigmented layer of the retina (retinal pigment epithelium or RPE) as well as the choroid cause an altered and abnormal diffusion of nutrients to the retina and RPE, possibly precipitating further RPE and retinal damage.[19] Animal studies show that oxidative stress–induced injury to the RPE results in an immune-mediated chronic inflammatory response, drusen formation, and RPE atrophy.[20]

Research has identified specific genetic changes that can lead to an inappropriate inflammatory response and set the stage for AMD onset.[21] Other studies looking at whether inflammatory markers predicted AMD risk found that higher levels of C-reactive protein (CRP) were predictive of AMD after controlling for genotype, demographic, and behavioral risk factors.[22,23]

**Phototoxicity.** Another risk factor for AMD is phototoxicity caused by exposure to blue and ultraviolet (UV) radiation, both of which adversely affect the functioning of RPE cells. Cultured human RPE cells are susceptible to apoptotic cell death induced by ultraviolet B (UVB) irradiation. Absorption of UV light by the innermost layer of the choroid can largely prevent the cytotoxic effect.[24] Exposure to sunlight without protective sunglasses is a risk factor for AMD.[25]

**Hypertension.** A study of 5875 Latino men and women identified a pronounced risk for wet AMD if diastolic blood pressure was high, or if individuals had uncontrolled diastolic hypertension.[26] Prolonged treatment of hypertension with a thiazide diuretic, however, was associated with a more significant incidence of neovascular AMD, possibly due to the known phototoxic effects of thiazide diuretics.[27]

**Low Carotenoid Intake.** Insufficient intake of the following carotenoids is linked to AMD: lutein, zeaxanthin, and meso-zeaxanthin. Lutein, zeaxanthin, and meso-zeaxanthin are carotenoids present in the retina and positively affect MP density.[28] Lutein and zeaxanthin help to prevent AMD by maintaining denser MP, resulting in less retinal tearing or degeneration.[29] The therapeutic efficacy of lutein and zeaxanthin in AMD is significant, according to the Lutein Antioxidant Supplementation Trial (LAST), which showed improvement in several symptoms accompanying AMD.[30]

Several studies show that low levels of certain B vitamins are associated with an increased risk for AMD. The Women's Antioxidant and Folic Acid Cardiovascular Study (WAFACS) in 5442 female health professionals showed that daily supplementation with folic acid, B6, and B12 resulted in significantly fewer AMD diagnoses compared to placebo.[31]

**High Fat Intake.** Higher intake of specific types of fat, rather than total fat, may be associated with a greater risk of advanced AMD. Diets high in omega-3 fatty acids, fish and nuts were inversely associated with AMD risk when intakes of linoleic acid (an omega-6 fatty acid) was low.[32]

A French study found that high total fat, saturated fat, and monounsaturated fat intake were all associated with an increased risk of developing AMD.[33] Eating red meat 10 or more times per week appears to increase risk for developing early AMD, while eating chicken more than 3 times per week may confer protection against the disease.[34]

High trans-fat consumption has been linked to an increased prevalence of late (more advanced) AMD in a study of 6734 individuals. In the same study, olive oil consumption offered a protective effect.[35]

**Ethnicity.** Studies in the United States indicate that a higher percentage of Caucasian Americans get macular degeneration compared to African Americans.[2]

## CONVENTIONAL AMD TREATMENTS

Dry-type macular degeneration develops gradually. Supplementation with antioxidants, lutein, and zeaxanthin has been suggested by the National Eye Institute and others to slow the progression of dry macular degeneration and, in some patients, improve visual acuity.[36]

Wet macular degeneration can develop more quickly. Patients require treatment soon after symptoms appear. There were no effective treatments for wet macular degeneration until recently. New drugs, called anti-vascular endothelial growth factor (anti-VEGF) agents, can promote regression of the abnormal blood vessels and improve vision when injected directly into the vitreous humor of the eye.[37–40] Photodynamic therapy, a systemic treatment used in oncology to eradicate early-stage cancer and reduce the tumor size in end-stage cancers, has also been used to treat wet AMD.[41]

**Anti-VEGF Medications.** Macugen®, Lucentis®, and Avastin® are among the newest conventional treatments for wet macular degeneration.

VEGF's main role is to induce new blood vessel formation. It also functions to increase inflammation and cause fluid to leak out of blood vessels. In wet macular degeneration, VEGF stimulates the formation of abnormal blood vessels in the macular area of the retina. Bleeding, leaking, and scarring from these blood vessels eventually causes irreversible damage to the photoreceptors as well as rapid vision loss if left untreated.

All anti-VEGF medications work in a similar fashion. They bind to and inhibit the biologic activity of VEGF. By preventing VEGF action, they effectively reduce and prevent the formation of abnormal blood vessels. They also reduce the amount of leakage and therefore reduce swelling in the macula. These actions lead to preservation of vision in patients with wet macular degeneration.

There are three anti-VEGF medications currently in use. Pegaptanib (Macugen®) selectively binds to a specific type of VEGF called VEGF 165, which is one of the most dangerous forms of VEGF.[37] Macugen® has been approved by the Food and Drug Administration (FDA) for treatment of wet AMD. It is administered via intraocular injection every 6 weeks.

Ranibizumab (Lucentis®) is also FDA-approved to treat wet macular degeneration. Lucentis® inhibits all forms of VEGF. Lucentis® is administered in monthly intraocular injections.

Bevacizumab (Avastin®) is similar to Lucentis® and works to inhibit all forms of VEGF. Avastin® is currently approved by the FDA for metastatic cancer (cancer that has spread to other parts of the body). This drug is commonly used but is not approved by the FDA for wet AMD. The cost of Avastin® is approximately 90% less than the other two agents.

Since VEGF has also been associated with poor prognoses in breast cancer, Avastin® was previously used as treatment. However, the FDA pulled approval of Avastin® for breast cancer treatment in November 2011 after review of four clinical studies.[42] These studies concluded that the drug does not prolong breast cancer patients' overall survival or significantly slow disease progression. Rigorous clinical trials for Avastin® are being performed by the National Eye Institute. Lucentis® is available free in the United Kingdom as long as patients meet certain criteria related to vision. Although the mechanisms of action of the anti-VEGF agents are similar, the success rates among treatments vary. When Macugen® was first approved, 70% of patients stabilized with no further severe visual loss.[43] Macugen® has not been found to improve vision. Lucentis® improved on the results of Macugen®: 95% of Lucentis® patients kept their vision, and nearly 40% of Lucentis® patients completing 1 year of treatment improved their vision to 20/40 or better.[39]

Because Avastin® is used off-label, and its makers do not plan to seek approval of the drug for AMD, it has not been as thoroughly investigated as Lucentis® or Macugen®.[44] However, many retina specialists believe that Avastin's® efficacy parallels that of Lucentis®.[39]

Lucentis®, Macugen®, and Avastin® are all administered via intraocular injection. In other words, these medications are injected directly into the eye. The injections are given after the surface of the eye has been cleansed and sterilized. Some doctors will give antibiotic drops prior to the injection. Some form of anesthesia is usually administered. This can be given in the form of drops or as a very small injection of anesthetic around the eye. A very fine needle is used and the actual injection takes only a few seconds.

A fourth intraocular anti-VEGF treatment, the VEGF Trap-Eye, approved in November 2011, appears to require fewer injections compared to Lucentis®, while still offering the same improvements in eyesight over a 1-year period. In trials of more than 2400 patients, VEGF Trap-Eye intraocular injections dosed every 2 months offered the same benefits as monthly Lucentis® dosing monthly.[45]

Possible complications are retinal detachment and the development of a cataract. High intraocular pressure usually follows the injection but generally resolves within an hour.

Possible adverse effects of intraocular injections occur in less than 1% of every 100 injections.[39] When adverse effects occur, however, they can be very serious and threatening to eyesight. One possible adverse reaction is a serious eye infection known as endophthalmitis, an inflammation of the internal tissues of the eyeball, which sometimes leads to loss of vision or severe damage to the eye.

Photodynamic therapy (PDT) is a systemic treatment used in oncology by a variety of specialists to eradicate premalignant and early-stage cancer and to reduce the tumor size in end-stage cancers. PDT involves three key components: a photosensitizer, light, and tissue oxygen.

Photosensitizing agents are drugs that become active when light of a certain wavelength is directed onto the anatomic area where they are concentrated. It is an approved treatment for wet macular degeneration, and is a more widely preferred treatment that takes advantage of certain unique properties of subretinal neovascular vessels.

Compared with normal blood vessels, neovascular tissue appears to retain the light-sensitive medicine used in photodynamic therapy. After the medicine—verteporfin (Visudyne®), for example—has been injected into a peripheral vein, it can detect abnormal blood vessels in the macula and attach itself to the proteins in the abnormal blood vessels. Laser light of specific wavelengths, which activates photosensitive drugs like verteporfin, is focused through the eye for about 1 minute. When verteporfin is activated by the laser, the abnormal blood vessels in the macula are destroyed. This happens without any damage to surrounding eye tissue. Because normal retinal vessels retain very little verteporfin, the abnormal subretinal vessels are selectively destroyed. Blood or fluid cannot leak out and damage the macula any further.[41]

While verteporfin PDT slowed wet AMD progression, newer anti-VEGF therapies have shown vision improvement in many patients. Combination therapies (PDT + corticosteroid + anti-VEGF) have shown some promise, particularly in certain classes of disease.[46]

**Laser Photocoagulation.** Laser photocoagulation (LP) is an effective treatment for wet-type AMD. However, LP is limited to the treatment of well-defined, or "classic" subretinal neovascularization, present in only 25% of those with wet-type AMD.[40] In eligible patients, LP is effective at preventing future vision loss, but it cannot restore or improve vision. In addition, choroidal neovascularization can recur after treatment and cause further vision loss.[47] LP has not worked well on atrophic (dry) AMD.

**Surgery.** Subretinal surgery has been attempted for AMD. Some surgeries were geared toward the removal of blood and the subretinal neovascular membrane. Another type of surgery attempted to physically displace the macula and move it onto a bed of healthier tissue. Overall, research studies show that the results of surgery are disappointing.[48] Vision has generally not improved after surgery.[49] Additionally, the frequency and severity of surgical complications were generally thought to be unacceptably high.

In late 2010, the FDA approved a device called the Implantable Miniature Telescope (IMT) to improve vision in some patients with end-stage AMD. The IMT replaces the natural lens through surgery in only one eye and provides 2× magnification. The other eye is used for peripheral vision. In the clinical trials upon which FDA approval was based, at 1 and 2 years post-surgery, 75% of patients had an improvement in their visual acuity of two lines of more, 60% improved their vision by three lines, and 40% had a four-line improvement on the eye chart.[50,51]

Each person may respond differently to the various conventional treatments available for macular degeneration. From a patient's perspective, it is very important to thoroughly understand wet macular degeneration and its treatment in order to be able to discuss a therapeutic plan with his or her doctor. A specific treatment plan should be tailored to each patient's needs and disease activity.

The advent of anti-VEGF therapies, for example, has been seen as a significant advancement for patients with wet macular degeneration. It is important to speak with a specialist regarding the benefits and side effects of anti-VEGF drugs to determine if they are appropriate for your specific case. It should be noted that there is some speculation, which is not supported by strong human data, that anti-VEGF macular degeneration treatments may exert systemic effects and negatively impact vascular health by "leaking" from the eye. It is, therefore, important to evaluate your cardiovascular health if you are receiving anti-VEGF treatment for macular degeneration. For instance, a person who recently had a heart attack or has extensive atherosclerosis may opt to avoid anti-VEGF treatments in favor of photodynamic therapy or laser photocoagulation. Individuals receiving anti-VEGF treatments should target an optimal cardiovascular health profile, which includes low-density lipoprotein (LDL) levels below 100 mg/dL, fasting glucose between 70 and 85 mg/dL, etc. For more tips on supporting your cardiovascular health, see the Atherosclerosis and Cardiovascular Disease protocol.

## EMERGING OPTIONS: HORMONE THERAPY

**DHEA.** Research has shown that the hormone dehydroepiandrosterone (DHEA) is abnormally low in patients with AMD.[52] DHEA has been shown to protect the eyes against oxidative damage.[53] Because the macula requires hormones to function, an emerging theory hypothesizes that low sex hormone levels in blood cause the retinal macula to accumulate cholesterol in an attempt to produce its own hormones.[54] The accumulation of cholesterol in macula may lead to the production of pathologic drusen and subsequent macular degeneration. An inverse association of female hormone with neovascular AMD was observed with current and former use of hormone replacement therapy among Caucasian and Hispanic women.[55] Restoring optimal hormone balance with bioidentical hormones may be an effective new treatment for both men and women. Clinical studies are underway to test this hypothesis and possible hormonal treatment options.

**Melatonin.** Melatonin is a hormone and strong antioxidant that scavenges free radicals. Several studies have shown that many areas of the eye have melatonin receptors.[56,57] In a clinical study, 100 patients with dry or wet AMD received 3 mg of melatonin at bedtime. The treatment prevented further vision loss. After six months, visual acuity had not diminished and the majority of patients had reduced pathologic macular changes upon examination.[58]

## DIETARY CONSIDERATIONS

**Soy.** Soy contains the phytonutrient genistein, which has documented antiangiogenesis properties postulated to be the result of inhibiting VEGF.[59] This property of inhibiting blood vessel growth is important in limiting abnormal ingrowth of choroidal blood vessels. In mice, genistein inhibited retinal neovascularization and expression of VEGF.[60]

**Food Rich in Omega-3 Fatty Acids.** Oily fish (eg, salmon, tuna, and mackerel) as well as flax seeds are important sources of omega-3 fatty acids, essential for protection against macular degeneration and other diseases.[61] A meta-analysis found that patients with a high dietary intake of omega-3 fatty acids had a 38% lower risk of late (more advanced) AMD. Additionally, an association was observed between eating fish two times a week and having a reduced risk of both early and late AMD.[62]

## Macular Pigments: Lutein, Zeaxanthin, and Meso-Zeaxanthin

The relationship between the density of macular pigment (MP) and the onset of AMD is well established. The MP is composed principally of three carotenoids: lutein, zeaxanthin, and meso-zeaxanthin. They represent roughly 36, 18, and 18%, respectively, of the total carotenoid content of the retina. They are found within the macula and surrounding tissues, including blood vessels and capillaries that nourish the retina.[63]

Lutein, zeaxanthin, and meso-zeaxanthin ensure proper functioning of the macula by filtering out harmful ultraviolet light and acting as antioxidants.[64,65] During the aging process, there is a decrease in levels of lutein and zeaxanthin; low levels of MPs are linked to AMD.[66] An autopsy study on donated eyes found that levels of all three carotenoids were reduced in those with macular degeneration compared to control subjects. The most significant finding, however, was the sharp decrease in meso-zeaxanthin in the macula of macular degeneration subjects.[67] This postmortem study helped confirm other studies indicating the importance of all three carotenoids in maintaining the structural integrity of the macula.[68] These carotenoids protect the macula and the photoreceptor cells beneath via their antioxidant properties and light-filtering capabilities.[61]

Intake of lutein and zeaxanthin is an important preventive measure, but may also reverse the degeneration process when it is ongoing.[30] Because lutein and zeaxanthin have the tissue-specific characteristic of all carotenoids, their natural tendency is to concentrate in the macula and retina. Consumption of foods rich in these substances is especially important, as they have a direct effect on macular pigment density—the denser the pigment, the less likely a retinal tear or degeneration will occur.[29] Fruits with a yellow or orange color (eg, mangoes, kiwis, oranges, and vegetables of the dark green leafy, orange and yellow varieties) are sources of lutein and zeaxanthin.[67]

Unlike lutein and zeaxanthin, meso-zeaxanthin is not found in the diet, but is needed to maintain youthful macular density.[69] Patients with macular degeneration have been shown to have 30% less meso-zeaxanthin in their macula compared to individuals with healthy eyes.[70] When taken as a supplement, meso-zeaxanthin is absorbed into the bloodstream and effectively increases macular pigment levels.[69]

# TARGETED NUTRITIONAL INTERVENTIONS

**Anthocyanidins and Cyanidin-3-Glucoside (C3G).** C3Gs are critical components of bilberry as well as being powerful antioxidants.[71,72] Positive results have been noted in many animal studies and some human studies using bilberry for macular degeneration as well as other eye disorders including diabetic retinopathy, retinitis pigmentosa, glaucoma, and cataracts.[73,74] C3G has been shown to improve night vision in humans by enabling the rods in the eye responsible for night vision to resume functioning faster.[75] In animal cells, C3G regenerated rhodopsin (the retinal complex that absorbs light).[71] The anthocyanidins in bilberry decrease vascular permeability by interacting with blood vessel collagen so as to slow down enzymatic attacks on the blood vessel wall. This may prevent the leakage from capillaries that is prevalent in neovascular AMD. Studies also show that bilberry increases oxidative stress defense mechanisms in the eyes.[74] There may be additional benefits by adding vitamin E.[76]

C3G, which is highly bioavailable, enhances other functions in the body.[77–79] Its potent antioxidant properties protect tissues against DNA damage, often the first step in cancer formation and aging of tissues.[80,81]

C3G protects endothelial cells against peroxynitrite-induced endothelial dysfunction and vascular failure.[82] In addition, C3G fights vascular inflammation by inhibiting inducible nitric oxide synthase (iNOS).[83] At the same time, C3G upregulates activity of endothelial nitric oxide synthase (eNOS), which helps maintain normal vascular function.[84] These effects on blood vessels are especially important in the retina, where delicate nerve cells depend on the single ophthalmic artery for their sustenance.

In animal models, C3G prevents obesity and ameliorates blood sugar elevations.[85] One way it does this is by increasing gene expression of the beneficial fat-related cytokine adiponectin.[86] Diabetics, of course, are predisposed to severe eye problems including blindness from elevated blood sugar levels.

C3G helps induce apoptosis (programmed cell death) in a number of human cancer lines, an important step in cancer prevention.[87,88] In a similar fashion (but via a different mechanism), C3G stimulates rapidly proliferating human cancer cells to differentiate so that they more closely resemble normal tissue.[89]

Finally, it was discovered that C3G is neuroprotective in experimental cellular models of brain function, helping to prevent the negative effects of the Alzheimer's-related protein amyloid beta on brain cells.[90]

**Grape Seed Extract.** Grape seed extract, a bioflavonoid, is a potent antioxidant. Plant-derived bioflavonoids are readily assimilated into the body when consumed. Bioflavonoids appear to protect retinal ganglion cells.[91] Studies conducted in fruit flies have revealed that grape seed extract attenuates the aggregation of pathologic proteins, which suggests a protective effect against macular degeneration and neurodegenerative disorders. Accordingly, eye health improved in fruit flies administered grape seed extract.[92] Similar experiments in diabetic animals indicate that grape seed extract limits the ocular blood vessel damage seen in diabetic retinopathy (degradation of the retina), which shares some pathologic characteristics with AMD.[93]

Compelling laboratory evidence demonstrates that grape extracts can inhibit angiogenesis in human cells.[94] This suggests that grape seed extract may suppress the aberrant blood vessel growth observed in wet AMD.

**Resveratrol.** Resveratrol is a potent polyphenolic antioxidant compound produced by grapes and other plants for protection against pathogens. In humans, it exerts a broad range of physiologic effects when ingested orally. Several studies have demonstrated cardioprotective properties of resveratrol, including endothelial protection and attenuation of oxidized-LDL-induced vascular damage.[94,95] In addition, emerging evidence indicates that resveratrol may combat macular degeneration and promote eye health via several mechanisms. In an animal model, resveratrol was able to stave off diabetes-induced vascular lesions.[96] Moreover, this same study showed that resveratrol was able to dampen VEGF signaling in mouse retinas, a key pathologic feature of AMD. Another study corroborated these results by showing that resveratrol inhibited angiogenesis and suppressed retinal neovascularization in mice prone to develop macular degeneration due to a genetic mutation.[97] Also, several laboratory experiments have suggested additional protective mechanisms of resveratrol in macular degeneration, including protecting retinal pigment epithelial cells from hydrogen peroxide-induced oxidative stress and light damage.[98,99]

Given these exciting initial findings regarding resveratrol and macular degeneration, along with its stellar track record in a variety of other conditions, Life Extension believes that individuals with AMD (especially the "wet" variety) may benefit from supplementation with resveratrol.

**Ginkgo Biloba.** *Ginkgo biloba* improves microcapillary circulation in the eye and slows deterioration of the macula.[100] By inhibiting platelet aggregation and regulating blood vessel elasticity, *Ginkgo biloba* improves blood flow through major blood vessels and capillaries. *Ginkgo* is also a powerful antioxidant.[101]

**Glutathione and Vitamin C.** Glutathione and Vitamin C are antioxidants found in high concentrations in healthy eyes and in diminished quantities in the eyes of AMD patients. Vitamin C aids glutathione synthesis in the eye. When combined with cysteine, an amino acid antioxidant, cysteine remains stable in aqueous solutions and is a precursor to glutathione synthesis. Vitamin C is important because it absorbs ultraviolet radiation, which contributes to cataracts.[36] Topical Vitamin C inhibited angiogenesis in an animal model of inflammatory neovascularization.[102]

**L-Carnosine.** L-carnosine is a naturally occurring antioxidant and antiglycation agent. Studies have shown that carnosine inhibits lipid peroxidation and free radical–induced cellular damage.[103] Topically applied N-acetyl-carnosine prevented light-induced DNA strand breaks and repaired damaged DNA strands,[104] as well as improved visual acuity, glare and lens opacification in animals and humans with advanced cataracts.[105,106]

**Selenium.** Selenium, an essential trace mineral, is a component of the antioxidant enzyme glutathione peroxidase, important in slowing the progression of AMD and other eye disorders including cataracts and glaucoma.[107,108] In mice, increased expression of glutathione peroxidase protected against oxidative-induced retinal degeneration.[109]

**Coenzyme Q10 (CoQ10).** CoQ10 is an important antioxidant that may protect against free radical damage within the eye.[110] Mitochondrial DNA (mtDNA) instability is an important factor in mitochondrial impairment culminating in age-related changes and pathology. In all regions of the eye, mtDNA damage is increased as a consequence of aging and age-related disease.[111] In one study, a combination of antioxidants including CoQ10, acetyl-L-carnitine, and omega-3 fatty acids improved the function of mitochondria in retinal pigment epithelium and subsequently stabilized visual functions in patients affected by early AMD.[112]

**Riboflavin, Taurine, and Lipoic Acid.** Riboflavin (B2), taurine, and R-lipoic acid are other antioxidants utilized to prevent AMD. Riboflavin is a B complex vitamin that reduces oxidized glutathione and helps prevent light sensitivity, loss of visual acuity, as well as burning and itching in the eyes.[113] Taurine is an amino acid found in high concentrations in the retina. A taurine deficiency alters the structure and function of the retina.[114] R- lipoic acid is considered a "universal antioxidant" because it is fat and water soluble. It also reduces choroidal neovascularization in mice.[115]

**B Vitamins.** Recent advances surrounding the causes of AMD have unearthed shared risk factors with cardiovascular disease (CVD) as well as similar underlying mechanisms, particularly elevated biomarkers of inflammation and CVD including C-reactive protein (CRP) and homocysteine.[116] Researchers have identified that elevated levels of homocysteine and low levels of certain B vitamins (critical to the metabolism of homocysteine), are associated with an increased risk of AMD and vision loss in older adults.[117] A strong study found that supplementing with folic acid, B6, and B12 can significantly reduce the risk of AMD in adults with cardiovascular risk factors.[31] The data, along with additional confirmatory studies, have convinced physicians to recommend B vitamin supplementation in patients with AMD. A study in more than 5000 women indicates that including folic acid (2.5 mg/day), B6 (50 mg/day) and B12 (1 mg/day) in the diet may prevent and reduce the risk of AMD.[31]

## Supplement Recommendations from the Age-Related Eye Disease Study (AREDs)

The largest and most important study of nutritional supplements in AMD is the Age-Related Eye Disease Study (AREDS). The AREDS demonstrated a reduction in the risk of progression to end-stage AMD when vitamins and zinc supplementation were given to patients with advanced forms of the disease. Thousands of patients were followed for over 6 years. The AREDS revealed significant improvements for patients with AMD and recommended antioxidants plus zinc for most patients with AMD, except those with advanced cases in both eyes. The AREDS formula consists of the following, which is to be taken daily: vitamin A (beta carotene), vitamin C, vitamin E, zinc, and copper.[118]

**DHA and EPA.** An 8-year trial of 2924 eligible AREDS AMD participants found that independent of AREDS supplementation, higher intakes of DHA and EPA were associated with a lower risk for progression to advanced AMD.[119]

**Zinc.** Following the revealing data from the AREDS, additional research on zinc has shown significant activity in treating dry-type AMD. In a clinical study, a zinc-monocysteine supplement significantly improved visual acuity and contrast sensitivity compared to placebo.[120]

## SUMMARY

There has been limited success within conventional medical treatment protocols to restore lost eyesight from either form of AMD. Leading researchers are documenting the benefits of more holistic approaches to AMD. Patients are encouraged to increase physical fitness, improve nutrition (including a reduction in saturated fats), abstain from smoking, and protect their eyes from excessive light. Dietary supplementation with trace elements, carotenoids, antioxidants, and vitamins is recommended for improving overall metabolic and vascular functioning. Early screening and patient education offer the most hope for reducing the debilitating effects of the disease.

### Life Extension Suggestions

- **Lutein**: 10–20 mg daily
- **Zeaxanthin**: 3–8 mg daily
- **Astaxanthin**: 6–12 mg daily
- **Cyanidin-3-glucoside** (C3G): 2–5 mg daily
- **Methyltetrahydrofolate** (MTHF): 1000–2000 mcg daily
- **Vitamin B6** (as pyridoxal 5'-phosphate): 100–200 mg daily
- **Vitamin B12** (as methylcobalamin): 1–5 mg daily
- **Beta carotene**: 25000 IU daily
- **Vitamin C**: 1000–2000 mg daily
- **Natural vitamin E**: 100–400 IU alpha-tocopherol and 200 mg gamma-tocopherol daily
- **Zinc**: 45–60 mg daily
- **Copper**: 2 mg daily
- **R-lipoic acid**: 300–900 mg daily
- **Selenium**: 200–400 mcg daily
- **Taurine**: 1000 mg daily
- **CoQ10** (as ubiquinol): 100–300 mg daily
- **N-acetyl-carnosine eye drops**: 1–2 drops, 1–4 times daily
- **Omega-3 fatty acids** (from fish): 2000–6000 mg daily
- **Ginkgo biloba** (standardized extract): 120–240 mg daily
- **Grape extract**: 150–300 mg daily
- **Bilberry** (standardized extract): 100–200 mg daily
- **Soy isoflavones**: 135–270 mg daily

The following *blood testing* resources may be helpful:

- Male and Female Panel
- Omega Score®
- Coenzyme Q10 (CoQ10)

In addition, the following pharmaceutical options should be discussed with your physician:

- **Lucentis**®
- **Macugen**®
- **Avastin**®

## REFERENCES

References available at: www.lef.org/dpt5/ch5

# 6

# *Allergies*

Allergies are a global public health menace.[1] More than 500 million people worldwide suffer from *food allergies*. More than 300 million, or about 5% of the global population, now suffer from *asthma*.[2] *Allergic rhinitis*, a risk factor for asthma, affects up to 30% of adults and 40% of children.[3]

Some scientists theorize that a potential cause of allergies in the modern world may be oversanitation. Excess utilization of antibiotics and less frequent exposure to microbes like bacteria and viruses during childhood may impair development of balanced immunity, causing hyper-reactivity to allergens later in life, a phenomenon known as the "hygiene hypothesis".[4,5]

Relieving allergy symptoms in hopes of improving quality of life is the primary goal of treatment. However, patients often report that their conventional medications fail to provide relief.[6,7] Also, *corticosteroids* and *beta-2-agonists*, drugs frequently used to treat allergic asthma, are fraught with potentially *deadly* side effects over the long-term.

Reliable *allergy testing* methods allow for a more guided treatment approach that includes identification and avoidance of troublesome allergens, as well as targeted *immunotherapy* with allergy shots, or via sublingual immunotherapy—an effective method underutilized in the United States, but which has been employed in Europe for decades.[8]

When you read this protocol, you will learn what causes allergies, how medical treatment can help relieve allergic reactions, and how allergy testing strategies can empower you to *significantly reduce* your allergic symptoms by identifying and avoiding the dietary or environmental culprits driving them. You will also read about several *natural* compounds with *immunomodulatory* properties that quell allergen-induced inflammatory responses to provide symptom relief.

## WHAT IS AN ALLERGY?

An allergy occurs when your immune system responds aggressively to a harmless environmental substance.

Common inhaled allergens include tree and flower pollen, animal dander, dust, and mold. Ingested allergens include medications (eg, penicillin) and foods such as eggs, peanuts, wheat, tree nuts, and shellfish. Nickel, copper, and latex can also cause allergies.[9,10]

These allergens can affect various parts of the body and elicit symptoms in the nasal passages (such as itchy, stuffy, and/or runny nose, postnasal drip, facial pressure and pain); mouth area (tingling sensation, swollen mouth and lips, itchy throat); eyes (swollen, itchy, red eyes); respiratory (wheezing, coughing, difficulty breathing, shortness of breath); skin (hives, rashes, swelling); and gastrointestinal (stomach cramps, vomiting, diarrhea). Symptoms can occur within minutes to days after exposure and can range from mild to severe.

The most severe form of allergic reaction is called *anaphylaxis*. It is a potentially deadly condition that results in respiratory distress and swelling of the larynx, often followed by vascular collapse or shock.[10] Anaphylaxis should be treated rapidly because death can occur within minutes or hours after the first symptoms appear. Many people prone to anaphylaxis carry self-injecting epinephrine pens in case of emergencies.

## WHAT CAUSES AN ALLERGIC RESPONSE?

The immune system normally functions to protect the body against viruses, bacteria, fungi, and other pathogens by targeting these substances for destruction upon recognition. However, an allergic response arises when your immune system mistakes harmless substances as potential pathogens and attacks them.

### TH1 AND TH2 IMMUNE RESPONSES IN ALLERGIES

*T lymphocytes* are immune cells that recognize foreign pathogens and also produce cell-signaling *cytokine* proteins, which facilitate immunological communication. The 2 main subsets of T cells—Th1 and Th2—complement one another to produce a comprehensive immune response against invading pathogens.

Th1 cytokines trigger the destruction of pathogens that enter the cells (such as viruses). They are also responsible for cell-mediated immune response and can perpetuate autoimmune reactions. Th2 cytokines destroy extracellular pathogens that invade the blood and other body fluids. As will be described below, an imbalance within the Th1–Th2 paradigm favoring Th2 underlies the increased susceptibility to allergies, called *atopy*, that some individuals experience.[11]

# A CLOSER LOOK AT THE IMMUNOLOGY OF AN ALLERGIC RESPONSE

According to the Th2 hypothesis of allergy, atopy results from an overproduction of Th2 cytokines in response to allergens. Atopic individuals are genetically predisposed such that they are more likely to overproduce Th2 cytokines and muster an insufficient Th1 response; the result of this imbalance is production of *antibodies* against normally innocuous environmental substances.[12]

The first time an allergen is encountered, the Th2 cytokines *interleukin-4* (IL-4) and/or *IL-13* alert *B cells* (components of the immune system responsible for antibody generation) to produce a particular type of antibody called *immunoglobulin E* (*IgE*); this process is called "sensitization."

Next, circulating IgE alerts other immune cells (*basophils* in the blood and *mast cells* in the skin and mucosal lining) that they should be ready to destroy the antigen in question if they detect it. IgE also triggers the formation of "memory" T cells, which are able to react much more quickly to future recognition of the same antigen.

Upon subsequent exposure to the same antigen, an atopic individual will have a dual response characterized by an immediate, or acute reaction within minutes, and a delayed, or late-phase reaction within the next 4–8 hours after exposure.[13]

## Acute Response

During an acute immune reaction, IgE antibodies, upon binding (crosslinking) a previously categorized antigen, provoke release of allergic mediators including *histamine*, *prostaglandins*, and *leukotrienes* from mast cells and basophils. These chemicals are responsible for the classic symptoms we think of in association with "allergy" (eg, itchy skin, runny nose, etc.).

This immediate IgE reaction responds to antihistamines and decongestants.[12]

## Late-Phase Response

After the acute response subsides, late-phase reactions can occur and produce long-term effects. The late-phase reaction manifests when an antigen is presented to a T cell (especially those already "primed" by IgE specific to that antigen) that then releases cytokines (primarily *IL-5*), which induce *degranulation* (release of allergic mediators) from another type of immune cell called an *eosinophil*.

For example, the pathogenesis of allergic rhinitis, atopic dermatitis and asthma, are thought to be influenced more by the late-phase immune reactions. In general, late-phase allergic reactions respond to anti-inflammatory agents such as corticosteroids.

Together, allergic mediators including histamine, leukotrienes, and interleukins cause a typical "allergy attack." In the skin, they cause itchy hives, rashes, and swelling. In the nasal cavities, these chemicals cause runny nose, tearing, burning or itching eyes, itching in the nose, throat, roof of the mouth, and eyes. The release of histamine and other mediators in the lungs cause muscles of the bronchial wall to tighten, become inflamed, and produce excessive mucus. This causes the symptoms of asthma—wheezing, difficulty breathing, and coughing. In the digestive system, histamine can cause vomiting, diarrhea, and stomach cramps.

# ALLERGIC DISORDERS

Epidemiologic studies revealed that the prevalence of allergic diseases has increased worldwide over the last few decades.[14-17] Allergic diseases include atopic dermatitis; allergic rhinitis; asthma; food, drug, and insect allergy; urticaria (hives); and angioedema (swelling beneath the skin).

Atopy, the genetic predisposition to producing IgE antibody in response to allergens, increases the risk of developing allergic disorders.[18,19] Having one allergic disorder significantly increases the risk of developing other allergic disorders.[20] Atopy is the strongest predisposing factor of asthma in children. Epidemiologic and experimental studies have shown that atopic disorders typically follow a natural history of manifestation or a progression of clinical signs, beginning with atopic dermatitis in infants and developing to allergic rhinitis and asthma in children.[21] This progression, called atopic march, may be influenced by shared genetic and environmental risk factors.[22]

## Atopic Dermatitis

Atopic dermatitis (AD) is a chronic inflammatory skin disorder that affects at least 15% of children and up to 10% of adults.[1] Studies among children reveal that AD develops very early in life. In fact, around 45% of affected children develop AD in the first 6 months of life, 60% develop it in the first year, and 85% before age 5 years. Further, more than half of affected children will continue to have AD beyond 7 years of age, and more than 40% will experience it through adulthood.[1]

Atopic dermatitis is often the first manifestation of allergic disease and many patients may develop allergic rhinitis and asthma later in life.[22] Eczematous rashes are dry, scaly, and itchy, and can become infected if left untreated. In infants and young children, the rashes appear on the face, neck, cheeks, and scalp. In older children and adults, eczema may appear on the folds of the forearms, the inner elbows, and behind the knees. Factors that make the symptoms worse include temperature, humidity, irritants, infections, food, inhalant and contact allergens, and emotional stress.[23] Atopic dermatitis can affect the development, personality, and quality of life of patients and their families.

Patients with atopic dermatitis have reduced skin barrier function. When vital skin lipids are lost, moisture escapes from the skin epidermis (top layer of the skin) and the skin becomes dry, causing cracks and microfissures to develop through which allergens and microbes can easily enter.[1] Soaking baths followed by an application of emollient (moisture-retaining lotion or salve) can help retain moisture and give the patient relief.

Topical corticosteroids are the standard treatment for atopic dermatitis. Low-potency corticosteroids help keep the symptoms under control and high-potency corticosteroids are used in severe flare-ups. Because of their potential adverse effects, high-potency corticosteroids should be used over short periods of time and topically only in areas that are lichenified (areas in which the skin has become leathery and thickened).[24]

## Allergic Rhinitis

Allergic rhinitis is an IgE-mediated inflammation of the nasal mucosa in response to outdoor and indoor allergens, the most common of which are pollens, dust mites, molds, and insects. Sensitization and subsequent exposure trigger a release of symptoms that include sneezing, runny or stuffy nose, teary eyes, and itchy nose, throat, or skin.[25] The nose becomes primed and hyper-reactive on repeated exposure to the allergen, and over time, the amounts of allergen needed to mount an immune response decreases.[1]

Allergic rhinitis is a major respiratory health problem that affects between 10–30% of adults and more than 40% of children worldwide. The prevalence of this disease is increasing. Allergic rhinitis negatively affects the patient's quality of life, school/work performance, and social interaction, and creates financial burden.[1] Allergic rhinitis is a risk factor for asthma,[26] and many patients with it also suffer from atopic dermatitis and conjunctivitis, and comorbidities that include sinusitis, nasal polyps, upper respiratory infections, sleep disorders, and impaired learning in children.[27] It can also develop 3–7 years later among patients with nonallergic rhinitis.[28]

Based on frequency and severity of symptoms, allergic rhinitis may be classified into (1) mild intermittent; (2) mild persistent; (3) moderate/severe intermittent; and (4) moderate/severe persistent.[29] Based on type of allergen, rhinitis is classified as perennial or seasonal, although patients can respond to both types of triggers. Symptoms can also last up to 4–9 months of the year.[25] Risk factors of allergic rhinitis in childhood include a family history of atopy, birth by cesarean section, exposure to cigarette smoke in infancy, endotoxin levels in house dust of inner city homes, and pollutants.[30]

Conventional treatment of allergic rhinitis usually begins with controlling exposure to the allergen(s), followed by use of intranasal corticosteroid sprays and nonsedating antihistamines. A survey of pediatric allergies in the United States[25] reported that parents and physicians consider nasal allergy medications as insufficient for relieving immediate and long-term symptoms and often have bothersome side effects. Some of the adverse side effects reported include nasal dryness, nose bleeds, and drowsiness from antihistamines.

## Asthma

Asthma is a life-long inflammatory disease characterized by airway hyperresponsiveness and airflow obstruction. In people with asthma, the inner lining of the airways become inflamed and the muscles surrounding the airways tighten up. Mucus glands in the airways secrete thick mucus. Together, these changes cause the airway to narrow and lead to difficulty breathing, shortness of breath, coughing, and wheezing.

Between 60 and 70% of asthma cases in children are allergic or atopic. Children with allergies have a 30% increased risk of developing asthma.[1] Genes play an important role in the susceptibility to develop asthma and several candidate genes have been identified in this regard.[31] Genes can impact a child's response to medications, and in particular, to beta-adrenergic agonists, glucocorticoids and leukotriene modulators.[2] Other factors that affect the development and severity of asthma include indoor allergen exposures, outdoor pollens, viral upper respiratory infections, exercise, foods, occupational history of the child and parents, environmental smoke, pollution, and exposure to day care.

Inhaled corticosteroids are anti-inflammatory medications for the treatment of persistent asthma. However, clinical control deteriorates within weeks to months once corticosteroid treatment is discontinued. The most effective long-term medications are long-acting inhaled beta-agonists,[1] but they come with potentially serious adverse effects.[2]

## Food Allergy

Food allergy is a global health burden; it is estimated to affect up to 10% of the population.[32] In the United States alone, food allergy is responsible for 200 anaphylaxis-related deaths and 2000 hospitalizations every year.[33]

The most common food allergens include cow's milk, eggs, peanuts, tree nuts, seafood, soy, and wheat. Symptoms of food allergy, which may occur following ingestion, inhalation, or contact, are mediated by IgE and non-IgE reactions. Upon sensitization of an allergen, IgE synthesis increases and elevated numbers of cytokines are produced in the serum and intestinal fluids.[34] IgE-mediated reactions occur within minutes to hours of exposure and include symptoms like angioedema (swelling of the inner layers of the skin), nausea and vomiting, swelling of the throat, hives, swelling and itchiness of the mouth area, diarrhea, and wheezing. Symptoms of non IgE-mediated reactions can occur hours to days later and may include constipation, atopic eczema, protein-induced enterocolitis syndrome, allergic proctitis or rectal inflammation, and Heiner syndrome (a pulmonary disease).[35]

The health of the gastrointestinal system plays a pivotal role in food allergies and food sensitivities. The gastrointestinal system acts as a semipermeable barrier, allowing only usable molecules into the bloodstream after food has been broken down. Studies have shown that allergen challenge in sensitized individuals can cause the intestinal walls to become more permeable.[36,37] When the intestinal wall has been weakened by infection or inflammation, the barrier function is compromised, allowing large molecules to pass through the intestinal wall and into the bloodstream.[34,38] Allergic sensitization can occur as the immune system responds to these abnormally large molecules, causing digestive complaints such as upset stomach or diarrhea, or symptoms such as joint pain and headaches.[38]

Healthy individuals host 100 trillion symbiotic bacteria that include *Lactobacillus*, *Clostridium*, *Bacteroidetes*, *Proteobacteria*, and *Bifidobacteria*.[39] Enteric bacteria modulate intestinal morphology; they also produce short-chain fatty acids, vitamins, ferment dietary fiber, and shape mucosal immunity.[40,41] Animal models have shown that enhancing or restoring intestinal commensal bacteria through supplementation (ie, supplemental probiotics)[42] can induce tolerance and prevent allergy. Evidence also suggests that a healthy population of intestinal bacteria can help reduce intestinal permeability.[43,44]

Probiotic bacteria include *Lactobacilli*, *Bifidobacteria*, and *Bacillus coagulans Saccharomyces boulardii* is a probiotic yeast.[45–48] Also, prebiotics, such as fructooligosaccharides, may be included to encourage the growth of beneficial bacteria.[49] Consuming plenty of dietary fiber each day supports intestinal microbiota as well.[50]

---

## IgG-MEDIATED "FOOD SENSITIVITIES"

A number of innovative doctors advocate an elimination diet based on *quantitative IgG antibody testing* for the relief of a wide array of patient complaints.[51] This involves assessing levels of IgG antibodies in a patient's blood using an ELISA method (described below) and then instructing the patient to eliminate any foods to which high levels of IgG4 antibodies are detected.

Innovative doctors suggest that this method can be effective for relieving ambiguous symptoms, such as headaches, fatigue, and mood imbalances when other causes cannot be identified. The postulated link is that IgGs, particularly IgG4, facilitate a *delayed reaction* to foods, which is often referred to as a "food sensitivity." These hypothesized IgG4-mediated "food sensitivities" are not the same as true IgE-mediated food allergies, and although some prominent alternative medical practitioners believe these to be separate and distinct phenomena, others disagree. IgG4-mediated food sensitivities are not a generally recognized phenomenon among mainstream medical professionals.

Clinical trials have noted improvements in patient symptoms with an elimination diet based on IgG4 testing. Mitchell and colleagues[52] found that when subjects who experienced frequent migraine-like headaches eliminated foods to which they produced high levels of IgG antibodies, headaches occurred less often at 4 weeks after initiating the diet, although by 12 weeks there was no difference.

In another trial, an IgG-based elimination diet slightly improved stool frequency in Crohn's disease patients.[53] Similarly, researchers found that levels of IgG against milk proteins correlated with self-reported gastrointestinal symptoms after consuming milk in subjects with abdominal symptoms.[54] Another research team showed that a 12-week, IgG-based elimination diet improved symptoms in patients with irritable bowel syndrome, and that better compliance with the elimination diet was associated with greater symptom improvement.[55]

---

# TESTS AND DIAGNOSIS FOR ALLERGIES

Proper diagnosis of allergy begins with a thorough medical history and physical examination. When a relationship between specific allergens and symptoms is suspected, allergy tests can be performed to identify the specific allergenic substances and treat the symptoms.

## Scratch or Skin Prick Test

This is the most commonly used allergy test. During this test, small amounts of suspected allergens are introduced on normal skin on the forearm or on the upper back using a small prick or needle. Redness, itching, and a raised wheal (welt) appear within 20 minutes if there is a positive reaction to an antigen. A common side effect is itchiness or hives around the wheal. Because it involves introduction of possible allergens, it does carry some risk, including the rare but serious occurrence of a life-threatening anaphylactic reaction.

## Radioallergosorbent Test (RAST)

This test evaluates the levels of specific IgE antibody and activity in serum. Like the skin test, the RAST provides allergen-specific information. The patient provides a blood sample at a clinic or laboratory. Because it is performed in the lab on serum only, there are no risks associated with this test. Common side effects are related to giving blood, such as minor pain or slight bruising.

## Enzyme-Linked Immunosorbent Assay (ELISA)

The ELISA is another method used to measure various levels of IgE. It provides an indirect determination of what materials a person may be allergic to. Like RAST, it carries no direct risk to the patient.

## Differential Leukocyte Count

The white blood cell count and differential is part of the *complete blood count* (CBC). The total number and types of white blood cells are measured. They generally include neutrophils, lymphocytes, monocytes, basophils, eosinophils, and bands. Eosinophils are often elevated with allergic reactions[56] This test is nonspecific and provides no information about specific allergenic substances.

## Elimination-Challenge Diet

The elimination-challenge diet is useful for detecting food allergies, but is very difficult to follow and requires diligence. This diet involves removal of common allergenic foods for at least 2 weeks—typically wheat, corn, soy, dairy, and so on. Overly processed foods, food dyes, and spices may also be eliminated. The patient then remains cognizant of symptoms for several weeks and slowly continues removing select food items until all symptoms of allergy disappear. The elimination diet is followed by a systematic reintroduction of possible triggers to the diet, one at a time, until symptoms reappear. Symptoms should be closely monitored.[57]

# PHARMACOLOGIC TREATMENTS FOR ALLERGY

Once an allergen has been identified, conventional therapy relies on avoidance of the allergen whenever possible and a diverse group of pharmaceuticals. The most common pharmaceuticals include the following:

## Antihistamines

This group of pharmaceuticals blocks the effect of histamine and reduces the signs and symptoms of asthma and allergy. Oral antihistamines can be used to treat nasal symptoms including congestion, sneezing, itchy or runny nose, and itchy, watery eyes. Antihistamines may also control skin flares and itching, and smooth muscle constriction in the lungs, which produces wheezing and aggravates asthma. Some antihistamine drugs may cause drowsiness and loss of coordination. Antihistamines are to be avoided in patients with high blood pressure or narrow angle glaucoma.

## Decongestants

These drugs cause small arterioles to constrict and decrease fluid and mucous secretion. Decongestants may be oral medications, nasal sprays, or eye drops. Active ingredients include pseudoephedrine, desoxyephedrine, oxymetazoline, and phenylephrine. Over-the-counter decongestants are frequently sold in combination products with antihistamines. Side effects may include increased blood pressure, arrhythmia, *heart attack*, anxiety, and dizziness.

## Glucocorticosteroids

These anti-inflammatory medications are taken orally, topically, inhaled into the lungs, or taken in nasal sprays. Intranasal corticosteroid sprays are used to treat allergic and nonallergic rhinitis with a minimal risk of systemic adverse effects. Relief can be expected after 7–8 hours of dosing but it may take 2 weeks before the drug becomes maximally effective. Inhaled corticosteroids are typically used as treatment in persistent moderate to severe asthma. It can reduce symptoms, decrease airway hyperresponsiveness and inflammation, and improve lung function. Topical corticosteroids are used to treat eczema. They are an effective first-line treatment, but they can inhibit the repair of skin cells and interfere with recovery in the long term.[1] Side effects can be serious if corticosteroids are taken orally over a long period of time.

## Leukotriene Antagonists

Leukotrienes are generated in mast cells and other white blood cells and contribute to the allergic response. Leukotriene antagonists are designed to inhibit leukotriene formation and are used to treat seasonal allergic rhinitis and mild persistent asthma.

## Cromolyn Sodium

Cromolyn is used as a nasal spray for rhinitis and inhaled for asthma and bronchospasm. It works by stabilizing mast cell membranes, preventing them from releasing histamine. It can prevent allergic rhinitis if used before symptoms start. However, cromolyn has fallen out of favor as a primary treatment option due to an inconvenient dosing regimen requirement (it must be taken 4 times daily) and the advent of effective, long-acting medications such as leukotriene receptor antagonists.

## Beta-Agonists

These are drugs that selectively activate beta-1- and beta-2-adrenergic receptors, causing smooth muscle relaxation and bronchodilation. There are 2 kinds of beta-agonists: long-acting B2-agonist (LABA) and short-acting B2-agonist (SABA). In combination with inhaled corticosteroids, LABAs improve symptoms, decrease nighttime asthma, and reduce the number of exacerbations.[1] SABAs can rapidly dilate the airways and improve breathing during an asthma attack. SABA should only be used as needed to reduce the risk of adverse side effects. The most common adverse effects associated with bronchodilators include nervousness, restlessness, and trembling. Albuterol and epinephrine are included in this category.

## Immunotherapy

Allergen-specific immunotherapy involves a gradual desensitization of the immune response. The patient receives increasing amounts of the specific antigen to induce the immune system to produce protective antibody. Treatment may be continued for ≥3 years. It is the only treatment that can reduce symptoms related to allergic rhinitis over time although there is a risk of side effects because of allergic reaction to the antigen that is intended to be therapeutic.

In the United States, immunotherapy is most frequently as a subcutaneous injection. However, European physicians have employed another form of immunotherapy for decades—*sublingual immunotherapy* or "allergy drops."[8]

Sublingual immunotherapy, in which small doses of allergen are delivered in a diluted solution under the tongue, works in the same way injectable immunotherapy does. Several comprehensive reviews have shown that sublingual immunotherapy is effective for reducing symptoms associated with allergic conditions including allergic rhinitis and allergic conjunctivitis.[58,59] Moreover, sublingual immunotherapy appears to be associated with fewer systemic reactions.[60] Data indicate that sublingual immunotherapy may be an alternative for those at high risk for anaphylactic reactions or those who do not wish to receive an antigen injection.

# USE OF PROBIOTICS

In order to prevent the development of childhood allergic diseases, an infant's immune system must mature from a Th2- to a Th1-dominated response through microbial contact soon after birth. In comparison with the time before antibiotics and common presence of infectious diseases, along with the widespread use of antimicrobial agents in consumer products like soap, individuals in modern times have reduced contact with microbes. In the theory known as the "hygiene hypothesis," scientists speculate that an antiseptic environment results in a lack of microbial stimulation to the gut immune system and causes an increase in allergic disease.[61,62] In fact, studies have shown that non-allergic children have higher levels of *Bifidobacteria* and *Lactobacilli* compared to allergic children.[63] The presence of these "harmless" probiotic bacteria in the intestinal biota seems to correspond with protection against allergy.

As defined by the World Health Organization, probiotics are "live microorganisms which, when administered in adequate amounts as part of food, confer a beneficial health effect by producing gut microflora on the host." [64]

Many randomized trials, clinical and experimental studies, and meta-analyses have been conducted on the efficacy of probiotics on the treatment or prevention of allergic diseases.

Randomized controlled trials (RCTs) showed that using probiotics provided significant clinical benefits to children with allergic rhinitis. Heat-killed or live *Lactobacillus casei* decreased the frequency and severity of nose and eye symptoms and improved the quality of life for children who were sensitized to house dust mites.[65,66] Among preschool children with seasonal allergic rhinitis, *L. casei* was also found to reduce symptoms and the number of episodes, and lessen the use of relief medications. The effect, however, was not statistically significant for asthma.[67] Similar positive effects were observed among children with pollen-sensitized allergic rhinitis who were treated with oral *Bacillus clausii* spores.[68]

Studies that examined the effects of probiotics at the level of the immune system also showed some positive effects. Supplementation with *L. gasseri* significantly reduced serum IgE specific to Japanese cedar pollen in children with seasonal allergies.[69]

Positive effects were also observed among patients who received *Bifidobacterium longum* BB536 supplement.[70] Moreover, BB536 seems to suppress Th-2 cell attraction and activation, suggesting that it may be effective in blunting the IgE-mediated allergic response.[71] In a 28-week clinical trial, BB536 favorably modulated intestinal microbiota, reducing the burden of allergens in subjects with cedar pollen allergies.[72] In an experimental model, a BB536 DNA oligodeoxynucleotide, shunted the cytokine profile in favor of Th1 and suppressed IgE levels, both markers of and contributors to a lessened allergic response.[73]

In 2 randomized controlled trials studying the clinical effects of *L. plantarum* No. 14 (LP14), eosinophil counts decreased immediately after intake in the group that took LP14, and the percentage of Th1 helper T cells increased after 6 weeks. LP14 also strongly induced the gene expression of Th1-type cytokines, indicating that probiotics are clinically effective in the management of seasonal allergic disease.[74]

A review of 13 randomized, controlled trials on the effectiveness of probiotics in the treatment or prevention of atopic dermatitis found that, regardless of IgE sensitization, *Lactobacillus rhamnosus* GG (LGG) and other probiotics were effective in preventing AD. Probiotics also reduced the severity of AD in half of the trials evaluated, although there was no significant change observed in the inflammatory markers.[75] One study demonstrated that skin severity scores were significantly lower in the group given heat-killed *L. paracasei*, and the placebo group used nearly double the amount of topical medicine during the study period.[76] Similar positive results were observed among preschool children with moderate to severe AD who were treated with a supplemental probiotics mixture. The absolute counts and percentages of CD lymphocyte subsets in the peripheral blood also decreased in the probiotic group.[77]

On the other hand, a randomized trial showed that prenatal treatment with LGG was not sufficient to prevent eczema among infants in the first year of life.[78]

In terms of preventing allergies, a meta-analysis of 6 studies reported significant benefits in infants at high risk of allergy who used probiotic supplements containing *L. rhamnosus*. A recent study[79] demonstrated that infants with suspected cow's milk allergy who were given partially hydrolyzed infant food supplemented with LGG had a higher probability of acquiring tolerance to cow's milk protein at 6 and 12 months compared with infants who were not given *LGG* supplementation. In addition, skin patch test responses were negative in all infants who acquired tolerance.

Clinical improvements have been reported among patients with allergic rhinitis and IgE-sensitized atopic eczema, but studies on the efficacy of probiotics in the management of asthma remain inconsistent. Possible reasons include differences in study designs, types of probiotics used and duration of probiotic supplementation, which limits the comparability of results.[80]

# NATURAL SUPPORT FOR ALLERGIES

## Vitamin D

In recent years, there has been an increased interest in the role that vitamin D plays in the immune system and, in particular, allergic diseases. It is known that vitamin D receptors are found in multiple tissues and cells in the human body, including mononuclear cells, T lymphocytes, and dendritic cells, which are important in the recognition of antigens. Vitamin D also has multiple cytokine-modulating effects and can decrease proliferation of both Th1 and Th2 cells, and lower the production of interleukins and interferons.[81] This vitamin has also been shown to have a role in airway remodeling, which may be important in understanding and treating asthma.[82] Molecular studies also provide evidence that vitamin D can modulate inflammatory responses, enhance antimicrobial peptide activity, and promote the integrity of the permeability barrier of the skin.[81]

Epidemiologic studies revealed that vitamin D deficiency is associated with an increased incidence of asthma and allergy symptoms,[83–85] higher IgE responses to food and environmental allergens in children and adults,[86] and severity of atopic dermatitis.[87] Similarly, children with well-controlled asthma were found to have higher levels of vitamin D,[88] and adults with chronic urticaria (hives) have lower vitamin D levels than controls.[89] A randomized controlled trial involving 45 atopic dermatitis patients provided evidence for the beneficial effect of vitamin D and E supplementation on clinical manifestations. Symptom scores significantly improved in the treatment groups for vitamin D, and vitamin E was associated with more favorable symptom scores.[90]

On the role of vitamin D in preventing asthma and atopic diseases, studies demonstrated that a woman's high intake of vitamin D during pregnancy lowers the risk of her child developing wheezing[91] or rhinitis at age 5.[92] This correlation was found in different populations, regardless of the amount of vitamin D intake. A prospective follow-up study showed conflicting results.

A recent longitudinal study demonstrated vitamin D as a predictor of asthma or atopy in later years. The study, involving 689 children from a cohort unselected for asthma or atopy who were examined at age 6 and again at age 14, showed that among male children, inadequate levels of vitamin D is a risk factor for developing atopy, bronchial hyperresponsiveness, and asthma. More importantly, vitamin D levels at age 6 were predictive of atopy/asthma-associated phenotypes at age 14 years.[93]

Although many epidemiologic studies over the past decade have clearly identified a link between vitamin D levels and asthma and/or atopic diseases, such studies have limitations and cannot establish causality. A clinical trial examining whether maternal supplementation with 4000 IU of vitamin D daily can reduce the incidence of asthma in their offspring during the first 3 years of life is currently underway. This trial will provide stronger evidence regarding the role of vitamin D in preventing allergies.[94]

## Vitamin E

Vitamin E is a fat-soluble vitamin that acts as a free-radical scavenger. It protects cell membranes and prevents damage to membrane-associated enzymes. Research suggests that vitamin E inhibits the activation of neutrophils—cells that contribute to respiratory inflammation in asthmatics.[95] Studies also indicate that vitamin E can influence and halt the proliferation of mast cells in culture,[96,97] suggesting a role for vitamin E in modulating allergies, atherosclerosis, cancer, and other diseases in which mast cells play a role.

Several studies provide evidence on the relationship between vitamin E intake and asthma or allergic diseases. A Japanese prospective study reported that low maternal vitamin E intake during pregnancy was associated with increased likelihood of wheezing in children younger than 2 years of age.[98] A Scottish birth cohort study reported that low alpha-tocopherol intake during the first trimester of pregnancy was associated with an increased risk of wheezing and asthma in 5-year-old children.[99] A case–control study reported that childhood asthma is associated with low dietary vitamin E intake,[100] and a 10-year prospective study of adult-onset asthma also reported similar findings.[101] In a clinical study of atopic dermatitis, patients randomly selected to orally receive 400 IU of vitamin E daily for 8 months reported remarkable improvement in facial erythema (redness) and lichenification (scaling and thickening of the skin). Eczematous lesions were also reportedly healed as a result of decreased itch sensation.[102]

Animal models have shown that supplementation with high-dose vitamin E reduced proliferation of splenic lymphocytes, the production of IL-4 and IL-5, and total serum IgE levels. Sneezing and nasal allergic response were also suppressed in the treatment group.[103] In a randomized controlled trial, patients with seasonal allergic rhinitis who received vitamin E supplementation during hay fever season experienced improvement in their symptoms.[104]

## Vitamin C

Vitamin C (ascorbic acid) increases the function of many immune cells, including T cells, phagocytes (which destroy pathogenic organisms), and others. As an antioxidant, ascorbic acid can protect cells from reactive oxygen species known to cause tissue damage and disease. Vitamin C has antihistamine properties[105] that can help relieve allergy symptoms, but the evidence is still controversial.

Early studies demonstrated that 2 g of vitamin C improve pulmonary function 1 hour after ingestion compared with a placebo,[106] and another study found a fivefold increase in bronchial hyperreactivity among those with the lowest intake of vitamin C.[107]

An animal model showed that high-dose vitamin C supplementation significantly decreased inflammation in the lungs.[108]

## Magnesium

Magnesium is utilized by every cell in the body and participates in energy metabolism and protein synthesis. Magnesium participates in at least 350 enzymatic processes within the body. Evidence from animal models indicates that magnesium plays a role in immune response, and that deficiency leads to increased inflammation.[109]

Results from randomized clinical trials showed that children and adults who were hospitalized for severe, acute asthma benefited from using intravenous (IV) magnesium sulfate.[110–113] One of these studies used a higher dose of magnesium sulfate (40 mg/kg) and observed a faster and more prolonged improvement in pulmonary function.[113] But one randomized study found no evidence that IV magnesium sulfate can treat moderate to severe asthma.[114]

A randomized study found that taking 200–290 mg of magnesium for 16 weeks significantly reduced the use of bronchodilators in children with mild to moderate asthma.[115] Similar beneficial effects of 12-week magnesium supplementation were found in a small study involving children with moderate persistent asthma treated with inhaled fluticasone.[116] More recently, long-term treatment with oral magnesium (170 mg twice a day for 6.5 months) in adults with mild to moderate asthma showed improvement in objective measures of bronchial reactivity and in subjective measures of asthma control and quality of life.[117]

## Fish Oil and Fatty Acids

Fish oils contain the omega-3 fatty acids docosahexaenoic acid (DHA) and eicosapentaenoic acid (EPA). EPA and DHA exert anti-inflammatory and antithrombotic (anticlotting) effects[118] because omega-3 fatty acids compete with arachidonic acid, which serves is converted into proinflammatory eicosanoids.[119–121] Studies suggest that fish oils reduce the production of inflammatory cytokines, such as interleukin-1, IL-2, and tumor necrosis factor, which are all involved in the allergic response. Additionally, lower levels of omega-3 fatty acids in the blood are associated with delayed-type hypersensitivity skin reactions in elderly malnourished subjects.[122]

In one study, an ointment containing DHA and EPA produced satisfactory results in 64 patients with refractory dermatitis.[123] A systematic review of maternal supplementation with omega-3 polyunsaturated fatty acids (n-3 PUFA) found evidence that they reduced the prevalence of childhood asthma, but supplementation during lactation did not prevent asthma or food allergy.[124] Intake of n-6 PUFA among 1002 pregnant Japanese females showed a tendency toward lesser allergic rhinitis in the children.[125]

Life Extension suggests that the omega-6 to omega-3 ratio should be kept below 4:1 for optimal health. More information on testing and optimizing your omega-6 to omega-3 ratio can be found in the *Life Extension Magazine* article entitled "Optimize Your Omega-3 Status."

## Butterbur

The perennial shrub butterbur (*Petasites hybridus*) is known to inhibit plasma histamine, leukotrienes, and the priming of mast cells in response to allergens.[126,127] Traditional Chinese medicine has used butterbur to treat asthma, migraine stress, and gastric ulcer.[128] Petasin, a pharmacologic compound extracted from the plant, has been commercialized as Ze 339 and approved in Switzerland as an antiallergic drug to treat seasonal allergic rhinitis.

A randomized controlled study found Ze 339 effective in improving asthma scores compared to placebo.[129] Other studies found the effect of Ze 339 comparable to cetirizine[130] and fexofenadine (antihistamine drugs).[131,132] A systematic review of 6 randomized controlled trials found that butterbur extract is effective as a nonsedative antihistamine for intermittent allergic rhinitis as well.[133] Ze 339 reduced allergic airway inflammation in the lungs of asthmatic animals and inhibited the production of Th2 cytokines, interleukins, and RANTES (regulated upon activation, normal T-cell expressed, and secreted), which facilitates infiltration of white blood cells during the inflammatory response.[134]

Extracts from the Japanese butterbur (*Petasites japonicus*), which contains a profile of active compounds similar to *Petasites hybridus*, inhibited eosinophil infiltration and reduced mucus secretion in an animal model of asthma. In cell culture studies, the extract inhibited the release of interleukins triggered by house dust mites,[135] suggesting that butterbur can suppress the pathogenesis of airway inflammation.

## Quercetin

Quercetin, one of the most common flavonoids found in a variety of foods such as red wine, green tea, and apples, has been studied for its ability to reduce the symptoms of allergies. It has been shown to inhibit leukotrienes, mast cells, and the release of histamine,[136] which makes it a good candidate for antiallergy therapy. Evidence also demonstrated that quercetin blunts the inflammatory response of immune cells upon antigen recognition.[137]

In an animal model of peanut allergy, quercetin completely stopped peanut-induced anaphylactic reactions after challenge. Histamine levels in quercetin-treated rats were significantly lower than the positive control group.[138] In guinea pigs sensitized with ovalbumin, a relatively low dose of quercetin reduced the hyperactivity of airways and caused significant bronchodilation.[139] Quercetin microemulsion treatment exhibited anti-inflammatory properties in a similarly designed murine model.[140]

Patients with nasal allergies treated with nasal spray containing quercetin and *Artemisia abrotanum* L experienced rapid and significant relief of nasal symptoms that was comparable to antihistamine preparations.[141] In 2 independent randomized, controlled studies among patients with pollen allergies, taking 100 mg of a quercetin-related compound for 8 weeks, significantly reduced nasal symptoms compared to placebo group.[142,143]

## Hesperidin Methyl Chalcone

Chemically similar to quercetin, the flavonoid hesperidin has been studied in a variety of contexts in both experimental models and in human clinical trials.[144] Its chalcone form was specifically studied in 99 atopic individuals in 1949. At daily doses ranging from 100–600 mg, hesperidin methyl chalcone provided complete relief of allergic symptoms in 35% of study participants; another 34% of the subjects achieved partial symptom relief.[145] More recently, hesperidin methyl chalcone has emerged as an effective treatment for chronic venous disorders.[146] Today, innovative doctors frequently suggest hesperidin methyl chalcone to patients with allergic symptoms and report clinical effectiveness.

## Rosmarinic Acid

Rosmarinic acid is a flavonoid found in various herbs such as basil, sage, mint, rosemary and *Perilla frutescens*. It is reported to have antioxidant, anti-inflammatory, antimicrobial, and antitumor effects.[147,148] Rosmarinic acid can also inhibit proinflammatory cytokines and chemokines and stabilize mast cells.[149,150] In animal models, cell cultures, and human studies, rosmarinic acid has shown potential as a natural therapeutic agent for asthma and allergic diseases.

Researchers demonstrated that daily treatment with rosmarinic acid from perilla leaf extract given orally to mice prevented allergic asthma caused by dust mite allergen. The investigators concluded that oral administration of perilla-derived rosmarinic acid may treat allergic asthma effectively by attenuating the production of cytokines and allergy-specific antibodies.[151] In another study, volatile rosemary extract significantly suppressed cytokines, eosinophils, and neutrophils in mice models of allergic asthma induced by house dust mites.[152] Similarly, rosmarinic acid effectively suppressed cytokines, chemokines, and IgE levels in murine models of atopic dermatitis.[148] It was also able to alleviate symptoms related to allergic rhinitis and allergic rhinoconjunctivitis in allergen-sensitized animal models.[153]

Oral supplementation with rosmarinic acid in patients with allergic rhinoconjunctivitis significantly relieved symptoms and inhibited eosinophils in nasal lavage fluid.[149] Another study demonstrated that perilla leaf extract enriched with rosmarinic acid is effective among humans suffering from seasonal allergic symptoms.[150] In this study, rosmarinic acid

inhibited the eye-related symptoms associated with seasonal allergies. In a randomized study on atopic dermatitis, patients given topical rosmarinic emulsions applied to the elbows twice a day for 8 weeks reported improvement in skin dryness and redness and general symptomatic relief.[154]

## Stinging Nettle

*Urtica dioica* acquired the common name "stinging nettle" because the leaves, flowers, seeds, and root contain different chemicals such as histamine, formic acid, acetic acid, and other irritants that cause mildly painful stings, itchiness, or numbness on contact.[155]

Historically, stinging nettle has been used to treat allergic rhinitis, but very few clinical studies have been conducted. In an open trial of 69 patients with allergic rhinitis, 58% of subjects who took 600 mg freeze-dried nettle leaf reported a relief in symptoms of rhinoconjunctivitis, and 48% found it more effective than over-the-counter medications.[156] Long-term use of the stinging nettle extract, IDS 30, was shown to have anti-inflammatory effects and to be effective in preventing chronic colitis in animal models.[157]

Recently, data from bioassay experiments revealed that bioactive constituents in nettle extract inhibit histamine receptors, inhibits enzymes involved releasing cytokines and chemokines that cause allergy symptoms, and reduces the production of allergy-specific prostaglandins. For the first time, these results provided a mechanistic understanding of the role of nettle extracts in reducing allergy and other inflammatory responses.[158]

## Spirulina

The term "spirulina" refers to the dried biomass of a species of cyanobacterium called *Arthrospira platensis*. It is widely consumed by humans as a dietary supplement and even used as a food source for some aquatic species and poultry.

Spirulina is a source of a variety micronutrients and phytonutrients; it is also, by weight, a good source of nonanimal protein.[159] Studies have shown that spirulina exerts a number of favorable biologic effects in both humans and animals when it is consumed as a food or a supplement.[159] Additionally, the U.S. Pharmacopeial Convention (USP) recently assigned a safety rating of "Class A" to spirulina, meaning that data support a high level of confidence regarding the safety of spirulina when used as a dietary supplement.[160]

Several trials have examined the role of spirulina in modulating the biology of allergic response.

Administered at 2000 mg per day, spirulina was shown by researchers to shift the T-cell profile away from Th2 in allergic rhinitis patients by inhibiting IL-4 signaling.[161] Upon analyzing their results, the scientists stated "this ... human feeding study ... demonstrates the protective effects of Spirulina towards allergic rhinitis."

A similarly designed clinical trial[162] corroborated previous findings by showing that "spirulina consumption significantly improved the symptoms and physical findings [in allergic rhinitis patients] compared with placebo including nasal discharge, sneezing, nasal congestion and itching."

To better explore the mechanisms by which spirulina blunts allergic reactions, researchers[163] studied its biological effects in a murine model of allergic rhinitis. They found that spirulina lowered IgE levels and, correspondingly, attenuated degranulation of nasal mast cells, resulting in suppressed histamine levels in serum. Another clinical trial reported very similar findings.[164]

## DHEA

Dehydroepiandrosterone (DHEA) and its metabolites are naturally present in humans and exert an array of actions throughout human physiology. DHEA has been studied in numerous contexts, and it is from these studies that the realization that DHEA possess considerable immunomodulatory action has arisen.

With respect to its immunologic properties, DHEA has been shown to promote balance between Th1 and Th2 cytokines and combat inflammatory responses.[165,166] Accordingly, researchers have carried these findings forward and examined the impact of DHEA on allergic reactions in clinical trials.

In one trial, immune cells were taken from subjects with asthma and cultured with or without DHEA. When DHEA was included, those immune cells produced less inflammatory cytokines and other allergic mediators, leading the investigators to conclude that "DHEA may be a useful therapy for asthma."[167] Another group[168] showed that nebulized (inhaled) DHEA-sulfate (DHEA-s, a major metabolite of DHEA) improved symptoms in patients with asthma.

Several lines of evidence support an anti-inflammatory role of DHEA in atopic individuals,[166] but levels of DHEA decline with advancing age. Supplementation with DHEA can restore blood levels of DHEA-s to youthful ranges. Individuals interested in reading more about DHEA should consult Life Extension's Male and Female Hormone Restoration Therapy protocols.

## Life Extension Suggestions

Initial strategies to reduce allergy symptoms should include avoiding known allergens as much as possible and ensuring that your environment is kept clean; regular vacuuming and use of an air purifier may help. Working with a qualified health care practitioner to identify allergens that you react to (using IgE antibody testing) and to initiate immunotherapy is an effective strategy for mitigating allergy symptoms. Many innovative doctors report that elimination diets based on quantitative IgG antibody testing are clinically effective for food allergies. In addition, the following natural compounds may help ease allergy symptoms:

- **Vitamin D:** 5000–8000 IU daily, depending on blood levels of 25-OH-vitamin D
- **Natural vitamin E:** 100–400 IU alpha-tocopherol and 200 mg gamma-tocopherol daily
- **Vitamin C:** 1000–2000 mg daily
- **Magnesium:** 140–500 elemental mg of highly absorbable magnesium
- **Fish oil** (with olive polyphenols): Providing 1400 mg EPA and 1000 mg DHA daily
- **Butterbur,** standardized extract: 75–150 mg daily
- **Rosmarinic acid:** 50–100 mg daily
- **Quercetin** (providing quercetin glycoside derivatives and free quercetin): 250–500 mg daily
- **Hesperidin methyl chalcone:** 100–600 mg daily
- **Stinging nettle** (leaf), standardized extract: 500–1500 mg daily
- **Spirulina:** 1000–2000 mg daily
- **DHEA:** Based on blood test results, doses typically range from 15–25 mg daily for women, and 25–75 mg daily for men.
- **Probiotics:** Per label instructions

In addition, the following blood testing resources may be helpful:

- Allergen Profile (IgE mediated)
- IgG antibody testing
- Omega Score®
- DHEA
- Vitamin D, 25-Hydroxy

## REFERENCES

References available at: www.lef.org/dpt5/ch6

# 7

# Alzheimer's Disease

Alzheimer's disease is a neurodegenerative disorder characterized by a decline in cognitive function that eventually leads to death.[1-4] Research in Alzheimer's disease has not yet identified a cure for the disease. Advanced age is a risk factor for development of Alzheimer's disease.[3,5]

With an increase in the aging population, the worldwide prevalence of Alzheimer's disease has increased remarkably and is expected to continue to do so. Estimates suggest that in the United States alone there will be 11–16 million individuals aged 65 and older diagnosed with Alzheimer's disease by 2050.[6,7]

Alzheimer's disease appears to be the consequence of several convergent factors, including *oxidative stress, inflammation, mitochondrial dysfunction*, and accumulation of *toxic protein aggregates* in and around neurons.[8-13] Emerging, intriguing research implicates *chronic infection* with several pathogenic organisms in the development and progression of Alzheimer's disease as well.[14] Moreover, age-related changes such as declining hormone levels and vascular dysfunction are thought to contribute to some aspects of Alzheimer's disease.[15-17]

Conventional pharmacologic interventions target symptoms, but fall short of addressing underlying, contributing factors for Alzheimer's disease. This results in a small reduction of symptoms, but does not halt or reverse disease progression.[18,19]

A comprehensive approach to Alzheimer's disease treatment is required that acknowledges and targets the many possible factors underlying the changes in brain structure and function that drive this complex condition.[18]

## THEORIES OF ALZHEIMER'S DISEASE

Research into the potential causes of Alzheimer's disease has been frustrating. A number of processes are believed to contribute to the cognitive decline observed in Alzheimer's disease. Brain deterioration in Alzheimer's disease is thought to begin decades before symptoms become evident. Outlined below are several factors postulated to contribute to Alzheimer's disease; each also represents a potential therapeutic target.[8,9]

### Senile Plaques

A prominent finding in Alzheimer's disease is that senile plaques, which are comprised of "clumps" of the protein fragment *amyloid beta*, accumulate and cause cellular damage in key areas of the brain, especially the hippocampus, which is involved in memory consolidation and spatial navigation.[20] Aggregates of amyloid beta have been shown to contribute to oxidative damage, excitotoxicity, inflammation, cell death, and formation of *neurofibrillary tangles* (NFTs).[21] However, therapies aimed solely at reducing amyloid beta have

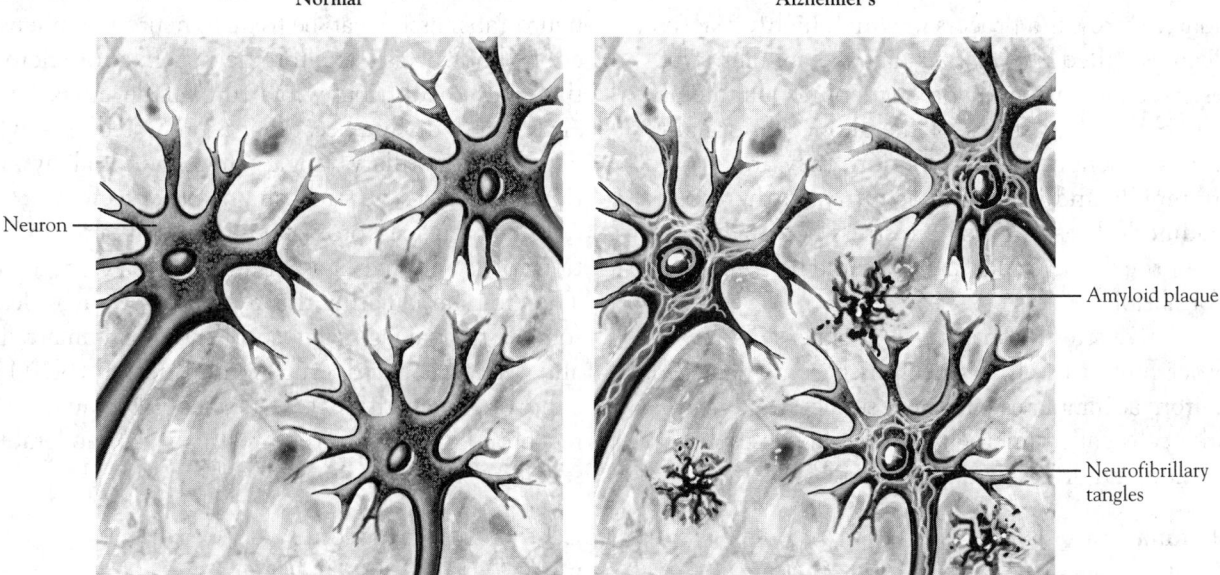

Normal Alzheimer's

Neuron

Amyloid plaque

Neurofibrillary tangles

Neurofibrillary tangles and amyloid plaques

proven disappointing, suggesting a more complex process is involved.[22–24]

## Neurofibrillary Tangles

Neurons contain a cellular skeleton made up of *microtubules*, secured in place by specialized proteins called *tau*. In Alzheimer's disease, microtubules disintegrate and tau proteins "clump" together to form aggregates called *neurofibrillary tangles* or NFTs. NFTs function much the same as amyloid beta aggregates in that they initiate several process that lead to cellular dysfunction and death. Whether amyloid beta or NFTs arise first in Alzheimer's disease is unclear, and this remains a heavily debated topic within the scientific community.[21,25]

## Acetylcholine Deficit

A theory once widely advocated, but which has proved to be disappointing at addressing underlying disease progression, is the cholinergic hypothesis. This view suggests that Alzheimer's disease is the consequence of insufficient synthesis of the neurotransmitter acetylcholine, which is fundamental in many aspects of cognition.[26,27]

Clinical trials have shown medications that support acetylcholine signaling reduce symptoms, but do not reverse or halt the disease. Therefore, inadequate cholinergic neurotransmission is now viewed as a consequence of generalized brain deterioration observed in Alzheimer's disease, rather than a direct cause. Nonetheless, drugs that modulate acetylcholine signaling are still a mainstay of symptomatic management of Alzheimer's disease.[26,27]

## Oxidative Stress

Oxidative stress is a process in which highly reactive molecules called *free radicals* damage cellular structures. Free radicals are byproducts of normal metabolism, but during states of metabolic abnormality such as mitochondrial dysfunction, they are created more rapidly and in greater quantity. In the case of Alzheimer's disease, oxidative stress both facilitates some of the damage caused by amyloid beta *and* spurs its formation.[28,29]

Oxidative stress propagates Alzheimer's disease via another route as well. As neurons become damaged, free iron accumulates on their surfaces and within nearby cells called microglia. Free iron causes radical formation and drives oxidative stress.[30]

## Inflammation

The inflammatory process appears to play an important role in the development of Alzheimer's disease. When high levels of amyloid beta accumulate in the brain, it activates the body's immune response, resulting in inflammation that damages neurons.[31] Part of the inflammatory response to amyloid beta appears to be facilitated by *tumor necrosis factor-alpha* (TNF-α).[32] TNF-α is a pro-inflammatory cytokine that is often found in high levels in serum and cerebral spinal fluid (CSF) of Alzheimer's patients; it represents a potential target for novel Alzheimer's disease therapies.[32–34]

## Mitochondrial Dysfunction

Mitochondria are the energy power plants of cells; they generate energy in the form of adenosine triphosphate (ATP), which is necessary for cellular function. Mitochondrial dysfunction has been implicated in many age-related diseases, including Alzheimer's disease.[35] One line of evidence that supports a link between Alzheimer's disease and mitochondrial dysfunction is the finding that ApoE4, a genetic variant associated with Alzheimer's disease and amyloid beta deposition within the brain, seems to play a role in disrupting mitochondrial respiratory chain function.[35–37]

Dysfunctional mitochondria are important mediators of amyloid beta toxicity.[38] Mitochondrial dysfunction contributes to an increased burden of oxidative stress as well, which itself is another mediator of amyloid beta toxicity. Mitochondrial dysfunction and oxidative stress then drive the formation of additional amyloid beta, creating a vicious, self-propagating cycle that ultimately leads to neuron death.[38]

## Excitotoxicity

Glutamate is the most abundant excitatory neurotransmitter in the brain and is necessary for normal brain function. However, too much glutamatergic neurotransmission can be toxic to neurons, a phenomenon known as "excitotoxicity." Excitotoxicity is thought to contribute to neuronal degeneration in Alzheimer's disease because it is promoted by amyloid beta, neurofibrillary tangles, mitochondrial dysfunction, and oxidative stress among other factors.[39]

Glutamate excitotoxicity is the result of overactivation of *N*-methyl-D-aspartate (NMDA) receptors. Therefore, modulating this receptor is a way to lessen some of the damaging effects of excess glutamate signaling. The Food and Drug Administration (FDA) has approved memantine (eg, Namenda®), an NMDA receptor blocker, for the treatment of moderate to severe Alzheimer's disease.[39]

## Loss of Sex Hormones

Evidence suggests that age-related loss of sex hormones–estrogen in women and testosterone in men–may contribute to Alzheimer's disease. Although the specific mechanisms are unclear, sex hormones appear to protect the brain against the development of Alzheimer's disease.[15,16] For example, declining estrogen and testosterone levels seem to be associated with increased amyloid beta and tau abnormalities.[40]

## Infections

An intriguing theory that remains largely unappreciated by the medical community is that chronic infection with a variety of pathogenic bacteria and/ or viruses may contribute to the development of Alzheimer's disease. Research indicates that some common pathogens are consistently detected in the brains of Alzheimer's patients. For example, a comprehensive analysis of studies found that *Spirochetes*, a family of bacteria, was detected in about 90% of Alzheimer's patients and was virtually absent in healthy age-matched controls. Further statistical evaluation revealed a high probability of a causal relationship between *Spirochetes* infection and Alzheimer's disease.[14]

*Spirochetes* and other bacteria can linger in the brain and drive inflammation and the formation of amyloid beta and neurofibrillary tangles, all of which are hallmarks of Alzheimer's disease.[14] Moreover, laboratory studies indicate that amyloid beta is an antimicrobial peptide, suggesting its formation could be an adaptive response to infectious organisms.[41] These and other findings have led some researchers to hypothesize that "early intervention against infection may delay or even prevent the future development of [Alzheimer's disease]."[42]

## RISK FACTORS FOR ALZHEIMER'S DISEASE

Several factors influence the risk of Alzheimer's disease. Some are modifiable, such as obesity and nutrient deficiencies, but others, such as carrying the ApoE4 gene, are not. A partial list of factors known to be associated with an increased risk of Alzheimer's disease follows[2,14,43–49]:

- Advancing age
- Family history of Alzheimer's disease
- Carrying the ApoE4 genetic variant
- Certain bacterial infections
- Vascular risk factors (eg, diabetes, atherosclerosis, high blood pressure, high cholesterol) appear to encourage development of phenomena associated

with Alzheimer's disease such as accumulation of amyloid beta[50]
- History of head trauma
- High homocysteine levels
- Nutrient deficiencies
- Silent strokes
- Central obesity (ie, high waist-to-hip ratio)

## DIAGNOSIS

Although autopsy provides a definitive diagnosis, there is no single test to definitively diagnose Alzheimer's disease in the living.[51,52] Alzheimer's disease is diagnosed by exclusion in the living. In other words, physicians must confirm that neurologic deficits are not being caused by other conditions (eg, vascular dementia). The standard diagnostic strategy comprises collection of detailed patient history data, standardized assessment of cognition and functional status (eg, mini-mental state examination), laboratory testing, and brain imaging examinations, such as magnetic resonance imaging (MRI), positron emission tomography imaging (PET), and single-photon emission computed tomography (SPECT).[20]

Discovering more specific biomarkers for Alzheimer's disease may lead to the development of more accurate diagnostic tools for early diagnosis.[20] Some genetic biomarkers that raise the risk of Alzheimer's disease have already been identified.[53,54]

## CONVENTIONAL TREATMENT

Conventional Alzheimer's disease treatment relies heavily on pharmacologic modulation of cholinergic and glutamatergic neurotransmission. This can result in symptomatic improvement, though the underlying progression of the disease is unaffected. Accumulation of amyloid beta and neurofibrillary tangles are challenging to target via pharmacologic means.[55]

### Acetylcholinesterase Inhibitors

Acetylcholinesterase inhibitors are typically first-line pharmacotherapy for mild to moderate Alzheimer's disease. They prevent the breakdown of acetylcholine, a chemical neurotransmitter in the brain, by inhibiting the enzyme *acetylcholinesterase*.

Tacrine, the first centrally acting cholinesterase inhibitor approved by FDA for the treatment of Alzheimer's disease, was withdrawn from the U.S. market, due to possible liver toxicity.[56–58] Cholinesterase inhibitors currently used in Alzheimer's disease include donepezil (Aricept®), rivastigmine (Exelon®), and galantamine (Razadyne®).[52] Although studies have repeatedly found that acetylcholinesterase inhibitors may reduce Alzheimer's symptoms, they do not halt or reverse the underlying disease process.[59,60]

## NMDA Receptor Blockers

Memantine (eg, Namenda®), an N-methyl-D-aspartate (NMDA) receptor antagonist (blocker), has been approved by the FDA for moderate to severe Alzheimer's disease.[61] Although memantine may help decrease formation of NFTs, NMDA receptor antagonists have also been linked to serious adverse effects, which appear to be worsened in combination with acetylcholinesterase inhibitors.[62]

## Additional Pharmacologic Therapies

**Nonsteroidal anti-inflammatory drugs (NSAIDs).** Evidence from population-based studies suggests beneficial effects of treatment with nonsteroidal anti-inflammatory drugs (NSAIDs) in Alzheimer's disease, although these effects have not been reproduced in clinical trials.[63] NSAIDs affect the pathology of Alzheimer's disease by inhibiting cyclooxygenase (COX) enzymes, which contribute to inflammation.

NSAIDs appear to prevent cognitive decline in older adults if started in midlife (prior to age 65) rather than late in life.[63,64] Unfortunately, NSAIDs, even at normal dosages, have been associated with significant adverse effects. Long-term use of NSAIDs is associated with gastrointestinal, kidney, and cardiovascular complications.[65–67] Low-dose aspirin, however, might be effective in reducing Alzheimer's incidence and side effects are relatively rare when only 81 mg per day are taken.

**Blood pressure–lowering drugs.** It has been hypothesized that treating cardiovascular risk factors might be an effective means of preventing or treating dementia syndromes, including Alzheimer's.[68] Specifically, elevated blood pressure during midlife appears to be associated with Alzheimer's development in late life. This effect may be caused by a link between high blood pressure and poor amyloid beta clearance from the brain.[69]

Drugs normally used to treat hypertension, including angiotensin-converting enzyme (ACE) inhibitors, angiotensin receptor blockers, and calcium channel blockers, have been considered as potential Alzheimer's therapies.[70] Some research suggests that these drugs mildly reduce cognitive decline, and may reduce risk of Alzheimer's development and progression.[71–73]

**Etanercept (Enbrel®).** Etanercept (Enbrel®), a biological inhibitor of the cytokine TNF-α, is approved for the treatment of certain inflammatory conditions (eg, rheumatoid arthritis, plaque psoriasis). When formulated as a perispinal injection and administered to Alzheimer's patients, preliminary research reports suggest that Enbrel® leads to sustained improvement in cognitive function that was evident within minutes.[32,74,75] Because preliminary findings using this novel therapeutic approach were encouraging, Life Extension Foundation® is currently sponsoring a clinical trial to further study the effects of perispinal injections of Enbrel in patients with mild to moderate Alzheimer's disease.

**Granulocyte colony-stimulating factor.** *Granulocyte colony-stimulating factor* (G-CSF) is a growth factor that stimulates production of certain white blood cells. It also supports the creation of new neurons in the brain and modulates cholinergic neurotransmission.[76] Lower levels of G-CSF have been identified in Alzheimer's patients compared to healthy individuals.[77] An animal model of Alzheimer's found that injections of G-CSF not only rescued compromised memory and cognitive functions, but also raised levels of acetylcholine.[78] A study at the University of South Florida seeks to evaluate the cognitive effects of administering G-CSF to Alzheimer's patients.[79]

**Brain-derived neurotrophic factor.** Brain-derived neurotrophic factor (BDNF), a signaling protein active in the brain, facilitates the growth of new neurons and synapses and also reverses neuronal atrophy. Since BDNF levels decline with age and Alzheimer's disease, administration of BDNF has been suggested as a potential therapy for memory loss.[80] Injecting BDNF into the brains of rodents and primates reversed synaptic damage, cell death, cognitive decline, and memory deficits.[81] Intensive research in rodents has led to the first promising clinical trials of intracerebral neurotrophin for Alzheimer's disease.[82]

**Lithium.** Lithium may be able to inhibit some fundamental processes that drive Alzheimer's disease. In one study, only 5% of elderly patients with bipolar disorder taking lithium were found to have Alzheimer's disease, compared with 33% of those not taking lithium.[83] Lithium has also been associated with a significant reduction in the levels of phospho-tau (a precursor to NFTs) in spinal fluid, which is characteristic of Alzheimer's disease.[84]

Several mechanisms could partly explain the link between lithium and reduction in Alzheimer's risk.

These include inhibition of cell death, support for the recycling of damaged cellular components, optimized mitochondrial function, and increased synthesis neuronal growth factors.[85]

**Selective estrogen receptor modulators.** Selective estrogen receptor modulators (SERMs) are drugs that either increase or decrease estrogen signaling, depending on the tissue type.[86] Currently, the most studied and clinically relevant SERMs are tamoxifen and raloxifene. Tamoxifen is best recognized as a potent antagonist (blocker) of estrogen action in breast tissue. However, low concentrations of tamoxifen have been noted to protect cultured neurons from amyloid beta and glutamate toxicity.[87] In postmenopausal women, raloxifene, at a dose of 120 mg per day, has been linked with reduced risk of cognitive impairment and development of Alzheimer's disease.[88]

**Vaccines.** Vaccines are being developed in hopes of clearing amyloid beta from the brains of Alzheimer's patients immunologically.[1] Initial research suggests a mechanistic possibility that this approach could work,[24] but many obstacles still impede the development of clinically effective vaccines for Alzheimer's disease.[89] For example, some studies suggest that simply eliminating amyloid beta may not be sufficient, and that targeting other aspects of Alzheimer's pathology in conjunction with amyloid beta vaccination may have a better chance of success.[90]

**Antibiotics.** As mentioned above, the theory that Alzheimer's disease could be cause by infectious organisms is gaining traction within the scientific community. Based on these findings, it has been proposed that antibiotics may represent a viable treatment for Alzheimer's disease.[14]

Early clinical trials have noted marked improvements in Alzheimer's patients following antibiotic treatment. In one such trial, 100 subjects with probable Alzheimer's disease were treated with the antibiotics doxycycline and rifampin for 3 months and followed for a year. At 6 months post-treatment, subjects who received antibiotics displayed significantly less cognitive decline than those who received a placebo, and the effect was even more pronounced at 12 months. Antibiotic recipients also showed less behavioral dysfunction at 3 months. The researchers concluded that "therapy with doxycycline and rifampin may have a therapeutic role in patients with mild to moderate [Alzheimer's disease]."[91] Another smaller trial found Alzheimer's patients treated with 100 mg daily of the antibiotic D-cycloserine

displayed significantly improved scores on a standardized assessment of cognitive function.[92]

Although larger trials with longer follow-up periods are needed to more thoroughly assess the therapeutic value of antibiotics in Alzheimer's disease, evidence continues to mount that the most common cause of dementia may be the result of an infection, and early treatment with inexpensive antimicrobial drugs might represent an advance in the management of this devastating condition.[14]

**Piracetam.** Piracetam has been studied in a wide-range of patient populations and has demonstrated small benefits in a variety of models of neurological disorders. Multiple mechanisms for the observable effects of piracetam on brain function have been proposed, though a precise description of its mode of action has yet to be elucidated. Preliminary studies suggest that piracetam may modulate the signaling of multiple neurotransmitter receptors, and improve neuronal membrane fluidity.[93,94]

A comprehensive review that assessed the efficacy of piracetam in older subjects suggests that the drug may provide appreciable benefits for cognitive dysfunction. The reviewers concluded that "the results of this analysis provide compelling evidence for the global efficacy of piracetam in a diverse group of older subjects with cognitive impairment."[95] Additionally, a piracetam analog called levetiracetam was shown to reverse synaptic and cognitive deficits in an animal Alzheimer's model.[96]

**Additional emerging therapies.** The following compounds hold promise, but more research is needed before their potential therapeutic value in Alzheimer's disease can be deciphered:

- *Rapamycin*[97] is an immunosuppressive drug that also improves removal of cellular debris, including amyloid beta, via enhancing a process called autophagy.

- *Secretase inhibitors* (used only in preliminary human trials)[98] target the enzymes that cleave amyloid precursor protein into amyloid beta fragments. In theory, blocking secretase activity would slow accumulation of amyloid beta.

# HORMONE REPLACEMENT THERAPY IN ALZHEIMER'S DISEASE

A potential strategy to modulate factors that underlie Alzheimer's disease is to target age-related depletion of sex hormones. Following menopause, women experience a rapid loss of estrogen and progesterone.

Similarly, men experience an age-related loss of testosterone, a condition known as androgen deficiency or hypogonadism. Since sex hormones have fundamental roles in neural health, hormone replacement therapy (HRT) is an intriguing therapeutic consideration in Alzheimer's disease.[16]

## Pregnenolone

In humans, the steroid hormone cascade begins with pregnenolone, a hormonal derivative of cholesterol. Subsequently, metabolic modification of pregnenolone gives rise to dehydroepiandrosterone (DHEA), which is then converted into estrogens, progesterone, and testosterone.[99,100] Aging is associated with a steep decline in the production of pregnenolone and other steroid hormones. French researchers have shown that pregnenolone directly influences acetylcholine release in several key brain regions. They also demonstrated pregnenolone's ability to promote new nerve growth.[101,102]

## Dehydroepiandrosterone

Dehydroepiandrosterone (DHEA) has neuroprotective effects and several studies indicate that patients with Alzheimer's disease have lower levels of DHEA than those without the disease.[103–105] In animal models, DHEA improved memory in rodents that overexpressed amyloid beta.[106]

## Estrogen

Estrogen is an important regulator of neural function. It has been reported to protect neurons from amyloid beta-mediated toxicity as well as to reduce neuronal death in cell culture.[107,108] However, the role of estrogen replacement therapy in brain protection is not entirely clear, and may be dependent on age at initiation.[109] One research team suggested that estrogen therapy could be beneficial when neurons are still healthy, but might exacerbate Alzheimer's disease once neurologic health is already compromised.[110] The Cache County Study reported that Alzheimer's risk was reduced with long-term HRT (>10 years) compared to short-term HRT,[111] suggesting that early initiation (near menopause) may be an important factor.[16,112]

## Progesterone

Like estrogen, progesterone levels decline during normal aging. Declining progesterone levels are linked with increased amyloid beta, increased NFTs, increased neuron death, and impaired cognition; all of which are associated with Alzheimer's disease.[16] Therefore, some scientific evidence suggests that progesterone may be effective for the prevention of degenerative brain diseases including Alzheimer's disease.[113]

## Testosterone

Unlike the sudden drop of female hormones that occurs during menopause, loss of testosterone is gradual in men, with bioavailable levels declining 2–3% annually from approximately 30 years of age.[16] Several studies have linked low testosterone to increased risk of Alzheimer's disease in men. In a clinical trial involving 16 male Alzheimer's patients and 22 healthy controls, 24 weeks of testosterone replacement therapy were associated with improved quality of life compared to placebo among those with Alzheimer's disease.[114]

## Melatonin

Endogenous melatonin not only helps regulate the sleep–wake cycle, but is a strong antioxidant.[115] Melatonin secretion within the brain declines with age and lower levels are associated with a higher degree of cognitive impairment.[116] Melatonin concentration is lower in Alzheimer's patients than in healthy people of the same age.[117] In animal studies, melatonin improved cognitive function and reduced oxidative injury and deposition of amyloid beta.[118] Additional studies have confirmed that melatonin protects brain cells from amyloid beta toxicity by impairing amyloid beta generation and slowing the formation of plaque deposits.[119] Melatonin has also been shown to reduce tau tangles and amyloid beta toxicity.[120]

# DIETARY AND LIFESTYLE MANAGEMENT STRATEGIES

Analysis of some dietary patterns indicates that dietary nutrient composition may affect the risk of developing Alzheimer's disease.[121]

## Mediterranean Diet

The Mediterranean diet has been shown to reduce the risk of Alzheimer's and other dementias in a host of studies. A recent review found a reduced risk of Alzheimer's among those whose dietary pattern included a higher intake of fruits, vegetables, fish, nuts, and legumes, as well as a lower intake of meats, high fat dairy, and sweets.[121] Another recent review of the literature noted a reduced risk of neurodegenerative diseases such as Alzheimer's, Parkinson's, and mild cognitive impairment, when patients were on a Mediterranean diet.[122]

Yet another review found that the Mediterranean diet reduced both the risk of Alzheimer's disease and the rate of progression from predementia syndromes to overt dementia. The researchers pointed out that the Mediterranean diet largely comprises individual foods (eg, fish, vegetable oils, nonstarchy vegetables, low-glycemic-index fruits, and red wine), independently proposed as potential protective factors against dementia and predementia.[123]

In one study, participants who most closely adhered to the Mediterranean diet, showed 28% lower risk of developing cognitive impairment over a 4.5-year period than those who were less adherent. Also, highly adherent participants with some cognitive impairment at the start of the study experienced 48% lower risk of developing Alzheimer's disease at follow-up (an average of 4.3 years later).[124]

The Mediterranean diet also appears to affect the mortality rate in Alzheimer's. For example, Alzheimer's patients whose adherence to the Mediterranean diet was greatest during a study period of 4.4 years were 76% less likely to die than those whose adherence was lowest. Alzheimer's patients who adhered to the Mediterranean diet to a moderate degree lived an average 1.3 years longer than those who adhered to the diet to the lowest degree. Patients who followed the diet very strictly lived, on average, 3.9 years longer.[125]

## Ketogenic Diet

The ketogenic diet, which involves a strict regimen of very high fat, moderate protein, and low carbohydrates, prompts the body to switch from its normal metabolic process of burning glucose to burning ketones. Ketones are substances produced when the body breaks down fat instead of glucose for energy. Initial research is being carried out to investigate the impact of the ketogenic diet on Alzheimer's development and progression.[126] In a transgenic mouse model, 43 days on a ketogenic diet resulted in ketone production and decreased amyloid beta levels.[127]

The ketogenic diet can cause adverse side effects (eg, increased cholesterol levels, kidney stones, and gastroesophageal reflux).[126]

## Low-Calorie Diet (Calorie Restriction)

Researchers reported that a low-calorie diet reduces the risk of mild cognitive impairment, which is the stage of memory loss between normal aging and overt dementia. Healthy study subjects between ages 70 and 89 were divided into 3 groups based on their normal daily caloric intake: 600–1526, 1526–2143, and 2143–6000 calories. Those in the highest

calorie group were almost twice as likely to develop mild cognitive impairment. This association was found to be dose-dependent; the risk increased gradually with the increase in calories.[128,129]

## Exercise

Regular exercise is associated with increases in brain-derived neurotrophic factor (BDNF), hippocampal neurogenesis, synaptic plasticity, brain volume, dendritic spines, and vascular function, as well as a reduction in cell death.[130,131] Research focusing on Alzheimer's patients found that those who exercised had reduced brain atrophy compared with those who did not.[132] As little as 3 minutes of very intense exercise has been shown to sharply raise BDNF levels, as well as produce a 20% improvement in memory.[133]

The benefits of exercise may be enhanced by consumption of omega-3 fatty acids and plant polyphenols.[131] Exercise and diets rich in omega-3 fatty acids have been shown to help normalize BDNF levels.[134,135]

# TARGETED NUTRITIONAL STRATEGIES

## Nutritional Interventions Studied in Alzheimer's

**Huperzine A.** Derived from the plant *Huperzia serrata*, huperzine A is an NMDA receptor blocker than can help prevent or reduce glutamate-mediated excitotoxicity.[136] It can also help block acetylcholinesterase, the enzyme that destroys acetylcholine, which is critical for cognition and memory. This mechanism of action is similar to that of several Alzheimer's drugs, such as donepezil and galantamine.[137] Some studies show that huperzine A may penetrate the blood–brain barrier, have greater bioavailability, and have longer duration of action than some pharmaceuticals.[138,139] Although not all studies on Huperzine show positive effects on cognition,[140] a review of previous studies revealed that doses of 300–500 mcg of huperzine A daily significantly improved the standardized cognitive test scores of Alzheimer's patients, and were slightly safer than some drug alternatives.[141]

**Lipoic acid.** This potent antioxidant has been shown to reduce inflammation, chelate metals, and increase acetylcholine levels in animal studies.[142,143] Although there have been only a few small human studies on lipoic acid in Alzheimer's, the results hold promise.

In one study, 9 patients with Alzheimer's or similar dementias took 600 mg of lipoic acid daily, for an average of 337 days. At the outset of the study, cognitive scores were declining continuously. By the end of the study, they had stabilized.[144] A second study extended this regime to 43 patients for 48 months and the disease progressed extremely slowly (compared with the typical disease progression rate seen in untreated patients).[145]

**Acetyl-L-carnitine (ALC).** ALC is an antioxidant that has been shown to correct acetylcholine deficits in animals and protect neurons from amyloid beta by supporting healthy mitochondria.[146–148] A group of researchers combined ALC with lipoic acid and found they could reverse some mitochondrial decay in aged animals. The same research group conducted a comprehensive review of 21 clinical trials of ALC in cases of mild cognitive impairment and mild Alzheimer's disease. They found significant benefit in the ALC group compared to placebo.[149]

ALC has been noted to reduce the effects of high homocysteine levels in mice (eg, deterioration of blood–brain barrier integrity, increased levels of amyloid beta, neurofibrillary tangle formation, and cognitive dysfunction).[150] Further, a small clinical trial among people with Alzheimer's disease showed that 3000 mg of ALC daily resulted in significantly less cognitive deterioration over a 1-year period.[151] Laboratory studies have found that ALC can reduce amyloid beta neurotoxicity by affecting amyloid precursor protein metabolism.[152]

**Panax ginseng.** Ginsenosides, steroid-like copounds in extracts of the plant *Panax ginseng* (*P. ginseng*), are believed to be the active chemicals that produce memory benefits.[153] A study that tested 200, 400, and 600 mg of *P. ginseng* in healthy patients without cognitive problems found that 400 mg produced the greatest benefit and boosted memory for 1–6 hours after dosing.[154] When higher dosages were tested in 58 Alzheimer's disease patients, 4.5 g of *P. ginseng* given daily over 12 weeks produced gradually increasing improvements, as compared to the 39 control patients whose cognitive abilities declined over the same period, although the improvements faded 12 weeks after discontinuation.[155]

**Vitamins C and E.** Vitamins C and E are well known for their antioxidant properties. Several studies have examined their combined potential in reducing the oxidative damage associated with Alzheimer's disease.[156,157] One observational study showed that supplementation with vitamins C (500 mg/day) and E (400 IU/day) was associated with reduced prevalence of Alzheimer's disease.[158]

Another team of researchers found that the combination of vitamin C and E was associated with a reduced risk of Alzheimer's disease, but neither supplement alone conferred substantial protection.[159] However, a placebo-controlled clinical trial found that high doses of vitamin E alone, up to 2000 IU daily, slowed the mental deterioration of Alzheimer's patients,[160] and in an animal model, vitamin C helped reduced amyloid beta aggregation.[161]

Deficiencies of vitamin E in Alzheimer's patients are associated with increased lipid peroxidation (oxidative deterioration of lipids), which appears to increase platelet aggregation.[162] Combination therapy with vitamins C and E has been shown to reduce lipid peroxidation in people with mild to moderate Alzheimer's disease.[163] A high intake of vitamins C and E may be associated with reduced incidence of Alzheimer's in the healthy elderly.[164]

One method by which vitamin E might protect Alzheimer's disease has to do with its relation to apolipoprotein E4 (apoE4). Researchers suspect that in people with the apoE4 phenotype, impaired antioxidant defense systems in neurons may increase oxidative damage.[165] Another theory suggests that vitamin E might be able to reduce the oxidative damage caused by large amounts of *inducible nitric oxide synthase*, a pro-oxidant that has been linked to progression of Alzheimer's.[166] Moreover, a recent study suggested that vitamin E may combat amyloid beta-induced oxidative stress, a characteristic of Alzheimer's disease.[167] (Note: Inducible *nitric oxide synthase* should not be confused with endothelial *nitric oxide synthase* that is needed to maintain healthy arterial function.)

**Ginkgo biloba.** Ginkgo biloba is an antioxidant that may serve as an anti-inflammatory agent, reduce blood clotting, and modulate neurotransmission.[168,169] In one study, ginkgo was tested on patients with mild to moderate Alzheimer's dementia. The results were inconsistent. However, in a subgroup of those patients with neuropsychiatric symptoms, 120–240 mg of ginkgo daily over 26 weeks significantly improved cognitive performance over placebo.[170] Another study found that ginkgo inhibited amyloid beta production in the brain.[171]

Ginkgo, if effectively combined with other brain-supporting nutrients, appears to offer a synergistic cognitive effect, resulting partly from its ability to improve cerebrovascular function.[172] Research has shown that combining ginkgo biloba with other nutrients such as phosphatidylserine, B vitamins, and vitamin E can deliver cognitive benefits to both animals and humans.[173,174] In addition, a study found that ginkgo extract can rescue neuronal cells from beta amyloid–induced cell death via a mechanism distinct from its antioxidant properties.[90] Ginkgo also appears to protect against Alzheimer's disease by inhibiting the formation of amyloid fibrils.[175] Finally, a review of 6 studies found that ginkgo benefits cognition and psychopathological symptoms, with no evidence of negative side effects.[176]

**Curcumin.** Curcumin is derived from the *Curcuma longa* (turmeric) plant. Many studies have suggested that curcumin may be an effective therapy for Alzheimer's because it exerts neuroprotective actions through numerous pathways including inhibition of amyloid beta, clearance of existing amyloid beta, anti-inflammatory effects, antioxidant activity, delayed degradation of neurons, and chelation (binding) of copper and iron, among others.[177-180]

Curcumin has been found to reduce cognitive dysfunction, neural synaptic damage, amyloid plaque deposition, and oxidative damage. It has also been found to modulate the levels of cytokines in brain neurons.[178,181] The anti-inflammatory effect of curcumin appears to result from a reduction of *nuclear factor-kappa B*, a nuclear transcription factor that regulates many genes involved in cytokine production.[182] Curcumin's ability to chelate toxic metals such as iron and copper and reduce their levels may also help prevent amyloid aggregation.[183] By inhibiting interaction with heavy metals (eg, cadmium and lead), curcumin may reduce cerebral deregulation.[178] Laboratory studies also suggest that curcumin is more effective at inhibiting accumulation of amyloid beta in animal brains than the over-the-counter NSAIDs ibuprofen and naproxen.[184] A clinical trial found that doses of regular curcumin ranging from 1 to 4 g daily were well tolerated and exerted anti-inflammatory effects and possibly reduced amyloid beta aggregation in 27 subjects with probable Alzheimer's.[185]

## Nutritional Interventions Studied in Cognitive Decline and Dementia

**Docosahexaenoic acid.** Docosahexaenoic acid (DHA), an omega-3 fatty acid found primarily in fish and fish oil, has been linked to cognitive function.[186] DHA constitutes 30–50% of the total fatty acid content of the human brain.[187] It has been shown to reduce amyloid beta secretion.[188] and increase phosphatidylserine levels.[189] Studies indicate that omega-3 fatty acids have the ability to inhibit early stages of neurofibrillary tangle formation,[190] and reduce amyloid plaque development.[191] An animal model revealed that fish oil supplementation may combat some of the negative effects of carrying the ApoE4 gene.[192] In a randomized study involving 485 individuals with age-related cognitive decline, 900 mg of DHA daily for 6 months resulted in a marked improvement in learning and memory tests.[193]

**Vinpocetine.** Vinpocetine, derived from the periwinkle plant, has neuroprotective properties and increases cerebral circulation.[194-196] It also protects against excitotoxicity.[197,198] Vinpocetine has been used as a drug in Eastern Europe for the treatment of age-related memory impairment.[199] In a controlled clinical trial, 10 mg of vinpocetine 3 times per day improved a variety of measures of cognitive function among subjects with vascular senile cerebral dysfunction.[200]

**Pyrroloquinoline quinone (PQQ).** PQQ is an important nutrient that stimulates the growth of new mitochondria in aging cells, and promotes mitochondrial protection and repair.[201,202] Mitochondrial decay contributes to many age-related diseases, including Alzheimer's.[203,204] Laboratory studies indicate PQQ may inhibit the development of Alzheimer's disease.[205-209] PQQ protects neurons from amyloid beta and the protein alpha-synuclein, which contributes to neurodegeneration in Parkinson's disease.[205,209]

Supplementation with 20 mg per day of PQQ resulted in improvements on tests of higher cognitive function in a group of middle-aged and elderly people.[210] These effects were significantly amplified when the subjects also took 300 mg per day of CoQ10.

**Phosphatidylserine (PS).** PS is a naturally occurring component of cell membranes. In a study conducted in Japan on 78 elderly people with mild cognitive impairment, supplementation with PS for 6 months resulted in significant improvements in memory functions.[211] In another study, 18 elderly subjects with age-related memory decline took 100 mg of PS 3 times daily for 12 weeks. Tests at 6 and 12 weeks showed cognitive gains compared to baseline measurements.[212] A group of researchers studied the safety and efficacy of phosphatidylserine-containing omega-3 fatty acids (PS-omega-3) in 8 elderly patients with memory complaints.[213] They found that PS-omega-3 had favorable effects on memory functions. Researchers are now finding that phosphatidylserine supplementation works optimally along with docosahexaenoic acid (DHA).[214]

**Glycerophosphocholine (GPC).** GPC is a structural component of brain cell membranes and a precursor to the neurotransmitter acetylcholine. In Alzheimer's disease, the concentration of GPC increases in the CSF due to the breakdown of cell membranes during neurodegeneration.[215] Supplementation with GPC and other nutritive substances like acetyl-L-carnitine, docosahexaenoic acid, α-lipoic acid and phosphatidylserine improves cognitive functions in mice.[216] A clinical trial on 261 patients with dementia of the Alzheimer's type showed improvement in cognitive symptoms with an acetyl-choline precursor.[217] A larger trial also revealed significant cognitive improvement when patients recovering from stroke were given 1000–1200 mg of alpha-GPC for 5 months.[218]

---

## LIFE EXTENSION STUDY: NUTRIENT COMPLEX MAY POSITIVELY IMPACT COGNITIVE PERFORMANCE

A 2012 study conducted by Life Extension Clinical Research, Inc. assessed the impact of daily dosing of a dietary supplement containing alpha-glyceryl phosphoryl choline (A-GPC), phosphatidylserine, vinpocetine, grape seed extract, wild blueberry extract, ashwagandha extract, and uridine-5'-monophosphate on cognitive performance in 40 middle-aged to elderly subjects with subjective memory complaints.

An online cognitive assessment tool (Computerized Neuropsychological Test) was used to assess the change in cognitive performance from baseline to day 30 and day 60; the Global Impression Improvement (CGI-I) scale provided an overall clinically determined summary measure.

Twenty-nine subjects completed the study with no significant adverse events being reported. Preliminary results revealed a statistically significant improvement in 3 tests: working memory (N-back), inspection time, and executive function. Based on the CGI-I Scale, improvement was noted after 30 days and 60 days of product dosing.

The study was presented at the Experimental Biology 2012 multidisciplinary scientific conference in San Diego, California, April 21–25, 2012.

---

## Additional Nutritional Support for Cognition

**Coffee and caffeine.** A review of several studies revealed that coffee consumption is associated with a reduced risk of Alzheimer's and Parkinson's diseases.[219] Long-term caffeine administration to mice can reduce brain amyloid beta deposition through suppression of beta- and gamma-secretase. An animal model showed that caffeine appeared to synergize with another coffee component to increase blood levels of *granulocyte colony-stimulating factor* (G-CSF). Both higher G-CSF levels and long-term administration of caffeinated coffee have been shown to enhance working memory.[220]

*Chlorogenic acid*, an antioxidant polyphenol present in coffee, has been shown to reduce blood pressure, systemic inflammation, risk of type 2 diabetes, and platelet aggregation.[220,221] In one study, when mice with impaired short-term or working memory were given chlorogenic acid, their cognitive impairment was significantly reversed.[222] Polyphenol availability varies with how long coffee beans are roasted and the roasting method itself. All roasting destroys some polyphenols, the most important being chlorogenic acid. However, there is a patented roasting process that returns polyphenol content back to the coffee beans allowing for a substantially increased polyphenol content compared to conventionally processed coffee.[223] Another excellent source of chlorogenic acid is *green coffee extract*.[224]

**Green tea.** The flavonoids in green tea, known as catechins, have been shown to possess metal-chelating (binding) properties, as well as antioxidant and anti-inflammatory effects.[30] Animal studies have demonstrated that the main flavonoid in green tea, epigallocatechin gallate (EGCG), along with other tea catechins, can decrease levels of amyloid beta in the brain,[225] and suppress amyloid beta-induced cognitive dysfunction and neurotoxicity.[226–228] Studies propose that green tea catechins also act as modulators of neuronal signaling and metabolism, cell survival-and-death genes, and mitochondrial function. Recently, population based studies have determined that intake of catechins in both green and black tea may reduce the incidence of Alzheimer's disease and dementia.[229]

**Resveratrol.** A polyphenol found in Japanese knotweed, red wine, and grapes, resveratrol has been shown to reduce amyloid beta levels, neurotoxicity, cell death, and degeneration of the hippocampus, as well as prevent learning impairment.[230] Several studies indicate that moderate consumption of red wine, in particular, is associated with a lower incidence of dementia and Alzheimer's disease.[231] Red wine also contains many phenolic antioxidant compounds that, research suggests, impede the pathological progress of Alzheimer's disease.[232] It has also been observed that stilbenoids–derivatives of resveratrol–lower amyloid beta peptide aggregation in Alzheimer's models.[233] Resveratrol has been shown to selectively neutralize detrimental clumps of amyloid peptides while leaving benign peptides intact as well.[234]

**Grape seed extract.** Grape seed extract contains potent antioxidants called proanthocyanidins.[235] In laboratory experiments, animal neurons were treated with grape seed extract before being exposed to amyloid beta. Unlike the untreated neurons that readily accumulated free radicals and subsequently died, the cells treated with grape seed extract were significantly protected.[236] In another animal study, administering grape seed polyphenols reduced amyloid beta aggregation in the brain and slowed Alzheimer's disease–like cognitive impairment.[237]

**Magnesium.** Magnesium is involved in the functioning of NMDA-type glutamate receptors, which are integral to memory processing.[238] Studies have found that imbalance of serum magnesium levels causes cognitive impairment.[239,240] Recently, scientists have discovered that a specially formulated magnesium compound called *magnesium-L-threonate* (MgT) boosts brain levels of magnesium more efficiently than other forms of magnesium. These higher brain levels of magnesium improved synaptic signaling, which is essential for proper neuronal and cognitive function, as well as enhanced long-term learning and memory. Testing of MgT on animals showed a substantial improvement in memory, especially long-term memory.[241]

**B vitamins.** High homocysteine levels, along with low levels of B vitamins (eg, folate, vitamin B12, and vitamin B6), have been associated with Alzheimer's disease and mild cognitive impairment.[242–244]

- **Vitamin B12.** In a study evaluating levels of vitamin B12 in patients with either Alzheimer's disease or another type of dementia, researchers found that lower B12 levels were linked to greater cognitive deterioration.[245] A population-based longitudinal study of people 75 or older without dementia found that those with low levels of vitamin B12 or folate had twice the risk of developing Alzheimer's disease over a 3-year period.[246]

- **Vitamin B6.** A study found that Alzheimer's patients after age 60 consumed a significantly lower amount of vitamin B6 compared to control subjects.[247] In addition, low vitamin B6 levels were associated with elevated numbers of lesions in the brains of patients with Alzheimer's disease.[248]

- **Folate.** Folate is needed for DNA synthesis.[46] In a study including 30 subjects with Alzheimer's disease, levels of folate in cerebrospinal fluid were significantly lower in patients with late-onset Alzheimer's disease.[249] Another longitudinal analysis of people aged 70–79 years found that those with either high levels of homocysteine or low levels of folate had impaired cognitive function. The link to cognitive impairment was strongest for low folate levels, leading researchers to suggest that folate might reduce the risk of cognitive decline.[250]

- **Niacin.** A study of more than 6000 people, conducted between 1993 and 2002, found that high levels of dietary niacin (vitamin B3) protected against Alzheimer's disease. The authors researched the dietary habits of initially healthy people aged ≥65 years. As the study progressed, some participants developed Alzheimer's disease and some remained healthy. Subjects with the highest intake of niacin had a 70% reduction in risk of cognitive decline.[251]

**Vitamin D.** The wide distribution of vitamin D receptors in the brain may be evidence for vitamin D's importance in neurological function.[252] Studies show that clearance of amyloid beta across the blood–brain barrier is promoted by adequate levels of vitamin D. Animal tests showed 1.3 times greater rate of amyloid beta elimination with vitamin D supplementation, pointing to a potential preventive effect against Alzheimer's disease.[253] Among nearly 500 women followed for 7 years, those in the highest quintile (1/5th) for vitamin D intake had a more than *75% reduction* in risk of developing Alzheimer's disease compared to those in the lowest quintile.[254]

**Coenzyme Q10.** Coenzyme Q10 (CoQ10) has been found to improve outcomes in several neurodegenerative disorders involving loss of mitochondrial function.[255,256]

Studies have shown that levels of CoQ10 are altered in Alzheimer's disease,[257] and supplementation has been suggested as part of an integrated approach to improve mitochondrial function in Alzheimer's disease.[258]

In one animal study, CoQ10 counteracted mitochondrial deficiencies in rats that had been treated with amyloid beta,[259] while in another experiment CoQ10 reduced the overproduction of amyloid beta.[260] Coenzyme Q10 was also shown to destabilize amyloid plaques in laboratory studies.[261]

Several clinical trials have evaluated the effects of synthetic CoQ10 analogs in Alzheimer's patients and shown good results. For example, a trial comparing tacrine, a pharmaceutical acetylcholinesterase inhibitor, to a CoQ10 analog among 203 Alzheimer's patients showed the CoQ10 analog was associated greater improvements on some standardized cognitive assessments.[262] Another trial revealed dose-dependent improvements on cognitive assessments in Alzheimer's patients receiving a CoQ10 analog compared to placebo. This trial also showed the CoQ10 analog to be safe and well tolerated.[263] Similarly, in a trial conducted on 102 Alzheimer's patients, a CoQ10 analog improved memory, attention, and behavior compared to placebo.[264]

**N-acetylcysteine.** N-acetylcysteine (NAC) is a precursor to glutathione, a powerful scavenger of free radicals in the body.[265,266] Glutathione deficiency has been associated with a number of neurodegenerative diseases.[267] One study showed that NAC significantly increased glutathione levels and reduced oxidative stress in rodents treated with a known free radical–producing agent.[267] Another study showed that glutathione-deficient mice were more vulnerable to neuronal damage from amyloid beta.[268] An animal model of Alzheimer's found that NAC alleviated oxidative damage and cognitive decline.[269]

**Ashwagandha.** Ashwagandha or *Withania somnifera* is a plant used in India to treat a wide range of age-related disorders.[270] A 2012 study using an animal model of Alzheimer's disease found that ashwagandha reversed accumulation of amyloid peptides and improved behavioral deficits.[271] Laboratory studies have shown that ashwagandha can regenerate neurites (ie, projections from nerve cells) and reconstruct synapses in severely damaged neurons.[272] In addition to its neuroprotective benefits, ashwagandha has been shown to mimic the action of the Alzheimer's drug donepezil, an acetylcholinesterase inhibitor.[273]

**Blueberry extract.** In 2005, scientists noted that the polyphenols present in blueberries reversed the cognitive and motor deficits caused by aging.[274] Blueberry extract stimulates neurogenesis and enhances neuronal plasticity (adaptability) in the hippocampus, the region of the brain chiefly affected by Alzheimer's disease.[275] In one study where researchers analyzed fruits and vegetables for their antioxidant capability, blueberries came out on top, scoring highest for its capacity to neutralize free radicals.[276]

**Luteolin.** Luteolin, a flavonoid found in fruits and vegetables (eg, green peppers, carrots, and celery), exhibited a protective effect against Alzheimer's disease in early research. When luteolin was administered to mice with Alzheimer's disease, there was a significant reduction in levels of amyloid beta. These mice also exhibited a reduction in the activity of glycogen synthase kinase 3, an enzyme that has been implicated in the development of amyloid beta and neurofibrillary tangles.[277]

**Multinutrient combinations.** Multinutrient deficiencies have been observed in people with Alzheimer's disease.[278,279] Recently, scientists found that individuals with higher serum levels of the biomarkers for vitamins B, C, D, and E, as well as for omega-3 oils most commonly found in fish–EPA and DHA–were less likely to exhibit brain shrinkage or reduced cognitive function.[280]

A human study of 14 individuals with early-stage Alzheimer's found that a formulation of multiple nutrients improved all measures of cognition, although the improvement in memory function was not statistically significant. The formulation comprised 400 mcg of folic acid, 6 mcg of vitamin B12, 30 IU of vitamin E, 400 mg of S-adenosylmethionine (SAM-e), 600 mg of N-acetylcysteine, and 500 mg of acetyl-l-carnitine. The cognitive improvement continued throughout the 12-month study.[281] In a study of 200 healthy middle-aged individuals with no cognitive or memory problems, those who were given a multivitamin for 2 months scored higher on cognitive function tests, showed less fatigue during extended cognitive challenges, achieved greater accuracy, and proved faster in mathematical processing, compared with the placebo-only group.[282]

## Life Extension Suggestions

**Nutritional Interventions Studied in Alzheimer's**
- **Huperzine A:** 200–800 mcg daily
- **R-lipoic acid:** 240–480 mg daily
- **Acetyl-L-carnitine:** 1000–3000 mg daily
- **Panax ginseng:** 400–1000 mg daily
- **Vitamin C:** 1000–2000 mg daily
- **Vitamin E:** 400 IU daily with at least 200 mg gamma-tocopherol
- **Ginkgo biloba,** standardized extract: 120 mg daily
- **Curcumin,** as highly absorbed BCM-95®: 400–800 mg daily

**Nutritional Interventions Studied in Cognitive Decline**
- **Fish oil,** with olive polyphenols: providing 1400 mg EPA and 1000 mg DHA daily
- **Vinpocetine:** 10–30 mg daily
  **Pyrroloquinoline quinone** (PQQ): 10–20 mg daily
- **Phosphatidylserine:** 100 mg daily

**Hormonal Support**
- **Pregnenolone:** 50–100 mg daily (depending on blood test results)
- **DHEA:** 15–25 mg daily for women; 25–75 mg daily for men (depending on blood test results)
- **Melatonin:** 0.3–5 mg before bed (sometimes up to 10 mg)
- **Testosterone replacement** in men to boost free testosterone levels to between 20–25 pg/mL
- **Estrogen and progesterone replacement** in women to increase blood levels to youthful ranges

**Additional Support**

- **Green coffee extract,** standardized to 50% chlorogenic acid: 400–1200 mg daily
- **Green tea extract,** standardized to 98% polyphenols: 725–1450 mg daily
- **Resveratrol:** 250 mg daily
- **Whole grape extract:** 150 mg daily
- **Magnesium:** 140 mg daily as magnesium-L-threonate and at least 100 mg daily as magnesium citrate
- **Vitamin B12:** 1000–5000 mcg daily
- **Vitamin B6:** 250 mg daily
- **Folate** (preferably as L-methylfolate): 400–1000 mcg daily
- **Niacin:** 50–600 mg daily

- **Vitamin D:** 5000–8000 IU daily; optimal blood levels of 25-OH-vitamin D are 50–80 ng/mL
- **Coenzyme Q10,** as ubiquinol: 100–300 mg daily
- **N-acetyl-cysteine (NAC):** 600–1800 mg daily
- **Ashwagandha extract:** 250 mg daily
- **Blueberry extract:** 375–750 mg daily
- **Luteolin:** 8 mg daily
- **S-adenosylmethionine** (SAMe): 200–1200 mg daily in divided doses

## REFERENCES

References available at: www.lef.org/dpt5/ch7

8

# Amnesia

Amnesia occurs when the portion of the brain responsible for retrieving stored memories is somehow compromised. This region of the brain is known as the limbic system, and it comprises the hippocampus, amygdala, and portions of the cortex. Besides retrieving memory, the limbic system is responsible for coordination of emotion and motivation, as well as some functions of the endocrine system.

People are amnesiac when the memory retrieval portion of the limbic system is not working properly, but there is otherwise no change in language, attention span, visual/spatial functioning, or motivation.

Memories are not actually stored in the limbic system or hippocampus. Rather, several areas of the brain are involved in memory; the type of information being assimilated determines where it is stored. For example, visual and auditory patterns are stored in the temporal lobe, whereas the parietal lobe stores language, speech, word usage, and comprehension.

## FORMS OF AMNESIA: DIFFERENT WAYS TO FORGET

There are 2 types of memory. Short-term or "working" memory stores information one needs to remember in the next few seconds, minutes, or hours (eg, a telephone number or driving directions). Long-term memory includes relational and procedural memory. Relational memory is concerned with relationships among objects and depends on the hippocampus. In amnesia, both relational and short-term memory may be impaired. Procedural memory represents memory for single objects or tasks (eg, riding a bicycle) and depends on cortical processors that remain intact in amnesia. This helps explain why amnesiacs often remember basic skills and motor function.

There are several forms of amnesia:

### Anterograde Amnesia

Anterograde amnesia, the most common, is characterized by the inability to store, retain, or recall new knowledge after the event that triggers the onset of amnesia. Patients in this state often cannot remember what they ate for their last meal or events from the immediate past. They may fill gaps in their memory with fabricated events (confabulation). This is the type of amnesia seen in dementia and Alzheimer's disease.

### Retrograde Amnesia

Retrograde amnesia is the loss of memories of events that occurred before the onset of amnesia. This is the form of amnesia most people think of when they hear the word amnesia. It often occurs after a head injury.

### Transient Global Amnesia

Transient global amnesia is a temporary loss of all memory, especially the ability to form new memories, with milder loss of past memories, going back several hours. This form is rare and seen mostly in older people. It usually dissipates within 24–48 hours. Transient global amnesia may be caused by migraine, small seizure(s) in the temporal lobe, or transient ischemic attack. Patients with this condition may become disoriented and repeatedly ask who they are, where they are, and what they are doing. Because this form of amnesia typically resolves on its own and only rarely recurs, there is no recommended treatment.

## CAUSES OF AMNESIA

There are many possible causes of amnesia. The most common include Alzheimer's disease, traumatic brain injury (head trauma), brain infection (such as encephalitis or meningitis), dementia, seizure(s), and stroke. Less common causes include a brain tumor or psychiatric disorder (eg, schizophrenia, depression, criminal behavior, or psychogenic amnesia). Psychogenic amnesia usually happens in close association with a stressful event that involves serious threat to life or health. Criminals frequently present with amnesia: reports indicate that 23–65% of murderers claim amnesia for their crimes.[1]

Amnesia can occur because of brain damage that interferes with memory storage, retrieval, or consolidation. What ultimately causes the memory loss—a failure to store memories or a failure to retrieve them—remains unclear. However, a study using rats suggested that memory loss is probably due to an error in memory retrieval, which explains why amnesiacs can usually recover their memories.[2]

Amnesia is also a symptom of Wernicke-Korsakoff syndrome. Wernicke-Korsakoff is caused by a severe thiamine (vitamin B1) deficiency due to chronic alcoholism or malnourishment. Thiamine is necessary for the body to process carbohydrates. Besides amnesia, symptoms of Wernicke-Korsakoff include confusion, loss of balance, drowsiness, and problems with vision (eg, double vision or rapid movement of the eye). In severe cases, memory loss may be accompanied by agitation and dementia. The standard treatment is intravenous thiamine, administered as soon as possible after symptoms become apparent. This therapy does not correct the condition, however, and recovery may be gradual and incomplete.

Drugs can lead to amnesia. These include recreational drugs such as cocaine, LSD, PCP, and mescaline. Several prescription medications, including aminophylline, barbiturates, bromide, digoxin, diuretics, isoniazid, methyldopa, and tricyclic antidepressants can also cause transient amnesia.[3] Any drug-related impairment is usually resolved once the drug is discontinued.

# NUTRITIONALLY SUPPORTING A HEALTHY MEMORY

Any neurologic disorder represents a challenge, not only for the patient and their family, but also for the treating physician. Patients with amnesia may be occasionally disoriented, and their symptoms may strongly resemble psychiatric disorders.[4] If amnesia is caused by an underlying condition such as Alzheimer's or dementia, physicians may prescribe drugs for that condition. Patients with these conditions are encouraged to read our Alzheimer's disease protocol for more detailed information.

Life Extension's approach to amnesia is based on the assumption that taking supplements shown to boost memory and brain function will help the amnesia. It is important to visit a physician if amnesia is present because amnesia usually occurs as a result of another condition. In most cases, the supplements discussed in this chapter have not been studied specifically for amnesia, rather researched more generally for their ability to enhance cognitive function, memory retention and recall, especially in the context of dementia and Alzheimer's disease.

There are several herbs, vitamins, and supplements that may help boost memory and provide support for the brain. These work through various mechanisms: enhancing cerebral blood flow, increasing neurotransmitter levels, reducing free radicals, and restoring cell membrane fluidity.

## Glyceryl Phosphoryl Choline

Glyceryl phosphoryl choline (GPC) is a form of choline that is naturally present in all the body's cells. Among aging adults, the rationale for GPC therapy goes back to the hypothesis developed more than 30 years ago that declining levels of acetylcholine, and a concurrent decrease in the number of neurons that are its intended target, are responsible for a range of cognitive deficits.[5] Acetylcholine is an essential neurotransmitter involved in muscle control, sleep, and cognition. By boosting acetylcholine levels in the brain, the hypothesis proposes, it may be possible to reverse cognitive deficits.[6]

Early clinical trials with GPC used daily dosages of 1200 mg. After an initial 2–4 weeks at this dose, some people reduced their dose to 600 mg daily. A daily dose of 300 mg may be appropriate for healthy young people.

## Ashwagandha

Ashwagandha is a medicinal plant used in India to treat a wide range of age-related disorders.[7–17] Its most remarkable effect may involve its ability to preserve the health of the aging brain.

## Phosphatidylserine

Phosphatidylserine is essential for brain health because it helps the brain use its fuel. By boosting glucose metabolism and stimulating production of acetylcholine, supplemental phosphatidylserine has been shown to improve the condition of patients experiencing age-associated memory impairment or cognitive decline.[18–22]

## Blueberries

Polyphenols are plant molecules with a remarkable array of characteristics, notably their potent antioxidant capabilities;[23] people with a high consumption of these molecules have lower rates of neurodegenerative disorders including Alzheimer's disease.[24] Blueberry polyphenol molecules can cross the vital blood-brain barrier, exerting their potent neuroprotection directly within the brain.[25]

Tufts University researchers have long pursued sources of antioxidant polyphenols as a means of preventing changes associated with the aging brain.[26,27] In 1999 they demonstrated that blueberries are potent sources of these neuroprotective polyphenols, improving rats' performance on a host of cognitive tasks, as well as enhancing the release of vital neurotransmitters from aged brain cells.[28]

In late 2008 neuroscientists at the University of South Florida discovered that blueberry extracts prevent the final steps in the formation of dangerous amyloid-beta proteins in Alzheimer's disease. They concluded that these findings could explain the recovery seen in supplemented animals and that supplementation could tip the scales away from formation of these destructive proteins in those at risk for Alzheimer's disease.[29]

## Grape Seed Extract

Molecules found in natural grape seed extracts include potent effectors like proanthocyanidins. The potent antioxidant activity of grape seed extract may be responsible for its reported neuroprotective effects, as observed in animal models of Alzheimer's disease.[30,31]

Recent research indicates that grape seed extract may play a specific role in protecting the brain by preventing the kind of neuronal toxicity experienced by patients with Alzheimer's disease. Korean scientists pretreated rat brain cells with grape seed extract in the laboratory before exposing the cells to amyloid-beta (amyloid-β), a toxic protein implicated in the formation of senile plaques in the brains of Alzheimer's patients. Untreated cells exposed to amyloid-β accumulated damaging reactive oxygen species (ROS) (free radicals) and underwent programmed cell death. However, the rat brain cells pretreated with grape seed extract were protected from the toxic effects of amyloid-β.[32]

Additionally, grape seed extract appears to protect rat brain cells and maintain the overall viability of the nervous system. Grape seed exerts these effects by modulating proteins implicated in cognitive disorders.[33]

## Pregnenolone and DHEA

Many studies have shown that hormone levels in the brain are closely tied to cognitive function and memory. Pregnenolone, the "master" sex hormone, is the first hormone in the cascade. It is derived from cholesterol. In the body, pregnenolone is converted into other important hormones, including dehydroepiandrosterone (DHEA), estrogens, progesterone, and testosterone.[34] Aging causes a sharp decline in pregnenolone production, and levels of the hormones for which it is a precursor tend to decline with age as well.[35–37]

DHEA levels have also been shown to decline with age, and patients with cognitive disorders such as Alzheimer's experience a steep decline in DHEA.[38] Like pregnenolone, DHEA is a neuroactive steroid that can help regulate brain function.[39] Animal studies have shown that DHEA interacts with amnesiac mice by stimulating the sigma-1 receptor in the brain, which is involved in memory. Other animal studies have shown that DHEA

improved short-term and long-term memory in a variety of amnesia models.[40]

## Fish Oil

One of the major building blocks of the brain, the omega-3 fatty acid docosahexaenoic acid (DHA) is critical for optimal brain health and function at all ages of life. Researchers are now finding that DHA provides brain-boosting benefits in aging adults.

A number of studies have shown that higher intakes of omega-3 oils significantly reduce the incidence of Alzheimer's disease as well as vascular dementia, and improve quality of life and memory in those affected by dementia.[41]

A study published in the Archives of Neurology examined 899 men and women over an average of more than 9 years to determine whether DHA had a protective effect against Alzheimer's and other forms of dementia.[42] Subjects with the highest DHA levels in their bloodstream had a marked 47% lower risk of developing all-cause dementia, and a modestly reduced risk of developing Alzheimer's disease.

Omega-3 fatty acids may also benefit those already suffering impaired cognitive function. In a study of the effects of DHA and EPA supplementation in patients with mild to moderate Alzheimer's disease who were undergoing pharmaceutical therapy, 6 or more months of omega-3 supplementation slowed the rate of cognitive decline in those with very mild Alzheimer's disease.[43]

## Coenzyme Q10 and Pyrroloquinoline Quinone

The decay of mitochondria in brain cells is a primary cause of all neurodegenerative disorders.[44,45] This deadly process begins when free radicals inflict damage to nerve cells.

Scientists believe that coenzyme Q10 (CoQ10) may hold promise in preventing or managing neurological conditions related to impaired energy production and oxidative stress, such as Huntington's disease, Friedrich's ataxia, amyotrophic lateral sclerosis (ALS), and Alzheimer's disease.[46,47] While research in these areas is still in the preliminary stages, CoQ10's ability to enhance energy production and quench oxidative stress may eventually help aging adults fend off a host of neurodegenerative disorders.

The critical role of pyrroloquinoline quinone (PQQ) across a range of biological functions has only gradually emerged. Like CoQ10, it is a micronutrient whose antioxidant capacity provides extraordinary defense against mitochondrial decay.

PQQ potently blunts the deadly effects of reactive oxygen species (ROS) in brain tissue, thereby helping to keep existing mitochondria intact.[48,49] There is strong evidence that PQQ also scavenges existing ROS,[50,51] which offers further promise in reducing the oxidant load on brain mitochondria. PQQ also stimulates the brain to produce healthy new mitochondria in a process known as mitochondrial biogenesis.[52]

Recent studies from Japan, where PQQ science is most advanced, show that a PQQ-supplemented diet improves learning ability in healthy animals.[53] When the animals were subjected to 48 hours of extreme oxidant stress to mimic accelerated aging, the PQQ-supplemented group showed better memory function than the control group, and that improvement was sustained long after the stress.

In humans, supplementation with 20 mg daily of PQQ resulted in improvements on tests of higher cognitive function in a group of middle-aged and elderly people.[54] These effects were significantly amplified when the subjects also took 300 mg daily of CoQ10.

## Acetyl-L-Carnitine

Acetyl-L-carnitine boosts the conversion of fats into energy in the mitochondria, helping to ensure that a plentiful energy supply is available for biochemical processes throughout the body. Because the brain requires abundant energy, this nutrient is especially crucial for peak brain energy and function.

Acetyl-L-carnitine alone is known to be neuroprotective, reducing the rate of nerve cell death in cultured cells exposed to some of the neurotoxic agents that are important in the development of Alzheimer's disease.[55] Studies of Alzheimer's patients have reported improvements in memory compared to patients receiving placebo.[56] Other studies have investigated the effectiveness of adding acetyl-L-carnitine to standard pharmaceutical treatments for Alzheimer's disease.

In a recent Italian study, Alzheimer's patients in the early phases of the disease took 2 g of acetyl-L-carnitine daily for 3 months. Response rates, as determined by a variety of functional and behavioral parameters, improved from 38% with standard acetylcholinesterase inhibitor drugs (such as Aricept®) alone to 50% with the addition of acetyl-L-carnitine.[57] Another placebo-controlled, double-blind study conducted at Stanford University concluded, "Acetyl-L-carnitine slows the progression of Alzheimer's disease in younger subjects."[58]

## Ginkgo Biloba

Ginkgo biloba leaf extract is the most widely sold phytomedicine in Europe, with 5 million prescriptions written in Germany alone every year for dementia. It has been used in Chinese medicine for thousands of years to treat respiratory ailments, improve circulation, aid digestion, and combat memory loss in the elderly.

In the United States, ginkgo is mostly used to aid mental acuity and memory, as well as an antioxidant. A review of 8 randomized studies demonstrated that ginkgo has modest effects on symptoms of dementia, including memory loss.[59] Another analysis of 50 articles examined the effect of ginkgo on cognitive function in patients with Alzheimer's. Four of the studies met criteria for adequate clinical trial design. Each study showed that Alzheimer's patients who received ginkgo experienced 10–20% improvement in standardized tests of attention, short-term memory, and reaction time compared to patients who took placebo. The reviewer reported that ginkgo's effects were comparable to the benefits of donepezil (Aricept®).[60] An analysis of 33 trials concluded that ginkgo appears safe and shows promising evidence of offering improvement in cognition and function.

## Vinpocetine

Vinpocetine (vinpocetine-ethyl apovincaminate) is a synthetic compound extracted from the seeds of the periwinkle plant (*Vinca minor*). It has been used widely in Hungary, Poland, and Germany for cerebral-related pathologies, and became available in the United States in 1998 as an herbal supplement. It has several pharmacological properties, including antioxidant, vasodilator, and neuroprotective benefits. Animal studies have shown that it crosses the blood-brain barrier and is absorbed by cerebral tissue.[61]

Vinpocetine is an effective scavenger of hydroxyl radicals,[62] and has been shown to inhibit lipid peroxidation in mouse brain tissue. It leads to enhanced cerebral circulation and decreased platelet aggregation.[63] It has also been found to have antioxidant properties comparable to vitamin E.[64]

A double-blind study testing vinpocetine's effect on short-term memory in 12 healthy women showed that those who took 40 mg 3 times daily for 2 days scored about 30% higher on short-term memory tests than the placebo group.[65] Another study demonstrated the effects of 30–60 mg of vinpocetine daily in patients with mild to moderate dementia. After 16 weeks, 21% of the treatment group reported their symptoms subsided, compared with 7% of the placebo group.[66]

A meta-analysis of 6 randomized, controlled trials involving 731 patients with degenerative cerebral dysfunction showed that vinpocetine was highly effective on cognitive and motor function.[67]

Memory endurance can be measured in the laboratory by the presence of electrical potentials. In lesioned brains of rats, reduced long-term memory was restored by vinpocetine as measured by the normalization of electrical potentials.[68]

## Huperzine A

Derived from the leaves of the Chinese club moss *Huperzia serrata*, huperzine A demonstrates beneficial characteristics similar to those of ginkgo. It acts like an antioxidant and has neuroprotective properties, including the ability to inhibit the breakdown of acetylcholine, an important neurotransmitter. Most of the studies examining huperzine A have been conducted in Alzheimer's patients.

Huperzine A has been shown to increase acetylcholine levels in rat brains. It also increases norepinephrine and dopamine. Several Chinese studies suggest that this herb may be as effective as tacrine and donepezil (medications which treat Alzheimer's disease) against Alzheimer's disease. A study in China[69] demonstrated a connection between huperzine A and improved cognitive function in dementia patients. Another study involved 50 Alzheimer's patients given huperzine A or placebo for 8 weeks. Significant improvement was reported in 58% of patients treated with huperzine A in terms of memory, cognitive and behavioral functions; only 36% of those taking placebo improved. No adverse side effects were reported.[70]

Clinical efficacy and safety of huperzine A in treatment of mild to moderate Alzheimer's was conducted in a randomized, placebo-controlled trial in China.[71] This study included 202 patients from various centers. One group received 400 mcg/day of huperzine A, and the other group received placebo. Seventy percent of the huperzine A group showed improvement in cognition, behavior, mood, and activities of daily life versus only 36% in the placebo group.

A study in rats[72] compared the effects of huperzine A, donepezil, and rivastigmine (current drugs for treating Alzheimer's) on cortical acetylcholine levels. Results showed that huperzine A was 8-fold more potent than donepezil and twice as potent as rivastigmine in increasing cortical acetylcholine levels with a longer lasting effect than either of them.

## Vitamins and Antioxidants

**Magnesium-L-threonate.** Researchers have found that a new, highly absorbable form of magnesium called magnesium-L-threonate concentrates more efficiently in the brain, rebuilds ruptured synapses, and restores the degraded neuronal connections observed in Alzheimer's disease and other forms of memory loss. In one study, just 24 days of oral supplementation with magnesium-L-threonate produced an increase in cerebrospinal magnesium sufficient to boost short- and long-term memory scores. Other forms of magnesium (such as magnesium chloride, magnesium citrate, magnesium glycinate, and magnesium gluconate) did not significantly elevate brain magnesium compared to the control group[73,74]

Another test on aging animals (rats) that had suffered memory decline showed that magnesium-L-threonate could reverse the kind of cognitive dysfunction that occurs in normal aging humans. The animals had magnesium-L-threonate added to their drinking water for 1 month. The findings showed an 18% improvement in short-term memory for those animals treated with magnesium-L-threonate. In a validated test for long-term memory, these same animals supplemented with magnesium-L-threonate exhibited 100% enhanced performance.[73]

**Vitamin E and vitamin C.** Vitamin E is lipid-soluble and interacts with cell membranes, traps free radicals, and disrupts the pathway that leads to cell damage.[75] It has also demonstrated (in animal models) the ability to reduce degeneration of hippocampal cells after cerebral ischemia.[76]

One study examined the effect of vitamins E and C on older women's performance on cognitive tests. Dietary information was collected from women older than age 70 who were not diagnosed with stroke. A total of 22 213 women were interviewed. Long-term, current users of vitamins E and C had significantly better performance than women who never used vitamin E or C. Higher mean scores were seen with increasing duration of use. Benefits were less consistent for women taking vitamin E alone. The researchers concluded that the specific use of vitamin E supplements, especially when combined with vitamin C, may be beneficial in maintaining cognitive function during later adult years.[77]

**Vitamins B1 and B12.** Vitamin B1 (thiamine) is water-soluble and necessary for the metabolism of proteins, carbohydrates, and fats. It has been shown to mimic acetylcholine in the brain,[78] which may account for its possible effects in Alzheimer's and other dementias.[79,80] Thiamine is also involved in nerve transmissions within cholinergic neurons, which are known to deteriorate in Alzheimer's disease.

A 1-year study involved 127 young adults given 15 mg thiamine with other B vitamins at dosages 10 times the recommended daily allowance. The most significant effect was enhanced cognitive function in women.[80] Another study involved 80 elderly women given 10 mg of thiamine daily for 10 weeks. Compared to the placebo group, those who took thiamine had significant increases in appetite, activity levels, energy intake, and general well-being, as well as improved sleep patterns and decreased fatigue.[81]

Symptoms of thiamine deficiency are varied and include memory loss, depression, weakness, insomnia, back pain, myalgia, weight loss, hypothermia, constipation, pain sensitivity, and dyspnea. It also manifests as Wernicke-Korsakoff syndrome, mentioned earlier.

Researchers have pursued the possible connection between B12 deficiency and dementia.[82] A review examined correlations between cognitive skills, homocysteine levels, and blood levels of folate, B6, and B12. The authors suggested that B12 deficiency might decrease levels of substances required for the metabolism of neurotransmitters.[83]

## Piracetam

Although not approved by the Food and Drug Administration (FDA) for use in the United States, piracetam is prescribed in Europe to treat amnesia, dementia, stroke, dyslexia, senility, and other cognitive problems. Developed more than 30 years ago by a Belgian company (UCB Laboratories), it is a derivative of the neurotransmitter gamma-aminobutyric acid and has been shown to restore cell membrane fluidity. At the neuronal level, it modulates neurotransmission and has neuroprotective and anticonvulsant properties.[84] One of its most interesting effects is the ability to promote the flow of information (via increased blood flow) between the right and left hemispheres of the brain in rats.[85] This may also account for piracetam's usefulness in treating dyslexia.[86]

One study suggests that piracetam may increase cholinergic receptors in the brain. Older mice were given piracetam for 2 weeks, and the density of muscarinic cholinergic receptors in the frontal cortex was measured. The older mice had 30–40% higher density of these receptors than before taking the drug.[87] Whether piracetam is beneficial for dementia or cognitive impairment has yet to be determined.[88] However, one study using high doses (8 g/day) demonstrated that piracetam might slow the progression of cognitive deterioration of Alzheimer's disease. It seemed to improve recent incident and remote memory.[89] For more information on piracetam, visit www.piracetam.info.

## Life Extension Suggestions

Life Extension's suggestions are based on the assumption that supplements have beneficial effects on cognitive function and memory. Supplements that have been shown to boost memory and brain function include the following:

- **Magnesium-L-threonate:** 6000 mg daily
- **Coenzyme Q10** (CoQ10) (ubiquinol form): 300 mg daily
- **Pyrroloquinoline quinone** (PQQ): 20 mg daily
- **Fish oil:** 2–6 g daily (minimum of 1400 mg EPA and 1000 mg of DHA)
- **Acetyl-L-carnitine:** 1500–3000 mg daily
- **Alpha-glyceryl phosphoryl choline** (A-GPC): 600 mg daily
- **Phosphatidylserine:** 100 mg daily
- **Pregnenolone:** 50 mg daily
- **Vinpocetine:** 20 mg daily
- **Grape seed** (procyanidin extract): 50 mg daily
- **Ashwagandha:** 125 mg daily
- **DHEA:** 15–75 mg daily, followed by blood testing after 3–6 weeks to ensure that youthful levels of this vital hormone are being maintained
- **Ginkgo biloba:** 120 mg daily
- **Huperzine A:** 50 mcg daily
- **Vitamin E:** 400 IU daily
- **Vitamin C:** 500–1000 mg daily
- **B-complex vitamins** containing:
  - **Thiamin,** 100 mg
  - **Riboflavin,** 50 mg
  - **Niacin,** 200 mg
  - **Vitamin B6,** 75 mg
  - **Folic acid,** 800 mcg
  - **Vitamin B12,** 1000 mcg
  - **Biotin,** 600 mcg
  - **Pantothenic acid,** 1000 mg
  - **Betaine free base,** 50 mg
  - **Choline,** 45 mg
  - **Inositol,** 250 mg
  - **Para-aminobenzoic acid,** 100 mg

In addition, the following blood testing resources may be helpful:

- Female Comprehensive Hormone Panel or Male Comprehensive Hormone Panel
- Omega Score®
- CoQ10 (coenzyme Q10)

## REFERENCES

References available at: www.lef.org/dpt5/ch8

# 9

# Amyotrophic Lateral Sclerosis (Lou Gehrig's Disease)

Amyotrophic lateral sclerosis (ALS) is a degenerative neuromuscular disease, also called Lou Gehrig's disease after the famous baseball player who died from this condition. ALS affects the nervous system and destroys motor neurons (nerve cells that help control movement) while sparing the abilities to see, hear, feel, touch, and taste. ALS is characterized by progressive dysfunction resulting in symptoms such as tripping, clumsiness, difficulty talking, slurred speech, muscle cramps, twitching, and ultimately, paralysis. The most common cause of death among ALS patients is respiratory failure, which occurs when nerve damage eventually affects the muscles that control breathing. The average survival time after being diagnosed with ALS is 3–5 years.[1]

There are 2 main forms of ALS: sporadic and familial. The sporadic form comprises 90% of all ALS cases. However, many scientists study the familial forms in order to try to understand the mechanisms of the disease. While familial ALS is typically caused by mutations in different genes (including a gene known as SOD1), researchers still do not completely understand the pathogenesis of sporadic ALS. Scientists are pursuing a number of theories including oxidative stress, glutamate toxicity, and mitochondrial dysfunction.[2–4] Other possible risk factors include viral infections[5] and environmental toxins.[6] The current consensus is that many factors may converge to cause the motor neuron damage typified by ALS.[4]

Conventional medicine, which has fared poorly in the treatment of ALS, attempts to lessen symptoms by slowing disease progression. Currently, the only drug approved by the Food and Drug Administration (FDA) for ALS patients is riluzole. Unfortunately, it has been shown to extend human life span by only 2–3 months.[7] By adding scientifically studied natural interventions to conventional therapies, one may be able to target pathogenic mechanisms of ALS from multiple angles in hopes of slowing disease progression and improving quality of life.

## POSSIBLE CAUSES OF ALS

### Superoxide Dismutase

Because SOD1 gene mutations can cause familial ALS, many researchers have studied this protein to determine how it plays a role in the death of motor neurons. SOD1 is a gene that codes for superoxide dismutase (SOD), an enzyme that helps convert superoxide radicals into less harmful molecules. Superoxide molecules are a form of free radical or reactive oxygen species, a class of molecules that can damage the DNA, proteins, and membranes of cells, causing them to die.[4] If SOD is either functioning poorly or is present in inadequate quantities, rampant oxidative stress driven by unabated superoxide molecules can damage tissue and contribute to disease.

Approximately 20% of familial cases and 2% of all ALS cases are linked to SOD1 gene mutations.[8–10] This suggests that the accumulation of superoxide molecules and other free radicals could contribute to ALS. In addition to increasing superoxide levels, SOD1 mutations can damage neurons in other ways. For example, mutant SOD1 produces abnormal SOD molecules, which are theorized to serve as the seed for large clusters of misfolded proteins that are toxic to neurons.[11,12]

### Oxidative Stress

Studies have found elevated levels of oxidative stress within the central nervous system as well as peripherally in ALS.[13–16] This suggests that motor neuron death in ALS is related to increased levels of reactive oxygen species. These conditions contribute to the neuronal death and muscle wasting common in ALS. Oxidative stress can be relieved by increasing the concentration of antioxidants such as beta-carotene,[17] vitamin C,[18] and vitamin E,[19] as well as the mineral selenium.[20] Many other supplements, such as coenzyme Q10, also have antioxidant properties.

### Glutamate Toxicity

Glutamate is an important neurotransmitter. Under normal conditions, its concentrations are tightly regulated. However, it appears the system regulating glutamate concentration in patients with ALS may be disturbed,[21] resulting in an accumulation of glutamate in the space (synapse) between cells.[22] This excess glutamate may excite nerve cells beyond their capacity resulting in nerve cell death. Patients with ALS have elevated levels of glutamate in their cerebrospinal fluid, support this hypothesis.[23,24] Mutant glutamate transport proteins are also associated with sporadic forms of ALS, further supporting the idea that elevated levels of glutamate-mediated excitation can kill motor neurons in ALS patients.[25–27] Some of the most powerful evidence supporting the critical role that glutamate plays in the pathology of ALS is the effectiveness of the medication riluzole, which inhibits glutamate's effects on the nervous system. It modulates the release of glutamate, thereby improving survival for ALS patients. Its effect, however, is modest, suggesting that excess glutamate is not the sole cause of the disease.

## Mitochondrial Dysfunction

The mitochondria provide energy for all cells, including neurons. Unfortunately, mitochondria also produce reactive oxygen species as a byproduct of energy generation. Mitochondrial dysfunction can result in the production of excessive amounts of superoxide, causing extensive cell damage and death. Accumulation of superoxide is prevented by SOD and other enzymes.[28]

There are a number of ways in which the mitochondria in motor neurons may become impaired in ALS.[29] In animal models of ALS, dysfunction of mitochondria in motor neurons occurs before any other observable pathologic changes, suggesting this is an early event in the progression of the disease.[30] Mutant forms of SOD appear to lead to mitochondrial dysfunction.[31] Studies of both human and animal neurons have found extensive mitochondrial dysfunction associated with ALS.[32–37] In addition, some patients with ALS appear to have impaired mitochondrial function in their muscle fibers.[38]

Animal models of ALS show abnormal transport of mitochondria in their motor neurons, which could further contribute to the progression of the disease.[39] Additionally, because proper mitochondrial function is so essential, other yet unidentified processes could be altered when mitochondrial health is impaired.[40] Along these lines, an emerging theory linking excitotoxicity and mitochondrial dysfunction suggests that an accumulation of lactate, a metabolic byproduct that is toxic (especially to nerve cells) at high concentrations may play a role in ALS progression.[41] This theory (also known as the *lactate dyscrasia* theory) proposes that mitochondrial dysfunction partly contributes to an accumulation of lactate in the junction of motor neurons and muscle cells (the neuromuscular junction [NMJ]) leading to death of both the nerve and muscle cells, thereby requiring the remaining muscle cells to work harder than normal to generate the force necessary for motor control. However, since lactate is a metabolic byproduct

and greater metabolic demand increases lactate production, the remaining muscle cells produce even more lactate than usual due to their increased workload, hastening the accumulation of lactate and exacerbating neuronal destruction and muscular atrophy. This theory also proposes that malfunction of an as yet undiscovered lactate shuttle within the NMJ may be a pathological feature of ALS, suggesting that supporting mitochondrial function may optimize lactate metabolism and combat the toxicity caused by accumulation of excess lactate. If this theory is correct, then combining drugs that inhibit lactate accumulation such as nizofenone.[42] with nutrients that support mitochondrial function (like coenzyme Q10 and pyrroloquinoline quinone (PQQ)) might be an effective therapy for ALS.

## Heavy Metals and Environmental Agents

The role of heavy metals in ALS is highly controversial. Since clusters of ALS patients have been found in certain geographical areas, researchers have searched for an underlying environmental theme such as heavy metal poisoning. For example, researchers have found that elevated levels of lead are associated with a higher risk of ALS.[43] Another toxin which has been identified as a potential mediator for ALS is mercury, although the link between mercury and ALS risk is not as clear.[44,45] These toxins can lead to subtle cellular changes such as interfering with the methylation of DNA.[46] Other studies however have failed to show a link between ALS and any of the common heavy metals.[47]

Beta-N-methylamino-L-alanine (BMAA), a neurotoxin made by certain bacteria may play an important role in the development of ALS. BMAA may be implicated in the high incidence of ALS in Guam, where these bacteria are commonly found in the seeds of the *Cycas circinalis* plant.[48]

Exposure to pesticides may also increase the risk of developing ALS.[49] Exposure to pesticides in the grass on playing fields is one theory put forth to explain the unusually high incidence of ALS in Italian soccer players.[50]

While there is good reason to think that neurotoxic agents like these may be somehow linked to degenerative brain and nerve conditions like ALS, researchers have been unable to meet the demanding scientific standard needed to establish a causal relationship.[49,51]

# DIAGNOSIS AND CONVENTIONAL TREATMENT OF ALS

Like many neuromuscular diseases, it can be difficult to make an early diagnosis of ALS. Depending on which muscle group is affected first, its symptoms vary from person to person and can include:

- Tingling in the fingers or toes
- Cramping in the arms or legs
- Trouble with tongue and facial movements, including chewing and swallowing

As the disease progresses, it spreads through the affected limb until eventually all muscle groups become involved. This spread into all muscle groups is the defining characteristic of ALS. In fact, the term *amyotrophy* refers to the atrophy (wasting) of muscle tissue, while lateral sclerosis refers to the hardening of the spinal column from the buildup of scar tissue.[52] The diagnosis of ALS is primarily a clinical one and requires the appearance of both upper (increased tone and reflexes) and lower (fasciculations and muscle atrophy) motor neuron involvement in many segments of the body. Electromyography, nerve conduction studies, and transcranial magnetic stimulation can all be used to support the diagnosis of amyotrophic lateral sclerosis.

Riluzole, the only FDA-approved drug for the treatment of ALS, blunts the effects of glutamate by decreasing its release and blocking the ability of glutamate to bind to its receptors, thereby decreasing the excitotoxicity that leads to cell death. Albeit small, its 2- to 3-month increase in survival time[7] indicates that controlling glutamate levels in the brain could be an essential component in fighting ALS and provides valuable information toward ultimately finding a more effective treatment for the disease.[53]

The remainder of conventional medical treatment for ALS patients focuses on relieving symptoms and improving quality of life. For example, noninvasive positive pressure ventilation is often used to help patients with ALS breathe, especially at night.[54,55] Physicians frequently recommend prescription medications to relieve painful muscle cramps (eg, carbamazepine and phenytoin),[56] excessive salivation (eg, atropine, amitriptyline, hyoscyamine, and injections of botulinum toxin into the salivary glands),[57–59] and other symptoms. ALS patients are often advised to engage in moderate exercise and seek physical therapy to maintain muscle strength and function. As the disease progresses, splints, braces, and wheelchairs are used to help with mobility. Also, higher toilet seats, headrests, and specialized utensils may help improve the quality of life for ALS patients.[60] Occupational and speech therapy help patients as their motor control gradually deteriorates.

# EMERGING MEDICAL THERAPIES

## Stem Cells

Stem cells, immature cells that can differentiate into specialized adult cells, may represent the next generation of ALS therapy.

However, due to federal restrictions on stem cell therapy as well as the difficulty of designing studies, very few trials have been conducted to date on the treatment of ALS with stem cells. Those that have been conducted, however, are encouraging and early trials show great promise. Researchers have found the following:

- Bone marrow–derived "stem-cell transplantation in the motor cortex delays ALS progression and improves quality of life."[61]
- Direct injection of bone marrow derived stem cells into the frontal motor cortex (a brain region) of human ALS patients is generally safe and well tolerated.[62]

Researchers have also experimented with the use of stem cells that express beneficial growth factors as a way of comprehensively treating ALS.[63,64] This therapy offers the potential to alter the course of ALS in afflicted patients.

## TAR DNA-Binding Protein 43 (TDP-43) and FUS (Fused in Sarcoma)

Research has identified the cellular protein TDP-43 as an important factor in the cause of ALS, especially the sporadic forms.[65] TDP-43 binds DNA and RNA in cells, including motor neurons. Aggregates of TDP-43 are found in the motor neurons of patients with ALS, suggesting that they may contribute to ALS pathogenesis. Identification of TDP-43's involvement in ALS rapidly fueled a breakthrough discovery of an additional causative mutation in the gene encoding another RNA/DNA binding protein called FUS (fused in sarcoma).[66,67] Because both of these proteins have been implicated in ALS, they may represent a novel pathway by which the motor neurons are damaged. This has also opened up the potential for gene therapy, allowing researchers to try to replace defective genes with functional ones, thus slowing or reversing the loss of motor neurons associated with ALS.[68,69] Researchers are also searching for ways to inhibit TDP-43 aggregation using chemicals such as methylene blue and latrepirdine.[70]

## IGF-1 and Growth Hormone

Insulin-like growth factor-1 (IGF-1) is a potent modulator of neuronal growth and function. This neurotrophic factor has the ability to protect neurons both in the central and peripheral nervous system. Researchers have examined the possibility in cell and animal models that IGF-1 could be an effective therapeutic treatment for ALS.[71] Human studies, however, have produced mixed results. Whereas one study found some slowing of the progression of ALS in patients treated with IGF-1 injections,[72] others found that subcutaneous (under the skin) injections are not effective in ALS patients.[73] However, the lack of effect with subcutaneous injections could be due to an inability to access the central nervous system. Intraspinal cord delivery has shown promise in animal models.[74] The use of retroviruses as a potential delivery method for administering IGF-1 to ALS patients has also shown promise.[75]

Similarly, growth hormone (GH) may be related to ALS, as one trial found that ALS patients had impaired GH secretion compared to healthy controls.[76] However, the potential therapeutic value of GH replacement therapy needs further investigation as a recent clinical trial found no improvement in ALS patients receiving GH compared to placebo.[77]

## Other Treatments

- Arimoclomol is an investigational drug that improves the expression of "heat shock proteins," thereby helping prevent the accumulation of misfolded proteins. Comprehensive in vivo and in vitro studies demonstrated its effect in the prevention of neuronal loss and promotion of motor neuron survival, even after the onset of symptoms. Clinical trials have reported good safety and tolerability.[78]

- Ceftriaxone, a commonly used antibiotic, may also be able to treat ALS by improving reuptake of glutamate. When used in an animal model of ALS, ceftriaxone delayed loss of neurons and muscle strength, thus increasing survival.[79]

- Dexpramipexole is under development by Knopp Neurosciences and Biogen Idec as a potential neuroprotective therapy for ALS.[80] While it has been shown to be safe and well tolerated,[81] more research needs to be done to determine its efficacy.

- Another new medication that is currently being studied in clinical trials is TRO19622.[82] TRO19622 is a cholesterol-like molecule and displays remarkable neuroprotective properties both in vitro and in vivo. TRO19622 is expected to preserve existing neuronal function by delaying or even stopping further progression of the disease. TRO19622 has been granted orphan drug designation status for the treatment of ALS in the United States. This status allows the opportunity to seek "fast track" review by the FDA.[83]

## NUTRITIONAL INTERVENTIONS

Adequate nutrition is crucial for ALS patients. As the disease progresses, patients gradually lose the ability to chew or swallow with ease. At the same time, the abdominal and pelvic muscles weaken, oftentimes resulting in depression. Patients often lose the ability and desire to eat, making malnutrition a common problem. The recognition that aggressive nutritional intervention is paramount among ALS patients has spurred ardent research efforts aimed at elucidating the potential therapeutic value of dietary supplementation.[22]

### Vitamins and Minerals

**Vitamin B12 (methylcobalamin).** Whereas ultrahigh (25 mg daily for 4 weeks) intramuscular doses of methylcobalamin (a form of vitamin B12) have been shown to slow muscle wasting,[84] low levels of vitamin B12 have been associated with nerve damage in many different animal models. One of the main problems associated with low levels of vitamin B12 is elevated levels of methylmalonic acid (MMA), which is toxic to neurons.[85] Low levels of vitamin B12 are also associated with poorly functioning peripheral nerves, which can be exacerbated by ALS.[86] Vitamin B12 can also prevent damage to the ophthalmic nerves by reducing MMA and homocysteine levels, both being associated with oxidative damage.[87] Low levels of vitamin B12 have also been associated with neuronal degeneration in other models.[88]

**Zinc.** Mutations to the copper/zinc superoxide dismutase gene are responsible for 2–3% of ALS cases. These mutations result in the SOD enzyme having a reduced affinity for zinc.[89] In fact, the loss of zinc from SOD1 results in the remaining copper in SOD1 becoming extremely toxic to motor neurons.[90] Altering zinc levels within the brain is being studied as a method for treating many different nervous system diseases, including ALS.[91] However, a study conducted at the Linus Pauling Institute found that large doses of zinc inhibit copper absorption, which can lead to anemia. In the study, researchers added a small dose of copper to animal ALS models receiving zinc and found that the copper prevented early death associated with high doses of zinc.[89] In summary, adding a small amount of copper to the subject's diets prevented this lethal anemia, suggesting that moderate amounts of zinc supplementation combined with small amounts of copper might help prevent neuron death in ALS.

## Herbal Supplements

**Ginseng.** In an animal model of ALS, ginseng was shown to significantly delay the onset of ALS symptoms.[92] An extract from the ginseng plant called ginsenoside has also been found to increase the expression of SOD1.[93] Ginseng and its extracts may also be able to protect motor neurons from apoptosis and membrane damage, further helping to slow the progression of ALS.[94]

**Ginkgo biloba.** Ginkgo biloba has antioxidant properties.[95] Additionally, it has been shown to promote healthy mitochondrial function.[40] During an in vitro study, it was found to protect against glutamate-induced excitotoxicity.[96] Ginkgo biloba also reduced weight loss in a mouse model of ALS.[97] Ginkgo biloba extract has been shown to protect neurons from death due to oxidative stress.[98]

## Additional Support

**Coenzyme Q10.** Coenzyme Q10 (CoQ10) acts as an antioxidant and is essential for proper mitochondrial function.[99] Human studies have found that ALS patients have a higher percentage of oxidized CoQ10 (ubiquinone), a condition the researchers blamed on oxidative stress caused by the disease.[100] Supplementation with ubiquinol, the reduced (nonoxidized) form of CoQ10 may ameliorate this problem, though no studies have tested this hypothesis. Several animal studies, including the following have supported the benefit of CoQ10 treatment in ALS:

- In an animal model of familial ALS, administration of coenzyme Q10 significantly extended life span and oral administration significantly increased CoQ10 concentrations in the brains and mitochondria of the test animals.[101]

As a result of these promising studies in mice, researchers have been testing the benefits of CoQ10 on humans with ALS. One phase II study did not find any substantial benefit of CoQ10 supplementation in patients with ALS.[102] However, more research still needs to be done as CoQ10 plays an important role in mitochondrial function and controlling oxidative stress—2 key components of ALS. In addition, it has been noted that high doses of CoQ10 are generally safe.[103]

**Acetyl-L-carnitine.** Acetyl-L-carnitine has been shown to improve mitochondrial function.[104–106] It appears to increase the growth and repair of neurons.[107,108] while protecting neurons from high levels of glutamate

when combined with lipoic acid.[109] Acetyl-L-carnitine also protects neuron cell cultures from excitotoxicity, one of the putative mechanisms of disease in ALS.[110] This supplement has also been found to reduce neuromuscular degeneration and increase life span in animal models of ALS.[111] In one animal study, the effects of acetyl-L-carnitine were increased when administered in conjunction with lipoic acid.[112]

**Lipoic acid.** Lipoic acid has been shown to have antioxidant properties as well as increase intracellular levels of glutathione.[113,114] It also chelates metals both in the test tube and in animal models.[115,116] As a result, lipoic acid supplementation might protect neurons from some of the changes that lead to ALS.[117] Furthermore, lipoic acid has been shown to protect cells against glutamate-induced excitotoxicity.[118] In one study, administration of lipoic acid improved survival in a mouse model of ALS.[119]

**Protein and amino acids.** Adequate protein intake is essential for patients with amyotrophic lateral sclerosis. Protein supplementation may help improve the nutritional status of ALS patients, thereby slowing the progression of the disease. A 2010 study found that patients with ALS taking whey protein supplements had improved nutritional and functional parameters as compared to the control group.[120] Some preliminary data suggest that whey protein may also directly protect motor neurons from oxidative stress, thus delaying the progression of ALS.[121] A Portuguese study suggested that dietary supplementation with amino acids may have some beneficial effects on the course of the disease.[122]

**Creatine.** In cells, creatine aids in the formation of adenosine triphosphate (ATP), the primary source of cellular energy. In multiple animal studies, creatine has been shown to provide protection against neurodegenerative diseases. For example, it has been suggested that creatine helps to stabilize cellular membranes.[123] Creatine may also lessen the burden of the excitotoxin glutamate in the brain, thus improving survival time in animals with ALS.[124] In human ALS patients, there is evidence to suggest that creatine may improve mitochondrial function.[125] In addition, a small preliminary study found that creatine supplementation improves muscle strength in ALS patients.[126] More recent research has confirmed that creatine can protect neurons from toxic processes such as those that drive the progression of ALS. Creatine, due to its antioxidant and anti-excitotoxic properties, has been found to have a significant therapeutic effect in mouse models of ALS.[127,128] However, human studies have yielded mixed results,[129] which may be due to insufficient sample size.[127] Creatine can cross the blood–brain barrier and gain access to the brain, a treatment that lowered levels of glutamate in the cerebrospinal fluid, which may help to protect the brain.[130]

**Glutathione and N-acetyl-cysteine.** The antioxidant glutathione is naturally synthesized by the body. Increasing glutathione levels could help prevent free radical damage to cells.[131] The glutathione precursor N-acetyl-cysteine (NAC) boosts blood levels of glutathione.[132] Patients with ALS tend to have higher levels of oxidized glutathione (glutathione that has already been used to protect the body from free radicals).[133] Increased levels of glutathione can also protect neurons from degeneration in models of ALS.[134] Interestingly, cell culture models have shown that ALS is associated with reduced glutathione levels due to mitochondrial dysfunction, and that reduced glutathione levels can result in elevated levels of glutamate.[135] Along with being a glutathione precursor, NAC has antioxidant activity of its own. In animal models of ALS, NAC administration has been shown to decrease motor neuron loss, improve muscle mass, and increase survival time and motor performance.[136,137] In addition, NAC supplementation can help thin mucous secretions in the oral cavity, which may make swallowing easier.[138]

**Green tea.** Green tea contains high concentrations of catechins, flavonoids with strong antioxidant properties.[139] Green tea extract has been demonstrated to have anti-inflammatory properties as well.[140] One of these catechins known as epigallocatechin-3-gallate (EGCG) is of particular interest in the context of ALS. EGCG and other catechins may be able to protect neurons from a variety of diseases.[141] EGCG has been found to protect cultures of motor neurons from death due to excessive levels of glutamate.[142] Motor neurons can also be protected from mitochondrial dysfunction with the addition of EGCG in culture.[143] EGCG can also bind to and inactivate iron, which may help protect motor neurons from the effects of ALS.[144] Epidemiologic data further support the following role of tea in its potential protection of neurons: green tea consumption reduces the risk of neurodegenerative diseases[145] and people who drink tea may have a lower risk of developing ALS.[146]

**Pycnogenol®.** Pycnogenol® is an extract of marine pine bark that includes procyanidins and phenolic acids.[147] It has been shown to have antioxidant properties,[147] as well as protective effects against glutamate excitotoxicity.[96] Pycnogenol® is a common complementary therapy option among ALS patients.[22] In addition, Pycnogenol® increased the levels of SOD produced in an animal study.[148]

**Resveratrol.** Resveratrol is a powerful antioxidant found in red grape skins and Japanese knotweed (*Polygonum cuspidatum*). Resveratrol has been found to suppress the influx of excitatory ions into some cell types, which is associated with reduced glutamate-induced cell toxicity.[149] Another way that resveratrol may target neurodegenerative diseases is by reducing oxidative stress, both on its own and by increasing the expression of SIRT1,[150] a stress-response gene associated with longevity and protection against a number of cellular assaults. Although it is not known what role this gene plays in ALS, increasing SIRT1 expression via resveratrol administration helps protect motor neurons from ALS in cell culture.[151,152] In addition, resveratrol can increase the activity of SOD in cells and protect them from apoptosis and oxidative stress.[153] Adding the cerebrospinal fluid from ALS patients to rat motor neuron cell cultures causes the cultured cells to die. One of the intriguing aspects of resveratrol is that it can protect the motor neuron cell cultures from death, which is something that riluzole, the only FDA-approved drug for ALS, cannot do.[154]

## Life Extension Suggestions

- **Comprehensive multivitamin/multinutrient formula:** per label instructions
- **Vitamin B12** (as methylcobalamin): 1–25 mg daily
- **Zinc:** 30–60 mg daily (with 2 mg of copper)
- **Ginseng extract:** 500–1000 mg daily
- **Ginkgo biloba,** standardized extract: 120 mg daily
- **Coenzyme Q10** (as ubiquinol): 100–400 mg daily, possibly higher depending on blood test results
- **PQQ** (pyrroloquinoline quinone): 20 mg daily
- **Acetyl-L-carnitine:** 1000–2000 mg daily
- **R-lipoic acid:** 240–480 mg daily
- **Whey protein:** 35 g daily, in a single serving
- **Creatine monohydrate:** 1.25 g daily
- **N-acetyl-cysteine:** 600–1800 mg daily
- **Green tea extract** (standardized to 98% polyphenols): 725–1450 mg daily
- **Pine bark extract** (as Pycnogenol®): 100 mg daily
- ***Trans*-resveratrol:** 100–500 mg daily

In addition, the following blood test may provide helpful information:

- Coenzyme Q10

## REFERENCES

References available at: www.lef.org/dpt5/ch9

# 10

---

# *Anxiety*

---

As nature intended it, anxiety serves a useful purpose. Characterized by the fear or worry that something bad will happen, *normal* anxiety occurs occasionally in response to situations that threaten our sense of security. This helps us avoid harm and remember not to put ourselves in the same potentially dangerous situation in the future. Anxiety is a normal *stress response* that has been conserved throughout human evolution and is evident in all other animals.

However, when anxiety occurs inappropriately in response to normal everyday events, it can become a debilitating condition known as *anxiety disorder*. Anxiety disorders cause a person to be constantly "primed," or "tense" in expectation of an impending threat to their physical or psychological well-being. Symptoms of anxiety disorders are often *chronic*, and can include difficulty concentrating, irritability, tense muscles, sleep disturbances, and trouble overcoming worries.

The conventional health care model typically attempts to alleviate anxiety with an array of psychoactive drugs that either mimic or manipulate neurotransmitter signaling. For instance, medications for anxiety might either increase the recycling of existing neurotransmitters or bind directly to neurotransmitter receptors and block or activate them, artificially altering mood. However, psychoactive drugs *fall short* of addressing the underlying causes of anxiety—hormonal and metabolic imbalances that emerge as our bodies attempt to adapt to *chronic* stress.

Recognizing and responding to underappreciated risk factors for anxiety disorders, such as *elevated homocysteine* and *sex hormone imbalances*, is an important aspect of any treatment regimen. Sadly, mainstream physicians often fail to address these subtleties, an oversight that undoubtedly contributes to the paltry 50% success rate of conventional anxiety treatments.

Anxiety is a *multifaceted disorder*, and must be addressed as such in order to achieve symptomatic relief. Clinical studies indicate that nutrients such as *omega-3 polyunsaturated fatty acids*, *magnesium*, and *adaptogenic herbs* like rhodiola can synergize with healthy eating habits and stress management techniques to effectively optimize the body's stress response mechanisms and support healthy neurological communication. Moreover, compounds such as *B vitamins* and *amino acids* can provide the *raw materials* the body needs to ensure proper neurotransmitter synthesis and signaling.

## PREVALENCE

Anxiety disorders affect about 40 million American adults, or about 18.1% of the U.S. adult population over 18 years of age.[1-3] Nearly 15% of adults will experience an anxiety disorder in their lifetime.[1-3] By comparison, only 14.8 million American adults, or about 6.7% of the U.S. adult population, suffer from major depression. However, depression and anxiety are very much interrelated.

For up to 90% of all cases, anxiety disorders generally develop early in life—before the age of 35 with the greatest risk of onset between ages 10 and 25.[1,4,5] Also, women are twice as likely as men to suffer from generalized anxiety disorder.[1,4,5] This last statistic suggests that an imbalance in female hormone levels during and after menopause, during menstruation, and after pregnancy may be tied to the etiology of anxiety. We will explore this connection in greater detail later in this protocol.

## TYPES OF ANXIETY DISORDERS

### Generalized Anxiety Disorder

Generalized anxiety disorder (GAD) is characterized by worry and tension in the absence of a real provoking environmental factor. A person with GAD is constantly apprehensive, anticipating disaster, and becoming overly concerned about their health, finances, and work without cause.

People with GAD are frequently unable to relax and battle insomnia and poor concentration. Other symptoms may include restlessness, fatigue, irritability, muscle tension, high blood pressure, and sleep disturbances. Many people with mild GAD often manage to maintain their careers and function socially. However, severe cases can lead to job failure and avoidance of social situations.

GAD affects almost 6.8 million American adults.[6] Physicians diagnose GAD based on the following criteria—an individual worrying excessively about everyday problems and exhibiting 3 or more GAD symptoms, on most days, for at least 6 consecutive months.[7]

## Panic Disorder

Panic disorder is characterized by sudden attacks of fear and the sense of impending doom. A panic attack can cause elevated heart rate, sweating, dizziness, fatigue, shortness of breath, nausea, chest pain, and feelings of being cold and numb. In many cases these physical symptoms exacerbate the panic attack as the person may feel like they are dying or in terrible physical danger.

Panic attacks are often unpredictable and come on suddenly, but can be triggered by exposure to stimuli associated with past trauma, such as driving through an intersection where the person was involved in a major car accident. Panic attacks typically last about 10 minutes. Episodes often appear without warning and with varying frequency. Panic disorder is very disabling, causing people to avoid places or situations that caused attacks before. As a result, people with panic disorder often lose their jobs or change their residence.

Nearly one third of people with panic disorder will become fearful of leaving their homes and develop *agoraphobia,* a fear of open spaces.

Panic disorder afflicts about 6 million Americans, and is also twice as common among women as men.[1] The clinical definition of panic disorder is when a person experiences recurrent, unexpected panic attacks, at least one of which is followed by one or more of the following: persistent concern about future attacks, worrying about the implications of the attack, and/or a significant change in behavior related to the attacks.[8]

## Obsessive-Compulsive Disorder

Obsessive-compulsive disorder (OCD) is characterized by persistent, upsetting thoughts (obsessions) that can lead to anxiety and the use of ritualistic actions (compulsions) in an attempt to alleviate this anxiety.[9,10]

A good example is a person obsessed with the presence of bacteria in the environment. In this case, a person with OCD may develop a compulsion to ritualistically and repetitively wash their hands, or engage in some other type of self-cleansing. The person with OCD does not find performing the ritual pleasurable, but it instead provides temporary relief from the anxiety.

While healthy people can demonstrate repetitive behaviors, such as double checking to see if the doors are locked, people with OCD perform rituals so repetitively that their behavior distresses them and can interfere with the performance of everyday tasks.

Approximately 2.2 million American adults suffer with OCD. Eating disorders, other anxiety disorders, and depression commonly accompany OCD. Recent research shows OCD affects men and women equally.[1]

## Phobias

Phobias are inexplicable and unjustifiable fears. Phobias may be a fear of certain objects or things. Social phobia, also known as social anxiety disorder, involves excessive self-consciousness and anxiety about everyday social situations. People with social phobia are chronically fearful of embarrassing themselves and being judged by others. They can experience dread weeks before a scheduled encounter or interaction, which may interfere with everyday activities. Physical effects associated with social phobia can include blushing, sweating, nausea, and difficulty speaking.

About 15 million Americans are affected by social phobias.[11] Other anxiety disorders and depression may accompany social phobia. The clinical definition of social phobia is when a persistent fear of social situations causes people to either avoid them or experience them with great anxiety.[12,13]

## Posttraumatic Stress Disorder

Experiencing or witnessing a traumatic or terrifying life event such as a serious accident, violent crime, or natural disaster can precipitate a posttraumatic stress disorder (PTSD). People with PTSD may either relive the event in nightmares or have disturbing recollections of it during waking hours. Ordinary events can trigger flashbacks that may result in a loss of reality, causing the person to believe the event is happening again.

PTSD affects more than 5 million Americans and can occur at any age.[1,14] Symptoms associated with PTSD can include an inability to sleep, hypersensitivity to external stimuli, feelings of detachment or numbness, and loss of memory surrounding the traumatic experience.

Physicians diagnosing PTSD consider whether the patient persistently re-experiences the traumatic event through memory, dreams, hallucinations, flashbacks, or physical reactions to internal or external triggers. For a diagnosis of PTSD, symptoms must be present for more than one month, but may occur years after the traumatic event.[1,14]

## RISK FACTORS AND ASSOCIATIONS

A variety of factors can increase the risk of anxiety disorder. Being female is a risk as it affects twice as many women than men. Age is another factor, with the greatest risk of onset affecting those between the ages of 10 and 25. Research shows children who are shy or likely to be the target of bullies are at a higher risk of developing anxiety disorders later in life. Anxiety disorders also tend to run in families, believed to have both a genetic and learned component. Lack of social connections, traumatic events, and certain medical conditions are also associated with an increased risk of anxiety disorders.

Anxiety can occur independently of or in conjunction with other psychiatric or medical conditions such as depression, chronic fatigue, cardiac disease, or respiratory compromise. Chronic anxiety is associated with a higher risk of illness and death from cerebrovascular and cardiovascular diseases such as hypertension, cardiac ischemia, and arrhythmias. Also, chronic anxiety predisposes people to a range of neurologic disorders.[15-17] People with anxiety disorders are less able to deal with life's occasional blows. Divorce, financial disaster, or other severe stressors may increase their risk of suicidal behavior.[18]

## Homocysteine and the Methylation Cycle

Homocysteine is an intermediary within a metabolic cycle known as *methylation*. Methylation reactions, relying largely on B-vitamin cofactors (particularly B6, B12, and folic acid), are critical for the proper synthesis of the neurotransmitters that play an important role in mood regulation.

As B-vitamin levels decline, the methylation cycle becomes impaired, leading to a concurrent increase in homocysteine levels (because it is no longer being recycled efficiently) and a disruption in neurotransmitter synthesis. The close relationship between neurotransmitter synthesis and homocysteine formation has led some researchers to suspect that there is a link between homocysteine and mood. Indeed, studies suggest that levels of homocysteine are an effective marker for B-vitamin status, and that changes in homocysteine levels correlate with changes in mood.

Interestingly, homocysteine levels have predicted duration of PTSD,[19] suggesting that lowering homocysteine levels through supplementation with B vitamins might reduce symptoms of mood disorders by freeing up metabolic resources involved in neurotransmission. Other studies have clearly tied genetic abnormalities such as a mutation in the folic acid-activating enzyme, MTHFR, to high homocysteine levels (and increased symptoms of mood disorders). This reinforces the notion that homocysteine metabolism is an important target in psychiatric imbalances.[20] Supplementation with homocysteine-lowering B vitamins was shown to relieve anxiety in 44 women with premenstrual anxiety.[21]

Another compound involved in the methylation cycle is *S-adenosylmethionine* (SAM-e). SAM-e functions to donate methyl groups into the methylation cycle, thereby facilitating the formation of neurotransmitters such as dopamine and serotonin. In clinical trials, SAM-e supplementation has been shown to be as effective as tricyclic antidepressants in treating depressive disorders.[22]

Given the role of healthy methylation in maintaining biochemical balances within the central nervous system, a target blood level of *less than 7–8 µmol/L* of homocysteine helps to ensure proper neurotransmitter metabolism and may balance mood during times of stress, depression, and anxiety.

## IMPAIRED STRESS RESPONSE: ANXIETY, DEPRESSION, AND THE HYPOTHALAMIC-PITUITARY-ADRENAL AXIS

Rarely does an anxiety disorder manifest itself alone. More typically, other mood disorders accompany it, particularly depression. In fact, depression and anxiety can both be viewed as manifestations of impaired stress response, the underlying physiologies of which are both very similar.

When an individual experiences a stressor, physical or emotional, internal or environmental, the body initiates a complex system of adaptive reactions to help cope with the stress. This reactive response involves the release of *glucocorticoids*, also known as stress hormones, which stimulate adaptive changes in a variety of bodily systems.

Under short-term circumstances, stress-induced changes prioritize functions involved in escaping danger such as redirection of blood flow to the muscles from most other body parts, dilation of pupils, and inhibition of digestion for energy conservation. During this time, fatty acids and

### Hypothalamic-pituitary-adrenal axis

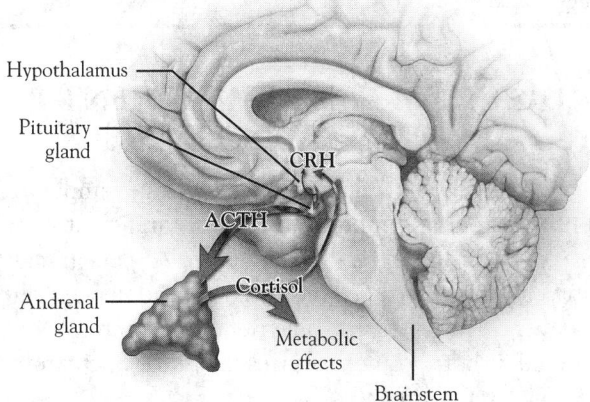

Hypothalamus

Pituitary gland

CRH

ACTH

Cortisol

Andrenal gland

Metabolic effects

Brainstem

glucose (blood sugar) are liberated from storage sites into the bloodstream where they are readily available for utilization by the muscles. This is known as the *fight-or-flight response*. This reactive and adaptive protection system originates in the brain. When a threat is perceived by the *hypothalamus* (a brain region), chemical signals are sent to the *pituitary gland* (another brain region). The pituitary gland then sends chemical signals to the *adrenal glands* (endocrine glands atop the kidneys), which in turn releases the stress hormone *cortisol*. Cortisol then goes on to initiate many of the physiologic changes that allow the organism to respond to the impending danger.

The fight-or-flight response is shared among nearly all animals in that the need to escape from imminent danger is paramount for the survival of the species. However, modern humans live in an environment filled with emotional stressors, such as financial worries, deadline pressures at work or school, as well as unnecessary physical stressors such as excessive caloric intake, obesity, and inactivity. All of these modern stressors *chronically activate* the *hypothalamic-pituitary-adrenal axis*, leading to adverse health consequences such as increased rates of cardiovascular disease, diabetes, and mood disorders like depression and anxiety.

The relationship between chronic stress, depression, and anxiety is complex and incredibly powerful. The chronic elevations in glucocorticoids (primarily cortisol) caused by excessive stressors in industrialized societies lead to actual *physical changes* in brain structure.

For example, dendrites, the branches of neurons that receive signals from other neurons, are shifted into less functional patterns upon chronic exposure to glucocorticoids. This has been documented in key brain regions associated with mood, short-term memory, and behavioral flexibility.[23] Furthermore, glucocorticoids cause receptors for the mood-regulating neurotransmitter *serotonin* to become less sensitive to activation.[24,25] Other detrimental effects of chronic stress include both increased susceptibility to neuronal damage and impaired neurogenesis, the process by which new neurons are "born."[23]

Interestingly, emerging research suggests that psychoactive drugs, like those used in anxiety and depression, may stabilize mood not only by acting on neurotransmitter levels, but by modulating the action of glucocorticoids receptors in the brain itself.[26] These new findings strongly support the idea that in order to alleviate mood disorders, controlling stress response is an important aspect of treatment. Indeed, several genetic and epidemiologic studies have linked excessive stress, and the inability to efficiently adapt to stress, to increased rates of anxiety and depression.[27,28]

# DIAGNOSIS AND TREATMENT OF ANXIETY DISORDERS

Because anxiety and depression may have similar or even overlapping symptoms, diagnosis and treatment of anxiety disorder can be difficult. A person can swing back and forth between anxiety and depression. However, as many of the same neural mechanisms are involved in both, sometimes treatment for one can be effective for the other.

While several screening tests are available to help determine the cause, type, and severity of anxiety, the diagnosis of anxiety disorders remains somewhat subjective and based on observation.[29] Once a doctor diagnoses an anxiety disorder, treatment will often integrate several approaches, including but not limited to diet and lifestyle changes, relaxation and massage therapy, psychotherapy, behavioral or cognitive-behavioral therapy, and drug intervention.

## Cognitive-Behavioral Therapy

Cognitive-behavioral therapy involves modifying thought patterns that influence anxiety and fear. It helps individuals recognize cognitive distortions, exaggerated and irrational thoughts that produce reactions such an anxiety and panic. Special tools then help the person detect distorted thinking and replace distorted thoughts with more accurate ones. Cognitive-behavioral therapy is a first-line treatment,[30,31] and is effective in treating all anxiety disorders.[30,31]

## Behavior Therapy

Behavior therapy uses several techniques such as diaphragmatic breathing exercises and exposure therapy. Diaphragmatic breathing teaches people how to control the physical signs of anxiety by taking slow, deep breaths to help control hyperventilation. Exposure therapy relies on small, progressive exposures to the frightening trigger, helping people build confidence and control anxiety.

## Drug Therapy

Drug therapy is often used in combination with psychotherapy to manage the biochemical and physiologic abnormalities that produce anxiety, including alterations in the levels of serotonin, norepinephrine, and cortisol (the stress hormone).

Drug therapy can present a number of problems, including poor success rates, side effects, withdrawal symptoms, the development of increased tolerance to the drug, and only acting on a small component of the neurologic mechanism involved in anxiety.

Pharmaceutical treatment of anxiety disorders involves manipulating or mimicking the action of neurotransmitters within the brain (typically GABA and serotonin, but sometimes dopamine and norepinephrine). However, these drugs usually do not resolve the overactivation of the hypothalamus-pituitary-adrenal axis that often underlies mood disorders.

Using medications to try to improve brain chemistry can offer relief, at least in the short term. However, medications do not restore normal levels of neurotransmitters or promote normal brain function. Instead, they manipulate the brain chemistry to achieve their desired effects.

Over time, the brain can get used to medications, resulting in them losing their effectiveness and requiring either higher doses or different drugs. Stopping them can frequently lead to withdrawal symptoms that feel worse than the original problem.

Types of drugs frequently prescribed to treat anxiety disorders include:

**Benzodiazepines.** Benzodiazepines act in part by modulating and extending the life of gamma-aminobutyric acid (GABA), an inhibitory (calming) brain neurotransmitter.[32] Benzodiazepines can relieve anxiety symptoms quickly. However, they can become habit forming. Some people develop a tolerance to them, requiring an increased dosage. When benzodiazepines are reduced or removed, some individuals can experience withdrawal symptoms, such as life-threatening seizures, confusion, memory loss, hyperanxiety, and reemergence of the original symptoms.[33] Commonly prescribed benzodiazepines include Valium® (diazepam), Xanax® (alprazolam), Klonopin® (clonazepam), and Ativan® (lorazepam).

While these drugs are highly effective in calming anxiety, they may also be habit-forming—a factor that dramatically limits their usefulness and possibly their long-term safety. Many benzodiazepines can also cause significant impairment, a highly undesirable effect.

*Azapirones* do not have the tolerance and dependency issues associated with benzodiazepines. These antianxiety drugs are partial serotonin receptor agonists. BuSpar® (buspirone) is an azapirone prescribed to treat general anxiety disorder. However, it may take several weeks before the effects of these drugs become apparent. Side effects can include nausea, headaches, and dizziness.

**Antidepressants.** Antidepressants are sometimes effective for treating anxiety, especially when it occurs in conjunction with depression. Types of antidepressant drugs include selective serotonin reuptake inhibitors (SSRIs) as well as the less common tricyclic antidepressants and monoamine oxidase inhibitors (MAOIs). These drugs can have significant side effects. In 2004, the U.S. Food and Drug Administration (FDA) announced that the most popular class of antidepressants, SSRIs, must carry a strong black-box warning advising patients of the dangers of increased suicide among adolescents using SSRIs. Popular SSRIs include Prozac® (fluoxetine), Zoloft® (sertraline), Luvox® (fluvoxamine), Paxil® (paroxetine), and Celexa® (citalopram).

**Beta-blockers.** Beta-blockers such as Inderal® (propranolol) or Tenormin® (atenolol) are used primarily to treat heart conditions. However, they are often prescribed for social phobia to help reduce heart palpitations as well as other physical symptoms of anxiety. Side effects can include sexual dysfunction, slow pulse, drowsiness, fatigue, dry mouth, numbness or tingling of fingers or toes, dizziness, diarrhea, nausea, weakness, and cold hands and feet.[34]

**Pregabalin.** Pregabalin is an anticonvulsant drug that is sometimes used to treat anxiety. Its effects become apparent quickly—some studies suggest within 1 week. Also, it appears to be effective in preventing a relapse of anxiety disorder,[35,36] as well as helping ease withdrawal symptoms after discontinuation of benzodiazepine therapy.[37] This drug often causes dizziness and drowsiness.

## ANXIETY AND HORMONES

Anxiety disorders affect twice as many women as men. Further, women experience more anxiety when they are pregnant, postpartum, premenstrual, and menopausal than at other times in life. This general observation has lead scientists to investigate a hormone-anxiety link.

By now, it is well known that most steroid hormones (eg, pregnenolone, estrogen, progesterone, testosterone, and DHEA) are neurologically active. In fact, large quantities of DHEA, estrogen, progesterone, and testosterone receptors are found in the brain. These hormones affect the brain in a number of ways, including regulation of mood.

A number of studies have linked abnormalities in hormone levels to various anxiety disorders.[38–41] Studies suggest that levels of estrogen and serotonin may be linked, both affecting a positive mood during menstruation in young women.[42] Likewise, the drop in estrogen during menopause, associated with reduced serotonin production, has a negative impact on mood and cognitive function.

Progesterone also plays a role in anxiety. In an animal study comparing a control group to mice lacking a progesterone receptor, researchers found progesterone decreased anxiety behavior through a mechanism similar to that of benzodiazepines—by acting on GABA receptors.[43] Another study found that while a single dose of progesterone given to animals decreased anxiety indicators during stress tests, the abrupt cessation of progesterone therapy increased measures of anxiety.[44]

In a placebo-controlled trial involving postmenopausal women, hormone replacement therapy using both estrogen and progesterone caused a marked reduction in anxiety, as well as improved sleep quality and better cognitive performance.[45]

## Bioidentical Hormone Replacement Therapy

Bioidentical hormone replacement therapy (BHRT) is an ideal method to restore youthful hormone levels for aging individuals. BHRT involves supplementation (usually) with either transdermal (topical) or oral preparations of hormones obtained from a compounding pharmacy. BHRT differs from conventional synthetic hormone replacement therapy (HRT) in that it relies on the use of *natural* hormones whose molecular structure exactly matches those of the hormones produced within the human body.

In a clinical trial conducted at the University of Texas, nearly 300 women with an average age of 52 years were treated with bioidentical progesterone and/or estrogen. After 6 months of BHRT, women aged 40–70 years experienced dramatic improvements in mood, including a 31% reduction in emotional ability, 37% reduction in irritability, 33% reduction in anxiety, and significant relief from night sweats and hot flashes. Moreover, of the women screened for heart attack or breast cancer an average of 1.9 years after beginning BHRT (21% of the cohort), *none* of them had either.[46]

Those who would like to learn more about the benefits of BHRT are encouraged to read the *Life Extension Magazine* article entitled "Bioidentical Hormones: Why Are They Still Controversial?"

Just as the female brain depends on healthy levels of estrogen and progesterone to function normally, the male brain depend on sufficient testosterone. Low testosterone levels can cause testosterone deficiencies in the brain, thereby impairing brain function leading to depression and anxiety.

In animal studies, mice with lower levels of testosterone displayed increased anxiety, supporting the idea that testosterone administration reduces anxiety.[47,48] In humans, increases in testosterone levels seen during DHEA therapy have been linked to reduced anxiety.[49] Laboratory studies indicate that activation of the androgen receptor by testosterone may reduce anxiety through interaction with GABA receptors.[50]

Normalizing hormone levels can be an integral part of managing anxiety disorders. Of course, it is also important to address the factors that cause hormonal imbalances in the first place. These include blood sugar dysregulation, oxidative stress, inflammation, and other disruptions in metabolic function leading to chronic stress, a condition that frequently results in both hormonal imbalances and anxiety disorders.

In addition to managing hormonal imbalances, it is important to examine the relationship between the stress hormone cortisol and DHEA (a building block for the sex steroid hormones). During times of prolonged stress, a greater proportion of cortisol is made compared to DHEA, with a high cortisol to DHEA ratio being a marker associated with anxiety disorder.[51] DHEA counteracts some of the negative impact of cortisol in the body. In a large follow-up study of Vietnam-era, U.S. army veterans, the ratio of cortisol to DHEA-sulphate was a strong predictor of all-cause mortality.[52] Having higher levels of cortisol and lower levels of DHEA-sulphate were linked with an increased risk of death due to any cause over a 15-year period.

Clinical studies have found DHEA supplementation to be particularly helpful in relieving anxiety in both schizophrenics and females with low hormone levels.[49,53] Life Extension suggests that males maintain DHEA blood levels of 350–490 µg/dL, while females maintain levels of 275–400 µg/dL.

It is important to note that all the major sex hormones are interrelated. Thus, people with anxiety may benefit from comprehensive hormone testing, and if necessary, a program of *bioidentical hormone replacement*. Those interested in learning more about hormone replacement therapy should read Life Extension's Female Hormone Restoration protocol and/or Male Hormone Restoration protocol.

---

## ANTIANXIETY HERBALS FOR MENOPAUSE SUPPORT

While St. John's wort can be taken by both men and women, it appears to be very effective in easing symptoms associated with women's hormonal fluctuations. Researchers found in a double-blind, randomized, placebo-controlled trial that *St. John's wort* reduces the duration and severity of hot flashes in premenopausal women.[54] In another study, St. John's wort improved the quality of life and alleviated sleep problems in symptomatic perimenopausal women aged 60–65.[55]

Researchers found in placebo-controlled studies that supplementing with 80 mg of red clover isoflavones per day for 90 days reduced anxiety in postmenopausal women.[56] Interestingly, red clover phytoestrogens were shown to lower both total and LDL (bad) cholesterol, triglycerides, and boost HDL (good) cholesterol in 40 postmenopausal women. In this study, there were no reported side effects of the red clover isoflavones.[57]

*Vitex* agnus-castus (chaste tree/berry), when taken over a 16-week period in combination with St. John's wort, reduced anxiety associated with premenstrual syndrome and menopause.[58] A metabolite of the isoflavone *daidzein* from soy has also been shown to reduce anxiety in premenopausal, perimenopausal, and postmenopausal women.[59] In healthy women of reproductive age, a preparation combining magnolia and phellodendron bark has been shown to reduce anxiety, in part by helping control cortisol levels.[60]

## LIFESTYLE CHANGES

People with anxiety disorders can take a number of steps to reduce their symptoms. For example, programs involving telephone-based exercise interventions have been shown to reduce anxiety in pregnant and postpartum women.[61]

Smoking, alcohol and caffeine consumption, lack of exercise and an increased body mass index (BMI) can all have a negative impact on the degree to which aging individuals experience anxiety.[62] Getting enough sleep and exercise, maintaining a healthy body weight, and moderating caffeine consumption on the other hand are recommended for reducing anxiety.[63,64]

Recent clinical trials demonstrate the benefit of yoga and tai chi. Most compelling was a study using brain scans showing a significant increase in thalamic GABA activity, which correlated to a better mood after the practice of yoga.[65] Tai chi and yoga have been shown to reduce anxiety and heart rate after each 20-minute session.[66] In one study, 2 months of yoga classes reduced stress symptoms in women with anxiety disorder.[67]

Music and massage therapy appear to be particularly helpful in reducing anxiety associated with postoperative stress and treatment for cancer.[68–70]

Healthy cooking and a nutritious diet are central to controlling anxiety.[71] In a study involving over 10,000 people, following a Mediterranean diet led to reductions in mood disorders.[72] When it is not always possible to have a well-balanced diet, nutritional supplementation can be an important lifestyle factor in the fight against anxiety.

## NATURAL THERAPIES TO BALANCE BRAIN CHEMISTRY

In general, a healthy diet is abundant in omega-3 fatty acids, organic fresh fruits and vegetables, and filtered water, and devoid of foods high in saturated fats and refined carbohydrates. This dietary pattern resembles the Mediterranean diet.

In addition, the following nutrients may support healthy stress response and help balance brain chemistry naturally.

### Amino Acids

When the brain produces a neurotransmitter, it starts with a raw ingredient—usually an amino acid from the diet or another chemical already present in the brain. Enzymes are then used to convert the amino acid into the needed brain chemical. By understanding this process in detail, we can take measures to ensure an ample supply of the raw ingredients and enhance the activity of the enzymes. There are various *cofactors* that help the enzymes work faster, such as B vitamins.

**L-tryptophan, L-tyrosine, and L-phenylalanine.** Insufficient intake of L-tryptophan, L-phenylalanine, or L-tyrosine are associated with increased symptoms of anxiety.[73–76] Supplementation with L-tryptophan or 5-hydroxytryptophan (5-HTP) has been shown to elevate brain serotonin levels and enhance both mood and one's sense of well being.[73,74,77]

*Vitamin B6, magnesium, and vitamin C*—nutrients already taken by most health-conscious people—are cofactors that facilitate the conversion of tryptophan to serotonin in the brain. As people age they produce more of an enzyme that degrades tryptophan, even if taking tryptophan supplements. *Lysine, niacinamide,* and anti-inflammatory nutrients such as *rosemary* have been shown to neutralize the effects of this enzyme and help preserve the synthesis of serotonin from tryptophan.

D,L-phenylalanine and L-tyrosine taken with a carbohydrate-rich meal can increase synthesis of dopamine and norepinephrine.[78] There are no reported adverse effects, but high doses should be avoided by pregnant women and individuals taking MAOIs.

**L-lysine and L-arginine.** An L-lysine deficiency has been shown to increase stress-induced anxiety in humans.[79,80] L-lysine binds to a serotonin receptor, acting as a serotonin antagonist by inhibiting serotonin reuptake in the synapse.[81] When presented with a stressful situation, supplementation with L-lysine and L-arginine reduced anxiety in human subjects.[82–84]

**Theanine.** Theanine, an amino acid found in green tea, produces a calming effect on the brain.[85–87] Theanine easily crosses the blood–brain barrier. It increases the production of GABA and dopamine and protects from damage the cells of the hippocampus, the seat of learning and memory in the brain.[88,89]

In an 8-week study involving 60 schizophrenic patients, 400 mg of theanine was added to standard antipsychotic therapy. The addition of theanine significantly reduced anxiety and improved several other measures of mood beyond what was achievable with pharmaceuticals alone.[90]

**S-adenosylmethionine (SAM-e).** SAM-e occurs naturally in the body. It is concentrated in the liver and brain and is a major methyl donor in the synthesis of hormones, nucleic acids, proteins, phospholipids, and catecholamine neurotransmitters such as dopamine and serotonin.[91] SAMe facilitates glutathione usage and maintains acetylcholine levels, helping to preserve cognitive function while aging and possibly attenuating neurodegeneration.

In an 8-week clinical study involving depressed individuals with HIV/AIDS, supplementation with up to 1600 mg of SAM-e considerably improved disposition on multiple standardized assessments. The effects of treatment with SAM-e became evident in as little as one week.[92]

## Minerals

**Magnesium.** Magnesium deficiency has been linked to anxiety disorders in several clinical studies. In fact, when researchers want to study anxiety disorder, they use mice that have been specifically bred to be magnesium deficient. This model is very effective at inducing anxiety.[93]

Several human trials have supported the link between magnesium deficiency and anxiety. When taken for one month in combination with a multivitamin, zinc, and calcium, magnesium dramatically decreased symptoms of distress and anxiety compared to a placebo.[94] Further, supplementation with magnesium and vitamin B6 effectively reduced premenstrual-related anxiety.[95] In a placebo-controlled study, dietary supplementation with magnesium reduced generalized anxiety disorder (GAD).[96] In community-based studies, a small reduction in mood disorders was seen in those with higher magnesium intakes.[97]

Groundbreaking research has recently shed light on a new preparation, *magnesium threonate*, which may overcome a long-standing obstacle in magnesium supplementation—blood–brain barrier permeability.

High magnesium levels in the brain have been linked with superior cognitive function. However, conventional magnesium supplements are not efficient in raising these levels because they do not penetrate the blood–brain barrier. Researchers at the Massachusetts Institute of Technology have shown that magnesium threonate effectively elevates magnesium levels inside the central nervous system. The scientists also discovered that magnesium threonate improves cognitive function significantly better than other forms of magnesium in laboratory animals.[98]

**Selenium.** Selenium has been shown to reduce anxiety. In double-blind randomized clinical trials, subjects given 100 mg of selenium daily for 5 weeks reported improved mood and less anxiety.[99,100] The same treatment regimen also reduced post-partum depression.[101] Selenium supplementation reduces anxiety in elderly hospitalized patients, cancer patients undergoing chemotherapy, and HIV patients receiving highly active antiretroviral therapy (HAART).[102–104]

The role of selenium in supporting positive mood is quite complex. Selenium is a critical component in a variety of important enzymes whose action can significantly impact overall health. For example, the enzymes that help synthesize thyroid hormones. In a selenium-deficient state, thyroid hormone synthesis may deteriorate, which can lead to poor mood and many other negative conditions.[105]

## Fatty Acids

**Omega-3 fatty acids.** The omega-3 fatty acids eicosapentaenoic acid (EPA) and docosahexaenoic acid (DHA) are necessary for proper brain function. The typical Western diet has an overly high ratio of inflammatory omega-6 fatty acids to anti-inflammatory omega-3 fatty acids. Omega-3 fatty acids have been shown to have a variety of health benefits, most recently being improved mood and reduced anxiety.[106–108]

In one double-blind, placebo-controlled, and randomized clinical trial, medical students were given either 2.5 g/day of omega-3 polyunsaturated fatty acids (PUFAs) or placebo capsules containing the fatty acid profile of a typical American diet. Compared to controls, those students receiving the omega-3 capsules showed a 20% reduction in anxiety.[109] In a double-blind, placebo-controlled study, omega-3 fatty acid supplementation for 3 months reduced anxiety and anger in substance abusers.[110] Reduced test anxiety and lower levels of the stress hormone cortisol have also been associated with omega-3 supplementation.[111]

Life Extension suggests that the omega-6 to omega-3 ratio should be kept below 4:1 for optimal neuropsychiatric and overall health. More information on testing and optimizing your omega-6 to omega-3 ratio can be found in the *Life Extension Magazine* article entitled "Optimize Your Omega-3 Status."

## Herbs and Botanical Medicine

Botanical herbs have been shown to manage many psychiatric disorders, including anxiety.[83,85,112–117] Being that the quality, composition, conditions for growth, and extraction processes of herbal products can vary greatly, care should be taken in choosing an herbal remedy.

The following herbs either have antianxiety effects or target key molecular sites associated with neurotransmitters in the central nervous system.

**St. John's wort** (*Hypericum perforatum*). St. John's wort is an aromatic perennial native to Europe, parts of Asia, and North and South America. The majority of controlled studies found it superior to placebo and similarly effective as standard antidepressant drugs.[118–120] St. John's wort has been shown to increase brain levels of serotonin in animals, operating through slightly different and more complex pathways than those of prescription SSRIs.[121,122] For instance, the combined antioxidant and anti-inflammatory properties of St. John's wort extract contribute to antidepressant affects through normalization of an overactive HPA axis.

While St. John's wort is known for its antidepressive affects, 2 recent studies also suggest that supplementation with this herb can reduce the anxiety associated with premenstrual syndrome (PMS).[123,124] St. John's wort is contraindicated for use during pregnancy, lactation, and exposure to strong sunlight, and should not be taken concurrently with antidepressant medication.[125]

**Ginkgo biloba.** Animals given ginkgo biloba demonstrated reduced anxiety in cognitive tests.[126,127] Several double-blind placebo-controlled studies showed that ginkgo biloba binds to and activates the GABA receptor, and like a benzodiazepine, reduces anxiety in patients with generalized anxiety disorders without side effects.[128,129]

**Valerian** (*Valeriana officinalis*). This temperate herb has been used for medicinal purposes since the time of Hippocrates. Components of valerian root have been shown in laboratory studies to bind to GABA receptors, increase the release of GABA, and decrease its reuptake.[130–133] Valerian root extracts were shown to have antianxiety effects in both rats and mice.[134–136] Valerian root extracts have also been shown to activate glutamic acid decarboxylase, an enzyme involved in the synthesis of GABA.[137]

In recent clinical studies, psychiatric rating scales have shown that a daily dose of 400–900 mg of extracts from valerian root is as effective as diazepam at reducing anxiety.[138–141]

**Lemon balm** (*Melissa officinalis*). Lemon balm is a member of the mint family, sometimes used as a culinary herb and flavoring agent. The plant also has several anxiolytic (antianxiety) actions.

In animal studies, extracts from lemon balm have been shown to suppress levels of stress hormones (glucocorticoids) while also promoting the growth of new neurons, a process called neurogenesis.[142] Moreover, lemon balm contains compounds that strongly suppress the breakdown of GABA, which may prolong the antianxiety effects of the neurotransmitter.[137]

Lemon balm has been shown to reduce anxious behavior in laboratory animals. In a human clinical trial, it significantly suppressed anxiety when combined with valerian root, another anxiolytic herb.[141,143]

*Rhodiola*. *Rhodiola rosea* is a known *adaptogen*, an herb that helps improve one's resistance to stress. It has also shown promise in alleviating anxiety disorder. Ten subjects receiving a daily dose of *Rhodiola rosea* extract for 10 weeks demonstrated significant improvement in symptoms of anxiety.[144] Another similar 10-week study found that a 340-mg daily dose of *Rhodiola rosea* extract significantly eased symptoms of generalized anxiety disorder.[145] Animal studies have found that compounds in *Rhodiola rosea* help ameliorate the anxiety associated with smoking cessation.[146]

**Ashwagandha** (*Withania somnifera*). Ashwagandha, or Indian ginseng, has long been used by Ayurvedic practitioners as a rejuvenating tonic. The herb has anti-inflammatory, antitumor, antistress, antioxidant, immunomodulatory, and rejuvenating properties.[147] In several studies, rodents treated with extracts of ashwagandha showed reduced anxiety when compared to a control group; and to a similar extent when compared to several benzodiazepine drugs.[148–150]

Ashwagandha has also been shown to reduce anxiety in humans.[151,152] In a clinical trial, patients with significant anxiety were divided into 2 groups, and for 12 weeks were provided either psychotherapy or treated with naturopathic treatment including ashwagandha. The ashwagandha treated group demonstrated a greater reduction in anxiety parameters.[153]

Our bodies are truly elegant in their design. This is especially apparent with brain function. A common element of this design is the brain's binary systems, wherein one chemical activates a process while its partner turns it off again. One example is *glutamate* and *GABA*, which together account for over 80% of brain activity. Glutamate accelerates brain activity (excitatory), while GABA puts the brakes on (inhibitory). Together, they keep the brain humming along at just the right pace—not too fast, not too slow.

If you have developed anxiety, then the balance of these 2 chemicals has been thrown off. As a result, the brain's activity level is turned up too high, at least in some areas. The balancing supplements for glutamate and GABA include but are not limited to the amino acids *GABA and L-theanine*, the antioxidant *NAC*, *vitamins B6 and D*, the minerals *magnesium and zinc*, and *omega-3 fatty acids*.

**GABA.** GABA, a neurotransmitter made from the amino acid glutamate, can be taken in the form of a dietary supplement. GABA is the chief inhibiting, or calming neurotransmitter in the brain, functioning as a

| Brain Chemical | Role in Neurotransmission and Stress Response | Nutritional Support |
|---|---|---|
| *Glutamate*, the excitatory chemical | Heightens overall brain activity | NAC, green tea, vitamin D3, magnesium, omega-3s |
| *GABA*, the inhibitory chemical | Slows overall brain activity | GABA, L-theanine, vitamin B6, zinc, inositol, herbal therapies |
| *Norepinephrine*, the arousal chemical | Raises level of alertness | Tyrosine, L-theanine, NAC, omega-3s, inositol |
| *Dopamine*, the reward chemical | Focuses attention and enhances pleasure and reward | Tyrosine, L-theanine, B vitamins, omega-3s, St. John's wort, ginkgo |
| *Serotonin*, the soothing chemical | Calms, regulates sleep and appetite, protects against stress | Tryptophan/5-HTP, DHEA, folic acid, vitamin B6, vitamin B12, vitamin D, omega-3s, St. John's wort |
| *CRH/cortisol*, the stress hormone | Prolonged elevation leads to fat storage, insulin resistance, degenerative brain disorders, memory loss, inflammation | DHEA, B vitamins, antioxidants, herbal adaptogens |

brake on the neural circuitry during stress. Low GABA levels are associated with restlessness, anxiety, insomnia, and a poor mood.[154–156] Clinical studies have shown that the use of GABA as a dietary supplement relieves stress, anxiety, and increases the production of alpha brain waves (associated with relaxation).[157–159]

**N-acetyl cysteine (NAC).** NAC shows promise for alleviating mood disorders through a variety of mechanisms. It acts as a precursor to glutathione, a potent cellular antioxidant that may help ease neuronal oxidative stress. Furthermore, in contributing to glutathione synthesis, NAC uses up excess glutamate stores. This might lessen the excitatory transmission triggered by glutamate.[160] Indeed, in at least one small clinical trial, a 6-month supplementation with NAC lead to a complete remission in depressive symptoms in 6 of 7 subjects, while placebo treatment lead to remission in only 2 of 7.[161]

**Vitamin D.** The impact of this hormone-like vitamin on mood disorders is complex. There are receptors for vitamin D throughout the brain, and animal data indicates that lower vitamin D signaling leads to increased anxious behavior.[162] There is a considerable association between low vitamin D levels and depression, but the connection with anxiety is less clear.[163] Nonetheless, maintaining a vitamin D level between

50–80 *ng/mL* is suggested for everyone to promote optimal health and protect against the ravages of aging.

## Life Extension Suggestions

**Amino acids** (provides raw materials needed to support neurotransmitter synthesis) (*Note:* Not all of these suggested amino acids will be of benefit in every case of anxiety. It is suggested to start at the low end of the dose range and increase or discontinue based on results.)

- **L-tryptophan or 5-HTP:** 1000–2000 mg tryptophan daily, or 50–150 mg, 5-HTP daily
- **L-tyrosine:** 500–1000 mg daily
- **L-phenylalanine:** 500–1500 mg daily
- **L-lysine:** 600–1800 mg daily
- **L-theanine:** 100–400 mg daily
- **L-arginine:** 800–2400 mg daily
- **GABA:** 700–2100 mg daily
- **N-acetyl cysteine:** 600–1800 mg daily

**Cofactors** (support the enzymes involved in hormone and neurotransmitter synthesis and metabolism)

- **B complex vitamins:** Per label instructions
- **Vitamin C:** 1000–2000 mg daily
- **Magnesium:** 500–2000 mg daily
- **Selenium:** 200–400 mcg daily
- **S-adenosylmethionine (SAM-e):** 400–1200 mg daily

**Fatty acids** (supports neuronal membrane health and proper neuronal communication)

- **Fish oil:** 2000–4000 mg daily

**Antianxiety herbals**

- **St. John's wort:** 300–600 mg daily
- **Ginkgo biloba,** standardized extract: 120–240 mg daily
- **Valerian,** standardized extract: 600–1200 mg daily
- **Lemon balm,** standardized extract: 300–600 mg daily

**Adaptogenic herbs** (help to increase resistance to stress)

- **Ashwagandha,** standardized extract: 125–250 mg daily
- **Rhodiola,** standardized extract: 250–500 mg daily

**General and hormonal support**

- **Vitamin D** (women and men): 5000–8000 IU daily (depending on blood test results)

- **DHEA** (women and men): 15–75 mg daily (depending on blood test results)
- **Soy isoflavones** (typically for women only): 50–150 mg daily
- **Vitex,** standardized extract: 20 mg daily
- **Rosemary leaf extract:** 100–200 mg daily

In addition, the following blood testing resources may be helpful:

- Male Panel with Hormone Add-On or Female Panel with Hormone Add-On

- Omega Score®
- Cortisol AM/PM

## REFERENCES

References available at: www.lef.org/dpt5/ch10

# 11

# Arrhythmias

Arrhythmias are abnormalities in heart rate or rhythm. They arise from disruption of the electrical conduction system within cardiac tissue, which must be properly synchronized to maintain normal heart rhythm. Arrhythmias often occur in people who have some form of underlying heart disease, such as coronary artery disease, but a healthy heart is not immune to abnormal heart rate or rhythm.[1-4]

There are 2 main categories of arrhythmias: *tachycardia*, in which the heart beats too fast, and *bradycardia*, in which the heart beats too slow. *Fibrillation*, in which the heart beats irregularly or "quivers," is an important heart rhythm irregularity sometimes classified as a subcategory of tachycardia.[1-6]

Arrhythmias are further classified depending on which part of the heart they affect; the two upper chambers of the heart are called *atria* and the two lower chambers are called *ventricles*.[4]

Some arrhythmias, such as *ventricular fibrillation*, can be immediately life-threatening because they impact the pumping action of the heart substantially enough to disrupt blood supply to the body, potentially leading to *sudden cardiac death*, one of the most common causes of death in the United States.[2,7-9] *Atrial fibrillation* is a common type of arrhythmia that is usually not life-threatening in its own right, but can dramatically increase risk of having a *stroke* because a blood clot can form within the fibrillating atria and then lodge in blood vessel(s) that supply the brain.[10-12] Still other arrhythmias, such as *premature ventricular contractions*, are fairly common and not usually considered significant health threats.[1,4]

*Conventional* arrhythmia treatment strategies rely on pharmaceutical treatment with drugs that often have potentially serious side effects, electrical synchronization procedures, or surgical procedures that work in a certain percentage of patients.

There are lifestyle considerations and several natural compounds including *magnesium* and *coenzyme Q10* that have been shown to support a healthy heart and reduce occurrence of arrhythmia.[13-21]

This protocol will explain types of arrhythmias, their causes, and how they affect the heart. Conventional treatment strategies, including medications and procedures, will be reviewed and some promising new antiarrhythmic drugs will be examined. The important, though sometimes neglected role of diet and lifestyle considerations in arrhythmia prevention and management will also be discussed, and data on a number of scientifically studied natural compounds that may help maintain a healthy heart rhythm will be presented.

## HOW THE HEART WORKS

The heart consists of 4 chambers: 2 upper chambers, called atria, which receive the blood, and 2 lower ones, called ventricles, which push the blood out from the organ. The atria and ventricles alternately contract and relax to pump blood through the heart and to the rest of the body.

A heartbeat originates as electrical impulses are generated and pass through a predetermined pathway in the heart. These electrical impulses originate in the *sinoatrial (SA) node*, which is a small mass of specialized tissue located in the right atrium; it is also known as the heart's pacemaker. This electrical impulse first causes the atria to contract and squeeze blood into the ventricles. It then passes through the *atrioventricular (AV) node* and triggers the ventricles to contract, which having just been filled with blood by the contracting atria, pump blood out to the rest of the body.[22]

A "normal" range for resting heart rate is approximately 60–100 beats per minute, with evidence

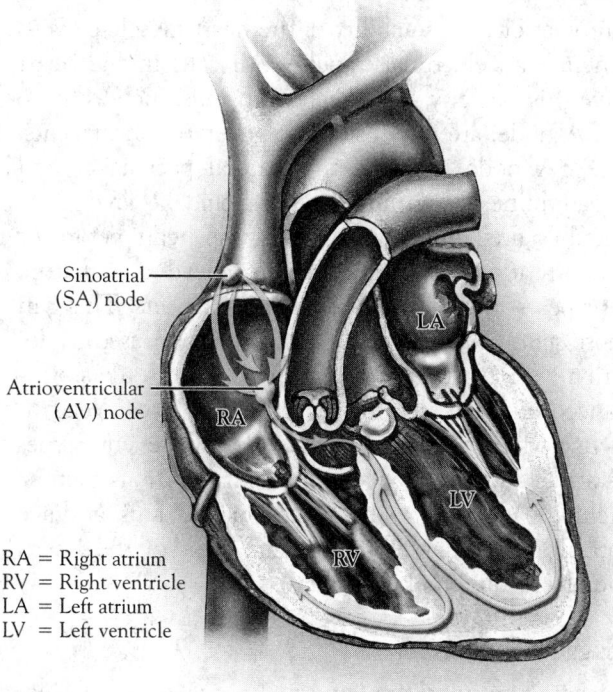

Sinoatrial (SA) node

Atrioventricular (AV) node

LA

RA

LV

RV

RA = Right atrium
RV = Right ventricle
LA = Left atrium
LV = Left ventricle

Heart Structure and Conduction System

suggesting that a heart rate at rest over 80 beats per minute may be cause for possible concern for underlying heart disease. For example, a study published in the *Journal of Epidemiology and Community Health* followed 50 000 healthy men and women over 20 years and found that for each increase of 10 heartbeats per minute, the risk of dying of a heart attack increased 18% among women and about 10% in men.[23] Any irregularities in the heart rhythm can affect the efficiency at which the heart pumps blood to the body, and may thereby lead to damage in various tissues and organs.[3,4]

The normal conduction of electric impulses and normal heart muscle contractions depend on the levels of various *electrolytes* in the body. Impulses are generated due to the movement of electrolytes through passages called "ion channels" that are present in the heart cells. Sodium, potassium, calcium, and magnesium are the chief ions required for generating electric impulses under normal circumstances. Inadequate levels of these ions prevent the proper formation of impulses, and/or their normal conduction, resulting in the development of arrhythmias. Most antiarrhythmic drugs act by modulating these ion channels.[24]

## DEVELOPMENT OF ARRHYTHMIAS

Mechanisms by which arrhythmias can develop include the following.[25]

### Enhanced or Suppressed Automaticity

Automaticity is the ability of the heart muscle cells to generate an electrical impulse. All cells in the heart have this capacity, but only certain cells, such as those in SA node, are responsible for generating heartbeats. The SA node is the heart's natural pacemaker and it determines when an impulse should be fired. Any impulses fired from elsewhere in the heart before or concurrently with SA node firing can lead to premature heartbeats or sustained abnormal heartbeats. This can cause *sinus node dysfunction (SND)*, a term used to describe various types of heart rhythm disorders. Enhanced automaticity, on the other hand, can lead to tachycardia (>100 beats/minute) and several types of atrial and ventricular arrhythmia. Various factors, including electrolyte imbalances, medications, and age can alter automaticity in specific areas of the heart, thereby leading to arrhythmias.

### Triggered Activity

Triggered activity, the abnormal propagation of electrical activity in individual heart cells, can lead to sustained abnormal heart rhythms.[26] Arrhythmias due to triggered activity are rare; when they occur, they are often due to problems in the ion channels in the heart muscle cells. They can also occur as a side effect of certain antiarrhythmic drugs such as digitalis.

### Reentry

Reentry is a common mechanism for the initiation of tachyarrhythmia (a rapid irregular heartbeat).[27] This happens when the electrical impulse travels backwards from the ventricles to the atria, initiating another heartbeat while the first heartbeat is still descending into the ventricles.

## TYPES OF ARRHYTHMIAS

Arrhythmias can be classified as follows.[3]

### Premature (Extra) Beats

Premature extra beats are a very common and mostly harmless type of arrhythmia. Those that occur in the atria are called premature atrial contractions (PACs), while those occurring in the ventricles are called premature ventricular contractions (PVCs).[28,29] Premature atrial contractions have been linked to excess consumption of caffeine and alcohol, the use of sympathomimetic medications (drugs that mimic the effects of sympathetic nervous system signaling molecules called catecholamines), and are sometimes present in people who have structural heart disease.[28] Premature ventricular contractions are often seen in the presence of structural heart disease, but they can also appear in the absence of any identifiable heart conditions.[29]

**Premature ventricular contractions.** Premature ventricular contractions (PVCs) are a transient ventricular arrhythmia that can cause the feeling of a "skipped beat" in the chest; they are typically benign in people without structural heart disease. PVCs are fairly common and are estimated to affect 1–4% of the general population, but they are much more common in the elderly, with a prevalence of 69% in individuals older than 75.[29,30]

Common causes of PVCs include electrolyte imbalance (eg, low levels of magnesium or potassium), ingestion of stimulants (eg, coffee), alcohol, and/or exercise.[31,32] While PVCs are typically asymptomatic, they can sometimes cause signs and symptoms such as palpitations, chest pain, and heart failure. However, in the absence of structural heart diseases, PVCs rarely develop into serious arrhythmias.[29–31]

- **PVC-induced cardiomyopathy.** PVC-induced cardiomyopathy is a condition in which the heart becomes enlarged and unable to pump blood efficiently due to very frequent PVCs. This condition is a diagnosis of exclusion (ie, any underlying heart disease causing frequent PVCs must first be ruled out). A treatment called *catheter ablation* is performed in patients with over 10 000–20 000 PVCs in a 24-hour period. This procedure involves using electrical impulses or extreme cold to destroy the abnormal heart tissue that is causing the PVCs; the intervention usually stops the PVCs.[2,30,33]

## Supraventricular Arrhythmias

Supraventricular arrhythmias start in the atria or in the atrioventricular node. Types of supraventricular arrhythmia include atrial fibrillation, atrial flutter, paroxysmal supraventricular tachycardia, and Wolff-Parkinson-White (WPW) syndrome.[2,28]

**Atrial fibrillation.** Atrial fibrillation is a common type of serious arrhythmia.[4] The incidence of atrial fibrillation increases with age, with 0.1% of individuals under 55 years and approximately 10% of those over 80 being affected.[11,34] Postoperative atrial fibrillation, a common form of atrial fibrillation, occurs in 25–40% of patients following cardiac surgery.[35]

Atrial fibrillation involves the fast and irregular contraction of the atria. In atrial fibrillation, the heart's electrical signals are not initiated in the SA node; instead, they start in another part of the atria or in the nearby pulmonary veins. As the electrical signals do not travel along the normal path, their spread throughout the atria occurs in a rapid and disorganized way. This causes the atria to fibrillate (quiver in an abnormal manner), and blood is not pumped into the ventricles the way it should be.[4] Atrial fibrillation is usually not life-threatening, but can be dangerous if it causes the ventricles to beat very fast.[4]

Atrial fibrillation has 2 major potential complications—*ischemic stroke* and *heart failure*.[4,36,37]

- **Ischemic stroke.** Ischemic stroke may develop due to the incomplete emptying of blood from the atria, which facilitates the formation of blood clots within the heart. These clots, if they travel to the brain, may cause an *ischemic stroke*. Anticoagulant medications (eg, warfarin [Coumadin®]) are typically used as a stroke-prevention strategy for patients with atrial fibrillation.

- **Heart failure.** Heart failure may occur if the heart is unable to pump enough blood to the body. This occurs if the ventricles do not completely fill with blood.

**Atrial flutter.** Atrial flutter, another common pathologic supraventricular tachycardia, occurs much less frequently than atrial fibrillation. Atrial flutter differs from atrial fibrillation in that the electrical signals move through the atria with a fast, but regular rhythm. Symptoms and complications of atrial flutter are similar to those of atrial fibrillation.[4,38]

**Paroxysmal supraventricular tachycardia.** Paroxysmal supraventricular tachycardia (PSVT), the most common supraventricular tachycardia, refers to a fast heart rate that occurs from "time to time." Symptoms of PSVT may begin and end suddenly. In PSVT, electrical signals can be transmitted in the reverse direction from the ventricles to the atria, causing extra heartbeats. PSVT may occur as a result of toxicity due to the medication digitalis, or in association with conditions such as WPW syndrome.

- **Wolff-parkinson-white syndrome.** WPW syndrome is a type of PSVT wherein the electrical signals travel along an extra pathway from the atria to the ventricles, thereby disrupting the timing of the signals and causing rapid beating of the ventricles. While WPW can be life-threatening, other types of PSVT are typically not life-threatening and can occur without symptoms.[28,38,39]

## Ventricular Arrhythmias

Ventricular arrhythmias are initiated in the ventricles and represent the most common cause of sudden cardiac death. They can be life-threatening and require emergency medical care. Normally, these arrhythmias occur in patients with structural heart problems, but they may sometimes occur in patients who lack evidence of cardiac disease.[40]

**Ventricular tachycardia.** Ventricular tachycardia is a fast (>100 beats/minute) but regular beating of the ventricles that can last from a few seconds to much longer. While mild episodes may not be life-threatening, continued ventricular tachycardia that lasts for more than a few seconds is dangerous and may evolve into ventricular fibrillation, which can be fatal.[4,31] It is important to keep in mind that individuals with ventricular tachycardia may sometimes have minimal symptoms.[2,31,41,42]

**Ventricular fibrillation.** As its name suggests, ventricular fibrillation (v-fib) makes the ventricles quiver due to disorganized electrical signals. When this happens, the heart is unable to pump blood to the body and death may occur within minutes. V-fib is treated by using a machine known as a "defibrillator" to deliver an electrical shock to the heart and restore its normal rhythm.[4]

## Bradyarrhythmias

Bradyarrhythmia, or slow heart rate, is defined in adults as a heart rate of less than 60 beats per minute. This may cause insufficient blood to reach the brain. Except for certain individuals, such as people who are very physically fit, in whom a slower heart rate can be normal, bradyarrhythmias may occur as a result of serious medical conditions (eg, heart attacks), medication(s) (eg, beta-blockers and calcium-channel blockers), hypothyroidism, and electrolyte imbalances in the blood.[4]

# SYMPTOMS OF ARRHYTHMIAS

Approximately one-third of people with arrhythmia do not exhibit any symptoms, preventing their timely diagnosis and treatment. For individuals who do have symptoms, these may include feelings of a racing or pounding heart, chest pain, shortness of breath, dizziness, lightheadedness, anxiety, fainting or near fainting, and reduced capacity to exercise, which can impair quality of life.[4,11] In some cases, symptoms can be dangerous and life-threatening, and may even lead to sudden cardiac death.[43]

---

## WHAT ARE PALPITATIONS?

Palpitations are sensations or feelings of a racing or pounding heart that may be felt in the chest, neck, or throat.[44] These may or may not be accompanied by an abnormal heart rhythm.[45] Typically they are harmless, and in up to 16% of cases no underlying cause can be found.[46,47] Palpitations can result from noncardiac causes such as anxiety, drug use, low blood sugar, electrolyte imbalance, or fever. Caffeine, alcohol, tobacco, and certain drugs can also lead to palpitations, as can panic attacks. Avoiding these triggers typically resolves the condition.[45,48]

When accompanied by dizziness or fainting, palpitations may indicate the existence of a more serious condition, such as tachyarrhythmia. However, most patients with arrhythmias do not report palpitations. Nonarrhythmia causes of palpitations include coronary heart disease and congestive heart failure.

An electrocardiogram can be used help determine the cause of palpitations. In cases where structural heart disease is absent, further monitoring of the heartbeat using a Holter monitor (instrument that records the heart rate over 24–48 hours) may be used to make a diagnosis.[46]

# CAUSES OF AND RISK FACTORS FOR ARRHYTHMIAS

## Conditions or Events That Affect the Heart

Arrhythmias are frequently associated with the following conditions or events that affect the structure or function of the heart.[2,3,31,32,49]

**Coronary artery disease.** The narrowing of arteries in coronary artery disease can lead to arrhythmias.[3,50–52]

**Congestive heart failure.** Congestive heart failure (deterioration of the heart's ability to pump blood) is associated with a high risk of sudden cardiac death from arrhythmia.[53,54]

**History of heart attack.** Some form of heart rhythm abnormality is present in over 90% of individuals who have had a heart attack.[31,55]

**Infectious myocarditis.** Infections that damage the heart (ie, infectious myocarditis) have been associated with some types of arrhythmia.[56,57]

**Cardiomyopathy.** A damaged or dysfunctional heart muscle (ie, cardiomyopathy) can cause arrhythmias.[58,59]

**Congenital heart defects.** Being born with certain heart malformations may lead to disturbances in the heart rhythm.[2,50,60]

## Indirect and Noncardiac Risk Factors for Arrhythmias

In addition to inherited and/or acquired structural/ functional heart problems, several other risk factors have well-established relationships with arrhythmias. These risk factors (such as cigarette smoking) may beget arrhythmias either by contributing to chronic structural or functional heart abnormalities over time, or temporarily altering the biochemistry of the body in such a way as to trigger a transient arrhythmia (such as from excessive intake of stimulants like caffeine).

**Imbalance of electrolytes.** Imbalanced blood levels of electrolytes such as sodium or potassium alter the excitability of the heart muscle and the conduction of the electrical impulses, and may lead to arrhythmias.[2]

**High blood pressure.** High blood pressure is thought to increase the thickness and stiffness of the left ventricular walls over time, which changes the way in which electrical impulses travel through the heart.[2]

**Obesity.** Obesity may increase risk of developing arrhythmia and lead to cardiac problems in several ways: it can affect the heart *indirectly*, by increasing lipid levels, blood pressure, and glucose intolerance; or *directly*, by increasing the blood volume, which elevates cardiac output and causes thickening of the heart muscle in the left ventricle.[61,62]

**Smoking.** The mechanisms that explain the link between smoking and arrhythmia are complex. It is thought that nicotine promotes the formation of excess fibrous tissue in the heart and increases susceptibility to stress hormones. Other constituents of tobacco smoke, such as carbon monoxide, along with oxidative stress, appear to play additional roles. Moreover, smoking causes coronary artery disease and chronic obstructive pulmonary disease, which independently predispose to arrhythmia.[63]

**Alcohol abuse.** Chronic alcohol use may lead to disease/dysfunction of the cardiac muscle and cause the heart to beat less efficiently.[2,64-66]

**Stress.** Acute emotional and psychological stress may trigger potentially deadly arrhythmias.[67-69]

**Diabetes.** Uncontrolled diabetes increases the risk of developing coronary artery disease and hypertension. In addition, episodes of low blood sugar may trigger arrhythmia.[2]

**Thyroid dysfunction.** Atrial fibrillation occurs in 10–15% of patients with hyperthyroidism, and low-serum thyroid stimulating hormone (TSH) concentrations are an independent risk factor for atrial fibrillation.[70,71]

**Stimulants.** Stimulants such as caffeine and certain prescription medications may lead to various types of arrhythmias. Certain illegal drugs, such as methamphetamine and cocaine, may lead to arrhythmias or sudden death due to ventricular fibrillation.[2,31]

**Oxidative stress.** Oxidative stress has been implicated in the development of ventricular tachycardia and fibrillation, particularly in situations wherein the blood supply to the heart is temporarily interrupted and then restored (eg, following a heart attack).[72]

**Performance sports.** Athletes are at increased risk for developing atrial fibrillation, a relatively common arrhythmia in the athletic community; it is more frequently seen in middle-aged than young athletes. Autonomic nervous system alterations, systemic inflammation, and increased atrial size are some of the factors thought to be involved.[73-75]

**Certain medications.** Certain medications including digoxin (Lanoxin®), tricyclic antidepressants, and antipsychotics can sometimes cause arrhythmias.[31] Other compounds that can induce arrhythmia are some antiemetics, antibacterial agents, anesthetics,

and bronchodilators. Even certain antiarrhythmia medications such as flecainide (Tambocor®), dofetilide (Tikosyn®), and sotalol (Betapace®) may induce or worsen other types of arrhythmia.[2,64-66]

# DIAGNOSIS

Cardiac arrhythmias can be diagnosed in a physician's office. By studying the characteristic wave pattern of a series of heartbeats, physicians can determine what kind of arrhythmia is present. The most common diagnostic tool is the electrocardiogram (ECG or EKG).[4]

Diagnosis may include one or more of the following tools.

## History and Physical Examination

The presence of heart disease or a history of heart disease, thyroid problems, or high blood pressure in the patient or in family members is associated with increased risk; family history of sudden death, diabetes, or other illness also increases risk.[4] Listening to the heart and measuring the rate and rhythm of the heartbeat, listening for heart murmurs, checking for swelling in the feet, and taking the pulse can all aid in the diagnosis of arrhythmias.[3]

## Electrocardiogram (ECG or EKG)

The ECG is a test that detects and records the heart's electrical activity.[2] An ECG may be performed at a doctor's office; however, if continuous monitoring is required, either a portable or implantable ECG monitor can be utilized.

**Portable ECG monitor.** If an arrhythmia is intermittent, a *portable ECG monitor* (eg, Holter monitor) that is attached to the patient may be employed. The Holter monitor can record the heart's electrical signals for 24–48 hours, after which the doctor may be able to detect the arrhythmia and reach a diagnosis.[46]

**Implantable loop recorder.** Another ECG monitoring method is an *implantable loop recorder*, a device that performs continuing ECG monitoring and can detect abnormal heart rhythms. The device is placed under the skin on the left chest area through minor surgery performed under local anesthesia. It can be used for as long as 12–24 months and allows prolonged continual monitoring.[4,76-78]

## Intracardiac Electrophysiology Study (EPS)

EPS is a procedure used to test the heart's electrical system. It is typically used in cases of serious arrhythmia to pinpoint the location and cause of the arrhythmia and to plan the therapeutic strategy. EPS involves directing a thin, flexible wire through a vein in the upper thigh/groin or arm to the heart to record the heart's electrical signals.[4]

## Echocardiography

Echocardiography is a test that uses sound waves for the dynamic visualization of the heart and to observe the flow of blood. It can provide information about the size and shape of the heart and its chambers and valves, and it can identify heart areas that do not function normally (such as areas with poor blood flow, areas that are not contracting normally, or areas with previous injury).[4]

## Stress Test

Some arrhythmias are triggered or worsened by exercise, and certain heart problems are easier to diagnose when the heart is working hard. The stress test involves testing for arrhythmias while the patient is exercising on a treadmill or a stationary bicycle. In patients who have difficulty exercising, the test involves being injected with a drug, such as adenosine, to stimulate the heart to mimic exercise. Heart activity is monitored during the test.[2,4,79]

## Coronary Angiography

This procedure uses dye and x-rays to visualize the inside of the coronary arteries.[4]

## Tilt Table Test

This test is recommended in patients who have fainting spells. Heart rate and blood pressure are measured while the patient is lying flat on a table. Subsequently, the table is tilted, and the heart and nervous system are monitored during the change in the angle.[2]

## Blood Tests

Thyroid hormone and electrolyte levels may be measured as abnormal levels are associated with increased risk of arrhythmia.[4]

---

## ELECTROMECHANICAL WAVE IMAGING–A NOVEL DIAGNOSTIC TECHNIQUE

Electromechanical wave imaging (EWI) is a newer noninvasive technique based on ultrasound imaging that can map the electrical circuitry of the heart. Unlike previously available diagnostic techniques, EWI can detect minute changes/deformations in the heart and be performed with real-time feedback. Moreover, this technique is adaptable to already existing ultrasound imaging machines.[80]

A study conducted on mice demonstrated the feasibility of EWI use as a noninvasive technique to visualize the electrical circuitry of the heart and enable the early detection of arrhythmias.[81,82] Additional exploratory experiments showed that EWI may be viable for mapping heart rhythms in canines and humans.[82,83]

EWI technology may enable doctors to precisely evaluate arrhythmias in real time, diagnose them, and design treatments appropriate for each patient.[82]

---

# CONVENTIONAL TREATMENT STRATEGIES

Several strategies are available for treating arrhythmias, and the approach varies depending on the type of arrhythmia. For bradycardia, or slow heart rate, a pacemaker can be implanted to help ensure the heart beats quickly enough. Tachycardias (fast heart rate) and fibrillations (irregular heart rate) can be treated with medications to slow the heart rate. A procedure called *cardioversion* uses electrical current, either synchronized or unsynchronized (defibrillation) with the cardiac cycle, to treat abnormally fast heart rate (tachyarrhythmia) or uncoordinated and irregular electrical activity in the heart (fibrillation). Another treatment option involves *ablation* of portions of heart tissue from which improper electrical signals are originating. In addition, since atrial fibrillation increases ischemic stroke risk, anticoagulant medications such as warfarin (Coumadin®) or dabigatran (Pradaxa®) are used to prevent blood clot formation in people with this arrhythmia.[2,84,85]

This section will outline several arrhythmia treatment considerations.

## Vagal Maneuvers

It may be possible to stop an arrhythmia that begins above the ventricles by using vagal maneuvers that affect the vagus nerve, which is a part of the nervous system responsible for controlling the heartbeats. Some examples of these maneuvers, which often cause the heart rate to slow, include holding your breath and straining (Valsalva maneuver), dunking your face in icy water, and coughing; a physician may be able to recommend other maneuvers to slow down a fast heartbeat.[4]

## Medications

Arrhythmias can be treated with a variety of medications. The type of arrhythmia present and the unique characteristics of each patient determine which type of drug should be used and how. Because the clinical assessment of arrhythmias and the algorithm that physicians employ to determine the best pharmacologic treatment strategy is complex, this protocol will not discuss all of the specific roles of drugs in the various types of arrhythmias. Rather, we will outline the basic classification of drugs that may be utilized as part of pharmacologic arrhythmia management. Individuals with any type of arrhythmia should consult with a physician experienced in arrhythmia management to be properly evaluated and treated.

A classification method called the *Vaughan-Williams system* is widely used to categorize antiarrhythmic agents based on their effects on the electrophysiologic system of the heart. This classification system characterizes antiarrhythmic drugs as follows[86–88]:

**Class I agents: sodium-channel blockers.** Class I antiarrhythmic agents are further subclassified as class IA, IB, or IC agents depending on how strongly they block sodium channels. Examples of class I agents include procainamide (Procanbid®), disopyramide (Norpace®), and flecainide (Tambocor®).

**Class II agents: beta-adrenergic blockers or "beta-blockers."** Some common beta-blockers are carvedilol (Coreg®), metoprolol (Lopressor®), and propranolol (Inderal®).

**Class III agents: potassium-channel blockers.** Drugs in this class include sotalol (Betapace®), dofetilide (Tikosyn®), and ibutilide (Corvert®).

**Class IV agents: calcium channel blockers.** A few common drugs that fall into this category include amlodipine (Norvasc®), diltiazem (Cardizem®), verapamil (Calan®).

**Other agents** There are several antiarrhythmic drugs whose mechanisms are complex and/or not fully understood; they are usually grouped into this category. One frequently used drug that falls into this category is digoxin.[89]

It should be noted that the *Vaughan-Williams system* has some considerable limitations because some drugs—such as amiodarone (which is typically considered a class III agent) for example—exhibit actions characteristic of more than one Vaughan-Williams class.[11] Therefore, physicians cannot rely solely on classification of antiarrhythmic agents in this manner when determining the best drug strategy for each patient.

## NEWER ALTERNATIVES TO AMIODARONE: BUDIODARONE AND DRONEDARONE

*Amiodarone* (Cordarone®) is one of the most frequently used antiarrhythmic agents because it effectively treats potentially deadly ventricular arrhythmias; it is also used in the management of atrial fibrillation.[90,91] However, it can cause some serious side effects, including the development of fibrous tissue in the lungs and thyroid dysfunction.[92,93] Therefore, a drug capable of delivering similar efficacy with fewer side effects would be a promising antiarrhythmic agent.[94]

One reason that amiodarone can cause significant side effects is that it remains in the body for a long time (ie, it has a very long half-life) and can build up in tissues.[94,95]

*Budiodarone* and *dronedarone* (Multaq®) are similar to amiodarone in both chemical structure and mechanism of action. However, they are metabolized more quickly than amiodarone, potentially resulting in less tissue accumulation and side effects.[95] Dronedarone was approved by the Food and Drug Administration (FDA) in 2009 for atrial fibrillation and atrial flutter; budiodarone is still undergoing trials as of the time of this writing.[96,97]

Clinical trials and data analyses have shown that both of these new drugs have efficacy and side effect profiles comparable or superior (at least in some aspects) to amiodarone.

### Dronedarone

In a comprehensive analysis of data from four trials involving nearly 6000 subjects with atrial fibrillation, treatment with *dronedarone* significantly reduced stroke risk compared to placebo treatment.[98] In another analysis, this time grouping data from 39 atrial fibrillation treatment trials, dronedarone was again shown to reduce stroke risk and produce fewer arrhythmic events than amiodarone, and amiodarone was shown to be associated with a higher mortality rate than dronedarone. However, dronedarone was not as efficacious at preventing recurrence of atrial fibrillation as amiodarone.[99]

Dronedarone is associated with increased risk of cardiovascular death, stroke, and heart failure in patients with *permanent* atrial fibrillation (ie, those who cannot be converted to normal heart rhythm). Therefore, the FDA does not advise that doctors prescribe dronedarone to this population.[100]

### Budiodarone

In a 12-week study, patients with atrial fibrillation and a previously implanted pacemaker who stopped taking antiarrhythmic agents for a period sufficient to "wash out" the drug from their systems were treated with *budiodarone* for 12 weeks. In the group receiving the highest dose of the drug (600 mg twice daily), atrial tachycardia/atrial fibrillation was reduced by 74%.[97]

Although more studies are needed before dronedarone and/or budiodarone can be asserted as unequivocally superior or inferior to amiodarone, data thus far suggest that these agents may become an important treatment consideration for select arrhythmia patients.

## Electrical Cardioversion

In some cases of arrhythmia, cardioversion (ie, the process of delivering an external electrical jolt through the chest to the heart) may be utilized to reset the heart to its normal rhythm. The machine used to deliver the electrical current is called a defibrillator.[31,101,102]

## Ablation Therapy

Another technique often employed to treat arrhythmias is *catheter ablation*. This procedure involves the insertion of a thin wire catheter into a blood vessel in the groin, arm, or neck, which is then guided to the heart. Radiofrequency energy is then delivered through the wire to generate heat and destroy (ablate) small sections of tissue in the heart responsible for triggering the arrhythmia.[103] Other ablation techniques include application of extreme cold (ie, "cryoablation") or high-frequency ultrasound through the catheter to destroy the arrhythmogenic tissue.[104,105]

## Implantable Devices

Treatment for heart arrhythmias may also involve the use of an implantable device. Several types of such devices are currently available.

**Pacemaker.** A pacemaker is an implantable, battery-operated device that is used in cases of slow or irregular heart rate. Implanting a pacemaker involves surgically placing the device under the skin, near the collarbone. An insulated wire connects the device to the right side of the heart, where it is permanently anchored. In cases of slow or abnormal heart rhythms, the device emits an electrical signal that stimulates the heart to beat at a normal rate. The device typically remains in a "switched-off" mode when the heartbeat is normal.[3,106]

**Implantable cardioverter-defibrillator.** In ventricular fibrillation, which is a potentially life-threatening disorder, an implantable cardioverter-defibrillator (ICD) may be placed near the left collarbone, similarly to a pacemaker. The ICD does not turn off and monitors heartbeats continuously. It acts as a pacemaker in cases of bradycardia and sends high-energy electrical impulses to reset the heart in cases of ventricular fibrillation or tachycardia.[3,7,107]

## Surgical Treatments

In some cases, surgery may be the recommended treatment for heart arrhythmias.

**Maze procedure.** This procedure involves making surgical incisions in the atria, which heal into carefully placed scars that force cardiac electrical impulses to travel along a preset pathway and cause the heart to beat efficiently. The resulting scars form boundaries and create a "maze" for electrical impulse to travel along. Rather than using a scalpel, scars can be created by using a "cryoprobe" to apply extreme cold or a radiofrequency device that applies heat. Since this procedure requires open-heart surgery, it is typically reserved for patients who do not respond to other types of treatment.[2,108]

**Coronary bypass surgery.** Coronary bypass surgery or coronary artery bypass graft (CABG) is performed in cases of severe coronary artery disease with frequent ventricular tachycardia. This procedure may help improve the blood supply to the heart and reduce the frequency of ventricular tachycardia.[2]

---

# STROKE PREVENTION IN ATRIAL FIBRILLATION

A major potential complication of atrial fibrillation is ischemic stroke that occurs as a result of blood stagnating and clotting in the fibrillating atria. The blood clot can then travel to the brain and lodge in a blood vessel, causing an ischemic stroke. Therefore, anticoagulant medications, which reduce the likelihood of blood clots forming, are an important stroke-prevention strategy in patients with atrial fibrillation.[103]

Without anticoagulants, the rate of ischemic stroke in patients with atrial fibrillation is approximately 5% per year. With anticoagulant therapy, the rate of stroke is reduced to less than 1.5%.[103,109] The most commonly used blood thinners include warfarin (Coumadin®), clopidogrel (Plavix®), and aspirin. Standard recommendations, including those by the American College of Chest Physicians, state that patients with atrial fibrillation at a lower risk of stroke should be prescribed a dose of aspirin ranging from 75 to 325 mg daily while patients at high risk should be prescribed warfarin.[109] Warfarin has a narrow therapeutic index, which refers to a very small dose range in which it is effective as an anticoagulant. Below this range, the compound is ineffective, and above these levels it is extremely toxic; therefore, patients on warfarin must be closely monitored.[110] However, not all patients are suitable candidates for warfarin therapy, in which case aspirin and clopidogrel may be used together to reduce stroke risk; although this combination increases bleeding (hemorrhage) risk and is not FDA-approved for prevention of stroke in individuals with atrial fibrillation.[111]

Other anticoagulant drugs include dabigatran (Pradaxa®), apixaban (Eliquis™),[110] and rivaroxaban (Xarelto™), all of which inhibit components of the blood coagulation cascade. Dabigatran inhibits a coagulation factor called *thrombin*, while the other three are direct inhibitors of factor Xa, a component of the coagulation cascade.[112] Dabigatran has been approved for the prevention of stroke, and research has found 150 mg of dabigatran twice daily may be superior to warfarin for stroke prophylaxis.[113] Based on clinical trials, all three drugs—dabigatran, apixaban, and rivaroxaban—significantly reduced the occurrence of hemorrhagic stroke as compared with warfarin.[112] Only dabigatran reduced the occurrence of ischemic stroke as compared with warfarin, but the other 2 compounds performed as well as warfarin.[110,112]

Advantages of Pradaxa® versus warfarin include:

- Rapid onset of action.
- Predictable, consistent anticoagulant effects.
- Low potential for drug–drug interaction.

- No requirement for anticoagulant blood test monitoring.
- Preliminary efficacy and safety advantages versus warfarin based on initial head-to-head, hard-endpoint data.
- No need to maintain low vitamin-K levels. Insufficient vitamin K promotes arterial calcification.

Disadvantages of Pradaxa® versus warfarin include:

- No antidote for reversal of over-anticoagulation effect. When too much warfarin is given and the patient's INR (International Normalized Ratio) indicates they are at risk for a major bleed (or are pathologically bleeding), vitamin K can be injected to immediately reverse warfarin's anticoagulant effect. If too much Pradaxa® is taken, there is no immediate antidote.
- No long-term safety data on Pradaxa® (the case with virtually all newly approved drugs).
- More expensive than warfarin.

# ALTERNATIVE THERAPIES AND DIETARY AND LIFESTYLE CONSIDERATIONS

## Acupuncture

Acupuncture refers to a procedure involving stimulation of a variety of points on the body using needles that are inserted manually.[114] A study that enrolled 80 patients with persistent atrial fibrillation was conducted to evaluate whether acupuncture treatment had any effects on recurrence rates and whether it was able to prevent arrhythmias. After patients had their normal heart rhythms restored via cardioversion, they were treated with amiodarone (Cordarone®), acupuncture, sham acupuncture (a procedure wherein acupuncture needles are inserted into the "wrong" points), or given no treatment. The results revealed that recurrence rates were lower in the acupuncture group (35%) than the sham (69%) or control (54%) groups.[115] The recurrence rates in patients treated with amiodarone were 27%. Analysis of data from eight separate studies showed that 87–100% of participants converted to normal heart rhythm after acupuncture treatment.[116]

## Mediterranean Diet

The Mediterranean diet has been shown to provide cardioprotective effects. A study conducted in 2011 sought to study the relationship between this type of diet, vitamin intake, and the incidence of arrhythmias. The study recruited 800 subjects, 400 of which had detected their first episode of atrial fibrillation. Low adherence to this diet was associated with the development of atrial fibrillation, and high adherence with spontaneous conversion back to normal electrical impulses in the heart. While further studies in a larger population are required to corroborate these findings, high adherence to a Mediterranean diet may potentially prevent atrial fibrillation episodes.[117]

## Lifestyle Changes

Other lifestyle measures that may reduce risk of arrhythmia include[20,117,118]:

- Adequate exercise[101]
- Maintaining a healthy body weight[119,120]
- Quitting smoking[101,121]
- Cutting back on caffeine[101,119,122,123]
- Cutting back on alcohol[101,119,123]
- Reducing stress[101,124]
- Avoiding stimulant medications (eg, pseudoepinephrine)[101]

# TARGETED NATURAL THERAPIES

## Omega-3/Fish Oil

Omega-3 fatty acids are important health-promoting lipids found in certain fish and other seafood as well as specific plant sources.[125,126] Fish oil contains eicosapentaenoic acid (EPA) and docosahexaenoic acid (DHA), two important omega-3 fatty acids for health.[125]

Several studies have shown that moderate consumption of fish oils/omega-3 fatty acids is heart-healthy and provides protection against arrhythmias, including atrial fibrillation and ventricular arrhythmias.[20,125] The omega-3 fatty acids potentially act by stabilizing the electrical activity in the heart through reduction of the sodium and calcium currents inside heart muscle cells.[20] A large study enrolled 11 324 people within 3 months after having an acute myocardial infarction and treated them with an omega-3 polyunsaturated fatty acid (PUFA) supplement by itself, vitamin E by itself, an omega-3 PUFA supplement together with vitamin E, or placebo. This study showed that 850 mg of EPA and DHA supplementation provided various cardiovascular benefits, mainly due to their antiarrhythmic effects; this included reduced nonfatal heart attack and nonfatal stroke rates, as well as reduced cardiovascular death.[20] A similar reduction in ventricular arrhythmia-related events was also noted in a subgroup analysis of 1014 patients with clinically diagnosed heart attack and diabetes who were treated with a combination of DHA, EPA, and alpha linolenic acid (ALA; a plant-based precursor of EPA).[126] Perhaps the most significant effects of omega-3 supplementation have been observed in patients with atrial fibrillation.[125] A study published in 2012 analyzed plasma levels of various omega-3 fatty acids in a population of

3326 individuals without history of atrial fibrillation or heart failure. The results showed that higher levels of omega-3 fatty acids and DHA were associated with a lower risk of atrial fibrillation in older patients.[21] However, not all studies have confirmed the beneficial effect of fish oil supplementation for the treatment of arrhythmias.[20,125,127] Additionally, caution should be exercised in patients with implantable defibrillator, as some studies show that there may be a slightly higher risk of sudden death in patients with an implantable defibrillator who are treated with fish oil supplements.[128,129]

## Magnesium and Potassium

As both magnesium and potassium are intricately involved in the heart's electrical stability, maintaining normal functional blood levels and ratios of each of these ions is important. Low concentrations of magnesium and potassium in the body are associated with increased risk of developing ventricular arrhythmias.[130]

**Magnesium.** Magnesium deficiency may result in congestive heart failure, hypertension, and angina.[17] The American Heart Association recommends administering magnesium sulfate intravenously (up to 2 g in 2 minutes) to treat some types of ventricular tachyarrhythmia. Oral magnesium oxide (15 mg/kg) added to a regimen of beta-blockers helped to improve some markers of imminent ventricular tachyarrhythmia, even in cases where the beta-blockers failed to make a difference on their own.[18] Additionally, oral magnesium (3 g daily for 30 days) improved symptoms of premature ventricular and supraventricular complexes in 93.3% of patients taking magnesium as compared with only 16.7% of patients administered placebo.[19]

**Potassium.** Potassium is important for the maintenance of cardiac electrical stability, and alterations (deficiency or excess) in serum potassium levels, such as can be induced by diuretic drugs, can contribute to the development of cardiac arrhythmias.[131-133] Assessing potassium levels via blood testing and increasing potassium intake via supplementation if levels are found to be low is an arrhythmia treatment consideration. In a study that enrolled 170 patients with symptomatic persistent atrial fibrillation, pretreatment with intravenous potassium/magnesium improved the success rate of achieving conversion to a normal heart rhythm.[130]

## Hawthorn

Hawthorn is a fruit-bearing shrub whose constituents have been used since the 1800s to support cardiovascular health.[134] Modern scientific inquiry has shown that hawthorn is rich in several antioxidant compounds such as flavonoids and anthocyanins, and that it may play a supportive role in several cardiovascular diseases.[134-136] It is thought that hawthorn supports heart and vascular health via modulation of ion (eg, potassium and calcium) channels, blood flow, inflammation, and oxygen utilization, as well as by scavenging damaging free radical molecules, which cause oxidative stress.[135,137]

In an animal model, infusions of hawthorn extracts reduced the number of arrhythmias compared to a control infusion following experimental deprivation and subsequent reinstitution of blood supply to the heart ("ischemia/reperfusion"), a paradigm that mimics some of the effects of a heart attack.[138] In another similarly designed animal model, long-term supplementation with a standardized hawthorn extract was associated with 6-fold fewer incidence of potentially deadly ventricular fibrillation following deprivation and subsequent reinstitution of blood flow to the heart.[139] A 24-week human clinical trial involving over 1000 patients with heart failure found that hawthorn supplementation improved heart function and reduced symptoms such as fatigue and palpitations. Supplementation also increased the amount of time subjects' heart rhythms remained normal.[140]

## Antioxidants

Oxidative stress and inflammation have been implicated in the development of atrial fibrillation, and this is particularly true in the case of postoperative atrial fibrillation.[141] Various studies have attempted to determine the usefulness of antioxidants in the treatment of atrial fibrillation.[142]

**N-acetyl-cysteine.** The beneficial effects of N-acetyl-cysteine (NAC) treatment are attributed to its antioxidant and anti-inflammatory properties.[141] Since oxidative stress has been implicated as a factor in postoperative atrial fibrillation, various trials have tried to assess the effectiveness of N-acetyl-cysteine (NAC) in preventing the condition. An analysis of data from eight separate trials that included a combined population of over 500 patients concluded that NAC supplementation may effectively reduce the incidence of postoperative atrial fibrillation.[35] In a trial conducted to study the effects of NAC treatment on postoperative atrial fibrillation, intravenous infusion of NAC was compared to a group receiving saline infusion. Postoperative atrial fibrillation was found in only 3 patients from the NAC-treated group, as compared with 12 patients from the saline group.[141]

**Vitamins C and E.** Vitamins C and E may also exert a protective effect against postoperative atrial fibrillation by virtue of their antioxidant properties. An analysis of data from 5 clinical trials that examined a total of 567 patients demonstrated that vitamin therapy caused a significant reduction in the incidence of postoperative atrial fibrillation and all-cause arrhythmia. This effect was independent of the type of surgery. There is also evidence of a synergistic effect between antioxidant vitamins and beta-blockers.[143] A separate study that enrolled 100 patients undergoing bypass surgery showed that a combination of oral vitamin C (2 g on the night prior to surgery and 2 g daily for 5 days thereafter) and a beta-blocker was more effective in preventing postoperative atrial fibrillation than the beta-blocker treatment alone. The incidence of postoperative atrial fibrillation was only 4% in the vitamin C group as compared with 26% in the control group.[144] Vitamin C treatment showed similar benefits in another study where a group of 44 patients receiving standard treatment following conversion to normal heart rhythm received either vitamin C or no additional treatment. Atrial fibrillation recurred in only 4.5% of the patients in the vitamin C group, as compared with 36.3% of the patients who did not receive any treatment.[145] Similarly, preoperative treatment with vitamin E for 28 days followed by vitamin C on days 27–29 reduced the incidence of arrhythmias in a group of 37 patients undergoing bypass surgery.[142]

**Resveratrol.** Resveratrol is a polyphenol found in grapes and Japanese knotweed (*Polygonum cuspidatum*) with antioxidant and anti-inflammatory properties. An animal model revealed that resveratrol can attenuate inflammatory responses and oxidative stress after myocardial infarction, which can lead to decreased inducibility of ventricular arrhythmias.[146] A preclinical study revealed that resveratrol treatment significantly suppressed myocardial infarction-induced ventricular arrhythmias and improved long-term survival. Resveratrol acts by a variety of mechanisms, and exerts its effects in a concentration-dependent manner, by inhibiting the calcium current, which reduces the intracellular calcium overload, or opening certain potassium channels.[147,148]

**Coenzyme Q10.** Coenzyme Q10 (CoQ10) is a powerful antioxidant and an important component of cellular energy production. A number of studies have revealed a therapeutic role for CoQ10 in conditions of impaired cardiac function, such as heart failure.[13,14] Animal data have shown that CoQ10 can exert powerful antiarrhythmic action following deprivation and subsequent reinstitution of blood flow to the heart.[15] Several clinical trials have revealed that CoQ10 possess antiarrhythmic action in situations of impaired cardiac function or metabolic disease such as type 2 diabetes. In a trial involving 27 diabetic individuals, CoQ10 supplementation was found to be beneficial in reducing premature ventricular contractions.[149] A trial involving 2500 heart failure patients found that 3 months of supplementation with 50–150 mg of CoQ10 daily was associated with an improvement in arrhythmia signs and symptoms in 62% of subjects.[16] Another trial evaluated the effects of CoQ10 supplementation (150 mg daily) for 7 days preceding scheduled coronary artery bypass grafting (CABG) procedures in 40 subjects who were divided to receive CoQ10 or act as a control group. Following CABG, CoQ10 supplementation was associated with lower markers of oxidative stress and significantly lower incidence of potentially deadly ventricular fibrillation.[150] In a controlled clinical trial among 144 subjects who had a heart attack, 28 days of supplementation with 120 mg of CoQ10 daily was associated with a 2.6-fold reduction in occurrence of arrhythmias. Moreover, subjects receiving CoQ10 also exhibited less evidence of oxidative stress, and levels of other antioxidants such as vitamins A, C, and E increased to a greater degree following heart attack in the group who received CoQ10 than those who received placebo.[151]

## Rhodiola

Rhodiola reduced the incidence of ventricular arrhythmias and increased the ventricular fibrillation threshold in an animal model of heart attack.[152] Preclinical research suggests the antiarrhythmic effect of rhodiola may be due to activation of opioid receptors.[153] Experimental preclinical research has demonstrated pretreatment with rhodiola improved several measures of heart cell health following induced ischemic injury.[154]

## Life Extension Suggestions

- **Vitamin D:** 5000–8000 IU daily; depending upon blood levels of 25-OH-vitamin D
- **N-acetyl-cysteine (NAC):** 600–1800 mg daily
- **Trans-Resveratrol:** 250 mg daily
- **Vitamin C:** 1000–2000 mg daily
- **Vitamin E:** 400 IU with at least 200 mg gamma-tocopherol daily
- **CoQ10 (as ubiquinol):** 200–400 mg daily
- **Fish oil (with olive polyphenols):** providing 1400 mg EPA and 1000 mg DHA daily

- **Potassium:** 99 mg daily (or more) when instructed to do so by a health care professional, based on blood test results
- **Magnesium:** 140 mg daily as magnesium-L-threonate plus 320 mg daily as magnesium citrate
- **Calcium:** 600–1200 mg daily
- **Hawthorn extract:** standardized to 60–300 mg daily of oligomeric polyphenols
- **Rhodiola extract** (root), standardized to 3% rosavins (7.5 mg): 250 mg daily

In addition, the following *blood tests* can provide helpful information:

- Vitamin D, 25-Hydroxy
- Chemistry panel (includes potassium levels)

- Red blood cell (RBC) magnesium
- Omega Score®

## REFERENCES

References available at: www.lef.org/dpt5/ch11

# 12

# Arthritis— Osteoarthritis

Osteoarthritis is a very common degenerative joint disease and a leading cause of disability. Affecting over 20 million in the United States alone, this progressive disease is characterized by structural damage and functional impairment within joints.[1-6]

Many interrelated factors—such as *obesity* and *oxidative stress*—work together in osteoarthritis to cause progressive, degenerative changes in weight-bearing joints including the knees, neck, lumbar spine, and hips, as well as the hands. A multifactorial approach is best when targeting osteoarthritis management.[7, 8]

Conventional medical treatment focuses on reducing load (eg, weight loss) and improving joint support (ie, enhancing muscle strength), as well as treating the pain and stiffness of osteoarthritis with acetaminophen and other non-steroidal anti-inflammatory drugs (NSAIDs).

However, these drugs expose arthritis sufferers to the risks of *liver and kidney damage*.[9] In addition, these drugs often offer only *incomplete/partial* relief,[10, 11] and treatment with acetaminophen and NSAIDs fails to help the body rebuild damaged joint cartilage.[12]

On the other hand, natural compounds like *undenatured type-II collagen* and *methylsulfonylmethane* (MSM) modulate fundamental aspects of osteoarthritis pathology, while others such as *krill oil* and *Boswellia serrata* target novel inflammatory pathways that can contribute to pain, swelling and joint degradation.[13-19]

Upon reading this protocol, you will learn about the critical medical factors of osteoarthritis, as well as learn about some *underappreciated, yet potentially dangerous side effects* of drugs often used to treat osteoarthritis pain. Additionally, you will discover several natural treatment strategies that have been shown to help support joint structure and function to provide *more* than just pain relief.

## UNDERSTANDING OSTEOARTHRITIS

### Normal Joint Anatomy and Function

The bones of the human skeletal system are connected by a complex series of joints, which connect two or more bones and allow for a wide variety of movements that would otherwise be impossible.[20]

In order to facilitate smooth joint movement, the surfaces of joints are lined by a low-friction, load-distributing, wear-resistant tissue called *articular cartilage*, which is composed of 65–80% water, collagen (fibrous proteins), proteoglycans, and chondrocytes (cells that produce cartilage).[21] In adults, damaged cartilage has a very limited capacity for self-healing due to blood supply limitations, and the relatively poor capacity of resident chondrocytes to migrate and proliferate.[22]

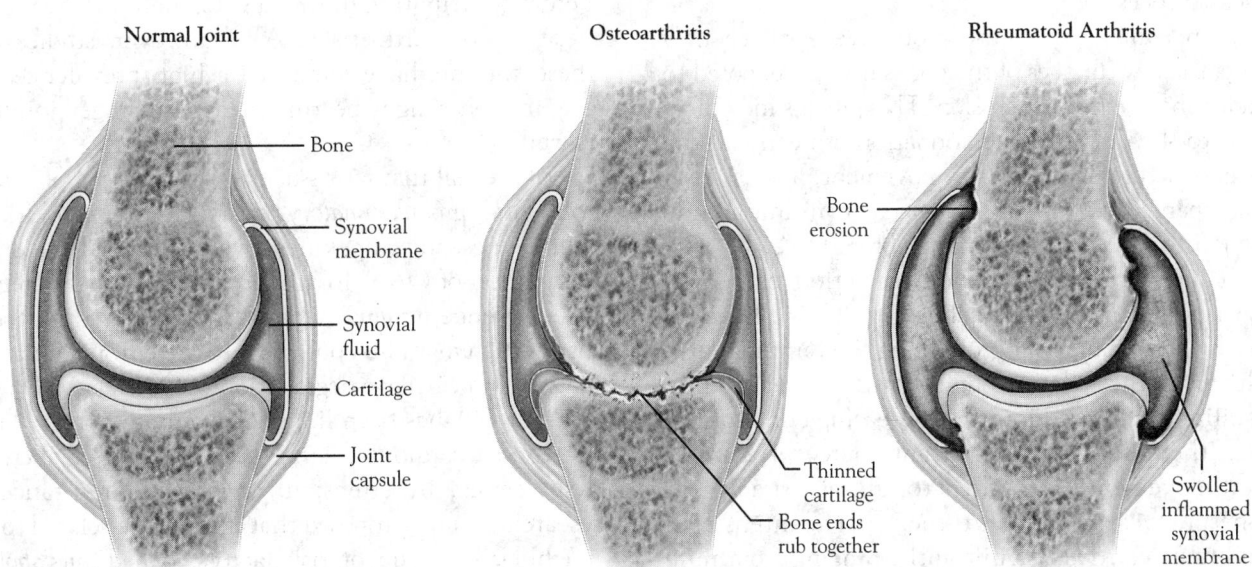

**Joint Anatomy**

Joints can be classified as synovial, fibrous, or combination joints, based on the presence or absence of a synovial membrane and the amount of motion that occurs in the joint.

Synovial joints allow a significant amount of motion and are composed of the following:

- Articular cartilage
- Subchondral bone
- Synovial membrane
- Synovial fluid
- Joint capsule

Normal articular surface of synovial joints consists of articular cartilage that protects the underlying subchondral bone by distributing large loads, maintaining low contact stresses, and reducing friction.

Synovial fluid supplies nutrients to the articular cartilage; it also absorbs shock from slow movements, as well as the elasticity required to absorb shock from rapid movements.

## Osteoarthritis Onset and Progression

Osteoarthritis (OA) can occur in any freely moving joint in the body, but it most commonly affects load- and stress-bearing joints like the knees, lumbar spine, and hips.[5]

At the onset of OA, where cartilage cells depart from their normal pattern of growth and differentiation, the outermost layer of articular cartilage begins to soften as its protein structure degrades. As OA progresses, this loss of protein content becomes more rapid, affecting deeper and deeper layers of cartilage.[21] Eventually, the entire protective layer of cartilage is destroyed as the chondrocytes become completely overwhelmed and unable to reverse the tissue damage.

Because cartilage does not contain free nerve endings, joint destruction is typically not associated with pain until it is considerably advanced. This is a major reason why OA tends to be diagnosed so late in the disease process.[11,23]

With a majority of the protective cartilage now gone, the raw surfaces of the bones become exposed to gradual bone-on-bone erosion. This process inevitably leads to the destruction/deformation of nearly all the joint structures involved in movement, and is often accompanied by *chronic inflammation* in and around the joint space (ie, synovial membrane).[21]

In many cases, the bone destruction caused by OA is followed by "remodeling," which is characterized by bone spurs that grow along the joint margins. Although these bony outgrowths are believed to stabilize the injured joint by increasing bone surface area, they are also a significant source of pain, as joint movement causes them to rub against adjacent bones, nerves, and/or soft tissue.[21,24] The intensity of symptoms can vary significantly, ranging from mild to severe.[25]

The pain caused by OA is typically worsened upon physical activity. As the disease progresses, however, patients may begin to report pain even when resting. Complaints of stiffness tend to occur more frequently in the morning, and often resolve shortly after awakening. However, any period of prolonged inactivity can cause this stiffness, which is sometimes referred to as "inactivity gelling."[26]

In cases of advanced OA, patients often report both physical and psychosocial disability. In fact, along with cardiovascular disease, OA causes more disability than any medical condition among the elderly.[27]

# OSTEOARTHRITIS CAUSES AND RISK FACTORS

Osteoarthritis (OA) arises as a result of a complex interplay of factors such as aging, mechanical forces, joint integrity, local inflammation, genetics, and congenital abnormalities.[11,28]

Risk factors for osteoarthritis include[4,8]:

- Advanced age
- Female gender
- Obesity
- History of physical labor
- High-impact sports
- Joint trauma
- Family history

## Obesity and Osteoarthritis

Because obesity increases the load and stress on many joints, it appears to be one of the most influential risk factors contributing to the development or advancement of osteoarthritis (OA).[8] However, studies of obese patients have identified a high prevalence of OA in non-weight-bearing areas (eg, finger joints) as well.[29]

Data reveal that fat tissue is a major source of catabolic and *proinflammatory mediators* (ie, cytokines, chemokines, and adipokines), which are implicated in the process of OA.[29] In addition, obese patients tend to experience *insulin resistance* and increased glucose load, which may also contribute to the chronic inflammation and cartilage degradation of OA.[30]

Since OA has been linked not only to obesity, but also other cardiovascular risk factors (eg, diabetes, dyslipidemia, hypertension, and insulin resistance), researchers have proposed that it might be related to a much larger group of risk factors, called "*metabolic syndrome*."[31,32]

Studies have shown that physical activity and diet programs (alone or in combination) are associated with a reduction in pain, as well as functional improvement among overweight or obese adults with OA.[33] In cases where patients are too obese to engage in physical activity, bariatric surgery has also been correlated with improvements in pain and function among patients with OA of the hip and knee.[34]

## Metabolic Factors Associated with Osteoarthritis

Several interrelated metabolic factors also contribute to osteoarthritis onset and progression, chief among which are *inflammation, mitochondrial dysfunction*, and *oxidative stress*.

- **Inflammation**—Osteoarthritis (OA), like many other age-related diseases, is tied to excessive inflammation.[35]

  Overindulgence in foods rich in proinflammatory *omega-6* fatty acids and insufficient intake of foods rich in anti-inflammatory *omega-3* fatty acids characterizes the dietary pattern of most modern, industrialized nations.

  *Arachidonic acid* (an omega-6 fatty acid) is the raw material used by the body to synthesize numerous inflammatory mediators, including *leukotriene B4, prostaglandin E2*, and *thromboxane A2*, all of which contribute to pain, swelling, and joint destruction.[36–38]

- **Mitochondrial dysfunction**—*Mitochondria* are the power cores of cells; they generate the energy that cells need to function. With age, mitochondrial function deteriorates, leading to a variety of negative consequences.[39–41]

  In the case of OA, *dysfunctional mitochondria* conspire with inflammation to augment joint destruction. One study found that the inflammatory propensity of chondrocytes was amplified when their mitochondria were dysfunctional. Specifically, mitochondrial dysfunction in chondrocytes is associated with increased reactive oxygen species production and activation of the "master-regulator" of inflammation, nuclear factor-kappa B (NF-κB).[39]

  Fortunately, adhering to a plant-based diet rich in dietary antioxidants, reduced in saturated fat, and balanced in omega-6 and omega-3 fats, such as the Mediterranean diet (see *Nutritional Interventions* section) may be an effective means of targeting several of the metabolic imbalances that affect OA.

- **Oxidative stress**—Oxidative stress, which is caused by *free radicals*, is known to be a factor in cartilage destruction and inflammation. These reactive molecules are also involved in pain perception.[42]

## HORMONES AND OSTEOARTHRITIS[46–55]

After the age of 50, more women are affected by osteoarthritis (OA) than men[11]; this female preponderance suggests that hormone abnormalities may influence the progression and development of the disease.[43]

The link between hormones and OA is further supported by evidence linking hormone (eg, estrogen) deficiencies to an increased risk of osteoarthritis.[44]

In addition, some evidence suggests that hormone replacement therapy can relieve symptoms of OA, especially among postmenopausal women.[45] As a result, Life Extension encourages OA patients to test for hormone deficiencies and correct them when identified.

Further information is available in the Female Hormone Restoration protocol.

## DIAGNOSIS

Osteoarthritis (OA) is diagnosed based on medical history and clinical examination.[8]

*Radiographic imaging* can aid in the diagnosis of OA. It involves the identification of a variety of anatomic abnormalities such as joint space narrowing, bone spurs, and joint bone deformity.[56] However, since many patients with joint abnormalities do not develop symptoms, a diagnosis of OA cannot be based solely on positive radiographic images. Likewise, patients with symptoms of OA may not display radiographic evidence.[11]

A newer method of imaging called delayed gadolinium-enhanced MRI of cartilage (dGEMRIC) provides information about cartilage quality and may offer an improved means of diagnosing OA in the early stages.[57] This method involves the intravenous injection of a negatively charged contrast agent, which then diffuses into articular cartilage over at least 2 hours. An increased concentration of contrast agent (in positively charged areas on the MRI scan) would be indicative of articular cartilage damage in that specific region.[58]

## CONVENTIONAL TREATMENT OPTIONS

Since there is no cure for osteoarthritis (OA), most available treatments are aimed at controlling pain and maintaining joint function.[12] If OA pain is unable to be controlled with less invasive measures like physical therapy and exercise, treatment options ranging anywhere from intermittent use of analgesics to total joint replacement surgery are available.[25]

## Physical Therapy/ Exercise

In most cases, osteoarthritis (OA) treatment should begin with the safest and least invasive therapies (eg, exercise).[59] This is because physical activity is associated with significant health benefits among OA patients (eg, preventing obesity, conserving physical function, and contributing to normal joint health).[60]

Exercise programs consisting of muscle strengthening and range-of-motion movements are associated with significant improvements in OA symptoms.[59] Similarly, aerobic activity can reduce pain and disability in people with OA of the knee.[61]

In patients who are either unable or unwilling to participate in vigorous exercise, walking for approximately 30 minutes per day, at least 3 days per week, can contribute to a reduction on OA symptoms.[62]

## Pharmacologic Treatment and Other Therapies

**Acetaminophen.** Acetaminophen is usually the first-line pharmacologic therapy in conventional medicine for osteoarthritis (OA).[9, 63] If acetaminophen is unsuccessful, the next pharmacological treatment level varies depending on patient-specific factors (eg, treatment success), but usually involves the use of one or more of the following options[63–65]:

- Topical nonsteroidal anti-inflammatory drugs (NSAIDs)
- Topical capsaicin
- Oral NSAIDs
- Intra-articular corticosteroid and hyaluronic acid injections
- Opioids

## THE POTENTIALLY LETHAL SIDE EFFECTS OF OVER-THE-COUNTER PAIN MEDICATIONS

In an effort to relieve suffering, many osteoarthritis (OA) patients turn to nonprescription over-the-counter (OTC) analgesics such as acetaminophen, aspirin, and other nonsteroidal anti-inflammatory drugs (NSAIDs).[66] However, since these drugs do not require a prescription, patients may incorrectly assume that they do not need to be as careful about safety as they would with a prescription analgesic. Therefore, it is important for patients to become educated about serious adverse side effects that can occur with popular nonprescription OTC analgesics.[67]

Acetaminophen is one of the most widely used analgesics in the United States. In 2008, approximately 25 billion doses of acetaminophen were sold in the United States alone.[68] Unintentional acetaminophen overdose is responsible for approximately 15 000 hospitalizations each year, and is the leading cause of acute liver failure in the United States.[9]

Patients taking acetaminophen should follow these recommendations[69]:

- Do not exceed a maximum dose of 4 g/day
- Remember that many prescription pain medications also contain acetaminophen.
- Recognize that acetaminophen is also called APAP, paracetamol, and acetyl-para-aminophenol.
- Do not use with other NSAIDs (without medical consultation), which increase the risk of kidney toxicity.
- Do not take with alcohol, which significantly increases the risk of liver toxicity.
- For those taking acetaminophen for pain relief, aggressive supplementation with hepato-protective nutrients such as *N-acetyl-cysteine* (NAC) and *milk thistle extract* may provide a means of reducing drug-induced liver damage.[70,71]

NSAIDs such as ibuprofen and naproxen are also associated with significant adverse effects such as gastrointestinal bleeding, peptic ulcer disease, high blood pressure, edema (ie, swelling), kidney disease, and heart attack.[72] For example, long-term use of NSAIDs can lead to impaired glomerular filtration, renal tubular necrosis, and eventual chronic renal failure by disrupting prostaglandin synthesis, which can impair renal perfusion.[73] Even in NSAID users without overt kidney dysfunction, subclinical irregularities in kidney function are often observed.[74]

Aspirin (a type of NSAID) is commonly used to treat minor aches and pains, as well as being recommended at low doses for heart protection and stroke prevention. Aspirin irreversibly inhibits an enzyme called cyclooxygenase-1 (COX-1) in platelets, which is why it poses a greater risk of bleeding (ie, hemorrhage) than other NSAIDs.[66] Therefore, patients taking aspirin should avoid the simultaneous use of anticoagulant drugs and/or alcohol (without talking to their doctor first). Aspirin can also cause mild side effects such as heartburn, nausea, vomiting, stomach ache, ringing in the ears, hearing loss, and rash.[2]

## NOVEL AND EMERGING THERAPIES

### Tanezumab

Tanezumab is an antibody that targets nerve growth factor (NGF), which plays a significant role in pain transmission.[75] Among patients with osteoarthritis (OA) of the knee, tanezumab was associated with a significant reduction in pain intensity.[76] However, in June 2010, the Food and Drug Administration (FDA) put all trials of tanezumab on hold because a significant number of patients taking this drug experienced an unusually rapid progression of joint bone necrosis.[77] Some researchers claim this bone necrosis occurred because of overuse of the joint (due to the potent analgesic effect of tanezumab). However, the

FDA is waiting for more information on the exact cause of this adverse effect before allowing trials to continue.[72-78]

## Stem Cells

*Autologous stem cell transplantation, which utilizes stem cells extracted from one's own body, as opposed to an embryo,* might *reverse* painful joint deterioration caused by *osteoarthritis* (OA). It involves using undifferentiated cells that can develop into almost any tissue— *new* cartilage, tendons, ligaments, and even bone—to replace damaged, arthritic joints.[79]

Unlike embryonic stem cells, mesenchymal stem cells (MSCs) have already differentiated to some extent, "committing" to develop into tissues such as bone, muscle, tendon, ligament, and cartilage. They can be found in abundance in bone marrow. Under the proper conditions, MSCs can be induced to *differentiate* into each of their potential specific tissue types, making them ideal for implanting into damaged joints and bones.[80]

By using MSCs from your own body (autologous), there is no risk of transplant rejection. There is even evidence that transplanted MSCs exert *anti-inflammatory, immune-modulating* influences within the joint.[81,82] This means they can theoretically outperform more traditional transplants, which run the risk of destruction by inflammation.

Two seminal reports presented the results of an early human case-report—an individual with a long history of chronic knee pain that proved unresponsive to surgery.[79,83]

The patient underwent successful harvest, expansion (through platelet-derived tissue factors), and transplant of his own MSCs into his damaged knee joint. The results were compelling—just 1 month after the injection the patient's cartilage surface had expanded by approximately 20%, a gain that was maintained at 3 months. The meniscus (cartilaginous tissue that provides structural support) was nearly 29% larger in volume at 3 months, indicating vigorous growth and remodeling of previously damaged tissue. The patient's pain level decreased as well.

## Apitherapy

Apitherapy, the use of bee venom for medicinal purposes, including relieving joint pain, can be dated back to at least the 5th century BC.[84] More recently, there have been numerous anecdotal reports of bee stings dramatically improving symptoms of OA.[85] Bee venom, when combined with acupuncture for the treatment of OA of the knee, was associated with a substantial analgesic effect compared to traditional (needle-only) acupuncture.[86] Researchers believe that the anti-inflammatory characteristics of bee venom can be attributed to mellittin, a component of bee venom that is one hundred times stronger than the inflammation-reducing hormone cortisone.[84]

# NUTRITIONAL INTERVENTIONS

Targeted nutritional interventions contain a variety of biologically active compounds known to positively influence cartilage degradation in osteoarthritis (OA). Unlike medications, nutritional interventions do not typically cause side effects, which may explain why nearly 1 out of every 5 OA patients uses alternative methods.[87]

## Joint Structure Support

**Glucosamine**—Glucosamine is a component of larger compounds called *glycosaminoglycans* and *proteoglycans,* which help trap water in the matrix of cartilage, providing it with the flexibility and resilience it needs to function properly.[88] In laboratory models, glucosamine has been shown to possess both anti-inflammatory and disease modifying effects in OA.[89] In addition, researchers believe that glucosamine may repair cartilage by stimulating synthesis of chondrocytes.[90] Glucosamine also plays a crucial role in maintaining joint lubrication.[88]

Commercial glucosamine preparations consist of either glucosamine *hydrochloride* or glucosamine *sulfate.*[91] When compared to placebo, high-quality clinical data indicate that glucosamine sulfate is superior for relieving the severity of OA symptoms.[92]

Although there remains some controversy in the conventional medical community over the effectiveness of glucosamine for osteoarthritis, most published studies show that glucosamine sulfate is effective and studies that have found otherwise have been limited by methodological flaws and dosing/ formulation inconsistencies.[11,89] Since glucosamine offers promise as structural support in osteoarthritis, additional research is planned.[4]

Because cartilage takes time to synthesize, and glucosamine is only one of its structural components, experts recommend up to 8 weeks of initial therapy before making an assessment concerning efficacy.[88]

**Chondroitin**—Chondroitin, which is a structural component similar to glucosamine, is believed to help in the management of OA due to its ability to maintain viscosity in joints, stimulate cartilage repair, and attenuate cartilage destruction.[14] Chondroitin has been shown to improve hand pain and stiffness in OA patients.[93] In addition, clinical trials have shown that chondroitin may have structure-modifying effects on OA of the fingers, as well as the knee.[94,95] Much like glucosamine, chondroitin has a delayed mode of action, thus requiring 2–3 weeks for therapeutic response.[94]

**Hyaluronic acid**—Hyaluronic acid (HA) is secreted by chondrocytes and used as a basic building block for cartilage synthesis. Researchers believe that HA is useful in the management of OA because it interferes with pain mediators and decreases the production of key enzymes (ie, metalloproteinases) responsible for digesting and destroying healthy cartilage tissue.[15] Hyaluronic acid intra-articular injections are used to treat OA of the knee. It has been linked to improvements in pain and functional status among OA patients,[96] especially when combined with other treatment strategies.[15]

Hyaluronic acid is typically administered intra-articularly; however, HA is absorbed orally much more efficiently when formulated with a phospholipid.[97]

Findings from an experimental trial show that orally administered hyaluronic acid improved the prognosis of horses that underwent joint surgery. In a blinded, placebo-controlled experiment involving 48 thoroughbreds, 30 days of postoperative use of oral hyaluronic acid significantly improved outcomes.[98, 99]

In a randomized, placebo-controlled, double-blind study of 20 human patients with OA of the knee, subjects received 80 mg of a specially formulated, orally ingested hyaluronic acid supplement called Hyal-Joint™ or a placebo daily for 8 weeks. The treatment group had a greater magnitude of improvement in bodily pain and social functioning.[100]

**Sulfur Compounds**—Sulfur containing compounds, such as *methylsulfonylmethane* (MSM), are commonly found in fruits, vegetables, and grains, as well as the human body.[101] Experts believe that these compounds may reduce peripheral pain and inhibit the degenerative changes of OA by stabilizing cell membranes and scavenging free radicals that can lead to inflammation. In clinical trials, MSM was able to reduce both pain and swelling among OA patients. It is well tolerated and not associated with any significant side effects.[16] Another study found that patients with OA of the knee taking MSM for 12 weeks demonstrated an improvement in pain and physical function.[102]

*Keratin* is another sulfur-rich compound[103] that supports joint health by supplying building blocks for joint repair, stimulating antioxidant enzymes, and acting as an antioxidant itself.[104,105] In a clinical evaluation, supplementation with solubilized keratin relieved OA pain more than placebo.[105]

**S-Adenosylmethionine**—S-adenosylmethionine (SAMe) is naturally occurring within the body and has been reported to possess both anti-inflammatory and analgesic effects. Clinical trials have shown that SAMe can reduce pain, stiffness, and increase functioning among patients with OA.[106,107] Moreover, SAMe has been found to be as effective—yet safer—than NSAIDs in the treatment of OA in some populations.[108] SAMe may achieve this by stimulating the production of cartilage through one of these potential mechanisms: modulating cellular growth/survival signals within joints, reducing inflammatory mediators, and/or increasing the production of antioxidants like glutathione.[109] SAMe is not found in food.[110]

## Anti-Inflammatory Nutrients

**Omega-3 Fatty Acids**—Omega-3 fatty acid supplementation is generally recommended for individuals consuming a typical Western diet (high in proinflammatory omega-6 fatty acids).[111,112] Increased levels of omega-6 fatty acids have been linked to the destruction of bone and cartilage among OA patients; supplementation with omega-3 fatty acids can combat this effect.[112] Omega-3 fatty acids have also been shown to reduce the amounts of certain proteins that are important in the pathology of OA.[113] In the clinical setting, the combination of omega-3 fatty acids with glucosamine was more effective at reducing morning stiffness and pain than glucosamine alone.[114]

**Krill**—Krill are cold water, shrimp-like crustaceans that are rich in omega-3 fatty acids.[115] In OA patients or those with related inflammatory conditions, supplementation with 300 mg of krill oil daily for 7 days reduced C-reactive protein (CRP)—a marker of inflammation—by more than 15% compared to placebo. By day 30, the reduction doubled to more than 30%. Additionally, 7 days of krill oil treatment reduced pain nearly 30%, stiffness more than 20%, and functional impairment almost 23%.[17]

**Undenatured Type-II Collagen**—Undenatured Type-II Collagen (UC-II) has received considerable attention as a therapeutic agent in OA.[116] Discoveries have revealed that gradual destruction of joints in OA leads to the exposure of joint collagen, which triggers an immune response that launches an autoimmune-like inflammatory attack on the joint.[117] UC-II functions as a "switch" to turn off this immune response. It does so by inducing what immunologists call specific oral tolerance—the desensitization of immune response to specific agents via an orally administered intervention.[118] Among OA patients, UC-II has been shown to significantly enhance daily activities and is not generally associated with any side effects.[116]

**Soy and Avocado Oil**—Avocado and soy unsaponifiable (ASU) mixtures may stimulate collagen synthesis and promote cartilage repair, as well as reduce circulating levels of proinflammatory cytokines, which are implicated in the pathology of OA.[119,120] A review of four clinical studies involving ASU treatments among OA patients found evidence for its use in reducing pain and improving function.[121] Among OA patients, ASU also significantly reduces the need to take NSAIDs.[122] ASU mixtures have been recommended by the American College of Rheumatology (ACR) and the European League Against Rheumatism (EULAR) for the symptomatic treatment of OA.[123]

**Curcumin**—Curcumin is a natural plant phenolic compound that has been shown to possess potent anti-inflammatory and antioxidant properties.[124] Research suggests that curcumin may represent a viable alternative to NSAIDs, and that it may complement the activity of some OA drugs.[125,126] Curcumin's effectiveness in OA may be due to its ability to attenuate nuclear factor kappa B (NF-κB) signaling, reduce the production of inflammatory mediators,[127,128] and interfere with cartilage destruction.[127] Curcumin has been recommended for the long-term complementary management of OA.[128,129]

**Ginger**—*Zingiber officinale* (ie, ginger) is related to curcumin. It has traditionally been used for a wide variety of medicinal purposes due to its antioxidant, antimicrobial, and anti-inflammatory properties.[130] Evidence suggests that ginger supplementation may reduce the subjective experience of pain, especially with respect to OA.[131] Clinical research has demonstrated that oral ginger extract can improve OA symptoms, and may be as effective as ibuprofen.[132] Interestingly, when applied topically in the form of a warm compress, ginger promotes relaxation and analgesia.[133]

**Boswellia**—*Boswellia serrata* is a tree commonly found in the hilly areas of India.[134] In the last two decades, the use of gum resins extracted from this tree has become popular among Western cultures.[135] This is because it is reported to possess beneficial anti-inflammatory, anti-arthritic, and analgesic properties.[134] Specifically, compounds in boswellia such as 3-O-acetyl-11-keto-ß-boswellic acid (AKBA) are inhibitors of the inflammatory enzyme 5-lipoxygenase (5-LOX).[136]

One of the first high-quality clinical studies involving the use of *Boswellia serrata* extract for the treatment of OA of the knee found that it was associated with a reduction in pain and swelling, as well as an improvement in function and range of movement. In addition, *Boswellia serrata* extract was well tolerated, and thus recommended for patients with OA of the knee.[137] A novel *Boswellia serrata* extract called Aflapin® has not only been shown to be clinically efficacious for reducing the symptoms of OA (eg, pain and function), but also appears to be able to fortify cartilage against damage and promote its repair.[18,19]

**Korean Angelica**—Decursinol is a medicinal compound found in the roots of the Korean flower *Angelica gigas Nakai* (Korean angelica).[45] It has been widely utilized in traditional Asian medicine as a treatment for pain associated with various conditions (eg, arthritis).[107] Laboratory evidence shows that an active constituent derived from Korean Angelica inhibits activation of nuclear factor-kappa B (NF-κB).[138] Decursinol may also act within the central nervous system to relieve pain.[139] One study found that co-administration of decursinol and acetaminophen resulted in synergistic pain-relieving effects. The authors of this study attributed the analgesic effect of decursinol to its ability to reduce the activity of the proinflammatory enzyme *cyclooxygenase*.[140]

**Proteolytic enzymes**—Numerous clinical studies have evaluated the efficacy of various preparations of proteolytic enzymes for conditions ranging from rheumatoid arthritis and muscular pain, to kidney disease and chronic airway disorders.[141,142] In one trial among 80 patients with OA of the knee, proteolytic enzymes were found to be as effective as the NSAID diclofenac for relieving pain and improving function.[143] Some early trials indicate that the proteolytic enzyme *bromelain* may be effective for relieving OA pain.[144]

One study reported that a supplement containing bromelain (90 mg, 3 times daily) was as effective as diclofenac (50 mg, twice daily) in improving the symptoms of osteoarthritis of the knee. Patients reported comparable reductions in joint tenderness, pain and swelling, and improvement in range of motion at the end of the study. The investigators found bromelain to be as good as diclofenac on a standard pain assessment scale and to be better than the drug in reducing pain at rest (by 41% for bromelain versus 23% for the drug), improving restricted function (by 10% for bromelain versus 0% for the drug), being rated by more patients in improving symptoms (24% for bromelain versus 19% for the drug), and being evaluated by more physicians as having good efficacy (51% for bromelain versus 37% for the drug). In summary, the investigators determined bromelain to be an effective and safe alternative to NSAIDs such as diclofenac for painful osteoarthritis.[145]

Experts generally advise consuming enteric-coated bromelain supplements to benefit from its anti-inflammatory effects.

**Vitamin D**—Vitamin D is a prohormone version of an important hormone called 1,25-dihydroxycholecalciferol or 1,25-dihydroxy vitamin D, also known as calcitriol.[146] Vitamin D, once converted into calcitriol, inhibits inflammation by regulating some of the genes responsible for producing proinflammatory mediators (ie, cytokines).[147] Evidence suggests that patients with osteoarthritis have lower blood levels of vitamin D than healthy controls[148]; this was especially true of younger osteoarthritis patients (ie, <60) in one study.[149]

Life Extension recommends routine vitamin D deficiency testing for all individuals with pain complaints. If vitamin D levels are low, vitamin D supplementation may result in significant improvements in pain.[150] Life Extension suggests that blood levels of 25-hydroxyvitamin D should be kept between 50 and 80 ng/mL for optimal health.

## Antioxidants

Oxidative stress is involved in OA-associated inflammation and pain.[7] Researchers have found that damaged human chondrocytes release free-radicals, which can exacerbate joint destruction.[150] Therefore, OA patients should maintain an adequate intake of antioxidants such as *astaxanthin* and *vitamin C*[151,152]; especially since antioxidant-deficient diets may increase the risk of OA.[153]

**Green Tea Extracts**—Epigallocatechin gallate (EGCG), the major and most biologically active component of green tea, was shown in an *in vitro* study to protect human chondrocytes from inflammatory damage.[154] This may be due to EGCG's ability to inhibit the expression of inflammatory mediators (eg, COX-2 and nitric oxide).[153] However, EGCG is only one of several green tea polyphenols (GTPs). A GTP mix has shown promise for managing symptomatic OA. An expert review on green tea's role in OA theorizes that GTP mixtures may be beneficial when used in combination with traditional OA treatments.[155]

## Additional Support

The following list of additional treatment options may be useful for managing the symptoms of OA.

- **Acupuncture**—Among OA patients, acupuncture is able to decrease pain levels and increase quality of life estimates. Experts believe that acupuncture achieves its analgesic effect by stimulating the body's natural opioid system and reducing the release of stress hormones.[88]

- **Boron**—Boron is an essential nutrient for healthy bones and joints. Evidence suggests that it is safe and effective for the treatment of OA.[156]

- **Niacinamide**—Niacinamide, a form of vitamin B3, has been shown to reduce inflammation, decrease consumption of anti-inflammatory medications, and increase joint mobility in OA patients.[157] One hypothesis suggests that it may have achieved these effects by modulating inflammatory pathways of joint destruction.[158]

- **Mineral Complex**—In a clinical study among OA patients, aquamin F (a seaweed-derived mineral mixture) was associated with an increased range of motion and walking distance. Its use in OA may also result in a decreased need for NSAIDs.[159] Most high quality *multivitamins* contain adequate concentrations of minerals.

- **Mitochondrial Support**—Resveratrol, and theoretically other nutrients that support mitochondrial health like *coenzyme Q10* (CoQ10) and *pyrroloquinoline quinone* (PQQ), may be able to ease inflammation and oxidative stress in chondrocytes. Mitochondrial dysfunction can increase inflammation in these cells, potentially impairing cartilage and joint function in OA.[39]

- **Topical Olive Oil**—In 2012, a 4-week-long clinical trial compared topical virgin olive oil to topical piroxicam, an NSAID, among 30 women aged 40–85 with osteoarthritis of the knee. From week 2 through 4, those randomized to the olive oil treatment reported less pain and greater physical function than those using piroxicam.[160]

- **Gamma Linolenic Acid**—GLA, a plant-derived omega-6 fatty acid, plays an important role in modulating inflammation throughout the body, especially when incorporated into the membranes of immune system cells.[161,162] It was noted that GLA regulates the inflammatory "master molecule" nuclear factor-kappa B (NF-κB), preventing it from switching on genes for inflammatory cytokines in cell nuclei.[163] While GLA has been shown to be effective among rheumatoid arthritis patients,[164] more research is needed to determine its effectiveness in OA.

## Life Extension Suggestions

### Joint Structure Support
- **Glucosamine sulfate**: 400–3200 mg daily
- **Hyaluronic acid** (as Hyal-Joint™): 40 mg daily
- **Methylsulfonylmethane** (MSM): 3000–6000 mg daily

- **Solubilized keratin**: 300 mg daily
- **Chondroitin sulfate**: 450–3600 mg daily
- **S-adenosylmethionine** (SAMe): 200–1200 mg daily in divided doses

## Nutrients to Ease Inflammation

- **Fish oil** (with olive polyphenols): providing 1400 mg EPA and 1000 mg DHA daily
- **Curcumin** (as highly absorbed BCM-95®): 400–800 mg daily
- **Boswellia serrata** (as highly absorbable Après-Flex™): 100 mg daily
- **Korean angelica extract** (as Decursinol-50™): 200 mg daily
- **Krill oil** (blended with astaxanthin and sodium hyaluronate): 350 mg daily
- **Ginger,** standardized extract: 150–300 mg daily
- **Undenatured type-II collagen (UC-II®):** 10 mg daily
- **Bromelain** (enteric coated): 500–1000 mg daily
- **Soy and avocado unsaponifiables**: per label instructions
- **Vitamin D**: 5000–8000 IU daily; depending on blood levels of 25-OH-vitamin

## Antioxidants

- **Green tea,** standardized extract: 725–1450 mg daily
- **Vitamin C**: 1000–2000 mg daily
- **N-acetyl-cysteine** (NAC): 600–1800 mg daily
- **Milk thistle,** standardized extract: 750 mg daily

## Additional Support

- **Multivitamin and mineral**: per label instructions
- **Capsaicin** (topical): per label instructions
- **Boron** (as calcium fructoborate as patented FruiteX B® OsteoBoron®): 1.5 mg daily
- **Gamma linolenic acid (GLA):** 300–600 mg daily
- **Pyrroloquinoline quinone (PQQ):** 10–20 mg daily
- **Coenzyme Q10** (as ubiquinol): 100–300 mg daily
- **Trans-resveratrol**: 100–500 mg daily

## REFERENCES

References available at: www.lef.org/dpt5/ch12

# 13

# Arthritis–Rheumatoid

Rheumatoid arthritis (RA) is a *systemic inflammatory disease* characterized by an *autoimmune response* that causes pain and disfigurement in peripheral joints. A dangerously underappreciated fact about RA is that it also significantly increases risk of *cardiovascular disease*. Because systemic inflammation hastens the onset of most age-related diseases, individuals afflicted with RA have a nearly 40% increased risk of *dying* compared to healthy people.[1–3]

Too often, conventional treatment strategies yield only marginal relief and fall pitifully short of mitigating the systemic risks that threaten the longevity of RA patients. Life Extension encourages both patients and physicians to view RA as a disease of the entire body, not just the joints. Initiating an aggressive cardiovascular risk reduction program should be as high a priority as relieving joint pain.

In this protocol, you will discover an advanced European drug delivery system that dramatically augments the efficacy and lessens the side effects of prednisone, a drug commonly used in the treatment of RA. You will also learn about *oral tolerance*—a unique, drug-free strategy that helps re-train the immune system to not attack the joints, as well as convenient blood tests and scientifically studied natural compounds that allow you to assess and target your cardiovascular risk.

## SYMPTOMS AND AFFECTED TISSUES

The prominent feature of RA is joint inflammation. Affected joints are usually swollen, warm, painful, and stiff. These symptoms typically worsen in the morning but, at least early in the disease process, can sometimes be eased by gentle movement. As the disease progresses, however, these symptoms often increase in severity until movement is severely impaired.

Inflammation associated with RA is systemic, meaning that it is not isolated to only those joints affected. RA tends to present symptoms in a symmetrical way. For example, if the joints of the right hand are inflamed, the joints of the left hand are likely to be inflamed as well.[4] While the hand and wrist joints are most often affected, other joints may be involved, including those of the feet and ankles, knees, hips, elbows, shoulders, and the cervical spine (ie, the neck).[5]

In general, the symptoms and severity of RA follow one of three patterns[6]:

- **Spontaneous remission:** The symptoms ultimately disappear, which occurs in <10% of patients with RA. This generally occurs only in patients whose blood tests are negative for a protein called rheumatoid factor (RF), an autoimmune mediator.

- **Relapsing/remitting disease:** The patient experiences periods of very severe symptoms called "flares," which are contrasted with episodes of mild or no

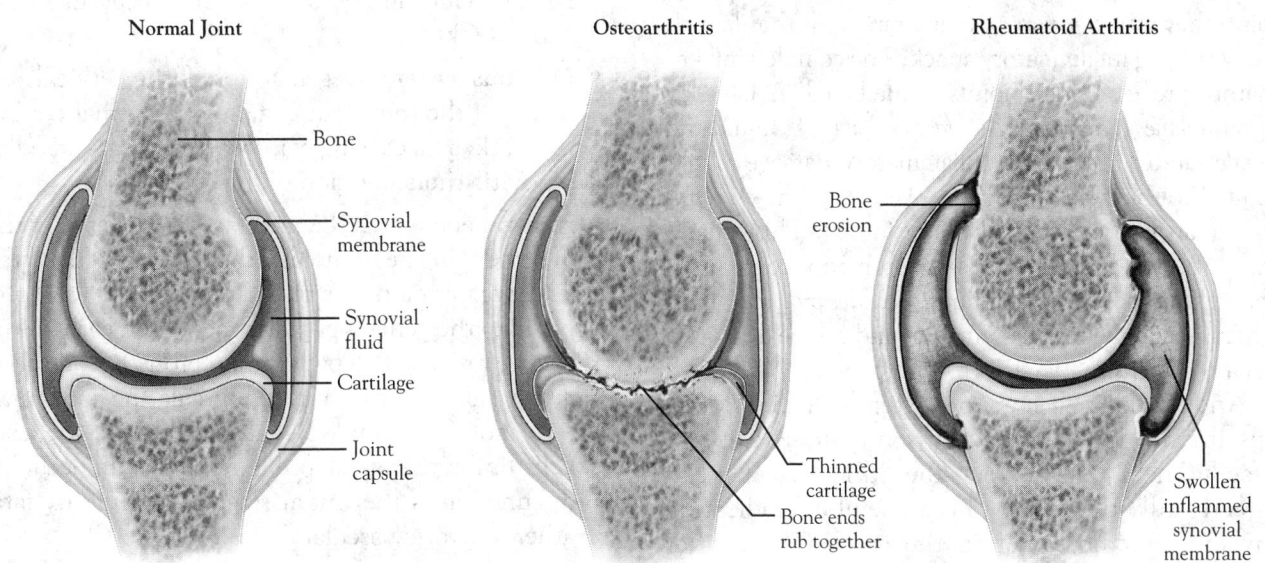

**Normal and arthritic joints**

symptoms. This pattern generally occurs early in the course of the disease.

- **Persistent and progressive disease:** Disease activity gets progressively worse. However, flares and periods of remission are not as dramatic as relapsing/remitting disease. This is the most common course of the disease.

During the course of the disease process, RA-mediated inflammation can cause permanent damage to several tissues in the body, especially the joints.[7]

# HOW AUTOIMMUNE INFLAMMATION DESTROYS JOINTS

In RA, the immune system mistakenly attacks healthy cells and tissues—predominantly the *synovium*, the soft tissue between the articular capsule (joint capsule) and the joint cavity of synovial joints. This immune mediated assault leads to the development of *pannus*, a destructive fibrous tissue within affected joints that erodes cartilage and exacerbates joint dysfunction.

RA damage is engendered by multiple components of the immune system, including *antibodies* and *killer T-cells*.

Antibodies are proteins secreted by *β-cells* that normally recognize and bind to invading microbes such as bacteria and viruses. By attaching to the invading microbe, they activate other components of the immune system to launch an inflammatory response, which destroys the cells.

In RA, antibodies mistakenly recognize "self" cells as invaders. Once antibodies attach to synovial cells in the joint, they attract a variety of immune cells that launch a devastating inflammatory attack. The complex inflammatory process within joints is mediated in large by the *cytokines tumor necrosis factor-alpha* (TNF-α) and *interleukin-6* (IL-6). The inflammatory damage is not limited to the synovium, but spills over to the *chondrocytes* (cartilage cells that cushion joints). This process raises the level of dangerous inflammatory compounds throughout the body, including *C-reactive protein* (CRP), which is a marker of inflammation and can be evaluated via a high-sensitivity CRP (hs-CRP) test.

Another kind of immune system cell that develops in the thymus and contributes to RA is the T-cell. One T-cell subtype—the "killer" T-cell—can directly kill other cells. This is useful in eradicating invading microbes, but in the case of RA, killer T-cells contribute to tissue damage by directly damaging joints and other affected organs.

An important pathological feature of arthritis is the exposure of *collagen* as a result of cartilage deterioration. When a joint is sufficiently damaged, collagen (a protein component of cartilage) becomes exposed to circulating immune cells, which attack it. This process promotes further inflammatory joint destruction.

Under normal circumstances, joint tissue can repair itself. However, joints may become permanently weakened and deformed if inflammation is severe, chronic, and occurs over many years as with RA.

## Inflammatory Damage Associated with Rheumatoid Arthritis Extends Beyond Joints

Once the immune system is activated against self-tissue, it sends inflammatory chemicals through the body resulting in widespread damage. For many patients it causes fatigue, malaise, and unexplained weight loss.

Other areas targeted by the immune system in RA can include the skin, lungs, eyes, blood, nervous system, heart, and bones. Signs and symptoms may include the following[4,5,8]:

- **Skin:** Nodules and ulcers on the surface of the skin occur in 50% of people with RA.[9]

- **Lungs:** RA may cause interstitial lung disease, resulting in a dry cough and shortness of breath that may worsen with physical activity; 20–30% of people with RA have some form of lung disease.[10]

- **Eyes:** Inflamed eyes are common and affect up to 25% of people with RA. Parts of the eye often targeted include the cornea, conjunctiva, and sclera (the white portion of the eye).

- **Blood:** Anemia and low iron levels often occur in RA and can cause fatigue, fast heartbeat, dizziness, and pale skin.

- **Nervous system:** Degeneration of the cervical vertebrae of the spine can compress the spinal cord in the neck area, causing pain on top of that caused by synovitis (inflammation of the synovium).

- **Heart:** People with RA are at a two-fold greater risk of developing heart disease, thus contributing to the 40% greater mortality rate of people with RA compared to the general population.[2,3] Even early in the disease process, RA patients are prone to *endothelial dysfunction* due to increased circulating inflammatory molecules. Endothelial cells are the delicate cells lining the inside of blood vessels. Endothelial dysfunction is the initial stage of potentially fatal atherosclerotic vascular disease.[11]

- **Bones:** People with RA have a significantly increased risk of bone fractures. Both the disease and medicine(s) used to treat RA (eg, corticosteroids) can cause bone loss, which increases the risk of bone fractures.[12]

- **Dyslipidemia:** People with RA are more likely to have dyslipidemia (elevated levels of cholesterol and triglycerides in blood).[13,14] One study showed dyslipidemia 10 years before the development of RA.[15] Therefore, it is important that people with both dyslipidemia and a family history of RA focus on prevention and monitor their health very closely. Dyslipidemia and endothelial dysfunction synergize to dramatically compromise the cardiovascular health of RA patients.

## DIAGNOSIS

The two important factors to consider when diagnosing RA are (1) whether inflammation is present, and (2) whether an autoimmune response is occurring. Inflammation can be measured with a variety of blood tests including hs-CRP (measures inflammation quantitatively) and an *erythrocyte sedimentation rate* (ESR) test (measures inflammation functionally).[7]

To help determine whether an autoimmune reaction is taking place, doctors often assess the levels of two proteins: rheumatoid factor (RF) and anticitrullinated protein antibody (ACPA), sometimes referred to as anticyclic citrullinated protein (anti-CCP). Both RF and ACPA are autoantibodies involved in the immune attack against self-tissue in RA.

A definitive diagnosis requires confirming synovitis due to RA in at least one joint and a total score of ≥6 by adding the individual criterion scores shown in Table 1.[16,17]

## CONVENTIONAL MEDICAL TREATMENT OF RHEUMATOID ARTHRITIS

The goal of RA treatment is to prevent and/or control joint damage, prevent loss of function, and decrease pain.[18] Early diagnosis and treatment are important for achieving the best possible outcome.[19,20]

To date, conventional medicine has relied on a mix of powerful pharmaceuticals designed to slow the disease process. While these drugs have been shown to provide relief for many patients, they may also cause side effects that can seriously reduce quality of life. Typically, treatment with one or more of the following types of prescription drugs begins as soon as the diagnosis is confirmed.

### Disease-Modifying Antirheumatic Drugs (DMARDs)

DMARDs decrease joint inflammation and slow the progression of joint damage.[21]

The two principal classes of DMARDs are *conventional* and *biologic*. Conventional DMARDs are chemically synthesized and suppress the immune system. Biologic DMARDs are genetically engineered to target specific molecules of the immune system.

Examples of conventional DMARDs include methotrexate, leflunomide, hydroxychloroquine, and sulfasalazine. Methotrexate (often the DMARD of

**Table 1.  Criteria for a Definitive Diagnosis of Rheumatoid Arthritis**[16,17]

| Criterion | Range Score | Score Calculation | Definition | Test |
|---|---|---|---|---|
| **Number and site of joints involved** | 0–5 | Add one point for each joint involved. | "Involved" means a joint is inflamed. | Physical exam, patient report, and/or imaging of the joint |
| **Serologic abnormality (abnormal blood test results)** | 0–3 | 0 = Normal<br>1 = Abnormalities are present at low levels<br>2 = Abnormalities are present at high levels | The presence (high or low levels) or absence of either RF or ACPA; high score is indicative of *autoimmunity*. | Blood test analyzed by laboratory |
| **Elevated acute-phase response** | 0–1 | 0 = Test is negative<br>1 = Test is abnormal | "Abnormal" means elevated CRP or high ESR; high scores indicate *inflammation*. | Blood test analyzed by laboratory |
| **Symptom duration** | 0–1 | 0 = Symptoms have persisted for <6 weeks<br>1 = Symptoms have persisted for ≥6 weeks | Symptoms that do not resolve within 6 weeks are indicative of RA. | Monitoring by doctor/patient report |

choice used to treat established RA) is sometimes used in combination with other drugs, including other DMARDs to reduce disease activity as much as possible.[22]

Biologic DMARDs are newer than conventional DMARDs. They are considered second-line drugs after conventional DMARDS for the treatment of RA. Examples of biologic DMARDs include drugs that target TNF-α (a potent proinflammatory mediator produced in large amounts in RA). Some anti–TNF-α drugs include adalimumab, etanercept, and certolizumab pegol. Since TNF-α orchestrates the inflammatory network that drives so many disease processes, some DMARDs are being used experimentally for conditions in which autoimmunity is not a central feature. For example, entanercept (Enbrel®) is being explored as a potential therapeutic agent for Alzheimer's disease.[23]

Another commonly prescribed biologic DMARD targeting β-cells (the immune cell that produces antibodies) is rituximab. Rituximab has been shown to reduce RA-related symptoms such as joint damage.[24,25] Other biologic DMARDs include abatacept, an inhibitor of T-cell activation, and tocilizumab, an antibody against the IL-6 receptor.[26]

## Glucocorticoids

Glucocorticoids suppress both inflammation and the activity of immune system cells. The most commonly used glucocorticoids today are prednisone and methylprednisolone (a more potent glucocorticoid than prednisone). When administered systemically, these drugs can be effective but can also cause side effects (eg, osteoporosis, eye disease, insomnia, weight gain, and increased susceptibility to infection), which can dramatically impact quality of life.[18,27] Even though glucocorticoids can be injected directly into the affected joint, the benefits of this delivery method are temporary.[18]

Doctors often use prednisone as a "bridging" therapy after patients are diagnosed with RA. This regimen includes the use of prednisone for 6 to 12 months to allow DMARDs to take effect.[7,28]

---

### CHRONOTHERAPY—EUROPEAN METHOD DRAMATICALLY REDUCES MORNING STIFFNESS IN RA

It is well known that the immune system displays diurnal variation; that is, it fluctuates depending on the time of day. Beginning around midnight, levels of the inflammatory mediators TNF-α and IL-6 rise sharply and peak in the early

morning hours.[29,30] This nocturnal inflammatory exacerbation underlies the early morning disease flares characteristic of RA and represents an opportunity for the emerging field of *chronotherapeutics*—biorhythmically targeted treatments.

Recently, a modified-release delivery method for *prednisone* has been developed. This form of prednisone is taken at bedtime (10 p.m.) and releases into the bloodstream at approximately 2 a.m. This is important because conventional prednisone formulations only suppress inflammation for a few hours, making it difficult to target inflammation late at night.

In clinical trials, this modified-release prednisone has been shown to dramatically reduce the duration of morning stiffness (–22.7% versus –0.4%) and suppress levels of the inflammatory mediator IL-6 (–29% versus no change) compared to conventional prednisone.[31,32] Modified-release prednisone also improved overall disease activity more than standard formulations of prednisone.

Unfortunately, the Food and Drug Administration (FDA) recently denied the request of a European drug maker to import a branded formulation of modified-release prednisone called Lodotra®.[33] However, after successfully achieving treatment goals in two RA clinical trials in the United States, the manufacturer of Lodotra®, Horizon Pharma, submitted a new drug application to the FDA in late 2011. As of 2011, U.S. approval is pending, but expected soon.

This advanced prednisone delivery system promises to fill a gap in current RA treatment regimens. By targeting nighttime inflammation and relieving morning disease flares, RA patients can hope to experience considerable improvement in their quality of life.

---

## Nonsteroidal Anti-Inflammatory Drugs (NSAIDs)

NSAIDs inhibit inflammation and reduce pain. This class of drugs operates by inhibiting the proinflammatory enzymes *cyclooxygenase-1* and *-2* (COX-1 and COX-2). Both of the COX enzymes convert *arachidonic acid* (an omega-6 fatty acid) into proinflammatory *prostaglandins*, which contribute to swelling and pain.

Selective COX-2 inhibitors were considered revolutionary when introduced—but then grave side effects were discovered.[7,34] The NSAID *rofecoxib* (Vioxx®) after being prescribed to tens of thousands of RA patients was removed from the market in 2004 when it was shown to significantly increase risk of heart attack and stroke. Other COX-2 inhibitors such as *valdecoxib* (Bextra®) were voluntarily removed from the market after studies revealed similar risks. Years before the public learned about the dangers of Vioxx® and Bextra®, Life Extension warned its members that taking these drugs would create lethal havoc in the body.[35] Currently, only one COX-2 inhibitor—Celebrex®—is available on the U.S. market.

The remaining NSAIDs on the market inhibit both the COX-1 and COX-2 enzymes. Unfortunately, these can lead to gastrointestinal side effects such as pain and bleeding because COX-1 is important for proper functioning of the gastrointestinal mucosa.

Additional NSAIDs include aspirin, naproxen, ibuprofen, and acetaminophen. Aspirin inhibits the aggregation of platelets (the components of blood that "clump together" and form a blood clot) more so than other NSAIDs. Taking low-dose aspirin may be beneficial for those at a higher risk of cardiovascular disease.[36] However, taking aspirin in combination with therapeutic doses of the common RA drug methotrexate may cause liver and kidney damage.[37]

## Statins

Because the chief cause of mortality among people with RA is cardiovascular disease, keeping cholesterol levels within a healthy range is an important component of treatment. Statin drugs have been shown to effectively lower cholesterol levels up to 16% as well as significantly reduce cardiovascular events (eg, heart attacks) in people with RA.[38,39]

Although statins are widely prescribed, they have many potential side effects including a breakdown of muscle tissue. Statins are also known to cause depletion of coenzyme Q10 (CoQ10), which is necessary for basic cell function. Patients taking statins should supplement with coenzyme Q10 to avoid depletion of this critical enzyme. Life Extension suggests that CoQ10 blood levels be kept in the range of 3–7 µg/mL.

## Stem Cells—A Developing Strategy for RA Treatment

Stem cells are unique in that they can either divide and reproduce or differentiate into specialized cells. The therapeutic potential of stem cells is a very hot topic in clinical research today. For example, scientists are testing ways to induce a stem cell to turn into normal nerve cells, and then implanting them to replace dead cells in people who have been paralyzed.

Stem cells can be treated in the laboratory to develop into cartilage, bone, and muscle cells, all of which can be damaged through RA-mediated inflammation.[43,44]

As of 2011, a total of 89 people with RA have received therapeutic stem cell transplants in hopes of causing disease remission or at a minimum, improvement. One study analyzed the result of high-dose chemotherapy in combination with a stem cell transplant in 7 patients with RA. Assessment of disease activity indicated that 5 (71.4%) of the patients clinically responded to this treatment, meaning that symptoms improved. However, stem cell transplants are associated with a treatment-related mortality (TRM) of approximately 5–10%. Therefore, this treatment is reserved for only the most severe cases.[45]

## RHEUMATOID ARTHRITIS AND THE GUT

Immunologic reactions to components of certain foods resemble the self-reactivity seen in RA. Therefore, it may be possible to calm the immune system by eliminating unnecessary

**Table 2.    Types of Conventional Medicines Used in Treatment of Rheumatoid Arthritis and Potential Side Effects**[10,18,21,27,40–42]

| Type | Drug | Potential Side Effects |
|---|---|---|
| **Conventional DMARDs** | Hydroxychloroquine | Eye damage |
| | Methotrexate | Liver/lung damage, decreased production of immune cells |
| | Leflunomide | Diarrhea, headache, hair loss, rash |
| | Sulfasalazine | Decreased production of immune cells |
| **Biologic DMARDs** | Anti-TNF | Injection site reaction, rash, infection |
| | Rituximab | Infusion reaction |
| | Abatacept | Infusion reaction, infection |
| | Anakinra | Injection site reaction, infections |
| | Tocilizumab | Low platelets and neutrophils, elevated cholesterol and triglycerides, infections |
| **Glucocorticoids** | Prednisone | Difficulty sleeping, increased appetite, mood changes |
| | Methyl-prednisolone | Difficulty sleeping, increased appetite, mood changes |
| | Cortisone | Difficulty sleeping, increased appetite, headache, sweating |
| **NSAIDs** | Acetaminophen Aspirin Ibuprofen Naproxen Coxibs (eg, Celecoxib) | Ulcers and bleeding in the gastrointestinal tract; potential kidney toxicity |

molecular triggers in foods. In a 12-week clinical trial, adherence to an allergen-restricted or allergen-free diet corresponded with symptomatic improvement for a small number of subjects.[127] This suggests that avoiding foods that result in elevated *IgG antibodies* in the blood may be an underappreciated method of relieving RA symptoms. Low-cost IgG blood testing allows RA patients to pinpoint potentially problematic foods and begin eating a diet that best suits their immunological profile.

### Oral Tolerance and Undenatured Type-II Collagen

Immune system T-cells are tasked with recognizing and distinguishing between "self" and "foreign" molecules. They do this by responding to very specific molecular shapes and 3-dimensional structures.[128] If T-cells in the blood are simply exposed without any "training" to a previously unrecognized protein structure (such as those found in joint collagen), they react violently and trigger a massive inflammatory response to destroy the protein.[129] Ingestion of a special type of undenatured type II collagen may help reduce immune reactivity in RA, a phenomenon called oral tolerance.[130–133]

# HORMONES AND RHEUMATOID ARTHRITIS

The role of steroid hormones in autoimmunity is evidenced by differences between men and women in both immune function and incidence of autoimmune disease. For example, estrogen actions tend to be proinflammatory, while progesterone, androgens, and glucocorticoids are anti-inflammatory.[46] Studies have documented low progesterone levels in women with autoimmune diseases, suggesting that a relative imbalance in favor of estrogen may contribute to immune reactivity in some female patients.[47] In RA and other autoimmune diseases, estrogen levels appear to be driven *too high* by actions of inflammatory mediators like TNF-α and IL-6.[48] In some studies, lower levels of testosterone have been observed in male patients with RA than in controls.[49] Testosterone and progesterone function to promote immune tolerance in males and females, respectively.[48] Therefore, ensuring adequate levels of progesterone to balance excess estrogen in women and sufficient levels of testosterone in men may modulate some underlying immunologic features of RA.[50,51] Medications used to treat RA symptoms have been shown to suppress sex hormone production as well, potentially compounding an existing hormone insufficiency or imbalance.[52]

While large-scale clinical trials have yet to evaluate the efficacy of *bioidentical hormone replacement therapy* in RA patients, Life Extension suggests that the potential for considerable benefit outweighs the minimal risk. Taking measures to achieve and

maintain optimal levels of sex hormones may soon emerge as an effective strategy for the symptomatic management of RA. Those interested in reading more about natural bioidentical hormone replacement therapy should review the Male or Female Hormone Restoration protocols.

The role and therapeutic potential of the hormone *dehydroepiandrosterone* (DHEA) in male and female RA patients is supported by a broad base of evidence. Between ages 25 and 75, levels of the multifunctional hormone DHEA decrease by approximately 80%.[53] Moreover, glucocorticoid therapy often employed in RA suppresses DHEA levels significantly.[54] The implications of low levels of DHEA may be considerable in RA, especially since DHEA counteracts the inflammatory cytokines TNF-α and IL-6 in the synovium. Conversely, local TNF-α suppresses DHEA levels in the synovium; thus, the relationship between anti-inflammatory effects of DHEA and proinflammatory effects of TNF-α is reciprocal in nature. In a 1-year, double-blinded, placebo controlled trial, 125 men and women aged 65–75 received 50 mg of DHEA daily. Treatment resulted in improved insulin sensitivity and lower levels of TNF-α and IL-6 in blood samples.[53] These results were maintained during an additional year of open-label continuation.

# NATURAL THERAPIES AND LIFESTYLE STRATEGIES FOR RHEUMATOID ARTHRITIS

### Fatty Acids

Polyunsaturated fatty acids (PUFAs), primarily those derived from marine sources, have been recommended for RA patients for many years because of their ability to reduce inflammation and bolster cardiovascular health while helping soothe the overactive immune system.[55]

There are two main types of dietary PUFAs: omega-6 and omega-3. Both are important for health. However, it is especially important to maintain the correct ratio of omega-6 to omega-3 in the diet. Research has shown that the typical American diet is composed of an omega-6 to omega-3 ratio as high as 25:1.[56] The ideal ratio, however, is about *4:1*, meaning that very few people are getting enough omega-3 fatty acid relative to the amount of omega-6.[57] A ratio so skewed toward omega-6 has the potential to be highly proinflammatory. Thus, it is essential for arthritis patients to get sufficient omega-3 fatty acids.

A number of trials have supported the benefit of RA patients consuming omega-3 fatty acids in the form of *fish oil*. These studies have shown that fish oil can help reduce the inflammation,[58] pain, and symptoms associated with RA. Eicosapentaenoic acid (EPA) and docosahexaenoic acid (DHA), typically derived from fish oil, have proven anti-inflammatory properties. The results of a study in which people with RA consumed 1800 mg EPA and 900 mg DHA daily for three months indicated that these fatty acids are effective in controlling morning stiffness, whereas those who received the placebo experienced worsening symptoms.[59]

Numerous clinical studies have supported the benefits of RA patients consuming fish oil.[60] In a study assessing joint tenderness and dose of NSAIDs required to control symptoms in people with well-established RA, those consuming fish oil experienced less joint pain and took lower doses of NSAIDs.[61] Data from a separate study indicated that consuming fish oil may *complement* the anti-inflammatory properties of acetaminophen.[62] Consuming fish oil also significantly reduced TNF-α and other proinflammatory cytokines.[63] Fish oil significantly improved cholesterol and triglyceride levels in people with RA as well, mitigating cardiovascular risk.[64]

*Krill oil* is a marine oil whose properties differ slightly from those of fish oil. In an animal model, krill oil "significantly reduced arthritis scores and swelling."[65] In a separate study of krill oil *combined* with *hyaluronic acid* and *astaxanthin*—both of which target proinflammatory agents in the body—arthritis patients reported a *55% pain reduction* in under 3 months; 63% of participants were entirely pain-free post-treatment.[66]

**Gamma-Linolenic Acid (GLA).** GLA is a beneficial omega-6 fatty acid found in oils from several different plants. Its heart healthy effects are well documented. In a study in which RA patients consumed 1400 mg GLA daily, their RA symptoms were significantly reduced, including number and severity of tender joints and degree of swelling.[67] A thorough review of clinical trials found that whereas consuming 1400 mg daily or more of GLA resulted in a significant improvement in RA related symptoms, lower doses (ie, 500 mg daily) did not appear effective.[68] Other studies have shown that the following GLA-rich oils may be beneficial in people with RA:

Blackcurrant seed oil (*Ribes nigrum*): A 24-week clinical trial involving people with RA compared the effects of blackcurrant oil to placebo and found that blackcurrant seed oil significantly improved RA related symptoms.[69]

Borage seed oil (*Borago officinalis*): Oil from the borage plant seed is rich in GLA. Borage seed oil was used as the source of GLA in the study testing the benefits of GLA in reducing RA symptoms.[67] Results from a comprehensive review indicate that borage seed oil is associated with improved clinical outcomes in people with RA.[70]

A recent clinical study found that RA patients consuming borage seed oil had decreased levels of total cholesterol, LDL, triglycerides, and increased HDL levels.[64] This effect is particularly beneficial for people with RA as they have a greater risk of heart disease than the general population.[2,3]

Evening primrose oil (*Oenothera biennis*): A review showed that primrose oil effectively reduced RA symptoms.[71] In one study, people with RA taking daily NSAID therapy consumed either 6 g per day of evening primrose oil or placebo. Those receiving daily doses of evening primrose oil experienced less morning stiffness after 3 months and less pain after 6 months.[72]

## Vitamins

**Vitamin D.** Vitamin D, which is synthesized when the skin comes into contact with ultraviolet light, plays an important immunomodulatory role and appears to appreciably ease RA symptoms. The results of a randomized clinical trial showed that RA patients taking a low dose of 1-25 dihydroxyvitamin D along with their disease-modifying antirheumatic drug (DMARD) therapy had significantly greater pain relief at 3 months compared with the group receiving DMARDs only.[73] Alarmingly, a recent Swiss trial found that 86% of 272 RA patients had deficient or insufficient levels of vitamin D.[74]

The vitamin D receptor (VDR), which binds vitamin D, is located on the surface of immune cells. Because immune cells play an important role in promoting inflammation in RA, it seems logical that vitamin D would also have a role in RA-mediated inflammation. Indeed, a recent study found that the VDR is important in limiting the inflammatory tendency of immune cells in a mouse model of RA.[75]

However, vitamin D does more than just arrest damaging immune cells; it also *supercharges* protective immune cells.

*T-reg* cells are specialized components of the immune system that help keep immunity *balanced*. If too few T-reg cells are present, the immune system becomes *overactive* as in autoimmune diseases like RA. Vitamin D increases the number of *protective* T-reg cells, restoring equilibrium to an overactive immune system.[76]

**Vitamin B6.** The prevalence of vitamin B6 deficiency is elevated in people with RA. This deficiency has been associated with more severe symptoms.[77] A study found that treatment with 100 mg daily of vitamin B6 reduced blood levels of TNF-α and other proinflammatory cytokines in people with RA.[78]

**Folate.** A folate deficiency is particularly common in people with RA being treated with methotrexate, as this drug depletes folate.[79] Therefore, folate supplementation may be beneficial for people with RA.

## Plants and Plant-Derived Compounds

**Andrographis.** Andrographolides, components extracted from the plant *Andrographis paniculata*, inhibit activity of the proinflammatory compound known as inducible *nitric oxide synthase* (iNOS). This helps exert a powerful anti-inflammatory effect.[80] Readers who are familiar with the vascular benefits of eNOS (endothelial NOS) should note that unlike eNOS, *iNOS* is proinflammatory and often involved in disease states where it is desirable to inhibit its actions.

Andrographolides suppress production of the *proinflammatory cytokines TNF-α and prostaglandin E2* (PGE-2), preventing their gene expression at multiple levels.[81,82] By doing so, they downregulate the chemical signaling pathways that cells use to "tell" each other to initiate the inflammatory response, which plays a key role in RA.[83]

Scientific analysis has further revealed that andrographolides operate "upstream" within the process of the inflammatory cascade by blocking the effects of the *proinflammatory* transcription factor *nuclear factor kappa-B* (NF-κB).[84]

NF-κB is found in almost all human cells. It plays a key role in cellular responses to stress, cytokines, free radicals, oxidized low-density lipoprotein (LDL), and bacterial or viral pathogens. Accordingly, its central role as a first responder to oxidative damage, infection, and toxin-induced stress links it to inflammation, cancer, and chronic disease.[85] NF-κB tightly regulates virtually all factors that are downstream in the inflammatory cascade, including cytokines known as *interleukins*, hormones known as *prostaglandins*, and *TNF-α*.

By blocking NF-κB, andrographolides inhibit production of a host of inflammatory mediators in one simple step.[86] As demonstrated in animal studies, they also permit *normal* activity of vital immune surveillance cells as they simultaneously suppress over-active inflammatory cells.[87]

This is a critical feature that distinguishes andrographolides from most antirheumatic drugs (DMARDS). Whereas andrographolides suppress inflammatory immune factors, DMARDs can suppress immune function in general resulting in an *increased risk of infection*.[88]

**Curcumin.** Curcumin is an antioxidant compound found in the spice turmeric and has potent anti-inflammatory and immunomodulatory properties. One laboratory-based study showed that curcumin reduces synovial inflammation.[89] Specifically, this study demonstrated that exposing inflamed synovial cells to curcumin not only reduced the inflammatory state of these cells, but suppressed the production of proinflammatory proteins and the activation of cells with inflammatory properties.

Curcumin also helps protect cartilage from inflammation-mediated destruction. A meta-analysis sought to examine the body of evidence concerning the effect of curcumin on chondrocytes, the cells that make up cartilage. The researchers concluded that curcumin not only helps prevent the degradation of cartilage induced by certain inflammatory proteins in the joint,[90] but it also helps promote cartilage regeneration.[91]

Curcumin may also help lower the dose of methotrexate required for therapeutic effects and drug-related liver toxicity. One study found that administering curcumin along with a very low, subtherapeutic dose of methotrexate in a mouse model of arthritis effectively treated the inflammation while reducing the level of drug-induced liver damage.[92] If as effective in humans, taking curcumin along with methotrexate would enable people with RA to take lower doses of methotrexate, thereby decreasing their risk of liver toxicity.

One small (18 people) but well-designed study found that consuming curcumin resulted in improved ambulation (increase in time) as well as a significant reduction in joint swelling and morning stiffness.[93] These results were corroborated by a larger clinical trial in which 45 RA patients were randomized to receive 50 mg of diclofenac sodium, 500 mg of a highly absorbable form of curcumin called BCM-95®, or both for 8 weeks. In this trial, curcumin alone and in combination with diclofenac sodium proved to be at least as effective as diclofenac sodium alone in easing RA disease activity, as measured by multiple standardized assessments. In addition, curcumin alone powerfully suppressed CRP (a marker of inflammation in the blood) by 52% from baseline, while diclofenac sodium alone only decreased CRP by 1.5%. The investigators of this trial remarked that "*Taken together, our present results provide a clear proof-of-principle for the superiority of curcumin, and the lack of any synergistic or additive efficacy when used in conjunction with diclofenac strongly favours the safe and effective application of curcumin alone in clinical settings for the management of rheumatoid arthritis, and other proinflammatory diseases including cancer in the future.*"[94]

**Quercetin.** Quercetin is a flavonoid compound rich in fruits and vegetables—especially apples, citrus fruits, parsley, sage, and onions. Quercetin strongly inhibits multiple components of the inflammatory process, including the COX enzymes that are targeted by NSAIDs.[95] Laboratory experiments with synovial cells have shown that although quercetin does not have an effect on the production of proinflammatory proteins, it directly reduces inflammation in the synovium as well as the activation of proinflammatory cells.[89]

A recent proof-of-concept study demonstrated decreased inflammation by utilizing bioengineering techniques to increase the bioavailability of quercetin in a rat model of RA. The investigators loaded quercetin into microspheres and delivered the microsphere-quercetin combination directly into the joint.[96] The microspheres enabled the quercetin to be released consistently over 30 days. Although additional human trials are needed, the data thus far support an anti-inflammatory role for quercetin in RA.

**Boswellia serrata extract.** Resin from the Boswellia genus of the Boswellia sacra tree contains a powerful anti-inflammatory compound called 3-acetyl-11-keto-β-boswellic acid (AKBA). Boswellia serrata extract (BSE) contains high levels of these boswellic acids, which are potent inhibitors of 5-lipoxygenase (5-LOX), a proinflammatory enzyme. 5-LOX leads to the production of inflammatory-producing leukotrienes. BSE may also have inhibitory effects on proinflammatory proteins like TNF-α.[97] These acids have even been shown to have immunomodulatory effects similar to NSAIDs.[98] A study investigating the effect of consuming BSE standardized to 30% AKBA on arthritis found that this extract significantly improved joint flexion, reduced swelling, and protected the joint from cartilage degradation induced by inflammation.[99] An improved extract called AprèsFlex™ (a.k.a. Aflapin®), which combines AKBA with other nonvolatile boswellia oils, demonstrated improved activity at a lower concentration when compared to other preparations standardized to the same percentage of AKBA.[100]

**Pomegranate.** Pomegranates contain a high concentration of polyphenols, which are compounds with strong antioxidant properties. Pomegranate seeds are either eaten in their natural form or processed to produce pomegranate juice. Alternatively, the active compounds can be extracted from the rest of the fruit's components.

One study tested the severity of inflammation and incidence of arthritis in mice fed a pomegranate extract in addition to their food. The mice in the pomegranate-fed group had a lower incidence of arthritis, and those who did get arthritis developed it later than normal (ie, delayed disease) as well as having reduced joint inflammation and damage.[101]

In a recent pilot study testing the efficacy of pomegranate extract in 6 people with RA, it was reported that the people consuming the extract had significantly fewer tender joints.[102] Expanding the sample size of patients studied will determine whether these effects are broadly applicable.

**Green tea.** The active ingredient in green tea is epigallocatechin 3-gallate (EGCG), which has been tested extensively for its health-promoting properties. EGCG has been shown to have significant anti-inflammatory and antioxidant effects as well as helping to optimize the lipid profile.[103]

Preclinical studies indicate that green tea may be effective in reducing inflammation in the joints of people with RA. For example, supplementing drinking water with green tea significantly reduced the severity of arthritis in a rat model of RA.[104] It was even effective in preventing the onset of arthritis in a mouse model of RA.[105]

**Ginger.** Ginger, the underground stem of the *Zingiber officinale* plant, has potent anti-inflammatory and antioxidant properties.[106] Ginger directly suppresses inflammation by inhibiting proinflammatory enzymes and blocking the production of proinflammatory proteins.[107] Furthermore, several investigators have reported that consuming ginger significantly prevented the onset of arthritis in rodent models of RA.[108–110]

***Nigella sativa* seeds**. These seeds are commonly called "black cumin" or "black caraway." Investigators have shown that consuming thymoquinone, the active compound of the seed oil, inhibited inflammation and prevented arthritis in a rat model of RA.[111]

A recent study compared the symptoms of RA patients receiving 500 mg of *Nigella sativa* oil twice daily for 1 month with those receiving placebo capsules. Remarkably, up to 40% (which varied approximately 10% based upon the disease activity scale used to assess symptoms) of people receiving *Nigella sativa* seed oil experienced an improvement in RA symptoms.[112]

**Beta-sitosterol and beta-sitosterol glucoside.** As suggested by some preliminary research, a proprietary 99:1 mixture of beta-sistosterol (BSS) and beta-sitosterol glucoside (BSSG) called Moducare® may modulate immunity in RA. In laboratory experiments, a BSS/BSSG blend has demonstrated an ability to balance immune cell function under varying conditions.[113,114] Two small pilot studies in human subjects have corroborated the in vitro data. In the first study, 17 ultramarathon runners were given either the BSS/BSSG mixture or placebo. After the race, when immune function is normally drastically altered, researchers assessed parameters of inflammation in both groups. In the group taking the BSS/BSSG mixture, it was noted that levels of immune cells rose while inflammatory mediators in the blood declined, suggesting that the mixture primed the immune system for defense while simultaneously suppressing excess inflammation.[115] In the second trial, 18 patients with active RA took either the BSS/BSSG mixture or placebo for 24 weeks. The mixture led to significant improvements compared to placebo in all of the following: measurable tender joint count, patient's assessment of pain, patient's global assessment of disease activity, and physician's global assessment of pain. Furthermore, erythrocyte sedimentation rate (ESR), an assessment of the inflammatory tendency of blood, decreased by 56%.[116]

## Endogenous Compounds

**SAMe.** S-adenosyl-L-methionine (SAMe) is a natural compound in the body that is necessary for many different physiological processes. SAMe has been shown to improve symptoms of osteoarthritis, liver disease, and even depression. Although most scientific research has focused on osteoarthritis, the mechanisms for SAMe suggest a role in RA. SAMe supports the production of the structural components of cartilage, which can be destroyed by the chronic inflammation of RA. The anti-inflammatory properties of SAMe suggest a supportive role for this compound in RA patients.[117]

A comprehensive review of several individual clinical studies found that SAMe relieved pain and improved joint function in people with osteoarthritis.[118] In fact, SAMe had similar analgesic and function improving effects as treatment with NSAIDs, but without the adverse effects.[119]

The common RA medicine methotrexate has been shown to inhibit cell signaling through the SAMe pathway.[120] Therefore, the cells in joint tissue may not process SAMe normally. This laboratory study suggests that people treated with methotrexate may benefit from SAMe supplementation.

**Glucosamine.** This compound is a precursor to *glycosaminoglycans*, components of larger molecules—proteoglycans—which are incorporated into cartilage. Proteoglycans are critical for healthy cartilage and proper cushioning of the joint because they draw water into the joint, acting as a lubricant. In addition, glucosamine seems to have some anti-inflammatory properties.[117]

Glucosamine has been shown to suppress production of the proinflammatory cytokine IL-8 in cells of the synovium.[121] Another study found that glucosamine was effective in significantly reducing RA symptoms despite no detectable differences in conventional markers of inflammation, such as CRP.[122]

**Chondroitin sulfate.** This compound is a structural component of cartilage. When taken as a supplement, it helps fight inflammation and supports the rebuilding of cartilage.[117] Chondroitin sulfate may be healthy for the heart as well. An animal model of atherosclerosis and chronic arthritis found that chondroitin sulfate prevented atherosclerotic lesions from developing.[66] These data, although very preliminary, raise the possibility that chondroitin sulfate may help fight the systemic inflammation present in RA that leads to joint and heart disease.

## Exercise

As with other rheumatic diseases, exercise is a critical component of maintaining muscle mass, supporting a healthy heart, and preventing joint damage as much as possible. Various types of exercises are beneficial for people with RA.

**Aerobic exercise.** Several studies have demonstrated that dynamic aerobic exercises such as swimming, walking, and bike riding not only improve overall health and quality of life in patients with RA but also reduce pain. Another benefit of dynamic exercise is the improvement in cardiovascular health, which is especially important for people with RA.[76] To date, no studies have reported that dynamic exercise has deleterious effects on disease activity or joint function.[123,124] Even high-intensity exercise has not been shown to lead to increased inflammation or joint damage.[125]

**Strength training.** Strength training (eg, weight lifting) involves applying resistance to various muscle groups to improve muscle strength. Similar to dynamic exercise, strength training reduced pain and improved function in people with RA.[126]

## Life Extension Suggestions

- **Fish oil** (with olive polyphenols and sesame lignans): providing 1400 mg EPA and 1000 mg DHA daily
- **Krill oil blend** (with astaxanthin and hyaluronic acid): 350 mg daily
- **Gamma linolenic acid** (with sesame lignans): 600–1400 mg daily
- **Vitamin D**: 5000–8000 IU daily depending on blood test results
- **Vitamin B6** (preferably as pyridoxal-5-phosphate): 75–105 mg daily
- **Folate** (preferably as L-methylfolate): 400–1000 mcg daily
- **Undenatured type-II collagen (UC-II®)**: 10 mg daily

- **Andrographis paniculata** (as PARACTIN® standardized extract): 150–300 mg daily
- **Curcumin** (as highly absorbed BCM95®): 400–800 mg daily
- **Quercetin**: 250–500 mg daily
- **Boswellia serrata** (as highly absorbed Apres-Flex™): 100 mg daily
- **Pomegranate** (standardized to 30% punicalagins): 400–800 mg daily
- **Green tea extract** (standardized to 98% polyphenols): 725–1450 mg daily
- **Ginger root extract**: 150–450 mg daily
- **DHEA**: 15–25 mg daily for women; 25–75 mg daily for men (depending on blood test results)
- **S-adenosyl-methionine (SAMe)**: 400–1200 mg daily
- **Glucosamine sulfate**: 2000 mg daily
- **Chondroitin sulfate**: 450–3600 mg daily
- **Beta-sitosterol/beta-sitosterol glucoside mixture (Moducare®)**: 20.2 mg–60.6 mg daily

In addition, the following blood tests can provide helpful information:

- **High-sensitivity C-reactive protein (hs-CRP)** (available in the Male or Female Panel)—Assesses systemic inflammation quantitatively
  - Optimal range: <1.5 mg/L for women; <0.55 mg/L for men
- **Erythrocyte sedimentation rate (ESR)**—A functional assessment of the inflammatory tendency of a blood sample
- **Rheumatoid factor**—Assesses the presence of antibodies indicating that an immune response against self-tissues is taking place

- **Coenzyme Q10 (CoQ10)**—Assesses blood levels of coenzyme Q10
  - Optimal range: 3–7 µg/mL
- **IgG antibodies**—Quantitatively assesses systemic immunoreactivity to foods
- **Omega Score®**—Assesses the blood fatty acid profile
  - Optimal range: omega-6 to omega-3 ratio <4:1
- **Vitamin D (25-hydroxy)**—Assesses vitamin D status
  - Optimal range: 50–80 ng/mL
- **DHEA** (available in the Male or Female Panel)
  - Optimal range: 350–490 µg/dL for men and 275–400 µg/dL for women
- **Free and Total Testosterone** (men) (available in the Male Panel)
  - Optimal ranges:
  - Free testosterone 20–25 pg/mL
  - Total testosterone: 700–900 ng/dL
- **Progesterone** (women) (available in the Female Panel)
  - Optimal ranges: 18–27 ng/mL at day 21 of menstrual cycle or 2–6 ng/mL for postmenopausal women using hormone replacement therapy
- **Estradiol** (women) (available in Female Panel)
  - Optimal ranges: 90–211 pg/mL at day 21 of cycle for premenopausal women or for postmenopausal using hormone replacement therapy

## REFERENCES

References available at: www.lef.org/dpt5/ch13

# 14

# Asthma

Asthma causes the airways of the lungs to swell and narrow, leading to wheezing, shortness of breath, chest tightness, and coughing.

It is distinguished by *bronchial hyper-responsiveness*, which is an exaggerated response of the airway characterized by swelling (edema) and infiltration of inflammatory immune cells.

*Allergens* and *inflammatory cytokines* are typical culprits involved in triggering asthmatic attacks.[1] Asthma symptoms include wheezing, chest tightness, shortness of breath, and coughing. The disease affects people of all ages, but often begins during childhood. In the United States, more than 22 million people have asthma.

Asthma therapies aim to reduce this inflammation and improve airway function. Conventional treatment modalities can effectively treat asthma in many cases; but for those with chronic, severe asthma, long-term use of *glucocorticoids* is linked to *detrimental side effects* such as *bone fractures* and *adrenal dysfunction*.[2,3]

An underutilized tool in the battle against asthma is blood testing for environmental and food allergens and for less conspicuous *food sensitivities* that may trigger inflammation. When potential triggers have been identified, many asthma patients may be able to improve their quality of life by avoiding exposures or eliminating foods to which their immune system is highly reactive.[4-7]

In this protocol, you will learn what causes asthma and how lifestyle and dietary choices can mitigate asthma exacerbations. You will also learn which medical treatments can help relieve symptoms and discover that emerging drug strategies appear promising. Lastly, you will read about several *natural compounds* that may complement conventional treatment strategies and target asthmatic inflammation from multiple angles.

## PATHOPHYSIOLOGY OF ASTHMA

**Airway Inflammation.** In those with asthma, cells and tissues within the airway are prone to inflammatory reactions against normally harmless substances. This inflammation can cause swelling, mucus production and lead to *airway narrowing*.[8]

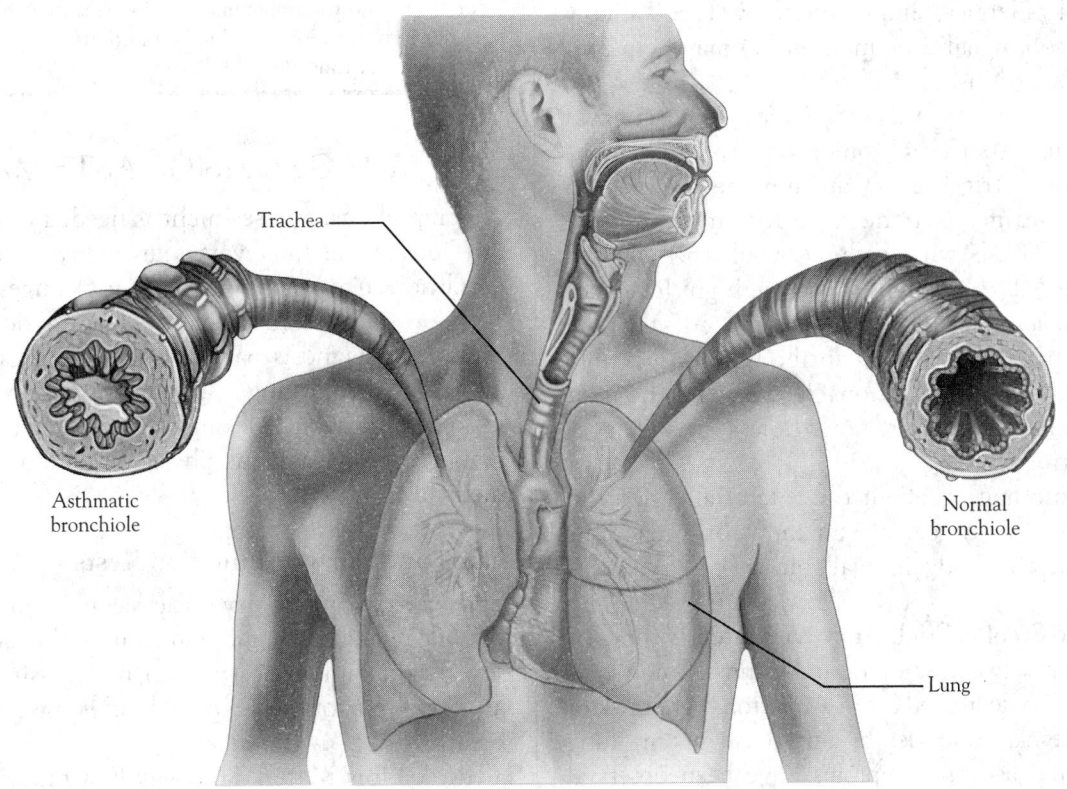

Trachea

Asthmatic bronchiole

Normal bronchiole

Lung

Normal and asthmatic airways

**Airway Narrowing.** Airway narrowing gives rise to asthma symptoms. When the airways are exposed to substances that trigger a reaction, *immunoglobulin E* (IgE) antibodies produced by *B-cells* help facilitate the release of inflammatory mediators including *histamine* and *leukotrienes* from *mast cells*. These mediators cause the airway smooth muscles to contract or spasm, triggering airway narrowing (ie, bronchoconstriction). Sensory nerves in the muscles become more sensitized, contributing to more bronchospasms.[9]

**Airway Remodeling.** Structural changes in bronchial tubes can occur with chronic and uncontrolled asthma attacks. For instance, epithelial cells (the layer of cells that line the airways and function as a barrier) can shed, allowing irritants or allergens to further penetrate into the inner muscle cells.[10–12] Sensory nerves can also become exposed leading to reflex neural effects on the airways.[13]

# CAUSES, TRIGGERS, AND RISK FACTORS

**Allergies and Sensitivities.** Allergies underlie many cases of asthma. An allergy is an inappropriate immune response against an innocuous compound. A wide variety of environmental allergens can cause an asthma attack,[4] including food allergies.[14]

For those whose asthma is associated with environmental allergies, immunotherapy (eg, "allergy shots" or sublingual immunotherapy) may help prevent exacerbations.[1,15,16]

In the case of *food sensitivities*, experimental research suggests that chronic, low-level inflammatory reactions triggered by an immune response to food particles may set the stage for airway inflammation.[6,7] Those with asthma would be wise to test to see if they are producing high levels of *IgG antibodies* toward any particular food(s). Some evidence suggests that IgG antibody testing is able to detect immune reactions less severe than an overt allergy, but that nonetheless may trigger inflammation.[6,7,17]

More information about the role of allergies and sensitivities in triggering inflammatory reactions throughout the body is available in the Allergies protocol.

**Tobacco Smoke.** Studies have consistently shown a relationship between smoking and asthma. Smoking is also related to decreased asthma control, higher risk of asthma attacks, and death. Improvements in lung function and asthma symptoms have been observed among those who quit smoking.[18]

**Occupational Exposure.** Occupations commonly associated with asthma include woodworking, detergent manufacturing, some health care professions, and baking.[19–21]

**Infections.** A variety of common viral infections acquired during infancy and early childhood appear to increase the risk of childhood wheezing episodes that may eventually lead to asthma.[8] In contrast, other evidence suggests that childhood exposure to microbial pathogens and foreign peptides may protect against the development of childhood asthma—a theory known as the *hygiene hypothesis*.[22,23]

**Medications.** Certain medications, including nonsteroidal anti-inflammatory drugs (NSAIDs) and ACE-inhibitors, can trigger an asthma attack in some people.[24]

**Exercise.** Exercise can trigger asthma exacerbations, so people with asthma should exercise with caution (NHLBI guidelines).

---

*Other medical conditions commonly associated with asthma* include chronic rhinitis, chronic sinusitis/rhinosinusitis, gastroesophageal reflux disease (GERD), obstructive sleep apnea, chronic obstructive pulmonary disease (COPD), hormonal disorders, obesity, depression, and anxiety. Stress has been associated with asthma as well.[25] These conditions may share some pathophysiologic mechanisms with asthma and may influence its expression. Associated diseases may also influence how a patient with asthma responds to treatment. Likewise, the asthmatic condition and the inflammatory processes in asthma may influence how these associated conditions develop or progress over time.[26,27]

---

# DIAGNOSIS OF ASTHMA

A comprehensive assessment is needed to differentiate between asthma versus an alternate disease or condition such as emphysema, early congestive heart failure or vocal cord problems. The physician makes a clinical diagnosis based upon symptoms, severity, and results from lung/respiratory function tests.[1] To make a thorough assessment and help the patient manage the disease, the physician obtains a detailed medical history.

## Lung and Airway Function Tests

**Spirometry.** Spirometry is the recommended method for diagnosing asthma. It measures the degree and severity of airflow obstruction by assessing the rate and amount of air expelled after taking a deep breath.[28]

**Peak Flow Meter.** The peak flow meter measures the maximum speed of air from forced expiration, known as peak expiratory flow (PEF). It measures the airflow through the bronchi and thus the degree of obstruction in the airways. This simple test can also be used to monitor asthma conditions in the home.[13]

# CONVENTIONAL TREATMENTS FOR ASTHMA

Asthma is treated pharmacologically in a stepwise fashion depending on severity of symptoms. Asthma medications include *quick-relief medications* used to treat acute symptoms of an asthma attack and *long-term control medications* used to prevent further exacerbations. The goal of treatment is to optimize long-term control so that quick-relief medications, which have many side effects, can be minimized or eliminated.[29]

## Quick-Relief Medications

**Short-Acting Beta-2 Agonists (SABAs).** SABAs cause bronchodilation of the smooth muscles of the airway. These drugs relieve breathlessness, chest tightness, and other acute symptoms of an asthma attack. SABAs are usually prescribed together with a maintenance medication. Intensity of treatment depends on severity of symptoms: up to 3 treatments at 20-minute intervals as needed. Side effects of bronchodilators include rapid heart rate, increased blood pressure, increased blood sugar levels, irregular heart rhythms, and a variety of other responses.[30] SABA medications include albuterol, levalbuterol, pirbuterol, bronkosol, isoproterenol, metaproterenol, and terbutaline. Use of SABA >2 days a week for symptom relief generally indicates inadequate control and the need to step up treatment (see *Stepwise Asthma Management* box).

**Corticosteroids.** Corticosteroids exert an immune-suppressing (ie, anti-inflammatory) effect and can be administered systemically for a short course in acute or severe asthma to ease airway inflammation.[31,32] However, systemic corticosteroids can lead to significant side effects including edema, osteoporosis, muscle weakness, chemical-induced diabetes, hypertension, adrenal gland dysfunction, cataracts, and glaucoma. They can also reduce calcium absorption from the gut and increase calcium loss from the kidneys.[3] To reduce the risk of these serious complications, the lowest dose possible should be taken to provide symptomatic control.[13]

**Theophylline.** Theophylline is a bronchodilator with modest anti-inflammatory properties. It can be used as an alternative stand-alone therapy for children older than 5 with persistent mild asthma. However, the toxic dose only slightly exceeds the effective dose, so patients must be carefully monitored.[33] Adverse effects include gastrointestinal symptoms, irregular heartbeat, seizures, and death.[34]

**Inhaled Anticholinergics.** The neurotransmitter acetylcholine contributes to bronchoconstriction. Therefore, blocking the binding of acetylcholine to its receptors in the airways with inhaled anticholinergics inhibits this action. Anticholinergic medications are sometimes added to SABAs and help promote bronchodilation during an acute exacerbation.[31]

## Long-Term Control Medications

**Corticosteroids.** Patients with asthma may require long-term use of inhaled corticosteroids.[31,32] Potential adverse local effects associated with inhaled corticosteroids include thrush, hoarseness, reflex cough, and bronchospasm.[34] Long-term use of high-dose inhaled corticosteroids is associated with osteoporosis and adrenal dysfunction.[3] Commonly used inhaled corticosteroids include beclomethasone, budenoside, and triamcinolone.

**Long-Acting Beta-2 Agonists (LABAs).** LABAs relax the airways and can provide up to 12 hours of bronchodilation.[33] They can be an add-on to long-term treatment for asthma that cannot be adequately controlled with inhaled corticosteroids alone. LABAs should not be used as stand-alone maintenance medications or to treat acute symptoms. The use of LABAs should be stopped if there is no response and the dose of inhaled corticosteroid is increased.[13] Studies have shown that LABAs can increase the risk of severe asthma attacks, asthma-related hospitalizations and death.[34] LABAs include salmeterol xinafoate and formoterol fumarate.

**Leukotriene Modifiers.** Leukotriene receptor antagonists (blockers) and inhibitors of leukotriene synthesis help prevent or reduce inflammation, mucus production, swelling, and airway tightening. They are less effective than inhaled corticosteroids and thus are commonly used as an add-on therapy for poorly controlled, persistent asthma and exercise-induced asthma.[35] Commonly used leukotriene modifiers include montelukast, zafirlukast, and zileuton.

**Mast cell stabilizers.** Mast cell stabilizers (eg, cromolyn and nedrocromil) prevent mast cells (a type of immune cell) from releasing histamine and related inflammatory mediators. These medications are very useful for preventing exercise-induced asthma when used prophylactically, but are not effective in treating an acute asthma attack. Mast cell stabilizers are also very safe but must be taken on a regular basis, even when free of symptoms.[36]

## STEPWISE ASTHMA MANAGEMENT

The *stepwise approach guidelines,* developed by the National Institutes of Health, are meant to assist clinical decision making and ensure that patient needs are met. The guidelines recommend consulting with an asthma specialist if step 4 or higher is required. Consider consultation at step 3. Advancement through these steps ("*stepping up*") is based on assessment of patient response to treatment while considering variables such as other medical conditions, adherence to treatment, and environmental factors (eg, level of allergens in the air). If the patient responds well to treatment and symptoms are well controlled for at least 3 months, then the physician may consider "*stepping down*" the patient to the next lower step in order to avoid medication side effects.

### Intermittent Asthma

#### Step 1

**Preferred:** Short-acting beta-2 agonists (SABAs) as needed

### Persistent Asthma

#### Step 2

**Preferred:** Low-dose inhaled corticosteroid (ICS)
**Alternative\*:** Cromolyn, leukotrine receptor antagonist (LTRA), nedocromil, or theophylline

#### Step 3

**Preferred:** Low-dose ICS + long-acting beta-2 agonist (LABA) or medium-dose ICS
**Alternative\*:** Low-dose ICS + LTRA or theophylline

#### Step 4

**Preferred:** Medium-dose ICS + LABA
**Alternative\*:** Medium-dose ICS + LTRA or theophylline

#### Step 5

**Preferred:** High-dose ICS + LABA
Note: Consider omalizumab for patients who have allergies.

#### Step 6

**Preferred:** High-dose ICS + LABA + oral systemic corticosteroid
Note: Consider omalizumab for patients who have allergies.

*\*If alternative treatment is used and response is inadequate, discontinue it and use the preferred treatment before stepping up.*

## NOVEL AND EMERGING ASTHMA THERAPIES

**Suplatast Tosilate.** The immunologic reaction to antigens is driven by two counterbalancing paradigms—*Th1* and *Th2*. In asthma, an imbalance favoring Th2

is observed.[37] Suplatast tosilate is a Th2 cytokine inhibitor that has been shown to ease inflammation in asthma and related allergic conditions.[38,39] Clinical trials with suplatast tosilate have been quite promising. Not only has suplatast tosilate been shown to be at least as effective as some traditional asthma drugs,[40] but it also improved lung function in asthmatic subjects who were already being treated with steroids[41,42] as well as subjects who did not respond to leukotriene receptor antagonists.[38] Unfortunately, suplatast tosilate is not approved in the United States, but is available in Japan as Tosilart® and IPD Capsules®.[43]

### Biological Agents

Biological agents (biologics) are protein-based products, which include antibodies and recombinant protein-based receptors. Examples include humanized monoclonal antibodies (antibodies manufactured in the laboratory from identical immune cells), which target specific antibodies or cytokines.

**Omalizumab (Xolair®).** Omalizumab, a monoclonal antibody that inhibits a key mediator of antigen sensitization called *immunoglobulin E* (IgE), is approved to treat asthma. Omalizumab's cost is high and hence is mainly prescribed for patients with severe, persistent asthma, which cannot be controlled even with high doses of corticosteroids. Adverse effects of omalizumab include severe allergic reactions and cancer.[44]

**Monoclonal Antibodies That Target Eosinophils.** Eosinophils are immune cells that accumulate in sites of asthmatic inflammation and release inflammatory mediators.[45,46] Interleukin-5 (IL-5) is a major regulator of eosinophil accumulation in tissues, and can modulate eosinophil behavior.[47] Several humanized monoclonal antibody therapies (eg, mepolizumab, benralizumab and reslizumab) have selected IL-5 as a potential target to prevent eosinophil-mediated inflammation in patients with asthma.[48] In one placebo-controlled trial, mepolizumab was associated with significantly fewer severe exacerbations of eosinophilic asthma than placebo over the course of 50 weeks.[49] Mepolizumab also significantly reduced the number of eosinophils in blood and sputum.[49,50] Another randomized, placebo-controlled trial found that intravenous infusions of reslizumab on poorly controlled eosinophilic asthma were generally well tolerated and reduced sputum eosinophil concentration, improved airway function, and trended toward greater asthma control compared to placebo.[51]

**Pitrakinra (Aerovant®).** Interleukin-4 (IL-4) is another important contributor to eosinophil-mediated inflammation.[52] In two independent randomized, double-blind, placebo-controlled trials using a drug called pitrakinra (Aerovant®) that blocks the effects of IL-4, researchers were able to significantly relieve asthma symptoms in 28 subjects with allergic asthma compared to 28 subjects who received a placebo.[53]

## Bronchial Thermoplasty

Bronchial thermoplasty is a therapy in which radio-frequency energy bursts are used to heat and destroy muscle tissue in the airway, thus hindering the ability of the bronchial tubes to constrict. It is used only for patients with severe refractory asthma. Results from clinical trials have shown that patients who underwent this procedure experienced fewer symptoms, enjoyed better quality of life and needed less emergency room visits.[54]

Although bronchial thermoplasty is relatively safe, patients have to be monitored during (for symptoms of asthma and other adverse events) and after treatment because exacerbations can occur up to 6 weeks following the final procedure. The U.S. Food and Drug Administration has approved bronchial thermoplasty for treatment of severe refractory asthma but a follow up of the Phase 4 trial study participants to determine long-term effects of the procedure is still pending.[54]

# LIFESTYLE MANAGEMENT FOR ASTHMA

Asthma needs to be managed even when symptoms are not present. According to the 2007 guidelines issued by the National Heart, Lung and Blood Institute,[55] people with asthma should educate themselves and have a clear *action plan* (regardless of severity) for the management of their asthma symptoms.

To effectively control and manage asthma in the long term, patients must be able to self-monitor their symptoms and recognize the warning sign(s) of an attack. They must also be able to respond quickly through timely use of medication(s) and/or other intervention(s). In addition, the patient must recognize and minimize contact with the specific asthma trigger(s) as well as manage other medical/health conditions that can exacerbate symptoms.

## Managing Asthma Triggers

People with persistent or seasonal asthma as well as a family history of allergies should have testing for airborne and food allergens. Because asthma and allergies frequently coexist, treating the allergy symptoms may improve asthma.[26] If possible, patients should reduce their exposure to known allergens at home, school,

work, or daycare. The patient's allergist can suggest specific ways to remove the offending allergen(s) and keep the area(s) allergy-free. More information is available in the Allergies protocol.

Patients with asthma are advised to exercise with caution because it can trigger an attack (NHLBI guidelines). They are also advised to avoid exertion when the level of air pollution is high as it can exacerbate exercise-induced asthma. Studies have shown, however, that supervised exercise and leisure-time physical activity reduced symptoms and improved the quality of life in some people with asthma.[56] Brief warm-ups and use of short-acting beta-2 agonist medications before exercise or vigorous activity may help prevent or alleviate asthma.[33]

Preliminary evidence shows that yoga and breathing exercises may also help manage asthma. However, more rigorous trials are needed to validate the evidence.[57,58]

## Managing Conditions Associated with Asthma

Treating conditions associated with asthma can help a patient manage and control the disease. Some evidence suggests that treating GERD may reduce asthma exacerbations and improve the quality of life for some asthma patients.[59] More information is available in the GERD protocol.

Proper rest and stress management are also important in reducing asthma attacks. Persistent asthma, especially if uncontrolled and severe, can bring about worry and anxiety in the patient. Likewise, evidence indicates that stress in general can precipitate and increase the risk of asthma attacks in children and adults.[60] More information is available in the Stress Management protocol.

## Dietary Considerations

It has been observed that people (regardless of health state) who eat fewer fruits and vegetables have weaker lungs. Also, asthma patients who ate less fruits and vegetables had more frequent attacks.[61]

Obesity is also associated with asthma.[26] Obese asthma patients who lost weight observed improvements in their respiratory symptoms and lung function.[62]

Also, evidence has revealed that a healthy, antioxidant rich diet may be protective against asthma. For instance, three studies found that children who followed a strictly *Mediterranean diet* (emphasizing plant-based foods such as fruits, vegetables, whole grains, legumes, and nuts, with limited intake of red meat) had lower risk of wheezing, diagnosis of asthma, and allergic rhinitis.[63–65] Adults who consumed Mediterranean-style foods were also seen to have improved control over asthma symptoms.[66] Also, apples may be protective against asthma. Several population studies have found that greater consumption of *apples* is associated with lower asthma incidence; polyphenols and other compounds present in apples are thought to convey the protection.[67,68]

# TARGETED NUTRITIONAL STRATEGIES

## Vitamin D

Vitamin D plays a crucial role in regulating a broad range of immune processes and anti-inflammatory reactions involved in asthma. Laboratory evidence from several animal models of allergic asthma suggest that vitamin D may play a role in reversing airway remodeling or airway inflammation in the asthmatic lung.[69,70] Evidence also suggests that vitamin D may protect against asthma exacerbations.[71] Studies among asthma patients found that low or deficient blood levels of vitamin D were associated with several indicators of asthma.[72–74]

Observational studies have shown that pregnant women with higher intakes of vitamin D had children with lower risks of wheezing and asthma compared to women with lower intakes of prenatal vitamin D.[75–77] Also, a longitudinal study on children with mild to moderate persistent asthma showed that low vitamin D levels were associated with higher risk of severe asthma exacerbations over a 4-year period.[78] Another study found that children who have low vitamin D levels at age 6 are more likely to have asthma at age 14 compared to children with higher vitamin D levels.[79]

In order to establish causality, intervention studies registered with the National Institutes of Health (clinicaltrials.gov) are underway to assess the ability of vitamin D to prevent or reduce the risk of asthma. Two randomized controlled clinical trials are ongoing to determine if maternal vitamin D supplementation can prevent childhood asthma (NCT00920621, NCT00856947). A clinical trial on adolescents and adults with asthma will test whether vitamin D supplementation affects the time of the first upper respiratory infection or severe exacerbation (NCT00978315). Another clinical trial on adults will test the effect of adding vitamin D to low-dose controller medications to prevent asthma symptoms and attacks (NCT01248065).

## Vitamin E

A number of studies have suggested that consuming antioxidants such as vitamins C and E, flavonoids, and selenium, among others reduces the bronchoconstriction associated with asthma.

Vitamin E is a collective name for a group of four tocopherols and four tocotrienols that possess antioxidant and anti-inflammatory properties. Studies have shown that vitamin E prevents the release of inflammatory cytokines, and specifically inhibits gene expression of IL-4.[80]

Studies have shown that asthma patients with higher vitamin E intakes had lower prevalence of wheezing, cough, and shortness of breath compared to those with lower intakes.[81] Some studies also report that low maternal vitamin E intake is associated with an increased risk of wheezing in infants and children,[82,83] and reduced lung function and increased risk of asthma in children 5 years old.[84] While one formal review of studies confirmed the protective effect of maternal vitamin E intake on wheezing,[85] another did not find evidence for an association between dietary intake of vitamin E and the risk of asthma.[86]

## Vitamin C

Population-based and experimental studies provide evidence for the link between low levels of vitamin C and asthma. An animal model has shown that supplementing with high-dose vitamin C at the time of allergy challenge decreased airway hyper-reactivity and lowered the number of inflammatory cells.[87]

One randomized controlled trial demonstrated the role of antioxidants in asthma. Children with persistent asthma who were supplemented with omega-3 fatty acids, vitamin C, or zinc experienced improved lung function. When children received all three nutrients, their lung function improved to an even greater extent than it did with the individual nutrients.[88] Another clinical trial of 8 asthmatic subjects found that those given 1500 mg of vitamin C daily for 2 weeks experienced significantly improved asthma symptom scores compared to subjects receiving placebo.[89]

## Polyunsaturated Fatty Acids

The two main groups of polyunsaturated fatty acids (PUFAs) include omega-3's and omega-6's. Typical sources of omega-3 fatty acids include fish oil, leafy green vegetables, nuts, and flaxseeds. Primary food sources of omega-6 fatty acids include vegetable oils like corn and sunflower oils, and nuts.

The Western diet has seen a decrease in consumption of foods rich in anti-inflammatory omega-3 fatty acids and an increase in proinflammatory omega-6 fatty acids, a trend that may have contributed to a rise in asthma and allergic diseases.[90] Observational studies report that higher intake of fish oil may be associated with lower risk of asthma,[91,92] while higher intake of margarine was associated with asthma.[93] Intervention studies also reported a potential benefit for the use of fish oil and omega-3 fatty acid supplements for asthma.[94,95]

## Probiotics

Evidence suggests that supplementation with beneficial bacteria—*probiotics*—may modulate components of the immune response and inflammatory processes.[96,97] Therefore, as asthma and allergy are intrinsically tied to inflammation, scientists have been interested in studying the effects of probiotics in people with asthma or other allergic diseases.

Probiotics have reliably shown positive effects in allergic rhinitis—a condition with allergic inflammation, similar to asthma. However, a clear therapeutic role of probiotics in adults with asthma needs to be further elucidated.[98] Probiotics have been shown to be effective among children with asthma.[99]

## Selenium

Studies have shown that people with chronic or severe asthma may suffer from a selenium deficiency.[100–102] Several studies have examined the use of selenium supplementation in asthma. One study found a decrease in corticosteroid use when patients were supplemented with 200 mcg daily.[103] while another study found significant clinical improvement with 100 mcg daily.[101] A 2007 study of 26 selenium-deficient, asthmatic patients revealed improvements in asthma-related quality of life and lung function measurements when deficiency was corrected with 200 mcg of selenium daily for 16 weeks.[104] Another randomized, controlled study revealed improvements in quality of life with no change in objective lung function measures.[105]

## Zinc

Large studies found that higher maternal intakes of zinc during pregnancy may protect against childhood wheezing and asthma.[83,84] Another study demonstrated that low levels of zinc in the sputum were associated with more episodes of wheezing, severe asthma, and decreased lung function.[106] Also, a study found that allergic mice exposed to cockroach allergen and supplemented with zinc had significantly lower cytokines in their airways, lower blood IgE levels, and decreased airway hyperresponsiveness.[107]

## Magnesium

Laboratory studies indicate that magnesium can relax bronchial smooth muscles.[108]

In a randomized, placebo-controlled trial, patients with mild to moderate asthma who received 340 mg of magnesium daily for 6.5 months were found to have significantly lower bronchial reactivity, improved lung function, and better asthma control and quality of life compared to the placebo group.[109] Two other trials among children with mild to moderate persistent asthma found similar benefits with magnesium supplementation.[110,111]

A recent comprehensive review of 16 clinical trials confirmed the benefit and safety of using intravenous magnesium sulfate in severe exacerbations.[112]

## Curcumin

Curcumin, a yellow pigment in the spice turmeric (found in curry powder), inhibits nuclear factor kappa-B (NF-κB), a protein involved in the production of inflammatory cytokines.[113] This was demonstrated in a laboratory animal model of asthma where treatment with curcumin reduced airway hyperresponsiveness, prevented the activation of NF-κB, and reduced the number of leukocytes (white blood cells) in lung fluid.[113]

## Lycopene

Researchers looking at the effects of lycopene (the red pigment found in tomatoes and some fruits) on asthma patients found that more than half of the patients supplemented with lycopene were significantly protected from exercise-induced asthma.[114] In animal models, lycopene supplementation suppressed the release of cytokines associated with the allergic response, suppressed the influx of eosinophils and mucus-secreting cells into the lung tissue and airways,[115] and suppressed airway hyper-responsiveness and inflammatory mediators.[116]

## Flavonoids

Flavonoids are polyphenols (found in fruits, vegetables, red wine, and tea) that have antioxidant and anti-inflammatory properties. Flavonoids have been associated with improved lung function.[117] The following flavonoids/ flavonoid-containing plants have been studied in the context of asthma:

- **Quercetin.** Part of quercetin's chemical structure is similar to cromolyn, a mast cell stabilizer sometimes used to treat asthma.[118] In one study, a high dietary intake of the flavonoids quercetin (found in wine, tea, and onions), naringenin (found in oranges and grapefruit), and hesperetin (found in oranges and lemons) was associated with a lower prevalence of asthma.[119] Several animal models of asthma have demonstrated the anti-inflammatory properties of quercetin. In one study, a single-dose oral administration of quercetin caused significant broncodilation, both in culture and *in vivo*.[120] In another study, oral administration of quercetin significantly reduced levels of the inflammatory cytokines IL-5 and IL-4 as well as inhibited mucus production in the lungs.[121] In yet another animal model, quercetin significantly inhibited all asthmatic reactions when it was administered before an asthma-inducing substance.[122]

- **Proanthocyanidin.** Proanthocyanidin is the main constituent of Pycnogenol®, an extract from the French maritime pine bark. Proanthocyanidin is a powerful antioxidant that neutralizes free radicals.[123] A randomized, placebo-controlled trial found that children with mild to moderate asthma who received Pycnogenol® for 4 weeks in addition to daily and/or rescue inhalers had significantly improved lung function and asthma symptoms compared to the placebo group. Also, the treatment group was able to reduce or discontinue use of rescue medication(s) more often than the control group.[124] Similar results were found in a more recent trial among adults with stable, controlled asthma who used Pycnogenol® as an adjunct compared to inhaled corticosteroid only or placebo.[125]

- **Ginkgo Biloba.** A flavonoid-rich extract of leaves of the *Ginkgo biloba* tree appears to be an effective asthma therapy.[126–128] In one study, ginkgo biloba extract was added to corticosteroids for 2 weeks. Researchers found that the sputum of patients on the ginkgo therapy had significantly less inflammatory cells compared to the drug-only or placebo groups, suggesting that ginkgo extract may relieve the airway inflammation associated with asthma.[128] In an animal model of asthma where an allergy challenge was followed by treatment with ginkgo, the extract inhibited the release of eosinophils in the lung tissue and mucus-secreting cells in the airways.[129]

## Butterbur

Butterbur (*Petasites hybridus*) is a perennial shrub used since ancient times to treat a variety of conditions. Four substances—petasin, isopetasin, S-petasin, and S-isopetasin—isolated from the plant can inhibit leukotrienes (inflammatory mediators associated with asthma).[130]

A few research teams have examined butterbur's effectiveness for asthma with encouraging results. In one open label trial of 64 adults and 16 children and adolescents, asthma patients were treated for

2 months with butterbur extract, followed by an optional 2-month treatment period. Data showed that all the measured symptoms improved throughout the study, and 40% of patients were able to reduce their intake of traditional asthma medications.[131] Another study found that butterbur therapy, in conjunction with inhaled corticosteroids, reduced asthma symptoms.[132]

Results from a laboratory animal model showed potential for S-petasin as a therapeutic agent for asthma. S-petasin, administered under the skin of allergen-challenged asthmatic animals, significantly slowed the production of inflammatory cells and mediators as well as relaxed the bronchial tubes, suggesting that S-petasin has both anti-inflammatory and bronchodilator properties.[133] An animal model testing butterbur extract observed similar anti-inflammatory effects on asthmatic mice.[134]

## Boswellia Serrata

Evidence suggests that compounds within the gum resin of the *Boswellia serrata* tree modulate the inflammatory process that drives asthma symptoms. Boswellia serrata inhibits leukotriene synthesis by blocking activity of the 5-lipoxygenase enzyme (5-LOX).[135] Moreover, it suppresses other enzymes (prostaglandin E synthase-1 and the serine protease cathepsin G) that, like 5-LOX, normally generate inflammatory compounds within the body.[136]

Two clinical trials have investigated the action of Boswellia serrata extract alone or in combination with other natural anti-inflammatory agents among people with asthma. First, 40 asthmatic subjects were randomized to receive either 300 mg of Boswellia serrata extract or placebo 3 times daily for 6 weeks.[137] While improvement was seen in only 27% of subjects receiving placebo, 70% of those receiving Boswellia serrata extract experienced improvements in symptoms, such as breathlessness, wheezing, and number of attacks. Those in the Boswellia group also exhibited decreased eosinophil count and lower erythrocyte sedimentation rate (ESR)—both measures of inflammation. In the second trial, 63 asthma patients took either a combination of Boswellia, curcumin, and licorice root or placebo 3 times daily for 4 weeks.[138] The herbal combination caused a significant decline in levels of LTC4 (an inflammatory leukotriene) and two markers of oxidative stress—malondialdehyde and nitric oxide. The scientists stated that a combination of Boswellia, curcumin, and licorice root "*has a pronounced effect in the management of bronchial asthma.*"

## Tylophora Indica (Tylophora Asthmatica)

*Tylophora indica* (*T. indica*) is a vine whose leaves have been studied as a potential therapy for asthma symptoms. In studies published in the late 1960s and early 1970s, *T. indica* relieved asthma symptoms more effectively than a control.[139-141] Unfortunately, no newer studies have rigorously evaluated *T. indica* as an asthma treatment. However, investigators recently pooled the data from the older trials and found that the treatment effect remained significant after adjustment for variables.[142] They concluded that "*Tylophora indica showed potential to improve lung function.*"

## Life Extension Suggestions

- **Butterbur**, standardized extract: 75–150 mg daily
- **Rosmarinic acid**: 50–100 mg daily
- **Quercetin** (providing quercetin glycoside derivatives and free quercetin): 250–500 mg daily
- **Curcumin** (as highly absorbed BCM-95®): 400–800 mg daily
- **Probiotics:** per label instructions
- **Vitamin D**: 5000–8000 IU daily; depending upon blood levels of 25-OH-vitamin D
- **Natural vitamin E**: 100–400 IU alpha-tocopherol and 200 mg gamma-tocopherol daily
- **Vitamin C**: 1000–2000 mg daily
- **Fish oil** (with olive polyphenols): providing 1400 mg EPA and 1000 mg DHA daily
- **Ginkgo biloba standardized extract:** 120 mg daily
- **Boswellia serrata extract** (standardized to 20% AKBA): 100 mg daily
- **Apple extract** (standardized to 50% polyphenols): 600–2400 mg daily
- **Tylophora indica** (Tylophora asthmatica): per label instructions
- **Lycopene:** 15 mg daily
- **Pycnogenol®:** 50–100 mg daily
- **Selenium:** 200 mcg daily
- **Calcium**: 200–1200 mg daily
- **Zinc:** 30 mg daily
- **Magnesium:** 140 mg daily as magnesium-L-threonate; 320 mg daily as magnesium citrate

In addition, the following *blood tests* may provide helpful information:

- Allergen profile (IgE mediated)
- IgG antibody testing
- Omega Score®
- Vitamin D, 25-Hydroxy

## REFERENCES

References available at: www.lef.org/dpt5/ch14

# 15

---

# Atherosclerosis and Cardiovascular Disease

---

Atherosclerosis and cardiovascular disease take a huge toll on our society. More than 81 million Americans suffer from some form of cardiovascular disease, making it the leading cause of death in the country. As of 2006, cardiovascular disease was responsible for at least one in every 2.9 deaths in the United States.[1]

Despite the fact that cardiovascular disease is the single most deadly disease in the United States, most individuals, including most mainstream physicians, have a flawed fundamental understanding of the disease. The fact is that long before any symptoms are clinically evident, vascular disease begins as a malfunction of specialized cells that line our arteries. These cells, called *endothelial* cells, are the key to atherosclerosis and underlying *endothelial dysfunction* is the central feature of this dreaded disease.

Not every person who suffers from atherosclerosis presents with the risk factors commonly associated with the condition, such as elevated cholesterol, but every single person with atherosclerosis has endothelial dysfunction. Aging humans are faced with an onslaught of atherogenic risk factors that, over time, contribute to endothelial dysfunction and the development of atherosclerosis.

Maturing individuals *must* address *all* of the underlying factors that contribute to endothelial dysfunction if they are striving to protect themselves from the ravages of vascular disease. Regrettably, mainstream medicine has failed to identify and correct *all* of the cardiovascular disease risk factors. This means that people wishing to stave off atherosclerosis must take matters into their own hands to ensure that all underlying causes are effectively neutralized.

In the antiquated view of mainstream medicine, blood vessels have been thought of as stiff pipes that gradually become clogged with excess cholesterol circulating in the bloodstream. The solution that physicians recommend most often is cholesterol-lowering drugs, which target only a very small number of the numerous factors that contribute to cardiovascular disease.

Conventional medicine's preferred method of reestablishing blood flow in clogged vessels is through surgery (coronary artery bypass graft surgery) or by insertion of catheters bearing tiny balloons that crush the plaque deposits against the arterial walls (angioplasty), followed by the implantation of tiny mesh tubes (stents) to keep the blood vessels open. However, the grafts used to reestablish blood flow often develop plaque deposits themselves. The same was true for balloon angioplasty; in their early years, up to half of all angioplasty procedures "failed" when the arteries gradually closed again. Even today, with the use of improved stents, the failure rate is considerable and many people have to undergo repeat angioplasty or even surgery.

---

## MAINSTREAM MEDICINE OVERLOOKS PROVEN ALTERNATIVE TO CORONARY STENTS AND BYPASS SURGERY: ENHANCED EXTERNAL COUNTERPULSATION

- Stable coronary artery disease and angina can cause disabling symptoms including shortness of breath, pressure or discomfort in the chest, exercise intolerance, and fatigue.
- A safe, effective, noninvasive therapy for the symptoms of coronary artery disease and angina is now available. Enhanced external counterpulsation (EECP) alleviates cardiac symptoms by enhancing coronary collateral circulation—alternate pathways by which blood can reach the heart muscle.
- The procedure is performed in a series of outpatient treatments, in which inflatable cuffs wrapped around the legs inflate and deflate in rhythm with the patient's heartbeat.
- More than 100 published studies show that EECP can effectively relieve symptoms of heart failure, increase exercise tolerance, reduce reliance on medication, and improve quality of life. Benefits of treatment can last up to five years.
- This novel therapy simulates the circulatory benefits of exercise, allowing patients to overcome symptoms and resume a healthy, active lifestyle.

To learn more about EECP, see "Doctors Ignore Proven Alternative to Coronary Stents and Bypass Surgery" in the June 2008 issue of *Life Extension Magazine*.

---

## ENDOTHELIAL DYSFUNCTION: THE UNDERLYING CAUSE OF ALL VASCULAR DISEASES

The cause and progression of vascular disease is intimately related to the health of the inner arterial wall. Blood vessels are composed of three layers. The outer

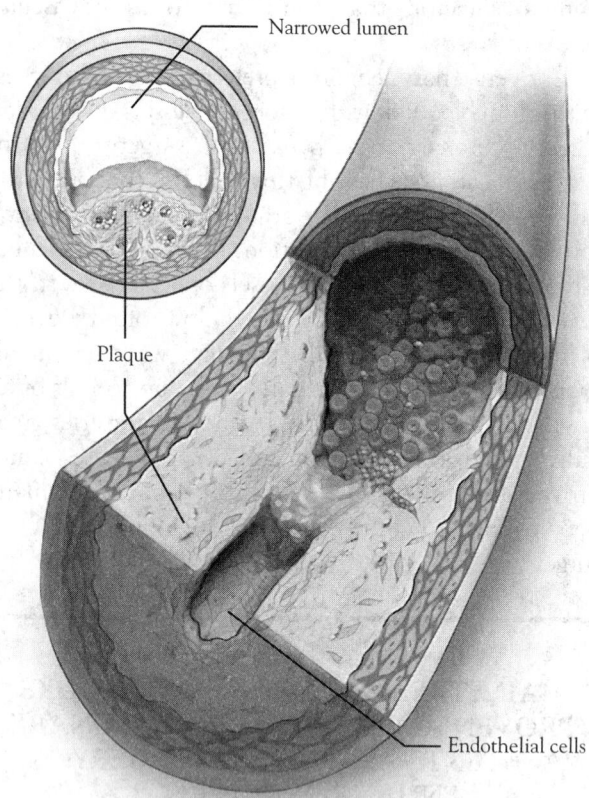

Atherosclerosis

layer is mostly connective tissue and provides structure to the layers beneath. The middle layer is smooth muscle; it contracts and dilates to control blood flow and maintain blood pressure. The inner lining consists of a thin layer of endothelial cells (the endothelium), which provides a smooth, protective surface. Endothelial cells prevent toxic, blood-borne substances from penetrating the smooth muscle of the blood vessel.

However, as we age, a barrage of atherogenic factors, if left unchecked, damage the delicate endothelial cells. This damage leads to endothelial dysfunction and ultimately allows lipids and toxins to penetrate the endothelial layer and enter the smooth muscle cells. This results in the initiation of an oxidative and inflammatory cascade that culminates in the development of plaque deposits. Subsequently, these plaques begin to calcify and, over time, become prone to rupture. If a plaque deposit ruptures, the result is often a deadly blood clot.

If people do not take steps to correct the endothelial dysfunction occurring in their aging bodies, the consequence will be a worsening of the epidemic of arterial disease that currently kills 35% of Americans and 30% of all people worldwide.[1] Sadly, mainstream

medicine continuously fails patients by prescribing drugs that address only a very small number of risk factors that contribute to the pathogenesis of vascular disease.

Numerous factors that directly contribute to endothelial dysfunction have been identified and aging individuals can easily assess their risk for vascular disease through blood testing. The results of these blood tests can then be used to develop targeted intervention strategies to modify levels of risk factors that do not fall within an optimal range. Atherogenic factors that all aging individuals *must* be aware of include:

- **Elevated low-density lipoprotein (LDL) cholesterol.** LDL is dangerous because it can penetrate the endothelial wall and contribute to the creation of *foam cells* that form the core of a plaque deposit. Oxidized LDL cholesterol (LDL that has been exposed to free radicals) within the endothelium also triggers an inflammatory process that accelerates vascular disease. Life Extension recommends keeping LDL cholesterol levels below 80 mg/dL.

- **Low high-density lipoprotein (HDL) cholesterol.** HDL protects against vascular disease by transporting cholesterol from the blood vessel wall back to the liver for disposal through a process known as *reverse cholesterol transport*. If HDL levels are low, then reverse cholesterol transport becomes inefficient, allowing for increased accumulation of cholesterol in the vessel wall. HDL levels of at least 50 to 60 mg/dL are recommended for optimal vascular protection.

- **Elevated triglycerides.** Triglycerides interact with LDL cholesterol to form a particularly dangerous subtype of LDL known as *small dense LDL*. Small dense LDL particles penetrate the endothelial layer and contribute to plaque formation much more efficiently than larger, more buoyant LDL particles. Life Extension recommends keeping fasting triglycerides below 80 mg/dL to limit the formation of small-dense LDL particles.

- **Oxidized LDL.** The oxidation of LDL results in severe vascular damage. Thousands of studies now reveal how oxidized LDL contributes to the entire atherogenic process from start to finish. Commercial blood tests are not yet available at affordable prices to measure oxidized LDL. Aging individuals should assume their endogenous antioxidant levels (superoxide dismutase, catalase, and glutathione) are being depleted and that the oxidation of their LDL is progressively worsening.[2] Many of the nutrient suggestions in this protocol afford considerable protection against LDL oxidation.

- **Hypertension.** High blood pressure is known to aggravate endothelial dysfunction and leading researchers have identified the endothelium as an "end organ" for damage caused by high blood pressure. Life Extension suggests a target optimal blood pressure of 115/75 mmHg (or lower).

- **Elevated C-reactive protein.** Inflammation is central to the endothelial dysfunction that underlies vascular disease. An effective way to measure inflammation is through a high-sensitivity C-reactive protein (CRP) blood test. Studies have shown that higher levels of CRP are associated with increased risk of stroke, heart attack, and peripheral vascular disease.[3-4] Stroke patients with the highest CRP levels are 2 to 3 times more likely to die or experience a new vascular event within a year than are patients with the lowest levels.[5]

- **Elevated Lp-PLA$_2$.** Like CRP, Lp-PLA$_2$ is a marker of inflammation. However, Lp-PLA$_2$ is a much more specific measure of vascular inflammation than CRP. Lp-PLA$_2$ is an enzyme secreted by inflamed vascular plaque. Thus the quantity of Lp-PLA$_2$ in circulation correlates with the amount of inflamed plaque in the blood vessels. Levels of Lp-PLA$_2$ above 200 ng/mL are indicative of heightened levels of vascular plaque buildup.

- **Elevated omega-6:omega-3 ratio.** High levels of proinflammatory omega-6 fatty acids relative to anti-inflammatory omega-3 fatty acids create an environment that fosters inflammation and contributes to vascular disease. It has been shown that lowering the omega-6:omega-3 ratio significantly decreases atherosclerotic lesion size and reduces numerous measures of inflammation.[6] Life Extension recommends maintaining a blood omega-6:omega-3 ratio of less than 4:1.

- **Elevated glucose.** High circulating levels of blood glucose (and insulin) cause microvascular damage that accelerates the atherogenic process, partly by contributing to endothelial dysfunction.[7] It has been shown that a fasting blood glucose level of greater than 85 mg/dL significantly increases risk of cardiovascular related mortality.[8] Life Extension suggests keeping fasting blood glucose levels below 86 mg/dL.

- **Excess Insulin.** As we age, we lose our ability to effectively utilize insulin to drive blood glucose into energy-producing cells. As glucose levels rise in the blood, the pancreas compensates by producing more insulin. As "insulin resistance" worsens, even more insulin is secreted in attempt to restore glucose control. Excess insulin is associated with a significantly greater risk of heart disease.[9] Life Extension suggests keeping fasting insulin below 5 µIU/mL.

- **Elevated Homocysteine.** High homocysteine levels damage endothelial cells and contribute to the initial pathogenesis vascular disease.[10] Homocysteine levels are associated with risk of heart disease.[11,12] To keep homocysteine-induced endothelial damage to a minimum, levels of homocysteine should be kept below 7 to 8 µmol/L.

- **Elevated Fibrinogen.** When a blood clot forms, fibrinogen is converted to fibrin, which forms the structural matrix of a blood clot.[13] Fibrinogen also facilitates platelet adherence to endothelial cells.[14] People with high levels of fibrinogen are more than twice as likely to die of a heart attack or stroke as people with normal fibrinogen levels.[15,16] In a review that included data for over 154000 patients, every 100 mg/dL increase in fibrinogen levels was associated with a significantly increased risk of developing coronary heart disease, stroke, and with vascular-related mortality. In one study, patients with the lowest one-third fibrinogen levels (mean 236 mg/dL) were much less likely to suffer a stroke, develop cardiovascular disease, or die of other vascular-related causes when compared to those with the highest one-third fibrinogen levels (mean 374 mg/dL).[17] This risk goes up even more in the presence of hypertension.[17a] Fibrinogen levels should be kept between 295 and 369 mg/dL.

- **Insufficient Vitamin D.** Vitamin D protects against vascular disease via several different mechanisms, including reducing chronic inflammatory reactions that contribute to the pathology of the disease. It has been shown that low vitamin D levels are associated with increased cardiovascular mortality.[18] Life Extension suggests maintaining a 25-hydroxy vitamin D blood level of 50–80 ng/mL.

- **Insufficient Vitamin K.** Vitamin K is essential for regulating proteins in the body that direct calcium to the bones and keep it out of the arterial wall. Low vitamin K status predisposes aging humans to vascular calcification,[19-21] chronic inflammation,[22] and sharply higher heart attack risks. Vitamin K blood tests assess levels of vitamin K to maintain healthy coagulation, but at this time are not used to identify optimal levels to reduce heart attack risk. However, there is a substantial amount of evidence suggesting that supplementation with vitamin K (as K1, MK-4, and MK-7) easily corrects the vitamin K deficits that are so common among Americans today.[24–28]

- **Low Testosterone and Excess Estrogen (in men).** Numerous studies link low testosterone (and excess estradiol) with increased heart attack and stroke risk.[29–32] Testosterone is intimately involved in the *reverse cholesterol transport* process, which *removes* cholesterol from the arterial wall by HDL. Excess *estrogen* is linked with higher C-reactive protein and a greater propensity for abnormal blood clots to form in arteries, causing a sudden heart attack or stroke.[33,34] Men should keep their free testosterone in a range of 20–25 pg/mL and their estradiol levels between 20 and 30 pg/mL.[35]

- **Insufficient CoQ10.** Supplemental CoQ10 alters the pathology of vascular diseases and has the potential for prevention of vascular disease through the inhibition of LDL cholesterol oxidation and by the maintenance of optimal cellular and mitochondrial function throughout the ravages of time and internal and external stresses. The attainment of higher blood levels of CoQ10 (>3.5 µg/mL) with the use of higher doses of CoQ10 appears to enhance both the magnitude and rate of clinical improvement.[36]

- **Nitric Oxide Deficit.** Nitric oxide is an important messenger molecule *required* for healthy cardiovascular function. Nitric oxide enables blood vessels to expand and contract with youthful elasticity and is vital to maintaining the structural integrity of the endothelium, thus protecting against vascular disease. Even when all other risk factors are controlled for, the age-related decline in endothelial nitric oxide too often causes accelerated vascular disease unless corrective measures are taken. Commercial blood tests are not yet available at affordable prices to assess nitric oxide status. Aging individuals should assume that they are developing a nitric oxide deficit in their inner arterial wall (the endothelium) and follow simple steps outlined in this protocol to protect themselves.[37–39]

### THE VAP™ TEST: MEASURING THE ATHEROGENIC POTENTIAL OF BLOOD LIPIDS

The Vertical Auto-Profile (VAP™) assesses subclasses of lipids that are known or emerging risk factors for cardiovascular disease, such as LDL particle size and lipoprotein(a).[40] This enables cardiologists and nutritionists to help high-risk patients identify these new risk factors for cardiovascular disease that are based on the amounts and sizes of cholesterol and other fat molecules that circulate in the blood. Comprehensive tests such as the VAP™ can provide the highly specialized information that doctors and patients need to make informed decisions about diet, lifestyle, supplements, and medication changes.

One of the chief advantages of the VAP™ method over other techniques of measuring lipid profiles is that it can determine not only the types of cholesterol particles (HDL, LDL, VLDL, and so on), but also their individual size and density.[41,42] That is vital because people who produce small, dense LDL particles, for example, are known to be at increased risk of heart disease.[42] The VAP™ test also measures lipoprotein(a), a particularly dangerous lipoprotein that can lead to heart attacks and strokes.

Knowledge of particle size and density is critical for determining the next steps in management of people who may have achieved their "target" lipid values, but who still have high-risk lipid particle types.[43] In essence, the VAP™ provides a "higher-resolution" picture of what is really going on in a person's lipid profile, allowing them to customize their management regimen. It can even help detect early risk factors in people who have apparently "normal" lipid profiles on older kinds of tests—according to K.R. Kulkarni, one of the experts who helped to develop the test, "because VAP™ measures so many different parameters of the lipid profile, it can identify patients at high risk for coronary heart disease who cannot be identified using the standard lipid profile."[44]

The VAP™ can be used to monitor the results of specific treatments, such as statin therapy,[45] to ensure that goals are being met. When the VAP™ uncovers hidden risk factors, additional approaches using diet, lifestyle, supplements, and certain drugs are advised.

### TARGETING VASCULAR DISEASE RISK FACTORS WITH NUTRITIONAL THERAPEUTICS

Scientific studies have revealed that several nutrients effectively protect against endothelial dysfunction caused by the atherogenic factors identified above. Unlike mainstream medicine's approach to treating atherosclerosis, which involves addressing only very few proven cardiac risk factors, a comprehensive nutritional regimen can be designed to target all risk factors that contribute to atherosclerosis.

### Omega-3 Fatty Acids

Studies have shown that omega-3 fatty acids combat the development and progression of vascular disease via multiple mechanisms, including lowering triglycerides, lowering blood pressure, improving endothelial function, and raising HDL levels.[46]

A team of researchers examined the correlation between tissue omega-3 fatty acid levels and measures of circulating Lp-PLA$_2$, a marker of inflammatory arterial plaque, in over 300 patients. They found a strong, independent, and inverse association between tissue omega-3 levels and circulating Lp-PLA$_2$. The researchers went on to conclude that intake of omega-3 fatty acids might reduce Lp-PLA$_2$ levels and reduce the risk of vascular disease.[47]

In another study involving 563 elderly men, 2.4 g per day of omega-3 fatty acid supplementation was found to improve arterial elasticity.[48]

In 16 patients with peripheral artery disease who were already being treated with conventional methods, the addition of 2 g daily of omega-3 fatty acids was shown to significantly improve endothelial function, as measured by brachial artery flow-mediated dilation (from 6.7% to 10.0%) and plasma soluble thrombomodulin (from 33.0 ng/mL to 17.0 ng/mL).[49] Similarly, another study found that when omega-3 fatty acids were combined with rosuvastatin, the combination improved endothelial dependent vasodilation (−1.42% to 11.36%) while rosuvastatin alone failed to improve endothelial function.[50]

## Propionyl L-Carnitine (PLC)

PLC has received attention for its ability to directly improve endothelial function. PLC passes across the mitochondrial membrane to supply L-carnitine directly to the mitochondria, the energy-producing organelles of cells. Carnitines are essential for mitochondrial fatty acid transport and energy production, which is important because endothelial cells and heart muscle cells burn fatty acids for 70% of their energy. By contrast, most other cells generate 70% of their energy from glucose and only 30% from fatty acids.[51]

In human studies, PLC produced significant improvement in maximum walking distance with claudication (sclerotic peripheral vascular disease) and had no major side effects.[52] Another study found that PLC significantly reduced homocysteine levels when administered intravenously to hemodialysis patients.[53]

Animal studies suggest that PLC may help prevent or decrease the severity of vascular disease. In rabbits fed a high-cholesterol diet, which normally induces endothelial dysfunction and subsequent atherosclerosis, supplementation with PLC resulted in reduced plaque thickness, markedly lower triglyceride levels, and reduced proliferation of foam cells.[54]

PLC also improves endothelial function by increasing nitric oxide production in animals with normal blood pressure and in animal models of hypertension. Nitric oxide is important because it helps keep arteries open. The increased nitric oxide production induced by PLC is related to its antioxidant properties; PLC reduces reactive oxygen species and increases nitric oxide production in the endothelium in the presence of the antioxidative enzymes superoxide dismutase and catalase.[55]

## L-Arginine

This amino acid has attracted attention for its ability to improve endothelial function. L-arginine serves as the precursor of nitric oxide in the endothelium.[56] To find out whether L-arginine improved arterial function in people with peripheral arterial disease, as well as determine an optimal oral dose, a group of researchers from the University of California-San Francisco looked at L-arginine's ability to improve walking distance and walking speed among people with peripheral arterial disease. The research group found in a pilot study of 80 patients that 3 g L-arginine daily improved both walking speed and distance.[57]

Another study looked at the effects of oral L-arginine in patients with stable coronary artery disease. The team found that L-arginine therapy of 10 g daily improved brachial artery dilation, a measure of endothelial function.[58]

## CoQ10

CoQ10 is critically important for vascular health, as it is directly involved in the production of ATP, the "energy currency" of the human body. Because the heart is a muscle that never rests, it needs a substantial amount of CoQ10. CoQ10 levels in heart tissue decline disproportionately with age. At age 20, the heart has a higher CoQ10 level than other major organs. At age 80 this is no longer true, with heart levels cut by more than half.[59] CoQ10 pioneer Karl Folkers,[59a] in agreement with other Japanese studies, found lower CoQ10 levels in patients with more severe heart disease and showed that CoQ10 supplements significantly raised blood and heart tissue levels of CoQ10 in these patients.

In addition to its involvement in energy production, CoQ10 is also a potent antioxidant. CoQ10 is the first line of defense against LDL oxidation; oxidized LDL is a major contributor to endothelial dysfunction.[60]

CoQ10, in combination with vitamins C, E, and selenium, was shown in a randomized controlled trial to significantly improve arterial elasticity in patients with multiple cardiovascular risk factors. The authors found that the antioxidant-induced increases in arterial elasticity were associated with improved glucose and lipid metabolism, as well as decreased blood pressure.[61]

In an animal study, CoQ10 supplementation was shown to improve endothelial function, as measured by thoracic aorta nitric oxide availability and blood pressure.[62]

## Pomegranate

For HDL to perform its vital functions, an enzyme called *paraoxonase-1* (PON-1) is attached to its surface. PON-1 serves to protect HDL from oxidation, which impairs its ability to protect arteries. As humans age, PON-1 levels markedly decline, thereby *reducing* the ability of HDL to protect against heart attack and stroke. This phenomenon helps explain the onset of *accelerated* atherosclerosis; where within a period of only a few years, an aging person's healthy arteries rapidly *occlude* with plaque. In addition to its ability to protect HDL against oxidation, PON-1 has also been shown to hydrolyze (break apart) *homocysteine* thiolactones, which are responsible for damage to blood vessels. So PON-1, on its own, is a blood vessel protector.[63]

Lipid peroxidation is a free radical reaction that severely damages cell membranes and is implicated in a host of degenerative diseases. PON-1 blocks destructive *lipid peroxidation* reactions, making it a crucial *enzyme* for aging humans to maintain.[64–67]

Research indicates that pomegranate and its extracts can significantly *elevate* levels of PON-1 activity in the body. Pomegranate does this through a number of distinct biomolecular pathways that include combating inflammation and LDL adhesion and favorably modulating gene expression. Pomegranate extracts reduce oxidation and inflammation largely through their effect on PON-1 activity, intervening at each step in the development of atherosclerosis.[68]

Researchers studied the effects of pomegranate on human subjects who consumed pomegranate juice for 2 weeks. The team found dramatic reductions in LDL "clumping" and retention in vessels, accompanied by a 20% increase in PON-1 activity.[69]

In atherosclerosis-prone mice supplemented with pomegranate, a 90% reduction in oxidation of LDL cholesterol was seen. Supplemented mice also developed atherosclerotic lesions *44%* smaller than controls, an effect attributed to reduction in the number of inflammatory foam cells.[69]

## Lipoic Acid

This naturally occurring antioxidant serves as a co-enzyme in energy metabolism of fats, carbohydrates,

and proteins. It can regenerate thioredoxin (an antioxidant protein), vitamin C, and glutathione, which in turn can recycle vitamin E. Lipoic acid also helps manage proper serum glucose levels in diabetic patients.[70] In animal studies, it has been shown to reduce endothelial dysfunction.[71] Human studies have found that lipoic acid improves endothelial function among people with metabolic syndrome.[72] Lipoic acid works best in combination with antioxidants, including vitamin E, coenzyme Q10, carnitine, and selenomethionine.[73]

## Garlic

Aged garlic extract has been studied for its ability to reduce inflammation and the damaging effects of cholesterol in the endothelium.[74] In one study of 15 men with coronary artery disease who were also being treated with statin drugs and low-dose aspirin, 2 weeks of supplementation with aged garlic extract significantly improved blood flow by improving endothelial function.[75]

Finally, high-dose garlic was studied in 152 individuals with clinically observable atherosclerotic plaque buildup. Over 48 months, the study participants experienced significantly less increase in plaque deposits than a control group, and a regression of plaque was seen in some participants, leading researchers to conclude that garlic had a "not only preventative but possibly also a curative role in arteriosclerosis therapy."[76]

## Ginkgo Biloba

Several studies have shown that ginkgo favorably alters endothelial function and reduces levels of oxidized LDL.[77–79] Ginkgo has also been shown to protect against the formation of foam cells.[80]

In a study involving eight patients who had recently undergone aortocoronary bypass surgery, supplementation with ginkgo biloba extract, 120 mg twice daily, was shown to reduce atherosclerotic plaque formation by 11.9% and reduce nanoplaque size by 24.4%. Furthermore, ginkgo increased levels of endogenous antioxidant enzymes and reduced levels of the dangerous oxidized LDL.[81]

In an animal model, researchers found that ginkgo was effective in reducing high homocysteine-induced intimal thickening, indicating a reversal in the atherosclerotic process.[82]

## Resveratrol

Experiments have shown that the benefits of resveratrol include improvements in the health of the endothelial tissue lining blood vessels.[83-86] One mechanism by which it does this is to facilitate the generation of endothelial progenitor stem cells, thereby providing the endothelium with fresh new cells.

Resveratrol benefits the circulatory system by eliciting a decrease in the oxidation of LDL, fostering decreases in platelet aggregation, and promoting relaxation of small blood vessels called arterioles.[87-90] Collectively, these mechanisms benefit the overall health of the cardiovascular system by reducing factors that contribute to the development of atherosclerosis and decreasing the likelihood of undesirable clotting, which, in turn, decreases the risk of stroke.[91] Furthermore, data indicate that resveratrol decreases the incidence of dangerous heart arrhythmias.[92]

## Quercetin

The so-called French paradox is the phenomenon of low rates of heart disease in a country known for its high intake of fatty foods. Recent research suggests that one of the reasons French people are protected from heart disease is a high intake of quercetin, a potent antioxidant and polyphenol found in red wine[93] and certain vegetables. Numerous studies have examined quercetin and found it to be both a powerful antioxidant and a stimulator of nitric oxide, which inhibits endothelial proliferation, a hallmark of atherosclerosis.[93]

In spontaneously hypertensive rats, quercetin, along with other bioflavonoids, preserved endothelial function by increasing nitric oxide and reducing blood pressure.[94]

A porcine study showed that quercetin has potent antioxidative properties and protects endothelial cells against induced dysfunction.[95] Quercetin and resveratrol may work particularly well together.

## Green Tea Extract

Green tea extracts, which are rich in natural antioxidants and antiplatelet agents, are routinely used in Asia to lower blood pressure and reduce elevated cholesterol. In studies of smokers, 600 mL green tea (not extract) was shown to decrease markers of inflammation and oxidized cholesterol, both of which are intimately involved in the development of atherosclerosis.[96]

A Japanese study of 203 patients found that the more green tea patients drink, the less likely they are to suffer from coronary artery disease.[97] This study supported an earlier study that found that greater green tea consumption was related to a reduced presence of coronary artery disease in Japanese men.[98]

## Vitamin C (Ascorbic Acid)

Vitamin C inhibits damage caused by oxidative stress. In cigarette smokers, daily supplementation with 500 mg vitamin C significantly decreased the appearance of oxidative stress markers.[99] Another study showed that supplementation with 500 mg vitamin C and 400 IU vitamin E daily reduced the development of accelerated coronary arteriosclerosis following cardiac transplantation.[100]

Vitamin C's benefits seem especially profound in people who suffer from both diabetes and coronary artery disease. One study demonstrated that, in this group, vitamin C significantly improved vasodilation.[101]

## Vitamin K

Vitamin K is steadily gaining attention for its ability to reduce vascular calcification and help prevent vascular disease.[102] Evidence for the ability of vitamin K to prevent calcification can also be found in an animal study in which researchers administered the anticoagulant warfarin to rats. Warfarin is known to deplete vitamin K. At the end of the study, all the animals had extensive calcification, suggesting they had lost the protective effect of vitamin K.[103]

A large study of more than 4800 subjects followed for 7–10 years in the Netherlands demonstrated that people in the highest one-third of vitamin K2 intake had a 57% reduction in risk of dying from vascular disease, compared to those with the lowest intake. Furthermore, their risk of having severe aortic calcification plummeted by 52%—a clear demonstration of the vitamin's protective effects.[104]

Another study by the same group showed that higher vitamin K2 intake was associated with a 20% decreased risk of coronary artery calcification.[105]

## Vitamin E

Vitamin E is often studied in conjunction with vitamin C for its potent antioxidant powers. It has been shown to decrease lipid peroxidation and inhibit smooth muscle cell proliferation, platelet aggregation, monocyte adhesion, oxidized LDL uptake, and cytokine production—all of which occur during sclerotic vascular disease.[106,107]

In cultured arterial endothelial cells, vitamin E increased the production of prostacyclin, a potent vasodilator and inhibitor of platelet aggregation.[108] Most vitamin E supplements come in the form of alpha tocopherol, but it is also important to supplement with around 200 mg of gamma tocopherol to gain vitamin E's comprehensive benefits.

Several studies show that patients with advanced cardiovascular disease exhibit normal plasma levels of alpha tocopherol but have substantially lower levels of gamma tocopherol.[109–111] In a 7-year follow-up study of more than 334,000 postmenopausal women with no previous heart disease, greater intake of dietary vitamin E—consisting predominantly of gamma tocopherol—was strongly associated with a lower risk of death from cardiovascular disease. The data did not appear to demonstrate a similarly protective role for supplemental alpha tocopherol.[112]

Numerous animal studies likewise suggest that gamma tocopherol may provide powerful protection for the heart. In laboratory rats, supplementation with gamma tocopherol reduced platelet aggregation and clot formation even more effectively than alpha tocopherol.[113] In addition, gamma tocopherol at physiologic doses was more effective than alpha tocopherol in enhancing the activity of superoxide dismutase (SOD), an antioxidant enzyme that may help reduce the risk of cardiac events.[114]

## Niacin

Niacin reduces very low-density lipoprotein (VLDL) particles. Less VLDL leads to less small-dense LDL (prone to oxidation and atherogenesis) and higher HDL.[115] Niacin also improves endothelial function and nitric oxide synthase activity.

Niacin's benefits are not limited to its influence on blood markers of vascular disease risk. It also reduces heart attack risk dramatically. The Coronary Drug Project was the first to establish that niacin is a powerful agent in lowering heart attack risk. When more than 1000 heart attack survivors were given 3000 mg of (immediate-release/crystalline) niacin daily for 6 years, the incidence of recurrent nonfatal heart attacks was reduced by 27%, and the number of strokes was reduced by 26%.[116]

## THE REMARKABLE LIFE-SAVING BENEFITS OF ASPIRIN

The benefits of aspirin are often overlooked in light of the numerous nutritional ingredients that convey cardioprotective effects. This is unfortunate because maturing individuals can utilize aspirin, along with these nutritional ingredients, to significantly enhance their defense against cardiovascular disease.

Studies indicate that aspirin may protect against heart disease in part by improving endothelial function. In a study involving 41 patients with hypertension and high cholesterol, 100 mg of aspirin daily was shown to lower both systolic and diastolic blood pressure and increase flow-mediated dilation, a marker of endothelial function.[117]

The heart depends on its coronary arteries for the oxygen supply that fuels this most vital of organs. Coronary heart disease occurs when normal blood flow through the arteries that feed the heart is slowed or interrupted by factors such as blood clots or plaque.

Preventing clots is another way that aspirin helps prevent heart attacks. By irreversibly blocking production of clot-promoting compounds known as thromboxanes, aspirin prevents platelets in the blood from latching on to each other and forming a clot. A platelet has a life span of 10 days, and aspirin irreversibly impairs the platelet's clotting ability. Aspirin helps blood flow more smoothly past any plaque that is narrowing an artery, and if a plaque ruptures, aspirin will reduce the likelihood of a clot clinging to it.[118]

Aspirin can also help prevent heart disease through its anti-inflammatory action. Inflammation participates in many disease processes in the body, including plaque accumulation in the arteries.[119] The growth of plaque can obstruct blood flow through the arteries. If a plaque ruptures due to inflammation, it can trigger a heart attack.

A 2003 meta-analysis examined aspirin's effects on primary heart-attack prevention (ie, the prevention of first heart attacks). In more than 55,000 men and women, aspirin use was associated with a 32% reduction in the risk of having a first heart attack, and with a 15% reduction in the risk of all major vascular events.[120]

A study presented at the 2005 meeting of the American Heart Association reported on the life-saving benefits of aspirin therapy. This study examined nearly 9000 women with stable heart disease, ranging in age from 50 to 79. During more than 6 years of follow-up, women taking aspirin were 25% less likely to die from heart disease and 17% less likely to die from any cause. Some women took 81 mg of aspirin daily, while others took 325 mg. The study authors stated that the 2 doses appeared to be similarly effective, but that higher doses of aspirin are associated with a greater risk of certain side effects, such as stomach bleeding.[121]

A meta-analysis published in 2006 examined the effects of aspirin therapy in preventing cardiovascular events in women and men. Examining data from more than 50,000 women, investigators determined that aspirin therapy was associated with a significant 12% reduction in cardiovascular events in women. Among more than 44,000 men, aspirin therapy produced a significant 14% reduction in all cardiovascular events and an even more impressive 32% reduction in heart attacks.[122]

According to the U.S. Preventive Services Task Force, aspirin's proven benefits are reason enough for people to start using it if they have at least a 6% chance of developing coronary heart disease in the next 10 years. By contrast, the American Heart Association recommends aspirin for people whose 10-year risk of developing coronary heart disease is 10% or higher, as long they have no medical contra-indications for taking the drug. A doctor can help you calculate your cardiovascular risk based on factors such as tobacco use, cholesterol, and blood pressure. You can also assess your cardiovascular risk by using online risk factor calculators available at the American Heart Association website.

Life Extension strongly recommends that people who have already had a heart attack (or other episode of heart disease) discuss aspirin therapy with their doctor as part of a strategy to prevent future problems. Life Extension also suggests that people with no previous history of cardiovascular disease—but who are nevertheless at high risk for heart disease—strongly consider aspirin therapy in consultation with their personal physician. The recommended dose for preventing heart-related problems is 81–325 mg daily. Speak with your doctor about your personal needs before beginning aspirin therapy.

# HORMONES AND CARDIOVASCULAR HEALTH

### Testosterone and Estrogen Balance (Men)

Recent studies suggest that testosterone-replacement may improve the symptoms of vascular disease. A placebo-controlled crossover study in men with ischemic heart disease and low testosterone levels reported that exercise time and the time to development of ischemic changes on a treadmill test were both increased with testosterone-replacement therapy.[123]

It has been shown that men with lower levels of testosterone have poorer endothelial function. In a study of 187 males, researchers found that men in the highest quartile of testosterone levels had 1.7-fold greater flow mediated dilation, a marker of endothelial function.[124]

In another study, researchers examined the correlation between testosterone levels and mortality in over 900 men with coronary heart disease. The team found that the mortality rate in patients with testosterone deficiency was 21%, while only 12% of subjects with normal testosterone levels died. The authors of the study concluded that "in patients with coronary

disease testosterone deficiency is common and impacts significantly negatively on survival."[125]

Researchers analyzed 30-day survival data for 126 men who had suffered a heart attack. All of the men who did not survive were found to have low total testosterone levels ($\leq$300 ng/dL). The team went on to conclude that "a low level of testosterone was independently related to total short-term [post-heart attack] mortality."[126]

Testosterone levels are also inversely associated with the development of coronary artery disease. In a study of men 45 years of age or younger, researchers found that subjects with diagnosed coronary artery disease had significantly lower levels of free testosterone than did healthy, age-matched controls. The researchers went on to caution that, based on their findings, "*a low level of free testosterone may be related to the development of premature coronary artery disease.*"[127]

Italian researchers compared plasma testosterone levels of 119 elderly men with isolated systolic hypertension to those of 106 nonhypertensive elderly men. All the study participants were 60 to 79 years old, nonobese, nondiabetic, and nonsmokers. The hypertensive men were found to have 14% lower levels of testosterone compared to the nonhypertensive men. In both the hypertensive and nonhypertensive men, low testosterone levels correlated with higher blood pressure values.[128]

In a study of over 11 000 men, followed for up to 10 years, baseline testosterone concentrations were inversely associated with cardiovascular and all-cause mortality. Men with total testosterone levels of 481 ng/dL or greater at baseline were significantly less likely to die of cardiovascular disease or any cause during the follow-up period compared to men with testosterone levels below 481 ng/dL. The correlation held even after adjustment for various other confounding factors. The authors of this study declared that "low testosterone may be a predictive marker for those at high risk of cardiovascular disease."[129]

A study published in the *Journal of the American Medical Association* (JAMA) measured blood estradiol (a dominant estrogen) in 501 men with chronic heart failure. Compared to men in the *balanced* estrogen quintile, men in the *lowest* estradiol quintile were 317% more likely to die during a 3-year follow-up, while men in the *highest* estradiol quintile were 133% more likely to die.[35]

The men in the *balanced* quintile—with the *fewest* deaths—had serum estradiol levels between 21.80 and 30.11 pg/mL. This is very similar to the optimal range that Life Extension has long recommended for aging men. The men in the highest quintile who suffered

133% increased death rates had serum estradiol levels of 37.40 pg/mL or *above*. The *lowest* estradiol group that suffered a 317% increased death rate had serum estradiol levels *under* 12.90 pg/mL.

For more information on optimizing male hormone levels in order to prevent not only vascular disease, but many other age-related diseases as well, see the Male Hormone Restoration protocol.

---

## TESTOSTERONE PROTECTS WOMEN TOO

Testosterone is often thought to be beneficial only for men. However, a study of nearly 3000 women reveals that maintaining optimal testosterone levels is important for females as well. After assessing testosterone levels at baseline, researchers found that over a 4.5-year follow-up period, women with the lowest levels of testosterone were more likely to experience a cardiovascular event and die of any cause than women with the highest testosterone. The authors concluded *"low baseline testosterone in women is associated with increased all-cause mortality and incident cardiovascular events independent of traditional risk factors."*[130]

---

## DHEA (Men and Women)

DHEA is a precursor to sex hormones such as testosterone and estrogen. Levels of steroid hormones, including DHEA, decline with the age-associated onset of a variety of medical conditions, including chronic inflammation, hypertension, and atherosclerosis. Higher levels of DHEA in humans are associated with lower levels of inflammatory biomarkers.[131]

A study showed that men with high levels of DHEA tended to have greater protection against aortic atherosclerosis progression.[132] Similarly, another study of 419 Japanese individuals found that those with the highest circulating levels of DHEA-sulfate (form of DHEA commonly measured on blood tests) were much less likely to have carotid atherosclerosis.[133]

Animal studies show a protective role for DHEA in preventing atherosclerosis. Providing DHEA to human vascular endothelial cells in culture increases nitric oxide synthesis, which boosts blood flow.[134]

## Progesterone (Women)

Several studies have determined that non-bioidentical progestin promotes the formation of atherosclerosis.[135,136] The story is quite different for bioidentical progesterone, where multiple animal studies have shown that bioidentical progesterone *inhibits* the process of atherosclerosis.[137,138] To illustrate, scientists fed postmenopausal monkeys a diet that is known to cause atherosclerosis for 30 months. The scientists then divided the monkeys into groups that received estrogen alone, estrogen plus non-bioidentical progestin, and a control group that did not receive hormones. The control group developed substantial atherosclerotic plaque. The administration of estrogen resulted in a 72% decrease in atherosclerotic plaque compared to the control group. Treatment with non-bioidentical progestin yielded disturbing results. The group that received estrogen combined with non-bioidentical progestin had a similar amount of atherosclerotic plaque as the control group, meaning that non-bioidentical progestin completely *reversed* estrogen's inhibitory effects on the formation of atherosclerosis.[139] In contrast, when the same investigators administered bioidentical progesterone along with estrogen, no such inhibition of estrogen's cardiovascular benefit was seen.[140]

In a trial published in the *Journal of the American College of Cardiology*, researchers studied postmenopausal women with a history of heart attack or coronary artery disease. The women were given estrogen in combination with either bioidentical progesterone or non-bioidentical progestin. After 10 days of treatment the women underwent exercise treadmill tests. Compared to the non-bioidentical progestin group, the amount of time it took to produce myocardial ischemia (reduced blood flow to the heart) on the exercise treadmill was substantially *improved* in the bioidentical progesterone group.[141]

## Estriol (Women)

Growing evidence suggests that *estriol* may offer benefits to the cardiovascular system. For instance, Japanese scientists found that a group of menopausal women given estriol for 12 months had a significant *decrease* in both systolic and diastolic blood pressure.[142] Another study compared the use of estriol for 10 months in 20 postmenopausal and 29 elderly women. Some of the elderly women had decreases in total cholesterol and triglycerides and an increase in beneficial HDL.[143]

To examine the effects of estriol on atherosclerosis, researchers conducted an experiment in which female rabbits were fed a high-cholesterol diet with or without supplemental estriol. The rabbits had their ovaries removed surgically to mimic menopause. Remarkably, the group receiving estriol had 75% *less* atherosclerosis than the group fed the high-cholesterol diet alone (without estriol).[144]

## Phytoestrogens (Women)

Following menopause, circulating levels of estrogen are depleted. Phytoestrogens are plant hormones with estrogenic activity. In postmenopausal women, phytoestrogens appear to have estrogen-like benefits such as protection against osteoporosis[145,146] and possibly hot flashes.[147] Phytoestrogens have also been shown to improve vascular function, which tends to decline with age. In one study, genistein, a phytoestrogen, provided in a daily 54-mg supplement for 1 year significantly improved endothelium-dependent vasodilation in postmenopausal women. Moreover, its benefits were as substantial as those observed in women receiving an estrogen-progestin regimen.[148]

For more information on optimizing female hormone levels in order to prevent not only cardiovascular disease but other age-related diseases as well, see the Female Hormone Restoration protocol.

# SUMMARY

Atherosclerosis is a serious threat to the health of a staggering number of individuals across the globe. Its progression has been linked to increased risk of heart attack, stroke, atrial fibrillation, and dementia, among other potentially fatal conditions. Since it may begin as early as childhood and aging has been identified as the greatest risk factor for its development, it is vital to combat this disease as early—and as aggressively—as possible. Unfortunately, if aging individuals leave the health of their arteries in the hands of mainstream medicine, they cannot expect conventional approaches to address all the risk factors that lead to atherosclerosis and cardiovascular disease.

Comprehensive blood testing helps aging individuals identify and target their specific risk factors, allowing for the development of a personalized, targeted treatment regimen that can be used to preserve and improve cardiovascular health.

In contrast to the methods of mainstream medicine, which address only very few heart disease risk factors, Life Extension has identified numerous scientifically validated ways by which aging individuals can improve the function of their endothelial cells and greatly reduce their risk of developing deadly atherosclerotic plaque buildup in their blood vessels.

## Life Extension Suggestions

Any program aimed at reducing the risk of vascular disease begins with comprehensive blood testing. This step is vital to designing a program that targets an individual's specific risk factors. Healthy adults should have their blood tested at least once a year. People who have vascular disease or a family history of vascular disease should have their blood tested

twice a year to monitor their progress. The following table summarizes optimal ranges for various blood levels.

| Blood Test | Conventional Medicine's Reference Range | Life Extension's Optimal Range |
|---|---|---|
| Fibrinogen | Up to 460 mg/dL | 295–369 mg/dL |
| C-reactive protein | Up to 4.9 mg/L | Less than 0.55 mg/L (men) Less than 1.5 mg/L (women) |
| Homocysteine | Up to 15 μmol/L | Less than 7–8 μmol/L |
| Cholesterol | Less than 200 mg/dL | 160–180 mg/dL |
| LDL | Less than 100 mg/dL | Less than 80 mg/dL |
| HDL | Greater than 40 mg/dL | Greater than 50-60 mg/dL |
| Triglycerides | Up to 199 mg/dL | Less than 80 mg/dL |
| Fasting glucose | 65–99 mg/dL | Less than 86 mg/dL |
| Fasting Insulin | Up to 24.9 μIU/mL | Less than 5 μIU/mL |
| Total testosterone (men) | 280–800 ng/dL | 700–900 ng/dL |
| Free testosterone (men) | 6.8–21.5 pg/mL | 20–25 pg/mL (LabCorp testing method) |
| Omega-6:omega-3 ratio | None established | Less than 4:1 |
| Lp-PLA$_2$ | Less than 200 ng/mL | Less than 200 ng/mL |
| CoQ10 | 0.37–2.20 μg/mL | At least 3.0 μg/mL (preferably higher) |
| 25-hydroxy vitamin D | 32–100 ng/mL | 50–80 ng/mL |

The following nutrients have been shown to improve and preserve endothelial function:

- **Folate** (as methyltetrahydrofolate)**:** 1000 mcg daily
- **Fish oil**: 3000–6000 mg daily
- **Vitamin B12** (as methylcobalamin)**:** 1000–2000 mcg daily
- **Propionyl-L-carnitine:** 1000–2000 mg daily
- **Standardized pomegranate extract**: 500–1500 mg daily
- **Trans-resveratrol:** 250–500 mg daily
- **Coenzyme Q10** (as ubiquinol): 200–400 mg daily
- **L-arginine:** 6000–12 000 mg daily (in 3 divided doses)
- **R-lipoic acid:** 150–300 mg daily
- **Aged garlic extract:** 1200 mg daily
- **Ginkgo biloba extract:** 120 mg daily
- **Green tea**, standardized extract**:** 725 mg daily
- **Quercetin:** 500–1000 mg daily (water-soluble quercetin)

- **Vitamin C:** 1000–3000 mg daily
- **Vitamin E:** 400 IU daily (with 200 mg gamma tocopherol)
- **Vitamin K:** 2100 mcg daily; providing K1, MK-4, and MK-7
- **Vitamin B6** (as pyridoxal 5'-phosphate): 100–300 mg daily
- **Niacin:** 1000–3000 mg daily
- **Aspirin:** 81–325 mg daily

In addition, bioidentical hormone therapy may be recommended, depending on blood testing results.

For more information on comprehensive blood testing, call 1-800-544-4440.

## REFERENCES

References available at: www.lef.org/dpt5/ch15

# 16

# Attention Deficit Hyperactivity Disorder (ADHD)

Attention deficit hyperactivity disorder (ADHD) is a distressing diagnosis for any parent to hear. It is well known that children with ADHD are at a disadvantage in school and that ADHD can have long-term effects. In addition, a number of powerful pharmaceuticals have been used to treat the condition.

Fortunately, newer findings in nutrition and wellness, and newer generations of pharmaceuticals, have been developed that can help children with ADHD gain control over their lives. The Life Extension Foundation has conducted an extensive survey of the scientific literature to uncover the safest and best approaches for families affected by this increasingly common condition.

ADHD is defined as a persistent lack of attention to tasks (attention deficit) and/or a lack of ability to control impulses and an increase in physical activity (hyperactivity) that is not typical of others at a similar stage of development.[1] ADHD is most prevalent in children and teens, although it can occur in adults. ADHD occurs in 3–6% of all children in the United States, with rates as high as 15% in some areas.[2]

According to the fourth edition of the American Psychiatric Association's Diagnostic and Statistical Manual of Mental Disorders (DSM-IV), ADHD is now the most commonly diagnosed childhood behavioral disorder. Boys with ADHD outnumber girls 3:1. Some children outgrow ADHD, but 60% continue to have symptoms into adulthood.[3]

## ADHD: A TYPICAL PROFILE

The behavior of children with ADHD is typically affected in many settings (eg, home, school, and with friends). The most prominent feature of ADHD is a consistent pattern of developmentally inappropriate levels of attention, concentration, distractibility, hyperactivity, and impulsivity. It is important to note that these problems must be inappropriate to a child's developmental level to be considered ADHD. One concern among physicians is rampant overdiagnosis of ADHD, in part because the condition has been so hard to define.

Children with attention deficits are unable to remain on task for extended periods of time. They may appear forgetful, in part because their inability to attend to information prevents them from understanding it in the first place. Such children may also have cognitive and language delays. Children with hyperactivity may fidget, have difficulty engaging in quiet activities, be excessively talkative, and always seem to be on the go. Children with impulse control problems may be impatient (eg, they may blurt out an answer before the question has been finished), have difficulty waiting their turn, and are often perceived to be intruding on others. All of these manifestations can cause difficulties in academic and social settings.[4]

It is common for children with ADHD to be misdiagnosed as having learning disorders because they often perform poorly on tests that require information processing and concentration.[5,6] There is also evidence that adults with ADHD are more likely to have a variety of addictive behaviors, among them alcoholism,[7] smoking,[8] and cocaine use.[9]

## WHAT CAUSES ADHD?

Although the exact cause(s) of ADHD are unknown, it is most likely due to an interaction of environmental, nutritional, and genetic factors with a strong focus on the interaction of multiple genes (genetic loading) that together cause ADHD.

There is some evidence that people with ADHD do not produce adequate quantities of certain neurotransmitters (eg, dopamine, norepinephrine, and serotonin). Some experts theorize that such deficiencies lead to self-stimulatory behaviors that can increase brain levels of these chemicals.[10–12]

There may also be some structural and functional abnormalities in the brain itself of children who have ADHD.[13,14] Evidence suggests that there may be fewer connections between nerve cells. This would further impair neural communication already impeded by decreased neurotransmitter levels.[15] Evidence from functional studies in patients with ADHD demonstrate decreased blood flow to those areas of the brain in which "executive function," including impulse control, is based.[16] There may also be a deficit in the amount of myelin (insulating material) produced by brain cells in children with ADHD.[17]

## DIAGNOSING ADHD

Establishing a diagnosis of ADHD is a considerable challenge, largely because of the lack of reliable and specific testing as well as firm criteria. ADHD has become a high-profile condition (which may result in it being both over- and under-diagnosed), depending on pressure from parents, teachers, and others. Although DSM-IV contains diagnostic criteria, they are often not followed by health professionals. Because of the lifelong implications of an ADHD diagnosis, most experts recommend a multidisciplinary team approach to diagnosis and treatment. Such an approach should involve physicians, child behavior experts, and parents. Nutritional experts may also be valuable members of the treatment team.

The core symptoms of ADHD in children are listed below. This list was adapted from the Centers for Disease Control and Prevention. It is important to note that the diagnosis of ADHD cannot be made unless the patient has experienced these symptoms in ways that are disabling for a 6-month period. The DSM-IV diagnosis includes:

I. Either A or B:

A. Six or more of the following symptoms of inattention have been present for at least 6 months to a point that is disruptive and inappropriate for developmental level:

1. Often does not give close attention to details or makes careless mistakes in schoolwork, work, or other activities.

2. Often has trouble keeping attention on tasks or play activities.

3. Often does not seem to listen when spoken to directly.

4. Often does not follow instructions and fails to finish schoolwork, chores, or duties in the workplace (not due to oppositional behavior or failure to understand instructions).

5. Often has trouble organizing activities.

6. Often avoids, dislikes, or does not want to do things that take a lot of mental effort for a long period of time (such as schoolwork or homework).

7. Often loses things needed for tasks and activities (such as toys, school assignments, pencils, books, or tools).

8. Is often easily distracted.

9. Is often forgetful in daily activities.

B. Six or more of the following symptoms of hyperactivity/impulsivity have been present for at least 6 months to an extent that is disruptive and inappropriate for developmental level:

**Hyperactivity**

1. Often fidgets with hands or feet or squirms in seat.

2. Often gets up from seat when remaining in seat is expected.

3. Often runs about or climbs when and where it is not appropriate (adolescents or adults may feel very restless).

4. Often has trouble playing or enjoying leisure activities quietly.

5. Is often "on the go" or often acts as if "driven by a motor."

6. Often talks excessively.

**Impulsivity**

1. Often blurts out answers before questions have been finished.

2. Often has trouble waiting his/her turn.

3. Often interrupts or intrudes on others (such as butts into conversations or games).

II. Some symptoms that cause impairment were present before age 7 years.

III. Some impairment from the symptoms is present in 2 or more settings (such as at school or work and at home).

IV. There must be clear evidence of significant impairment in social, school, or work functioning.

V. The symptoms do not happen only during the course of a pervasive developmental disorder, schizophrenia, or other psychotic disorder. The symptoms are not better explained by another mental disorder (such as a mood disorder, anxiety disorder, dissociative disorder, or personality disorder).

## MIND–BODY APPROACHES

A number of behavioral and self-awareness strategies have been found to have some effect on improving symptoms of ADHD, and potentially reducing the amount of stimulant medications required. These include basics such as establishing household and school routines, avoiding information and stimulus overload,[18,19] and maintaining good eye contact, as well as techniques that require more practice and specific training (eg, meditation and some forms of biofeedback).

In addition, there is preliminary evidence that vigorous exercise may have a role in managing some features of ADHD, especially in boys. This may be related to exercise-induced increases in dopamine activity.[20]

## CONVENTIONAL MEDICAL TREATMENT

In addition to behavioral management, medical treatment of ADHD includes stimulant and nonstimulant drugs.

### Stimulant Drugs

Effective prescription drugs are primarily the so-called stimulant drugs. These agents are known to increase concentrations of a variety of brain neurotransmitters, most importantly dopamine, and exert a calming effect on people who have ADHD. Since dopamine enhances signaling between nerve cells that are involved in task-specific activities and also decreases "noise" or "nonsense signaling," increased concentrations of dopamine are thought to help individuals stay focused and on task.

Despite their limitations, stimulants are still considered first-line treatment for ADHD. They are effective in 70–80% of patients. Stimulants are highly effective at alleviating core ADHD symptoms (eg, inattention, hyperactivity, or impulsivity). Original stimulant preparations had very short periods of action that could result in dramatic rises and falls in drug levels. Newer long-acting preparations have been developed to even out these swings.

Even with the newer formulations, some adverse effects are inevitable. Long-term effects, although unusual, can occur. There is some evidence, for example, that long-term use of stimulants, especially methylphenidate (Ritalin®), can cause a delay in growth.[21] It is understandable that many parents are hesitant to give their young children this medication.

While they are effective, stimulant drugs are members of the amphetamine class, which means they can have significant adverse effects and hold some potential for abuse. Unfortunately, methylphenidate has gained popularity as a recreational drug, especially among adolescents and college students. While methylphenidate paradoxically acts as a calming drug among people diagnosed with ADHD, it acts as a stimulant among people who do not have ADHD. Surveys have indicated that more than 90% of college students and adolescents who abuse prescription drugs identified methylphenidate as their drug of choice.[22]

### Nonstimulant Drugs

The negative effects of stimulant drugs have led to an intensive search for better alternatives. Atomoxetine is the first nonstimulant drug approved by the Food and Drug Administration (FDA) for treatment of ADHD and the only agent approved by the FDA for treatment of ADHD in adults.

Atomoxetine therapy for ADHD controls symptoms, maintains remission, has comparable efficacy with methylphenidate, a favorable safety profile, and noncontrolled substance status.[23] Atomoxetine is safe and well tolerated.[24] It effectively reduces ADHD symptoms and improves social functioning in school-aged children, adolescents, and adults. As with stimulant medications, atomoxetine should be used with caution in patients with hypertension or a cardiovascular disorder.[23]

In addition to atomoxetine, other drugs that increase brain concentrations of dopamine and/or serotonin have been used with varying degrees of success. Among these are the anticonvulsant gabapentin,[25] dopamine-enhancing antidepressant bupropion,[26] wakefulness-promoting modafinil,[27] and acetylcholinesterase inhibitor donepezil, which increases brain levels of acetylcholine. Studies, however, have cast doubt on donepezil's effectiveness.[28]

## ENVIRONMENTAL AND DIETARY CONSIDERATIONS

Considerable controversy continues to surround the question of the degree to which environmental toxins and dietary factors contribute to ADHD.[29] Overt toxicity from contaminants and pollutants such as mercury and polychlorinated biphenyls (PCBs) is known to cause a wide spectrum of behavioral disorders,[30] although the effects of more subtle exposures are less clear.

Similarly, several theories have advanced regarding the association between dietary components (eg, simple sugars) and ADHD, but again, convincing evidence is lacking.[31] Dietary manipulations such as the Feingold elimination diet (in which one or several categories of food is carefully excluded) have been tried, but with no success in treating ADHD.[32]

Likewise, although allergies to foods or food additives have been proposed as a cause of ADHD,[33,34] there is little scientific basis for this idea. Oligoantigenic diets aim to reduce the number and variety of food-based allergens that children might be exposed to. A few small trials have shown some benefit in carefully selected groups of children.[35] Because oligoantigenic diets aim to eliminate large categories of food on which growing children may depend, they should be undertaken only in careful collaboration with a physician. Allergy testing has rarely proved helpful in treating ADHD.

## Role of Dietary Sugar

Despite a great deal of attention in the popular press, there has been no convincing evidence that dietary sugar is causal in ADHD.[32] In a 1985 study, children with ADHD were shown to have lower adrenaline levels after sugar intake than control children.[36] The implications of this study are not clear. However, other studies have suggested that some children with ADHD may have food sensitivities that include sugar. The authors of these studies conclude that diet modification is an important part of ADHD management.[37] Whatever the outcome of this debate, there is little doubt about whether dietary sugar is beneficial in a child's diet. It is linked to tooth decay, obesity, and other health conditions. Therefore, it is probably wise for all children to limit or completely avoid dietary sugar.

# NUTRITIONAL THERAPY

As previously mentioned, ADHD is most likely caused by multiple factors, including nutritional issues. Children with ADHD may have specific nutrient deficiencies that aggravate their condition. As researchers learn more about the intersection between diet and behavioral disorders, the case for nutritional intervention among children with ADHD becomes more compelling. In the future, it is almost certain that this multifactorial disease will be treated on multiple fronts, including nutritional intervention.[38] Already, many progressive parents and physicians are turning to comprehensive health-care options to battle this frustrating condition.

## Essential Fatty Acids

A growing body of scientific literature is helping parents and doctors better understand the link between fatty acids and behavioral disorders such as ADHD. The ratio between omega-3 and omega-6 fatty acids (eg, arachidonic acid) seems especially important. Eicosapentaenoic acid (EPA) and docosahexaenoic acid (DHA) are omega-3 fatty acids found in flaxseed oil and cold-water fish. In the typical Western diet, we tend to consume more omega-6 fatty acids relative to omega-3 fatty acids. The ratio of omega-3 to omega-6 fatty acids has been

shown to influence the development of neurotransmitters and other chemicals that are essential for normal brain function. Increased intake of omega-3 fatty acids has been shown to reduce the tendency toward hyperactivity among children with ADHD.[39]

Several studies have examined the role of essential fatty acids in ADHD, with very encouraging results:

- In a pilot study, children with ADHD were given flaxseed oil, which is rich in alpha-linolenic acid. In the body, alpha-linolenic acid is metabolized into EPA and DHA. At the end of the study, researchers found that the symptoms of children with ADHD given the flaxseed oil improved on all measures.[40]

- Another study examined the effects of flaxseed oil and fish oil, which provide varying degrees of omega-3 fatty acids, on adults with ADHD. The patients were given supplements for 12 weeks. Their blood levels of omega-3 fatty acids were tracked throughout the 12 weeks. Researchers found that high-dose fish oil increased omega-3 fatty acids in the blood relative to omega-6 fatty acids. An imbalance between arachidonic acid and omega-3 fatty acids is considered a risk factor for ADHD.[41]

- One study compared 20 children with ADHD who were given a dietary supplement (that included omega-3 fatty acids) to children with ADHD who were given methylphenidate. The dietary supplement was a mix of vitamins, minerals, essential fatty acids, probiotics, amino acids, and phytonutrients. The groups showed almost identical improvement on commonly accepted measures of ADHD.[38]

- Finally, a study has also indicated that children with ADHD benefit from the intake of a combination of essential fatty acids and vitamin E.[42]

## Magnesium and Vitamin B6

Combining magnesium and vitamin B6 has shown promise for reducing symptoms of ADHD. Vitamin B6 has many functions in the body, including assisting in the synthesis of neurotransmitters and forming myelin, which protect nerves. Magnesium is also very important; it is involved in more than 300 metabolic reactions. At least three studies have demonstrated that the combination of magnesium and vitamin B6 improved behavior, decreased anxiety and aggression, and improved mobility among children with ADHD.[43-46]

## Iron

Iron deficiency may be implicated in ADHD,[47] although supplementation studies have shown minimal or no effects.[48] Because of the potential toxicity of iron supplements, parents should consult their children's pediatrician before beginning supplementation.

## Zinc

Zinc is a cofactor for the production of neurotransmitters, fatty acids, prostaglandins, and melatonin, and indirectly affects the metabolism of dopamine and fatty acids. However, the role of zinc in ADHD is still emerging. While numerous studies have shown that children with ADHD are often deficient in zinc, researchers have not determined that a zinc deficiency causes ADHD or that treatment with zinc can improve symptoms of ADHD.[49,50] Two Turkish studies, however, have tested zinc therapy among children with ADHD with positive results. In these studies, children were randomized to groups that received either zinc or placebo. In one study, the conditions of children who took zinc for 6 weeks improved.[51] In the second study, zinc as the sole therapy resulted in significant improvements compared to placebo.[52]

## Acetyl-L-carnitine

Acetyl-L-carnitine, a form of L-carnitine, is responsible for transporting fatty acids into the mitochondria. It has been associated with a host of positive health benefits, including reducing impulsivity. In an animal model of ADHD, acetyl-L-carnitine was shown to reduce the impulsivity index.[53]

## Phosphatidylserine

Phosphatidylserine, a critical component of cell membranes, plays a role in nerve cell signaling. Phosphatidylserine has been found to improve memory and concentration in adults[54]; one report found that it significantly improved attention and learning in children with ADHD.[29]

## Neurotransmitter Support

A new technique related to magnetic resonance imaging (MRI) is proton magnetic resonance spectroscopy (1H-MRS), which reveals important information about chemical compounds in different brain areas. Recent studies using 1H-MRS suggest that choline, creatine, glutamate, and other specific compounds may play a role in ADHD. Choline is one of the building blocks of acetylcholine, an important neurotransmitter involved in memory. Glutamate and glutamine are amino acids involved in the production of GABA (gamma-aminobutyric acid), a neurotransmitter that inhibits certain nerve impulses and may affect hyperactivity.

In one study, 1H-MRS analysis showed that children with inherited and structural features linked to poor memory had lower concentrations of creatine-phosphocreatine and choline-containing compounds, whereas creatine and N-acetyl aspartate were associated with good memory, reflecting differences in energy metabolism in the frontal lobes of the brain.[55]

However, a 1H-MRS study of ADHD showed a mild increase in the ratio of choline to creatine on one side of the striatum, a deep brain region in which about one quarter of the nerve cells were lost or severely dysfunctional. The investigators concluded that neurotransmission involving acetylcholine was mildly hyperactive.[56]

In another 1H-MRS study, 8 children with ADHD but without learning disabilities had increased glutamate-to-glutamine ratios in both frontal areas, and increased N-acetyl aspartate and choline in the right frontal area, compared to 8 controls.[57]

Investigators from Venezuela found diminished blood levels of the amino acids glutamine and phenylalanine in ADHD patients. They hypothesized that this imbalance could cause alterations in amino acid metabolism and transport to the brain, which might alter central nervous system function. Their findings support the theory that ADHD represents a disorder of the inhibitory neurotransmission system.[58]

Choline supplementation is theoretically more beneficial for diminished memory and learning than for other ADHD symptoms (eg, hyperactive and impulsive behavior). Choline has an unpleasant taste, so children may prefer DMAE (dimethylaminoethanol), a supplement that increases brain levels of choline.[59] DMAE may speed up production of acetylcholine in the brain, and has been used to treat reduced attention span, learning and reading problems, hyperactivity, and poor coordination associated with ADHD.[60,61]

## Additional Nutrients and Hormones

**Melatonin.** Melatonin is a hormone secreted at night by the pineal gland. It participates in multiple body processes, including regulation of the sleep–wake cycle. Because many children and adults with ADHD also have sleep problems, melatonin can be an important part of integrative therapy. By some estimates, up to 25% of children with ADHD also have sleep disorders. However, conventional therapy treats hyperactivity but neglects the sleep disorder.[62] In one study of 27 children with ADHD and insomnia, 5 mg of melatonin, combined with sleep therapy, helped reduce insomnia.[63]

**Dehydroepiandrosterone (DHEA).** DHEA is an important neuroactive steroid hormone that may be involved in ADHD. However, researchers are still trying to understand the relationship. ADHD is associated with low blood levels of DHEA, its principal precursor pregnenolone, and its principal metabolite dehydroepiandrosterone-sulfate (DHEA-S). Higher blood levels of these neurosteroids are associated with fewer symptoms.[64] Furthermore, a study of adolescent boys with ADHD showed that DHEA levels rise after a 3-month course of methylphenidate treatment, which implies that DHEA somehow plays a role in the drug's effectiveness.[65]

**Ginkgo biloba and ginseng.** A combination of ginkgo biloba and ginseng has been studied for its ability to improve symptoms among patients with ADHD. In a study of 36 children ranging in age from 3 to 17 years, a combination of Ginkgo biloba and American ginseng was administered twice daily on an empty stomach for 4 weeks. At the end of the study, more than 70% of patients had experienced improvement on a widely used measure of ADHD symptoms.[66]

**L-theanine.** Research has shown that the amino acid L-theanine, found in green tea, is more effective than a common prescription drug in promoting relaxation by increasing levels of serotonin and dopamine, and blocking the binding of L-glutamic acid to glutamate receptors.[67–69]

**Pycnogenol®.** A few case studies suggest that some ADHD patients may benefit from Pycnogenol®, an extract of French maritime pine bark and a potent antioxidant, which supports blood vessel dilation and provides cellular protection.[70] Children given a daily dose of 1 mg/kg of body weight (about 0.5 mg/lb) of this pine bark extract for 4 weeks showed significant improvements in multiple standard measures of ADHD.[71]

## Life Extension Suggestions

The following lifestyle changes may be helpful:

- **Diet.** Aim for a well-balanced diet. Avoid unnecessary simple sugars. Use specific elimination diets only in partnership with a physician. People observing elimination diets are likely to need supplementation with vitamins, minerals, and possibly other nutrients.
- **Exercise.** Moderate to vigorous physical activity is beneficial for all children, but especially for children with behavior disorders. Try moderate-intensity activity for 30 minutes almost every day and a minimum of 30 minutes of vigorous activity 3–4 days per week.
- **Mind–body techniques.** Try massage, biofeedback, and meditation. Avoid information overload. Some children with ADHD benefit from predictable, rigid schedules.

In addition, the following nutrients may be helpful. Please note that the dosages provided below are for adults.

- **Zinc:** 15–30 mg daily
- **EPA/DHA:** 1400 mg daily of EPA and 1000 mg daily of DHA
- **Vitamin E:** 400 IU daily of alpha-tocopherols and at least 200 mg daily of gamma-tocopherols
- **Magnesium:** 160–500 mg daily
- **Vitamin B6:** up to 250 mg daily
- **Acetyl-L-carnitine:** 1000–2000 mg daily
- **Melatonin:** 300 mcg–5 mg daily
- **DHEA:** 15–75 mg daily; have blood tested after 3–6 weeks to determine optimal levels
- **Ginkgo biloba:** 120 mg daily
- **American ginseng:** 500 mg daily
- **Choline:** 250 mg daily as cytidine 5'-diphosphate choline
- **Glutamine:** 500–1000 mg daily
- **Phenylalanine:** 500 mg daily
- **L-theanine:** 200 mg daily
- **Phosphatidylserine:** 100 mg daily
- **Pycnogenol:** 75–100 mg daily

## REFERENCES

References available at: www.lef.org/dpt5/ch16

# 17

---

# *Autoimmune Diseases*

---

Autoimmune diseases are characterized by the body's immune responses being directed against its own tissues, causing prolonged inflammation and subsequent tissue destruction. Autoimmune disorders can either cause immune-responsive cells to attack the linings of the joints (resulting in rheumatoid arthritis) or trigger immune cells to attack the insulin-producing islet cells of the pancreas (leading to insulin-dependent diabetes mellitus).

A healthy immune system recognizes, identifies, remembers, attacks, and destroys bacteria, viruses, fungi, parasites, cancer cells, or any health-damaging agents not normally present in the body. A defective immune system, on the other hand, wreaks havoc throughout the host by directing antibodies against its own tissues.

Any disease in which cytotoxic cells are directed against self-antigens in the body's tissues is considered autoimmune in nature. Such diseases include, but are not limited to, celiac disease, Crohn's disease, pancreatitis, systemic lupus erythematosus, Sjögren's syndrome, Hashimoto's thyroiditis, and other endocrinopathies. Allergies and multiple sclerosis are also the result of disordered immune functioning.

## AGING

Age is recognized as an important factor in the appearance of autoimmune disease. In a paper that appeared in *The Lancet* in 1992; investigators assessed the difference in physiologic chemistry between healthy centenarians and unhealthy 60- and 70-year-olds. The most striking difference was that the healthy centenarians had very low levels of autoantibodies to their thyroid, adrenal, pituitary, and hypothalamus.[1] This has led some people to speculate that autoimmunity is the result of environmental exposure to foreign substances. Thus, the immune system may also be suppressed or weakened as a result of lifestyle factors (ie, intake of alcohol, caffeine, tobacco, drugs, sugar, poor diet, and lack of sleep) that are not associated with a degenerative disease. These lifestyle factors can have a substantial effect on the trends of autoimmune diseases.

As we age, our autoimmune system declines in its effectiveness due in large part to oxidative damage caused by the recurrent presence of significant amounts of free radicals. In addition, proteins can become glycated, that is, a sugar molecule is attached to the protein. The accumulation of these glycated proteins in the body affects the immune system because the immune system sees them as altered proteins with different structure and function.[2-4] Regarding these substances as foreign, the immune system develops antibodies against them. The possibility of becoming allergic to oneself, with the associated autoimmunity and inflammation, increases as one accumulates these damaged glycated proteins.

The body is made up largely of proteins, so its health depends on its freedom from damage (as through oxidation or glycation) as well as its timely removal as part of normal protein turnover. The body's antioxidant system and other lines of defense cannot completely protect proteins. Nature's second line of defense is the body's system for repairing or removing damaged proteins. While some protein repair mechanisms exist, it is difficult for the body to repair most protein damage. Yet, it is essential to efficiently remove aberrant and unneeded proteins to fully protect against autoimmune diseases.

Methods to protect against excessive protein glycation will be discussed later in this protocol.

## BASIC PATHWAYS OF AUTOIMMUNE DYSFUNCTION

Autoimmune diseases tend to be viewed as separate entities. A broader perspective, however, may reveal that shared mechanisms are the cause of disease, rather than just its byproduct. If this perspective were applied, patients would benefit (before the development of irreversible tissue damage) from improved therapies and early intervention. Majid Ali has long considered that there must be a single initial common pathway to all disease, including immune dysfunction.

One consideration is the continued exposure to heavy metals and environmental pollution that overload the immune system. On a daily basis, we battle with pesticides, herbicides, chemical fertilizers, industrial wastes, cigarette smoke, and automobile exhaust. Our air, water, and food (in particular) are full of toxic substances. There is no doubt that these toxins play a role in immune dysfunction. Even substances considered by most people as safe impair immune function. Sugar consumption in all forms (glucose, fructose, and sucrose) will impair the ability of white cells to destroy biological agents. This effect begins within a half-hour of consumption and lasts for 5 hours. After 2 hours, immune function is reduced by 50%.[5,6]

Oxidative stress plays a role in autoimmune diseases. It can be compared to a piece of metal rusting and results from the action of damaging molecules (ie, free radicals), which are a natural byproduct of the body's metabolism. The electrically charged free radicals attack healthy cells, causing them to lose their structure and function, and eventually destroying them. Free radicals are not only produced by our bodies, but are also ingested from toxins and pollution in the air we breathe.

Chronic systemic inflammation is related to several autoimmune disorders, such as lupus, rheumatoid arthritis, Sjögren's syndrome, and fibromyalgia (see separate protocols on these topics). Inflammation can be traced to destructive cell-signaling chemicals known as cytokines, which contribute to many degenerative diseases.[7] In rheumatoid arthritis, excess levels of proinflammatory cytokines, such as tumor necrosis factor-alpha (TNF-α), interleukin-6 (IL-6), interleukin 1(b) (IL-1b), and/or leukotriene B4 (LTB4), are known to cause or contribute to the inflammatory syndrome that ultimately destroys joint cartilage and synovial fluid. Certain nutritional supplements and low-cost prescription medications will often lower cytokine levels and control the inflammatory state.

# NUTRITIONAL SUPPLEMENTS TO IMPROVE AUTOIMMUNE HEALTH

The autoimmune system needs a good nutritional foundation (over a long period of time) to alleviate or reverse lifestyle autoimmune dysfunction and assist with combating fully developed autoimmune diseases. The fundamental causal basis for autoimmune system boosting was shown in an early study designed to measure the serum concentrations of vitamin E, beta-carotene, and vitamin A in patients prior to developing rheumatoid arthritis or systemic lupus erythematosus. Two to 15 years after the volunteer patients had originally donated their blood to the serum bank (1974), the serum samples were assayed for vitamin E, beta-carotene, and vitamin A. Those patients who developed rheumatoid arthritis or lupus showed lower serum concentrations of vitamin E, beta-carotene, and vitamin A in 1974; those with the lowest serum level of beta-carotene in 1974 were the most likely to develop rheumatoid arthritis later in life.[8] This indicates the long-term importance of maintaining adequate vitamin status for the prevention of autoimmune diseases.

## Slowing the Damage to Healthy Protein

Carnosine, a dipeptide amino acid found naturally in the body, helps slow the formation of glycated protein end products. Recall that glycated protein may be unrecognizable to the immune system, thereby triggering an autoimmune attack. Since the normal removal of damaged protein declines with aging, slowing the development of protein crosslinking (glycation) may help to reduce an autoimmune reaction. In addition to its antiglycation effects, carnosine has been found to modulate immune system neutrophils, thus suppressing a response.[9]

## Reducing Inflammation

A study found that fish oil containing *vitamin E* delayed the onset of autoimmune diseases in autoimmune-prone mice.[10] Another study on the effects of vitamin E deficiency found that dietary components that provide antioxidant effects may contribute to the treatment of inflammatory/autoimmune diseases.[11]

Supplementation with *omega-3 essential fatty acids (EFAs)* from fish, flaxseed, or perilla oils—along with borage oil, evening primrose oil, or black currant seed oil, which contain the essential omega-6 fatty acid *gamma-linolenic acid (GLA)*—can alleviate many symptoms of autoimmune disease through their anti-inflammatory activity. Docosahexaenoic acid (DHA) extracted from fish oil may be as effective as some prescription medications in reducing inflammation.

*Dehydroepiandrosterone (DHEA)* is a prosteroidal hormone that decreases with age. Decreases in DHEA levels have been linked to a number of chronic and degenerative diseases, including cancer, coronary artery disease, depression, stress disorders, and neurologic functioning.[12] As a result of aging, immunity may become compromised due to dysregulation of cellular hormones (cytokines and growth factors) that govern immune response. Too much or too little of various cytokines produces disease states or compromised responses to various challenges.

In aging animals, the addition of DHEA has normalized deranged cytokine levels, including the primary inflammatory factor interleukin-6 (IL-6).[13] In the aged test animals, serum IL-6 was elevated 9-fold from normal. After administration of DHEA or dehydroepiandro-sterone-sulfate (DHEA-S), IL-6 dropped to within 15% of youthful levels. In the same studies, it was shown that antibodies directed toward oneself rose 5-fold with aging, but fell by over 50% after 2 weeks on DHEA-S.[14]

In a study of 10 women with the autoimmune disease Sjögren's syndrome, all were shown to have decreased serum concentrations of DHEA-S and an increased cortisol/DHEA-S ratio compared with healthy controls.[15]

Rheumatoid arthritis is an autoimmune disorder in which the body attacks its own tissues as though they were foreign invaders. *Boswellia* may also offer relief to autoimmune-related rheumatoid arthritis patients. *Boswellia* can help reduce immune cells that encourage inflammation, while increasing the number of immune cells that inhibit inflammation.[16] Studies indicate that boswellia's ability to modulate the immune system and inhibit inflammatory activity may help improve the symptoms of rheumatoid arthritis and other autoimmune conditions.[17]

## Reducing Free Radical Damage

Antioxidants are a broad group of compounds that destroy or neutralize free radicals in the body; thus, they protect against oxidative damage to cells caused by normal aging or daily exposure to pollutants and toxic substances. Antioxidants are found naturally in healthy food, especially fruits and vegetables. The most effective antioxidants include *vitamin C, vitamin E, green tea extract, beta-carotene, grape seed-skin extract, coenzyme Q10 (CoQ10),* and *selenium.*

**Vitamin C.** Vitamin C may be the most important water-soluble antioxidant, having the ability to scavenge both reactive oxygen and nitrogen radicals. In controlled studies, vitamin C has demonstrated anti-atherogenic, anticarcinogenic, antihistaminic, and immunomodulatory benefits.

**Vitamin E.** Vitamin E is a fat-soluble, essential nutrient for humans. Increased risk for coronary artery disease, Alzheimer's disease, and cancer has been associated with vitamin E deficiency.

**Green tea.** Green tea belongs to the flavonoid family. Green tea catechins are potent free radical scavengers that have demonstrated anticarcinogenic, anti-inflammatory, antiatherogenic, and antimicrobial activity.

**Beta-carotene.** Beta-carotene is a dietary precursor to vitamin A. Beta-carotene has demonstrated immuno-modulatory effects in male nonsmokers and increased lymphocyte counts in healthy male smokers. Beta-carotene's antioxidant activity may prevent oxidative damage to DNA and inhibit lipid peroxidation.

**Grape seed-skin extract.** Grape seed-skin proanthocyanidins have demonstrated several antioxidant activities, including inhibiting the oxidation of damaging LDL cholesterol. Other research has shown tumor-, cardio-, and liver-protective benefits.

**Coenzyme Q10 (CoQ10).** CoQ10 has shown antioxidant activity within the mitochondria and cellular membrane. CoQ10 levels decline with aging and are strongly related to increased cardiovascular disease, especially congestive heart failure. Supplemental CoQ10 has shown usefulness in treating periodontal disease and boosting energy levels.

**Selenium.** Selenium is a trace mineral that is essential for healthy immune function. Selenium provides protection to immune cells from stress-induced oxidative damage and neutralizes the effects of some toxic metals. Low dietary intake of selenium is associated with cardiovascular disease and certain cancers.

## Modulating the Immune System

The immune system functions because of adequate amounts of circulating antibodies. Antibodies are proteins with a unique concave region (combining site) in which they can combine with foreign proteins (antigens). Antigens are most often surface molecules found on the membrane of invading or diseased cells. After the antigen and antibody combine, the new complex produces a number of changes that inactivate or kill the invading cell. This function is known as humoral or antibody-mediated immunity. Lymphocytes are the most numerous cells of the immune system and are responsible for antibody production. B cells are lymphocytes that produce humoral immunity.

T cells are lymphocytes formed in the thymus shortly before and after birth. When T cells come into contact with foreign antigens, the antigen binds to protein on the surface of the T cell, making it sensitized. Sensitized T cells destroy invading pathogens by releasing a specific and toxic poison to the cells of bound antigens. T cells can also indirectly destroy toxic invaders by releasing a substance that attracts macrophages to the area that will ingest and destroy (phagocytose) the pathogen. This function is known as cell-mediated immunity. T cells regulate natural killer cell activity and the body's inflammatory response to disease.

In a healthy body, circulating antibodies attack and destroy pathogenic invaders by means of humoral or cell-mediated immunity. In autoimmune disease, circulating antibodies seek, attack, and destroy self-antigens found in healthy tissue (see Table 1 for examples).

## Table 1: Autoimmune Classification

| Disease | Antibody Action on |
| --- | --- |
| Myasthenia gravis | Acetylcholine receptors |
| Graves' disease | Thyroid-stimulating hormone receptor |
| Thyroiditis | Thyroid |
| Insulin-resistant diabetes | Insulin receptor |
| Asthma | Beta-2 adrenergic receptors |
| Juvenile insulin-dependent diabetes | Pancreatic islet cells |
| Pernicious anemia | Gastric parietal cells |
| Addison's disease | Adrenal cells |
| Idiopathic hypoparathyroidism | Parathyroid cells |
| Spontaneous infertility | Sperm |
| Premature ovarian failure | Interstitial cells, corpus luteum cells |
| Pemphigus | Intercellular substance of skin |
| Primary biliary cirrhosis | Mitochondria |
| Autoimmune hemolytic anemia | Erythrocytes |
| Idiopathic thrombocytopenic purpura | Platelets |
| Idiopathic neutropenia | Neutrophils |
| Vitiligo | Melanocytes |
| Osteosclerosis and Ménière's disease | Type II collagen |
| Chronic active hepatitis | Nuclei of hepatocytes |
| Goodpasture's syndrome | Basement membranes |
| Rheumatoid arthritis | Gamma globulin, virus-related antigens |
| Sjögren's syndrome | Nuclei and centromeres |
| Systemic lupus erythematosus | Nuclei, DNA, RNA, erythrocytes, etc. |
| Scleroderma | Nuclei and centromeres |
| Polymyositis | Nuclei, RNA |

T cells can further divide into helper lymphocytes (Th) and cytotoxic (Tc) or suppressor cells. In response to a foreign pathogen, T cells secrete communication molecules known as lymphokines, cytokines, interleukins, and interferons. T-helper cells assist B cells and further divide into 2 special lines of defense: Th1 and Th2. When one of these lines (Th1 or Th2) over-expresses, an opportunity for immune dysregulation occurs, resulting in either a hyperimmune response causing autoimmune disease or a hypoimmune response leading to uncontrollable infection. Sterinol, a combination of natural plant sterols and sterolins, modulates the function of T cells by enhancing their ability to divide. They further promote interleukin-2 and gamma-interferon without enhancing Th2 helper cells that promote inflammation and produce more antibodies. Conventional drug treatment inhibits the entire immune response. Sterolins, however, modulate the immune response and are able to reverse immune abnormality at the disease site.[18,19]

Alkylglycerols are derived from *shark liver oil*. Studies indicate that the activation of protein kinase C, an essential step in cell proliferation, can be inhibited by alkylglycerols. Although the mechanism of anti-proliferative and immunomodulatory action is unknown, hormonal action of both the autocrine and paracrine systems has been suggested.[20] Alkylglycerols have been promoted for use in immune system stimulation. However, benefits have been reported in those suffering from asthma, lupus, rheumatoid arthritis, and other autoimmune disorders.

L-carnitine, an amino acid known to improve conditions associated with low cellular energy, has been shown to reduce the impairment of immune function caused by the consumption of dangerous fats.[21] This beneficial action is attributed to L-carnitine's ability to lower serum lipids (fats) by enhancing the transport of beneficial fatty acids into the cell's mitochondria, where they are used to produce energy. *Acetyl-L-carnitine* is the form of carnitine utilized more efficiently in the mitochondria.

Mounting evidence suggests that *vitamin D* may be a critical *missing link* in virtually all autoimmune diseases, including lupus. Vitamin D is capable of *modulating* the activity of immune cells. Studies have identified widespread vitamin D *deficiency* in lupus patients.[22,23] For example, one study found that *1.2%* of lupus patients had adequate vitamin D levels compared to 45% of healthy controls.[24] Another found that *lower* vitamin D levels were linked with more *aggressive* lupus autoimmunity.[25]

Scientists have discovered how to provide natural immunological support using immune-protective proteins found in hen's eggs. This development promises to deliver substantial immune enhancement at a fraction of the cost of medications,[26] which is good news for all of us as we age—and great news for those whose immune systems are particularly vulnerable (eg, cancer or HIV/AIDS patients).

### Supporting the Gastrointestinal Tract

Intestinal permeability is often disrupted by health conditions such as rheumatoid arthritis, Crohn's disease, pancreatic dysfunction, and food allergies. Aging, stress, medications, and alcohol consumption also alter permeability, compromising the barrier that separates food and intestinal bacteria from the rest of the body.

Poor intestinal motility and peristalsis can change beneficial bacterial flora by altering the natural flow of nutrients available to them. These same factors can add to the overgrowth of abnormal bacteria and the byproducts they produce, leading to the absorption of antigenic substances into the bloodstream. Immune-related disease is associated with antigenic substances produced by intestinal flora. To correct the problem, bacterial balance must be restored through the use of supplemental *probiotics* and prebiotics that feed the beneficial bacteria. Species of bifidobacteria and lactobacilli may help restore microfloral balance and stabilize intestinal permeability. Fructooligosaccharides (FOS) are simple sugars that are the preferred nutrient for lactobacilli and bifidobacteria (with the exception of the bifidum species).

Certain nutritional supplements are used by intestinal cells for growth and function. They include:

- *L-glutamine*, a nonessential amino acid that increases the number of cells in the small intestine along with the number and height of villi on those cells

- *Butyric acid*, a short-chain fatty acid that enhances function and integrity in the large intestine and is an anticancer agent

- The fatty acids *DHA* (from fish oil) and *GLA* (from borage oil), which decrease inflammation and improve intestinal functioning

## Reducing Stress

Stress is a major risk factor in developing disease. Even prolonged low-level stress stimulates the adrenal glands to produce cortisol, which in excess impairs immune function. Lack of proper rest and sleep, depression, and emotional disturbance contribute to immune dysfunction. In addition, there is a connection between the limbic system (ie, the part of the brain that gives rise to emotion) and immune function. Therefore, to balance the immune system, one must balance the mind and emotions. Biofeedback, guided imagery, yoga, deep breathing, musical participation, positive affirmations, meditation, and prayer all help maintain balance.[27-31]

A supplemental approach to stress reduction would be obtained from *Garum Armoricum extract*, which contains a class of unique polypeptides that act as precursors to endorphins and other neurotransmitters. These polypeptides exert a regulatory effect on the nervous system enabling an individual to adapt to mentally and physically stressful conditions.[32] Another antidote to stress is an amino acid found in green tea called *theanine*. Although theanine creates a tranquilizing effect on the brain, it appears to increase concentration and focus thought.[33] DHEA supplementation is the most effective way of blocking the effects of excess cortisol secretion.

## Improving Liver Health

The liver plays a critical role in all aspects of metabolism and health. It is important in the synthesis and secretion of albumin (a blood-clotting protein), storage of glucose, and synthesis of vitamins and minerals. Because the liver has a major role in the purification and clearance of waste products, drugs, and toxins, disease states may be improved by supporting liver function. The herb *milk thistle* and its components silymarin and silibinin have 2 therapeutic mechanisms. First, they alter the structure of the outer cell membrane of the hepatocyte to prevent penetration of liver poison into the interior of the cell. Second, they stimulate the action of nucleolar polymerase A, resulting in an increase in ribosomal protein synthesis, thus stimulating the regenerative ability of the liver and the formation of new hepatocytes.[34,35]

## Life Extension Suggestions

Autoimmune diseases may be greatly improved by strengthening the immune system with nutritional supplements and by making healthy lifestyle changes in diet and stress management. Treatment protocols may include prescription drugs as well as the following nutrients.

### Easing Inflammation
- **Omega-3 fatty acids (EPA and DHA):** 1400 mg of EPA, 1000 mg DHA daily
- **Gamma-linolenic acid:** 300–600 mg daily
- **DHEA:** 15–25 mg daily for women, and 25–75 mg daily for men (depending on blood test results)
- **Boswellia:** 100 mg daily, standardized to 20% 3-O-acetyl-11-keto-β-boswellic acid (AKBA) (20 mg)

### Protect Against Oxidative Stress
- **Vitamin C:** 1000–4000 mg daily
- **Natural vitamin E:** 100–400 IU alpha-tocopherol and 200 mg gamma-tocopherol daily
- **Green tea extract**, standardized to 98% polyphenols: 725–1450 mg daily
- **Beta-carotene:** 25000 IU daily
- **Grape seed extract:** 100 mg daily
- **CoQ10:** 100–200 mg daily
- **Selenium** (SeMSc): 200 mcg daily

### Protect from Glycation
- **L-carnosine:** 500–1500 mg daily

**Immunologic**
- **Shark liver oil:** 1000 mg daily containing 200 mg alkylglycerols
- **Plant sterols:** 20 mg daily
- **Vitamin D:** 5000–8000 IU daily based on blood results

**Intestinal Support**
- **Probiotics:** per label instructions
- **L-glutamine:** 1–2 g daily
- **Butyric acid or butyrate enemas:** as prescribed by a doctor

**Managing Stress**
- **Garum Armoricum:** 210–420 mg daily
- **L-Theanine:** 100–400 mg daily

**Liver Support**
- **Milk thistle:** 750 mg providing 600 mg silymarin, 225 mg silibinin, and 60 mg isosilybins

## REFERENCES

References available at: www.lef.org/dpt5/ch17

# 18

---

# *Bacterial Infections*

---

The fight against bacterial infection represents one of the high points of modern medicine. The development of antibiotics in the 1940s offered physicians a powerful tool against bacterial infections that has saved the lives of millions of people. However, because of the widespread and sometimes inappropriate use of antibiotics, strains of bacteria have begun to emerge that are antibiotic-resistant. These new, stronger bacteria pose a significant threat to general health and welfare—and a challenge to researchers.

Bacterial infections can be caused by a wide range of bacteria, resulting in mild to life-threatening illnesses (such as bacterial meningitis) that require immediate intervention. In the United States, bacterial infections are a leading cause of death in children and the elderly.[1] Hospitalized patients and those with chronic diseases are at especially high risk of bacterial infection.[2] Common bacterial infections include pneumonia, ear infections, diarrhea, urinary tract infections, and skin disorders.

Under normal circumstances, people are protected from bacterial infections by a healthy immune system. Thus, maintaining the healthiest immune profile possible will help reduce the risk of bacterial infection. For more comprehensive information on the immune system and general nutritional strategies to support healthy immune function, see the Immune System Strengthening protocol. The present protocol focuses specifically on bacteria and approaches to staving off bacterial illness.

## RISK FACTORS FOR BACTERIAL INFECTIONS

Although every human being is exposed to innumerable bacteria, some of us are at higher risk of infection than others. Besides a weakened immune system, there are other risk factors for bacterial infection and illness.

### Age

Individuals at either end of the age spectrum (neonates and the elderly) are at increased risk of bacterial infections.[3,4] Neonates are most susceptible to infections by pathogens such as *Escherichia coli*.[5,6] People older than 60 years are susceptible to lower respiratory tract infections caused by *Streptococcus pneumoniae* (*S. pneumoniae*).

### Nutritional Status

The human body requires a balanced diet that provides nutrients, minerals, and vitamins for a functional and effective immune response.[6] Immune function is impacted by factors including hormonal status, age, and nutritional status.[7] Malnutrition results in a depressed immune system that raises the risk of infection.

### Genetic Predisposition

Scientists have long known that some people have a genetic predisposition to bacterial infection.[8] The Human Genome Project, which recently completed a map of the entire human genome, increased our ability to locate specific genes related to infectious disease susceptibility.[9] Ultimately, researchers hope to use genetic testing to identify people who are at increased risk of infectious diseases, and then design drug therapies that target specific genetic defects that are expressed in conjunction with diseases.[10]

## FORMS OF BACTERIAL INFECTIONS

Bacteria are associated with many illnesses and conditions. Some of the more common are listed in subsequent sections.

### Respiratory Infections

**Upper respiratory tract infections.** Upper respiratory tract infections are a leading cause of time lost from work and school.[11] Bacteria account for up to 25% of upper respiratory tract infections. Group A streptococci are responsible for 95% of the cases of strep throat in the United States.[12,13] Strep throat is most common in children and adolescents (aged 3–18 years). Other pathogens include *Haemophilus influenzae*.[14,15]

**Otitis media.** Middle ear infections are the most common bacterial infections in children in the United States. By the age of 3 years, two-thirds of American children have had at least one episode of otitis media, and the other third has had 3 or more episodes. *S. pneumoniae* is the most frequent cause.[16]

**Lower respiratory tract infections.** Common lower respiratory tract infections include acute, chronic, and health care-associated pneumonia and bronchitis.[7,17] *S. pneumoniae* is the most frequent cause of community-acquired lung infections and pneumonia. Lower respiratory tract infections can occur in both healthy and immunocompromised individuals.

**Tuberculosis (TB).** An estimated 15 million people in the United States are infected with *Mycobacterium tuberculosis*.[18,19] Of these, however, far fewer will actually develop clinically evident disease. Whether TB infection will progress to disease depends on a person's nutritional status. TB occurs disproportionately in poorer populations. Infection is more likely to occur in people aged 15–25 years and older than 60 years, people with HIV, or people who have been incarcerated for longer than 6 months.[20] In prisons in particular, overcrowding and the frequent movement of prisoners between cells is a factor in the spread of infection.[21] It is important to note that the antibiotics used as first-line treatments in TB, such as Isoniazid, are known to cause vitamin B6 deficiencies.[22]

## Gastrointestinal Infections

Infectious diarrhea is a leading cause of morbidity and mortality worldwide.[23,24] In the United States, 100 million people are affected by acute diarrhea every year. Most diarrhea is viral (not bacterial) in origin, but bacteria remain an important cause. Nearly half of patients with acute diarrhea must restrict activities, 10% consult physicians, 250 000 require hospitalization, and approximately 3000 die. Common bacterial pathogens that cause diarrhea include *Campylobacter* species, *Salmonella*, *Shigella*, and *E. coli* O157:H7.

**Campylobacter jejuni.** *C. jejuni* is the most common cause of bacterial diarrhea in the United States. The Centers for Disease Control and Prevention (CDC) estimate that more than 1 million Americans are affected yearly. Previously, most cases of bacterial diarrhea were caused by *Salmonella*, but the increased use of antibiotics in poultry and cattle feed has been linked to the increasing incidence of drug-resistant *C. jejuni*.[25–27] Transmission occurs via exposure to contaminated food (especially chicken) and water, or contact with infected animals (especially cats and puppies).[28]

**Salmonella.** Salmonellosis is the second most frequent cause of bacterial disease in the United States. In 2002, more than 44 000 cases were reported to the CDC. Mild infections often are undiagnosed or unreported, so incidence may be 30 or more times greater than reported.[29] Infections with *Salmonella* species include diarrhea, fever, and abdominal cramps.[2] The elderly, infants, and people with impaired immune systems are at greater risk of severe disease. Transmission occurs via exposure to contaminated food (especially eggs) or water, or contact with infected animals (reptiles).[1,30]

**Shigella.** *Shigella* species infection causes a watery or bloody diarrhea with abdominal pain, fever, and malaise. An estimated 448 240 cases occur in the United States yearly. Groups at highest risk in the United States are children in child care centers, individuals in custodial institutions, and international travelers.[11,29]

**Escherichia coli O157:H7.** *E. coli* O157:H7 is associated with a severe diarrheal disease called hemolytic uremic syndrome. It has caused several nationally prominent outbreaks of food poisoning. An estimated 73 000 cases are reported in the United States annually.[30] Transmission occurs through contaminated hamburger meat, apple cider, and fruits and vegetables.[11]

**Helicobacter pylori.** *H. pylori* is the most common chronic infection in humans.[31,32] Acute infection causes abdominal pain, weight loss, nausea, and vomiting. *H. pylori* is the major cause of gastritis and peptic ulcers in adults and children.[33] *H. pylori* impairs absorption of nutrients, altering the balance of iron, vitamin B12, folic acid, alpha-tocopherol, vitamin C, and beta-carotene.

## Skin Infection

Skin infections include impetigo, boils, carbuncles, cellulitis, and complications from burns.[29,34] Common pathogens include *Staphylococcus aureus*, group A *streptococci*, and *Pseudomonas aeruginosa*.[35–37] Impetigo, a skin infection caused mostly by group A *streptococci*, can cause severe kidney inflammation, sometimes resulting in kidney failure.

## Health Care-Associated Infection

Hospital-acquired and health care-related infections comprise an increasing threat to patient safety and health in the United States.[38,39] In the United States, infections encountered in the hospital or a health care facility affect more than 2 million patients, cost $4.5 billion, and contribute to 88 000 deaths in hospitals annually.[40,41]

Urinary tract infections (UTIs) are the most common, followed by pneumonias, skin and soft tissue infections, and invasive bloodstream infections. Surgical wound infections account for 20–30% of cases, but contribute to as many as 57% of extra hospital days and 42% of extra costs. *Staphylococcus epidermidis*, *S. aureus*, *Enterococcus faecium*, *Enterococcus faecalis*, *E. coli*, *Enterobacter* species, and *P. aeruginosa* are common pathogens in wound infections.[38,42]

## WHAT ARE BACTERIA?

Bacteria are microscopic, single-celled organisms found in air, water, soil, and food. They live on plants, insects, animals, pets, and even in the human digestive system and upper respiratory tract. There are thousands of kinds of bacteria, but only a few actually cause disease in humans.

Bacteria are frequently identified by their shape, makeup of cell walls, and ability to grow in air. They can be round (such as *staphylococci* or *streptococci*), rod-shaped (such as *bacillus or E. coli*), or corkscrew-shaped (*Borrelia* species). In most cases, bacteria have cell walls that provide a target for many antibiotics (antibiotics easily identify bacteria).[29]

They are also classified by their color after a Gram stain is applied. Gram-positive bacteria stain blue, while Gram-negative bacteria stain pink.

Gram-negative bacterial cell walls contain a substance known as lipopolysaccharide (LPS), a highly inflammatory chemical that provokes an immune response in the human body. LPS is responsible for triggering the overreaction of the host immune system, which results in the release of oxygen and nitrogen species, cytokines, and other proinflammatory mediators.

## CONVENTIONAL TREATMENTS FOR BACTERIAL INFECTIONS: ANTIBIOTICS AND RESISTANT BACTERIA

Antibiotics are the mainstay of bacterial treatment.[43] The goal of these drugs is to kill invading bacteria without harming the host. Antibiotic effectiveness depends on mechanism of action, drug distribution, site of infection, immune status of the host, and bacteria resistance factors.[43,44]

Antibiotics work through several mechanisms. Some (such as vancomycin and penicillin) inhibit formation of bacterial cell walls. Erythromycin, tetracycline, and chloramphenicol interrupt protein synthesis. Still others inhibit bacterial metabolism (sulfa drugs) or interfere with DNA synthesis (ciprofloxacin, rifampin) and/or cell membrane permeability (polymyxin b).[30]

When antibiotics were discovered in the 1940s, they were incredibly effective in bacterial infection treatment. Over time, however, many antibiotics have lost effectiveness against common bacterial infections because of increasing drug resistance.[45,46] Bacteria may be naturally resistant to different classes of antibiotics or may acquire resistance from other bacteria through exchange of resistant genes. Indiscriminate, inappropriate, and prolonged use of antibiotics have selected out the most antibiotic-resistant bacteria.[47,48] Antibiotic-resistant strains

have emerged in hospitals, long-term care facilities, and communities worldwide.[49–51]

For example, S. *aureus* is a common bacterial pathogen that causes pneumonia and skin and urinary tract infections, as well as blood and surgical site infections. Some strains that are resistant to all current antibiotics, including vancomycin, have emerged in the United States and Japan. Antibiotic-resistant organisms lead to increased hospitalizations, health costs, and mortality.[35,41,45,52–56]

Besides increased drug resistance, high-dose and prolonged antimicrobial therapy can eliminate helpful bacterial flora and predispose people to infection.[57,58] A common adverse effect of antibiotics is diarrhea, which can lead to loss of essential vitamins and minerals, especially vitamin K, magnesium, and zinc.[59–62] Other adverse effects of antibiotic therapy include vitamin deficiencies, seizures, allergic shock (in people who are allergic to antibiotics), autoimmune disease, decreased platelets, kidney injury, drug–drug interaction, and death.[44]

### WHAT YOU HAVE LEARNED SO FAR

- Bacteria can be found colonizing every surface of our environment(s), and some even live inside our digestive, respiratory, and genitourinary tracts. Bacteria can be beneficial or harmful to human health.
- A compromised immune system raises the risk of infection from harmful bacteria. Also, advanced age, genetic predisposition, or compromised nutritional status can raise the risk of bacterial infection.
- Bacteria can cause a wide range of illnesses, from gastrointestinal upset and skin disorders to life-threatening illnesses that require immediate attention. Dangerous bacteria that cause illness include *Streptococcus* species, *E. coli*, and *Salmonella*. Bacterial illnesses include diarrhea, respiratory illness, and pneumonia.
- The mainstay of bacterial infection treatment is antibiotics. While antibiotics work in the majority of cases, indiscriminate use of antibiotics has resulted in the emergence of drug-resistant bacteria.
- A healthy immune system and proper nutritional status can help stave off bacterial infection or improve the immune response to infection. An inflammatory immune response to bacterial infection can result in further injury to cells and tissues.

## NUTRITIONAL APPROACHES TO BACTERIAL INFECTIONS: A HEALTHY IMMUNE SYSTEM

Nutritional deficiencies can affect immune response and increase susceptibility to infection. In turn, infection further aggravates nutritional deficiencies by increasing metabolic demands, decreasing nutrient intake, or blocking absorption from the gut.[63–65] Nutritional and dietary supplements stimulate immune response and may result in fewer infections, particularly in the elderly and in malnourished, critically ill individuals.[66]

Some dietary supplements have been shown to enhance immune function.

## Phytonutrients

Phytonutrients are plant-derived, naturally occurring compounds thought to have curative, preventive, and nutritive value.[67,68] The major immune-boosting components in fruits, vegetables, and herbs are flavonoids and carotenoids, which are antioxidants that protect cells from oxidative damage.[68,69] Flavonoids have a number of powerful complementary and overlapping effects, including modulation of detoxification enzymes, stimulation of the immune system, reduction of platelet aggregation, modulation of cholesterol synthesis, reduction of blood pressure, and antioxidant and antibacterial effects.[69,70] Carotenoids may boost the immune system to fight bacteria by increasing the number of white blood cells.[67,69]

## Alkylglycerols

Alkylglycerols are found in shark liver oil as well as cow, sheep, and human breast milk. They are thought to act as immune boosters against infectious diseases. They have no known adverse effects at relatively high dosages of 100 mg 3 times daily.[71]

## Whey Protein

Whey protein is a rich source of essential amino acids. Compared with other protein sources, whey contains a higher concentration of branched-chain amino acids, which are important for tissue growth and repair. Additionally, whey is rich in the sulfur-containing amino acids cysteine and methionine, which enhance the body's antioxidant protection by bolstering synthesis of glutathione, an important free radical scavenger.[72] Other constituents of whey include beta-lactoglobulin, lactoferrin, and immunoglobulins, all of which support the immune system.[73]

## Fighting Bacteria

In addition to immune-boosting supplements, a number of nutrients have shown antibacterial activity, especially when it comes to inhibiting bacterial infection. While large-scale human studies have yet to be conducted on many antibacterial nutrients, the existing animal studies show considerable promise with these agents.

**Bee propolis and honey.** Before antibiotics, honey was used to treat bacterial wound infections.[74–76] Bee propolis has antibacterial and anti-inflammatory properties. In vitro laboratory studies have shown activity against TB, *H. pylori*, skin ulcers, and colitis.[77–79]

**Bromelain.** Bromelain (a digestive enzyme derived from the pineapple plant) has been used for centuries as a folk remedy for digestive problems and to promote wound healing. It has been proposed as a digestive aid and shown immunomodulatory properties.[80] In animal studies, bromelain has been effective against *E. coli* by disrupting the bacteria's ability to adhere to mucosal lining in the digestive wall.[81,82]

**Cranberry juice.** Cranberry juice can be an effective therapy for bacterial urinary tract infections, both to manage infection and reduce recurrence.[83,84] A study demonstrated *conclusively* that cranberry proanthocyanidins provoke disabling alterations in the fimbriae and other surface properties of the *E. coli* bacterium, vastly diminishing its capacity to attach *specifically* to the surface of the cells lining the urinary tract.[85]

The bacteriostatic effect of cranberry and its extracts have been well documented.[84,86] In 2009, a group of researchers compared antibiotics head-to-head with daily supplements of cranberry extract in women suffering from recurrent infection.[87] Cranberry extract (500 mg) and antibiotics (100 mg trimethoprim) were shown to be almost equally effective in preventing urinary tract infections.

**Hibiscus.** *Hibiscus sabdariffa* contains a range of powerful compounds that prevent *E. coli* from adhering to the walls of the urinary tract. In a double-blind, placebo-controlled clinical trial, women taking hibiscus experienced a reduction in UTIs.[88] Sixty-one women participated in the 6-month study, and 59 women completed the entire study. All of them had a history of frequent UTIs (more than 4 per year, including one or more in the 3 months prior to the start of the study). The women were randomly assigned to one of three groups and received a daily dose of 200 mg of hibiscus extract standardized to 90% polyphenols, 200 mg of hibiscus extract standardized to 60% polyphenols, or placebo. Compared to the control group, women taking the hibiscus concentrations experienced a 77% decrease in infections, as well as overall improvement in urinary comfort.

**Oil of oregano.** Oregano oil has been used for centuries in Far Eastern and Middle Eastern cultures to treat respiratory infections, chronic inflammation, urinary tract infections, dysentery, and jaundice. Laboratory studies in which the oil was applied directly to food-borne pathogens showed that oregano oil has strong antibacterial properties.[89] Medicinal oregano grows wild in mountainous areas of Greece and Turkey. It has a high mineral content that enhances its therapeutic benefits, including calcium, magnesium, zinc, iron, potassium, copper, boron, and manganese. This oil is considered safe for humans and may be used in conjunction with antibiotics to fight bacterial infection.[90]

**Thyme.** Thyme, another essential herbal oil, has shown antibacterial properties. For example, thyme has been demonstrated to inhibit many strains of *E. coli*, including *E. coli* O157:H7.[91] It has also been very effective in preventing the growth of *Listeria*.[92]

**Ginger.** The characteristic odor and flavor of ginger root come from a volatile oil composed of shogaol and gingerols. Gingerols have been investigated for analgesic, sedative, antipyretic, antibacterial, and gastrointestinal tract motility effects. They have been found to inhibit Gram-positive and Gram-negative bacteria.[93–95]

**N-acetyl-cysteine.** N-acetyl-cysteine (NAC) may help fight *H. pylori* infections, both because of its ability to interfere with the oxidant-inflammation connection, and also because of its potential to travel deep into the gastric mucous layer beneath which the organisms hide.[96]

NAC markedly inhibits growth of *H. pylori* both in culture dishes and in live mice, helping to reduce the total load of organisms present.[96] It also powerfully regulates gene expression in stomach lining cells, reducing hydrogen peroxide production induced by *H. pylori*, and decreasing activation of NF-κB and subsequent release of inflammatory cytokines.[97,98] In human trials, NAC improves eradication rates of *H. pylori* produced by standard treatment with antacids and antibiotics when given at doses of 1200 mg per day.[99,100]

## Enhancing Your Immune System While Fighting Bacteria

The nutrients vitamin A, beta-carotene, folic acid, vitamin B12, vitamin C, vitamin D, riboflavin, iron, copper, zinc, and selenium have both antioxidant activity and immunomodulating functions that affect the course and outcome of bacterial infections.[101–103] In general, people taking multivitamin and multimineral supplements report significantly fewer infectious illnesses. In one small study, efficacy was highest in individuals with type 2 diabetes.[104]

**Glutamine.** Glutamine helps build and maintain muscles, modulates pH, and contributes to a healthy digestive system.[105] It is also an important precursor to glutathione, a natural antioxidant. Glutamine has been shown to help boost immune function through white blood cell respiration and production of messenger chemicals used by the immune system.[106]

**Vitamin A.** Low levels of vitamin A have been associated with increased susceptibility to bacterial infection, and vitamin A supplementation has been suggested to decrease days of work lost to infection.[101,104,107] Vitamin A appears to be important in mucosal immune responses in the respiratory and gastrointestinal tracts.[108] The effect may be primarily from stabilizing the membranes of mucosal cells and enhancing white blood cell function.[109] Vitamin A has been studied in dosages up to 75 000 IU daily for up to 12 months (in the context of skin cancer) with no appreciable toxicity.[110]

**Vitamin E.** Vitamin E improves immune function in the elderly. Supplementation with vitamin E (alpha-tocopherol) has been documented to increase levels of anti-inflammatory chemicals and decrease levels of proinflammatory proteins.[102] Vitamin E enhances the immune system through its ability to protect immune cells from free-radical attack, which preserves membrane integrity and fluidity.[111]

**Zinc.** Many studies have shown that zinc deficiency is associated with impaired immune function.[112–115] A combination of zinc and selenium may enhance immunity and protect against infections, especially in the elderly. A review article of published studies showed that elderly individuals taking modest doses of a multivitamin and multimineral dietary supplement containing zinc and selenium had fewer days on antibiotics and fewer infections than counterparts who did not take zinc-containing multivitamins or supplements.[116]

**Garlic.** Crushed garlic has potent antibacterial effects.[117–120] It fights infection by enhancing immune cell activity and inhibiting bacteria and other microorganisms.[121,122] The compound in garlic that produces antibacterial activity is known as allicin.[117,120] Allicin is released when intact cells of a garlic clove are cut or crushed. There is evidence that garlic is effective against antibiotic-resistant strains of *Staphylococcus* species, pneumonia-causing bacteria, and antibiotic-resistant strains of *H. pylori*.[123–125]

**Goldenseal.** Goldenseal (a member of the buttercup family) has been used topically to treat eye and skin irritations and orally to treat infections.[126] Berberine, the main active ingredient in goldenseal, prevents bacteria from adhering to epithelial cells,[127] inhibits the intestinal secretory response of cholera and *E. coli* toxins, and normalizes intestinal mucous membranes after damage from cholera.[128]

**Licorice.** Licorice is derived from the root of the *Glycyrrhiza* species. Glycyrrhizin is converted by intestinal flora to glycyrrhetinic acid, which has immunomodulating activity. In laboratory studies, glycyrrhetinic acid has demonstrated powerful effects against *H. pylori* gastritis and ulcers.[129,130] Studies have shown that, in humans, adverse effects begin at daily dosages of 100 mg.[131]

**Lactoferrin.** Lactoferrin (a component of whey) increases good microflora (such as *Bifidobacterium bifidum*) and decreases bad bacteria, resulting in a desirable intestinal flora environment that is essential for optimal health, immunity, and disease resistance. Lactoferrin is a powerful antimicrobial able to inhibit a wide range of pathogenic bacteria and other microbes.[132–136] The mechanism appears to lie with lactoferrin's ability to bind iron, as it is known to have an extremely high affinity for this metal.[137–139] It is referred to as hololactoferrin in its iron-bound form and apolactoferrin in its iron-depleted form. Studies have found that the apolactoferrin form has the most powerful effects as an antimicrobial agent.[140–143]

Other organisms inhibited by lactoferrin include Gram-positive and Gram-negative bacteria, yeasts, and some intestinal parasites such as *Vibrio cholerae*, *E. coli*,[144] *Shigella flexneri*, *S. epidermidis*, *P. aeruginosa*, and *Candida albicans*.[143,145–147]

Lactoferrin may be especially useful as an adjuvant therapy for antibiotics. One study looked at the synergistic effect between lactoferrin and vancomycin. Researchers found that lactoferrin lowered vancomycin resistance in some bacteria.[148]

**Probiotics.** Probiotics are bacterial cultures contained in yogurt, buttermilk, cheese, kefir, sauerkraut, or dietary supplements that contain friendly bacteria (such as *Lactobacillus*, *Bifidobacterium*, *Eubacterium*, and *Propionibacterium* species) normally present on skin and in vaginal, urinary, and intestinal tracts. These bacteria are essential to the proper function of the vaginal, urinary, and digestive tracts.[114,149,150]

Probiotics assist immune function by inhibiting harmful bacterial growth, promoting good digestion, maintaining proper pH, and enhancing immune function.[151] Probiotics produce bacteria-inhibiting substances (natural antibiotics) and prevent harmful bacteria from attaching to vaginal, urinary, and intestinal tract mucosal linings.[152,153] Probiotics have demonstrated an ability to suppress *H. pylori* in vitro.[154–158] They may be useful in preventing acute infectious diarrhea,[23] urinary tract infections,[159,160] and restoring vaginal flora.[161]

Antibiotics often destroy friendly bacteria on skin and in urinary, vaginal, and intestinal tracts. Probiotics can be used to recolonize and restore natural floral balance in organ and body systems after antibiotic treatment.[58,162,163]

**Tea catechins.** Tea (black, green, or oolong) is a good source of free-radical scavenging antioxidants.[164] Other infection-fighting chemicals were heightened in cells of tea drinkers, leading researchers to conclude that drinking tea primed the immune system to fight infection.[165,166]

These results have been borne out in many clinical studies. Elements of tea, called catechins, have been widely studied for their ability to prevent bacterial infection. One such study examined catechins' ability to prevent infection in the prostate gland in rats. This condition, known as chronic bacterial prostatitis, is extremely common in men. Researchers found that tea catechins were able to reduce both bacterial growth and inflammation in the rats' prostate glands. Moreover, the catechins worked well as an adjuvant therapy for ciprofloxacin, the standard antibiotic treatment for this condition. Researchers suggested that tea catechins, which have shown additional antibacterial effects and synergistic properties with antibiotics, be considered to help manage chronic bacterial prostatitis.[167]

In another interesting study, researchers infused plastic film with tea catechins, and then tested this surface for antibacterial properties. They found that the catechin-infused film was significantly resistant to bacteria such as *E. coli* and suggested that implants and catheters made from catechin-infused plastic might be able to help reduce infection during invasive procedures.[168]

Catechins are thought to boost immunity by enhancing resistance to infection and selectively modulating the formation of cytokines, which are associated with inflammation, among other things. Researchers have also hypothesized that hydrogen peroxide generated by the catechins may also be responsible for its antibacterial properties.[169] In a laboratory study of immune cells taken from heavy smokers, tea catechins were shown to help the immune cells recover their function.[170]

**Beta-glucan.** Numerous substances including polysaccharides, lymphokines, and peptides activate the defensive properties of macrophages. A polysaccharide called beta-glucan not only enhances macrophages' ability to recognize and subdue microbial invaders, but also increases their ability to communicate with other cellular defenders of the immune system.

At Brigham and Women's Hospital in Boston, researchers found that the compound enhances antibiotic efficacy in rats infected with antibiotic-resistant bacteria. Rats with intra-abdominal sepsis due to antibiotic-resistant bacteria—namely *Escherichia coli* or *Staphylococcus aureus*—were given a type of beta-glucan (PGG glucan) that enhances the function of macrophages and neutrophils. Researchers looked at beta-glucan's ability to work in partnership with antibiotics to decrease mortality of the rats. "Results of these studies demonstrated that prophylaxis with PGG glucan in combination with antibiotics provided enhanced protection against lethal challenge with *Escherichia coli* or *Staphylococcus aureus* as compared with the use of antibiotics alone," wrote the researchers.[171]

Canadian scientists have demonstrated that beta-glucan confers protection against deadly anthrax infection in animals. For example, in mice that received beta-glucan for 1 week prior to infection with anthrax bacteria, survival increased from 50% to 100%. When beta-glucan was administered only after infection had occurred, survival rates increased from 30% to 90% in the treatment groups. "These results demonstrate the potential for [beta-glucan] immune modulators to provide a significant degree of protection against anthrax," the researchers concluded.[172] Similar results against other pathogens have been reported by other researchers.[173–175]

**Andrographis.** Healers in Asia and India have long prescribed the bitter herb *Andrographis paniculata* for the treatment of ailments ranging from infections and inflammation to colds and fevers.[176] Researchers have isolated a number of the herb's active ingredients. Chief among these are andrographolides, which are phytochemicals that are believed to exert their effects, in part, on tissues of the blood cell-producing bone marrow and/or spleen.

**Hyperimmune egg extracts.** Agricultural scientists long ago discovered that they could immunize hens against germs that threaten humans. This immunity was then passed on by the hen to her egg.[177–179] Concentrated protein extracts from those so-called "hyperimmune eggs" confer some immunity to humans who consume them.[180,181]

Patients with cystic fibrosis (CF) are especially at risk for colonization of their lungs with *Pseudomonas*

*aeruginosa* (PA), an organism that thrives in overly viscous mucous secretions. PA infection is in fact the major cause of death and disability in cystic fibrosis patients.[182] Among cystic fibrosis patients who gargled with a hyperimmune egg preparation from hens immunized against PA, none became chronically colonized with the organism, while 24% of control subjects did.[182]

Hyperimmune egg may also be effective for other less serious, but more common respiratory tract infections. There was a reduction in symptoms among people with both acute and chronic bacterial sore throat when they used a hyperimmune egg-containing throat spray, compared with placebo-treated subjects.[183]

## Life Extension Suggestions

Bacterial infections are occasionally life-threatening health concerns. Older and newly emerging antibiotic-resistant infections are an increasing danger for children, the elderly, and people who have chronic diseases. Bacterial infections can disrupt normal intestinal flora, reduce nutrient and mineral supplies, and compromise immune responses. A healthy immune system can prevent or neutralize bacterial infections.

When dealing with a possible bacterial infection, it is impossible to tell, short of laboratory tests, which pathogen is causing the problem. Therefore, it is important to visit a physician for proper testing and, if necessary, to obtain prescription antibiotics. In addition, many nutrients have been shown to help strengthen the immune system and inhibit bacterial infection. Nutrients that have been demonstrated to inhibit bacterial activity or enhance the immune system include the following:

- **Comprehensive multinutrient formula:** per label instructions
- **Vitamin E:** 400 IU daily (with 200 mg gamma-tocopherol)
- **Vitamin D:** 5000–8000 IU daily, depending on blood test results
- **Vitamin A**, as beta-carotene: 5000 IU daily
- **Lactoferrin**, providing 95% of apolactoferrin: 300 mg daily
- **Oregano oil:** 400–1000 mg of essential oils daily
- **Aged garlic extract:** 600–1200 mg daily
- **Shark liver oil** (containing 260 mg of active alkylglycerols): 1000 mg daily
- **Bromelain:** 500 mg before each meal
- **L-arginine:** 900 mg daily
- **L-glutamine:** 1000–2000 mg daily

- **Cranberry extract:** 500 mg daily
- **Hibiscus,** standardized extract: 200 mg daily
- **Probiotics,** containing *Lactobacillus* and *Bifidobacterium* strains: per label instructions
- **Whey protein isolate:** 20–40 g daily in divided doses
- **Green tea,** standardized extract: 725 mg daily
- **Garlic bulb powder,** standardized to 12 mg allicin: 1200–4800 mg daily with meals (for current infections)
- **N-acetyl-cysteine** (NAC): 600–1200 mg daily

- **Beta-glucan,** highly purified beta 1,3/1,6 glucan: 100–600 mg daily 30 minutes before a meal
- **Andrographis extract:** 25–150 mg daily 30 minutes before a meal
- **Hyperimmune egg extracts:** per label instructions

## REFERENCES

References available at: www.lef.org/dpt5/ch18

# 19

# Balding and Hair Loss

Hair shedding is part of a normal hair-growth cycle. At any given time, 90% of scalp hair is in a 2- to 6-year growth phase; 10% is in a 2- to 6-month dormant phase. When the dormant phase ends, hair is shed. New hair subsequently emerges from these follicles. Throughout a normal growth cycle, many hairs are shed. Loss of 50 to even 100 hairs daily is not cause for alarm. Noticeable thinning indicates significant hair loss or balding. Hair loss and balding are not life-threatening, but can cause emotional distress.

Hair loss results from aging, genetic predisposition, thyroid imbalance, eating disorders, illness, hormonal effects of birth control pills, pregnancy, menopause, and certain medications. The most common cause of hair loss is a hereditary condition known as androgenetic alopecia (AGA). Balding runs in families.[1]

Hair loss caused by AGA in men and women is characterized by a gradual shrinking of hair follicles which shortens the life cycle of hair. As the growth cycle phase progressively shortens, newly grown hair is shorter and thinner until new hair growth eventually ceases entirely. Hair thinning conditions can be treated. Consult a physician or dermatologist for an evaluation to determine the cause of thinning hair.[2]

## EPIDEMIOLOGY AND GENETICS

Genetic or hereditary hair loss does not discriminate between sexes or races. Approximately 40 million men (or 2 out of 3 men) in the United States have significant hair loss. About 25% have some form of balding by age 30, and 65% begin to bald by age 60. In women, the number affected by pattern-type hair loss is slightly less: about 30 million or 1 in 4. Thinning hair can occur anytime between ages 25–45, but most commonly hair loss presents after age 40. Hair loss occurs in about 25% of premenopausal women and in 38% of postmenopausal women.

## TYPES AND CAUSES OF HAIR LOSS

### Male Pattern Baldness

Male pattern balding, the most common type in men, usually starts at the temples and gradually recedes to form an "M" shape. Hair on the top of the head thins. Over time, hair takes on a horseshoe-shaped pattern. Some males have only a receding hairline or bald spots at the crown. Hair remaining in the balding areas is long, thick, and pigmented. It then changes into fine, nonpigmented hair that grows at a slow rate. Males losing their hair during the mid-teen years are likely to become completely bald on top of their heads.[3]

Androgenetic alopecia (AGA) is a major factor in male pattern baldness. AGA is attributed to androgens, hormones that are responsible for male characteristics. AGA has 3 causal factors: advanced age, an inherited tendency to early baldness, and overabundance of dihydrotestosterone (DHT). DHT, which is derived from testosterone, is the most potent androgen in the hair follicle. Testosterone is metabolized into DHT by 5-alpha-reductase, an enzyme produced in the prostate, adrenal glands, and scalp. DHT (and perhaps other androgens) causes hair follicles to shrink and enter a permanent dormant state. DHT triggers synthesis of transforming growth factor-beta2 (TGF-$\beta$2), which suppresses epithelial cell proliferation and eventually leads to apoptotic cell death.[4] TGF-$\beta$2 is directly responsible for significant hair loss on a cellular level. Using combination therapy (with current DHT and androgen inhibitors) to combat the effects of TGF-$\beta$2 may have a significant role in treating hair loss.[5]

### Female Pattern Baldness

Female pattern baldness (or diffused thinning) is caused by aging, genetic susceptibility, and androgens.[5] Female pattern baldness usually begins about age 30. It becomes more noticeable by age 40 and can be quite evident following menopause. Female pattern baldness usually causes hair to thin all over the head. It rarely progresses to near or total baldness. Female pattern baldness causes permanent hair loss.

### Telogen Effluvium

Telogen effluvium is an abnormal loss of hair caused by alteration of a normal hair cycle. In telogen effluvium, a large proportion of hair enters the dormant phase and hair shedding is greater than normal.[6] Telogen effluvium can follow a case of flu, emotional stress,[7] or can occur after a pregnancy. Hormonal changes in pregnancy can cause increased numbers of hair follicles to remain in a growth phase. After pregnancy, an increased proportion of these hairs enter a dormant phase, a temporary self-correction that increases hair shedding.[8] This condition is seen when birth control pills are stopped.[9]

## Chemotherapeutic Hair Loss

Cancer chemotherapy causes hair cells to stop dividing, a usually transient condition.[10] Hair can fall out for 3–4 months before growing back. When a drug is prescribed, ask your physician if a side effect is hair loss. Side effects of all prescription drugs are listed in the *Physicians' Desk Reference*. Pharmacists also have this information.

## Alopecia Areata

Alopecia areata is a highly unpredictable, autoimmune skin condition that causes loss of scalp hair, facial hair, and hair elsewhere on the body. It affects approximately 1.7% of individuals (more than 4.7 million people) in the United States.[11] In alopecia areata, affected hair follicles are mistakenly attacked by an individual's immune system (white blood cells) and the hair growth stage is arrested. Alopecia areata typically begins with one or more small, round, smooth bald patches on the scalp. It can progress to total scalp hair loss (alopecia totalis) or total body hair loss (alopecia universalis).[12] Alopecia areata affects males and females of all ages and races. Onset often begins in childhood when it can be emotionally devastating. Alopecia areata is not life-threatening, but is life-altering. Its sudden onset, recurrent episodes, and unpredictable course have profound psychological impact.

## Trichotillomania

Trichotillomania is a psychological disorder (an impulse control disorder). Impulse control disorders are characterized by an uncontrollable urge (or impulse) to harm oneself or others. Trichotillomania patients repetitively pull hair out at the root of the scalp, eyebrows, eyelashes, or chronically scratch or brush their hair. Trichotillomania affects 1–2% of the population, primarily children. Girls are more likely to be affected than boys.

## Scarring Alopecia

Scarring alopecia describes skin scarred by burns, x-ray therapy, skin cancer, or severe injury that results in hair loss.

## Other Causes of Hair Loss

Hair loss can occur from damage caused by hair styling processes and products as well as from twisting and pulling hair. Certain skin conditions cause hair loss and baldness. Hair loss can be caused by oral medications, including cholesterol-lowering drugs, Parkinson's medications,[13] antiulcer drugs,[14] anticoagulants,[15] anti-arthritics,[16,17] drugs derived from vitamin A,[18] anticonvulsants,[19] antidepressants,[20] beta-blockers, antithyroid agents,[21] and anabolic steroids.

# ANATOMY AND PHYSIOLOGY (STRUCTURE AND FUNCTION)

Each hair originates in a deep pouch-like structure in the epidermis (hair follicle) that penetrates the dermis. A hair root extends down into the hair follicle and widens into an indented bulb at its base. Extending into the indentation is the papilla (center of hair growth), which contains capillaries and nerves that supply hair. Newly dividing cells at the base of the hair multiply, forcing cells above them upward. As cells move upward, they gradually die and harden into a hair shaft. A hair shaft has 2 layers: cuticle and cortex. The cuticle (outer layer) consists of flat, colorless, overlapping cells. The cortex (inner layer) contains pigment and keratin, a tough protein. The cortex forms the bulk of a hair shaft. Coarse hair (eg, scalp hair) contains an additional inner core (medulla). Hair is lubricated by sebaceous glands located in hair follicles. Illness or stress can lessen pigment secretion and cause hair shafts to whiten. Age-related whitening is genetically determined. Hair color is determined by pigment and air spaces in the cortex and medulla. Hair color and texture are inherited characteristics. Human scalp hairs generally shed every 2–4 years; body hairs shed more frequently.[22]

# PATHOPHYSIOLOGY

In the scalp, a hair growth cycle has 3 main phases: anagen, catagen, and telogen. The anagen phase typically lasts 3–5 years. On a healthy scalp, hair numbers approximately 100 000 and 90% of the follicles are continually in the anagen phase of hair growth. The catagen phase follows the end of the growth period when a follicle begins to become dormant. The telogen phase is a dormant or resting period lasting 3–4 months. When the dormant phase ends, an old hair falls out. A hair follicle then returns to the anagen phase and a new hair begins to grow.[23]

An average rate of hair growth is about half an inch per month depending on hair follicles and age of an individual. On average, 50–60 scalp hairs are lost daily in a normal hair growth cycle and new hairs begin to grow from these follicles. Hair loss begins when less new hair begins the regrowth stage.

# ETIOLOGY

In male pattern baldness, scalp hair in affected areas becomes shorter, finer, and less pigmented with successive growth cycles. Androgenic alopecia is thought to be associated with the presence of dihydrotestosterone (DHT), a metabolite of testosterone. Eunuchs have low levels of testosterone and do not lose scalp hair; and men with a genetic deficiency of 5-alpha-reductase (the enzyme that converts testosterone to DHT) do not have male pattern baldness.[24]

# CONVENTIONAL TREATMENT OPTIONS

## Traditional Approaches

A biopsy may be required to determine baldness type. A biopsy ascertains if hair follicles are normal.

Conventional choices can be used to treat hair loss: take better care of the scalp, use minoxidil (Rogaine®) and/or Proscar®, have hair transplants or a scalp reduction, or have hair replaced nonsurgically.

Successful prevention and treatment of accelerated hair loss necessitates treating factors that are involved in contributing to the hair-loss process (excluding the genetic component).

## Antiandrogens

DHT (the male hormone dihydrotestosterone) is associated with premature hair loss. A wide variety of anti-androgens are used to prevent or reverse premature hair loss: progesterone, spironolactone (Aldactone®), flutamide (Eulexin®), finasteride (Proscar®), cimetidine (Tagamet®), Serenoa repens (Permixon®), and cyproterone acetate (Androcur/Diane®). The most effective antiandrogens are oral finasterides (Propecia®, Proscar®).

In hair-loss, an immune reaction caused by male hormones (eg, DHT) has perhaps the most significant role. Stimulated by androgens, the immune system targets hair follicles in genetically susceptible areas and causes premature hair loss characteristic of male pattern baldness.[25]

## Growth Stimulators

Topical oxygen free-radical scavengers such as superoxide dismutases (SODs) (enzymes that counter excessive free-radical activity) are potent hair-growth stimulators. SOD inhibits oxygen radicals, may inhibit a localized immune response implicated in hair loss, and offsets damage and inflammation.[26] Unless immunologic factors involved in the hair loss process are

effectively treated, potential for significant hair regrowth may be very limited.

Available agents (eg, Rogaine®) stimulate some degree of hair growth in some individuals, but cannot by themselves produce healthy hair and cosmetic benefits. A multimodal approach is required that combines antiandrogens, autoimmune-system protective agents, oxygen free-radical inhibitors, and other hair-growth stimulators to halt hair loss and generate hair regrowth.

## Finasteride

Finasteride (Proscar®) was originally developed to treat benign prostatic hyperplasia (BPH). It is available by prescription in 5-mg tablets. Finasteride (Propecia®) is approved by the Food and Drug Administration (FDA) for hair loss treatment. It is available by prescription in 1-mg tablets for men. Propecia® cannot be taken by women. Finasteride was once thought to be useless for androgenic alopecia treatment because it primarily affected 5-alpha-reductase, the type-2 DHT-producing enzyme. However, finasteride in doses as low as 0.2 mg daily maximally decrease scalp, skin, and serum DHT levels.[27]

Finasteride can produce visible hair growth in most men with mild-to-moderate alopecia and can stop hair loss in a majority of patients. Finasteride (1 mg daily over 5 years) was well-tolerated, produced durable improvement in scalp hair growth, and slowed further hair loss progression that occurred with no treatment.[28] The most common side effect is decreased sexual desire or lowered amount of ejaculate (<2%, although men receiving placebo experienced the same side effects). Initial results of the Prostate Cancer Prevention Trial produced concerns that finasteride might promote prostate cancer. Finasteride was thought to reduce incidence of prostate cancer in men older than 55 by one researcher; trial participants who developed prostate cancer had slightly more high-grade tumors.[29]

## Dutasteride

Dutasteride (GG745), similar to Propecia®, blocks enzymatic conversion of testosterone to DHT. Unlike finasteride, dutasteride blocks 2 enzymes that create DHT rather than one and may be a more potent treatment for hair loss.[30]

## Azulfidine

Azulfidine is an anti-inflammatory sulfa drug used to treat autoimmune disorders (eg, rheumatoid arthritis and Crohn's disease). It is used in alopecia areata. In a clinical trial, azulfidine completely reversed alopecia areata in 23% of participants. Although some regrowth occurred in other participants, the majority had no effect.[31]

## Minoxidil

Originally used to treat high blood pressure, minoxidil is now widely used as a topical solution applied twice daily to treat male pattern baldness. It may improve hair growth in 10–20% and slow hair loss in 90% of users. How minoxidil acts is unclear, but when effective, it appears to prolong the growing phase in the hair growth cycle, enlarge follicles, and cause dormant follicles to grow. Minoxidil may take 4 months or longer to produce results. Treatment is relatively expensive and must be continued indefinitely. When minoxidil is stopped, regrown hair falls out. Newly grown hair may not be as long or thick as normal hair. Minoxidil is more effective in young men and men with recent-onset hair loss.[32]

## Hair Transplantation

Early hair grafting techniques were somewhat crude, often leaving a "patchwork" appearance. Newer techniques transplant productive hair follicles from a donor area on the scalp to a balding area. Hair follicles are commonly taken in plugs of 1 or 2 hairs (micrografts) from the sides or back of the head and moved to the front and/or top, slowly reconstructing a hairline. Larger plugs of up to 10 hairs can be used. Donor sites with full hair produce more successful transplants. The flap technique transplants larger areas of hair from the sides and back of the scalp to the top of the head. Some scarring at the donor site may result. Transplanted follicles can be permanent or last only a few years.

## Scalp Reduction

Balding scalp areas can be surgically removed to decrease an appearance of baldness. Scalp reduction is usually used in conjunction with grafts or flaps. Prior to reduction, the scalp may be stretched to expand areas of hair growth. Effectiveness of scalp reduction depends on degree of hair loss and scalp elasticity.

# NUTRITIONAL THERAPY

A healthy, low fat diet high in fiber, fresh fruit, and vegetables can have a major role in inhibiting hair loss associated with aging and genetics. In Asian countries, where vegetables are prevalent in standard dietary practices, pattern type hair loss is rarely observed. Botanically based nutrients may prevent hair follicles from entering a permanent dormant state. Nutritional supplements can provide some benefit.

## Comprehensive Multinutrient Formula

A comprehensive multinutrient formula containing a unique combination of vegetable, fruit, and herbal extracts, as well as amino acids, vitamins, minerals, and special antioxidants is essential in maintaining healthy cells via physiologic processes separate from traditional antioxidants. Consumption of these types of nutrients is based on research from prestigious medical centers.

## L-Lysine

A U.S. patent has been issued for L-lysine (an amino acid) for treatment of various types of hair loss, including androgenetic alopecia. L-lysine inhibits 5-alpha-reductase.[33]

## L-Arginine

Hair follicles use nitric oxide to maintain and promote new hair growth. L-arginine is required to produce nitric oxide.[34]

## Saw Palmetto

Saw palmetto (Serenoa repens) is a palm-like plant that is native to North America. An extract derived from saw palmetto berries contains fatty acids and sterols. Saw palmetto is commonly used to treat benign prostatic hyperplasia because it inhibits testosterone's action on the prostate. Extracts of saw palmetto block 5-alpha-reductase, reduce DHT uptake by follicles, and block binding of DHT to androgen receptors. The liposterolic extract of saw palmetto combined with beta-sitosterol (a phytosterol common to many plants and grains) produced marked improvement.[35]

## Green Tea Extract

Topical agents such as finasteride inhibit type II 5-alpha-reductase in hair follicles. Agents from tea (catechins, [–]epigallocatechin-3-gallate, and [–]epicatechin-3-gallate) affect type-I, 5-alpha-reductase activity responsible for converting testosterone to DHT. All tea is derived from the same plant species, but types and varieties differ according to where and how the plants are grown and how the tea is produced. Catechins in green tea leaves are more potent. Black pekoe is allowed to dry and ferment, but green tea is not, thereby preserving catechin integrity.[36]

## Proanthocyanidins and Procyanidins

Proanthocyanidins and procyanidins (specifically oligomeric proanthocyanidins [OPCs]) are a class of flavonoids found in woody plants. Two common sources of OPCs are grape seeds (*Vitis vinifera*) and white pine (*Pinus maritima*, *P. pinaster*). Procyanidin B-2 and procyanidin B-3, which directly stimulate epithelial cell growth and check the growth-inhibiting effect caused by TGF-beta2, are of specific interest. Supplementing with 100–200 mg proanthocyanidins daily in the form of OPCs from grape seed extract is suggested for adults.[37]

## Bioenhanced Tocotrienol Complex

Using a supplement with *tocotrienols* can be pivotal in addressing the various physiologic mechanisms that lead to thinning hair.[38] A natural, orally administered, bioenhanced tocotrienol complex can be taken to support *youthful hair* thickness and growth. In an unpublished study involving 30 volunteers who took tocotrienol supplements for 8 months, nearly all the subjects showed significant improvement in hair thickness and density.[38]

## Complementary Topical Treatment

Peter Proctor has developed a unique, nonprescription, multi-ingredient hair formula for balding. Proctor's formula includes 3-carboxylic acid pyridine-N-oxide (NANO, known as "natural" minoxidil), with natural hair protection and the following hair growth agents: endothelium-derived relaxing factor (EDRF) enhancers, SODs, and free-radical scavengers. Zinc sulfate and copper peptides are antiandrogens that enhance production of EDRF.[39,40] This liquid product, which may be used as a shampoo, can be applied to the scalp as follows: 8–10 drops once or twice daily on thinning areas.

For a really serious hair loss problem, you may need to try Proctor's most potent formula, which contains an array of natural hair growth protectors combined with several drugs compounded into a cream. This European hair formula is available by prescription and contains topical antiandrogens that increase EDRF levels and oxygen free-radical scavengers. These agents are combined with the following drugs: minoxidil, phenytoin (Dilantin), tretinoin (Retin-A) and spironolactone. The European hair formula is available by prescription from a compounding pharmacy. Call (713) 960-1616 for details.

## SUMMARY

Several factors lead to hair loss in men and women, most notably androgenic alopecia, an inherited condition. Treatment is available. Early treatment produces better results. Balding is a cosmetic condition, usually resulting from genetic influences, aging, skin conditions, or certain medications. The most common forms of balding are male and female pattern balding. Baldness has no cure. Oral prescription drugs (eg, Propecia® and Proscar®) and over-the-counter preparations (eg, minoxidil) have benefits. Most hair-growth drugs prevent hair loss better than they regrow hair. Taking aggressive steps today helps maintain healthy hair.

Hair loss has many causes, including aging, genetic predisposition, thyroid imbalance, eating disorders, illness, hormonal effects of birth control pills, pregnancy, and menopause, as well as certain medications and medical treatments. There is no single "cure" for baldness. A product that is effective for one individual may provide only limited results for another. Combining traditional treatments with nutritional supplements and natural topical solutions improves chances of inhibiting pattern hair loss.

## Life Extension Suggestions

### Conventional Therapy

- At the first sign of thinning hair, consult a dermatologist to determine the cause.
- Ask your physician if any prescription drug you take causes temporary hair loss.
- Ask your physician about drugs that may revive hair growth.

### Lifestyle Modification

- Maintain a healthy diet that is low in fat and rich in whole foods.

### Nutritional Supplements

- **L-lysine:** 700 mg daily
- **L-arginine:** 900 mg 2 times daily
- **Saw palmetto:** 160 mg 2 times daily
- **Green tea extract:** 725 mg daily
- **Grape seed extract:** 100–200 mg daily
- **Comprehensive multinutrient formula:** Per label instructions
- **Bioenhanced tocotrienol complex:** 50 mg tocotrienols 2 times daily

## REFERENCES

References available at: www.lef.org/dpt5/ch19

# 20

# *Bell's Palsy*

Bell's palsy is a mysterious condition in which one half of the face abruptly becomes paralyzed. This sudden paralysis may be preceded by pain behind one ear for 1–2 days, but it usually occurs quickly.

People with Bell's palsy might experience a number of uncomfortable symptoms, including total paralysis or pronounced weakness on one side of the face. The weak side typically becomes flat and expressionless, and affected people might feel a heaviness or numbness in their faces (even though normal sensation remains). Other symptoms include a drooping appearance on the affected side of the face and impairment of tear and saliva function.

If the upper part of the face is involved, affected people may have problems with their eyes. Because they are unable to close their eyes, dryness is a problem. In extreme cases this dryness can result in eye damage or even blindness. To help prevent these problems, some physicians recommend the use of paper tape at night to keep the affected eye closed and lubricated. In addition, people with Bell's palsy may experience loss of taste or abnormally enhanced hearing because the muscle that stretches the eardrum is paralyzed.

Most people with Bell's palsy (about 80%) recover within a few weeks or months. Among those who do not recover fully, the affected side of their face may continue to be weak and droop. About 1 in 60 people will experience Bell's palsy at some point in their lifetime. It can occur at any age, but is most common between the age of 15 and 60.[1]

Bell's palsy is associated with presence of the herpes simplex virus 1 (HSV1), which suggests that reactivation of this virus in the facial nerve might be responsible for the condition.[1] According to the herpes theory, about 80% of Bell's palsy cases are caused by reactivation of HSV1 or varicella zoster (a member of the herpes family). HSV1 is most commonly associated with oral lesions, as opposed to HSV2, which is most commonly associated with genital lesions. Varicella zoster is responsible for chicken pox in children and shingles in adults. The herpes virus can be transported to the facial nerve, where it may remain dormant until it activates and causes Bell's palsy.[2] Although this theory has yet to be proven, supporting evidence is strong enough that Bell's palsy is often treated with antiviral drugs (eg, acyclovir, famciclovir, and valacyclovir) used to kill the herpes virus. To date, although viral DNA has been found in the facial nerves of patients with Bell's palsy, no studies have actually found actively replicating herpes viruses.[3] Those interested in learning more about the implications and varieties of herpes viruses should read Life Extension's Herpes and Shingles protocol.

Other infectious diseases that may be associated with Bell's palsy include Lyme disease, the common cold, hepatitis C, influenza, HIV, typhoid fever, and tuberculosis.[1]

No single test can diagnose Bell's palsy. Instead, physicians diagnose the condition by first excluding other possible causes of facial paralysis (eg, cancer, leukemia, bacterial infections, stroke, multiple sclerosis, head trauma, and other disorders). There are two classic characteristics of Bell's palsy that help guide diagnosis[4,5]:

1. The symptoms have a quick onset.
2. It affects the entire half of the face (while stroke or cerebral tumor usually cause paralysis below the eye).

During the diagnosis, a few tests might be ordered to help exclude other conditions, including blood tests to check for diabetes, HIV, bacterial infection, and Lyme disease. In some cases, an x-ray might be ordered to check for a tumor in the head.

## THE DISEASE COURSE

In about 80% of cases, Bell's palsy resolves completely within 3 months. However, 15% of patients will experience facial asymmetry, and 5% will show persistent neurologic impairment or disfigurement.[2,6]

Besides antiviral drugs, the standard treatment for Bell's palsy is corticosteroids (eg, prednisone). Corticosteroids have been shown to reduce inflammation of the facial nerve, which minimizes compression and damage,[7] although a few studies have found that steroids are ineffective.[8] Some studies have also suggested that antivirals are effective only if prescribed early in the disease process.[9]

In severe cases, surgical treatment might be recommended, although surgery is associated with a high risk of hearing loss, and many clinicians recommend against it. The surgery used to treat Bell's palsy is known as decompression surgery. It is used to relieve pressure on the affected facial nerve.

A number of alternative or complementary therapies have been studied for Bell's palsy. Many people believe that facial massage will help relieve the condition, although there is evidence that facial massage will not help.[10] Acupuncture combined with exercise therapy has been shown to increase therapeutic effect, with a cure rate of 66.7% among people on combined therapy compared with a cure rate of 46.7% in the control group.[11]

Vitamin B12 has also been documented to improve the symptoms of Bell's palsy. In one study, three groups of patients were tested: one received methylcobalamin (vitamin B12), one received corticosteroids, and the third received methylcobalamin in combination with corticosteroids. At the end of the study, the patients in both methylcobalamin groups showed greater improvement in their symptoms than those in the corticosteroid group.[12]

Other supplements have attracted attention in Bell's palsy but have not been subjected to rigorous scientific testing. Some people with Bell's palsy report symptom relief from omega-3 fish oils, a natural anti-inflammatory that may work by relieving nerve inflammation.[13]

## Life Extension Suggestions

- **Methylcobalamin:** 5 mg sublingual lozenges. A suggested dose is 40–80 mg daily until symptoms subside.
- **Omega-3 fish oil:** 1400 mg EPA and 1000 mg DHA daily

## REFERENCES

References available at: www.lef.org/dpt5/ch20

# 21

# Benign Prostatic Hyperplasia (BPH)

Benign prostatic hyperplasia or "BPH" is a condition of prostate gland enlargement often leading to bothersome urinary symptoms.[1–5] It primarily affects older men: about 25% of men in their 40s have BPH, but this increases to more than 80% between the ages of 70 and 79. According to 2007 data, BPH is responsible for 1.9 million doctor visits and more than 202 000 trips to the emergency department.[6]

Benign prostatic hyperplasia can cause significant urinary symptoms in men. In fact, more than 50% of men in their 60s and approximately 90% of men over the age of 80 have lower urinary tract obstruction due to prostate enlargement. This causes symptoms such as a weak urinary stream, urinary hesitancy (delay in initiating urination), involuntary cessation of urination, straining to void, and a feeling of incomplete emptying of the bladder. Blockage of the urethra, the "tube" through which urine leaves the body, by the prostate can also affect the bladder. This may result in increased urinary frequency/urgency, need to urinate during the night, bladder pain, painful urination, and/or incontinence.[6]

Sex hormones exert significant influence over BPH development and progression. While many men are aware of a pro-growth role of a testosterone metabolite called DHT (*dihydrotestosterone*) in prostatic hyperplasia, few know that *estrogen* may also contribute to BPH.[7,8] Aging in men is associated with an increase in the activity of an enzyme called aromatase, which converts testosterone into estrogen.[9] Some research suggests increased estrogen levels in prostate tissue may promote hyperplasia.[7,10–14]

This protocol will discuss the underlying causes of BPH and review conventional treatments along with their drawbacks. In addition, we will review several scientifically studied natural therapies that may ease BPH symptoms, as well as a novel medical therapy that may provide relief to BPH sufferers who have failed to respond to conventional therapy.

## PROSTATE FUNCTION AND CAUSES OF BPH

The main function of the prostate is to facilitate male fertility. This is accomplished through the liquid volume of ejaculate, rich in fructose, which functions as a fuel source for sperm, and also contains a protein called prostate-specific antigen (PSA). PSA is believed to help liquefy the ejaculate and promote sperm motility.[15]

The development of BPH is a multifactorial process. As men age, prostate cell growth becomes less well controlled by cell signaling activity. Also, the cells in the prostate become less responsive to signals that induce apoptosis or "programmed cell death." This results in an overabundance of cells in the prostate, also known as prostate hyperplasia.[15]

This breakdown in cellular regulation that occurs with aging allows prostate cells to proliferate and promote the formation of additional tissue. This additional tissue is smooth muscle, and this tends to increase the overall muscle tone of the prostate, which can contribute to blockage of the urinary tract.[15]

**Normal versus Enlarged Prostate**

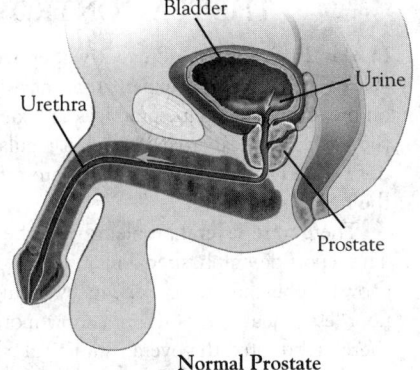

**Normal Prostate**

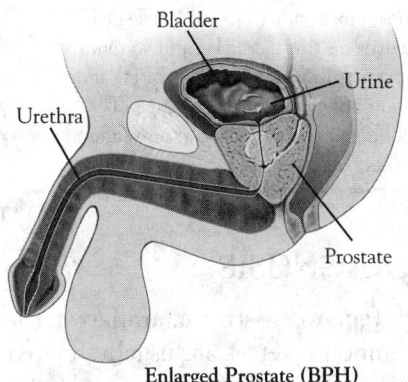

**Enlarged Prostate (BPH)**

Imbalanced hormone levels contribute to BPH. A derivative of testosterone (ie, *dihydrotestosterone* [DHT]) stimulates growth of the prostate. DHT is derived from testosterone via conversion by the enzyme *5α-reductase,* which is an important pharmacologic target for BPH therapies.[16] In addition, high levels of insulin-like growth factors and inflammatory markers (eg, C-reactive protein) can also contribute to BPH.[6,15]

Furthermore, ethnic differences have been reported, such as lower rates of BPH and prostate surgery among Asian men relative to Caucasian men. Furthermore, one study reported higher rates of moderate-to-severe lower urinary tract symptoms among Afro-Caribbean men relative to Caucasian men, whereas other studies have shown similar rates of BPH diagnosis and hospitalization among Afro-Caribbean men and Caucasian men.[15]

## ESTROGEN AND BPH

*Estrogens* appear to contribute to prostate tissue growth and may represent an underappreciated piece of the BPH puzzle.[7,8]

As men age, estrogen (eg, estrone and estradiol) levels appear to increase. Aromatase, an enzyme which converts testosterone into estrogen, also increases with age in men.[9] BPH risk also increases with age and studies have identified high concentrations of estradiol in cells from hyperplastic prostates.[11–13] Further investigations into the action of estrogen receptors in prostate cells led one group of researches to conclude that "*estrogens … may contribute at some level to the etiology of the most prevalent prostatic diseases including … BPH.*"[17]

Therefore, based on these and other findings, Life Extension suggests that aging men strive to maintain estradiol blood levels between 20 and 30 pg/mL for optimal prostatic and overall health.

A potentially useful strategy to help aging men control estradiol levels is to take an aromatase inhibiting drug like anastrazole (Arimidex®). One study showed that men 60 or older with low testosterone levels who took anastrazole for 12 months exhibited a reduction in serum estradiol levels without significant increases in BPH symptoms.[14] However, evidence is inconsistent regarding the efficacy of aromatase inhibitor therapy in BPH, as these drugs can increase DHT levels.[18] Fortunately, there are *5-alpha reductase*-inhibiting drugs like Avodart® and finasteride that can block DHT formation and thus neutralize this factor behind so many cases of prostatic enlargement. Men who have BPH, and whose estradiol levels are above the optimal range of 20–30 pg/mL, are encouraged to discuss use of aromatase inhibiting drugs with their health care provider.

## DIAGNOSIS

Symptoms of BPH (eg, weak stream, urinary hesitance, incomplete emptying, etc.) are usually related to obstruction of the urinary tract. Severity of the symptoms can be measured using the American Urological Association Symptom Index (AUASI), a widely used questionnaire that quantifies the severity of lower urinary tract blockage symptoms.[19] The International Prostate Symptom Score, or IPSS,[20] is another questionnaire often used for quantifying symptoms of BPH in research studies.

The first step in evaluating patients with BPH-related symptoms includes a complete overview of the patient's general medical, neurologic, and urologic history, as well as their fluid and caffeine consumption, to rule out other causes of urinary tract symptoms. Medications should also be reviewed, since diuretics and antihistamine drugs may cause urinary symptoms.[6]

Next, a digital rectal exam (DRE) is performed and PSA levels are measured.[6] PSA levels are important because while BPH is associated with some elevation of PSA levels, a very high or quickly rising PSA level can be a sign of prostate cancer. For example, in one study, the median PSA value in patients with BPH was 1.8 ng/mL, whereas the median PSA value among patients with prostate cancer was 13.2 ng/mL.[21] Still, PSA levels are not a perfect measure since levels can be normal in men with prostate cancer. Therefore, the DRE (digital rectal exam) is also important, both to help rule out prostate cancer (a smooth prostate accessible by rectal examination is less likely to be cancerous than one with hard nodules and irregularities) and to determine the size of the prostate. Classification of the prostate size as "normal," "big," and "very big" can help determine therapy. Measuring urine flow rates using uroflowmetry can also help assess bladder outflow obstruction.[15] Additional testing, such as free PSA and PSA velocity, also helps to differentiate BPH from prostate cancer. For more information see the *Life Extension Magazine* article titled "Life Saving Advances in Prostate Cancer Testing."

## THE PSA CONTROVERSY

In May 2012, the U.S. Preventive Services Task Force (USPSTF), a panel of experts that makes recommendations on preventive medicine practices to health care providers in the United States, proclaimed that regular PSA testing should not be used as a screening tool for prostate cancer based on their analysis.[22]

There were several problems with the USPSTF analysis. The report de-emphasized a major, high-quality trial that showed robust mortality benefits by including trials of poor/lesser quality that did not show mortality benefits, and therefore, diluted the overall statistical effect of the higher-quality trial on mortality (benefit) in their analysis.

This high-quality trial was the European Randomized Study of Screening for Prostate Cancer (ERSPC), which randomized 182 000 men aged 50–74 from seven countries to PSA testing every 2–7 years (depending on center and year) or to usual care. A prespecified analysis of 162 243 men aged 55–69 found that screening was associated with 20% reduction in prostate cancer-specific mortality, for an estimated 1410 men undergoing PSA screening.[23]

After publication of the main ERSPC results, a participating center (Göteborg, Sweden) reported their results separately. This site determined that a PSA screening threshold of 2.5–3.0 µg/L every 2 years in 20 000 men aged 50–64 years decreased risk for prostate cancer-specific mortality by 44% after a median of 14 years.[24]

Poor-quality trials included by the USPSTF in their analysis statistically diluted the beneficial effect observed in the higher-quality ERSPC trial in their overall assessment. Several lesser/poor-quality trials found no difference between screening-invited and control groups in prostate cancer-specific mortality risk.[25,26] Major methodologic flaws in these trials included failure to adequately control for randomization and/or poor allocation blinding, poor attempts to capture lost data points, and so on. One trial even used an exorbitantly high PSA cut-point—10 µg/L—as a screening threshold.[25]

Life Extension advocates the use of PSA screening to prevent prostate cancer deaths, with an important caveat—PSA results should be tracked and monitored over time (ie, PSA velocity) with less emphasis being placed on individual test results. Life Extension issues a cautionary advisory whenever PSA levels exceed 1.0 µg/L. A level of, say 1.4, should be closely followed with PSA blood tests every 6–12 months to carefully track any consistent increase indicative of an early stage prostate tumor that may be treatable with lifestyle changes and medications with low side-effect profiles.

Life Extension has examined this issue in detail. For more information, see the *Life Extension Magazine* multipart series titled "The PSA Controversy."

# CONVENTIONAL TREATMENT

Conventional BPH treatments typically depend on the severity of the patient's symptoms. In men with mild or asymptomatic BPH, watchful waiting is appropriate, which includes an annual physical examination and completion of the AUASI.[6]

## Pharmacologic Treatment

Pharmacologic treatment options can be employed for men who have moderate-to-severe (AUASI score ≥ 8) and/or bothersome symptoms after consideration of the risks and benefits.[6] Currently, 4 different classes of medications and/or surgery are used to treat BPH.

**α1-andrenergic receptor blockers.** Increased smooth muscle tone in the prostate is responsible, at least in part, for some of the urinary symptoms associated with BPH.[15] Smooth muscle tone is regulated by α1-adrenergic receptors, which respond to levels of certain hormones in the body. One BPH treatment option includes α1-adrenergic receptor blocker medications, since the α1A subtype of these receptors is thought to be the main regulator of smooth muscle tone in the neck of the bladder and prostate.[27] Treatment with α1-adrenergic receptor blockers is generally considered first-line therapy for symptomatic BPH,[28] even though some of these drugs were initially developed as high blood pressure treatments.[27]

There are many different α1-adrenergic receptor blockers, and the 4 most prescribed—alfuzosin (Uroxatral®), terazosin (Hytrin®, Zyasel®), doxazosin (Cardura®, Carduran®), and tamsulosin (eg, Flomax®)—all effectively increase urinary flow rate and relieve BPH symptoms. However, these medications also have side effects, such as low blood pressure and dizziness, although tamsulosin may have a reduced risk of these side effects.[27] Furthermore, these medications do not prevent BPH progression and are usually only effective for up to 4 years.[28]

**5α-reductase inhibitors.** Medications in the 5-α-reductase inhibitor class block the conversion of testosterone to dihydrotestosterone, helping to shrink the prostate and prevent further growth.

Finasteride (Proscar®, Propecia®) and dutasteride (Avodart®) are two 5α-reductase inhibitors approved by the Food and Drug Administration (FDA). Both medications are capable of reducing prostate size by as much as 25% and can reduce AUASI scores by 4–5 points in men with large prostates.[6] Combining α1-adrenergic receptor blockers with 5α-reductase inhibitors may increase the benefits for men with BPH.[29]

Medications in the 5α-reductase inhibitor class are associated with significant sexual side effects, including decreased libido, impotence, reduced ejaculate volume, and problems with ejaculation.[6,29] In addition, some men experience breast enlargement and tenderness. Although sexual side effects associated with 5α-reductase inhibitors tend to decrease over time,[29] some men experience persistent diminished libido, erectile dysfunction, and depression when using these drugs.[30]

Some important considerations should be taken into account when choosing between finasteride and dutasteride in the management of BPH. First, there are 2 variants (ie, *isoforms*) of the 5α-reductase enzyme: type 1 and type 2; both are present in prostate tissue. However, evidence suggests that the type 1 isoform may be more active in malignant prostate tissue.[31] This is significant because dutasteride inhibits both type 1 and 2 isoforms, whereas finasteride inhibits only type 2. This means that dutasteride may more effectively control growth of cancerous tissue than finasteride. Since several studies suggest the two drugs confer similar benefits and risks in BPH, dutasteride appears to be a better choice as it might also provide some cancer protection.[32–36]

**Antimuscarinics.** Many men with BPH also have an overactive bladder, which can cause symptoms such as urinary urgency and incontinence.[28] Antimuscarinic drugs block muscarinic receptors in the detrusor muscle. This muscle contracts and squeezes the bladder to facilitate urination, and remains relaxed otherwise, allowing the bladder to stretch and fill. Activation of muscarinic receptors stimulates contraction of the detrusor muscle. Pharmacologic blockade of these receptors decreases the incidence of overactive-bladder symptoms of BPH.[6]

Many antimuscarinic drugs have been approved to treat symptoms of overactive bladder, including darifenacin (Enablex®), tolterodine (Detrol®), fesoterodine (Toviaz®), trospium chloride (Sanctura®), oxybutynin (Ditropan®), and solifenacin (Vesicare®).[6] Combining antimuscarinic medications with α-adrenergic blockers can improve BPH symptoms, particularly the number of times patients need to urinate during the day and night as well as episodes of urinary urgency.[37] However, there is insufficient evidence that these medications are effective when used as a single therapy for individuals with predominantly storage problems.[6]

One concern with these medications is that they can cause increased urinary retention, although studies in men with good emptying (post-voiding residual urine volume less than 250 mL) have not identified any adverse effects associated with urinary retention. However, caution should be used in men with incomplete bladder emptying.[37] Common side effects associated with these medications include dry mouth, dry eyes, and constipation.[6]

**Phosphodiesterase-5 inhibitors.** Men with lower urinary tract symptoms sometimes experience erectile dysfunction, which has led some researchers to speculate that the two symptoms may be linked.[38] Phosphodiesterase inhibitors are used to treat erectile dysfunction, but may also relieve lower urinary tract symptoms in men with BPH.[6]

These medications may work via several mechanisms. One postulated mechanism is that phosphodiesterase-5 inhibitors block a signaling pathway that causes smooth muscle contraction. They may also increase levels of nitric oxide, a compound that relaxes smooth muscles in the lower urinary tract. They have also been proposed to decrease hyperactivity of the autonomic nervous system affecting the bladder, prostate, and penis.[39]

A comprehensive review found that phosphodiesterase-5 inhibitors alone effectively treat lower urinary tract symptoms and erectile dysfunction, and that treatment with both phosphodiesterase-5 inhibitors and alpha-blockers leads to a small improvement in flow rates in men with BPH. This class of medication may even be effective in patients without erectile dysfunction.[40] Tadalafil (Cialis®) is the only medication of this class that has been FDA-approved for treating urinary symptoms. It can cause headaches, flushing, indigestion, back pain, and nasal congestion, and may lead to low blood pressure when combined with α1-adrenergic blockers or organic nitrates (eg, nitroglycerin).[6]

## Surgery

BPH can also be treated surgically. The purpose of surgery is to either remove the prostate or reduce its size, thereby relieving the lower urinary tract symptoms.

Two minimally invasive treatments—transurethral needle ablation of the prostate and transurethral microwave thermotherapy—have been developed to treat BPH, although there is some uncertainty regarding which patients will respond well, and more studies need to be done to evaluate the effectiveness of these treatments. More invasive procedures can be used for patients with moderate-to-severe symptoms of BPH, particularly for patients who have not responded to pharmacologic therapy.[41]

*Transurethral prostatectomy (TURP)*, a procedure in which the prostate is endoscopically removed, is the benchmark surgical therapy for BPH.[41] Endoscopic procedures involve insertion of fine surgical and viewing devices directly into the patient's body through small incisions; this type of surgery is less invasive than traditional "open" surgery. However, approximately 14% of men who undergo TURP will become impotent.[42] This procedure can also cause transurethral prostatectomy syndrome, a serious complication in which fluid used to irrigate the surgical area enters the intravascular space. This can result in cardiopulmonary (heart and lung) complications (eg, high or low blood pressure, slow heart rate, irregular heartbeat, respiratory distress, shock), hematologic and renal (blood and kidney) systems (eg, excess ammonia in the blood, electrolyte disturbance, anemia, acute renal failure), and the central nervous system (eg, nausea/vomiting, confusion/restlessness, blindness, twitches/seizures, lethargy/paralysis, dilated/nonreactive pupils, coma), as well as death.[43] Other complications include voiding failure, urinary tract infections, and bleeding during or after surgery.[44]

Men with very large prostates may benefit from an *open prostatectomy*, in which the entire prostate is removed, but this treatment can result in significant blood loss, incontinence, impotency, pain, and longer hospital stays.[41]

*Transurethral laser therapy* is another surgical option that is gaining momentum. This treatment option may reduce the length of stay in the hospital, although more information regarding the safety of this therapy is needed.[41] The adoption of laser-based operations for BPH has led to more cases of BPH being treated surgically.[45]

## INTRAPROSTATIC BOTULINUM TOXIN INJECTIONS—AN EMERGING BPH THERAPY

Botulinum toxin is a bacteria-derived neurotoxin that relaxes muscles by preventing certain neurotransmitter (acetylcholine) signals. Since lower urinary tract symptoms are attributable in part to excessive smooth muscle contraction around the bladder and prostate in men, scientists have hypothesized that injecting botulin toxin directly into the prostate may relax those muscles and relive some urinary symptoms.[46]

In a preliminary trial, 10 men with lower urinary tract symptoms suggestive of BPH received intra-prostatic injections of botulinum toxin. Significant improvements were noted, including a nearly 50% reduction of urinary symptoms assessed by a standardized assessment, a significant reduction in PSA levels and prostate volume, and a 42% reduction in frequency of nighttime urination. The investigators in this study concluded that "[i]ntraprostatic injection of Botulinum-A may be an effective and safe treatment for symptomatic BPH in selected patients whose medical treatment has faced failure and are poor surgical candidates."[47] Another similarly designed study on 10 men with BPH demonstrated similar efficacy: "Intraprostatic [purified botulinum neurotoxin] injection induces prostate shrinkage and is effective in men with BPH."[48] A slightly larger study (34 men with BPH who failed medical treatment) published in September 2012 reported very similar findings.[49]

## DIETARY AND LIFESTYLE CONSIDERATIONS

There are many ways men can reduce their risk of developing urinary symptoms associated with BPH.

### Low Fat Diet

A diet high in fat can increase the risk of developing BPH. A 2008 study found that men who received more than 38% of their calories from fat are nearly one-third more likely to develop BPH than men who received less than 26% of their calories from fat.[50] These findings suggest that lowering one's overall fat intake may help reduce the risk of developing BPH.

### Eating Vegetables

Studies have found that men who eat more vegetables are less likely to develop BPH.[50,51] In particular, vegetables rich in beta-carotene, lutein, and vitamin C are associated with a decreased risk of BPH.[51]

### Weight Loss and Blood Sugar Control

There is a direct relationship between body weight and prostate size. Obese men are more likely to develop symptoms of BPH; greater weight, BMI, and waist circumference are all associated with a higher incidence of BPH. One study found that obese men are 3.5 times as likely to develop BPH as normal weight men. Men with diabetes mellitus are likely to have increased prostate volume, and have a two-fold higher risk of BPH compared to men with normal blood sugar control.[52]

### Exercise

Regular physical exercise decreases the risk of developing BPH. One study found that men who regularly engage in strenuous physical activity as part of their job have a 30–40% lower risk of developing BPH. Even regular walking can reduce one's risk of developing BPH. For example, men who walk 2–3 hours per week have a 25% lower risk of developing BPH.[52]

## TARGETED NUTRITIONAL INTERVENTIONS

Treatment of BPH with plant-derived compounds dates back to the 15th century BC in Egypt and natural therapies comprise approximately 50% of all treatments for BPH in Italy.[53]

### Saw Palmetto

Saw palmetto, also known as *Serenoa repens* (*S. repens*) or *Sabal serrulata* (*S. serrulata*), is the most widely used phytotherapeutic treatment for BPH.[53,54] It has been documented as a treatment for swollen prostate glands since the 1800s.[53] Saw palmetto has been found to be effective in treating the lower urinary tract symptoms of BPH. Evidence suggests that saw palmetto has similar efficacy to finasteride and tamsulosin, two medications used to treat BPH.[55] Saw palmetto extract appears to inhibit the activity of the 5α-reductase enzyme. It may also have anti-inflammatory properties and a tendency to promote apoptosis of prostate cells.[55,56]

A pilot study examining the effects of 320 mg of saw palmetto extract found that this herbal treatment reduced BPH symptoms by over 50% after 8 weeks of treatment.[55] Another study found a combination of saw palmetto and stinging nettle root extract to be as effective as finasteride at treating BPH.[57] However, a review of studies found that saw palmetto was not significantly better than placebo.[58] But differences in methodologic quality of the studies included in this review limit the interpretation of the results.

Saw palmetto has not been reported to cause any significant side effects. A study found no difference in the rate of serious and nonserious symptomatic adverse events between saw palmetto and placebo.[59] Most studies examining the benefits of saw palmetto for BPH have used doses of 320 mg daily.[60] Saw palmetto is rich in phytosterols, including beta-sitosterol, and this may contribute to its therapeutic effects.[61]

## Beta-Sitosterol

Beta-sitosterol belongs to a family of plant-derived compounds chemically similar to cholesterol. These compounds are called *phytosterols*. The impact of human intake of phytosterols has been studied in a variety of contexts, including cardiovascular disease and cancer.[62–66] A beneficial role for phytosterols, and beta-sitosterol in particular, in prostate conditions is supported by a considerable body of research in both laboratory and clinical settings.[67–74]

A comprehensive review of four studies comprising data on 519 men with BPH showed that beta-sitosterol improved urinary symptoms and flow measures.[69] A clinical trial in which men with symptomatic BPH consumed beta-sitosterol or placebo for 6 months, and were then followed for another 12 months, gave men the option to discontinue therapy after 6 months, or continue. Those men who chose to continue taking beta-sitosterol showed stable results on standardized prostate/urinary symptom and quality of life assessments at the 18-month follow-up, while men who chose not to continue therapy experienced a decline in some of the prostate/urinary scores.[75] In another clinical trial, 200 men with symptomatic BPH were randomized to receive either 20 mg of beta-sitosterol 3 times daily or placebo for 6 months. Men who took beta-sitosterol experienced greater improvements on 2 standardized assessments of prostate/urinary symptoms than men who took a placebo. Beta-sitosterol recipients also experienced improvements in peak urine flow rate and residual urinary volume; these parameters were unaffected by the placebo.[74] These results were corroborated in a later study of similar design, but which employed a higher dose of beta-sitosterol (130 mg daily). Men who took beta-sitosterol in this study not only experienced improvements in

standardized prostate/urinary symptom assessments over placebo, but also in quality of life.[73] In a clinical trial on 127 men with BPH, a combination of saw palmetto, beta-sitosterol, vitamin E, and rye flower pollen extract was superior to placebo in improving urinary frequency at night and during the day and also led to more significant improvements on a standardized prostate/urinary symptom assessment.[76]

## Pygeum Africanum

*Pygeum africanum* (*P. africanum*), also known as African plum, is used as a treatment for BPH in Europe.[77] *P. africanum* may prevent the proliferation of cells within the prostate.[77,78] A review of studies examining the effects of African plum on BPH found that it provides moderate relief from urinary symptoms.[60,79] The typical dose used in studies is between 75–200 mg daily.[60]

## Rye Pollen

Rye pollen extract (also called *Secale cereale*) is made by first subjecting the pollen to bacterial degradation, followed by further extraction using organic and water solvents.[77] It is commonly used in Japan, Argentina, and parts of Western Europe.[60] Laboratory studies have shown that the water-soluble portion of the extract inhibits growth of prostate cells.[77] Studies of its efficacy have found that rye pollen extract reduces nighttime urination.[60] One study found that the use of 320 mg of honeybee-collected pollen extract improved urinary flow rate.[80] Another study found that rye pollen extract reduced BPH symptoms, shrank prostate size, and increased urinary flow over the course of 4 years.[81]

## Urtica Dioica ("Stinging Nettle")

Stinging nettle root extracts have shown effectiveness as natural therapeutics for BPH.[82,83] A study found that a combination of saw palmetto and 120 mg of stinging nettle extract was as effective as finasteride in the treatment of BPH; the herbal combination also had fewer side effects than finasteride.[57] Another study showed that stinging nettle alone had beneficial effects in patients with symptomatic BPH.[84] This finding is supported by animal studies showing that stinging nettle extract reduced the size of the prostate, weekly urine output, and PSA levels, perhaps by disrupting prostate cell growth.[83]

## Isoflavones and Lignans

Plant-derived compounds called *isoflavones*, which are abundant in soybeans, and *lignans*, which are abundant in flax and Norway spruce, modulate estrogen signaling in the human body via interaction with estrogen receptors. Thus, these compounds are sometimes classified as *phytoestrogens*. Isoflavones and lignans have been investigated for their anticancer effects, but their ability to affect hormone-responsive tissues appears to influence the prostate.[85]

Evidence suggests that isoflavones may inhibit testosterone-mediated prostate cell growth.[85] These compounds were also shown to block the activity of 5α-reductase, the enzyme that converts testosterone to dihydrotestosterone (DHT), which promotes prostate growth.[86] One study suggested that men with BPH may have lower dietary intake of soy isoflavones than men with healthy prostates, as determined by lower prostate tissue concentrations of *genistein*, a potent isoflavone.[87] Genistein levels may also correlate with the size of the prostate in BPH: men with small-volume BPH have been found to have higher levels of genistein in their prostate tissue than men with large-volume BPH.[88]

Supplementation with soy isoflavones has been found to reduce PSA levels in men with prostate cancer.[85] In addition to preventing prostate cell proliferation, isoflavones may increase programmed cell death (ie, apoptosis) in low-to-moderate grade tumors from prostate cancer patients.[89] Another study found that isoflavones are very well tolerated.[90]

Lignans have also been evaluated as a treatment for BPH, and one study found that a flaxseed lignan extract reduced both BPH symptoms and the grade of lower urinary tract symptoms experienced by some patients.[20]

## Pumpkin Seed Oil

Pumpkin seeds (*Cucurbita pepo*) have been used in folk medicine as a treatment for urinary problems caused by an enlarged prostate.[91] Compounds in pumpkin seeds may interfere with the action of dihydrotestosterone, which stimulates prostate cell growth.[92] Studies in animal models of BPH have found that pumpkin seed oil blocks testosterone-mediated prostate growth.[92,93] Pumpkin seed oil's effects were greater in animal models when the oil was combined with phytosterols.[91]

Similar results have also been found in human studies. For example, one study found that pumpkin seed oil reduced BPH symptoms in Korean men and also improved their urinary flow rate. This study also found that a combination of pumpkin seed oil and saw palmetto reduced PSA levels.[94]

## Lycopene

Lycopene is a carotenoid occurring abundantly in tomatoes. Men with higher lycopene levels in their blood, suggesting greater dietary lycopene consumption, are less likely to develop prostate cancer.[95] One laboratory experiment found that lycopene inhibited the growth of normal human prostate cells.[96] Another study suggested that lycopene supplementation may decrease the growth of prostate cancer.[97]

## Fatty Acids

Healthy fats, such as eicosapentaenoic acid (EPA), docosahexaenoic acid (DHA), and gamma-linolenic acid (GLA), exhibit a wide range of beneficial effects on the human body and may support prostate health.[98]

Flaxseed oil and fish oil are rich sources of essential fatty acids.[99,100] A pilot study found that flaxseed supplementation, combined with a low-fat diet, lowered PSA levels in men who were scheduled to have a repeat prostate biopsy. This special diet also reduced the rate of prostate cell proliferation.[101] Another study found that the essential fatty acids gamma-linolenic acid (GLA) and eicosapentaenoic acid (EPA), and their metabolites, suppressed the activity of 5α-reductase.[102]

## Additional Support

Several other dietary constituents may also be able to protect against BPH, although more studies are needed.

***Boswellia serrata.*** *Boswellia serrata* is an African tree whose bark yields an oily, resinous extract that has been used in traditional medicine.[103] Compounds in Boswellia resin, particularly acetyl-11-keto-β-boswellic acid (AKBA), have potent anti-inflammatory properties.[104] Inflammation plays a role in the development of BPH and is associated with an increase in BPH symptoms.[105,106] Several studies indicate that AKBA may slow growth of prostate cancer cells and induce apoptosis.[107–109] Although studies have yet to formally evaluate the effect on Boswellia in men with BPH, its documented anti-inflammatory and cancer-fighting properties suggest it may deliver some benefits in this population.

**Selenium.**  Selenium is a mineral the body needs in small quantities[110]; however, increased selenium intake may help prevent BPH. A study found that a combination of selenium, lycopene, and saw palmetto was more effective than saw palmetto alone at preventing hormone-dependent prostate growth.[111] Another study found that higher serum levels of selenium were associated with a reduced risk of BPH.[112]

**Garlic.**  Garlic has anti-inflammatory, anticancer, and antioxidant effects, all of which may help prevent the development of BPH and prostate cancer. Although its mechanism of action is not clear, several animal and cell culture studies have suggested that garlic may be beneficial for BPH. In addition, combining garlic with other foods beneficial for the prostate, such as olive oil and tomatoes, may enhance its effects.[113]

**Beta-carotene and vitamin C.** Increased intake of beta-carotene and vitamin C is associated with a decreased risk of having BPH requiring surgical treatment.[114]

## Life Extension Suggestions

- **Saw palmetto extract,** standardized to 85–95% total fatty acids and sterols (272 mg): 320 mg daily
- **Flower pollen extract (Secale cereale):** 252 mg daily
- **Pumpkin seed oil extract,** standardized to 85% total fatty acids (170 mg): 200 mg daily
- **Stinging nettle extract** (root): 240 mg daily
- **Pygeum extract** (bark): 100 mg daily
- **Lycopene:** 10 mg daily
- **Beta-sitosterol:** 180 mg daily
- **Boswellia serrata extract,** standardized to 20% 3-O-acetyl-11-keto-β-boswellic acid (AKBA) (14 mg): 70 mg daily
- **Lignans from Norway spruce and flaxseed:** 20 mg daily

- **Soy isoflavones:** 135 mg (including 28 mg genistein) daily
- **Fish oil** (with olive polyphenols): providing 1400 mg EPA and 1000 mg DHA daily
- **Gamma-linolenic acid (GLA):** 300–600 mg daily
- **Vitamin C:** 1000–2000 mg daily
- **Beta-carotene:** 4500 IU daily
- **Lutein:** 15 mg daily
- **Selenium:** 200–400 mcg daily
- **Garlic extract,** standardized to 10 000 ppm allicin potential (12 mg): 1200–4800 mg daily

In addition, the following *blood tests* may be helpful:

- Male Comprehensive Hormone Panel (includes PSA, total and free testosterone, DHEA-S, DHT, and estradiol). Life Extension recommends that men complete the male comprehensive hormone panel annually to monitor hormone and PSA levels.
- C-reactive protein (CRP)

## REFERENCES

References available at: www.lef.org/dpt5/ch21

# 22

# *Blood Clot Prevention*

You may not know it, but if you are over 50 the greatest threat to your continued existence is the formation of *abnormal* blood clots in your arteries and veins.

The most common form of *heart attack* occurs when a blood clot (thrombus) blocks a coronary artery that feeds your heart muscle. The leading cause of *stroke* occurs when a blood clot occludes, or obstructs, an artery supplying blood to your brain. Formation of vascular blood clots is also a leading cause of death in *cancer* patients because cancer cells create conditions that favor clotting.

While normal blood clots are a natural part of healing, *abnormal* arterial and venous blood clots are a significant cause of death and disability.[1]

The good news is that health-conscious individuals already take a wide variety of nutrients through their diet and supplement program that drastically *reduce* their risk of developing *thrombosis*, which is the medical term for an abnormal vascular blood clot.

Certain individuals, however, have underlying medical conditions that predispose them to developing thrombotic events. These include atherosclerosis, mechanical heart valves, atrial fibrillation, venostasis, blood clotting disorders, and cancer. These individuals must take special precautions to protect against thrombosis.

Conventional medicine offers drugs proven to reduce thrombotic risk via specific mechanisms. These drugs fail, however, to neutralize the broad array of mechanisms that can induce a thrombotic event, which is why a comprehensive thrombosis-prevention program is so critically important to those at high risk.

This protocol first discusses some technical details about thrombosis, the conventional drugs that doctors prescribe, and important blood tests to consider. It then reveals little-known methods of inhibiting a multitude of thrombotic risk factors that mainstream doctors overlook.

Life Extension believes patients succumb to thrombotic events, even when taking powerful anti-coagulation drugs such as warfarin, because their doctors failed to suppress the many *other* underlying risk factors that cause abnormal clots to form inside a blood vessel.

## THE FLAWS OF MAINSTREAM THERAPIES

The most effective means of blood clot management is *prevention*. For high-risk patients, mainstream prophylaxis against thrombosis and its complications often includes powerful anti-clotting medications. These require careful monitoring and inconvenient dietary restrictions.

Conventional medications used to prevent blood clots, such as *warfarin (Coumadin®)*, increase the potential for serious bleeding as well as the risk of mortality from traumatic injuries.[2] Moreover, warfarin may lead to significant long-term side effects, such as increased risk of *atherosclerosis* and *osteoporosis*.

Life Extension has identified a strategy to reduce the detriments of long-term warfarin therapy. Judicious use of *vitamin K2* has been shown in *peer-reviewed studies* to *reduce* the fluctuation in coagulation status associated with warfarin therapy. This notion runs contrary to that of conventional medicine, whose best advice is to totally eliminate vitamin K from the diet during warfarin therapy, an *outdated* guideline that *compromises vascular and skeletal health*.

Next-generation anticoagulant medications that overcome these vascular and skeletal risks are emerging, yet they still lack sufficient data from clinical trials to solidify them as first-line treatments. The most promising of these new drugs is *dabigatran (Pradaxa®)*; however, early trials indicate that dabigatran may be more effective for reducing stroke risk in patients with atrial fibrillation.[3,4]

Life Extension emphasizes that optimal thrombosis risk reduction can never be viewed in isolation, but must encompass a *global strategy*. Measures to reduce the risk of blood clots include reducing chronic inflammation, maintaining healthy body weight, reducing cholesterol, suppressing homocysteine levels, and lowering blood pressure. Additionally, the use of scientifically studied nutrients to target abnormal *platelet aggregation* can intervene in the thrombotic process *before* it causes a life-threatening medical emergency.

## WHAT IS A BLOOD CLOT?

A normal blood clot consists of a "clump" of blood-borne particles that have become "stuck" together inside a blood vessel; this usually occurs at the site of a blood vessel injury and is part of the normal healing process. However, clotting also can occur in areas where blood flow is slow or stagnant, such as in a blood vessel occluded, or obstructed, by atherosclerotic plaque. A blood clot that develops in a blood vessel or the heart and remains there is called a *thrombus*, while a blood clot that has broken loose and floats freely through the circulatory system is called an *embolus*.

Blood clots are made up of:

- **Platelets.** Small fragments of larger cells called *megakaryocytes*, platelets circulate through the blood and carry important substances such as proteins and other cellular signaling molecules. A platelet has a life span of about 7–10 days.
- **Red blood cells.** The most common type of blood cell, red blood cells transport oxygen from the lungs and distribute it to all tissues in the body.
- **White blood cells.** The cells of the immune system, white blood cells originate in the bone marrow as stem cells that differentiate into various types of immune cells.
- **Fibrin.** A web-like proteinaceous gel, fibrin binds the other components of the clot together.

## THROMBOTIC DISEASE

A clot formation can be especially dangerous if it blocks blood flow to organs or tissues. For example, blockage of the coronary arteries (the blood vessels that directly supply oxygen to the heart muscle itself) can result in myocardial infarction (a heart attack), and death of heart muscle tissue.

An unstable thrombus can break away from the vessel wall and cascade freely through the bloodstream. This thrombus can become problematic if it becomes wedged in a blood vessel too small to allow its passage, obstructing blood flow and impairing oxygen delivery to tissue. This blockage is called an embolism. Cerebral embolism is one such example— an embolism in the small arteries of the brain can cause an embolic stroke.

*Arterial thrombosis* is associated with several life-threatening complications. Clots in the veins (*venous thrombosis*) of the legs are relatively common, and pose a significant risk of forming emboli that can travel to the lungs, causing a potentially fatal *pulmonary embolism*.

## COMPLICATIONS OF THROMBOSIS

**Conditions caused by *arterial* thrombosis** (blockage of arteries that carry oxygen-rich blood from the heart to other tissues):

- **Stroke**: Either slow-developing caused by thrombi, or rapid-onset caused by embolism.
- **Transient ischemic attack (TIA)**: A "mini-stroke" without tissue death.
- **Myocardial infarction (heart attack)**: Blockage of the coronary arteries that supply oxygen to the heart muscle.
- **Pulmonary embolism**: Life-threatening blockage of arteries in the lungs, starving the body of oxygen. Some estimates place the incidence of pulmonary embolism at more than 180 000 new cases per year, making it the third most common life-threatening cardiovascular disease in the United States.[5] A blood clot that leads to pulmonary embolism often forms in the legs as deep vein thrombosis (DVT), but can also form in the atrium in those with atrial fibrillation. In about 40% of cases, the origin of the emboli is unknown.[6]
- **Angina pectoris**: Reduction of blood supply to the heart, typically resulting in severe chest pain.

**Conditions caused by *venous* thrombosis** (blockage of veins that carry oxygen-poor blood back to the heart):

- **Deep vein thrombosis (DVT)**: A clot formed in a deep vein, usually in the legs; quite common. Data suggest that the lifetime risk of DVT is about 5%.[7] Unstable clots formed from DVT have the potential to break free and travel to the artery that supplies deoxygenated blood to the lungs, where they can cause a potentially fatal pulmonary embolism. Damage from DVT can also lead to post-thrombotic syndrome, a condition typified by leg pain, heaviness, swelling, or ulceration. More than one-third of women with DVT develop post-thrombotic syndrome.[8]
- **Portal vein thrombosis**: A rare blockage of the vein that carries blood from the abdomen to the liver. Portal vein thrombosis is relatively uncommon and usually associated with liver disease.[9]
- **Renal vein thrombosis**: A blockage of the vein that drains blood from the kidney. This type of thrombosis is relatively uncommon and often associated with trauma to the abdomen.

## RISK FACTORS FOR THROMBOSIS

The risk factors for thrombosis are believed to increase clotting through one or more of these 3 mechanisms: altering or damaging the blood vessel lining (endothelium), impairing or slowing the flow of blood, or promoting a state that favors excess coagulation (hypercoagulation).

### Alteration or Damage to the Blood Vessel Lining (Endothelium)

Alteration of the blood vessel lining (endothelium) produces areas of disturbance that are not necessarily tears, but may nonetheless mimic the physiology of vascular injury, thus encouraging the recruitment of platelets and the clotting process. Selected factors that pose a risk to endothelial cell health follow.

**Abnormal blood lipids.** Abnormal blood lipids, particularly elevated total cholesterol, LDL (low-density lipoprotein) cholesterol, triglycerides, and low HDL (high-density lipoprotein) cholesterol, pose a risk to endothelial cell health. Blood lipid values outside of optimal ranges (see Table 1) are one of the risk factors for *atherosclerosis*, which causes arterial plaques on blood vessel walls. Clots can form on or near the lipid-rich arterial plaques in vessel walls, disrupting blood flow and increasing heart attack or stroke risk. Scientific strategies for cholesterol risk reduction are available in Life Extension's Cholesterol Management protocol.

**Elevated high-sensitivity C-reactive protein (hsCRP).** hsCRP is an indicator of inflammation and blood vessel injury; high levels are predictive of future risk of heart attack or stroke.[10] CRP also exerts several prothrombotic activities, and may be associated with risk of venous thrombosis.[11]

**Hypertension.** Sustained high blood pressure compromises the integrity of the endothelium, and can cause endothelial activation and initiation of clotting.[12] For optimal endothelial protection and blood clot prevention, a target blood pressure of *115/75 mmHg* is suggested. Those with blood pressure higher than the optimal range are encouraged to read Life Extension's High Blood Pressure protocol.

**Elevated glucose.** Elevated blood glucose levels, even those that remain in the lab-normal range, may significantly increase the risk of developing a blood clot. In fact, a clinical study involving patients with coronary artery disease (CAD) found that patients with fasting glucose levels above 88 mg/dL had greater platelet-dependent thrombosis than those with levels below 88 mg/dL. The authors of this study remarked: "The relationship is evident even in the range of blood glucose levels considered normal, indicating that the risk associated with blood glucose may be continuous and graded. These findings suggest that the increased CAD risk associated with elevated blood glucose may be, in part, related to enhanced platelet-mediated thrombogenesis."[13]

Life Extension suggests that fasting glucose levels be kept at *70–85 mg/dL* to limit glucose-induced platelet aggregation and to promote optimal overall health.

**Excess abdominal body fat.** Abdominal obesity, also known as android obesity, consists of excessive deposition of fat tissue around the trunk of the body (eg, the belly). The fatty tissue around the trunk is prone to secrete inflammatory chemicals and cause high blood sugar and hypertension, all factors that pose dire risk to the health of endothelial cells. Maintaining an ideal body weight is critical to reducing thrombosis risk.

**Elevated homocysteine.** Elevated homocysteine has been associated with a 60% increase in venous thrombosis risk for each 5 µmol/L increase in concentration.[14] Homocysteine damages the endothelium, increases endothelial cell and platelet activation, and lowers fibrinolytic (clot breakdown) activity.[15] Life Extension recommends keeping homocysteine levels *below 7-8 µmol/L* for optimal health (Table 1); guidelines for doing so are discussed in the Homocysteine Reduction protocol.

**History of vascular events of disease.** History of stroke, transient ischemic attack, heart attack, or coronary artery disease all indicate a susceptibility to arterial thrombosis and are among the strongest predictors of future thrombotic events.

> **Note:** *In addition to these factors listed above, additional discussion of risk factors that compromise endothelial health (and therefore increase risk for thrombosis) can be found in the* Life Extension Magazine *article titled, "How to Circumvent 17 Independent Heart Attack Risk Factors."*

## Interrupted Blood Flow

Interrupted blood flow stimulates thrombosis by allowing the localized accumulation of circulating platelets and clotting factors and by increasing the probability of clotting reactions. Risk factors include the following.

**Sedentary behavior.** Sedentary behavior, either as inactive lifestyle or due to extended immobilization such as during hospitalization or long-distance travel, is a risk factor for interrupted blood flow.[16] According to the CDC, adults aged 18 years and older should engage in *at least* 2.5 hours of moderate-intensity aerobic exercise each week, and full-body strength training at least twice a week. Even greater health benefits are available through 5 hours of moderate-intensity aerobic exercise each week combined with full-body strength training 2 or more days a week.

**Surgeries of the lower extremities.** Surgeries of lower extremities (hip, knee, ankle) increase thrombosis risk either due to trauma to the veins during surgical manipulation, or immobilization during recovery.[17] Without treatment, the incidence of deep vein thrombosis following total hip or total knee replacement surgery is as high as 40–60%.[18]

**Atrial fibrillation.** Atrial fibrillation, the most common type of abnormal heart rhythm, can lead to blood pooling in the heart and subsequent clot formation in the left atrium, increasing stroke risk 5-fold.[19]

## Hypercoagulation

Hypercoagulable states, sometimes called thrombophilias, are conditions in which the nature or composition of the blood encourages coagulation. Some hypercoagulable states are inherited disorders that increase the activity of clotting factors or reduce the activity of natural anticoagulants. Some of the more common nongenetic hypercoagulable states include the following.

**Thyroid disorders.** Thyroid disorders, which alter the balance of clotting factors and anticoagulants, can increase the risk of thrombosis. Hyperthyroidism (high thyroid function) increases the risk of thrombosis due to disruption of the clotting process, such as increased production of clotting factors, increased thrombin activity, and reduced rate of fibrinolysis (clot breakdown).[20] Hyperthyroidism also can increase blood volume, which can lead to high blood pressure and cardiac arrhythmias, both of which are risk factors for thrombosis.[21] In hyperthyroid patients, the incidence of arterial thrombosis, especially cerebral thrombosis, is 8–10%.[22] Hypothyroidism (low thyroid function) also increases the risk of thrombosis. Hypothyroid patients cannot clear clotting factors from the blood as quickly, have elevated levels of fibrinogen, and have reduced rates of fibrinolysis.[23]

**Elevated plasma fibrinogen.** Elevated plasma fibrinogen, the main coagulation protein, may result from a variety of conditions such as smoking, thyroid disorders, or infection.[24] A comprehensive review of observational studies estimated that a 98 mg/dL reduction in fibrinogen concentration would lead to a relative risk reduction of 80% in coronary heart disease.[24]

**Pregnancy.** Pregnancy shifts the balance of hemostatic factors toward coagulation and enhances the activation of platelets, especially in pre-eclampsia (pregnancy-associated hypertension), which may affect 2–4% of pregnancies.[25]

**Cancer.** Cancer can increase risk of venous thrombosis four- to seven-fold, especially in metastatic cancers or those in which the infiltration of tumors or compression of blood vessels disrupt blood flow.[26] Pancreatic, brain, and gastric cancers especially increase the risk of thrombosis.[26]

Blood clots may be predictive of cancer risk as well. In a case–control study involving nearly 60 000 patients, the likelihood of developing any cancer within 6 months of diagnosis of venous thromboembolism (VTE) was 420% higher than that of the general population.[27] Particularly, cancer of the ovary was more than 700% more likely, while non-Hodgkin's lymphoma and Hodgkin's disease were 500–600% more likely within a year of VTE.

Tumors exert a number of prothrombotic effects on the blood, as does chemotherapy itself.[28] Unfortunately, once cancer has progressed sufficiently to cause a blood clot, it is usually in an advanced stage, and the survival rate of patients diagnosed with cancer within 1 year of VTE is poor.[29]

Alarmingly, the close link between cancer and thrombogenesis appears to be underappreciated by conventional physicians. A small survey of oncologists revealed that 27% believed cancer patients were not at increased risk for clotting.[28] Similarly, another survey found that the majority of oncologists use thromboprophylaxis in cancer patients very rarely, despite the fact that VTE is a leading cause of death in this population.[30]

Additional risk factors include age, female sex, smoking, and obesity; additionally, surgery can increase thrombosis risk.

**Table 1: Recommended Blood Values and Pressure to Reduce Thrombosis Risk**[31]

| Blood Test | Standard Reference Range | Optimal |
|---|---|---|
| Total cholesterol | 100–199 mg/dL | 160–180 mg/dL |
| LDL cholesterol | 0–99 mg/dL | Under 70–100 mg/dL |
| HDL cholesterol | over 39 mg/dL | Over 50–60 mg/dL |
| Fasting triglycerides | 0–149 mg/dL | Under 80 mg/dL |
| Fasting glucose | 65–99 mg/dL | 70–85 mg/dL |
| Homocysteine | 0–15 µmol/L | Under 7–8 µmol/L |
| Fibrinogen | 150–450 mg/dL | 295–369 mg/dL |
| TSH | 0.45–4.5 µIU/mL | 1.0–2.0 µIU/mL |
| CRP | 0–3.0 mg/L | Men: under 0.55 mg/L |
| | | Women: under 1.5 mg/L |
| Blood pressure | Hypertension: over 139/89 mmHg | 115/75 mmHg |

TSH, thyroid-stimulating hormone; LDL, low-density lipoprotein; HDL, high-density lipoprotein; CRP, C-reactive protein; µU/dL, microunits per deciliter; mg/dL, milligrams per deciliter; µmol/L, micromoles per liter; mg/L, milligrams per liter; mmHg: millimeters of mercury.

# BLOOD CLOTTING MECHANISMS

*Hemostasis*, a process that maintains the blood in a free-flowing state and helps stop bleeding during injury, is critical for survival. Blood clotting or *coagulation* is necessary to repair not only large injuries to blood vessels, but also the thousands of microscopic internal tears that happen daily under normal circumstances. Without a proper hemostatic response, the smallest of vessel injuries would lead to fatal hemorrhage (bleeding).

However, if the intricate balance among hemostatic mechanisms is disturbed, the tendency for a clot to become pathologic dramatically increases. The steps below briefly outline key aspects of the clotting process. This list also highlights points at which some drugs and natural compounds can combat derangement of the clotting system and offset thrombosis risk.

Normal blood clotting is a complex process, consisting of the following major phases: (1) *vasoconstriction*, (2) temporary blockage of a break by a *platelet plug*, and (3) blood *coagulation*, or formation of a clot that seals the hole until tissue repair occurs.

Four steps that summarize clot formation and also highlight key areas that pharmaceutical drugs and some natural compounds target in order to impede clotting are discussed in following sections.

1. **Vasoconstriction:** *Endothelial damage* occurs, leading to neurogenic vessel constriction and decreased blood flow near the site of injury. This creates a local environment that favors clotting. Examples of injuries that may initiate the clotting process include rupture of an atherosclerotic plaque and homocysteine-induced endothelial damage.

   a. Damage to the endothelium liberates subendothelial *collagen* and *tissue factor* (factor III), which initiate the *intrinsic* and *extrinsic* clotting pathways, respectively, in the immediate area (details in Secondary Hemostasis section).

   - *Intervention:* Polyphenolic antioxidants, such as *punicalagins* from *pomegranate*, oligomeric procyanidins from *grape seed*, and trans-*resveratrol*, protect endothelial cells against injury and help maintain flexibility of blood vessels.

## Primary Hemostasis

2. **Platelet Adhesion and Activation**

   b. As circulating platelets pass by the site of vessel wall injury, receptors on their surfaces bind to exposed collagen and membrane proteins on activated endothelial cells, causing adhesion of platelets at and around the site of injury. This adhesion is mediated by von Willebrand factor and P-selectin.

   - *Intervention: Curcumin*, a bioactive compound derived from the spice turmeric, acts to suppress P-selectin expression and limits platelet adhesion by this mechanism.[32]

   c. Binding of the surface receptors leads to several molecular events that "activate" the platelets, causing release of *adenosine diphosphate (ADP)* from secretory granules within the platelet.

   - *Intervention:* Bioactive compounds in *garlic* work to suppress platelet granule release.[33]

   d. ADP binds to surface receptors called *P2Y1* and *P2Y12* on nearby platelets. This binding causes increased synthesis of *thromboxane A2* (TXA2) via conversion of the inflammatory omega-6 fatty acid *arachidonic acid* by the enzyme *cyclooxygenase-1 (COX-1)*.

   - *Intervention: Aspirin* inhibits the activity of COX-1 for the entire lifespan of the platelet, which is about 7–10 days.

   - *Intervention:* The omega-3 fatty acids *EPA* and *DHA* from *fish oil* counteract the synthesis of TXA2 by competing with omega-6 fatty acids as substrates for the COX enzyme.[34]

   e. Binding of P2Y1 and P2Y12 by ADP also causes the expression of another surface receptor, called *glycoprotein IIb/IIIa (GPIIb/IIIa)*. The significance of GPIIb/IIIa will be examined in the "platelet aggregation" section.

   - *Intervention:* The "blood thinning" drugs *Plavix®* (*clopidogrel*) and Ticlid® (ticlopidine) block ADP from binding to the P2Y12 receptor for the entire lifespan of the platelet, which is about 7–10 days. The drug Effient® (prasugrel) is a reversible inhibitor of P2Y12; its effects last about 5–9 days.

   f. Additional factors, including newly synthesized thromboxane A2, increase expression of the surface receptor GPIIb/IIIa as well.

   g. This process of platelet activation is self-propagating among platelets that happen to be near each other, and near the site of blood vessel wall injury.

3. **Platelet Aggregation**

   h. Following the activation of platelets, the expressed GPIIb/IIIa surface receptors bind a circulating protein called *fibrinogen*, which comprises about 4% of total blood protein.

- *Intervention:* The B-vitamin *niacin*, which is well known for being heart healthy, exerts some of its cardioprotective actions by lowering plasma fibrinogen levels, thus attenuating the proclivity for platelets to aggregate and form a clot.[35,36]

- *Intervention:* *Vitamin C* also appears to lower plasma fibrinogen levels, as suggested by some clinical trials and epidemiologic studies.[37,38]

i. Fibrinogen can bind GPIIb/IIIa receptors on adjacent platelets, linking them together in a process known as *platelet aggregation*.

- *Intervention:* *Tomato bioactives* inhibit the function of GPIIb/IIIa, thereby blocking platelets from (1) binding circulating fibrinogen, and (2) binding to each other.[39]

j. In a matter of *seconds* after vessel wall damage, platelet adhesion, activation, and aggregation culminate in the formation of a *platelet plug*, temporarily sealing off the injury.

## Secondary Hemostasis

4. **Coagulation:** Simultaneously to the formation of the platelet plug, *tissue factor* and *collagen* that were liberated upon vessel wall injury initiate 2 separate but related *coagulation pathways*.

k. Collagen interacts with *factor XII* to initiate the *intrinsic coagulation cascade*.

l. Concurrently, tissue factor interacts with *factor VII* to initiate the *extrinsic coagulation cascade*.

m. Both the intrinsic and extrinsic pathways converge into the *common pathway*, which, through a complex series of interactions, converts *prothrombin* (factor II) into an enzyme called *thrombin*. This process is locally self-propagating via a process known as *amplification*, in which thrombin feeds back into the intrinsic pathway to drive further conversion of prothrombin.

n. Thrombin then acts upon circulating fibrinogen to convert it into *fibrin*.

- *Intervention:* *Heparin* is a naturally occurring anticoagulant that enhances the action of *antithrombin*, a glycoprotein that suppresses the ability of thrombin to convert fibrinogen to fibrin, thus slowing the coagulation process. Heparin is helpful when administered

during medical emergencies involving atrial fibrillation and deep-vein thrombosis (DVT).

Rarely, some individuals develop a condition called heparin-induced thrombocytopenia (HIT) after receiving heparin. This is due to genetic differences in the immune response of these patients. Patients who develop HIT can be treated more safely with a new heparin alternative called fondaparinux.

- *Intervention:* *Dabigatran (Pradaxa®)* is a *direct thrombin inhibitor*. Dabigatran directly inhibits the action of thrombin, preventing it from converting fibrinogen to fibrin.

o. Individual fibrin particles associate with one another to form polymers, which themselves associate into a web-like gel that traps circulating white blood cells, red blood cells, and additional platelets.

- The widely used anticoagulant drug *warfarin (Coumadin®)* interferes in several steps along both the intrinsic and extrinsic coagulation pathways by inhibiting the activity of *vitamin K*.

- Vitamin K is required for activation of a number of factors (*II, VII, IX, X, protein C, and protein S*) involved in coagulation. Vitamin K facilitates *carboxylation reactions* required to activate these coagulation factors. After vitamin K successfully "carboxylates" a coagulation factor, it transitions to a less active form. In order for vitamin K to carboxylate additional coagulation factors, it must be *recycled* into its active form; this is accomplished by an enzyme called *vitamin K epoxide reductase*. Warfarin inhibits vitamin K epoxide reductase and impairs the recycling of vitamin K, thus slowing activation of factors required for coagulation.

p. The fibrin gel and included blood cells and platelets then fuse with the platelet plug to reinforce the injury and completely seal it off until tissue repair can begin.

## Fibrinolysis

After clotting and coagulation is complete (usually between 3–6 minutes after injury), the trapped platelets within the clot begin to retract. This causes the clot to shrink, and pulls the edges of the injury closer together, squeezing out any excess clotting factors. Then the process of vessel repair can begin. Once healing is complete, the unneeded clot is dissolved and removed by a process called *fibrinolysis*.

Fibrinolysis involves the cleavage ("cutting") of the fibrin mesh by the enzyme *plasmin* to release the trapped blood cells and platelets, allowing the clot to "dissolve."

q. An enzyme called *tissue plasminogen activator (TPA)* converts the inactive protein *plasminogen* into the active *plasmin*, which then cleaves the fibrin web.

  • *Intervention:* In some medical emergencies involving an embolic event, such as embolic stroke, pulmonary embolism, and myocardial infarction (heart attack), *TPA* can be administered intravenously to dissolve the blood clot and improve clinical outcome. TPA should be administered as soon as possible after an embolic event for maximum benefit.

  • *Intervention: Nattokinase*, a fermentation product from soy, is an enzyme that has been shown to increase the fibrinolytic activity of plasma in laboratory studies.[40]

## REGULATION OF COAGULATION DURING HEALTHY CONDITIONS

In the absence of a blood vessel injury, platelet activation and coagulation cascades must be kept in check or the risk for thrombotic disease increases. Several factors disable blood clotting when it is not needed:

**Protein C and protein S.** These proteins associate with another protein called *thrombomodulin*, produced by healthy endothelial cells, to form a complex that blocks the activation of factor V and hence the conversion of prothrombin to thrombin.

  • Interestingly, the action of the protein C/S complex depends on *vitamin K*. Therefore, vitamin K is not only critical for optimal coagulation when blood vessel injury has occurred, but it is also needed to limit the formation of thrombi during healthy conditions. *Adequate vitamin K intake is paramount in ensuring hemostatic balance at all times.*

**Antithrombin.** The liver produces this small protein and it is found in relatively high concentrations in blood plasma. It inhibits the activation of several coagulation factors and remains constantly active to limit thrombotic disease risk. When clotting is needed to repair an injury, the coagulation cascade initiated by the exposure of collagen and tissue factor overwhelms antithrombin and clotting is able to proceed.

As previously noted, the anticoagulant heparin dramatically increases antithrombin activity. When administered intravenously, heparin can cause the anticoagulatory tendency of antithrombin to inhibit the clotting cascade, thus slowing clot formation.

**Tissue factor pathway inhibitor.** This polypeptide blunts the ability of the extrinsic pathway to activate thrombin under healthy conditions. However, as with antithrombin, vessel wall injury overwhelms this coagulation inhibitor by liberating large amounts of tissue factor, allowing coagulation to proceed.

**Plasmin.** Healthy endothelial cells secrete *tissue plasminogen activator*, an enzyme that converts *plasminogen* into plasmin. Plasmin breaks down the fibrin web that holds clots together. Therefore, plasmin is constantly contributing to *fibrinolysis* by breaking down any clots that are not needed.

**Prostacyclin (PGI2).** This fatty acid derivative is produced by healthy endothelial cells and by platelets via the action of the *cyclooxygenase-2* enzyme. PGI2 counteracts the action of thromboxane A2, thereby suppressing platelet activation during healthy conditions. PGI2 also acts as a *vasodilator* to help maintain free blood flow during healthy conditions.

**Nitric oxide (NO).** NO is a signaling molecule involved in a vast array of biochemical functions. During healthy conditions, the endothelium produces NO via an enzyme called *endothelial nitric oxide synthase (eNOS)*. eNOS contributes to vasodilation, thus reducing the risk of thrombosis.

## CONVENTIONAL THERAPIES FOR BLOOD CLOTS AND THROMBOSIS RISK REDUCTION

Two classes of pharmaceutical drugs reduce the risk of thrombosis and its complications, *antiplatelet drugs* and *anticoagulants*. Reserved for emergency situations, a third class called *thrombolytics/fibrinolytics* break up blood clots and limit tissue damage; tissue plasminogen activator (Activase®) and urokinase (Abbokinase) are 2 examples.

### Antiplatelet Drugs

Antiplatelet drugs inhibit platelet activation and aggregation, an early step in the clotting process. Several classes of antiplatelet drugs inhibit platelet aggregation and activation at a different point in platelet metabolism.

The most common antiplatelet drug is *aspirin*. It inhibits the enzyme *cyclooxygenase* (COX), which is responsible for synthesizing thromboxane A2.[41] Thromboxane A2 is a factor secreted by platelets to recruit other platelets to the site of injury during the initial stages of the clotting process. The cyclooxygenase inhibitory effect of aspirin is permanent for the life of the platelet (about 7–10 days). Aspirin has been shown effective in preventing complications of several disorders, including hypertension, heart attack, and stroke.[42] Importantly, ibuprofen can attenuate the COX inhibitory action of aspirin in platelets; therefore, if low-dose aspirin is being taken preventively, ibuprofen for pain relief should be taken at least 8 hours apart from aspirin to ensure maximum effectiveness.

Interestingly, aspirin also inhibits the COX enzyme in endothelial cells, but does not exert an irreversible action here. Unlike platelets, endothelial cells contain DNA and RNA and can therefore synthesize new COX enzymes even after aspirin has bound to existing COX enzymes. This dichotomy of aspirin action in platelets versus endothelial cells is significant because the COX enzyme is critical for the synthesis of the antiplatelet, vasodilatory compound *prostacyclin* (PGI2). Healthy endothelial cells secrete prostacyclin to counteract the action of TXA2 and ensure that a clot does not continue to grow and occlude the blood vessel.

The difference between endothelial cell biology and platelet biology also explains why low-dose aspirin is cardioprotective. Low-dose aspirin does not impair endothelial secretion of prostacyclin because these cells quickly synthesize new COX enzymes and overwhelm low concentrations of aspirin. However, platelets do not synthesize new COX so that aspirin, even in low concentrations, suppresses platelet-derived TXA2 until new platelets arise from the bone marrow. Thus, low-dose aspirin is effective for reducing the risk of pathologic clot formation while maintaining optimal endothelial function.

Aspirin's inhibition of COX also helps explain its potential in cancer reduction as observed in several studies.[43–46] Several types of cancers (particularly breast, prostate, and colon) overproduce the proinflammatory enzyme COX-2, which appears to play a role in increasing the proliferation of mutated cells, tumor formation, tumor invasion, and metastasis.[47,48] COX-2 may also contribute to drug resistance in some cancers, and its expression in cancer has been correlated with a poor prognosis.[48]

A second group of commonly prescribed antiplatelet drugs, including clopidogrel (Plavix™), prasugrel (Effient™), and ticagrelor (Brilinta™), are characterized by their ability to bind to the surface of platelets and block the P2Y12 ADP receptor, inhibiting the platelet from becoming activated. Clopidogrel, the most widely prescribed antiplatelet, is more effective than aspirin in its ability to reduce the aggregation of platelets.[49] Clopidogrel activity can be enhanced when combined with aspirin,[50] and this combination has been tested for its efficacy, safety, and cost effectiveness for a variety of clinical applications. In some cases, the combination represents a significant improvement over clopidogrel alone.

In patients with acute coronary syndrome, the CURE trial (Clopidogrel in Unstable angina to prevent Recurrent Events) demonstrated that combining clopidogrel and aspirin resulted in a 20% reduction in risk of cardiovascular death, heart attack, or stroke, as compared to aspirin alone after a one year follow up. However, those in the clopidogrel group had an increased risk of bleeding.[51] Similar results were also observed in the COMMIT trial (Clopidogrel and Metoprolol in Myocardial Infarction Trial), in which short-term combination therapy (4 weeks) lowered risk of heart attack, stroke, and death in patients with a previous heart attack (9% risk reduction).[52] In both trials the benefits of the combination therapy outweighed the moderate cost increase in treatment. However, for other applications, such as prevention of heart attack in high-risk individuals without established cardiovascular disease, or in the treatment of stable coronary artery disease, treatment with aspirin alone has proven safer and more cost effective than combination therapy.[53,54]

Other clinically important oral antiplatelets include dipyridamole (Persatine™) and cilostazol (Pletal™), which are platelet phosphodiesterase inhibitors. These drugs are used less frequently as large-scale clinical trials have not proved them to be more effective than aspirin and Plavix®.

## Anticoagulants

Anticoagulants inhibit the transformation of fibrinogen into fibrin, one of the last steps in the clotting process that stabilizes a thrombus.

Warfarin has a lengthy list of interactions that can increase the risk of bleeding (*hemorrhage*). More than 205 pharmaceutical, nutritional, and herbal medicine interactions have been identified for warfarin. Some medications that can potentially interact with warfarin include aspirin, cimetidine, lovastatin, thyroid hormones, and oral contraceptives. Foods and nutritional ingredients such as onions, garlic, ginger, CoQ10, fatty fish, and vitamin E have been reported to increase the risk of bleeding when combined with warfarin; however, many of these reports are anecdotal and may not represent significant concerns.[55,56] Many nutritional ingredients that "thin the blood" do so by different mechanisms than warfarin. For instance, rather than interfering with coagulation they may inhibit platelet aggregation, a different step in blood clot formation.

While it is prudent to follow a conservative approach regarding warfarin's potential for interaction with a variety of pharmaceutical and nutritional agents, being overly cautious may cause potential cardiovascular health benefits to go unrealized.

In fact, warfarin combined with conventional antiplatelet drugs has been studied already in patients at high risk for thrombosis.[57] Additional evidence suggests warfarin can be combined safely with antiplatelet nutrients, such as garlic,[58] as long as one takes these nutrients responsibly. The most important considerations for individuals who wish to take this approach are monitoring and awareness; patients must work closely with their health care practitioner and undergo regular blood testing to measure coagulant activity (see Testing Clotting Function section).

Two other oral anticoagulants have been approved recently in the United States for use under very specific circumstances: *rivaroxaban (Xarelto™)*, an inhibitor of the clotting factor Xa as a prophylaxis against clotting after orthopedic surgery; and *dabigatran (Pradaxa™)*, an inhibitor of thrombin, for stroke prevention in patients with atrial fibrillation.[1]

Both of these newer therapies may have significant benefits over warfarin and related anticoagulants that interfere with vitamin K metabolism. First, they both inhibit clotting factors that do not depend on vitamin K, so they are less sensitive to dietary fluctuations of vitamin K intake. In trials, neither dabigatran nor rivaroxaban exhibited major interactions with other foods or medications.[59] Unlike warfarin, these medications do not need regular blood test monitoring of coagulant status or repeat dosage adjustment.[60] In clinical trials, both treatments were at least as effective as warfarin for reducing stroke risk in patients with atrial fibrillation, and preventing/treating deep vein thrombosis, with a reduced risk of bleeding.[61–63]

Of these 2 drugs, dabigatran appears more promising. For example, in a major hard-endpoint study of Pradaxa® (dabigatran) versus warfarin (the RE-LY trial), Pradaxa® was superior for anticoagulant efficacy at 150 mg 2 times a day with similar major bleeding risk as warfarin treatment (when patients maintained their INR 2.0–3.0).

The INR (international normalization ratio) is a test that evaluates the clotting tendency of blood. A normal INR reading is 0.8–1.2, but in patients predisposed to abnormal vascular blood clotting (such as those with mechanical heart valves or atrial fibrillation), physicians seek to boost INR to 2.0–3.0, which reduces clotting propensity. Increasing INR to this higher level (2.0–3.0) also increases bleeding risk. When Pradaxa® was used at a lower dose of 110 mg 2 times daily, it showed similar efficacy to warfarin but with reduced major bleeding risk. The *advantages* of Pradaxa® versus warfarin include:

- Rapid onset of action.
- Predictable, consistent anticoagulant effects.
- Low potential for drug–drug interaction.
- No requirement for anticoagulant blood test monitoring.

- Preliminary efficacy and safety advantages versus warfarin based on initial head-to-head, hard-endpoint data.

*Disadvantages* of Pradaxa® versus warfarin include:

- No antidote for reversal of over anti-coagulation effect. When too much warfarin is given and the patient's INR indicates they are at risk for a major bleed (or are pathologically bleeding), vitamin K can be injected to immediately reverse warfarin's anticoagulant effect. If too much Pradaxa® is taken, there is no immediate antidote.

- No long-term safety data on Pradaxa® (the case with virtually all newly approved drugs).

- More expensive than warfarin.

Overall, preliminary results suggest benefit (versus warfarin), but larger/longer studies must be conducted before definitive conclusions can be drawn. Some data hints that dabigatran may work best in combination with aspirin due to paradoxical platelet-activating effects associated with dabigatran.[4] A recent comprehensive review of pooled data from 7 clinical trials involving over 30 000 subjects found that dabigatran users were statistically 33% more likely to suffer a heart attack or acute coronary syndrome than users of warfarin, enoxaparin (Lovenox®), or placebo.[64] The investigators concluded that "[t]he overall benefit and risk balance of dabigatran use appears to be favorable in patients with [atrial fibrillation] because of reduction in ischemic stroke. However, the cardiac risk of dabigatran should be investigated further, especially if it is used in populations at high risk of [heart attack] or [acute coronary syndrome]."

## VITAMIN K AND WARFARIN

Besides its dualistic role in coagulation (recall that the coagulation factors II, VII, IX, and X are vitamin K-dependent, but so are the antithrombotic factors protein C and S), vitamin K is central to bone and vascular health as well. Just as several coagulation factors must undergo vitamin K-dependent carboxylation before they become active, a number of proteins involved in bone formation and stability require this same activation; warfarin can disable these proteins too, leading to compromised bone integrity. Moreover, a protein in blood vessels, *matrix GLA protein*, works to keep blood vessels flexible by inhibiting calcification of vascular cells (eg, "hardening" of the arteries). Matrix GLA protein must also be carboxylated by vitamin K to function properly; thus, vitamin K epoxide reductase inhibition can compromise vascular elasticity.

Tragically, there is poor appreciation within mainstream medicine for enhanced risk of conditions associated with vitamin K antagonist treatment, including vascular calcification,[65] lower bone mineral density,[66] and osteoporotic fracture.[67]

Many conventional physicians have been reluctant to supplement a warfarin regimen with low-dose vitamin K in order to stabilize coagulation time and guard against long-term detriment associated with vitamin K-antagonist therapy. Peer-reviewed scientific literature indicates that this strategy can decrease dangerous fluctuations in coagulant status during warfarin treatment (as measured by wide variations in prothrombin time [PT] standardized for the international normalized ratio [INR]).[68,69]

There are several potential reasons for fluctuating INR values during warfarin treatment, including genetic polymorphisms in vitamin K-related genes, interactions with other drugs, and dietary vitamin K intake.[70] Unstable anticoagulation has been associated with diets low in vitamin K,[68] and a strong association between variations in INR and highly variable vitamin K intake exist.[69] Consistent intake of a low dose of vitamin K, with appropriate adjustment of warfarin dosage, has been shown in several studies to stabilize INR values. This is likely due to maintenance of constant body stores of the vitamin and minimizing the effects of dietary fluctuations.[71]

In a small, open-label crossover study, 9 patients (average age 50 years) with a history of unstable INR received 500 mcg/day of vitamin K for 8 weeks. In 5 of the 9 patients, variability in INR decreased (as measured by the reduction in viability between INR measurements at several time points) and achieved a therapeutic range within an average of 14 days. On average, warfarin doses were increased by 50% to achieve a stable INR value during the vitamin K supplementation.[72]

The amount of time that INR stays within a therapeutic range (called the TTR) is another measurement of INR variability. On average, patients on coumarin anticoagulant therapy only maintain their INR within the therapeutic range 50–60% of the time, despite careful monitoring.[73] Three studies have shown that combination therapy of vitamin K and coumarin anticoagulants can significantly increase TTR, especially in patients with unstable coagulation control. A small study[74] compared 2 groups of 35 patients on warfarin therapy with fluctuating INR values receiving 150 mg vitamin K1 or a placebo daily for 6 months. Variability in the test group decreased at the end of the study compared to the control group, and the amount of time patients maintained their INR in the therapeutic range increased by 13%.

In a second study, 2 groups of 100 patients on a coumarin anticoagulant were assigned to receive either 100 mcg vitamin K1 or placebo. Unlike previous studies, however, this study was not limited to patients with unstable control of anticoagulation. Compared to the control group, patients receiving vitamin K showed a 3.6% increase in TTR.[75]

A larger study of 400 patients from 2 anticoagulation clinics were randomized to receive a placebo or 100, 150, or 200 mcg of vitamin K once daily with their coumarin anticoagulant for a period between 6 and 12 months. Although this study also was not limited to patients with a history of unstable INR, the results showed that doses of 100 or 150 mcg increased the amount of time patients had an INR within the therapeutic range (by 2.1% and 2.7%, respectively), compared to the control group. Moreover, these patients had twice the chance of maintaining their INR within the therapeutic range for extended periods of time.[76]

Vitamin K supplementation in those taking warfarin should be conducted under careful supervision by a health care practitioner.

*Heparin* is a natural anticoagulant that stimulates the activity of antithrombin III and prevents the assembly of fibrinogen molecules into fibrin. Several heparin derivatives, including low-molecular-weight heparin, unfractionated heparin, and fondaparinux (a synthetic heparin derivative) are also clinically important. Heparin and its derivatives are given by injection.[1]

Other potential therapies currently being investigated make use of thrombolytic (clot-dissolving) agents. These include: the co-administration of a clot-dissolving thrombolytic drug and an anticoagulant (warfarin) for deep vein thrombosis treatment; directly infusing the thrombolytic drug *tissue plasminogen activator* (tPA) into clots in the brain (through a minimally invasive surgical technique) or clots in the leg (by injection)[77,78]; and the administration of red blood cells coated with tPA to patients, which increases the lifetime of the drug and reduces the likelihood that it will cause excess bleeding.[79]

## TESTING CLOTTING FUNCTION

Several different lab tests assess clotting function. The appropriateness of each test depends on several variables (ie, which type of "blood-thinning" medication the person is taking, if the person has any genetic predispositions to clotting dysfunction, etc.). A health care practitioner should help determine the test most appropriate in each situation.

**Clot-based assays** test the time it takes for a sample of blood plasma to clot. They are used to test the function of the latter stages of clotting (fibrin formation). Different types of clot-based assays exist to test for deficiencies in different parts of the coagulation cascade. (Recall that there are three "pathways" involved in secondary hemostasis: intrinsic, extrinsic, and common pathways.)

- **Prothrombin time (PT test or PT/INR)** measures the time (in seconds) it takes for a blood sample to clot after the addition of a platelet activator inhibitor and a clotting factor (tissue factor). The PT test is most often used to monitor coagulation status during *warfarin therapy*. This test is useful for assessing factor VII activity.

  Due to variation in laboratory methodology, the results of this test are reported as the international normalized ratio (INR), which can correct for this variability. Conditions that affect coagulation (like vitamin K deficiency or warfarin use) prolong clotting time, while those that affect platelet activity (like taking aspirin) have no effect on the test.

  A target INR range of 2.0–3.0 is typically recommended for individuals being treated with anticoagulant medication.

  Because the PT test does *not* reveal *antiplatelet* activity, patients on combination warfarin/antiplatelet therapy with either antiplatelet drugs and/or antiplatelet nutrients should undergo regular *bleeding time tests* and PT tests. By using these two tests in concert, a balanced program of conventional anticoagulant therapy plus antiplatelet drugs and/or antiplatelet nutrients can be uniquely tailored to an individual.

- **Activated partial thromboplastin time (aPTT)** is a related test that measures clotting in response to various clotting factors; specifically, the aPPT test does *not* measure factor VII activity (ie, this test focuses on the intrinsic pathway). This test is typically used to measure the efficacy of *heparin* on clotting (heparin prolongs the aPTT time) but other anticoagulants can increase aPTT clotting time as well.

**Platelet function assays** test the ability of platelets to become activated or aggregate, which occurs in the initial stages of the clotting process. They are less sensitive to the effects of coagulation factors. In other words, platelet function assays test primary hemostasis, while coagulation assays test secondary hemostasis.

- **The bleeding time test** is a simple test in which blood pressure is maintained by use of a blood pressure cuff while small cuts or "pricks" are made on the fingertip or lower arm. The time for bleeding to stop (a measurement of platelet plug formation) is measured. A normal result is 1–9 minutes, depending on which method is used.
- **Light transmittance aggregometry (LTA)** is a standard technique in which platelet-rich plasma is exposed to an aggregating agent (like collagen or ADP), and the clumping of platelets is measured by their ability to block the transmission of light. This technique can be used to monitor the efficacy of antiplatelet drugs, or can detect genetic platelet defects such as von Willebrand disease.
- **The platelet function analyzer (PFA)** is a relatively new instrument that measures the effect of an aggregating agent (collagen, ADP, or others) on platelet aggregation in conditions simulating arterial blood flow. As platelets flow through the instrument, they are forced through a small opening (simulating a vessel tear), and the time for a thrombus to form over the opening (called closure time) is reported. Some local labs typically offer this test, and those interested in having the PFA test should discuss it with their physicians.

**Platelet count** determines whether blood platelets fall within a healthy range (about 150 000–400 000 platelets per microliter), although it does not determine whether the platelets are functioning properly.[80,81]

# DIETARY APPROACHES TO REDUCE THROMBOSIS RISK

The successful nutritional approach to reduce thrombosis risk does not depend solely on a set of "antithrombotic nutrients." Rather, Life Extension supports a multifactorial approach that includes nutrition and lifestyle interventions to reduce the risk of thrombosis. These include abnormal blood lipids, chronic inflammation, hypertension, elevated plasma homocysteine, and obesity.

## Reducing Platelet Activation and Aggregation

Platelet activation and aggregation occurs via a complex, multifactorial process. Several natural ingredients can target varying steps involved in clot formation, and a diversified regimen can provide multiple defenses against aberrant clotting.

**Olive.** Olive (*Olea europaea*) has a history of use against high blood pressure, atherosclerosis, and diabetes.[82] The leaves contain the active iridoid compounds oleuropein and oleacein,[83] which are thought to be responsible for its blood pressure-lowering and cholesterol-lowering properties demonstrated in recent human trials.[84]

In laboratory tests, olive leaf extract also demonstrated antiplatelet activity in blood isolated from healthy male volunteers.[85] High-oleuropein extracts from olive tree wood also inhibit aggregation of human platelets in laboratory tests, especially those from type II diabetic patients.[86] Hydroxytyrosol and hydroxytyrol acetate, two metabolites of oleuropein that are found in olive fruit and oil, have well-established anti-inflammatory and antiplatelet activities in laboratory tests and in animal models.[87]

Phenolic-rich olive oil preparations have demonstrated decreases in the production of proinflammatory and prothrombotic factors in human studies as well.[88,89] Hydroxytyrosol acetate inhibits platelet aggregation with an efficacy similar to aspirin in vitro using whole-blood samples from healthy volunteers.[90] Hydroxytyrosol-rich extracts (25 mg/day) for 4 days reduced production of the prothrombotic factor thromboxane A2 in a pilot trial of five diabetic adults.[91] High-fat diets rich in olive oil lowered the plasma levels of several clotting factors in a larger study of 20 healthy young adults.[92]

**Tea.** Tea consumption has established protective effects on cardiovascular health; reductions in risk of coronary heart disease and stroke from tea consumption have been confirmed through the analyses of several population studies.[93] Purified green tea polyphenols, such as EGCG, increase clotting time in rats and reduce platelet aggregation in isolated human platelets.[94]

Human trials of tea consumption and thrombosis risk have had mixed results. While short-term consumption (2 weeks) of green tea showed no measurable effect of platelet activity,[95] longer-term studies showed modest improvements in platelet function.[96] The most promising results have been observed in a randomized, blinded trial of tea consumption; 6 weeks of black tea consumption (4 cups/day) in 37 healthy volunteers significantly reduced platelet activation, as measured by the presence of platelet aggregates.[97] Tea catechins and the flavonoid quercetin have demonstrated synergistic reductions in platelet adhesion, activation, and aggregation in vitro.[98]

**Quercetin.** Quercetin has demonstrated success inhibiting platelet aggregation. Single doses of quercetin glucosides, the naturally occurring form of quercetin (150 or 300 mg), from food sources and higher quality dietary supplements were able to significantly inhibit collagen-induced platelet aggregation in one small human study.[99] However, long-term supplementation with 1 g/day of quercetin aglycone (the form typically found in lower-quality dietary supplements) for 28 days had no significant effect on platelet aggregation in healthy human volunteers.[100] It should be noted that the plasma concentrations of quercetin in the former study (successful) were significantly higher than in the latter at the time of aggregation measurements, suggesting that quercetin glucosides are absorbed more efficiently than quercetin aglycone. Quercetin from food sources (onions) have shown positive trends on platelet aggregation.[101]

**Salvia.** Salvia is a diverse genus of plants encompassing hundreds of species, many with ornamental, culinary, or medicinal importance. *Salvia miltiorrhiza* (red sage or danshen) is one of the most versatile Chinese herbal drugs, used for hundreds of years in the treatment of cardiovascular diseases,[102] and still widely used as standard thrombolytic treatment in Chinese hospitals.[103] Salvianolic acids A and B, water-soluble polyphenols from *S. miltiorrhiza* root, are responsible for its observed antiplatelet activity in animal models[104] and in blood samples from healthy human volunteers.[105]

The seeds of *Salvia hispanica* (chia) are rich in protein and the omega-3 fatty acid α-linolenic acid. In a small study of 27 patients with type II diabetes, whole chia seed (15 g/1000 kcal of intake) for 12 weeks showed significant reductions in plasma fibrinogen and the platelet adhesion protein von Willebrand factor (vWF). Small reductions in additional cardiovascular risk factors (systolic blood pressure and high-sensitivity, C-reactive protein) were also observed.[106]

**Resveratrol.** Resveratrol has several effects on blood platelets as determined in vitro (using human platelets) and in animal models, including inhibition of platelet adhesion and aggregation, reduction in secretion of clotting factors from platelets, and inhibition of cyclooxygenase, the proinflammatory enzyme involved in platelet activation.[107,108] Plasma resveratrol from consumption of red or white wine increases the release of nitric oxide from platelets in healthy volunteers, inhibiting their activation.[109] In an experimental study, resveratrol was able to suppress the detrimental effects of homocysteine on platelet aggregation and free radical generation.[110]

**Grape seed extract.** Grape seed extract contains oligomeric procyanidins that support cardiovascular

health through vasodilation and an increase in nitric oxide production.[111] They have significantly reduced blood pressure in human trials.[112] Grape seed extract also exhibits antithrombotic activity in animals[113] and in platelets isolated from healthy human volunteers.[114] This may be related to an anti-inflammatory effect.[115]

In a small, 8-week study of 17 postmenopausal women taking 400 mg/day of flavonoid-rich grape seed extract, a significant (23%) lengthening of clotting time compared to the control was observed on day 1 of the study. (Increased clotting time indicates reduced platelet activation and aggregation.) After 8 weeks, the difference in clotting time was not as significant, but trended higher in the test group.[116] Similar short-term reductions in platelet activity also were observed in a study of 23 male smokers.[117] When combined with grape skin polyphenols, grape seed extracts demonstrated better antiplatelet properties than either extract alone in animal models as well as human platelets.[118]

**Tomatoes.** Tomatoes contain several nutrients with established protective effects on the cardiovascular system. Lycopene has demonstrated hypotensive activity in humans,[119] and several human trials indicate a cholesterol-lowering effect.[120] One mechanism by which lycopene may limit platelet aggregation is by activating cyclic-GMP, a signaling molecule involved in vessel dilation.

Tomatoes also exert potent antiplatelet activity in laboratory tests.[121] The antithrombotic compounds of tomato are small molecules found within its water-soluble fractions, which are also high in soluble sugar content. Removal of these sugars increases the concentration of tomato actives and stimulates their inhibition of platelet aggregation by up to 50 times.[122]

Two studies examined the effects of these standardized tomato extracts on platelet function in healthy human volunteers. High-dose (18 g, equivalent to six whole tomatoes) and low-dose (equivalent to two tomatoes) standardized tomato extracts both exhibited significant reductions in platelet aggregation up to 6 hours after ingestion.[122,123] Standardized bioactives from tomato suppress platelet adhesion and aggregation by reversibly inhibiting P-selectin and GPIIb/IIIa, two receptors necessary for clot formation.[122,123]

**Pomegranate.** Pomegranate contains several bioactive antioxidant polyphenols, including the unique tannins *punicaligins*. Pomegranate juice consumption has been associated with significant decreases in blood pressure in hypertensive subjects[124,125] and decreases in LDL cholesterol oxidation.[126] Pomegranate juice polyphenols also function as vasodilators by supporting endothelial function, and as inhibitors of angiotensin-converting enzyme, an enzyme associated with high blood pressure. Two weeks of pomegranate juice consumption (50 mL/day) reduced platelet aggregation by 11% in a small study of 13 healthy individuals.[127] In a human clinical trial, pomegranate juice consumption was shown to prolong clotting time as little as 6 hours after consumption.[128]

**Garlic.** Garlic's (*Allium sativum*) promotion of cardiovascular health has been substantiated by several human trials, particularly its blood pressure-lowering activity[129] and its ability to induce favorable blood lipid profiles.[130] In cell models, garlic extracts inhibit platelet aggregation by reducing ion signaling involved in platelet activation, and by increasing synthesis of c-GMP, a vasodilator. Garlic bioactives also promote endothelial nitric oxide release and enhance fibrinolysis.[131,132] Moreover, garlic inhibits the COX-1 and COX-2 enzymes, which suppresses TXA2 levels.[133]

The antithrombotic activity of garlic has also been the subject of several human trials in both healthy subjects and patients with cardiovascular disease, using aged extracts,[134] water extracts,[135] or garlic oil.[136] Garlic demonstrated reductions in platelet aggregation in each of the studies.

**Fish oil.** Fish oil is a source of omega-3 fatty acids, eicosapentaenoic acid (EPA), and docosahexaenoic acid (DHA), which are essential for several metabolic processes. Studies of tens of thousands of moderate- and high-risk cardiovascular disease patients demonstrated the ability of fish oil to reduce plasma triglycerides, blood pressure, and the risk of cardiovascular mortality.[137] Several human studies observed the antithrombotic activities of fish oil,[138] due in part to its ability to reduce the production of the platelet aggregator thromboxane A2, a metabolite of the inflammatory omega-6 fatty acid arachidonic acid.

Fish oil consumption decreases platelet activation[139] and aggregation[140] and plasma fibrinogen levels.[141] In type 2 diabetic patients, the pooled data from 3 human trials of 159 participants demonstrated a reduction in plasma fibrinogen by 32 mg/dL, and platelet aggregation by more than 10%.[142]

**Capsaicinoids.** Capsaicinoids (capsaicin and dihydrocapsaicin) are the major pungent constituents of chili peppers from the genus *Capsicum*. Regular intake of chili peppers delays oxidation of serum lipids, and lowers and improves insulin and glucose profiles following a meal, both of which contribute to reducing

the risk of cardiovascular disease.[143] In animal models, capsaicin reduces platelet aggregation.[144] An early study attributed the reduced plasma fibrinogen and increased fibrinolytic activity of native Thai individuals, compared to Americans living in Thailand, to the amounts of capsaicin in their diets.[145] In laboratory tests, both capsaicin and dihydrocapsaicin reduced platelet aggregation and reduced the activity of clotting proteins in blood samples from 6 healthy patients.[146]

**Ginger.** Ginger has been shown to inhibit platelet aggregation and to decrease platelet thromboxane production in laboratory tests.[147] Both raw and powdered preparations reduced platelet aggregation in small human trials.[148] Five grams per day of fresh ginger for 7 days inhibited thromboxane production in 7 healthy volunteers,[149] while two additional studies (a single dose of 2.5 g dried powder in 10 healthy volunteers and 10 g dried powder per day for 3 months in 30 patients with coronary artery disease) demonstrated inhibition of platelet aggregation.[150,151] Doses lower than 2.5 g had no effect in human trials.[152]

**Curcumin.** Curcumin has a variety of protective roles in cardiovascular health, reducing oxidative stress, inflammation, and the proliferation of vascular smooth muscle cells and monocytes (immune cells that contribute to atherosclerosis in the presence of oxidized LDL cholesterol). Human trials revealed the effects of curcumin on reducing lipid peroxidation[153,154] and plasma fibrinogen,[155] both factors in the progression of atherosclerosis.[156] Another mechanism by which curcumin inhibits platelet aggregation is through dampening expression of *P-selectin*, an adhesion molecule expressed on both activated endothelial cells and platelets that mediates aggregation between these 2 cell types.[32] P-selectin also recruits leukocytes to the forming thrombus.

In eight subjects with abnormally high plasma fibrinogen, 20 mg of curcumin for 15 days reduced fibrinogen levels by nearly 50%.[155] Experiments using human platelets or whole blood have demonstrated curcumin's ability to inhibit platelet aggregation.[157]

## Suppressing Fibrinogen Levels

**Niacin/nicotinic acid.** Niacin/nicotinic acid (vitamin B3) is an essential nutrient with important effects throughout human metabolism. At dosages substantially above the Recommended Dietary Intake (RDI), niacin reduces risk factors for cardiovascular disease, and reduces cardiovascular events and mortality.[158] Some of this risk reduction is due to niacin's ability to significantly raise HDL cholesterol by up to 35%,[159] and reduce the amount of small, low-density lipoprotein (LDL) particles, a risk factor for atherosclerosis.[160]

Niacin also lowers plasma fibrinogen levels, a risk factor for cardiovascular disease. In the multicenter *Arterial Disease Multiple Intervention Trial* (ADMIT), patients with peripheral arterial disease (PAD) who were randomized to niacin (initially 100 mg a day, raised to 3000 mg/day over the 12-month study) saw an average reduction of fibrinogen by 48 mg/dL (~13.5%), as well as a reduction in prothrombin time, a measure of blood clotting.[35] Similar reductions in plasma fibrinogen (–54 mg/dL, ~15%) were observed in a 6-week study of men with elevated triglycerides.[36]

**Vitamin C.**   Vitamin C may suppress fibrinogen levels, as suggested by some association studies. A study involving more than 3200 men in the United Kingdom found those with the higher plasma levels of vitamin C also had lower levels of fibrinogen and superior endothelial function.[38] Likewise, a study of 96 aging men and women found that an increase of dietary vitamin C of 60 mg daily, or the equivalent of about one orange, was associated with a reduction in fibrinogen that was estimated to cause a 10% reduction in risk of ischemic heart disease.[37]

In an animal model, vitamin C was shown to reduce levels of von Willebrand factor and fibrinogen, suggesting inhibition of platelet adhesion and aggregation. Moreover, vitamin C was able to reduce blood pressure in this study.[161]

An experimental study found that incubation of fibrinogen molecules with vitamin C in vitro caused functional changes to fibrinogen, which may be associated with an impaired capacity for binding the surface of platelets.[162]

## Promoting Fibrinolysis (Clot Breakdown)

**Nattokinase.**   Nattokinase is a fibrinolytic enzyme (an enzyme that breaks down fibrin clots) found in natto, a soy fermented by the bacteria *Bacillus subtillis*. The bacteria produce the enzyme—nattokinase is not a metabolite of soy. In laboratory tests it reduces platelet aggregation and blood viscosity,[163] and enhances the fibrinolytic activity of plasma in animal models.[40]

At a dose of 4000 fibrinolysis units (FUs) per day, nattokinase has been shown to reduce circulating fibrinogen and clotting factors (which are independent risk factors for cardiovascular disease) in patients undergoing dialysis or with cardiovascular disease, and in healthy volunteers.[164] It was also able to reduce the frequency of deep vein thrombosis in 94 high-risk individuals on extended airline flights when combined with *pine bark extract*, or pycnogenol.[165] Nattokinase

also has been shown to reduce blood pressure in hypertensive individuals, which may be attributed to its ability to lower blood viscosity.[166]

**Ethanol.**   Ethanol (drinking alcohol) in low doses reduces thrombotic risk by modifying platelet function and reducing platelet aggregation. As little as a half glass of red wine daily provides enough ethanol to reduce thrombotic risk. However, higher doses of ethanol increase the risk for clotting substantially.[167] All types of ethanol consumed in moderation (two drinks or less daily for men and one drink or less daily for women) should reduce thrombotic risk, but red wine also provides beneficial polyphenols such as quercetin.

## Life Extension Suggestions

Life Extension's suggestions for blood clot prophylaxis rely upon a multifactorial approach that optimizes benefit and minimizes the risk of serious complications from thrombosis. This involves regular blood testing to assess biomarkers in the blood known to be associated with endothelial dysfunction and a hypercoagulable state, such as homocysteine, blood lipids (eg, cholesterol, triglycerides), C-reactive protein, and thyroid hormone. Also recommended is direct measurement of the tendency for blood hypercoagulability, such as prothrombin time (PT), activated partial thromboplastin time (aPTT), platelet count, and fibrinogen level. Reduction of thrombosis risk also involves making nutritional and lifestyle choices consistent with the most current research on arterial and venous thrombosis risk reduction.

It should be noted that the majority of the natural ingredients below interact with *platelets* to modulate the clotting process. Therefore, tests that measure secondary hemostasis, such as PT and aPTT, *cannot* be used as benchmarks to assess the impact that these supplements have on your clotting parameters. Instead, the bleeding time test should be used to assess how "thin" your blood is as a result of your supplementation regimen.

### Reducing Platelet Activation and Aggregation
• **Green tea,** standardized extract: 725–1450 mg daily
• **Quercetin** (providing quercetin glycosides): 500–1000 mg daily
• *Trans*-**resveratrol**: 250–500 mg daily
• **Grape extract** (seed and skin): 150 mg daily
• **Lycopene**: 15 mg daily

- **Pomegranate,** standardized to 30% punicalagins: 500 mg daily
- **Garlic** (aged garlic extract): 1200–2400 mg daily
- **Fish oil** (with olive polyphenols): 1400 mg EPA and 1000 mg DHA daily
- **Flax seed oil:** 1000–3000 mg daily (optional if fish oil is taken)
- **Olive leaf,** standardized extract: 250–1000 mg daily (optional if olive polyphenols are obtained in fish oil or possibly other sources such as high dietary sources of olive oil)
- **Black tea,** standardized extract: 350 mg daily
- **Capsaicin** (from cayenne), supplying 40 000–100 000 heat units (HUs): per label instructions
- **Ginger,** standardized extract: 150–450 mg daily
- **Curcumin** (as highly absorbed BCM-95®): 400–800 mg daily

### Suppressing Fibrinogen Levels
- **Niacin:** 500–2500 mg daily
- **Vitamin C:** 1000–2000 mg daily

### Promoting Fibrinolysis (Clot Breakdown)
- **Soy natto extract:** (supplying 2000 fibrinolytic units [FUs] of nattokinase): 100–200 mg daily

- **Ethanol** (drinking alcohol): Up to two servings daily for men and one serving daily for women

In addition, the following blood testing resources may be helpful:

- Chemistry Panel/CBC
- C-reactive protein (CRP)
- Thyroid stimulating hormone (TSH)
- Homocysteine
- Fibrinogen
- International Normalized Ratio (INR)

### REFERENCES

References available at: www.lef.org/dpt5/ch22

**Table 1** shows the standard reference ranges and optimal levels recommended by the Life Extension Foundation® for blood parameters associated with risk of thrombosis or its complications.

# 23

# *Blood Disorders (Anemia, Leukopenia, and Thrombocytopenia)*

Like any part of the body, blood can be afflicted with diseases and disorders that can compromise your health. Disorders of the blood range from mild, with no symptoms, to life-threatening medical emergencies.

Most of the blood consists of plasma. Plasma is mostly water and contains dissolved salts and proteins, as well as hormones, electrolytes, fats, sugars, minerals, and vitamins. Other components of blood follow:

- **Red blood cells.** Red blood cells are responsible for carrying oxygen from the lungs to all other cells in the body, and transporting carbon dioxide back to the lungs. Red blood cells are produced in the bone marrow. Each red blood cell has a life cycle of about 120 days, at which point they wear out and are destroyed in the spleen. Red blood cells are able to transport oxygen because of hemoglobin, an iron-containing molecule that binds to oxygen. About 90% of each red blood cell is hemoglobin, and each molecule of hemoglobin can carry 4 molecules of oxygen.[1]

- **White blood cells.** White blood cells are the backbone of the immune system. They fight infection by engulfing invading organisms or abnormal cells. There are 5 basic kinds of white blood cells: neutrophils, monocytes, lymphocytes, eosinophils, and basophils. Neutrophils are the most common form of white blood cell and are responsible for fighting infection.

- **Platelets.** Platelets are responsible for blood clotting. They circulate constantly in the bloodstream. In the event of an injury, platelets gather (aggregate) at the injured site and begin a chemical reaction that results in a blood clot. Abnormal platelet function may result in increased bleeding or the formation of dangerous blood clots where they do not belong, which can cause a heart attack or stroke.

This protocol reviews 3 blood disorders—anemia (low red blood cells), leukopenia (low white blood cells), and thrombocytopenia (low platelets). The protocol addresses how these disorders are diagnosed, conventionally treated, and how to support healthy red blood cells, white blood cells, and platelets with nutrition.

## ANEMIA

Anemia is a common blood disorder characterized by a decrease in the amount of red blood cells, or a decrease in the capacity of red blood cells to transport oxygen. This results in a lack of oxygen reaching the body's cells and tissues. Referred to as the "hidden hunger" by the World Health Organization, anemia poses significant health risks worldwide. It affects 2–15% of people in the United States.[2] Women are about twice as likely to be anemic as men. This is especially true of premenopausal women; 4–8% of premenopausal women have iron deficiency anemia.[2,3]

Anemia is associated with poor health outcomes. In patients who have had a heart attack, anemia sharply increases mortality,[4] and is a strong predictor of overall mortality in the elderly. Over a 5-year period, anemic people aged 70–79, 80–89, and 90–99 were 28%, 34%, and 48%, respectively, more likely to die than people of the same ages who were not anemic. Stroke is commonly associated with anemia.[5]

### Symptoms of Anemia

Anemia is associated with the following symptoms[2]:

- Weakness and fatigue
- Irritability
- Shortness of breath
- Headaches
- Sore tongue and bleeding gums
- Pallor
- Nausea and loss of appetite
- Faintness and dizziness
- Confusion and dementia
- Increased heart rate
- Heart failure (in severe cases)

### Classifications of Anemia

Depending on its cause, anemia is generally classified in 3 ways: excessive bleeding, decreased red blood cell production, or increased red blood cell destruction.

**Excessive bleeding.** This form of anemia occurs when a person loses too much blood, either because of an injury (acute anemia) or chronic disease. When the body loses a large amount of blood, it reacts by pulling water from surrounding tissues into blood vessels to maintain a healthy blood pressure. This dilutes the blood, lowering the proportion of red blood cells.

Excessive bleeding can result in very serious anemia, depending on the nature of the injury. Acute anemia that involves the rapid loss of great volumes of blood can result in heart attack or stroke.[6] However, anemia related to chronic conditions, such as recurrent nosebleeds or ulcers in the stomach, develops more slowly and may not be as obvious. This type of anemia sometimes occurs as a result of cancer, especially colon cancer.

Chronic blood loss can cause a deficiency in iron. Iron deficiency anemia is the most common form of anemia,[7,8] affecting about 2 billion people worldwide.[9] It results in decreased red blood cell production. Because it can take several months to deplete the body's supply of iron, it might take a long time for symptoms to develop. Iron deficiency anemia caused by blood loss is one of the most common forms of anemia in the United States.[6] In women, this condition is frequently related to excessively heavy menstrual bleeding; in men, it is often related to gastrointestinal bleeding.

**Decreased red blood cell production.** Red blood cells are manufactured in the bone marrow. This process relies on various nutrients, including iron, vitamin B12, and folic acid, as well as smaller amounts of vitamin C, riboflavin, and copper. Also, the production of red blood cells is stimulated by a hormone called erythropoietin. Deficiencies in any of these nutrients or in erythropoietin can result in anemia. Other forms of anemia include:

- **Pernicious anemia (vitamin B12 deficiency).** It is estimated that 300 000–3 million people in the United States have a vitamin B12 (cobalamin) deficiency.[10] Vitamin B12 deficiency is rarely related to a dietary deficiency. Rather, vitamin B12 relies on intrinsic factor (a protein generated by cells in the stomach) to be bound to vitamin B12 and then absorbed in the ileum (the last segment of the small intestine). People who lack intrinsic factor cannot use available vitamin B12, meaning that anemia can develop even if large amounts of vitamin B12 are consumed. Besides a lack of intrinsic factor, pernicious anemia can be caused by Crohn's disease, stomach surgery, or a strict vegetarian diet. Breast-fed infants of vegan mothers are particularly at risk of vitamin B12 deficiency.

- **Folic acid deficiency anemia.** Folic acid is abundant in green leafy vegetables. Because many people in industrialized countries do not eat enough vegetables, folic acid deficiency is more common than pernicious anemia. Folate deficiency is found in malnourished individuals (especially alcoholics), infants who are fed only cow milk, pregnant women, and adults over age 60. It can also be caused by diseases that affect absorption in the small intestine, including Crohn's disease.

- **Anemia of chronic disease.** Anemia is associated with various chronic diseases and conditions, including infections, inflammatory diseases, and cancers that affect the ability of the body to produce red blood cells.[11,12] Diseases or conditions that are associated with anemia include cancer,[13,14] HIV/AIDS,[15] and testosterone deficiency.[16,17] In patients with cancer or HIV/AIDS, anemia is associated with increased mortality.[18,19] Testosterone deficiency can cause anemia because the hormone helps stimulate kidneys and bone marrow to produce erythropoietin and stem cells. Symptoms of testosterone deficiency include decreased libido, impotence, infertility, fatigue, and decreased muscle mass and strength.[20]

Additionally, aplastic anemia is a rare form of anemia that occurs when bone marrow fails to produce all 3 types of blood cells: red blood cells, white blood cells, and platelets. Causes of aplastic anemia include autoimmune diseases, viruses, or chemicals (eg, benzene or pesticides) (see the Metabolic Detoxification protocol for more information). Symptoms include frequent infections (white blood cells are reduced), fatigue (red blood cells are reduced), and bleeding (platelets are reduced).

**Increased red blood cell destruction.** If the rate of red blood destruction is more rapid than the creation of new red blood cells, hemolytic anemia occurs. This form of anemia is less common than the other two. Hemolytic anemia can result from infection, certain drugs, autoimmune disorders (in which the body attacks and destroys its own red blood cells), and inherited disorders (eg, sickle cell anemia or thalassemia).

Additionally, an enlarged spleen can result in anemia. The spleen is responsible for destroying old red blood cells; an enlarged spleen can increase the rate of red blood cell destruction beyond the body's ability to manufacture new red blood cells.

Sickle cell anemia is the most common inherited blood disorder in the United States, affecting 1 in 500 African Americans and 1 in 2000 Hispanics of Caribbean or South or Central American descent.[21] In this disease, the red blood cells are abnormally shaped (resembling boomerangs), and their blood-carrying capacity is reduced. These cells are fragile and break up as they travel through blood vessels, resulting in a reduced red blood cell count.

Thalassemia occurs when there is an imbalance in the production of one of the amino acid chains that make up hemoglobin. Many people with thalassemia also have mild anemia.

Autoimmune disorders can cause anemia if the body identifies red blood cells as invader pathogens and attacks them. In most people, the cause of autoimmune anemia is unknown.[6]

## Diagnosing Anemia

Anemia is typically diagnosed with a complete blood count (CBC) test. Anemia is defined as a decreased number of red blood cells, decreased quantity of hemoglobin, or lowered hematocrit (the ratio of red blood cells to whole blood). The following table shows the reference ranges for these measurements.

### Reference Ranges for Blood Indicators

| Indicator | Men | Women |
|---|---|---|
| Red blood cell count | 4.10–5.60 ($\times10^6$/µL) | 3.80–5.10 ($\times10^6$/µL) |
| Hemoglobin | 12.5–17.0 (g/dL) | 11.5–15.0 (g/dL) |
| Hematocrit | 36–50% | 34–44% |

If initial blood tests analyzing hemoglobin, red blood cell count, or hematocrit indicate anemia, additional testing should be done to determine the cause of anemia.[11] Additional tests may include the following:

**Stool tests.** If a person has symptoms of anemia and noticed bleeding, a physician may test for the presence of blood in the stool, which can indicate chronic bleeding that would cause anemia.

**Iron deficiency tests.** Iron deficiency is best diagnosed by blood testing.[22] Additionally, physicians may test for levels of transferrin (a protein that carries iron) or ferritin (a protein that stores iron).

**Other tests.** Laboratory tests for vitamin B12 anemia are usually based on low serum vitamin B12 levels or elevated serum methylmalonic acid and homocysteine levels.[23] Similarly, folic acid levels can be measured to detect a folic acid deficiency.

## Managing Anemia

Management of anemia depends on the cause. If anemia is caused by chronic bleeding, for example, the goal is to stop the bleeding; the anemia may then resolve on its own. For instance, in patients with HIV/AIDS, anemia can be treated by temporarily suspending treatment with the antiretroviral drugs used to attack the virus. In extreme cases of acute blood loss, a transfusion may be necessary to raise the red blood cell count.

In some cases, anemia is treated by prescribing erythropoietin, a hormone that stimulates red blood cell production. Erythropoietin is a very expensive drug that is sometimes used to treat severe anemia caused by chemotherapy, certain anti-HIV drugs, testosterone deficiency, or chronic kidney failure. Erythropoietin, taken along with iron, may help reduce the need for a red blood cell transfusion. It is particularly important to supplement erythropoietin with iron because erythropoietin causes the iron to be utilized to form new red blood cells. A poor result may occur if an iron supplement is not prescribed concurrently with erythropoietin.

If the anemia is caused by a genetic disorder (such as sickle cell anemia), blood transfusions may be used to raise the red blood cell count while other drugs are prescribed to treat the genetic disorder itself.

## Nutritional Support

Some forms of anemia respond well to nutritional therapy, including anemia caused by iron deficiency or folic acid deficiency.

**Iron.** In the United States, dietary iron deficiency is rare because of a diet high in iron-rich foods such as red meat, beans, egg yolks, whole-grain products, nuts, seafood, iron-fortified cereals, dark green leafy vegetables, and dried fruit. However, some people in the United States have a higher need for iron, including children, pregnant or menstruating women, strict vegetarians, and long-distance runners.

Oral iron supplements are available to treat iron deficiency anemia. However, gastrointestinal malabsorption syndromes may require the intramuscular or intravenous injection of iron dextran (Imferon) by a physician. Iron protein succinate (sold as a drug in Germany) may be the most effective oral treatment of iron deficiency anemia. This form of iron has been evaluated in multicenter clinical trials to determine efficacy and tolerability.[24]

The following effects were seen in anemic adults after only 60 days:

- 23% increase in percentage of red blood cells (hematocrit)
- 30% increase in blood oxygen-carrying capacity (hemoglobin)
- 6% increase in total number of red blood cells

One new and novel approach to iron supplementation is the use of ferritin (a protein involved in the storage of iron and found naturally in foods like beans). Newer studies have shown that ferritin supplementation may be able to boost iron levels without the side effects associated with iron supplementation.[25] In one study, a ferritin complex was shown to be effective in children who had anemia caused by hemodialysis.[26]

**Vitamin C.** Research indicates that vitamin C (ascorbic acid) promotes the absorption of iron, while preventing its oxidation.[27,28] Along with enhancing iron's absorption in the digestive tract, vitamin C influences production of erythrocytes (red blood cells).[29]

**Folic acid.** The recommended daily requirement of folate is difficult to obtain from food sources alone. Symptoms of folic acid deficiency may include diarrhea and other gastrointestinal problems. Because supplementation with folic acid can mask a vitamin B12 deficiency, folic acid and vitamin B12 should be taken together.

Anemia caused by folic acid deficiency normally responds quickly to oral folic acid and vitamin B12 supplementation. Anticonvulsants, antituberculosis drugs, alcohol, and oral contraceptives have been associated with low serum levels of folate.[30]

**Vitamin B12.** In pernicious anemia, the body lacks intrinsic factor, which is needed to carry vitamin B12 from the digestive tract into the bloodstream. This condition often affects the gastrointestinal tract and the nervous system, with symptoms ranging from weakness to vertigo and angina. Vitamin B12 is available as a supplement in multiple forms, including cyanocobalamin and methylcobalamin. The conventional treatment for pernicious anemia is an intramuscular injection of cyanocobalamin, often followed by lifelong supplementation with vitamin B12.

One study, however, showed that subjects given 1500 mcg daily of oral methylcobalamin for 1–3 months experienced prompt correction of their anemia, with recovery of neurological disturbances observed after 1 month and recovery of hemoglobin and serum concentrations within 2 months. These results imply that orally administered methylcobalamin may be as effective as traditional vitamin B12 injections for treatment of pernicious anemia.[31] If, however, red blood cell levels fail to respond to treatment with methylcobalamin, conventional treatment should be sought.

**Copper, zinc, and selenium.** Trace minerals can be an adjunctive nutritional therapy to reduce the effect of anemia on normal red blood cell function. Copper, zinc, and selenium are used in biochemical processes such as cellular utilization of oxygen, DNA and RNA reproduction, maintenance of cell membrane integrity, and sequestration of free radicals.[32]

**L-carnitine.** Patients with anemia caused by end-stage renal disease respond to therapy with L-carnitine. In one study, L-carnitine therapy increased hematocrit and decreased resistance to erythropoietin.[33]

**Testosterone therapy.** Anemia associated with testosterone deficiency can be addressed with testosterone replacement therapy, which can stimulate erythropoietin production and increase hematocrit. Potential candidates for testosterone replacement therapy should undergo a complete physical examination including a complete medical history and hormone profile.[34] Dehydroepiandrosterone (DHEA) is available as a supplement and can be metabolized into other sex hormones, including testosterone.

## LEUKOPENIA

Leukopenia is a diminished white blood cell count. When white blood cells are depleted, the immune system is weakened and people are at increased risk of infection. Leukopenia is associated with diseases, medications, and genetic deficiencies.

The most common form of leukopenia is neutropenia, or a reduced number of neutrophils. Neutrophils comprise about 45–75% of the total white blood cell count. They are responsible for fighting bacterial, fungal, viral, and parasitic infections. Neutropenia is associated with increased risk of bacterial infections. If not treated during the early infectious phase, and if the level of neutrophils falls too low, septic shock and death often occur.[35,36]

Diagnosis is dependent on a CBC test. Neutropenia in adults is defined as an absolute neutrophil count of less than 500 cells per microliter (μL) of blood. However, even a neutrophil count of less than 1000 cells/μL can raise the risk of infection.[6]

Treatment of neutropenia depends on the cause and any associated conditions. Neutropenia can occur when the neutrophils are destroyed faster than they are created (eg, by an autoimmune response), or when the production of neutrophils in the bone marrow is reduced (eg, cancer, influenza, and vitamin B12 or folic acid deficiencies). Neutropenia is also associated with radiation treatment that has affected the bone marrow. In fact, the most common cause of neutropenia is drugs or therapies that are used to fight cancer or autoimmune disorders. Other drugs that have been associated with neutropenia are antibiotics (including penicillin) and antiretroviral drugs used in the treatment of HIV/AIDS. Drug-induced neutropenia can often be reversed by discontinuing use of the drug.

It is possible to resolve neutropenia associated with other conditions by addressing the underlying health concern. For instance, bacterial neutropenia may be treated with broad-spectrum antibiotics, while a fungal infection caused by neutropenia may be treated with antifungals. For viral infections such as herpes, the use of acyclovir is common.[37]

If neutropenia is caused by a genetic disease or chemotherapy, it will typically be treated with granulocyte colony-stimulating factor and other bone marrow-derived growth factors.[38,39] These drugs, approved by the Food and Drug Administration (FDA), stimulate the production of neutrophils by increasing the number of bone marrow–neutrophil precursors.[39] Additionally, melatonin has been shown to reduce neutropenia in patients who have undergone chemotherapy to treat cancer.[40]

If neutropenia is caused by an autoimmune disorder, it may be treated with glucocorticoids, cyclosporine, or granulocyte colony-stimulating factor.[41,42]

Additionally, vitamin E may be recommended for patients with chemotherapy-induced neutropenia. In a study of 49 women undergoing chemotherapy for breast cancer, neutropenia was common. Ingestion of vitamin E or multivitamins resolved the condition.[43]

# THROMBOCYTOPENIA

Under normal circumstances, the blood contains about 150 000–350 000 platelets/µL. These platelets are involved in blood clotting. They circulate constantly in the bloodstream, looking for damaged areas. In response to an injury in a blood vessel, the platelets respond by sticking to the site and clumping together (platelet aggregation). This aggregation begins the clotting that prevents further bleeding.[44]

Thrombocytopenia occurs when the platelet count falls too low. At levels of 20 000–30 000 platelets/µL, bleeding can occur in response to relatively minor

trauma. At platelet counts less than 20 000/µL, spontaneous bleeding can occur, which increases the risk of bleeding that can result in shock and death.[45]

Like other blood disorders, thrombocytopenia can occur when the body either does not produce enough platelets, or too many platelets are destroyed. Thrombocytopenia is associated with leukemia or lymphoma, aplastic anemia, vitamin B12 or folic acid deficiency anemia, an enlarged spleen, infectious diseases (eg, HIV/AIDS), and massive blood transfusions.

Two diseases occur because of increased destruction of platelets.

## Idiopathic Thrombocytopenic Purpura (ITP)

This disease occurs when antibodies attack and destroy the body's platelets for unknown reasons. In children, ITP can be an acute condition that occurs after infection. Acute ITP is rare in adults. More common is chronic ITP, a condition that may persist for years and most frequently affects women aged 20–40 years. If symptoms (such as bleeding or easy bruising) are present, a physician may prescribe prednisone to be taken for 4–6 weeks.

## Thrombotic Thrombocytopenic Purpura (TTP)

TTP is a life-threatening disease that occurs when small blood clots form suddenly throughout the body. It can result in cardiac hemorrhage and death.[46] TTP occurs more often in women and is associated with pregnancy, metastatic cancer, chemotherapy, HIV/AIDS, and some prescription drugs (eg, ticlopidine). Patients with TTP experience kidney failure or decreased kidney function, fever, and neurological problems. The most common treatment is fresh frozen plasma (FFP) exchange, which is associated with a 90% survival for this once-fatal disease. Other therapies include vitamin E, kidney dialysis, and transplant.[47]

# SUPPORTING HEALTHY BLOOD CELLS THROUGH NUTRITION

A number of nutrients have been studied for their ability to promote healthy blood and fight diseases of the blood cells, including thrombocytopenia and leukopenia. These nutrients include the following:

## Antioxidant Vitamins

In a series of animal studies, supplementation with vitamins C, E, and A was investigated to find out their effects on thrombocytopenia. Vitamins C, E, and A each diminished coagulation activation induced by surgery, and diminished thrombocytopenia.[48] Fewer deaths occurred after surgery in study animals pretreated with these vitamins.[49] The antioxidant effect of these vitamins is believed to diminish development of free radicals and thereby diminish platelet cell destruction.[50]

## Blueberry, Green Tea, Carnosine, and Vitamin D

Stimulating the healthy growth of stem cells is a critical component of every antiaging program. Studies have shown that specific nutrients can encourage the growth or proliferation of stem cells in one's body, thus promoting regeneration and healing.

In a groundbreaking study, scientists took several nutrients known for their health and cognition-enhancing benefits and studied their effects, alone and in combination, on the proliferation of bone marrow and hematopoietic cells (which are capable of generating all cell types of the blood and immune system).[51] The researchers found a dose-related effect of blueberry, green tea, catechin, carnosine, and vitamin D3 on the proliferation of human bone marrow. Furthermore, combinations of these nutrients stimulated bone marrow proliferation by as much as 83%, compared with only 48% in a control group, which received granulocyte colony-stimulating factor.[51]

## Omega-3 Fatty Acids

Dietary supplementation with omega-3 is associated with prolonged platelet viability, decreased platelet activation (and aggregation), and diminished production of free radicals. In a study comparing fish oil consumption to placebo, platelet survivability was shown to be significantly longer and platelet activation was diminished.[52] The results of this clinical study suggest that fish oil supplementation rich in omega-3 polyunsaturated fatty acids increases platelet survivability by decreasing cell loss due to platelet activation.

The extended platelet life span induced by omega-3 fatty acids may also be due to reduced generation of free radicals. In a study examining the effects of omega-3 on free radical production in neutrophils, the amount of free radical production was significantly lower in the group supplemented with omega-3.[53] Lipid peroxidation, a process that results in death of white blood cells and platelets, is promoted by free radical formation. Omega-3 diminishes free radical formation,[53] and therefore diminishes destruction of platelets and white blood cells.

## Shark Liver Oil

Shark liver oil is rich in a class of compounds known as alkylglycerols, which occur naturally in various mammalian tissues, including most organs responsible for producing blood cells. While most studies have focused on the ability of shark liver oil to fight cancer, it has also been shown to boost immunity by stimulating production of neutrophils and activating macrophages (another type of white blood cell).[54]

## Copper and Zinc

Leukopenia and thrombocytopenia can be caused by copper deficiency, which reduces production of red blood cells, white blood cells, and platelets. Effective copper replacement reverses leukopenia within 2 months.[55]

Zinc deficiency can result in leukopenia.[56] These findings are supported by murine studies in which a limited zinc diet was provided. Moderate zinc deficiency occurs in disorders such as sickle cell anemia, renal disease, and gastrointestinal disorders. The short-term use of zinc supplementation boosts the immune system and appears to protect against opportunistic infections.[56]

## Melatonin

A number of studies have shown that melatonin can enhance blood health by supporting production of blood platelets and neutrophils.

In a pilot study, 3 patients with ITP were given melatonin for up to 46 months. All patients had an initial response after 1 month of treatment, and disease progression subsequently diminished. There were no manifestations of toxicity in any of the study subjects.[57] A follow-up case study of a patient with refractory ITP, which typically has a poor prognosis, showed that melatonin was able to successfully manage the symptoms of severe bleeding.[58] Melatonin has also been shown to enhance the production of platelets and resolve thrombocytopenia in a variety of patients.[59]

Scientists have delved into researching melatonin's ability to protect patients with cancer by boosting the health of bone marrow, among other benefits. Studies have reported that melatonin may decrease thrombocytopenia and neutropenia in patients with cancer.[60]

## Life Extension Suggestions

### Supporting Vitamin B12's Role in Red Blood Cell Formation

- **Vitamin B12:** 2000–4000 mcg daily, orally or sublingually, in the form of methylcobalamin (Note: If blood tests do not show rapid improvement, consult your physician about vitamin B12 injections.)

- **Zinc:** 30 mg daily
- **Copper:** 2–3 mg daily
- **Selenium:** 200 mcg daily

### Supporting Folic Acid's Role in Red Blood Cell Formation

- **Folic acid:** 1600 mcg daily
- **Vitamin B12:** 2000–4000 mcg daily, sublingually
- **Zinc:** 30 mg daily
- **Copper:** 2–3 mg daily
- **Selenium:** 200 mcg daily

### Supporting Iron's Role in Red Blood Cell Formation

- **Iron:** 300 mg of iron protein succinate, equivalent to 15 mg of elemental iron per capsule daily
- **Zinc:** 30 mg daily
- **Copper:** 2–3 mg daily
- **Selenium:** 200 mcg daily

### To Help Maintain Healthy Blood (Including Healthy Platelets and White Blood Cells)

- **Shark liver oil:** 500–1000 mg (containing 20% alkylglycerols, 100–200 mg) daily
- **Vitamin C:** 2000 mg daily
- **Vitamin E:** 400 IU daily
- **Vitamin A:** 3000 IU daily
- **Green Tea extract:** 725 mg daily
- **Vitamin D:** 5000–8000 IU daily (depending on blood test results; optimal levels are between 50 and 80 ng/mL)

- **L-carnosine:** 500–1500 mg daily
- **Blueberry extract:** 500–2000 mg daily
- **Zinc:** 30–60 mg daily
- **Copper:** 2–3 mg daily
- **Selenium:** 200 mcg daily
- **Folate and vitamin B12:** 800 mcg of folate and 300 mcg of vitamin B12 daily
- **Fish oil:** Two 600-mg softgel capsules of eicosapentaenoic acid (EPA) and docosahexaenoic acid (DHA) twice daily (for a total of 2400 mg daily)
- **Melatonin:** 20 mg daily
- **DHEA:** 15–75 mg daily, followed by blood tests in 3–6 weeks

In addition, the following blood test may provide helpful information:

- **Anemia Panel** (including chemistry profile, complete blood count [CBC], ferritin, total iron-binding capacity [TIBC], vitamin B12, folate, and reticulocyte count)

### REFERENCES

References available at: www.lef.org/dpt5/ch23

# 24

# Blood Testing

Too often, people fall victim to a disease that could have been prevented if their blood had been tested once a year.

For instance, we know that prescription drugs can cause liver and kidney problems, but other factors (alcohol, over-the-counter drugs, excess niacin, hepatitis C) can make a person susceptible to liver or kidney damage. These conditions often smolder for years until a life-threatening medical crisis occurs. Because of a phenomenon known as "individual variability," some people are especially vulnerable to liver and kidney damage. However, a blood chemistry test can easily detect an underlying problem in time to take corrective action.

The average person older than age 60 takes several prescription drugs daily to treat or prevent chronic medical conditions. According to the American Medical Association, adverse reactions to prescription drugs are either the fourth, fifth, or sixth leading cause of death in the United States.[1] The American Medical Association emphasizes that these deaths occur even though the doctors prescribing the drugs are supposed to be monitoring their patients to prevent such drug-induced deaths. The problem is that cost-conscious health maintenance organizations and hurried physicians are not mandating blood tests that would detect drug-induced tissue damage in time to prevent disability and death. If you are taking certain prescription medications, regular blood testing is mandatory according to the drug labeling, yet doctors routinely fail to prescribe the recommended blood tests, and their patients too often pay the "ultimate" price.

The reason most people consider blood testing is to ascertain their risk factor(s) for cardiovascular disease. Published studies consistently show that various cholesterol fractions (HDL, LDL) and triglycerides can contribute to heart attack and stroke. Most people do not realize that significant changes can occur in their blood fat levels over the course of a single year, meaning that an earlier test may not accurately reflect their current serum lipid status.

Since 1983, Life Extension has advocated regular medical testing for the purpose of optimizing your personal life extension program.

## THE IMPORTANCE OF ACHIEVING YOUTHFUL BLOOD TEST READINGS

When physicians review blood test results, their primary concern is any result that falls outside the normal laboratory reference range. The problem is that standard reference ranges usually represent "average" populations rather than the optimal level required to maintain good health. It now appears that most standard reference ranges are too broad to adequately detect health problems or prescribe appropriate therapy on an individual basis. This is especially true when these reference ranges are relied on to treat a patient with a serious medical disorder.

An example of flawed reference ranges can be seen in blood tests used to assess thyroid status. A long-standing controversy rages over the best way to diagnose thyroid deficiency. Most conventional doctors rely on thyroid blood tests whereas alternative physicians look for signs and symptoms of thyroid deficiency. A 2002 article published in the *Lancet* challenged conventional medical wisdom regarding the use of standard reference ranges in diagnosing and treating thyroid deficiency. According to the researchers, the problem with thyroid blood tests may be faulty reference ranges that fail to reflect what an optimal thyroid hormone level should be in a particular individual.[2]

Thyroid-stimulating hormone (TSH) is the standard blood test used to determine thyroid gland hormone output. When a deficiency in thyroid hormone occurs, the pituitary gland releases TSH to signal the thyroid gland to produce more hormones.

When the TSH level is in the "normal range," doctors usually assume that the thyroid gland is secreting enough thyroid hormone. The question raised by the *Lancet* article's authors, however, was whether the current reference range for TSH reflects optimal thyroid hormone status.

The TSH reference range used by many laboratories is 0.35–5.50 µIU/mL. A higher TSH level indicates a thyroid hormone deficiency (because the pituitary gland is over-signaling TSH to compensate for low levels of thyroid hormone in the blood). Any result >5.50 µIU/mL alerts a doctor to a thyroid gland problem and the possibility that thyroid hormone therapy may be warranted.

The TSH reference range is so broad that most doctors will interpret a TSH reading as low as 0.35 to be as normal as 5.50. The difference between 0.35 and 5.50, however, is 15.7-fold, a range of values far too great to indicate optimal or even normal thyroid function.

A review of published findings about TSH levels reveals that readings greater than 2.0 may indicate health problems relating to insufficient thyroid hormone output. One study showed that individuals with TSH values greater than 2.0 have an increased risk of developing clinically significant thyroid deficiency during the next 20 years.[3] Other studies show that TSH values greater than 1.9 indicate risk of autoimmune disease of the thyroid gland.[4]

A more startling study showed that a TSH value >4.0 increases the likelihood of heart disease in postmenopausal women.[4] Another study showed that administration of thyroid hormone lowered cholesterol in people with TSH ranges of 2.0–4.0, but had no cholesterol-lowering effect in those whose TSH value was in the 0.2–1.9 range.[5] It also showed that in people with elevated cholesterol, TSH values ≥2.0 could indicate that a thyroid deficiency is the culprit, causing excess production of cholesterol, whereas TSH levels ≤1.99 would indicate normal thyroid hormone status.

Doctors routinely prescribe cholesterol-lowering drugs to people without properly evaluating their thyroid status. Based on the evidence presented to date, it might make sense for doctors to investigate a thyroid deficiency (based on a TSH value >1.9) before resorting to cholesterol-lowering drugs.

In a study to evaluate psychological well-being, impairment was found in people with thyroid abnormalities who were nonetheless within "normal" TSH reference ranges.[6]

The authors of the *Lancet* study stated, "The emerging epidemiological data begin to suggest that TSH concentrations above 2.0 (mU/L, milliunit per liter) may be associated with adverse effects."

The authors prepared a chart based on previously published studies that provides guidance when interpreting the results from TSH blood tests. Here are 3 highlights from their chart that may be useful in understanding what TSH values really mean:

- TSH value greater than 2.0: increased 20-year risk of thyroid deficiency and increased risk of thyroid-induced autoimmune attack[3]
- TSH value greater than 4.0: greater risk of heart disease[4]
- TSH value between 2.0 and 4.0: cholesterol levels decline in response to thyroxine (T4) therapy[5]

Despite these intriguing findings, the *Lancet* authors stated that more studies were needed to define an optimal TSH range, suggested as 0.2–2.0 instead of 0.2–5.5 (µIU/mL). *Note: These optimal reference ranges are now expressed in µIU/mL, so the ideal range according to this epidemiological data is 0.35–2.1 µIU/mL.*

If you have depression, heart disease, high cholesterol, chronic fatigue, poor mental performance, or any of the many other symptoms associated with thyroid deficiency, you may want to ask your doctor to "defy the reference ranges" and try a different thyroid replacement therapy.

# THE RISK OF FOLLOWING STANDARD REFERENCES RANGES

Standard laboratory reference ranges represent average populations and not optimal levels. In the 1960s, for instance, the upper reference range for cholesterol was 300 mg/dL (milligrams per deciliter). This number was based on a statistical calculation indicating that a total cholesterol as high as 300 mg/dL was "normal." Of course, it was also considered "normal" for men to have fatal heart attacks at a relatively young age. As knowledge about the risk of heart attack and high cholesterol has increased, the upper limit reference range gradually dropped to 200 mg/dL.[7,8]

Blood test reference ranges are not the only measures that fail to provide physicians and patients with optimal numbers. For example, high blood pressure (hypertension) is defined medically as a blood pressure reading of 140/90 (read as "140 over 90") or greater. However, a diastolic blood pressure reading (the second number in a blood pressure reading—90 in this example) higher than 80 mmHg (millimeters of mercury) is associated with an increased risk of stroke. A high percentage of people older than age 60 have diastolic readings higher than 80 mmHg, and this is the age group most vulnerable to stroke.[9] If your physician checks your blood pressure and says it is "normal," Life Extension (LE) advises you to ask what the optimal range is. Optimal blood pressure is defined as 115/75. In fact, the risk of cardiovascular disease doubles with each increase of 20/10 mmHg, starting at 115/75 mmHg. It is important to know that midlife hypertension predisposes people to stroke later in life, so keeping blood pressure readings within optimal ranges is important at any age.

## Standard Hormone Reference Ranges May Be Antiquated

Conventional medicine tends to neglect hormone imbalances that develop in men and women as they grow older. The result is that aging people suffer a variety of miseries that are correctable and preventable with simple hormone adjustments.

Aging men, for instance, often suffer from excess production of insulin and estrogen, with simultaneous deficiencies of free testosterone and dehydroepiandrosterone (DHEA). The standard reference ranges for all 4 of these hormones are so wide that most men would fall into the so-called normal category. Standard reference ranges indicate that dangerously high insulin and estrogen levels are "normal" in older men (but so are heart attack, stroke, cancer, benign prostate enlargement, weight gain, type 2 diabetes, kidney impairment, and a host of other diseases associated with excess insulin and estrogen). The same standard reference ranges for free testosterone and DHEA show that very low levels are perfectly "normal" for aging men. It is no coincidence that aging men with low testosterone and DHEA levels have high rates of depression, memory loss, atherosclerosis, senility, impotence, cholesterol, abdominal obesity, fatigue, and many other diseases related to low blood levels of testosterone and DHEA.[10-22]

Standard reference ranges have failed aging people because they are adjusted to reflect age. Since it is normal for an aging person to have imbalances of critical hormones, standard laboratory reference ranges do not flag dangerously high levels of estrogen and insulin or deficient levels of testosterone, thyroid, and DHEA. The following table compares standard and optimal hormone and TSH blood reference ranges for 60-year-old men.

| Hormone | Standard Reference Range | Life Extension's Optimal Range |
|---|---|---|
| DHEA | 51.7–295.0 μg/dL | 350–490 μg/dL |
| Insulin (fasting) | 2.6–24.9 μIU/mL | <5 μIU/mL |
| Free testosterone | 6.6–18.1 pg/mL | 20–25 pg/mL |
| Estradiol | <54 pg/mL | 20–30 pg/mL |
| Thyroid stimulating hormone | 0.45–4.50 μIU/mL | 1–2 μIU/mL |

## DEFYING THE REFERENCE RANGES

Traditional medical thinking accepts that imbalances of life-sustaining hormones are normal in aging people. Traditional practitioners almost never test hormone levels because they think that nothing should be done to restore hormone profiles to youthful ranges. For more specific information on optimizing hormone levels, turn to the following protocols: Male Hormone Restoration, Female Hormone Restoration, Thyroid Regulation, and DHEA Restoration Therapy.

## THE MOST IMPORTANT BLOOD TESTS

Life Extension suggests that a basic battery of tests be performed annually. The recommended male panel consists of a complete blood count (CBC)/chemistry test, homocysteine, free testosterone,

estradiol, prostate-specific antigen (PSA), and DHEA. The recommended female panel consists of a CBC/chemistry test, estradiol, progesterone, free testosterone, DHEA, and homocysteine.

In addition to these special male and female panels, the following tests are especially important for men and women over age 40: fasting insulin, fibrinogen, thyroid stimulating hormone (TSH), and free triiodothyronine (T3). If a serious abnormality is detected—such as elevated blood glucose (sugar), hormone imbalance, or high cholesterol—testing should be repeated more often than annually to determine the benefits of any therapy you are using to correct the potentially life-shortening abnormality.

Life Extension also recommends consulting a physician regarding any other test(s) that may be appropriate for your individual condition. The following list describes individual tests and ranges that can be used to assess health and longevity. If your physician is unwilling to prescribe these tests, or if commercial laboratory prices are beyond your budget, we provide information at the end of this protocol about the availability of low-cost mail order blood testing.

## ALPHABETICAL LISTING OF BLOOD TESTS

### ABO Grouping and Rh (D) Typing

This test is used to determine blood grouping and Rh typing. The possible blood types are O positive, O negative, A positive, A negative, B positive, B negative, AB positive, and AB negative.

### Alpha 1 Antitrypsin (Serum)

This test is used to detect hereditary decreases in the production of alpha1-antitrypsin (AAT). Decreased or nearly absent levels of AAT can be a factor in chronic obstructive lung disease and liver disease. Elevated levels of AAT can be an indication of inflammatory states (eg, rheumatoid arthritis, bacterial infection, vasculitis, or neoplasia).

*Reference range: 90–200 mg/dL*

### Amino Acid Profile (Quantitative)

This panel evaluates 41 amino acids and is used to monitor body functions and nutritional status. Increased amino acid concentrations in plasma may reflect inherited metabolic abnormalities, as in tyrosinemia or phenylketonuria.

### Apolipoprotein A-1

This test is used to evaluate survival rate or risk factors for patients with myocardial infarction and peripheral vascular diseases. APO A-1 deficiency states include Tangier disease, HDL deficiency, and hypoalpha-lipoprotein anemia. Apolipoprotein levels may be a better indicator of atherogenic risks than high-density lipoprotein (HDL), low-density lipoprotein (LDL), and very-low-density lipoprotein (VLDL) measures.

Reference ranges
**Men:** *110–180 mg/dL*
**Women:** *110–205 mg/dL*

## B-Type Natriuretic Peptide

This test is used to support the finding of congestive heart failure.

*Reference range: 0–100 pg/mL*

## Beta-Carotene

This test is used to confirm carotenoderma and detect fat malabsorption and depressed carotene levels that may be found in cases of steatorrhea.

*Reference range: 10–85 μg/dL*

## Cancer Antigen (CA-15-3)

The CA 15-3 antigens are tumor-associated serum markers, most specifically for breast tissue, available for monitoring various types of malignancies, evaluating response to therapy, and possibly indicating recurrence.

*Reference range: 0.0–32.4 U/mL*

## Cancer Antigen (CA-27.29)

This test is used to monitor metastatic carcinoma of the breast. CA-27.29 is a useful measurement in the monitoring of both the course of disease and the response to therapy because there is a direct correlation between the changing levels of CA-27.29 and clinical status.

*Reference range: 0–38.6 U/mL*

## Cancer Antigen (CA-125)

CA-125 is a tumor marker for monitoring disease progression in ovarian cancer. It is most useful in monitoring progression or recurrence in cases of known ovarian carcinoma.

*Reference range: 0–32 U/mL*

## Candida Antibodies Qualitative

This test is used to diagnose systemic candidiasis. This test is qualitative, and if candida antibodies are found, you have had or now have a candida infection.

## Carbohydrate Antigen (CA-19-9)

This test is used to monitor gastrointestinal, pancreatic, liver, and colorectal malignancies. This test may also be positive in patients with non-neoplastic

disease, inflammatory disease of the bowel, cirrhosis, and autoimmune conditions.

*Reference range: 0–37 U/mL*

## Carcinoembryonic Antigen (CEA)

This tumor marker is used to determine the extent of disease and its prognosis in cancer patients (especially those with gastrointestinal or breast cancers). It can also be used to monitor the disease and its treatment.

*Reference range:*
*Nonsmoker: <2.5 ng/mL*
*Smoker: <5.0 ng/mL*

## Chemistry Panel/CBC

This panel is a comprehensive blood evaluation including the following tests:

### *Chemistry Panel*

**Glucose (fasting).** This test directly measures glucose levels and is commonly used in the evaluation of diabetes.

*Reference range: 65–99 mg/dL*
*LE's optimal range: 70–85 mg/dL*

**Uric acid.** This test is used in the evaluation of gout or recurrent urinary calculus.

*Reference range:*
**Men** *(18 years and older): 3.7–8.6 mg/dL*
**Women** *(18 years and older): 2.5–7.1 mg/dL*
*LE's optimal range: 3–7 mg/dL*

**BUN (blood urea nitrogen).** This test is used to measure liver function and to indirectly assess renal function and glomerular filtration rate.

*Reference range: 5–26 mg/dL*

**Creatinine.** This is a renal function test used to estimate glomerular filtration rate and to follow progression of renal disease.

*Reference range:*
**Women** *(15 years and older): 0.57–1.00 mg/dL*
**Men:** *0.76–1.27 mg/dL*
*LE's optimal range: <1.5 mg/dL and ideally <1.1 mg/dL*

**BUN/creatinine ratio.** This test is used to diagnose impaired renal function. With creatinine, BUN is used to monitor patients on dialysis.

*Reference range: 8:1–27:1*

**Sodium.** This routine test is used to evaluate and monitor fluid and electrolyte balance and therapy.

*Reference range: 135–144 mmol/L*

**Potassium.** This routine test is used to evaluate and monitor electrolyte balance and is especially important for cardiac patients.

*Reference range: 3.5–5.2 mmol/L*

**Chloride.** This test by itself does not provide adequate information. However, as part of a multiphasic testing for electrolytes, it can give an indication of acid-base balance and hydration status.
*Reference range: 97–108 mmol/L*

**Carbon dioxide.** This test is used to assist in the evaluation of pH and electrolyte status.
*Reference range: 20–32 mmol/L*

**Calcium.** This test is used to evaluate parathyroid function and calcium metabolism.
*Reference range:*
*18–59 years old: 8.7–10.2 mg/dL*
*>59 years old: 8.6–10.2 mg/dL*

**Phosphorus.** This test is used to measure serum phosphorus levels. An imbalance could indicate the possibility of any number of conditions.
*Reference range for people aged 12–60 years: 2.5–4.5 mg/dL*

**Total protein/albumin/globulin.** This test is used to assist in the diagnosis of many diseases that affect blood proteins as a whole or one single fraction of protein.
*Reference range:*
*Total protein: 6.0–8.5 g/dL*
*Albumin: 3.5–5.5 g/dL*
*Globulin: 1.5–4.5 g/dL*

**Albumin/globulin ratio.** This test is used to evaluate renal disease and other chronic diseases.
*Reference range: 1.1:1–2.5:1*

**Bilirubin.** This test is used to evaluate liver function.
*Reference range:*
*Total Bilirubin: 0.1–1.2 mg/dL*

**Alkaline phosphatase.** This test is used to detect and monitor liver or bone disease.
*Reference range: 25–150 IU/L*

**LDH (lactic dehydrogenase).** This test measures the intracellular enzyme LDH, which when present in the blood, supports the diagnosis of injury or disease.
*Reference range: 100–250 IU/L*

**AST (SGOT).** This test is used to evaluate the possibility of coronary occlusive heart disease or liver disease.
*Reference range: 0–40 IU/L*

**ALT (SGPT).** This test is used to identify liver disease and to distinguish between liver and red blood cell hemolysis as the source of jaundice.
*Reference ranges:*
**Men:** *0–55 IU/L*
**Women:** *0–40 IU/L*

**Iron.** This test is used to evaluate many diseases, including iron deficiency anemia and hemochromatosis.
*Reference range:*
**Women:** *35–155 μg/dL*
**Men:** *40–155 μg/dL*
*LE's optimal range: 40–100 μg/dL*

## Lipid Profile

**Cholesterol.** This test is used to determine the risk of developing coronary heart disease and hyperlipidemias.
*Reference range: 100–199 mg/dL*
*LE's optimal range: 160–180 mg/dL*

**Triglycerides.** This test is used to identify the risk of developing coronary heart disease or when disorders in fat metabolism are suspected.
*Reference range: 0–149 mg/dL*
*LE's optimal range: <80 mg/dL*
*Pre-existing cardiovascular disease: <60 mg/dL*

**HDL cholesterol.** This test measures alpha lipoprotein and is used to predict heart disease.
*Reference range: 40–59 mg/dL*
*LE's optimal range: ≥50 mg/dL*

**LDL cholesterol.** This test measures beta lipoproteins and is also used to predict heart disease.
*Reference range: 0–99 mg/dL*
*LE's optimal range: <100 mg/dL*
*Pre-existing/high risk cardiovascular disease: <70 mg/dL*

**Ratio of total cholesterol to HDL cholesterol.** This test is used to determine the risk of coronary heart disease.

| Reference Ranges: | Men | Women |
|---|---|---|
| *1/2 average risk* | *3.4* | *3.3* |
| *Average risk* | *5.0* | *4.4* |
| *2× average risk* | *9.6* | *7.1* |
| *LE's optimal range:* | *<3.4* | *<3.4* |

## CBC (Complete Blood Count) with Platelets and Differential

This is a series of tests of the peripheral blood that provides a variety of information about the blood components.

**White blood cell count**
*Reference range: 4.0–10.5 x10E3/uL*

**Red blood cell count**
*Reference ranges:*
**Men:** *4.1–5.6 x10E6/uL*
**Women:** *3.8–5.10 x10E6/uL*

**Hemoglobin**
*Reference ranges:*
**Men:** *12.5–17.0 g/dL*

**Women:** *11.5–15.0 g/dL*
*LE's optimal range: Upper end of reference range*

## Hematocrit

*Reference ranges:*
**Men:** *34–50%*
**Women:** *34–44%*
*LE's optimal range: Upper end of reference range*

## Red Blood Cell Indices

- **Mean corpuscular volume**
  *Reference range: 80–98 fL*

- **Mean corpuscular hemoglobin**
  *Reference range: 27–34 pg*

- **Mean corpuscular hemoglobin concentration**
  *Reference range: 32–36 g/dL*

## Red Blood Cell Distribution of Width

*Reference range: 11.7–15.0%*

## Differential count

*Reference ranges:*
*Polyneutrophils: 1.8–7.8 x10E3/uL*
*Lymphocytes: 0.7–4.5 x10E3/uL*
*Monocytes: 0.1–1.0 x10E3/uL*
*Eosinophils: 0.0–0.4 x10E3/uL*
*Basophils: 0.0–0.2 x10E3/uL*

## Platelet count

*Reference range: 140–415 x10E3/uL*

## Cortisol A.M.–P.M.

This test is to measure adrenal function. It is used to diagnose adrenocortical insufficiency or hypersecretion and Cushing's syndrome and is also useful in detecting malfunction of the hypothalamic axis.
*Reference ranges:*
A.M.: *6.2–19.4 µg/dL*
P.M.: *2.3–11.9 µg/dL*

## Coenzyme Q10 (CoQ10)

This test is used to check the blood level of CoQ10 and will enable more precise dosing for anyone seeking to achieve and maintain high levels of this critical antioxidant. Coenzyme Q10 is produced by the human body and is necessary for the basic functioning of all cells. It is known to be highly concentrated in heart muscle cells due to the high energy requirements of this cell type.
*Reference ranges: 0.37–2.20 µg/mL*

*LE's optimal range: 3–7 µg/mL: At least 3 µg/mL for general health; at least 4 µg/mL for cardiovascular*

issues; and up to 7 µg/mL for maximal anti-aging and neurodegenerative protection

## C-Peptide

This test is used to evaluate diabetics and monitor insulinoma.
*Reference ranges: 1.1–5.0 ng/mL*

## C-Reactive Protein (CRP) (Cardiac) (High Sensitivity)

This test is used to assess risk of cardiovascular and peripheral vascular disease.
*Reference ranges:*
*Low risk: <1.0 mg/L*
*Average: 1.0–3.0 mg/L*
*High risk: >3.0 mg/L*
*LE's optimal ranges:*
**Men:** *<0.55 mg/L*
**Women:** *<1.5 mg/L*

## Cystatin-C

This test is used to evaluate kidney function. It has also been suggested that cystatin-C might predict the risk of developing chronic kidney disease, thereby signaling a state of 'preclinical' kidney dysfunction.
*Reference ranges: 0.53–0.95 mg/L*
*LE's optimal range: <0.91 mg/L*

## Cytokine Panel

This panel is used to find the source of chronic inflammation after a high CRP reading or the persistence of any chronic inflammatory condition. This panel measures interleukin-1 beta (IL-1b), interleukin-6 (IL-6), interleukin-8 (IL-8), and tumor necrosis factor-alpha (TNF-α). Each is described separately.

## D-Dimer

This test is a very specific confirmatory test for disseminated intravascular coagulation (DIC). It is also used for the detection of deep vein thrombosis, acute myocardial infarction, and unstable angina. The fragment D-dimer assesses both thrombin and plasmin activity.
*Reference range: 0.0–0.4 µg/mL*

## Dehydroepiandrosterone (DHEA) Sulfate

This test is used to determine female infertility, amenorrhea, or hirsutism and to aid in the evaluation of excess androgen/adrenocortical disease, including congenital adrenal hyperplasia and adrenal tumors.
*Reference ranges:*
**Men:**
*15–19 years: 70.2–492.0 µg/dL*

20–24 years: 211.0–492.0 µg/dL
25–34 years: 160.0–449.0 µg/dL
35–44 years: 88.9–427.0 µg/dL
45–54 years: 44.3–331.0 µg/dL
55–64 years: 51.7–295.0 µg/dL
65–74 years: 33.6–249.0 µg/dL
>74 years: 16.2–123.0 µg/dL
LE's optimal range: 350–490 µg/dL
**Women:**
15–19 years: 65.1–368.0 µg/dL
20–24 years: 148.0–407.0 µg/dL
25–34 years: 98.8–340.0 µg/dL
35–44 years: 60.9–337.0 µg/dL
45–54 years: 35.4–256.0 µg/dL
55–64 years: 18.9–205.0 µg/dL
65–74 years: 9.4–246.0 µg/dL
>74 years: 12.0–154.0 µg/dL
LE's optimal range: 275–400 µg/dL

## Deoxypyridinoline (Dpd) Cross-Link Test

This test can be used to assess bone resorption rates in healthy individuals and in those with enhanced risk of developing metabolic bone disease. Dpd can be used to monitor antiresorptive therapies (which may include bisphosphonates) and osteoporosis.

*Reference range: 2.3–7.4 nmol Dpd/mmol creatinine*

## Dihydrotestosterone

This test measures serum concentrations of dihydrotestosterone, which is closely related to testosterone levels, but are lower and may indicate hypergonadism or hirsutism.

*Reference ranges:*
**Men:** 30–85 ng/dL
**Women:** 4–22 ng/dL
*LE's optimal range:*
**Men:** 30–50 ng/dL

## Epstein-Barr Virus (EBV) Acute Infection

This test is used to diagnose a suspected EBV infection (infectious mononucleosis).

| EBV Interpretation | VCA-IgG | VCA-IgM | EA-IgG | EBV-NA |
|---|---|---|---|---|
| Susceptible: | – | – | – | – |
| Acute infection: | + | + | ± | – |
| Convalescent phase: | + | ± | ± | + |
| Chronic or reactivated: | + | – | + | ± |
| Old infection: | ± | – | – | + |
| Antibody present: | + | | | |
| Antibody absent: | – | | | |

## ESR Westergren Sedimentation Rate (ESR, Sed Rate Test)

The ESR is a nonspecific test used to detect illness associated with acute and chronic infection, inflammation (collagen-vascular diseases), advanced neoplasm, and tissue necrosis or infarction.

*Reference ranges:*
**Men:**
0–50 years: 0–15 mm/hour
50 years and older: 0–20 mm/hour
**Women:**
0–50 years: 0–20 mm/hour
50 years and older: 0–30 mm/hour

## Estradiol

This test is used to assess hypothalamic and pituitary functions, menopausal status, and sexual maturity. In males it is helpful in the assessment of gynecomastia or feminization syndromes.

*Reference ranges:*
**Men:** 7.6–42.6 pg/mL
**Women:**
　Follicular: 12.5–166.0 pg/mL
　Ovulation: 85.8–498.0 pg/mL
　Luteal: 43.8–211.0 pg/mL
　Postmenopausal: <6.0-54.7 pg/mL
*LE's optimal ranges:*
**Men:** 20–30 pg/mL
**Women:**
Premenopause: varies with time in cycle, max 528 pg/mL
Menopause:
　To ameliorate symptoms: 30–50 pg/mL
　Typical with Bi-est: 80–100 pg/mL
　Restore menstrual cycle: 90–211 pg/mL

## Estriol

This test provides an objective assessment of placental function and fetal normality in high-risk pregnancies. Estriol is the major estrogen in the pregnant female.

*Reference range:*
*Men or nonpregnant women: <2.0 mg/dL*

## Estrogens Total

Estrogen measurements are used to evaluate sexual maturity, menstrual and fertility problems in females. This test is also used in the evaluation of males with gynecomastia or feminization syndromes. In pregnant women, it is used to indicate fetal-placental health. In patients with estrogen-producing tumors, it can be used as a tumor marker.

*Reference ranges:*
**Men**:
*40–115 pg/mL*
*LE's optimal range: 40–77 pg/mL*
**Women**:
*Day 1–10: 61–394 pg/mL*
*Day 11–20: 122–437 pg/mL*
*Day 21–30: 156–350 pg/mL*
*Postmenopausal: <40 pg/mL*
*LE's optimal range:*
*Postmenopausal: 75–200 pg/mL (with HRT)*

## Estrone

This test is used to evaluate postmenopausal bleeding due to peripheral conversion of androgenic steroids. Increased estrone levels may be associated with increased levels of circulating androgens and their subsequent peripheral conversion.

*Reference ranges:*
**Men**: *12–72 pg/mL*
**Women**:
*Follicular phase: 37–138 pg/mL*
*Midcycle peak: 60–229 pg/mL*
*Luteal phase: 50–114 pg/mL*

## Factor VIII Activity

This test is used to evaluate levels of coagulant factor VIII. A deficiency in factor VIII is known as hemophilia A. Elevated levels are associated with a significantly increased risk of ischemic heart disease and with the development of the geriatric syndrome of frailty.

## Fasting Glucose and Insulin

These 2 tests are used to determine elevated levels of glucose and insulin. Excess glucose and insulin are implicated in many age-related diseases, such as type 2 diabetes, hypertension, heart disease, and stroke, and are a hallmark of mammalian aging. *Please note:* These tests require a fasting blood level, meaning that a 12-hour fast is required before the collection of a blood sample. Each of these tests is described separately.

**Glucose.** This test is used to detect diabetes mellitus and evaluate carbohydrate metabolism disorders including alcoholism. It is also used to evaluate acidosis, ketoacidosis, dehydration, coma, hypoglycemia, insulinoma, and neuroglycopenia.

**Insulin.** This test is primarily used to measure insulin evaluation in individuals with fasting hypoglycemia. Insulin levels tend to be inappropriately elevated in individuals with insulin-secreting tumors. Fasting hypoglycemia in association with

markedly elevated serum insulin levels is considered the determining factor for insulinoma. Insulin levels can be useful in predicting susceptibility to the development of type 2 diabetes, although C-peptide has largely supplanted insulin measurement for this role.

## Female Panel

The female panel consists of a chemistry panel, CBC, free testosterone, total testosterone, DHEA-S, estradiol, progesterone, homocysteine, TSH, Vitamin D 25-Hydroxy, and cardiac CRP. Each of these tests is described separately.

## Ferritin

This test is used to evaluate iron reserves in the body and to determine iron deficiency anemia or iron overload.

*Reference ranges:*
**Men:** *22–322 ng/mL*
**Women:** *10–291 ng/mL*
*LE's optimal range: 50–150 ng/mL*

## Follicle-Stimulating Hormone (FSH) and Luteinizing Hormone (LH)

This test is used in the determination of menopause and is integral in the evaluation of suspected gonadal failure.

| FSH | Reference Ranges: | LH | Reference Ranges: |
|---|---|---|---|
| **Adult Men:** | | **Adult Men:** | |
| | | 20–70 years: | 1.5–9.3 mIU/mL |
| >15 years: | 1.4–18.1 mIU/mL | >70 years: | 3.1–34.6 mIU/mL |
| LE's optimal Range: | 1.4–14 mIU/mL | LE's optimal Range: | 0.5–9.3 mIU/mL |
| **Women:** | | **Women:** | |
| Follicular phase: | 2.5–10.2 mIU/mL | Follicular phase: | 1.9–12.5 mIU/mL |
| Ovulatory peak: | 3.4–33.4 mIU/mL | Ovulatory peak: | 8.7–76.3 mIU/mL |
| Luteal phase: | 1.5–9.1 mIU/mL | Luteal phase: | 0.5–16.9 mIU/mL |
| Postmenopausal phase: | 23.0–116.3 mIU/mL | Postmenopausal phase: | 5.0–52.3 mIU/mL |
| | | Contraceptives | 0.7–5.6 mIU/mL |

## Fructosamine

This test is used to evaluate diabetic control. Fructosamine, rather than glucose level, is an index of longer-term control.

## Gamma Glutamyl Transpeptidase

This test is a sensitive indicator of hepatobiliary disease (obstructive jaundice, intrahepatic cholestasis, or pancreatitis). It is also used as an indicator of chronic and heavy alcohol abuse.

*Reference range: 0–65 IU/L*

## Glucose (Serum) (Fasting)

This test is used to detect diabetes mellitus. It is used to evaluate carbohydrate metabolism disorders including alcoholism. It is also used to evaluate acidosis, ketoacidosis, dehydration, coma, hypoglycemia, insulinoma, and neuroglycopenia. Please note: These tests require a fasting blood level, meaning that a 12-hour fast is required before the collection of a blood sample.

*Reference ranges:*
*Normal: <100 mg/dL*
*Prediabetic: 100–125 mg/dL*
*Diabetic: >126 mg/dL*
*LE's optimal range: 70–85 mg/dL*

## Glucose (2-Hour Postprandial)

Normally, your blood glucose levels increase slightly after you eat. This increase causes your pancreas to release insulin so that your blood glucose levels do not get too high. Blood glucose levels that remain high over time can damage your eyes, kidneys, nerves, and blood vessels. This test measures blood glucose exactly 2 hours after eating.

*Reference ranges:*
*Normal: <140 mg/dL*
*Prediabetic: 140–199 mg/dL*
*Diabetic: >200 mg/dL*
*LE's optimal range: <120–125 mg/dL is ideal; acceptable up to 140 mg/dL*

## Human Chorionic Gonadotropin (HCG) Beta Subunit, Pregnancy

This test is used to detect the beta subunit of HCG, providing a sensitive, specific test for the detection of early pregnancy, ectopic pregnancy, or threatened abortion.

## HCG Beta Subunit, Quantitative (Cancer)

This test is used to detect a tumor marker for certain cancers.

*Reference ranges:*
*Negative: <10 mIU/mL*
*Borderline: 10–20 mIU/mL*
*Positive: >20 mIU/mL*

## Heavy Metals Profile I, Blood

This test is used to monitor exposure to arsenic, lead, and mercury.

*LE's optimal range: As low as possible*

## *Helicobacter (Campylobacter) pylori,* Immunoglobulin M

This test is used as an aid in the diagnosis of *H. pylori* infection and gastric and duodenal disease.

*Reference ranges:*
*Negative: <0.8 U/mL*
*Equivocal: 0.8–1.19 U/mL*
*Positive: >1.19 U/mL*

## Hemoglobin A1C

This test is most frequently used to assess glucose control in insulin-dependent diabetic patients whose glucose levels are very labile.

*Reference range: 4.8–5.6%*
*Increased risk for diabetes: 5.7–6.4%*
*Diabetes: >6.5%*
*Glycemic control for adults with diabetes: <7.0%*
*LE's optimal range: <4.5%*

## Hepatitis Panel (A, B, C), Acute

This test is used as a comprehensive panel for detecting markers for hepatitis A, B, and C virus infections and is used for all stages of infection.

*Reference range: Negative or positive*

## Hepatitis B Surface Antibody, Qualitative

This test is useful for evaluation of possible immunity in individuals who are at increased risk of exposure to hepatitis B.

*Normal range: Negative or positive*

## Hepatitis C Virus Antibody

This test is used to assess exposure to hepatitis C virus infection.

*Reference range: Negative or positive*

## Homocysteine

This test is intended for use in screening patients who may be at risk for heart disease and stroke. Homocysteine has been shown to be an independent risk factor for the premature development of coronary artery disease and thrombosis.

*Reference range:*
**Men:** *4.3–11.4 μmol/L*
**Women:** *3.3–10.4 μmol/L*
*LE's optimal range: <7–8 μmol/L*

Studies have shown that even moderate levels of homocysteine pose an increased risk for arteriosclerosis.

## Insulin (Fasting)

This test is used for insulin measurement in patients with fasting hypoglycemia or hyperglycemia. High fasting insulin is a sign of insulin resistance and the start of type 2 diabetes or metabolic syndrome.

*Reference range: 2.6–24.9 μIU/mL*
*LE's optimal range: <5 μIU/mL*

## Interleukin-1 beta (IL-1b)

This test is used to identify elevated levels of interleukin-1 beta, which have been implicated in sepsis, cachexia, rheumatoid arthritis, chronic myelogenous leukemia, asthma, psoriasis, inflammatory bowel disease, anorexia, AIDS, physical stress, anxiety and panic disorders, and graft-versus-host disease associated with bone marrow transplants. Higher-than-normal levels of IL-1b have been associated with a significant increased risk of myocardial infarction independent of cardio-CRP levels.

*Reference range:*
*IL-1B: <2.9 pg/mL*

## Interleukin-6 (IL-6)

This test is used to identify elevated levels of interleukin-6. Elevated IL-6 serum or plasma levels may occur in sepsis, autoimmune diseases, lymphomas, AIDS, alcoholic liver disease, tumor development, Alzheimer's disease, and in concert with infections or transplant rejection. Elevated levels of IL-6 may be associated with an increased risk of heart attack or stroke.

*Reference range:*
*IL-6: 0–14 pg/mL*

## Interleukin-8 (IL-8)

This test is used to identify elevated levels of IL-8. Elevated concentrations are observed in psoriasis, rheumatoid arthritis, chronic polyarthritis, tumor development, and hepatitis C.

*Reference range:*
*IL-8: 7.8 pg/mL*

## Iron and Total Iron Binding Capacity (TIBC)

This test is used in the diagnosis of anemia. TIBC levels are often used to monitor the course of patients receiving hyperalimentation.

*Reference range: 40–180 μg/dL*
*LE's optimal ranges: Iron: 40–100 mg/dL;*
*TIBC: 250–420 mg/dL*

## Insulin-Like Growth Factor I

This test is used to determine acromegaly, in which somatomedin-C and insulin-like growth factor is increased. It is also used to evaluate hypopituitarism. Low values may indicate hypopituitarism, malnutrition, diabetes mellitus, Laron dwarfism, hypothyroidism, maternal deprivation syndrome, pubertal delay, cirrhosis, hepatoma, anorexia nervosa, nonfunctioning pituitary tumors, constitutional delay of growth, and some cases of short stature. High values occur with adolescence, true precocious puberty, pregnancy, obesity, pituitary gigantism, acromegaly, and diabetic retinopathy.

*Reference ranges:*
*20 years: 127–424 ng/mL*
*21–25 years: 116–358 ng/mL*
*26–30 years: 117–329 ng/mL*
*31–35 years: 115–307 ng/mL*
*36–40 years: 109–284 ng/mL*
*41–45 years: 101–267 ng/mL*
*46–50 years: 94–252 ng/mL*
*51–55 years: 87–238 ng/mL*
*56–60 years: 81–225 ng/mL*
*61–65 years: 75–212 ng/mL*
*66–70 years: 69–200 ng/mL*
*71–75 years: 64–188 ng/mL*
*76–80 years: 59–177 ng/mL*
*81–85 years: 55–166 ng/mL*

## Lipase

This test is used to diagnose pancreatitis or inflammatory bowel disease. An injured or diseased pancreas will produce abnormal amounts of this enzyme.

*Reference range: 0–59 U/L*

## Lipoprotein (a)

This test is used to measure excess small dense lipoprotein. Elevated lipoprotein (a) is a strong indicator of premature coronary disease and atherosclerotic vascular disease and is associated with increased risk of cardiac death in patients with acute coronary syndromes and coronary bypass procedures.

*Reference ranges: 0–30 mg/dL*
*Desirable: <20mg/dL*
*Borderline High Risk: 20–30 mg/dL*
*High Risk: 31–50 mg/dL*
*Very High Risk: >50 mg/dL*

## Magnesium (Serum)

This test is used to evaluate magnesium levels. Decreased levels of magnesium have been associated with cardiac arrhythmias, hypocalcemia, hypokalemia, long-term hyperalimentation, intravenous therapy, diabetes mellitus (especially during treatment of keto-acidosis), alcoholism and other types of malnutrition, malabsorption, hyperparathyroidism, dialysis, pregnancy, and hyperaldosteronism. Magnesium deficiency produces neuromuscular disorders causing weakness, tremors, tetany, and convulsions. Renal loss of magnesium occurs with cis-platinum therapy. Increased magnesium levels relate mostly to individuals in renal failure or with Addison's disease. Marked increases may be found in individuals who take magnesium salts (eg, antacids, which contain magnesium) or magnesium-containing cathartics and in pregnant woman with severe preeclampsia or eclampsia who are receiving magnesium sulfate as an anticonvulsant. High magnesium levels are manifested in decreased reflexes, somnolence, and heart block.

*Reference range: 1.6–2.6 mg/dL*

## Magnesium (RBC)

This test is used to evaluate magnesium deficiency.

*Reference range: 4.2–6.8 mg/dL*

## Male Panel

This panel consists of a chemistry panel, CBC, free testosterone, total testosterone, DHEA-S, PSA, estradiol, homocysteine, cardiac CRP, TSH, and Vitamin D 25-Hydroxy. Each of these tests is described separately.

## Male Hormone Modulating Profile

This panel consists of a male panel plus progesterone, FSH, and LH. Each of these tests is described separately.

## Osteocalcin

This test is used to evaluate bone disease characterized by increased bone turnover. Osteocalcin has been found to be elevated in Paget disease of the bone, cancer accompanied by bone metastases, primary hyperparathyroidism, and renal osteodystrophy. Osteocalcin levels may also be used to monitor therapeutic results.

*Reference ranges:*
**Men:** *3.2–39.6 ng/mL*
**Premenopausal Women:** *4.9–30.9 ng/mL*
**Postmenopausal Women:** *9.4–47.4 ng/mL*

## Parathyroid Hormone, Intact

This test is used in diagnosing parathyroid disease, diagnosing and monitoring other diseases of calcium homeostasis, and monitoring patients undergoing renal dialysis.

| Intact Parathyroid Hormone | Calcium | Interpretation |
|---|---|---|
| 12–65 pg/mL | 8.5–10.6 mg/dL | Normal |
| >65 pg/mL | >10.6 mg/dL | Primary Hyperparathyroidism |
| >65 pg/mL | <10.6 mg/dL | Secondary Hyperparathyroidism |
| <65 pg/mL | >10.6 mg/dL | Nonparathyroid hypercalcemia |
| <12 pg/mL | <8.5 mg/dL | Hypoparathyroidism |
| 12–65 pg/mL | <8.5 mg/dL | Nonparathyroid hypocalcemia |

## Pregnenolone

This test is used to determine ovarian failure, hirsutism, adrenal carcinoma, and Cushing's syndrome.

*Reference ranges:*
**Men:** *10–200 ng/dL*
**Women:** *10–230 ng/dL*
*LE's optimal range:*
**Men:** *125–175 ng/dL; max 200 ng/dL*
**Women:** *130–180 ng/dL; max 230 ng/dL*

## Progesterone

This test is used to establish the presence of a functional corpus luteum, or luteal cell function, confirm body temperature for occurrence of ovulation, obtain indication of day of ovulation, evaluate the functional state of corpus luteum in infertile patients, assess placental function during pregnancy, and evaluate ovarian function.

*Reference ranges:*
**Men:** *0.2–1.4 ng/mL*
**Women:**
  *Follicular: 0.2–1.5 ng/mL*
  *Luteal: 1.7–27.0 ng/mL*
  *Ovulation: 0.8–3.0 ng/mL*
  *Menopausal: 0.1–0.8 ng/mL*
  *LE's optimal ranges:*
**Men:** *approximately 1–1.2 ng/mL*
**Women:**
  *Still having menstrual cycle: 18–27 ng/mL (at ~day 21)*
  *Menopause: 2–6 ng/mL*
  *Max: 27 ng/mL*

## Prolactin

This test is used to assess inappropriate lactation and is also useful in the detection of prolactin-secreting pituitary tumors. Elevated prolactin is associated with anovulation and amenorrhea. Prolactin can also be elevated in hypothyroidism when TSH is high. Some studies indicate that elevated prolactin may promote breast and prostate cancer growth.

*Reference ranges:*
**Men**: *2.1–17.7 ng/mL*
   *LE's optimal range: 2.1–5 ng/mL*
**Women**: *2.8–29.2 ng/mL*
   *LE's optimal range: 2.8–7 ng/mL*
   *Nonpregnant: 2.8–29.2 ng/mL*
   *Pregnant: 9.7–208.5 ng/mL*
   *Postmenopausal: 1.8–20.3 ng/mL*

## Prostate-Specific Antigen (PSA)

PSA is produced by normal, hyperplastic, and cancerous prostatic tissue. Serum PSA has been found to be the most sensitive marker for monitoring patients with prostate cancer and to enhance efficacy in monitoring progression of disease and response to therapy.
   *Reference range: 0–4.0 ng/mL*
   *LE's optimal range: 0–2.5 ng/mL*

## PSA Free-to-Total Ratio

This test is used in men to measure the percentage of free PSA relative to the amount of total PSA. This ratio helps determine the probability of prostate cancer. The lower the percentage of free PSA, the higher the possibility of prostate cancer. In the following table, the percentages given under each age group are the percentages of men with cancer whose percentage of free PSA falls within the given range.
   *Reference range: 0–4.0 ng/mL*

| Free PSA | 50–64 Years | 65–75 Years |
|---|---|---|
| 0.00–10.00% | 56% | 55% |
| 10.01–15.00% | 24% | 35% |
| 15.01–20.00% | 17% | 23% |
| 20.01–25.00% | 10% | 20% |
| >25% | 5% | 9% |

## Prothrombin Time

This test is used to evaluate the adequacy of the extrinsic system and common pathway in the clotting mechanism. Prothrombin time testing provides a control for long-term anticoagulant therapy, which usually involves the use of a coumarin derivative (eg, Coumadin®).

## Partial Thromboplastin Time

This test is used to evaluate the intrinsic coagulation system. It is also used to monitor heparin therapy to aid in detecting classical hemophilia A, Christmas disease, and congenital deficiencies of Factors II, V, VIII, IX, X, XI, and XII. Partial thromboplastin time is also used to screen for the presence of dysfibrinogenemia, disseminated intravascular coagulation, liver failure, congenital hypofibrinogenemia, vitamin K deficiency, congenital deficiency of Fitzgerald factor, congenital deficiency of prekallikrein, high molecular weight kininogen, and circulatory anticoagulant.

## Reticulocyte Count

This test is used to evaluate erythropoietic activity, which increases in acute and chronic hemorrhage and in hemolytic anemias. It is also used to evaluate erythropoietic response to antianemic therapy.

## Reverse T3

This test is useful in evaluating thyroid function and metabolism and is also used to evaluate euthyroid sick patients with low T3 concentrations.
   *Reference range: 90–350 pg/mL*

## Rheumatoid Arthritis Factor

This test is used in the differential diagnosis and prognosis of arthritic disorders.
   *Reference range: Negative: <10.0 IU/mL*

## Selenium

This test is used to monitor selenium deficiency and occupational exposure. Because selenium is a very important supplement for the extension of life, optimal levels are in the upper half of the normal range.
   *Reference ranges:*
   *Environmental Exposure: 79–326 μg/L*
   *Normal range: 46–143 μg/L*

## Sex Hormone Binding Globulin

This test is used to monitor sex hormone binding globulin levels that are under the positive control of estrogens and thyroid hormones and suppressed by androgens. Decreased levels are found in hirsutism, virilism, obese postmenopausal women, and women with diffuse hair loss. Increased levels are present in hyperthyroidism, testicular feminization, cirrhosis, male hypogonadism, pregnancy, prepubertal children, and women using oral contraceptives.
   *Reference ranges:*
   **Men** *(20–49 years): 16.5–55.9 nmol/L*
   **Men** *(>49 years): 19.3–76.4 nmol/L*
   **Women** *(20–49 years): 24.6–122.0 nmol/L*
   **Women** *(>49 years): 17.3–125.0 nmol/L*
   *LE's optimal ranges:*
   **Men:** *approximately 30–40 nmol/L, max 56 nmol/L (20–49 years) and 76 nmol/L (>49 years)*
   **Women:** *approximately 60–80 nmol/L, max 110 nmol/L (20–49 years) and 125 nmol/L (>49 years)*

*Postmenopause, no HRT: approximately 35–55 nmol/L, max 69 nmol/L*

## Sex Hormone Profile

This is a test for estradiol, progesterone, and free testosterone.

## Somatomedin-C

This is a screening test to identify patients with growth hormone deficiency, pituitary insufficiency, and acromegaly.

*Normal ranges:*
*Age (years):*
*21–25: 116–358 ng/mL*
*26–30: 117–329 ng/mL*
*31–35: 115–307 ng/mL*
*36–40: 109–284 ng/mL*
*41–45: 101–267 ng/mL*
*46–50: 94–252 ng/mL*
*51–55: 87–238 ng/mL*
*56–60: 81–225 ng/mL*
*66–70: 75–212 ng/mL*
*71–75: 64–188 ng/mL*
*76–80: 59–177 ng/mL*
*81–85: 55–166 ng/mL*

## T3 Uptake

This is a thyroid function test for the diagnosis of hypothyroidism or hyperthyroidism.

*Reference range: 24–39%*

## Testosterone (Free with Total)

Testosterone testing is used to evaluate androgen excess or deficiency related to gonadal function, adrenal function, or tumor activity. Testosterone levels in men may be helpful for the diagnosis of hypogonadism, hypopituitarism, Klinefelter syndrome, and impotence (low values). Testosterone levels in women may be requested to investigate the cause of hirsutism, anovulation, amenorrhea, virilization, masculinizing tumors of the ovary, tumors of the adrenal cortices, and congenital adrenal hyperplasia (high values).

Most circulating testosterone is bound to sex hormone-binding globulin (SHBG). A smaller amount is bound to albumin, and an even smaller proportion exists as free (bioavailable) hormone.[23] All non-SHBG-bound testosterone is referred to as free testosterone, while all bound and non-bound testosterone is referred to as total testosterone. When measuring testosterone levels, it is critical to determine both free and total testosterone to better understand the cause of any observed symptoms of deficiency.[24]

*Reference ranges:*

**Free Testosterone:**
  **Men**:
  *20–29 years: 9.3–26.5 pg/mL*
  *30–39 years: 8.7–25.1 pg/mL*
  *40–49 years: 6.8–21.5 pg/mL*
  *50–59 years: 7.2–24.0 pg/mL*
  *60+ years: 6.6–18.1 pg/mL*
  **Women:**
  *20–59 years: 0.0–2.2 pg/mL*
  *60+ years: 0.0–1.8 pg/mL*
  *LE's optimal range:*
  **Men:** *20–25 pg/mL*
  **Women:** *1–2.2 pg/mL*

**Total Testosterone:**
  **Men**: *348–1197 ng/dL*
  **Women (20–49 years)**: *8–48 ng/dL*
  **Women (>49 years)**: *3–41 ng/dL*
  *LE's optimal range:*
  **Men**: *700–900 ng/dL*
  **Women**: *35–45 ng/dL, max: 48 ng/dL*

## Thrombin and Antithrombin III

These 2 tests are used to evaluate the intrinsic coagulation system. They can determine heparin effect, warfarin anticoagulant therapy, liver failure, and Disseminated Intravascular Coagulation (DIC).

**Thrombin.** This test is used to evaluate the fibrinogen-to-fibrin reaction. It is used to determine severe hypofibrinogenemia, dysfibrinogenemia, and the presence of heparin-like anticoagulants. Thrombin levels are used to confirm and monitor DIC and fibrinolysis and can be used to monitor therapy with heparin. This test can also be used to monitor fibrinolytic therapy.

**Antithrombin III.** This test is used to evaluate the hypercoagulable state, fibrinogenolytic state, and response to heparin. Antithrombin deficiency is associated with severe cirrhosis, chronic liver failure, DIC, thrombolytic therapy, pulmonary embolism, nephrotic syndrome, or postsurgical state (especially liver transplant or partial hepatectomy).

## Thyroid Antithyroglobulin Antibody

This test is used to detect and confirm autoimmune thyroiditis and Hashimoto's thyroiditis.

*Reference range: 0-40 IU/mL*
*LE's optimal range: <5 IU/mL*

## Thyroid Stimulating Hormone (TSH)

This is a function test for thyroid disease to differentiate between primary and secondary hypothyroidism.

Some doctors believe that any TSH levels greater than 2.0 mIU/mL should be considered suspect for subclinical hypothyroidism if symptoms are present.

*Reference range: 0.46–4.50 μIU/mL*
*LE's optimal range: 1–2 μIU/mL*

## Thyroxidine (T4) Total

This is one of the first tests done in assessing thyroid function. It is used to diagnose thyroid function and to monitor replacement and suppressive therapy.

*Reference range: 4.5–12.0 μg/dL*
*LE's optimal ranges:*
**Men:** 8.5–10.5 μg/dL
**Women** (<60 years): 9–11 μg/dL
**Women** (>60 years): 8.5–10.7 μg/dL

## Thyroxine (T4) Free, Direct

This test is used to evaluate thyroid function in patients who may have protein abnormalities that could affect total T4 levels. It is also used to diagnose thyroid function and monitor replacement and suppressive therapy.

*Reference range: 0.82–1.77 ng/dL*
*LE's optimal range: upper 3rd of range*

## Tri-Iodothyronine (T3)

This is a test for thyroid function used particularly in the diagnosis of T3 thyrotoxicosis and hyperthyroidism.

*Reference range: 85–205 ng/dL*

## Tri-Iodothyronine (T3) Free

This test is used to evaluate thyroid function and assess abnormal binding protein disorders.

*Reference range: 2.0–4.4 pg/mL*
*LE's optimal range: 3.4–4.2 pg/mL*

## Troponin 1

This test is used to detect cardiac injury, predict mortality in unstable cases of angina, and serve as a marker for perioperative myocardial infarction.

*Reference range: <1.0 ng/mL*

## Tumor Necrosis Factor-alpha (TNF-α)

This test is used to identify elevated levels of tumor necrosis factor-alpha. TNF-α levels may be elevated in sepsis, cachexia, AIDS, hepatitis C, transplant rejection, various infectious, and autoimmune diseases.

*Reference range: <8.1 pg/mL*

## Urinalysis, Routine

This test is used to detect abnormalities in urine and diagnose and manage renal disease and metabolic disease, urinary tract infection and neoplasm, systemic diseases, and inflammatory or neoplastic disease.

## VAP™ Test

The VAP™ cholesterol test provides a more comprehensive lipoprotein analysis and better assesses the risk of coronary heart disease than a conventional lipid profile. It provides a direct measurement of total cholesterol, LDL-C, HDL-C, VLDL-C, Lp(a), and triglycerides as well as the qualitative assessment of LDL particle size, HDL subfractions (HDL2-C and HDL3-C), and VLDL subfractions (VLDL 1+2-C, VLDL3-C, and IDL-C). Further, the VAP™ cholesterol test provides information relating to emerging risk factors for metabolic syndrome.

## Vitamin B12 and Folate

This test measures the amount of vitamin B12 and folic acid in the blood. It is used to evaluate for malnutrition and macrocytic or megaloblastic anemia and to diagnose congenital absence of transcobalamin II or cobalophilin.

*Reference ranges:*
*B12: 211–946 pg/mL*
*Folic Acid: >5.4 ng/mL*

## Vitamin D

This test is used to rule out vitamin D deficiency as a cause of bone disease. It can also be used to identify hypercalcemia.

*Reference range: 32–100 ng/mL*
*LE's optimal range: 50–80 ng/mL*

# HOW TO ORDER BLOOD TESTS

The blood tests discussed in this protocol are available through Life Extension National Diagnostics, Inc. For ordering information, call 1-800-208-3444 anytime toll-free or visit us online at www.lef.org. You can order blood tests by mail or by calling (800) 208-3444. All tests must be prepaid. As soon as you place your order, you will be sent a package containing information regarding the location of the nearest blood-drawing stations, a Request for Phlebotomy form, and a Test Requisition form.

At your convenience, you can then take the Request for Phlebotomy and Test Requisition forms to the designated blood-drawing station in your area. A phlebotomist will draw the appropriate specimens of your blood. You (or your physician) will be mailed your test results. These results will show whether you have any abnormalities. If the results show abnormalities, make sure you show them to your physician. Your physician can determine if you have any serious problems and if so, what can be done about them.

# 25

---

# *Brain Tumor*

---

The National Cancer Institute (NCI) and the American Cancer Society (ACS) estimated that 22 020 primary malignant brain tumors would be diagnosed in 2010.[1] The American Brain Tumor Association, since they count both malignant and benign brain tumors, predicted twice as many cases.[2] Secondary brain tumors, which originate elsewhere in the body, outnumber primary tumors 4:1, so add another 100 000 cases a year to get an idea of the total number of people who will be diagnosed with brain cancer each year.[3]

The medical treatment of primary brain tumors typically consists of 2 steps: surgical excision followed by combined radiation and chemotherapy. For advanced or high-grade tumors, the benefit of these therapies seems small. "After conventional treatments, the survival rate for patients with astrocytomas or glioblastomas is about 50% at 1 year, 25% at 2 years, and 10–15% at 5 years."[4] Thus, many patients wisely seek complementary therapies hoping to improve their odds.

The risk factors for brain tumor are almost unknown, although there are hints that suggest early exposure to certain chemicals might play a role.

In 2010, the Fred Hutchinson Cancer Research Center in Seattle reported that children who develop brain tumors are likely both to have been exposed to higher than average amounts of pesticides and to have been born with a reduced ability to detoxify these chemicals.[5,6]

Other studies also point to chemical exposure as a potential risk factor. The children of women who had high exposure to beauty products are at increased risk for brain tumors.[7] Personal hair dye use increased risk in one study. Using brown hair dye for 20 years, for example, almost quadrupled risk of glioma in women.[8] Individuals who engage in a hobby that involves using glue are at 18 times the average risk.[9]

A 2009 review found that people who used cell phones for at least 10 years had a 2.4-fold greater risk of developing an acoustic neuroma in the ear to which they routinely held their phone, but had no change in risk for other types of cancer.[10]

The idea that nitrosamines in processed meats may increase the risk of glioma has been circulating for several decades,[11] yet a July 2010 paper found only a modest increase in risk in people who ate large amounts of nitrosamines compared to those who ate very little.[12]

There are no tests to predict risk of brain cancer, or steps we can take to prevent it. Our focus is on preventing recurrence, or at least slowing down the disease.

## BRAIN TUMOR NUTRITIONAL PROTOCOL

### Hormones and Brain Tumors

**Vitamin D.** Vitamin D deficiency that occurred before birth may have set the stage for brain tumor formation later in life. Vitamin D deficiency during gestation causes long-term effects on brain development.[13]

Vitamin D remains important after birth, as it activates chemical pathways, in particular the sphingomyelin pathway, which kills glioblastoma cells.[14] Vitamin D3, the chemical form of vitamin D made in the skin and sold as a nutritional supplement, calcitriol (1,25-dihydroxy vitamin D), the active form of vitamin D, and various chemical analogs and metabolites of vitamin D, have all been shown to inhibit growth and trigger apoptosis in neuroblastoma and glioma cells.[15–18]

A 2009 report on brain tumor death statistics from Finland alludes to the benefit of vitamin D. Mortality from brain tumors is highest in patients who were diagnosed and underwent surgery during the late winter, particularly from February to March. This is the time of year when vitamin D levels are at their lowest.[19] Similar seasonal variations in cancer survival rates are seen for lung,[20] breast,[21] and colon cancer.[22] The explanation tendered in all these studies is that in the winter people have lower vitamin D levels and are less capable of fighting the cancer.

Another data analysis from Spain revealed a direct correlation between latitude and brain cancer incidence. The higher the latitude, that is the farther from the Equator someone lives, the greater their risk for brain cancer.[23] The farther people live from the Equator, the lower their vitamin D levels.[24]

**Melatonin.** Melatonin is often suggested for treating various forms of cancer, particularly breast, lung, and colorectal cancers. Lissoni has conducted repeated studies demonstrating that patients with advanced cancers given melatonin survive longer than patients receiving a placebo.[25]

There is growing evidence suggesting that melatonin may be useful in treating primary brain tumors. An in vitro experiment showed that melatonin, at physiologic concentrations, inhibits growth of neuroblastoma cells.[26] A 2006 paper published in *Cancer Research* reported that melatonin stopped the growth of gliomas that had been implanted into rats.[27] As a result, some researchers suggest melatonin might be useful in treating glioma.[28]

The strongest evidence for the use of melatonin in brain cancer is in treating pituitary tumors. Melatonin given to rats inhibits the chemical-induced formation of pituitary tumors.[29] Giving melatonin to rats with pituitary tumors halts tumor growth and triggers apoptosis, especially if the tumor secretes prolactin.[30]

## Vitamins and Minerals

**Folic acid and 5-MTHF.** To be of use in the body, natural folate from food and folic acid from supplements must be converted into the active form, 5-MTHF (5-methyltetrahydrofolate), by the enzyme 5,10-methylenetetrahydrofolate reductase (MTHFR). In certain people the gene that codes for this enzyme produces a less effective enzyme. In some studies, the risk for glioma in these people is increased by about 23% while meningioma risk is more than doubled.[31–33]

People can compensate for this genetic problem by taking a supplement of active 5-MTHF and bypassing the need for the MTHFR enzyme.

A German study compared survival times of patients with glioblastoma multiforme with their MTHFR gene variants. Those patients who were best able to convert folate into its active form survived for about 13 months. Those with the less effective MTHFR genes survived for only 7 months.[34] This suggests that supplementing with the active form of folate might be helpful.

**Selenium.** Selenium is another antioxidant that patients with brain tumors should consider. Many oncologists fear that any nutritional supplement classified as an antioxidant will interfere with the ability of radiation or chemotherapy to kill cancer cells. Although this theory sounds logical, there is little published evidence to support it.

In the case of selenium, a 2004 paper in the journal *Anticancer Research* reports a "radiosensitizing effect" on glioma cells.[35] Exposing brain cancer cells to selenium makes them more sensitive to, and more likely to die after, radiation therapy.

Selenium also inhibits growth and invasion, and induces apoptosis in various types of brain tumor cells, including malignant cell lines.[36,37]

**Vitamin E.** Vitamin E is another antioxidant of particular interest in connection with brain cancer. According to a 2005 study, alpha-tocopherol-succinate enhances chemotherapy treatment of drug-resistant glioblastoma cells, increasing effectiveness.[38]

A researcher from Tufts University described the use of vitamin E in treating glioblastoma multiforme in a 2004 article in the *Journal of Nutrition*. "Glioblastoma multiforme is the most common and aggressive brain cancer in humans and resists all forms of therapy. Vitamin E (succinate) induces apoptosis in glioblastoma cells in a dose-related manner; we find that a 48-h exposure to 50 µmol/L vitamin E results in a 15% increase in apoptosis in the glioblastoma cells over control. Pretreatment with vitamin E may have a potential role in sensitizing glioblastoma to radiotherapy."[39]

## Botanical or Herbal Extracts

**Berberine.** Berberine is an alkaloid found in various different medicinal herbs. Probably the most popular herb containing berberine is goldenseal (*Hydrastis canadensis*), followed by Oregon grape (*Berberis aquifolium*) and Chinese Isatis (*Isatis tinctoria*).

A 1990 study tested the tumor-killing effect of berberine compared to the chemotherapy drug BCNU (*carmustine*) in both glioma cell cultures and in rodents implanted with tumors. Berberine alone produced a 91% kill rate in cell cultures, compared to 43% for BCNU. Combining berberine with BCNU yielded a kill rate of 97%.[40]

A 1994 paper described in vitro experiments using berberine alone, or in combination with laser treatments, on glioma cells. The combination was especially effective, suggesting "the possibility of berberine as a photosensitive agent."[41]

A 2004 paper tells us that berberine increases the benefit of radiation treatment by making glioblastoma cells more sensitive to radiation damage, without affecting healthy brain cells.[42] A similar effect is seen in lung cancer wherein berberine sensitizes lung tumor cells to radiation.[43,44]

Berberine slows the spread of nasopharyngeal carcinoma, decreasing motility of the tumor cells.[45] Berberine inhibits gene expression and enzyme activity necessary for glioblastoma and astrocytoma growth.[46] It also inhibits an enzyme called arylamine N-acetyltransferase (NAT). NAT may initiate cancer and has been correlated with the carcinogenic effect of heterocyclic aromatic amines, the kind of chemicals formed when red meat is cooked.[47]

The scientific understanding of how berberine actually works continues to advance. A 2007 description suggested that berberine acts "through several ways, such as regulating apoptotic gene expression, suppressing the formation of tumor angiogenesis [and] blocking signal transduction pathway."[48] A 2008 study explained that berberine triggers apoptosis in glioblastoma cells through the mitochondrial caspases pathway.[49] As of 2009, research reported that berberine kills glioma cells through several mechanisms: "Cytotoxicity is attributable to apoptosis mainly through induced G2/M-arrested cells, in an ER-dependent manner, via a mitochondria-dependent caspases pathway regulated by Bax and Bcl-2."[50] In 2010, explanations for action expanded to include the inhibition of NF-κB and the reduction of a series of chemicals that help cancer cells to survive, including one called survivin.[51] Survivin slows down apoptosis, allowing tumor cells to survive. Healthy cells do not produce survivin but cancer cells typically do.[52]

Several hundred published papers suggest that berberine is effective against not only brain tumors but a range of cancers. In the last few months alone, several interesting papers have been published. Among their conclusions are: berberine prevents cell growth and induces apoptosis in breast cancer cells[53,54]; berberine is cytotoxic to cervical cancer cells[55]; berberine inhibits cell growth in pancreatic cancer cells by inducing DNA damage[56]; and berberine triggers cellular suicide in tongue cancer.[57]

**Boswellia.** The resin from *Boswellia serrata* also has an important role in treating brain cancer. *Boswellia* is commonly used for treating inflammation because it acts as an NF-κB inhibitor. It is neuroprotective, anti-inflammatory, and reduces anxiety.[58]

One important use of *Boswellia* is in the treatment of traumatic brain injuries. *Boswellia* decreases the brain swelling from glioblastoma, allowing a decrease in the use of *prednisone* and thus reducing its side effects.[59]

*Boswellia* inhibits hippocampal neurodegeneration and exerts a beneficial effect on functional outcome after closed head injury, as evidenced by reduced neurological severity scores and improved cognitive ability in an object recognition test.[60]

A 2006 paper reports that *Boswellia serrata* was gaining importance in the treatment of edema surrounding tumors and other chronic inflammatory diseases. This study suggested that *Boswellia* might be considered as an alternative to corticosteroids in reducing cerebral peritumoral edema.[61]

Finding ways to reduce or replace steroid use in the treatment of brain tumors is important, since steroid drugs may protect brain tumor cells. According to a 2000 article in *Neuroscience*, "glucocorticoids are often used in the treatment of gliomas to relieve cerebral edema, the inhibition of apoptosis by these compounds could potentially interfere with the efficacy of chemotherapeutic drugs."[62]

A 2006 study reported that steroids interfere with glioma cell apoptosis.[63] Steroids block the cancer-killing action of *camptothecin*, a chemotherapy drug used in treating glioma.[64]

*Boswellia* may be doubly useful for primary brain tumors. Studies published in 2000[65] and 2002[66] tell us that in addition to helping reduce cerebral swelling around the tumor, *Boswellia* also kills glioblastoma cells in a dose-dependent manner.

*Boswellia* is also useful for treating secondary brain tumors. In 2007, researchers reported using *Boswellia* to treat a patient with breast cancer metastasis to the brain. Familiar with the German research on using *Boswellia* in the treatment of primary brain tumors, the team tried it with these secondary brain tumors and reported benefit. After 10 weeks of *Boswellia* treatment in combination with radiation treatment, all signs of brain metastases on the patient's CT scans had disappeared.[67]

**Curcumin.** Curcumin is extracted from turmeric rhizomes (*Curcuma longa*), a plant that has been eaten for thousands of years. As of this writing, the National Institute of Health's website, PubMed, lists 1335 published papers on curcumin and cancer in the peer-reviewed scientific literature.

A growing number of these studies focus specifically on using curcumin in connection with brain cancer. A 2006 paper tells us curcumin suppresses growth of glioblastoma by triggering the apoptotic pathways that destroy glioblastoma cells.[68] Curcumin turns off the signals in the cells that protect glioblastoma cells from apoptosis, allowing the suicide process to destroy the cancer cells.[69,70]

Curcumin has a similar action against other brain tumor types, including medulloblastoma cells and pituitary cancers.[71,72] Curcumin inhibits pituitary cancer from forming.[73] It also slows growth of pituitary tumors and inhibits production of excess pituitary hormones by tumors.[74,75]

Curcumin's mechanisms of action are complex. It acts through multiple pathways, interfering with cancer growth and stimulating cancer destruction.[76] Curcumin decreases glial cell line-derived neurotrophic factor (GDNF), a chemical that promotes tumor migration and invasion.[77,78] It also acts as an angiogenesis inhibitor.[79]

An article in *Brain Research* confirms that curcumin crosses the blood–brain barrier, thus reaching the brain and any tumor cells there.[80]

A study published in the *Journal of Neurochemistry* reported that curcumin sensitized glioma cells to several of the chemotherapy drugs often utilized to treat brain cancers (*cisplatin, etoposide, camptothecin,* and *doxorubicin*) as well as to radiation. "These findings support a role for curcumin as an adjunct to traditional chemotherapy and radiation in the treatment of brain cancer."[81]

Curcumin has long been known for poor bioavailability, requiring high doses to achieve desired blood levels. A novel curcumin formulation, BCM-95®, has been developed. It delivers up to 7 times more bioactive curcumin to the blood than earlier curcumin formulations. Human evidence for the increased bioavailability of BCM-95® was published in a 2008 study in the *Indian Journal of Pharmaceutical Science*.[82] An earlier animal trial was published in *Spice India* in 2006.[83]

## Other Natural Ingredients

**Quercetin.** Quercetin enhances glioma cell death.[84] While killing cancer cells, quercetin protects healthy brain cells.[85]

An especially interesting study tested a combination of quercetin and the chemotherapy drug *temozolomide* (Temodar®) on astrocytoma tumor cells. Temozolomide is commonly used for the treatment of glioma in conjunction with radiation therapy. This drug typically kills brain tumor cells by triggering a process called autophagy, while quercetin promotes necrosis in a dose-dependent manner. This study reported for the first time that quercetin combined with temozolomide was much more effective in inducing apoptosis, programmed cell death, in glioma cells than was either substance alone. To quote the authors, "Our results indicate that quercetin acts in synergy with temozolomide and when used in combination rather than in separate pharmacological application, both drugs are more effective in programmed cell death induction. Temozolomide administered with quercetin seems to be a potent and promising combination which might be useful in glioma therapy."[86]

**Resveratrol.** Resveratrol also strongly inhibits brain tumor cells.[87–89] Quercetin and resveratrol, when taken together "presented a strong synergism in inducing senescence-like growth arrest. These results suggest that combining these polyphenols can potentiate their antitumoral activity, thereby reducing the therapeutic concentration needed for glioma treatment."[90]

**Green tea and coffee.** People who drink 5 cups per day of tea or coffee are 40% less likely to get glioma.[91]

A 2006 study informed us that the EGCG in green tea reduces the radio-resistance of glioblastoma cells potentially increasing the benefit of the standard radiation and chemotherapy treatment of this cancer.[68]

Caffeine, found in significant quantities in coffee and green tea, inhibits migration of glioblastoma cells and increases survival.[92] It also makes glioma cells more sensitive to ionizing radiation and chemotherapy.[93] Caffeine enhances the effect of temozolomide in radiation treatments.[94]

At least part of the explanation for these benefits is that coffee is a peroxisome proliferator-activated receptor (PPAR) gamma agonist.[95] PPAR gamma agonists inhibit brain tumor growth and possibly even brain cancer stem cells.[96,97]

**Sulforaphane.** Sulforaphane is one of the active compounds in cruciferous vegetables, especially broccoli, responsible for their anticancer action.

Sulforaphane activates "multiple molecular mechanisms for apoptosis in glioblastoma cells following treatment."[98]

Resveratrol and sulforaphane act synergistically against brain tumor cells. A 2010 article states, "Combination treatment with resveratrol and sulforaphane inhibits cell proliferation and migration, and reduces cell viability. Resveratrol and sulforaphane may be a viable approach for the treatment of glioma."[99]

# A DIET FOR BRAIN CANCER

There are 2 specific diets that should be considered for treating brain tumors, either separately or in combination.

## Ketogenic Diet

The ketogenic diet is a very high-fat, high-protein, and extremely low-carbohydrate diet typically used to treat epilepsy.[100]

Without carbohydrates, the body shifts from using glucose to ketones for energy. Healthy brain cells can utilize either glucose or ketones. Brain tumor cells can only burn glucose. The theory is that switching to ketones for energy starves brain tumor cells.

A 2007 study tested this theory on mice implanted with malignant brain tumors. The treatment group was fed a drink high in fat and protein that was designed to cause ketosis in children with epilepsy, and the control group was fed a low-fat, high-carbohydrate diet. The ketone-producing diet decreased growth of the brain tumors from 35–65%, depending on the tumor line, and significantly enhanced health and survival compared to the control group, which was on the low-fat, high-carbohydrate diet.[101]

In 1995, doctors from Case Western Reserve reported treating 2 young girls suffering from astrocytomas with low-carbohydrate ketogenic diets. One of the girls had a favorable clinical response without reported disease progression for 12 months at the time of publication.[102]

In April 2010, a case report was published describing an older female patient treated for glioblastoma multiforme with an initial 2-day water fast followed by a ketogenic diet and then simply a caloric-restricted diet. The tumor regressed during treatment, getting smaller on subsequent scans from January until July, at which point the patient stopped following the diet. The tumor returned 10 weeks later.[103]

At this point, the evidence supporting the management of brain cancer through a ketogenic diet is intriguing, and the risks are minimal.[104]

### Caloric Restriction

Caloric restriction also appears to slow brain tumor growth. A 2002 study reported experiments on mice with brain tumors. Compared to mice that were not restricted in their food intake, the brain tumors in mice on a calorie-restricted diet grew slower, were less dense, and displayed less angiogenesis (building new blood vessels to feed the tumor). The tumor cells in the caloric-restricted mice were more likely to undergo apoptosis.[105]

A July 2010 paper confirmed the benefit in mice with glioblastoma multiforme. Caloric restriction was effective in reducing malignant brain tumor growth and invasion.[106]

Caloric restriction, although it may put the body into ketosis, is thought to act differently than the ketogenic diet. Hunger puts a mild stress on the body. Mild stress is, in turn, hypothesized to create a *hormetic* reaction that awakens protective mechanisms within the body, stimulating the individual cells to fight the cancer.[107]

Researchers at Boston College are now investigating the simultaneous implementation of both of these dietary strategies by using a caloric-restricted ketogenic diet against brain cancer.[108]

## SUMMARY

Given the inadequacy of standard medical treatment in controlling high-grade malignant brain tumors, this approach of co-treating brain tumors with brain tumor-specific diet and nutritional supplementation, in addition to the medical oncology standard of care, is an option that offers hope to those afflicted with brain tumors.

Because of the synergistic effects between various anticancer nutrients and phytochemicals, the Life Extension Foundation recommends use of a wide variety of these substances rather than attempting to rely on large doses of single nutrients to fight cancer.

## ANTIDEPRESSANTS AND BRAIN TUMORS

People with brain tumors should be selective about antidepressants.

There is a chemical made in the brain called *glial cell-line derived neurotrophic factor* (GDNF). It typically aids the survival of neurons after injury. The problem is that it also helps brain tumor cells survive, and, in particular, gliomas. It also helps tumor cells migrate and invade surrounding brain tissue.[77,78,109]

Many antidepressants increase GDNF and thus may help tumor cells survive treatment. A 2007 paper reported that amitriptyline, a tricyclic antidepressant, did so.[110] Serotonin itself increases GDNF.[111] Antidepressants classified as selective serotonin reuptake inhibitors (SSRIs), which increase serotonin levels in the brain, may therefore increase GDNF, increasing tumor survival and helping it spread farther into the brain.

While SSRIs might pose a problem, certain tricyclic antidepressants may be useful in treating brain tumors. A 2010 paper reported the effects of several tricyclic antidepressants on the cellular respiration rates of malignant glioma cells. Lowered cellular respiration rates are an indirect measure of increased apoptosis. *Clomipramine* (Anafranil®) was the most potent inhibitor of cellular respiration in glioma cells. Of even more interest, combining clomipramine with the steroid drug *dexamethasone* had a synergistic effect, increasing cell death rates even further.[112] This research is still in its early stages. In the future, though, doctors may prescribe specific antidepressants during brain cancer treatments with the intention of increasing tumor cell death.

## STEROID MEDICATIONS AND BRAIN TUMORS

Steroids are a potential problem in patients with brain cancer. Almost all patients who undergo surgery or radiation treatment will be prescribed some form of steroid medication, such as prednisone, as part of their treatment. These drugs are needed to reduce brain swelling. The problem is that these drugs may inhibit apoptosis in glioma cells, preventing cancer cell death. A 2000 paper concluded, "Since glucocorticoids are often used in the treatment of gliomas to relieve cerebral edema, the inhibition of apoptosis by these compounds could potentially interfere with the efficacy of chemotherapeutic drugs."[62] Steroids also block the chemotherapy drug *camptothecin* from killing glioma cells.[64]

Patients should be cautious in using these drugs. Concomitant use of curcumin and *Boswellia* may act to reduce inflammation, reducing the necessity for steroids.

## Life Extension Suggestions

- **Vitamin D3:** 5000 IU daily. Blood levels of vitamin D3 should be monitored and kept at 50–80 ng/mL on any 25(OH)D3 serum test.
- **Melatonin:** 10–20 mg before bed each night
- **Selenium:** 200 mcg daily
- **Vitamin E succinate** (alpha-tocopherol-succinate): 400 IU daily
- **Berberine:** 500–1000 mg daily
- **Boswellia:** 500–1000 mg daily

- **Curcumin** (BCM-95®): 400–1200 mg daily
- **Quercetin:** 1000 mg daily
- **Green tea extract:** 700–2100 mg of EGCG daily
- **_Trans_-resveratrol:** 500 mg daily
- **Sulforaphane:** 60–90 mg daily

## REFERENCES

References available at: www.lef.org/dpt5/ch25

# 26

# *Breast Cancer*

Most women share a fear of developing breast cancer. This is not an unfounded fear when considering that, except for lung cancer, breast cancer is the most common cancer found in women, accounting for one of every 3 diagnoses. However, men are also affected by breast cancer. In 2002, the American Cancer Association estimated that 1500 men would be diagnosed with breast cancer, and 400 would die as a result. In 2001, an estimated 192 200 American women were diagnosed with breast cancer and 39 600 women died of the disease.

## WHAT IS BREAST CANCER?

Breast cancer occurs when cells in the breast tissue divide and grow without control. The cell cycle is the natural mechanism that regulates the growth and death of cells. When the normal cell regulators malfunction and cells do not die at the proper rate, there is a failure of cell death (apoptosis); therefore, cell growth goes unchecked. As a result, cancer begins to develop as cells divide without control, accumulating into a mass of extra tissue called a tumor. A tumor can be either noncancerous (benign) or cancerous (malignant). As a tumor grows, it elicits new blood vessel growth from the surrounding normal healthy tissues and diverts blood supply and nutrients away from this tissue to feed itself. This process is termed "angiogenesis," meaning the development (genesis) of new blood vessels (angio). Unregulated tumor angiogenesis facilitates the growth of cancer throughout the body.

Cancer cells have the ability to leave the original tumor site, travel to distant locations, and recolonize. This process is called metastasis and it occurs in organs such as the liver, lungs, and bones. Both the bloodstream and lymphatic system (the network connecting lymph nodes throughout the body) serve as ideal vehicles for the traveling cancer. Although these traveling cancer cells do not always survive beyond the tumor, if they do survive, the cancer cells will again begin to divide abnormally and create tumors in each new location. A person with untreated or treatment-resistant cancer may eventually die of the disease if vital organs such as the liver or lungs are invaded, overtaken, and destroyed.

Cancerous tumors in the breast usually grow slowly. It is thought that by the time a tumor is large enough to be felt as a lump, it may have been growing for as long as 10 years. This has lead to the belief that undetectable spread of tumor cells (micrometastasis) may have already occurred by the time of the diagnosis. Therefore, preventive measures such as a healthy balanced diet and lifestyle, nutritional supplementation, and exercise are of primary importance against the development of cancer. Early diagnosis is the best way to reduce the risk of dying from breast cancer. This can be accomplished by monthly self-breast exams, annual clinical breast exams, and screening mammography. If breast cancer is detected, a multimodality approach incorporating nutritional supplementation, dietary modification, detoxification, and one or more of the following may be considered: surgery, chemotherapy, radiation, hormone therapy, or vaccine therapy.

## RISK FACTORS

A wide variety of factors may influence an individual's likelihood of developing breast cancer; these factors are referred to as risk factors. The established risk factors for breast cancer include: female gender, age, previous breast cancer, benign breast disease, hereditary factors (family history of breast cancer), early age at menarche (first menstrual period), late age at menopause, late age at first full-term pregnancy, obesity, low physical activity, use of postmenopausal hormone replacement therapy, use of oral contraceptives, exposure to low-dose ionizing radiation in midlife, and exposure to high-dose ionizing radiation early in life.

Correlated risk factors for breast cancer include never having been pregnant, having only one pregnancy rather than many, not breast feeding after pregnancy, diethylstilbestrol (DES), certain dietary practices (high intake of fat and low intakes of fiber, fruits, and vegetables), tobacco, smoking, abortion, breast trauma, breast augmentation, large breast size, synthetic estrogens, electromagnetic fields, use of nonsteroidal anti-inflammatory drugs (NSAIDs), and alcohol consumption. Alcohol is known to increase estrogen levels. Alcohol use appears to be more strongly associated with risk of lobular carcinomas and hormone receptor–positive tumors than it is with other types of breast cancer.[1]

A novel growth inhibitor recently identified as estrogen downregulated gene 1 (EDG1) was found to be switched off (downregulated) by estrogens. Inhibiting EDG1 expression in breast cells resulted in increased breast cell growth, whereas over-expression of EDG1 protein in breast cells resulted in decreased cell growth and decreased anchorage-independent growth, supporting the role of EDG1 in breast cancer.[2]

Regular screening is especially important for women who are at high risk of breast cancer. A woman can be placed in a high-risk category if she possesses either a single factor that greatly increases her risk or a combination of lesser factors that together increase her risk.

Single factors that can place a woman in a high-risk category include a personal history of breast cancer, carcinoma in situ, atypical hyperplasia, and exposure to high doses of ionizing radiation in childhood or young adulthood (eg, for treatment of Hodgkin's disease).[3-5] A family history of breast cancer, especially in a mother, sister, or daughter, or a particular genetic mutation can also place a woman at high risk of breast cancer. In addition, research on genetic markers for breast-cancer risk has pinpointed a number of genes, 2 of which (BRCA1 and BRCA2) are associated with a markedly elevated risk of breast and ovarian cancer. As many as 60–80% of women with mutations in either of these 2 genes may develop breast cancer in their lifetimes.[6-8]

There are also several moderate risk factors for breast cancer, which occurring together can place a woman at high risk. They include having a first period (menarche) before age 12, not bearing a child, and having a first child after age 30. It is recommended that women at high risk for breast cancer have annual clinical breast examinations more frequently than women at average risk.

## ANATOMY OF THE BREAST

The breast is composed mainly of fat (adipose tissue) and breast tissue, along with connective tissue, nerves, veins, and arteries. Breast tissue is a complex network known as the mammary gland. Within the mammary gland, there are 15–20 lobes or compartments separated by adipose tissue. Within each lobe are several smaller compartments called lobules.

Lobules are composed of grapelike clusters of milk-secreting glands termed alveoli, which are found embedded in connective tissue. Spindle-shaped cells called myoepithelial cells, whose contractions help propel milk toward the nipple, surround the alveoli. There are about 1 million lobules contained within each breast.[9] The lobules are connected by tiny ducts that are joined together (much like a grape stem) into increasingly

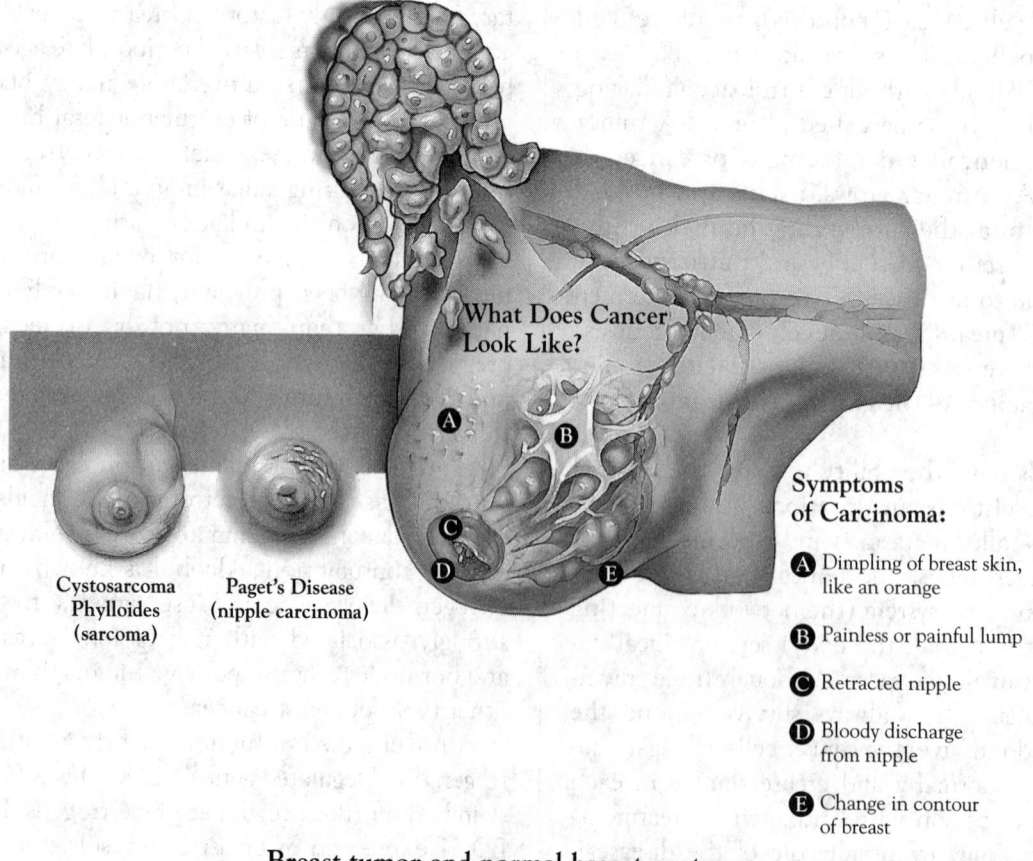

What Does Cancer Look Like?

Cystosarcoma Phylloides (sarcoma)

Paget's Disease (nipple carcinoma)

**Symptoms of Carcinoma:**

Ⓐ Dimpling of breast skin, like an orange

Ⓑ Painless or painful lump

Ⓒ Retracted nipple

Ⓓ Bloody discharge from nipple

Ⓔ Change in contour of breast

**Breast tumor and normal breast anatomy**

larger ducts. Within each breast there are 5–10 ductal systems, each with its own opening at the nipple.

Surrounding the nipple is a darkly shaded circle of skin called the areola. The areola appears rough because it contains modified sebaceous (oil) glands. These glands secrete small amounts of fluid to lubricate the nipple during breastfeeding.

Of all breast cancers, about 80% originate in the mammary (lactiferous) ducts, while about 20% arise in the lobules.[10] One of the most important distinctions to understand is the difference between invasive breast cancer and carcinoma in situ.

## TYPES OF BREAST CANCER

### Invasive Cancer

When abnormal cells from within the lobules or mammary ducts break out into the surrounding tissue the condition is referred to as invasive breast cancer. However, this term does not necessarily mean that metastases have been found anywhere beyond the breast.

### Carcinoma In Situ

Carcinoma in situ is referred to as precancerous condition because it can increase the risk of developing cancer. When abnormal cells grow within the lobules or mammary ducts and there is no sign that the cells have spread into the surrounding tissue or beyond, the condition is called carcinoma in situ. The term in situ means "in place."

Noninvasive cancer is grouped into 4 subcategories, based on how the cells grow relative to each other within the center of the milk duct:

- **Solid:** There is wall-to-wall cell growth.
- **Cribriform:** There are holes between groups of cells, making it look like Swiss cheese.
- **Papillary:** The cells grow in fingerlike projections, toward the inside of the duct.
- **Comedo:** There are areas of "necrosis," which is debris from dead cells; this indicates that a tumor is growing so fast that some tumor cells die because there is insufficient blood supply.

There are 2 main categories of carcinoma in situ: ductal carcinoma in situ (DCIS) and lobular carcinoma in situ (LCIS).

**Ductal carcinoma in situ.** Mammary ducts are hollow to allow fluid to pass through. However, with DCIS, excess cells grow inside the mammary ducts. DCIS is not invasive cancer. It is a precancerous condition that has the potential to develop into breast cancer. DCIS is, however, a risk factor for breast cancer.

**Lobular carcinoma in situ.** The lobules of the breast tissue have open space inside them much like the mammary ducts. LCIS is the growth and accumulation of large numbers of abnormal cells within the lobules. LCIS is often referred to as lobular neoplasia in situ. LCIS is not a direct cancer precursor. The abnormal cells found inside the lobules are not likely to mutate into cancer. LCIS is, however, a risk factor for breast cancer.

## SPECIAL MANIFESTATIONS OF CANCER

### Paget's Disease of the Nipple

Paget's disease is a rare, slowly growing cancer of the nipple. Paget's disease is usually associated with in situ or invasive cancer. One of the biggest problems with Paget's disease of the nipple is that its symptoms appear to be harmless. It is frequently thought to be a skin inflammation or infection, leading to unfortunate delays in disease detection, diagnosis, and treatment. Symptoms of Paget's disease include persistent redness, itching, oozing, crusting, and fluid discharge from the nipple or a sore on the nipple that does not heal. Typically, only one nipple is affected. Treatment and prognosis for the disease are directly related to the type and extent of the underlying cancer.

### Inflammatory Breast Cancer

Inflammatory breast cancer (IBC) is a rare and aggressive form of invasive breast cancer that is usually not detected by mammograms or ultrasounds. IBC usually grows in nests or sheets rather than as a confined solid tumor and can be diffuse throughout the breast with no palpable mass. The cancer cells clog the lymphatic system just below the skin, resulting in lymph node involvement. Increased breast density compared to prior mammograms should be considered suspicious.

However, the main symptoms of IBC are breast swelling, inflammation, pink, red, or a dark colored area (erythema), sometimes with texture similar to the skin of an orange (peau d'orange), ridges and thickened areas of the breast skin, an area of the breast that is warm to the touch, what appears to be a persistent bruise, itching (pruritus) that is unrelenting and unaffected by medicated creams and ointments, increase in breast size over a short period of time, nipple flattening, retraction, or discharge, breast pain that is not cyclic in nature and may be constant or stabbing, or swollen lymph nodes in the armpit or above the collar bone. Since many of these symptoms mimic a breast infection, doctors frequently treat inflammatory breast cancer merely as an infection. When symptoms do not improve after antibiotic treatment for the suspected "infection," only then is the inflammatory breast cancer diagnosed.

IBC has an extremely high risk of recurrence and a very poor prognosis. It is the most lethal form of breast cancer. To improve the chances of survival, it is important that symptoms are recognized early, resulting in an immediate diagnosis and treatment. Chemotherapy is usually begun within days of diagnosis. Without treatment, chances of 5-year survival for individuals with inflammatory breast cancer are very poor. With treatment, about 50% of patients will be living 5 years after diagnosis.

# BREAST DISEASES

There are a variety of breast diseases, ranging from infections to excessive cell growth (neoplasms). Unfortunately, many breast diseases mimic the symptoms of cancer and therefore require tests and possibly surgical biopsy to obtain an accurate diagnosis. The majority of biopsies are found to be benign (noncancerous) forms of breast disease. While most breast diseases are not dangerous in themselves, they may increase the risk of developing breast cancer. Hyperplasia, cysts, fibroadenomas, and calcifications are the common benign breast diseases.

## Calcifications

Calcifications are randomly scattered residues of calcium, that in older women, may have left the bones to appear in other parts of the body (eg, joints or breasts). Microcalcifications are small, tight clusters of tiny calcifications in the ducts that can be seen on a mammogram and may indicate a precancerous or cancerous condition.

## Cysts

Cysts are sacs filled with fluid; they are almost always benign. Although most are too small to feel, approximately a third of women aged 35–50 have cysts in their breasts. If large enough, cysts may feel like lumps in the breast. Normally, cysts are left untreated. However, if a cyst becomes painful, it can be aspirated or drained of its fluid. Some women may prefer to have a cyst removed if, after being aspirated repeatedly, it continues to recur.

Cysts are not associated with an increased risk of cancer; yet, they are more common in women as they approach menopause and occur much less frequently after menopause.[11] What causes cysts to develop is unknown; however, certain dietary factors, such as the intake of caffeine have been proposed as possible risk factors for the development of breast cysts.

## Fibroadenomas

Fibroadenomas are a type of benign lump most commonly found in younger women. They are usually not removed since they pose no risk. If a fibroadenoma is large, uncomfortable, and produces a lump, it may be removed. In older women, fibroadenomas are generally removed to ensure that they are not malignant tumors. Fibroadenomas do not pose an increased risk of cancer.

## Hyperplasia

Hyperplasia is not a precancerous condition. It is the excessive accumulation or proliferation of normal cells typically found on the inside of the lobules or the ducts in the breast tissue. Hyperplasia is associated with approximately a two-fold risk of breast cancer.

## Atypical Hyperplasia

Atypical hyperplasia occurs when excess cells in the lobules or ducts are abnormal. This condition falls between hyperplasia (too many normal cells) and carcinoma in situ (too many abnormal cells). However, atypical hyperplasia is associated with an approximately 3.5–5 times increased risk of developing breast cancer.[12–14]

# TYPES OF STANDARD SCREENING TECHNIQUES

In order to detect breast cancer at its earliest, most treatable stage, the importance of regular monthly breast self-exams and yearly clinical breast exams cannot be overemphasized. Mammography, sonography, contrasting magnetic resonance imaging (MRI) and digital infrared thermal imaging are all viable diagnostic tools, which will be discussed later in this protocol. Having regular breast-cancer screening exams is considered the single most effective way to lower the risk of dying from breast cancer.

"Early-stage" invasive cancer is considered very treatable because the tumor is relatively small and the cancer cells have not spread to the lymph nodes. However, when a tumor has become very large or has spread to other organs (such as the liver, lungs, or bones), it is considered "advanced-stage" invasive cancer and is far less treatable.

Breast cancer was thought to grow in an orderly progression from a small tumor in the breast tissue to a larger tumor. The cancer was believed to then travel from the breast into the adjacent lymph nodes, spreading throughout the distant nodes and finally metastasizing in other areas of the body. However, a growing body of research now contends that cancer cells are capable of traveling from the breast throughout the blood and lymphatic systems very early in the course of the disease. This strengthens the rationale for early detection and treatment.

## Breast Self-Exam

A breast self-exam provides an opportunity to detect tumors that may develop in the time between yearly clinical breast exams. To increase a woman's chances of detecting a small tumor at a time when it may be more responsive to treatment, a breast self-exam should be performed monthly, usually 2–3 days after menstruation. For women with irregular periods, it is important to remember to perform a monthly exam on the same day each month. Keep in mind that prior to menstruation or during pregnancy, breasts may be somewhat lumpy or more tender than usual.

By performing self-exams once a month, women can become familiar with the normal appearance and "feel" of their breasts, increasing the likelihood of recognizing changes such as thickening, lumps, or spontaneous nipple discharge. Because breast tissue normally has a bumpy texture, it may feel lumpy. However, there can be a great deal of individual variation. If a breast has lumpiness throughout, then it is probably just the normal contours of the breast tissue and in most cases is no cause to worry. Dominant lumps are firmer than the rest of the breast and are of more concern. When a dominant lump is found, there is an increased risk that it may be cancer, even though cysts and fibroadenomas can cause similar lumps. Any time a woman discovers a lump that feels dominant, it should be checked by a medical professional.

*How to do breast self-exam:*

1. Lie down. Flatten your right breast by placing a pillow or towel under your right shoulder. Place your right arm behind your head. Examine your right breast with your left hand.

2. Use the pads, not the tips, of the middle 3 fingers on your left hand. With fingers flat, press gently using a circular, rubbing motion and feel for lumps. In small, dime-sized circles without lifting the fingers, start at the outermost top edge of your breast and spiral in toward the nipple.

3. Press firmly enough to feel the different breast tissues, using 3 different pressures. First, light pressure to just move the skin without jostling the tissue beneath, then medium pressure pressing midway into the tissue, and finally deep pressure to probe more deeply down to the ribs or to the point just short of discomfort.

4. Completely feel all of the breast and chest area up under your armpit, up to the collarbone, and all the way over to your shoulder to cover breast tissue that extends toward the shoulder.

5. Gently squeeze both nipples and look for discharge.

After you have completely examined your right breast, examine your left breast using the same method with your right hand. You may want to examine your breasts or do an extra exam while showering. It is easy to slide soapy hands over your skin and feel anything unusual. You should also check your breasts in a mirror, looking for any change in size or contour, dimpling of the skin, or spontaneous nipple discharge.

## Clinical Breast Exam

Clinical breast exams are physical examinations to check the appearance and "feel" of the breasts for signs of lumps. A physician, nurse practitioner, or other trained medical staff person will examine the breasts, both when the woman is sitting upright and when she is lying down.

Clinical breast exams are an important part of breast cancer screening. For younger women, clinical breast exam may have an advantage over mammography; mammography images can be more difficult to read in some younger women because of their dense breast tissue. For this reason, clinical breast exams are generally started much earlier than mammograms.

## Mammography

Mammography is an x-ray technique used to locate small or indistinctly shaped breast lumps that may not be felt during an exam. A mammogram takes about 15 minutes and consists of compressing each breast individually between 2 plates to make an x-ray image. Afterwards, a radiologist will read the film and look for any signs of abnormal tissue.

X-ray images appear in gradations of black, gray, and white depending on the density or hardness of the tissue. For example, since bone is especially dense, it appears white on an x-ray, while fat appears dark gray. Cancerous tumors and some other noncancerous abnormalities appear as a lighter shade of gray. Unfortunately, this may pose a problem because normal, dense breast tissue may appear light gray on a mammogram. Breast density changes with age. Younger women have proportionately more breast tissue than fat and therefore denser breasts, making mammograms difficult to interpret. In older women's breasts, density dissipates with age, leaving breasts that are composed mostly of fat. A mammogram that shows the light gray patch of a tumor or lesion surrounded by the dark gray image of fat tissue is most easily recognized.

Cysts and fibroadenomas appear as circular or oval patches with stark outer edges on x-rays, allowing a radiologist to identify where the border of the benign abnormal tissue ends and the surrounding normal tissue begins. On an x-ray, the core cancerous cells appear as a light patch, while the cancer cells that invade the surrounding tissue create a fuzzy or spiky appearance along the outer edge (called "spiculated"), producing an image with no clear borders.

There is growing controversy regarding the safety and efficacy of mammography. The National Cancer Institute clearly states on their website "Being exposed to radiation is a risk factor for breast cancer."[15] Further, both low-filtered (30-kVp) x-rays and mammography x-rays have mutagenic effect on mammalian cells. A re-evaluation of the risk assessment of mammography, especially for familial predisposed women is recommended. People with known increased risk of breast cancer, particularly those with a familial predisposition, are advised to be cautious and avoid early and frequent mammography exposure. Alternative examination methods should be considered for women with an inherited increased risk of breast cancer.[16]

There is evidence that high-quality mammography may reduce breast cancer mortality in women aged 50–69. In fact, the risk of radiation-induced breast cancer decreases with increasing age at radiation exposure.[17] There has been difficulty in establishing the benefit of screening mammography in younger women. This difficulty has been attributed to both the technical limitations introduced by younger women's dense breast tissue and to differences in breast cancer biology in younger women. Equally, women with inherited increased risk for breast cancer may gain no benefits from early screening.

The false positive rate ranges from 2.6–15.9%.[18] False positives usually result in additional diagnostic tests, which can include an additional x-ray examination, or a biopsy, which is the removal of a small portion of breast tissue for microscopic examination. A portion of the population's mammograms are misread as false negatives. A false negative mammogram occurs when the mammogram is read as "normal" or "negative" although a malignancy is present. Screening mammograms from a population-based screening registry estimated a missed detectable cancer rate of 29%.[19] Other studies report a missed detectable cancer rate by mammograms of approximately 12–37%.[20]

Regardless of the high rates of false-positives and false-negatives, x-ray mammography is still considered the gold standard of breast cancer screening since it can detect tumors at an early stage when they are small and responsive to treatment. Most physicians recommend annual mammograms for women over 40, and for those at high risk with a family history of breast cancer.

## Ultrasound

Ultrasound, also known as sonography, is an imaging method that utilizes very-high frequency sound waves to produce a picture that outlines the breast without exposure to ionizing radiation. During a sonogram (also known as echogram), sound waves are transmitted through the breast. Depending on the nature of the breast tissue, the sound waves are reflected back or are transmitted through the tissue being examined. The pictures generated are the results of such echoes; they are picked up and translated by a computer resulting in the ultrasound image. Breast ultrasonography can be used to evaluate breast problems found during a mammogram or a physical exam.

Ultrasound is useful for some breast masses. It can be used to determine if a breast mass is solid (and more likely to be malignant) or if it is cystic and filled with fluid (and more likely to be benign). The ultrasound facilitates analysis by enabling the radiologist to guide a needle to biopsy a solid mass or to remove fluid if it is a cystic fluid-filled mass. The limitation of both mammography and ultrasound is that both have diagnostic features, which depend primarily on structural distinction and anatomical variation of a tumor from the surrounding breast tissue. These limitations make distinguishing benign microcalcifications from malignancies nearly impossible.

## Magnetic Resonance Imaging

Magnetic resonance imaging (MRI) of the breast is an imaging method consisting of a high-field (1.5 Tesla) magnet with dedicated breast coils linked to a computer. The most useful MRI breast examination combines a contrast material (known as gadolinium DTPA), magnetization, and radio waves to provide detailed pictures of an area inside the breast by a computer without the use of radiation. Every MRI produces hundreds of images of the breast from side-to-side, top-to-bottom, and front-to-back.

MRI is the most sensitive imaging modality for detection of breast cancer.[21,22] Unfortunately, an MRI cannot always accurately distinguish between cancer and benign (noncancerous) breast conditions. Like ultrasound, MRI cannot detect microcalcifications. MRI is, however, effective in evaluating dense breast tissue and may be useful in screening younger women at high risk for breast cancer due to a predisposing family history of breast cancer.

MRI can be used to evaluate women who have had augmentation or breast enlargement surgery using implants. In such context, MRI is an excellent tool for imaging the augmented breast, including the breast implants itself, and the surrounding tissue, since abnormalities or signs of breast cancer are sometimes obscured by the implant. In contrast, the x-rays used in mammography are not able to penetrate silicone or saline implants sufficiently to image the overlying or underlying breast tissue. Compared to mammography or ultrasound, MRI is more accurate in women with augmented breasts.

## Thermography

Digital infrared thermal imaging, also known as thermography, is a painless, noninvasive diagnostic technique, which does not involve any radiation exposure. This technology at one time appeared promising but lost favor about 20 years ago. However, with new ultrasensitive high-resolution digital infrared devices, its efficacy has been improved. Infrared imaging software utilizes high precision pixel temperature measurements that can detect minute temperature variations related to blood flow and demonstrate abnormal blood flow patterns associated with the initiation and progression of a chaotic tumor vasculature (blood flow system). Angiogenesis is a key factor that facilitates the growth of cancer, and it is this biological feature of cancer on which thermography is based. Due to thermography's sensitivity to blood flow and metabolic changes, it can detect tumors at a smaller size than mammography.

Unfortunately, there are no studies involving the detection of breast cancer that compare the accuracy of digital infrared thermal imaging to that of mammography, ultrasound, and MRI. However, studies have been conducted to evaluate the accuracy of mammography versus ultrasound versus MRI. In a study that screened 192 women at high risk for breast cancer, cancer was detected in 9 patients. Mammography and ultrasound detected 6 of the 9 cases of cancer whereas MRI detected all 9 cases of breast cancer.[21]

Another study comparing the accuracy of these 3 modalities screened 196 women at high risk for hereditary breast cancer and detected a total of 6 cases of invasive breast cancer. Mammography detected 2 of the 6 cases, ultrasound detected 3 of the 6, and MRI detected all 6 cases.[22]

## TYPES OF ABNORMAL SCREENING FINDINGS

Typically, a clinical breast exam or mammogram will show no sign of disease. However, for some women, the test results will prove to be abnormal, and they will need to have additional tests to determine whether

they have cancer. Which tests are performed depends on a number of factors, such as the type of abnormality found and the age of the woman. Usually the follow-up tests begin with the least invasive methods, such as an ultrasound or second mammogram, and progress, if necessary, to the more invasive methods, such as a needle or surgical biopsy. A biopsy should spare the tissue, removing just enough tissue to make a diagnosis without being unnecessarily invasive. A woman should not rush from one abnormal screening mammogram or clinical breast exam to a major invasive surgical procedure or to treatment for breast cancer. Following the series of tests outlined in the sections that follow may help avoid unnecessary procedures.

### From a Clinical Breast Exam

A lump called a palpable mass is the most common abnormal finding from a clinical breast exam. The first determination that must be made is whether the mass is solid or fluid-filled. Most likely, if it is fluid-filled, the mass is a cyst. Simple fluid-filled cysts are not cancerous and can be left untreated in many cases. However, complex cysts contain both solid tissue and fluid and may need additional examination to assure they are not cancerous. Solid masses, on the other hand, are potentially cancerous.

**For individuals age 30 and older.**   The general approach to follow up a palpable mass involves further examination of the mass with a diagnostic mammogram, ultrasound, or needle biopsy. Mammography with or without an ultrasound is often the first choice. However, a person with a mass that is likely not cancerous may choose to begin follow-up with a needle biopsy. Instead of an initial needle biopsy, most individuals with a palpable mass begin follow-up tests with a mammogram and/or ultrasound of the mass. This imaging may help avoid a needle biopsy by identifying a mass as a simple cyst, complex cyst, or a suspicious mass that could be cancerous.

### Needle Biopsy

A needle biopsy is the insertion of a thin, hollow needle into a breast mass to ascertain if fluid can be drawn out (aspirated). If fluid can be aspirated, this indicates that the mass is a cyst. If the cyst is completely reduced after being aspirated and does not return after 2–3 months, then no further treatment is required. If the mass is not completely reduced after being aspirated or if it later returns, then additional steps are necessary to rule out cancer, including another needle biopsy, an ultrasound examination, or surgical removal of the mass.

If fluid is not aspirated during the initial needle biopsy, this is an indication that the mass is solid, and an examination of the tissue removed during the needle biopsy will determine the next step. If the mass is found to be a fibroadenoma, then the woman has a choice to make: have it removed or have it closely monitored. Removal involves surgery, but can determine definitively whether or not there is any cancer present.

If the initial needle biopsy results are unclear, then the mass will be examined with mammography and/or ultrasound, followed by either another needle biopsy or a surgical biopsy. However, if the initial needle biopsy reveals cancer, then treatment should begin at once.

**For individuals under age 30.** In this age group, the follow-up is slightly different because most individuals with a palpable mass have a very low rate of breast cancer. Follow-up of a palpable mass usually begins with observing the mass for a duration of 1–2 menstrual cycles (in women) to see if it persists or disappears. During this follow-up period, clinical breast exams should not be performed in the week before or during a woman's menstrual period because cysts can become enlarged during menstruation. If the mass remains after the observation period, then an ultrasound or needle biopsy will be performed. If a woman has a strong family history of cancer (eg, 2 or more immediate family members with cancer), there is increased risk of breast cancer, and an ultrasound or needle biopsy may be performed without waiting.

### Other Abnormal Findings from a Clinical Breast Exam

In addition to a palpable mass, other potentially abnormal findings during a clinical breast exam include thickening within the breast, changes to the skin, and nipple discharge. Any of these abnormal findings require a follow-up to assure that they are not signs of cancer.

### Abnormal Findings from a Mammogram

Nonpalpable lesions are tissue abnormalities that generally are either too small to be detected during a clinical breast exam or are spread out in such a way that there is no lump even if the mass is large. Nonpalpable lesions are typically found by mammogram.

First, the radiologist compares the mammogram with previous (or baseline) abnormal mammograms. Next, the radiologist will perform a diagnostic mammogram, focusing on the area where there appears to be abnormal tissue. An ultrasound of the area may also be performed.

The next step will be determined based on the findings from the diagnostic mammogram and ultrasound. If the lesion is clearly not cancer (eg, a simple cyst), there is no further follow-up necessary. If the lesion

appears likely to be benign (eg, a fibroadenoma), a repeat mammogram at 6 months and follow up at the physician's discretion is required.

A suspicious lesion can be cancerous; therefore, the next step is to perform a biopsy of the lesion using stereotactic fine needle aspiration or core needle biopsy (both will be discussed later in this protocol). If the biopsy findings do not agree with the mammogram findings, both procedures must be repeated. If the findings are in agreement, a diagnosis can be made. If the lesion is found to be cancerous, treatment should commence immediately. If the lesion is benign, a follow-up mammogram should be performed within a year. If the follow-up mammogram reveals nothing abnormal, then a woman can return to her normal schedule of mammograms and clinical breast exams. If a lesion is a particular type of benign breast disease (eg, atypical hyperplasia), the lesion should be excised and examined for the presence of cancer. If cancer is found, treatment should commence immediately. If no cancer is found, then a woman can return to her normal screening schedule.

## TYPES OF BIOPSIES

Two general categories of biopsies are used to diagnose breast cancer. These are:

1. Needle biopsies, which include core needle biopsy and fine needle aspiration.
2. Open biopsies, which include excisional biopsy (including wire localization) and incisional biopsy.

### Core Needle Biopsy

Core needle biopsy, or cutting needle biopsy, is a method of procuring tissue samples from the breast using a thin, hollow needle. Palpable lumps can be biopsied in a doctor's office using local anesthetic. Using the fingertips to isolate the lump, the doctor makes a small nick in the skin, inserts a needle, and removes a sample of the tissue from the suspicious area. A pathologist, who microscopically evaluates the breast tissue and/or lymph nodes removed during biopsy or surgery for cancer, then examines the tissue sample.

For nonpalpable areas that cannot be felt to be sampled, the procedure is more involved and will likely be performed in a hospital or outpatient clinic because of the need for special equipment to locate and accurately sample the correct area. An ultrasound or special three-dimensional mammography (ie, stereotactic mammography) is used.

A core needle biopsy using stereotactic mammography entails first placing a woman on her stomach on a mammography table with the affected breast fitted through a hole in the table. The breast is compressed so that it will remain in place to record an accurate image. Calculations are made based on this image, and a biopsy device containing a needle automatically takes a number of tissue samples from the affected area in the breast. Multiple samples increase the chances of an accurate diagnosis. This procedure involves little pain because the device inserts and removes the needle very quickly.

A core needle biopsy using ultrasound entails a women lying on her back and the doctor holding an ultrasound transducer against the breast. The transducer makes an image of the area to be sampled, allowing the doctor to follow the needle as it enters the breast and reaches the abnormal area. The needle is then inserted by hand and a sample of tissue is removed.

The core needle biopsy provides several advantages. It supplies specific information about a tumor, such as whether it is in situ or invasive. It is accurate, quick, relatively inexpensive, only mildly uncomfortable, and does not involve surgery.

There are disadvantages to the core needle biopsy. The most important is that the core needle biopsy can produce false negative results. False negatives may occur if the needle misses the tumor and instead takes a sample of normal tissue. This can impact a woman's chances for long-term survival because the undiagnosed cancer may go untreated. Furthermore, the samples taken may not provide complete information about a tumor; a tumor may be diagnosed as being in situ instead of invasive. Taking multiple tissue samples can help limit this potential problem.

### Fine Needle Aspiration

Fine needle aspiration (FNA), also known as fine needle biopsy, is a method of procuring cell samples using a very thin needle. Although FNA can be performed on both palpable lumps as well as nonpalpable areas found by mammogram, FNA is recommended only for use on palpable lumps. The key to an accurate diagnosis is the removal of an adequate number of cells from the suspicious area. With nonpalpable lesions, however, FNA can frequently remove insufficient samples of cells, especially compared to core needle biopsy.

For palpable lumps, FNA can be done in a doctor's office. During the procedure, the doctor will locate and isolate the lump with the fingertips, insert a very thin needle attached to a syringe, and draw out (or aspirate) a sample of cells. The needle is so thin that there is little pain and no anesthetic is needed. The whole procedure takes only a few minutes. Then the sample cells will be sent to a doctor or a cytopathologist who specializes in examining individual cells for a diagnosis.

The advantages of FNA are that it is quick, relatively inexpensive, only mildly uncomfortable, and does not involve surgery. FNA is an excellent method of diagnosing cancer when it is performed on a palpable lump by an experienced doctor and analyzed by an experienced cytopathologist.

There are several disadvantages to using the FNA procedure. FNA is not recommended for nonpalpable lesions. Even for palpable masses, FNA may not remove enough cells for the cytopathologist to be able to make an accurate diagnosis. In addition, false negatives occur in about 0–4% of FNA procedures performed on palpable lesions.[5] As a result, a woman having an FNA may need to have a more definitive biopsy, such as a core needle or excisional biopsy, to ensure that the palpable lesion is not cancerous.

Another drawback of FNA is that while it can be used to determine if cells are cancerous, it cannot distinguish in situ cancers from invasive cancers. However, these 2 types of cancers are generally treated differently via surgery. Finally, FNA requires an experienced breast cytopathologist to accurately analyze the sample of cells, a type of physician that not all hospitals or medical centers will have on staff.

### Excisional Biopsy

An excisional biopsy is the most accurate method for diagnosing breast cancer. It is also referred to as "lumpectomy" or "partial mastectomy." An excisional biopsy is performed by a surgeon and generally done under a local anesthetic, meaning the area to be operated on is desensitized, but the patient remains awake. During the procedure, the surgeon makes an incision in the breast and removes the entire suspicious area and a small amount of surrounding normal tissue. Most women are able to have a biopsy and return home the same day.

### Wire Localization for Nonpalpable Lesions

A nonpalpable lesion is difficult to locate during an excisional biopsy. Therefore, a radiologist uses a mammography or ultrasound image for direction and a surgeon inserts a very thin wire into the breast as a guide to identify the breast tissue that requires removal. The surgeon then removes the abnormal tissue. This procedure is called wire localization or needle localization.

Once the nonpalpable mass is removed, the tissue is immediately x-rayed. This allows the surgeon and radiologist to match the suspicious areas on a woman's mammogram with those in the biopsy tissue. If the areas do not match, the surgeon has 2 options. One option is for the surgeon to make an additional attempt to remove the correct tissue. The other option is to wait and rebiopsy at another time when the area has been targeted a second time using the wire localization technique.

## Frozen Sections

Immediately after the tumor is removed from the breast, a frozen section is usually performed. This process entails freezing a portion of the biopsied tissue and then quickly cutting a thin slice for the pathologist to analyze under the microscope. In the past, if a biopsy came back as positive for cancer, surgical treatment was performed immediately. Currently, biopsies are prior to and separate from the definitive surgery. However, immediate results using frozen sections can help alleviate a woman's anxiety.

A high percentage of false negatives may be produced with frozen sections. Therefore, frozen section results are only preliminary and need to be confirmed by a routine fixed sample, which takes about 2 working days to analyze.[5]

## Excisional Biopsy as a Surgical Treatment

The primary function of an excisional biopsy is to diagnose cancer. However, it can also serve as definitive surgery by removing the cancerous tumor from the breast. Definitive surgery consists of the removal of the entire tumor plus a surrounding amount of normal tissue (a margin) and possibly the axillary lymph nodes.

The pathologist will then inspect the tumor margins. If normal tissue surrounds the entire tumor (which is termed clean or uninvolved or negative margins), the surgery is considered definitive and no additional surgery is needed. If there is insufficient normal tissue surrounding the tumor ("dirty" or involved or positive margins), additional surgery is required to remove the remaining tumor.

The excisional biopsy has many advantages over a needle biopsy. It provides a larger sample size, ensuring far fewer false negative results, and provides accurate information on factors such as tumor size, tumor grade, and the presence of estrogen receptors, all of which are key factors in deciding on a treatment plan.

The excisional biopsy has some disadvantages. It is a far more extensive procedure than a needle biopsy. If a large amount of tissue is removed, the appearance and feel of the breast may also be changed. An excisional biopsy is also expensive and has a longer, more painful recovery period.

## Incisional Biopsy

Incisional biopsy is a surgical procedure done most often on women with advanced-stage cancer whose tumors are too large to be removed as an initial treatment. Only a portion of the tumor is removed, providing a sufficient amount of tissue to procure information essential for developing a treatment plan.

# PROGNOSTIC AND PREDICTIVE FACTORS

Once cancer is diagnosed, there are several tests performed on lymph node or tumor tissue that can be useful in determining a woman's prognosis and assessing the most effective treatment for her specific breast cancer. The issue of which factors are the most reliable at determining a woman's prognosis and predicting her outcome to certain treatments is perpetually under study. As research progresses, certain factors will fall in and out of favor. Only when found to be accurate and reliable does a factor become a part of standard practice. Commonly assessed prognostic and predictive factors include lymph node status, tumor size and grade, type of cancer, hormone receptor status, proliferation rate, and HER2/neu (also known as erbB2 expression).

## Axillary Lymph Nodes

Lymph nodes are simply small clumps of immune cells acting as filters for the lymphatic system. Like the circulatory system, the lymphatic system runs throughout the body carrying fluid, cells, and other material. When breast cancer spreads, the first places it usually goes is to the axillary lymph nodes in the armpit. The best prognosis is when the cancer remains localized within the breast. Once the cancer spreads beyond the breast, the prognosis worsens.

There are 2 ways to determine node status. The first method consists of palpating the axillary lymph nodes during a physical examination. If the nodes are enlarged, it is possible that cancer has spread. This method, while fast and convenient, is not very accurate. It has both a 30% false negative and a 30% false positive rate.[5]

The second method is removal of the nodes from under the armpit in a procedure called an axillary dissection. The nodes are then examined to determine whether or not they contain cancer. This procedure may be performed at different stages of a woman's treatment. However, a standard axillary dissection is typically performed during removal of the breast tumor, and approximately 10–25 lymph nodes are also removed from tissue layers under the armpit.

When an excisional biopsy serves as definitive surgery, the axillary dissection may be performed at the same time or as a separate procedure. Many surgeons now try to perform both procedures together to eliminate the need for separate surgery, anesthesia, and recovery. However, regardless of when the procedure is performed, the node samples are sent to a pathologist for analysis. If the samples do contain cancer, the pathologist will carefully note the number of cancerous nodes as well as their order and location, from proximal (closest to the breast) to distal (farthest away from the breast).

## The Sentinel Node Biopsy

The sentinel node biopsy is a procedure that finds and removes the first (or sentinel) node from the tumor site and examines it to see if it contains cancer cells. If the sentinel node is cancer free, it is likely that the other axillary nodes are cancer free as well.[23] However, if the sentinel node is positive for cancer, there is a strong likelihood that other nodes may also be involved, and a standard axillary dissection may be required.[24]

In order to locate the sentinel node, a colored dye and/or radioactive-labeled tracer is injected into the breast near the tumor. A device called a scintillation counter determines which lymph node is the first node to take up the dye or tracer. This node is then surgically removed and sent to a pathologist for examination.

The advantages of this procedure are that, when done correctly, it is accurate, less traumatic, and allows axillary dissections to be done on only those women whose sentinel nodes present positive for cancer.

The disadvantages of the procedure are that it is fairly new, not widely available, and its accuracy depends in large part on the training of the surgeon doing the procedure.[25] Several ongoing clinical trials will ultimately determine whether sentinel node biopsy becomes part of the standard diagnostic procedure for breast cancer.[25–28] However, the integration of sentinel node biopsy into contemporary clinical practice is underway.[29]

## Tumor Size and Lymph Node Status

Based on numerous studies, there appears to be a strong correlation between tumor size and lymph node involvement. Research demonstrates that the larger the breast tumor, the more likely it is that the lymph nodes will be positive for cancer.[30] One study of 644 women with tumors 2 cm or smaller found that only 11% of the women with tumors 0.1–0.5 cm in size had axillary lymph node involvement. However, when tumors 1.7–2.0 cm were found, more than 40% of the women had axillary lymph node involvement. The prognosis for breast cancer is related to the size of the tumor. Tumor size can be determined by touch during a physical examination, through imaging with an ultrasound or mammography, or most accurately through postsurgical examination of the tumor. In general, the larger the tumor size, the poorer the prognosis.

## Tumor Grade

The grade of a tumor is used to determine how fast a cancer may spread to the lymph nodes or other areas of the body. A pathologist microscopically examines biopsied tissue, determining how closely the cancer cells resemble normal tissue. The less the tumor cells resemble normal tissue, the higher the tumor grade. The pathologist will also assess the rate of cancer cell division. Rapidly dividing cells indicate accelerated tumor growth and therefore a higher tumor grade. Tumor grades are determined as grade 1, or low; grade 2, or medium; and grade 3, or high. Tumor grade is considered directly related to prognosis: the higher the grade, the poorer the prognosis.

## Hormone Receptors

An important aspect in any reproductive cancer is whether the tumor growth is hormonally driven. Often breast tumors require hormones for growth, that is, a hormonally responsive tumor. The hormones attach to their receptor sites and promote cell proliferation. Hormone receptor-positive tumors consist of cancer cells with receptor sites for estrogen, progesterone, or both. The receptor status of a tumor is determined by testing tissue removed during a biopsy. Breast cancer can be categorized by its receptor status, which can be estrogen receptor-positive (ER+), estrogen receptor-negative (ER–), progesterone receptor-positive (PR+), progesterone receptor-negative (PR–), or any combination thereof. Both estrogen and progesterone are naturally occurring hormones that the body produces in varying amounts throughout one's lifetime. These hormones are essential for many other physiologic functions, such as bone integrity, which will be discussed later in this protocol.

Treatment to block the hormones from attaching to the tumor receptor sites may slow or stop the cancer's growth. The drug most often used in this type of treatment is tamoxifen, which is very effective against receptor-positive cancers. Tamoxifen will be discussed extensively later in this protocol.

## HER2 Gene Overexpression

HER2 (human epidermal growth factor receptor 2) is a gene found in every cell of the human body; its purpose is to help a cell divide. The HER2 gene tells a cell to form the HER2 protein on the cell surface. HER2 protein then receives a signal to send a message to the center of the cell, or the nucleus, that it is time to divide. The HER2 protein is also called the HER2 receptor.

Each healthy breast cell contains 2 copies of the HER2 gene, which contribute to normal cell function. When a change occurs that causes too many copies of the HER2 gene to appear in a cell, the gene, in turn, causes too many HER2 proteins, or receptors, to appear on the cell surface. This is referred to as HER2 protein overexpression. Patients considered HER2-positive have cancer that grows and spreads more rapidly.

HER2 protein overexpression affects about 25% of breast cancer patients and results in a more aggressive form of the disease and earlier disease reappearance; in these cases, the disease may not be as responsive to standard therapies. The HER2 status of a tumor is determined by testing tissue removed during a biopsy.

Herceptin may be considered by breast cancer patients whose tumors overexpress the HER2 gene.[31]

## P53 Gene Mutation

The p53 protein is a tumor suppressor encoded by the p53 gene, whose mutation is associated with approximately 50–60% of human cancers. The p53 gene acts as the guardian of DNA and, in the event of DNA damage, it performs several crucial functions. The p53 gene acts as a checkpoint in the cell cycle inducing growth arrest (halting the cell cycle) by increasing the expression of the p21 gene. It initiates DNA repair. If DNA can be repaired, the p53 gene prevents apoptosis (programmed cell death); if DNA cannot be repaired, it initiates apoptosis. The p53 protein also plays a role in the transcription ("reading") of DNA by binding to and initiating the expression of multiple genes.

When a mutation in the p53 gene occurs, one amino acid is substituted for another and p53 loses its ability to block abnormal cell growth. Indeed, some mutations produce a p53 molecule that actually stimulates cell division and promotes cancer. These cancers are more aggressive, more apt to metastasize, and more often fatal.

People inheriting only one functional copy of the p53 gene from their parents are predisposed to cancer in early adulthood. Usually several independent tumors develop in a variety of tissues. This is a rare condition known as Li-Fraumeni syndrome. The p53 gene has been mapped to chromosome 17p13, and mutations in the p53 gene are found in most tumor types and contribute to the molecular events that lead to tumor formation.

Since the hallmark of cancer is the unchecked proliferation of cells, the role of p53 is critical. The question then becomes, if the p53 gene is a built-in tumor suppressor, why does cancer still develop? The answer is that the p53 molecule can be inactivated in several ways. As discussed earlier, in some families p53 mutations are inherited and family members have a high incidence of cancer. More often, the p53 molecule is inactivated by an outside source.

In the cell, p53 protein binds DNA, which in turn stimulates another gene to produce a protein called p21 that interacts with a cell division-stimulating protein (cdk2). When p21 binds with cdk2, the cell cannot pass through to the next stage of cell division. Mutant p53 can no longer bind DNA in an effective way, and as a consequence the p21 protein is not made available to act as the "stop signal" for cell division.

Thus, cells divide uncontrollably and form tumors. DNA tumor viruses, such as the human adenovirus and the human papilloma virus can bind to and inactivate the p53 protein function, altering cells and initiating tumor growth. In addition, some sarcomas amplify another gene, called mdm-2, which produces a protein that binds to p53 and inactivates it, much the way the DNA tumor viruses do.

The amount of information that exists on all aspects of p53 normal function and mutant expression in human cancers is vast, reflecting its key role in the pathogenesis of human cancers. It is clear that p53 is just one component of a network of events that culminate in tumor formation.

## Ras Mutation

Ras oncogenes often govern the regulation of cancer cell growth. The ras family is responsible for modulating the regulatory signals (mitogen activated protein kinase [MAPK] signal transduction cascade) that govern the cancer cell cycle and proliferation. The Ras protein also plays a role in initiating a number of other signal transduction cascades, including phosphoinositide (PI) kinase, and the activation of protein kinase C (PKC). Inhibition of Ras protein action is important because ras induces the expression of the MDM2 gene, whose protein serves to inhibit the activity of the p53 protein. In this way, ras activity reduces the ability of the p53 protein to induce cell death (apoptosis) in cancer cells. Mutations in genes encoding ras proteins have been intimately associated with unregulated cell proliferation of cancer. Further, since ras protein plays an important role in multiple signal transduction pathways and is overexpressed in a large number of cancers, the inhibition of ras is now considered a goal in cancer treatment.[32]

## BRCA1 and BRCA2 Mutations

BRCA1 and BRCA2 are familial (inherited) gene mutations that have been linked to breast cancer. BRCA1 is a tumor suppressor gene located on the long arm of chromosome 17, and BRCA2 is located on chromosome 13. Tumor suppressor genes play a role in regulating cell growth. When one copy of BRCA1 is inherited in a defective (mutant) form, a woman is predisposed to breast and ovarian cancer. However, BRCA1 mutations do not appear critical for the development of the majority of breast and ovarian cancers. Development of cancer in either organ involves a number of additional mutations, at least one of which involves the other copy (allele) of BRCA1. A woman who inherits one mutant allele of BRCA1 from either her mother or father has a greater than 80% risk of developing breast cancer during her life. While it appears that a high number of currently identified high-risk families have mutations in either the BRCA1 or BRCA2 genes, hereditary breast cancer accounts for only about 5% of all cases of breast cancer.

Testing tumors in women with breast cancer for the BRCA1 gene could increase the effectiveness of chemotherapy dramatically. Cancer cells with functional BRCA1 are highly resistant to one type of chemotherapy but extremely sensitive to another. In laboratory tests, tumor cells react differently to anticancer agents depending on the BRCA1 gene activity. A functioning BRCA1 gene made tumor cells more than 1000 times more sensitive to drugs such as Taxol® and Taxotere, which work by blocking the final stage of cell division. The same cells, however, were 10–1000 times more resistant to drugs like cisplatin that work by damaging DNA within tumors. Assessing a tumor's BRCA1 status may be invaluable in deciding which type of chemotherapy to use.

The BRCA1 gene plays an important role in stopping the development of cancer, and women who inherit a damaged version of this gene have a high risk of developing breast cancer. BRCA1 may also get "switched off" in as many as 30% of tumors, even in patients who inherit a normal version of the gene.

## Aggressive Tumors

Certain tumors may be classified as aggressive based on a number of prognostic factors, such as tumor type, size, and grade. Typically, an aggressive tumor is one that under microscopic examination shows signs of fast growth and has a high grade. Because aggressive tumors have a greater chance of spreading to other areas of the body and returning after treatment, they are often treated more intensively. One example of an aggressive tumor is inflammatory breast cancer.

## Staging

Cancer is classified into stages, which determine treatment and prognosis. There are a number of methods for staging breast cancer. The most widely used is the TNM classification (Tumor, Nodes, Metastases). TNM takes into account the size of the tumor (T), number of cancerous lymph nodes (N), and whether or not the cancer has spread to other areas of the body (metastasis) (M). The stage of cancer is usually determined twice: first is clinical staging, which is based on results from a physician's physical exam and tests such as mammography; second is pathologic staging, which is based on direct examination of the lymph nodes and a tumor removed during surgery.

## Tumor Size

| | |
|---|---|
| **TX:** | Tumor size cannot be assessed |
| **T0:** | No tumor can be found |
| **Tis:** | Only carcinoma in situ |
| **T1:** | Tumor is 2 cm or smaller |
| | **Subcategories of T1:** |
| **T1mic:** | Very small tumor (0.1 cm or smaller) |
| **T1a:** | Tumor is larger than 0.1 cm, but no larger than 0.5 cm |
| **T1b:** | Tumor is larger than 0.5 cm, but no larger than 1 cm |
| **T1c:** | Tumor is larger than 1 cm, but no larger than 2 cm |
| **T2** | Tumor is larger than 2 cm, but no larger than 5 cm |
| **T3** | Tumor is larger than 5 cm |
| **T4** | Tumor is any size, but has expanded past the breast tissue to the chest wall or skin |
| | **Subcategories of T4:** |
| **T4a:** | Tumor has expanded to chest wall |
| **T4b:** | Tumor has expanded to skin |
| **T4c:** | Tumor has expanded to both chest wall and skin |
| **T4d:** | Presence of inflammatory carcinoma |

## Lymph Node Status

| | |
|---|---|
| **NX:** | Nodes cannot be evaluated. This can happen if, for example, they have been removed previously |
| **N0:** | Axillary nodes do not have cancer |
| **N1:** | Axillary nodes have cancer, but can be moved |
| **N2:** | Axillary nodes have cancer and are fixed to each other or the chest wall (cannot be moved) |
| **N3:** | Internal mammary nodes have cancer |

## Distant Metastases

| | |
|---|---|
| **MX:** | Distant metastases cannot be assessed |
| **M0:** | No distant metastases |
| **M1:** | Distant metastases |
| | **In Situ Cancer** |
| **Stage 0:** | TisN0M0 |
| | **Early-Stage Invasive Cancer** |
| **Stage 1:** | T1N0M0 |
| **Stage 2a\*** | T0N1M0 |
| | T1N1M0 |
| | T2N0M0 |
| **Stage 2b\*** | T2N1M0 |
| | T3N0M0 |
| | **Advanced Stage Invasive Cancer** |
| **Stage 3a:** | T0N2M0 |
| | T1N2M0 |
| | T2N2M0 |
| | T3N1M0 |
| | T3N2M0 |
| **Stage 3b:** | T4, any N, M0 |
| | Any T, N3, M0 |
| | **Metastatic Breast Cancer** |
| **Stage 4:** | Any T, any N, M1 |

*\* Although classified here as "early stage," prognosis can be poor for some stage 2 cancers, particularly those with multiple lymph node involvement.*

# TESTS FOR DISTANT METASTASES

Cancer cells have the ability to leave the original tumor site, travel to distant locations, and metastasize in areas of the body such as the liver, lungs, or bones. The process of metastasis is dynamic and requires an optimal environment in order for a tumor cell to proliferate, invade surrounding tissues, be released into the circulation, adhere to blood vessels in the liver, invade the liver, proliferate, and establish its own blood supply (tumor angiogenesis). This complex process requires interaction of tumor cells with the microenvironment of the liver to the extent that the tumor cell can utilize the growth factors and blood vessels of the liver in order to grow.

In addition to tests for prognostic and predictive factors, women diagnosed with node-positive breast cancer will require a number of tests to confirm that the cancer has not spread to other areas of the body, such as the lungs, liver, and bone. Only about 6% of women when first diagnosed with breast cancer have distant metastases.[33] Most women found to have metastases have previously been treated for the disease and are experiencing a recurrence.

Symptoms such as shortness of breath, chronic cough, weight loss, and bone pain may indicate distant metastases. However, only after specific tests can the occurrence of distant metastasis be confirmed or ruled out. The 3 primary tests performed are blood tests that check for liver and/or bones metastasis, bone scans to test for bone metastasis, and x-ray/CT scans to test for chest, abdomen, and liver metastasis. Based on the results of the primary tests and the symptoms the woman experiences, further testing may be required. Common tests for distant metastases follow:

## X-rays

An x-ray is a test in which an image is created using low doses of radiation reflected on film paper or fluorescent screens providing an image of specific areas. The films created by x-rays show different features of the body in various shades of gray. The darkest images are those areas that do not absorb x-rays well; the lighter images are dense areas (like bones) that absorb more of the x-rays. To enhance visibility, some x-ray exams will use a contrasting solution that can be swallowed, injected intravenously into the circulatory system, or given by an enema to locate or confirm possible metastases.

## Computer Axial Tomography (CAT or CT) Scan

This procedure combines the use of a digital computer together with a rotating x-ray device to create detailed cross-sectional images, or "slices," of the different organs and body parts. This procedure may or may not involve injecting an intravenous contrasting solution into the circulatory system. It does, however, always involve exposure to ionizing radiation. A CAT scan has the unique ability to image a combination of soft tissue, bone, and blood vessels and can assist in locating possible metastasis.

## Magnetic Resonance Imaging (MRI)

MRIs involve no ionizing radiation and can be used for precise imaging of any organ suspected of having metastases. This is a special imaging technique used to image internal structures of the body, particularly the soft tissues. An MRI image is often superior to a normal x-ray image. In an MRI exam, the patient passes through a tunnel surrounded by a magnet, which polarizes hydrogen atoms in the tissues and then monitors the summation of the energies within living cells. A computer tracks the magnetism and produces a clear picture of the tissues, particularly soft tissues. Images are very clear and are particularly good for soft tissue, brain, and spinal cord, joints, and abdomen. These scans may be used for detecting some cancers or following their progress.

## Positron Emission Tomography

Positron emission tomography (PET) is a highly specialized imaging technique using short-lived substances such as simple sugars (glucose), which are labeled with signal emitting tracers (18-fluoro-deoxyglucose [18-FDG]) and injected into the patient. A scanner records the signals these tracers emit as they travel through the body and collect in various organs targeted for examination. Although all cells use glucose, more glucose is used by cells with increased metabolism such as tumor cells, which use more glucose than neighboring cells; thus, they are easily seen on the PET scan. PET uses a camera that produces powerful images to reveal metastasis that other imaging techniques cannot detect. This technique is very sensitive in deciphering and picking up active cancer cells or tumor tissue but does not measure size. PET can follow the course of cancer through the body and accurately show the extent of the disease. PET can differentiate between normal tissue, scar tissue, and malignant cancerous tissue.

## Ultrasound

Very-high-frequency sound waves are used to produce an image of many of the internal structures in the body without exposure to ionizing radiation. This is highly operator-dependent and thought to be useful in diagnosis but not particularly accurate in the assessment of tumor response. For the latter, CT or MRI scans are more accurate. Intraoperative ultrasonography is useful in the detection of liver metastases.

## Bone Scan

A bone scan is a nuclear medicine study of the body skeleton used to look for cancer, stress fractures, and other bone or joint problems. It does not measure bone density and is not used to diagnose osteoporosis. This procedure uses a radioisotope tracer (Technetium-99m MDP or HDP) injected intravenously into the circulatory system. This radioactive compound localizes in the bone and the distribution of the radioactivity in the body is recorded by the radionuclide scanner (better known as a gamma or scintillation camera), producing an image of the tracer's distribution in the skeletal system. This recording can reveal the presence of bone metastases.

## Bone Density

Since excessive bone breakdown releases tumor growth factors into the bloodstream that can fuel cancer growth, a bone density scan and a test that can be used to assess bone resorption rates should be regularly performed for cancer patients. All bone density scan measurements, with the exception of ultrasound, use small doses of radiation to determine the amount of bone present.

## Deoxypyridinoline

The deoxypyridinoline (DPD) cross-links urine test (Pyrilinks-D) can be used to assess bone resorption rates; this test should be done every 60–90 days to detect bone loss in patients with cancer that has a proclivity to spread to bone. A QCT bone density scan should be done annually. Every cancer patient should take a bone-protecting supplement to protect against excess bone breakdown. For information regarding maintaining bone integrity, refer to the protocol Cancer Treatment: The Critical Factors.

## Quantitative Computed Tomography

Quantitative computed tomography (QCT) densitometry (often referred to as a QCT bone density scan) is a method used to measure bone mass. The principle underlying QCT densitometry and other bone mass measurements (such as DXA) is that calcified tissue will absorb more x-rays than surrounding tissue so that the CT density measurement can be used to measure total bone mass within a sample of tissue. With proper technique, precision for the conventional (2D) method is 2–3%, and about 1% for 3D QCT, so monitoring patients at yearly intervals yields clinically useful results. Only QCT isolates the metabolically active bone

for analysis. The QCT examination is performed on any modern CT scanner and takes approximately 10 minutes. Insurance companies and Medicare may reimburse for QCT examinations.

## Dual X-ray Absorptiometry

Dual x-ray absorptiometry (DXA) was previously known as DEXA, dual energy x-ray absorptiometry. Low-dose x-rays of 2 different energies are used to distinguish between bone and soft tissue, giving an accurate measurement of bone density at these sites. However, DXA also includes aortic calcification and osteophytes in the calculation of bone mineral. Lateral DXA has been shown to have a sensitivity intermediate between the high sensitivity of QCT and the somewhat lower one of conventional DXA (used for detection of osteoporosis). It uses 4–10 times the radiation exposure, is less precise, and the study time is increased compared to conventional DXA/QDR.

## Blood Tests

A variety of blood tests can assess the health of different organs and systems in your body. "Cancer marker" tests can detect possible cancer activity in the body. If cancer is present, it can produce specific protein in the blood that can serve as a "marker" for the cancer. CA 15.3 is the name of a protein used to find breast and ovarian cancers, although it is important to note that there may be insufficient quantities of this protein present in the blood to ensure early-stage breast cancer detection. Creatine-kinase-BB serves as a marker for breast, ovarian, colon, and prostate cancers. CEA (carcinoembryonic antigen) is a marker for the presence of colon, lung, and liver cancers, and a marker for secondary breast and ovarian cancer sites. CA125 may signal ovarian cancer and secondary breast and colorectal cancer sites. TRU-QUANT and CA 27.29 are other examples of proteins associated with the recurrence of breast cancer (more information on tumor markers will follow). Blood tests should evaluate for the presence of anemia or hepatic dysfunction, both of which can be consequences of the patient's underlying cancer.

## TREATMENT OF BREAST CANCER

In the past 20 years, many strides have been made to improve the treatment of breast cancer. Some of the trauma associated with breast cancer treatment has been reduced because of increased early detection through mammography, surgery options that conserve much of the breast, and the increasing long-term survival rate. The treatment goal is to rid the body of the cancer as completely as possible and prevent the cancer from returning. This is usually accomplished by utilizing multimodalities, including surgery, anticancer drugs (chemotherapy), irradiation, hormone therapy, nutritional supplementation, and diet modification.

Surgery and radiation therapy are considered local treatments. They focus on eliminating cancer from a limited or local area, such as the breast, chest wall, and axillary nodes. Chemotherapy, hormone therapy, nutritional supplementation, and diet modification are considered systemic therapy. In systemic therapy, the entire body is treated in order to eradicate any cancer cells that may have spread from the breast tumor to other areas of the body.

Treatment depends on many factors, such as age, tumor stage, and estrogen receptor status. However, deciding on a particular treatment is both a personal and a medical choice. Each treatment option has risks and benefits. Therefore, the type of treatment a woman chooses should be based on an understanding of how these risks and benefits relate to one's personal values and lifestyle.

## Localized Treatment

**Surgery.** Breast cancer surgery strives to completely remove the tumor from the breast. However, surgery may also include the removal of one, some, or all of the axillary lymph nodes. Following surgery, both the tumor and/or lymph nodes are sent to a pathologist for examination to determine the stage of the breast cancer so the physician and patient can decide what additional treatment may be required after surgery.

There are 2 basic types of surgery for breast cancer: breast-conserving surgery and total mastectomy.

- **Breast-conserving surgery.** Breast-conserving surgery consists of the removal of the breast tumor and some surrounding normal tissue. This procedure can be referred to as a lumpectomy, wide excision, or partial-radical mastectomy. During the operation, axillary lymph nodes may also be removed.

    During breast-conserving surgery, the patient is usually given general anesthetic, causing unconsciousness. The surgeon then opens the breast and removes the tumor and a small amount of normal tissue. The surgeon then sutures together the edges of the incision, trying to keep the breast as normal looking as possible.

    If axillary lymph nodes are removed, the surgeon will also open the area under the armpit on the same side as the affected breast, removing about 10–15 lymph nodes. However, if a sentinel node biopsy is performed, only 1–3 lymph nodes are removed and used to assess node status.

Breast-conserving surgery can be done on palpable tumors (tumors that the physician is able to feel) as well as tumors that are not palpable but can be located by mammography. In the case of tumors that are not palpable, a radiologist will insert a very thin wire into the area of the tumor in the breast during a mammogram. This procedure is called wire localization or needle localization (discussed earlier). The wire remains in the breast until the surgery and serves as a guide for the surgeon.

The tumor and lymph nodes removed during surgery are sent to a pathologist who will assess the tumor margins to determine whether there is an adequate amount of normal tissue surrounding the tumor. This margin of normal tissue helps indicate whether or not the entire tumor was removed. If clean, uninvolved, or negative margins are found, this indicates that only normal tissue remains at the edges of the tissue removed and no additional surgery is needed. If normal tissue does not completely surround the tumor, the margins are considered "dirty," "involved," or "positive." Additional surgery will then be done to obtain adequate margins.[34]

A second breast-conserving operation is usually done if the tumor margins are found to be "dirty." This surgery is called a re-excision. If it does not achieve negative margins, a total mastectomy may be recommended.

- **Total mastectomy.** A total mastectomy procedure entails the removal of the entire breast. This may include an axillary dissection as well. For women who have decided to have breast reconstruction, this procedure will directly follow the mastectomy surgery.

    A total mastectomy is done under general anesthetic. During the operation, all of the breast tissue is removed, including the nipple. For women considering breast reconstruction during or sometime after surgery, as much skin as possible is left intact in order to cover the implant. If a woman is not having reconstruction or is having it at a later time, the skin in the area is sewn together and a drainage tube is inserted so fluid from the healing wound can drain away.

    The pathologist will evaluate the breast tissue and lymph nodes. The results of these tests will help determine which adjuvant therapy will be used.

- **Luteal phase surgery.** Studies have suggested that premenopausal women who have their breast-conserving procedure or mastectomy done during the later part of their menstrual cycle (during the *luteal phase*) may have a better outcome after surgery. However, researchers are still assessing the benefits to "timing surgery."[35,36]

**Radiation therapy.** Radiation therapy (also known as radiotherapy) is considered a local treatment for breast cancer that uses targeted, high-energy x-rays to impede cancer cells' ability to grow and divide. The aim of radiation therapy is to rid the breast, chest, and axillary lymph nodes of cancer by using high-energy x-rays. For women with early-stage breast cancer, radiation therapy is most often performed following breast-conserving surgery. It is believed that after conserving surgery, there may still be microscopic cancer in the breast undetectable to the naked eye. Therefore, to reduce the chance of recurrence, radiation therapy is necessary to eliminate any remaining cancer.

Radiation therapy may also be used on the axillary lymph nodes and chest wall following total mastectomy. Radiation therapy usually commences several weeks after surgery. However, it may be postponed if a patient is receiving chemotherapy first. (For more information regarding radiation therapy, please see the Cancer Radiation Therapy protocol.)

## Adjuvant Treatment

The goal of an adjuvant treatment is to systemically eliminate any cancer cells or micrometastases that may have spread from the breast tumor to other parts of the body as well as to eliminate any microscopic cancer cells that may remain in the local breast/lymph node area. These therapies are referred to as adjuvant, meaning "in addition to," because they are used with surgery and radiation. It is called adjuvant systemic therapy because the entire system of the body is treated. Several types of adjuvant systemic treatments are used for early-stage breast cancer: chemotherapy and hormone therapy are well established conventional adjuvant therapies; nutritional supplementation and diet modification may be incorporated in any conventional adjuvant treatment plan.

Except for some women with very small tumors (<1 cm) and with lymph nodes that do not have cancer, adjuvant therapy is usually recommended for women with early-stage breast cancer. Which therapies, and in what combination, depends on many things, such as the woman's age, whether the tumor has estrogen receptors, and the number of positive lymph nodes.

**Chemotherapy.** Chemotherapy uses drugs that can be taken in oral form or injected intravenously to kill cancer cells; sometimes, a combination is used. However, intravenous drugs are usually given in a hospital or doctor's office. Depending on the drugs used, chemotherapy is administered once or twice a month for 3–6 months. Sometimes the range might be extended to 7 or 8 months. Chemotherapy usually begins 4–6 weeks after the final surgery and is administered in a combination of 2 or 3 drugs that have been found to be the most effective. Unfortunately, chemotherapy drugs have many side effects that can damage or destroy normal healthy tissue throughout the body.

Although the exact schedule depends on the specific drugs used, drugs may be given on day 1 of a 3-week cycle or there may be a period of 1–2 weeks on the drugs, followed by a period of about 2 weeks off the drugs. This cycling allows the body a chance to rest and recover between treatments; however, it also gives the cancer cells an opportunity to rest, recover, and possibly mutate into a type of cancer that is chemotherapy-resistant. An entire course of chemotherapy lasts about 4–6 months, depending on the drugs used. Recent studies indicate that a more efficacious approach would be to lower the dose of conventional chemotherapy agents, reschedule their application, and combine them with agents designed to interfere with cancer's ability to produce new blood vessels (antiangiogenic agents).[37]

This lower-dose approach, known as "metronomic dosing," uses a dosing schedule as often as every day. An amount as low as 25% of the maximum tolerated dose (MTD) in combination with antiangiogenesis agents targets the tumor endothelial cells making up the blood vessels and microvessels feeding the tumor. Tumor endothelial cells can be killed with much less chemotherapy than tumor cells, and the side effects to healthy tissue and the patient in general are dramatically reduced.[38]

While chemotherapy is an effective treatment for many women, it is associated with a number of well-known and traumatic side effects, such as hair loss, and exhausting bouts of nausea and vomiting, which many patients find difficult to tolerate. (For more information on chemotherapy, please refer to the Chemotherapy protocol.)

**Hormone therapy.** Breast tumors often require hormones for growth, which poses a unique problem because the hormones involved in tumor growth are either estrogen, progesterone, or both. Estrogen and progesterone are naturally occurring and necessary hormones, produced mainly in the ovaries and adrenal glands in varying amounts throughout a woman's lifetime. These hormones are essential for many physiologic functions, such as bone integrity, which will be discussed later in this protocol.

Hormone receptor–positive tumors can consist of cancer cells with receptor sites for estrogen, progesterone, or both. The hormones attach to receptor sites and promote cell proliferation. Hormone therapy blocks the hormones from attaching to the tumor receptor sites and may slow or stop the cancer's growth. The drug most often used in this type of endocrine therapy is tamoxifen, with a response rate of 30–60%. Other therapies are sometimes used, such as aromatase inhibitors (that inhibit the conversion of precursors to estrogens) or oophorectomy (the removal of the ovaries).

The effective role of some newer hormonal therapies in the treatment of both pre- and post-menopausal women with early-stage breast cancer has been studied. Hormonal therapy with goserelin, either with or without tamoxifen, has been endorsed as an alternative to chemotherapy for young women with hormone-sensitive disease since it is equally effective and better tolerated. Twenty-five percent of all women diagnosed with breast cancer are premenopausal; of these women, approximately 60% have hormone-sensitive tumors.

While chemotherapy kills cancer cells by destroying all rapidly dividing cells in the body, goserelin suppresses the supply of estrogen from the ovaries, which stimulates the cancer cells to grow. This is achieved by inhibiting production of another hormone called luteinizing hormone (LH), which stimulates the ovaries to make estrogen. Since many breast cancers grow more rapidly in the presence of estrogen, this can help to reduce tumor growth.

Tamoxifen prevents estrogen from stimulating cancer cell growth by blocking estrogen receptors in the cancer cells. Cutting off the cancer's supply of estrogen provides an effective alternative method of combating the disease and avoids the distressing side effects of chemotherapy. Based on evidence from adjuvant studies, hormonal therapy with goserelin is better tolerated and equally effective as an alternative to chemotherapy. This gives physicians and patients a real choice in treatment following initial surgery.[39]

- **Tamoxifen (Nolvadex®).** Tamoxifen is an antiestrogenic drug used to treat women whose tumors are estrogen- or progesterone-receptor positive. This endocrine therapy blocks the female hormone estrogen from binding to the tumor cells. Tamoxifen has been the gold standard hormonal agent used for the treatment of breast cancer for more than 8 years. It is a prototype for a class of compounds called selective estrogen receptor modulators (SERMs) of breast cancer, but is also an effective primary treatment for advanced disease. Women with early-stage breast cancer who take tamoxifen have, on average, a 25% proportional increase in their chances of surviving 5 years after diagnosis.

  Tamoxifen does not work equally well in all women. As the name implies, estrogen receptor-negative tumors do not have estrogen receptors, and therefore do not respond to tamoxifen. A phase 3 study of 2691 high-risk cancer patients tested the effectiveness of tamoxifen with both pre- and

post-menopausal subsets of receptor-negative and receptor-positive tumors. Both the 5-year disease-free and overall survival in patients with receptor-positive tumors treated with the addition of tamoxifen to chemotherapy was significantly higher than with chemotherapy alone, while no such advantage in disease-free or overall survival was found in receptor-negative patients. Further, in the receptor-positive postmenopausal group, the addition of tamoxifen showed a significant improvement in both disease-free and overall survival. However, in the premenopausal receptor-negative patients tamoxifen led to a worse outcome, as indicated by the significantly reduced survival rate.[40] Women with estrogen receptor-negative tumors may receive chemotherapy instead of tamoxifen.

Therefore, for the patient whose breast cancer's growth is estrogen-dependent, tamoxifen can keep estrogen from these cells, slowing or stopping their growth. Tamoxifen is a pill taken daily for 5 years. To date, studies do not show any benefit to taking tamoxifen for longer than 5 years.[36] Studies show that the use of tamoxifen as a postsurgical adjuvant therapy can reduce the chances of the cancer reoccurring.

Tamoxifen has a host of side effects, including hot flashes, weight gain, mood swings, abnormal secretions from the vagina, fatigue, nausea, depression, loss of libido, headache, swelling of the limbs, decreased number of platelets, vaginal bleeding, blood clots in the large veins (deep venous thrombosis), blood clots in the lungs (pulmonary emboli), cataracts,[41] and the side effect of the greatest concern—endometrial cancer.[5]

Studies have shown an increase of early-stage endometrial cancer (cancer of the lining of the uterus) among women taking tamoxifen, and the risk increases if the drug is taken for more than 5 years. Endometrial cancer is usually diagnosed at a very early stage and is usually curable by surgery. The studies have also shown an increased risk of uterine sarcoma (a rare cancer of the connective tissues of the uterus) among women taking tamoxifen. Unusual vaginal bleeding is a common symptom of both of these cancers. The treating physician should be notified immediately if vaginal bleeding occurs.

- **Raloxifene.** Raloxifene is a drug similar to tamoxifen. It is a SERM that blocks the effect of estrogen on breast tissue and breast cancer. It is currently in the testing phase to assess its effectiveness in reducing the risk of developing breast cancer. Pending testing completion, this drug is not recommended as hormonal therapy for women diagnosed with breast cancer.

- **Toremifene (Fareston®).** This antiestrogen drug, which is closely related to tamoxifen, may be an option for postmenopausal women with breast cancer that has metastasized. Fareston® is a type of antiestrogen medication used in tumors that are estrogen receptor-positive or estrogen receptor-unknown.

   Some patients treated with antiestrogens who have bone metastasis may experience a tumor flare with pain and inflammation in the muscles and bones that will usually subside quickly. Blood calcium level should be monitored because tumor flare can cause a raised level of calcium in the blood (hypercalcemia) with symptoms of nausea, vomiting, and thirst. Often a short stay in the hospital is necessary until calcium levels have been reduced or treatment may need to be stopped. Fareston® is being studied in clinical trials for use in earlier stages of breast cancer.

- **Anastrozole (Arimidex®), letrozole (Femara®), and exemestane (Aromasin®)** Anastrozole (Arimidex®), letrozole (Femara®), and exemestane (Aromasin®) are 3 hormonal therapy drugs referred to as aromatase inhibitors. Aromatase is the enzyme that converts male hormones (testosterone) into female hormones (estrogens) in postmenopausal women. Premenopausal women get most of their estrogen from the ovaries. But postmenopausal women still have estrogen in their bodies, and it is this conversion to estrogen of androgens coming from adrenal glands in the body that needs to be interrupted so the breast cancer cells no longer have estrogen to stimulate their growth. Unlike tamoxifen, which slows the growth of breast cancer by preventing estrogen from activating its receptor, anastrozole blocks an enzyme needed for the production of estrogen, inhibiting the conversion of precursors to estrogens, and is effective in hormone receptor-positive breast cancers. Anastrozole is currently an option for women whose advanced breast cancer continues to grow during or after tamoxifen treatment.

   Studies are ongoing to compare tamoxifen and anastrozole as adjuvant hormonal therapies. Anastrozole (Arimidex®) was better than tamoxifen at preventing the recurrence of breast cancer in a study conducted in 381 centers in 21 countries, involving 9366 patients, and examining 3 treatment arms: tamoxifen alone, tamoxifen in combination with other therapy, and anastrozole alone. The trial results showed that women taking anastrozole experienced fewer side effects than women taking tamoxifen. However, women taking tamoxifen experienced fewer musculoskeletal disorders. The study was only conducted for a relatively short period of time, 2 years, and the long-term effects (5 years and beyond) are not yet known. Longer-term studies are needed to assess both the benefits and risks of this therapy. However, more recent studies have showed anastrozole to be slightly superior to tamoxifen.[42]

   In a primary trial of 33 months, anastrozole was superior to tamoxifen in terms of disease-free survival (DFS), time to recurrence (TTR), and incidence of contra-lateral breast cancer (CLBC) in adjuvant endocrine therapy for postmenopausal patients with early-stage breast cancer. After an additional follow-up period of 47 months, anastrozole continued to show superior efficacy.

   When compared with tamoxifen, anastrozole has numerous advantages in terms of tolerability. Endometrial cancer, vaginal bleeding and discharge, cerebrovascular events, venous thromboembolic events, and hot flashes all occurred less frequently in the anastrozole group. However, musculoskeletal disorders and fractures continued to occur less frequently in the tamoxifen group. The study concluded that the benefits of anastrozole are likely to be maintained in the long term and provide further support for the status of anastrozole as a valid treatment option for postmenopausal women with hormone-sensitive early-stage breast cancer.[43]

   The biological basis for the superior efficacy of neoadjuvant letrozole versus tamoxifen for postmenopausal women with estrogen receptor-positive locally advanced breast cancer was investigated. Letrozole inhibited tumor proliferation more than tamoxifen. While the molecular basis for this advantage was complex, it appeared to include a possible tamoxifen agonist effect on the cell cycle in both HER1/2+ and HER1/2- tumors. Letrozole seems to inhibit tumor proliferation more effectively than tamoxifen independent of HER1/2 expression status.[44]

   Letrozole (2.5 mg per day) and anastrozole (1 mg per day) were compared as endocrine therapy in postmenopausal women with advanced breast cancer previously treated with an antiestrogen. Letrozole was significantly superior to anastrozole in the overall response rate (ORR) and both agents were well tolerated. Advanced breast cancer is more responsive to letrozole than anastrozole as a second-line endocrine therapy, as letrozole has the greater aromatase-inhibiting activity.[45] These results support previous studies which showed that letrozole (Femara®) was significantly more potent than anastrozole (Arimidex®) at inhibiting aromatase activity in vitro and inhibiting total body aromatization in patients with breast cancer.

A once a day oral dose of Femara® lowered the risk of breast cancer recurrence by 43% in 5000 older women who had already completed 5 years of treatment with tamoxifen. After just over 2 years, 207 women had a recurrence of cancer–75 in the Femara® group and 132 in the placebo group. There were 31 deaths in women receiving Femara® and 42 deaths in women receiving placebo. Compared with placebo, Femara® therapy after the completion of standard tamoxifen treatment significantly improved disease-free survival. This is a significant finding because in more than 50% of women treated for breast cancer, the cancer recurs 5 or more years after the original diagnosis.[46]

Possible side effects of aromatase-inhibitor drugs include those associated with menopausal-like estrogen deficiency, such as hot flashes, night sweats, menstrual irregularity, depression, bone or tumor pain, pulmonary embolism (a blood clot in the lung), musculoskeletal disorders, and generalized weakness.

- **Megestrol acetate.** Megestrol acetate (Megace®) is another drug used for hormonal treatment of advanced breast cancer, usually for women whose cancers do not respond to tamoxifen or have stopped responding to tamoxifen. Megestrol acetate is a man-made substance called progestin that is similar to the female hormone progesterone.

  As with other therapies, there are reported side effects, including an increase in appetite causing weight gain, fluid retention causing ankle swelling, and nausea at the onset of therapy, which usually subsides. In rare cases, allergic reactions, jaundice, and raised blood pressure have been reported.

- **Oophorectomy** Oophorectomy is surgery in which the ovaries are removed, therefore eliminating the body's main source of estrogen and progesterone in premenopausal women. Prior to the advent of antiestrogen drugs, an oophorectomy was commonly used to treat breast cancer in premenopausal women.

  Occasionally this procedure is still used in premenopausal women. However, chemotherapy drugs can alter the ovaries and reduce estrogen production. Tamoxifen may block any remaining estrogen effect on cancer cells, allowing many women to avoid surgery.

**Trastuzumab (Herceptin).** Trastuzumab (Herceptin) is an anticancer drug therapy for women with HER2-positive metastatic breast cancer. This monoclonal antibody therapy differs from traditional treatments, such as chemotherapy and hormone-blocking therapy. Herceptin works by specifically targeting tumor cells that overexpress the HER2 protein. A monoclonal antibody blocks the receptors and prevents activation of genes that induce cell division, thereby slowing tumor growth.

The reported side effects are chills, diarrhea, nausea, weakness, headache, vomiting, and possible damage of the heart muscle, anemia, and nerve pain. Trastuzumab can be used alone or in combination with the drug paclitaxel (Taxol®) and is prescribed for metastatic breast cancer.

**Paclitaxel (Taxol®).** Paclitaxel (Taxol®) belongs to the group of medicines called antineoplastics (anticancer drugs) that interfere with the growth of cancer cells and eventually destroy them. Because the growth of normal cells may also be affected by paclitaxel, side effects can occur. Some side effects may not occur until months or years after the medicine was used.

Side effects include neutropenia (decreased white blood cell count), anemia (decreased red blood cell count), thrombocytopenia (decreased platelet count), increased risk of infection, fatigue, bruising, hemorrhage, rash, itching, redness, hives, facial flushing, chest pain, difficulty breathing, high or low blood pressure, decreased heart rate, lightheadedness, dizziness, increased perspiration, shortness of breath, headache, numbness or tingling of the hands and/or feet, muscle aches, bone pain, mouth ulcers (sores), alopecia (loss or thinning of scalp and body hair), decreased appetite, diarrhea, nausea, vomiting, skin burns and ulcers, nail changes, hot flashes, and vaginal dryness.

# NATURAL THERAPIES FOR TREATMENT OF BREAST CANCER

## Indole-3-Carbinol

The stronger form of estrogen, estradiol, can be converted into the weaker form, estriol, in the body without using drugs. Estriol is considered to be a more desirable form of estrogen. It is less active than estradiol, so when it occupies the estrogen receptor, it blocks estradiol's strong "growth" signals. Using a natural substance, the conversion of estradiol to estriol increased by 50% in 12 healthy people.[47] Furthermore, in female mice prone to developing breast cancer, the natural substance reduced the incidence of cancer, and the number of tumors significantly. The natural substance was indole-3-carbinol (I3C).

Indole-3-carbinol (I3C) is a phytochemical isolated from cruciferous vegetables (broccoli, cauliflower, Brussels sprouts, turnips, kale, green cabbage, mustard seed, etc.). I3C given to 17 men and women for 2 months reduced the levels of strong estrogen and increased the levels of weak estrogen. More importantly, the level of an estrogen metabolite associated with breast and endometrial cancer—16 alpha-hydroxyestrone—was reduced by I3C.[48]

When I3C changes "strong" estrogen to "weak" estrogen, the growth of human cancer cells is inhibited by 54–61%.[49] Moreover, I3C provoked cancer cells to self-destruct (kill themselves via apoptosis). Induction of cell death is an approach to suppress carcinogenesis and the prime goal of cytotoxic chemotherapy. The increase in apoptosis induced by I3C before initiation of new tumor development may contribute to suppression of tumor progression. Nontoxic I3C can reliably facilitate apoptosis (12-week treatment in rats); thus, this phytonutrient may become a standard adjunct in the treatment of breast cancer.[50]

I3C inhibits human breast cancer cells (MCF7) from growing by as much as 90% in culture; growth arrest does not depend on estrogen receptors.[51] Furthermore, I3C induces apoptosis in tumorigenic (cancerous) but not in nontumorigenic (noncancerous) breast epithelial cells.[52]

I3C does more than just turn strong estrogen to weak estrogen. 16-a-Hydroxyestrone (16-OHE) and 2-hydroxyestrone (2-OHE) are metabolites of estrogen in addition to estriol and estradiol. 2-OHE is biologically inactive, while 16-OHE is biologically active; that is, like estradiol, it can send "growth" signals. In breast cancer, the dangerous 16-OHE is often elevated, while the protective 2-OHE is decreased. Cancer-causing chemicals change the metabolism of estrogen so that 16-OHE is elevated. Studies show that people who take I3C have beneficial increases in the "weak" estriol form of estrogen and also increases in protective 2-OHE.

African-American women who consumed I3C, 400 mg for 5 days, experienced an increase in the "good" 2-OHE and a decrease in the "bad" 16-OHE. However, it was found that the minority of women who did not demonstrate an increase in 2-OHE had a mutation in a gene that helps metabolize estrogen to the 2-OHE version. Those women had an 8 times higher risk of breast cancer.[49]

**I3C stops cancer cells from growing.** Tamoxifen is a drug prescribed to reduce breast cancer metastases and improve survival. I3C has modes of action similar to tamoxifen. I3C inhibited the growth of estrogen receptor-positive breast cancer cells by 90% compared to 60% for tamoxifen. The mode of action attributed to I3C's impressive effect was interfering with the cancer cell growth cycle. Adding tamoxifen to I3C gave a 5% boost (95% total inhibition).[53]

In estrogen receptor-negative cells, I3C stopped the synthesis of DNA by about 50%, whereas tamoxifen had no significant effect. I3C also restored p21 and other proteins that act as checkpoints during the synthesis of a new cell. Tamoxifen showed no effect on p21. Restoration of these growth regulators is extremely important. For example, tumor suppressor p53 works through p21 that I3C restores. I3C also inhibits cancers caused by chemicals. If animals are fed I3C before exposure to cancer-causing chemicals, DNA damage and cancer are virtually eliminated.[53]

A study on rodents shows that damaged DNA in breast cells is reduced 91% by I3C. Similar results are seen in the liver.[54] Female smokers taking 400 mg of I3C significantly reduced their levels of a major lung carcinogen. Cigarette chemicals are known to adversely affect estrogen metabolism.[55]

There is no proven way to prevent breast cancer, but comprehensive scientific evidence supports phytochemicals such as I3C.[56] The results from a placebo-controlled, double-blind, dose-ranging chemoprevention study on 60 women at increased risk for breast cancer demonstrated that I3C at a minimum effective dosage (300 mg per day) is a promising agent for breast cancer prevention.[57] The results of a single-blind phase I trial which studied the effectiveness of I3C in preventing breast cancer in nonsmoking women who are at high risk of breast cancer are awaited. The rationale for this study is that I3C, ingested twice daily, may be effective at preventing breast cancer.

I3C was found to be superior to 80 other compounds, including tamoxifen, for anticancer potential. Indoles, which downregulate estrogen receptors, have been proposed as promising agents in the treatment and prevention of cancer and autoimmune diseases such as multiple sclerosis, arthritis, and lupus. Replacement of all the chemically altered estrogen drugs, such as tamoxifen, with a new generation of chemically altered indole drugs that fit in the aryl-hydrocarbon (Ah) receptor and regulate estrogen indirectly may prove beneficial to cancer patients.[58] An I3C tetrameric derivative (chemically derived) is currently a novel lead inhibitor of breast cancer cell growth, considered a new, promising therapeutic agent for both estrogen receptor-positive and estrogen receptor-negative breast cancer.[59]

A summary of studies shows that indole-3-carbinol (I3C) can:

- Increase the conversion of estradiol to the safer estriol by 50% in healthy people in just 1 week.[47]

- Prevent the formation of the estrogen metabolite, 16 alpha-hydroxyestrone, that prompts breast cancer cells to grow[60] in both men and women in 2 months.[61]

- Stop human cancer cells from growing (54–61%) and provoke the cells to self-destruct (apoptosis).[49]

- Inhibit human breast cancer cells (MCF7) from growing by as much as 90% in vitro.[62]

- Inhibit the growth of estrogen receptor-positive breast cancer cells by 90%, compared to tamoxifen's 60%, by stopping the cell cycle.[53]

- Prevent chemically induced breast cancer in rodents by 70–96%. Prevent other types of cancer, including aflatoxin-induced liver cancer, leukemia, and colon cancer.[63]

- Inhibit free radicals, particularly those that cause the oxidation of fat.[64]

- Stop the synthesis of DNA by about 50% in estrogen receptor-negative cells, whereas tamoxifen had no significant effect.[51]

- Restore p21 and other proteins that act as checkpoints during the synthesis of a new cancer cell. Tamoxifen has no effect on p21.[51]

- Virtually eliminate DNA damage and cancer prior to exposure to cancer-causing chemicals (in animals fed I3C).[63]

- Reduce DNA damage in breast cells by 91%.[54]

- Reduce levels of a major nitrosamine carcinogen in female smokers.[55]

**How to use I3C.** While evidence is compelling, it is too soon to know exactly how effective I3C will be as an adjuvant breast cancer therapy.

Suggested dosage: Take one 200-mg capsule of I3C twice per day, for those under 120 lb. For those who weigh more than 120 lb, three 200-mg capsules per day are suggested. Women who weigh over 180 lb should take four 200-mg I3C capsules per day.

*Caution:* Pregnant women should not take I3C because of its modulation of estrogen. I3C appears to act both at the ovarian and hypothalamic levels, whereas tamoxifen appears to act only on the hypothalamic-pituitary axis as an antiestrogen. Both I3C and tamoxifen block ovulation by altering preovulatory concentrations of luteinizing hormone (LH) and follicle stimulating hormone (FSH).[65] The reported aversion to cruciferous vegetables by pregnant women may be associated with their ability to change estrogen metabolism. Estrogen is a necessary growth factor for the fetus.

## Apigenin

Apigenin, a flavone (ie, a class of flavonoids) present in fruits and vegetables (eg, onions, oranges, tea, celery, artichoke, and parsley) has been shown to possess anti-inflammatory, antioxidant, and anticancer properties. Many studies have confirmed the cancer chemopreventive effects of apigenin.[66]

Apigenin stimulates apoptosis in breast cancer cells.[67] A 2012 study showed that apigenin slowed the progression of human breast cancer by inducing cell death, inhibiting cell proliferation, and reducing expression of a gene associated with cancer growth (Her2/neu). In another study, it was noted that blood vessels responsible for feeding cancer cells were smaller in apigenin-treated mice compared to untreated mice. This is significant because smaller vessels mean restricted nutrient flow to the tumors and may have served to starve the cancer as well as limit its ability to spread.[68]

Apigenin has been proven to have a synergistic treatment effect when combined with the chemotherapy drug paclitaxel.[69] In a study, apigenin increased the efficacy of the chemotherapy drug 5-Fluorouracil against breast cancer cells.[70]

## Astragalus

Astragalus, an herb used for centuries in Asia, has exhibited immune-stimulatory effects. Astragalus potentiates lymphokine-activated killer cells.[71] One study found that astragalus could partially restore depressed immune function in tumor-bearing mice,[72] while another concluded that "astragalus could exhibit anti-tumor effects, which might be achieved through activating the ... anti-tumor immune mechanism of the host."[73]

It was observed in a clinical trial that astragalus inhibited the proliferation of breast cancer cells. Authors of the study stated, "The antiproliferation mechanisms may be related to its effects of upregulating the expressions of p53...."[74] Similar findings were noted in a previous experiment.[75]

## Blueberry

Blueberries are rich in anthocyanins (ie, dark pigments in fruits) and pterostilbenes (ie, antioxidant closely related to resveratrol). The anticancer effects of blueberries are mediated by multiple mechanisms:

**Blueberry extracts block DNA damage.** Damage to cellular DNA underlies most forms of cancer. By preventing such damage, blueberry extracts can block the malignant transformation of healthy cells.[76]

**Blueberry extracts inhibit angiogenesis.** Rapidly growing cancers recruit new blood vessels to meet their ravenous appetites for nutrients and oxygen. Blueberry inhibits new tumor blood vessel growth, known as angiogenesis.[77,78]

**Blueberry extracts trigger cancer cells' suicide.** If normal cells replicate too fast, they are programmed to die through apoptosis. Cancerous cells, by contrast, ignore that programming, constantly doubling their population unchecked. Blueberry components restore normal programming and induce apoptosis in cells from a variety of cancers, putting the brakes on their rapid growth.[79-83]

**Blueberry extracts stop excessive proliferation.** Uncontrolled cell reproduction results in formation of dangerous tumors, as cells ignore the normal signals to stop growing. By restoring normal cellular signaling, blueberry extracts stop such out-of-control proliferation.[80,84,85] In an experimental breast cancer cell line, blueberry significantly reduced breast cancer cell proliferation, leading researchers to state that "blueberry anthocyanins ... demonstrated anticancer properties by inhibiting cancer cell proliferation and by acting as cell antiinvasive factors and chemoinhibitors."[86] In rats with experimentally induced breast cancer, the volume of new breast tumor formation was reduced by 40% in the group of rats supplemented with blueberry compared to the control group.[87]

**Blueberry extracts slow tumor spread by invasion and metastasis.** Solid cancers produce matrix metalloproteinases, which are "protein-melting" enzymes that help them invade adjacent tissues and that enable them to metastasize. Blueberry extracts block matrix metalloproteinases, thereby inhibiting cancer invasion and metastasis.[88,89] In one experiment published in 2011, blueberry extract was administered to mice with breast cancer. Compared to the control group, tumor volume was 75% lower in mice fed blueberry extract. Moreover, mice fed blueberry extract developed 70% fewer liver metastases and 25% fewer lymph node metastases compared to the control group.[90]

## Chrysin

Breast cancers that are estrogen-receptor positive can grow and be exacerbated in the presence of estrogen in the body. One aim of drug therapy for estrogen receptor-positive breast cancer is to decrease the levels of estrogen in the body. To that end, drugs used to block the enzyme (ie, aromatase) that converts testosterone into estrogen (ie, aromatase inhibitors) are widely used in women with estrogen receptor-positive breast cancer. Chrysin, a flavonoid, is a natural aromatase inhibitor.[91,92]

## Coffee

Coffee, especially brews enriched with chlorogenic acid, protect cells against the DNA damage that leads to aging and cancer development.[93-95] Growing tumors develop the ability to invade local and regional tissue by increasing their production of "protein-melting" enzymes called matrix metalloproteinases. Chlorogenic acid—present in coffee—strongly inhibited matrix metalloproteinase activity.[96,97]

A 2011 study reported that postmenopausal women who drank 5 cups of coffee daily exhibited a 57% decreased risk of developing *estrogen receptor-negative* (non–hormone-responsive) breast cancer.[98] Chlorogenic acid and other polyphenols are the likely beneficial agents in such cancers.[99]

## Curcumin

Curcumin is extracted from the spice turmeric and is responsible for the orange/yellow pigment that gives the spice its unique color. Turmeric is a perennial herb of the ginger family and a major component of curry powder. Chinese and Indian people, both in herbal medicine and in food preparation, have safely used it for centuries.

Curcumin has a number of biological effects in the body. However, one of the most important functions is curcumin's ability to inhibit growth signals emitted by tumor cells that elicit angiogenesis (growth and development of new blood vessels into the tumor).

Curcumin inhibits the epidermal growth factor receptor and is up to 90% effective in a dose-dependent manner. It is important to note that while curcumin has been shown to be up to 90% effective in inhibiting the expression of the epidermal growth factor receptor on cancer cell membranes, this does not mean it will be effective in 90% of cancer patients or reduce tumor volume by 90%. However, because two-thirds of all cancers overexpress the epidermal growth factor receptor and such overexpression frequently fuels the metastatic spread of the cancer throughout the body, suppression of this receptor is desirable.

Other anticancer mechanisms of curcumin include:

- Inhibition of the induction of basic fibroblast growth factor (bFGF). bFGF is both a potent growth signal (mitogen) for many cancers and an important signaling factor in angiogenesis.[100]

- Antioxidant activity. In vitro it has been shown to be stronger than vitamin E in prevention of lipid peroxidation.[101,102]

- Inhibition of the expression of COX-2 (cyclooxygenase 2), the enzyme involved in the production of prostaglandin E2 (PGE-2), a tumor-promoting hormone-like agent.[103]

- Inhibition of a transcription factor in cancer cells known as nuclear factor-kappa B (NF-κB).

Many cancers overexpress NF-κB and use this as a growth vehicle to escape regulatory control.[104,105]

- Increased expression of nuclear p53 protein in human basal cell carcinomas, hepatomas, and leukemia cell lines. This increases apoptosis (cell death).[106]

- Increased production of transforming growth factor-beta (TGF-beta), a potent growth inhibitor, producing apoptosis.[107,108] TGF-beta is known to enhance wound healing and may play an important role in the enhancement of wound healing by curcumin.[109,110]

- Inhibition of PTK (protein tyrosine kinases) and PKC (protein kinase C). PTK and PKC help relay chemical signals through the cell. Abnormally high levels of these substances are often required for cancer cell signal transduction messages. These include proliferation, cell migration, metastasis, angiogenesis, avoidance of apoptosis, and differentiation.[111,112]

- Inhibition of AP-1 (activator protein-1) through a nonantioxidant pathway. While curcumin is an antioxidant,[113] it appears to inhibit signal-transduction via protein phosphorylation, thereby decreasing cancer-cell activity, regulation, and proliferation.[114]

Based on the favorable, multiple mechanisms listed above, higher-dose curcumin would appear to be useful for cancer patients to take. However, as far as curcumin being taken at the same time as chemotherapy drugs, there are contradictions in the scientific literature. Therefore, caution is advised. Please refer to the Chemotherapy protocol before considering combining curcumin with chemotherapy.

Curcumin's effects are a dose-dependent response, and a standardized product is essential. The recommended dose is four 900-mg capsules 3 times per day, preferably with food.

## Green Tea

As a tumor grows, it elicits new capillary growth (angiogenesis) from the surrounding normal tissues and diverts blood supply and nutrients away from the tissue to feed itself. Unregulated tumor angiogenesis can facilitate the growth of cancer throughout the body. Antiangiogenesis agents, including green tea, inhibit this new tumor blood vessel (capillary) growth.

Green tea contains epigallocatechin gallate EGCG, a polyphenol that helps block the induction of vascular endothelial growth factor (VEGF). Scientists consider VEGF essential in the process of angiogenesis and tumor endothelial cell survival. It is the EGCG fraction of green tea that makes it a potentially effective adjunct therapy in the treatment of breast cancer. In vivo studies have shown green tea extracts to have the following actions on human cancer cells[115,116]:

- Inhibition of tumor growth by 58%
- Inhibition of activation of nuclear factor-kappa beta
- Inhibition of microvessel density by 30%
- Inhibition of tumor-cell proliferation in vitro by 27%
- Increased tumor-cell apoptosis 1.9-fold
- Increased tumor endothelial-cell apoptosis 3-fold

The most current research shows that green tea may have a beneficial effect in treating cancer. While drinking green tea is a well-documented method of preventing cancer, it is difficult for the cancer patient to obtain a sufficient quantity of EGCG anticancer components in that form. Standardized green tea extract is more useful then green tea itself because the dose of EGCG can be precisely monitored and greater doses can be ingested without excessive intake of liquids. A suggested dose for a person with breast cancer is 5 capsules of 350-mg lightly caffeinated green tea extract 3 times daily with each meal. Each capsule should provide at least 100 mg of EGCG. It may be desirable to take a decaffeinated version of green tea extract in the evening to ensure that the caffeine does not interfere with sleep. Those sensitive to caffeine may also use this decaffeinated form.

However, there are benefits to obtaining some caffeine. Studies show that caffeine potentiates the anticancer effects of tea polyphenols, including the critical EGCG. Caffeine will be discussed in further detail later in this protocol.

## Conjugated Linoleic Acid (CLA)

Conjugated linoleic acid (CLA) found naturally, as a component of beef and milk, refers to isomers of octadecadienoic acid with conjugated double bonds. CLA is essential for the transport of dietary fat into cells, where it is used to build muscle and produce energy. CLA is incorporated into the neutral lipids of mammary fat (adipocyte) cells, where it serves as a local reservoir of CLA. It has been proposed that CLA may be an excellent candidate for prevention of breast cancer.[117] Low levels of CLA are found in breast cancer patients, but these do not influence survival. Nevertheless, it has been hypothesized that a higher intake of CLA might have a protective effect on the risk of metastasis.[118]

CLA was shown to prevent mammary cancer in rats if given before the onset of puberty. CLA ingested during the time of the "promotion" phase of cancer development conferred substantial protection from further development of breast cancer in the rats by inducing cytotoxicity (ie, cell kill) of pre-cancerous lesions.[119] It was determined that feeding CLA to female rats while young and still developing conferred life-long protection against breast cancer. This preventative action was achieved by adding enough CLA to equal 0.8% of the animal's total diet.[120]

CLA inhibits the proliferation of human breast cancer cells (MCF-7), induced by estradiol and insulin (but not EGF). In fact, CLA caused cytotoxicity when tumor cells were induced with insulin.[121] The antiproliferative effects of CLA are partly due to their ability to elicit a p53 response that leads to growth arrest.[122] CLA elicits cell killing effects in human breast tumor cells through both p53-dependent and p53 independent pathways according to the cell type.[123] Refer to the Cancer Treatment: The Critical Factors protocol for more information on determining the p53 status of cancer. The effects of CLA are mediated by both direct action (on the epithelium) as well as indirect action through the stroma.

The growth suppressing effect of CLA may be partly due to changes in arachidonic distribution among cellular lipids and an altered prostaglandin profile.[124] Intracellular lipids may become more susceptible to oxidative stress to the point of producing a cytotoxic effect.[125] CLA has the ability to suppress arachidonic acid. Since arachidonic acid can produce inflammatory compounds that can promote cancer proliferation, this may be yet another explanation for CLA's anticancer effects.

Life Extension's recommendation for CLA is a dose of 3000–4000 mg daily, which is approximately 1% of the average human diet. The suggested amount required to obtain the overall cancer-preventing effects is only 3000–4000 mg daily in divided doses.

CLA may work via a mechanism similar to that of some antidiabetic drugs not only by enhancing insulin-sensitivity, but also by increasing plasma adiponectin levels, alleviating hyperinsulinemia, and protecting against cancer.[126] A number of human cancer cell lines express the PPAR-gamma transcription factor, and agonists for PPAR-gamma can promote apoptosis in these cell lines and impede their clonal expansion both in vitro and in vivo. CLA can activate PPAR-gamma in rat adipocytes, possibly explaining CLA's antidiabetic effects in Zucker fatty rats. A portion of CLA's broad-spectrum anticarcinogenic activity is probably mediated by PPAR-gamma activation in susceptible tumor.[127]

However, CLA's anticarcinogenic effects could not be confirmed in one epidemiologic study in humans.[128]

**Note:** *The term PPAR-gamma is an acronym for peroxisome proliferator–activated receptor-gamma. A PPAR-gamma agonist such as Avandia®, Actos®, or CLA activates the PPAR-gamma receptor. This class of drug is being investigated as a potential adjuvant therapy against certain types of cancer.*

## Caffeine

Caffeine occurs naturally in green tea and has been shown to potentiate the anticancer effects of tea polyphenols. Caffeine is a model radio-sensitizing agent thought to work by abolishing the radiation-induced, G2-phase checkpoint in the cell cycle. Caffeine can induce apoptosis of a human lung carcinoma cell line by itself and can act synergistically with radiation to induce tumor cytotoxicity and cell growth arrest. The cancer cell killing effect of caffeine is dependent on the dose.[129]

Caffeine enhances the tumor cell killing effects of anticancer drugs and radiation. A preliminary report on radiochemotherapy combined with caffeine for high-grade soft tissue sarcomas in 17 patients (treated with cisplatin, caffeine, and doxorubicin after radiation therapy) determined complete response in 6 patients, partial response in 6 patients, and no change in 5 patients. The effectiveness rate of caffeine-potentiated radiochemotherapy was therefore 17%, and contributed to a satisfactory local response and the success of function-saving surgery for high-grade soft tissue sarcomas.[130]

In a randomized, double-blind placebo-controlled crossover study, the effects of caffeine as an adjuvant to morphine in advanced cancer patients was found to benefit cognitive performance and reduce pain intensity.[131]

Cancer patients should note that one study demonstrated that caffeine reduced the cytotoxic effect of paclitaxel on human lung adenocarcinoma cell lines.[132]

To ascertain the inhibitory effects of caffeine, mice at high risk of developing malignant and nonmalignant tumors (SKH-1) received oral caffeine as their sole source of drinking fluid for 18–23 weeks. Results revealed that caffeine inhibited the formation and decreased the size of both nonmalignant and malignant tumors.[133]

In cancer cells, p53 gene mutations are the most common alterations observed (50–60%) and are a factor in both carcinomas and sarcomas. Caffeine has been shown to potentiate the destruction of p53-defective cells by inhibiting p53's growth signal. The effects of this are to inhibit and override the DNA damage-checkpoint, and thus kill dividing cells. Caffeine uncouples cell-cycle progression by interfering with the replication and repair of DNA.[134-137]

Caffeine inhibits the development of Ehrlich ascites carcinoma in female mice.[138] Topical application of caffeine inhibits the occurrence of cancer and increases tumor cell death in radiation-induced skin tumors in mice.[139] Caffeine inhibits solid tumor development and lung experimental metastasis induced by melanoma cells.[140]

Consumption of coffee, tea, and caffeine was not associated with breast cancer incidence in a study of 59 036 Swedish women (aged 40–76 years).[141]

## Lignans

Lignans are found in high concentrations in flaxseed and sesame. Once consumed, lignans are converted in the intestines into enterolactone. Enterolactone has been shown to inhibit angiogenesis and promote cancer cell apoptosis.[142,143]

Enterolactone inhibits the aromatase enzyme, which converts testosterone into estrogen.[144,145]

Researchers conducted an analysis of breast cancer risk and dietary lignan intake in 3158 women. They determined that premenopausal women with the highest lignan intake had a 44% reduced risk of developing breast cancer.[146]

Thirty-two women awaiting surgery for breast cancer were randomized to receive either a muffin containing 25 g of flaxseeds or no flaxseed (control group). Postoperative analysis of the cancerous tissue revealed that markers of tumor growth were reduced by 30–71% in the flaxseed group versus no reduction in the control group.[147] Scientists concluded that "dietary flaxseed has the potential to reduce tumor growth in patients with breast cancer."

In order to examine the relationship between dietary lignan intake and breast cancer, researchers assessed the diets of 1122 women in the 1–2 years before breast cancer diagnosis. They noted that postmenopausal women with the highest dietary intake of lignans had a 71% decreased risk of death from breast cancer.[148]

## Melatonin

One of the most important supplements for a breast cancer patient is the hormone melatonin. Melatonin inhibits human breast cancer cell growth[149] and reduces tumor spread and invasiveness in vitro.[150] Indeed, it has been suggested that melatonin acts as a naturally

occurring antiestrogen on tumor cells, as it downregulates hormones responsible for the growth of hormone-dependent mammary tumors.[151]

A high percentage of women with estrogen receptor-positive breast cancer have low plasma melatonin levels.[152] There have been some studies demonstrating changes in melatonin levels in breast cancer patients; specifically, women with breast cancer were found to have lower melatonin levels than women without breast cancer.[153] Normally, women undergo a seasonal variation in the production of certain hormones, such as melatonin. However, it was found that women with breast cancer did not have a seasonal variation in melatonin levels, as did the healthy women.[154]

Low levels of melatonin have been associated with breast cancer occurrence and development. Women who work predominantly at night and are exposed to light, which inhibits melatonin production and alters the circadian rhythm, have an increased risk of breast cancer development.[155] In contrast, higher melatonin levels have been found in blind and visually impaired people, along with correspondingly lower incidences of cancer compared to those with normal vision, thus suggesting a role for melatonin in the reduction of cancer incidence.[156]

Light at night, regardless of duration or intensity, inhibits melatonin secretion and phase shifts the circadian clock, possibly altering the cell growth rate that is regulated by the circadian rhythm.[157] Disruption of circadian rhythm is commonly observed among breast cancer patients[158,159] and contributes to cancer development and tumor progression. Circadian rhythm alone is a statistically significant predictor of survival time for breast cancer patients.[160]

Melatonin differs from the classic antiestrogens such as tamoxifen in that it does not seem to bind to the estrogen receptor or interfere with the binding of estradiol to its receptor.[161] Melatonin does not cause side effects, such as those caused by the conventional antiestrogen drug tamoxifen. Furthermore, when melatonin and tamoxifen are combined, synergistic benefits occur. Moreover, melatonin can increase the therapeutic efficacy of tamoxifen[162] and biological therapies such as IL-2.[163]

How melatonin interferes with estrogen signaling is unknown, although recent studies suggest that it acts through a cyclic adenosine monophosphate (cAMP)-independent signaling pathway.[151] It has been proposed that melatonin suppresses the epidermal growth factor receptor (EGF-R)[164] and exerts its growth inhibitory effects by inducing differentiation ("normalizing" cancer cells).[165] Melatonin directly inhibits breast cancer cell proliferation[166] and boosts the production of immune components, including natural killer cells (NK cells) that have an ability to kill metastasized cancer cells.

In tumorigenesis studies, melatonin reduced the incidence and growth rate of breast tumors and slowed breast cancer development.[167] Furthermore, prolonged oral melatonin administration significantly reduced the development of existing mammary tumors in animals.[168]

In vitro experiments carried out with the estrogen receptor-positive human breast cancer cells (MCF-7 cells) demonstrated that melatonin, at a physiologic concentration (1 nM) and in the presence of serum or estradiol (a) inhibits, in a reversible way, cell proliferation; (b) increases the expression of p53 and p21WAF1 proteins and modulates the length of the cell cycle; and (c) reduces the metastatic capacity of these cells and counteracts the stimulatory effect of estradiol on cell invasiveness. Further, this effect is mediated, at least in part, by a melatonin-induced increase in the expression of the cell surface adhesion proteins E-cadherin and beta (1)-integrin.[169]

Melatonin can be safely taken for an indefinite period of time. The suggested dose of melatonin for breast cancer patients is 3–50 mg at bedtime. Initially, if melatonin is taken in large doses, vivid dreams and morning drowsiness may occur. To avoid these minor side effects, melatonin may be taken in low doses nightly and the dose slowly increased over a period of several weeks.

## Pomegranate

Pomegranate, which is rich in antioxidants, has gained widespread popularity as a functional food (ie, has health benefits). The health benefits of the fruit, juice(s), and extract(s) have been studied in relation to a variety of chronic diseases, including cancer.[170,171]

Researchers discovered that consumption of whole pomegranate seed oil and juice concentrate[172] resulted in dramatic growth inhibition of estrogen-dependent breast cancer cells. The same study showed inhibition of tumor formation in rodent cells exposed to known breast carcinogens. Using different methods, another research group found a 42% reduction in tumor formation with whole pomegranate juice polyphenols and an 87% reduction with pomegranate seed oil.[173]

Pomegranate seed oil is a potent inhibitor of aromatase, the enzyme that converts testosterone into estrogen.[174] This enzymatic *blockade* contributes to pomegranate seed oil's ability to inhibit growth of estrogen-dependent breast cancer cells. Pomegranate extract has also been shown to enhance the effects of the estrogen blocking drug tamoxifen, with the authors of a study stating that "pomegranate combined with tamoxifen may represent a novel and a powerful approach to enhance and sensitize tamoxifen action."[175] Pomegranate also increases apoptosis, even in cancer cells that lack estrogen receptors.[172]

Cancer cells need to grow new blood vessels to support their rapid growth and tissue invasion (angiogenesis). They typically do this by ramping up production of a variety of growth factors, including VEGF and inflammatory interleukins. Pomegranate seed oil powerfully inhibits production of VEGF while upregulating production of migratory inhibitory factor (MIF) in breast cancer cells. In a laboratory model of vessel growth, these modulations translated into a significant decrease in new blood vessel formation.[176] Pomegranate seed oil's capacity to block breast cancer development was also demonstrated in an organ culture model of mouse breast cancer.[173] Treating the glands with pomegranate seed oil prior to exposure to a powerful carcinogen resulted in a 87% reduction in the number of cancerous lesions compared with controls.

Pomegranate seed oil contains a number of unique chemical constituents with potent biological effects. Punicic acid, an omega-5 polyunsaturated fatty acid that inhibits both estrogen-dependent and estrogen-independent breast cancer cell proliferation in lab cultures,[177] also induced apoptosis at rates up to 91% higher than those in untreated cell cultures—effects which appear to be related to fundamental regulation of cancer cell signaling pathways.[177]

## Polysaccharide K (PSK)

PSK, which is a specially prepared polysaccharide extract from the mushroom *Coriolus versicolor*, has been studied extensively in Japan where it is used as a nonspecific biological response modifier to enhance the immune system in cancer patients.[178–180] PSK suppresses tumor cell invasiveness by downregulating several invasion-related factors.[181] PSK has been shown to enhance NK cell activity in multiple studies.[182–185]

In a study investigating the use of PSK in women with stage 2 breast cancer, postoperative participants received tamoxifen with PSK (3 g daily) or tamoxifen alone. The 5-year survival was 89.9% in the PSK group compared to 86.9% in the group receiving tamoxifen only.[186]

## Pterostilbene

Pterostilbene, a polyphenol found in blueberries, grapes, and in the bark of the Indian kino tree, is closely related to resveratrol (but with unique attributes). Pterostilbene's mechanisms of action include blocking enzymes that activate carcinogens,[187,188] inducing apoptosis[189] and cell cycle arrest,[190] and enhancing nitric oxide-induced cell death.[191]

Researchers observed that pterostilbene markedly inhibited the growth of breast cancer cells in the laboratory by inducing apoptosis and cell cycle arrest.[190]

## Quercetin

Quercetin is a flavonoid found in a broad range of foods, from grape skins and red onions to green tea and tomatoes. Quercetin's antioxidant and anti-inflammatory properties protect cellular DNA from cancer-inducing mutations.[192] Quercetin traps developing cancer cells in the early phases of their replicative cycle, effectively preventing further malignant development and promoting cancer cell death.[193] Furthermore, quercetin favorably modulates chemical signaling pathways that are abnormal in cancer cells.[194,195]

In breast cancer cells, quercetin induces apoptosis and cell cycle arrest.[196,197] Quercetin inhibited the growth of tumors[198] and prolonged survival of mice with breast cancer.[199]

## Se-Methylselenocysteine

Se-methylselenocysteine (SeMSC), a naturally occurring organic selenium compound found to be an effective chemopreventive agent, is a new and better form of selenium. SeMSC is a selenoamino acid that is synthesized by plants such as garlic and broccoli.

Methylselenocysteine (MSC) has been shown to be effective against mammary cell growth both in vivo and in vitro[200] and has significant anticancer activity against mammary tumor development.[201] Moreover, SeMSC was one of the most effective selenium chemoprevention compounds and induced apoptosis in human leukemia cells (HL-60) in vitro.[202] Exposure to MSC blocks expansion of cancer colonies and premalignant lesions at an early stage by simultaneously modulating pathways responsible for inhibiting cell proliferation and enhancing apoptosis.[203]

SeMSC has been shown to:

- Produce a 33% better reduction of cancerous lesions than selenite
- Produce a 50% decrease in tumor development
- Induce cell death (apoptosis) in cancer cells
- Inhibit cancer-cell growth (proliferation)

- Reduce density and development of tumor blood vessels
- Downregulate VEGF (vascular endothelial growth factor)[200,201,203–206]

Unlike MSC, which is incorporated into protein in place of methionine, SeMSC is not incorporated into any protein, thereby offering a completely bioavailable compound. In animal studies, SeMSC has been shown to be 10 times less toxic than any other known form of selenium. Breast cancer patients may consider taking 400 mcg of SeSMC daily.

## Sulforaphane

Sulforaphane, which is an isothiocyanate, is most highly concentrated in broccoli as well as other cruciferous vegetables (eg, Brussels sprouts, cabbage, and cauliflower).

Sulforaphane detoxifies potential carcinogens, promotes apoptosis, blocks the cell cycle required for cancer cell replication, prevents tumor invasion into healthy tissue, enhances natural killer cell activity, and combats metastasis.[207–210] Research has also demonstrated that sulforaphane is among the plant chemicals most potently capable of blocking the cancer-producing effects of ultraviolet radiation.[211]

It has been observed that sulforaphane activated apoptosis[212] and inhibited the proliferation of breast cancer cells in culture.[213,214] The binding of estrogen hormones to estrogen receptor *alpha* promotes *breast cell proliferation*, which can promote the progression of breast cancer. Researchers have also noted that sulforaphane downregulates the expression of estrogen receptor alpha in breast cancer cells.[213]

In another clinical trial, mice injected with breast cancer cells developed 60% less tumor mass when treated with sulforaphane compared to untreated mice.[215]

## Coenzyme Q10 (CoQ10)

CoQ10 is synthesized in humans from tyrosine through a cascade of 8 aromatic precursors. These precursors require 8 vitamins, which are vitamin C, B2, B3 (niacin) B6, B12, folic acid, pantothenic acid, and tetrahydrobiopterin as their coenzymes.

Since the 1960s, studies have shown that cancer patients often have decreased blood levels of coenzyme Q10.[216–218] In particular, breast cancer patients (with infiltrative ductal carcinoma) who underwent radical mastectomy were found to have significantly decreased tumor concentrations of CoQ10 compared to levels in normal surrounding tissues. Increased levels of reactive oxygen species may be involved in the consumption of CoQ10.[219] These findings sparked interest in the compound as a potential anticancer agent.[220] Cellular and animal studies have found evidence that CoQ10 stimulates the immune system and can increase resistance to illness.[220–222]

CoQ10 may induce a protective effect on breast tissue and has demonstrated promise in treating breast cancer. Although there are only a few studies, the safe nature of CoQ10 coupled with this promising research of its bioenergetic activity suggests that breast cancer patients should take 100 mg up to 3 times a day. It is important to take CoQ10 with some kind of oil, such as fish or flax, because dry powder CoQ10 is not readily absorbed.

In a clinical study, 32 patients were treated with CoQ10 (90 mg) in addition to other antioxidants and fatty acids; 6 of these patients showed partial tumor regression. In one of these cases, the dose of CoQ10 was increased to 390 mg; within 1 month the tumor was no longer palpable, and within 2 months the mammography confirmed the absence of tumor. In another case, the patient took 300 mg of CoQ10 for residual tumor (post nonradical surgery) and within 3 months there was nonresidual tumor tissue.[223] This overt complete regression of breast tumors in the latter 2 cases coupled with further reports of disappearance of breast cancer metastases (liver and elsewhere) in several other cases[216] demonstrates the potential of CoQ10 in the adjuvant therapy of breast cancer.

There are promising results for the use of CoQ10 in protecting against heart damage related to chemotherapy. Many chemotherapy drugs can cause damage to the heart,[224–227] and initial animal studies found that CoQ10 could reduce the adverse cardiac effects of these drugs.[217,228–232]

*Caution:* Some studies indicate that CoQ10 should not be taken at the same time as chemotherapy. If this were true, it would be disappointing, because CoQ10 is so effective in protecting against adriamycin-induced cardiomyopathy. Adriamycin is a chemotherapy drug sometimes used as part of a chemotherapy cocktail. Until more research is known, it is not possible to make a definitive recommendation concerning taking CoQ10 during chemotherapy. For more information, see the Chemotherapy protocol.

## EPA and DHA

Dietary polyunsaturated fatty acids (PUFAs) of the omega-6 (n-6) class, found in corn oil and safflower oil, may be involved in the development of breast cancer, whereas long chain (LC) omega-3 (n-3) PUFAs, found in fish oil can inhibit breast cancer.[233]

A case control study examining levels of fatty acids in breast adipose tissue of breast cancer patients has shown that total omega-6 PUFAs may be contributing to the high risk of breast cancer in the United States and that omega-3 PUFAs, derived from fish oil, may have a protective effect.[233]

A higher omega-3:omega-6 ratio ([n-3]:[n-6] ratio) may reduce the risk of breast cancer, especially in premenopausal women.[234] In a prospective study of 35 298 Singapore Chinese women aged 45–74 years, it was determined that high levels of dietary omega-3 fatty acids from marine sources (fish/shellfish) were significantly associated with reduced risk of breast cancer. Furthermore, women who consumed low levels of marine omega-3 fatty acids had a statistically significant increased risk of breast cancer.[235]

Omega-3 fatty acids, primarily eicosapentaenoic acid (EPA) and docosahexaenoic acid (DHA) found naturally in oily fish and fish oil, have been consistently shown to retard the growth of breast cancer in vitro and in animal experiments, inhibit tumor development and metastasis. Fish oils have antiproliferative effects at high doses, which means they can inhibit tumor cell growth, through a free radical-mediated mechanism, while at more moderate doses omega-3 fatty acids inhibit Ras protein activity, angiogenesis, and inflammation. The production of pro-inflammatory cytokines can be modified by dietary omega-3 PUFAs.[236]

High consumption of fatty fish is weakly associated with reduced breast cancer risk.[234] Flaxseed, the richest source of alpha-linoleic acid inhibited the established growth and metastasis of human breast cancer implanted in mice. This effect was found to be due to its downregulation of insulin-like growth factor I (IGF-1) and epidermal growth factor receptor (EGF-R) expression.[237] The recommended dosage is to consume a fish-oil concentrate supplement that provides 3200 mg of EPA and 2400 mg of DHA daily in divided doses.

## Vitamins A, D, and E

Vitamin A and vitamin D3 inhibit breast cancer cell division and can induce cancer cells to differentiate into mature, noncancerous cells. Vitamin D3 works synergistically with tamoxifen (and melatonin) to inhibit breast cancer cell proliferation. The vitamin D3 receptor as a target for breast cancer prevention was examined. Preclinical studies demonstrated that vitamin D compounds could reduce breast cancer development in animals. Furthermore, human studies indicate that both vitamin D status and genetic variations in the vitamin D3 receptor (VDR) may affect breast cancer risk. Findings from cellular, molecular, and population studies suggest that the VDR is a nutritionally modulated, growth-regulatory gene that may represent a molecular target for chemo-prevention of breast cancer.[238]

Daily doses of vitamin A at 350 000–500 000 IU were given to 100 patients with metastatic breast carcinoma treated by chemotherapy. A significant increase in complete response was observed; however, response rates, duration of response, and projected survival were only significantly increased in postmenopausal women with breast cancer.[239]

Breast cancer patients may take 4000–6000 IU of vitamin D3 every day. Water-soluble vitamin A can be taken in doses of 100 000–300 000 IU every day. Monthly blood tests are needed to make sure toxicity does not occur in response to these high daily doses of vitamin A and vitamin D3. After 4–6 months, the doses of vitamin D3 and vitamin A can be reduced.

Vitamin E is the term used to describe 8 naturally occurring essential fat-soluble nutrients: alpha-, beta-, delta-, and gamma-tocopherols plus a class of compounds related to vitamin E called alpha-, beta-, delta-, and gamma-tocotrienols. Vitamin E from dietary sources may provide women with modest protection from breast cancer.

Vitamin E succinate, a derivative of fat-soluble vitamin E, has been shown to inhibit tumor cell growth in vitro and in vivo.[240,241] In estrogen receptor-negative human breast cancer cell lines, vitamin E succinate inhibited growth and induced cell death. Since vitamin E is considered the main chain breaking lipophilic antioxidant in plasma and tissue, its role as a potential chemopreventive agent and its use in the adjuvant treatment of aggressive human breast cancers appears reasonable. Those with estrogen receptor-negative breast cancers should consider taking 800–1200 IU of vitamin E succinate per day. Vitamin E supplementation, 800 IU daily for 4 weeks, was shown to significantly reduce hot flashes in breast cancer survivors.[242]

*Caution:* When taking doses of vitamin D3 in excess of 1400 IU per day, regular blood chemistry tests should be taken to monitor kidney function and serum calcium metabolism. Vitamin E has potential blood thinning properties; individuals taking anticoagulant drugs should inform their treating physician if supplementing with vitamin E and have their clotting factors monitored regularly.

## Tocotrienols

When vitamin E was isolated from plant oils, the term tocopherols was used to name the initial 4 compounds that shared similar structures. Their structures have 2 primary parts—a complex ring and a phytyl (long-saturated) side chain—and have been designated as alpha-, beta-, delta-, and gamma-tocopherol. Tocopherols (vitamin E) are important lipid-soluble antioxidants that can protect the body against free radical damage.

However, there are 4 additional compounds related to tocopherols—called tocotrienols—that are less widely distributed in nature. The tocotrienol structure, 3 double bonds in an isoprenoid (unsaturated) side chain, differs from that of tocopherols. While tocopherols are found in corn, olive oil, and soybeans, tocotrienols are concentrated in palm, rice bran, and barley oils.

Tocotrienols elicit powerful anticancer properties, and studies have confirmed tocotrienol activity is much stronger than that of tocopherols.[243]

Tocotrienols provide more efficient penetration into tissues such as the brain and liver. Because of the double bonds in the isoprenoid side chain, tocotrienols move freely and more efficiently within cell membranes than tocopherols, giving tocotrienols greater ability to counteract free radicals. This greater mobility also allows tocotrienols to recycle more quickly than alpha-tocopherol. Tocotrienols are better distributed in fatty cell membranes and demonstrate greater antioxidant and free-radical-scavenging effects than that of vitamin E (alpha-tocopherol).[244,245]

Tocotrienol's antioxidant function is associated with lowering DNA damage, tumor formation, and cell damage. Animals exposed to carcinogens that were fed corn oil- or soybean oil-based diets had significantly more tumors than those fed a tocotrienol-rich palm oil diet. Tocotrienol-rich palm oil did not promote chemically induced breast cancer.[246]

Tocotrienols possess the ability to stimulate the selective killing of cancer cells through programmed cell death (apoptosis) and to reduce cancer cell proliferation while leaving normal cells unaffected.[247] Tocotrienols are thought to suppress cancer through the isoprenoid side chain.

Isoprenoids are plant compounds that have been shown to suppress the initiation, growth, and progression of many types of cancer in experimental studies.[248] They are common in fruits and vegetables, which may explain why diets rich in these foods have consistently been shown to reduce the incidence of cancer.

Isoprenoids induce cell death (apoptosis) and arrest cell growth in human breast adenocarcinoma cells (MCF-7).[249] Isoprenoids may suppress the mevalonate pathway, through which mutated Ras proteins transform healthy cells into cancer cells. Mutated ras is the most common cellular defect found in human cancers. The mevalonate pathway escapes regulatory control in tumor tissue but remains highly sensitive to regulation by tocotrienols. Tocotrienols are at least 5 times more powerful than farnesol, the body's regulator of the mevalonate pathway. Interestingly, human breast cancer cells have been shown to respond very well to treatment with tocotrienols.[250]

Tocotrienols cause growth inhibition of breast cancer cells in culture independent of estrogen sensitivity and have great potential in the prevention and treatment of breast cancer.[251]

In vitro studies have demonstrated the effectiveness of tocotrienols as inhibitors of both estrogen receptor-positive (estrogen-responsive) and estrogen receptor-negative (nonestrogen-responsive) cell proliferation. The effect of palm tocotrienols on 3 human breast cancer cells lines, estrogen-responsive and estrogen-nonresponsive (MCF7, MDA-MB-231, and ZR-75-1), found that tocotrienols inhibited cell growth strongly in both the presence and absence of estradiol. The gamma- and delta-fractions of tocotrienols were most effective at inhibiting cell growth, while alpha-tocopherol was ineffective. Tocotrienols were found to enhance the effect of tamoxifen.[252]

Delta-tocotrienol was shown to be the most potent inducer of apoptosis (programmed cell death) in both estrogen-responsive and estrogen-nonresponsive human breast cancer cells, followed by gamma- and alpha-tocotrienol (beta-tocotrienol was not tested). Interestingly, delta-tocotrienol is more plentiful in palm tocotrienols than in tocotrienols derived from rice. Of the natural tocopherols, only delta-tocopherol showed any apoptosis-inducing effect, although it was less than one-tenth of the effect of palm and rice delta-tocotrienol.[253]

Tocotrienols effectively arrested the cell cycle and triggered cell death of mammary cancer cells (from mice) whereas tocopherols (alpha, gamma, and delta) did not cause inhibition of tumor cell growth. Highly malignant cells were most sensitive to the antiproliferative effects of tocotrienols, whereas less aggressive precancerous cells were the least sensitive.[254]

Tocotrienols were found to be far more effective than alpha-tocopherol at inhibiting breast cancer cell growth. Tocotrienols in combination with tamoxifen proved more effective than either compound alone in both estrogen-responsive and nonresponsive breast cancer cells. The synergism between tamoxifen and tocotrienols may reduce the risk of adverse side effect from tamoxifen.[255]

Tocotrienols are considered important lipid-soluble antioxidants, with potent anticancer and anti-inflammatory activity. Therefore, a daily dose of 240 mg of tocotrienols should be considered as an adjuvant breast cancer therapy.

# PREVENTING BREAST CANCER CELL METASTASIS

Breast cancer cells frequently metastasize to the bone, where they cause severe degradation of bone tissue. Metastatic cancer affects more than half of all women during the course of their disease. Bone metastases are a significant cause of morbidity due to pain, pathologic fractures, hypercalcemia (abnormally high levels of calcium in blood plasma), and spinal cord compression. The bisphosphonates, including alendronate (Fosamax®), tiludronate (Skelid®), pamidronate (Aredia®), etidronate (Didronel®), risedronate (Actonel®), ibandronate, and zoledronic acid (Zometa®), are a class of drugs that protect against the degradation of bone, primarily by inhibiting osteoclast-mediated bone resorption (bone breakdown).

Bisphosphonates are analogs of a naturally occurring compound, called pyrophosphate, which serves to regulate calcium and prevent bone breakdown. Bisphosphonates are a major class of drugs used for the treatment of bone diseases as they have a marked ability to inhibit bone resorption. Bisphosphonates are considered standard care for tumor-associated hypercalcemia and have been shown to reduce bone pain, improve quality of life, and delay and reduce skeletal events.[256,257]

## Bone Remodeling

The renewal of bone is responsible for bone strength throughout our life. Old bone is removed (resorption) and new bone is created (formation). This process is called bone remodeling. Healthy bone is continually being remodeled. Two main types of cells are responsible for bone renewal: the osteoblasts involved in bone formation and the osteoclasts involved in bone resorption. There are several stages involved in bone remodeling. The first is activation. This process involves preosteoclasts that are stimulated and differentiated under the influence of cytokine and growth factors to mature into active osteoclasts. The next step is resorption, in which osteoclasts digest mineral matrix (old bone). The third step is reversal, which ends resorption and signals for the final phase, formation. During this stage, osteoblasts are responsible for bone matrix synthesis (collagen production). Two other noncollagenous proteins are also formed: osteocalcin and osteonectin, together they form new bone.

## Bone Metastases Affects Remodeling

In patients with bone metastases, bone resorption by the osteoclasts is increased and exceeds bone reformation. Calcium lost from the bones appears in increased amounts in the patient's blood serum and urine. This increase in bone resorption may result in pain, bone fractures, spinal cord compression, and hypercalcemia.

Normally, the activity of the osteoclasts and osteoblasts is well balanced, with the osteoclasts cleaning out the fatigued bone and the osteoblasts rebuilding new bone. In metastatic cancer, there is increased osteoclast activity caused by factors called osteoclastic activating factors (OAFs). These OAFs, released by tumor cells, include parathyroid hormone-related peptide (PTHrP), growth factors, and cytokines.

Among the known inhibitors of osteoclast activity, the bisphosphonates are the most promising drugs available (by prescription) to women with breast cancer who have a high risk of advancing cancer. Bisphosphonates interrupt the "vicious cycle" of bone metastases. Bisphosphonates inhibit bone turnover directly by decreasing resorption of bone and inhibiting the recruitment and function of osteoclasts.

Bisphosphonates may stop bone metastases from occurring if they are included at the onset of cancer diagnosis and treatment.[40] Bisphosphonates may delay the occurrence of bone metastases in women with breast cancer who do not have metastases.

In patients with bone metastases, bisphosphonates are useful as an adjuvant therapy to decrease bone pain, fractures, hypercalcemia, and progression of bone metastases.[258] Treatment with bisphosphonates can also prevent the destruction of bone by cancer metastases and reduce the progression of metastatic tumors. A new bisphosphonate, risedronate, slows the progression of bone metastases in breast cancer patients, either by inhibiting the resorption of bone, which reduces the release of tumor growth factors, or inhibiting the adhesion of breast cancer cells to bone matrix.[258]

In women with early and advanced breast cancer and bone metastases, the use of bisphosphonates (oral or intravenous) in addition to hormone therapy or chemotherapy reduced bone pain, the risk of developing a fracture, and increased the time to a fracture.[259] Monthly infusions of pamidronate in 382 women with stage 4 breast cancer and bone metastases significantly reduced the incidence and prolonged the median time of skeletal complications.[260]

Bisphosphonates are now third generation and are often used in the treatment of lytic bone metastasis.

They inhibit the osteoclast activity that causes elevation of the blood calcium level and osteolytic bone weakening. Osteolytic holes form as the cancer degrades the bone, making it prone to fracture.[261] The bisphosphonates, zoledronate and ibandronate, manage tumor-induced hypercalcemia, Paget's disease of the bone, and multiple myeloma-associated bone resorption. These bisphosphonate drugs are 3 orders of magnitude more potent than the first-generation drugs: etidronate, clodronate, and tiludronate. Patients newly diagnosed with lytic bone metastasis of breast cancer are offered bisphosphonate therapy, such as intravenous zoledronate or pamidronate every 3–4 weeks, as long as it proves effective. Oral clodronate offers equivalent results but is less well-tolerated.

Women with primary breast cancer who receive chemotherapy, hormone therapy, aromatase therapy, or oophorectomy may experience ovarian failure or early menopause, leading to a loss of bone mineral density.

The mechanisms by which tumor cells degrade bone involve tumor-cell adhesion to bone, as well as the release of compounds from tumor cells that stimulate osteoclast-induced bone degradation. Bisphosphonates inhibit cancer-cell adhesion and inhibit osteoclast activity. By preventing tumor-cell adhesion, bisphosphonates are useful agents for the prophylactic treatment of patients with cancer that is known to preferentially metastasize to bone.

There is evidence that growth factors, such as insulin-like growth factor and transforming growth factor, are released when the bone matrix is degraded. These growth factors could stimulate tumor-cell proliferation throughout the body and may activate cancer cells to the degraded bone ripe for clonal development, which may be a reason that early use of bisphosphonates significantly improved survival and may ward off metastasis.

Based on the mounting research, it is strongly recommended that the use of bisphosphonates be considered at onset of breast cancer treatment to potentially stop bone metastases from developing. Patients are urged to discuss the use of bisphosphonates with their physicians.

*Note: Administration of bisphosphonate therapy should be accompanied by an adequate intake of a bone supplement that supplies all the raw materials to make healthy bone. These include calcium, magnesium, boron, silica, vitamin D, and vitamin K. Do not take vitamin K with Coumadin or other anticoagulant drugs or blood thinners.*

## Bone Loss and Fatty Acids

While people often use omega-3 fatty acids to reduce the inflammation associated with arthritis, these fatty acids may actually help prevent bone loss. French researchers found in a group of 105 patients that high levels of pro-inflammatory omega-6 fatty acids were strongly associated with bone loss. However, the use of omega-3 supplements—360 mg per day of EPA and 240 mg per day of DHA–appeared to decrease production of proinflammatory prostaglandin E2 in bone and significantly stopped bone loss.[262]

## Hormone Therapy and Metastasis

In primary breast cancer, estrogen receptor status represents an important prognostic factor, and therefore has a profound impact on the type of therapy employed. Yet, there is little research into the estrogen receptor expression of disseminated breast cancer cells even though these cells are the main targets in adjuvant therapy.

A small pilot study involving 17 patients evaluated the estrogen receptor expression profile on disseminated epithelial cells in bone marrow, one of the preferential organs for manifestation of distant metastases in breast cancer. Eleven patients (64.7%) were found to have estrogen receptor-positive primary carcinomas. Of those eleven, only 2 patients revealed estrogen receptor-positive epithelial cells in bone marrow. Additionally, one of these 2 patients expressed both estrogen receptor-positive and estrogen receptor-negative epithelial cells in bone marrow. Although in both of these cases the estrogen receptor-positive epithelial cells in bone marrow derived from estrogen receptor-positive primary tumors, in this small patient cohort none of the prognostic ally relevant clinical and pathologic factors tested (ie, TNM classification, grading, and estrogen receptor status in primary breast cancer) correlated with the estrogen receptor status in bone marrow. A striking discrepancy between estrogen receptor expression in primary breast cancers and the corresponding disseminated epithelial cells in bone marrow was found. This suggests either the selective dissemination of estrogen receptor-negative tumor cells into the bone marrow or a negative impact of the bone marrow microenvironment on epithelial estrogen receptor expression. While further research is required before conclusions can be drawn, this phenomenon might influence therapeutic effects of antihormonal treatment.[263]

# DIETARY AND OTHER CONSIDERATIONS

## Diet

Cancer has an appetite for sugar and requires sugar for survival. Sugar plays an active role in reducing the immune response and energizes cancer, as tumors are primarily obligate glucose metabolizers.

There is a relationship between lactic acid, insulin, and angiogenesis. In tumors, hypoxic conditions occur through both inflammation, which reduces blood flow, and the chaotic development of blood vessels within tumors. These hypoxic conditions alter the pathways by which immune cells and tumor cells burn fuel (glucose) for energy, creating excessive lactic acid. In an oxygen-rich (aerobic) environment, glucose is burned in an efficient process that produces a maximum amount of energy and a minimal amount of lactic acid. However, tumor cells in chronic hypoxic conditions produce excessive lactic acid and inefficient utilization of glucose. Thus, there is a vicious cycle in which the reduced energy output stimulates the tumor cells to burn more glucose, which in turn produces more lactic acid. Tumor cells consume glucose at a rate of 3–5 times higher than normal cells, creating a highly stimulated glycolysis (glucose-burning) pathway.

This glucose consumption can waste the cancer patient's energy reserves, and the increased production of lactic acid can stimulate increased production of angiogenic factors. The macrophage-mediated angiogenesis creates a complex interplay between opposing regulators. Insulin plays an active role in promoting angiogenesis. Insulin is a growth factor that stimulates glycolysis and the proliferation of many cancer-cell lines through tyrosine kinase growth factors.[264] In cancer patients, elevated levels of insulin are common in cancerous tissue and blood plasma. Obesity and early stages of type 2 non-insulin-dependent diabetes mellitus (NIDDM) have been implicated as risk factors in a variety of cancers.

Based on cancer's sugar dependency, a sugar-deprivation diet is strongly recommended. An effective tool in eliminating sugar from the diet is the glycemic index. The index is a list that rates the speed at which foods are digested and raise blood sugar levels. The ratings are based on the rate at which a measured amount of pure glucose affects the body's blood sugar curve. Glucose itself has a rating of 100, and the closer a food item is to a rating of 100, the more rapidly it raises blood glucose levels. Foods with a low glycemic index, such as vegetables, protein, and grains, are suggested (refer to the Obesity and Weight Loss protocol for specific information about low-glycemic foods).

With regard to depleting sugar from the diet, the following should be considered:

- Limit or avoid all white foods, including (but not limited to) sugar, flour, rice, pasta, breads, crackers, cookies, and so on.

- Read labels. Sugar has many names (brown sugar, corn syrup, honey, molasses, maple syrup, high-fructose corn syrup, dextrin, raw sugar, fructose, polyols, dextrose, hydrogenated starch, galactose, glucose, sorbitol, fruit juice concentrate, lactose, brown rice syrup, xylitol, sucrose, mannitol, sorghum, maltose, and turbinado, to mention a few).

- Limit all fruit juices; per glass they contain the juice of many pieces of fruit, a large amount of fructose (fruit sugar), but no fiber. Instead, infrequently eat low-glycemic-rated fruit in small portions.

Natural compounds have also been reported to inhibit the cancer-promoting effects of insulin. For example, vitamin C has been reported to increase oxygen consumption and reduce lactic acid production in tumor cells. In addition, some natural compounds may help reduce insulin production by reducing insulin resistance. Insulin resistance occurs when cells are no longer sensitive to insulin and thus more insulin is produced in an effort to reduce glucose levels. Insulin resistance has been implicated as a risk factor for breast cancer, and diets high in saturated fats and omega-6 fatty acids promote insulin resistance. Although the exact pathway is unknown, it is thought that the mechanism of action is via chronic activation of PKC. Some of the known natural compounds that can reduce insulin resistance include omega-3 fatty acids, curcumin, flavonoids, selenium, and vitamin E.

As discussed earlier in the protocol, estrogen is a growth factor for most breast cancers. High-fat diets and associated increases in fat tissue can increase estrogen availability in a number of ways:

- Fat tissue is a major source of estrogen production in postmenopausal women. Therefore, there is an association between high body weight and decreased survival in breast cancer patients.

- Obesity and possibly insulin resistance can decrease the levels of sex hormone binding globulin (SHBG) in both men and women and increase breast cancer risk or cancer progression. This is an important factor in estrogen-dependent breast cancer cells because it is adequate levels of SHBG that act as an antiproliferative and provide an antiestrogenic effect.

- Obesity can alter liver metabolism of estrogen, allowing the retention of high estrogen byproducts with high estrogenic activity within the body.

- High-fat diets may reduce the amount of estrogen excreted in feces. In contrast, low-fat/high-fiber diets can reduce circulating estrogen.

Another consideration when discussing diet and breast cancer is the reduction of dietary estrogen. Several foods contain naturally occurring hormones (found in animal sources); synthetic hormones that can mimic estrogen in the human body (found in commercially packaged meat, poultry, and dairy products); or naturally estrogenic properties that can encourage the body's production of estrogens (natural foods such as soy). Regardless of the source, try to avoid all commercial animal products (including, but not limited to meats, poultry, and dairy). Also, avoid the use of soft plastic food-storage products that can give off large amounts of polymers (eg, by leaching into food contents), thought by environmentalists and some researchers to be a possible cause of breast cancer.

In order to reduce estrogen, a breast cancer patient should consider increasing dietary intake of fish high in omega-3 fatty acids, whey, eggs, and nuts, occasionally including hormone-free poultry and hormone-free, low-fat dairy products.

## BLOOD TESTING

Monthly blood tests should include complete blood chemistry, with tests for liver function and serum calcium levels, prolactin, parathyroid hormone, and the tumor marker CA 27.29 (or CA 15.3). Additional blood tests to consider are the CEA and GGTP tests. These tests monitor the progress of therapies used and also detect toxicity from high doses of vitamins A and D3. The patient should insist on obtaining a copy of their blood workups every month.

## SUMMARY

When considering breast cancer treatment options, physicians and patients alike must sort through an overwhelming amount of information. This protocol attempts to simplify complicated scientific research and bring to the forefront the most up-to-date, multimodality approach to cancer treatment. It integrates surgery, anticancer drugs, irradiation, hormone therapy, nutritional supplementation, and diet modification in a comprehensive approach to counteract breast cancer.

As discussed in this protocol, cancer growth is based on many complicated interactions via numerous physiologic pathways within the body. Despite the huge strides in scientific research, there are still many unanswered questions regarding cancer's growth and development. What we do know is that there is overwhelming research supporting an integrated approach to the treatment of cancer. Additionally, research supports using nutritional supplementation to improve the efficacy of chemotherapy drugs and radiotherapy (see the Chemotherapy and Cancer Radiation protocols for more information). In fact, combining certain supplements can create a synergism that can effectively block or impede certain cancer pathways.

Therefore, the following supplementation regimen is suggested. Please read the entire protocol before considering this regimen because there are certain cautions to consider. As always, consult your physician before beginning any nutritional supplementation regimen.

## Life Extension Suggestions

- **Apigenin:** 20–50 mg daily
- **Astragalus:** 2000–4000 mg daily
- **Blueberry:** 900–1800 mg daily
- **Chrysin:** 1000–2000 mg daily
- **Coffee:** 400 mg, 3 times daily
- **Cruciferous vegetable extract:** containing at least 80–160 mg of indol-3-carbinol (I3C) daily
- **Curcumin:** 400 mg, 3 times daily (as highly absorbable BCM-95®)
- **Lightly caffeinated green tea extract:** Three 725-mg capsules, 2 times daily with meals. Use decaffeinated green tea extract if you are sensitive to caffeine or want to use a less-stimulating version with the evening dosage.
- **CLA or CLA with guarana:** 3000–4000 mg daily of CLA and about 300 mg of guarana early in the day
- **Lignans:** 75–125 mg daily
- **Melatonin:** 3–50 mg at bedtime
- **Pomegranate:** 280–375 mg daily of punicalagins
- **Powders** (broccoli, cabbage, and other cruciferous vegetables that provide sulforaphane and other cancer-fighting plant extracts): 1–2 tbsp daily
- **PSK** (from the mushroom *Coriolus versicolor*): 3 g daily
- **Pterostilbene:** 1–3 mg daily
- **Quercetin:** 1000–3000 mg daily
- **Se-methylselenocysteine:** 200–400 mcg daily
- **Sulforaphane:** 400–1600 mg daily of a broccoli extract
- **CoQ10** (as ubiquinol): Three 100-mg softgels in divided doses. Note the caution stated in this protocol.
- **EPA/DHA** (with sesame lignans): 2–4 g daily. Take with nonfiber meals.
- **Vitamin D3:** 4000–6000 IU taken daily with monthly blood testing to monitor for toxicity. Reduce dosage at 6 months.
- **Water-soluble vitamin A:** 100000–300000 IU daily with monthly blood testing to monitor for toxicity. Reduce dosage at 6 months.
- **Vitamin E:** succinate (tocopheryl succinate), 1200 IU daily
- **Gamma tocopherol:** at least 359 mg of gamma E-mixed tocopherols daily
- **Vitamin C:** 4000–12000 mg throughout the day
- **Gamma linolenic acid (GLA):** 299–1495 mg daily
- **Whey protein concentrate-isolate:** 30–60 g daily in divided doses
- **Calcium:** 1000–1200 mg daily
- **Magnesium:** 200–1000 mg daily
- **Vitamin K:** 10 mg daily
- **Silicon:** 6 mg daily
- **Multinutrient formula:** per label instructions

**Reminder:** Bisphosphonate (injectable Zometa® or Aredia®) drug therapy is strongly encouraged for all breast cancer patients as well as aromatase-inhibitor therapy (Arimidex®, Femara®, or Aromasin®) if appropriate.

**Note:** *If chemotherapy and/or radiation are being considered, refer to the Chemotherapy and Cancer Radiation protocols. Also refer to the protocols titled Cancer Treatment: The Critical Factors and Cancer Adjuvant Therapy.*

## FOR MORE INFORMATION

Contact the American Cancer Society, 1 (800) ACS-2345.
Sources for National Cancer Institute Information:

- Cancer Information Service, (800) 4-CANCER (1-800-422-6237); TTY (for hearing impaired callers), (800) 332-8615
- NCI Online/Internet, use http://cancer.gov to reach the NCI website.
- CancerMail Service. To obtain a contents list, send e-mail to cancermail@cips.nci.nih.gov with the word "help" in the body of the message.

## STAYING INFORMED

This protocol raises many issues that are subject to change as new data emerge. Furthermore, cancer is still a disease with unacceptably high mortality rates, and none of our suggested regimens can guarantee a cure.

Life Extension is constantly uncovering information to provide to cancer patients. A special website has been established for the purpose of updating patients on new findings that directly pertain to the published cancer protocols. Whenever Life Extension discovers information that may benefit cancer patients, it will be posted on the website www.lefcancer.org.

Before utilizing this cancer protocol, we suggest checking www.lefcancer.org to see if any substantive changes have been made to the recommendations described herein. Based on the sheer number of newly published findings, there could be significant alterations to the information you have just read.

## REFERENCES

References available at: www.lef.org/dpt5/ch26

# 27

# *Bronchitis (Acute)*

Acute bronchitis is one of the most common reasons people in the United States seek medical care. It is important to distinguish episodes of acute bronchitis from the chronic bronchitis, which is associated with chronic obstructive pulmonary disease (COPD). For more information on COPD, see the Chronic Obstructive Pulmonary Disease (COPD) protocol.

During an episode of acute bronchitis, the tissue(s) lining the bronchi become irritated and inflamed, causing increased secretion of mucus and a narrowing of the airways. This produces the characteristic cough.[1] For many people, the cough itself becomes an aggravating factor and worsens their condition.

Up to 95% of acute bronchitis cases are caused by viral infection, with most of the rest caused by environmental irritants. The most common viral causes are influenza, parainfluenza, and common cold viruses. In many cases (up to 70%), antibiotics are prescribed for acute viral bronchitis, making it one of the leading situations in which antibiotics are misused. Accordingly, the American College of Physicians and the U.S. Centers for Disease Control and Prevention have issued guidelines aimed at stopping physicians from automatically prescribing antibiotics to patients with acute bronchitis. According to these 2 organizations, the only form of bronchitis that should be treated with antibiotics is pertussis (whooping cough). However, because of the risk of acute bronchitis being caused by certain bacteria, some physicians will also prescribe antibiotics to certain patients to prevent further infection.

Unfortunately, there is little that can be done to stop an episode of acute bronchitis once it begins. The most common recommendation for treatment is to wait for the inflammation to subside naturally, which will relieve the coughing and other symptoms. In very severe cases, a physician might recommend medications that limit coughing, reduce mucus production, and open airways. However, many of these medications have unpleasant side effects.

Life Extension's approach to acute bronchitis is based on 2 simple ideas:

1. The best defense is a good offense. Since acute bronchitis is usually caused by viral infection, every effort should be made to prevent exposure to these viruses from progressing to a full-blown infection. Life Extension has developed an aggressive program to help avoid infections by these common viruses. To read about this program in detail, see the Influenza and Common Cold protocols, or refer to the section at the end of this protocol. It is important that people act quickly if they suspect they are coming down with a viral infection.

2. Although no medication or dietary supplement has been shown to specifically inhibit acute bronchitis, it may be possible to reduce symptoms by attacking the underlying cause of the condition, namely inflammation and its associated free radical damage and mucus production. Many nutrients have been shown to possess powerful anti-inflammatory and antioxidant capabilities.

## DIAGNOSING AND TREATING ACUTE BRONCHITIS

Diagnosing acute bronchitis can be somewhat complicated because of the many conditions it resembles. Patients with acute bronchitis typically show up at the physician's office with a productive cough and signs of bronchial obstruction, including wheezing and breathlessness. Other symptoms may include chest pain and hoarseness. Fever is rarely associated with acute bronchitis, so if a fever is present in addition to a cough, the diagnosis is likely to be influenza or pneumonia. Other conditions that may be accompanied by a chronic cough (and are sometimes mistaken for acute bronchitis) include postnasal drip syndrome, asthma, and gastroesophageal reflux disease (GERD).

It is important to note that in nonsmokers, acute bronchitis should generally not be treated with antibiotics. These drugs are ineffective against the viruses that typically cause acute bronchitis, and their overuse leads to antibiotic-resistant pathogens. If therapy is warranted, physicians will likely suggest medications that control symptoms of acute bronchitis, such as coughing and mucus production. Pain relievers such as aspirin or nonsteroidal anti-inflammatories may be used, along with over-the-counter nasal decongestants. Cough suppression is not considered a primary treatment goal; the cough will resolve as the inflammation subsides and the bronchi heal.

People with acute bronchitis are also advised to drink plenty of fluids to help thin the mucus and hydrate the body. Expectorants, or medications that thin mucus, may also be recommended. The only antiviral drugs of value are those that specifically treat influenza virus in patients whose bronchitis is caused by this virus. There is some evidence that anti-influenza drugs can reduce the unnecessary use of antibiotics. Bronchodilators (which open airways) are rarely prescribed, except to adults who are wheezing and have evidence of restrictive airway disease.[2]

Whether treated or not, acute bronchitis will typically resolve on its own as the inflammation of the bronchi gradually subsides and the airways open again. Nevertheless, the condition is aggravating and painful while it persists, so early intervention—at the first sign of symptoms of viral infection—is important to prevent acute bronchitis. More information on Life Extension's aggressive early intervention programs for the common cold and influenza can be found elsewhere in this protocol. Life Extension also advocates that people practice good "viral hygiene" by washing their hands as frequently as possible and avoiding coming into close contact with infected people.

# ANTIOXIDANT THERAPY

Antioxidants, which combat free radicals and reduce oxidative stress, are important weapons in the fight against respiratory infection(s). During an infection, the immune system is activated to produce inflammatory cytokines and increase free radical production.[3] The oxidative stress caused by increased free radical production enhances the inflammation already present, leading to a self-reinforcing cycle of inflammation and free radical production.

## Vitamin C

Although few clinical trials have addressed antioxidants and acute bronchitis, it is logical that people suffering from inflammation of the bronchi and elevated free radical damage would benefit from a strong antioxidant defense. There is good evidence that large doses of vitamin C can interfere with viral infections at the first sign of symptoms,[4] thus reducing one's risk of developing acute bronchitis.

- In one study, investigators examined cold and flu symptoms in 2 groups of students. The control group was given conventional pain relievers and decongestants, while the treatment group was given hourly doses of 1000 mg vitamin C for the first 6 hours and then 3 times per day thereafter. Flu and cold symptoms in the treatment group decreased 85% compared with the control group.[4]

- In a randomized, double-blind study, older patients hospitalized with acute respiratory infections (bronchitis and bronchopneumonia) were given 200 mg of vitamin C daily. Upon evaluation 2 and 4 weeks after admission, significant increases in vitamin C concentration in plasma and white cells were noted, even in the presence of acute respiratory infection. Patients were further evaluated by a clinical scoring system based on primary symptoms of their respiratory illness. Those receiving vitamin C fared significantly better than those receiving placebo.[5]

## Vitamin E

Evidence from animal and human studies also shows that vitamin E, a powerful antioxidant, plays an important role in immune system maintenance. Even marginal deficiencies in vitamin E may predispose individuals to viral infections by reducing immune response. Therefore, supplying the body with additional antioxidants could reduce oxidative stress and enhance immune function.[6] A recent review has proposed that supplementation with antioxidants may improve or exert a protective effect upon lung health.[7]

## N-Acetylcysteine

N-acetylcysteine (NAC) is a precursor of glutathione, an important internal antioxidant. NAC has been in clinical use for more than 30 years as a mucolytic drug. NAC is routinely used to boost antioxidant levels and dissolve mucus in people suffering from respiratory ailments.[8]

In a randomized study of 24 bronchitis patients with an average age of 66, the addition of 600 mg NAC twice daily to standard therapy improved symptoms and quality of life.[9] Other investigators have shown that administration of NAC reduces episodes of influenza and influenza-like illnesses, especially in older high-risk individuals.[10]

## Inflammation and Additional Nutritional Support

**Omega-3 fatty acids.** Inflammation that produces symptoms is the defining feature of acute bronchitis. Many nutrients have been shown to reduce inflammation by interfering with the cascade of chemical reactions that causes inflammation. Among the best known are omega-3 fatty acids. These essential fatty acids have been shown to decrease the production of bronchorestrictive leukotrienes by reducing the production of arachidonic acid. Some researchers believe that this effect explains why Eskimos, who consume a lot of these fatty acids via a diet rich in cold-water fish, experience less lung disease than other populations.[11]

**Boswellia.** *Boswellia serrata* (frankincense) is a traditional antiarthritic in Ayurvedic medicine. Its anti-inflammatory properties have been attributed to the specific inhibition of the 5-lipoxygenase (5-LOX) enzyme and reduction in the production of proinflammatory leukotrienes by boswellic acids, a constituent of the Boswellia gum resin.[12] In addition to inhibiting 5-LOX and blocking the biosynthesis of harmful inflammatory leukotrienes,[13] boswellic acids decrease the activity of another proinflammatory enzyme, human leukocyte elastase (HLE). HLE is associated with various respiratory illnesses linked by inflammation.[14] To date, the only anti-inflammatory compounds that inhibit both HLE and 5-LOX are those derived from Boswellia.

**Curcumin.** Curcumin, which is derived from the common spice turmeric, is also a natural anti-inflammatory. This supplement is a natural inhibitor of nuclear factor kappa beta, which mediates most inflammatory processes in the body. Curcumin has shown promise in protecting lung tissue against inflammation induced by chemical and infectious agents in the laboratory.[15] Although there are no human trials examining curcumin in acute bronchitis, its antioxidant and anti-inflammatory properties make it a logical therapy.

**Bromelain.** Bromelain, an extract of the pineapple plant, has also demonstrated anti-inflammatory and mucolytic properties.[16] Bromelain is a collective term for enzymes found in pineapple fruit, stem, and leaves. These enzymes are proteolytic, meaning they break down protein into its constituent peptides and amino acids. Bromelain has been found to be a mucolytic (ie, a compound that breaks down mucus).[17] A recent review noted that bromelain may offer therapeutic benefits to individuals with bronchitis and sinusitis.[16]

## LIFE EXTENSION'S FLU AND COMMON COLD PROGRAM

Because acute bronchitis is so often caused by the flu virus and common cold, a summary of Life Extension's flu and common cold prevention program is presented here. For a more complete description, please see the appropriate protocols. At the first sign of infection, consider taking the following supplements. This program is not meant for long-term use because of the high doses. Follow these recommendations for only a few days.

### Vitamin C

Megadoses of vitamin C (1000 mg hourly for the first 6 hours and 3 times daily thereafter) administered during or after influenza infection decreased influenza symptoms in a large group of students.[4]

### Vitamin E

Both human and animal studies have shown that vitamin E can help fight influenza infection by boosting the immune system.[18,19] Animal studies have shown that vitamin E, in conjunction with other antioxidants, can help protect against the flu by reducing the oxidative damage associated with the virus.

- After being infected with the influenza virus, aged mice fed a diet supplemented with vitamin E had significantly lower pulmonary viral levels and maintained their body weight, unlike control mice or mice fed with other antioxidants. Levels of proinflammatory cytokines, including interleukin-6 and tumor necrosis factor-alpha, were lowest in the group supplemented with vitamin E.[20]

- Vitamin E was shown to reduce viral activity in the lungs of middle-aged mice after exposure to influenza.[21]

- Supplementation with vitamin E before infection helped protect the lungs of mice against lipid peroxidation.[22]

### Selenium and Zinc

A combination supplement containing selenium and zinc can reduce the severity of flu infection.

- In one study, seniors receiving an experimental formula of zinc, selenium, fermentable oligosaccharides (a kind of sugar that enhances beneficial bacteria), and structured triacylglycerides for 183 days showed signs of enhanced immune function and had fewer days of upper respiratory symptoms.[23]

- A 2-year supplementation program of vitamins and micronutrients showed that selenium and zinc significantly reduced infections in elderly residents of nursing homes[24] and enhanced the residents' immune response to influenza vaccination.[25]

Mice deficient in selenium are more susceptible to influenza infection.[26] In selenium-deficient mice, the proinflammatory response is stronger and the immune response weaker than in mice with an adequate level of selenium.[27] Moreover, the genome of viruses in selenium-deficient mice shifts toward more virulent, resistant strains.[28]

Zinc has also been studied extensively for its ability to inhibit viruses (eg, rhinovirus) that cause the common cold.[29-32]

## Lactoferrin

Lactoferrin is a subfraction of whey and has antiviral, antimicrobial, anticancer, and immune-enhancing effects. Lactoferrin is concentrated in the saliva, where it comes into direct contact with pathogens and kills or suppresses them through a variety of mechanisms.[33,34] Lactoferrin may stimulate macrophages, which in turn may help induce cell-mediated immunity.[35] Lactoferrin is present naturally in many mucous membrane secretions, suggesting an innate antimicrobial function.[35,36] A recent study showed that lactoferrin inhibits viral infection by interfering with the ability of certain viruses to bind to cell receptor sites.[37]

## Elderberry Extract

Studies show that a black elderberry extract has antiviral properties against 10 strains of influenza virus. In a double-blind, placebo-controlled, randomized study, elderberry extract reduced the duration of influenza symptoms by 1–2 days.[38,39]

## Green Tea

Green tea has been shown to inhibit bacteria and viruses, as well as stimulate the immune system. Black tea and extracted components, such as catechin and saponins,[40] inhibit influenza virus growth, infectivity, and symptoms.[41,42] In a cell culture study, the active ingredients in green tea were found to be powerful inhibitors of all varieties of influenza virus.[43]

## Garlic

Garlic has been valued for centuries for its medicinal properties. Garlic, and its active component, allicin, have a wide spectrum of antifungal, antibacterial, and antiviral action. Garlic benefits the immune system by increasing the number of natural killer cells and the killer activities of spleen cells.[44,45] One recent study tested an allicin-containing garlic supplement on a group of 146 volunteers for 4 months. Half the group took one garlic capsule daily while the other half received a placebo. The placebo group had 63% more infections than the group that took the garlic capsule. Even more significant, those who took garlic capsules

and who did catch a cold experienced symptoms for an average of only 1.52 days, compared with 5.01 days for the placebo group.[46] Aged garlic has also been shown to have antiviral properties (particularly against influenza B)[47] and immunomodulatory effects.[45]

## Dehydroepiandrosterone and Melatonin

The hormones dehydroepiandrosterone (DHEA) and melatonin have been shown to bolster the body's immune response.[48-51] Taking higher-than-usual doses (200–400 mg) of DHEA in the morning and higher-than-usual doses (10–50 mg) of melatonin before bedtime would appear to be logical approaches to battling a viral infection.

## Vitamin D

Vitamin D upregulates the expression of antimicrobial peptides.[52] Secreted by immune cells throughout the body, antimicrobial peptides damage the outer lipid membrane of infectious agents (including influenza viruses), rendering them vulnerable to eradication. This provides a definitive biological mechanism to explain why vitamin D confers such dramatic protection against common winter illnesses and protects against bacterial, fungal, and viral infections.

## Cimetidine

The antiviral drug cimetidine (Tagamet®) is an over-the-counter drug used to treat heartburn. It also has potent immune system-boosting effects that can drastically reduce the duration of certain viral infections. Because cimetidine is safe for most people to take, 800–1000 mg taken at night (or 200 mg 3 times/day and 400 mg at night) can help boost the immune system in the event of exposure to influenza. Cimetidine in 200-mg tablets can be purchased over the counter. The directions in over-the-counter package inserts indicate that it is safe to take as much as 800 mg cimetidine daily. Some published studies state that up to 1000 mg cimetidine daily is safe.[53]

## Life Extension Suggestions

By staying healthy and avoiding viral infection and environmental pollutants, your chances of contracting acute bronchitis will be greatly reduced. Acute bronchitis is more common during the winter months—the flu and cold season—than at other times. Common-sense strategies to prevent acute bronchitis include ensuring appropriate and thorough hand washing, to avoid exposure to viruses and reducing exposure to such irritants as air pollution, tobacco, and smoke.[54]

## Immune System Support

- **Cimetidine:** 800–1000 mg daily
- **Garlic:** 9000 mg once or twice daily (consume food after ingesting this amount of garlic to reduce esophageal burning)
- **Aged garlic extract:** 800 mg daily
- **DHEA:** 200–400 mg daily in the morning
- **Lactoferrin:** 1200 mg daily
- **Zinc:** Two 24-mg lozenges every 2 hours while awake. This is a very high dosage of zinc and is toxic if taken for long periods. Take this much zinc only for a few days.
- **Melatonin:** 10–50 mg at bedtime
- **Vitamin C:** 6000 mg daily (1000 mg every hour for the first 6 hours), and then 3000 mg daily (1000 mg several hours apart)
- **Vitamin E:** 400 IU daily
- **Green tea extract:** 725 mg daily (A decaffeinated form is available for people who are sensitive to caffeine.)
- **Selenium:** 200 mcg daily
- **Elderberry extract:** 30 mg, 3 times daily
- **Vitamin D:** 5000–8000 IU daily; depending on blood levels of 25-OH-vitamin D

## Nutrients to Ease Inflammation and Provide Antioxidant Support

- **Vitamin C:** 2000–3000 mg daily
- **Vitamin E:** 400 IU daily, with at least 200 mg gamma tocopherol
- **NAC:** 600–1800 mg daily
- **Fish oil,** (with olive polyphenols): providing 1400 mg EPA and 1000 mg DHA daily
- **Gamma linolenic acid (GLA):** 900–1800 mg daily
- **Curcumin,** as highly absorbed BCM95®: 400–800 mg daily
- **Bromelain:** 500 mg several times daily on an empty stomach
- **Boswellia serrata,** as highly absorbed Apres-Flex™: 100 mg daily

## REFERENCES

References available at: www.lef.org/dpt5/ch27

# 28

# *Caloric Restriction*

Caloric restriction (CR) is a general strategy for improving well-being and life span. It is more than a simple limitation of calories for maintenance of body weight; CR is the dramatic reduction of caloric intake to levels that may be significantly (up to 50% in some cases) below that for maximum growth and fertility, but nutritionally sufficient for maintaining overall health ("undernutrition without malnutrition").[1] It remains one of the most researched and successful approaches to life extension in laboratory settings. Although the effects of CR on health are diverse, its mechanisms are not fully understood, and are thought to involve the activation of survival mechanisms that have been evolutionarily conserved to protect organisms from stress.

The idea of extending health span (the period of healthy living before the onset of age-related disease) and life span by lowering food intake is not a new one. Louis Caranaro's 16th-century bestseller antiaging book suggested that longevity would come to those who ate only enough to sustain life. Benjamin Franklin supported the concept of abstinence as a defense against disease two centuries later.[2] But it was the work of McCay in the 1930s that first demonstrated that reducing calories below the level required for maximum fertility, while avoiding malnutrition, could extend the mean and maximum lifespan of laboratory rats by ≥40%.[3] In the years following that seminal work, the health and longevity effects of CR have been observed in a wide range of organisms, ranging from single-celled *Saccharomyces*, to primates and humans.

The practical challenge of long-term or lifetime CR has recently generated interest in caloric restriction mimetics (CRMs), an alternative to CR that may provide the prolongevity benefits without an actual reduction in caloric intake.[4] CRMs are a broad class of compounds and interventions that may promote life- and health-span by a diversity of mechanisms, ranging from induction of genes that protect against stress, to antioxidation and anti-inflammation.

## CALORIC RESTRICTION IN ANIMALS AND NONHUMAN PRIMATES

Seventy-five years of research have determined that the longevity and health effects of CR are a broad biological phenomenon that has been observed in species from three kingdoms of life (Animalia, Fungi, and Protoctista).[5] Both the mean and maximum life spans of yeast (*Saccharomyces cerevisiae*), rotifers, nematodes (*Caenorhabditis elegans*), fruit flies (*Drosophila melanogaster*) and medflies, spiders, fish (guppies, zebrafish), rodents (hamsters, rats, mice), and dogs have been extended significantly by decreasing normal caloric consumption by 30–40%.[6] Recently, the effects of CR on life span have been observed in nonhuman primates. The rhesus monkey (*Macaca mulatta*) is an excellent model for the study of human aging, exhibiting many physiologic and biochemical similarities to humans.[7] Unlike other animal aging models, the rhesus monkey also allows the study of brain atrophy, a characteristic of human aging that does not occur in smaller mammals.[8] With an average life span of about 27 years in captivity,[9] the rhesus also is suitable for determining the effects of CR on maximal lifespan.

Studies of CR effects on 3 separate rhesus colonies are currently underway; results from two have been published. A 20-year study conducted at the Wisconsin National Primate Research Center suggests that CR of baseline diet by 30% may slow aging in the rhesus, as gauged by two indicators of aging retardation: delays in mortality and in the onset of age-associated diseases (particularly diabetes, cancer, cardiovascular disease, and neurologic impairment; the most prevalent age-related diseases in humans).[10] At study entry, the animals (46 males and 30 females) were at adult age (7–14 years); at the time the study was published (20 years later), nearly 3 times as many control monkeys had died of age-related causes than CR monkeys (37% vs. 13%). The CR monkeys appeared to be biologically younger than their normal-fed counterparts, and not surprisingly, had lower body and fat mass. Sarcopenia (age-related muscle loss) was attenuated in the CR group. CR monkeys were also free of diabetes (compared to 5/38 control animals) or glucose intolerance (compared to 11/38 control animals). Incidence of cardiovascular disease, all cancers, and adenocarcinoma of the gastrointestinal tract (the most common cancer in rhesus monkeys[11]) was reduced by half in the CR group. Calorie restriction resulted in preservation of brain volume in the caudate, putamen and insula, areas that are classically involved in regulation of motor and executive function. The effects of CR on maximum lifespan have yet to be determined for this colony, as animals in both groups are still living.

A smaller study at the University of Maryland tracked 8 CR rhesus monkeys and 109 ad-libitum (free-fed) controls over a period of 25 years, and produced many of the same observations.[12,13] Ad-libitum fed animals died at 25 years of age compared to a median survival of 32 years in the CR group. CR also reduced hyperinsulinemia (elevated circulating insulin) and the frequency of age-associated diseases.

Although the available data are limited, these two studies do implicate that the health span and lifespan benefits of CR that have been observed in rodents and lower animals may also extend to primates and possibly humans.

## CALORIC RESTRICTION IN HUMANS AND INCREASED LIFESPAN

Assessing the effects of dietary interventions on human lifespan is a difficult endeavor; with average life expectancies of 75 and 80 years for men and women, respectively,[14] any prospective study would likely necessitate several generations of researchers to carry out. Therefore, human aging studies must rely on surrogate measures (biomarkers) of aging. Reduced body temperature and lowered fasting insulin levels are robust markers of CR and slowed aging in rodents and rhesus monkeys.[15]

Dehydroepiandrosterone sulfate (DHEA-S), which declines in both rhesus monkeys and humans during normal aging, may be important in health maintenance and may serve as another potential longevity marker.[16] DHEA-S, a product of the adrenal glands and the most abundant circulating steroid hormone, serves as the precursor to the sex steroids (androgens and estrogens). Increased DHEA-S levels in monkeys on CR are associated with survival.[17] Similarly, data from the Baltimore Longitudinal Study of Aging (BLSA)[18] suggest that long-lived humans exhibit some of the same physiologic and biochemical changes that accompany caloric restriction in animals. In the study, human survival rates were highest in those with low body temperatures, low levels of circulating insulin; and high DHEA-S levels.[19]

While there is yet no direct evidence of human lifespan extension by CR, there has been limited observational and clinical data that suggest a connection. In the 1970s, the Japanese island of Okinawa was reported to contain up to 40 times as many centenarians as other Japanese communities, which was suggested to result from CR. (The caloric intake of adults and children in Okinawa was 20% and 40% lower than mainland counterparts, respectively.[20]) Two decades earlier, a small study revealed that 60 healthy seniors receiving an average of 1500 kcal/day for a period of 3 years had significantly lowered rates of hospital admissions and a numerically lowered death rate than an equal number of control volunteers.[21]

## CALORIC RESTRICTION IN HUMANS MITIGATES DISEASE RISK

There is a growing body of evidence suggesting that CR may reduce disease risk factors, which may have a direct influence on health span (and indirectly increase lifespan). Several observational studies have tracked the effects of CR on lean, healthy individuals, and have demonstrated that moderate CR (22–30% decreases in caloric intake from normal levels) improves heart function, reduces markers of inflammation (C-reactive protein, tumor necrosis factor [TNF]), reduces risk factors for cardiovascular disease (elevated LDL cholesterol, triglycerides, blood pressure), and reduces diabetes risk factors (fasting blood glucose and insulin levels).[22–25] CR in healthy individuals has also been associated with reductions in circulating insulin-like growth factor-1 (IGF-1), and cyclooxygenase II (COX-2),[26] all of which may be indicative of a decreased risk of certain cancers. Epidemiologic data show an association between higher plasma IGF-1 concentrations and a greater risk of breast,[27] prostate,[28] and colon cancers.[29] COX-2, in addition to its role in inflammation, can promote the growth and spread of tumors.[30–32]

Preliminary results from the Comprehensive Assessment of Long-Term Effects of Reducing Intake of Energy (CALERIE)[33] are reproducing many of the metabolic and physiologic responses to CR observed in rodents and monkeys.[34] To better elucidate the effects of CR in humans, the National Institute on Aging (NIA) is sponsoring a multisite randomized human clinical study to assess the safety and efficacy of 2 years of CR in nonobese but overweight healthy individuals. Researchers of the Pennington CALERIE group have followed 48 overweight (average BMI 27.5), middle-aged (average age 37) individuals for 6 months adopting one of 4 protocols: (1) 25% caloric restriction (CR group), (2) 12.5% CR with an additional 12.5% caloric expenditure from exercise (CREX group), (3) very low-calorie diet (890 kcal/day) until 15% weight reduction, followed by a diet of sufficient calories to maintain this weight (VLCD group), or

(4) control. Not surprisingly, all three intervention groups demonstrated reduced body weight, visceral (abdominal) fat, and fat cell size,[35,36] as well as reduced liver fat deposits.[37] Fat loss was not significantly different between the CR and CREX groups (24% total fat, 27% visceral fat).[38] All three intervention groups also demonstrated reductions in DNA damage.[39] Only the CR and CREX groups, however, were able to improve two markers of longevity (reduced body temperature and reduced fasting plasma insulin), as well as reduce cardiovascular risk factors (LDL-C, triglycerides, and blood pressure). C-reactive protein was reduced only in the CREX group.[40] Circulating thyroid hormone (T3) concentrations were lower in the CR and CREX groups.[41] Under conditions of CR, reduction in circulating thyroid hormone and body temperature suggests the normal adaptation of the body to lower energy intake and expenditure; similar reductions in T3 and metabolic rate have been observed in other human and animal CR studies.[42] The CR groups also exhibited increases in the amount of mitochondria (the cellular sites of energy production), and increased expression of two genes (TFAM and PGC-1α) that are indicative of mitochondrial biogenesis, the formation of new mitochondria.[43] Mitochondrial loss and dysfunction may be responsible for some of the most potent effects of the aging process.[44]

Similar results have been observed from the CALERIE studies at Washington University on a separate group of 50- to 60-year-old, non-obese overweight (average BMI 27) volunteers after 1 year of either CR (3 months of 16% CR followed by 9 months of 20% CR) or exercise training of equivalent energy expenditure (ie, expending 20% of daily caloric intake).[45] CR improved cardiovascular parameters (left ventricular diastolic function, diastolic and systolic blood pressure),[46] lowered C-reactive protein and insulin resistance,[47] and lowered circulating thyroid hormone T3[48] and fasting plasma insulin.[49]

CR in this second, older volunteer population was not without some negative consequences: compared to the exercise-only group, CR demonstrated decreases in muscle mass, strength, and aerobic capacity.[50,51] The CR group also demonstrated significantly more loss of bone mineral density (BMD) at the spine, hip, and femur (interochanter) than either the exercise-only or control groups, which was observable by month 3 of the study.[52] It should be noted that in the younger CALERIE study group, there was no significant differences in BMD in any of the groups at month 6.[53] The potential of losses in aerobic capacity and BMD stress the importance of exercise in CR protocols.

The CALERIE group at the Jean Mayer-USDA Human Nutrition Center on Aging at Tufts University compared the effects of CR diet composition (high glycemic vs. low glycemic load) in 29 healthy overweight adults provided with 30% calorie restricted meals for 6 months, followed by self-monitored restriction for an additional 6 months. Clinical indicators (fasting serum triglycerides, cholesterol, insulin) were significantly reduced in both groups at 6 and 12 months, but were not different between groups.[54] There was no significant difference in weight loss or energy expenditure between the high glycemic (HG; 60% of calories from carbohydrates) and low glycemic (LG; 40% of calories from carbohydrates) groups, but the LG group lost significantly more fat mass, and retained more fat-free mass.[55] The LG group also demonstrated greater declines in CRP during the first 6 months of the CR protocol.[56] While these data indicate that the overall reduction in energy intake, and not diet composition, may be a more important determinant of weight loss and its associated CR health benefits, it does suggest additional benefits of LG diets. By their very nature, LG diets can limit postprandial ("postmeal") elevations in blood glucose, aiding in the maintenance of the target 2-hour postmeal level of <140 mg/dL, which the International Diabetes Federation suggests may lower the risk of several diseases, including cancer, cognitive impairment, cardiovascular disease, and retinopathy.[57]

## MECHANISMS OF CALORIC RESTRICTION

The mechanism(s) of CR has not been definitively determined, although theories abound. Possible mechanisms include protection from oxidative damage, increased cellular repair, reduction in the production of catabolic cytokines, such as the inflammatory molecules TNF and interleukin-6 (IL-6), and increases in energy (ATP) production.[58]

The free-radical theory of aging proposes that cumulative oxidative damage during the course of normal metabolism compromises cellular function and causes aging.[59,60] The observation that CR inhibits oxidative damage to lipids, DNA, and protein support a role of antioxidation as a CR mechanism.[61-64] Levels of endogenous antioxidants (glutathione) and antioxidant enzymes (superoxide dismutase, catalase, glutathione-S-transferase) are also protected by CR from age-related decline in animal models.[65-67] CR also stimulates DNA repair.[68]

While inflammation is a complex, well-orchestrated process that is designed to limit injury and promote repair, uncontrolled or chronic inflammation can have the opposite effect; chronic inflammation has been implicated in a range of age-related diseases. Age-related increases in the production of proinflammatory enzymes, cytokines, and adhesion molecules may also accelerate aging through the increase in reactive oxygen and nitrogen species (ROS and RNS) and subsequent oxidative damage. In cell culture and animal models, CR has been shown to attenuate the inflammatory response by suppressing the production of pro-inflammatory proteins (interleukins 1B, 6, and TNF) and prostaglandins ($E_2$, $I_2$).[69] CR has reduced the activity of the inflammatory enzyme COX-2 in rats[70] and humans,[71] and has suppressed COX-derived free-radical production in rats.[72]

Autophagy is a major repair process for cellular damage,[73] one which has been associated with positive effects on longevity.[74] During autophagy, intracellular components such as damaged or unnecessary cellular machinery or aggregated proteins are engulfed by organelles called autophagosomes and degraded within lysosomes (organelles that digest cellular wastes). Autophagy also represents an important mechanism for cell survival during nutrient deprivation.[75] Recent studies have revealed that age-related reductions in autophagy in rats are slowed by CR.[76,77]

CR has been shown to increase efficiency of the mitochondrial energy production while decreasing the generation of reactive oxygen species, the undesirable by-product of this process.[78,79]

At the genetic level, CR has been shown to stimulate the production of several factors that are involved in nutrient sensing and insulin signaling, notably the proteins PGC-1α and SIRT1. PGC-1α (peroxisome proliferator-activated receptor γ coactivator-1α) is often described as the master regulator of mitochondrial biogenesis. Among its many functions, PGC-1α turns up (upregulates) the expression of genes in the cell nucleus that encode mitochondrial enzymes.[80] Additionally, PGC-1α stimulates the replication of mitochondrial DNA, a necessary step in mitochondrial biogenesis.[81,82] The enzyme SIRT1, the founding member of the sirtuin gene family, has been of considerable interest in the last decade: acting as a "metabolic sensor," SIRT1 may increase mitochondrial activity,[83] improve glucose tolerance,[84] and extend lifespan in experimental models.[85] CR also reduces the production of mTOR (mammalian target of rapamycin), an enzyme that responds to levels of insulin and IGF-1, to control cell growth and division. mTOR is abnormally elevated in many cancers,[86] and its inhibition has been found to slow aging in yeast, nematodes, and mice.[87]

CR may attenuate some of the detrimental changes in gene expression that accompany the aging process. Aging in rats is accompanied by changes in expression of genes associated with increased inflammation and stress, and decreased apoptosis and DNA replication; CR reversed many of these changes.[88] CR reduces the expression of nuclear factor kappa beta (NF-κB), a key mediator of inflammation. NF-κB senses cellular threats (such as free radicals or pathogens) and responds by activating other inflammatory genes. NF-κB activity is enhanced in many tissues during the aging process.[89] By reducing NF-κB, CR in turn reduces the expression of other proinflammatory genes, including IL-1B, IL-6, TNFa, COX-2, and inducible nitric oxide synthase (iNOS).[90]

An attempt to resolve the seemingly disparate mechanisms of CR on life extension and health promotion has suggested that a unified process (hormesis) may also be at work.[91] Hormesis is classically described as a phenomenon in which the response to a chemical or physical agent is different depending in the degree of its intensity[92]; for example, a cell might respond positively to caloric restriction (low intensity) but negatively to frank starvation (high intensity). In the context of aging, hormesis is characterized by the beneficial effects of cellular responses to the mild stress of caloric restriction, which stimulates maintenance and repair processes.[93] In this manner, a significant, sustained reduction of calories below a certain threshold may activate several genes that sense the nutrient deprivation (such as sirtuins, PGC-1α, or mTOR), which turn off cell growth, and switch on processes that protect or repair the cell (which, in turn, may increase antioxidant capacity and attenuate inflammation).

## PRACTICING CALORIC RESTRICTION WITH OPTIMUM NUTRITION (CRON)

Although CR has in the past been defined as a 30–40% reduction in calorie intake (as determined by daily energy expenditure) there is no "official" definition of caloric restriction,[94] and newer investigations have revealed CR benefits can still occur at less-restrictive caloric intakes. Based on our current knowledge of CR, its definition may someday be not simply based on a restriction "value," but rather a combination of anticipated gene expression patterns and physiological changes. As demonstrated in the examples above, CR protocols that have demonstrated significant results over a range of caloric intakes and durations, with and without the inclusion of exercise. Extremely low caloric intakes (only 550 kcal/day) have been used for very short durations (6 weeks) with dramatic results in obese individuals: insulin sensitivity increased by 35%, CRP decreased by half, and liver triglycerides decreased by 60%.[95,96] However, maintenance of extreme CR for longer periods of time, for instance 45% CR for 6 months has resulted in several negative side effects including anemia, muscle wasting, neurologic deficits, and edema.[97] Although the comprehensive CALERIE studies were designed for CR of 16–25% and have demonstrated short-term success, when compliance is considered, the actual degree of CR in the groups may have been closer to 11.5%.[98]

The frequency of meals is not important for CR, at least in animal models. Lifespan extensions in rodents have been observed at meal frequencies ranging from 6 times per day to 3 times per week.[99,100] "Every-other-day-feeding" (EOD), which was initially thought to be distinct from CR, may actually function as a mild CR, and demonstrates a lower incidence of diabetes, and lower fasting blood glucose and insulin concentrations.[101] It is unclear whether meal frequency affects the benefits of CR in humans. While reduced meal frequency to one meal per day, consuming sufficient calories to maintain body weight in healthy, normal-weight, middle-aged adults demonstrated significant increases in blood pressure and LDL-C,[102] this effect was not observed in non-obese overweight individuals following an EOD approach to CR.[103]

The duration of a CR plan depends on its anticipated outcomes. Although controlled longevity data are unavailable for humans, one could imagine that, based on human observational data and the wealth of animal studies, that life extension through CR requires a lifetime commitment. However, reduction in body fat mass, cardiovascular disease and diabetes risks are observable even within the abbreviated timescales of the CALERIE studies (6–12 months), as are certain markers of slowed aging, such as mitochondrial biogenesis and reduced DNA oxidative damage. Even short periods (21–48 days) of fasting or caloric/dietary restriction (such as religious fasts) can have favorable effects on blood lipids, insulin sensitivity, and biomarkers of oxidative stress.[104,105] Short-term CR has also been validated by gene expression data, in which alterations in the expression of age-related genes including those involved in inflammation, apoptosis, and DNA expression could be observed after only 4 weeks of CR in mice.[106]

While there is no defined composition of the CR diet, the potentially significant reduction in caloric intake necessitates the consumption of nutrient-dense foods, and the avoidance of "empty" calories from foods such as white flour and refined sugar. It is also imperative that the intake of essential micronutrients, such as vitamins, minerals, essential fatty acids and essential amino acids, are carefully monitored, and added back to the diet if necessary. Even a carefully chosen CR diet may not be nutritionally complete. In studies of 4 popular, published diet plans that limited calories to 1100–1700 per day, including the National Institutes of Health and American Heart Association–recommended "DASH diet" (Dietary Approaches to Stop Hypertension), all were found to be on average only 43.5% sufficient in RDIs for 27 essential micronutrients values, and deficient in 15 of them.[107] While hunger cannot realistically be eliminated during a dedicated CR diet, there are dietary strategies to reduce hunger such as sufficient fiber consumption (increasing fiber intake to 35 g/day had a significant effect on satiation and adherence to the CR protocol in the CALERIE study[108] and consumption of "fast" proteins, like whey, that are rapidly absorbed and quickly signal satiety.[109,110]

## CALORIC RESTRICTION MIMETICS

Maintaining a dramatically reduced caloric intake over the long term can be very demanding. Few people are willing to reduce their caloric consumption by the 30–40% to meet the classic CR definition,[111] and even the less restrictive protocols (16–25%) used in human interventions have not been met with full compliance.[112] The search for an alternative or complement to CR has involved the identification or development of compounds that mimic some of the physiologic or gene-expression changes associated with CR, without the requirement of lowered caloric intake or loss of body weight. While many compounds can be broadly interpreted as CR mimetics (CRMs), a more focused definition of CRM would be a compound or intervention that mimics the metabolic, hormonal, or physiologic effects of CR without reducing long-term food intake, while stimulating maintenance and repair processes, and producing CR-like effects on longevity and reduction of age-related disease.[113]

### Green Tea, Ginko Biloba, and Curcumin

Several compounds have been investigated as CRMs, with encouraging preliminary results in animal models. Tetrahydrocurcumin (a curcumin metabolite) and green tea polyphenols have both demonstrated increases in average and maximum lifespans in mice.[114]

The effects were observed when the mice received treatments by month 13 (if given later in life, the treatments had no effect on lifespan), and in the case of green tea extract, the treatment had no effect on body weight. An investigation of ginkgo biloba on cognitive behavior in male Fischer rats revealed an unexpected, statistically significant increase in average lifespan when compared to controls (26.4 vs. 31.0 months).[115] The National Institute on Aging (NIA) Aging Intervention Testing program,[116,117] a multicenter study on longevity-enhancing compounds, has already identified life-extending or CRM activities in rapamycin[118,119] and aspirin[120] in rodents, and is currently testing other potential compounds including medium chain triglycerides, caffeic acid esters, and curcumin.[121]

## Resveratrol and Pterostilbene

Stress-induced plant compounds can stimulate stress responses in other species; this cross-species hormesis is called xenohormesis.[122] Xenohormesis may have evolved as an early warning in animals about impending changes in the environment (such as scarcities in the food supply), allowing them to adapt accordingly. The most familiar of these stress-inducing compounds is resveratrol, well-known for its presence in grape skin, but also present at detectable levels in several plant species. Resveratrol simulates caloric restriction[123] in the absence of actual nutrient deficiency by activating sirtuins (SIRT1 is the human homolog), and has been shown to increase lifespan in fungi, nematodes, flies, fish, and mice.[124] SIRT1 also suppresses NF-κB (and the inflammatory cytokines and enzymes NF-κB activates), lending resveratrol anti-inflammatory activity in cell culture and animal models.[125–127] High-dose resveratrol reduced IGF-1 levels in healthy human volunteers, a chemopreventive activity that is also associated with CR.[128] Pterostilbene, a methylated analogue of resveratrol from blueberries, similarly attenuates inflammation in a CR-like manner, reducing NF-κB signaling and COX-2 activities in cell culture.[129,130]

## Fisetin, Quercetin, and Theaflavins

Other plant-derived polyphenolic compounds (such as catechins, curcumin, or flavonoids) may also have xenohormesis activities as well; it has been suggested that the majority of health benefits from plant phytochemical consumption might not be from their antioxidant properties, but rather by a CR-like modulation of stress-response pathways.[131] Fisetin, quercetin, proanthocyanidins, and theaflavins are examples of compounds that have inherent chain-breaking antioxidant chemistries, but appear to exert profound health effects unrelated to their ability to quench free radicals. Fisetin and quercetin have both been shown to stimulate SIRT1,[132] a central activity of CR. In vitro, fisetin, like CR, reduced mTOR signaling,[133] NF-κB activation and COX-2 gene expression,[134] and activated antioxidative and detoxifying gene pathways (Nrf2).[135] Fisetin has also been shown to increase lifespan in *Saccharomyces*[136] and *Drosophila*.[137] Quercetin, in addition to proanthocyanidins from grape seed, have also been shown to reduce the production of inflammatory cytokines, and the expression of vascular endothelial growth factor (VEGF),[138] which may prevent tumors from recruiting blood vessels. This same chemoprotective activity has been observed in rats under CR.[139] Theaflavins are flavan-3-ols from black tea that are produced during the oxidation (fermentation) of tea leaves. Aside from their suppression of NF-κB and inflammatory cytokines in vitro and in mice[140] and their induction of apoptosis in cancer cells,[141] theaflavins also stimulate the longevity factor Forkhead box 1 (FOXO1) in invertebrate and mammalian cells.[142]

## Metformin and Cinnamon

The glucoregulatory agent metformin can produce many of the gene expression changes found in mice on long-term caloric restriction. In particular, it can decrease the expression of chaperones (ie, a set of proteins), which in addition to their other functions can reduce apoptosis (self-destruction of damaged or malignant cells) and promote tumorgenesis.[143] Metformin has increased mean lifespan in the worm *C. elegans*.[144] Along with the related antidiabetic biguanide drugs phenformin and buformin, metformin extended the mean lifespan of mice by up to 37.9% and their maximum life span by up to 26% in multiple studies[145], while significantly decreasing the incidence and size of mammary tumors.[146] These effects on spontaneous tumor incidence, however, were limited to female animals.[147] Metformin's CR-like effects are possibly due to influence on insulin or IGF-1 signaling. This mechanism may also explain the lifespan extension properties of the glucoregulatory herb *Cinnamomum cassia* (cinnamon bark) in the *C. elegans*.[148]

## Fish Oil

Fish oil, while not a CRM, appears to increase the efficacy of CR at preventing free radical damage; fish oil feeding with 40% CR in mice demonstrated synergistic reductions in thiobarbituric acid reactive substances (TBARS, a marker of lipid peroxidation), and was more effective at reducing inflammatory markers (COX-2 and iNOS expression) than CR or fish oil alone.[149]

## Branched-Chain Amino Acids and Pyrroloquinoline quinone (PQQ)

The branched-chain amino acids (leucine, isoleucine, and valine) exhibit several CR-like properties, particularly related to mitochondrial biogenesis. Leucine increased mitochondrial mass in cultured human myocytes (muscle cells), and activated genes associated with CR (PGC-1α and SIRT-1).[150] Elevations in CR gene expression were observed in mouse cardiomyocytes using a mixture of all three BCAAs.[151] The BCAAs have also extended lifespan in *Saccharomyces*[152] as well as in mice[153] when supplied above normal dietary levels. Similarly, pyrroloquinoline quinone (PQQ), a bacterial electron carrier[154] and cofactor for several bacterial enzymes (and at least one mammalian enzyme[155]) increased mitochondrial DNA content and stimulated oxygen respiration (both indicative of biogenesis) in cultured mouse hepatoma cells through the activation of the CR gene PGC-1α.[156]

## WHAT YOU NEED TO KNOW ABOUT CALORIC RESTRICTION

Caloric restriction (CR), a significant, sustained reduction of caloric intake from baseline levels, is the most thoroughly and successfully researched method for lifespan and health span extension in a broad range of animals and nonhuman primates.

In many cases, the reduction of caloric intake by 30–40% in animal models has resulted in longevity increases by ≥40%.

Although there is not yet direct human evidence of lifespan extension in humans from CR, results of the NIA-funded CALERIE study have shown significant reductions in risk factors for disease (cardiovascular disease, diabetes, some cancers), from moderate CR.

CR in humans reduces fasting insulin levels and lowers resting body temperature, which are two biomarkers for aging reversal.

Although CR has classically been defined as a long-term 30–40% reduction in calories, some CR health benefits in humans have been observed at less-restrictive caloric reductions (16–25%) over short time periods (weeks to months).

CR may work by reducing oxidative damage, increasing cellular repair, lowering production of inflammatory cytokines, or by hormesis, a mild stress that may stimulate cellular protection.

Several compounds may mimic the effects of CR without requiring a reduction in calories; these include resveratrol, metformin, green tea polyphenols, aspirin, pyrroloquinoline quinone (PQQ), and branched-chain amino acids.

## Life Extension Suggestions

- **Curcumin** (as highly absorbed BCM-95®): 400–800 mg daily
- **Green tea,** standardized extract: 725–1450 mg daily
- *Trans*-**resveratrol:** 250 mg daily
- *Trans*-**pterostilbene:** 3 mg daily
- **OPCs** (from grape seed extract): 50 mg daily
- **Black tea,** standardized extract: 300 mg daily
- **Fisetin:** 48 mg daily
- **Omega-3 fatty acids** (from fish oil): 2000–4000 mg daily
- **Vitamin D3:** 5000–8000 IU daily
- **Quercetin:** 150–400 mg daily
- **Ginkgo biloba,** standardized extract: 120–240 mg daily
- **CoQ10** (as ubiquinol): 100–300 mg daily
- **Pyrroloquinoline quinone** (PQQ): 10–20 mg daily
- **Branched chain amino acids** (BCAAs): 2400–4800 mg daily
- **Whey protein isolate:** 20–40 g daily
- **Cinnamon extract** (bark): 175-525 mg daily

## REFERENCES

References available at: www.lef.org/dpt5/ch28

# 29

# Cancer Adjuvant Therapy

The good news is that many of the 4 million people being treated for cancer in America will survive the disease and go on to live full and productive lives.

While the numbers that survive are far too low (about 44%), many of the more than 1500 daily cancer deaths occur because patients and their families are unaware of the depth of the resources currently available. Unfortunately, some die avowing that they would never resort to natural medicine, while others are interested but lack the expertise to implement the program to their best advantage. Regrettably, some turn to alternative care fairly late in the course of the disease process, weakening the probability of recovery.

Mainstream medicine (relying on surgery, chemotherapy, and radiation) may initially appear successful, but the indications of the disease process are less often addressed. Conventional cancer treatments are not for those individuals who are frail in body or spirit. For the past 30 years, cancer therapies have experienced tremendous setbacks because of an associated toxic response, resulting in significant numbers of treatment-induced deaths rather than disease-induced fatalities. Awareness regarding historic numbers of unsuccessful outcomes has forced patients to look for alternatives to bolster survival odds. Many who use alternative therapies report doing so without their oncologist's knowledge, fearful of criticism or rejection by a physician.[1]

The University of Texas M.D. Anderson Cancer Center (Houston) found that 99.3% of patients had heard of complementary medicine, and 68.7% of patients reported having used at least one unconventional therapy.[1] About 75% of the patients surveyed, however, yearned for more information concerning complementary medicine and about one-half of those participating in the survey wanted the information to come from their physician.

Until most recently, major medical schools granted only a few hours to nutritional education out of the hundreds of academic hours required to complete medical school. The exclusion began when Abraham Flexner (commissioned to correct inequities occurring

in medical schools) penned the Flexner Report of 1910. His contribution, titled *Medical Education in the United States and Canada*, closed smaller medical schools, and forced those that survived to adopt a uniform curriculum that excluded nutritional courses. Thus, some physicians emerged from medical schools scoffing at the concept of nutrition influencing health or overcoming disease.

Sir William Osler (1849–1919), chief physician at the Johns Hopkins School of Medicine, drilled into students that medical research must be validated and replicated to be good medicine. This led to controlled experiments (as randomized, controlled trials) that became the backbone of mainstream medicine. Nutritional protocols often used multiple nutrients, a difficult model to apply in clinical trials. Testing a single nutraceutical denied the patient full support of nutritional pharmacology, an injustice when treating a seriously ill patient. In addition, trials are expensive to conduct and early natural healers (by and large) did not represent an affluent subset of society.

But, ever so slowly, the medical scene is being revolutionized. According to the American College for Advancement in Medicine, physicians (in many cases) are showing eagerness to learn more about natural medicine and how to best implement it into their practice.[2] Scientists, teaching at nutritional seminars, report attendees are often medical doctors, a vast departure from years past.

## PREVENTING AND CONTROLLING CANCER

While some individuals will be reading this protocol looking for help managing a malignancy, others will be focusing on prevention and recurrence. The alphabetical list that follows provides quick guidelines for structuring a program, highlighting major nutrients in the prevention and treatment of cancer.

These guidelines should not be implemented individually in aggressive cancers without careful consultation of the remainder of the material. Cancer patients (and physicians) should be deliberate about reading the entirety of this protocol in order to avoid missing information that could prove to be life-saving.

**Note:** *It is important that the reader also consult protocol titled Cancer Treatment: The Critical* ^ors.

The dosages required for treating cancer considerably larger than those required (as on the tion) can change the effects that a nutr body. The risk is multidirectional. Overdosing or underdosing, as well as a lack of patient awareness regarding the full potential of natural pharmaceuticals, hampers recovery.

## THE CRITICAL IMPORTANCE OF SCHEDULED BLOOD TESTS

It is important to measure the successes or losses in regard to treatment-associated tumor response. Evaluating tumor markers in the blood or tumor imagery provides a basis for calculating regression of the disease. In addition, tumor markers provide direction for introducing other therapies if failures are evidenced.

**Table 1:  Type of Cancers and Tumor Marker Used for Assessment**

| Type of Cancer | Tumor Marker Blood Test |
|---|---|
| Ovarian cancer | CA 125, CK-BB |
| Prostate cancer | PSA, PAP, prolactin, testosterone |
| Breast cancer | CA 27.29, CEA, alkaline phosphatase, and prolactin (or CA 15-3 rather than CA 27.29) |
| Colon, rectum, liver, stomach, and other organ cancers | CEA, CA 19-9, AFP, TPS, and GGTP |
| Pancreatic cancer | CA 19.9, CEA, and GGTP |
| Leukemia, lymphoma, and Hodgkin's disease | LDH, CBC with differential, immune cell differentiation and leukemia profile |

It is also important to evaluate the effectiveness of immune-boosting therapies and guard against anemia and therapeutic toxicities. At a minimum, a monthly complete blood chemistry (CBC) test that includes assessment of hematocrit, hemoglobin, and liver and kidney function should be done in all cancer patients undergoing treatment.

An immune cell test should be performed bimonthly, measuring total blood count, CD4 (T-helper), CD4/CD8 (T-helper-to-T-suppressor) ratio, and NK (natural killer) cell activity. Also consider tests measuring cortisol levels (Cortisol [am and pm]) and HCG (human chorionic gonadotropin), a hormone that may be elevated 10–12 years prior to a diagnosis of cancer. For information regarding test availability, call (800) 208-3444.

## COMPLEMENTARY THERAPIES

When prescribing the various complementary cancer therapies, it is not possible to endorse one supplement, hormone, drug over another. We have provided as much evidence as space allows so that patients and their physicians can evaluate what approach may be suited for the individual situation.

A great deal of effort has been made to identify therapies that are substantiated in published scientific literature or that provide a cancer patient with the opportunity to experiment with cutting-edge treatment strategies. The focus of our effort has been to identify potentially lifesaving therapies that have been overlooked by mainstream oncology. We also attempt to discuss both positive and negative studies when applicable.

Life Extension can assume no responsibility for outcome, apart from a self-assigned duty to stay abreast of the most promising of therapies and to share the data with members. No guarantees (expressed or implied) accompany the material; neither is the information intended to replace medical advice. As always, each reader is urged to consult professional help for medical problems, especially those involving cancer. All supplements, drugs, and hormones are listed alphabetically and not in order of importance.

### Aloe

Scientists conducted a study comparing the use of aloe in combination with chemotherapy versus chemotherapy alone. They recruited 240 participants with solid metastatic tumors and randomized the participants to receive chemotherapy with or without aloe. The group treated with chemotherapy and aloe had significantly higher rates of tumor regression and disease control, achieving a 44% increase in response to therapy and 25% better disease control over chemotherapy alone.[3]

Fifty individuals with advanced cancers were randomized to receive melatonin or melatonin plus aloe. Survival at 1 year was 37.5% in the melatonin plus aloe group compared to 15.4% for the group receiving only melatonin.[4]

### Alpha-Lipoic Acid

Alpha-lipoic acid is a powerful antioxidant that regulates gene expression and preserves hearing during cisplatin therapy. Lester Packer (scientist and professor at the Berkeley Laboratory of the University of California) refers to lipoic acid as the most powerful of all the antioxidants; in fact, Packer says that if he were to invent an ideal antioxidant, it would closely resemble lipoic acid.[5] Alpha-lipoic acid claims anticarcinogenic credits because it independently scavenges free radicals, including the hydroxyl radical (a free radical involved in all stages of the cancer process and linked to an increase in the likelihood of metastasis).

Lipoic acid increases the efficacy of other antioxidants, regenerating vitamins C and E, coenzyme Q10, and glutathione for continued service. In fact, lipoic acid boosts the levels of glutathione by 30–70%, particularly in the lungs, liver, and kidney cells of laboratory animals injected with the antioxidant. In addition, glutathione tempers the synthesis of damaging cytokines and adhesion molecules by influencing the activity of nuclear factor kappa B (NF-κB), a transcription factor.[6]

**Note:** *A great deal of material relating to NF-κB is presented in the protocol Cancer Treatment: The Critical Factors.*

Lipoic acid can downregulate genes that accelerate cancer without inducing toxicity. So responsive are cancer cells that laboratory-induced cancers literally soak up lipoic acid, a saturation that increased the life span of rats with aggressive cancer by 25%.[7]

Alpha-lipoic acid was preferentially toxic to leukemia cells lines (Jurkat and CCRF-CEM cells). The selective toxicity of lipoic acid to Jurkat cells was credited (in part) to the antioxidant's ability to induce apoptosis (programmed cell death). Lipoic acid activated (by nearly 100%) an enzyme (caspase) that kills leukemia cells.[8] Other researchers showed that lipoic acid acted as a potentiator, amplifying the antileukemic effects of vitamin D. It is speculated that lipoic acid delivers much of its advantage by inhibiting NF-κB and the appearance of damaging cytokines.[9,10] Finding that lipoic acid can differentiate between normal and leukemic cells charts new courses in treatment strategies to slow or overcome the disease.[5]

As with all antioxidants, the appropriateness of using lipoic acid with chemotherapy arises. Animal studies indicate that alpha-lipoic acid decreased side effects associated with cyclophosphamide and vincristine (chemotherapeutic agents) but did not hamper drug effectiveness.[11] More recently, a combination of alpha-lipoic acid and doxorubicin resulted in a marginally significant increase in survival of leukemic mice.[12] Nonetheless, the definitive answer regarding coupling antioxidants with conventional cancer therapy is complex. Factors, such as type of malignancy, as well as the nature of the cytotoxic chemical and even the time of day the agents are administered, appear to influence outcome.

To its credit, lipoic acid appears able to counter the hearing loss and deafness that often accompanies cisplatin therapy. Depreciated hearing occurs as free radicals, produced as a result of treatment, plunder the inner ear; lipoic acid preserves glutathione levels and thus prevents deafness in rats.[13]

A suggested lipoic acid dosage for healthy individuals is 150–300 mg a day. Degenerative diseases usually require larger dosages (sometimes as much as 500 mg 3 times a day).

## Apigenin

Apigenin, a flavone (ie, a class of flavonoids) that is present in fruits and vegetables (eg, onions, oranges, tea, celery, artichoke, and parsley), has been shown to possess anti-inflammatory, antioxidant, and anticancer properties. Many studies have confirmed the cancer chemopreventive effects of apigenin.[14]

**Ovarian cancer.** Cancer cells need an increased blood supply to support growth and reproduction. Test tube and animal studies have found that apigenin inhibits blood vessel growth (angiogenesis) in human ovarian cancer cells, blocking production of two main signaling molecules required to stimulate vessel growth.[15,16] In addition, apigenin inhibited proliferation of ovarian cancer cells[17,18] and metastasis of ovarian cancer in mice.[19]

**Pancreatic cancer.** In a 2008 study, apigenin was applied to human pancreatic cancer cells in culture to determine its effect on the cells' uptake of glucose. Researchers concluded that apigenin deprived cancer cells of glucose, which supports their aggressive growth, by downregulating vital glucose-transporting proteins in cancer cells—effectively starving cancer cells of their food source.[20] In laboratory testing, apigenin inhibited the proliferation of pancreatic cancer cells.[21] In addition, in test tube and animal studies, apigenin enhanced the effectiveness of the chemotherapy drug gemcitabine against pancreatic cancer.[22,23]

**Breast cancer.** Apigenin stimulates apoptosis in breast cancer cells.[24] A 2012 study showed that apigenin slowed the progression of human breast cancer by inducing cell death, inhibiting cell proliferation, and reducing expression of a gene associated with cancer growth (Her2/neu). In another study, it was noted that blood vessels responsible for feeding cancer cells were smaller in apigenin-treated mice compared to untreated mice. This is significant because smaller vessels mean restricted nutrient flow to the tumors and may have served to starve the cancer as well as limit its ability to spread.[25]

Apigenin has been proven to have a synergistic treatment effect when combined with the chemotherapy drug paclitaxel.[26] In a study, apigenin increased the efficacy of the chemotherapy drug 5-Fluorouracil against breast cancer cells.[27]

**Lung cancer.** Apigenin inhibits expression of vascular endothelial growth factor (VEGF) and angiogenesis in lung cancer cells.[28] It was observed in a study that apigenin suppressed the proliferation of lung cancer cells and increased their susceptibility to antitumor drugs.[29]

**Colon cancer.** Apigenin may prove effective against colon cancer as well. Researchers concluded that apigenin stimulated apoptosis in colon cancer cells[30] and inhibited colon cancer cell growth.[31] In an animal study, apigenin significantly decreased the incidence of metastasis in rats with colon cancer.[32]

A clinical trial evaluated the effects of apigenin and EGCG (a component of green tea) in individuals after surgical removal of colon cancer. The treatment group received apigenin (20mg) and EGCG (20mg) for 2–5 years, while the control group did not. There were no recurrences of colon cancer in the treatment group compared to 20% in the control group. Furthermore, only 7% of the treatment group developed precancerous polyps compared to 27% of the control group.[33]

**Leukemia.** Apigenin has shown to induce apoptosis in leukemia cells.[34,35] In addition, apigenin inhibited the growth of human leukemia cells and induced these cells to differentiate (they became healthy mature cells).[36,37] Topoisomerases are enzymes involved in many aspects of leukemic cell DNA metabolism (such as replication). In one study, apigenin was shown to inhibit topoisomerase-catalyzed DNA irregularities.[38]

**Prostate cancer.** In an animal experiment, prostate cancer cells were transplanted into apigenin-fed mice. Administering apigenin to mice—either before or after transplantation—inhibited the volume of prostate cancer cells in a dose-dependent manner by as much as 59% and 53%, respectively.[39]

## Arginine

Various scientists have attempted to describe the complex role of arginine in cancer biology and treatment. L-arginine is the common substrate for 2 enzymes, arginase and nitric oxide synthase. Arginase converts L-arginine to L-ornithine, a pathway that can increase cell proliferation. Nitric oxide synthase converts L-arginine to nitric oxide (NO), a conversion process with uncertain effects regarding cancer.

A positive study conducted by a team of German researchers showed that arginine contributed significantly to immune function by increasing levels of white blood cells. Scottish scientists added that dietary supplementation with arginine in breast cancer patients enhanced NK cell activity and lymphokine

cytotoxicity.[40] (Lymphokines are chemical factors produced and released by T lymphocytes that attract macrophages to a site of infection or inflammation in preparation for attack.) Various researchers have shown that increasing arginine increases neutrophils (white blood cells that remove bacteria, cellular debris, and solid particles), significantly upgrading host defense.[41]

Apart from enhancing immune function, arginine increases a number of amino acids, creating the possibility of an amino acid imbalance. Oversupplying some amino acids while undersupplying others is thought to destabilize the tumor. All cells, both healthy and diseased, have amino acid requirements; if not met, the cell is significantly disabled.[41] Amino acid manipulation has been applied in oncology for decades with varying degrees of success.

Interesting studies have emerged regarding arginine or arginine analogs in cancer treatment. For example, infusions of arginine significantly reduced the incidence of liver and lung metastasis in laboratory mice. Earlier research found that supplemental arginine altered the number of tumor-infiltrating lymphocytes in human colorectal cancer, offering important implications for new strategies in cancer treatment.[42] Though many factors are involved (including appropriate dosages), Japanese researchers found that arginine-induced apoptosis in pancreatic (AR4-2J) cells, inhibiting cell proliferation.[43]

The 2 faces of arginine, however, cloud dosing with confidence. The role of NO, a molecule synthesized from arginine, remains controversial and poorly understood. While a few reports indicate that the presence of NO in tumor cells or their microenvironment is detrimental to tumor-cell survival, and subsequently their metastatic potential, a large body of data suggests that NO actually promotes tumor progression. Illustrative of its fickleness, NO was recently identified as a downstream regulator of prolactin, an inhibitor of apoptosis. However, arginine stimulated proliferation of prolactin-dependent Nb2 lymphoma cells in laboratory rats.[44] In addition, NO production (by murine mammary adenocarcinoma cells) promoted tumor-cell invasiveness, whereas introducing NO inhibitors resulted in an antitumor, antimetastatic profile.[45]

Ambiguity and nonconformity reduce arginine's role at the present time to adjunctive support with either traditional cancer treatment or fish oil supplementation. A heartening report regarding arginine, fish oil, and doxorubicin therapy appears in this protocol in the section titled Essential Fatty Acids.[46] Nonetheless, the diverse biological properties of L-arginine demand further careful studies, clarifying chemopreventive advantages and endangerments.[47]

## Astaxanthin

Astaxanthin is a red-orange carotenoid pigment derived from microalgae and fish. By quenching free radical production in oxidatively stressed tissues, astaxanthin has been found to prevent DNA damage,[48] which is required to initiate many forms of cancer. By subduing inflammatory mediators such as COX-2 and NF-κB, astaxanthin may prevent cancer promotion, the step that allows potentially cancerous cells to blossom into full-blown tumors.[49] By supporting healthy intercellular communication, astaxanthin may improve tissue resistance to cancers.[50] Also, by impairing enzymes like matrix metalloproteinases (MMPs) that cancer cells use to break down tissue barriers, astaxanthin may help prevent tumor invasion and metastatic spread.[49]

Astaxanthin has shown beneficial effects in preventing colon, breast, and bone cancers in a variety of animal models.[51-53] Laboratory studies demonstrate that astaxanthin has multiple beneficial effects on the immune system, boosting function of natural killer cells that patrol for abnormally developing cells that could turn cancerous.[54-56]

## Astragalus

Astragalus, an herb used for centuries in Asia, has exhibited immune-stimulatory effects. Astragalus potentiates lymphokine-activated killer cells.[57] One study found that astragalus could partially restore depressed immune function in tumor-bearing mice,[58] while another concluded that "astragalus could exhibit anti-tumor effects, which might be achieved through activating the... anti-tumor immune mechanism of the host."[59]

**Liver cancer.** In a laboratory experiment, astragalus inhibited the growth of hepatocellular carcinoma cells.[60] A 2012 study demonstrating that astragalus significantly inhibited tumor growth in mice with hepatocellular carcinoma.[61]

**Leukemia.** Astragalus has also shown to be beneficial against leukemia. It was observed in a clinical trial that astragalus-induced apoptosis in a chronic myeloid leukemia cell line.[62]

**Stomach cancer.** In a 2012 study, researchers demonstrated that astragalus induced apoptosis and downregulated VEGF in gastric cancer cells. They concluded that astragalus "has the potential to be further developed into an effective chemotherapeutic agent in treating advanced and metastatic gastric cancers."[63]

**Breast cancer.** It was observed in a clinical trial that astragalus inhibited the proliferation of breast cancer cells. Authors of the study stated, "The antiproliferation mechanisms may be related to its effects of upregulating the expressions of p53."[64] Similar findings were noted in a previous experiment.[65]

**Colon cancer.** In mice with colon cancer, the administration of astragalus produced a reduction in tumor volume comparable to the conventional chemotherapeutic drug 5-fluorouracil. The authors of this study stated, "These results indicate that astragalus saponins could be an effective chemotherapeutic agent in colon cancer treatment, which might also be used as an adjuvant in combination with other orthodox chemotherapeutic drugs to reduce the side effects of the latter compounds."[66]

**Chemotherapy.** Astragalus administered by injection has shown to significantly improve quality of life in individuals with advanced lung cancer receiving chemotherapy.[67] In tumor-bearing mice, astragalus reduced kidney damage caused by the chemotherapy drug cisplatin.[68] A study was conducted to observe the effects of astragalus injection on the efficacy and toxicity of chemotherapy in 120 individuals with unspecified cancer. Compared to the control group, the astragalus group showed a reduced likelihood of disease progression, as well as a lower incidence of reductions in white blood cell and platelet counts. The authors of the study concluded that "astragalus injection supplemented with chemotherapy could inhibit the development of tumor, decrease the toxic-adverse effect of chemotherapy, elevate the immune function of organism and improve the quality of life in patients."[69]

**Lung cancer.** In a 2003 study, individuals with advanced lung cancer received injectable astragalus. The 1-year survival rate was 46.8% in the astragalus group compared to 30% in the control group.[70] In 2006, researchers conducted a review to evaluate evidence from trials using astragalus-based herbal medicine combined with platinum-based chemotherapy in patients with advanced non–small cell lung cancer. The researchers identified 12 studies with a total of 940 subjects that reported a 33% decreased risk of death at 1 year in those receiving astragalus-based Chinese herbal combinations compared to chemotherapy alone. Additionally, nine studies were identified with a total of 768 subjects that reported a 27% decreased risk of death at 2 years in favor of those receiving astragalus-based Chinese herbal combinations compared to chemotherapy alone.[71]

## Blueberry

Blueberries are rich in anthocyanins (ie, dark pigments in fruits) and pterostilbenes (ie, antioxidant closely related to resveratrol). The anticancer effects of blueberries are mediated by multiple mechanisms:

**Blueberry extracts block DNA damage.**   Damage to cellular DNA underlies most forms of cancer. By preventing such damage, blueberry extracts can block the malignant transformation of healthy cells.[72]

**Blueberry extracts stop excessive proliferation.** Uncontrolled cell reproduction results in formation of dangerous tumors, as cells ignore the normal signals to stop growing. By restoring normal cellular signaling, blueberry extracts stop such out-of-control proliferation.[73–75] In an experimental breast cancer cell line, blueberry significantly reduced breast cancer cell proliferation, leading the researchers to state that "blueberry anthocyanins...demonstrated anticancer properties by inhibiting cancer cell proliferation and by acting as cell anti-invasive factors and chemoinhibitors."[76] In rats with experimentally induced breast cancer, the volume of new breast tumor formation was reduced by 40% in the group of rats supplemented with blueberry compared to the control group.[77]

**Blueberry extracts prevent development of precancerous lesions.**   Many cancers, such as those of the colon and cervix, begin as "precancerous" lesions, or areas of abnormal, but not yet malignant cell growth. Blueberry compounds sharply reduce the number of abnormal tissues by as much as 94% in the case of colon cancer.[78,79] In a 2006 study, blueberry reduced the formation of precancerous colon tumors in rats by 30% compared to controls.[80]

**Blueberry extracts inhibit angiogenesis.**   Rapidly-growing cancers recruit new blood vessels to meet their ravenous appetites for nutrients and oxygen. Blueberry inhibits new tumor blood vessel growth, known as angiogenesis.[81,82]

**Blueberry extracts slow tumor spread by invasion and metastasis.**   Solid cancers produce matrix metalloproteinases, which are "protein-melting" enzymes that help them invade adjacent tissues and that enable them to metastasize. Blueberry extracts block matrix metalloproteinases, thereby inhibiting cancer invasion and metastasis.[83,84] In one experiment published in 2011, blueberry extract was administered to mice with breast cancer. Compared to the control group, tumor volume was 75% lower in mice fed blueberry extract. Moreover, mice fed blueberry extract developed 70% fewer liver metastases and 25% fewer lymph node metastases compared to the control group.[85]

**Blueberry extracts trigger cancer cells' suicide.**   If normal cells replicate too fast, they are programmed to die through apoptosis. Cancerous cells, by contrast, ignore that programming, constantly doubling their population unchecked. Blueberry components restore normal programming and induce apoptosis in cells from a variety of cancers, putting the brakes on their rapid growth.[73,86–89]

**Blueberry can protect against the damaging effects of chemotherapy.**   In a 2007 study, mice were given the chemotherapeutic drug 5-fluorouracil, which resulted in significant reductions in red blood cell, white blood cell, and platelet counts. The mice fed a blueberry extract experienced a 1.2-fold increase in red blood cells and a 9-fold increase in white blood cells compared to mice treated with 5-fluorouracil alone.[90] Additionally, 2 studies investigated the ability of blueberry to protect against the toxicity of the chemotherapeutic drug doxorubicin. This drug is frequently prescribed to women with breast cancer. Doxorubicin toxicity can lead to heart damage. In comparison to the control groups, both studies found that rats fed blueberry experienced significantly less heart damage with doxorubicin administration. Blueberry also mitigated hematological toxicity by restoring depressed levels of red blood cell, hemoglobin, and bone marrow cell counts.[91,92]

## Carotenoids

Carotenoids have antioxidant activity, inhibit cellular proliferation, and offer protection against numerous types of malignancies. Carotenoids, acting as immune enhancers and free-radical scavengers, are important substances in oncology. When using carotenoids for antioxidant and cancer protection, it appears wise to use mixed carotenoids, that is, alpha-carotene, lycopene, zeaxanthin, canthaxanthin, beta-cryptoxanthin, and lutein rather than emphasizing only beta-carotene.

The following illustrate the benefits of mixed carotenoids:

- Lycopene offers targeted protection against cancers arising in the prostate,[93] pancreas,[94] digestive tract,[95] and colon.[96]

- The *American Journal of Clinical Nutrition* added that individuals seeking broad-spectrum colon protection should also include lutein-rich foods in their diet (spinach, broccoli, lettuce, tomatoes, oranges, carrots, celery, and greens).[97]

- Canthaxanthin, a less well-known carotenoid, was shown to induce apoptosis and inhibit cell growth in both WiDR colon adenocarcinoma and SK-MEL-2 melanoma cells.[98]

- Researchers showed that the risk of breast cancer approximately doubled (2.21-fold) among subjects with blood levels of beta-carotene in the lowest quartile, compared with those in the highest quartile. The risk of breast cancer associated with low levels of other carotenoids was similar, that is, a 2.08-fold increased risk if lutein is deficient and a 1.68-fold greater risk if beta-cryptoxanthin is lacking.[99] A Swedish study found that menopausal status has an impact on the protection delivered by carotenoids. Analysis showed that lycopene was associated with decreased breast cancer risk in postmenopausal women, but in premenopausal women, lutein offered greater protection.[100]

- Leukoplakia (an often precancerous condition marked by white thickened patches on the mucous membranes of the cheeks, gums, or tongue) is responsive to spirulina, a source of proteins, carotenoids, and other micronutrients.[101] An inverse relationship between beta-carotene and thyroid carcinoma was observed in both papillary and follicular carcinomas.[102] A high dietary intake of beta-carotene appears a protective (though modest) factor for the development of ovarian cancer.[103]

- Lastly, Japanese researchers showed that all the carotenoids inhibited hepatic (liver) invasion, probably through antioxidant properties.[104]

Men who consume 10 or more servings of tomato products per week reduce their risk of prostate cancer by about 35%. The American Chemical Society in August 2001 reported that 32 (largely African-American) patients diagnosed with prostate cancer and awaiting radical prostatectomy were placed on diets that included tomato sauce, providing 30 mg a day of lycopene. After 3 weeks, mean serum prostate-specific antigen (PSA) concentrations fell by 17.5%, oxidative burden by 21.3%, DNA damage by 40%, while programmed cell death increased three-fold in cancer cells.[105] Part of lycopene's protection involves the ability of carotenoids to counteract the proliferation of cancer cells induced by insulin-like growth factors.[106]

Beta-carotene exhibited a radioprotective effect among 709 children exposed to radiation inflicted by the Chernobyl nuclear accident. For example, the Chernobyl accident showed that irradiation increases the susceptibility of lipids to oxidative damage and that natural beta-carotene may act as an in vivo lipophilic antioxidant or radio-protective agent.[107] Therefore, using beta-carotene following radiotherapy may reduce the tissue damage caused during treatment.

Beta-carotene, perhaps the most controversial of the family of carotenoids, has come under attack several times in the past. For example, smokers who received synthetic beta-carotene (as a prophylactic) in the CARET study had a higher rate of lung cancer and death than smokers not supplemented. In fact, the study was terminated by the National Cancer Institute (NCI) because of the widespread discrepancy between the 2 groups. The CARET study is not new, but because it still concerns beta-carotene users, we will attempt to explain the unexpected results of the study.

Packer described the subjects as "walking time bombs." Many were victims of asbestos exposure or heavy smoking. The form of beta-carotene selected for the study (synthetic versus natural) was also cited as another possible explanation for the negative outcome.

Leo Galland (practitioner and director of the Foundation of Integrated Medicine, New York City), also explains that high-dose beta-carotene (25 000 IU a day) administered to smokers results in a particular pattern of metabolism.[108] The process is orchestrated as cytochrome p450 enzymes (phase 1 detoxification system) are summoned into action by tars in cigarette smoke. As beta-carotene is acted on by cytochrome p450, oxidized end products are formed, as well as toxic derivatives.

Simultaneously, vitamins C and A, as well as glutathione, are depleted, severing antioxidant protection. This sequence can damage DNA and increase the likelihood of lung cancer, particularly in an environment with initially high oxidative stress, a profile common to smokers. Without full spectrum antioxidant support, the single dose of beta-carotene produces an oxidative environment rather than one of protection.

**Note:** *As one free radical is neutralized by an antioxidant, another oxidant may be formed. It is well established that vitamin C can serve as a pro-oxidant through the formation of ascorbyl radicals. It is also known that this radical is quenched by vitamin E to yield a tocopheryl radical, which in turn is reduced by the conversion of glutathione to glutathione disulfide. Thus, the full spectrum of antioxidants is preferable, rather than emphasizing single antioxidants.*

Beta-carotene is largely considered nontoxic even at high doses; for example, some nonconventional cancer therapies recommend large amounts of carrot juice. One large glass of carrot juice can contain 100 000–200 000 IU of provitamin A or carotene. The problem with carrot juice is that it is loaded with fructose (sugar). Cancer cells feed on sugar, and drinking carrot juice may induce an insulin spike that could potentially fuel cancer cell propagation.

Cancer patients should consider natural beta-carotene supplements in lieu of carrot juice. Suggested phytonutrient dosages are from 9–20 mg of sulphoraphane, 10–30 mg a day of lycopene, and 15–40 mg of lutein, along with a mixed carotenoid blend that includes alpha- and beta-carotene.

*Note: The section titled "What should cancer patients eat?" (appearing later in this protocol) contains a discussion regarding the value of sulphoraphanes in the diet.*

## Chrysin

Breast cancers that are estrogen-receptor positive can grow and be exacerbated in the presence of estrogen in the body. One aim of drug therapy for estrogen-receptor-positive breast cancer is to decrease the levels of estrogen in the body. To that end, drugs used to block the enzyme (ie, aromatase) that converts testosterone into estrogen (ie, aromatase inhibitors) are widely used in women with estrogen-receptor-positive breast cancer. Chrysin, a flavonoid, is a natural aromatase inhibitor.[109,110]

## Cimetidine (Tagamet®)

Histamine (H2) receptor antagonists (such as cimetidine) became popular in the late 1970s to treat gastrointestinal ulcers and other benign conditions of the stomach, esophagus, and duodenum. In 1985, Life Extension announced that cimetidine had merit as a cancer adjunct. Since then, many studies have been published encouraging the use of cimetidine as a means of disabling tumors and expanding survival rates.[111,112]

Cimetidine impacts cancer by way of a three-pronged mechanism including (1) inhibition of cancer cell proliferation, (2) stimulation of lymphocyte activity by inhibition of T-cell suppressor function, and (3) inhibition of histamine's activity as a growth factor.[113]

In a Japanese study, a total of 64 colorectal cancer patients (who had earlier undergone surgery) were evaluated for the effects of cimetidine on survival and disease recurrence. The cimetidine arm of the study received 800 mg a day of cimetidine along with 200 mg a day of the chemotherapy drug 5-fluorouracil (5-FU); the control group received only 5-FU. The treatment was initiated 2 weeks following surgery and terminated 1 year later. Strikingly beneficial effects were noted: The 10-year survival rate for patients treated with cimetidine/5-FU was 84.6%, whereas that of the control group (5-FU alone) was only 49.8%.[114]

The effect of cimetidine on a particularly aggressive form of colon cancer (Dukes grade C) was investigated. The cumulative 10-year survival rate of the cimetidine-treated group was consistently 84.6%, whereas that of the control group was only 23.1%. (Less virulent cancers—Dukes A or B—responded less well to cimetidine treatment.)[114]

Cimetidine treatment is particularly effective in patients whose tumors express higher levels of Lewis A and Lewis X antigens (ie, breast and pancreatic cancers, as well as about 70% of colon cancers). Lewis A and Lewis X antigens are cell surface ligands that adhere to a molecule in the blood vessels called E-selectin. (Ligand comes from the Latin word *ligare*, meaning that which binds.)

The adhesion of the cancer cell to vascular endothelial cells expressing E-selectin is a key step in invasion and metastasis. Cimetidine improved patient outcome presumably by inhibiting the expression of E-selectin, thus abolishing the binding site for continued cancer growth and metastasis. The 10-year cumulative survival rate of the cimetidine group displaying Lewis antigens was 95.5%, whereas the control group was only 35.1%.[114] Note that patients are well-advised to undergo Lewis antigen determinations for optimal therapy and a more favorable outcome. Contact Impath Laboratories at 521 West 57th Street, New York, NY 10019, (800) 447-8881, for information regarding testing.

Researchers recently unearthed another mechanism through which cimetidine offers cancer protection. Cimetidine enhanced cell-mediated immunity by improving suppressed dendritic cell function.[115] Dendritic cells capture foreign invaders and carry the antigen to lymph nodes and spleen. The "hand-delivered" antigen shows the immune system exactly what it has to fight. A more in-depth explanation regarding dendritic cells appears in the protocol titled Cancer Vaccines and Immunotherapy.

The growth inhibitory effects of cimetidine were assessed on 5 cell lines derived from human brain tumors of different tissue types and grades of malignancy. Each cell line was treated with cimetidine 24 hours before analysis. Cimetidine significantly inhibited cell proliferation in 3 of 5 cell lines, which indicates the apparent dependence of these cells on histamine stimulation.[116]

Because we do not wish the reader to interpret positive material as a universal ameliorant for all cancers, the following findings are noted:

• Fred Hutchinson Cancer Research Center researchers explored whether cimetidine exerted a cancer-preventive effect on prostate and breast cancers by tracking 48 512 individuals in 1977–1995. Unfortunately, the study concluded that cimetidine did not influence the risk of female breast cancers; in addition, the researchers concluded that there was little evidence to support the previously hypothesized preventive effect of cimetidine on the risk of prostate cancers.[117]

- In multiple myeloma patients, cimetidine reduced by about 30% the bioavailability of melphalan (Alkeran®), the standard treatment for the disease.[118]

- A total of 132 male rats were evaluated for immune status after ingesting cimetidine to forestall a diagnosis of gastric cancer. In the cimetidine-fed group, 19 of 48 developed cancer, versus 12 of 43 in the control group. The Norwegian researchers concluded that cimetidine had no significant immune-modulating effects on the development of gastric cancer in rodents.[119]

While cimetidine is not efficacious in cancer prevention, it shows efficacy in treating certain cancers. A suggested cimetidine dosage for cancer patients is 800 mg (taken at night). Do not supplement with cimetidine without physician awareness; the drug can interact with several medications (such as digoxin, theophylline, phenytoin, warfarin, and lidocaine), increasing or decreasing drug potency.

## Clodronate

Clodronate is a bisphosphonate that inhibits cell proliferation and the threat of metastasis. Clodronate reduced the incidence and number of metastasis in bone and viscera (organs enclosed in the abdominal, thoracic, or pelvic cavity) in high-risk breast cancer patients by 50%[120] (see also Journal Club on the Web).

Between 1990 and 1995, 302 patients (median age 51 years) with primary breast cancer and tumor cells in the bone marrow (the presence of which is a risk factor for the development of distant metastasis) were randomly assigned to receive 1600 mg a day of oral clodronate for 2 years or standard follow-up without clodronate supplementation.[120] At the conclusion of the trial, bone metastases were detected in 12 (8%) of the clodronate group versus 25 (17%) of the control group. The mean number of bony metastases per patient was 3.1 in the clodronate group versus 6.3 in the nontreated group. Visceral metastasis was observed in 13 (8%) versus 27 (19%) of controls; 6 patients (4%) died in the clodronate group, compared to 22 (15%) in the untreated group. Researchers concluded that clodronate opposed metastasis by altering the binding capacities of adhesion molecules on tumors and bone cells. Women with existing metastatic breast cancer (who added

bisphosphonates to their regimen) reported less bone pain and fewer fractures with treatment.

The bisphosphonates (particularly zoledronic acid) appear to be effective against the skeletal complications of multiple myeloma, reducing vertebral fractures and pain. In the early phase of metastasis to bone, tumor cells activate osteoclasts, cells that break down and resorb bony tissue. This favors tumor growth, as growth factors are released when bone is degraded. Bisphosphonates inhibit the development of monocytes into osteoclasts (cells that digest and remove bone) and promote osteoclast death.

In addition, bisphosphonates restrain the production of bone-resorbing cytokines such as interleukin-6, an inflammatory marker for myeloma prognosis. Lastly, bisphosphonates directly affect myeloma by inducing apoptosis of malignant plasma cells. The biochemical effects of zoledronic acid continued for as long as 8 weeks after a single administration,[121] but myeloma mortality was not decreased by bisphosphonates.[122,123] Typically, a synergism (a cooperative effort) exists between bisphosphonates and cytotoxic agents, increasing chemotherapy's effectiveness.

The standard dose of clodronate for treating cancer is 800 mg taken twice daily, although double this dosage has been used safely. Breast cancer patients may consider a 3- to 5-year regimen of clodronate or other bisphosphonate therapy. Blood tests to measure serum calcium levels and kidney function are required 10 days after beginning clodronate and every 1–2 months thereafter. Persons who are pregnant or who have severe renal insufficiency requiring dialysis should avoid clodronate.

**Note:** *Newer bisphosphonate drugs such as Zometa®, Actonel®, Fosamax®, and Aredia®, more potent than clodronate, are now approved by the Food and Drug Administration (FDA), readily available in the United States, and covered by most health insurance plans. Prophylactic bisphosphonate therapy is highly recommended for cancers with a propensity to metastasize to bone, such as prostate and breast cancers. Most cancer patients should be on bisphosphonate therapy since any amount of bone breakdown releases growth factors that fuel cancer cell growth. Refer to Cancer Treatment: The Critical Factors for more information about bisphosphonate drugs approved in the United States.*

## Coenzyme Q10 and Statin Drugs

Statins, a class of cholesterol-lowering drugs, have been shown to inhibit the activity of Ras oncogenes. Ras oncogenes are involved in the regulation of cell growth, modulating the signals that govern the cancer cell cycle. Mutations in genes encoding Ras proteins have been closely associated with unregulated cell proliferation, a hallmark of cancer (refer to the protocol Cancer Treatment: The Critical Factors to read more about Ras oncogenes).

Numerous studies have shown the value of statin drugs in a cancer regimen, and the benefit escalates when a statin is combined with a nonsteroidal anti-inflammatory drug (NSAID). People who regularly used NSAIDs lowered their risk of colon cancer by as much as 50%; when lovastatin was added to a cyclo-oxygenase 2 (COX-2) inhibitor, the rate of cell death of 3 colon cancer cell lines increased up to five-fold.[124]

The statin's mode of operation, however, raises concern. Statin drugs reduce cholesterol synthesis in the liver by inhibiting the activity of 3-hydroxy-3-methylglutaryl coenzyme A (HMG-CoA) reductase. HMG-CoA reductase is required for the conversion of HMG-CoA to mevalonic acid, a step in cholesterol synthesis.[125] Inhibiting HMG-CoA reductase results in lower amounts of cholesterol being produced. Disruption of the cascade also interferes with the synthesis of coenzyme Q10 (CoQ10), creating a potential tradeoff regarding advantages and disadvantages gathered from statin usage.[125,126]

The impact on CoQ10 levels when taking statin drugs can be significant. For example, patients taking CoQ10, who later started lovastatin, lowered their CoQ10 levels by 44-75%. The problems associated with drug-related suppression of CoQ10 escalate when age-associated decline in serum CoQ10 levels are also present. A CoQ10 deficiency of 25% is linked with illness in animals and a deficit of 75% with death.[127,128] Administering adequate amounts of CoQ10 with a statin drug allows the cancer patient the value of the drug without the risks imposed by depletion of the coenzyme.

In 1997, Life Extension suggested that cancer patients ask their oncologist to consider lovastatin (80 mg a day) as adjunct therapy. The recommendation was based on scientific studies indicating lovastatin interfered with the cancer cell cycle and appeared to encourage apoptosis.[129] Lovastatin, sold under the name Mevacor®, is a fat-soluble statin drug, as are Zocor® and Lipitor®. Water-soluble statin drugs such as Pravachol may not work as effectively against cancer as the fat-soluble varieties, although one study showed that Pravachol induced significant benefits to a group of primary liver cancer patients.[130]

One of the concerns associated with low levels of CoQ10 is an increased risk of developing cancer. CoQ10 has been reported to be effective in inhibiting the progression of cancers and metastasis, even in

patients for whom all conventional treatment failed.[131,132] CoQ10, acting as a nonspecific stimulant to the immune system, increases blood levels of T lymphocytes and improves the T4–T8 lymphocyte ratio.[133] Contrast this with the energy loss and immune suppression associated with conventional cancer therapies.

Karl Folkers, a pioneer in CoQ10 exploration, reported that in a study of blood levels of CoQ10 in 116 breast cancer patients, 23.1% had blood levels of CoQ10 below 0.5 µg/mL. The incidence of breast cancer cases with levels below 0.6 µg/mL was 38.5%, higher percentages than observed in healthy women. A subsequent study reported in the *Journal of Clinical Pharmacology and Therapeutics* showed a statistically significant relationship between the level of CoQ10 deficiency and breast cancer prognosis.[134,135]

*Molecular Aspects of Medicine* reported the results of an 18-month study conducted in Denmark involving 32 breast cancer patients.[136] The patients had complicated medical profiles; that is, some had involvement in axillary lymph nodes and others had distant metastasis. The patients all received antioxidant therapy, consisting of vitamins C, E, and beta-carotene, select minerals and trace minerals, along with essential fatty acids, and 90 mg of CoQ10 a day. Their treatment was an integrated approach that also included surgery, radiation therapy, and chemotherapy. The survival rate during the 18-month study was 100%; a follow-up evaluation at the 24-month interval indicated all participants were still alive, although the expected deaths were 4 at 18 months and 6 at 24 months. All 32 of the enrollees in the study reported improvement in quality of life, stabilization of weight, a withdrawal from pain medications, and no signs of further distant metastases; 6 of the 32 patients showed apparent partial remissions.

Patients ($n = 15$) with myeloma showed a mean CoQ10 blood level of 0.67 ± 0.17 µg/mL. The incidence of a CoQ10 blood level below 0.7 mcg/dL was 53.3%, which is higher than the 24.5% found among a group of nonmyeloma patients.[134] Individuals with bloodborne tumors are often saddened with the scarcity of nutritional material relevant to their type of cancer. When links are found, patients and physicians should take special note. The full clinical implication of this finding remains to be explored.

Patients, with and without cancer, report a decrease in the incidence of infection while taking CoQ10.[137] This is particularly important to the cancer patient, who often faces additional challenges because of a suppressed immune system. Another extremely important characteristic of CoQ10 is its antioxidant potential, stabilizing cell membranes and preserving cellular integrity.[138]

One of the most potent chemicals used in cancer chemotherapy treatment is Adriamycin® (doxorubicin). A significant consequence of this drug is cardiac damage, especially in older patients with established heart disease. Italian researcher Mario Ghione discovered a depletion of CoQ10 in the diseased hearts of animals after long-term Adriamycin® administration. When CoQ10 was given to a group of mice before Adriamycin® therapy, 80–86% survived; a control group (receiving Adriamycin® but without CoQ10) had only a 36–42% survival rate.[139,140]

Dosage suggestions are 90–390 mg a day of CoQ10, taken with some fat to enhance absorption. The *American Journal of Health-System Pharmacy* reported that liver enzymes could become elevated when taking 300 mg of CoQ10 a day for extended periods of time.[141] Also, *Folia Microbiologica* reported that mice injected with human small cell lung cancer cells and then given high doses of CoQ10 had a diminished response to radiation therapy compared to the nonsupplemented group.[142] Food sources of CoQ10 include mackerel, salmon, and sardines along with beef, peanuts, and spinach.

## Coffee

Coffee, especially brews enriched with chlorogenic acid, protect cells against the DNA damage that leads to aging and cancer development.[143–145] Growing tumors develop the ability to invade local and regional tissue by increasing their production of "protein-melting" enzymes called matrix metalloproteinases. Chlorogenic acid—present in coffee—strongly inhibited matrix metalloproteinase activity.[146,147]

In a 2004 study, coffee induced cell cycle arrest and apoptosis in liver cancer cells, while significantly reducing tumor growth and lung metastasis in rats with liver cancer.[148] In addition, chlorogenic acid induced apoptosis in chronic myelogenous leukemia cells.[149]

Studies are demonstrating an association between higher coffee consumption and a reduced risk of various cancers. In one study, researchers reported that men who drank over *6 cups of coffee daily* had an *18%* lower risk of prostate cancer and a *40%* lower risk of aggressive prostate cancer.[150] This effect was noted for decaffeinated as well as caffeinated coffee, indicating that compounds other than caffeine are responsible for this preventive effect.

"Heavy" coffee drinking has been associated in multiple studies with as much as a *57%* reduction in colon cancers.[151–155] Coffee and its constituents target specific cancer cell–signaling systems to suppress colon cancer formation and metastasis.[156]

A 2011 study reported that postmenopausal women who drank *5 cups of coffee daily* exhibited a *57%* decreased risk of developing *estrogen-receptor negative* (non–hormone-responsive) breast cancer.[157] Chlorogenic acid and other polyphenols are the likely beneficial agents in such cancers.[158]

Individuals who consumed more than *3 cups of coffee daily* had a *40% lower* risk of oral, pharyngeal, and esophageal cancers compared to those who drank one cup of coffee or less daily.[159]

Researchers noted that consumption of *one cup of coffee daily* was associated with a *42%* lower risk of liver cancer.[160] Additionally, consuming at least one cup daily reduced the risk of death due to liver cancer by *50%* compared to nondrinkers.[161]

Women with the highest coffee intake were *30%* less likely to develop endometrial cancer than those who consumed none.[162]

## Conjugated Linoleic Acid

Conjugated linoleic acid (CLA) is a trace fatty acid that inhibits tumor formation and metastasis, suppresses arachidonic acid, and encourages apoptosis. Researchers at the Roswell Park Cancer Institute (Buffalo, New York) showed that CLA, derived mainly from dairy products, reduced the incidence of breast cancer.[163] Animal experiments showed that only 50% of rats feeding on CLA butter developed mammary tumors when exposed to high doses of known carcinogens, compared to 93% of the rats deprived CLA. This research demonstrated for the first time that CLA in foods is biologically active and that a food can offer significant protection against cancer.[164]

*Anticancer Research* published supporting data that CLA (in both test tube and animal models) demonstrates strong antitumor activity. Particularly gratifying effects were observed regarding inhibition of growth and metastatic spread of transplantable mammary tumors in severely immune deficient mice. The mice were fed CLA for 2 weeks prior to inoculation with human breast adenocarcinoma cells (107 MDA-MB468) and throughout the trial. CLA completely abolished the spread of breast cancer cells to the lungs, blood, and bone marrow. These results indicate that CLA blocks the local growth and spread of human breast cancer via mechanisms independent of the immune system.[163,165,166]

The effects of CLA and beta-carotene were assessed on white blood cell (lymphocyte) and macrophage function. CLA alone increased lymphocyte numbers and their cell killing ability. Conversely, CLA inhibited interleukin-2 (IL-2) production (a desirable cytokine) and suppressed the ability of macrophages to destroy foreign material. When given together, CLA and beta-carotene interacted in an additive manner to increase lymphocyte production and their cytotoxicity. In addition, beta-carotene was able to overcome the inhibitory action of CLA on the phagocytic activity of macrophages.[167]

**Note:** *The Melanoma Center at the University of Pittsburgh Cancer Institute showed a potential role for histamine in cancer immunotherapy. A phase 2 trial of IL-2 versus IL-2 and histamine in patients with metastatic melanoma demonstrated a trend toward a superior survival benefit from IL-2 and histamine for all patients enrolled and a statistically significant survival benefit for patients with hepatic metastasis.[168]*

The effect of 3 different diets on the local growth and metastatic potential of human prostatic carcinoma cells (DU-145) in severely immune-deficient mice was studied. Animals were fed either a standard diet or diets supplemented with 1% linoleic acid (LA) or 1% CLA for 2 weeks prior to inoculation with cancer cells and throughout the 14-week study. Mice receiving the LA-supplemented diet displayed significantly higher body weight, lower food intake, and increased local tumor load as compared to the other 2 groups of mice. Mice fed the CLA-supplemented diet exhibited not only smaller local tumors, but also a significant reduction in lung metastasis.[169] It was estimated that CLA inhibited the formation of premalignant lesions by approximately 50%, while increasing apoptosis in diseased cells.[170]

CLA, in a dose-related fashion, has an ability to suppress arachidonic acid (AA). Since AA produces inflammatory mediators that can promote cancer at initiation and progression, CLA's ability to stifle AA elevates its status as a chemopreventive.[171,172]

In 1996, Life Extension was in the forefront recommending CLA; after evaluating the results of numerous studies, Life Extension presented the promising anticarcinogenic nature of CLA to members. Relatively small doses (3–4 g of CLA) are effective. For example, young female rats (still maturing) fed 0.8% of their diet from CLA achieved long-term protection against breast cancer. The dose of 0.8% correlates positively to the recommended daily dosage of 3–4 g endorsed by Life Extension. A dose of six 1000-mg CLA capsules (76%) each day is suggested for cancer patients; pregnant and lactating women should avoid CLA.

## Cyclooxygenase-2 (COX-2) Inhibitors (Naturally Occurring)

The following compendium drawn (in part) from *Beyond Aspirin*[173] underscores herbs that inhibit COX-2,

an enzyme intricately involved in the cancer process. Natural compounds usually have many mechanisms of action; thus, the protective mechanisms common to the herb often extend beyond enzyme inhibition and are described herein. Because of the synergism of herbs, combinations are often of greater value than a single herb. The COX-2–cancer connection is thoroughly discussed in the protocol Cancer Treatment: The Critical Factors.

**Berberine-containing herbs (goldenseal, barberry, goldthread, and Oregon grape).** Berberine, strong and bitter in taste and found in various herbs, delivers anti-inflammatory properties via COX-2 inhibition.[174] Kaempferol, a constituent of berberine, is a strikingly active inhibitor of COX-2 activity.[173,175] Berberine is unique, having the ability to inhibit COX-2 activity without involving the beneficial COX-1 enzyme. Berberine, perhaps by impacting the production of cyclooxygenase, influences the development of cancers at various sites:

- Berberine is effective against bladder cancers.[176]

- Berberine suppressed colon carcinogenesis and inhibited COX-2 without COX-1 inhibition. The COX-2 enzyme is abundantly expressed in colon cancer cells and plays a role in tumorigenesis. The berberine-COX-2 connection appears to best explain the mechanism of berberine's anti-inflammatory and antitumor-promoting effects.[173,174]

- Berberine induced apoptosis in human leukemia cells.[177]

- Berberine inhibited the development of skin tumors.[178]

- Berberine has potent antitumor activity against human and rat malignant brain tumors.[179] Studies using goldenseal, which contains the alkaloid berberine, showed average cancer kill rate of 91% in rats, over twice that seen in BCNU (a standard chemotherapy agent for brain tumors). Rat studies used 10 mg/kg of berberine.

A suggested dose is three 250-mg capsules of goldenseal each day. The preparation should be standardized to provide 5% hydrastine. Various respected herbalists suggest that goldenseal should be cycled (rotated with other herbals) rather than routinely administered. Goldenseal contains the alkaloids berberine, hydrastine, and canadine.

**Feverfew (Tanacetum parthenium).** The anti-inflammatory traits of feverfew have an ability to inhibit the COX-2 enzyme.[180] According to researchers[173] feverfew contains a lactone, or chemical compound called parthenolide. Parthenolide, in turn, contains a variant of methylene-gamma-lactone (MGL) that interacts with macrophages. The white blood cell-lactone interaction suppresses a critical protein process, a repression that ultimately inhibits the COX-2 enzyme. In addition, feverfew contains apigenin (a flavonoid) and melatonin, both COX-2 inhibitors.[181]

Researchers at Children's Hospital Medical Center (Cincinnati, Ohio) explained another of parthenolide's anti-inflammatory traits; that is, its ability to inhibit NF-κB, the predecessor of a number of potentially damaging cytokines.[182] Recall that as inflammation is reduced, the risks of many degenerative diseases decrease as well (turn to the protocol titled Cancer Treatment: The Critical Factors to read about the cytokine–cancer connection).

In addition, feverfew inhibits 5-lipoxygenase, an enzyme that metabolizes AA. A byproduct of this metabolism (hydroxy-eicosatetraenoic acid or HETE) feeds cancer cells and promotes angiogenesis, the development of new blood vessels. Agents that inhibit the production of lipoxygenase should be of particular interest to individuals taking COX-2 inhibitors; as the COX-2 enzyme is inhibited, 5-lipoxygenase enzymes become activated.[183]

A suggested dosage is 1–2 capsules of feverfew a day, standardized to contain 600 mcg of parthenolide. Pregnant and lactating women should avoid feverfew, as well as those showing allergic sensitivities.

**Ginger (Zingiber officinalis).** From the scores of biologically active components contained in ginger, some are specific for inhibiting COX-2 and others for inhibiting 5-lipoxygenase, enzymes responsible for the formation of proinflammatory agents (prostaglandin E2 and leukotriene B4) from AA. Ginger safely modulates COX-2 activity but also brings balance to COX-1 (an enzyme responsible for gastric mucosal integrity) in a manner vastly superior to synthetic NSAIDs.[173,184]

As COX-2 and 5-lipoxygenase are repressed, 2 distinct metabolic pathways are inhibited, one leading to the synthesis of prostaglandins and the other leading to the production of HETEs. Prostaglandin E2 (PGE2) (produced from COX-2-arachidonic acid interactions) promotes cellular proliferation, and 5-HETE is considered indispensable fuel for tumor growth (prostate in particular).

It has been speculated that therapeutic dosages of ginger inhibit PGE2 by up to 56%. As ginger slows down 5-lipoxygenase and 5-HETE production, cell death is stimulated in both hormone responsive and nonresponsive human prostate cancer cells.[185,186] Leukotrienes, produced by lipoxygenase, are considered

1000 times more reactive than histamine. Ginger has more 5-lipoxygenase inhibitors than any other botanical source.[173]

Ginger may also be useful in overcoming nausea that accompanies chemotherapy and toxicity associated with the breakdown products of cancerous tissue. James Duke, distinguished botanist and author, has high regard for ginger, adding that it has a major advantage over other antiemetics because of its safety profile. Ginger's antioxidant activity adds another plus to a booming list of anticancer credits. A suggested dosage is 2 g of ginger a day.

**Green tea.** Salicylic acid, the main anti-inflammatory component of aspirin, is a naturally occurring compound found in green tea, having COX-2–inhibiting qualities. The polyphenols and flavonoids contained in green tea are also COX-2 inhibitors.[187]

Mayo Clinic researchers showed that green tea consumption inhibited cancer growth.[188] They identified the green tea polyphenol EGCG (epigallocatechin gallate) as the most potent inhibitor of cancer cell proliferation. Japanese researchers pinpointed the types of cancer most responsive to green tea (breast, esophageal, liver, lung, skin, and stomach) by surveying cancer-free individuals who consumed 4–6 cups of green tea a day.

The odds ratio of stomach cancer decreased to 0.69 with a high intake of green tea (≥7 cups a day).[189] Another study conducted in Yangzhong (a region in China with a high incidence of chronic gastritis and gastric cancer) showed the amount and duration of green tea consumption governed the rate of stomach cancer. Frequent long-term green tea drinkers had approximately 50% less risk of developing gastric cancer compared to individuals consuming little or no tea.[190] Green tea reduces the damaging effects of nitrites in the acidic environment of the stomach with greater efficiency than vitamin C.

The growth of non-Hodgkin's lymphoma cells, transplanted in mice, was reduced by 50% when green tea was a part of the animal's diet. Cyclophosphamide, a chemotherapeutic drug, administered at the maximum tolerable dose, was unable to replicate similar benefits.[191] Part of green tea's anticancer profile includes an antimutagenic factor that helps DNA replicate accurately.[192]

PGE2 is thought to stimulate tumor promotion in precancerous and cancerous cells.[191,193] Of 14 subjects, 10 (71%) demonstrated a response to green tea, as evidenced by at least a 50% inhibition of PGE2 in rectal mucosa.

EGCG appears to normalize the cell growth cycle and prompt apoptosis in cancer cells by inhibiting NF-κB, a growth vehicle that cancer cells use to escape cell regulatory control.[194] EGCG strongly and directly inhibits telomerase, an enzyme (normally dormant from birth) that delivers immortal status to cancer cells.[195]

Cigarette smokers who drink green tea have a 45% lower risk of lung cancer compared to non-tea drinkers. Even though Japan has one of the highest numbers of smokers in the world, they have one of the lowest rates of lung cancer of any developed nation; a protection thought to be delivered by green tea.

The number of anticarcinogens, antioxidants, and antiproliferative agents found in green tea (carotenoids, chlorophyll, polysaccharides, vitamins C and E, and numerous flavonoids) explains why some researchers advocate using a broad-spectrum extract, replicating the plant's total constituents. Considering the vastness of green tea's anticancer effects, incorporating green tea into the diet (5–10 cups a day; or five 350-mg capsules, 3 times a day of a 95% polyphenol extract) would appear to be wise for individuals concerned with cancer.

**Curcumin.** Worldwide clinical trials have chiseled out a definite place for curcumin in oncology. Among them are New York Presbyterian Hospital and the Weill Medical College, which reported that curcumin, a curcuminoid found in turmeric, directly inhibited the COX-2 enzyme.[196] So excited are various oncologists regarding curcumin that the potent anti-inflammatory has been classed as a potential third-generation cancer chemopreventive agent.

Curcumin inhibited thromboxane A2 (TxA2), a highly unstable, biologically active compound created by COX from AA.[173,197] Unless controlled, TxA2 promotes tumor endothelial cell migration (metastasis) and angiogenesis. By inhibiting TxA2, curcumin reduces the tumor's blood supply and lessens the threat of metastasis.[198,199] Curcumin is effective at inhibiting 5-lipoxygenase and subsequently HETE, a survival factor for prostate, breast, and pancreatic cancers.[173,186,200,201]

The following list illustrates the depth of curcumin's defenses against cancer:

- **Colon.** Curcumin inhibited chemically induced carcinogenesis in the colon when administered at different stages of the cancer process. Laboratory rats, administered curcumin during either initiation or late in the premalignant phase, had a lesser incidence and fewer numbers of invasive malignant colon tumors.[202] Also, by inhibiting COX-2-arachidonic acid interactions, curcumin suppresses prostaglandins responsible for inflammatory processes.[203] Chronic inflammation has for decades been regarded as a cause of colon cancer.[204]

- **Antioxidant activity.** Curcumin inhibits or possibly even reverses oxidative damage by scavenging and neutralizing free radicals. By defusing the hydroxyl and superoxide radicals and breaking oxidative chain reactions, curcumin protects DNA with greater efficiency than lipoic acid, vitamin E, or beta-carotene.[201,205,206]

- **Breast cancer.** Curcumin inhibits the growth of multiple breast cancer cell lines,[207] particularly those that result from exposure to environmental estrogens such as chemicals and pesticides.[208] Also, curcumin, estrogen, and estrogen mimickers gain entry into the cell through the aryl hydrocarbon receptor. Because curcumin competes for entry, it can crowd out damaging materials.[209] According to researchers, curcumin blends well with other cancer inhibitors. For example, a curcumin-isoflavonoid combination suppressed the growth of estrogen receptor-positive cancer cells up to 95%.[208]

- **Oral tumors.** Curcumin inhibits oral squamous cell carcinoma more effectively than either genistein or quercetin.[210] Only cisplatin, a platinum-based chemotherapy drug, was more effective.

- **Skin tumors.** Curcumin inhibits skin tumors. When applied topically, curcumin reduces skin inflammation and inhibits local swelling.[211]

- **Prostate cancer.** Curcumin was able to decrease the proliferative potential of androgen-independent prostate cancer cells—and cells of other androgen-dependent cancers—largely by encouraging apoptosis. Moreover, a significant decrease in microvessel density, the sustaining blood supply of a tumor, was also observed.[212]

- **Leukemia.** Curcumin-induced apoptotic cell death in promyelocytic leukemia HL-60 cells at concentrations as low as 3.5 μg/mL.[213]

- **Protein kinase C (PKC) and epidermal growth factors (EGF).** Curcumin was proclaimed "potentially useful" in developing antiproliferative strategies to control tumor growth by suppressing the activity of protein kinase C (PKC).[214] As the activity of PKC is slowed down, tumor proliferation is halted.[215] PKC transmits signals from the epidermal growth factor receptor (EGF-R), a cycle that ultimately encourages the growth of tumors. Conversely, cancers awaiting EGF stimulation are dealt a severe blow if this pathway is severed. Curcumin blocked the activation of EGF by 90%.

- **p53 potentiator.** Curcumin increases expression of healthy nuclear p53 protein in human basal cell carcinomas, hepatomas, and leukemia cell lines.[216]

- **Tumor necrosis factor-alpha (TNF-α).** Researchers at the University of Kentucky showed that

TNF-α acts as a catalyst in cytokine production, stimulating interleukin-6 (IL-6) and -8 (IL-8) and activating NF-κB.[217] Curcumin inhibits TNF-α, thus blocking TNF-α, NF-κB pathways, and the emergence of proinflammatory cytokines.[201,218,219]

- *Helicobactor pylori (H. pylori).* Exposure of gastric epithelial cells to the ulcer-causing bacterium *H. pylori* (considered a potential gastric and pancreatic carcinogen) induces secretion of IL-8. IL-8 plays a pivotal role in the development of cancer. The more virulent *H. pylori*, the greater the production of IL-8. *H. pylori* strains that fail to induce IL-8 secretion do not activate NF-κB, while all IL-8 inducing strains activate the transcription factor. Curcumin is capable of inhibiting NF-κB and completely suppressing IL-8. By restraining essential players in the development of *H. pylori*, curcumin diminishes the risks of both gastric and pancreatic cancer.[220,221]

Although the benefits of curcumin are impressive, curcumin is poorly assimilated. This means that while the digestive tract and liver profit, the remainder of the body may be denied benefit. Administering 2000 mg of curcumin showed that very little reached the bloodstream. This dilemma is amendable by adding a small amount of piperine (a component of black pepper) to curcumin, increasing bioavailability by 2000%.[222] However, it is possible that piperine in combination with prescription drugs could increase the bioavailability of the drug. Therefore, it is recommended that curcumin (containing piperine) be taken 2 hours apart from prescription medications.

Healthy people typically take 900 mg of curcumin each day. Cancer patients often take as much as four 900-mg capsules 3 times a day for a 6- to 12-month period, reducing the dosage thereafter. Individuals with biliary tract obstruction should avoid curcumin because it enhances biliary flow from the liver. High doses of curcumin should not be taken on an empty stomach to protect against gastric irritation.

**Note:** *The question ultimately arises as to whether curcumin is appropriate during chemotherapy. A recent study from the University of North Carolina (Chapel Hill) showed that curcumin reduced the effectiveness of chemotherapy in breast cancer patients by inhibiting reactive oxygen species.[223] Refer to the Chemotherapy protocol to read more about the advisability of taking curcumin during conventional treatment.*

## Dimethyl Sulfoxide

In August 1995, Julian Whitaker relayed his own experience with dimethyl sulfoxide (DMSO), when a basal cell carcinoma (about the size of a dime) appeared on his ear. A dermatologist recommended surgical removal of the cancerous portion and a skin graft replacement. Instead, Whitaker made a paste from shark cartilage, vitamin C, and DMSO and applied the mixture to the lesion daily. Within 3.5 weeks, the basal cell had completely disappeared. Stanley Jacob, professor at the Oregon Health Sciences University (Portland) suspected DMSO was the hero, although Whitaker has confidence in the full formula.[224]

The Sealy Center for Molecular Sciences reported that DMSO, administered either before or 15 minutes after TNF-α, blocked 80% of NF-κB. By suppressing TNF-α and NF-κB, DMSO broke an inflammatory cascade that otherwise terminates in an onslaught of potentially damaging cytokines.[225]

DMSO is an excellent transporter of other therapies into cancerous cells. In fact, many offshore cancer clinics consider it the standard for all patients who are undergoing various therapies.

## Essential Fatty Acids

Essential fatty acids (EFAs) block arachidonic acid, inhibit COX-2 enzyme, regulate cell division and inhibit adhesion, prevent cachexia, potentiate traditional cancer therapies, and suppress the activity of proinflammatory cytokines. As a result of the current fat phobia, over 80% of Americans consume inadequate amounts of essential fatty acids (especially omega-3 fatty acids). Physicians report that this scarcity is contributing to epidemic proportions of degenerative diseases, including cancer.[226] The omega-6 to omega-3 fatty acid ratio typically seen may be as high as 20:1, whereas the optimal ratio may be nearer 1:1.[227] EFAs, although not manufactured by the body, perform vital functions that prevent and control cancer.

- As enzymes metabolize AA, the byproducts of the metabolism fuel the cancer process.[228] Oxidized AA is, in fact, considered a primary initiator of cancer.[173] One gram of omega-3 fatty acids blocks 10 g of AA.[183]

- The COX-2 enzyme (interacting with AA) can cause excess production of PGE2, promoting cancer cell growth. Eicosapentaenoic acid (EPA) and docosahexaenoic acid (DHA) (derived from alpha-linolenic acid or fish oil) are effective COX-2 inhibitors.[229]

- Fish oil is the most documented supplement to suppress (up to 90%) a cascade of damaging cytokines, including TNF-α and IL-1.[230] It should be noted that psychological stress induces the production of proinflammatory cytokines, such as TNF-α, IL-6, and IL-10. Increasing omega-3 fatty acids lessened the proinflammatory response to psychological stress.[231] For information regarding a blood test to obtain a cytokine profile, call (800) 208-3444.

- Women with high levels of alpha-linolenic acid in breast tissue have a 60% lower risk of breast cancer compared to women with low levels.[232,233] Jeffrey Bland, esteemed scientist and teacher, reported a supportive study involving 500 (C3H) mice prone to breast cancer. The mice were divided into 10 groups of 50 animals and evaluated regarding the impact of various dietary oils on the occurrence of cancer. One-tenth of the animals received standard chow and served as a control group; another group received standard chow plus benzanthracene, a carcinogen. The other 8 groups received isocaloric diets along with the cancer inducer; the variable was the type of fat (not the amount) fed in conjunction with the chow. Eight oils were evaluated: tallow, fish, corn, primrose, safflower, linseed oils, and two others. At the conclusion of the study, 8 of the 10 groups (400 animals) were dead with mammary cancer. The 100 survivors were animals fed omega-3–rich oils. The study was repeated using different types of oils and varying amounts of the cancer inducer. The end results were the same. Researchers postulated that the advantage of omega-3 fatty acid was the oil's ability to reduce inflammatory mediators, those signaling tumor progression and metastasis.[234]

- Epidemiologic and experimental studies suggest that oils rich in omega-3 fatty acids lessen the risk of colon cancer. A relatively small fraction of alpha-linolenic-rich perilla oil (25% of total dietary fat) provided an appreciable beneficial effect in reducing cancer risk.[235]

- Low EFA status results in a lack of oncogene control with a shift toward cell proliferation.[183] EFAs also regulate the adhesiveness of cancer cells, including cell-cell and cell-matrix adhesions.[236]

- Fatty acids, particularly EPA, inhibited the growth of 3 human pancreatic cancer cell lines (MIA PaCA-2, PANC-1, and CFPAC), suggesting therapeutic benefit to pancreatic cancer patients.[237]

- Omega-3 fatty acids prevent cachexia (the muscle wasting and weight loss that occurs in some cancer patients irrespective of proper nutritional intake). Controlling the symptoms common to cachexia (anorexia, abnormal macronutrient metabolism, and fatigue) improves quality of life and extends periods of remission.[238]

- Researchers found DHA and EPA cytotoxic to myeloma cells *in vitro*.[239] Individuals who regularly consume fish and cruciferous vegetables appear to lessen their risk of developing multiple myeloma.[240]

Thirty-two dogs with stage 3 lymphoma and their response to a dietary and chemotherapeutic regime were evaluated. All of the animals were fed identical diets, but they received varying types of oils. For example, one group received menhaden fish oil (rich in omega-3 fatty acid) and arginine, while the control group received soybean oil.[46] The animals also received doxorubicin every 3 weeks.

As DHA and EPA levels increased in the test group, the animals experienced longer disease-free intervals and subsequently increased survival time. Dogs receiving the supplemented diet lived about 700 days; animals receiving the soybean oil lived only about 400 days. The time until relapse was also significant: 425 days in the treatment group versus 275 days in the control group.

> **Note:** *Since fish oil increases the effectiveness of chemotherapeutic agents, the animals receiving the menhaden oil realized an additional advantage over the soybean-treated animals.*[241]

Suggested dosages for various EFAs: Take six 1000-mg capsules a day of perilla oil, which provide 550–620 mg of alpha-linolenic. Flaxseed oil in 1000-mg softgels is a rich source of omega-3 fatty acids. Take 7 softgels a day. A preventive dose of a fish oil concentrate is 4000 mg a day (2800 mg of EPA/DHA).

## Garlic (*Allium sativum*)

Garlic is inhibitory to a number of malignancies, minimizes damage imposed by known carcinogens, and boosts the immune system. No plant has the medicinal history, spanning as many cultures, of garlic. Garlic, in fact, appears to be the quintessential medicine/food, having influence on simplistic diseases from common colds to degenerative diseases. For centuries the Chinese have used garlic-containing herbal formulas to treat tumors, but scientists were challenged to find the mechanism that rendered it efficacious.

Among those dedicated to validating garlic is Benjamin Lau. Focusing on cancer biology and immunology, Lau was motivated by an epidemiologic study reported by the People's Republic of China. The study compared 2 large populations in the Shandong Province: Cangshan County and Qixia County.[242] Residents of Cangshan County experienced the lowest death rate due to stomach cancer (3 per 100000), regularly consuming about 20 g of garlic a day; the people of Qixia had a 13-fold higher stomach cancer death rate, eating garlic only rarely. It appears that lowering nitrite concentrations may be the protective mechanism resulting in fewer numbers of gastric cancers. Jhinzou Liu, a Chinese biochemist, found garlic "much more effective than vitamin C" in keeping nitrosamines, potentially carcinogenic compounds, from forming.

Garlic's anticarcinogenic effects are not restricted to gastric malignancies.

- Garlic (administered intralesionally to mice) was significantly more effective than BCG (bacillus Calmette-Guerin), a weakened form of the tuberculosis bacilli, in treating bladder cancer.[243]

- Garlic extract reduced the incidence of breast cancer (in mice) by 70–90%.[244]

- Diallyl disulfide, a sulfur compound, induced apoptosis in non–small cell lung cancer cells[245]; diallyl sulfide, a component of garlic oil, inhibited liver carcinogenicity following carcinogenic exposure[246]; S-allyl cysteine, a derivative of aged garlic extract, inhibited human neuroblastoma cell growth in vitro[247]; allixin, one of the compounds of aged garlic extract, inhibited the development of skin cancer[248]; and diallyl sulfide was highly inhibitory during the initiation phase of esophageal cancer.[249]

- S-allyl cysteine (SAC) inhibited proliferation and cell growth of 9 human and murine melanoma cell lines, producing positive results without side effects.[250] Of equal importance, garlic modulated major cell differentiation markers of melanoma. As the cell shows distinguishable characteristics (differentiation), it eventually loses its uncontrollable propensity to divide.

- S-allyl cysteine and diallyl sulfide reduced colonic damage and the incidence and frequency of colon tumors if administered 3 hours prior to each carcinogenic injection. Colonic damage was inhibited by 36% and 47%, respectively.[251] Michael Wargovish (Houston) claims that diallyl sulfide is one of the most active chemopreventive agents known.

S-allyl cysteine (SAC) appears to be able to overcome the adverse side effects (heart and liver damage) associated with the chemotherapeutic agent doxorubicin. Doxorubicin resulted in a 58% mortality rate among laboratory mice; SAC reduced doxorubicin-induced mortality to 30%.[252] Weight loss, typical with doxorubicin, was reduced from 13% to 9% with SAC.

Certain garlic constituents possess antioxidant properties, while other constituents act as oxidants. The latter case is strikingly demonstrated when human hemoglobin is mixed with extracts from fresh garlic and from dried raw garlic powder products. The hemoglobin-garlic extract mixtures turn dark, and their spectra reveal the oxidation of hemoglobin to methemoglobin. Contrarily, extracts from aged garlic do not cause oxidative changes.

When t-butylhydroperoxide, a free-radical generator and oxidant, is used to oxidize red blood cells, it results in rupturing of the cells and darkening of the hemoglobin. An extract of aged garlic, added to the red blood cell suspension prior to the addition of the oxidant, minimized oxidation and cell rupture.[253] Since many cancer therapies produce free radicals in an attempt to kill cancer cells, researchers concluded that garlic could offer significant protection against treatment-induced tissue damage.

Another benefit of garlic to the cancer patients is its effect on enhancing immune function. Here are a few of the numerous studies relating to garlic's effect on immune cells:

- Garlic stimulates proliferation of lymphocytes, those cells comprising 25% of total white blood cells that carry out the principal responsibilities of the immune system.[254]

- Garlic quickens macrophage phagocytosis, a process by which microorganisms and cellular debris are engulfed and destroyed.[255]

- Fraction 4 (F4), a protein isolated from aged garlic extract, enhanced the cytotoxicity of human lymphocytes. Although F4 alone increased cytotoxicity, the effect was amplified when F4 was combined with suboptimal doses of IL-2. F4 is an efficient immune potentiator and may be used for immune therapy.[256]

T-helper/T-suppressor ratios converted to normal among a small group of AIDS (acquired immune deficiency syndrome) patients supplementing with garlic. Thrombocytopenia (a reduction in platelet count) is often therapy resistant in individuals with AIDS. Yet, platelet numbers have been reported to increase, sometimes greater than 100000, during 4 months of garlic supplementation. Although AIDS is not cancer, this feared disease has forced researchers and clinicians to look closely at the immune system.[257]

Research suggests that garlic preparations are not equal in pharmacologic value. While raw garlic juice, heated garlic juice, dehydrated garlic powder, and aged garlic extract all significantly enhanced natural killer cell numbers and activity, only aged garlic extract and heated garlic juice inhibited the growth of tumor cells in mice.[258]

Abdullah evaluated the percentage of tumor kill using raw and aged garlic. Raw garlic killed 139% of tumor cells compared to an untreated group, while aged garlic killed 159%.[259]

*Note: Defining the most efficacious type of garlic is confounding. Some physicians and clinicians report greater gains from odorous garlic supplementation. If garlic is part of your nutritional program, experiment with different varieties, assessing both subjective and objective improvements. It is highly possible that different metabolic types respond differently to various forms of garlic.*

Evaluating hundreds of garlic users, however, it should be noted that garlic thins the blood, and for some individuals (particularly those using anticoagulants) it is essential to abstain from or to watchfully monitor supplementation coagulation status.

Therapeutic factors contained in garlic include magnesium, selenium, 17 amino acids, 33 sulfur compounds, and vitamins B1, A, and C, as well as germanium. Germanium has been shown to induce production of interferon, enhance natural killer cell activity, and activate macrophage activity in experimental animals.[260]

## Glutamine

Glutamine increases NK cell activity, decreases PGE2 synthesis, inhibits tumor growth, stabilizes weight loss, and reduces incidence of stomatitis and infection. Tumors typically have high concentrations of glutamine; thus, physicians have been reluctant to add supplemental glutamine to a cancer protocol. However, oral glutamine (1 g per kg of body weight a day administered to rats) upregulated tissue glutathione (a powerful antioxidant) by 25% and increased natural killer cell activity 2.5-fold. PGE2 synthesis (a proinflammatory prostaglandin that fuels tumor growth) decreased and tumors were inhibited by 40%.[261]

When glutamine accompanied either chemotherapy or radiotherapy, it protected the host and actually increased the selectivity of therapy for the tumor. This was evidenced among a group of rats (receiving methotrexate, cyclophosphamide, or cisplatin) whose tumor reduction nearly doubled with glutamine supplementation.[262,263]

Researchers also observed that glutamine decreased progression of tumor formation in rats implanted with mammary tumors, suggesting oral glutamine may be useful as a chemopreventive in breast cancer.[264] Oral glutamine maintained lymphocyte numbers and protected the gut of esophageal cancer patients during radio/chemotherapies.[265]

Glutamine typically stabilizes weight loss by preserving intestinal function and allowing better nutrient absorption. Subsequently, glutamine prolongs survival by slowing down catabolic wasting, a disorder characterized by weight loss, diminished muscle mass, and loss of body fat. Fewer incidences of stomatitis (a generalized inflammation of the oral mucosa) and bouts of infection help reduce the number of days spent in a hospital.[266] Harvard University research showed that glutamine supplementation decreased medical expenses of leukemia patients undergoing bone marrow transplants by $21 095 per patient.[267] (The retail cost of glutamine is $10.00 per day.)

A suggested glutamine dosage is ≥2 g a day taken on an empty stomach. Glutamine is regarded as nontoxic, but cancer patients contemplating higher dosages should do so only after consulting with a health care provider.

## Inositol Hexaphosphate (IP-6)

Inositol hexaphosphate (IP-6) activates natural killer cells, promotes differentiation, supports p53 activity, and normalizes the cell cycle by modifying signal transduction pathways. IP-6, a promising anticancer compound sold as a nutritional supplement, is a combination of inositol (a B vitamin) and phytic acid, also known as inositol hexaphosphate. According to A. Shamsuddin, who introduced IP-6 after more than 15 years of research, it works by enhancing the body's ability to defend itself against cancer, making it of equal importance as either a cancer preventive or therapeutic agent.

Inositol hexaphosphate is a sugar, very much like glucose, except it has 6 phosphates attached to its molecules. Every animal and plant species tested had varying levels of IP-6, but the highest amounts were found in rice, about 2% by weight: 100 g of rice provide approximately 2 g of IP-6, but even that amount is not readily available. Since the body is dependent on digestive enzymes to break it down, only a meager amount is actually absorbed from foodstuffs. Thus, IP-6 in encapsulated or bulk forms should be of special interest to cancer patients and those desiring protection against cancer.

The following chemotherapeutic properties are assigned to the immune modulator:

- IP-6 activates natural killer cells, cells that work without antibody participation.[268]

- IP-6 decreases cellular proliferation.[269,270] Illustrative of its potential, IP-6 reduced large intestinal cancer (by regulating cell proliferation) in F344 rats even when the treatment was begun 5 months after carcinogenic induction.[271]

- IP-6 promotes differentiation ("normalization") of cancer cells, that is, an unspecialized, atypical cell structure assumes the likeness of the tissue of origin, indicating the virulence of the malignancy is waning.[272] IP-6 was shown to inhibit growth and induce differentiation in HT-29 human colon cancer cells, making it valuable as an adjunctive treatment in colon cancer. IP-6 also strongly inhibited growth and induced differentiation in human prostate cancer cells (PC-3) in both in vitro and in vivo studies.[273]

- IP-6 has been effective against every cancer cell tested.[274,275]

- After inducing cancer in laboratory animals, IP-6 administered either orally or by injection at the site of the tumor, or intraperitoneally, resulted in tumors two-thirds smaller than the controls. As tumors reduced in size, survival rate increased.[271]

- IP-6 increases expression of the tumor suppressor gene p53 by up to 17-fold. p53 acts on cells under stress, such as those with DNA damage, reducing proliferation and encouraging apoptosis. When cancer arises, a mutation in p53 is commonly involved. Lastly, since loss of p53 function increases cancer cells' resistance to chemotherapeutic agents, the stimulating action of IP-6 on p53 makes it an attractive adjuvant chemotherapeutic agent.[274,276]

Toxicity studies (dating back to 1958) showed that a daily dose of 9 g of IP-6 for 3 years resulted in side effects, including lesser incidences of kidney stones and fatty liver, as well as lower cholesterol levels. It is important to note that IP-6 does not kill cancer cells, as most anticancer agents do; thus, hair loss and immune suppression do not occur. A suggested dosage of 1–3 g a day is adequate for most individuals. For those requiring larger doses, a powder is available (1 scoop twice daily is equivalent to 16 capsules, supplying about 6.4 g of IP-6).

## Lactoferrin

Lactoferrin is immunoregulatory, inhibits angiogenesis, and binds iron. Perhaps one of the most promising therapeutic uses of lactoferrin, a milk protein with bacteriostatic properties, may be as a nontoxic, anticancer agent. Lactoferrin, a minor fraction of whey, results in a significant reduction in the incidence of esophageal, lung, bladder, and colon cancer in laboratory rats.[277–279]

Since evidence indicates milk products protect against colon cancer, researchers speculate that bovine lactoferrin, a natural ingredient in milk, may be the chemoprotective agent.[280] Rats treated with a carcinogen and supplemented with 2% bovine lactoferrin for 36 weeks had a reduced incidence of colon cancer (27% of that observed in a control group; rats receiving 0.2% bovine lactoferrin reduced incidence to 46%).

A remarkable 43% reduction in spontaneous lung metastasis (compared to controls) occurred after implanting colon carcinoma 26 (Co 26 Lu) in lactoferrin-treated laboratory animals.[281]

In addition to inhibiting angiogenesis (the vascular network that sustains the tumor), lactoferrin maintains the integrity of the immune system.[279,282] Typically, bovine lactoferrin prompts an increase in the number of natural killer cells, as well as the cytotoxicity of white blood cells.[281] The antibiotic, anti-inflammatory, and immune-modulating properties of lactoferrin appear active against the gastritis-, ulcer-, and cancer-inducing bacterium *Helicobacter pylori*.[283]

Lactoferrin, a natural iron-binding protein, scavenges free radicals in fluids and inflamed areas, suppressing free radical mediated damage. It decreases the availability of iron in neoplastic cells, depriving them of an iron supply.[284,285]

The suggested dosage is 300–900 mg a day of the superior apolactoferrin (iron-depleted) form of lactoferrin. Lactoferrin is a natural component of cows' and human mothers' milk, but is also found in the milk of sheep, goats, and pigs.

## Lignans

Lignans are found in high concentrations in flaxseed and sesame. Once consumed, lignans are converted in the intestines into enterolactone. Enterolactone has been shown to inhibit angiogenesis and promote cancer cell apoptosis.[286,287]

**Liver cancer.** Lignans inhibited the growth and metastasis of liver cancer in rats.[288]

**Breast cancer.** Enterolactone inhibits the aromatase enzyme, which converts testosterone into estrogen.[289,290]

Researchers conducted an analysis of breast cancer risk and dietary lignan intake in 3158 women. They determined that premenopausal women with the highest lignan intake had a 44% reduced risk of developing breast cancer.[291]

Thirty-two women awaiting surgery for breast cancer were randomized to receive either a muffin containing 25 g of flaxseeds or no flaxseed (control group). Postoperative analysis of the cancerous tissue revealed that markers of tumor growth were reduced by 30–71% in the flaxseed group versus no reduction in the control group.[292] Scientists concluded that "dietary flaxseed has the potential to reduce tumor growth in patients with breast cancer."

In order to examine the relationship between dietary lignan intake and breast cancer, researchers assessed the diets of 1122 women in the 1–2 years before breast cancer diagnosis. They noted that postmenopausal women with the highest dietary intake of lignans had a 71% decreased risk of death from breast cancer.[293]

**Prostate cancer.** Cancer cells utilize the tyrosine kinase enzymes to fuel their rapid growth. In one study, metastatic prostate cancer cells were shown to overexpress tyrosine kinases by 10- to 100-fold as compared to normal prostate epithelial cells.[294] Enterolactone inhibits the tyrosine kinase enzyme.[295]

The 5-alpha reductase enzyme converts testosterone into a potent metabolite called dihydrotestosterone (DHT). DHT provokes a stimulatory effect on prostate cancer cells. Enterolactones have been shown to inhibit 5-alpha reductase, thus reducing levels of DHT.[296]

In a study evaluating the relationship between prostate cancer and dietary lignans, results showed a 34% reduced risk of prostate cancer in the group consuming the highest amount of enterolactone-precursor lignan foods.[297]

In another study, men with the highest blood levels of enterolactone were 82% less likely to have prostate cancer compared to men with the lowest blood enterolactone levels.[298] A similar study showed that men with the highest blood enterolactone levels were 60% less likely to have prostate cancer compared with men with the lowest levels.[299]

In an animal model, lignans were fed to mice with prostate cancer. The results demonstrated a 360% greater apoptotic index (programmed cell death) in the mice fed lignans compared with the control group. The control group displayed a 260% greater tumor volume compared to the mice fed lignans.[300]

**Colon cancer.** One study documented that a high intake of lignans was associated with a 47% reduced risk of colorectal adenomas, which are colon polyps considered to be precursors to colon cancer.[301] In another study, lignan-fed mice experienced a 33% reduction in the number of colon adenomas compared to the control group.[302] In addition, it has been observed that enterolactones induced apoptosis and inhibited growth of colon cancer cells.[303]

**Uterine cancer.** When researchers assessed lignan intake and cancer status among nearly 1000 women, they concluded that postmenopausal women with the highest dietary lignan intake experienced a 43% lower risk of developing uterine cancer.[304] Also, lignans have reduced the incidence of uterine cancer in rats.[305]

## Lycopene

Lycopene, a carotenoid found in high concentrations in many fruits and vegetables (eg, tomatoes), has been shown to be associated with decreased risk of chronic diseases such as cardiovascular disease and cancer.[306]

**Prostate cancer.** Research has focused on the use of lycopene in men with prostate cancer. In a clinical trial investigating the preoperative effects of lycopene in patients undergoing a prostatectomy, 15 men received lycopene at 15 mg twice daily for 3 weeks prior to surgery versus 11 that received none (control). Results indicated that the cancer was confined within the prostate with no cancer present at the surgical margins (both excellent prognostic factors) in 73% of the men taking lycopene versus 18% of the control group. Moreover, 84% of the lycopene group had smaller tumors (<4 ml) compared to only 45% of the control group.[307]

In a study of 20 men with metastatic prostate cancer, each man received 10 mg daily of lycopene for 3 months.[308] One achieved a complete response (defined as a reduction of PSA [to <4] and the absence of any sign of the disease for 8 weeks); and 6 patients (30%) had a partial response (defined as a 50% reduction in PSA and alleviation of other symptoms such as bone pain if present). The disease remained stable in 10 patients (50%) and progressed in 3 (15%). In addition, 63% (10 of 16) with bone pain (from bone metastasis) were able to reduce their daily use of pain-suppressing drugs.[308]

In another study of metastatic prostate cancer patients, 50% were castrated and given 4 mg of lycopene daily while the other half were castrated only (control group).[309] Castration (surgical removal of the testes) dramatically reduces testosterone levels and was a treatment for those with metastatic prostate cancer. Currently, the use of drugs has replaced castration as a means to greatly reduce testosterone levels in the body. After 2 years, 40% of the control group achieved a PSA of less than 4 ng/mL compared to 78% in the castration plus lycopene group. Also, bone scans showed no evidence of bone metastasis in 30% of the lycopene group compared to 15% of the control group. Additionally, the lycopene group experienced a 9% improvement in survival compared to the control group. The authors of the study concluded, "Adding lycopene to orchidectomy (castration) produced a more reliable and consistent decrease in serum PSA level; it not only shrinks the primary tumor but also diminishes the secondary tumors, providing better relief from bone pain and lower urinary tract symptoms, and improving survival compared with orchidectomy alone."

In yet another study, lycopene given at 30 mg per day resulted in a stabilization of PSA in 95% of men with a rising PSA after their initial treatment.[310]

**Brain cancer.** A clinical trial examined the effects of lycopene in patients with high-grade gliomas, with 64% being glioblastoma multiforme.[311] The study participants were randomized to receive radiation therapy with or without lycopene at 8 mg daily. Researchers observed that 28% of the lycopene group achieved a complete response compared to 8% of the control group. Also, 16% of the lycopene group achieved a partial response compared to 8% of the control group. They also noted that the disease continued to progress in 68% of the control group compared to only 44% of the lycopene group. The authors concluded, "lycopene may have potential therapeutic benefit in the adjuvant management of high-grade gliomas."

It has also been observed that lycopene inhibits the proliferation and progression of breast, colon, and oral cancer cells in test tube studies.[312–316]

## Melatonin

Melatonin is an immune modulator that increases the survival time of most cancer patients. Some cancer patients are now taking melatonin, an immune-modulating neurohormone, as part of a comprehensive, nontoxic cancer treatment. The cone-shaped pineal body, a small but crucial gland located in the brain, produces melatonin, a hormone that influences sexual maturation but also appears to play an important role in cancer.

Melatonin supplementation appears to restore circadian rhythms, which diminish or disappear with age. When melatonin's circadian rhythm is abolished, the aging process is accelerated, life span is shortened, and an increase in spontaneous tumors occurs.[317] It has been shown that when the defense system is compromised due to disrupted rhythms, tumors grow 2–3 times faster.[318]

Melatonin also protects and restores normal blood-cell production caused by the toxicity of conventional treatments; a profile shared with the FDA-approved drug Neupogen®, a granulocyte colony-stimulating factor (G-CSF), and Leukine®, a granulocyte-macrophage colony-stimulating factor (GM-CSF). A combination of melatonin and low-dose IL-2 neutralizes treatment-induced lymphocytopenia, a decrease in the numbers of lymphocytes in the peripheral circulation of cancer patients.[319]

Researchers found the best way to amplify the antitumoral activity of low dose IL-2 is by not coadministering another cytokine but rather cosupplementing with the immune-modulating neurohormone melatonin.[320] This is hopeful news for a subset of cancer patients, because melatonin has been shown to cause tumor regression in neoplasms non-responsive to IL-2.[317]

The Division of Radiation Oncology of the San Gerardo Hospital (Milan) developed the following protocol for 80 patients with advanced metastatic tumors.[320] The patients were randomized to receive 3 million IU of IL-2, 6 days a week, for 4 weeks or IL-2 plus 40 mg a day of melatonin. A complete response was achieved in 3 of 41 patients treated with IL-2 plus melatonin and in none of the patients receiving only IL-2. A partial response occurred in 8 of 41 patients treated with IL-2 plus melatonin and in 1 of 39 patients treated with IL-2. Tumor regression rate was significantly higher in patients using IL-2 and melatonin compared to those receiving IL-2 (11/41 versus 1/39). The survival rate at 1 year was higher in patients treated with IL-2 and melatonin than in the IL-2 group (19/41 versus 6/39). Lymphocytic populations were consistently higher when melatonin accompanied the treatment and thrombocytopenia (a decrease in the number of circulating platelets) occurred less frequently.

For patients with bloodborne cancers, an IL-2/melatonin combination is also promising. Twelve patients (nonresponsive to standard therapies) evaluated the efficacy and tolerability of a combination of low-dose IL-2 plus melatonin in advanced malignancies of the blood, including non-Hodgkin's lymphoma, Hodgkin's disease, acute myelogenous leukemia, multiple myeloma, and chronic myelomonocytic leukemia. IL-2 was given 6 days a week for 4 weeks, along with oral melatonin (20 mg a day). Cancer was stabilized and did not progress in 8 of 12 (67%) participants for an average duration of 21 months. An additional benefit accrued as the melatonin/IL-2 therapy was well-tolerated.[321]

Nonresectable brain metastasis remains an untreatable disease. Because of melatonin's cytostatic action (the ability to suppress the growth of cells) and its anticonvulsant activity, the pineal hormone may prove effective in the treatment of brain metastasis. In a study to test the theory, 50 patients with inoperable brain metastasis were given supportive care or supportive care plus 20 mg of melatonin nightly. Freedom from brain tumor progression and survival rates at 1 year were higher in patients who were treated with melatonin compared to those who received only supportive care.[322,323] Even when melatonin was unable to stop the progression of advanced, metastatic disease, it improved the performance status of patients (see Table 2).

Low melatonin levels play a role in escalating rates of breast cancer. As melatonin levels decrease, the secretion of estrogen increases. Nighttime production

**Table 2:   Summary of Studies Using Melatonin (Lissoni's Phase 2 Randomized Clinical Trial Results)**

| Tumor Type | Patient Number | Basic Therapy | Melatonin Dose | 1-Year Survival Melatonin | Placebo | Level of Significance |
|---|---|---|---|---|---|---|
| Metastatic non–small cell lung | 63 | Supportive care only | 10 mg | 26% | <1% | <0.05 |
| Glioblastoma | 30 | Conventional radiotherapy | 10 mg | 43% | <1% | <0.05 |
| Metastatic breast | 40 | Tamoxifen | 20 mg | 63% | 24% | <0.01 |
| Brain metastases | 50 | Conventional radiotherapy | 20 mg | 38% | 12% | <0.05 |
| Metastatic colorectal | 50 | IL-2 | 40 mg | 36% | 12% | <0.05 |
| Metastatic non–small cell lung | 60 | IL-2 | 40 mg | 45% | 19% | <0.05 |

*Compiled by Cancer Treatment Centers of America and published in the March 2002 issue of Life Extension Magazine.*

of melatonin inhibits the body's secretion of estrogen and decreases the proliferation of human breast cancer cells. Conversely, exposure to light during the night decreases melatonin production and increases cumulative lifetime estrogen levels, a sequence that may increase the risk of breast cancer.

In fact, 2 current studies show that women who work night shifts may increase their risk of breast cancer up to 60%. Blind women have a significantly lower risk (36% less) of breast cancer than normally sighted women because of consistently higher levels of melatonin.[324] Women, who are classed as only visually impaired, realize no protective effects in regard to breast cancer.

It appears that melatonin may also reduce the number of estrogen receptors on breast cancer cells. Since estrogen effectively feeds the growth of hormone-responsive breast tumors, reducing the receptors might slow tumor growth. *Science News* reported that the amount of melatonin required to inhibit breast cell proliferation appears no greater than the amount commonly present in human blood at night.[325,326]

Electromagnetic fields (EMFs) are another inhibitor of melatonin production. There is evidence that ELF (extremely low frequency) magnetic fields can act at the cellular levels to enhance breast cancer cell proliferation by blocking melatonin's natural oncostatic action. The mechanism(s) of action is unknown and may involve modulation of signal transduction events associated with melatonin's regulation of cell growth.[327]

Melatonin delivers another anticancer perk through its antioxidant values. Physicians who once credited glutathione and vitamin E as being antioxidants of choice have now given special honor to melatonin. The neurohormone appears to protect against tumors by shielding molecules (especially DNA) from oxidative stress. Melatonin exerts its antioxidant properties by detoxifying the highly reactive hydroxyl radical, as well as singlet oxygen, hydrogen peroxide, and peroxynitrite anions.[328]

A typical dose for a healthy individual is 300 mcg–6 mg each night. Cancer patients often take between 3–20 mg each night.

## Modified Citrus Pectin

Modified citrus pectin (MCP) retards cancer growth and metastasis. MCP, also known as fractionated pectin, is a complex polysaccharide obtained from the peel and pulp of citrus fruits. Through pH and temperature modifications, the pectin is broken down into shorter, nonbranched, galactose-rich, carbohydrate chains. The shorter chains dissolve more readily in water, making them better absorbed than ordinary, long-chain pectin. The short polysaccharide units afford MCP its ability to access and bind tightly to galactose-binding lectins (galectins) on the surface of certain types of cancers. By binding to lectins, MCP is able to powerfully address the threat of metastasis.[329]

In order for metastasis to occur, cancerous cells must first bind or clump together; galectin is thought responsible for much of cancer's metastatic potential by providing the binding site.[330–332] MCP appears small enough to access and bind tightly with galectins, inhibiting (or blocking) aggregation of tumor cells and adhesion to surrounding tissue.[333] Deprived of the capacity to adhere, cancer cells fail to metastasize.

Men with prostate cancer who took 15 g of MCP a day had a slowdown in the doubling time of their PSA levels. (Lengthening of doubling time represents a decrease in the rate of cancer growth.) Interestingly, rats injected with prostate adenocarcinoma and given MCP (in drinking water) showed a significant reduction in metastasis (compared to control animals), although the primary tumor was unaffected. According to Kenneth Pienta (leader of the Michigan Cancer Foundation), MCP may be the first oral method of preventing spontaneous prostate cancer metastasis.[331,332]

As with prostate adenocarcinoma, research shows that metastasis of breast cancer cell lines requires aggregation and adhesion of the cancerous cells to tissue endothelium in order for it to invade neighboring structures.[334] To test the antiadhesive properties of MCP, researchers evaluated (in an in vitro model) breast carcinoma cell lines MCF-7 and T-47D. The study concluded that MCP countered the adhesion of malignant cells to blood vessel endothelium and subsequently inhibited metastasis.[335] MCP decreased metastasis of melanoma to the lung by more than 90% in laboratory animals.[336]

Because MCP is a soluble fiber, no pattern of adverse reaction has been recorded in the scientific literature, apart from a self-limiting loose stool at high doses. MCP dosages are usually expressed in grams, with a typical adult dose ranging from 6–30 g divided throughout the day. MCP's apparent safety and proven antimetastatic action, and the lack of other proven therapies against metastasis, appear to justify its inclusion in a comprehensive orthomolecular anticancer regimen.[333] The dosage for MCP is about 15 g a day.

## N-Acetyl-Cysteine

N-acetyl-cysteine (NAC) is an anticarcinogenic and antimutagenic agent; it inhibits IL-6 as well as invasion and metastasis of malignant cells. NAC is the acetylated precursor of the amino acids L-cysteine and reduced glutathione. Historically, it is used as a mucolytic agent in respiratory illnesses as well as an antidote for acetaminophen hepatotoxicity, but more recently its credits have grown. Animal and human studies have shown it to be a powerful antioxidant and a potential therapeutic agent in the treatment of cancer.[337,338]

The biological value of NAC is attributed to its sulfhydryl group, while its acetyl-substituted amino group offers protection against oxidative and metabolic processes.[339,340] In vitro studies showed NAC to be directly antimutagenic and anticarcinogenic; in vivo, NAC inhibited mutagenicity of a number of mutagenic materials.[341,342]

NAC has both chemopreventive and therapeutic potential in malignancies arising in the lung, skin, breast, liver, head, and neck.[338,343] NAC is effective in inhibiting tumor cell growth in melanoma, prostate cells, and astrocytoma cell lines (the latter is a primary tumor in the brain).[344–346] Neovascularization (new blood vessel growth) is crucial for tumor mass expansion and metastasis. NAC inhibited invasion and

metastasis of malignant cells by up to 80% by preventing angiogenesis.[347]

A number of cancers express IL-6 and other potentially dangerous cytokines. NAC inhibited (in a dose-dependent manner) the synthesis of IL-6 by alveolar macrophage.[348,349]

Peak plasma levels of NAC occur approximately 1 hour after an oral dose; 12 hours after dosing, it is undetectable. Despite a relatively low bioavailability (4–10%), research has shown NAC to be clinically effective.[350] A suggested NAC therapeutic dosage is usually in the range of 600 mg per day.

## Panax Ginseng

Panax ginseng, also known as Korean ginseng, has been used in China for thousands of years as a popular remedy for various diseases including cancer.[351]

**Melanoma.** In a clinical trial, panax ginseng extract was shown to inhibit cell proliferation and induce apoptosis of melanoma cells in culture.[352] Panax ginseng extract also inhibited the formation of blood vessels to tumors in mice with melanoma, as well as inhibiting lung metastasis.[353,354] In another study of mice with melanoma, panax ginseng extract inhibited lung metastasis and improved survival.[352]

**Stomach cancer.** A study demonstrated the effects of panax ginseng in patients with stomach cancer. After surgery for stage 3 stomach cancer, patients received chemotherapy with or without panax ginseng. The 5-year survival rate was 76.4% in the panax ginseng group compared to 38.5% for the control group.[355]

**Colon cancer.** Panax ginseng extract induced apoptosis in colon cancer cells[356] and inhibited metastasis in rats and mice with colon cancer.[357,358]

**Leukemia.** Researchers observed that panax ginseng extract suppressed growth in human promyelocytic leukemia cells by inducing apoptosis.[359,360] Also, the ability of vitamin D to induce differentiation (ie, the process by which cancer cells transform into cells that appear to be normal to a greater degree, and therefore less aggressive) of leukemic cells was enhanced by panax ginseng.[361]

**Ovarian cancer.** In a study, panax ginseng extract increased survival in mice with ovarian cancer.[362] Similar findings were observed when panax ginseng was combined with the chemotherapy drug cisplatin; panax ginseng increased survival to a greater extent than the group receiving cisplatin alone.[363]

**Radiation therapy.** Laboratory studies have demonstrated the ability of ginseng to reduce damage caused by radiation on healthy cells.[364,365] In an experiment with mice exposed to radiation, panax ginseng offered protection against radiation-induced toxicity.[366] In another study, panax ginseng extract administered to mice exposed to radiation increased the number of bone marrow and spleen cells.[367]

**Chemotherapy.** Cancers can develop resistance to chemotherapy drugs. Multidrug resistance, the principal mechanism by which many cancers develop resistance to chemotherapy drugs, is a major factor in the failure of many forms of chemotherapy.[368] P-glycoprotein—expressed within cancer cells—confers multidrug resistance by transporting chemotherapy drugs out of cancer cells. Researchers observed that panax ginseng extract reversed P-glycoprotein-induced multidrug resistance, which resulted in increased accumulation of chemotherapy drugs within cancer cells.[369] Also, panax ginseng extract enhanced the anticancer effects of the chemotherapy drug mitomycin C in stomach cancer cells[370] and potentiated the antitumor effects of the chemotherapy drug cisplatin in mice with ovarian cancer.[363]

## Pomegranate

Pomegranate, which is rich in antioxidants, has gained widespread popularity as a functional food (ie, has health benefits). The health benefits of the fruit, juice(s), and extract(s) have been studied in relation to a variety of chronic diseases, including cancer.[371,372]

**Prostate cancer.** Pomegranate and its extracts suppress virtually every phase of prostate cancer development.[373] Pomegranate extracts powerfully suppressed proliferation, growth, invasion, and blood vessel formation of *human prostate cancer cells* in test tube studies as well as when implanted in experimental animals.[374–377] Pomegranate juice also helps stimulate cancer cells to undergo apoptosis.[378–380] Dramatic *synergistic effects* were discovered by Israeli researchers, who found that extracts from various parts of the whole fruit acted in concert to block prostate invasion.[381]

Pomegranate seed oil sharply inhibits proliferation of a number of human prostate cancer lines through changes in the cell growth cycle, inducing apoptosis, and suppressing cancer cell invasion.[374] Pomegranate oil also acts in synergy with other pomegranate components, suppressing prostate cancer proliferation and metastatic potential more effectively than each component alone.[381]

Related research has demonstrated that by modulating gene expression, pomegranate downregulated production of androgens (male hormones) and the androgen receptors that many prostate cancers need

to survive and grow.[382] In fact, scientists have found that pomegranate is effective at inhibiting both androgen-dependent *and* androgen-independent cancers of the prostate.[383]

In a landmark clinical trial,[384] researchers studied men who had already undergone surgery or radiation treatment for prostate cancer, but nevertheless had rising levels of prostate-specific antigen (PSA), the serum marker of tumor growth or reoccurrence. Men drank 8 oz of pomegranate juice daily, and the researchers measured the time it took for their PSA levels to double. The longer the doubling time, the more slowly the disease was progressing. The average PSA doubling time increased dramatically and significantly with pomegranate supplementation, rising from 15 months at baseline to 54 months. In other words, the PSA doubling time was less one and a half years before supplementation and four and a half years after supplementation.

In a similar study conducted at the Prostate Cancer Research Program at Johns Hopkins, men with a rising PSA after their initial treatment for prostate cancer received a pomegranate extract for up to 18 months.[385] Results showed that the median PSA doubling time increased from 11.9 months at baseline to 18.5 months after treatment. PSA doubling time increases of over 100% from baseline were also observed in 43% of patients.

**Breast cancer.** Researchers discovered that consumption of whole pomegranate seed oil and juice concentrate[386] resulted in dramatic growth inhibition of estrogen-dependent breast cancer cells. The same study showed inhibition of tumor formation in rodent cells exposed to known breast carcinogens. Using different methods, another research group found a 42% reduction in tumor formation with whole pomegranate juice polyphenols and an 87% reduction with pomegranate seed oil.[387]

Pomegranate seed oil is a potent inhibitor of aromatase, the enzyme that converts testosterone into estrogen.[388] This enzymatic *blockade* contributes to pomegranate seed oil's ability to inhibit growth of estrogen-dependent breast cancer cells. Pomegranate extract has also been shown to enhance the effects of the estrogen blocking drug tamoxifen, with the authors of a study stating that "pomegranate combined with tamoxifen may represent a novel and a powerful approach to enhance and sensitize tamoxifen action."[389] Pomegranate also increases apoptosis, even in cancer cells that lack estrogen receptors.[386]

Cancer cells need to grow new blood vessels to support their rapid growth and tissue invasion (angiogenesis). They typically do this by ramping up production of a variety of growth factors, including VEGF and inflammatory interleukins. Pomegranate seed oil powerfully inhibits production of VEGF while upregulating production of migratory inhibitory factor (MIF) in breast cancer cells. In a laboratory model of vessel growth, these modulations translated into a significant decrease in new blood vessel formation.[390] Pomegranate seed oil's capacity to block breast cancer development was also demonstrated in an organ culture model of mouse breast cancer.[387] Treating the glands with pomegranate seed oil prior to exposure to a powerful carcinogen resulted in a 87% reduction in the number of cancerous lesions compared with controls.

Pomegranate seed oil contains a number of unique chemical constituents with potent biological effects. Punicic acid, an omega-5 polyunsaturated fatty acid that inhibits both estrogen-dependent and estrogen-independent breast cancer cell proliferation in lab cultures,[391] also induced apoptosis at rates up to 91% higher than those in untreated cell cultures—effects which appear to be related to fundamental regulation of cancer cell signaling pathways.[391]

**Colon cancer.** Pomegranate seed oil has been shown to *suppress experimentally induced colon cancer* in laboratory rats.[392] Inflammation is a powerful trigger for colon cancers, and pomegranate extract directly suppresses inflammatory cell signaling in colon cancer cells via several mechanisms involving modulation of gene expression.[393] Ellagic acid, produced in the colon from ellagitannins in pomegranate juice, induces apoptosis in colon cancer cells.[394]

**Lung cancer.** Pomegranate extract provides significant protection against experimentally induced lung cancer. Researchers observed that 8 months of pomegranate supplementation reduced lung tumor formation by 66% in mice exposed to lung carcinogens.[395] Another study found that pomegranate fruit extract inhibited the formation of tumor growth in mice implanted with lung cancer cells, leading the authors to conclude that "pomegranate fruit extract can be a useful chemopreventive/chemotherapeutic agent against human lung cancer."[396]

## Proteolytic Enzymes

Proteolytic enzymes are comprised of a group of enzymes that break down, or digest proteins. Papain, trypsin, and chymotrypsin are proteolytic enzymes that have commonly been used in cancer studies.

**Radiation therapy.** Several studies have demonstrated the ability of proteolytic enzymes to decrease the side effects of radiation therapy. In one clinical trial, 100 individuals with head and neck cancer received radiation therapy with or without proteolytic enzymes. Proteolytic enzymes reduced the severity of acute side effects from radiation therapy. Also, the proteolytic enzyme group experienced a 41% reduction in mucositis (a painful inflammation and ulceration of the mucous membranes caused by radiation), 50% reduction in skin reactions, and 36% reduction in difficulty swallowing.[397] Commenting on the effects of proteolytic enzymes, the authors stated, "There was significant protection against acute side effects of radiation therapy in the study arm. Not only was the severity of acute side effects less but the duration was shorter and the time to onset was also delayed."

Another study of head and neck cancer patients compared radiation therapy plus proteolytic enzymes (consisting of trypsin, papain, and chymotrypsin) to radiation therapy alone (control group). While mucositis and skin reactions were present in almost all patients in both groups, the severity of these symptoms were substantially lower in the proteolytic enzyme group. With regard to mucositis, 76% of the proteolytic enzyme group experienced the mildest form compared to 8% of the control group. Also, 72% of the proteolytic enzyme group experienced the mildest form of skin reactions compared to 12% of the control group.[398]

A group of patients with uterine or cervical cancer received radiation therapy with or without proteolytic enzymes (consisting of papain, trypsin, and chymotrypsin). The proteolytic enzyme group experienced a reduction in skin reactions (42%), vaginal mucosal reactions (35%), and genitourinary symptoms (33%).[399]

**Multiple myeloma.** Researchers observed that proteolytic enzymes taken for greater than 6 months decreased the risk of death in patients with multiple myeloma by 60%. Median survival of stage 3 patients was 83 months for the proteolytic enzyme group compared to 47 months for the control group.[400]

Proteolytic enzymes were also found to offer substantial improvements to women with lymphedema after breast cancer surgery.[401,402]

## Protein-Bound Polysaccharide K (PSK)

PSK, which is a specially prepared polysaccharide extract from the mushroom *Coriolus versicolor*, has been studied extensively in Japan where it is used as a nonspecific biological response modifier to enhance the immune system in cancer patients.[403–405] PSK suppresses tumor cell invasiveness by downregulating several invasion-related factors.[406] PSK has been shown to enhance NK cell activity in multiple studies.[407–410]

**Stomach cancer.** Several studies have investigated the use of PSK with stomach cancer. In one study, stomach cancer patients received postoperative PSK with or without chemotherapy. The 5-year survival was 73% in the PSK group compared to 60% in chemotherapy alone group.[411] In a similar trial, the 5-year survival rate for postoperative stomach cancer patients was 71.7% for the group receiving chemotherapy plus PSK compared to 58.5% for the group receiving chemotherapy alone.[412]

In a study comparing the use of chemotherapy with or without PSK in stage 3 stomach cancer patients, subjects received 3 g daily of PSK (treatment group) for at least 1 year after surgery. A dramatic difference in survival was noted between the 2 groups, with a 3-year overall survival of 62.2% in the treatment compared to only 12.5% in the chemotherapy alone group.[413]

**Lung cancer.** In another clinical trial, individuals with stages 1–3 lung cancer received radiation therapy with or without PSK. Researchers observed that the 5-year survival was 39% in the PSK group compared to 17% in the control (stages 1 and 2) and 26% in the PSK group compared to 8% in the control (stage 3).[414] Similar results were obtained by these same researchers in a previous study.[415]

**Colon cancer.** A group of colon cancer patients were randomized to receive chemotherapy with or without PSK. After 2 years of supplementation, the PSK group had a 10-year survival of 81.9% compared to 50.6% without PSK.[416] In a similar trial, colon cancer patients received chemotherapy alone or combined with PSK (3 g daily) for 2 years. The 5-year survival for stage 3 colon cancer patients receiving PSK was 75% compared to 46% in the group receiving chemotherapy alone.[417]

PSK was also shown to improve survival in colorectal cancer patients over age 70. After surgery, individuals were given chemotherapy plus PSK or chemotherapy alone. The 3-year survival rate was 80.8% in the PSK group and 52.8% in the group that did not receive PSK.[418]

**Breast cancer.** In a study investigating the use of PSK in women with stage 2 breast cancer, postoperative participants received tamoxifen with PSK (3 g daily) or tamoxifen alone. The 5-year survival was 89.9% in the PSK group compared to 86.9% in the group receiving tamoxifen only.[419]

**Uterine/cervical cancer.** In a clinical trial that evaluated the effects of PSK in individuals with uterine or cervical cancer, study participants received postradiation therapy PSK (3 g daily) for 2 weeks per month. The 5-year survival in those with stage 3B cancer who received PSK was 65% compared to 49% in those not receiving PSK.[420]

**Leukemia.** The coriolus mushroom has demonstrated antileukemic effects. In one study, coriolus suppressed the proliferation of leukemic cells by greater than 90%.[421] Other studies have confirmed these findings with the mechanism of action mediated via apoptosis.[422,423]

**Chemotherapy.** PSK has been shown to provide protection against chemotherapy toxicity. Peripheral neuropathy (ie, nerve damage often occurring in the hands and feet) is a common side effect experienced by colon cancer patients receiving the chemotherapy drugs oxaliplatin, leucovorin, and 5-fluorouracil. Researchers observed grade 2 or grade 3 peripheral neuropathies in only 4% of colon cancer patients receiving these chemotherapy drug with PSK,[424] which is in stark contrast to a 38.4% incidence in those receiving the chemotherapy drugs without PSK.[425]

## Pterostilbene

Pterostilbene, a polyphenol found in blueberries, grapes, and in the bark of the Indian Kino Tree, is closely related to resveratrol (but with unique attributes). Pterostilbene's mechanisms of action include blocking enzymes that activate carcinogens,[426,427] inducing apoptosis,[428] cell cycle arrest,[429] and enhancing NO-induced cell death.[430]

It has been observed that pterostilbene suppresses formation of precancerous cells in the colons of carcinogen-exposed animals.[79] In a 2010 study, researchers investigated the effects of pterostilbene in rats exposed to a potent carcinogen. They observed that the incidence of colon cancer was 67.8% in the group of rats fed pterostilbene versus 87.5% in the control group. Moreover, the number of tumors per rat was 66% lower in the pterostilbene group compared to the control group.[431]

Researchers also observed that pterostilbene markedly inhibited the growth of breast cancer cells in the laboratory by inducing apoptosis and cell cycle arrest.[429] In addition, pterostilbene inhibited the growth of melanoma, lung cancer, and pancreatic cancer cell lines,[432–434] and prevented the metastasis of melanoma cells to the liver in laboratory animals.[434]

## Quercetin

Quercetin is a flavonoid found in a broad range of foods, from grape skins and red onions to green tea and tomatoes. Strong evidence from epidemiologic studies demonstrates that people with the highest quercetin intake have substantially reduced risks for many of the leading causes of cancer death, including:

- **Lung cancer.** The top cause of cancer deaths, a 51% overall risk reduction, and a 65% reduction among smokers.[435]

- **Colon cancer.** The second top cause of cancer deaths, a 32% reduction in risk.[436]

- **Stomach cancer.** A 43% overall risk reduction and an 80% reduction in risk among female smokers.[437]

Quercetin's antioxidant and anti-inflammatory properties protect cellular DNA from cancer-inducing mutations.[438] Quercetin traps developing cancer cells in the early phases of their replicative cycle, effectively preventing further malignant development and promoting cancer cell death.[439] Furthermore, quercetin favorably modulates chemical signaling pathways that are abnormal in cancer cells.[440,441]

A clinical trial of quercetin in patients with various cancer types demonstrated a decrease in activity of enzymes required for tumor growth in 9 of 11 patients studied.[442] Two patients with advanced cancers that failed to respond to standard chemotherapy experienced significant drops in chemical tumor markers during the study.

**Colon cancer.** Colon cancer involves chronic inflammation in the intestinal tract. It has been observed that quercetin reduces the amount of fat oxidation and inflammation of the intestine in animal studies,[443,444] which reduces the incidence of tumors in lab animals as well as tumor size and the number of tumors per animal.[445] Quercetin also decreases the number and size of precancerous lesions called "aberrant crypt foci."[446]

In 2006, scientists studied patients suffering from familial adenomatous polyposis, a hereditary condition in which hundreds of premalignant polyps develop and eventually turn malignant. All patients treated with curcumin and quercetin experienced a decrease in polyp number (60.4%) and size (50.9%) after 6 months of supplementation.[447]

**Lung cancer.** Quercetin inhibits the growth of lung cancer cells.[439,448] In one experiment, laboratory rats were treated with quercetin (25 mg/kg body weight) before exposure to benzo(a)pyrene, a powerful environmental carcinogen found in cigarette smoke, charbroiled foods, and automobile (particularly diesel) exhaust, making it among the most common pollutants in the environment. While untreated rats developed lung cancers, those supplemented first with quercetin showed no such findings.[449]

**Liver cancer.** The liver is the prime organ responsible for receiving and detoxifying the bulk of environmental toxins it is exposed to daily. As a result, liver cells are at the epicenter of toxin-induced cancer development. Studies show that quercetin increases the production of protective proteins and enzymes in liver cells, blocks the cancer replicative cell cycle, and reduces toxin-induced DNA mutations.[450,451]

**Prostate cancer.** Quercetin blocks the androgen receptors used to sustain growth by prostate cancer cells.[452] Researchers noted that quercetin inhibited the growth of highly aggressive prostate cancer cells by 69%, with a concomitant greater than 50% upregulation of tumor-suppressor genes and a 61–100% downregulation of cancer-promoting oncogenes.[453] Quercetin also inhibits the migration and invasiveness of prostate cancer cells.[454]

**Breast cancer.** In breast cancer cells, quercetin induces apoptosis and cell cycle arrest.[455,456] Querctin inhibited the growth of tumors[457] and prolonged survival of mice with breast cancer.[458]

**Chemotherapy.** Quercetin potentiates the anticancer activity of the chemotherapy drug Adriamycin® against breast cancer cells[458–460] by increasing concentrations of Adriamycin® within cancer cells.[461] In mice with breast cancer, combining quercetin with Adriamycin® led to long-term, tumor-free survival, whereas mice failed to be cured when treated with Adriamycin® alone.[462] Interestingly—when given together with quercetin—Adriamycin® inflicted substantial DNA damage to cancer cells. However, normal cells were protected against the DNA damaging effects of Adriamcyin®.[460] This effect cannot be understated, as the main problem associated with the use of chemotherapy is that it inflicts damage to normal cells as well as cancer cells.

Quercetin enhances the anticancer activity of the chemotherapy drug cisplatin.[463] The concomitant administration of quercetin and cisplatin reduced tumor growth to a significantly greater degree than cisplatin alone in mice with lung cancer.[464]

## Reishi

The active constituents of reishi mushroom include polysaccharides, a unique protein named LZ-8, and triterpenes.[465–467] Among its broad-spectrum immune-boosting effects are the following:

- Reishi promotes specialization of dendritic cells and macrophages, which are essential in allowing the body to react to new threats, vaccines, and cancer cells.[468–472]

- Reishi's effects on dendritic cells have been proven to boost the response to tetanus vaccine; the mushroom's proteins are also under investigation as "adjuvants" to emerging cancer DNA vaccines and other immune-based cancer treatments.[469,473–475]

- Reishi polysaccharide triggers growth and development of bone marrow, where most immune cells are born; following bone marrow eradication by chemotherapy, reishi increased production of both red and white blood cells.[476]

- Reishi increases numbers and functions of virtually all cell lines in the immune system, such as natural killer cells, antibody-producing B cells, and the T cells responsible for rapid response to a new or "remembered" antigen.[470,477,478]

Laboratory and animal studies confirm that reishi stimulates an appropriate anticancer immune response while quashing a cancer-promoting inflammatory one. A few small human studies have demonstrated reishi's ability to enhance immune function in patients with advanced cancers.[479–481]

Reishi polysaccharides provide immune-boosting function to circulating cancer-killing white blood cells of various types.[466] They also fight new blood vessel development required by solid tumors to support their rapid growth and expansion.[466]

Triterpenes from reishi provide important anti-inflammatory effects that both reduce the likelihood of a new cancer forming and take away the inflammatory stimuli that promote early cancer development.[482]

These mechanisms, combined with their unique antioxidant characteristics, allow reishi mushrooms to fight many different types of cancers, most notably those of the gastrointestinal tract (liver and colon) and reproductive system (breast and prostate).[482–490]

Reishi extracts have also proven useful in inducing cell death in various "white blood cell cancers" such as lymphoma, leukemia, and multiple myeloma.[491] In each of these cancer types, reishi mushroom extracts have been shown to prevent new tumors from arising, and in many cases to shrink existing tumors or precancerous masses.[492–495] These effects, because they may stop a tumor in its tracks before it ever reaches a detectable or dangerous size, can be considered successful cancer prevention by immunosurveillance.[492,493]

## Resveratrol

Resveratrol influences cancer at initiation, promotion, and progression stages. Resveratrol is one of a group of compounds (called phytoalexins) that are produced in plants during times of environmental stress, such as adverse weather or insect, animal, or pathogenic

attack. Resveratrol has been identified in more than 70 species of plants, including mulberries and peanuts, and the skins of red grapes, which are a particularly rich source.[496] According to Pezzuto, "Of all the plants we've tested for cancer chemopreventive activity, this one [resveratrol] has the greatest promise."[497]

Resveratrol was effective against cancer during all 3 phases of the cancer process: initiation, promotion, and progression. For example, resveratrol displayed antimutagenic and antioxidant activity, providing greater protection against DNA damage than vitamins C, E, or beta-carotene. Resveratrol restored glutathione levels, considered by some as the most essential of antioxidants.[496] It increased levels of a phase 2 detoxifying enzyme (quinone reductase), an enzyme responsible for metabolically disassembling carcinogens.

Resveratrol inhibited the activity of cyclooxygenase-2 (COX-2), reducing the inflammatory response in human epithelial cells.[498] Upregulation of COX-2 is associated with the physical manifestations of various human cancers, as well as other inflammatory disorders. Since inflammation is closely linked to tumor promotion, substances with potent anti-inflammatory activities are thought to exert chemopreventive effects, particularly in the promotion stage of the disease.

Resveratrol prompted differentiation of human promyelocytic leukemia cells. The development of preneoplastic lesions in mouse mammary glands was inhibited by resveratrol.[499–501]

The following studies illustrate the many pathways resveratrol employs to inhibit cancer:

- Italian researchers recently determined that resveratrol exhibited a protective role against colon carcinogenesis, with the defense attributed to changes occurring in Bax protein, which encourages apoptosis, and p21 expression.[502] Reduced Bax activity is associated with resistance to cytotoxic therapy.[503] p21 is able to arrest the cell cycle at the G1 phase by inhibiting DNA replication.[504] Suppressing the growth cycle allows for a critical phase in cellular development referred to as differentiation, that is, an abnormal cell becomes more normal.

- Resveratrol appears a promising anticancer agent for both hormone-dependent and hormone-independent breast cancers. At high concentrations, resveratrol caused suppression of cell growth in 3 breast cancer cell lines: estrogen-receptor (ER)-positive KPL-1 and MCF-7 and ER-negative MKL-F. Growth inhibition was credited in part to upregulation of Bax protein and activation of caspase-3 (a key mediator of apoptosis in mammalian cells).

Resveratrol was also able to lessen the growth stimulatory effects of linoleic acid, a fatty acid frequently overconsumed in Western diets.[505]

- Resveratrol significantly reduced tumor volume (42%), tumor weight (44%), and metastasis (56%) in mice with highly metastatic Lewis lung carcinoma. Resveratrol was able to inhibit angiogenesis and reduce oxidative stress.[506,507]

- Wine polyphenols (catechin, epicatechin, quercetin) including resveratrol may be effective against prostate cancer. Prostate cancer cell lines (LNCaP and DU145) produce high concentrations of NO; PC3 produces low concentrations. Researchers propose that the antiproliferative effects of polyphenols are due to their ability to adjust NO production.[508] Grape extract, a rich source of resveratrol, inhibited prostate cancer growth up to 98% in a dose- and time-dependent manner.[509]

- Resveratrol appears to be promising in the control of acute monocytic leukemia.[510] Resveratrol induced apoptotic cell death in human leukemia cells (HL60)[511] and stopped the growth of lymphocytic leukemia cells during the S-phase of the growth cycle (the time of DNA replication).[512]

- Resveratrol inhibits NF-κB, thus inhibiting cell proliferation and cytokine production.[513] The inhibition of cytokine production by resveratrol was found to be irreversible.

If using pure resveratrol, the suggested dosage is 7–50 mg a day. Beware of diluted supplements that provide very little active resveratrol. At the time of this writing, there were only a few sources of pure high-potency resveratrol available as dietary supplements.

## Selenium

Selenium is protective against many types of cancers, promotes apoptosis, is a powerful antioxidant, and improves quality of life during aggressive cancer therapies. Many animal studies have been conducted to evaluate the effects of super nutritional levels of selenium on experimental carcinogenesis using chemical, viral, and transplantable tumor models. Two-thirds of these studies found that high levels of selenium reduced the development of tumors at least moderately (14–35% compared to controls) and, in most cases, significantly (by >35%).[514]

The impact of selenium supplementation on basal cell carcinoma was studied on 1312 subjects (18–80 years of age, 75% of whom were men).[515] Within 6–9 months, the group receiving 200 mcg a day of selenium realized about a 67% increase in plasma selenium levels. The nonsupplemented group, although judged "normal" in regard to plasma selenium levels, experienced twice the rate of cancer as those receiving selenium. Researchers concluded that higher amounts of dietary selenium than the amount recommended by the FDA are needed to prevent cancer.

Although the study failed to show the effectiveness of selenium in altering the course of either basal or squamous cell carcinoma, selenium impacted the incidence of other types of malignancies with amazing success. The overall reduction in cancer incidence was 37% in the selenium-supplemented group; a 50% reduction in cancer mortality was observed over a 10-year period.[515]

The following are the site-specific reductions in cancer incidence observed in the study: colorectal cancers (58%), lung cancer (46%), and prostate cancer (63%). A selenium deficiency appears to increase the risk of prostate cancer four- to five-fold. It was determined that as the male population ages, selenium levels decrease, paralleling an increase in prostate cancer.[516]

The data are compelling regarding the usefulness of selenium's protective effects against cancer:

- Selenium-enriched broccoli is protective against chemically induced mammary and colon cancer in rats.[517]

**Note:** *While selenium is contributing to the lower incidence of malignancy, the anticancer effects of broccoli should also be factored into the defense. Read the section in this protocol titled "What should cancer patients eat?" for valuable information regarding dietary factors affecting patient outcome.*

- The relationship between serum levels of selenium and the development of upper digestive tract cancer was examined.[518] The relative risk of esophageal cancer was 0.56 in individuals in the highest quartile of selenium level compared with those in the lowest quartile. The corresponding relative risk of gastric cardia cancer was 0.47. Based on the data, it was concluded that 26.4% of esophageal and gastric cardia cancers are attributable to low selenium levels.

- Adding selenium to salt resulted in a significant reduction in the incidence of cancer.[514]

- A significant increase in apoptosis and a decrease in DNA synthesis in breast cancers cells (MCF-7 and SKBR-3) occurred with selenium supplementation.

The selenium benefit was just as impressive in cancers of the lung (RH2), small intestine (HCF8), colon (Caco-2), and liver (HepG2). Prostate cancers (PC-3 and LNCaP) as well as colon cancer (T-84), although initially less affected by supplementation, became responsive when selenium was coadministered with Adriamycin® or Taxol®.[519] This study suggests that selenium potentiates the anticancer effects of chemotherapy. Selenium supplementation in patients undergoing radiation therapy for rectal cancer improved quality of life and reduced the appearance of secondary cancers.[520]

- It appears that selenium acts as an immunologic response modifier, normalizing every component of the immune system.[521,522]

A suggested selenium dosage is 200 mcg a day. The optimal dose for cancer patients is unknown at this time, but suggestions have ranged from 200–400 mcg a day depending on the selenium content of the soil. Foods considered good sources of selenium include Brazil nuts, grains, onions, tomatoes, broccoli, chicken, eggs, garlic, liver, seafood, and wheat germ. Americans typically consume 60–100 mcg of selenium a day from dietary sources.

## Silibinin

Silibinin (from milk thistle) has antioxidant activity, increases sensitivity to chemotherapy while reducing its side effects, assists in arresting the growth of cancer, promotes differentiation, inhibits COX-2 enzyme, and suppresses NF-κB. Fourteen years ago, Life Extension introduced silymarin, a hepatoprotective herb, to members. The major active constituent of silymarin is silibinin, a long-recognized antioxidant with more recently ascribed anticarcinogenic traits. Silibinin inhibits the growth of various cancer cell lines and acts synergistically with cisplatin and doxorubicin, common chemotherapeutic drugs, improving their efficacy. By arresting tumor cell division at a strategic stage, silibinin appears to make tumor cells more sensitive to chemotherapy. Also, the harsh side effects associated with cytotoxic chemicals are less damaging when silibinin is utilized.[523]

Milk thistle is described as an adaptogenic herb. For example, it encourages new cell growth where repair is needed but arrests cell division in tumor tissue; it increases the activity of certain enzymes but inhibits others. Milk thistle inhibits COX-2.[524]

*Note: See the section in this protocol titled "Cyclooxygenase-2 (COX-2) Inhibitors (Naturally Occurring)" for other nutraceuticals capable of*

*inhibiting the COX-2 enzyme. Also, refer to the section on Cyclooxygenase Inhibitors in the protocol titled Cancer Treatment: The Critical Factors to learn more about the connection between COX-2 and cancer.*

Silibinin arrests cell growth in the early phase of the cycle known as G1, a period of growth before DNA replication. Silibinin discourages cell growth by inhibiting various kinase enzymes (those playing a pivotal role in regulatory mechanisms), enabling a critical stage in cellular development referred to as differentiation. Differentiated cells abandon their primitive façade and assume the physical likeness and behavioral patterns of healthy cells. In fact, silibinin caused differentiation of a significant number of malignant prostate cells to more normal cells, while simultaneously decreasing PSA levels.[525]

Silibinin inhibits growth of drug-resistant breast and ovarian cancer lines. It binds to type 2 estrogen–binding sites, an action that turns off the proliferative effects of the cell.[526] In addition, silymarin inhibited the secretion of VEGF (an angiogenic factor) by malignant cells, thwarting the formation of cancer's vascular network.[527]

Silymarin potently suppressed NF-κB, but did not affect TNF-α-induced NF-κB, demonstrating a pathway-dependent inhibition by silymarin. It appears the inhibitory effect of silymarin on NF-κB activation is associated with its liver-protecting properties. Suppression of NF-κB, a key regulator in inflammatory and immune reactions, significantly improves the anticarcinogenic status of silymarin.[528]

Silymarin/silibinin is remarkable medicine for the liver. Numerous studies show that milk thistle is effective in treating virtually every type of liver disease, including cirrhosis and alcohol or chemical-induced liver damage.[529,530] So worthy is the herb in protecting against life-threatening toxins that individuals poisoned by the Amanita mushroom survived when silibinin was utilized.[531] A healthy liver is essential to detoxification, a process key to restoring health to cancer patients.

Standardized milk thistle extract usually consists of 35% silibinin, whereas the silymarin concentrate used in Europe contains a minimum of 80% silibinin. Life Extension suggests the highly beneficial 80% silibinin extract.

## Soy

Soy is protective against certain malignancies, appears to be an alternative to signal transduction–inhibiting drugs, and inhibits angiogenesis, cell proliferation, and metastasis.

Legumes, including the soybean, contain bioactive compounds classified broadly as phytoestrogens as opposed to estrogens. Phytoestrogens are nonsteroidal and can actually inhibit steroids such as aromatase. Most have little or no estrogenic activity. When others have such activity, it is usually beneficial and specific to a certain tissue. For example, some soy isoflavones (a type of phytoestrogen) benefit bone but do not affect the kidney. In pharmacology terms, this is called a selective estrogen receptor modulator (SERM). A compound in soy, genistein, is a natural SERM. Tamoxifen and raloxifene are chemical SERMs.[532]

Studies suggest that the reason different estrogens have different effects on different tissues is because there is more than one type of estrogen receptor. So far, 3 variations of the estrogen receptor have been found: one alpha and two betas. They share similar estrogen structure. The estrogen receptor-beta (ERb) may suppress the action of the estrogen receptor-alpha (ERa)—at least in cancer cells.[533–535] Also, growth-promoting estrogens such as estradiol activate ERa. Phytoestrogens preferentially activate the ERb, which is repressive.[536] For this reason, phytoestrogens have been characterized as good estrogens, and whatever estrogenic effect they have (which is estimated to be 1000–10000 times weaker than estradiol, where it exists) may be nullified by their inhibition of estrogen synthesis and repression of the receptor that allows estradiol into the cell.[537]

In normal tissue, the 2 estrogen receptors apparently work together to control both the amount and the use of estrogen in the body. It has been demonstrated that some types of cancer cells lose one type of estrogen receptor, leaving the control mechanism inoperable.[538,539] This has been demonstrated in prostate cancer. Some types of prostate cancers do not express their ERa and some lose beta. This is why some will respond to estrogen and stop growing and others will stop growing when an antiestrogen, such as genistein or tamoxifen is added.

The loss or gain of estrogen receptors occurs because of methylation abnormalities that occur in DNA.[540] DNA methylation abnormalities are caused by 3 known factors: poor diet (ie, a diet lacking in methylation factors including folate and vitamins B6 and B12), chemicals, and age.

Phytoestrogens include many diverse plant compounds, including resveratrol from grapes,[541] curcumin from roots,[542] and polyphenols from tea leaves.[543] It is a very broad category that is further broken down into dozens of classifications such as flavonoids and flavones. The anticancer effects of phytoestrogens are the subject of dozens of scientific studies.[544]

**Soy isoflavones.** Soy contains phytoestrogens known as isoflavones, including daidzein, coumestrol, and genistein. Isoflavone supplements contain a mixture of many different types of these compounds. Interest in their anticancer potential stems from the lower occurrence of hormone-related cancers in Asians who eat a lot of soy. It is doubtful that the low rates of breast, prostate, and other hormonally related cancers are due solely to soy, but studies show that compounds isolated from soy have significant anticancer effects.[545]

**Prostate cancer.** The most dangerous aspect of prostate cancer is metastasis (spreading to other areas). Prostate cancer can be controlled if it can be limited to the prostate gland. Unfortunately, many men with prostate cancer have undetected metastases.

Genistein has powerful and specific effects against the spread of prostate cancer. Genistein significantly activated 832 genes in prostate cancer cells, 13 of which are related to metastasis.[546–548]

Genistein downregulated multiple genes that dissolve surrounding tissue to enable metastasis and invasion of surrounding tissue, and downregulated genes that create new tumor blood vessels. Genistein also affected genes important in stopping the cell cycle, differentiation, apoptosis, and cell signaling communication.[546]

Genistein has "potent antiproliferative effects" against human prostate cells[549] and inhibits metastasis.[550] Genistein is one component of soy. Soy has powerful effects in the prevention and eradication of prostate cancer. Diverse components of soy have different effects against prostate cancer cells. Genistein blocks an enzyme that destroys an anticancer vitamin D metabolite in cancer cells.[551]

Prostate cancer is a hormone-related cancer. In a study mice were fed 3 different soy products: soy protein without isoflavones, soy phytochemical concentrate (a combination of genistein, daidzein, glycitein, and other compounds), and genistein. All 3 feeds had a positive effect on hormones as they relate to prostate cancer growth. The androgen receptor, which correlates with tumor weight, was reduced 42% by soy protein. Genistein reduced serum dihydrotestosterone, a form of testosterone associated with hyperplasia and cancer, and caused a 57% reduction in tumor growth. Soy phytochemical concentrate inhibited the overall growth of prostate cancer by 70%. Soy phytochemical concentrate also stopped metastases to lymph nodes and lung. Cell death was induced, and angiogenesis was significantly inhibited.[552]

Healthy, normal rodents fed genistein for 2 weeks at a dietary level had significant reductions in androgen and the 2 estrogen receptors.[553] Minimizing the number of hormone receptors reduces levels of cell growth-promoting hormones in the prostate gland. The levels of phytoestrogens in 25 men with and without benign prostatic hyperplasia (BPH), a noncancerous overgrowth of prostate cells, were examined. Genistein levels in men with BPH were significantly lower than in those without BPH.[554] Adding genistein to prostate tissue taken from men with BPH stops the prostate cancer growth.[555]

Various soy diets have significant effects against prostate cancer compared to a casein (milk protein) diet. Soy significantly reduced insulin-like growth factor (IGF-1), a protein that helps tumors create blood vessels. Blood vessel density and tumor cell proliferation were decreased. Cell death was increased. Dietary soy works through "a combination of direct effects on tumor cells and indirect effects on tumor neovasculature" (blood vessels).[556] The cell-killing effects of soy components are important not only for men who have been diagnosed with prostate cancer, but for healthy men as well.

Prostate-specific antigen (PSA) is elevated in men with prostate enlargement. PSA is regulated by androgens. Genistein and its precursor, biochanin A, markedly decrease PSA in prostate cancer cells by inactivating testosterone.[557] A study of rats showed a 38% decline in PSA, along with a significant reduction in metastases when genistein was given subcutaneously.[550,558]

The ability of genistein to reduce cellular proliferation in men with elevated PSA is currently under investigation. In addition, the ability of supplemental soy to lower PSA and kill cancer cells in men with localized prostate cancer is being studied. The ability of soy isoflavones to modulate hormones and cancer-related proteins in men with prostate cancer is also being studied.

Population-based studies have shown that men with high levels of soy and other isoflavones in their blood have the lowest risk of prostate cancer. In a study on men from Japan, China, and the United States, it was shown that legumes, including soy, reduce the incidence of prostate cancer by 38%. Eating yellow-orange vegetables reduces it 33%, and cruciferous vegetables reduce it 39%. These findings are consistent across ethnicities, indicating that isoflavones, not genes, are responsible for the reductions in risk.[559] An analysis of data collected from 12 395 Seventh-Day Adventist men indicates that more than one serving per day of soy milk can reduce the risk of prostate cancer 70%.[560]

**Note:** *Seventh-Day Adventists are vegetarians; meat is a known risk factor for prostate cancer.*

*Maintaining a vegetarian diet may have contributed to the low rates of prostate cancer.*

Genistein downregulates proteins that enhance prostate cancer growth, including HER2/neu. Genistein has no adverse toxicity, and the amount needed to reduce the proteins by half is achieved with supplemental genistein or a diet high in soy products. Genistein inhibits EGF signaling pathway suggesting that this phytoestrogen may be useful in both protecting against and treating prostate cancer.[561]

Soy isoflavones clearly work against prostate cancer through several mechanisms, including modulating hormones, blocking metastasis, interfering with cell signaling, stopping cell growth, inducing cell death, and possibly activating and deactivating cancer-related genes.

**Breast cancer.** Soy phytoestrogens help to prevent and control hormone-related breast cancer.[562,563] It is especially beneficial for Western women, who are exposed to a comparatively high level of environmental estrogens. Soy is antiestrogenic. It prevents the conversion of estrone to 17-beta-estradiol. Estrone fuels the growth of breast cancer, whereas estriol is a weaker estrogen. Genistein causes cancer cells to metabolize estradiol to estrogenically weaker or inactive metabolites.[564]

Soy phytoestrogens naturally activate the receptor, known as ERb, which in turn suppresses the activation of ERa and allows growth-promoting estradiol into cancer cells.[565] ERa is the receptor referred to as "estrogen receptor positive"; "estrogen-receptor-negative" breast cancer cells contain estrogen ERb. Estrogen-receptor-positive cells have lost their beta receptors during the events leading to breast cancer. Normal cells have both types of estrogen receptors.

Genistein naturally activates ERb, inhibiting cell proliferation. Activating the beta-receptor downregulates the alpha-receptor, or estradiol-activated, receptor. This negates estradiol's cancer-promoting effects.

The consumption of soy reduced the risk of having ERa-positive breast cancer by 56%, whereas the effect on both types of breast cancer was 30%.[566]

Genistein interferes with cancer's ability to grow blood vessels. A direct link between alpha-receptors and angiogenesis has been discovered in estrogen receptor positive cancer cells (MCF-7). These cells have too many alpha-receptors and not enough beta-receptors. When estradiol attaches to the alpha-receptors, it activates a protein that promotes the formation of new blood vessels.[539] Genistein blocks the formation of new blood vessels.[567,568] Furthermore, genistein prevents vitamin D from being degraded by cancer cells.[551]

In a study on estrogen receptor positive breast cancer cells (MCF-7), genistein competed successfully with estradiol for access to the cells, and once inside, blocked estradiol from inducing cell growth. In a study on Japanese women who drank soy milk containing 100 mg of isoflavones a day, estrone and estradiol levels fell by almost 30%.[569]

Breast cancer cells have elevated levels of enzymes that produce estradiol. One of the enzymes, known as 17-beta-hydroxysteroid dehydrogenase type 1 (17HSD1), causes the conversion of "weak estrogen" (estriol) to "strong estrogen" (estrone) and helps cancer cells grow. A variant known as 17HSD2 does the opposite. Breast cancer cells have elevated amounts of 17HSD1 and insufficient 17HSD2.[570] Studies show that if cancer cells are treated with genistein, 17HSD2 will be made, and "strong estrogen" (estradiol) will be converted to "weak" (estriol).[571] A woman with breast cancer may have the same level of estrogen in her blood as a woman without breast cancer. The elevated estradiol levels occur inside cancer cells where abnormalities create imbalances in enzymes. Such 17HSDvariances favor the accumulation of estrogen for cell growth.

Genistein also inhibits an enzyme that is elevated in breast cancer cells known as "aromatase."[572,573] Aromatase helps convert testosterone to estrogen. Elevated male hormones, enlarged prostate, and abnormal cell growth do not promote prostate cancer in mice that lack aromatase.[574]

Asian women get early protection by eating soy their entire lives.[575] The genistein in soy promotes more differentiated tissue in the breast, which leaves less tissue that can become cancerous. Soy isoflavones decrease density in the breast enabling easier detection of cancer by mammogram.[576] A serving of tofu every week decreases the risk of breast cancer by 15%.[577] It is well-established that when Asian women abandon their traditional diet, their risk of breast cancer escalates. It is important to realize, however, that while it has been proven that soy components have direct and powerful effects against cancer cells, it cannot be assumed that soy alone is responsible for the reduced risk of hormone-related cancers in Asians. There are many aspects of the Asian diet that undoubtedly play a role, including the low consumption of animal fat. Green tea is another component of the Asian diet that has proven anticancer effects. A polyphenol from black tea has no effect on prostate cancer cells. However, when combined with genistein, it stops proliferation.[578]

HER2/neu and EGFR are both related to breast cancers resistant to treatment with tamoxifen and other therapies.[579] Genistein blocks an enzyme that promotes the proliferation of cancer cells. Because protein tyrosine kinases activate other cancer-promoting factors, genistein is a very attractive candidate for the prevention and treatment of various types of cancer. A dietary amount of the soy compound genistein significantly delayed the appearance of the HER2/neu-type cancer. It did not, however, reduce tumor size or number in this study.[580]

It is important to note that DDT and other chlorine-related chemicals activate tyrosine kinases (TK), including HER2/neu-related ones in human cancer cells. Although DDT was banned decades ago, Americans are still being exposed to it. Genistein and other isoflavones block the activation of TK by DDT and related estrogen-mimicking chemicals, but tamoxifen does not.[208,581]

A mouse study shows that increasing amounts of genistein retard cancer growth, in accordance with the cell studies.[582] The animals must be implanted with estradiol to make the cancer cells grow.[583–585] When mice are fed the equivalent of what Asians usually consume in their diets, the appearance of a genetic type breast cancer (as opposed to a chemically induced one) is significantly delayed by genistein, soy isoflavones, and daidzein, another soy compound.[580]

Studies in monkeys, the closest animal model to humans, show that soy phytoestrogens impede the proliferation of cells responsive to estrogen. "Soybean phytoestrogens are not estrogenic at dietary doses."[586] Statistics on the rate of hormone-related cancers in Asians prove that soy is extremely beneficial against hormone-related cancers in humans. They show that people who eat large amounts of soy products have the lowest levels of strong estrogen in their bodies and the lowest rates of breast and prostate cancers.

**Soy and other types of cancer.** Soy has powerful anticancer effects that do not involve hormones. Genistein inhibits a chemical reaction used by many different types of cancer cells to multiply and spread. Compounds that can do this are called tyrosine kinase (TK) inhibitors. Dozens of studies in different types of cancer cells show that genistein is a powerful and effective TK inhibitor.

- **Glioma.** Glioma cancer cells have very high TK activity, which correlates with cancer growth. Several in vitro studies show that genistein inhibits the growth of glioma.[587–589] Genistein also enhances the effectiveness of the chemotherapeutic drugs carmustine and camptothecin with a 40% decrease in growth and a 50% increased killing effect in some cells.[589,590] The amount of genistein needed to enhance the effectiveness of carmustine is not high. The appropriate amount of genistein can be obtained by following the supplement program recommended in the Soy Dosing and Precautions section.

- **Bladder cancer.** Genistein's ability to inhibit TK may be of great benefit in keeping bladder cancer localized. In Asia, the incidence of invasive bladder cancer is much lower than in the United States, leading some researchers to investigate the effects of soy. Invasive bladder cancers have high levels of a protein known as epidermal growth factor receptor (EGFR), which enables the cancer to invade muscle. EGFR is activated by TK and can be reversed by genistein.[591]

   The effects of genistein, soy protein isolate, and soy phytochemical concentrate on human bladder cancer cells and bladder cancer were studied in mice. The 3 soy products reduced tumor volume 40%, 37%, and 48%, respectively. They blocked tumor blood vessel formation and induced tumor cell death, stopping the cells from growing at the G2-M part of the cell cycle.[567]

   A mixture of isoflavones work better than a single soy compound for bladder cancer. In a study on 7 different cell lines, genistein plus isoflavones inhibited tumor growth and induced cell death at levels obtainable through the diet or soy supplements. Both genistein and combined isoflavones exhibited a significant tumor suppressor effect in vivo. These results justify the potential use of soybean isolate as a practical chemoprevention approach for patients with urinary tract cancer.[592]

- **Stomach cancer.** The effects of soy products on 10 different types of human gastrointestinal cancer cells found that genistein and biochanin A (a genistein precursor) strongly inhibited proliferation of stomach, colon, and esophageal cancers.[593] Data from a study involving over 30 000 people was analyzed and it was found that people who eat the most soy products reduced their risk of stomach cancer by half compared to those who eat the least.[569]

- **Melanoma.** Studies on the effects of genistein on human melanoma cancer cells showed that genistein is a powerful inhibitor of the growth of this cancer and that it stops the cell cycle as effectively as the chemotherapeutic drugs Adriamycin® and etoposide.[594]

   Studying melanoma in mice revealed that genistein reduces the blood supply to lung tumors and has an additive effect with the drug cyclophosphamide. In laboratory rodents, genistein can reduce the growth of tumors by half through supplements and/or diet.[595]

- **Lung cancer.** Genistein has several actions against small cell and non–small cell lung tumors.

In a study in which Lewis lung cancer was transplanted into mice, genistein reduced the tumor colonies by half, and genistein plus cyclophosphamide reduced them by 90%.[568] Several studies show that genistein stops lung cancer cells from growing and induces cell death.[596–598] Genistein inhibits enzymes that help lung cancer cells to proliferate and spread.[599] Genistein upregulates tumor suppressor genes p53 and p21.[600] Genistein reverses the multidrug resistance-associated protein, a protein that makes lung cancer cells resistant to daunorubicin, doxorubicin, etoposide, and vinblastine.[601,602]

Researchers in Japan analyzed information from 333 people with lung cancer. They found that eating tofu every day reduced the risk of lung cancer 45% in men and 86% in women.[603]

- **Colon cancer.** Soy has anticancer effects against cells that line the digestive tract. For this reason, it may have beneficial effects against different types of digestive tract cancers. Researchers looking at how 3 different types of human colon cancer cells react to soy confirmed that colon cancer is susceptible to soy's anticancer effects.[604] Some colon cancers may be estrogen dependent. Estradiol activates 4 kinase enzymes in colon cancer cells, 2 of which are tyrosine dependent and therefore potentially susceptible to genistein. Genistein blocks at least one of these enzymes and retards cell growth.[605] Genistein also suppresses the growth of nonestrogen-dependent colon cancer cells, which also respond to treatment with tamoxifen.[606]

   In a study that investigated how tamoxifen, genistein, and estradiol affect intestinal cells, genistein and tamoxifen emerged as the strongest inhibitors of cell proliferation, inhibiting TK and inducing the death of cancer cells.[607] Genistein reverses resistance to doxorubicin and other chemotherapeutic drugs in at least one type of colon cancer by a "novel drug resistance pathway."[608] However, a study in mice showed that soy isoflavones may not counteract a bad diet. Mice fed a Western high-fat, low-fiber, and low-calcium diet developed colon cancer despite isoflavones in their food.[609] Soy could not reverse colon cancer (whereas rye lignans could) in mice on high-fat diets.[610]

- **Thyroid cancer.** Soy may have beneficial effects against thyroid cancer. In 608 cases of people with thyroid cancer, it was observed that those who consumed soy compounds (ie, genistein and daidzein) in their diet reduced their risk of this cancer by one-third. However, adding soy flour or protein to a Western diet was not effective.[611]

- **Leukemia.** A few studies have been done on human leukemia cells treated with genistein. Of 9 compounds tested, genistein showed the strongest inhibitory effects against human promyelocytic leukemia (HL-60) cells. All 9 compounds are found in miso.[612] In human leukemia cells resistant to chemotherapy, genistein was able to reverse the drug resistance almost completely.[613] The antiproliferative effect of genistein against human leukemia was significantly augmented by vitamin D analogs.[614]

**Free-radical scavenging effects.** The antioxidant effects of soy were the focus of much of the early research on how soy prevents cancer. The powerful free-radical scavenging effects of soy compounds and how they impact cancer continue to emerge.

Soy has an additive effect with vitamin E; it lowers rather than elevates estrogen levels in women and androgen levels in men.[615] Damage to DNA caused by certain types of free radicals is strongly inhibited by genistein and other soy compounds.[616,617] This helps prevent cancer. Dietary amounts significantly lower free-radical damage.[617,618]

In addition to blocking free-radical damage, soy phytoestrogens also block inflammation, a contributor to cancer growth, notably in the colon.[617,619]

The effects of genistein against the activation of EGFR by free radicals were demonstrated. In this study, genistein reversed the free-radical activation of EGFR in normal cells.[620] The benefits of genistein against oxidative stress are evident from a study on brain cells exposed to hydrogen peroxide. Free radicals generated by this oxidant degrade phospholipids and activate enzymes, which are crucial for memory and other brain functions. Genistein, through its ability to inhibit a tyrosine kinase enzyme that sets off the reaction, rescues cells from damage.[621]

**Soy precautions and dosage.** While the data are persuasive regarding the chemoprotective effects of soy, many questions remain. Some nutritionally based oncologists do not permit soy in their patients' regime. Others believe that soy should be avoided by everyone and have launched massive public relations campaigns to discredit soy and discourage even moderate consumption by healthy people.

Breast cancer patients should avoid soy until their estrogen receptor status has been determined. Estrogen receptor alpha-positive breast cancer patients may benefit from genistein, while beta–receptor positive breast cancer patients' tumors cells may proliferate faster in response to genistein. It has been suggested that patients avoid soy supplements 1 week prior to, during, and 1 week after radiation therapy, although

new studies appearing in the Cancer Radiation Therapy protocol indicate a potential benefit to using soy isoflavones during radiation therapy.

Some people believe that soy is toxic to the thyroid gland, yet this may be a concern only in cases of iodine deficiency.[622] Some of the more credible arguments deal with soy-based infant formulas.[623]

There are a number of human clinical studies being conducted on the use of soy to both prevent and treat cancer (http://clinicaltrials.gov/ct/search?term=soy). When the findings of these studies are published, perhaps more definitive recommendations can be made about soy supplements. Based on the information available to us as of this writing, those concerned about cancer may consider these guidelines: a suggested dosage is five 700-mg capsules 4 times a day of a soy extract providing a minimum of 40% isoflavones. For prevention purposes, as little as 135 mg of a 40% soy isoflavone extract once a day may be adequate.

## Sulforaphane

Sulforaphane, which is an isothiocyanate, is most highly concentrated in broccoli as well as in other cruciferous vegetables (eg, Brussels sprouts, cabbage, and cauliflower).

Sulforaphane detoxifies potential carcinogens, promotes apoptosis, blocks the cell cycle that is required for cancer cell replication, prevents tumor invasion into healthy tissue, enhances natural killer cell activity, and combats metastasis.[624–627] Research has also demonstrated that sulforaphane is among the plant chemicals most potently capable of blocking the cancer-producing effects of ultraviolet radiation.[628]

Sulforaphane also possesses the ability to prevent toxin-induced cancers. When researchers studied people in the Chinese province of Qidong (where liver cancer rates are among the highest in the world, in part due to exposure to foods contaminated with the fungal carcinogen aflatoxin),[629] they noted that consumption of a tea produced from broccoli sprouts resulted in decreased urinary markers of aflatoxin-damaged DNA in subjects with high levels of sulforaphane in their urine.

**Leukemia.** In a clinical trial, sulforaphane enhanced the efficacy of imatinib (a drug used in the treatment of chronic myelogenous leukemia) against leukemia cells.[630] It has also triggered apoptosis in leukemia cells.[631]

**Colon cancer.** Sulforaphane induces apoptosis in colon cancer cells.[632,633] Sulforaphane inhibited the formation of colon tumors in an animal model.[634] Another study with mice with colon cancer found that in comparison to untreated controls, mice treated with sulforaphane experienced a 70% reduction in tumor weight.[632]

**Breast cancer.** It has been observed that sulforaphane activated apoptosis[635] and inhibited the proliferation of breast cancer cells in culture.[636,637] The binding of estrogen hormones to estrogen receptor alpha promotes breast cell proliferation, which can promote the progression of breast cancer. Researchers have also noted that sulforaphane downregulates the expression of estrogen receptor alpha in breast cancer cells.[636]

In another clinical trial, mice injected with breast cancer cells developed 60% less tumor mass when treated with sulforaphane compared to untreated mice.[638]

**Chemotherapy.** Sulforaphane also shows promise as an adjuvant to chemotherapy. When added to the chemotherapy drug oxaliplatin, sulforaphane improved the ability of the drug to kill colon cancer cells.[639]

**Radiation therapy.** When head and neck cancer cells were treated with sulforaphane and subsequently irradiated, researchers observed that the combination therapy resulted in a stronger inhibition of cell proliferation than each treatment method alone.[640]

## Theanine

Theanine increases efficacy of chemotherapeutic drugs. Researchers speculate that drinking 1 cup of green tea favors a positive mental attitude and increases the efficacy of chemotherapy. However, components of green tea have been identified (caffeine, epigallocatechin gallate [EGCG], flavonoids, and theanine) that better explain the chemotherapeutic advantage beyond its soul-soothing effects.[641]

Japanese researchers focused specifically on theanine and its influence on the antitumor activity of Adriamycin®. In vitro, theanine inhibited the outflow of Adriamycin® from cancerous cells, increasing concentrations within the cell by almost three-fold. An increase in Adriamycin® concentrations was not observed in normal tissues, suggesting theanine protects healthy organs, such as the heart and liver.[642] Illustrative of the enhancing qualities of theanine, injecting Adriamycin® into ovarian sarcoma-bearing (M5076) mice did not inhibit tumor growth, whereas a combination of theanine and Adriamycin® reduced tumor weight 62%.[643]

When theanine was added to pirarubicin, intracellular concentrations of pirarubicin increased 1.3-fold and the overall therapeutic efficacy of the drug increased 1.7-fold.[644] Satisfying results were also found when theanine was used with Idarubicin (IDA), which is highly toxic to bone marrow and an antileukemia agent similar to doxorubicin. Risk factors permitted only about one-fourth of the standard IDA dose to be used in combination with theanine. However, theanine reduced toxicities and increased IDA antitumor activity, rendering the chemotherapeutic agent a possibility for the treatment of leukemia.[645]

Part of theanine's anticancer effects can be attributed to mimicking glutamate, an amino acid that potentiates glutathione. Glutathione detoxifies chemotherapeutic agents, barricading chemicals from cells, and inhibiting tumor cell kill. Theanine is structurally similar to glutathione and crowds out glutamate transport into tumor cells. Cancer cells (in confusion) erringly take in theanine and theanine induces glutathione production. Glutathione (derived from theanine) does not detoxify like natural glutathione, and instead blocks the ability of cancer cells to neutralize cancer-killing agents. Deprived of glutathione, cancer cells cannot remove chemotherapeutic agents, and the tumor cell dies as a result of chemical poisoning.[646]

Administered with doxorubicin, the suggested dose of theanine is 500–1000 mg a day, although no human studies have been conducted with chemotherapy and theanine.

## Thymus Extract

Thymus extract improves T-cell response and regulates the activity of cytokines. The thymus gland was at one time removed as an unnecessary appendage. It is an essential organ of the immune system, increasing stamina, energy, well-being, and the ability to ward off infections and cancer. Since 1965, when Burnet was awarded the Nobel Prize for demonstrating the endocrine function of the thymus gland, medical interest has focused on the thymus. It is now largely accepted that the thymus gland plays a central role in the mammalian immune system.

The immune system is made up of B cells that protect against bacterial and viral infections and T cells that guard against viral and fungal infections, as well as cancer. This powerful body of cells normally treats a developing cancer as foreign tissue, destroying aberrant cells before rapid multiplication occurs.

The effectiveness of T-cell–mediated immunity depends on the activity of T lymphocytes (T cells), which are programmed by proteins from the thymus gland. Immature (naïve) T-4 cells do not function properly until programmed by thymic proteins. As new T lymphocytes migrate from the bone marrow to the thymus, they are programmed to distinguish between self-tissue (the host) and nonself tissue (an invading pathogen).

The thymus gland, a lymphoid organ situated in the anterior superior mediastinum, reaches its maximum weight near puberty and then undergoes involution, or degenerative change, shrinking to about one-sixth of its original size. By the age of 40, the thymus gland is scarcely functional in many individuals; therefore, the essential thymus-provided protein is no longer available to program T-4 cells. More than 20 years ago, thymic protein A was isolated and purified from bovine thymus cells (by Terry Beardsley, an immunologist). Beardsley patented a technology to grow thymus cells in the laboratory and then purify a specific thymus protein (thymic protein A) that helps T cells to mature with immune competency. The active ingredient in thymic protein A is the precise thymus protein that programs the T-4 lymphocytes to locate abnormal cells and then directs T-8 killer cells to destroy them.

Three types of cells emerge from the thymus: T-4 helper cells (master regulators), T-8 cytotoxic killer cells (guided by T-4 helper cells to attack and destroy invading cells), and T-8 suppressor cells. T-4 helper cells regulate many key functions, including the activity of IL-2 and interferon.

High-dose thymosin, a humoral factor secreted by the thymus, in conjunction with intensive chemotherapy was administered to 21 patients with advanced lung cancer. Ordinarily, patients with late stage lung cancer live about 240 days; the median survival rate more than doubled (500 days) among patients receiving thymosin. Some of the thymosin-treated group were alive and disease-free 2 years after treatment.[647]

Blood tests to measure the immune response are extremely valuable when detailing either a preventive or a therapeutic program to fight cancer. While determining T lymphocyte numbers is important, assessing their activity is even more crucial. It is possible for a person with a total count of 1000 T-4 cells to have only 50% of these cells activated by the thymus. It is important that the patient know the degree of immune impairment in order to structure a corrective program. Tests to evaluate the activity of the immune system are performed at the Immuno-Science Laboratory (Los Angeles, California), (310) 657-1077.

## Vitamin A

Vitamin A offers protection against radiation-induced tissue damage, downregulates telomerase activity, and is involved at almost every juncture of cancer control. Retinoids induce cell differentiation, control cancer growth and angiogenesis, repair precancerous lesions, prevent secondary carcinogenesis and metastasis, and act as an immunostimulant. After FAR therapy (5-fluorouracil-retinol palmitate with radiation and

surgery), the disease-specific, 5-year survival was nearly 50% in various head and neck cancers.[648] Retinoids, at pharmacologic levels, assist in preventing the appearance of secondary tumors following curative therapy for epithelial malignancies.

It is well-established that a vitamin A deficiency (in laboratory animals) correlates with a higher incidence of cancer and an increased susceptibility to chemical carcinogens. This is in agreement with epidemiologic studies, which indicate that individuals with a lower dietary vitamin A intake are at a higher risk of developing cancer.[649] The chemotherapeutic possibilities surrounding vitamin A are plentiful.

Two vitamin A analogs currently in large chemoprevention, intervention trials, or epidemiologic studies are all-trans-retinoic acid (ATRA) and 13-cis-retinoic acid (13-cis-RA).

*Note: Retinoic acid is biologically active in 2 forms: all- trans- retinoic acid and 9-cis-retinoic acid. Vitamin A and 13-cis-RA are converted to these biologically active forms.*

Thirty-two women with previously untreated cervical carcinoma (ages 14–60) were treated for at least 2 months using oral 13-cis-RA (1 mg per kg body weight a day) and alpha-interferon subcutaneously (6 million units daily). Sixteen of the women (50%) had major reactions, including 4 complete clinical responses. Remission occurred in 15 of the patients within 2 months and in one patient within 1 month; toxicity to treatment was described as manageable.[650] The positive results were replicated in other studies using a similar model.[651,652]

The role of 13-cis-RA on a human prostate cancer cell line (LNCaP) was studied. It was found that 13-cis-RA significantly inhibited PSA secretion and the ability to form new tumors. It was also noted that tumors that appeared (having escaped 13-cis-RA inhibition) were smaller compared to tumors in nontreated animals.[653] During the course of 13-cis-RA therapy, prostate cancer cells became more differentiated; that is, they resembled (microscopically) normal prostate cells.

A combination of phenylbutyrate and 13-cis-RA as a differentiation and antiangiogenesis strategy against prostate cancer was evaluated. Phenylbutyrate, considered nontoxic, is used to arrest tumor growth and induce differentiation of premalignant and malignant cells. Tissue examination of tumors showed decreased cell proliferation and increased apoptosis, as well as reduced microvessel density in animals treated with

13-cis-RA and phenylbutyrate; tumor growth was inhibited by 82–92%. In contrast, researchers reported 13-cis-RA and phenylbutyrate, when used singularly, were suboptimal in terms of clinical benefit.[654]

A pilot study conducted at M.D. Anderson Cancer Center found ATRA alone ineffective as a long-term treatment for chronic myelogenous leukemia (CML). Only 4 of 13 subjects showed a transient, nonsustaining indication of an antileukemic effect.[655] However, combinations of therapeutic agents that included ATRA were promising in the treatment of CML. The combination included alpha-interferon plus ATRA, which reduced proliferation 50–60%.[656]

Cisplatin (a popular chemotherapeutic agent) shares a similar chemotherapeutic profile with ATRA (the ability to induce cytotoxicity through apoptosis). A combination of ATRA and cisplatin-induced apoptosis in significantly more cancer cells, particularly in ovarian and head and neck carcinomas, than either drug alone.[657] A combination of ATRA and IL-2 showed therapeutic value in treating resistant metastatic osteosarcoma, a malignant tumor of the bone.[658]

For decades, researchers have searched for ways to minimize the damage to the heart during Adriamycin® therapy. Adriamycin®, although relatively effective, damages the heart muscle. Several animal studies indicated that supplemental vitamin A reduced Adriamycin®-induced inflammation and preserved heart tissue. Vitamin A appears not only to counter Adriamycin® damage, but also to increase survival in animals.[659] Vitamin A extends similar protection to patients using cisplatin, a drug often used for bladder and ovarian cancer, as well as small cell carcinoma.

Radiation-induced lung injury frequently limits the total dose of thoracic radiotherapy that can be delivered to a patient undergoing treatment, restricting its effectiveness. Animal studies suggest that supplemental vitamin A may reduce lung inflammation after thoracic radiation and modify radiotherapy damage to the lungs.[660]

Vitamin A (in dosages of 25 000 IU a day) offers significant protection against radiation-induced tissue damage. Various cancer patients use more than 100 000 IU of a water-soluble vitamin A liquid a day, a dosage that must be supervised by a physician. Do not supplement with vitamin A if the cancer involves the thyroid gland or if the liver is damaged. Good food sources of vitamin A include liver and fish liver oils, green and yellow fruits and vegetables such as apricots, asparagus, broccoli, cantaloupe, carrots, collards, papayas, peaches, pumpkins, spinach, and sweet potatoes. High-potency, water-soluble vitamin A is available as a dietary supplement.

## Vitamin C

Vitamin C (ascorbic acid) has a chemotherapeutic effect on many cancers, promotes collagen production, sequestering the tumor, and reduces the toxicity of conventional therapies. Linus Pauling, winner of the Nobel Prize for chemistry in 1954 and the Nobel Prize for Peace in 1963, believed strongly that vitamin C could play an important role in cancer treatment. Pauling suggested 10 g of vitamin C a day for patients with advanced cancer for whom conventional treatments had ceased to be of benefit.[661] Over an 8-year period, 500 patients with varying stages and types of cancer were treated with vitamin C therapy. Those receiving 10 g of vitamin C a day improved their state of well-being, as measured by increased appetite and mental alertness, as well as a decreased need for pain-killing drugs. A retrospective analysis showed that those using vitamin C lived considerably longer than those not supplemented.

Various clinics are using intravenous vitamin C and with positive results. Hugh Riordan, recognized as a world authority on this procedure, practices from Wichita, Kansas, at the Center for the Improvement of Human Functioning International. Riordan's vitamin C story began in 1984 when he treated his first cancer patient; a 70-year-old renal cell carcinoma patient with metastasis to the lung and liver, using injectable vitamin C. Renal cell carcinoma has only a 5% response rate.

The initial treatment began with 15 g of vitamin C administered intravenously 2 times a week; showing excellent tolerance, the vitamin C dosage was increased to 30 g twice weekly. Within 6 weeks, the patient showed a favorable response to treatment and at the 12-week interval was pronounced tumor-free. The patient lived 14 additional years and died of congestive heart failure with no evidence of tumors.

In light of the favorable initial response to intravenous (IV) vitamin C, ascorbic acid was investigated. Vitamin C is preferentially toxic to tumor cells, that is, it kills tumor cells but not normal cells.

In low doses, vitamin C assumes the nature of an antioxidant; in high dosages, vitamin C changes roles and becomes a prooxidant, inducing peroxide production. Tumor cells have a relative catalase deficiency, an enzyme necessary to detoxify hydrogen peroxide to water and oxygen. A 10- to 100-fold difference in catalase concentrations exists between tumor cells and normal cells. Without the protection of catalase, peroxide accumulates in cancerous cells, along with aldehydes (toxic byproducts of the reaction), causing death to malignant cells. On the other hand, normal, healthy tissues have the protection of the detoxification enzyme and are spared destruction by peroxide and aldehyde. Vitamin C, a virtually nontoxic nutrient,[662] could cause a transient diarrhea if not absorbed properly.

Vitamin C is safe compared to standard chemotherapeutics and has an ability to preserve immune function. Many patients succumb, not because of cancer, but rather from a postchemotherapeutic toxicity, resulting from a damaged immune system. Vitamin C protects the immune system. Vitamin C is preferentially toxic to many types of cancer cells, including 20 different melanoma cell lines. Ovarian cell lines are more susceptible to vitamin C-induced toxicity than pancreatic cells. Breast cancer appears to be one of the most responsive cancers to IV vitamin C.

Much higher concentrations of vitamin C are required to kill cancer cells than originally thought, about 600 mg/dL. Also, as the density of the cells increases, the efficacy of vitamin C decreases. It is extremely difficult to reach vitamin C concentrations greater than 200 mg/dL even when administered intravenously.[663] To increase the sensitivity of tumor cells to vitamin C, other approaches need to be employed.

Alpha-lipoic acid, a water- and lipid-soluble antioxidant that recycles vitamin, enhances the toxic effect of ascorbic acid. Lipoic acid decreases the dose of vitamin C required to kill tumor cells from 700 to 120 mg/dL.[663] Vitamin C toxicity is further enhanced by 1000 mcg of vitamin B12, which forms cobalt ascorbate, a benign but cancer-cell-toxic agent. Vitamin K, selenium, quercetin, niacinamide, biotin, and grape seed extract are also regarded as potentiation factors.

The goal is to achieve and maintain 400 mg/dL of vitamin C in the plasma. At this concentration, every cancer cell line so far tested has been found to be sensitive to vitamin C. After reaching an ascorbic acid peak, as occurs during infusion, the level returns to near baseline levels 24 hours after the IV infusion.

Vitamin C has an ability to increase collagen production. Vitamin C is required for the hydroxylation of proline, which in turn is required for collagen production. Vitamin C has the ability to inhibit enzymes that degrade or break down the extracellular matrix. Vitamin C dramatically increased the collagen within tumor cells, an act that tended to immobilize the cells.

Vitamin C (supported by lipoic acid) has been used as a cancer therapy. It is strongly advised that patients contact a physician trained in administering infusions and monitoring progress. By giving vitamin C intravenously,

doctors can achieve a blood saturation that far exceeds that attained by administering vitamin C orally (200% versus 2%). A high dose of vitamin C is critical to achieve tumor cell kill.

A Hickman line allows large doses of vitamin C to be self-administered at home on a daily to weekly basis over a period of months, modulating down or up in frequency according to response. Otherwise the treatment can be administered as an outpatient. Contraindications to vitamin C therapy are few but include individuals with kidney failure and on dialysis, as well as those with hemochromatosis. Also, physicians should screen patients for a red blood cell glucose-6 phosphate dehydrogenase deficiency, a rare condition whose presence can lead to a hemolytic crisis involving red blood cell breakdown.

Large doses of vitamin C should be reached gradually to establish tolerance. For example, 15 g for one or two sessions and then 50–100 g if necessary. The exact dose is determined by the individual's plasma saturation immediately after an infusion. The therapy should not be stopped abruptly because a rebound effect could result in scurvy. Patients should allow weeks or even months to wean off the treatment, with oral vitamin C therapy used on the days between infusions.

A 10-year research project using high-dose IV vitamin C has been completed. While a number of orthomolecular physicians are using IV vitamin C therapy, it is recommended that Riordan's protocol become the backbone of the therapy. Instructions are available to physicians on request from the center.[664]

Center for the Improvement of Human Functioning

3100 North Hillside Avenue

Wichita, KS 67219

(316) 682-3100

Other chemotherapeutic credits awarded to vitamin C include:

- Vitamin C prolongs the lives of animals undergoing conventional cancer treatment by protecting normal cells against chemotherapy-induced toxicity; in tandem, vitamin C increases the cytotoxicity targeted at the cancer.[665,666] When 5-FU was administered together with vitamin C, the tumor cell kill rate was boosted from 38 to 95.5%. X-ray therapy decreased cancer growth 72%, but adding vitamin C to the regime decreased cancer growth by 98.2%. Full-spectrum antioxidants rather than isolated nutrients are suggested.[667,668]

- Infection with *H. pylori* increases the risk of developing stomach cancer[669] as well as pancreatic cancer.[221]

High doses of vitamin C inhibit the growth of *H. pylori*, both in vitro and in vivo.[670] A study showed vitamin C levels to be consistently low in individuals with the *H. pylori* infection.[671]

- Frequent intake of vitamin C from food and supplement sources was associated with a protective effect against multiple myeloma, particularly among Caucasians. African Americans benefited less from ascorbic acid intake.[240]

- NF-κB is a central mediator of altered gene expression during inflammation and is implicated in cancer. Vitamin C inhibited the activation of NF-κB by multiple stimuli, including IL-1 and TNF-α.[662]

It should be re-emphasized that oral vitamin C does not bestow equal benefits compared to intravenous vitamin C. If a patient with a solid tumor elects to use oral vitamin C, ascorbic acid buffered with sodium may produce better results. If the cancer is blood-borne (leukemia, lymphoma, or myeloma), ascorbic acid crystals buffered with calcium appears to offer greater efficacy. The majority of the patients use 6–12 g a day. Food sources of vitamin C are berries, citrus fruits, papayas, and pineapple, as well as tomatoes, broccoli, Brussels sprouts, dandelion and mustard greens, peas, red peppers, and spinach.

## Vitamin D

Vitamin D promotes differentiation, inhibits angiogenesis, and regulates cell division. Current recommendations to avoid natural sunrays to thwart the possibility of deadly melanoma may be allowing other endangerments. For more than 50 years, medical literature has affirmed that regular sun exposure is associated with a substantial decrease in death rates from certain types of cancers. It is estimated that moderate sun exposure without sunscreen—enough to stimulate vitamin D production but not enough to damage the skin—could prevent 30 000 cancer deaths in the United States each year.[672] The most damaging of the sun's rays occur between the hours of 10 a.m. and 3 p.m. and are thus the hours demanding the greatest watchfulness.

Evidence points to a prostate, breast, and colon cancer belt in the United States, which lies in northern latitudes under more cloud cover than other regions.[673] Certain regions in the United States, such as the San Joaquin Valley cities and Tucson and Phoenix, Arizona; Albuquerque, New Mexico; El Paso, Texas; Miami, Jacksonville, Tampa, and Orlando, Florida have a lower incidence of breast and bowel cancers. Conversely, New York; Chicago; Boston; Philadelphia; New Haven, Connecticut; Pittsburgh; and Cleveland, Ohio have the highest rates of breast and intestinal cancer of the 29 major cities in the United States. The greater hours of year-round sunlight correlate to a lower rate of breast and intestinal cancer in the United States.

Vitamin D is formed in the skin of animals and humans by the action of shortwave UV light, the so-called fast-tanning sunrays. Precursors of vitamin D in the skin are converted into cholecalciferol, a weak form of vitamin D3, which is then transported to the liver and kidneys where enzymes convert it to 1,25-dihydroxy-cholecalciferol, the more potent form of vitamin D3.[674] Although vitamin D exists in 2 molecular forms, vitamin D3 (cholecalciferol) found in animal skin and vitamin D2 (ergocalciferol) found in yeast, vitamin D3 is believed to exhibit more potent cancer-inhibiting properties and is therefore the preferred form.

Dark-skinned people require more sun exposure to produce vitamin D, because the thickness of the skin layer (the stratum corneum) affects the absorption of UV radiation. Black human skin is thicker than white skin and thus transmits only about 40% of the UV rays needed for vitamin D production. Darkly pigmented individuals who live in sunny equatorial climates experience a higher mortality rate from breast and prostate cancer when they move to geographic areas that are deprived of sunlight exposure in winter months.[674,675]

Women with polymorphisms (genetic variations) of the vitamin D receptor gene may be less able to benefit from the nutrient. There is some evidence that vitamin D receptor gene polymorphisms play a role in the breast cancer[676]; however, more recent studies do not support this evidence.[677]

Identifying the at-risk groups through the assessment of genetic variations in the vitamin D receptor appears to be a forthcoming tool for planning intervention strategies.

Human leukemia cells cultured in the presence of vitamin D exhibited a reduced rate of tumor growth when injected into mice. Cells grown in vitamin D3 failed to form detectable tumors in 11 of 12 inoculated mice.[678] The anticarcinogenic properties of vitamin D confronts multiple stages of cancer development, including apoptosis, differentiation, angiogenesis, and metastasis, as well as regulating the cell growth cycle.[679]

Since vitamin D can cause calcium to be released from bones (a condition referred to as hypercalcemia), large doses of vitamin D cannot be used in patients whose medical history or genetics puts them at increased risk. Using a combination of Vitamin D3 and vanadium (a metallic element) enables vitamin D to retain its anticancer activity and vanadium addresses the problem of hypercalcemia.[680]

Rats were supplemented with vanadium or vitamin D3 or both vanadium and D3 4 weeks prior to induced liver cancer and continued thereafter until the 20th week. After 20 weeks of supplementation, the vitamin D3-vanadium combination had significantly reduced the number and size of abnormal hepatic nodules. The combination also showed an additive effect, reducing the number and size of hyperplastic nodes from 83.3 to 37.5%. In addition, vanadium effectively blocked the entry of calcium into cells.

A modified form of vitamin D (referred to as a deltanoid) delays the onset and reduces the number of skin cancers in laboratory mice. The microscopically altered structure of vitamin D produced a potentially effective cancer therapeutic. The vitamin D analog retains its anticancer profile but diminishes the threat of hypercalcemia. The most effective of 4 analogs tested was a doubly modified hybrid compound containing fluorine.[681]

During one study, mice painted with a chemical substance, inducing cancerous tumors were concurrently the animals were given the deltanoid. After 20 weeks, the fluorine-containing analog had reduced the incidence of tumors more than 28%, while the actual number fell 63%.[682] Deltanoids are in the early stages of development and, unfortunately, it may take 10 years before they become available.[683] It is possible that deltanoids could lessen the need for hormone treatments or aggressive chemotherapy. Patients could theoretically stay on the treatment for the remainder of their life to keep the cancer from advancing.

Studies indicate that moderate or severe hypovitaminosis D was present in 66% of patients taking daily vitamin D in amounts less than the recommended dosage for their age. Adults may need a minimum of 5 times the RDA (recommended dietary allowance), or 1000 IU daily, to protect against cancer.[684] Therapeutic dosages of vitamin D typically range from 800–4000 IU a day. Monthly kidney function blood tests (creatine, BUN, etc.) should be performed if daily vitamin D intake exceeds 1400 IU. These tests are included in most standard blood chemistry tests that cancer patients regularly perform to guard against anemia and overt immunosuppression.

Food sources of vitamin D include egg yolks, organ meats, fortified dairy products, butter, cod liver oil, and cold-water fish, such as salmon, herring, and mackerel. Vitamin D enhancers are vitamins A and C, calcium, magnesium, phosphorus, and choline. Antagonists are mineral oil, phenobarbital, and laxatives.

## Vitamin E

Vitamin E is an antioxidant that can protect smokers, reduces radiation damage, potentiates chemotherapy, and inhibits many types of cancers. The inhibitory role of vitamin E in the growth of a number of human tumor cells, as well as its defensive functions in overcoming treatment-induced toxicity have been examined. The impact of vitamin E (perhaps acting through its antioxidant strengths) is significant, as evidenced by the following studies:

- After examining 29 000 male smokers in Finland, researchers found that high blood levels of alpha-tocopherol reduced the incidence of lung cancer by approximately 19%. The relationship appears stronger among younger persons and among those with less cumulative smoke exposure. These findings suggest that high levels of alpha-tocopherol, if present during the early critical stages of tumorigenesis, may inhibit lung cancer development.[685]

- A combination of vitamin E and pentoxifylline (PTX), a drug that inhibits abnormal platelet aggregation, allowing more blood to reach irradiated areas, resulted in a 50% regression of superficial radiation-induced fibrosis (the proliferation of fibrous connective tissue) in half of the patients studied.[686,687] A suggested dosage is 800 mg a day of PTX and 1000 IU per day of vitamin E.

- An antimelanoma effect obtained from vitamin E succinate in vivo has been reported.[688,689]

- Gamma-tocopherol inhibits COX-2 activity, demonstrating anti-inflammatory properties.[690,691]

- The use of vitamin E, in combination with vitamins A and C, led to a four-fold reduction in p53 mutations.[692] This is an extremely important finding because p53 mutations indicate a more malignant, aggressive form of cancer.

- Men with a high intake of vitamin E are 65% less likely to develop colorectal adenomas (precursors to colon cancer) compared to men with low vitamin E intake.[693]

- Lower morbidity and mortality from prostate cancer were reported in men taking 50 mg of synthetic alpha-tocopherol daily. Subsequent testing determined gamma-tocopherol to be superior, however, to alpha-tocopherol in terms of tumor cell inhibition.[694] Men in the highest fifth of the distribution for gamma-tocopherol had a five-fold reduction in the risk of developing prostate cancer compared to those in the lowest fifth. In addition, statistically significant protection from high levels of selenium and alpha-tocopherol occurred only when gamma-tocopherol concentrations were also high.[695]

- Vitamin E's mode of efficacy in regard to prostate protection: Vitamin E interferes with 2 proteins (the receptor for testosterone and prostate-specific antigen [PSA]). The fewer androgen receptors there are on a prostate cancer cell, the less capable the remaining receptors are of turning on genes that stimulate prostate cancer growth and progression. PSA serves as a good marker molecule for androgen receptor activity.[696]

- Tocotrienols, quite similar to a tocopherol (but for the addition of an unsaturated tail in its chemical structure), accumulate in adipose tissues, including mammary glands. If a cell becomes diseased, the tocotrienol is prepared for action, ready to inhibit growth and regulate aberrant cellular activity at onset. Curiously, the more cancerous the cell, the more susceptible it is to tocotrienols. Scientists apparently have been focusing on the wrong form of vitamin E (the tocopherols), which show little protection against breast cancer. Tocotrienols appear to inhibit proliferation of human breast cancer cells by as much as 50%.[697] Results suggest that tocotrienols are effective inhibitors of both estrogen receptor-negative and estrogen receptor-positive cells and that combination with tamoxifen should be considered as a possible improvement in breast cancer therapy. This strategy could significantly reduce the amount of tamoxifen required to affect the cancer.[698]

- Cortisol (associated with poorer survival) and IL-6 (a negative marker for various cancers) were significantly lower in laboratory animals that received alpha-tocopherol before a cortisol-IL-6 challenge.[699]

A suggested vitamin E dosage is 400–1200 IU a day of alpha-tocopherol together with gamma E tocopherol. For optimal results, use 80% alpha-tocopherol and 20% gamma-tocopherol. A tocotrienol dosage is 240 mg each day. Good food sources of vitamin E are cold-pressed vegetable oils, wheat germ, eggs, dark green vegetables, nuts, brown rice, and butter.

## Vitamin K

Vitamin K is a growth regulator, promotes apoptosis, and decreases proinflammatory cytokines. A novel form of vitamin K that appears extremely promising in the treatment of primary liver cancer, a type notoriously resistant to chemotherapy has been discovered by scientists at the University of Pittsburgh Cancer Institute (UPCI). The research published in the *Journal of Biological Chemistry* described an innovative approach to treat, and possibly prevent cancer by triggering apoptosis.[700]

The UPCI team found that a vitamin K analog, Compound 5 (CPD5), causes an imbalance in the normal activity of enzymes that controls the addition or removal of small molecules (phosphate groups) from proteins inside cells. Specifically, CPD5 blocks the activity of enzymes (protein-tyrosine phosphatases) that normally remove phosphate groups from selected proteins inside liver cancer cells. CPD5, however, does not interfere with another group of enzymes called protein tyrosine-kinases, which add phosphate groups to the same proteins. The result is an excess of tyrosine-phosphorylated proteins, which triggers a variety of activities within cells, including the shutting down and subsequent death of the cell.

It may be possible to remove some individuals from liver transplant waiting lists if CPD5 is as effective in humans as it is experimentally. However, the vitamin K compound is not limited to killing liver cancer; in tissue culture the compound was also effective against melanoma and breast cancers. Although the new vitamin K is not in clinical testing at this time, clients and physicians may contact the UPCI's Cancer Information and Referral Service at 412-647-2811 for periodic updates regarding the treatment. Inquirers can also visit the University's website at http://www.upci.upmc.edu.

Vitamin K compounds inhibited IL-6 production by lipopolysaccharide-stimulated fibroblasts, which are recognized as rich sources of cytokines.[701] This finding has significant anticancer implications because overexpression of IL-6 is intricately involved in the inflammatory process, bone resorption, activation of telomerase, and cancer proliferation. A suggested vitamin K dosage is 10 mg a day. Interesting research relating to the use of vitamin K concurrent with anticoagulant therapy (not usually a recommended practice) appears in the protocol Atherosclerosis and Cardiovascular Disease in the section dedicated to vitamin K.

## OTHER FACTORS AFFECTING PATIENT OUTCOME

### What Should Cancer Patients Eat?

For a cancer patient who appreciates the importance of a properly planned diet, the task is daunting. The diversity of the population minimizes the likelihood of a universal diet; nonetheless, most diets are hyped as being nutritionally correct for everyone. This section explores dietary variables, conceding that many generalities exist, such as eat organic when available and eat on schedule to avoid blood glucose swings. Select foods characterized by color and texture. Avoid synthetic and refined foods: white flour products and sugar as well as trans fats (those fats altered by overheating, hydrogenation, and refining). Avoiding well-done meats and exposure to heterocyclic amines (formed during high temperature cooking) eliminates another significant cancer source.[702]

Tumors are primarily obligate glucose metabolizers, meaning they require sugar for survival. Even though the brain normally uses high amounts of glucose, hepatomas (a tumor of the liver) and fibrosarcomas (a sarcoma that contains fibrous connective tissue) consume roughly as much glucose as the brain. Some Americans continuously satisfy cancer's appetite, ingesting as much as 295 pounds of sugar a year.

Nobel laureate Otto Warburg discovered in 1955 that cancer cells use glucose for fuel. But glucose accomplishes another strategic maneuver that strongly favors the cancer: it immobilizes internal defenses, the actions of the immune system. A study involving 10 healthy human volunteers assessed fasting blood glucose levels and the phagocytic index of neutrophils, a type of white blood cell. Glucose, fructose, sucrose, honey, and orange juice all significantly decreased the capacity of neutrophils to engulf bacteria. A diet structured away from sugars deprives cancer of its energy and increases the reliability of the immune response.

Jeff Bland advises selecting foodstuffs low on the glycemic index to avoid gratifying the tumor's appetite. The glycemic index lists the relative speed at which different foods are digested and raise blood sugar levels. Each food is compared to the effect of the same amount of pure glucose on the body's blood sugar curve. Glucose itself has a glycemic index rating of 100. Foods that are broken down and raise blood glucose levels quickly have higher ratings. The closer to 100, the more the food resembles glucose. The lower the rating, the more gradually that food affects blood sugar levels.

Common foods have the following glycemic ratings: baked potatoes, 95; white bread, 95; mashed potatoes, 90; chocolate candy bar, 70; corn, 70; boiled potatoes, 70; bananas, 60; white pasta, 55; peas, 50; unsweetened fruit juice, 40; rye bread, 40; lentils, 30; soy, 15; green vegetables and tomatoes, <15.

**Note:** *The glycemic index should not be relied on without factoring in the glycemic load, which is the glycemic index of a food times its carbohydrate content in grams, a concept developed at Harvard School of Public Health in 1997. Carrots, for instance, have a high glycemic index, but a very low glycemic load. This means that carrots consumed in moderation usually do not present a problem. Refer to the Obesity and Weight Loss protocol for complete information about the glycemic index load.*

An admonition, based more on folk medicine than scientific certainty, to avoid the white foods (all sugar-containing foods, as well as rice, and white flour and flour-based products) appears to have validity when applied to the glycemic index. A diet structured principally around carbohydrates that promotes hyperglycemia (high blood sugar level) and hyperinsulinemia (high blood insulin level) provides an environment that feeds the fire of cancer. High blood insulin levels drive protein tyrosine kinase (leading to cell division) and high blood glucose metabolically feeds cancer cells. On the other hand, a diet centered on fiber-, vitamin-, and mineral-rich foods that cause no blood glucose rise or insulin rush is an excellent target for healthy eating.

The diseases such as obesity and diabetes mellitus (often characterized by hyperinsulinemia) are associated with an increased risk of endometrial, colorectal, and breast cancers. The mechanisms underlying insulin-mediated neoplasias appear to include enhanced DNA synthesis (with the resultant tumor cell growth), inhibited apoptosis, and an altered sex hormone milieu. The reduced insulin levels seen with physical activity, weight loss, and a high-fiber diet may in fact account for the decreased cancer incidence observed in individuals who maintain normal glucose and insulin levels.[703] Note that reducing blood insulin levels may result in remarkable improvements in men with prostate disease, with a concurrent drop in PSA levels.[704]

Unfortunately, glucose modulation is an underutilized component of cancer treatment. Some aspects of traditional treatments actually contribute to higher blood levels of glucose. For example, consider hospital meals, often favoring sugar-based foodstuffs. In addition, if the patient is on an IV solution, the infusion is largely dextrose based, feeding the cancer and perpetuating its growth.

The American Cancer Society believes that 30% of all cancers are due to inadequate consumption of vegetables and fruits. About 91% of Americans fail to achieve target recommendations, that is, 5 vegetable servings a day or 2–3 pounds a week. Asians who consume from 15–20 servings of fruits and vegetables a day have a much lower incidence of some cancers.

Vegetables of the cruciferous family isolate the anticarcinogenic constituents of *Brassica* plants. Glucosinolates (appearing in cruciferous vegetables) can inhibit, retard, or even reverse experimental multistage carcinogenesis.[705] As enzymatic processes hydrolyze glucosinolates, isothiocyanates are released, including sulphoraphane. Sulphoraphane wields a strong arm against cancer, promoting apoptosis, inducing phase 2 detoxification enzymes, increasing p53 and participating in the regulatory mechanisms of the cell's growth cycle. Necrosis (localized death of diseased tissues) is typically observed after prolonged exposure to elevated doses of sulphoraphane.

For the past several years, researchers at Johns Hopkins University have urged the inclusion of broccoli sprouts in the diet. According to Paul Talalay, broccoli sprouts have 20–50 times more anticancer sulphoraphanes than grown vegetables.[706] Eating a few tablespoons of sprouts daily can supply the same amount of chemoprotection as 1–2 pounds of broccoli eaten weekly.[707]

Broccoli sprouts contain a chemical that kills *H. pylori*, even in antibiotic-resistant conditions. The release of anticarcinogenic chemicals from *Brassica* vegetables is a sequential process that occurs as the plant tissue is broken down. Indole-3-carbinol (I3C), a product of cruciferous metabolism, is referred to as a secondary metabolite, meaning it is not found in a preformed state in the vegetables. Rather, I3C is formed after myrosinase (an enzyme inherent to the plant) is exposed to a phytochemical in the vegetable (glucobrassicin), a glucosinolate that subsequently delivers I3C. This occurs only when vegetable cells are crushed or eaten, a process known as enzymatic hydrolysis. I3C, thus formed, is then broken down in the presence of stomach acid to various byproducts including diindolylmethane (DIM), another powerful defense against cancer.[708] It appears highly possible that the breakdown products of I3C may be delivering as much protection as I3C itself.[708–710]

An undesirable effect is the conversion of estrone to a carcinogenic material called 16-alpha hydroxyestrone that damages DNA and inhibits apoptosis. The ratio of 2-hydroxyestrone to 16-hydroxyestrone indicates a woman's risk for developing breast and ovarian cancer. Levels of 2-hydroxyestrone are typically higher in women who do not get cancer; 16-hydroxyestrone is higher in women with cancer. When breast cancer cells are treated with I3C (in vitro), 90% of cells undergo growth inhibition, whether the cells are estrogen positive or negative.[108]

Broccoli (500 g for 12 days) increased the average 2-alpha-hydroxyestrone:16-alpha-hydroxyestrone ratio.[711] Hence, consuming vegetables rich in I3C gives hope that as 2-hydroxyestrone increases, cancers will be decreased in both men and women. The ability of I3C to neutralize estrogen metabolites as well as to block aflatoxin (a mycotoxin that promotes prostate cancer) makes cruciferous vegetables equally important to men.

By inhibiting protein kinases and other growth factors, restoring p21 activity, and encouraging apoptosis, I3C appears an effective chemopreventive/

therapeutic agent against many types of malignancies.[712,713] Evidencing its benefits, I3C reduced the incidence of cervical cancer from 76% to 8% in laboratory mice,[714] and administered together with tamoxifen, I3C inhibited the growth of estrogen-dependent human MCF-7 breast cancer more effectively than either agent used alone.[715]

If vegetables providing I3C are in short supply in the diet, I3C capsules are available. For those under 120 pounds, one 200-mg capsule taken 2 times a day is suggested; those at 120–180 pounds could take 200 mg 3 times a day, while those over 180 pounds could take four 200-mg capsules a day.

## Cholesterol (Can It Be Too Low?)

Hypocholesterolemia (abnormally low levels of cholesterol) has been shown in several epidemiologic studies to be related to increased mortality from human cancer. Cholesterol and triglyceride levels in 135 patients with squamous cell and small cell lung carcinoma were evaluated. All lung cancer patients had higher rates of hypocholesterolemia as well as lower triglyceride levels compared to a healthy control group. Total cholesterol concentrations were lower in both histological types, but triglyceride levels were lower only in patients with squamous cell lung cancer.[716]

An article in *Hematology and Oncology* reported that 90% of 83 patients with acute myeloid leukemia were hypocholesterolemic.[717] Additionally, another article in the *European Journal of Haematology* reported that remission in acute myelogenous leukemia was associated with a significant increase in cholesterol levels in those patients with low cholesterol concentrations or high leukocyte counts at diagnosis.[718]

Various reports have emerged showing that low cholesterol levels are associated with higher death rates (particularly among elderly people), from cancer and infection.[719,720] These findings raise concerns regarding hypocholesterolemic drug therapy and diet manipulation to drastically lower cholesterol levels in a subset of the population.

## STRESS AND CANCER

Few events are as stressful as a diagnosis of cancer. As the stress level increases, the outpouring of the adrenal cortex hormone (cortisol) also increases. Women with breast cancer who had abnormal cortisol rhythms survived an average of 3.2 years, while those with normal rhythms survived an average of 4.5 years (more than a year longer). The difference in survival times began to emerge about 1 year after the cortisol testing and continued for at least 6 additional years.[721]

Animal studies, mostly involving rats, demonstrated stress as a causal factor in cancer. The onset of cancer appears similarly allied in humans, with the immune system highly responsive to emotional pitfalls. It is well established that when the individual is emotionally challenged, cancer has a significant advantage.[722]

Psychobiologist Shamgar Ben-Eliyahu has been working for the past decade on stress, tumor development, and the activity of NK cells.[723] Considering all immune system cells, NK cells show the strongest activity in preventing metastasis and the strongest response to stress. Even short-term stress decreases NK-cell activity in laboratory animals, significantly increasing the risk of certain types of cancer and metastasis. Gender plays a significant role in the NK cell response to stress, with men more adversely affected than women.[724] The stress of abdominal surgery promotes the growth of cancerous tumors in rats, a sequence thought to be orchestrated by NK cell suppression.[725]

High levels of neuropeptide-gamma are observed in the bloodstream of depressed individuals, an elevation synonymous with immune suppression.[726,727] Macrophages (pathogen scavengers) have receptor sites that attract endorphins (mood enhancers with analgesic traits). With the right emotional programming, white blood cells swim through the bloodstream with determination; conversely, under stress, immune competence falters, and the immune attack becomes lethargic.

Breast cancer patients with the most anxiety had a weaker immune response and were less equipped to fight the disease. The following stress-associated situations and personality types are associated with breast cancer: (1) use of denial or repression as a coping strategy, (2) an experience of separation or loss, (3) history of stressful life experiences, (4) tendency toward melancholy and hopelessness (this trait has, since antiquity, been associated with uterine and breast cancers), and (5) a personality type characterized by conflict avoidance. It is theorized that the genes that cause one to avoid conflict are the same genes that increase susceptibility to cancer.[728,729]

Also, psychological stress induces the production of proinflammatory cytokines, such as TNF-α, IL-6, and IL-10,[231] which play a role in malignancies.

The effect of chronic stress on the immune system of 116 recently treated breast cancer patients found (reproducibly) that stress levels significantly predicted (1) lower NK cell activity, (2) diminished response of NK cells to interferon-gamma, and (3) decreased proliferation of lymphocytes (ie, white

blood cells considered the army of the immune system.)[730] Oncologists often suggest stress management (eg, meditation, yoga and breathing exercises, guided imagery, or spirituality) to help bring about calm.

Because the cells responsible for cancer surveillance work best in an environment favoring confidence and calm, it is important that the message springing from our thoughts and transmitted to cells is commensurate with healing. Fright, pessimism, and melancholy send uncertain instructions and the cells respond with a feeble effort. The enduring message (fear or assurance, despair or hopefulness, laughter or tears) reflects our hour-to-hour psyche and sets the tone for health victories or failures. Expect little more from your body than the quality of your thoughts at this very moment: "As a man thinks in his heart, so is he" (Proverbs 23:7).

## SUMMARY

The drugs, hormones, and nutrients discussed in this protocol have documented mechanisms of action that may benefit the cancer patient. The objective of implementing an adjuvant regimen consisting of multiple agents is to increase the odds of achieving a long remission. Once a remission is achieved, preventing recurrence and secondary cancers becomes a lifetime commitment.

Few oncologists aggressively seek to prevent recurrence once the primary disease appears to have been eradicated. However, the regrettable facts are that colonies of cancer cells can remain dormant in the body for years or decades before reappearing as full-blown disease that is highly resistant to treatment. This has been documented in autopsy studies of people who died of diseases other than cancer but nonetheless showed significant residual metastatic tumors in their bodies.

In too many cases, breast cancer, melanoma, or other cancer reemerges that was supposed to have been cured. Scientists speculate that the body has natural anticancer control mechanisms that may diminish with age and exposure to physical and emotional stress factors. It is thus important for cancer patients to be vigilant in maintaining an inhospitable environment for cancer cells to propagate and protecting against age-associated immune dysfunction.

Table 3 summarizes several natural cancer adjuvant therapies. In addition to the agents listed here, a number of other potential adjuvant approaches are discussed in this protocol. For long-term control of cancer, some cancer patients attempt to incorporate as many of these adjuvant approaches as are tolerable

## Table 3: Cancer Adjuvant Therapy

| Nutrient | Preventive Dose | Cancer Adjuvant Dose |
|---|---|---|
| Apigenin | 10–25 mg daily | 20–50 mg daily |
| Astaxanthin | 2–4 mg daily | 6–12 mg daily |
| Astragalus | 500 mg daily | 2000–4000 mg daily |
| Blueberry | 180–450 mg daily | 900–1800 mg daily |
| Chrysin | 500 mg daily | 1000–2000 mg daily |
| Curcumin | 400 mg daily of a BCM–95® extract with food | 800–3600 mg daily of a BCM–95® extract with food |
| Coenzyme Q10 | 100 mg daily with food | 200–400 mg daily with food |
| Coffee | 400 mg, 3 times daily | 400 mg, 3 times daily |
| EPA-DHA fatty acids | 2000–4000 mg daily of fish oil concentrate supplying 700–1400 mg EPA and 500–1000mg DHA with food | 4000–8000 mg daily of fish oil concentrate supplying up to 2800 mg EPA and 2000 mg DHA with food |
| Garlic | 600 mg daily with food | 1200–4800 mg daily with food |
| Gamma tocopherol | 200–250 mg daily with food | 400–1000 mg daily with food |
| GLA (gamma-linolenic acid) | 300 mg daily with food | 700–900 mg daily with food |
| Grape seed extract | 100 mg daily | 300 mg daily |
| Green tea extract | 300–350 mg daily of EGCG | Up to 3000 mg daily of EGCG |
| Cruciferous vegetable concentrate | 1 tbsp daily | 1–4 tbsp daily |
| Indole-3-carbinol (I3C) | 80–160 mg daily | 200–600 mg daily |
| Lignans | 25–50 mg daily | 75–125 mg daily |
| Lycopene | 10 mg daily with food | 15–45 mg daily with food |
| Melatonin | 300 mcg–3 mg before bed | 10–50 mg between 8–10pm |
| Panax ginseng | 100 mg daily of standardized to contain 4–7% ginsenosides | 200–600 mg daily of standardized to contain 4–7% ginsenosides |
| Pomegranate | 80–120 mg daily of punicalagins | 280–375 mg daily of punicalagins |
| Proteolytic enzymes | 1–2 pills daily on an empty stomach of a formula containing pancreatin, papain, trypsin, and chymotrypsin | 2–10 pills, 3 times daily on an empty stomach of a formula containing pancreatin, papain, trypsin, and chymotrypsin |
| PSK (*Coriolus versicolor*) | 600–1200 mg daily of a 40% polysaccharide extract | 3000 mg daily of a 40% polysaccharide extract |
| Pterostilbene | 0.25–3 mg daily | 1–3 mg daily |
| Quercetin | 500 mg daily | 1000–3000 mg daily |
| R-dihydro-lipoic acid | 150–250 mg daily on an empty stomach | 600–1200 mg daily on an empty stomach |
| Reishi | 980 mg daily of standardized to contain 13.5% polysaccharides and 6% triterpenes | 980–3000 mg daily of standardized to contain 13.5% polysaccharides and 6% triterpenes |
| Selenium | 200 mcg daily with food | 200–600 mcg daily with food |
| Silibinin | 225 mg daily | 225–450 mg daily |
| Sulforaphane | 400–800 mg daily (broccoli extract) | 400–1600 mg daily (broccoli extract) |
| Vitamin C | 1000–3000 mg daily | 4–12 g daily |
| Vitamin D3 | 2000–10 000 IU daily with food, based on individual blood testing. Optimal blood levels of vitamin D are 50–80 ng/mL | 2000–10 000 IU daily with food, based on individual blood testing. Optimal blood levels of vitamin D are 50–80 ng/mL |

and affordable. Others pick and choose which drugs, hormones, and supplements they want to consume over the long term.

Patients should read Life Extension's other cancer protocols, with special attention given to Cancer Treatment: The Critical Factors. If surgery, radiation, or chemotherapy is being considered, please refer to these specific protocols: Cancer Surgery, Cancer Radiation, and Chemotherapy.

**Note:** *While it would be wholly inappropriate for Life Extension to steer individuals in decisions of omission or commission regarding therapies, it would be equally improper to shun responsibility. Because we are challenged by a professional and moral commitment to assist in overcoming appalling statistics, we have discussed some controversial issues in this protocol. We look forward to new findings to better substantiate optimal therapeutic approaches.*

## STAYING INFORMED

This cancer protocol raises many issues that are subject to change as new data emerge. Furthermore, cancer is still a disease with unacceptably high mortality rates, and none of our suggested treatment regimens can guarantee a cure.

Life Extension is constantly uncovering information to provide the cancer patient with more ammunition to battle their disease. A special website has been established for the purpose of updating patients on new findings that directly pertain to the cancer protocols published in this book. Whenever Life Extension discovers information that points to a better way of treating cancer, it will be posted on the website, www.lefcancer.org.

Before utilizing the cancer protocols in this book, we suggest that you log on to www.lefcancer.org to see if any substantive changes have been made to the recommendations described in this protocol. Based on the sheer number of newly published findings, there could be significant alterations to the information you have just read.

Alternatively, call 1-800-226-2370 and ask a health advisor if your topic of interest has been updated on the website, www.lefcancer.org.

## REFERENCES

References available at: www.lef.org/dpt5/ch29

# 30

---

# *Cancer Radiation Therapy*

---

Along with surgery and chemotherapy, radiation therapy (radiotherapy) is one of the most important methods of cancer treatment. At least 50% of all cancer patients will receive radiotherapy at some stage during the course of their illness. It is currently used to treat localized solid tumors, such as cancers of the skin, brain, breast, or cervix, and can also be used to treat leukemia and lymphoma.[1]

Most types of radiation do not attack cancer cells specifically, and therefore cause injury to normal tissues surrounding the tumor. The adverse effects are a major factor limiting the success of radiation treatment. However, proton therapy and CyberKnife® therapy are technologically advanced forms of radiotherapy that cause little damage to normal tissue because they focus intensely on the tumor.

The effectiveness of radiation therapy can be enhanced by both radiosensitizers, such as genistein, curcumin, green tea, and hyperthermia, and radioprotectors, such as ginseng, glutathione, whey protein, and shark liver oil. Overall, the use of specific nutritional supplements, drugs, and other strategies may prevent and help alleviate and treat the side effects caused by radiation, thereby improving the effectiveness of radiotherapy.

## PRINCIPLES OF RADIATION THERAPY (RADIOTHERAPY)

Radiation therapy is the treatment of cancer with ionizing radiation. Radiation works by damaging the DNA (genetic material) within the tumor cells, making them unable to divide and grow. Radiation is often given with the intent of destroying the tumor and curing the disease (curative treatment). However, although radiation is directed at the tumor, it is inevitable that the normal, noncancerous tissues surrounding the tumor will also be damaged by the radiation.[2] The goal of radiation therapy is to maximize the dose to tumor cells while minimizing exposure to normal, healthy cells.[3]

Because no single therapy can provide complete treatment for a patient with a solid tumor, radiotherapy is often used in combination with surgery or chemotherapy to improve the chances of a successful treatment outcome. Sometimes radiation is used to relieve symptoms, such as pain or seizures; this is called palliative treatment.[4]

## WHAT IS IONIZING RADIATION?

Radiation used for cancer treatment is called ionizing radiation because it forms ions (ie, atoms that have acquired an electric charge through the gain or loss of an electron) as it passes through a tissue.[5] Ions can cause cell death or genetic change either directly or indirectly. The direct effect causes a change in the molecular structure of biologically important molecules, most likely DNA. The indirect action of radiation occurs when it interacts with water molecules in the cells, resulting in the production of highly reactive and unstable free radicals or reactive oxygen species (ROS), which immediately react with any biomolecules in the surrounding area, producing cellular damage.[6]

This damage can lead to cell death by 2 mechanisms.[7] The first process, known as apoptosis, results in cell death within a few hours of radiation.[8] The second mechanism is radiation-induced failure of cell division and the inhibition of cellular proliferation, which in turn leads to cell death. Several enzymatic and nonenzymatic antioxidant defense mechanisms exist in cells and prevent excessive damage through the scavenging and inactivation of these ROS.[9]

## TYPES OF RADIATION THERAPY

### External Beam Radiation Therapy

External beam radiation therapy (EBRT) creates a radiation beam and aims it at the tumor. The radiation adequately covers the tumor but minimizes the dose to the nontumor normal tissues. Radiation is given in fractions rather than as a single dose, and the use of this fractionated radiotherapy allows normal cells time to repair between each radiation session, protecting them from injury.

Conventional fractionation in the United States is 1.8–2 Gray (Gy) per day, administered 5 days a week for 5–7 weeks, depending on the particular clinical situation. (The Gray is a unit of measure of absorbed radiation dose.) While this schedule is strictly for the convenience of physicians trying to maintain a normal work week, the relatively long intervals between doses of radiation may allow cancer cells (as well as normal cells) to recover and regrow.

A number of different radiotherapy schedules have been suggested to overcome this problem.[10] In hyperfractionation, the time between fractions is reduced from 24 hours to 6–8 hours to enhance the toxic effects on tumor cells,[11] while still preserving an adequate time interval for the recovery of normal cells. Continuous hyperfractionated accelerated radiation therapy (CHART) is an intense schedule of treatment, in which multiple daily fractions are administered within a short period of time. Clinical studies have shown benefits of altered fractionation over conventional treatment for several cancers, including head and neck cancer[12] and nonoperable lung cancer.[13]

## Proton Beam Radiation Therapy

This is one of the most precise and sophisticated forms of external beam radiation therapy available. The advantage of proton radiation therapy over x-rays is its ability to deliver higher doses of shaped beams of radiation directly into the tumor while minimizing the dose to normal tissues. This leads to reduced side effects and improved survival rates.[14] As of 2002, more than 32 000 patients around the world had received part or all of their radiation treatment by proton beams.

There are approximately 19 proton treatment centers worldwide. Two major hospital-based facilities in the United States that regularly treat patients with proton beams (often fractionated) are Loma Linda University Medical Center in southern California (LLUMC Proton Treatment Center) and the Northeast Proton Treatment Center at Massachusetts General Hospital in Boston. The IU Health Proton Therapy Center (formerly Midwest Proton Radiotherapy Institute) in Bloomington, Indiana (http://iuhealthprotontherapy.org/) treats children and adults with certain brain tumors, as well as those with tumors that are close to vital organs and therefore cannot be treated successfully using traditional methods.

The efficacy of proton beam radiation therapy has been clinically proven[15] in prostate,[16,17] lung,[18] hepatocellular,[19] and uveal melanoma[20-22]; sarcomas of the skull base and cervical spine[23]; optic pathway gliomas[24]; astrocytomas[25]; benign meningioma[26]; nonresectable rectal, esophageal,[27] and liver cancers[28]; head and neck cancers, including thyroid cancer[29,30]; and more.

## Intensity-Modulated Radiation Therapy

Intensity-modulated radiation therapy (IMRT) creates a shaped radiation beam, delivering high doses of radiation to the tumor and significantly smaller doses of radiation to the surrounding normal tissues.[31,32] This may result in a higher cancer-control rate and a lower rate of side effects.[33,34]

IMRT has been used successfully in the treatment of several types of cancer, including prostate,[35] cervical,[36] nasopharyngeal,[37] and pediatric cancers.[38]

## Brachytherapy

Brachytherapy can be used for many types of cancers, but it is most commonly used to treat prostate cancer[39] and gynecologic cancers, such as cervical or uterine cancer.[40] Brachytherapy usually involves the insertion of devices around or within the tumor to hold radioactive sources or seeds. Radioactive isotopes, such as cesium, are then inserted into the delivery device, either temporarily or permanently, allowing for the slow delivery of a high dose of radiation to the interior of the tumor.[41]

## Radioimmunotherapy

Radioimmunotherapy (RIT), one of the newest developments in the treatment of non-Hodgkin's lymphoma,[42] has achieved a high tumor response rate (up to 80%) in several clinical trials.[43] Radioimmunotherapy uses drugs called monoclonal antibodies, which have a radioactive isotope attached to them. This is targeted to the surface of a cancer cell, destroying it. Radioimmunotherapy can be used (in a targeted fashion) to treat single cells that have spread around the body.[44] Because the radiation does not concentrate in any one area of the body, radioimmunotherapy does not cause side effects commonly seen with external beam radiation therapy. The most significant side effect associated with radioimmunotherapy may be a temporary drop in white blood cell or platelet count.[45]

## Stereotactic Body Radiation Therapy

Stereotactic body radiation therapy (SBRT) is a standard form of treatment for primary and metastatic brain cancer.[46] It is delivered using a machine called a gamma knife, which uses converging beams of gamma radiation that meet at a central point within the tumor, where they add up to a very high, precisely focused dose of radiation in a single fraction. Due to this precision, the cancer can be located in an area of the brain or spinal cord that might normally be considered inoperable.[47]

## CyberKnife®

CyberKnife® is a noninvasive, precise radiation technique that can deliver concentrated and accurate beams of radiation to any site in the body. This system combines robotics and advanced image guidance cameras to locate the tumor's position in the body and deliver highly focused beams of radiation that converge at the tumor, avoiding normal tissue. It is a successful method used to treat spinal tumors[48] or tumors at other critical locations that are not amenable to open surgery or radiation, as well as to treat medically inoperable patients.[49] It can also be used to treat benign tumors and lesions in a previously irradiated site, or to boost standard radiotherapy.[50,51]

## Three-Dimensional Conformal Radiation Therapy

Three-dimensional conformal radiation therapy (3D-CRT) is a technique that uses imaging computers to precisely map the location of a tumor.[52] The patient is fitted with a plastic mold or cast to keep the body part still so that the radiation can be aimed more accurately from several directions. By aiming the radiation more precisely at the tumor, it is possible to reduce radiation damage to normal tissues surrounding the tumor by up to 50%.[53]

# RADIATION THERAPY VERSUS MEDICAL X-RAYS (DIAGNOSTIC IMAGING)

Although diagnostic x-rays provide great benefits, including the earlier detection of cancers and the possibility of early treatment, their use is associated with small increases in cancer risk.[54] One study estimated that cancer risk due to diagnostic x-rays varied 0.6–3% in the 15 developed countries studied.[55]

Therefore, it is prudent to avoid unnecessary x-ray procedures. Up to 30% of chest x-rays may not be necessary.[56] Unnecessary computed tomography (CT) examinations may result in increased radiation exposure.[57,58] The cumulative risk of cancer mortality from CT examinations in the United States is about 800 radiation-induced cancer deaths per 1 million examinations in children under the age of 15.[59]

Mammography (chest x-ray) uses low-dose x-rays to create a detailed image of the breasts. Although there is some controversy regarding mammography's effectiveness in reducing breast cancer mortality, successful treatment is linked to early diagnosis, as mammography can often show changes in the breast before they can be detected by manual examination.[60]

The effective radiation dose from a mammogram is about the same as the average person receives from background radiation over a 3-month period.[61]

At present, the consensus view is that the benefits of screening women over 50 years of age with yearly or twice-yearly mammograms substantially outweighs the associated risks due to radiation exposure.[62] However, there appears to be no significant benefit for women under the age of 40, and there may be harm for women under 30 due to the danger of cancer developing after exposure to radiation.[63] Therefore, the main area of controversy concerns women between the ages of 40 and 49.

## Typical Effective Doses From Diagnostic Medical Exposures in the 1990s

| Diagnostic Procedure | Typical Effective Dose in Millisieverts (mSv) | Equivalent Number of Chest X-rays | Approximate Equivalent Period of Natural Background Radiation* |
|---|---|---|---|
| **X-ray examinations:** | | | |
| Limbs and joints (except hip) | <0.01 | <0.5 | <1.5 days |
| Chest (single PA film) | 0.02 | 1 | 3 days |
| Skull | 0.07 | 3.5 | 11 days |
| Thoracic spine | 0.7 | 35 | 4 months |
| Lumbar spine | 1.3 | 65 | 7 months |
| Hip | 0.3 | 15 | 7 weeks |
| Pelvis | 0.7 | 35 | 4 months |
| Abdomen | 1.0 | 50 | 6 months |
| Intravenous urogram (IVU) | 2.5 | 125 | 14 months |
| Barium swallow | 1.5 | 75 | 8 months |
| Barium meal | 3 | 150 | 16 months |
| Barium follow-through | 3 | 150 | 16 months |
| Barium enema | 7 | 350 | 3.2 years |
| CT head | 2.3 | 115 | 1 year |
| CT chest | 8 | 400 | 3.6 years |
| CT abdomen or pelvis | 10 | 500 | 4.5 years |

*(Continued)*

Typical Effective Doses From Diagnostic Medical Exposures in the 1990s—cont'd

| Diagnostic Procedure | Typical Effective Dose in Millisieverts (mSv) | Equivalent Number of Chest X-rays | Approximate Equivalent Period of Natural Background Radiation* |
|---|---|---|---|
| **Radionuclide studies:** | | | |
| Lung ventilation (Xe-133) | 0.3 | 15 | 7 weeks |
| Lung perfusion (Tc-99m) | 1 | 50 | 6 months |
| Kidney (Tc-99m) | 1 | 50 | 6 months |
| Thyroid (Tc-99m) | 1 | 50 | 6 months |
| Bone (Tc-99m) | 4 | 200 | 1.8 years |
| Dynamic cardiac (Tc-99m) | 6 | 300 | 2.7 years |
| PET head (F-18 FDG) | 5 | 250 | 2.3 years |

*In the United Kingdom, average background radiation = 2.2 mSv per year. Regional averages range from 1.5 to 7.5 mSv per year.*

# RADIATION: A CAUSE OF CANCER?

The link between radiation and cancer was first recognized by studying atomic bomb survivors in Japan.[64] Some cases of leukemia are related to radiation exposure and usually develop within a few years of exposure, peaking at 5–9 years after exposure, then slowly declining.[54,64] The development of other types of cancer after radiation exposure can take much longer to occur. Most cancers do not occur until 10 years after radiation exposure and some are diagnosed 15 or more years later.[65]

## WHAT YOU HAVE LEARNED SO FAR

- Radiation therapy is one of the primary methods currently used to treat cancer.
- Radiation therapy involves targeting the tumor with a beam of ionizing radiation, leading to the death of tumor cells through either the production of ROS or from direct DNA damage.
- Radiation cannot selectively target the tumor; therefore, normal cells within the radiation field suffer damage, leading to potentially serious side effects.[66]
- Ionizing radiation is used in many diagnostic techniques, such as mammography and CT scans.
- Radiation is a potent carcinogen that can give rise to a second radiation-induced cancer.

# STRATEGIES TO OPTIMIZE RADIOTHERAPY RESPONSE

## Tumor Gene Analysis

An examination of the genetic material of tumor cells often reveals differences between the cells that can be manipulated therapeutically. For example, the tumor suppressor gene p53 is the most frequently mutated gene in human tumors,[67] and tumors containing wild type p53 (p53 that is not mutated) are associated with a significantly better prognosis when treated with radiation.[68,69] However, this is not a universal finding.[70]

Results of the largest known biomarker study of prostate cancer patients treated with radiation therapy indicate that the presence of a protein biomarker called Ki-67 is a significant predictor of outcome in men treated with both radiation and hormones.[71] When a tumor cell tests positive for Ki-67, the tumor is actively growing, and the greater the proportion of prostate tumor cells with Ki-67, the more aggressive the cancer.[72] Ki-67 can be measured by a test offered by Genzyme Genetics (www.GenzymeGenetics.com).

## Guarding Against Anemia

Anemia is one of the most common blood abnormalities of cancer. In patients with solid tumors, the incidence of anemia has been reported to vary between 45% in those with colon cancer up to 90% in patients with small-cell lung cancer.[73] An association between hemoglobin level and controlling tumor growth and survival has been identified for a large number of cancers, including breast,[74] cervical,[75] and head and neck cancers.[76]

Cancer patients with low hemoglobin levels do not respond as well to radiotherapy as nonanemic patients[77] due to impairment of oxygen transport to tumor cells.[78] Hemoglobin values measured during treatment are believed to be predictive of outcome.[79]

Treatment outcome might be improved by correcting anemia (low hemoglobin levels).[80] Nutritional supplements that may help correct anemia include melatonin, folic acid, and vitamin B12; for more information, refer to the Blood Disorders (Anemia, Leukopenia, and Thrombocytopenia) protocol. The use of erythropoietin (sold under the drug brand name Procrit®) with minimal iron supplementation,[81] or blood transfusions[82] may be required in some cases. Erythropoietin is a growth factor that produces a steady, sustained increase in hemoglobin levels.[83,84]

## Measurement of Tumor Oxygen Levels

Low tumor oxygen levels (hypoxia) and anemia in the patient are associated with increased risk of spread (metastasis) and recurrence,[85,86] especially for cervical cancers, head and neck cancers, and soft tissue sarcomas.[87,88] Hypoxia presents a problem for radiotherapy because radiation's ability to kill cancer cells (ie, radiosensitivity) rapidly decreases in areas of oxygen depletion, as free radicals cannot be produced due to limited oxygen supply.[89]

Tumor oxygen levels are usually measured by the use of electrodes inserted directly into the tumor.[90,91] If a tumor is found to be hypoxic, strategies to improve oxygen levels could be employed to improve radiotherapy,[92] or alternatively, radiotherapy may be reconsidered.

Tumor hypoxia has been exploited in cancer treatment.[93] A number of chemical agents, such as misonidazole, that preferentially sensitize hypoxic cells to radiation have been developed and tested in the clinic, particularly for the treatment of head and neck cancers.[94] However, some have poor clinical effectiveness.[95] A number of approaches (eg, carbogen and nicotinamide [ARCON]) have been introduced and are now in clinical trials.[96]

Hypoxia is also implicated in the activation of angiogenic cytokines—especially vascular endothelial growth factor (VEGF)—that are necessary for the growth of new tumor blood vessels,[86,97] and thus tumor growth. Angiogenic inhibitors seek to interrupt the process of angiogenesis (the creation of new blood vessels) to prevent new tumor blood vessel formation, whereas vascular (blood vessel)-disrupting agents aim to cause direct damage to the existing tumor blood supply.[98] Lead agents of both categories (eg, Combretastatin A-4) have now advanced into clinical trials.[99]

Silymarin/silibinin inhibits VEGF secretion in a range of human cancer cell lines, in concentrations that should be clinically feasible.[100] Other naturally derived agents that impede cancer-induced angiogenesis include green tea polyphenols, fish oil, selenium, copper restriction, and curcumin.[101]

## Hyperbaric Oxygen Therapy

Following the identification of hypoxia as a possible source of radiation resistance, a major effort was made to solve the problem through the use of hyperbaric oxygen. Hyperbaric oxygen therapy (HBOT) is a mode of therapy in which the patient breathes pure, 100% oxygen at pressures 2–3 times greater than normal atmospheric pressure.[102] The concentration of oxygen normally dissolved in the bloodstream is thus raised many times above normal (up to 2000%).

This hyperoxygenation provides immediate support to poorly perfused tumor tissue in areas of compromised blood flow.[103] These include radiation-damaged tissue that has lost blood supply and is oxygen deprived due to scarring and narrowing of the blood vessels within the area treated.[104] Healing is dependent on oxygen delivery to the injured tissues, and HBOT provides a better healing environment, leads to the growth of new blood vessels, and also helps to eradicate anaerobic bacteria that may cause infection via toxin inhibition and inactivation.[104,105]

Hyperbaric oxygen has been used to treat normal tissue injury caused by radiation therapy in several sites, including the head and neck,[106] pelvis,[107] breast,[108] prostate,[109] and brain,[110] with few serious side effects.

In a study of 45 patients with radiation-induced late side effects, the majority showed improvement in their condition after either HBOT alone or HBOT followed by other surgical or medical procedures.[111] In particular, osteoradionecrosis (necrosis, or death of the bone following radiotherapy) appeared to be highly responsive to HBOT.[112] This condition usually involves the lower jaw in a minority (8%) of head and neck cancer patients treated with radiation therapy, is difficult to treat, leads to intense pain and fracture, and makes oral feeding impossible.[113]

However, the use of HBOT is not widespread, partly because it is cumbersome and difficult in practice and partly because many of the studies to date have involved small numbers of patients.[114,115] Larger trials are needed to investigate the true efficacy of HBOT.

## Breathing Oxygen During Radiotherapy

The inhalation of oxygen during radiotherapy may increase the radiation kill effect on the tumor by counteracting areas of hypoxia-based radioresistance, and thus improve overall survival. Stage 2 cervical cancer patients, with squamous cell carcinoma, who received oxygen (normobaric) during all radiotherapy sessions had significantly improved loco-regional cancer control.[116]

Patients with stage 3 (7%) and stage 4 (93%) advanced squamous cell carcinomas of the head and neck who breathed pure, normobaric oxygen for 15–20 minutes during irradiation had improved mean survival time (15.8 versus 11.8 months) and 3-year survival (19% versus 2%), respectively ($p < 0.05$). Thus, breathing normobaric oxygen before and during radiation therapy could increase the effectiveness of conventional radiotherapy for advanced squamous cell carcinomas of the head and neck.[117]

## Radioprotectors/Radiosensitizers

Researchers are investigating 2 types of drugs that may increase the effectiveness of radiation therapy.[118] Radiosensitizers make tumor cells more susceptible to radiation damage, while radioprotectors protect normal tissues from the damaging effects of radiation, allowing a higher dose of radiation to be directed at the tumor.

Radiosensitizers are chemicals that increase the damaging effects of radiation if administered simultaneously. Two types of radiosensitizers have been used in conjunction with radiation therapy:

1. *Halogenated pyrimidines,* such as bromodeoxyuridine, which depend on the amount of drug incorporated in the cell.[119] As tumor cells divide more rapidly than the surrounding normal cells, they take up more of the radiosensitizer.

2. *Hypoxic cell sensitizers,* which increase the radiosensitivity of only those cells located in areas of low oxygen.[120] As many tumors contain large regions of hypoxic cells compared to normal tissues, these drugs are able to produce a differential effect, that is, they are toxic to hypoxic cells only.

**Amifostine.** Amifostine (Ethyol®) has been approved by the Food and Drug Administration (FDA) specifically for use as a radioprotector. It is approved for the prevention of xerostomia (dry mouth) in head and neck cancer patients treated with radiation therapy.[121] Adequate hydration is critical before amifostine administration (given intravenously once daily as a 3-minute infusion starting 15–30 minutes before standard fraction radiation therapy).

The 2 major side effects of amifostine that cause treatment discontinuation are vomiting and transient low blood pressure (hypotension),[122] and these adverse effects limit its wide acceptance.

**Ginseng.** Ginseng has several beneficial effects on blood vessels.[123] In experimental studies, ginseng was shown to be a promising radioprotector,[124] that is, it may protect normal healthy tissue from damage during radiation therapy.[125,126] In a clinical study, ginseng polysaccharide injection improved immune function in nasopharyngeal carcinoma patients during radiotherapy.[127]

**Glutathione.** Glutathione is a natural antioxidant synthesized from the amino acids glutamine, cysteine, and glycine.[128] A severe reduction in glutathione content can predispose cells to oxidative damage. When tumor cells are irradiated, either lethal damage can occur and the cells die, or the damage can be modified via DNA repair and not lead to permanent cell death.

Cancer cells have higher glutathione levels than the surrounding normal healthy cells. Therefore, selective tumor depletion of glutathione presents a promising strategy in cancer management. Dietary glutamine supplementation lowers glutathione levels in tumor cells,[129,130] but increases production in normal tissues. Furthermore, glutamine supplementation decreases the toxicity of radiation therapy.[131,132]

**Whey protein.** Whey protein is an effective and safe cysteine donor for glutathione replenishment.[129,133] Radiation therapy is known to cause immunosuppression.[134] Cysteine is the critical limiting amino acid for intracellular glutathione synthesis.[135] The amino acid precursors to glutathione present in whey might increase glutathione concentration in relevant tissues, stimulate immunity, and detoxify potential carcinogens.[135] Glutathione stimulation is thought to be whey's primary immune-modulating mechanism.[136]

**Alkylglycerols.** Alkylglycerols are active ingredients of shark liver oil. They have been widely used for the treatment of cancer in Scandinavian countries,[137] and research suggests their use may result in a lower incidence of normal tissue radiation damage.[138] Although their protective mechanism is not fully understood,[139] they cause increased tumor cell death (apoptosis) and have many beneficial effects on the immune system, including the stimulation of neutrophils and macrophages.[140] Doses of shark liver oil up to 100 mg, 3 times daily can be taken with no unfavorable side effects.[141]

**Hyperthermia with radiotherapy.** Hyperthermia is the artificial elevation of the temperature of a tissue. Tumor cells can be selectively killed by temperatures of 40–44°C as compared with normal cells[142] because of improved tissue oxygenation and a consequent temporary increase in radiosensitivity.[143]

Numerous studies have shown that the combination of hyperthermia and radiation therapy improves clinical outcomes, particularly in breast cancer, melanoma, head and neck tumors, cervical cancer, and glioblastoma.[144]

Normal tissue toxicity with hyperthermia only results if the tissue temperature exceeds 44 °C for more than 1 hour.[145] The toxicity from superficial hyperthermia is usually a skin burn; for deep-seated tumors, a subcutaneous fat or muscle burn may occur, which heals spontaneously.[142]

**Phytochemicals.** Phytochemicals such as epigallocatechin-3 gallate (EGCG) found in green tea, curcumin, and genistein have been shown to enhance the radiation-induced death of cancer cells in addition to restraining tumor growth in animal models.[146,147] They also have antioxidant properties and can therefore neutralize the detrimental effects of ROS on normal cells.[148]

**EGCG.** EGCG (mainly derived from green tea) may increase the efficacy of radiation therapy by decreasing the activity of VEGF.[149] VEGF acts as a crucial survival factor for tumor cells.[150]

**Soy isoflavones.** Soy isoflavones, including genistein, daidzein, and glycitin (mainly derived from soybean), have been found to slow cancer growth in experimental animal studies.[147] Genistein significantly enhances the radiation effect (that is, acts as a radiosensitizer) for cervical cancer cells.[151]

**Sulforaphane.** Sulforaphane, which is an isothiocyanate, is most highly concentrated in broccoli as well as in other cruciferous vegetables (eg, Brussels sprouts, cabbage, and cauliflower). When head and neck cancer cells were treated with sulforaphane and subsequently irradiated, researchers observed that the combination therapy resulted in a stronger inhibition of cell proliferation than each treatment method alone.[152]

**Curcumin.** Curcumin, a natural antiproliferative compound for many types of tumor, is extracted from the spice turmeric.[153] Curcumin blocks the nuclear factor-kappa beta (NF-κB) activation process.[154] The maintenance of appropriate levels of NF-κB activity is crucial for normal cell division, and NF-κB activation is involved in the enhanced growth properties observed in several cancers.[155] Curcumin can sensitize squamous cell carcinoma cells to the ionizing effects of radiation.[156] In prostate cancer cell lines, curcumin is a potent radiosensitizer and acts by overcoming the effects of radiation-induced prosurvival gene (bcl-2) expression.[157]

# PREVENTING AND COUNTERACTING ADVERSE EFFECTS OF RADIOTHERAPY

## Antioxidant Use and Radiation Therapy

A survey of cancer patients found that 63% use vitamins and herbs (including antioxidants), and the majority combine them with conventional therapies.[158] Critics argue that excessive nutrient-derived antioxidant use during radiation therapy could, in theory, protect cancer cells against the damaging effects of ROS or oxidants, which are formed by radiation. This could occur by the antioxidants directly scavenging ROS or repairing cellular damage in tumor cells.[159] However, this theory has never been confirmed by clinical studies, and antioxidants can have protective effects that have nothing to do with oxidation.[160]

Furthermore, there is no controversy surrounding physician-prescribed antioxidants such as amifostine (Ethyol®), an FDA-approved orphan drug for the prevention of xerostomia (dry mouth) in head and neck cancer patients undergoing radiation treatment. Amifostine has been clearly shown to reduce the incidence of side effects (xerostomia and mucositis) in patients receiving head and neck irradiation.[161] It has also been used in combination with radiation therapy in the treatment of lung, prostate, breast, cervical, and esophageal cancer patients, with much success. The problem with amifostine is that it causes intolerable nausea, vomiting, diarrhea, and abdominal cramping, which limits its use.

Supplemental antioxidant use is further supported because they may help protect normal cells from the increased damage and side effects caused by radiation therapy.[162] Moreover, it has been shown that levels of antioxidants are decreased in cancer patients in response to radiation therapy.[163] Thus, supplementation with dietary antioxidants (such as vitamins C and E) may improve the efficacy of radiation therapy by increasing tumor response and decreasing some of its toxicity on normal cells.[164]

Dietary antioxidants (including vitamin E, vitamin C, and selenium) as well as antioxidant enzymes found within cells (eg, superoxide dismutase and glutathione peroxidase) can help maintain an appropriate balance between the desirable and undesirable effects of ROS formed by radiation therapy.[165]

In several clinical radiotherapy studies, supplementation with the antioxidants vitamin E, selenium, and melatonin during treatment was shown to improve the efficacy of radiation therapy by decreasing radiation toxicity in normal cells and enhancing the immune response.[164,166,167]

Many clinical studies (detailed herein) have shown that antioxidant supplementation (with vitamins C and E, N-acetylcysteine [NAC], glutamine, and glutathione) both before and during radiotherapy prevents normal tissue complications,[168–175] thus improving radiotherapy outcomes.

Overall, the data suggest that careful, sensible use of the antioxidants outlined herein may be helpful in improving the outcome of radiation therapy. Natural antioxidants (such as tocopherols, ascorbic acid, squalene, and lecithin) are present in most plant-based foods[176] and in fruit, fish, herbs, and cereals.[177]

**Vitamin A.** Radiation therapy effectiveness is increased when combined with vitamin A, which is thought to be due to an increased immune response against the tumor.[178] Vitamin A (8000 IU taken orally twice daily for 7 weeks) appeared to be very effective in the treatment of radiation-induced anorectal damage in a patient with human immunodeficiency virus (HIV) infection.[179]

In a randomized, double-blind trial comparing retinol palmitate (vitamin A, 10 000 IU taken orally for 90 days) to placebo, oral retinol palmitate significantly reduced the rectal symptoms of radiation proctopathy in 19 patients 6 months after pelvic radiotherapy.[180]

**Vitamin C.** Experimental studies show that radiation treatment reduces the level of vitamin C in the body.[181] Conversely, studies of mice have shown that supplementing vitamin C at high doses preferentially radiosensitizes tumors while offering some protection to normal tissues.[182]

**Vitamin E.** Vitamin E has been recognized as one of the most important antioxidants. Tocopheryl succinate (dry powder vitamin E) enhanced radiation damage to ovarian and cervical cancer cells in culture, while protecting healthy cells.[183]

Vitamin E and selenium have been reported to have an increased beneficial effect when used in combination.[184] A study of rats showed that pretreatment with both selenium and vitamin E for 4 weeks before radiation gave some protection against radiation-induced intestinal injury.

**Selenium.** A large number of selenium derivatives have been studied for their radioprotective effects.[185] Selenium is a very efficient scavenger of ROS and a radiosensitizer, with a very low toxicity profile.[186]

Supplementation with 200 mcg daily of sodium selenite for 8 weeks, beginning on the first day of standard treatment (surgery and/or radiation) for squamous cell carcinoma of the head and neck, resulted in a significantly enhanced immune response during and after therapy.[166]

**Coenzyme Q10.** Coenzyme Q10 (CoQ10), a mitochondrial enzyme, has been shown to have a therapeutic benefit in cancer patients at doses of 90–390 mg daily. A decrease in distant metastasis[187] and increase in long-term survival[188] have been noted in breast cancer patients. However, a study of mice indicated that CoQ10 reduced the effect of radiation therapy when used at a dose equivalent to 700 mg in humans; therefore, as a precaution, a dose of 100–400 mg a day should not be exceeded.[189]

**Melatonin.** Melatonin is the chief secretory hormone of the pineal gland. Melatonin reduces oxidative damage from the production of free radicals.[190] Several studies indicate that melatonin functions as a radioprotector,[191] reducing the toxic effects of radiation on mammalian cells.[192] In experiments and animal models, administration of melatonin has inhibited the growth and division of several types of cancer cells, particularly breast cancer and melanoma cells.[193,194]

Several reports indicate that melatonin administration improves quality of life for many cancer patients.[195] Patients with glioblastoma generally experience a poor survival rate, which is typically less than 6 months. A radio-neuroendocrine approach utilizing radiotherapy with melatonin supplementation (20 mg daily) in patients with untreatable glioblastoma showed that the likelihood of survival at 1 year was significantly higher in those who received melatonin with radiotherapy (6 of 14 patients alive) versus radiotherapy alone (1 of 16 patients alive).[196] A reduction in radiation-induced toxicity was also observed in the melatonin-treated group.

Melatonin reduces gamma radiation-induced primary DNA damage in human white blood cells (lymphocytes).[197] It has been suggested that supplementing with an adjuvant therapy of melatonin may benefit cancer patients who are suffering from toxic therapeutic regimens such as radiotherapy and/or chemotherapy, and may alleviate symptoms caused by radiation-induced organ injuries.[198]

## Preventing Normal Tissue Complications

The goal of radiation therapy is to deliver a precisely measured dose of ionizing radiation to a defined tumor area, with as little damage as possible to surrounding healthy, noncancerous tissue.[2] However, a number of patients undergoing radiation therapy will experience a range of side effects, which may lead to an interruption of treatment or limiting the dose of radiation.[199]

Radiation's effects on normal tissues are commonly divided into 2 categories: "early" and "late" reactions. Early, or acute effects occur within a few days or weeks of irradiation.[200] Late effects appear after a period of months or years and occur predominantly in slowly growing tissues such as the lungs, kidneys, heart, liver, and central nervous system.

The size of the radiation treatment field, the dose per fraction, and the total dose of radiation received are important factors associated with these effects.[3]

**Heart damage.** The use of 3D-conformal radiation therapy (3D-CRT) reduces the dose and volume of radiation exposure to the heart.[31] However, significant risks remain, and cardiovascular abnormalities may result following radiation therapy.[201] Hodgkin's disease survivors treated with chest radiation therapy are at increased risk of death as a result of cardiovascular disease.[202] Women treated with radiation therapy following mastectomy for left-sided breast cancer, which involves exposure of the heart, have been shown to have an increased frequency of cardiovascular disease.[203]

In a small trial of a mixture of antioxidants—including *vitamin E* (600 mg), *vitamin C* (1 g), and *NAC* (200 mg)—taken during treatment, researchers sought to determine the mixture's ability to prevent heart damage during chemotherapy and radiation therapy. No patient taking the antioxidant mixture had a decrease in ejection fraction (the amount of blood pumped out of the heart during each heartbeat) of greater than 10%. By contrast, in the control group, in which 4 of 6 patients were treated with radiation therapy and 2 of 7 patients underwent chemotherapy, the ejection fraction reduction was greater than 10%, indicative of a weakened heart.[175]

**Gastrointestinal mucositis (inflammation of the gut lining).** More than 70% of patients treated for cancer of the prostate, bladder, and other malignancies in the pelvic region develop acute inflammatory small intestinal changes.[204] Acute enteritis or proctitis (inflammation of the intestine or rectum, respectively) is characterized by diarrhea, abdominal pain, and tenesmus (fecal urgency with cramp-like rectal pain) that usually starts during the second week of radiation therapy and resolves within 2 weeks of completing treatment.[205] In 5–10% of patients, serious gastrointestinal problems may occur, including bowel obstructions and bleeding.[206]

Both *glutamine*[207] and *arginine*[208] are amino acids that have an important role in maintaining mucosal growth and function. Supplementation with these amino acids before or after abdominal irradiation appears to decrease the likelihood of both acute and chronic effects on the lower intestine,[169,171,173] but not all studies have shown benefits.[209,210] Oral glutamine supplementation may enhance radiation therapy by protecting normal tissues from (and sensitizing tumor cells to) radiation damage.[211] In one study, oral glutamine supplementation (30 g/day) reduced gut permeability

and protected lymphocytes in patients with esophageal cancer during radiochemotherapy.[212]

Patients receiving 1200 mg of intravenous *glutathione* (diluted in normal saline solution) 15 minutes before pelvic irradiation suffered less post-therapy diarrhea (28%, compared to 52% for controls) and were more likely to complete their treatment without interruption than a control group (71%, compared to 52%).[168]

Several studies have reported a positive effect of *HBOT* in patients with chronic radiation cystitis or proctitis (inflammation of the bladder or rectum, respectively).[213] Radiation-induced hemorrhagic cystitis can be treated successfully with HBOT; it is well tolerated even in patients debilitated by advanced cancer and blood loss. Long-term remission is possible in most patients, and re-treatment effectively manages recurrent bleeding.[214,215]

*Short-chain fatty acids* and *butyrate* are derived from the bacterial fermentation of unabsorbed carbohydrates within the colon.[216] They are readily absorbed in the large bowel and are beneficial in treating colitis (inflammation of the bowel).[217] A small study of 7 patients who had received previous radiation therapy (for an average of 23 months before the study) examined the use of short-chain fatty acid enemas (administered twice daily for 4 weeks) for the treatment of proctitis (inflammation of the rectum) and found a significant decrease in rectal bleeding.[218] This was confirmed in another study of 20 patients who presented with proctitis within 3 weeks of completing radiation therapy. Half were treated daily with one 80-mL sodium butyrate enema (80 mmol/L) and half with a sodium chloride placebo over a 3-week period.[219] All patients treated with butyrate reported a significant improvement in their symptoms compared to only 3 patients in the placebo group who reported a slight improvement.

**Hair loss.** Radiation therapy can cause hair loss (alopecia), but only in the area being treated.[220] Hair loss is usually temporary and regrowth is evident within a few weeks after completion of therapy.

*Melatonin* has been reported to have a beneficial effect on hair growth in animals.[221] Furthermore, a study of 40 women suffering from alopecia sought to determine whether topically applied melatonin influences hair growth. A melatonin solution (0.1%) or placebo was applied to the scalp daily for 6 months. Positive results were obtained in the melatonin-treated group.[222]

**Liver damage.** Hepatocellular carcinoma is a common malignancy, and 3D-CRT is increasingly used in treatment as part of multimodal therapy.[223] However, one of the most frequently encountered complications following such treatment is radiation-induced liver disease, occurring in approximately 18% of patients.[224] Patients present with fatigue, rapid weight gain, and in rare cases, jaundice, approximately 4–8 weeks after treatment.[225] Radiation-induced liver disease leads to the deterioration of liver function, and up to half of radiation-induced liver disease patients may die from this complication.[226]

*Silymarin*, a flavonoid complex found in the herb milk thistle, is frequently used in the treatment of liver disease.[227,228] It functions as an antioxidant,[229] maintains cellular glutathione content,[230] and has a low toxicity profile.[231] A study of rats found that an intravenous injection of silymarin (50 mg/kg) 30 minutes before a single dose of radiation protected against radiation-induced liver disease.[232] Silymarin is well tolerated and produces a small increase in glutathione and a decrease in lipid peroxidation in peripheral blood cells in certain patients.[233] Treatment with silymarin (600 mg/day) was found to reduce the lipoperoxidation of cell membranes and insulin resistance.[234]

**Hypersensitivity reactions: skin/fibrosis.** Acute radiation dermatitis (inflammation of the skin) is a common side effect of radiotherapy. Dermatitis includes redness (erythema) and dry or moist peeling skin (desquamation). It has been estimated that 87% of all women undergoing radiation therapy for breast cancer will develop some degree of radiation dermatitis.[235] Severe radiation dermatitis can be painful, may lead to infections, and can cause permanent scarring.

No standard treatment has been recommended for the prevention of radiation-induced dermatitis, although several therapies have been suggested.[236,237] Several dressing types used to treat radiation dermatitis can provide a moist healing environment that is optimal for cell migration across the wound, thereby shortening healing time.[238]

Topical agents such as corticosteroid creams and other products, including *aloe vera* gel or *trolamine* (Biafine®), are commonly prescribed at the onset of radiation dermatitis or at the beginning of radiotherapy.[239,240] Biafine® is a water-based emulsion that has been used in France since 1973 to alleviate symptoms of radiation dermatitis.[235,241]

*Calendula*, derived from the marigold flower, has purported anti-inflammatory properties and is often used for wound healing. A trial found that calendula was significantly better than Biafine® in preventing mild-to-severe acute radiation dermatitis in breast cancer patients, as well as in providing pain relief.[242] Patients applied the preparation to the irradiated skin at least twice a day at the onset of radiation therapy and continued this until completion of treatment.

In clinical trials, the application of aloe vera gel was no better than placebo or aqueous cream in reducing radiation-induced dermatitis.[243,244] However, aloe vera gel added to soap has a protective effect for patients who received higher cumulative radiation doses, prolonging the time to detectable skin damage from 3–5 weeks.[245]

*Dexpanthenol (vitamin B5) creams* have been shown to improve acute radiotherapy skin reactions in some,[246] but not all studies.[247]

NAC is capable of stimulating radioprotective cytokines.[248] The application of gauze soaked in 10% NAC for 15 minutes before radiation therapy was associated with more rapid healing of skin reactions and less use of pain relievers compared to an untreated control group.[172]

Unsaturated essential fatty acids (EFAs) are necessary for the production of prostaglandins (inflammatory modulators) and play an important role in maintaining cell membrane structure by regulating membrane fluidity.[249] The ability of EFAs containing both *gamma-linolenic acid* (GLA) and *eicosapentaenoic acid* (EPA) to modify radiation-induced skin reactions was studied in pigs.[250] Oral administration of 3 mL of oil daily for 4 weeks before and up to 16 weeks after irradiation significantly reduced both acute and late radiation skin damage. Prospective studies suggest that prostaglandins have great potential in minimizing the adverse effects of radiotherapy on normal tissue. The potential use of misoprostol, a PGE(1) analogue, before irradiation may be considered in the prevention of radiation-induced side effects.[251]

*Radiation-induced fibrosis*, a serious late effect of radiotherapy, is mainly characterized by changes in the connective tissue involving excessive extracellular matrix deposition and hyperactive fibroblasts.[252] A combination of pentoxifylline (Trental®), a methylxanthine derivative structurally related to theophylline and caffeine, and vitamin E (alpha tocopherol) may be effective in treating radiation-induced fibrosis.[253] Pentoxifylline promotes healing and relieves pain following radiation damage,[254] and vitamin E was used for its ability to scavenge ROS.[255] Twenty-two patients who developed radiation-induced fibrosis following radiotherapy for breast cancer were treated with 800 mg/day of pentoxifylline and 1000 IU/day of vitamin E. The area of radiation-induced fibrosis was significantly reduced when these patients were examined after 6 months, with no adverse effects reported.[256] For more information, see the section of this protocol on pulmonary toxicity.

**Lymphedema.** Lymphedema is an accumulation of protein-rich fluid that results in swelling of the underlying skin. It may occur in the arm following radiotherapy for breast cancer due to the interruption of axillary (armpit) lymphatic drainage or because of axillary lymph node dissection, axillary radiation, or both. It results in pain, decreased stretching ability of tissue around the joints, and increased weight of the extremity.[257] The reported incidence of lymphedema varies, with rates of 2–24% reported in a review of breast cancer patients[258] and 22–56% for the head and neck region.[259]

Several nonpharmacologic options are available for managing lymphedema,[260] including the use of graded compression garments[261] and pneumatic compression pumps.[262]

Arm exercises may also help to control the symptoms caused by lymphedema, by strengthening the muscle-pumping action and consequently increasing lymph flow. Many clinicians encourage patients to continue exercising 2–3 times a day for 6 months, then daily for life.[263] Scrupulous skin care should be followed and maintenance of an ideal body weight should be encouraged, as obesity is a contributing factor for the development of lymphedema.[264]

Clinical studies have shown a beneficial effect of *selenium* in treating lymphedema at different locations.[265,266] Forty-eight patients were evaluated either 10 months (upper limb) or 4 months (head and neck) after the end of radiotherapy. Patients received 500 mcg of sodium selenite per day over 4–6 weeks. Approximately 80% of patients showed a significant improvement in their lymphedema and quality of life.[267]

Other investigators concluded that *sodium selenite* represents a suitable adjuvant treatment of secondary lymphedema. Treatment with sodium selenite (1000 mcg daily for 3 weeks) can be instituted immediately after treatment and before wound healing when manual lymphatic decongestion therapy cannot be applied.[268]

**Kidney toxicity (nephrotoxicity).** The kidney is one of the most radiosensitive organs at risk of developing damage after abdominal irradiation. Radiation nephropathy takes various forms, the most common of which, acute radiation nephritis, presents as azotemia (dangerously high levels of nitrogen waste products in the bloodstream), hypertension, and anemia, starting at 6–12 months following treatment.[269] If left untreated, this can lead to renal failure, and survival on chronic dialysis is poor.[270]

Dietary protein restriction is effective in treating various chronic kidney diseases,[271] although care must be taken to maintain adequate nutrition.[272]

All-trans retinoic acid (a vitamin A–like drug) exacerbates radiation nephropathy, possibly by inhibiting renal nitric oxide production, and its use should be restricted during renal irradiation.[273]

**Nerve toxicity (neurotoxicity).** The nervous system is particularly sensitive to radiation therapy, and radiation-induced neurotoxicity can involve the central nervous system and peripheral nervous system.[274]

Radiation therapy for skull-base, orbital, and sinus tumors invariably involves the irradiation of brain tissue.[275] Following brain irradiation, acute toxicity may cause headaches, dizziness, fatigue, and problems with speech.[276] Corticosteroids are useful in relieving a number of these acute complications, but should be used only as long as medically necessary, as they may have side effects. Early physical therapy can prevent lymphedema, frozen shoulder, and atrophy (muscle wasting).

**Radiation necrosis.** Radiation necrosis (tissue ulceration) and cognitive dysfunction are the main late complications of brain irradiation. Radiation necrosis may occur from 6 months to 2 years following treatment,[277] and is caused primarily by blood vessel damage.[278] Up to 20% of patients receiving stereotactic radiosurgery and 80% undergoing interstitial brachytherapy will develop symptoms of radiation necrosis.[279]

This is a serious condition with symptoms that vary from fatigue to dementia, and may require surgical intervention.[280] Nonsurgical treatments that have been clinically investigated include steroids, heparin, low-iron diets with iron chelators, pentoxifylline, and HBOT.[281,282] HBOT is important in the treatment and healing of soft tissue radiation necrosis, particularly of the brain.[110,283,284]

The use of pentoxifylline is deemed safe and effective in preventing radiation necrosis, particularly in the prevention of radiation-induced lung toxicity.[285] At an oral dose of 400 mg three times daily, pentoxifylline has a protective effect against radiation necrosis complications, possibly by reducing platelet aggregation and preventing tumor necrosis factor–mediated inflammation.[286,287]

Osteoradionecrosis (see the earlier section of this protocol on hyperbaric oxygen therapy) is a late adverse effect of radiation therapy that does not resolve spontaneously. In a preliminary study, a combination of pentoxifylline (800 mg daily), tocopherol (vitamin E 1000 IU daily), and clodronate (Bonefos®, 1600 mg daily) was of clinical benefit, with more than 50% regression of progressive osteoradionecrosis observed at 6 months in 12 patients.[254,288] In another study, this same regimen completely reversed severe progressive osteoradionecrosis when administered daily for 3 years.[289]

**Oral complications.** Between sixty and ninety percent of head and neck cancer patients receiving standard radiation therapy will develop inflammation of the lining of the mouth (mucositis),[290] which usually improves within a few weeks after completing treatment.[291]

One of the most important factors that predisposes someone to oral mucositis is preexisting oral or dental disease.[292] Oral mucositis can lead to secondary complications, including infection, poor nutritional intake, and xerostomia (dry mouth). Several treatment interventions have been suggested for preventing and treating oral mucositis, although no effective treatment currently exists.[293,294]

Maintaining good oral hygiene is important in preventing mucositis, and it is particularly important to instigate this at least a week before starting radiation therapy.[295] Patients should brush twice daily with a soft-bristled tooth brush, floss daily, and rinse the mouth once daily with normal saline (1/2 teaspoon of salt in 8 oz of water) or sodium bicarbonate (baking soda or Alka-Seltzer®).[296]

A trial of head and neck cancer patients indicated that oral *glutamine* (16 g in 240 mL of normal saline, 4 times daily during radiation) may significantly reduce the duration and severity of oral mucositis during radiotherapy.[170]

*Honey* reduces the symptoms of mucositis. Forty patients diagnosed with head and neck cancer were divided into 2 groups. One group was advised to take 20 mL of pure honey 15 minutes before, 15 minutes after, and 6 hours after radiotherapy. In the honey-treated group, symptomatic mucositis was reduced significantly, and there was either no change in weight or positive weight gain compared to the control group.[297]

*Antibiotics* supplied either as a topical pastille or paste may be beneficial in preventing mucositis.[298,299] The overgrowth of certain yeast and bacteria, which occurs following radiation therapy, may be important in the progression of this condition.[300] Head and neck cancer patients who were given a pastille containing amphotericin, polymyxin, and tobramycin to suck 4 times daily were significantly less likely to develop the most serious form of mucositis than those who

received a placebo.[301] However, this beneficial finding has not been seen in all studies using antibiotics.[302,303]

Alternatively, the flower *Matricharia camomile* may be beneficial in reducing mucositis during radiotherapy[304] due to its antibacterial properties.[305] In a study in which Kamillosan® (a camomile preparation) oral rinse was given to patients receiving radiation therapy and chemotherapy, mucositis was less severe than expected.[305]

*Proteolytic enzymes* have anti-inflammatory properties and are effective in reducing normal tissue reactions such as oral[306] and gastrointestinal mucositis.[307] They function by reducing cytokine levels.[308] In one clinical study, 53 patients were given 3 tablets, 3 times a day, containing papain (100 mg), trypsin (40 mg), and chymotrypsin (40 mg). The treatment was started 3 days before radiation therapy and continued until 5 days after completion of treatment.[309] Both mucositis and skin reactions were significantly reduced in the enzyme-treated group compared to controls.

*Beta-carotene* (75 mg daily) during radiation therapy for advanced squamous cell carcinoma of the mouth markedly reduced the incidence of severe mucositis without causing noticeable side effects.[174]

Damage to the salivary glands is another common adverse effect of radiotherapy. Reduced saliva production can cause chronic dry mouth. This is a significant problem for cancer patients, with a reported prevalence of 29–77%.[310] Xerostomia can greatly impair a patient's ability to speak, chew, swallow, and taste, and therefore is often accompanied by a loss of appetite and weight, leading to adverse effects on quality of life.[311]

To manage this condition, some patients use artificial saliva substitutes, but most patients find them inadequate.[312] Salivary gland dysfunction after therapeutic radiation is a difficult, if not impossible condition to reverse, although some evidence suggests that patients with this condition should be considered for HBOT.[111] The use of noncinnamon or mint-based sugar-free drops, chewing gum, fresh pineapple chunks, or frequent sips of water to maintain adequate hydration has been suggested to stimulate salivary flow.[313]

**Poor appetite and cachexia.** Patients undergoing radiotherapy for cancer of the head and neck or gastrointestinal tract are at higher risk of developing malnutrition.[314] Malnutrition increases the risk of infections and treatment toxicities, and decreases the response to treatment.[315]

Cachexia is treated by attempting to increase nutritional intake and inhibit muscle and fat wasting. This is done by manipulating the metabolism with various pharmacologic agents and by treating the causes of reduced food intake, such as nausea and vomiting.[316] (For more information, see the protocol titled Catabolic Wasting.) Diets that include the omega-3 fatty acids *EPA* and *docosahexaenoic acid* (*DHA*),[317] melatonin,[318] and vitamin supplements (*alpha-lipoic acid*, 300 mg/day; *carbocysteine lysine salt*, 2.7 g/day; *vitamin E*, 400 IU/day; *vitamin A*, 30 000 IU/day; *vitamin C*, 500 mg/day),[319] have shown promise in some, but not all[320] studies undertaken.

**Pulmonary toxicity.** The lung is among the most radiosensitive organs, and therefore the risk of severe side effects seriously compromises treatment outcome. Radiation pneumonitis (inflammation of the lung) is a common acute side effect occurring in 5–30% of patients treated for lung cancer 1–6 months after radiotherapy.[321] Radiation therapy-induced fibrosis is associated with scarring of the lung and typically occurs months to years after radiotherapy.

The amino acids *taurine* and *L-arginine* may protect against radiation-induced lung fibrosis by reducing production of collagen, a protein implicated in the fibrotic process.[322]

The drug pentoxifylline downregulates the production of proinflammatory cytokines, particularly tumor necrosis factor-alpha (TNF-$\alpha$), and may therefore protect against radiation-induced, cytokine-mediated damage.[323] In a clinical trial, 64 patients with non–small-cell lung cancer were randomly divided into a pentoxifylline (400 mg, 3 times/day) plus radiotherapy group or a radiotherapy-only group.[324] Following treatment, patients in the pentoxifylline-plus-radiotherapy group had significantly longer survival and time to relapse.

A potentially important determinant of lung toxicity risk may be vitamin A nutritional status. Human studies have linked low vitamin A intake and/or reduced serum retinol levels with an increased risk of lung dysfunction.[325] Low levels of vitamin A have been found in human lung tissues obtained from patients undergoing lung resection.[326] Retinoids may exert their effects by modulating inflammatory cytokines and growth factors.[327] Experimental animal studies suggest that supplemental *vitamin A* may reduce lung inflammation after thoracic radiation and may be an important radioprotective agent in the lung.[328]

**Nausea and vomiting.** Radiation-induced nausea and vomiting typically occur within 24 hours of treatment, and over 80% of patients undergoing radiation of the upper body will develop symptoms of nausea and vomiting.[329,330] If untreated, nausea and vomiting

can cause physiologic changes, including dehydration, electrolyte imbalance, malnutrition, and cachexia.[331]

The use of 5-hydroxytryptamine (5-HT3)-receptor antagonists, such as granisetron (Kytril®), is the current "gold standard" in treating nausea and vomiting resulting from radiation therapy.[330]

Hypnosis effectively treated anticipatory nausea in pediatric[332] and adult cancer patients.[333] Clinical research found acupuncture to be effective for nausea in cancer patients, whether it be postoperative nausea or chemotherapy-induced nausea.[334–336] Acupuncture may also reduce radiation-induced symptoms.[337–339]

**Second cancers.** Although long-term survival following treatment for primary cancer has increased significantly, one of the most serious side effects of cancer treatment is the induction of a new tumor.[340] Second cancers account for up to 10% of all cancer diagnoses.[341] A study of patients with primary cancer in adulthood showed a 1.3-fold increased risk of developing a second cancer from radiation therapy.[342]

The increased risk of second malignancy usually, although not exclusively, occurs in the radiation field. The risk is dose dependent and appears to be higher when radiation exposure occurs at a younger age. The latency period is long; for example, secondary leukemia usually develops 1–10 years after radiotherapy, whereas an interval of more than 6 years and often decades is usual for solid tumors.[343]

A large number of studies have evaluated the risk of solid tumors following radiotherapy for Hodgkin's disease.[344,345] Survivors of Hodgkin's disease appear to face a 2–4% greater risk of second malignancy per person per year.[343]

Overall, it should be noted that the risk of second cancers is generally low, and the benefit of radiation therapy for patient survival outweighs the risk of developing a second tumor.[346]

**Sexual dysfunction.** Erectile dysfunction occurs in 7–84% of prostate cancer patients treated with radiation, even with the development of advanced radiation techniques such as proton beam therapy and 3D-CRT, which spare more normal tissue.[347]

Sixty patients presenting with erectile dysfunction 39 months after radiation treatment for prostate cancer were enrolled in a 12-week study to determine the efficacy of sildenafil citrate (Viagra®). Patients reported a significant increase in erectile function, with only mild side effects, at a dose of 100 mg taken 1 hour before sexual activity.[348]

Vaginal stenosis (narrowing) occurs in up to 88% of women undergoing brachytherapy for gynecologic cancers.[349] The time of onset of stenosis varies widely, from 6 weeks to several years after treatment.[350] Stenosis leads to thinning of the vaginal mucosa, scarring, and eventually scar tissue.[351] This results in shortening and narrowing of the vagina, leading to dyspareunia (pain during intercourse) and sexual dysfunction.[352]

Several treatment options have been suggested to manage radiation injuries of the vulva and vagina.[353] Proper personal hygiene is crucially important in managing acute vulva skin reactions.[354] Dilatation of the vagina either through the use of vaginal dilators or regular sexual intercourse should be performed to help prevent stenosis. Use of dilators should start before or immediately upon completion of treatment and continue indefinitely.[350]

**Stroke.** Although head and neck cancer is the fifth most common cancer, most people are not familiar with this type of cancer.[355] The mortality rate for those diagnosed with head and neck cancer (which does not include brain tumors) is high.[356]

Radiation therapy is an important part of treating many different head and neck tumors, and is often used after surgery.[357] Lethal radiation necrosis to the brain is one potential side effect.[358]

Another danger of radiation therapy to the head is increased risk of stroke.[359] A study of head and neck cancer patients who received radiation therapy found that stroke rates were 5 times greater than expected.[360] This elevated stroke risk was found many years after administration of radiation. The average time between radiation treatment and stroke was 10.9 years, but the increased risk of stroke persisted for 15 years after radiation therapy.

For cancer patients treated with radiation therapy who later die from a stroke, the official cause of death is stroke, even though the cancer radiation therapy probably caused the stroke. This is an example of how cancer cure statistics are misleading. The government contends that radiation therapy is curing cancer patients, yet long-term radiation side effects cause many deaths that are not attributed to cancer.

The government claims that more cancer victims are living beyond 5 years, but ignores the fact that the toxic therapies often used to eradicate cancer can themselves cause premature death.[361]

(The authors of this study do not recommend that head and neck cancer patients refuse radiation therapy, as it often adds years to their lives. Patients who have received radiation therapy to the head or neck should take extra precautions to reduce their risk of stroke.)

# DIETARY AND LIFESTYLE CONSIDERATIONS

Radiation therapy can change nutritional needs and alter the body's absorption and use of food.[362] Common cancer symptoms and toxic effects of radiation treatment include fatigue, anorexia, weight change, nausea, vomiting, pain, and changes in taste and bowel habits.[362]

Some researchers have suggested a low-fat (10% of calories from fat) and high-fiber (25–30 g from vegetables and fruits) diet be consumed during and after cancer treatment.[363] Such a diet can interfere with tumor growth by reducing tumor-stimulating signals.[364] Lifestyle changes that should be encouraged include quitting smoking, reducing consumption of caffeine and alcoholic beverages, exercising daily, and reducing stress levels.[365]

## Diet

Dietary changes such as the use of low-residue and elemental diets are suggested for those patients undergoing pelvic radiotherapy, as they place less strain on the digestive system than do conventional diets.[366] Several studies have investigated the following dietary interventions in those undergoing pelvic radiotherapy.[366]

**Dietary fat.** Dietary fat regimens, using 20–40 g of fat per day, significantly reduced diarrhea and the frequency of bowel motions.[367] There was no difference in stool frequency or use of antidiarrhea medication through dietary lactose restriction.[368]

**Probiotics.** The use of probiotics has a positive effect on gastrointestinal toxicity.[369] Probiotics refer to "friendly" bacteria that contribute to the health of the gastrointestinal tract. Twenty-four female patients suffering from gynecologic malignancies all received dietary counseling recommending a low-fat, low-residue diet during their radiotherapy. Half the patients also received 150 mL of a fermented milk product supplying at least $2 \times 10^9$ *Lactobacillus acidophilus* bacteria daily and 6.5% lactulose as substrate for the bacteria. The results indicated significantly reduced diarrhea in the group receiving probiotics, although with increased flatulence.[370]

**Elemental diets.** Elemental diets are liquid diets consisting of essential amino acids, glucose, vitamins, and necessary minerals.[371] Nutrients are usually in digested form so they do not stress the digestive system. The use of an elemental diet during radiotherapy[372] resulted in a statistically significant decrease in the incidence and severity of acute diarrhea.[373,374] In one favorable study, the elemental diet began 3 days before radiation therapy and was continued until completion. Patients were also placed on a modified diet that recommended low fiber, moderate fat intake, and adequate proteins and carbohydrates.[373]

**Micronutrient supplementation.** Micronutrient supplementation in patients with proctitis (inflammation of the rectum) has been previously outlined.[179] A study of 19 patients treated with pelvic radiotherapy for more than 6 months examined whether vitamin A could reduce the resulting radiation-induced proctitis.[180] Ten patients received 10 000 IU of oral vitamin A for 90 days, after which 7 patients reported a significant improvement in symptoms, compared to only 2 of 9 placebo-treated patients who reported improvement.

In a pilot study, 20 patients with chronic radiation proctitis due to previous pelvic irradiation took vitamin E (400 IU, 3 times daily) and vitamin C (500 mg, 3 times daily) supplements for up to 1 year. Significant improvements were reported in the side effects of bleeding and diarrhea, but not pain.[375] However, in another study in which the same doses were administered, all symptoms subsided following 6–12 weeks of treatment.[376]

## Exercise

Fatigue is a major determinant of quality of life and is present in as many as 50–70% of patients with cancer at diagnosis.[377] Several studies have investigated fatigue during radiation therapy for both breast[378] and prostate cancer.[379] The initiation of radiation therapy is accompanied by significant increases in fatigue.[380] However, levels of fatigue tend to return to pretreatment levels within several weeks of completing treatment.[381]

A number of studies have examined the therapeutic value of exercise during cancer treatment.[362,382] A trial was performed to determine whether aerobic exercise would reduce the incidence of fatigue and prevent deteriorating physical function during radiotherapy for localized prostate carcinoma.[383] Those men who followed advice to rest if they became fatigued demonstrated a slight deterioration in physical function and a significant increase in fatigue at the time of radiotherapy. By contrast, a home-based, moderate-intensity walking program produced a significant improvement in physical function, with no significant increase in fatigue.

An exercise program of walking (self-paced walks of 20–30 minutes, 4–5 days per week) was evaluated in participants who were to receive radiation therapy after surgery for breast cancer.[384] Before radiation therapy, patients were assigned to either the exercise intervention group or a control group. Those who underwent the walking program experienced significantly less fatigue on the completion of radiation therapy than those in the control group.

## FOR MORE INFORMATION

The complications related to radiation can be acute (such as low blood cell counts) and chronic (gastrointestinal, pulmonary, neuropathic, and cardiac). For more information on some of the topics outlined in this protocol, see the following protocols:

- Blood Disorders (Anemia, Leukopenia, and Thrombocytopenia)
- Catabolic Wasting
- Complementary Alternative Cancer Therapies
- Cancer Adjuvant Therapy
- Erectile Dysfunction
- Neuropathy (Diabetic)

For general information on all aspects of radiation therapy, see http://www.cancerlinksusa.com/radiation.htm.

### Proton Therapy Centers in North America

- The Loma Linda University Medical Center (LLUMC), California. LLUMC sponsors Prolit, a proton therapy literature database.
- Northeast Proton Therapy Center at Massachusetts General Hospital in Boston.
- Particle Therapy Co-operative Group (PTCOG) and the PTCOG publication Particles.
- Midwest Proton Radiotherapy Institute, Bloomington, Indiana.
- Proton Radiation Therapy at TRIUMF Vancouver, Canada. Pion Therapy is also available.
- UC-Davis, California. The Berkeley Eye Program.

### Life Extension Suggestions

For optimal results, the majority of these supplements or dietary changes should be introduced before starting radiation treatment. Refer to the text for a more detailed explanation of the dose and duration of the specific supplements.
- **R-lipoic acid**: 300 mg daily
- **Beta-carotene**: 25 000 IU
- **Coenzyme Q10**: 100–400 mg daily
- **Curcumin**: up to 3.2 g daily
- **Panax ginseng** (Siberian): 200–1000 mg daily
- **Green tea extract**: 725 mg, 3 times daily

- **Proteolytic enzymes**: papain (100 mg), trypsin (40 mg), and chymotrypsin (40 mg): 3 days before radiation therapy and continuing until 5 days after completion of treatment
- **Kamillosan**: 10 drops in 1 oz of water, 3 times daily (http://www.smallflower.com/)
- **L-arginine**: 900 mg daily
- **L-glutamine**: 20–40 g administered before starting radiation therapy
- **Melatonin**: up to 20 mg daily
- **Multivitamin/multimineral supplement** (without copper): per label instructions
- **N-acetylcysteine**: 200–600 mg daily
- **Omega-3 fatty acids**: 1–2 g daily
- **Probiotics**: $2 \times 10^9$ *Lactobacillus acidophilus* daily
- **Pure honey**: 20 mL, 15 minutes before, 15 minutes after, and 6 hours after radiotherapy
- **Selenium**: 200–1000 mcg daily
- **Silymarin**: 150–600 mg daily
- **Soy extract**, containing 50 mg of isoflavones: twice daily
- **Sulforaphane**: 400–1600 mg daily of a broccoli extract
- **Taurine**: 1000 mg daily
- **Vitamin A**: 8000–30 000 IU daily
- **Vitamin C**: 500 mg, 3 times daily
- **Vitamin E**: 400–1200 IU daily
- **Whey protein isolate**: 20 g daily

## REFERENCES

References available at: www.lef.org/dpt5/ch30

# 31

# Cancer Surgery

Surgical removal of the primary tumor has been the cornerstone of treatment for most types of cancer. The rationale for this approach is straightforward—if you can get rid of the cancer by removing it from the body, then a cure can likely be achieved. Unfortunately, this approach does not take into account that following surgery, the cancer will frequently metastasize (spread to different organs). Quite often the metastatic recurrence is far more serious than the original tumor. In fact, for many cancers it is the metastatic recurrence, and not the primary tumor that ultimately proves to be fatal.[1]

A growing body of scientific evidence has revealed that cancer surgery can increase the risk of metastasis.[2] Even though this contradicts conventional medical thinking, the facts are undeniable.

A complicated sequence of events must occur in order for cancer to metastasize.[2] Isolated cancer cells that break away from the primary tumor must first breach the connective tissue immediately surrounding the cancer. Once this occurs, the cancer cell enters a blood or lymphatic vessel. To gain entry, the cancer cell must secrete enzymes that degrade the basement membrane of the blood vessel.[3] This is vitally important for the metastatic cancer cell as it uses the bloodstream for transport to other vital organs of the body (ie, the liver, brain, or lungs) where it can form a new deadly tumor.

Traveling within the bloodstream can be a hazardous journey for cancer cells. Turbulence from the fast moving blood can damage and destroy the cancer cell. Furthermore, cancer cells must avoid detection and destruction from white blood cells circulating in the bloodstream.

To complete its voyage, the cancer cell must adhere to the lining of the blood vessel where it degrades through and exits the basement membrane of the blood vessel. Its final task is to burrow through the surrounding connective tissue to arrive at its final destination, the organ. Now the cancer cell can multiply and form a growing colony, serving as the foundation for a new metastatic cancer.

We now see that cancer metastasis is a complicated and difficult process. Fraught with peril, very few freestanding cancer cells survive this arduous journey.[2]

In a groundbreaking study, researchers reported that cancer surgery itself can greatly reduce the cancer cell's obstacles to metastasis.[2] Cancer surgery can produce an alternate route of metastasis that bypasses natural barriers. During cancer surgery, the removal of the tumor almost always disrupts the structural integrity of the tumor and/or blood vessels feeding the tumor. This can lead to either an unobstructed dispersal of cancer cells into the bloodstream or seeding of these cancer cells directly into the chest or abdomen.[4-7] This surgery-induced "alternate route" can greatly simplify the path to metastasis.

To illustrate, a study compared the survival of women with breast cancer who had surgery to that of women with breast cancer who did not have surgery. As expected, surgery substantially improved survival in the early years. However, further analysis of the data revealed that the surgery group had a spike in their risk of death at 8 years that was not evident in the nonsurgery group.[8]

Given these findings, a worthwhile strategy to protect against the increased risk of metastasis would be to examine all of the mechanisms by which surgery promotes metastasis, and then create a comprehensive plan that counteracts each and every one of these mechanisms.

## WHAT YOU NEED TO KNOW: CANCER SURGERY

- Surgical removal of cancer typically provides the best chance of disease-free survival.
- Since metastatic disease is often deadlier than the original tumor, it is important to utilize preventive strategies to prevent cancer metastasis.
- A growing body of evidence suggests that cancer surgery itself may increase the risk of metastasis (spread to other areas) via numerous mechanisms including increasing cancer cell adhesion, suppressing immune function, promoting angiogenesis (growth of new blood vessels from pre-existing vessels), and stimulating inflammation.
- Choose surgeons and anesthesiologists who utilize advanced techniques that may reduce metastatic risk.
- Certain nutrients and drugs are associated with reduced risk of metastasis.

## SURGERY INCREASES CANCER CELL ADHESION

One mechanism by which surgery increases the risk of metastasis is by enhancing cancer cell adhesion.[9] Cancer cells that break away from the primary tumor utilize adhesion to boost their ability to form metastases in distant organs. These cancer cells must be able

## Cancer Metastasis

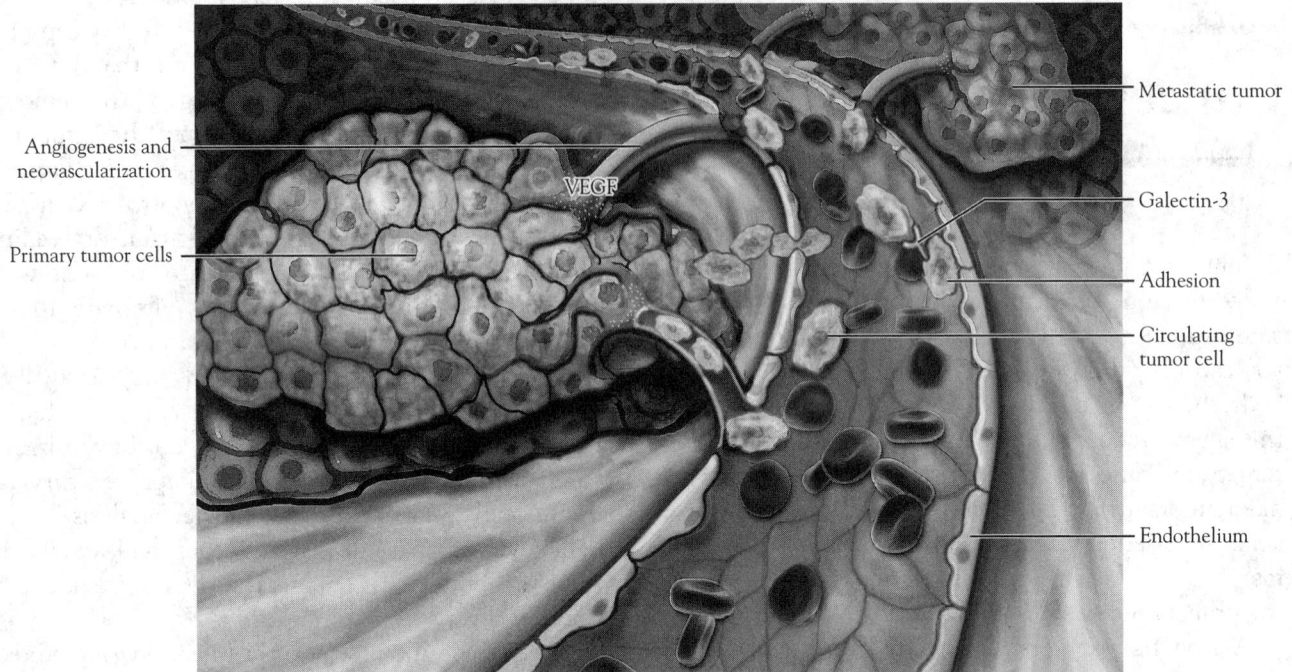

Angiogenesis and neovascularization

Primary tumor cells

VEGF

Metastatic tumor

Galectin-3

Adhesion

Circulating tumor cell

Endothelium

to clump together and form colonies that can expand and grow. It is unlikely that a single cancer cell will form a metastatic tumor. Cancer cells use adhesion molecules (which are present on the surface of cancer cells), such as galectin-3, to facilitate their ability to clump together.[10] Cancer cells circulating in the bloodstream also make use of galectin-3 surface adhesion molecules to latch onto the lining of blood vessels.[11] The adherence of circulating tumor cells (CTCs) to the blood vessel walls is an essential step for the process of metastasis. A cancer cell that cannot adhere to the blood vessel wall will just continue to wander through the bloodstream, incapable of forming metastases. Eventually, white blood cells circulating in the bloodstream will target and destroy the CTCs. If the CTCs successfully bind to the blood vessel wall and burrow their way through the basement membrane, they will then utilize galectin-3 adhesion molecules to adhere to the organ to form a new metastatic cancer.[10]

## COMBATING CANCER CELL ADHESION

Research has shown that cancer surgery increases tumor cell adhesion. In one experiment that mimicked surgical conditions, scientists reported that the binding of cancer cells to the blood vessel walls was increased by 250%, compared to cancer cells not exposed to surgical conditions.[12] A natural supplement called modified citrus

pectin (MCP) can help neutralize the surgery-induced increase in cancer cell adhesion. Citrus pectin—a type of dietary fiber—is not absorbed into the intestine. However, modified citrus pectin has been altered so that it can be absorbed into the blood and exert its anticancer effects. Modified citrus pectin inhibits cancer cell adhesion by binding to galectin-3 adhesion molecules on the surface of cancer cells, thereby preventing cancer cells from sticking together and forming a cluster.[13] Modified citrus pectin can also inhibit circulating tumor cells from latching onto the lining of blood vessels. This was demonstrated by an experiment in which modified citrus pectin blocked the adhesion of galectin-3 to the lining of blood vessels by 95%. Modified citrus pectin also substantially decreased the adhesion of breast cancer cells to the blood vessel walls.[13]

In one study, rats were injected with prostate cancer cells. One group received the modified citrus pectin while the other (control group) did not. Lung metastasis was noted in 50% of the modified citrus pectin group versus 93% in the control group. Even more noteworthy was that the modified citrus pectin group had an 89% reduction in the size of the metastatic colonies compared to the control group.[14] In a similar experiment, mice injected with melanoma cancer cells that were fed modified citrus pectin experienced a greater than 90% reduction in lung metastasis compared to the control group.[15]

In a human trial, 10 men with recurrent prostate cancer received 14.4 g daily of modified citrus pectin.

After one year, a considerable improvement in cancer progression was noted as determined by a rate reduction in the prostate-specific antigen (PSA) level.[16] This was followed by a study in which 49 men with various types of prostate cancer were given modified citrus pectin for a 4-week cycle. After 2 treatment cycles, 22% of the men experienced a stabilization of their disease or improved quality of life; 12% remained stable for more than 24 weeks. The authors of the study concluded that "MCP seems to have positive impacts especially regarding clinical benefit and life quality for patients with far advanced solid tumor."[17]

Cimetidine, commonly known as Tagamet®, is a drug historically used to alleviate heartburn. A growing body of scientific evidence has revealed that cimetidine also possesses potent anticancer activity. Cimetidine inhibits cancer cell adhesion by blocking the expression of an adhesive (cancer cells latch on) molecule called E-selectin on the surface of cells lining blood vessels.[15] By preventing the expression of E-selectin, cimetidine significantly limits the ability of cancer cell adherence to the blood vessel walls.

In a study supporting the potential anticancer effects of cimetidine, 64 colon cancer patients received chemotherapy with or without cimetidine (800 mg per day) for one year. The 10-year survival rate for the cimetidine group was almost 90% versus 49.8% for the control group. For patients with a more aggressive form of colon cancer, the 10-year survival was 85% in those treated with cimetidine compared to 23% in the control group.[18] The authors of the study concluded that "taken together, these results suggested a mechanism underlying the beneficial effect of cimetidine on colorectal cancer patients, presumably by blocking the expression of E-selectin on vascular endothelial [lining of blood vessels] cells and inhibiting the adhesion of cancer cells." These findings were supported by another study with colorectal cancer patients wherein cimetidine given for just 7 days at the time of surgery increased 3-year survival rate from 59–93%.[19]

This combination regimen of 14 g of modified citrus pectin and 800 mg of cimetidine, taken at least 5 days before surgery, may be followed for a year or longer to reduce metastatic risk.

## PREVENTING SURGERY-INDUCED IMMUNE SUPPRESSION

The immune system is essential in combating cancer. Natural killer (NK) cells are a type of white blood cell that seeks out and destroys cancer cells. Research has shown that NK cells can spontaneously recognize and kill a variety of cancer cells.[20]

In a study examining NK cell activity in women shortly after surgery for breast cancer, it was reported that low levels of NK cell activity were associated with an increased risk of death from breast cancer.[21] In fact, reduced NK cell activity was a better predictor of survival than the actual stage of the cancer itself. In another study, colon cancer patients with a reduced NK cell activity before surgery had a 350% increased risk of metastasis during the following 31 months.[22]

The likelihood of surgery-induced metastasis requires the immune system to be highly active and vigilant in seeking out and destroying renegade cancer cells during the perioperative period (the time immediately before, during, and after surgery). Numerous studies have documented that cancer surgery results in a substantial reduction in NK cell activity.[6,7,23,24] In an investigation, NK cell activity in women having surgery for breast cancer was reduced by over 50% on the first day after surgery.[23] A group of researchers stated that "we therefore believe that shortly after surgery, even transitory immune dysfunction might permit neoplasms [cancer] to enter the next stage of development and eventually form sizable metastases."[7]

The surgical procedure itself reduces NK activity. In other words, NK cell activity becomes impaired when it is most needed to fight metastasis. With that said, the perioperative period presents a window of opportunity to actively strengthen immune function by enhancing NK cell activity. Fortunately, numerous nutraceutical (eg, dietary supplements, herbal products), pharmaceutical, and medical interventions known to enhance NK cell activity are available to the person undergoing cancer surgery.

One prominent natural supplement that can increase NK cell activity is PSK (protein-bound polysaccharide K), a specially prepared extract from the mushroom *Coriolus versicolor*. PSK has been shown to enhance NK cell activity in multiple studies,[25–28] thereby improving survival in cancer patients. For example, 225 patients with lung cancer received radiation therapy with or without PSK (3 g/day). For those with stage 3 cancer, 26% taking PSK were alive after 5 years versus 8% not taking PSK. PSK more than doubled the 5-year survival rate in those individuals with stage 1 (39%) or stage 2 (17%) cancer.[29]

A group of colon cancer patients were randomized to receive either chemotherapy alone or chemotherapy with PSK, which was taken for 2 years. The group receiving PSK had a 10-year survival rate of 82% versus 51% in the group receiving chemotherapy alone.[30] In a similar trial, the 5-year survival rate was 75% in the PSK group as compared to 46% in the group receiving chemotherapy alone.[31] Research has confirmed that PSK also improves survival in cancers of the breast, stomach, esophagus, and uterus.[32–35]

Other nutraceuticals that have been documented to increase NK cell activity are garlic, glutamine, IP6 (inositol hexaphosphate), and lactoferrin.[36–40] One experiment in mice with breast cancer found that glutamine supplementation resulted in a 40% decrease in tumor growth paired with a 2.5-fold increase in NK cell activity.[39]

Scientists in Germany explored the effects of mistletoe extract on NK cell activity in 62 patients undergoing surgery for colon cancer. The participants were randomized to receive either an intravenous infusion of mistletoe extract immediately before general anesthesia or general anesthesia alone. Measurements of NK cell activity were taken before and 24 hours after surgery. The group receiving anesthesia alone experienced a 44% reduction in NK cell activity 24 hours after surgery. The scientists reported that the group receiving mistletoe did not experience a significant decrease in NK cell activity after surgery. They went on to conclude that "perioperative infusion of mistletoe extracts can prevent a suppression of NK cell activity in cancer patients."[41]

Pharmaceuticals used to increase NK cell activity include interferon-alpha and granulocyte-macrophage colony-stimulating factor. These drugs were shown to prevent surgery-induced immune suppression when given perioperatively.[42,43] Another immune-boosting drug to consider in the perioperative setting is interleukin-2.[44]

## HEIGHTENING IMMUNE SURVEILLANCE WITH CANCER VACCINES

Using vaccines for cancer is the same as using vaccines for infectious diseases, except that tumor vaccines target cancer cells instead of a virus. Another distinguishing feature of tumor vaccines is that they are autologous, that is, they are produced from a person's own cancer cells and removed during surgery. This is a critical distinction since there can be considerable genetic differences between cancers. This highly individualized cancer vaccine greatly amplifies the ability of the immune system to identify and target any residual cancer cells present in the body. Cancer vaccines provide the immune system with the specific identifying markers of the cancer that can then be used to mount a successful attack against metastatic cancer cells.

Autologous cancer vaccines have been studied extensively, with the most encouraging results noted in randomized, controlled clinical trials including more than 1300 colorectal cancer patients in which tumor vaccines were given after surgery. These trials reported reduced recurrence rates and improved survival.[45] Unlike chemotherapy, which can cause severe side effects and toxicity, cancer vaccines are a gentle therapy with proven long-term safety.[46]

In a landmark study reported in 2003, 567 individuals with colon cancer were randomized to receive either surgery alone or surgery combined with vaccines derived from their own cancer cells. The median survival for the cancer vaccine group was over 7 years (66.5% 5-year survival rate) compared to 4.5 years (45.6% 5-year survival rate) for the group receiving surgery alone.[47] This difference in 5-year survival rates clearly displays the power of individually tailored cancer vaccines to greatly focus a person's own immunity to target and attack residual metastatic cancer cells.

## CANCER SURGERY, ANGIOGENESIS, AND METASTASIS

Angiogenesis (the formation of new blood vessels) is a normal and necessary process for childhood growth and development as well as wound healing. Unfortunately, cancers use this otherwise normal process in order to increase blood supply to the tumor. Because tumors cannot grow beyond the size of a pinhead (ie, 1–2 mm) without expanding their blood supply, the formation of new blood vessels supplying the tumor is a requirement for successful metastasis.[48,49]

The primary tumor produces antiangiogenic factors that serve to limit the growth of metastatic cancer elsewhere in the body[50–53] by inhibiting the formation of new blood vessels to potential sites of metastasis. Unfortunately, the surgical removal of the primary cancer also results in the removal of these antiangiogenic factors, and the growth of metastasis is no longer inhibited. With these restrictions lifted, it is now easier for small sites of metastatic cancer to attract new blood vessels that promote their growth.[54] Indeed, these concerns were voiced by researchers who declared that "removal of the primary tumor might eliminate a safeguard against angiogenesis and thus awaken dormant micrometastasis [small sites of metastatic cancer]."[7]

As it turns out, the surgery causes another angiogenic effect. After surgery, levels of vascular endothelial growth factor (VEGF) (factors that increase angiogenesis) are significantly elevated. This can result in an increased formation of new blood vessels supplying areas of metastatic cancer. A group of scientists asserted that "after surgery, the angiogenic balance of pro- and anti-angiogenic factors is shifted in favor of angiogenesis to facilitate wound healing. Especially levels of vascular endothelial growth factor (VEGF) are persistently elevated. This may not only benefit tumor recurrence and the formation of metastatic disease, but also result in activation of dormant micrometastases."[2]

Various nutrients have been shown to inhibit VEGF. These include soy isoflavones (genistein), silibinin (a component of milk thistle), epigallocatechin gallate (EGCG) from green tea, and curcumin.[55-60]

In one experiment, EGCG, the active constituent of green tea, was administered to mice with stomach cancer. EGCG reduced the tumor mass by 60% and the concentration of blood vessels feeding the tumor by 38%. In addition, EGCG decreased the expression of VEGF in cancer cells by 80%. The authors of the study concluded that "EGCG inhibits the growth of gastric cancer by reducing VEGF production and angiogenesis, and is a promising candidate for antiangiogenic treatment of gastric cancer."[55]

In a survey of curcumin's antiangiogenic effects, researchers noted that "[c]urcumin is a direct inhibitor of angiogenesis and also downregulates various proangiogenic proteins like vascular endothelial growth factor." Additionally, they remarked that "cell adhesion molecules are upregulated in active angiogenesis and curcumin can block this effect, adding further dimensions to curcumin's antiangiogenic effect." In conclusion, they commented that "[c]urcumin's effect on the overall process of angiogenesis compounds its enormous potential as an antiangiogenic drug."[43]

## THE CHOICE OF SURGICAL ANESTHESIA CAN INFLUENCE METASTASIS

The traditional protocol is general anesthesia during surgery followed by intravenous morphine (for pain control) after surgery. However, this may not be the optimal approach for preventing surgery-induced metastasis. At a time when immune function is already suppressed, morphine further weakens the immune system by diminishing NK cell activity.[61] Surgical anesthesia has also been shown to weaken NK cell activity.[62] One study found that morphine increased angiogenesis and stimulated the growth of breast cancer in mice. The

researchers concluded that "these results indicate that clinical use of morphine could potentially be harmful in patients with angiogenesis-dependent cancers."[63]

Given the inherent problems associated with the use of morphine and anesthesia, researchers have explored other approaches to surgical anesthesia and pain control. One approach is the use of conventional general anesthesia combined with regional anesthesia (anesthesia that affects a specific part of the body). The benefits achieved with this approach are twofold: the use of regional anesthesia reduces the amount of general anesthesia required during surgery, and it decreases the amount of morphine needed after surgery for pain control.[54]

In one experiment, mice with cancer received surgery with either general anesthesia alone or combined with regional anesthesia. The scientists reported that the addition of regional anesthesia "markedly attenuates the promotion of metastasis by surgery." Regional anesthesia reduced 70% of the metastasis-promoting effects of general anesthesia alone.[64]

In another study, doctors compared NK cell activity in patients receiving general or regional anesthesia for abdominal surgery. NK cell activity dropped substantially in the general anesthesia group, while it was preserved at preoperative levels in the group receiving regional anesthesia.[65] In a pioneering study, 50 women having breast cancer surgery with general and regional anesthesia were compared to 79 women having breast cancer surgery and receiving general anesthesia followed by morphine. The type of regional anesthesia used was called a paravertebral block, which involves the injection of a local anesthetic around the spinal nerves between the vertebral bones of the spine. After nearly 3 years, dramatic differences were noted between the 2 groups. Only 6% of patients who received regional anesthesia experienced a metastatic recurrence compared to 24% in the group that did not receive regional anesthesia. In other words, women who received regional and general anesthesia had a 75% decreased risk for metastatic cancer. These findings led researchers to proclaim that regional anesthesia for breast cancer surgery "markedly reduces the risk of recurrence of metastasis during the initial years following surgery."[54]

In yet another study, surgeons concluded that regional anesthesia "can be used to perform major operations for breast cancer with minimal complications. Most importantly, by reducing nausea, vomiting, and surgical pain, paravertebral block [regional anesthesia] markedly improves the quality of operative recovery for patients who are treated for breast cancer."[66]

A group of researchers announced that "as regional [anesthesia] techniques are easy to implement, inexpensive, and do not pose a threat greater than general anesthesia, it would be easy for anesthesiologists to implement them, thus reducing the risk of disease recurrence and metastasis."[54]

Those requiring medication for pain control after surgery can consider asking their doctor for tramadol instead of morphine. Unlike morphine, tramadol does not suppress immune function.[67] On the contrary, tramadol has been shown to stimulate NK cell activity. In one experiment, tramadol prevented the suppression of NK cell activity and blocked the formation of lung metastasis induced by surgery in rats.[68]

## LESS INVASIVE SURGERY REDUCES RISK OF METASTASIS

Surgery places an enormous physical stress upon the body. There is considerable scientific evidence supporting the belief that less invasive surgeries, and therefore less traumatic, pose a decreased risk of metastasis. Laparoscopic surgery, performed by making a small incision in the abdomen, is one type of minimally invasive surgery.

In a study comparing laparoscopic to open surgery in colon cancer patients receiving a partial colectomy (removal of the colon), the laparoscopic group had a 61% decreased risk of cancer recurrence coupled with a 62% decreased risk of death from colon cancer. The surgeons concluded that laparoscopic colectomy is more effective than open colectomy for treatment of colon cancer.[69] A long-term (median time ~8 years) follow-up of these patients reported a 56% decreased risk of death from colon cancer following laparoscopic surgery as compared to traditional open surgery.[70]

Minimally invasive surgery has produced substantial improvements in survival rates for lung cancer patients. Video-assisted thoracoscopic surgery (VATS) was compared to traditional open surgery for removing lung tumors (lobectomy). The 5-year survival rate from lung cancer was 97% in the VATS group compared to 79% in the open surgery group.[71]

A group of surgeons commented that minimally invasive surgery for lung cancer "can be performed safely with proven advantages over conventional thoracotomy [chest surgery] for lobectomy: smaller incisions, decreased postoperative pain, decreased blood loss, better preservation of pulmonary function, and earlier return to normal activities. The

evidence in the literature is mounting that VATS may offer reduced rates of complications and better survival."[72]

## ADMINISTERING CHEMO AND RADIATION THERAPIES PRIOR TO SURGERY

A group of doctors studied the use of combined radiation and chemotherapy prior to surgery for individuals with esophageal cancer. Twenty-six cancer patients received surgery alone, while 30 received radiation and chemotherapy followed up by surgery. The group receiving combined treatment had a 5-year survival rate of 39% compared to 16% in the group treated with surgery alone.[73]

In another study comparing treatment with surgery alone to treatment with chemotherapy (both directly before and after surgery) in patients with stomach or esophageal cancer, the 5-year survival rate for the group receiving surgery and chemotherapy was 36% compared to 23% in the group receiving surgery alone.[74]

Research also supports the use of chemotherapy and radiation therapy during the critical perioperative period. In one study, 544 patients with stomach cancer received combined chemotherapy and radiation shortly after surgery. Survival comparisons were made with a similar group of 446 patients with stomach cancer treated with surgery alone. The group treated with surgery alone had a median survival of only 62.6 months compared to 95.3 months in the combination group.[75]

## INFLAMMATION AND METASTASIS

Cancer surgery causes an increased production of inflammatory chemicals such as interleukin-1 and interleukin-6.[76–78] These chemicals are known to increase the activity of cyclooxygenase-2 (COX-2). A highly potent inflammatory enzyme, COX-2 plays a pivotal role in promoting cancer growth and metastasis by stimulating the formation of new blood vessels feeding the tumor.[79,80] It also increases cancer cell adhesion to the blood vessel walls,[81] thereby enhancing the ability of cancer cells to metastasize.

This was evident in an article that reported levels of COX-2 in pancreatic cancer cells to be 60 times greater than in normal pancreatic cells.[82] Levels of COX-2 were 150 times higher in cancer cells from individuals with head and neck cancers compared to normal tissue from healthy volunteers.[83] This was further supported when 288 individuals undergoing surgery for colon cancer had their tumors examined for the presence of COX-2. With other factors being controlled, the group whose cancers tested positive for the presence of COX-2 had a 311% greater risk of death compared to the group whose cancers did not express COX-2.[84] A subsequent study in lung cancer patients found that those with high tumor levels of COX-2 had a median survival rate of 15 months compared to 40 months in those with low levels.[85]

Given these findings, researchers began investigating the anticancer effects of COX-2 inhibitor drugs. Although initially used for inflammatory conditions (ie, arthritis), COX-2 inhibitor drugs have been shown to possess powerful anticancer benefits. For example, 134 patients with advanced lung cancer were treated with chemotherapy alone or combined with Celebrex® (a COX-2 inhibitor). For those individuals with cancer expressing higher amounts of COX-2, treatment with Celebrex® dramatically prolonged survival.[86] Treatment with Celebrex® also slowed cancer progression in men with recurrent prostate cancer.[87]

In a groundbreaking study, the incidence of bone metastases in breast cancer patients receiving COX-2 inhibitors for at least 6 months (following the initial diagnosis of breast cancer) was compared to the incidence in breast cancer patients not taking a COX-2 inhibitor. Those taking a COX-2 inhibitor were almost 80% less likely to develop bone metastases than those not taking a COX-2 inhibitor.[88]

Nonsteroidal anti-inflammatory drugs (NSAIDs), such as aspirin and ibuprofen, are COX-2 inhibitors. The widespread use of NSAIDs for pain and arthritis has created an ideal environment in which to examine whether these drugs can prevent cancer. Large-scale studies have documented a substantial reduction in cancer risk with the use of NSAIDs. A comprehensive review of 91 published studies reported that long-term use of NSAIDs (primarily aspirin) produced risk reductions of 63% for colon cancer, 39% for breast cancer, 36% for lung cancer, 39% for prostate cancer, 73% for esophageal cancer, 62% for stomach cancer, and 47% for ovarian cancer. The authors concluded that "this review provides compelling evidence that regular intake of NSAIDs that block COX-2 protects against the development of many types of cancer."[89]

A number of nutritional and herbal supplements are known to inhibit COX-2. These include curcumin, resveratrol, vitamin E, soy isoflavones (genistein), green tea (EGCG), quercetin, fish oil, garlic, feverfew, and silymarin (milk thistle).[57,90–97]

Scientists created an experimentally induced increase in COX-2 activity in human breast cells, which was completely prevented by resveratrol. Resveratrol blocked the production of COX-2 within the cell, as well as blocking COX-2 enzyme activity.[92]

## Life Extension Suggestions

**Note:** *These products are to be used for cancer surgery recovery and preparation and are not intended to prevent, cure, or treat cancer.*

Begin taking the following supplements at least 5 days prior to surgery, discontinue taking the supplements the day of the surgery, and resume taking the supplements 1 day after surgery (unless otherwise directed by your physician).

It is suggested to take these supplements for approximately 1 month after surgery.

- **Glutamine:** 3000 mg daily without food
- **IP6** (inositol hexaphosphate): 1–3 g daily
- **Lactoferrin:** 300–900 mg daily
- **PSK** (protein-bound polysaccharide K [coriolus]): 3000 mg daily
- **Cimetidine:** 800 mg before bedtime
- **Modified citrus pectin:** 14–30 g daily without food
- **Soy isoflavones** (genistein): 100–200 mg daily with food
- **Silibinin** (component of milk thistle): 500–600 mg daily
- **EGCG** (from green tea): 650–1000 mg daily
- **Curcumin (as highly absorbable BCM-95®):** 400 mg daily with food *or* 2500 mg daily with food of a regular curcumin supplement. Different formulations of curcumin vary in their absorption and bioavailability. These differences in absorption can affect suggested doses.
- **Resveratrol:** 20–25 mg before surgery; increase to 100–250 mg 2 weeks after surgery
- **Quercetin:** 500–1000 mg daily

Due to their blood-thinning effects, avoid the following supplements for 2 weeks prior to surgery and begin taking 2 weeks after surgery:

- **Garlic:** 1200–2400 mg daily with food
- **Fish oil:** 4000 mg daily with food
- **Vitamin E:** 400–800 IU daily with food
- **Feverfew:** 250 mg daily

### Prescription Drugs

Pharmaceuticals prescribed prior to surgery depend on the status of the individual cancer patient.

Patients with low white blood count are typically treated with granulocyte colony–stimulating growth (GCF) factors such as Neupogen® (300–480 µg daily) or Neulasta® (6 mg), which lasts 3 weeks. Other pharmaceutical compounds that have shown benefits for cancer patients undergoing surgery are interferon alpha and interleukin-2.

## REFERENCES

References available at: www.lef.org/dpt5/ch31

# 32

---

# Cancer Treatment: The Critical Factors

---

In order to derive the greatest potential benefit from any cancer treatment regimen, both patients and physicians must respect and adapt to the complex and multidimensional nature of each individual's unique cancer. Sadly, the mainstream medical establishment treats the majority of cancer cases with a one-size-fits-all strategy that may deprive many patients of a greater chance of successful treatment.

Implementing strategies to address each of the *ten critical factors of cancer treatment* identified in this Life Extension protocol provides an evidenced based approach that will:

- Aid physicians in determining which medical therapies are most likely to be effective for each individual's unique cancer

- Pharmacogenomically and nutrigenomically target multiple biochemical pathways known to be aberrant in many cancers

- Provide a more thorough prognostic analysis that can help physicians make informed decisions about how aggressive treatment should be, and to properly inform their patients about the state of their health

- Educate patients about some potential side effects associated with conventional cancer treatment options, and what they can do to minimize risk

In this protocol, Life Extension will discuss the following *ten critical steps* that may increase the likelihood of a successful outcome in the treatment of many cancers.

1. Evaluating the molecular biology of the tumor cell population

2. Analyzing the patient's living tumor cells to determine sensitivity or resistance to chemotherapy

3. Circulating tumor cell testing

4. Inhibiting the cyclooxygenase enzymes (COX-1 and COX-2)

5. Suppressing Ras oncogene expression

6. Correcting coagulation abnormalities

7. Maintaining bone integrity

8. Inhibiting angiogenesis

9. Inhibiting the 5-lipoxygenase (5-LOX) enzyme

10. Inhibiting cancer metastasis

Of critical importance to treatment-naïve patients is implementing as many of these ten critical steps as can safely be done concurrently with conventional therapy. In newly diagnosed patients who have not yet been treated, the objective is to eradicate the primary tumor and metastatic cells with a multi-pronged "first-strike therapy" so that residual tumor cells are not given an opportunity to evolve survival mechanisms that make them resistant to further treatments.

## STEP ONE: EVALUATING THE MOLECULAR BIOLOGY OF THE TUMOR CELL POPULATION

Throughout this protocol, you will see terminology relating to the molecular aspects of the cancer cell. When we use the term *molecular*, we are referring to specific characteristics of cancer cells such as:

- Tumor-promoting genes (oncogenes)

- Tumor suppressor genes

- Receptors or docking sites on the cell membrane where communication with proteins occurs

- Cellular differentiation—the degree of aggressiveness of the cancer cell (poorly differentiated cancer cells are more aggressive, while highly differentiated cells are less aggressive)

These individual variations—the unique biology of the cancer cell—help to explain why a particular therapy may be highly effective for some cancer patients but fail for others.

People typically think of their disease based on the organ it affects (eg, lung cancer or colon cancer). The problem with that rationale is that not all cancers are the same, even if they affect the same organ. With the advent of advanced molecular diagnostic profiling, the specific strengths and vulnerabilities of each patient's cancer can be identified in order to design an individually tailored treatment program.

It is critically important to obtain a description of the type of cells that populate your tumor. Not only does this assist the oncologist in recommending the most effective conventional therapy, but it also helps determine what adjuvant nutritional and/or off-label drug therapies to consider. The human eye can serve to provide the most basic information about a cancer cell through the microscopic examination of the cell's general characteristics. Taking this one step further is evaluation by an *immunohistochemistry* test. This test detects markers of diagnostic value on and within the cell surface, through the application of colored dye or stains. In order to perform this and other tests, it is necessary for a sample of your tumor to be sent to a specialized laboratory.

GENZYME provides a comprehensive range of customized analyses to help cancer specialists correctly identify difficult-to-diagnose tumors, establish prognosis in many cancers (including breast, prostate, and colon), and determine optimal treatment. By providing this information, GENZYME starts treatment on the right course and helps avoid unnecessary and potentially ineffective therapies. GENZYME performs more specialized analyses for cancer than any other laboratory in the world.

When a person has cancer, the physician confronts a chain of pressing questions: What type of cancer is it? Where did it originate? Which treatments are most likely to be effective? GENZYME can help clinicians with answers to many of these questions.

As far as diagnosis is concerned, many cancers defy classification by visual examination. In fact, the diagnosis of "metastatic cancer of unknown primary site" accounts for 2–6% of cancer diagnoses.[1] In a majority of these difficult cases, GENZYME's medical expertise and advanced technologies lead to an accurate diagnosis.

Visual examination of tumors provides very little information about their growth rate or the type of treatment to which they will respond. GENZYME's prognostic expertise can accurately evaluate the aggressiveness of the cancer, and predict the effects of therapy.

Cancers have traditionally been treated as follows: if one therapy proves ineffective, then try another until a successful therapy is found or all options are exhausted. GENZYME helps to eliminate the need for this trial-and-error method by providing individualized information to help determine the optimal therapy before initiating treatment. This can save the patient time and money and most importantly, it may provide a better opportunity for first-strike eradication.

GENZYME provides highly sensitive patient monitoring for the follow-up care of many cancers. For example, GENZYME can determine whether certain types of lymphomas have recurred before they can be detected by any other method. The earlier tumor recurrence is detected, the greater the likelihood of therapeutic success.

Typically, within 48 hours after receiving a specimen, GENZYME returns the stained slides along with a thorough and detailed case report to a physician. Your oncologist can also consult with a member of the GENZYME staff by phone. Contact information for GENZYME follows: (800) 447-5816, www. genzymegenetics.com.

## How to Implement Step One

Make certain that your surgeon sends a specimen of your tumor to GENZYME for immunohistochemistry testing. Be sure to follow the instructions that GENZYME provides for proper shipping of the surgical specimen. You may have to pay out of pocket for this test because not all insurance plans reimburse for it. Please note that this test may not be of benefit to all cancer patients. While it provides a basis for improved treatment, not all cancers are effectively treated with current therapies.

## STEP TWO: DETERMINE SENSITIVITY OR RESISTANCE TO CHEMOTHERAPY

When a person is prescribed a treatment for their cancer, they might assume that the treatment was chosen based on the uniqueness of their cancer. For instance, when a woman with early-stage breast cancer is told that her chemotherapy treatment regimen will consist of the drugs Adriamycin® (doxorubicin), Cytoxan® (cyclophosphamide), and Taxol® (paclitaxel) (ACT), she might think this treatment was individually tailored for her cancer. In actuality, ACT is a standard chemotherapy protocol given to breast cancer patients. This one-size-fits-all approach to breast cancer treatment would work well if superior results were obtained from this routine practice. Sadly, this has not been the case.

The one-size-fits-all approach to prescribing chemotherapy has failed to improve survival for the vast majority of women with breast cancer. In a shocking study of women with breast cancer over the age of 50 who had cancer present in their lymph nodes, standard chemotherapy regimens were shown to increase 10-year survival by only 3%.[2,3] Other studies have determined that standard chemotherapy does not improve survival in women with estrogen-receptor–positive breast cancer.[4,5]

A critical flaw of the one-size-fits-all approach rests in treating all breast cancers as if they are the same. Although traditional oncology does make distinctions in a few obvious qualities, such as size of the cancer, lymph node status, and estrogen receptor status, we now know there can be substantial individual differences in cancer cell genetics among those with "similar" breast cancers. These differences can dramatically influence the response to treatment. A powerful illustration of the lack of appreciation for individual differences in cancer treatment was clearly revealed in a landmark study published in the *New England Journal of Medicine* in 2007. Researchers compared women with lymph node–positive breast cancer who received ACT chemotherapy to those who did not receive chemotherapy.[6] Their HER2 status was also determined—which refers to a genetic characteristic of the cancer. The researchers discovered that the group of women who were HER2 negative and estrogen receptor positive did not benefit at all from taking Taxol®. The ramifications of this study are immense, as a large percentage of women with breast cancer fall into this category. In recognition of the failure of Taxol® to benefit this large group of women with breast cancer, oncologist Anne Moore, professor of clinical medicine at the Weill Medical College, Cornell University, stated, "The days of 'one size fits all' therapy for patients with breast cancer are coming to an end."[7]

A further indictment of the one-size-fits-all approach was prominently displayed in a study published in the *Journal of the National Cancer Institute* in 2008. In this investigation,[8] scientists measured the effectiveness of an anthracycline-based chemotherapy regimen in 5354 women with early-stage breast cancer. Anthracyclines are a class of chemotherapy drugs of which Adriamycin® is a key member. The authors determined that women with early-stage breast cancer who were HER2-negative derived absolutely no benefit from taking Adriamycin® or other anthracycline drugs. Given that approximately 80% of breast cancers are HER2 negative,[7] these results suggest that only 1 of 5 women with breast cancer may benefit from these considerably toxic drugs. For example, in a large-scale study, 5% of patients treated with Adriamycin® developed congestive heart failure.[9]

Breast cancer is not the only type of cancer in which resistance to chemotherapy may impair treatment; in fact, all cancers may display interindividual variability in chemosensitivity. For example, assessing expression of a chemoresistance protein (IGFBP2) in leukemia patients helped identify those who were likely to respond to standard chemotherapy, and those who were not.[10]

If chemotherapy is being considered, it is crucial to ascertain which chemotherapy drugs will have the highest probability of being effective against your

particular cancer. Rational Therapeutics performs chemosensitivity testing in the laboratory on living cancer cells to determine how they respond when exposed to various drugs.

Rational Therapeutics was founded in 1993 by Robert Nagourney, a prominent hematologist and oncologist. Rational Therapeutics pioneers cancer therapies that are specifically tailored for each individual patient, and is a leader in individualized cancer strategies. With no financial ties to outside health care organizations, recommendations are made without financial bias.

Rational Therapeutics develops and provides cancer therapy recommendations that have been designed scientifically for each patient. Following the collection of living cancer cells obtained at the time of biopsy or surgery, Rational Therapeutics performs an ex-vivo analysis of programmed cell death (EVA-PCD) functional profile on your tumor sample to measure drug activity (sensitivity and resistance). Ex-vivo analysis means that your living tumor cells are maintained outside of your body for the purpose of determining which drug or drug combination most effectively induces cell death in the laboratory. Each patient is highly individualized with regard to his or her sensitivity to chemotherapy drugs. Your responsiveness to chemotherapy is as unique as your fingerprints. Therefore, this test will help to determine which drug(s) will be most effective for you. Rational Therapeutics then makes a treatment recommendation based on these findings.

Rational Therapeutics provides custom-tailored, assay-directed therapy based on the response of a specific tumor in the laboratory. This eliminates much of the guesswork prior to undergoing potentially toxic side effects of chemotherapy regimens that could prove to be of little value against an individual's cancer. Contact information for Rational Therapeutics: Rational Therapeutics, 750 East 29th Street, Long Beach, CA 90806, (562) 989-6455, http://www.rationaltherapeutics.com/.

## How to Implement Step Two

Contact Rational Therapeutics so that your surgeon can follow the precise instructions required to send a living specimen of your tumor for chemosensitivity testing. It is important that your surgeon carefully coordinate with Rational Therapeutics in order to ensure that your cells arrive in a viable condition. You may have to pay for this test yourself because your insurance may not reimburse for it. Please note that this test may not be of benefit to all cancer patients. While it provides a basis for improved treatment, not all cancers are effectively treated with current therapies.

# STEP THREE: CIRCULATING TUMOR CELL TESTING

Circulating tumor cell (CTC) testing involves the detection of cancer cells in the bloodstream. These circulating tumor cells are the "seeds" that break away from the primary site of cancer and spread to other parts of the body. Understanding circulating tumor cells is critically important since it is the spread of cancer to other parts of the body—and not the primary cancer—that is very often responsible for the death of a person with cancer.

Historically, medical science has been focused on the primary tumor, basing treatment decisions on the specific genetic characteristics of the primary cancer cells—which assumes that the metastatic cancer cells are genetically identical to the primary tumor. This assumption might be ill-advised, as research has demonstrated that metastatic cancer cells can be genetically dissimilar from the primary tumor as they become more highly differentiated.

In an illuminating study conducted with metastatic breast cancer patients, researchers compared the genetic composition of the cancer cells that had formed distant metastasis to the genetic composition of the corresponding cancer cells in the primary breast tumor. The findings were alarming—in 31% of the comparisons, the genetic composition of the metastatic cancer cells differed almost completely from that of the primary breast tumors.[11] Amazingly, further analysis revealed that none of the pairs of primary breast tumors with its corresponding metastatic cancer were identical. Based on these findings, the authors remarked that "because metastatic cells often have a completely different genetic composition, their phenotype [biological behavior], including aggressiveness and therapy responsiveness, may also vary substantially from that seen in the primary tumors," leading to their conclusion that "the resulting heterogeneity [genetic variability] of metastatic breast cancer may underlie its poor responsiveness to therapy...." To further support the evidence that metastatic cancer cells can vary genetically from the primary tumor, two additional studies of breast cancer patients have demonstrated that CTC can be HER2 positive while the primary breast tumor can be HER2 negative.[12,13]

This research suggests that directing treatment towards the cancer cells of the primary tumor can, in some cases, fail to destroy the circulating tumor cells.

For this reason, focusing on the metastatic cancer cells could potentially lead to better results.

CTC testing has been shown to improve prognostic accuracy. German scientists studied 35 women with nonmetastatic breast cancer who had their levels of CTC measured before they had received any treatment for their cancer.[14] Seventeen tested positive for CTC, while 18 tested negative for CTC. The group that tested negative for CTC had a median overall survival of 125 months. The group with ≥5 CTC present in their blood sample had a median overall survival of only 61 months. In a related study, researchers at the M.D. Anderson Cancer Center, University of Texas, measured CTC in 151 women with metastatic breast cancer.[15] These patients were also evaluated for other prognostic cancer markers, such as hormone receptor status, CA 27.29, and HER2 status. Those who had 5 or more CTC per blood sample had a median overall survival of 13.5 months. The median overall survival for those with <5 CTC per blood sample was over 29 months. The researchers also discovered that the presence of ≥5 CTC in a blood sample had the highest predictive value compared to all other tumor markers. The researchers went on to state that "circulating tumor cells have superior and independent prognostic value..."

Furthermore, recent research indicates that CTC evaluation can be used to predict prognosis for men with prostate cancer. Researchers at Thomas Jefferson University compared the levels of CTC in 37 men with metastatic prostate cancer.[16] Their findings were remarkable—for the men with ≥5 CTC per blood sample, the median overall survival was only 8.4 months. For those with <5 CTC, the median overall survival was 48 months. Yet another study measured CTC in 55 men with a rising PSA after surgery for prostate cancer.[17] A rising PSA after surgery is strongly predictive of prostate cancer recurrence.[18] Radiation therapy was administered to 15 patients. Sixty percent of those who were CTC-positive had progression of their disease during radiation therapy, while there were no disease progression in the CTC-negative group. Additional studies have confirmed these results.[19,20]

One of the most exciting potential uses of CTC technology is to allow doctors to evaluate treatment effectiveness during the early phase of therapy. With regard to chemotherapy, doctors have often had to wait at least a few months before they can assess the effectiveness of treatment. This inability to evaluate a treatment's efficacy during the early phase of therapy can have disastrous consequences for the person with cancer. Those 3 months of waiting to know if the treatment is working can make the difference between altering therapy to reflect the lack of response, or continuing with an ineffective treatment and allowing the cancer to progress. This waiting may become a thing of the past, as recent studies have demonstrated that CTC testing can reliably predict the response to treatment during the early phase of therapy. In an important study,[21] 163 women with metastatic breast cancer were tested for CTC at 4 different times during the course of treatment. The first measurement of CTC was taken approximately 4 weeks after treatment had begun. At the first measurement the researchers discovered that those patients with <5 CTC per sample had a median overall survival of >18.5 months. Those with ≥5 CTC per sample had a median overall survival of only 7 months. Additionally, 66% of those with ≥5 CTC per sample had died after 1 year, compared to only 19% of those who had <5 CTC per sample. Thus, as early as 4 weeks into therapy, CTC testing determined which patients were not responding and whose cancer would continue to progress with ineffective treatment. The authors of this study concluded that "detection of elevated CTC at any time during therapy is an accurate indication of subsequent rapid disease progression and mortality for metastatic breast cancer patients."

In a study published in the *Journal of Clinical Oncology* in 2008, 430 patients with metastatic colon cancer had CTC testing before and 3–5 weeks after the initiation of treatment with chemotherapy.[22] For patients who initially started with ≥3 CTC detected in their blood sample, if they converted to <3 CTC, then the median survival was 11 months. However, if they continued to have ≥3 CTC on follow-up testing, then the median survival was only 3.7 months. For patients whose cancers were deemed to be nonprogressing by imaging studies, median survival was 18.8 months if they had <3 CTC on follow-up testing, whereas those with ≥3 CTC on follow-up testing had a median survival of only 7.1 months. The authors concluded that "the number of CTCs before and during treatment is an independent predictor of ... overall survival in patients with metastatic colorectal cancer. CTCs provide prognostic information in addition to that of imaging studies."

CTC testing can also predict the likelihood of recurrence after initial cancer treatment. In 2006, scientists in Spain measured the presence of CTC in 84 high-risk breast cancer patients after they received initial chemotherapy.[23] The researchers found dramatic differences in the relapse rates between those whose blood samples tested positive for CTC, as compared to those who tested negative. The group testing positive

for CTC had a 269% increased risk of relapse, and a 300% increased risk of death, compared to the group testing negative. Further analysis showed a striking 53-month difference in the time to relapse between the groups. In a related study, German scientists in 2008 studied 25 women with breast cancer that had not metastasized.[24] They measured CTC levels before and after the patients received chemotherapy. The results showed that relapse occurred in only 9% of patients whose CTC levels indicated a decline, no change, or minor increase when compared to baseline CTC levels. There was a substantially higher relapse rate of 40% in the group with a CTC increase at the end of therapy.

Given that CTC can be the seeds that eventually form metastatic disease, then CTC analysis provides medical science with an excellent opportunity to examine the genetic features of these cancer cells before metastasis occurs, when treatment is far more likely to be successful. In addition to detecting the presence and quantity of CTC in the bloodstream, recent advances in technology now allow the examination of CTC for a large number of tumor cell markers and genetic expressions. The information obtained from this analysis can provide vital insight as to which chemotherapy drugs are best suited to exploit the genetic weaknesses of the CTC, as well as which chemotherapy agents are likely to be powerless against the genetic strengths of the CTC.

The following examples illustrate the benefits of CTC analysis of tumor markers and genetic expressions. Chemotherapy drugs can exert their therapeutic effects by inhibiting essential enzymes within the cancer cell. The overexpression of these enzymes—called drug targets—can enhance the tumor destructive effects of these drugs. Adriamycin® (doxorubicin) is a prime example of this mechanism of action. The main drug target for Adriamycin® is topoisomerase 2. Studies have demonstrated that those patients with cancers expressing higher levels of topoisomerase 2 can benefit from treatment with Adriamycin®.[25] Conversely, patients with cancers that produce smaller amounts of topoisomerase 2 are less likely to respond to Adriamycin®. Cancer cells also have the ability to produce enzymes that convert chemotherapy drugs into less potent forms, which weakens the antitumor activity of these drugs. 5-FU is commonly used in the treatment of breast and colon cancer. DPD is an enzyme that degrades 5-FU to an inactive metabolite. Cancer cells expressing higher levels of DPD can be resistant to 5-FU. One study of colorectal cancer patients treated with 5-FU revealed that those with high DPD levels had significantly *shorter overall survival* compared to patients with low DPD expression.[26]

As an added benefit, genetic analysis of CTC can inform us as to which natural supplements might be best indicated. For instance, NF-κB promotes the growth of cancer. Curcumin is an inhibitor of NF-κB.[27] So, a person whose cancer is expressing high levels of NF-κB might consider including curcumin as part of their supplement program.

Some cancers are able to produce GSTpi, which confers resistance to multiple chemotherapy drugs. Ellagic acid—from pomegranate—inhibits GSTpi.[28] Supplementation with ellagic acid may be wise if CTC analysis demonstrates over production of GSTpi.

## How to Implement Step Three

To test for the presence and quantity of CTC in your blood, speak with your physician regarding the Veridex CellSearch CTC test. You may also order quantitative CTC tests for breast, colon, and prostate cancer from Life Extension at 800-226-2370, or on the web at www.lef.org.

> **Note:** *Qualitative CTC testing is most feasible with any kind of* carcinoma (*eg, lung, colon, breast, ovary, cervix, prostate, stomach, gastric, esophagus, liver, etc.*), mesothelioma, *or* melanoma.

It is also possible to test for *synovial sarcoma.* However, other types of sarcoma (eg, liposarcoma, leiomyosarcoma, chondrosarcoma, etc.) gave lower success rates for isolation of tumor cells (<50%).

Testing *central nervous system* tumors (eg, glioblastoma) is limited, because in the majority of cases isolating CTCs is not successful, since these tumors rarely shed tumor cells into the bloodstream.

*Hematological cancers* (eg, Hodgkin- or non-Hodgkin lymphomas, B-cell lymphomas, myelogenous and lymphocytic leukemias) can be assayed as well. Please note that we cannot test for T-cell cancers at all. Testing for multiple myeloma (MM) is not recommended since low detection rates in MM have been observed.

For a molecular analysis of your CTC, contact the International Strategic Cancer Alliance at 610-628-3419 to arrange for a blood specimen to be obtained and shipped for testing. Note that this test is qualitative and will not provide the number of CTC present in your blood. You may have to pay out of pocket for this test because not all insurance plans reimburse for it. Please note also that this molecular analysis test of circulating tumor cells may not be of benefit to all cancer patients. While it provides a basis for improved treatment, not all cancers are effectively treated with currently available therapies.

## STEP FOUR: INHIBITING THE CYCLOOXYGENASE ENZYMES (COX-1 AND COX-2)

Inflammation plays a pivotal role in the formation and progression of cancer. There are many inflammatory pathways in the body. The cyclooxygenase (COX-2) enzyme is a particular inflammatory pathway that has been the focus of research in the realm of oncology. Initially, scientists believed COX-2 was merely an inducible response to inflammation. It is now speculated that COX-2 performs biological functions in the body, particularly in the brain and kidneys as well as the immune system. COX-2 becomes troublesome when upregulated (sometimes 10- to 80-fold) by proinflammatory stimuli (interleukin-1, growth factors, tumor necrosis factor, and endotoxins). When overexpressed, COX-2 participates in various pathways that could promote cancer (ie, angiogenesis), cell proliferation, and the production of inflammatory prostaglandins.[29–31]

A growing body of research has documented the relationship between COX-2 and cancer:

- An article in the journal *Cancer Research* showed that COX-2 levels in pancreatic cancer cells are 60 times greater than in adjacent normal tissue.[32]

- Solid tumors contain oxygen-deficient or hypoxic areas (a reduced oxygen supply to a tissue below physiologic levels). Hypoxia promotes upregulation of COX-2 and angiogenesis, and establishes resistance to ionizing radiation.[33]

- Within the nonsteroidal anti-inflammatory drug (NSAIDs) class is a subclass referred to as COX-2 inhibitors (cyclooxygenase inhibitors). COX-2 inhibitors were popularly prescribed to relieve pain but now have found a place in oncology. It began when scientists recognized that people who regularly take NSAIDs lowered their risk of colon cancer by as much as 50%.[34]

- The *Journal of the American Medical Association* reported that a 9.4-year epidemiologic study showed that COX-2 upregulation was related to more advanced tumor stage, tumor size, and lymph node metastasis as well as diminished survival rates among colorectal cancer patients.[35] With more regular use of aspirin (a COX-2 inhibitor), the risk of dying from the disease decreased.[36,37] The journal *Gastroenterology* reported additional encouragement, showing that three different colon cell lines underwent apoptosis (cell death) when deprived of COX-2; when lovastatin was added to the COX-2 inhibitor the kill rate increased another 5-fold.[38]

The benefits observed with COX-2 inhibitors extend beyond colon protection to the cardiovascular system, where they help sustain endothelial cell function.[39]

- A groundbreaking study published in 2009 revealed that breast cancer patients treated with COX-2 inhibitors had a greatly reduced risk of bone metastases. In this investigation, the incidence of bone metastases were recorded in breast cancer patients who were not treated with a COX-2 inhibitor, as well as in individuals who received a COX-2 inhibitor for at least 6 months following the diagnosis of breast cancer. The findings were astounding— those who were treated with a COX-2 inhibitor were 90% less likely to develop bone metastases than those who were not treated with a COX-2 inhibitor.[40]

- In another study, 134 patients with advanced lung cancer were treated with chemotherapy alone or combined with Celebrex® (a COX-2 inhibitor). For patients with cancers expressing increased amounts of COX-2, treatment with Celebrex® dramatically prolonged survival.[41]

- Celebrex® slowed cancer progression in men with recurrent prostate cancer.[42,43]

- Celebrex® prevented weight loss and improved quality of life in individuals with head and neck cancers.[44]

- Regular intake of OTC NSAIDs produced highly significant composite risk reductions of 43% for colon cancer, 25% for breast cancer, 28% for lung cancer, and 27% for prostate cancer. Furthermore, in a series of case control studies, daily use of a selective COX-2 inhibitor, either celecoxib or rofecoxib, significantly reduced the risk for each of these malignancies. The evidence is compelling that anti-inflammatory agents with selective or nonselective activity against cyclooxygenase-2 (COX-2) have strong potential for the chemoprevention of cancers of the colon, breast, prostate, and lung. Results confirming that COX-2 blockade is effective for cancer prevention have been tempered by observations that some selective COX-2 inhibitors pose a risk to the cardiovascular system.[45]

Life Extension recognizes the value of COX-2 inhibitors in cancer treatment. Some progressive oncologists include COX-2 inhibitors in their anticancer protocols, but the numbers are still relatively few. The risks associated with traditional NSAIDs include gastrointestinal perforation, ulceration, and bleeding, and less frequently, renal and liver damage, but the benefits for certain cancer patients may outweigh these risks.

A number of natural COX-2 inhibitors are discussed in the protocol titled Cancer Adjuvant Therapy.

Like COX-2, the COX-1 enzyme also catalyzes (mediates) the conversion of certain fatty acids into inflammatory end products in some cell types. Cancer cells are sometimes genetically altered in such a way that causes them to express higher levels of COX-1; this has been observed in several types of cancer including ovarian, colon, and head and neck cancers.[46–48] Moreover, selectively inhibiting COX-1 with experimental compounds has demonstrated a marked reduction in viability of colon cancer cells and ovarian cancer cells.[48,49]

Experimental studies on breast cancer cells revealed that simultaneous inhibition of both COX-1 and COX-2 might exert a synergistic effect to combat cancer cell growth.[50] The authors of this study concluded that "[t]he significant and additive effects exhibited by the combination of COX-1 and -2 inhibitors and their effects on cell cycle suggest that these agents could become an effective treatment modality for carcinoma of the breast."

*Aspirin* is an NSAID, but its actions are unique in that it selectively inhibits COX-1 activity while modulating the expression of COX-2.[51] The net result of this dualistic action is diminished production of harmful metabolites via COX-1 and a reduction in total COX-2 activity. Since both COX-1 and COX-2 are drivers of inflammatory cancer cell growth, aspirin is an important yet underappreciated anticancer drug.

At the forefront of the growing field of research into aspirin's role as a cancer fighter is Peter Rothwell at Oxford University. Having specialized primarily in cardiovascular medical research, he and his colleagues had at their disposal a trove of information compiled from eight massive studies examining the effect of aspirin therapy on cardiovascular health.

Among the most compelling of their findings:

- Aspirin reduced the overall risk of death from cancer by approximately *20%*.

- Most of that benefit was due to a *30–40%* reduction in deaths occurring after *5 years* of daily aspirin intake.

- The reduction in deaths due to solid cancers was maintained for *20 years* in studies in which data were available for that period of time.

- These effects were consistent across *all* populations studied, despite diversity in health histories.

- A dose of just *75 mg* daily was all that was required for the protective effect—higher doses did not increase the benefit.

- The reduction in cancer deaths increased with age: peak effects were observed in people aged *55-64* and remained high in those *65 years or older*.

- The effect of aspirin on reducing risk of fatal cancers was powerful enough to contribute to a *significant reduction in mortality rates from all causes*.

The data correlating aspirin therapy with *colon cancer* prevention proved particularly compelling. Rothwell's team saw a 24% reduction in the risk of developing colon cancer over a 20-year period in patients who took aspirin daily and a 35% reduction in the risk of dying from colon cancer. The most potent preventive benefit was observed in cancers of the *upper* colon (the ascending and transverse colon).[52]

Separate observational studies have suggested a preventive effect for cancers of the *esophagus, stomach, lung, breast,* and *ovaries*.[53-55] A 2010 study revealed that men taking regular aspirin supplements attained a 10% reduction in prostate cancer risk compared to men who took no aspirin.[56] Another study showed a risk reduction of 24% in long-term users (>5 years), and 29% in daily aspirin users.[57]

## How to Implement Step Four

- Take a low-dose aspirin each day.
- Ask your physician to prescribe one of the following COX-2–inhibiting drugs:

Lodine XL 1000 mg once daily

Celebrex®, 100–200 mg every 12 hours

**Note:** *The use of Lodine and Celebrex® has been associated with an increased risk of heart attack and stroke. The anticancer benefits of these drugs have to be weighed against increased cardiovascular risks. Using aspirin in combination with a COX-2 inhibitor may increase the risk for bleeding, but also reduce cardiovascular risks. Consult with your physician before combining aspirin with a COX-2 inhibitor.*

## STEP FIVE: SUPPRESSING RAS ONCOGENE EXPRESSION

The family of proteins known as Ras plays a central role in the regulation of cell growth. It fulfills this fundamental role by integrating the regulatory signals that govern the cell cycle and proliferation.

Defects in the Ras-Raf pathway can result in cancerous growth. Mutant Ras genes were among the first oncogenes identified for their ability to transform cells into a cancerous phenotype (ie, a cell observably altered because of distorted gene expression). Mutations in one of three genes (H, N, or K-Ras) encoding Ras proteins are associated with upregulated cell proliferation and are found in an estimated 30–40% of all human cancers. The highest incidences of Ras mutations are found in cancers of the pancreas (80%), colon (50%), thyroid (50%), lung (40%), liver (30%), melanoma (30%), and myeloid leukemia (30%).[58-64]

The differences between oncogenes and normal genes can be slight. The mutant protein that an oncogene ultimately creates may differ from the healthy version by only a single amino acid, but this subtle variation can radically alter the protein's functionality.

The Ras-Raf pathway is used by human cells to transmit signals from the cell surface to the nucleus. Such signals direct cells to divide, differentiate, or even undergo programmed cell death (apoptosis).

A Ras gene usually behaves as a relay switch within the signal pathway that instructs the cell to divide. In response to stimuli transmitted to the cell from outside, cell-signaling pathways are activated. In the absence of stimulus, the Ras protein remains in the "off" position. A mutated Ras protein gene behaves like a switch stuck on the "on" position, continuously misinforming the cell, instructing it to divide when the cycle should be turned off.[65,66] Researchers have known for some time that injecting anti-Ras antibodies, specific for amino acid 12, cause a reversal of excessive proliferation and a transient alteration of the mutated cell to one of a normal appearance.[67] Recently, scientists have taken advantage of the high frequency at which K-ras is mutated in several types of cancer by developing vaccines that trigger the immune system to attack cells harboring this mutant protein. For example, a 2011 study found that patients with resected pancreatic cancer were much more likely to be alive 10 years postvaccination (20%) than those who did not receive the vaccine (0%).[68]

To establish new methods for diagnosing pancreatic cancer, K-Ras mutations were examined in the pancreatic juice of pancreatic cancer patients. Pancreatic juice was positive for K-Ras in 87.8% (36/41) of patients.[69] When combined with p53 mutations in the stool and CA 19-9 (a blood marker for pancreatic cancer), it may be possible to identify the disease much earlier than by conventional diagnostic methods.[70]

Greater understanding regarding the activity of mutant Ras genes opens exciting avenues of treatment. Researchers found that precursor Ras genes must undergo several biochemical modifications to become mature, active versions. After such maturation, the Ras proteins attach to the inner surface of the cell's outer membrane where they can interact with other cellular proteins and stimulate cell growth.

The events resulting in mature Ras genes take place in three steps, the most critical being the first, known as the farnesylation step. A specific enzyme, farnesyl-protein transferase (FPTase), speeds up the reaction. One strategy for blocking Ras protein activity has been to inhibit FPTase. Inhibitors of this enzyme block the maturation of Ras protein and reverse the cancerous transformation induced by mutant Ras genes.[66]

A number of natural substances impact the activity of Ras oncogenes. For example, limonene is a substance found in the essential oils of citrus products. Limonene has been shown to act as a farnesyl transferase inhibitor. Administering high doses of limonene to cancer-bearing animals blocks the farnesylation of Ras, thus inhibiting cell replication.[71,72] Curcumin inhibited the farnesylation of RAS, and caused cell death in breast cancer cells expressing RAS mutations.[73,74]

Japanese researchers examined the effects of vitamin E on the presence of K-Ras mutations in mice with lung cancer. Prior to treatment with vitamin E, K-Ras mutations were present in 64% of the mice. After treatment with vitamin E, only 18% of the mice expressed K-Ras mutations.[75] Vitamin E decreased levels of H-Ras proteins in cultured melanoma cells.[76] A study conducted at Mercy Hospital of Pittsburgh also showed that diallyl disulfide, a naturally occurring organosulfide from garlic, inhibits p21 H-Ras oncogenes, displaying a significant restraining effect on tumor growth.[77]

Researchers at Rutgers University investigated the ability of various green and black tea polyphenols to inhibit H-Ras oncogenes. The Rutgers team found that all the major polyphenols contained in green and black tea except epicatechin showed strong inhibition of cell growth.[78] Investigators at Texas A&M University also found that fish oil decreased colonic Ras membrane localization and reduced tumor formation in rats. In view of the central role of oncogenic Ras in the development of colon cancer, the finding that omega-3 fatty acids modulate Ras activation could explain why dietary fish oil protects against colon cancer.[79]

Statins are a class of popular cholesterol-lowering drugs. Mevacor® (lovastatin), Zocor® (simvastatin), and Pravachol (pravastatin) are statin drugs shown to inhibit the activity of Ras oncogenes.[80] Statin drugs block the HMG-COA reductase enzyme, which depletes cells of farnesyl pyrophosphate. This results in a reduction of activated farnesylated Ras.[81]

Illustrative of the potential of statin therapy, patients with primary liver cancer were treated with either the chemotherapeutic drug 5-FU or a combination of 5-FU and 40 mg/day of pravastatin.[82] Median survival increased from 9 months, among patients treated with only 5-FU, to 18 months when using 5-FU combined with the statin drug pravastatin (Pravachol). In 2008, German researchers studied the effects of pravastatin in patients with advanced liver cancer.[83] A total of 131 patients received chemoembolization alone, while 52 patients received chemoembolization plus pravastatin (20–40mg). During the observation period of up to 5 years, 23.7% of the patients treated with chemoembolization alone had survived, compared to a 36.5% survival for the chemoembolization and pravastatin group. Median survival was 12 months for the chemoembolization-only group, while the pravastatin group had a median survival of 20.9 months.

Statin drugs are known to deplete coenzyme Q10 (CoQ10) levels; therefore, those taking a statin drug should supplement with CoQ10. For a detailed explanation, see the Coenzyme Q10 section in the Cancer Adjuvant Therapy protocol.

Individuals with cancer should consider an immunohistochemistry test of their cancer tissue for mutated ras genes at GENZYME Laboratories (see Step One of this protocol), a recommendation the Life Extension first made in 1997; Life Extension strongly believes all cancer patients should undergo immunohistochemical testing to determine Ras status.

## How to Implement Step Five

Ask your physician to prescribe one of the following statin drugs to inhibit the activity of Ras oncogenes:

- Mevacor® (lovastatin)
- Zocor® (simvastatin)
- Pravachol (pravastatin)

**Note:** *Statin drugs may generate adverse side effects. Physician oversight and careful surveillance with monthly blood tests (at least initially) to evaluate liver function, muscle enzymes, and lipid levels are suggested.*

In addition to statin drug therapy, consider supplementing with the following nutrients to further suppress the expression of Ras oncogenes:

- Curcumin, as highly absorbed BCM-95® extract: 400–800 mg daily
- Fish oil: 2100 mg of EPA and 1500 mg of DHA daily with meals
- Green tea, standardized extract: 725–1450 mg of EGCG daily
- Aged garlic extract: 2400 mg daily with meals
- Vitamin E: 400–1000 IU of natural alpha tocopherol along with at least 200 mg of gamma-tocopherol daily with meals

## STEP SIX: CORRECTING COAGULATION ABNORMALITIES

Both experimental and clinical data have determined that coagulation disorders are common in patients with cancer. Many cancer patients reportedly have a hypercoagulable state, with recurrent thrombosis (blood clot) due to the impact of cancer cells and chemotherapy on the coagulation cascade.[84] Pulmonary embolism (blood clot in the lung) is a particular problem for patients with pancreatic and gastric cancer, colon cancer, and ovarian cancer.[85] Thus, momentum is building for anticoagulant therapy through reports, the vast majority of which are derived from secondary analyses of clinical trials on the treatment of thromboembolism.

Research on low-molecular-weight heparin (LMWH)—an anticoagulant—shows promise in regard to increasing cancer survival rates. Data comparing unfractionated heparin to LMWH indicate that LMWH is equally beneficial if not more beneficial to cancer patients in terms of survival. The improved life expectancy gathered from anticoagulant therapy is not solely a result of the reduced complications from thromboembolism, but also from enzyme interactions, cellular growth modifications, and antiangiogenic factors.[86,87] It appears that heparin inhibits the formation of cancer's vascular network by binding to angiogenic promoters (ie, basic fibroblast growth factor and VEGF).[88]

Another important aspect of anticoagulant therapy involves breaking down fibrin, a coagulation protein found in blood. Cancers employ various strategies to utilize fibrin for their own benefit. For example, fibrin covers cancer cells with a protective coat, hindering recognition by the immune system. In addition, fibrin relays a signal to the cancer to initiate angiogenesis—the growth of new blood vessels. As fibrin encourages a healthy vascular network and tumor growth increases, it sets the stage for metastasis.

German scientists evaluated whether cancer fatalities in women with previously untreated breast cancer were reduced using LMWH therapy. The study showed that breast cancer patients receiving LMWH had a lower rate of mortality during the first 650 days following surgery, compared to women receiving unfractionated heparin. The survival advantage was apparent after even a short course of therapy.[89] In another study of 300 breast cancer patients, none of the trial participants developed metastasis while receiving anticoagulant therapy, although 37 (12.3%) died from the disease.[90]

Similar advantages were evidenced among small-cell lung cancer patients undergoing heparin therapy in conjunction with conventional treatments. When subjects were treated with heparin they enjoyed a better prognosis, with greater numbers of complete responses, longer median survival, and higher survival rates at 1, 2, and 3 years compared to patients who did not receive heparin.[91]

A comprehensive analysis of the data pertaining to all studies published on the impact of heparin treatment on survival in cancer patients determined that treatment with heparin (both unfractionated heparin and LMWH) decreased the risk of death by 23%, compared to those who did not receive heparin.[92]

### How to Implement Step Six

Ascertain if you are in a hypercoagulable state by having your blood tested for prothrombin time (PT), partial thromboplastin time (PTT), and D-dimers. A hypercoagulable state is suggested if the shortening of the PT and PTT are seen in conjunction with elevation of D-dimers (see Table 1).

If there is any evidence of a hypercoagulable (prethrombotic) state, ask your physician to prescribe the appropriate individualized dose of low-molecular-weight heparin (LMWH). Repeat the prothrombin blood test every 2 weeks.

## STEP SEVEN: MAINTAINING BONE INTEGRITY

Some types of cancer (ie, breast, prostate, and multiple myeloma) have a proclivity to metastasize to the bone.[93,94] The result may be bone pain, which also may be associated with weakening of the bone and an increased risk of fractures.[95,96]

**Table 1:  Lab Tests for Hypercoagulability**

| Tests Routinely Available | Results If Hypercoagulable | Tests Requiring Dedicated Coagulation Laboratory | Results If Hypercoagulable |
|---|---|---|---|
| Protime (PT) | Less than normal | Alpha-1 antitrypsin (A1AT) | Elevated |
| Partial thromboplastin time (PTT) | Less than normal | Euglobulin clot lysis time (ECLT) | Prolonged |
| Platelet count (part of CBC) | Elevated | Factor VIII levels | Elevated |

Patients with prostate cancer have been found to have a very high incidence of osteoporosis or osteopenia even before the use of therapies that lower testosterone levels.[97] In settings such as prostate cancer, when excessive bone loss is occurring, there is a release of bone-derived growth factors, such as TGF-beta-1, which has been associated with aggressive prostate cancer.[98] In turn, prostate cancer cells produce substances such as interleukin-6 (IL-6), which causes effects the further breakdown of bone.[85,88] Thus, a vicious cycle results: bone breakdown, the stimulation of prostate cancer cell growth, and the production of interleukin IL-6 and other cell products, which leads to further bone breakdown.

The administration of any of the drugs called bisphosphonates, such as Aredia®, Zometa®, and Fosamax® or Actonel® can be used to stop this vicious cycle. These agents inhibit excessive bone breakdown and favor bone formation.[99–103]

The problem that prostate and breast cancer patients face is that bisphosphonate therapy is usually only prescribed for preexisting bone metastasis. If bisphosphonates were administered to those with cancer preventively, then the risk of bone metastasis could theoretically be reduced,[104] although not all studies substantiate this. A study published in 2008 revealed that premenopausal women with early-stage breast cancer (ie, no bone metastasis) given Zometa® experienced a trend toward decreased bone metastasis and greater survival.[105] A subsequent study found an improvement in survival in women with breast cancer who were 5 years past menopause who took Zometa® preventively. However, premenopausal and perimenopausal women did not experience a survival benefit.[106]

Other studies have documented the ability of Zometa® to prevent the onset of bone metastasis. In one study, patients with advanced solid tumors and no evidence of bone metastases were randomized to receive Zometa® or no further treatment. After 12 months, 60% of those receiving Zometa® were free of bone metastasis, compared to only 10% in the control group. After 18 months, 20% of those in the Zometa® group were free of bone metastasis, compared to only 5% in the control group.[104] Zometa®

has also been shown to benefit those with multiple myeloma when given preventatively, by improving survival and reducing the risk of bone metastasis.[107]

The benefits of Zometa® in women with breast cancer are not limited to the prevention of bone metastasis. Many women with breast cancer are given a drug called an aromatase inhibitor. This class of drugs comprises estrogen blockers, frequently used in place of tamoxifen in postmenopausal women with estrogen receptor positive breast cancer. Aromatase inhibitors can cause bone loss and can increase the risk of osteoporosis. In addition to preventing bone metastasis, Zometa® has also been shown to protect against the loss of bone density from the use of aromatase inhibitors.[108]

**Note:** *Bisphosphonate drugs have potentially serious adverse effects. The use of bisphosphonate drugs has been associated with an increased risk of osteonecrosis of the jaw (death and decay of the jaw bone). The incidence of osteonecrosis of the jaw during therapy with Zometa® was found to be 1.3%.[109] This risk is considerably greater in those who had major dental work (ie, tooth extraction) performed during bisphosphonate use. Individuals should avoid undergoing tooth extractions during therapy with Zometa®. Individuals who use bisphosphonate medications under a physician's guidance can help reduce their risk of osteonecrosis of the jaw by receiving a dental examination and undergoing any necessary dental procedures such as tooth extractions before initiating drug therapy.[110] Those taking bisphosphonate drugs should also take bone-protecting minerals like calcium, magnesium, and boron, along with vitamins D and K.*

Additionally, people treated with Zometa® have an increased risk of atrial fibrillation, or irregular heart rhythm causing the heart to pump blood less efficiently, potentially resulting in pulmonary edema (fluid in the lungs), congestive heart failure, stroke, or death. A study showed that 2.5–3% of patients taking bisphosphonates developed atrial fibrillation and 1–2% developed serious atrial fibrillation, with complications including hospitalization or death.[111]

It should be noted that 6.9% of individuals treated with Zometa® experienced kidney toxicity. Zometa® should be used with caution in those with preexisting kidney disease and is contraindicated in those with severe kidney disease.[109]

New research has produced an alternative to Zometa® for the treatment of bone metastasis. Denosumab (Xgeva®) is a monoclonal antibody that inhibits osteoclastic-mediated bone resorption by binding to osteoblast-produced RANKL. By reducing RANKL binding to the osteoclast receptor RANK, bone resorption and turnover decrease.[112] Denosumab has recently been shown to be more effective than Zometa® in the treatment of bone metastasis. In one study, 1904 men with prostate cancer and bone metastasis were randomized to receive Zometa® or Denosumab. The time it took for a subsequent bone metastasis–related event (ie, fracture, spinal cord compression, or radiation/surgery to bone) was longer in the denosumab group, demonstrating the superiority of denosumab over Zometa®.[113]

Denosumab was also compared to Zometa® in women with breast cancer with bone metastasis. This trial found that Denosumab was superior to Zometa® in delaying the time to bone metastasis–related events.[114] Unfortunately, osteonecrosis of the jaw is also a side effect of treatment with Denosumab. Indeed, the incidence of osteonecrosis of the jaw was slightly higher with Denosumab compared to Zometa®. As with Zometa®, renal toxicity has been associated with the use of Denosumab.

A COX-2 inhibitor drug presents another option for the prevention of bone metastasis. As discussed in Step Four of this protocol: Inhibiting COX-2 Enzyme, breast cancer patients treated with a COX-2 inhibitor drug had a 90% reduced risk of developing bone metastases compared to those not treated with a COX-2 inhibitor.

Life Extension advises that the status of bone integrity should be evaluated periodically by means of a quantitative, computerized tomography bone-mineral-density study, called QCT. At the very least, this should be done annually. We prefer to use the QCT scan over the standard DEXA scan since the QCT is not affected by arthritis or calcifications in blood vessels that are commonly seen in individuals over age 50. It is fairly common to see patients with a normal DEXA scan and yet the QCT scan will be blatantly abnormal. The radiation exposure with QCT is only marginally greater than with DEXA scan.

QCT testing sites possibly near you can be found via Mindways, Inc. at (877) 646-3929 or Image Analysis at (800) 548-4849.

Tests that assess bone breakdown are inexpensive and involve a simple urine collection. One such accurate test of bone resorption is called DPD (deoxypyridinoline). This test provides information on excessive bone breakdown. The deoxypyridinoline (DPD) cross-links urine test can be ordered through Life Extension by calling 1-800-226-2370.

## How to Implement Step Seven

If you have a type of cancer with a proclivity to metastasize to the bone (ie, multiple myeloma, breast, or prostate), consider speaking to your oncologist regarding Zometa or Denosumab. If either of these medications is contraindicated, then consider the COX-2 inhibitor drug Celebrex®. Please see Step Four of this protocol for a complete discussion of COX-2 inhibition.

One must always weigh the risks versus the benefits when evaluating a given treatment. This is certainly the case when considering the use of Zometa®, Denosumab, or Celebrex® for the prevention of bone metastasis. Given the excellent prognosis and low risk of bone metastasis, Life Extension *does not* recommend the use of Zometa®, Denosumab, or Celebrex® for women with stage 1 and stage 2A breast cancer. With higher risk cancer, the benefits of these medications likely outweigh the risks. Life Extension recommends the use of medications for the prevention of bone metastasis in women with stage 2B, stage 3, or stage 4 breast cancers.

With regard to prostate cancer, a large percentage of men will be cured with surgery or radiation. Treatment failure is easily detected by a rising PSA after initial treatment. Furthermore, it usually takes several years for bone metastasis to form once a rising PSA has detected treatment failure. This prolonged time frame for the formation of bone metastasis allows for the use of proactive therapies once treatment failure has been detected by a rising PSA. For this reason, Life Extension recommends the use of medications for the prevention of bone metastasis *only* when treatment failure has been detected by a rising PSA after initial treatment. An exception to this recommendation would be men with osteoporosis receiving androgen-deprivation therapy for their initial treatment. Androgen-deprivation therapy can result in further loss of bone density. Given that Zometa® can protect against the loss of bone density, the benefits of using this medication may outweigh the risks in men with osteoporosis receiving long-term androgen deprivation therapy.

Since excessive bone breakdown releases growth factors into the bloodstream that can fuel cancer cell growth, the DPD urine test should be done every 60–90 days to detect bone loss. A QCT bone density scan should be done annually. If either of these tests indicates bone loss, ask your physician to initiate bisphosphonate therapy.

To support bone integrity, the use of bone-supporting nutrients is highly recommended. These include optimal amounts of *vitamin K*, *vitamin D*, *calcium*, *magnesium*, *boron*, and *silica*. See the Osteoporosis protocol for a detailed discussion of the use and dose of these nutrients for bone support.

## STEP EIGHT: INHIBITING ANGIOGENESIS

Angiogenesis—the growth of new blood vessels—is critical during fetal development but occurs minimally in healthy adults. Exceptions occur during wound healing, inflammation, following a myocardial infarction, in female reproductive organs, and in pathologic conditions such as cancer.[115,116]

Angiogenesis is a strictly controlled process in the healthy adult human body, a process regulated by endogenous angiogenic promoters and inhibitors. Judah Folkman, the father of the angiogenesis theory of cancer stated, "Blood vessel growth is controlled by a balancing of opposing factors. A tilt in favor of stimulators over inhibitors might be what trips the lever and begins the process of tumor angiogenesis."[117]

Solid tumors cannot grow beyond the size of a pinhead without inducing the formation of new blood vessels to supply the nutritional needs of the tumor.[118] Since rapid vascularization and tumor growth appear to occur concurrently, interrupting the formation of new blood vessels is paramount to overcoming the malignancy.[119]

Tumor angiogenesis results from a cascade of molecular and cellular events, usually initiated by the release of angiogenic growth factors. At a critical phase in the growth of a cancer, signal molecules are secreted from the cancer to nearby endothelial cells to activate new blood vessel growth. These angiogenic growth factors diffuse in the direction of preexisting blood vessels, encouraging the formation of new blood vessel growth.[120,121] VEGF and basic fibroblast growth factors are expressed by many tumors and appear to be particularly important for angiogenesis.[122]

A number of natural substances, such as curcumin, green tea, N-acetyl-cysteine (NAC), resveratrol, grape seed-skin extract, and vitamin D have antiangiogenic

properties. For further discussion, see the Cancer Adjuvant Therapy protocol.

The Food and Drug Administration (FDA) has approved an antiangiogenesis drug called Avastin® (bevacizumab), but it has demonstrated severe side effects and often only mediocre efficacy. Several other drugs inhibit angiogenesis as secondary mechanisms and are sometimes utilized in cancer therapy. These included sorafenib, sunitinb, pazopanib, and everolimus. These options should be discussed with a healthcare professional because these drugs may cause considerable side effects, and are only FDA approved for specific types of cancer.

### How to Implement Step Eight

There are clinical trials using other antiangiogenesis agents. Log on to www.cancer.gov/clinicaltrials to find out if you are eligible to participate.

Several nutrients have demonstrated potential antiangiogenesis effects.

- Green tea, standardized extract: 725–1450 mg daily
- Curcumin (as highly absorbed BCM-95®): 400–800 mg daily
- Vitamin D: 5000–8000 IU daily (depending on blood levels)
- Grape extract (seed and skin): 150–300 mg daily
- N-acetyl cysteine: 600–1200 mg daily
- Trans-resveratrol: 250 mg daily

## STEP NINE: INHIBITING THE 5-LIPOXYGENASE (5-LOX) ENZYME

As discussed in step four of this protocol, Inhibiting the Cyclooxygenase-2 (COX-2) Enzyme, the scientific literature has demonstrated that inflammation plays a pivotal role in the formation and progression of cancer.

The 5-lipoxygenase (5-LOX) enzyme is another inflammatory enzyme that can contribute to the formation and progression of cancer. Arachidonic acid—a saturated fat found in high concentrations in meat and dairy products—promotes elevation of the 5-LOX enzyme. A growing number of studies has documented that 5-LOX directly stimulates prostate cancer cell proliferation via several well-defined mechanisms.[123–131] In addition, arachidonic acid is metabolized by 5-LOX to 5-HETE, a potent survival factor that prostate cancer cells utilize to escape destruction.[126,132–135]

In response to arachidonic acid overload, the body increases its production of enzymes like 5-lipooxygenase

(5-LOX) to degrade arachidonic acid. Not only does 5-LOX directly stimulate cancer cell propagation,[136–146] but the breakdown products that 5-LOX produces from arachidonic acid (such as leukotriene B4, 5-HETE, and hydroxylated fatty acids) cause tissue destruction, chronic inflammation, and increased resistance of tumor cells to apoptosis (programmed cell destruction).[147–153]

Based on studies showing that consumption of foods rich in arachidonic acid is greatest in regions with high incidence of prostate cancer,[136,147,154,155] scientists sought to determine how much of the 5-LOX enzyme is present in malignant versus benign prostate tissues. Using prostate biopsy samples, the researchers found that 5-LOX levels were an astounding 6-fold greater in malignant prostate tissues compared to benign tissues. This study also found that levels of 5-HETE were 2.2-fold greater in malignant versus benign prostate tissues.[156] The scientists concluded this study by stating that selective inhibitors of 5-LOX may be useful in the prevention or treatment of patients with prostate cancer.

As the evidence mounts that consuming saturated fats increase prostate cancer risk, scientists are evaluating the effects of 5-LOX on various growth factors involved in the progression, angiogenesis, and metastasis of cancer cells. One study found that 5-LOX activity is required to stimulate prostate cancer cell growth by epidermal growth factor (EGF) and other cancer cell proliferating factors produced in the body. When 5-LOX levels were reduced, the cancer cell stimulatory effect of EGF and other growth factors was diminished.[147]

In a mouse study, an increase in 5-LOX resulted in a corresponding increase in vascular endothelial growth factor (VEGF), a key growth factor that tumor cells use to stimulate new blood vessel formation (angiogenesis) into the tumor. 5-LOX inhibitors were shown to reduce tumor angiogenesis along with a host of other growth factors.[157] Chronic inflammation is tightly linked to the induction of aberrant angiogenesis used by cancer cells to facilitate the growth of new blood vessels (angiogenesis) into tumors.[158]

In both androgen-dependent and androgen-independent human prostate cancer cell lines, the inhibition of 5-lipoxygenase (5-LOX) has consistently been shown to induce rapid and massive apoptosis (cancer cell destruction).[136,154,159–162]

As humans age, chronic inflammatory processes can cause the overexpression of 5-LOX in the body. Excess 5-LOX may contribute to the development and progression of prostate cancer in aging males.[163]

Based on the cumulative knowledge that 5-LOX can promote the invasion and metastasis of prostate cancer cells, it would appear advantageous to take aggressive steps to suppress this lethal enzyme. A critical approach to decreasing 5-LOX activity in the body is to decrease the consumption of saturated and omega-6 fats that contain high concentrations of arachidonic acid and high glycemic carbohydrates that contribute to arachidonic acid formation. Another worthwhile approach is to supplement with fish oil, which reduces 5-LOX activity in the body.[164,165] Studies show that lycopene and saw palmetto extract also help to suppress 5-LOX.[159,166–179] The suppression of 5-LOX by these nutrients may partially account for their favorable effects on the prostate gland.

Specific extracts from the boswellia plant selectively inhibit 5-lipoxygenase (5-LOX).[180,181] In several well-controlled human studies, boswellia has been shown to be effective in alleviating various chronic inflammatory disorders.[156,182–190] Scientists have discovered that the specific constituent in boswellia responsible for suppressing 5-LOX is AKBA (3-O-acetyl-11-keto-B-boswellic acid). Boswellia-derived AKBA binds directly to 5-LOX and inhibits its activity.[70] Other boswellic acids only partially and incompletely inhibit 5-LOX.[181,191]

Researchers have discovered how to obtain an economically viable boswellia extract standardized to contain a greater than 20% concentration of AKBA. A novel boswellia extract has been developed that is 52% *more* bioavailable compared to standard boswellia extracts,[192,193] thus providing a greater opportunity to suppress deadly 5-LOX and other cancer-promoting byproducts of arachidonic acid. This more bioavailable AKBA extraction discovery was patented and given the trademark name AprèsFlex™.

## How to Implement Step Nine

Decrease the consumption of saturated and omega-6 fats that contain high concentrations of arachidonic acid, such as meats, dairy products, and egg yolks, along with high-glycemic carbohydrates.

Consider supplementing with the following nutrients to suppress 5-LOX enzyme activity:

- AprèsFlex™: 100–400 mg daily
- Fish oil: 2100 mg of EPA and 1500 mg of DHA daily with meals
- Lycopene: 30 mg daily with meals
- Curcumin (as highly absorbed BCM-95®): 400–800 mg daily

# STEP TEN: INHIBITING CANCER METASTASIS

The surgical removal of the primary tumor has been the cornerstone of treatment for the great majority of cancers. The rationale for this approach is straightforward: if you can get rid of the cancer by simply removing it from the body, then a cure can likely be achieved. Unfortunately, this approach does not take into account that after surgery the cancer will frequently metastasize (spread to different organs). Quite often, the metastatic recurrence is far more serious than the original tumor. In fact, for many cancers, it is the metastatic recurrence—and not the primary tumor—that ultimately proves to be fatal.[194]

One mechanism by which surgery increases the risk of metastasis is by enhancing *cancer cell adhesion*.[195] Cancer cells that have broken away from the primary tumor utilize adhesion to boost their ability to form metastases in distant organs. These cancer cells must be able to clump together and form colonies that can expand and grow. It is unlikely that a single cancer cell will form a metastatic tumor, just as one person is unlikely to form a thriving community. Cancer cells use adhesion molecules—such as *galectin-3*—to facilitate their ability to clump together. Present on the surface of cancer cells, these molecules act like Velcro® by allowing free-standing cancer cells to adhere to each other.[196]

Cancer cells circulating in the bloodstream also make use of galectin-3 surface adhesion molecules to latch onto the lining of blood vessels.[197] The adherence of circulating tumor cells (CTC) to the blood vessel walls is an essential step for the process of metastasis. A cancer cell that cannot adhere to the blood vessel wall will just continue to wander through the bloodstream incapable of forming metastases. Unable to latch onto the wall of the blood vessel, these circulating tumor cells become like "ships without a port" and are unable to dock. Eventually, white blood cells circulating in the bloodstream will target and destroy the CTC. If the CTCs successfully bind to the blood vessel wall and burrow their way through the basement membrane, they will then utilize galectin-3 adhesion molecules to adhere to the organ to form a new metastatic cancer.[196]

Regrettably, research has shown that cancer surgery increases tumor cell adhesion.[198] Therefore, it is critically important for the person undergoing cancer surgery to take measures that can help to neutralize the surgery-induced increase in cancer cell adhesion.

Fortunately, a natural compound called *modified citrus pectin* (MCP) can do just that. Citrus pectin—a type of dietary fiber—is not absorbed from the intestine. However, modified citrus pectin has been altered so that it can be absorbed into the blood and exert its anticancer effects. The mechanism by which modified citrus pectin inhibits cancer cell adhesion is by binding to galectin-3 adhesion molecules on the surface of cancer cells, thereby preventing cancer cells from sticking together and forming a cluster.[199] Modified citrus pectin can also inhibit circulating tumor cells from latching onto the lining of blood vessels. This was demonstrated by an experiment in which modified citrus pectin blocked the adhesion of galectin-3 to the lining of blood vessels by an astounding 95%. Modified citrus pectin also substantially decreased the adhesion of breast cancer cells to the blood vessel walls.[199]

After these exciting findings in animal research, modified citrus pectin was then put to the test in men with prostate cancer. In this trial, 10 men with recurrent prostate cancer received modified citrus pectin (14.4 g/day). After 1 year, a considerable improvement in cancer progression was noted, as determined by a reduction of the rate at which the prostate-specific antigen (PSA) level increased.[200] This was followed by a study in which 49 men with prostate cancer of various types were given modified citrus pectin for a 4-week cycle. After two cycles of treatment with modified citrus pectin, 22% of the men experienced a stabilization of their disease or improved quality of life; 12% had stable disease for more than 24 weeks. The authors of the study concluded that "MCP (modified citrus pectin) seems to have positive impacts especially regarding clinical benefit and life quality for patients with far advanced solid tumor."[201]

In addition to modified citrus pectin, a well-known over-the-counter medication can also play a pivotal role in reducing cancer cell adhesion. *Cimetidine*—commonly known as *Tagamet®*—is a drug historically used to alleviate heartburn. A growing body of scientific evidence has revealed that cimetidine also possesses potent anticancer activity.

Cimetidine inhibits cancer cell adhesion by blocking the expression of an adhesive molecule—called *E-selectin*—on the surface of cells lining blood vessels.[202] Cancers cells latch onto E-selectin in order to adhere to the lining of blood vessels.[202] By preventing the expression of E-selectin, cimetidine significantly limits the ability of cancer cell adherence to the blood vessel walls. This effect is analogous to removing the Velcro® from the blood vessels walls that would normally enable circulating tumor cells to bind.

Cimetidine's potent anticancer effects were clearly displayed in a report published in the *British Journal of*

*Cancer* in 2002. In this study, 64 colon cancer patients received chemotherapy with or without cimetidine (800 mg/day) for 1 year. The 10-year survival for the cimetidine group was almost 90%. This is in stark contrast to the control group, which had a 10-year survival of only 49.8%. Remarkably, for those patients with a more aggressive form of colon cancer, the 10-year survival was 85% in those treated with cimetidine compared to a dismal 23% in the control group.[203] The authors of the study concluded, "Taken together, these results suggested a mechanism underlying the beneficial effect of cimetidine on colorectal cancer patients, presumably by blocking the expression of E-selectin on vascular endothelial [lining of blood vessels] cells and inhibiting the adhesion of cancer cells." These findings are supported by another study with colorectal cancer patients wherein cimetidine given for just 7 days at the time of surgery increased 3-year survival from 59–93%.[204]

Another major contributor to cancer metastasis is immune dysfunction, primarily that which occurs immediately following a surgical procedure such as removal of a primary tumor.[205] Specifically, surgery suppresses the number of specialized immune cells called natural killer (NK) cells, which are a type of white blood cell tasked with seeking out and destroying cancer cells.

To illustrate the importance of NK cell activity in fighting cancer, a study published in the journal *Breast Cancer Research and Treatment* examined NK cell activity in women shortly after surgery for breast cancer. The researchers reported that low levels of NK cell activity were associated with an increased risk of death from breast cancer.[202] In fact, reduced NK cell activity was a better predictor of survival than the actual stage of the cancer. In another alarming study, individuals with reduced NK cell activity before surgery for colon cancer had a 350% increased risk of metastasis during the following 31 months.[206]

One prominent natural compound that can increase NK cell activity is PSK (*protein-bound polysaccharide K*), a specially prepared extract from the mushroom *Coriolus versicolor*. PSK has been shown to enhance NK cell activity in multiple studies[207,208] PSK's ability to enhance NK cell activity helps to explain why it has been shown to dramatically improve survival in cancer patients. For example, 225 patients with lung cancer received radiation therapy with or without PSK (3 g/day). For those with more advanced stage 3 cancers, more than 3 times as many individuals taking PSK were alive after 5 years (26%), compared to those not taking PSK (8%). PSK more than doubled 5-year survival in those individuals

with less advanced stage 1 or 2 disease (39% versus 17%, respectively).[209]

In a 2008 study, a group of colon cancer patients were randomized to receive chemotherapy alone or chemotherapy plus PSK, which was taken for 2 years. The group receiving PSK had an exceptional 10-year survival of 82%. Sadly, the group receiving chemotherapy alone had a 10-year survival of only 51%.[210] In a similar trial reported in the *British Journal of Cancer*, colon cancer patients received chemotherapy alone or combined with PSK (3 g/day) for 2 years. In the group with a more dangerous stage 3 colon cancer, the 5-year survival was 75% in the PSK group. This compared to a 5-year survival of only 46% in the group receiving chemotherapy alone.[211] Additional research has shown that PSK improves survival in cancers of the breast, stomach, esophagus, and uterus as well.[212–214]

## How to Implement Step Ten

The following three novel compounds have shown efficacy in inhibiting several mechanisms that contribute to cancer metastasis. It is especially important to consider these compounds during the perioperative period (period before and after surgery), because a known consequence of surgery is an enhanced proclivity for metastasis.

- Modified citrus pectin: 15 g daily, in 3 divided doses
- Cimetidine: 800 mg daily, in 2 divided doses
- *Coriolus versicolor*, standardized extract: 1200–3600 mg daily

## Life Extension Suggestions

Of critical importance to treatment-naïve patients is implementing as many of these *ten critical steps* as can safely be done concurrently with conventional therapy. In newly diagnosed patients who have not yet been treated, the objective is to eradicate the primary tumor and metastatic cells with a multi-pronged "first-strike therapy" so that residual tumor cells are not given an opportunity to evolve survival mechanisms that make them resistant to further treatments. Omitting any of the following ten steps may provide an opening for residual cancer cells to mutate in a way that makes them very difficult to treat a second time.

### Step One: Evaluating Tumor Cell Population

Make certain your surgeon sends a specimen of your tumor to GENZYME for immunohistochemistry testing. Be sure to follow the instructions that GENZYME provides for proper shipping of the surgical specimen. Contact information for GEN-ZYME: (800) 447-5816; www.genzyme.com.

### Step Two: Determine Sensitivity or Resistance to Chemotherapy

Contact Rational Therapeutics so that your surgeon can follow the precise instructions required to send a living specimen of your tumor for chemosensitivity testing. It is important that your surgeon carefully coordinate with Rational Therapeutics in order to ensure that your cells arrive in a viable condition.

Contact information for Rational Therapeutics: (562) 989-6455; www.rationaltherapeutics.com.

### Step Three: Circulating Tumor Cell Testing

For a molecular analysis of your CTC, contact the International Strategic Cancer Alliance at 610-628-3419 to arrange for a blood specimen to be obtained and shipped for CTC testing.

To test for the presence and quantity of CTC in your blood, speak with your physician regarding the Veridex CellSearch CTC test. You may also order this test from Life Extension at 800-226-2370.

### Step Four: Inhibiting the Cyclooxygenase Enzymes (COX-1 and COX-2)

- Take a *low-dose (81 mg) aspirin* daily.
- Ask your physician to prescribe one of the following COX-2 inhibiting drugs:
  Lodine XL 1000 mg once daily, or
  Celebrex®, 100–200 mg every 12 hours

**Note:** *The use of Lodine and Celebrex® has been associated with an increased risk of heart attack and stroke. The anticancer benefits of these drugs have to be weighed against increased cardiovascular risks. Using aspirin in combination with a COX-2 inhibitor may increase the risk for bleeding; speak with your physician before combining aspirin with a COX-2 inhibitor.*

### Step Five: Suppressing Ras Oncogene Expression

Ask your physician to prescribe one of the following statin drugs to inhibit the activity of Ras oncogenes:

- Mevacor® (lovastatin)
- Zocor® (simvastatin)
- Pravachol (pravastatin)

**Note:** *Statin drugs may generate adverse side effects. Physician oversight and careful surveillance with monthly blood tests (at least initially) to evaluate liver function, muscle enzymes, and lipid levels are suggested.*

In addition to statin drug therapy, consider supplementing with the following nutrients to further suppress the expression of Ras oncogenes:

- Curcumin, as highly absorbed BCM-95® extract: 400–800 mg daily

**Note:** *Different curcumin formulations will differ in their absorption and bioavailability. These differences in absorption can affect the suggested doses. For example, one type of curcumin—called BCM-95®—has been shown in studies to be approximately 7 times more bioavailable than traditional curcumin preparations.*[215]

- Fish oil: 2100 mg of EPA and 1500 mg of DHA daily with meals
- Green tea, standardized extract: 725–1450 mg of EGCG daily
- Aged garlic extract: 2400 mg daily with meals
- Vitamin E: 400–1000 IU of natural alpha tocopherol along with at least 200 mg of gamma-tocopherol daily with meals

### Step Six: Correcting Coagulation Abnormalities

Ascertain if you are in a hypercoagulable state by having your blood tested for prothrombin time (PT), partial thromboplastin time (PTT), and D-dimers. A hypercoagulable state is suggested if the shortening of the PT and PTT are seen. (See Table 1)

If there is any evidence of a hypercoagulable (prothrombotic) state, ask your physician to prescribe the appropriate individualized dose of low-molecular-weight heparin (LMWH). Repeat the prothrombin blood test every 2 weeks.

Also, refer to Life Extension's Blood Clot Prevention protocol for more information.

### Step Seven: Maintaining Bone Integrity

If you have a type of cancer with a proclivity to metastasize to the bone (ie, breast or prostate), ask your physician for a bisphosphonate drug before evidence of bone metastasis occurs.

Because excessive bone breakdown releases growth factors into the bloodstream that can fuel cancer cell growth, the DPD urine test should be done every 60–90 days to detect bone loss. A QCT bone density scan should be done annually. The radiation exposure with QCT is only marginally greater than with DEXA scan. If either of these tests indicates bone loss, ask your physician to initiate bisphosphonate therapy and make sure you take plenty of bone building nutrients like *vitamin K, calcium, magnesium, boron, silica,* and *vitamin D*.

**Note:** *The use of bisphosphonate drugs has been associated with an increased risk of osteonecrosis of the jaw. This risk is considerably greater in those who had major dental work performed during bisphosphonate use. Those using bisphosphonates should speak with their physician before undergoing major dental work. The use of bisphosphonate drugs has been associated with an increased risk of atrial fibrillation. The anticancer effects of these drugs have to be weighed against the increased risks of osteonecrosis of the jaw and atrial fibrillation.*

### Step Eight: Inhibiting Angiogenesis

There are clinical trials using antiangiogenesis agents. Call (800) 422-6237 or log on to www.cancer.gov/clinicaltrials to find out if you are eligible to participate.

Several nutrients have demonstrated potential antiangiogenesis effects such as green tea extract and curcumin.

- Green tea, standardized extract: 725–1450 mg daily
- Curcumin (as highly absorbed BCM-95®): 400–800 mg daily
- Vitamin D: 5000–8000 IU daily (depending on blood levels)
- Grape extract (seed and skin): 150–300 mg daily
- N-acetyl cysteine: 600–1200 mg daily
- Trans-resveratrol: 250 mg daily

### Step Nine: Inhibiting the 5-lipoxygenase (5-LOX) Enzyme

Decrease the consumption of saturated fats that contain high concentrations of arachidonic acid, such as meats, dairy products, and egg yolks.

Consider supplementing with the following nutrients to suppress 5-LOX enzyme activity:

- AprèsFlex™: 100–400 mg daily
- Fish oil: 2100 mg of EPA and 1500 mg of DHA daily with meals
- Lycopene: 30 mg daily with meals
- Curcumin (as highly absorbed BCM-95®): 400–800 mg daily

### Step Ten: Inhibiting Cancer Metastasis

The following three novel compounds have shown efficacy in inhibiting several mechanisms that contribute to cancer metastasis. It is especially important to consider these compounds during the perioperative period (period before and after surgery), because a known consequence of surgery is an enhanced proclivity for metastasis.

- Modified Citrus Pectin: 15 g daily, in 3 divided doses
- Cimetidine: 800 mg daily, in 2 divided doses
- *Coriolus versicolor*, standardized extract: 1200–3600 mg daily

Life Extension oncology health advisors are available to provide clarification on any of the steps in this protocol; they can be reached at 800-226-2370.

### REFERENCES

References available at: www.lef.org/dpt5/ch32

# 33

# Cancer Vaccines and Immunotherapy

Cancer immunotherapies, including cancer vaccines, are novel investigational cancer therapies. In contrast to chemotherapy and radiotherapy regimens that are often associated with severe side effects, cancer immunotherapy stimulates the body's immune system and natural resistance to cancer, thus offering a gentler means of cancer treatment that is less damaging to the rest of the body. Surgery is generally (but not always) performed, prior to immunotherapy, to remove most of the tumor.[1,2] Vaccination or immunotherapy prompts the immune system to kill residual cancer cells that persist after surgery and could result in the cancer recurring.

The status of the patient's immune system is the key physiologic factor affecting the outcome of cancer immunotherapy. However, each individual's immune status is in turn affected by several factors (including age, tumor-induced and surgery-associated immunosuppression, and nutritional status) that need to be assessed, and some require continuous monitoring for the successful application of immunotherapeutic regimens. Immune cells play a central role in mediating the effects of immunotherapy, and specific nutritional supplements that enhance immune cell function can be effective in preparing patients for immunotherapy or vaccination.[3]

Therapeutic cancer vaccines developed for melanoma, renal cell carcinoma, and colorectal cancer have shown benefits in phase 3 trials by extending the disease-free survival period (before relapse) and overall survival. In addition, several immunotherapy clinical trials have been performed for metastatic breast cancer and non-Hodgkin's lymphoma.

## THE IMMUNE SYSTEM AND CANCER

Evidence showing the role of the immune system in detecting and killing cancer cells has been available for some time.[4–10] This knowledge has been used in developing immunotherapies to bolster the immune system's natural capacity to counteract cancer cells.

## How the Immune System Detects Cancer Cells

Cancer cells display abnormal proteins (antigens) on their surface, and the immune system can detect and destroy cancer cells because of these proteins.[11,12] (An antigen is a substance that causes the immune system to make a specific immune response.)

The immune system has an innate ability to resist cancer development; however, in most cases, the immune system fails due to a series of sophisticated strategies that tumor cells use to evade immune detection. These strategies range from methods designed to hide tumor cells, to active incapacitation of immune cells by tumor-produced agents that lower the immune system's responses, which are known as immunosuppressive agents.[13–18] Therefore, a prerequisite to successful cancer immunotherapy is the implementation of strategies to boost the immune system's natural resistance to cancer.

T cells and B cells (lymphocytes) are immune system cells responsible for what is known as *specific immunity*.[19–21] By contrast, other immune cells (eg, eosinophils, natural killer (NK) cells, and macrophages) generate nonspecific responses to infections by bacteria and parasites.[22,23] T cells and B cells respond only when they detect specific markers that identify infected cells.[19–21]

## A Role for the Immune System in Cancer Control

The role of the immune system in counteracting the development of cancer was initially supported by individual clinical case reports. Groundbreaking work in the late 1800s by a New York surgeon, William Coley, noted that some cancer patients who were simultaneously suffering from bacterial infections had regression of their tumors.[4,5] He concluded that, in trying to fight off the bacterial infection, the patients' immune systems had become highly activated and that this had given them some resistance to the tumor. Coley later concocted a crude vaccine preparation, called "Coley's toxins," that was made up of killed bacteria. While some of Coley's patients enjoyed complete tumor regression, the responses were somewhat varied and his work was initially regarded with skepticism.[4,5]

However, research has produced a considerable body of scientific evidence documenting the immune system's role in controlling cancer growth. For example, cancer occurs more frequently in individuals with weakened immune systems.[8,9,24] In addition, some types of cancer undergo spontaneous regression, again adding weight to the notion that the immune system is naturally able to fight cancer.[7] Furthermore, cancer patients often have specific antibodies (proteins that bind to antigens) circulating in their blood, again demonstrating that the immune system can detect tumor cells and mount a specific response[6] that also involves specific T cells, or T lymphocytes.[10,25,26]

## How Tumors Escape Immune Detection

Under normal circumstances, all cells display segments of their proteins on their surface. Upon infection with a viral or bacterial agent, cells display on their surface sample segments from these foreign proteins.[19–21] T cells and B cells patrolling the body for foreign invaders seek and destroy any cells that display these foreign proteins on their surface. These proteins are called antigens, substances that can stimulate a specific immune response or activity.

In cancer, the tumor cell also displays a sample of its abnormal proteins on its surface, which can signal the immune system that it is no longer a normal, healthy cell. These protein segments—either from proteins overproduced in the cancer cell or from viral or bacterial proteins that infected the cell and caused the cancer—act as red flags and attract the attention of T cells and B cells.[27] Tumor cells evade immune detection by failing to display protein segments (antigens) on their surface, thus, in effect, hiding from immune cells.[13,15]

In aggressive cases, tumor cells can also evade immune detection by producing agents that reduce immune cell activity.[14,16–18] Alternatively, the immune system may not be able to cope with a tumor's rapid growth if the initial immune response to the tumor is not sufficient to reject or control it completely. Despite the immune system's natural ability to detect and kill cancer cells, in most circumstances the immune system fails to control tumor growth. The goal of immunotherapy is to specifically target tumor antigens as a means of killing cancer cells.[11,12] Table 1 shows some tumor antigens (substances that stimulate an immune response) that form the basis of cancer vaccines in clinical studies.

## Table 1: Tumor Antigens Form the Basis of Vaccines in Clinical Development

| Tumor Antigen | Cancer |
| --- | --- |
| Carcinoembryonic antigen (CEA) | Colon, breast, lung, pancreatic |
| Prostate-specific antigen (PSA) | Prostate |
| Tyrosinase protein | Melanoma |
| Human papillomavirus nucleoproteins | Cervical |

## WHAT YOU HAVE LEARNED SO FAR

- The immune system has a natural ability to detect and kill cancer cells; however, tumors that develop in the presence of a competent immune system evolve complex immune-evasion strategies to avoid destruction and removal of the tumor.
- Not all tumors are naturally programmed to alert the immune system and mount an immune response, due to loss or coverage of cell surface antigens.
- The goal of immunotherapy is to produce antitumor effects through activation of the patient's immune system or through patient supplementation with natural substances, and thus to ultimately destroy the cancer.
- Therapeutic cancer vaccines are used to boost the immune system as a way to control established cancer. Preventive cancer vaccines are used to vaccinate people against infectious agents known to cause cancer.
- Surgery is often performed to remove most of the tumor before cancer immunotherapy or vaccination, which should then eliminate any persisting tumor cells that would grow or spread.
- For each individual, immune system status is the key factor that will affect the success of cancer vaccine therapy.
- Cancer patients preparing to undergo immunotherapy should ensure optimal immune system function through adequate nutrition and the use of nutritional supplements.

# TYPES OF IMMUNOTHERAPY

## Monoclonal Antibody (mAb)

Monoclonal antibodies target specific tumor antigens, such as tumor growth factors, and can enhance the immune response against cancer. Many monoclonal antibodies (eg, Herceptin®) have other anticancer activities such as biological response modification and signal transduction inhibition, which slow or prevent cancer growth signals. Monoclonal antibody therapies for various cancers are outlined in Table 2.

**Herceptin®.** Approximately 25–30% of breast cancer patients exhibit an excess of the protein HER-2/neu (a member of the human epidermal growth factor receptor family), which can be measured in the blood via its extracellular domain.[28] HER2/neu-positive breast cancer cells are associated with aggressive disease and decreased overall survival.

Herceptin® (trastuzumab) is the first monoclonal antibody that "targets" the HER2/neu protein on human cancer cells. This drug, which is approved for the treatment of metastatic breast cancers that are HER2-positive,[29] provides a median overall response rate of 23%.[30] Herceptin® attaches to HER2 present on cancer cells, thus preventing cancer proliferation and inducing cancer cell death (apoptosis). Herceptin® is also a biological response modifier and

## Table 2: Targeted Therapies

| Drug | Molecular Target | Mechanism of Action | Cancer Type | References |
|---|---|---|---|---|
| Herceptin® (trastuzumab) | HER2/neu (human epidermal growth factor receptor) | mAb, BRM, STI | Breast (metastatic) | Baselga et al[31] |
| Erbitux™ (cetuximab) | EGFR (epidermal growth factor receptor) | mAb, BRM, STI | Colorectal (advanced), head and neck, and pancreatic | Bonner et al[216], Moroni et al[217], Xiong et al[218] |
| Tarceva® (erlotinib) | EGFR-TKI (epidermal growth factor receptor-tyrosine kinase inhibitor) | mAb, BRM, STI | Non–small cell lung and pancreatic (advanced) | Johnson et al[219], Moore[220] |
| Iressa® (gefitinib) | EGFR-TKI | BRM, STI | Non–small cell lung (restricted access) | Fukuoka et al[221] |
| Avastin™ (bevacizumab) | Humanized antibody to VEGF (vascular endothelial growth factor) | BRM, anti-angiogenic | Colorectal (metastatic), clear-cell renal carcinoma (metastatic) | Hainsworth et al[222], Jubb et al[223] |
| Rituxan® (rituximab) (see protocol on Lymphoma) | Monoclonal antibody to CD20, a B-cell antigen | mAb, BRM | B-cell non-Hodgkin's lymphoma (NHL) | van Heeckeren et al[224] |
| Thalidomide | Anti–TNF-α (tumor necrosis factor-alpha) | Antiangiogenic, TNF modifier | Multiple myeloma, renal cell carcinoma (not FDA approved; restricted to clinical trials) | Rajkumar et al [225], Srinivas et al[226] |

*mAb, monoclonal antibody; BRM, biologic response modifiers; STI, signal transduction inhibitors.*

a mediator of antibody-dependent cell-mediated cytotoxicity via natural killer cells and monocytes.[31] Because Herceptin® damages the heart, an echocardiogram and complete blood count are usually monitored.

## Cytokine Therapy

Cytokines such as interleukin-2 and the interferons (alpha, beta, and gamma) have been used clinically in cancer patients.

**Interleukin-2 (IL-2).** IL-2 is naturally produced in the body by T cells after activation by antigen, but it can also be given as a drug (immunotherapy). Clinical use of IL-2 counteracts the immunodeficiency state caused by the tumor and conventional treatments. IL-2 does not directly affect cancer cells; rather, its effects result from its ability to stimulate immune reactions in the body. Used as immunotherapy for metastatic melanoma (7% complete response) and kidney cancer (9% complete response), IL-2 can mediate durable regression (ie, prevent cancer recurrence).[32] However, a significant side effect of IL-2 therapy is vascular leak syndrome.[33]

Various IL-2 dosing schedules and combinations with interferon alpha (IFN-α) have been tested in patients with advanced melanoma. Response rates reported with IL-2 alone or in combination with IFN-α vary from 10–41%, with a small but significant proportion of durable responses.[34] High-dose

IL-2 immunotherapy is useful in patients with metastatic renal cell carcinoma, and even in highly selected dialysis patients.[35,36] IL-2 combined with thalidomide can produce durable, active responses in patients with metastatic renal cell carcinoma.[37]

Treatment of skin and soft-tissue melanoma metastases by injection of IL-2 directly into the tumors resulted in complete response in 62.5% of patients (the longest remission lasting 38 months) and partial response in 21% of patients.[38]

Preoperative immunotherapy with IL-2 in pancreatic cancer patients achieved a positive effect on postoperative complications and increased 2-year survival (33% in the treated group compared to 10% in the control group).[39]

**Interferon.** Interferons (IFNs) are produced naturally in the body in response to viral infections, but they can also be given as a drug (immunotherapy). Interferon alfa has immunomodulatory, antiangiogenic, antiproliferative, and antitumor properties[40] against leukemia (CLL, CML, and HCL)[41,42] and lymphoma,[43] and in combination with other anticancer agents, against breast cancer.[44] Adjuvant high-dose interferon alfa-2b is approved for all melanoma patients with intermediate- and high-risk disease, but it benefits only 20–30% of patients and its use is limited due to its toxicity.[45] A favorable outcome in patients with high-risk melanoma treated with adjuvant interferon alfa-2b appears to depend on the development of autoimmunity during or after treatment.[46] Adverse reactions to interferon therapy include flu-like symptoms of fever, chills, fatigue, and muscle aches.

## Gene Therapy

Cancer gene therapy has provided preliminary results through phase 1 clinical trials. In advanced breast cancer or melanoma patients, gene therapy with MetXia-P450 (a novel recombinant retroviral vector that encodes the human cytochrome P450 type 2B6 gene) was safe, well tolerated, and produced an antitumor response, suggesting it merits further clinical assessment.[47]

In mesothelioma patients, gene therapy with intrapleural adenoviral (Ad) vector encoding the herpes simplex virus thymidine kinase "suicide gene" (Ad.HSVtk/ganciclovir) was safe, well tolerated, and resulted in long-term durable responses in 2 patients, which may have been due to induction of antitumor immune responses. The researchers hypothesize that approaches aiming to enhance the immune effects of adenoviral gene transfer (ie, with the use of cytokines) may lead to increased numbers of therapeutic responses in otherwise untreatable pleural (lung) cancers.[48]

## CANCER VACCINES

In contrast to chemotherapy and radiotherapy, cancer vaccines are not associated with any serious side effects. Cancer vaccines and the immune system have the ability to mount and amplify antigen-specific antitumor responses.[49,50] These activities cannot be produced by chemotherapy or radiotherapy. Once the immune system generates T cells specific for a particular antigen, a group of "memory cells" that remember this antigen will remain in the body, and in the event of a second threat from that antigen, an immune response will be mounted much faster than the first one.[49,50]

Phase 1 clinical studies assessing the safety of cancer vaccines have shown them to be associated with no toxicities outside reports of mild flu-like symptoms, irritation at the vaccination site, and fatigue.[51-53]

## TYPES OF CANCER VACCINES

### Preventive Cancer Vaccines

Preventive cancer vaccines are being developed as a means of preventing cancers caused by chronic viral, bacterial, and parasitic infections that are associated

with up to 20% of all cancer cases, including cervical and liver cancers.[54,55]

## Therapeutic Cancer Vaccines

Most cancer vaccines are therapeutic, in that they are intended to treat existing cancer rather than to prevent it.[56,57] The cancer patient would initially undergo surgery to remove most of the tumor. Vaccination would then be undertaken to generate a specific immune response capable of clearing any residual cancer, thus preventing relapse,[57-59] and extending the period of remission or survival in the patient.

The manner in which therapeutic cancer vaccines are used in the clinic is summarized in Table 3.

---

### HOW CANCER VACCINES WORK

The immune system is capable of both specific and nonspecific responses against tumor cells. However, successful cancer vaccines must stimulate the immune system to act largely in a tumor-specific fashion.

A successful cancer vaccine would present tumor antigens to immune cells and activate CD4 (also known as helper T cells) and CD8 T cells (also known as cytotoxic or killer T cells). CD8 T cells become activated and directly kill the tumor cells[20] while CD4 T cells are indirectly activated by dendritic cells and macrophages[60] to produce messengers (cytokines) that boost CD8 (killer) T-cell activity.[61]

B cells are immune cells that produce antibodies to human tumors.[62,63] Cancer immunotherapy that generates a good antibody response produces a better clinical outcome for the patient.[64,65]

The immune system also has a range of nonspecific tools that can be stimulated into action by cancer vaccines, including natural killer cells and macrophages.[22,23]

---

The 2 main categories of therapeutic cancer vaccines are *whole-cell vaccines* (self [autologous], donor [allogenic], or dendritic cell) and *synthetic protein antigens* (soluble vaccines).

**Whole-cell vaccines.** Whole-cell vaccines use inactivated whole tumor cells as the vaccine given to the cancer patient. These inactivated tumor cells have a range of abnormal tumor proteins to which the patient's immune cells respond by generating an antitumor immune response and attacking any cancer cells persisting after surgery. Using the whole tumor cell

### Table 3: Use of Therapeutic Cancer Vaccines in the Clinic

| Stage 1 | Cancer diagnosis |
|---------|------------------|
| Stage 2 | Surgery to remove accessible tumor |
| Stage 3 | Vaccination |
| Stage 4 | Patient monitoring |

as a vaccine eliminates the problem of having to identify the various key antigens, most of which remain unknown.

- **Self versus donor (autologous versus allogenic) vaccines.** The tumor cells used in whole-cell vaccines can be derived from the patient's own (self or autologous) tumor[66] after it has been removed during surgery. Alternatively, these tumor cells can be obtained from a tumor sample removed from another individual (donor or allogenic) with the same cancer type.[67]
- **Dendritic cell vaccines.** Dendritic cells are finger-like cells that pick up proteins from tumor cells (antigens) or invading organisms (bacteria, viruses, and parasites), and process and present them to young lymphocytes,[68,69] which then initiate immune responses.[70,71]

  Dendritic cell–based cancer vaccines, prepared from blood samples taken from the cancer patient,[69,72] have been used to treat prostate cancer,[73] colorectal cancer,[74] non–small cell lung cancer,[75] breast cancer,[76] and B-cell cancers.[77–79] Dendritic cells pulsed with tumor cells (lysate) are partially efficient in triggering effective antimelanoma immunity in stage 4 patients.[80] Dendritic cell cancer vaccines are safe and well tolerated in humans.

**Synthetic protein antigens.** Synthetic protein antigens are mass-produced synthetic versions of abnormal proteins displayed by tumors, and can generate immune responses capable of destroying cells in the body that display these antigens.[81] This type of vaccination is given to patients with immune system boosters (adjuvants) or other messengers to further enhance immune system activity.[81] Dendritic cells, which coordinate the function of immune cells, are often used as a vehicle to deliver these synthetic proteins to the immune system.[82]

# CLINICAL STUDIES USING DIFFERENT TYPES OF CANCER VACCINES

## Melanoma

Melanoma is perhaps the cancer that has been the central focus of cancer vaccine research.

**Synthetic proteins.** Proteins that have been identified as tumor antigens for melanoma include tyrosinase, MART-1 (also known as Melan A), gp100,[83] and products of the MAGE gene family.[84,85] These proteins are not unique to melanoma cells, but are normal body proteins that are overproduced by melanoma cells and therefore called melanoma-associated antigens.[83]

Vaccines made up of MART-1, tyrosinase, and gp100 synthetic proteins were successfully used to vaccinate melanoma patients and induced objective tumor regression in all patients.[83] Other melanoma cancer vaccines have used synthetic MAGE proteins and have been noted to cause complete tumor regression in some patients.[86,87]

**Gangliosides (GM2, GM3, GD2, and GD3).** Gangliosides are cell surface molecules that are abnormally displayed or overproduced by all tumors. They are linked to an increased ability of tumors to spread, or metastasize,[88,89] and to poor clinical outcomes.[90] Therefore, they represent targets for vaccine-generated immune responses. Indeed, vaccination with purified gangliosides, prepared from laboratory-grown melanoma cells, showed that they were capable of generating an immune response in melanoma patients.[91]

Another clinical study has shown that vaccination of melanoma patients (after surgery to remove skin, lymph node, and other metastases) with a concoction containing GM3, GD3, GM2, and GD2 generated strong immune responses that were associated with increased disease-free survival.[92] The successful use of ganglioside cancer vaccines is supported by improved survival of stage 3 melanoma patients who were treated with a GM2 vaccine following surgery to remove most of the tumor.[93]

**Heat shock proteins (HSPs).** Heat shock proteins are abundant cell proteins known as molecular chaperones because they guide the assembly and eventual loading of proteins, prepared within the cell, into the external structures on which they are displayed to immune cells guarding the body.[94,95] Heat shock proteins from tumor cells therefore contain the perfect sample of tumor antigens for that particular tumor type and have proved effective as a basis for cancer vaccines, particularly for melanoma and renal cell carcinoma.[96–98]

A phase 3 trial was performed with 300 patients with stage 4 melanoma using heat shock protein (gp96)-peptide complexes derived from the patients' own tumors (given once weekly for the first 4 weeks and every other week thereafter). The patients with skin and lymph node disease survived an estimated median of 626 days compared to 383 days in the control group.[99]

## Non-Hodgkin's Lymphoma

Other vaccine approaches (eg, anti-idiotype) have demonstrated clinical benefit in the treatment of non-Hodgkin's lymphoma,[100–102] and are being assessed for multiple myeloma treatment.[103]

## Pancreatic, Lung, Colorectal, Breast, and Ovarian Cancers

*Carcinoembryonic antigen* (CEA) is a glycoprotein (a protein attached to sugar groups) that is normally produced by cells only during fetal development. However, it is grossly overproduced by almost 50% of all human cancers,[104–106] including colon, rectal, breast, ovarian, lung, pancreatic, and gastrointestinal tract cancers.[105,107] Indeed, CEA can be detected in blood samples from cancer patients, and is therefore used to monitor cancer therapy and progression.[105]

CEA loaded into dendritic cells and used as a cancer vaccine generated (CD4 and CD8) antitumor responses that were associated with disease stabilization.[82,108,109] CEA delivered to the cancer patient's immune system (by a poxvirus) brought about disease stabilization in up to 37% of treated patients.[108] A CEA-based vaccine (ALVAC-CEA) developed using vaccinia virus has also been shown to be safe in humans and capable of generating specific antitumor immune responses.[105]

## Breast and Ovarian Cancers

Sialyl-Tn (STn) is a carbohydrate that is overproduced by several types of cancer cells, including breast, ovarian, colorectal, gastric, and pancreatic cancer cells.[110] As a result, this tumor-associated antigen is a good candidate for a therapeutic vaccine for these cancers.

A STn-based cancer vaccine called Theratope®, developed by a Canadian company (Biomira Inc.), is effective in the treatment of breast and ovarian cancer patients.[111,112] In a clinical setting, this vaccine was safe and was associated with reduced risk of relapse (longer remission period) or death.[111,112]

## Enhancing Immunotherapy Responses

**Boosters for the immune system.** Tumor cells used as vaccine are often manipulated to produce and secrete messengers such as IL-2 and granulocyte macrophage colony stimulating factor (GM-CSF), which directly activate immune cells.[113–115] In the clinical setting, vaccines are often administered with immune system boosters (adjuvants), such as bacillus Calmette-Guerin (BCG) and DETOX, to make the immune system more responsive to the presented antigens.[116–118]

# CANCER VACCINES IN CLINICAL TRIALS (PHASE 3)

A variety of candidate cancer vaccines showed promise in early (phase 1 and 2) clinical studies.[73,87] However, most failed to translate this success to the larger phase 3 studies that examine the impact of the vaccine-induced immune response on the period of remission (or disease stabilization) enjoyed by the patient, and on overall survival. The former is also referred to as disease-free survival or progression-free survival.[119] Consequently, when making a balanced assessment of cancer vaccines as a treatment option, it is important to focus on vaccines that have reached phase 3 studies. With the exception of lung cancer, therapeutic cancer vaccines have progressed to phase 3 clinical studies for all the major cancer types.

## Renal Cell Carcinoma

A cancer vaccine for renal cell carcinoma has been tested in a phase 3 setting using autologous (self-donated) cancer cells and lysates (prepared by breaking down cancer cells).[2,120] This study involved 558 renal cell carcinoma patients who were vaccinated (six injections in the skin once a month) with the autologous tumor cell vaccine after surgery.[2] After 70 months of follow-up, the progression-free survival of vaccinated patients was 67.8% compared to 59.3% in nonvaccinated patients.[2] These results support the use of this renal cell carcinoma vaccine following surgery (removal of a kidney) in renal cell carcinoma cases not larger than 2.5 cm.[2]

## Melanoma

Several types of cancer vaccines for melanoma have progressed to phase 3 clinical assessment, including ganglioside and whole-cell (allogenic and autologous)–based vaccines.[117,118,121]

A whole-cell melanoma vaccine (CancerVax/Canvaxin) has been tested in a phase 3 clinical trial by comparing the outcomes of 935 vaccinated patients (after surgery) and 667 nonvaccinated patients.[121,122] The 5-year overall survival of vaccinated patients was 49% compared to 37% in the nonvaccinated group of patients.[122]

Melacine, a melanoma cancer vaccine prepared from allogenic (donor) tumor cells, has also progressed to phase 3 clinical evaluation.[118,123] This vaccine is given to patients with an immunologic booster and has been shown to confer vaccinated patients with survival benefits.[118]

A ganglioside-based vaccine, developed for melanoma treatment and administered with an adjuvant, was initially shown to induce antibodies that could clear melanoma cells.[117] However, evaluation of this vaccine in phase 3 studies produced somewhat disappointing results, as a standard treatment of high-dose interferon therapy generated better results in relation to relapse-free survival and overall survival.[124]

## Colon Cancer

Cancer vaccines for colorectal cancer that have progressed to phase 3 clinical studies have focused on the use of CEA proteins and whole-cell autologous (self) tumor cells.[1,116,125] An autologous tumor cell vaccine used in combination with BCG as an adjuvant (immune booster) has been tested in a study of 412 stage 2 and 3 colorectal cancer patients who had undergone surgery to remove most of the tumor.[116] Vaccinations were given 4 weeks after surgery and patients who received this treatment showed benefits in disease-free survival and overall survival.[116]

## Breast Cancer

The vaccine Theratope® (manufactured by Biomira Inc.), based on the tumor-associated antigen STn, is currently being evaluated in a large phase 3 study of 1000 metastatic breast cancer patients.[110,126] Findings from this study have yet to be published.

> **Note:** Biomira Inc., a pharmaceutical company, does not treat patients. However, Biomira provides vaccines to physicians at various cancer clinics in North America and Europe where government-approved clinical trials are ongoing. The vaccines are provided only to physicians who are currently involved in vaccine exploration and who have extensive experience with these agents. To speak to Biomira's Medical Information Assistant, call (877) 234-0444, ext. 500.

## Prostate Cancer

Provenge®, a dendritic cell-based vaccine for prostate cancer, is being evaluated in phase 3 clinical studies by the U.S. company Dendreon.[127] This vaccine involves loading synthetic prostate cancer cell proteins (recombinant protein antigens) into the patient's dendritic cells (grown in the laboratory) and administering them as vaccine. Clinical studies have shown that this vaccine has activity in patients with hormone-independent prostate cancer.[128] More recent media reports (NewsRX.com) have indicated that this vaccine improved survival in men with advanced prostate cancer in phase 3 studies; however, these results have not yet been published in the scientific literature.

## Blood (Hematologic) Cancers

The National Cancer Institute is currently overseeing a large phase 3 clinical study using an idiotype-based vaccine given to patients with follicular lymphoma after they have undergone chemotherapy.[129]

# FACTORS AFFECTING IMMUNE SYSTEM STATUS

## Age

While cancer is more common in the elderly,[130] immune strength gradually declines with age and can pose a problem for the successful use of immunotherapy in the elderly.[131,132] Although age-related decline in immune status is a natural feature of the immune system, it is also aggravated by lifestyle factors such as diet.[133] Therefore, nutritional supplements to boost immune function may have even more significance in elderly cancer patients than in young adults.

## Tumor-Induced and Surgery-Associated Immunosuppression

Two types of immunosuppression affect the successful outcome of immunotherapy: immunosuppression from the tumor and that associated with surgery to remove the tumor. Tumor-induced immunosuppression, due to the production of immunosuppressive factors by cancer cells, is overcome by surgical removal of the tumor mass,[134] and thus creates an environment in which immune cells can better respond to immunotherapy. However, the process of surgery and the associated use of particular anesthetic and analgesic drugs also dampen immune cell function, again reducing the effectiveness of any immunotherapy used.[135] It is recommended that anesthetic and analgesic drugs be carefully selected to minimize immunosuppression, and that patients prepare for surgery by optimizing nutritional and immune status.[136]

## Nutritional Status

The production of immune-suppressing (immunosuppressive) agents by cancer cells presents a significant obstacle to cancer immunotherapy.[14,17] Excessive production of proinflammatory cytokines and reactive oxygen species may damage the immune system, resulting in adverse immunotherapy outcome and cancer progression.

Therefore, nutritional supplements that improve the function of key immune cells will affect the efficacy of immunotherapy and could also be used to prepare patients for immunotherapy.[3]

The impact of nutrition on the function of immune cells that play a key role in the efficacy of cancer immunotherapy is well established.[137,138] Studies of cancer patients demonstrate that nutritional supplements can play a role in restoring immune status depleted by cancer and surgery to normal levels that would be more responsive to immunotherapy treatment.[3]

# NUTRITIONAL THERAPY

Although the direct effect of nutritional supplements on the effectiveness of cancer immunotherapy has yet to be clinically evaluated, the impact of nutrition, particularly micronutrients, on immune cell function (ie, immunonutrition) is central to the success of any cancer treatment.[137,138] Several nutrients are able to modulate immune response and counteract inflammatory processes. Zinc, omega-3 fatty acids, and glutamine all act differently to modulate immune response, but all appear to have the potential to protect against cancer progression.[139]

Immunonutrition has gained recognition as an adjuvant cancer therapy and should be an integral part of cancer immunotherapy, particularly against cancers associated with chronic inflammation,[140] as it has beneficial effects on patient outcomes, enhances the immune response, and improves the prognosis of cancer patients.[141]

Cells of the immune system that are essential for the success of cancer vaccines include:

- Dendritic cells
- CD4 T cells (lymphocytes)
- CD8 T cells (lymphocytes)
- B cells (lymphocytes)
- Natural killer (NK) cells
- Macrophages
- Neutrophils

Micronutrients that have been established as being essential to the optimal function of these immune cells include zinc, vitamins C and E, folic acid, and glutamine.[137,142]

## Zinc

Zinc supplements improve immune cell function.[143,144] Indeed, diets lacking in zinc are linked to reduced CD4 and CD8 T-cell function.[138] While deficiencies in zinc also compromise the function of natural killer cells, macrophages, and neutrophils,[143] this impairment of the immune system can be reversed by dietary zinc supplements.[138,143] Zinc supplements should, however, be carefully monitored, as excessive intake (over 100 mg per day) is counterproductive and reverses any benefits seen with the suggested doses of 20–50 mg per day.[137,145,146]

Zinc supplements of 50 mg per day improve the structure of Langerhans' cells (a type of dendritic cell found in the skin epidermis) by endowing them with a more dendritic (or finger-like) structure that improves their mobility and thus their ability to pick up antigens and transport them to lymphocytes.[146]

## Astragalus

Astragalus, an herb used for centuries in Asia, has exhibited immune-stimulatory effects. Astragalus potentiates lymphokine-activated killer cells.[147] One study found that astragalus could partially restore depressed immune function in tumor-bearing mice,[148] while another concluded that "astragalus could exhibit anti-tumor effects, which might be achieved through activating the...anti-tumor immune mechanism of the host."[149]

## Antioxidants (Vitamins C and E)

Supplementing the diet of colorectal cancer patients with high doses of vitamin E (750 mg per day) for 2 weeks increased lymphocyte numbers and improved the lymphocytes' ability to produce messengers (IL-2 and interferon gamma) that are associated with the type of immune response required to destroy cancer cells.[3] Therefore, high-dose vitamin E supplements may be considered to support the use of cancer vaccines and immunotherapy. Long-term supplementation at lower doses of 100–200 mg per day has improved immune function.[137,150]

Vitamin C supplements also improve immune function and protect lymphocytes against damage.[151,152]

## Folic Acid

Deficiencies in folic acid impair the immune system by reducing the ability of CD8 T cells to divide and increase in number.[153] In addition, low levels of folic acid lead to genetic instability in lymphocytes and increased cell death, or apoptosis.[153,154] However, the impairment of lymphocyte function can be restored by folic acid supplements.[153]

## Vitamin B12

Vitamin B12 plays a key role in immune function, as B12 deficiencies in humans lead to low numbers of CD8 T cells and impair the activity of natural killer cells.[155] These cells are essential for the cytotoxic arm of the immune system, which in turn is essential for destroying cancer cells. Supplementing with B12 restores CD8 T-cell numbers and natural killer cell activity.[155]

## Vitamin B6

Deficiencies in vitamin B6 impair the immune system and are associated with a reduced ability of lymphocytes to produce messengers (cytokines) required for sustained immune activation.[156]

## Selenium

Selenium supplements (100 mcg per day) improve immune cell function by increasing the cells' ability to produce messengers (cytokines) associated with the type of immune responses required to clear tumor cells.[157]

## Glutamine

Glutamine supplements (30 g per day) sustain immune cell function.[158] Clinical studies have shown glutamine supplements to be particularly effective in counteracting immunosuppression associated with surgery,[142,159] and thus to be of benefit to patients undergoing an immunotherapy/vaccination regimen after surgical removal of the tumor.

## Ginseng

The medicinal herb ginseng improves immune cell function.[160] Of particular importance to the successful use of cancer vaccines is the ability of ginseng products to drive the development of dendritic cells that are essential for successful cancer vaccination.[161]

## Melatonin

Melatonin hormone supplements (20 mg per day, at bedtime) improve lymphocyte function and have been tested in clinical studies of blood cancers.[162,163]

## Garlic

Garlic extracts boost the activity of natural killer cells against tumor cells.[164]

## Mushroom Extracts

Extracts from various mushrooms boost immune cell function.[165] In particular, active hexose-correlated compound (AHCC) improves the function of natural killer cells and confers benefits to liver cancer patients after surgical removal of the tumor.[166]

## Polysaccharide-K

Polysaccharide-K (PSK), which is a specially prepared polysaccharide extract from the mushroom *Coriolus versicolor*, has been studied extensively in Japan where it is used as a nonspecific biological response modifier to enhance the immune system in cancer patients.[167–169] PSK suppresses tumor cell invasiveness by downregulating several invasion-related factors.[170] PSK has been shown to enhance NK cell activity in multiple studies.[171–174]

## Reishi

The active constituents of reishi mushroom include polysaccharides, a unique protein named LZ-8, and triterpenes.[175–177] Among its broad-spectrum immune-boosting effects are the following:

- Reishi promotes specialization of dendritic cells and macrophages, which are essential in allowing the body to react to new threats, vaccines, and cancer cells.[178–182]

- Reishi's effects on dendritic cells have been proven to boost the response to tetanus vaccine; the mushroom's proteins are also under investigation as "adjuvants" to emerging cancer DNA vaccines and other immune-based cancer treatments.[179,183–185]

- Reishi polysaccharide triggers growth and development of bone marrow, where most immune cells are born; following bone marrow eradication by chemotherapy, reishi increased production of both red and white blood cells.[186] Reishi polysaccharides provide immune-boosting function to circulating cancer-killing white blood cells of various types.[176]

- Reishi increases numbers and functions of virtually all cell lines in the immune system, such as natural killer cells, antibody-producing B cells, and the T cells responsible for rapid response to a new or "remembered" antigen.[180,187,188]

Laboratory and animal studies confirm that reishi stimulates an appropriate anticancer immune response while quashing a cancer-promoting inflammatory one. A few small human studies have demonstrated reishi's ability to enhance immune function in patients with advanced cancers.[189–191]

## Omega-3 Fatty Acids

The ratio of omega-3 and omega-6 polyunsaturated fatty acids (PUFAs) modulates the inflammatory response. Inflammatory cells typically contain high levels of arachidonic acid and low levels of omega-3 PUFA.[192,193] Increasing omega-3 fatty acid intake antagonizes arachidonic acid levels in inflammatory cell membranes, and decreases the amount of arachidonic acid that is available for production of proinflammatory arachidonic acid-derived mediators.[194]

Omega-3 PUFA may have indirect immunomodulatory activity mediated through tumor necrosis factor-alpha (TNF-$\alpha$) and nuclear factor-kappa beta (NF-$\kappa$B) production.[195] Administration of omega-3 fatty acids before and after surgery (prior to immunotherapy) may have a favorable effect on outcome by lowering the magnitude of inflammatory response and preventing immune suppression.[196] Fatty fish such as salmon, mackerel, tuna, and herring are good sources of long-chain omega-3 PUFA.

# TRACKING YOUR PROGRESS

## Monthly Blood Tests

A range of blood tests and other diagnostic procedures can be used to monitor the effectiveness of cancer immunotherapy. Results from these tests provide information required to assess the effectiveness of this new treatment modality.

The following tests are essential for monitoring the effectiveness of immunotherapy.

**Tumor antigen profile.** Determining the antigens (abnormal proteins) produced by each tumor is important in assessing the use of cancer vaccines or other forms of immunotherapy as a treatment choice. Tumor antigen profile should also be monitored during immunotherapy, as the tumor can develop variations that stop the display of these antigens as a means of escaping detection.

**Immune cell function.** The function of lymphocytes is monitored during cancer immunotherapy by a variety of techniques. These include proliferation assays to assess their ability to expand in response to activation, and cell-kill (cytotoxic) assays to assess the ability of CD8 lymphocytes to kill tumor cells.[197-199]

**Prostate-specific antigen (PSA).** PSA can be detected in blood samples from prostate cancer patients and has been established as a reliable marker for disease progression or patient response to therapy.[200,201] Prostate cancer patients treated with cancer vaccines in clinical studies showed reductions in their PSA levels.[202,203]

**Carcinoembryonic antigen (CEA).** Monitoring of serum levels of CEA is recommended for colorectal cancer patients as a marker for disease progression or response to treatment.[204]

**Angiogenesis markers.** Angiogenesis is the process of forming new blood vessels, which is essential for tumors to spread to other parts of the body. Increased levels of the angiogenic factor vascular endothelial growth factor (VEGF) in the blood of cancer patients serves as a robust indicator of disease progression and can be used to monitor response to treatment with cancer immunotherapy.[205-207] Circulating endothelial cells, detectable in the blood of cancer patients, are increased and have also been established as another indicator of disease progression.[208,209]

**Growth factors.** Serum levels of the growth factors pleiotrophin (PTN) and fibroblast growth factor-2 (FGF-2) are increased in prostate cancer patients and can be used as a marker for disease progression or response to therapy.[210]

**Immunosuppressive agents.** Levels of tumor-produced immunosuppressive agents (eg, interleukin-10 [IL-10][17] and transforming growth factor-beta [TGF-β][14]) can be detected in patients' serum and used to check for disease progression or response to treatment.

**X-rays and scans.** X-rays and scans can be used to monitor the response or progression of disease during cancer immunotherapy.

**Physical examination.** Regular physical examinations can detect changes in body mass and enlarged lymph nodes that may be signs of disease progression.[204]

# FOR MORE INFORMATION

Cancer immunotherapy patients may wish to read the following protocols and design a program that addresses the full range of their cancer problems:

- Cancer Adjuvant Therapy
- Complementary Alternative Cancer Therapies
- Cancer Surgery
- Immune System Strengthening
- Blood Disorders (Anemia, Leukopenia, and Thrombocytopenia)
- Blood Testing

The National Cancer Institute Clinical Trials Database lists and describes ongoing clinical trials at various locations throughout the United States. This can be accessed at the website http://cancertrials.nci.nih.gov or by calling the Cancer Information Service at (800) 4-CANCER.

## Life Extension Suggestions

Patients should ask their physicians for assistance in obtaining information on ongoing cancer vaccine and other immunotherapy clinical studies, and the criteria for subject enrollment and participation. Immunotherapy patients should consult their physicians before starting to use any nutritional supplements while receiving treatment. In addition, if using nutritional supplements, they should ask their physicians for assistance in ensuring the implementation of blood tests and diagnostic procedures that are essential in monitoring the effectiveness of any adjuvant therapy for cancer.

Some guidelines for using nutritional supplements with immune-boosting cancer therapies include:

- **Zinc:** 20–50 mg daily[145,146]
- **Astragalus:** 2000–4000 mg daily
- **Vitamin C:** 120 mg daily[145]
- **Vitamin E:** 800 IU of d-alpha tocopheryl succinate daily for 2 weeks[3]; 400 IU daily for long-term use[137,150]
- **Folic acid:** 800 mcg daily[211]
- **Vitamin B12:** 7 mcg daily[211]
- **Vitamin B6:** 2.1–2.7 mg (one B-complex capsule) daily[212]
- **Selenium:** 100 mcg daily[157]
- **Glutamine:** 30 g daily[158]
- **Ginseng, panax:** 100 mg daily[213]
- **Melatonin:** 20 mg daily at bedtime[163]
- **Garlic:** 250 mg daily[214]
- **Mushroom extract** (active hexose-correlated compound): 3 g daily[166]
- **PSK:** 3000 mg daily of a 40% polysaccharide extract
- **Reishi:** 980–3000 mg daily standardized to contain 13.5% polysaccharides and 6% triterpenes
- **Fish oil** (containing EPA): 4.7 g daily[215]

Note that most cancer patients take higher doses of vitamin C (2000–20000 mg/day), selenium (200–400 mcg/day), vitamin B6 (100–750 mg/day), and vitamin B12 (100–300 mcg/day). These doses are considerably higher than the doses used in the studies cited above.

## BLOOD TEST AVAILABILITY

Tests for PSA, CEA, selenium, vitamin B12, and folate serum levels are available via Life Extension/ National Diagnostics, Inc., and may be ordered by calling (800) 544-4440 or by ordering online at http://www.lef.org/bloodtest/.

Tumor antigen profile can be determined via Genzyme Genetics (http://www.genzymegenetics.com) and may be ordered by a physician by calling (800) 966-4440.

Tests for immune cell function, serum growth factor levels, and immunosuppressive agents (IL-10) are available at UCLA's Jonsson Comprehensive Cancer Center (http://www.cancer.mednet.ucla.edu/).

X-rays, scans, and physical examinations can be arranged through your physician.

## REFERENCES

References available at: www.lef.org/dpt5/ch33

# 34

# Carpal Tunnel Syndrome

Carpal tunnel syndrome (CTS) is caused by the compression of the median nerve, which runs through a small channel in the wrist on the palm side. Under normal circumstances, there is very little pressure on the median nerve because the carpal tunnel is inflexible. It is surrounded by bone on 3 sides and a tough ligament on the fourth side.

People with CTS experience numbness, tingling, and pain in the first 3 fingers of the affected hand (or hands). The pinky finger is usually spared, which often provides a valuable clue in the diagnosis of the condition.

CTS is the most common peripheral nerve compression syndrome, affecting about 2.1 million American adults.[1,2] It tends to be more prevalent among women than men. Any activities that involve highly repetitive use of the hands, especially flexion of the fingers, can result in CTS. People at risk include those who use computers, as well as carpenters, grocery checkers, assembly-line workers, meat packers, violinists, pianists, and mechanics. Hobbies such as gardening and needlework can sometimes bring on the symptoms, while sports such as rowing, golf, tennis, downhill skiing, archery, competitive shooting, and rock climbing also place pressure on the hand and wrist joints. In addition, the syndrome can be caused by underlying disorders that affect the carpal tunnel, including arthritis, thyroid problems, gout, and diabetes. Finally, pregnant women are at risk of developing CTS.

The nerve compression associated with CTS is due to fibrous bands of tissue that form inside the carpal tunnel, squeezing the median nerve. Although CTS is linked to repetitive stress, the underlying cause—which would explain why some people suffer from it and others do not—is unknown. Newer research has uncovered some of the chemical changes that occur in response to mechanical injury among people who suffer from CTS. Although CTS is technically a non-inflammatory condition (because there is no systemic inflammation and the immune system is not activated), it is characterized by localized increases in many proinflammatory chemicals in the tissue of the carpal tunnel itself.

Researchers have discovered that prostaglandin-2, vascular endothelial growth factor, and interleukin-6 are all elevated in the carpal tunnel tissue of people with CTS. These inflammatory factors act directly on tissue by increasing the ability of fluids and small molecules to cross from the blood into the tissue itself, and they may stimulate the growth of fibroblasts, which are responsible for forming scar tissue.[3] However, levels of interleukin-1, a proinflammatory chemical, are the same in people with CTS and people without the condition, which implies that those with CTS do not have a full-blown, systemic inflammatory response. Instead, evidence suggests that the underlying cause of CTS may be an increase in specific local inflammatory factors in response to mechanical stress that causes increased vascular permeability and perfusion (or movement of fluid through the tissues of the carpal tunnel), which leads to the deposition of scar tissue (fibrosis) that characterizes CTS.[4-7]

Researchers have also uncovered evidence that the condition may be linked to inherited anatomy in the wrist. People with family members who suffer from CTS in both hands are more likely to develop the condition themselves, suggesting there may be a genetic influence or that familial similarities in the size and anatomy of the wrists may cause a predisposition for CTS.[8]

## SYMPTOMS AND DISEASE PROGRESSION

The early symptoms of CTS typically include tingling or burning in the parts of the hand that receive innervation from the median nerve. These include the palm and the palmar sides of the middle 3 fingers, as well as the palm side of the wrist. Pain may also radiate up the arm to the shoulder and sometimes the neck, causing stiffness. These symptoms are caused by an increased volume of tissue in the carpal tunnel.[9,10]

In many cases, patients complain of waking in the middle of the night with pain and a feeling that the whole hand is asleep. Careful investigation usually shows that the little finger is unaffected because the ulnar nerve rather than the median nerve services that finger.

This can be a key piece of information in making the diagnosis. If you awaken with your hand asleep, pinch your little finger to see if it is numb. Other complaints include numbness or growing weakness while using the hand for gripping activities, such as sweeping and hammering, or during repetitive finger flexion activities, such as typing.

As the condition worsens, daytime paresthesia (a sensation of prickling or tingling of the skin) can become common. The prickling is aggravated by activities such as typing, playing piano, using a computer mouse, driving, holding a book or phone, and combing hair. In long-standing or severe cases of CTS, the muscle group at the base of the thumb might degenerate due to loss of nerve supply, diminishing manual dexterity. This condition may cause difficulty with daily activities such as buttoning clothes and holding small objects. Pain and tingling can also occur in the forearm, elbow, shoulder, and neck. If the condition is allowed to progress, the muscles supplied by the median nerve in the hand may become weak and degenerate. This results in an inability to bring the thumb into opposition with the other fingers, hindering the grasp.

In advanced stages of CTS, the individual nerve cells making up the median nerve can lose their protective layers of myelin. Disruption of the myelin sheath results in impaired conduction of nerve impulses and eventually leads to damage of the axons themselves, producing potentially permanent nerve injury.[11]

## UNDERLYING DISEASES AND CONDITIONS CONTRIBUTING TO CTS

The following diseases and underlying conditions are associated with CTS.

### Tendonitis

CTS can arise from irritation and inflammation of the tenosynovium, a slippery substance covering the tendons. Different types of arthritis can directly cause inflammation of the tenosynovium, including rheumatoid arthritis, osteoarthritis, reactive arthritis, and tendonitis. Repetitive stress injuries can also cause tendonitis.

### Pregnancy

CTS was found in 28% of pregnant women in their third trimester, although 80% of the pregnant women with CTS were asymptomatic.[12] The condition usually subsides after delivery, although new mothers who maintain a flexed wrist posture while feeding or holding their babies may be prone to CTS.[13]

### Diabetes

Diabetes is also associated with several musculoskeletal disorders of the hand that can be debilitating, including CTS. Maintaining good glycemic control improves or prevents the development of these hand conditions.[14]

## DIAGNOSIS OF CTS

In most cases, CTS is diagnosed by the presence of symptoms and specific sensitivities to movement. The following tests may be used to confirm the diagnosis.

### Phalen's Test

Phalen's test, or wrist flexion, checks for pain, tingling, or numbness that may suggest carpal tunnel problems.

### Tinel's Test

Tinel's test, in which the doctor taps the inner wrist directly over the median nerve, may produce pain, tingling, or numbness and may result in a diagnosis of CTS.

### Nerve Conduction Study

Nerve conduction studies may be conducted in some cases to measure how quickly nerve impulses are conducted through the nerve. These tests allow physicians to detect CTS very early in the disease course.

### Magnetic Resonance Imaging (MRI) Scan

MRI studies may be performed in selected, atypical cases when symptoms may not match classic CTS or there is concern about another diagnosis.

## CONVENTIONAL TREATMENTS FOR CTS

The treatment of CTS is dictated by the cause, duration, and amount of compression of the median nerve. If the disease is secondary to another problem, such as arthritis or gout, treatment of the primary condition will often resolve the CTS.

In most cases caused by repetitive stress or whose cause is unknown, treatment usually relies on a combination of medications and lifestyle changes, such as splinting and avoidance of activities that aggravate the condition. Splints, available in pharmacies, may be helpful in milder cases. They keep the wrist extended and allow limited use of the fingertips.

Physicians may prescribe nonsteroidal anti-inflammatory drugs (NSAIDs) to reduce pain, diuretics to relieve pressure, and vitamin B6. There is controversy, however, over the effectiveness of NSAIDs, which also have potentially serious side effects, and diuretics. While NSAIDs are effective for short-term flare-ups, long-term results with NSAIDs have been poor.[15] Oral steroids may also be prescribed.[16]

For people who do not respond to the initial treatment, injections of corticosteroids directly into the carpal tunnel may be recommended. Newer research has shown that a single injection of methylprednisolone, at doses up to 60 mg, may be effective at long-term relief and that a second injection may not be necessary.[17,18] A single injection is best because it avoids the complications associated with corticosteroid injections, including nerve damage and relapse.

In the most severe cases, surgery to relieve pressure in the carpal tunnel is also an option. During surgery, the carpal ligament (the "roof" of the carpal tunnel) is surgically separated to relieve the pressure. Alternatively, the procedure can be performed endoscopically to reduce recovery time and the size of the surgical wound.

For moderate cases, in which surgery is not required, or for patients who have not responded to aggressive medical intervention or surgery, 2 additional treatments—low-level laser acupuncture and transcutaneous electrical nerve stimulation—may be recommended. They are often used together. During low-level laser acupuncture, a red laser penetrates the shallow acupuncture points of the hand. A trained acupuncturist or doctor must perform this procedure. Additional acupuncture points may be treated on the forearm or up to the shoulder area, according to the distribution of radiating pain.[19]

In addition to medication and surgery, people with CTS can use a number of strategies to improve their condition, including the following:

1. Take more frequent breaks from the pain-causing movement.

2. Wear wrist splints at work or at home at night during sleep. Wearing splints at night is important because fluid redistributes throughout the body while people recline, increasing in volume in the upper part of the body and producing increased pressure in the carpal tunnel.

3. Wear a forearm brace, a narrow cuff worn just below the elbow that reduces fluid content in the carpal tunnel.

4. Use cooling pain gel on the wrist. Many of these gels contain methyl salicylate, an aspirin-like substance. Before regular use, consult with your physician about possible drug interactions.

5. Have another person massage your neck, shoulders, and back to relieve tension in the forearm and wrist.

6. Use a wrist rest in front of your keyboard and keep your keyboard level, not elevated, at your computer workstation.

7. Some larger companies offer ergonomic consultation for their employees.[20] If it is available, make use of it.

## LIFESTYLE CHANGES FOR CTS

A wealth of clinical data confirms that lifestyle changes can help ease the suffering of those afflicted with CTS. However, there is no single "magic potion" or change that will work for everyone. People with CTS should consider the suggestions below to determine what works for them.

1. When sleeping, cock the wrists upward instead of bending them downward to minimize pressure in the carpal tunnel. A splint will help maintain this position.

2. At home or work, minimize repetitive hand movements when possible.

3. Alternate between activities or tasks to reduce the strain on the body.

4. When using the wrists, keep them straight and let the arms and shoulders share the stress.

5. Use the whole hand or both hands to pick up an item.

6. Avoid holding an object the same way for a long time.

7. Adjust your desk, chair, and keyboard so you are in the best possible position: back straight, feet flat on the floor or resting on a footrest, knees level with or slightly lower than your hips, shoulders in a neutral position (neither forward nor back), elbows bent at a 90-degree angle, forearms parallel to the floor, and wrists straight.

8. Take breaks at least once an hour to rest, shake your hands, massage the palms and backs of your hands, and do a few stretches and loosening movements of the shoulders and arms before settling back to work.

9. Keep hands warm, with gloves if necessary.

10. Get regular aerobic exercise such as walking or swimming.

11. Cut down on caffeine and smoking, which may reduce blood flow to your hands. Nerve tissue is the most sensitive to reduced blood flow.

12. If your work requires using tools, avoid holding an object or tool the same way for a long time.

13. Minimize time using vibrating tools. If that is not possible, stop frequently and follow the warm-up program below.

According to a report published by the American Academy of Orthopaedic Surgeons, a simple warm-up routine such as the following may greatly reduce the incidence of CTS.

- Hold your hands in front of you as if pushing on a wall. Count to 5.
- Relax your wrists and fingers.
- Make tight fists with both hands.
- Bend both fists downward. Count to 5.
- Repeat each step 10 times.
- Then shake arms loosely while they are hanging at your sides.

## NUTRITIONAL THERAPY TO REDUCE PRESSURE

Nutritional approaches to CTS are based on reducing pressure in the carpal tunnel and relieving pain.

### Vitamin B6

Although more studies are needed, evidence suggests that vitamin B6 has a place in treatment of CTS and should be considered as a nutritional therapy.[21]

If CTS is severe, nutritional therapies are unlikely to reverse it. However, while surgery will take pressure off the nerve, it does not correct for nutritional deficiencies. Likewise, steroid injections will not correct vitamin B deficiencies.

Vitamin B6, given in conjunction with vitamins B1 and B12, has a pain-killing effect that is due to inhibition of the body's natural pain conduction system. Studies have shown that vitamin B6 is effective in relieving the pain associated with CTS, and there is evidence that B6 deficiency may cause CTS.[22,23] One study, which noted the controversy surrounding the use of NSAIDs and nighttime splints, recommended that 200 mg vitamin B6 daily be included in treatments for CTS.[23]

Vitamin B6, however, should be used with caution since high doses over the long term can cause damage to the central nervous system or neuropathy (damage to peripheral nerves).

There is evidence that vitamin B6 will not work properly except in combination with adequate amounts of other B vitamins. In one individual, vitamin B2 use for 5 months caused "nearly complete disappearance" of CTS.[24]

### Enzymes

Serrapeptase (or serratiopeptidase), a proteolytic enzyme, shows promise in the treatment of CTS. This proteolytic enzyme, which digests protein, is produced by bacteria in the gut of silkworms and digests their cocoons. When this enzyme is isolated and coated in the form of a tablet, it has been shown to reduce swelling.[25] Significant improvement in electrophysiologic parameters was reported in patients with CTS who received serratiopeptidase daily for 6 weeks.[26]

### Nutrition to Relieve Inflammation

Although people with CTS do not have elevated markers of systemic inflammation, there is no doubt that localized inflammation in the wrist contributes to their condition. Thus, any nutrient that reduces inflammation might be able to help relieve the symptoms of CTS. Unfortunately, however, few natural anti-inflammatories have been studied in the context of CTS. Most research has been directed toward surgery or pharmaceuticals rather than nutritional approaches. Nevertheless, the following nutrients have been shown to reduce inflammation in other diseases.

**Fish oil.** Fish oil is rich in omega-3 fatty acids. These fats have shown anti-inflammatory effects in a number of diseases, including cancer, atherosclerosis, and autoimmune disorders.[27] Fish oil works by downregulating the levels of proinflammatory cytokines, which are shown to be elevated in people with CTS.[28] Among people with arthritis, which is also characterized by localized inflammation, fish oil, in conjunction with vitamins A, C, E, and selenium, can reduce inflammation and provide an important defense against the oxidative stress that occurs in inflamed joints.[29] Oxidant stress within the joints has also been implicated in CTS.[30]

**Curcumin.** A component of the spice turmeric, curcumin has well-known anti-inflammatory properties. A review of 300 scientific papers on curcumin found that it can inhibit proinflammatory cytokines and that significant curative effects have been observed in experimental animal models of a number of diseases, including atherosclerosis, cancer, diabetes, intestinal diseases, and many others.[31]

**Ginger.** The anti-inflammatory properties of ginger have been known for centuries, and studies have shown clearly that ginger extracts can reduce inflammatory cytokines.[32,33] Specifically, ginger has been shown to reduce the inflammation associated with joint disorders such as arthritis.[34,35]

## Life Extension Suggestions

- **Vitamin B6:** 200 mg daily. Caution should be exercised, however, because high doses of vitamin B6 have been linked to neuropathy.
- **Serrapeptidase enzyme:** 5 mg twice daily between meals
- **Fish oil:** 4000 mg daily, containing at least 1400 mg eicosapentaenoic (EPA) acid and 1000 mg docosahexaenoic acid (DHA)

- **Ginger extract:** 1000 mg daily
- **Curcumin** (as highly absorbed BCM-95®): 400–800 mg daily
- **Vitamin A:** 10000–25000 IU daily
- **Vitamin E:** 400 IU alpha-tocopherol and 200 mg gamma-tocopherol daily
- **Selenium:** 200 mcg daily

## REFERENCES

References available at: www.lef.org/dpt5/ch34

# 35

# Catabolic Wasting

Catabolic wasting (cachexia) is a clinical wasting syndrome characterized by unintended and progressive weight loss, weakness, and low body fat and muscle. At least 5% of body weight is lost. Cachexia is not caused by poor appetite and nutritional intake, but rather a metabolic state in which a "breaking down" rather than "building up" occurs in bodily tissues, no matter how much nutritional intake occurs. Additionally, whether a patient receives oral or intravenous nutrition makes no difference. The patient simply cannot gain weight, so eating more is not a solution.

It is estimated that half of all cancer patients experience catabolic wasting, with a higher occurrence seen in cases of malignancies of the lung, pancreas, and gastrointestinal tract. The syndrome is equally common in acquired immune deficiency syndrome (AIDS) patients and can also be present in bacterial and parasitic diseases, rheumatoid arthritis, and chronic diseases of the bowel, liver, lungs, and heart. It is usually associated with anorexia (ie, loss of appetite) and can manifest as a condition in aging or as a result of physical trauma. Catabolic wasting diminishes quality of life, worsens the underlying condition, and is a major cause of death.

## CACHEXIA AND CANCER

Researchers previously believed that cancer increased metabolic demand (stolen protein), produced toxins, and suppressed appetite, resulting in malnutrition. New research, however, shows that although cancer may raise resting metabolic rate, improved nutrition does not alleviate the symptoms of anorexia, chronic nausea, early satiety, and changes in taste that make even favorite foods unpalatable to some cancer patients. The view of clinicians is that bodily wasting is the result of a combined action of tumor products and host immune factors—cytokines, in particular—that lead to poor appetite, muscle wasting, and an altered metabolism. The cytokines interleukin-1 (IL-1), interleukin-6 (IL-6), interferon-gamma, tumor necrosis factor-alpha (TNF-α), and brain-derived neurotrophic factor appear to increase and play a role in the progression of cachexia in cancer, as well as in other diseases associated with bodily wasting.

Other metabolic alterations associated with the syndrome are hyperglyceridemia, lipolysis, and accelerated protein turnover, all leading to a loss of fat mass and body protein. The dysregulation of metabolic processes produces a negative energy balance.

Clinicians are currently treating cancer-related catabolic wasting with a variety of interventions, including nutritional supplementation, administration of cytokine inhibitors, steroids, hormones, cannabinoids, and thalidomide. Gemcitabine, a chemotherapeutic drug, has shown clinical benefits in treating cachexia. Newer nutritional interventions with megestrol acetate derivatives, gamma-receptor agonists, amino acid manipulations, myostatin inhibitors, and uncoupling protein modifiers is currently being explored. Further research must be done to investigate gender differences in relation to pathophysiology and therapy.

There is some evidence that the drug hydrazine sulfate may help cancer patients gain weight and improve the cachectic state. The drug is by prescription and should be given by a complementary physician familiar with its use, as it can be toxic. The dose is usually 60 mg daily. Narcotic painkillers or benzodiazepine anxiety-reducing agents cannot be given concomitantly.

## CACHEXIA AND HIV

Bodily wasting is a common manifestation of human immunodeficiency virus (HIV), occurring at any state of infection and indicative of disease progression. Malnutrition, a result of appetite loss, is commonly due to nausea and vomiting. Weakness and diarrhea are often present as well. Persons with HIV may also experience malabsorption of nutrients due to enteric infections associated with the disease, even if they consume sufficient calories.

The effects of malnutrition are thought to contribute to increased immune suppression including a reduction in T-lymphocyte helper and suppressor cells, altered phagocytic functions, and decreased killer-cell activity, leading to opportunistic infections and cancers. Pro-inflammatory cytokines IL-1, IL-6, and TNF have been cited in many studies as potential causes of wasting. Most people with advanced HIV and AIDS have some degree of wasting.

To reverse weight loss, appetite stimulants, anabolic agents (such as growth hormone or testosterone), cytokine inhibitors, and hormones are often prescribed. Megestrol acetate and dronabinol (which contains the active ingredient in marijuana) are approved for the treatment of wasting. Thalidomide, which aids in the healing of aphthous ulcers of the mouth and esophagus, is now available.

## DIAGNOSIS

Unfortunately, the cachectic state is all too apparent to any observer. In severe chronic disease with the development of multiple organ failure, some degree of malabsorption of nutrients probably contributes to the cachectic state. The entire picture is reflected in a continuing decline of the serum albumin as the illness progresses. Conversely, an increase in serum albumin suggests an improvement in the nutritional state. As long as a patient consumes nutrition by mouth, optimizing the state of digestive secretions is probably advisable, although there may not be clinical studies demonstrating this. The Heidelberg test reflects this environment and can be used to ascertain the need for either hydrochloric acid or pancreatic enzyme supplementation.

## RESISTANCE

Resistance or strength training is defined by resisting, lifting, and lowering weights. Resistance exercise training for a period of 8–12 weeks results in significant increases in muscle mass, muscle strength, and muscle function. Even in cases where dietary protein intake falls below recommended daily allowances, the anabolic effect of resistance training appears to improve energy intake and protein use, allowing nitrogen retention.[1] Resistance training has been shown to improve muscle strength and functioning in people with disease-causing muscle wasting and in healthy, but frail elderly people.[2] Resistance exercise training is cost-effective, noninvasive, and a means to improve the quality of life—and as such, should be considered as an adjunct treatment modality.

## APPETITE STIMULANTS

Appetite stimulants have been used in both HIV and cancer patients with wasting syndrome.

Marinol® (dronabinol) is a synthetic version of the active ingredient in marijuana, 9-tetrahydro-cannibol (THC). Marinol® can be prescribed by a physician and taken orally. Results have been mixed as a treatment for nausea and vomiting due to chemotherapy. As an appetite stimulant, however, results are more encouraging. In a study of 139 people with HIV, Marinol® significantly improved appetite, body weight,

mood, and decreased nausea and vomiting compared to those on placebo.[3] Side effects from Marinol® may include heightened awareness, a sense of well-being, and elation. Dizziness, drowsiness, muddled thinking, and anxiety are also possible side effects.

Megace® is a synthetic progesterone used to stimulate appetite in people with wasting syndrome caused by HIV or advanced stages of cancer. It is also used as a therapy in women with breast cancer, interfering with the action of estrogen on cancer cell receptor sites. Although an increase or stabilization of weight may be seen after 6 weeks at the therapeutic dose of 800 mg daily, most of the gain will be in fat. A lower therapeutic dose along with resistance training will help to promote more muscle mass. Megace® has a low incidence of adverse side effects when taken as directed.

## TESTOSTERONE

Testosterone, a natural anabolic steroid, can help place patients in a positive nitrogen balance. Dosages of 100–200 mg weekly can be given to most men and women. Consideration can be given to DHEA (see the DHEA Restoration Therapy protocol) and pregnenolone as well. The intravenous administration of vitamins (25–50 g of vitamin C, 2–3 times weekly, in particular) may be helpful.

Testosterone supplementation in male HIV patients with wasting syndrome has been shown to increase lean body mass at daily doses of 200 mg administered intramuscularly. The most significant results were seen in combination with resistance weight training. In a study, 54 men were given testosterone or placebo and placed on a 12-week exercise training program or no training at all. Lean body mass and muscle increased in those undergoing training and testosterone therapy. Levels of beneficial HDL cholesterol increased in those training, but fell in those supplementing with testosterone. Viral load fell in those taking the hormone.[4]

Consideration should be given to "adrenal support." Patients with catabolic wasting should be assumed to have some degree of adrenal fatigue from the stress of chronic disease (see the Adrenal Disorders [Addison's Disease and Cushing's Syndrome] protocol).

*Warning:* The possibilities discussed above have not been thoroughly studied with respect to potentially worsening cancer (if cancer is the source of the cachectic state). It is suggested that you discuss any potential treatment with a physician practicing complementary medicine prior to initiating therapy.

# TARGETED NATURAL INTERVENTIONS

## Fish Oil

Depletion of muscle and adipose tissue in cancer cachexia appears to arise not only from decreased food intake, but also from the production of catabolic factors (eg, TNF and other autoimmune cytokines) secreted by certain tumors. Experiments with a cachexia-inducing tumor in mice showed that when part of the carbohydrate calories in their diet was replaced by fish oil, host body weight loss was inhibited. The catabolic-inhibiting effect occurred without an alteration of either the total calorie consumption or nitrogen intake.[5]

Fish oil concentrate was found to inhibit tumor-induced lipolysis directly.[6] The catabolic fat loss-preventing effect of fish oil arose from an inhibition of the elevation of cyclic AMP (adenosine monophosphate, a nucleotide involved in energy metabolism) in fat cells. The increased protein degradation in the skeletal muscle of catabolic animals was also inhibited by fish oil; this effect was due to the inhibition by fish oil of muscle prostaglandin E2 production in response to a tumor-produced proteolytic factor. Thus, reversal of cachexia by fish oil in this mouse model results from its capacity to interfere with tumor-produced catabolic factors.[7] Similar factors have been detected in human cancer cachexia.

Studies show that the docosahexaenoic acid (DHA) fraction of fish oil is the best documented supplement to suppress the inflammatory cytokines involved in the catabolic process such as TNF-α, IL-6, IL-1β, and prostaglandin E2.[8–18] Catabolic wasting patients should consider taking a combination of gamma-linolenic acid (GLA) and primarily the DHA fraction of fish oil. Both GLA and DHA significantly suppress inflammatory cytokines.[13,19–22]

## Glutamine

Glutamine has been one of the most intensively studied nutrients in the field of nutrition support in recent years. Animal studies show that glutamine is effective against catabolic stress.[23–25] Glutamine supplementation was shown to improve organ function, survival, or both in most published studies. These studies also have supported the concept that glutamine is a critical nutrient for the gut mucosa and immune cells.[24–27]

Molecular and protein chemistry studies define the basic mechanism involved in glutamine action in the gut, liver, other cells and organs.[25] Double-blind prospective clinical investigations suggest that glutamine-enriched diets are generally safe and effective in catabolic patients.[28] Intravenous glutamine has been shown to increase plasma glutamine levels, exert protein anabolic effects, improve gut structure and function, and reduce important indices of disease (eg, infection rates and length of hospital stay) in selected patient subgroups.[29]

Glutamine is the most abundant free amino acid in the human body. In catabolic stress situations, such as after surgical operations or trauma and during sepsis, glutamine is rapidly transported to organs and blood cells. This results in an intracellular depletion of glutamine in the muscles and the ensuing catabolic wasting effect.[30] Increasing evidence suggests that glutamine is a crucial substrate for immunocompetent cells. Glutamine depletion decreases the proliferation of lymphocytes, possibly by arresting a critical phase of the growth cycle of the cells.[31]

Glutamine is a precursor for the synthesis of glutathione and stimulates the formation of heat-shock proteins.[32] Moreover, there are suggestions that glutamine plays a crucial role in the stimulation of intracellular protein synthesis.[33] Experimental studies revealed that glutamine deficiency causes a necrotizing enterocolitis—an inflammation of the small intestine and colon, leading to cell death—and increases the mortality of animals subjected to bacterial stress.[34]

A clinical human study involving bone-marrow transplant patients demonstrated, after supplementation with glutamine, a decrease in the incidence of infections and a shortening of hospital stay. In critically ill patients, parenteral glutamine reduced nitrogen loss and caused a reduction of the mortality rate.[31] In surgical patients, glutamine invoked an improvement of several immunologic parameters.[35] Moreover, glutamine exerted a nutritional (tropic) effect on the intestinal mucosa, decreased the intestinal permeability, and thus may prevent the translocation of bacteria.

Glutamine is an important metabolic substrate of rapidly proliferating cells. It influences cellular hydration (molecular water content) state and has multiple effects on the immune system, intestinal function, and protein metabolism.[29] In several disease states, glutamine may become an indispensable nutrient supplement. Catabolic wasting patients should consider supplementing with 2000 mg of glutamine daily.

## Whey Protein

Scientists have examined the impact of whey protein concentrate on preventing or treating catabolic wasting, immune dysfunction, and cancer. A study involving HIV-positive men fed whey protein concentrate found dramatic increases in glutathione levels, with most men reaching their ideal body weight.[36] In another study, when different groups of rats were given a powerful carcinogen, those fed whey protein concentrate showed fewer tumors and reduced tumor masses.[37] Whey appears to inhibit the growth of breast cancer cells at low concentrations. In one clinical study, when cancer patients were fed whey protein concentrate at 30 g per day, some patients' tumors showed a regression.[38]

The research using whey protein concentrate has led researchers to a discovery regarding the relationships between cancerous cells, whey protein concentrate, and glutathione. Glutathione is an antioxidant that protects the body against harmful compounds. It was found that whey protein concentrate selectively depletes cancer cells of their glutathione, thus making them more susceptible to cancer treatments, such as radiation and chemotherapy.[38,39] It has been found that cancer cells and normal cells will respond differently to nutrients and drugs that affect glutathione status.

The concentration of glutathione in tumor cells is higher than that in normal cells surrounding the tumor. This difference in glutathione status between normal cells and cancer cells is believed to be an important factor in the resistance of cancer cells to chemotherapy. Research has shown that cancer cells subjected to whey proteins were depleted of their glutathione and their growth was inhibited, although normal cells had an increase in glutathione and increased cellular growth. These effects were not seen with other proteins.

The researchers concluded, "Selective depletion of tumor glutathione may, in fact, render cancer cells more vulnerable to the action of chemotherapy and eventually protect normal tissue against the deleterious effects of chemotherapy."

Whey protein also appears to play a direct role in bone growth. Researchers found that rats fed whey protein concentrate showed increases in bone strength and bone protein (eg, collagen). Whey protein was found to stimulate total protein synthesis, DNA content, and increased hydroxyproline content of bone cells in a dose-dependent manner.

It should be noted that not all whey protein concentrates are created equal. Processing whey protein to remove the lactose and fats, but without losing its biological activity, takes special care by the manufacturer. The protein must be processed under low-temperature and low-acid conditions so as not to denature it. Maintaining the natural state of the protein is essential to its biological activity.

Whey protein has the highest biological value rating of any protein. When the biological value is high, that means protein is absorbed, used, and retained better in the body. High biological values also are associated with tissue sparing. Thus, whey protein concentrate can be beneficial for people with catabolic wasting diseases.

## Plant-Based Protein

For vegetarians or those limiting their animal protein intake, plant-based protein is a viable option. Plant-based protein contains more glutamine than whey or egg protein, with comparable branched chain amino acid (BCAA) values to whey, egg, and casein. It also contains more arginine than these 'gold standard' animal proteins. Arginine is essential for nitric oxide synthesis, which promotes healthy endothelial function and blood vessel dilation and relaxation.[40]

## Creatine

The muscle atrophy commonly seen in older adults comes mainly from a loss of fast-twitch (type 2) muscle fibers recruited during high-intensity movements (eg, weight lifting and sprinting). These are the fibers most profoundly affected by the dietary supplement creatine. Various studies have found that creatine helps increase strength and lean body mass in older adults participating in resistance exercise training.[41–43] According to one research group, creatine supplementation in older adults may help attenuate age-related loss of muscle strength as well as improve one's ability to perform functional living tasks.[42]

## Vitamin D

While scientists have long known that vitamin D plays an important role in bone health, studies suggest that it is also essential for maintaining muscle mass in aging people. Vitamin D helps preserve the type 2 muscle fibers that are prone to atrophy in the elderly. Scientists noted that vitamin D helps support both muscle and bone tissue. Also, that low levels of vitamin D seen in older adults may be associated with poor bone formation and muscle function. Thus, ensuring adequate vitamin D intake may help reduce the incidence of both osteoporosis and sarcopenia (age-related loss of lean muscle mass, strength, and functionality) in aging people.[44]

## Other Nutritional Supplementation

Conjugated linoleic acid (CLA), a fatty acid, has anticatabolic properties. This has been demonstrated in laboratory mice injected with endotoxin to produce a catabolic response. Seventy-two hours after feeding with linoleic acid, the mice presented body weights similar to controls. The researchers concluded that conjugated linoleic acid prevented anorexia in endotoxin-injected test subjects.[45] The suggested dose of CLA for a person in a catabolic state is two 1000-mg capsules taken 2 times a day.

The amino acid arginine, in combination with hydroxyl-methylbutyrate (HMB) and glutamine, increased fat-free mass in patients with stage 4 cancer when given at a dose of 14 g per day.[46] Additional amino acid supplementation should include 2400 mg of L-carnitine and at least 1200 mg of leucine, isoleucine, and valine.

*Warning:* Some nutritionists are concerned about the use of high doses of glutamine or arginine in cancer patients. Because glutamine and arginine promote cellular growth, the concern is that these amino acids could cause cancer cells to grow faster. Scientific studies, however, show that glutamine and arginine provide beneficial effects to cancer patients. Only one study on breast cancer patients hinted at a risk for arginine supplementation.

## Life Extension Suggestions

- **Glutamine:** 2000 mg daily
- **Gamma-linolenic acid (GLA):** 1300 mg daily
- **Omega 3 fatty acids from fish oil:** 1400 mg of EPA and 1000 mg of DHA daily
- **Conjugated linoleic acid (CLA) blend** (containing a minimum of 78% CLA): 2000 mg twice daily
- **Biologically active whey protein:** 30–60 g daily
- **Plant protein blend** (containing pea protein isolate, artichoke protein, and brown rice protein concentrate): 1 scoop daily
- **Arginine:** 10–20 g daily in divided doses
- **L-carnitine:** 200–400 mg daily in divided doses
- **Comprehensive multinutrient formula:** per label instructions
- **Consider growth hormone, DHEA, and/or testosterone replacement therapy**
- **Branched chain amino acids (BCAAs)**, containing at least 1200 mg of L-leucine, 600 mg of L-isoleucine, and 600 mg of L-valine: once daily
- **Creatine:** 1000–2000 mg daily
- **Vitamin D3:** 5000–8000 IU daily, depending on blood levels of 25-OH-vitamin D

## REFERENCES

References available at: www.lef.org/dpt5/ch35

# 36

# Cataracts

A cataract, which is clouding of the eye lens that reduces the amount of incoming light, results in deteriorating vision. Cataracts are often described as being similar to looking through a waterfall or waxed paper. Daily functions such as reading or driving a car may become difficult or impossible. Eyeglass prescriptions may require frequent changes. An estimated 200 million people worldwide have cataracts.

Minor lens opacities at birth may never progress to cataract in adulthood, while others progress to a degree requiring surgery or causing blindness. Factors that influence vision and cataract development include age, nutrition, heredity, medications, toxins, health habits, sunlight exposure, and head trauma. Hypertension, kidney disease, diabetes, or direct trauma to the eye can also cause cataracts.

Cataract surgery is common in the United States, with over 1.5 million done yearly. Annual costs associated with cataract treatment are estimated to be over $3.4 billion.[1,2] Because 60% of people who qualify for Medicare already have cataracts, cataract surgery costs Medicare more than any other medical procedure.[3]

The most common type of cataract is nuclear cataract, which occurs when proteins of the nucleus (center) degenerate and darken, causing light to scatter. Cortical cataracts, the second most common type, occurs in the cortex (or periphery) of the lens. Cortical cataracts form when the order of fibers in the cortex is disturbed and the gaps fill with water and debris, thus altering the pathophysiology of light by scattering and/or absorbing it. Posterior subcapsular cataracts, the least common type, affect the back of the lens.

## EPIDEMIOLOGY AND GENETICS

Estimates are that 20.5 million Americans older than 40 years (representing 17.2% of the U.S. population) have a cataract in at least one eye and 6.1 million (5.1%) have had cataract surgery to remove a lens (aphakia) or replace a lens with an artificial lens (pseudophakia).[4] There is evidence that genetics plays a role in the formation of cataracts, especially congenital cataracts.[5] Cataracts have shown to be more prevalent among older individuals. By age 80 years, more than 50% of the U.S. population either have a cataract or have had cataract surgery.[6] Due to the growing elderly population, the number of individuals with a cataract could climb to 30.1 million by the year 2020; of these, 9.5 million would be expected to have aphakia or pseudophakia.[4]

## RISK FACTORS

Identification and awareness of risk factors for cataracts could have an important benefit. Estimates are that if cataract onset could be delayed by 10 years, the number of cataract surgeries could be reduced annually by 45%.[2] Risk factors include:

### Gender

In the United States, women have a significantly higher age-adjusted prevalence of cataracts, with 58% of cataract cases.[4] Women have a higher risk for most types of cataracts,[7] although evidence suggests estrogen may protect against cataract formation.[8] The antiestrogen drug tamoxifen (used to block estrogen receptors) increases risk of cataracts when taken long term.[9]

### Education Status and Socioeconomic Factors

Risk for cataracts is greater among individuals with lower socioeconomic status or educational level. This is attributed to increased exposure to conditions inducing cataract development (eg, nutritional deficiencies from poor diet, increased exposure to disease, and poor general health).[2]

### Exposure to Excessive Sunlight

Geographical areas with more hours of sunlight have a greater prevalence of cataracts, showing an association between ultraviolet B irradiation and cataract formation.[10]

### Exposure to Radiation

Exposure to x-rays or gamma radiation is a risk factor for cortical and posterior subcapsular cataracts in humans. Radiologists routinely minimize exposing the lens to ionizing radiation; if not possible, however, cataracts frequently develop and require surgical treatment.[11]

### Nutrition

A diet lacking a high intake of antioxidants (particularly vitamins A, C, and E) fails to protect the lens from cataract formation.[12,13]

## Smoking and Alcohol

There is an increased risk of nuclear cataracts among smokers.[14,15] Risk for all cataract types increase with heavy alcohol consumption.[7]

## Diabetes

Diabetics are more likely to develop cortical opacities or require cataract surgery.[16]

## Corticosteroids

Corticosteroid use is associated with posterior subcapsular cataracts.[17]

## Genetics

Lens-specific genes include gene-encoding proteins for growth and transformation of lens fiber cells (cystallins) and mediation of cellular respiration and metabolism, such as major intrinsic polypeptide (MIP) and certain connexins.[18,19] Mutations in lens-specific genes are associated with hereditary cataracts, possibly through a mechanism that produces a protein interfering with normal proteins, thus disrupting normal function and cataract formation.[20]

Numerous hereditary syndromes manifest cataracts as a characteristic feature. Gene mutations are identified for some syndromes: Lowe's syndrome, neurofibromatosis type 2, galactosemia, and Werner syndrome.[21,22] In most diseases, identifying the genes responsible for cataract development offers no explanation as to why cataracts manifest.[20] A better understanding of biochemical and molecular mechanisms underlying cataract formation may provide more information.[5,23]

# SYMPTOMS AND DISEASE PROGRESSION

## Symptoms

**Decreased visual acuity.** Declining visual acuity (ie, a measure of eyesight sharpness and focus) is one of the first signs of cataracts. Measurement of visual acuity is most commonly used to detect changes in visual function caused by cataracts (and other conditions) over time.[24] An individual with a cataract will often notice worsening vision that requires frequent changes to a stronger lens correction. Visual acuity testing uses the Snellen Visual Acuity Chart.

A Snellen test is not always the best measure of cataracts or the best indicator for surgery. Clinically, visual acuity can remain high despite age-related lens opacities. The Snellen test may not always reflect visual disabilities occurring under less than ideal (clinical) circumstances, as with contrast sensitivity.[24]

The Preferred Practice Pattern of the American Academy of Ophthalmology recommends Snellen acuity tests as the best indicator of surgery with respect to functional and visual needs, environment, and risk factors.[25]

**Reduced contrast sensitivity.** Common complaints are loss of ability to see objects in bright sunlight and being blinded by strong lights at night, such as oncoming headlights.[26] All cataracts lower contrast sensitivity, but do so most severely in posterior subcapsular cataracts. Cataracts that reduce contrast sensitivity normally occur within the pupil diameter.

**Glare.** Even minor degrees of lens opacity produce glare due to the scatter of light toward the front of the lens. All cataract types can cause glare, especially cortical and posterior subcapsular. Patients with glare symptoms frequently have poorer vision in daylight conditions and when driving. Unlike contrast sensitivity reduction, some glare can be produced by opacities not within the pupil diameter.[24]

**Myopic shift.** The natural aging process in the human lens produces a progressive shift toward hyperopia (ie, farsightedness). When a cataract is forming in the nucleus of the lens, clouding of the lens changes the way light bends (or refracts). This produces greater nearsightedness (a myopic shift). Myopic shift enables an aging person who previously needed reading glasses to read without corrective lens. This phenomenon, called "second sight," is indicative of hardening of the lens nucleus, a predictor of a developing nuclear cataract.[27]

**Double vision and color shift.** Other common signs of cataracts are monocular diplopia (double vision in one eye) and change in color vision. Monocular diplopia occurs with lens opacities, particularly cortical spoke cataracts. In cortical spoke cataracts, water clefts form radial wedge shapes that contain a fluid with a lower refractive index than the surrounding lens. All light entering the lens is not bent to the same extent, producing double or multiple images. There may be a perception of haloes around light.[28]

Color shift is produced by a lens that is more absorbent at the blue end of the spectrum, causing color perception to fade. Color shift is common with nuclear cataracts. Patients are usually not aware of a defect in color perception, although it becomes apparent after cataract surgery when they readjust to normal color perception.[6]

## Disease Progression

**Observation and assessment.** Cataracts are usually observed and assessed with a slit lamp biomicroscope (ie, a microscope with 2 eyepieces). Different magnifications combined with a strong light are focused into a slit to examine the eye. Slit lamp examination measures visual acuity and amount of light scattered in the eye.[27] Cataracts can be detected with a funduscope, an optical instrument that inspects the retina. Retinal blood vessels are blurred by light scattering caused by opacity in the lens.

**Lens clouding.** Disease progression in all types of cataract is indicated by increased lens opacity, although opacity manifests differently in each type.

**Nuclear cataract.** In nuclear cataracts, lens density initially increases in the central lens nucleus. Opacity follows producing color changes that begin by clear changing to yellow, and to brown at more advanced states.[29]

**Cortical cataract.** Changes in transparency involve the periphery (or cortex) of the lens. Water gets into the lens cortex and creates pockets under the lens capsule called vacuoles. The vacuoles gradually lengthen into ray-like spaces and fill with fluid that is first transparent and later opaque. Vacuoles begin at the periphery and gradually spread toward the center, taking on an appearance of wedges or spokes. Because cortical cataracts begin at the periphery, vision may not be affected at first, but eventually visual acuity decreases.[29]

**Posterior subcapsular cataract.** Cataracts form in front of the posterior capsule (ie, lens casing at the back of the lens) as a cluster of swollen cells. These cataracts develop as independent, isolated entities, but are associated with cataract formation in nuclear or cortical regions. Granules and vacuoles in front of the posterior capsule are signs of posterior subcapsular cataracts. Although uncommon, progression and severity can be more extreme than other types.[29]

**Cataract classification.** Cataracts are classified as immature, mature, and hypermature. A lens with remaining clear areas is an immature cataract. A mature cataract is completely opaque. A hypermature cataract has a liquefied surface that leaks through the capsule. The leaking material can cause inflammation in other eye structures.[6]

# ETIOLOGY AND MECHANISMS OF ACTION

## Cataract

Cataract (ie, any type of opacification of the lens) is considered clinically significant when opacification interferes with visual function. Decreased lens transparency results in increased light scattering as light passes through the lens to the retina where diminished focus of light impairs vision. Cataract adversely impacts vision by light absorption in a less transparent lens.

The underlying mechanism for cataracts involves: disruption of the structure of lens fiber cells, increases in protein aggregation, or cytoplasm dysfunction in the lens cell.[30]

## Age-Related Cataracts

Each type of age-related cataract has a specific mechanism that leads to their development. These include oxidative damage, protein aggregation, breakdown of glutathione, damage to fiber cell membranes, protein breakdown, elevated calcium, abnormal lens epithelial cell migration, or aberrant changes in lens fiber cells.

## Nuclear Cataract

Nuclear cataracts show increased oxidative damage to lens proteins and lipids causing protein-to-protein interactions that result in aggregation and increase light scattering.[31] A lens with a cataract has increased interaction between crystallins and lens fiber cell membranes.[32]

Evidence suggests a strong connection between aging and increased oxidized glutathione in the lens nucleus indicative of an imbalance between protein and lipid oxidation, and glutathione-dependent reduction.[33,34] Nuclear cataract formation may be caused by separation of lens cell cytoplasm (a jelly-like substance) into protein-rich and protein-poor liquid phases, accounting for the opacity.[35,36]

## Cortical Cataract

Cortical opacities start in small regions of the lens periphery. Opacity may spread around the circumference of the lens. The following mechanisms may initiate the cortical cataract: damage to the fiber cell plasma membrane, loss of protective molecules (eg, glutathione), excessive breakdown of proteins (proteolysis), and damage to systems responsible for calcium homeostasis. These factors are interrelated because any one of them leads to the others in the initial formation of cortical cataracts.[20]

Loss of calcium homeostasis spreads opacification around the lens periphery and towards the nucleus. In cortical cataracts, calcium levels are elevated in damaged cells.[37] Elevated calcium leads to proteolysis, protein aggregation, and light scattering.[38]

## Posterior Subcapsular Cataract

Posterior subcapsular cataracts are caused by environmental stresses such as ultraviolet light, diabetes, and drug ingestion.[2,39] Light scattering occurs in a cluster of swollen cells at the back of the lens, beneath the lens capsule. Because opacity produced by the cell cluster is within the optical axis (or line of sight), these cataracts can be particularly debilitating. Posterior subcapsular cataracts are associated with abnormal migration of lens epithelial cells or aberrant changes in lens fiber cells at the back of the lens.[40]

# ANATOMY AND PHYSIOLOGY (STRUCTURE AND FUNCTION)

## The Lens

A lens is formed from specialized epithelial cells during embryonic development. The epithelium is a sheet of cube-shaped cells covering the anterior surface of the lens near the cornea. The major part of the lens consists of concentric layers of elongated fiber cells. The outermost shells of fiber cells extend from beneath the epithelium to the posterior lens surface near the vitreous body. The lens is one centimeter from front to back, surrounded by the capsule (ie, an elastic matrix of cells produced during embryonic development by secretions from epithelial and fiber cells on the lens surface).[41]

In an adult lens, only a few epithelial cells replicate, proliferating slowly, producing new fiber cells that elongate and accumulate crystallins (lens proteins). Crystallins give the lens its refractive power to focus light on the retina.[42] During maturation, layers of fiber cells build up.[43]

After the elongation process, a differentiation begins that degrades all intracellular, membrane-bound organelles.[44] As generations of fiber cells go through this process, mature fiber cells are buried deeper within the lens. The lens increases in size and cell number throughout life.[45] Because protein synthesis stops with organelle degradation, mature fiber cells are more stable than cells having other functions in the body.[46]

## Zonules

Zonules (ie, inelastic microfibrils that suspend the lens) are located above and below the lens in the anterior part of the lens and extending into the lens capsule. Zonules are inelastic compared to other fibrils in the body (eg, in the skin and arterial walls), but stretch enough to create tension responsible for altering lens curvature. This is required for accommodation (ie, process of focusing on objects at different distances).[47]

## Refractive Properties of the Lens

Refractive properties of the lens result from high concentration of crystallins in the cytoplasm of lens fiber cells and curvature of the lens. Lens crystallins are water-soluble proteins in lens fibers that provide a high refractive index. The lens is able to focus light on photoreceptors in the retina.[48] In a healthy lens, refractive error is caused by abnormalities in corneal curvature or length of the ocular globe, but rarely from defects in the curvature or refractive index of the lens itself.[20]

An essential component of lens transparency is a high concentration of lens crystallins and minimization of light scattering and absorption. Light passes through the lens because of the regular structure of lens fibers, an absence of membrane-bound organelles, and small, uniform spaces between the cells. This reduced light scattering is due to short-range interactions among densely packed crystalline molecules.[49]

# PATHOPHYSIOLOGY

## Nuclear Cataract Formation

Cataract formation (especially in nuclear cataracts) is caused by oxidative stress that occurs in all biological systems, particularly the lens. Oxidative stress and generation of free radicals results from normal activity of mitochondria and other metabolic processes.[50] Oxidation is controlled by an environment of reducing agents. Reducing agents produced in the mitochondria neutralize free radicals.

Production of reducing agents requires energy output, a challenge for the deeper lens fiber cells that lack mitochondria. The enzyme systems in deeper cells are less active because they were synthesized decades earlier.[20] These central lens fiber cells are delicately balanced between being damaged by oxidation of membrane lipids and cytoplasmic protein, and being protected by reducing agents transported from epithelial cells and immature lens fiber cells near the surface. Transport of reducing agents is difficult because there is little space between lens fiber cells. Movement is by diffusion.[51]

Another challenge is maintenance of protein stability for many decades. Once a lens is formed, proteins are synthesized in outer fiber cells close to the surface. Proteins deeper in the lens generated during embryogenesis have to last 100 years or more. Accumulated damage to these proteins reduces enzymatic activity and increases protein aggregation, a component of cataract formation.[30]

## Cortical Cataract Formation

Unlike nuclear cataracts, cortical cataracts show disorganization of fiber cell structure. Causes of cortical cataracts include loss of calcium balance, protein breakdown and aggregation, and diminished antioxidant protection (from glutathione). There is evidence for a genetic cause of cataract formation.[52] There is no overall explanation why initial damage is restricted to the center of affected cells or why the preferred location of cortical cataracts is the lower half of the lens.[53]

## Posterior Subcapsular Cataract Formation

Posterior subcapsular cataracts are less common and occur with the other 2 types. A "pure" posterior subcapsular cataract is uncommon, occurring in only 10% of cases.[54]

An important risk factor in posterior subcapsular cataract development (and cortical cataracts) is exposure to excessive x-ray or gamma-radiation.[55] Mechanisms that initiate cellular or molecular dysfunction are poorly understood.[20]

## CONVENTIONAL TREATMENT

No successful anticataract drug is available. Research continues on possible anticataract agents, including nonsteroidal anti-inflammatory drugs (NSAIDs) such as salicylic acid and ibuprofen. Animal trials have tested the effects of aldose reductase inhibitors. High levels of aldose reductase (an enzyme) are associated with diabetic cataracts. No clinical trials have demonstrated these substances have any convincing anticataract effect.[56]

## Surgical Removal and Intraocular Lens Implantation

The most common treatment is surgical removal of the cataract and replacement with an artificial lens. Phacoemulsification and extracapsular extraction are widely used surgical procedures. In phacoemulsification, a small incision is made in the cornea. A probe vibrating with ultrasound waves then emulsifies the cataract and the fragments are removed by suction. The lens capsule is left in place to provide support for a lens implant.[57]

If a cataract has advanced to an extent that phacoemulsification cannot effectively break up the lens, the preferred alternative is extracapsular extraction, requiring a larger incision so the lens nucleus is removed in one piece through the open lens capsule. The softer lens cortex is vacuumed out, leaving the shell in one piece.[57]

After the cataract is removed, an artificial lens is implanted into the empty lens capsule. This implant, an intraocular lens (IOL), is made of plastic, acrylic, or silicone. An IOL requires no care and becomes a permanent part of the eye. Early IOLs were rigid plastic and the incision required several sutures. IOLs currently used are flexible, allowing a smaller incision that requires no sutures. Flexible IOLs are folded by a surgeon and inserted into the capsule. Reading glasses will be required after surgery.[57]

## Secondary Cataracts

A common complication of extracapsular cataract extraction is formation of secondary cataracts. Secondary cataracts occur because lens epithelial cells migrate under the IOL to the posterior capsule that has been denuded of cells by surgery. These cells are then abnormally transformed into a mass of fiber-like cells (globular clusters) or fibrotic plaques, which scatter light, degrade visual images, and cause secondary cataract formation.[20] Secondary cataracts develop postoperatively in 50% of cases.[57]

A common, effective method for secondary cataract removal uses a laser procedure called yttrium aluminum garnet (YAG) capsulotomy. A YAG laser delivers tiny, rapid bursts of energy that pass through the front of the eye and IOL. When the laser beam reaches the posterior capsule, it makes a tiny opening. Light can then pass into the vitreous body and reach the retina. Enough of the posterior capsule is left to hold the IOL in place.[57]

## ENDOCRINOLOGY AND BIOCHEMISTRY (REGULATION AND METABOLISM)

### Energy Sources

The lens has no direct blood supply; therefore, its oxygen concentration is lower than most parts of the body.[58] The lens depends on glycolytic metabolism to produce much of the adenosine triphosphate (ATP) (ie, the energy currency of the body) and reducing agents for metabolism.[59]

Glycolysis is the process by which sugars (like glucose) are metabolized to produce ATP. When glycolysis occurs in differentiated lens fiber cells deep within the lens, the absence of oxygen (anaerobic glycolysis) only allows 10% of available energy to be conserved. Glucose comes from the aqueous humor, the fluid sac between the lens and cornea. Energy from glucose is derived from (aerobic) oxidative pathways in superficial lens fiber cells and epithelial cells containing mitochondria. In animal studies, 50% of the ATP produced by epithelial cells came from oxidative metabolism; glycolysis accounted for almost all ATP produced in most lens fiber cells.[59]

## Oxidative Damage: Protective Biomechanisms

**Glutathione.** Although the oxygen level within the lens is very low, the lens still derives a substantial proportion of ATP from mitochondrial (aerobic) oxidative phosphorylation, which creates free radicals as an unwanted byproduct. Glutathione provides the most important protection against damage from free radical and other oxidants.[60] Glutathione is a very small specialized protein (a tripeptide) consisting of 3 amino acids: glutamic acid, cysteine, and glycine. Glutathione is concentrated within the lens and readily oxidized by damaging oxidants. Those oxidants are chemically reduced (neutralized) as glutathione is chemically oxidized in cytoplasm of cells within the lens. When glutathione levels decline in the epithelial cells (or entire lens), cell damage and cataract formation can occur unabated.[61]

Lens epithelial cells and superficial lens fiber cells synthesize glutathione. Additional glutathione is transported into the lens from the aqueous humor.[62] Oxidized glutathione can be regenerated (ie, reduced) by the enzyme glutathione reductase, which uses the coenzyme reduced nicotinamide adenine dinucleotide phosphate (NADPH). NADPH is the cofactor derived from the dietary or supplemental B-vitamin niacin (niacinamide or vitamin B3).[60] Regeneration of reduced glutathione from oxidized glutathione is especially important because it is the chemically reduced form of glutathione that is effective in neutralizing (chemically reducing) free radicals. Glutathione is unique in its ability to regenerate its chemically reduced state by simply finding an electron donor. This cycle allows one molecule of glutathione to continually act as a free radical scavenger.

Reduced glutathione diffuses into lens fiber cells, moving toward the lens center, while oxidized glutathione moves toward the lens surface. Impediment of diffusion in an older lens is a possible cause of nuclear cataract.[34] The rate of diffusion between superficial and deeper layers of the lens decrease with age. Consequently, proteins and lipids in nuclei of older lens are more affected by oxidative stress.

**Vitamin C.** Ascorbic acid (vitamin C) protects the lens from oxidative damage. In the aqueous humor, ascorbic acid reaches concentrations that are 30–50 times the levels in blood. Ascorbic acid is found in substantial quantities within the lens and surrounding ocular tissues.[63] Dehydroascorbate (the oxidized form of ascorbic acid) can enter the lens through a glucose transporter. It is then reduced by glutathione-dependent processes.[64] Ascorbic acid reacts readily with free radicals and other oxidants in the aqueous humor and lens, preventing damage to lens proteins, lipids, and nucleic acids.

# DIETARY AND LIFESTYLE CHANGES

Recommendations include increased consumption of vegetables and fruits, "good fats" found in oily fish (eg, salmon and tuna), whole grains, and legumes, and minimal consumption of saturated fats and cholesterol.[65] Consuming foods rich in the carotenoids lutein and zeaxanthin is especially important.

Wear protective eyewear and avoid the following risk factors:

- Smoking

- Excessive alcohol consumption

- Exposure to sunlight (particularly UV radiation)

- Excessive exposure to x-ray and gamma irradiation

# NUTRITIONAL THERAPY

## Protection from Free Radical Damage

The benefits of dietary supplements for cataracts are widely documented. Free radical action, directly linked to cataracts, is a major cause of damage to eyes and cataract formation.[66] Numerous studies have documented the effects of supplements, including their ability to reduce free radical damage and reverse damage in some cases.[67,68]

**Glutathione.** A healthy eye contains glutathione in very high concentrations, whereas low levels adversely affect the eye.[69] Glutathione maintains water balance in the lens. It is synthesized in the lens (and elsewhere) and is essential to normal metabolism.[41,60] Glutathione can benefit lens function by:

- Preserving the physicochemical integrity of proteins in the lens.[34]

- Maintaining action of the sodium–potassium transport pump and molecular integrity of lens fibers (protein)[34]

- Maintaining molecular integrity of lens fiber membranes and acting as a free radical scavenger to protect membranes and enzymes from oxidation[68]

- Preventing free radical–induced photochemical generation of harmful byproducts[64]
- Reactivating oxidized vitamin C, which improves antioxidant capability in the lens[70]

**Vitamin C.** Vitamin C (ascorbic acid) is essential for normal ocular metabolism and occurs in the lens at a concentration 30–50 times higher than blood. This concentration is second only to the central nervous system and adrenal cortex. Vitamin C is found in high concentrations in eyes of animals active during daylight hours; low concentrations are found in nocturnal animals.[71] Prior to cataract formation, vitamin C concentrations significantly drop.[72,73] Vitamin C provides protective benefits for the lens by:

- Protecting the lens from photochemical oxidation.[74]
- Helping increase levels of glutathione[75]
- Supporting delicate membranes regulating transport of nutrients and ions (minerals and electrolytes) into the lens[63]
- Protecting against damaging ultraviolet (UV) radiation and visible light[76]
- Protecting against superoxide radical, $O_2^-$ (known to be extremely destructive in every cell)[77]

**Vitamin B2.** Vitamin B2 (riboflavin) is a required precursor to the cofactor, reduced flavin adenine dinucleotide (FADH) used by glutathione reductase, which in the lens enzymatically reduces, and thereby, activates glutathione; and makes that glutathione available for the enzyme glutathione-selenium peroxidase, which chemically reduces peroxide free radicals to harmless water. Deficiency of glutathione creates a faulty antioxidant defense system in the lens.[78]

Light, especially UV light, destroys riboflavin and FADH. Most B vitamins, because they are not stored, must be replaced daily. Riboflavin deficiency is a prime cause of photosensitivity, making the eye more sensitive to UV damage. A daily dose of 50–150 mg of riboflavin reduces this photosensitivity.[79]

**Selenium and vitamin E.** Low plasma levels of vitamin E increase the risk of lens opacities.[80] Selenium works with alpha-lipoic acid to increase cellular concentrations of glutathione, which protects the eye lens from free radical damage.[77]

**Alpha-lipoic acid.** Supplementation of animals with alpha-lipoic acid prevents cataract formation resulting from inhibition of glutathione synthesis. Alpha-lipoic acid reduced cataract formation by 40% and protected the lens from losing vitamins C, E, and glutathione. Unsupplemented animals lose these nutrients.[81]

**N-acetyl-cysteine and garlic.** A combination of diallyl disulfide (a major organosulfide in garlic oil) and N-acetyl-cysteine (NAC) prevented cataract development in animals.[82] NAC assists in glutathione production because it is a source of cysteine, one of the 3 amino acids in this tripeptide.[83]

**Melatonin.** Melatonin is an antioxidant that can impede cataract development. In animals, melatonin potently inhibited cataract formation due to free radical scavenging or stimulation of glutathione production.[84] Melatonin production slows after age 40 years; by age 60 years, virtually no melatonin is produced at a time when most cataracts develop.

## Lens Protein Protection

**Vitamin B6.** Vitamin B6 (pyridoxine) is essential for amino acid and protein metabolism, vitamin B12 absorption, and proper synthesis of nucleic acids. Its coenzyme is required for many amino acid reactions and related metabolic functions. Vitamin B6 is suggested for nutritional support for cataract patients.[85]

**Acetyl-L-carnitine.** Acetyl-L-carnitine is an amino acid that maintains cellular metabolism of fatty acids. During aging, mitochondria (energy-producing organelles within the cell) begin to deteriorate, resulting in accumulation of cellular debris and eventual cell death. Acetyl-L-carnitine can diminish advanced glycation end product (AGE) damage that leads to cataract formation.[86] Acetyl-L-carnitine can acetylate (deactivate) potential glycation sites on crystallins and protect them from glycation-mediated protein damage.[87]

**Aminoguanidine.** Aminoguanidine inhibits AGEs and may treat diabetic cataracts. In moderately and severely diabetic rats, aminoguanidine inhibited cataracts only in moderately diabetic rats.[88] Blood sugar control is important so antiglycating agents such as aminoguanidine can protect against cataract.

> **Note:** *Although aminoguanidine has been safely used throughout the world for decades, clinical experience is limited in the United States. Aminoguanidine has not been approved by the U.S. Food and Drug Administration. Aminoguanidine should be taken under the supervision of a physician. It can inhibit vitamin-B6 uptake so co-administration of B6 is suggested.*

## Lens Metabolism Support

**Bioflavonoids.** Bioflavonoids are powerful inhibitors of the enzyme aldose reductase.[70] If aldose reductase activity falls, sorbitol is not synthesized. This reduces the accumulation of water in the lens.[89] The bioflavonoids quercetin, myrcetin, and kaempferol (from limes) specifically inhibit diabetic cataracts.[73] Gingko is a widely used flavonoid that maintains microcirculation to the eye and inhibits free radicals.[90]

**Inositol.** Inositol nicotinate is a B vitamin that occurs in high concentrations in the lens. Inositol exhibits antioxidant properties, resulting in the quenching of reactive oxygen and scavenging of glucose.[91] Inositol works best when taken with B-complex vitamins. A suggested dose of inositol is 250 mg daily.[92]

**Carnosine.** Carnosine inhibits formation of AGEs and protects normal proteins from the toxic effects of existing AGEs.[93,94] Eye drops containing N-acetyl-L-carnosine (NAC) can delay vision senescence in humans: effective in 100% of primary senile cataract cases and 80% of mature senile cataract cases. NAC, which enters the aqueous and lipid parts of the eye, prevents and repairs light-induced breaks to DNA strands.[95] NAC eye drops are approved for human use in Russia for the treatment of many eye diseases.

## Ocular Environment Support

**Carotenoids.** Carotenoids are fat-soluble, yellowish pigments found in some plants, algae, and photosynthetic bacteria. Carotenoids are light-gathering pigments that provide protection from the toxic effects of oxygen free radicals and singlet oxygen, which are generated in the presence of light and oxygen.[96] Lutein, zeaxanthin, and meso-zeaxanthin are carotenoids found in high concentrations in the macula of the retina.[97,98] Lutein and zeaxanthin protect the eye from age-related macular degeneration and cataract formation.[67] Lutein is derived from dark green, leafy vegetables (spinach, broccoli, kale, and collard greens). Zeaxanthin is found in yellow fruits and vegetables (corn, peaches, and mangoes). The Nurses' Health Study examined the impact of 12 years of carotenoid consumption on cataract formation in more than 77 000 female nurses over the age of 45 years. After controlling for factors such as age and smoking, women with the highest intake of zeaxanthin and lutein had a 22% lower risk of cataract extraction (defined as cataracts severe enough to require surgical removal). More frequent intake of spinach and kale—two foods rich in lutein—was also linked to a moderately lower risk of cataract.[99]

Unlike lutein and zeaxanthin, meso-zeaxanthin is not found in the diet, but usually converted in the retina from ingested lutein.[100] If taken as a supplement, meso-zeaxanthin is absorbed into the bloodstream and effectively increases macular pigment levels.[101]

**Coenzyme Q10.** Coenzyme Q10 (CoQ10) is an antioxidant that provides protection from free radical damage in the eye.[102] A combination of antioxidants including CoQ10, acetyl-L-carnitine, polyunsaturated fatty acids (PUFAs), and vitamin E improved mitochondrial function (linked to age-related macular degeneration) in retinal pigment epithelium.[86] Mitochondrial dysfunction in lens epithelial cells and superficial fiber cells of the eye may lead to oxidative stress and cataract formation. Mitochondrial dysfunction occurs throughout the body and produces damaging reactive oxygen species thought to cause aging and disease.[103]

**Potassium and magnesium.** A lens with cataracts has decreased concentrations of potassium and magnesium. Potassium and magnesium are often deficient in aging humans. Supplementation with 400 mg of elemental potassium and 800 mg of elemental magnesium increases availability of these minerals to the lens and protects the arterial system.[104]

**Ginkgo and bilberry.** Ginkgo biloba extract is an antioxidant, increases circulation to the optic nerve, and exhibits potential anticataract ability.[78,90] Bilberry (from *Vaccinium myrtillus* fructus) is a proanthocyanidin historically used for eye conditions, including glaucoma, cataracts, age-related macular degeneration, diabetic retinopathy, and retinitis pigmentosa.[78] Ginkgo biloba and bilberry may restore microcapillary circulation.[86]

## Life Extension Suggestions

- **High potency multivitamin/multinutrient formula** providing N-acetyl-cysteine, selenium, inositol, vitamins B2, B6, C, and E, bioflavonoids, and other antioxidants
- **N-acetyl-carnosine eye drops**: 1–2 drops, 1–4 times daily
- **Carnosine**: 500–1500 mg daily
- **Zeaxanthin**: 3–8 mg daily
- **Lutein**: 10–20 mg daily
- **Meso-zeaxanthin**: 1 mg daily
- **Vitamin C**: 500 mg daily
- **Vitamin B2**: 50–150 mg daily
- **Selenium**: 200–400 mcg daily
- **Natural vitamin E**: 100–400 IU alpha-tocopherol and 200 mg gamma-tocopherol daily

- **Vitamin B6**: 50–250 mg daily
- **Magnesium**: 500–1500 mg daily
- **Glutathione**: 50–500 mg daily
- **R-lipoic acid**: 210–420 mg daily
- **N-acetyl-cysteine**: 600 mg daily
- **Melatonin**: 300 mcg–3 mg at bedtime
- **Acetyl-L-carnitine arginate**: 320–960 mg daily
- **Coenzyme Q10**: 100–200 mg daily
- **Potassium**: 99 mg daily (or more) when instructed to do so by a health care professional based on blood test results

- **Ginkgo biloba**: 120 mg daily
- **Bilberry**: 100 mg daily
- **Garlic**: 1200 mg providing daily
- **UV-blocking sunglasses**

## REFERENCES

References available at: www.lef.org/dpt5/ch36

# 37

# Cervical Dysplasia

Cervical dysplasia is characterized by abnormal (dysplastic) cells in the cervix. Extending into the vagina, the cervix is the lowest part of the uterus. Although cervical dysplasia does not produce symptoms itself, it is potentially dangerous because it can progress to cervical cancer, the second-most common type of cancer in women, especially among younger women.[1-3]

Since the introduction of the Pap smear in 1941, the death rate from cervical cancer has dropped significantly because of early detection of cervical dysplasia. In developing countries, where Pap smears are not as common as in industrialized countries, cervical dysplasia is reported to be the leading cause of cancer in women.[4] Worldwide, cervical cancer accounts for 11.6% of cancers in women.[3,5]

In more than 99% of cases, cervical cancer and cervical dysplasia are caused by the human papillomavirus (HPV), the virus that causes genital warts.[6] HPV is very common: the lifetime risk of a woman contracting genital HPV is estimated to be 80%.[7] It is transmitted through sexual intercourse. The virus may be present without symptoms, making it possible for carriers to transmit it unknowingly.

The vast majority of women with HPV will not develop cervical dysplasia or cancer.[2,5] There are many variations of the virus, and some forms carry a higher risk for the development of cancer than others, especially HPV16 and HPV18.[8] HPV is often difficult to detect because it rarely causes symptoms. Only about 1% of women with HPV have visible genital warts,[9] which adds to the importance of regular Pap smears.

The goal of cervical dysplasia treatment is reducing the risk of its progression to cervical cancer. This risk reduction may be accomplished through dietary modification, supplementation, and possibly by chemoprevention through the use of medical or chemical modifiers.[3,10,11] Fortunately, there is hope on the horizon. Because of lifestyle changes, the prevalence of Pap smears, and exciting research into HPV vaccines, cervical cancer rates are expected to continue dropping in the industrialized world.

## CLASSIFICATION AND SCREENING FOR CERVICAL DYSPLASIA

Cervical dysplasia is commonly referred to as cervical intraepithelial neoplasia (CIN). It is often classified by the degree of penetration of abnormal cells into the tissue lining (epithelium):

- CIN I describes the involvement of the basal third of the epithelium.
- CIN II involves the basal two thirds of the epithelium.
- CIN III involves more than two thirds of the epithelium.

A diagnosis of cervical dysplasia does not necessarily mean that cervical cancer will develop. In fact, up to 74% of women with mild CIN will naturally regress to normal within 5 years.[12] Of those cases that do progress, only a minority of women will actually develop cancer.

- Only 1% of women with CIN I who experience progression will progress to severe dysplasia or worse.[12]
- Among patients with CIN II, 16% will advance to severe dysplasia within 2 years and 25% within 5 years.
- An overall progression rate of severe dysplasia (CIN III) to cervical cancer has been observed in 12–32% of patients.[13,14]

Pap smears are the standard tool used to screen women for cervical dysplasia or cancer. During a Pap smear, cells are scraped from the cervix and then evaluated microscopically. About 5–7% of Pap smears yield abnormal findings.[15]

One major problem with screening is poor follow-up testing among women with abnormal Pap smears. In most cases, an abnormal Pap smear requires a follow-up test in a few months. However, an estimated 10–61% of women with abnormal Pap smears do not undergo follow-up testing.[16] Factors associated with noncompliance include an elementary education, prior surgery, additional diseases, consumption of medications for chronic conditions, and family illness.[17]

In general, according to the American Cancer Society's 2002 screening guidelines:

- Women should begin cervical cancer screening no later than 3 years after beginning vaginal intercourse but no later than 21 years of age.
- Cervical cancer screening should be performed annually with regular Pap tests or every 2 years with liquid-based Pap tests.

- A woman 30 years of age or older with 3 consecutive normal Pap smears may elect to be screened every 2–3 years.

- Women who have undergone hysterectomy can elect to discontinue Pap smears if the surgery was not performed to treat cervical cancer or precancer. Women with an intact cervix post hysterectomy should undergo screening until at least age 70.

- A woman older than age 70 may choose to discontinue Pap smear screening after 3 prior normal Pap smears and no abnormal results in the preceding 10 years.

## RISK FACTORS FOR PROGRESSION

While it may take years for cervical dysplasia to progress to cancer, the cancer can quickly spread throughout the body once established. If left untreated, cervical cancer has a relatively high mortality rate, although the survival rate for properly treated early-stage cervical dysplasia and cervical cancer is high.

Early symptoms of cervical cancer, such as altered vaginal discharge and abnormal vaginal bleeding, are rare. Advanced cervical cancer may present with pelvic, back, or leg pain, leaking of urine or feces from the vagina, loss of appetite, weight loss, and bone fracture.

Not all cases of cervical dysplasia progress into cancer.[2] Rather, it appears that certain factors may hasten the progression from cervical dysplasia to cervical cancer:

### Decreased Methylation

DNA hypomethylation is significantly associated with the grade of CIN.[18,19]

### Multiple HPV Types

One study showed a significantly increased risk of CIN in women with several HPV subtypes.[20]

### Viral Load

A high level of the virus is a significant risk factor for CIN.[20–27]

### High-Risk HPV Variants

Certain virus strains are an independent risk factor for cervical dysplasia.[28,29]

### Persistence of HPV Infection

Persistent infection with HPV increases the risk of cervical cancer.[26,30]

### Smoking

Smoking is a serious independent risk factor for advanced cervical dysplasia.[31] Passive cigarette smoking via a spouse also has been associated with a higher incidence of high-grade squamous intraepithelial lesions.[32] Women with abnormal Pap smears absolutely should avoid smoking.

### Obesity

In one large study, fewer overweight and obese women (78% in each group) underwent cervical cancer screening with Pap smears.[33] Because this group of women have a higher mortality rate for cervical cancer compared with women of normal weight, special attention should be paid to increasing screening among overweight and obese women.

### Number of Sexual Partners

The number of sexual partners increases the risk of cervical dysplasia,[28] perhaps by increasing the chances of encounters with HPV strains.

### Multiple Pregnancies

Multiple pregnancies have been cited as a possible risk factor for cervical dysplasia.[8,28,34]

### Lower Socioeconomic Status and Lack of Pap Smears

Women with a lower educational level may avoid follow-up Pap smears.[17] Additionally, those with lower socioeconomic status may lack access to appropriate health care.

### Diethylstilbestrol (DES)

DES was given to expectant mothers from the late 1930s until 1970 to prevent early delivery. However, many mothers were unaware that the drug was being administered to them; sometimes it was given with a vitamin supplement. Unfortunately, it resulted in increased cervical cancer in female offspring. Current research regarding the use of DES focuses on the effects of the drug in granddaughters and grandsons of those who received it.[35]

### Compromised Immune Function

Women with medical conditions that affect the immune system are at greater risk for cervical dysplasia. These conditions include HIV, systemic lupus erythematosus, and transplanted organs.[36–40]

### Other Sexually Transmitted Diseases

One study concluded that the presence of other sexually transmitted diseases, such as Herpes simplex virus and Chlamydia trachomatis, can cause dysplasia to progress to cervical cancer.[41,42] However, other studies failed to show an association between these sexually transmitted diseases and cervical cancer progression.[43,44]

# CONVENTIONAL TREATMENT OF CERVICAL DYSPLASIA AND CANCER

## Cervical Dysplasia

The success rate of treating early-stage cervical dysplasia is extremely high. During treatment, a physician will attempt to remove the abnormal cells through a variety of methods, including cryotherapy, or freezing the cells to destroy them.

Alternatively, a procedure called loop electrosurgical excision may be performed. During this procedure, a thin wire loop with an electrical current is used to remove a cone-shaped piece of tissue. Women treated with loop excision are likely to convert to HPV-negative status, which eliminates the risk for HPV-related cervical dysplasia and cancer.[45] If a larger area of the cervix contains abnormal cells, a gynecologist may perform a surgical procedure called cervical conization to remove all the abnormal cells.

In case of high-grade CIN, or if previous surgeries left too little cervical tissue, a hysterectomy may be recommended.[46] In rare advanced cases, all the organs of the pelvis can be removed in a procedure called pelvic exenteration. Except for hysterectomy or pelvic exenteration, the surgical choices typically allow a woman to carry a child in future pregnancies.

## Cervical Cancer

Sometimes radiation or chemotherapy is required in addition to surgery for cancers that are recurrent or have spread beyond the pelvis. Survival rates depend on the stage of the cancer. With treatment, 5-year survival rates are 80–85% for cervical and uterine tumors, 60–80% for tumors involving the upper part of the vagina, 30–50% for tumors still retained in the pelvis, and 14% when cancer has invaded the bladder or rectum or metastasized outside the pelvis.

---

## VACCINES AND ANTIVIRALS: HOPE FOR THE FUTURE?

Recently, media attention has focused on possible vaccines for cervical cancer. Although these vaccines are still in the development stage, a vaccine for low-grade dysplasia will likely be available soon.[47]

Large-scale trials have shown that developmental vaccines have reduced the rate of HPV infection and CIN.[48,49] One factor that may complicate a successful vaccination program is a lack of vaccines in developing countries (where vaccines are most needed); another is a lack of vaccines that are specific to certain types of HPV.[50]

However, given their early record, it appears that vaccines may soon offer hope of dramatically reducing the rate of HPV infection and in turn, the rates of cervical dysplasia and cervical cancer.

---

## WHAT YOU HAVE LEARNED SO FAR

- Cervical dysplasia is a proliferation of abnormal cells in the lining of the cervix.
- Cervical dysplasia left untreated may develop into cervical cancer.
- Cervical cancer is the second-most common type of cancer in women.
- Early detection and treatment of cervical cancer are highly effective. The mortality rate for untreated cervical cancer is 95% within 2 years.
- The survival rate for properly treated early-stage cervical cancers is 70–100%.
- Virtually 100% of cases of cervical dysplasia and cervical cancer are the result of HPV.
- The lifetime risk of contracting a genital HPV infection is about 80% in women.
- Not all women with HPV will develop dysplasia or cancer of the cervix.
- Only 1% of women with HPV develop external warts.
- Dysplasia does not cause symptoms.
- The lack of symptoms in dysplasia, infrequent screening, and various risk factors sometimes allow cervical dysplasia to develop into cervical cancer.
- The Pap smear is the standard screening tool to detect dysplasia.

---

# NUTRIENT SUPPORT FOR A HEALTHY CERVIX

Since as far back as 1981, statistically significant differences in levels of vitamins A, C, and beta carotene have been noted between women with cervical dysplasia and healthy controls.[51,52] Other nutrients studied in cervical dysplasia include folate, zinc, and vitamins B6, B12, and E. Changes in diet and nutritional supplementation can reduce the odds of developing cervical cancer.[2,53,54]

## Vitamin A

Vitamin A deficiency has been observed in women with various grades of CIN, and higher levels of vitamin A have been shown to help reduce the risk of progression to cervical cancer.[6,8,55–57] Vitamin A deficiencies have been linked to CIN among Southwestern American Indian women[6] and HIV-positive women.[58] Vitamin A also may have a protective effect for black women in the early stages of CIN.[59]

In two studies of women with CIN, a 3-fold to 4.5-fold higher risk of cervical cancer development was seen in those with a low level of vitamin A.[60,61] More severe stages of cervical dysplasia were associated with an even lower level of vitamin A.[55] Conversely, high levels of vitamin A were associated with cervical dysplasia regression, particularly in those who were HPV16-positive.[29]

## B vitamins

Numerous studies have also shown vitamin B deficiencies among women with cervical dysplasia.

**Vitamin B1.** In women with high- and low-grade squamous intraepithelial lesions of the cervix, the level of vitamin B1 was decreased in those with CIN. Progression of cervical dysplasia was associated with reduced levels of vitamin B1.[62]

**Vitamin B2.** Low levels of vitamin B2 have been associated with an increased risk of low- and high-grade CIN.[8,62] Interestingly, vitamin B2 deficiency has been associated with oral contraceptive use.

**Vitamin B6.** Cervical squamous intraepithelial lesions have been associated with a vitamin B6 deficiency.[63]

**Vitamin B12.** Low levels of vitamin B12 have been associated with both low- and high-grade squamous cervical lesions, as well as with HPV persistence.[19,62,64] However, another study did not show an association between vitamin B12 and women who were either positive or negative for HPV.[65]

**Folic acid.** Insufficient intake of folate is associated with increased risk for cervical dysplasia.[8,19,62,66–72] Interestingly, folate deficiency can be misdiagnosed as cervical dysplasia because their characteristics are similar.[73,74]

Other theories to explain the connection between folate deficiency and cervical dysplasia include the increased demand for folate associated with pregnancy and oral contraceptive use.[74,75] This increased demand results in a folate deficiency in the cervical tissue, which could increase the risk of CIN.[76]

One study suggests that folate deficiency could cause chromosomal damage, such as that seen in cervical cancer, as a result of impaired DNA synthesis or repair.[77] Additional studies state that folate status may be involved in early stages of CIN but not in advanced disease.[4,71]

## Vitamin C

Increased incidence of cervical dysplasia has been found with low levels of vitamin C (ascorbic acid) in several studies.[4,8,67,78–83]

## Antioxidants

In general, antioxidant status has been closely linked to cervical dysplasia. Many studies have found low levels of antioxidants in women with various grades of cervical dysplasia. These antioxidants include alpha-tocopherol, gamma-tocopherol, beta-carotene, lutein, lycopene, canthaxanthin, alpha- and beta-cryptoxanthin, coenzyme Q10, and glutathione.[20,30,31,79,84–87] However, the relationship between reduced antioxidant levels and cervical dysplasia is poorly understood. It could be that lower antioxidant levels contribute to development of the condition, or conversely, the disease might cause reduced antioxidant levels as the body seeks to fight the disease. In either case, patients with cervical dysplasia should consider supplementing with a robust antioxidant program.

## Minerals

Cervical dysplasia patients have also been found to have abnormal levels of minerals, including copper, selenium, and zinc. Studies have shown that patients with cervical dysplasia and invasive cancers have lower levels of selenium and zinc and a higher level of copper.[29,86,88,89] Ferritin, an iron-storing protein, has been shown to have a protective effect against cervical dysplasia.[90]

## Cumin

Finally, the spice cumin has been demonstrated in animal studies to reduce the likelihood of developing cervical cancer.[53]

## Melatonin

Melatonin may help suppress rapid cell growth and mutation, but this association is still being studied, and some studies have found melatonin to have no effect on certain cancer lines.[91,92] Nevertheless, melatonin is commonly used by patients with cervical dysplasia.[93] One study found that melatonin inhibits the growth of cervical cancer cells in laboratory cultures after 48 hours of treatment.[94]

Researchers are also looking at variations in melatonin levels among patients with cervical dysplasia. One study revealed lowered melatonin secretion in endometrial cancer patients but not in those with squamous cervical cancer.[95]

## WORKING TO FIGHT OFF CERVICAL CANCER

It is fortunate that most cases of cervical dysplasia will not progress to cancer, and if detected, cervical dysplasia is relatively easily treated. If cervical dysplasia progresses to cervical cancer, the treatment options are similar: cryosurgery (ie, freezing the cancer) or loop electrosurgical excision. If they are treated early enough, it is possible for many women with early-stage cervical cancer to bear children. Advanced cancer that has spread beyond the cervix can require hysterectomy, radiation treatment, or chemotherapy.

While an abnormal Pap smear is reason to carefully adhere to any regimen of follow-up testing and treatment under the care of a physician, studies show that certain nutrients also have an ability to fight cervical cancer. Research on cervical cancer has focused on agents that have low toxicity and display activity against HPV-positive cell lines.[96] The following chemical compounds are under investigation:

### Indole-3-Carbinol

Indole-3-carbinol, a plant compound from cruciferous vegetables like broccoli and cauliflower, has been studied in connection with the management of CIN. The effectiveness of this plant compound has been documented in small clinical trials.[97,98] Indole-3-carbinol reduces the formation of 16-alpha-hydroxyestrone, a suspected carcinogen, which in high levels is associated with a greater risk of cervical cancer.[99]

### Vitamin A

Retinoids, the natural and synthetic forms of vitamin A, inhibit the growth of epithelial cells through transforming growth factor beta.[100] Additionally, retinoids have been reported to support the differentiation of cells (thereby preventing abnormal cervical cancer cells), as well as to affect the immune response of cells.[101,102]

### Coenzyme Q10

Coenzyme Q10 is used by cells for growth and maintenance and as an antioxidant. Some studies have suggested coenzyme Q10 stimulates the immune system. Low levels have been found in certain cancers. Studies suggest the usefulness of coenzyme Q10 in adjuvant therapy in cervical cancer, especially in conjunction with alpha- and gamma-tocopherols.[84]

### Green Tea

A study of 51 patients showed a reduction of 69% of cervical dysplasia lesions in patients who received green tea extracts as either an ointment or capsule.[103]

### Blueberry Extract

Blueberries may slow the growth of cancer cells. In 2001, University of Mississippi researchers conducting in vitro tests found that blueberry and strawberry extracts were remarkably successful in slowing the growth of 2 aggressive cervical cancer cell lines and 2 fast-replicating breast cancer cell lines, with the blueberry extract performing best against the cervical cancer cells.[104]

### Melatonin

In animal studies, this hormone is reported to prevent the proliferation of errant cells as well as to help prevent mutation of cells and the breakage of chromosomes.[91] In lab studies, growth of cervical cancer cells diminished within 48 hours of administration of melatonin.[94]

### Turmeric (curcumin)

Turmeric is effective in regulating cell development, cell division, and programmed cell death.[105-115] Regarding cervical cancer, turmeric affects the transcription of the high-risk variant HPV18 as well as other cellular transcription responses.[116] Finally, turmeric combined with the chemotherapeutic agent vinblastine is effective against resistant cervical cancer.[117,118]

### Life Extension Suggestions

High-potency multivitamin that includes the following:

- **Vitamin A:** 500 IU acetate and 4500 IU beta-carotene daily
- **Vitamin C:** 1000–3000 mg daily
- **Folate,** preferably as L-methylfolate: 400–1000 mcg daily
- **Vitamin B6,** preferably as pyridoxal-5-phosphate: 75–105 mg daily
- **Vitamin B12:** 300–600 mcg daily
- **Selenium:** 200 mcg daily
- **Zinc:** 30 mg daily
- **Melatonin:** 3–10 mg nightly
- **Curcumin,** as highly absorbed BCM-95®: 400–800 mg daily
- **Vitamin E,** as high gamma-tocopherol mix with sesame lignans: 359 mg daily
- **Indole-3-carbinol:** 80–160 mg daily
- **Coenzyme Q10,** as ubiquinol: 100–200 mg daily with food
- **Blueberry extract:** 500–2000 mg daily
- **Green tea extract:** 725 mg daily

### REFERENCES

References available at: www.lef.org/dpt5/ch37

# 38

---

# *Chemotherapy*

---

Cancer cells are everything we would like healthy cells to be: They quickly adapt to toxic environments, readily alter themselves to assure their continued survival, and utilize biologic mechanisms to promote cellular immortality. All of these factors make cancer an extremely difficult disease to treat.

Chemotherapy drugs have a high rate of failure because they usually kill only specific types of cancer cells within a tumor or the cancer cells mutate and become resistant to the chemotherapy. Cancer chemotherapy could save more lives if the latest scientific findings were incorporated into clinical medicine.

What concerns us is that respected cancer journals are publishing articles that identify safer and more effective treatment regimens, yet few oncologists are incorporating these synergistic methods into their clinical practice. Cancer patients often suffer through chemotherapy sessions that do not integrate the latest scientific findings. Our objective is to provide the patient with more options to discuss with their oncologist and bring about multimodality approaches to improve the probability of a successful outcome.

It is impossible to design a single chemotherapy protocol that is effective against all types of cancer. The oncologist might need to administer several chemotherapy drugs at varying doses because tumor cells express survival factors with a wide degree of individual cell variability. This protocol conveys the findings from published scientific studies so that a cancer patient will have a logical basis to augment the effects of chemotherapy and also reduce the potential for side effects.

## HOW DOES CHEMOTHERAPY WORK?

According to the National Cancer Institute, almost all normal cells grow and die in a controlled way through a process called *apoptosis*. Cancer cells, on the other hand, keep dividing and forming more cells without a control mechanism to induce normal apoptosis.

Anticancer drugs destroy cancer cells by stopping them from growing or dividing at one or more points in their growth cycle. Chemotherapy may consist of one or several cytotoxic drugs that kill cells by one or more mechanisms. The chemotherapy regimen chosen by most conventional oncologists is based on the type of cancer being treated. As you will read later in this protocol, there are factors other than the type of cancer that can be used to determine the ideal chemotherapy drugs that should be used to treat an individual patient.

The goal of chemotherapy is to shrink primary tumors, slow tumor growth, and kill cancer cells that may have spread (metastasized) to other parts of the body from the original, primary tumor. However, chemotherapy kills both cancer cells and healthy normal cells. Oncologists try to minimize damage to normal cells and to enhance the cell killing (cytotoxic) effect on cancer cells. Too often, unfortunately, this delicate balance is not achieved.

Clinical studies show that certain types of cancer chemotherapy prolong survival and increase the percentage of patients achieving a remission. A partial remission is defined as 50% or greater reduction in the measurable parameters of tumor growth as may be found on physical examination, radiologic study, or by biomarker levels from a blood or urine test. A complete remission is defined as complete disappearance of all such manifestations of disease. The goal of all oncologists is to strive for a complete remission that lasts a long time—a durable complete remission, or CR. Unfortunately, the vast majority of remissions achieved are partial remissions. Too often, these are measured in weeks to months and not in years. Some types of cancer do not show any meaningful response to chemotherapy.

## CHOOSING THE BEST CHEMOTHERAPY DRUGS TO KILL YOUR TUMOR

It is highly desirable to know what drugs are effective against your particular cancer cells before these toxic agents are systemically administered to your body. A company called Rational Therapeutics, Inc., performs chemosensitivity tests on living specimens of your cancer cells to determine the optimal combination of chemotherapy drugs.

Robert Nagourney, a prominent hematologist/oncologist, founded Rational Therapeutics, Inc. in 1993. Rational Therapeutics pioneers cancer therapies that are specifically tailored for each individual patient. This company is a leader in individualized cancer strategies. With no economic ties to outside health care organizations, recommendations are made without financial or scientific prejudice.

Rational Therapeutics develops and provides cancer therapy recommendations that have been designed scientifically for each patient. Following the collection of living cancer cells obtained at the time of biopsy or surgery, Rational Therapeutics performs an ex-vivo apoptotic (EVA) assay on your tumor sample to measure drug activity (sensitivity and resistance). This will determine exactly which drug(s) will be most effective for you. They then make a treatment recommendation. The treatment program developed through this approach is known as assay-directed therapy.

At present, medical oncologists, according to fixed schedules, prescribe chemotherapy. These schedules are standardized drug regimens that correspond to specific cancers by type or diagnosis. These schedules, developed over many years of clinical trials, assign patients to the drugs for which they have the greatest statistical probability of response.

Patients with cancers that exhibit multidrug resistance will likely receive treatments that are wrong for them. A failed attempt at chemotherapy is detrimental to the physical and emotional well-being of patients, financially burdensome, and may preclude further effective therapies.

Rational Therapeutics' EVA assay uses living tumor cells to determine which drug or drug combination induces apoptosis in the laboratory. Each patient is highly individualized with regard to sensitivity to chemotherapy drugs. A patient's responsiveness to chemotherapy is as unique as their fingerprints.

Rational Therapeutics, leading the way in custom-tailored, assay-directed therapy, provides personal cancer strategies based on the tumor response in the laboratory. This eliminates much of the guesswork prior to the patient undergoing the potentially toxic side effects of chemotherapy regimens that could prove to be of little value against their cancer. Rational Therapeutics may be contacted at:

Rational Therapeutics, Inc.

750 East 29th Street

Long Beach, CA 90806

Telephone: (562) 989-6455; Fax: (562) 989-8160

Web site: www.rationaltherapeutics.com

In addition to the EVA chemosensitivity testing, we advocate immunohistochemistry testing of your tumor to provide additional data that will assist in making treatment decisions. The importance of the immunohistochemistry test is described in the Cancer Treatment: The Critical Factors protocol. The immunohistochemistry test can be done if your physician sends a specimen of your tumor to a specialty laboratory called GENZYME (www.genzymegenetics.com). GENZYME can be reached by calling (800) 447-5816. GENZYME also performs chemosensitivity testing of living tumors (fresh specimens). Because many chemotherapy patients' primary tumors were previously removed or irradiated, GENZYME can perform the immunohistochemistry test with a frozen or paraffin-preserved tissue sample that is accessible through the pathology laboratory that examined your previous tumor(s).

## Inhibiting the Cox-2 Enzyme

Some progressive oncologists are prescribing cyclooxygenase-2 (COX-2) inhibitor drugs along with chemotherapy to improve the odds of successful treatment. COX-2 is an enzyme that many types of cancers use in order to propagate. COX-2 and its byproducts such as prostaglandin E2 (PGE2) have been shown to help fuel the growth of cancers such as colon, pancreas, estrogen-negative breast, prostate, bladder, and lung cancer.

Since chemotherapy can cause gastrointestinal bleeding, careful physician monitoring is needed when using a COX-2 inhibiting drug such as Celebrex®. Caution is urged for those with known kidney disease, poor heart-lung function, liver disease, or susceptibility to stress-induced ulcers. The protocol titled Cancer Treatment: The Critical Factors contains a detailed description of the connection between COX-2 and cancer and why inhibiting the COX-2 enzyme is so important in treating many cancers.

In 1996, Life Extension recommended that most cancer patients take a COX-2 inhibiting drug because of solid evidence that cancer cells use the COX-2 enzyme to sustain their rapid division. In 1996, Americans had to import a COX-2 inhibitor named nimesulide from other countries because this class of drug was not widely available in the United States.

Experiments in laboratory animals suggest that drugs such as Celebrex® could help cure cancer, especially if combined with chemotherapy or radiation.[1-3] There are 100 separate cancer studies involving COX-2 inhibitors going on worldwide at this time.

Doctors are predicting that COX-2 inhibiting drugs may become standard therapy in 5–10 years. There was adequate evidence in 1996, however, to recommend COX-2 inhibiting drugs available to cancer patients. There are 2 potent COX-2 inhibiting drugs on the American marketplace. You may ask your physician to prescribe one of the following COX-2 inhibitors:

- Lodine XL, 1000 mg once a day or
- Celebrex®, 200–400 mg every 12 hours

## Controlling Cancer Cell Growth

A family of proteins known as ras oncogenes often governs the regulation of cancer cell growth. The Ras family is responsible for modulating the regulatory signals that direct the cancer cell cycle and rate of proliferation. Mutations in genes encoding Ras proteins have been intimately associated with unregulated cell proliferation, that is, cancer.

There is a class of cholesterol-lowering drugs known as statins that has been shown to inhibit the activity of Ras oncogenes. Some of these cholesterol-lowering drugs are lovastatin, simvastatin, and pravastatin.[4-9]

In advanced primary liver cancer (hepatoma or hepatocellular carcinoma), patients who received 40 mg of pravastatin survived twice as long compared to those who did not receive this statin drug.[10] Interestingly, statins are also associated with the preservation of bone structure and improvement in bone density.[11-13]

Some types of cancer (breast and prostate) have a proclivity to metastasize to the bone.[14,15] This results in bone pain that also may be associated with weakening of the bone and an increased risk of fractures.[16,17] Patients with prostate cancer, for example, are found to have a very high incidence of osteoporosis even before the use of therapies that lower the male hormone testosterone.[18,19]

In prostate cancer, when excessive bone loss is occurring, there is a release of bone-derived growth factors—for example, TGF-β1 (transforming growth factor-beta 1)—that stimulate the prostate cancer cells to grow further.[20,21] In turn, prostate cancer cells elaborate substances such as interleukin-6 (IL-6) that facilitate the further breakdown of bone.[22,23] Thus, a vicious cycle results: bone breakdown-stimulation of prostate cancer cell growth that results in production of IL-6 and other cell products, which leads to further bone breakdown. When there is a breakdown of bone, the growth factors released can fuel cancer cell growth. (All cancer patients should refer to the Osteoporosis protocol to read about how to optimally maintain bone integrity and prevent the release of these cancer cell growth factors. The Prostate Cancer protocol has an extensive discussion about the importance of maintaining bone integrity.)

As far as statin drug dosing, higher amounts than are required to lower cholesterol are suggested for a period of several months. Cancer patients, for instance, have used 80 mg per day of lovastatin (Mevacor®). This should be considered during chemotherapy in some cases. A monthly SMAC/CBC blood test is also recommended while taking a statin drug to monitor liver function. A rare potential side effect that can occur with the use of statin drugs is a condition known as rhabdomyolysis in which muscle cells are destroyed and released into the bloodstream. If muscle weakness should occur, alert your doctor so you can have a creatine kinase (CK) test to determine if muscle damage has occurred.

## Combining a COX-2 Inhibitor with a Statin Drug and Chemotherapy

Depending on the type of cancer, a logical approach would be to combine a statin (such as Mevacor®) with a COX-2 inhibitor and the appropriate dosing of chemotherapy.

Mevacor® augmented up to 5-fold the cancer-killing effect of the COX-2 inhibitor Sulindac.[24] In this study, 3 different colon cancer cell lines were induced to undergo apoptosis by depriving them of COX-2. When Mevacor® was added to the COX-2 inhibitor, the kill rate increased 5-fold.

Physician involvement is essential to mitigate potential side effects of these drugs. Those who are concerned about potential toxicity should take into account the fact that the types of cancers that these drugs might be effective against have extremely high mortality rates. Please note that the use of statin drugs and COX-2 inhibitors for cancer is considered an off-label use of these drugs. You may ask your doctor to prescribe one of the following statin drugs to inhibit the activity of Ras oncogenes:

- Mevacor® (lovastatin), 40 mg twice per day or
- Zocor® (simvastatin), 40 mg twice per day or
- Pravachol (pravastatin), 40 mg once per day

In addition to statin drug therapy, consider supplementing with the following nutrients to further suppress the expression of Ras oncogenes:

- Fish Oil Capsules: 2400 mg of EPA and 1800 mg of DHA daily
- Green Tea Extract: 1500 mg of tea polyphenols daily
- Aged Garlic Extract: 2000 mg daily

# SHOULD ANTIOXIDANTS BE TAKEN AT THE SAME TIME AS CHEMOTHERAPY?

There is a controversy as to whether cancer patients should take antioxidant supplements at the same time that cytotoxic chemotherapy drugs are being administered.

Proponents of antioxidants point to human studies showing that antioxidant supplements protect healthy cells from the damaging effects of chemotherapy drugs.

Chemotherapy drugs can cause lethal heart muscle damage in a small percentage of cancer patients. Antioxidants such as vitamin E, coenzyme Q10 (CoQ10), N-acetyl-cysteine (NAC), glutathione, retinoids, ginkgo biloba, and vitamin C have been shown to specifically protect against chemotherapy-induced heart muscle damage.[25-33] Other antioxidants have been shown to protect kidneys, bone marrow, and the immune system against chemotherapy toxicity.

Those who argue against antioxidant supplementation during chemotherapy are concerned that antioxidants will protect cancer cells against free-radical-induced destruction. Chemotherapy drugs work by varying mechanisms to induce cellular death. Some chemotherapy drugs kill cells by inflicting massive free-radical damage, while other chemotherapy drugs interfere with different cellular metabolic processes in order to eradicate cancer cells (and healthy cells as well). Depending on the type of cytotoxic drug used, however, antioxidants may confer protection to cancer cells during active chemotherapy.

The difficulty in reaching a consensus is that there are no controlled human or animal studies comparing the effects of various chemotherapy drugs, with and without antioxidants, against different cancers. The issue is complicated by studies showing that certain nutrients are associated with improved survival in cancer patients.

One problem is that there are little data to indicate whether supplements that have been shown to benefit the cancer patient should be taken during active chemotherapy. In other words, we know that antioxidants protect against chemotherapy side effects and may improve long-term survival in cancer patients, but not whether they lower the odds of achieving a long-term remission when administered during active chemotherapy.

Cancer patients contemplating cytotoxic chemotherapy are thus faced with a dilemma: they can take antioxidant nutrients to protect their healthy cells against the toxic effects of chemotherapy, or avoid all antioxidants during chemotherapy to possibly improve the chances that the chemotherapy drugs will kill enough cancer cells to induce a complete response or cure.

To further complicate matters, certain supplements have proven mechanisms that could augment the cytotoxic efficacy of chemotherapy. For instance, curcumin has been shown to suppress growth factors that cancer cells use to escape eradication by chemotherapy drugs. (A complete description of curcumin's potential synergistic benefits with chemotherapy drugs appears later in this protocol.) The problem is that curcumin is also a potent antioxidant, and one animal study shows that curcumin could interfere with the cancer cell-killing effect of certain chemotherapy drugs. The scientists who authored this study pointed out that while curcumin has demonstrated potent effects in preventing cancer, its use during active chemotherapy is questionable because of its ability to protect cells against the type of molecular damage inflicted by these chemotherapy drugs.[34]

Critics of this study point out that the low dose of curcumin used in this animal study was adequate to provide antioxidant protection to the cancer cells, but not high enough to suppress growth factors that enable cancer cells to escape regulatory control by the chemotherapy drugs. It was also pointed out that not all chemotherapy drugs kill cancer cells by generating free radicals. This means that curcumin may not hinder other chemotherapy drugs, as evidenced by remarkable tumor regressions found in other animal studies and human case histories.

Due to the multiple molecular complexities of this issue and the lack of specific in vivo studies, cancer chemotherapy patients are faced with choosing one of the 2 options discussed in following sections.

## Option One

Two weeks prior to the initiation of a chemotherapy regimen, discontinue all antioxidant supplements until 2–3 weeks after the last chemotherapy session. Most chemotherapy sessions are scheduled to last for 6–8 weeks.

The risk in depleting your body of antioxidants is that healthy cells will not be as well protected against the toxic effects of chemotherapy. This means that depending on the chemotherapy drug used, you could experience organ damage. You may also have increased immune impairment that could weaken your ability to fight the cancer. The toxic side effects of chemotherapy drugs can be the direct cause of death in some patients. Those who choose to deplete their bodies of certain antioxidants will also lose the potential benefit that these nutrients may have on cancer calls. These nutrients help prevent cancer cells from developing escape mechanisms that enable them to develop resistance to chemotherapy and other anticancer drug(s). The potential benefit is that the chemotherapy drug(s) might work better if these antioxidants are not present.

## Option Two

Continue taking antioxidant supplements recommended in this and the Cancer Adjuvant Therapy protocol before, during, and after the chemotherapy is administered.

The risk is that these antioxidants could interfere with the cell-killing effects of the chemotherapy drugs. This is no small risk because cancer patients who need chemotherapy usually have only one opportunity to eradicate enough cancer cells to experience a long-term remission or cure. Cancer cells not killed by the first round of chemotherapy may become highly resistant to future rounds.

As stated earlier, it is important to note that not all chemotherapy drugs function by inducing free-radical damage to the cancer cells. In fact, many cytotoxic chemotherapy drugs function by alternative toxic actions such as interfering with DNA/RNA synthesis (the antimetabolites), disrupting the microtubular network (microtubule inhibitors), and inhibiting chromatin function (topoisomerase inhibitors). To help a cancer patient understand the mechanism of action of common cytotoxic chemotherapy drugs, we have provided Table 1.

Based on the information provided in Table 1, it might appear that one could make a determination

### Table 1: How Different Chemotherapy Drugs Kill Cancer Cells

| Drug | Trade Name | Mechanism of Action |
|---|---|---|
| *Chemotherapy drugs that kill cancer cells by inflicting free-radical damage* | | |
| **Alkylating agents** | | Free-radical damage |
| Busulfan | Myleran | |
| Carboplatin | Paraplatin | |
| Carmustine | BiCNU | |
| Chlorambucil | Leukeran | |
| Cisplatin | Platinol | |
| Cyclophosphamide | Cytoxan | |
| Ifosfamide | Ifex | |
| Procarbazine | Matulane | |
| **Anthracyclines** | | Free-radical damage |
| Bleomycin | Blenoxane | |
| Doxorubicin | Adriamycin® | |
| Daunorubicin | Cerubidine | |
| Epirubicin | Ellence | |
| Mitomycin C | Mutamycin | |
| **Plant alkaloids** | | Free-radical damage |
| Teniposide | Vumon | |
| VP-16 | Etoposide | |
| *Chemotherapy drugs that kill cancer cells by other mechanisms* | | |
| **Antimetabolites** | | Inhibition of DNA/RNA synthesis |
| Asparaginase | Elspar | (Analog of the vitamin folic acid) |
| Azacitidine | Mylosar | |
| Cladribine | Leustatin | |
| Cytarabine | Cytosar | |
| Fludarabine | Fludara | |
| Fluorouracil | Adrucil | |
| Hydroxyurea | Hydrea | |
| Mercaptopurine | Purinethol | |
| Methotrexate | Abitrexate | |
| Pentostatin | Nipent | |
| Raltitrexed | Tomudex | |
| Thioguanine | Lanvis | |
| **Topoisomerase inhibitors** | | Inhibition of chromatin function |
| Bleomycin | Blenoxane | Inhibition of topoisomerase II |
| Dactinomycin | Cosmegen | Inhibition of topoisomerase II |
| Daunorubicin | Cerubidine | Inhibition of topoisomerase II |
| Doxorubicin | Adriamycin | Inhibition of topoisomerase II |

*(Continued)*

**Table 1: How Different Chemotherapy Drugs Kill Cancer Cells—cont'd**

| Drug | Trade Name | Mechanism of Action |
|---|---|---|
| Epirubicin | Ellence | Inhibition of topoisomerase II |
| Etoposide | Vepesid | Inhibition of topoisomerase II |
| Gemcitabine | Gemzar | Inhibition of topoisomerase I |
| Idarubicin | Idamycin | Inhibition of topoisomerase II |
| Irinotecan | Camptosar | Inhibition of topoisomerase I |
| Mitoxantrone | Novantrone | Inhibition of topoisomerase II |
| Plicamycin | Mithramycin | Inhibition of topoisomerase II |
| Teniposide | Vumon | Inhibition of topoisomerase II |
| Topotecan | Hycamtin | Inhibition of topoisomerase I |
| **Microtubule inhibitors** | | **Inhibition of chromatin function** |
| Docetaxel | Taxotere | |
| Paclitaxel | Taxol | |
| Teniposide | Vumon | |
| Vinblastine | Velban | Mitotic arrest through binding of |
| Vincristine | Oncovin | microtubules and spindle precursors |
| Vinorelbine | Navelbine | Mitotic arrest through binding of |
| VP-16 | Etoposide | microtubules and spindle precursors |

as to whether to take antioxidants based on the type of chemotherapy drug(s) used. Regrettably, there are other pathways (in addition to those listed) by which chemotherapy drugs induce cancer cell apoptosis that could be interfered with by taking the wrong dose of antioxidants. As already indicated, it is not possible to reach a scientific consensus as to which option to choose, that is, antioxidants or no antioxidants during active chemotherapy. There are too many variables such as the type of cancer, category of chemotherapy drug(s), molecular makeup of the cancer cells, individual variability, and so on, to provide a conclusive recommendation for or against antioxidant supplementation during chemotherapy.

Cancer patients often take antioxidant supplements based on published studies showing that antioxidants help prevent cancer. Although some nutrients have been shown to reverse precancerous lesions, antioxidants alone are not a cure once cancer develops. There is persuasive evidence, however, that certain antioxidant supplements are effective in the adjuvant treatment of cancer. In other words, these supplements may help conventional therapies work better. What is missing is evidence of the effects of antioxidants in cancer patients undergoing aggressive chemotherapy.

## MAKING CHEMOTHERAPY DRUGS WORK MORE EFFECTIVELY

The dose-delivery schedule of chemotherapy drugs can determinate their efficacy in killing cancer cells and the degree of toxicity to the patient. Conventional chemotherapy treatment often uses a maximum tolerated dose (MTD) of chemotherapeutic drugs, typically administered on a schedule that varies from once a week to every 21 days, allowing a period of rest so that healthy tissue has a chance to recover. Unfortunately, while the MTD schedule is convenient for oncologists, allowing them to squeeze more patients each month into their chemotherapy unit, the rest period enables cancer cells to recover and develop survival mechanisms such as new blood vessel growth into the tumor. This means that when the next high dose of chemotherapy is given 7–21 days later, the cancer cells have become more resistant. The administration of the MTD also exposes healthy tissues to more damage.

Some studies indicate that a better approach would be to lower the dose of conventional cytotoxic agents, reschedule their application, and combine chemotherapy drugs with antiangiogenesis agents to effectively interfere with cancer's various growth pathways and inhibit the production of blood vessels[35] (http://www.cancer.gov/clinicaltrials/developments/anti-angio-table).

This lower-dose approach, known as metronomic dosing, uses a dosing schedule as often as every day or alternates different chemotherapy drugs every other day instead of administering them all together the same day. An amount as low as 25% of the MTD, sometimes given on alternative days in combination with various signal transduction pathway inhibitors, targets the endothelial cells making up the vessels and microvessels feeding the tumor. Tumor endothelial cells then die with much less chemotherapy than cancer cells and the side effects to healthy tissue and the patient in general are dramatically reduced.[36]

During standard chemotherapy, the typical 21-day rest period is enough to allow the tumor endothelial cells a chance to recover. However, with tighter chemotherapy dose scheduling, the slowly proliferating endothelial cells are unable to recover. In one study, mice were given the chemotherapeutic drug vinblastine at doses far below the MTD. This dose had little effect on tumor growth in the mice. A second group of mice was given the drug DC101 that inhibits the formation of new blood vessels into tumors (by blocking the induction of vascular endothelial growth factor [VEGF]). In the DC101 group of mice, tumor growth was slowed, as it was with the vinblastine, but then tumor growth resumed. However, in a third group of mice, a combination of the 2 drugs, at the low dose, resulted in full regression of the tumors with no recurrence for 6 months.[37]

The administration of low doses of conventional chemotherapy drugs on a frequent basis with no breaks enables these drugs to invoke an antiangiogenesis effect, particularly when combined with a tumor endothelial cell-specific antiangiogenic drug.[38,39] There are clinical studies using antiangiogenic drugs (http://www.cancer.gov/clinicaltrials/developments/anti-angio-table). As will be described later in this protocol, certain dietary supplements have also been shown to interfere with angiogenesis.

At the time of this writing, a number of animal studies suggested that chemotherapy drugs could work better if the dosing schedule were changed. Human studies are ongoing, meaning it will be difficult to convince an oncologist to incorporate metronomic dosing instead of the standard MTD. While we cannot definitively recommend metronomic (lower dose/more frequent administration) chemotherapy at this time, the results of new human studies on this subject will be posted at www.lefcancer.org.

## GOING BEYOND CHEMOTHERAPY

Conventional chemotherapy drugs too often show limited efficacy. Yet there is evidence indicating that the cancer cell-killing effects of these drugs can be enhanced if additional compounds are administered to the patient.

One approach is to inhibit the overexpression of receptor sites on cancer cells, which enables these cells to bind to growth factors that allow them to become resistant to the cell-killing effects of the chemotherapy drugs. Cancer cells use these signal transduction pathways as growth vehicles to escape natural regulatory control and protect themselves against the cytotoxic effects of cancer drugs. The utilization of these signal transduction inhibitors enhances the potential effect of low(er) dosing of chemotherapeutic drugs.

Another therapeutic target is the endothelial cells that form new blood vessels. The process by which new blood vessels are formed is called angiogenesis, and cancer cells initiate blood vessel proliferation in order to fuel rapid growth.[36] Agents that interfere with the formation of new blood vessels are an important part of a comprehensive treatment strategy.

Because cancer cells are stimulated to produce new blood vessels in response to a low-oxygen environment (hypoxia), boosting the oxygen-carrying capacity of blood, as discussed earlier, is critically important.

### Inhibiting Signal Transduction Pathways

All cells, both normal and cancerous, have molecular receptor sites on their surface. These sites are much like locks that may be opened or activated only by the correct molecular key. Once opened or activated, a chain of biochemical events occurs specific to that receptor. Cytokine growth factors are a class of substances that stimulate cell growth by a variety of mechanisms.

An example of such a pathway is the binding of transforming growth factor-alpha (TGF-α) to the epidermal growth factor receptor (EGFR) site. Such a binding is a growth pathway for many cancers, causing rapid cell proliferation. The overexpression of this pathway is also implicated in tumor cells that are resistant to cytotoxic drugs (including the interferons).

Interference with this pathway at the EGFR site can effectively shut down overexpression and the subsequent cell proliferation, making the cancer much more vulnerable to therapy. Blocking the EGFR has been shown to inhibit tumor growth by interfering with cancer cell repair, tumor invasion, metastasis, and angiogenesis.[40,41]

Drugs that inhibit the EGFR showed promise in early studies but failed in recent clinical trials when combined with cytotoxic chemotherapy drugs. One of these EGFR inhibiting drugs is Iressa®. One reason that Iressa® and a similar-acting drug named Erbitux® failed in human clinical studies is that an inadequate combination and dosing schedule of chemotherapy drugs may have been used to kill the cancer cells. Drugs such as Iressa® will not cure cancer by themselves, but they could be of benefit if metronomic-dosing chemotherapy were used and/or during immune-augmentation therapy if they were used with drugs such as alpha interferon.

The objective of blocking the signal transduction pathway is to prevent cancer cells from mutating in a way that enables them to avoid destruction.

**Natural signal transduction inhibitors.** As noted, molecular evidence and animal studies suggest that agents that inhibit certain growth signals used by cancer cells might work synergistically with metronomic cycled chemotherapy or be useful as postchemotherapy agents along with immune-augmentation therapy.

There are natural signal transduction inhibitors available, but because most of them are potent antioxidants, some cancer patients may choose to wait 2–3 weeks after chemotherapy ends to start using them.

*Soy (genistein) extract* is known to inhibit the EGFR via an interference with the TGF-α pathway.[42]

Genistein is also known to block the induction of the basic fibroblast growth factor (bFGF), a potent growth and angiogenic factor in cancers such as renal cell carcinoma and malignant melanoma.[43] Additionally, genistein is known to block induction of the VEGF considered essential for angiogenesis and tumor endothelial cell survival.[44]

The blockade of the overexpression of the EGFR and inhibition of the signaling pathways, bFGF and VEGF, is dose-dependent response. Soy genistein may be an effective adjuvant to conventional or metronomic chemotherapy, but human clinical studies are lacking, which is unfortunately the case with most nonpatented natural therapies. There is a controversy about the use of soy as a cancer treatment. A complete description of the pros and cons of high-dose genistein therapy can be found in the Cancer Adjuvant Therapy protocol.

*Curcumin*, an extract of the spice turmeric, is synergistic with genistein and inhibits angiogenic growth signals emitted by tumor cells. Curcumin acts via a different mechanism than genistein to inhibit the EGFR but is up to 90% effective in a dose-dependent manner. It is important to note that while curcumin has been shown to be up to 90% effective in inhibiting the expression of the EGFR on cancer cell membranes, this does not mean that it will be effective in 90% of cancer patients or reduce tumor volume by 90%. Because two-thirds of all cancers, however, overexpress the EGFR and such overexpression frequently fuels the metastatic

spread of cancer throughout the body, the suppression of this receptor is desirable.

Curcumin has a number of other antiangiogenic properties that appear to be synergistic with metronomic dosing chemotherapy. These potential synergistic and/or additive mechanisms include:

- Inhibition of the induction of bFGF. bFGF is both a potent mitogen (growth signal) for many cancers and an important signaling factor in angiogenesis.[45]
- Inhibition of the induction of hepatocyte growth factor (HGF), overexpression is involved in hepatocellular (liver cell-related) carcinoma.[46]
- Inhibition of the expression of COX-2, the enzyme involved in the production of PGE-2, a tumor-promoting prostaglandin.[47]
- Inhibition of a transcription factor in cancer cells known as nuclear factor-kappa B (NF-κB). Many cancers overexpress NF-κB and use this as a growth vehicle to escape regulatory control.[48]
- Increased expression of nuclear p53 protein in human basal cell carcinomas, hepatomas, and leukemia cell lines, which increases apoptosis.[49]

## Inhibiting Angiogenesis

Angiogenesis provides nourishment for the tumor's rapid propagation. Antiangiogenesis agents inhibit this new tumor blood vessel growth and are being studied as potential cancer therapies. As noted, genistein and curcumin have demonstrated molecular effects involved in the inhibition of new blood vessel growth into tumors. An extract from green tea may also be an effective antiangiogenesis agent.

The primary action of *green tea* is through its catechin, epigallocatechin gallate (EGCG), which blocks the induction of VEGF, considered essential in angiogenesis and tumor endothelial cell survival. In vivo studies have shown green tea extracts to have the following actions on human colon cancer cells:

- Inhibited tumor growth by 58%
- Inhibited microvessel density by 30%
- Inhibited tumor cell proliferation by 27%
- Increased tumor cell apoptosis 1.9-fold
- Increased tumor endothelial cell apoptosis 3-fold[50]

The optimal dose of green tea, soy, and curcumin as well as when they should be taken will be discussed later in this protocol. Please note that EGCG is a powerful antioxidant, as are other polyphenols found in green tea. Some chemotherapy patients may choose to wait 3 weeks after chemotherapy has ended to initiate green tea (EGCG) supplementation.

## Why Agents That Inhibit Angiogenesis and Block Signal Transduction Are Failing

Based on the multiple favorable mechanisms listed, higher-dose curcumin would appear to be useful for cancer patients. There are contradictions in scientific literature concerning curcumin intake at the same time as chemotherapy drugs. Some studies indicate enhanced benefit, whereas other studies hint at reduced benefit and even potential toxicity. The anticancer drug cisplatin is strongly enhanced with curcumin,[51] yet cisplatin kills cancer cells by generating free radicals, and curcumin is an antioxidant. Another study showed that low-dose curcumin inhibited camptothecin-, mechlorethamine-, and doxorubicin-induced apoptosis of several different human breast cancer cells. This same study showed that curcumin inhibited cyclophosphamide-induced breast tumor regression in an in vivo animal model.[34] Another in vitro study involving curcumin's concomitant use with the chemotherapy drug Irinotecan indicated potential toxicity,[52] yet chemotherapy drugs are inherently toxic.

Whether high-dose curcumin is beneficial or detrimental depends on the type and dose of the chemotherapeutic drug used, kind of cancer cell, and dose of curcumin. Until more definitive information is published, we prefer to err on the side of caution and recommend that chemotherapy patients wait 3 weeks after their last dose of chemotherapy before taking high doses of curcumin.

Pharmaceutical companies are investing billions of dollars to develop drugs proven to interfere with cancer cell growth. Unfortunately, these drugs have failed to extend survival in late-stage cancer patients. In some of these clinical studies, tumor shrinkage is observed, but the patients still die. Experts remain convinced, however, that these drugs will eventually play a significant role in the treatment of cancer.

One reason these drugs are not working is they usually suppress only one of the growth factors that cancer cells use to escape regulatory control. Scientists know of more than 20 growth factors used by tumors. Late-stage breast cancer cells, for example, may express as many as 6 different growth factors that induce angiogenesis. Cancer cells emit these growth factors to draw new blood vessels into tumors and/or overexpress the EGFR.

Human studies have tested angiogenesis inhibitors or EGFR blockers on late-stage patients whose cancer cells have mutated to become highly resistant. If these drugs were tested earlier in the disease process, some physicians believe they would work better. One problem is that the Food and Drug Administration (FDA) restricts the testing of new cancer drugs to only patients who have failed all other proven therapies. Regrettably, we know that cancer cells mutate each time they are exposed to a new therapy. By testing new cancer drugs only on patients who have failed previous therapy, a tremendous burden of efficacy is being placed on these new compounds, that is, these drugs are expected to kill cancer cells in their most aggressive stages.

Some experts note that ultimately successful treatment using antiangiogenesis and signal transduction blockers may depend on the use of a multidrug cocktail, one that would block all known growth factors used by cancer cells. That would parallel the success in treating AIDS (acquired immune deficiency syndrome), in which several antiviral drugs that work by different mechanisms are combined into cocktails that have turned the condition into a manageable disease for some people.

Based on current knowledge, it would appear logical to simultaneously test a wide range of angiogenesis inhibitors and signal transduction pathway blockers on early-stage cancer patients. Such testing might be considered at the time that other cytotoxic therapies are administered or shortly thereafter.

The potential advantage of combining high potency genistein, curcumin, and green tea extracts is that they have been shown to suppress a wide variety of growth factors used by cancer cells. Considering the enormous cost of testing drugs that work in similar ways to genistein, curcumin, and green tea, it is doubtful that these nonpatented natural agents will be tested on cancer patients in the near future. The cancer patient is thus faced with deciding whether or not to incorporate these natural agents into their overall treatment program based on the data currently available.

## MITIGATION OF CHEMOTHERAPY SIDE EFFECTS

Cancer chemotherapy is known to produce severe side effects such as heart muscle damage, gastrointestinal damage, anemia, nausea, and lethal suppression of immune function.

Nutrients and hormone therapies can be used to mitigate the toxicity of chemotherapy. Bolstering the immune system may help alleviate or reduce the severity of the complications associated with chemotherapy. As discussed earlier in this protocol, however, using natural antioxidants to protect against chemotherapy side effects could possibly reduce the cancer cell-killing efficacy of the cytotoxic drug(s). Regrettably, there are no survival studies to verify the long-term effects of using natural therapies to mitigate the toxic effects that chemotherapy inflicts on healthy normal cells. In other words, we know that certain nutrients can protect normal cells against the immediate toxic effects of chemotherapy, but we do not know if this protection extends to cancer cells in such a way as to diminish cancer cell death.

For those who choose to use antioxidants to protect against chemotherapy side effects, supplementation with these nutrients should be initiated several days or even weeks before any planned chemotherapy is begun and should continue well after chemotherapy has been completed.

## Vitamins E, C, and N-Acetyl-Cysteine

Vitamins E, C, and N-Acetyl-Cysteine (NAC) can protect against heart muscle toxicity for cancer patients undergoing high doses of chemotherapy. A controlled study examined the effects of these nutrients on cardiac function in a group of chemotherapy and radiation patients. One group was given supplements of vitamins C, E, and NAC, while the other group was not supplemented. In the unsupplemented group, left ventricle function was reduced in 46% of the chemotherapy patients compared to those who took the supplements. Furthermore, none of the patients from the supplement group showed a significant fall in overall ejection fraction, but 29% of the nonsupplement group showed reduced ejection fraction.[53]

Vitamin C improved the antineoplastic activity of the chemotherapeutic drugs doxorubicin, cisplatin, and paclitaxel in human breast carcinoma cells. Patients reported improved appetite while taking vitamin C, as well as a reduced need for painkillers.

Vitamin E has been shown to protect against cardiomyopathies induced by chemotherapy. Vitamin E has also been used in combination with vitamin A and CoQ10 to reduce the side effects of the chemotherapy drug Adriamycin® (doxorubicin). Vitamin E is complementary to chemotherapy in that it boosts the effectiveness of these drugs. One study showed enhanced efficacy of both 5-FU and doxorubicin against human colon cancer cells with vitamin E supplementation.[54]

**Note:** *Fluorouracil, or 5-FU, is an antineoplastic agent used in the palliative management of certain cancers.*

The mechanism of action of vitamin E appears to be the induction of the tumor suppressor protein p21. The dry powder succinate form of vitamin E appears to be most beneficial to cancer patients. The more common acetate form has proven ineffective in slowing cancer cell growth in some test tube studies, whereas natural dry powder vitamin E succinate has shown efficacy.[55]

Still another study specifically suggested that cancer patients treated with Adriamycin® should supplement with vitamins A, E, and selenium to reduce its toxic side effects.[56]

## Astragalus

Astragalus is a medicinal herb that has been used for centuries in Asia. Astragalus administered by injection has shown to significantly improve quality of life in individuals with advanced lung cancer receiving chemotherapy.[57] In tumor-bearing mice, astragalus reduced kidney damage caused by the chemotherapy drug cisplatin.[58] A study was conducted to observe the effects of astragalus injection on the efficacy and toxicity of chemotherapy in 120 individuals with unspecified cancer. Compared to the control group, the astragalus group showed a reduced likelihood of disease progression as well as a lower incidence of reductions in white blood cell and platelet counts. The authors of the study concluded that "astragalus injection supplemented with chemotherapy could inhibit the development of tumor, decrease the toxic-adverse effect of chemotherapy, elevate the immune function of organism, and improve the quality of life in patients."[59]

## Blueberry

Blueberries are rich in anthocyanins (ie, dark pigments in fruits) and pterostilbenes (ie, antioxidant closely related to resveratrol). In a 2007 study, mice were given the chemotherapeutic drug 5-FU, which resulted in significant reductions in red blood cell, white blood cell, and platelet counts. The mice fed a blueberry extract experienced a 1.2-fold increase in red blood cells and a 9-fold increase in white blood cells compared to mice treated with 5-FU alone.[60] Additionally, 2 studies investigated the ability of blueberry to protect against the toxicity of the chemotherapeutic drug doxorubicin. This drug is frequently prescribed to women with breast cancer. Doxorubicin toxicity can lead to heart damage. In comparison to the control groups, both studies found that rats fed blueberry experienced significantly less heart damage with doxorubicin administration. Blueberry also mitigated hematologic toxicity by restoring depressed levels of red blood cell, hemoglobin, and bone marrow cell counts.[61,62]

## Coenzyme Q10 (CoQ10)

CoQ10 is used with vitamin E to protect patients from chemotherapy-induced cardiomyopathies. CoQ10 is nontoxic even at high dosages and has been shown to prevent liver damage from the drugs mitomycin C and 5-FU. Adriamycin-induced cardiomyopathies have been prevented by concomitant supplementation with CoQ10.

*Caution:* Some studies indicate that CoQ10 should not be taken at the same time as chemotherapy. If this were true, it would be disappointing because CoQ10 is so effective in protecting against Adriamycin-induced cardiomyopathy. Adriamycin® is sometimes used as part of a chemotherapy cocktail. Until more research is known, it is not possible to make a definitive recommendation of whether to take CoQ10 during chemotherapy.

## Selenium

Selenium has been used in combination with vitamins A and E to reduce the toxicity of chemotherapy drugs, particularly Adriamycin®.[56,63] The synergistic effect of vitamin E and selenium together to enhance the immune system is greater than either alone. A new form of selenium, Se-methylselenocysteine (SeMSC) (ie, a naturally occurring selenium compound found to be an effective chemopreventive agent), is a selenoamino acid synthesized by plants such as garlic and broccoli. SeMSC has been shown to induce apoptosis in certain ovarian cancer cells[64] and to be effective against breast cancer cell growth both in vivo and in vitro.[65] SeMSC has also demonstrated significant anticarcinogenic activity against mammary tumorigenesis.[66]

Moreover, SeMSC is one of the most effective chemopreventive compounds, inducing apoptosis in leukemia HL-60 cell lines.[67] Some of the most impressive data suggest that exposure to SeMSC blocks clonal expansion of premalignant lesions at an early stage. This is achieved by simultaneously modulating certain molecular pathways responsible for inhibiting cell proliferation and enhancing apoptosis.[68]

Unlike selenomethionine, which is incorporated into protein in place of methionine, SeMSC is not incorporated into any protein, thereby offering a completely bioavailable compound for preventing cancer. Therefore, 200–400 mcg of SeMSC a day is suggested for cancer patients. Note that selenium also possesses antioxidant properties, so its use

before, during, or immediately after chemotherapy could theoretically inhibit the actions of certain chemotherapy drugs.

## Whey Protein

Glutathione balance is very important for the cancer patient. Glutathione is an antioxidant that protects normal cells from toxic chemotherapy drugs. Glutathione levels in cancer cells are very high and act to protect against the destructive actions of chemotherapy and radiation. Whey lowers cancer cell glutathione levels, allowing the chemotherapy and radiation to be more effective at destroying cancer cells but not normal cells.

Tumor cell glutathione concentration may be among the determinants of the cytotoxicity of many chemotherapeutic agents and radiation. An increase in glutathione concentration in cancer cells appear to be at least one of the mechanisms of acquired drug resistance to chemotherapy. Whey proteins used in combination with glutathione appear to reduce concentrations of glutathione in cancer cells, thereby making them more vulnerable to chemotherapy while maintaining or even increasing glutathione levels in normal healthy cells.

Cancer cells had reduced glutathione levels in the presence of whey protein while at the same time normal cells had increased glutathione levels with increased cellular growth of healthy cells. Selective depletion of tumor glutathione may render malignant cells more vulnerable to the action of chemotherapeutic agents.[69]

Glutathione production in cancer and healthy cells is negatively inhibited by its own synthesis. Because glutathione levels are higher in cancer cells, it is believed that cancer cells would reach a level of negative-feedback inhibition for glutathione production more easily than normal cells.

Chemotherapy patients should consider taking 30–60 g per day of whey protein concentrate (in divided doses) 10 days before initiation of chemotherapy, during chemotherapy, and at least 10 days after the chemotherapy session is completed.

**Note:** *If blood testing shows that chemotherapy has suppressed the immune system, patients should insist that their oncologists use the appropriate immune restoration drug(s) as outlined later in this protocol.*

Whey protein concentrate selectively depletes cancer cells of glutathione, making them more susceptible to cancer treatments such as radiation and chemotherapy.[70,71]

## Shark Liver Oil (Not Shark Cartilage)

Chemotherapy causes a reduction in blood cell production. A natural therapy to restore healthy platelet production is 5 capsules a day of standardized shark liver oil, containing 200 mg of alkylglycerols per capsule. Shark liver oil can boost the production of blood platelets. Studies have shown the immune-enhancing capabilities of shark liver oil.[72]

*Caution:* Shark liver oil capsules should be taken at a dose of 5 capsules containing 200 mg of active alkylglycerols for a maximum duration of 30 days. A complete blood count (CBC) and platelet count should be obtained weekly to monitor the effectiveness of shark liver oil and prevent against excessive platelet production, that is, values greater than 400000. Platelet counts exceeding 400000 have been associated with increased risk of thrombosis and hemorrhage.

## Melatonin

Melatonin has been shown to protect against chemotherapy-induced immunosuppression. Melatonin mediates the toxicity of chemotherapy and inhibits free radical production.[73] In a randomized study to evaluate the effect of melatonin on the toxicity of chemotherapy drugs, patients receiving melatonin with chemotherapy had lower incidences of neuropathies, thrombocytopenia, stomatitis, alopecia, malaise, and vomiting. The appropriate dose of melatonin was between 30–50 mg at bedtime.[74,75] Adding melatonin to a chemotherapy regimen may prevent some toxic effects of the chemotherapy drugs, especially myelosuppression (suppression of blood cells production in bone marrow) and neuropathies (abnormality of nerve functioning both within and outside the central nervous system).

It is important to understand that melatonin protects against thrombocytopenia. If melatonin is considered, it should be started before chemotherapy is initiated. Melatonin may also be an especially effective and safe therapy to correct thrombocytopenia, a condition characterized by a decrease in the number of blood platelets. In patients who randomly received chemotherapy alone or chemotherapy plus melatonin (20 mg each evening), thrombocytopenia was significantly less frequent in those treated with melatonin.[76]

Malaise and lack of strength were also significantly less frequent in patients receiving melatonin. Finally, stomatitis (inflammation of the mouth area) and neuropathy were less frequent in the melatonin group. Alopecia and vomiting were not influenced.[75]

Administration of melatonin during chemotherapy may prevent some chemotherapy-induced side effects, particularly myelosuppression and neuropathy.

Oncologists often prescribe drugs that work in a similar way as melatonin to protect the immune system. Leukine®, for instance, is a granulocyte/macrophage colony-stimulating factor drug that can restore immune function debilitated by toxic cancer chemotherapy drugs. If you are on chemotherapy and your blood tests show white blood cell immune suppression, you should request the appropriate immune restoration drug (such as Leukine® or Neupogen®) from your medical oncologist.

Studies have shown that melatonin specifically exerts colony-stimulating activity and rescues bone marrow cells from apoptosis induced by cancer chemotherapy compounds. The number of granulocyte/macrophage colony-forming units has been shown to be higher in the presence of melatonin; the dose used was between 30–50 mg nightly.[77–79]

Melatonin enhances the anticancer action of interleukin-2 (IL-2) and reduces IL-2 toxicity when used in combination. Melatonin used in association with IL-2 cancer immunotherapy has been shown to have the following actions:

1. Amplification of IL-2 biological activity by enhancing lymphocyte response and antagonizing macrophage-mediated suppressive events

2. Inhibition of production of tumor growth factors that stimulate cancer cell proliferation by counteracting lymphocyte-mediated tumor cell destruction

3. Maintenance of a circadian rhythm of melatonin, which is often altered in human neoplasms and influenced by cytokine injection

The subcutaneous administration of 3 million IU a day of IL-2 and high doses of melatonin (40 mg each evening orally) has appeared to be effective in tumors resistant either to IL-2 alone or to chemotherapy. The dose of 3 million IU a day of IL-2 is a low dose, while serious toxicity normally begins at 15 million IU a day.

European oncologists have treated numerous end-stage solid tumor patients with the melatonin/IL-2 combination. The conclusion drawn from clinical studies is that melatonin protects against IL-2 toxicity and synergizes with the anticancer action of IL-2.[80] The combination strategy was shown to be a well-tolerated therapy to control tumor growth.

In the largest clinical study to date, the effects of melatonin were evaluated in 1440 patients with untreatable advanced solid tumors. One group received supportive care alone, while the other group received supportive care plus melatonin. In a second study, the influence of melatonin on the efficacy and toxicity of chemotherapy was evaluated in 200 metastatic patients with chemotherapy-resistant tumors. These patients were randomized to receive chemotherapy alone or chemotherapy plus melatonin. In both studies, 20 mg of melatonin were given orally at night. The frequency of cachexia, asthenia, thrombocytopenia, and lymphocytopenia was significantly lower in patients treated with melatonin compared to those who received supportive care alone.

Moreover, the percentage of patients with disease stabilization and the percentage 1-year survival rate were both significantly higher in patients concomitantly treated with melatonin than those treated with supportive care alone. The objective tumor response rate was significantly higher in patients treated with chemotherapy plus melatonin than those treated with chemotherapy alone. In addition, melatonin induced a significant decline in the frequency of chemotherapy-induced asthenia, thrombocytopenia, stomatitis, cardiotoxicity, and neurotoxicity. These clinical results demonstrate that melatonin may be successfully administered in the supportive care of untreatable advanced cancer patients and for the prevention of chemotherapy-induced toxicity.[76]

**Melatonin precautions.** Life Extension introduced the world to melatonin in 1992, and it was Life Extension that issued the original warnings about who should not take melatonin. These warnings were based on preliminary findings, and in 2 instances, Life Extension was overly cautious.

First, we suggested that prostate cancer patients might want to avoid high doses of melatonin. However, subsequent studies indicated that prostate cancer

patients could benefit from moderate doses of melatonin, although Life Extension still advises prostate cancer patients to have their blood tested for prolactin. Prolactin is a hormone secreted by the pituitary gland. Its role in men has not been demonstrated, yet in women, prolactin promotes lactation after childbirth.

Melatonin could possibly elevate prolactin secretion, and if this were to happen in a prostate cancer patient, the drug Dostinex (0.5 mg twice weekly) could be used to suppress prolactin so that melatonin could continue to be taken (in moderate doses of 1–6 mg each night). Note that the starting dose of Dostinex is 0.125 mg twice per week. If well tolerated, increase to 0.25 mg twice per week. If again well tolerated after 2 weeks, then increase to 0.5 mg twice per week while checking morning fasting prolactin levels.

Some physicians initially thought that ovarian cancer patients should not take melatonin, but a study in *Oncology Reports* indicated that high doses of melatonin may be beneficial in treating ovarian cancer. In this study, 40 mg of melatonin along with low doses of IL-2 were given nightly to 12 advanced ovarian cancer patients who had failed chemotherapy. While no complete response was seen, a partial response was achieved in 16% of patients and a stable disease was obtained in 41% of the cases.[81] This preliminary study suggested that melatonin is not contraindicated in advanced ovarian cancer patients. It is still not known what the effects of melatonin are in leukemia; therefore, leukemia patients should use melatonin with caution.

## Polysaccharide-K (PSK)

PSK, which is a specially prepared polysaccharide extract from the mushroom *Coriolus versicolor*, has been

## Table 2: Summary of Studies Using Melatonin

**Lissoni's Phase 2 Randomized Clinical Trial Results**

| Tumor Type | Patient Number | Basic Therapy | Melatonin Dose | 1-Year Survival Melatonin | 1-Year Survival Placebo |
|---|---|---|---|---|---|
| Metastatic Non–small cell lung | 63 | Supportive Care Only | 10 mg | 26% | Under 1% |
| Glioblastoma | 30 | Conventional Radiotherapy | 10 mg | 43% | Under 1% |
| Metastatic breast | 40 | Tamoxifen | 20 mg | 63% | 24% |
| Brain metastases | 50 | Conventional Radiotherapy | 20 mg | 38% | 12% |
| Metastatic colorectal | 50 | IL-2 | 40 mg | 36% | 12% |
| Metastatic non–small cell lung | 60 | IL-2 | 40 mg | 45% | 19% |

*Compiled by Cancer Treatment Centers of America and published in the March 2002 issue of Life Extension Magazine.*

studied extensively in Japan where it is used as a non-specific biological response modifier to enhance the immune system in cancer patients.[82–84]

PSK has been shown to provide protection against chemotherapy toxicity. Peripheral neuropathy (ie, nerve damage often occurring in the hands and feet) is a common side effect experienced by colon cancer patients receiving the chemotherapy drugs oxaliplatin, leucovorin, and 5-FU. Researchers observed grade-2 or -3 peripheral neuropathies in only 4% of colon cancer patients receiving these chemotherapy drug with PSK,[85] which is in stark contrast to a 38.4% incidence in those receiving the chemotherapy drugs without PSK.[86]

## Protecting Immune Function

Cancer patients using cytotoxic chemotherapy drugs should ask their oncologist to place them on FDA-approved immune-protective medications concurrently with chemotherapy. Leukine®, in particular, partially restores immune cell production lost due to the toxic effects of chemotherapy. The primary benefit of Leukine® is to stimulate macrophage production to prevent bacterial infection in the chemotherapy patient. Macrophages also engulf cancer cells and assist in their destruction by the immune system.[87] In one study, patients with refractory (resistant to treatment) solid tumors treated with standard chemotherapy and Leukine® had a 33.3% objective response rate versus 15% with chemotherapy alone.[88]

The timing of administration of colony-stimulating drugs such as Leukine® is crucial. The oncologist should not wait until there are toxic bone marrow effects to prescribe Leukine®. The administration of Leukine® should be timed to be initiated 24–48 hours after the last round of chemotherapy in order to prevent a dangerous nadir (precipitous decline) in immune cells (granulocytes). Proper administration of Leukine® can dramatically reduce immune damage that chemotherapy inflicts on the body and increase the cancer cell-killing efficacy of conventional chemotherapy drugs.

## Enhancing Immune Function

Alpha-interferon and/or IL-2 are immune cytokines (regulators) that should be considered by some cancer patients. Interferon directly inhibits cancer cell proliferation and has been used in the therapy of hairy cell leukemia, Kaposi's sarcoma, malignant melanoma, and squamous cell carcinoma. IL-2 allows for an increase in the cytotoxic activity of natural killer (NK) cells. An oncologist must carefully administer these drugs because they can produce temporary side effects. A significant side effect of interferon is that it can leave some patients temporarily debilitated, which is one reason why interferon has not become popular.

A cancer patient has to weigh the benefit of achieving complete tumor eradication in relation to the debilitation occurring during the time of active therapy. A typical dose of alpha-interferon is 3 million IU administered by self-injection daily for 2 weeks. To mitigate the debilitating effects, most patients take interferon for 2 weeks and then skip 2 weeks. IL-2 has been self-administered by subcutaneous injection in the dose of 3–6 million IU per day for 5–6 days each week.

**Note:** *Interferon has been shown to work on squamous cell carcinomas but not on common adenocarcinomas.*

Retinoic acid (vitamin A) analog drugs enhance the efficacy of some chemotherapy regimens and reduce the risk of secondary cancers. These vitamin A analog drugs have been shown to work well when taken in conjunction with alpha-interferon. Ask your oncologist to consider prescribing vitamin A analog drugs such as Accutane (13-cis-retinoic acid) or Vesanoid (all-trans retinoic acid). The use of a retinoid drug therapy depends on your type of cancer. Some cancers have historically responded well to retinoid drug therapy while others have not. See the tumor cell testing recommendations in the protocol Cancer Treatment: The Critical Factors to help determine whether retinoid drug therapy is appropriate. Your oncologist must carefully prescribe the use and dosage of potentially toxic retinoid drugs such as Accutane.

Some cancer patients produce too many T-suppressor cells that shut down optimal immune function. The administration of drugs such as cimetidine helps prevent cancer cells from prematurely shutting down the immune system. Cimetidine, also known as Tagamet®, is an over-the-counter medication that blocks the action of histamine on stomach cells and reduces stomach acid production. An immune cell blood test will reveal the status of your T-helper cells, T-suppressor cells, and natural killer (NK) cell count and activity. A suggested cimetidine-dosing regimen is 800 mg each night. Cimetidine also interferes with metastasis by blocking the expression of an adhesion molecule known as E-selectin that enables cancer cells to bind to blood vessel walls and start metastatic colonies.

*Caution:* Cimetidine may increase the toxicity of certain chemotherapy drugs. Cimetidine increased blood concentrations of the drug epirubicin used to treat breast cancer,[89] while cimetidine combined with 5-FU dramatically improved survival in certain types of colon cancer.[90] If you are taking cimetidine, tell your oncologist so that the dose of your chemotherapy drug can be adjusted if necessary.

## Anti-Nausea Drugs for Chemotherapy Patients

Nausea is one of the most common and difficult aspects of chemotherapy for cancer patients. Nausea can have secondary effects on cancer patients by interfering with their eating habits during and immediately after chemotherapy.

Drugs to mitigate chemotherapy-induced nausea include Kytril®, Megace®, and Zofran®. The high cost of some of these drugs has kept many cancer patients not covered by insurance from obtaining one of these potentially beneficial drugs. If you are receiving chemotherapy and experiencing nausea, you should be able to demand that any HMO, PPO, or insurance carrier pay for this class of drug. These drugs may enable a cancer patient to tolerate chemotherapy long enough for it to be effective.

An interesting study evaluated glutathione and vitamins C and E for their antinausea properties. Glutathione and vitamins C and E significantly reduced cisplatin-induced vomiting in dogs. The antinausea activity of antioxidants was attributed to their ability to react with free radicals generated by cisplatin. Ginger extract has also been shown effective in reducing nausea symptoms.[91]

**Aprepitant (Emend®).** Chemotherapy-induced acute and delayed nausea and vomiting (CINV) can occur with either an initial chemotherapy cycle or repeated chemotherapy cycles. Cisplatin is a commonly used chemotherapy drug known to cause CINV in most patients who receive it. Cisplatin is used to slow or stop cancer cell growth in patients with metastasized testicular and ovarian tumors who have already had surgical and/or radiotherapy procedures. It is used in patients with metastasized ovarian tumors who are unresponsive to standard chemotherapy, but have not yet received cisplatin.

Patients with advanced transitional-cell bladder cancer that is no longer controlled by surgery and/or radiotherapy also receive cisplatin. The drug is given intravenously in cycles, often in combination with other chemotherapy drugs. Severe CINV usually occurs within 1–4 hours after administration and symptoms can continue for 24 hours or persist for up to a week. A delayed form can occur in patients who had no nausea when cisplatin was initially administered. This form begins 24 hours or more following cisplatin chemotherapy. The symptoms of cisplatin CINV are so debilitating that some patients refuse further chemotherapy treatment.

On March 26, 2003, aprepitant (Emend®) received FDA approval. Aprepitant is a drug to be used in combination with other antinausea/antivomiting drugs to prevent CINV. Standard antinausea therapy for CINV is dexamethasone (Decadron®, a corticosteroid) and ondansetron (Zofran®, a 5-HT3 or serotonin receptor antagonist). However, aprepitant works in combination with these antinausea drugs by targeting a different family of receptors in the brain associated with nausea called the NK1 receptors (neurokinin 1). A typical combination treatment regimen directed by a treating physician follows:

- Day 1: 125 mg of aprepitant orally 1 hour before chemotherapy, 32 mg of ondansetron intravenously before chemotherapy, and 12 mg of dexamethasone orally.
- Days 2–4: 80 mg of aprepitant orally on days 2 and 3 only, and 8 mg of dexamethasone orally in the morning on days 2–4.

Aprepitant (Emend®) is the first NK1 blocking drug to be approved by the FDA. FDA approval was based on the results of studies including over 1000 cancer patients who received chemotherapy that caused CINV.[92–94] In these studies, when compared to symptoms in patients who received standard CINV medicines, the symptoms of CINV were reduced significantly when aprepitant was included with the standard medicines.

In a phase 3 study (520 patients; multicenter, randomized, double-blind, placebo-controlled; endpoint of complete response) that evaluated patients for 5 days after chemotherapy, 72.7% of the patients using aprepitant had complete response on days 1–5 (no nausea and vomiting; no rescue therapy). This response was significantly higher than the 52.3% response in the standard therapy group.[93] A similar phase 3 study evaluated 523 patients for efficacy and 568 patients for safety for 5 days following high-dose cisplatin chemotherapy. During the 5 days after chemotherapy, patients in the aprepitant group had a complete response of 62.7% versus 43.3% in the standard therapy group. Incidence of adverse events was similar in both groups (72.8% versus 72.6%). In the aprepitant group, complete response ranged from 82.8% on day 1 to 62.7% on days 2–5 versus 68.4% on day 1 and 46.8% on days 2–5 for the standard therapy group.[94]

Another phase 3, double-blind study (endpoint of complete response) enrolled 202 patients and observed them for 6 chemotherapy cycles. The group receiving aprepitant (125 mg before cisplatin and 80 mg on days 2–5 versus 375 mg/250 mg) reported a complete response of 64% versus 49% for the group receiving standard ondansetron/dexamethasone treatment. After cycle 6, the aprepitant group still had a complete response of 59% compared to 35% in the standard therapy group.[92] Researchers conducting these 3 studies concluded that aprepitant plus a standard regimen of odansetron and dexamethasone consistently provided superior protection from CINV compared to standard therapy alone.[92,94,95] Additionally, de Wit et al.[92] concluded that aprepitant provided sustained protection against CINV over multiple cycles of chemotherapy when existing drugs often become less effective.

A multi-center, randomized, double-blind, placebo-controlled study seeking to define the most appropriate dose regimen of oral aprepitant (375 mg/250 mg versus 125 mg/80 mg versus 40 mg/25 mg versus standard therapy) was conducted in 376 patients with cancer who were receiving initial cisplatin. (While the study was ongoing, aprepitant 375 mg/250 mg was discontinued resulting from pharmacokinetic data obtained that indicated an apparent interaction with dexamethasone.) The authors concluded that an aprepitant 125 mg/80 mg regimen added to a standard regimen of intravenous ondansetron and oral dexamethasone had the most favorable benefit-to-risk profile.[96] Possible drug interactions with aprepitant include some chemotherapies, birth control pills (reduces effectiveness), blood thinners (Coumadin®), and other drugs (eg, Orap®, Seldane®, Hismanal®, and Propulsid®) as well as nonprescription and herbal products.[97]

# NATURAL APPROACHES TO ENHANCING CHEMOTHERAPY EFFICACY

## Fish Oil

Fish oil may enhance the effectiveness of cancer chemotherapy drugs. A study compared different fatty acids on colon cancer cells to see if they could enhance mitomycin C, a chemotherapy drug efficacy. Eicosapentaenoic acid (EPA) concentrated from fish oil was shown to sensitize colon cancer cells to mitomycin C.[98] It should be noted that fish oil also suppresses the formation of prostaglandin E2, an inflammatory hormone-like substance involved in cancer cell propagation.

In another study, a group of dogs with lymphoma were randomized to receive either a diet supplemented with arginine and fish oil or soybean oil alone. Dogs on the fish oil and arginine diet had a significantly longer disease-free survival time than dogs on the soybean oil.[99]

## Caffeine

The use of caffeine in combination with chemotherapy has been shown to enhance the cytotoxicity of chemotherapy drugs. Caffeine occurs naturally in green tea and has been shown to potentiate the anticancer effects of tea polyphenols. In SKH-1 mice at high risk of developing malignant and nonmalignant tumors, oral administration of caffeine (as sole source of drinking fluid for 18–23 weeks) inhibited the formation and decreased the size of both nonmalignant and malignant tumors.[100]

p53 gene mutations are the most common genetic alterations observed in cancer patients, occurring in 50–60%, including those with carcinomas and sarcomas. Caffeine has been shown to potentiate the destruction of p53 defective cells by inhibiting growth in the G2 phase. This ability of caffeine is important because the basis of many anticancer therapies is to damage tumor DNA and destroy the replicating cancer cells. Caffeine uncouples tumor cell-cycle progression by interfering with the replication and repair of DNA.[101–104]

## Panax Ginseng

Panax ginseng, also known as Korean ginseng, has been used in China for thousands of years as a popular remedy for various diseases, including cancer.[105] Cancers can develop resistance to chemotherapy drugs. Multidrug resistance, the principal mechanism by which many cancers develop resistance to chemotherapy drugs, is a major factor in the failure of many forms of chemotherapy.[106] P-glycoprotein—expressed within cancer cells—confers multidrug resistance by transporting chemotherapy drugs out of cancer cells. Researchers observed that panax ginseng extract reversed P-glycoprotein-induced multidrug resistance, which resulted in increased accumulation of chemotherapy drugs within cancer cells.[107] Also, panax ginseng extract enhanced the anticancer effects of the chemotherapy drug mitomycin C in stomach cancer cells[108] and potentiated the antitumor effects of the chemotherapy drug cisplatin in mice with ovarian cancer.[109]

## Quercetin

Quercetin is a flavonoid found in a broad range of foods, from grape skins and red onions to green tea and tomatoes. Quercetin's antioxidant and anti-inflammatory properties protect cellular DNA from cancer-inducing mutations.[110] Quercetin traps developing cancer cells in the early phases of their replicative cycle, effectively preventing further malignant development and promoting cancer cell death.[111] Furthermore, quercetin favorably modulates chemical signaling pathways that are abnormal in cancer cells.[112,113]

Quercetin potentiates the anticancer activity of Adriamycin® against breast cancer cells[114-116] by increasing concentrations of Adriamycin® within cancer cells.[117] In mice with breast cancer, combining quercetin with Adriamycin® led to long-term, tumor-free survival, whereas mice were failed to be cured when treated with Adriamycin® alone.[118] Interestingly, when given together with quercetin, Adriamycin® inflicted substantial DNA damage to cancer cells. However, normal cells were protected against the DNA damaging effects of adriamcyin.[115] This effect cannot be understated, as the main problem associated with the use of chemotherapy is that it inflicts damage to normal cells as well as cancer cells.

Quercetin enhances the anticancer activity of the chemotherapy drug cisplatin.[119] The concomitant administration of quercetin and cisplatin reduced tumor growth to a significantly greater degree than cisplatin alone in mice with lung cancer.[120]

## Sulforaphane

Sulforaphane, which is an isothiocyanate, is most highly concentrated in broccoli as well as other cruciferous vegetables (eg, Brussels sprouts, cabbage, and cauliflower). Sulforaphane shows promise as an adjuvant to chemotherapy. When added to the chemotherapy drug oxaliplatin, sulforaphane improved the ability of the drug to kill colon cancer cells.[121]

## Theanine

L-theanine is a unique amino acid, naturally occurring in green tea, shown in one study to enhance Adriamycin® concentration in tumors 2.7-fold and reduce tumor weight 62% over controls, whereas Adriamycin® by itself did not reduce tumor weight.[122] Adriamycin® is an anthracycline antibiotic having a wide spectrum of antitumor activity. Additionally, L-theanine was shown to reverse tumor resistance to certain chemotherapeutic drugs by forcing more of the drug to stay inside the tumor. It does not, however, increase the amount of drug in normal tissue, which sets it apart from other drugs designed to overcome multidrug resistance.[123]

**Theanine makes chemotherapy work.** In 1999, researchers performed a study testing the use of theanine in conjunction with a drug similar to doxorubicin known as idarubicin. The use of idarubicin has been tried in drug-resistant leukemia cells, but it caused toxic bone marrow suppression.

Researchers wanted to see if theanine would cause the drug idarubicin to work. In the first experiment, about one-fourth of the standard dose of idarubicin was used. At this dose, the drug usually does not work, and it also does not cause toxicity. When combined with theanine, however, idarubicin worked but still without toxicity. Tumor weight was reduced 49% and the amount of drug in the tumors doubled. In the next experiment, theanine was added to the usual therapeutic dose of idarubicin. Theanine increased the effectiveness of idarubicin and significantly lessened usual bone marrow suppression. Leukocyte loss was reduced from 57% to 37%.[124]

Part of theanine's activity can be attributed to its mimicking of glutamate, an amino acid that potentiates glutathione. Theanine crowds out glutamate transport into tumor cells. Cancer cells (in confusion) erringly take in theanine, and theanine-created glutathione results. Glutathione (created by theanine) does not detoxify like natural glutathione; instead, it blocks the ability of cancer cells to neutralize cancer-killing agents. Deprived of glutathione, cancer cells cannot remove chemotherapeutic agents, and the cell dies as a result of chemical poisoning.[125]

## SUMMARY

Chemotherapy drugs have a high rate of treatment failure. Twenty years of clinical trials using chemotherapy on advanced lung cancer patients yielded survival improvement of only 2 months. While new chemotherapy regimens appear to be improving survival, when these same regimens are tested on a wider range of cancer patients, the results have been disappointing. Oncologists at a single institution may obtain a 40–50% response rate in a tightly controlled study, but when these same chemotherapy drugs are administered in a real-world setting, the response rates decline to 17–27%.

New approaches beyond chemotherapy are required. There have been few clinical trials, however, to determine if adjuvant approaches actually improve survival in cancer patients. In fairness, it should be noted that lymphomas (Hodgkin's, non-Hodgkin's, and Burkitt's), myeloma, hairy cell leukemia, and chronic lymphocytic and certain other types of leukemia are all responding better to chemotherapy than 30 years ago. Also, depending on the timing of treatment, certain institutions are achieving better results with breast and early-stage lung cancers.

Our objective in conveying this large body of data is to provide chemotherapy patients with a better opportunity to beat cancer and minimize toxic side effects. We advocate that you follow a protocol based on a wide range of individual considerations, including the results of chemosensitivity and immu-nohistochemistry testing recommended at the beginning of this protocol. Information on your tumor cells obtained by these tests will help determine therapies most likely to work for you. In addition to these tumor cell tests, and based on your particular medical situation, you and your health care team will need to design a program specific to your needs and tolerances. The following is an outline of the steps described in this protocol:

1. Decide on an appropriate chemotherapy regimen. Chemosensitivity and immunohistochemistry tumor cell tests can help you and your physician make a more informed decision.

2. Based on tumor type, consider asking your physician to prescribe a COX-2 inhibiting drug, such as Lodine.

3. Based on findings from the immunohistochemistry test, if your tumor expresses the K-Ras oncogene, consider high-dose statin drug therapy such as lovastatin (80 mg per day).

4. The following supplements might help block growth signals used by cancer cells to escape eradication by chemotherapy. These supplements have also displayed antiangiogenesis properties. Some of these supplements may be best initiated 3 weeks after cessation of chemotherapy if one believes that antioxidants will protect cancer cells from the effects of chemotherapy drug(s):

   • Soy extract (40% isoflavones), five 675-mg capsules taken 4 times per day. Note that isoflavones from soy have antioxidant properties.

   • Curcumin (as highly absorbed BCM-95®): 400–800 mg daily

*Warning:* Use caution when combining curcumin with other chemotherapy drugs. Do not take curcumin with the chemotherapy drugs Irinotecan, Camptosar, or CPT-11. Watch for NSAID-like side effects such as gastric ulceration because curcumin is a COX-2 inhibitor. Do not take curcumin if you have a biliary tract obstruction. Also note that curcumin is a potent antioxidant.

   • Green tea extract, two or three 725-mg capsules with meals. Each capsule should be standardized to provide a minimum of 200 mg of EGCG. It is the EGCG fraction of green tea that has shown the most active anticancer effects. These are available in a decaffeinated form for persons who are sensitive to caffeine or want to take the less stimulating decaffeinated green tea extract capsules in the evening dose. Note that green tea is a potent antioxidant.

5. To possibly enhance the efficacy of certain chemotherapy drugs:

   • Fish oil, 4000–8000 mg daily of a fish oil concentrate supplying up to 2800 mg EPA and 2000 mg DHA

   • Panax ginseng, 200–600 mg daily standardized to contain 4–7% ginsenosides

   • Quercetin, 1000–3000 mg daily

   • Sulforaphane, 400–1600 mg daily of a broccoli extract

   • L-theanine, five 100-mg capsules twice per day

6. The following natural supplements may reduce side effects and healthy tissue damage caused by chemotherapy. All of these supplements except shark liver oil, PSK, and astragalus are potent antioxidants:

   • Vitamin E, 400 IU per day of vitamin E succinate

   • Vitamin C, 4000–12 000 mg throughout the day

   • Astragalus, 2000–4000 mg daily

   • Blueberry, 900–1800 mg daily

   • Coenzyme Q10 (as ubiquinol): 100–300 mg daily

   • Melatonin, 3–50 mg at bedtime. Dose may be reduced after chemotherapy ends if too much morning drowsiness occurs. After several months, most cancer patients take 3–20 mg of melatonin at bedtime.

   • PSK (from the mushroom *Coriolus versicolor*), 3 g daily

   • Se-methylselenocysteine (SeMSC), 200–400 mcg daily

   • Whey protein concentrate isolate, 30–60 g in divided doses daily

**Note:** *Cancer patients undergoing chemotherapy should consider taking whey protein concentrate at least 10 days before beginning therapy, during therapy, and then for at least 30 days after completion of therapy.*

   • Shark liver oil, 200 mg alkyglycerols, 5 capsules daily for 30 days

   • Digestive enzyme capsules may reduce the gas and bloating associated with high soy intake.

7. Ask your oncologist to consider prescribing immune-enhancing drugs suggested in this protocol, such as Leukine® and alpha interferon or IL-2 (along with a retinoid drug).

For more information on specific types of cancer, see the following protocols: Breast Cancer, Cancer Radiation Therapy, Cancer Surgery, Colorectal Cancer, Leukemia, Lymphoma, Pancreatic Cancer, and Prostate Cancer. We suggest you check www.lefcancer.org regularly for the latest updates regarding cancer chemotherapy and related subjects.

## ADDITIONAL INFORMATION ON CANCER TREATMENT

After reading this protocol, please refer to Cancer Treatment: The Critical Factors. It contains important additional information for the chemotherapy patient that we do not want to duplicate in this protocol section. Cancer patients may want to refer to the other protocols in this edition or visit our website at www.lef.org or www.lefcancer.org.

## FOR MORE INFORMATION

U.S. Department of Health and Human Services, Public Health Service, National Institutes of Health National Cancer Institute, Bethesda, MD 20892 and NIH Publication No. 94-1136.

## STAYING INFORMED

This protocol raises many issues that are subject to change as new data emerge. Furthermore, cancer is still a disease with unacceptably high mortality rates, and none of our suggested regimens can guarantee a cure.

Life Extension is constantly uncovering information to provide to cancer patients. A special website has been established for the purpose of updating patients on new findings that directly pertain to the published cancer protocols. Whenever Life Extension discovers information that may benefit cancer patients, it will be posted on the website www.lefcancer.org.

Before utilizing this cancer protocol, we suggest that you check www.lefcancer.org to see if any substantive changes have been made to the recommendations described herein. Based on the sheer number of newly published findings, there could be significant alterations to the information you have just read.

## REFERENCES

References available at: www.lef.org/dpt5/ch38

# 39

---

# *Cholesterol Management*

---

Emerging research into underappreciated aspects of cholesterol biochemistry has revealed that cholesterol *levels* account for only a portion of the cardiovascular risk profile, while the *properties* of the molecules responsible for transporting cholesterol through the blood, called *lipoproteins,* offer important insights into the development of *atherosclerosis.*

In fact, the *size* and *density* of lipoproteins are important factors for cardiovascular risk—for example, large, buoyant LDL ("bad cholesterol") particles are much *less dangerous* than small, dense LDL particles; likewise large, buoyant HDL ("good cholesterol") particles offer greater vascular protection than smaller, more dense HDL. The development of advanced lipid testing strategies that take the importance of lipoprotein particle size into consideration, such as the *Vertical Auto Profile (VAP)* or *NMR (nuclear magnetic resonance)* tests, allow a far deeper assessment of cardiovascular risk than a conventional lipid profile utilized by most mainstream medical practitioners.

Furthermore, metabolic processes, such as *oxidation* and *glycation,* modify the functionality of lipoproteins, transforming them from cholesterol transport vehicles into *highly reactive* molecules capable of damaging the delicate *endothelial cells* that line arterial walls. This endothelial damage both initiates and promotes atherogenesis. Scientifically supported natural interventions can target the formation of these modified lipoproteins and help avert deadly cardiovascular diseases such as *heart attack* and *stroke.*

The pharmaceutical industry has been very successful in promoting cholesterol reduction with statin drugs as essentially the most important strategy for reducing cardiovascular risk. However, although the use of *pharmaceutical treatment* has saved lives, Life Extension has long recognized that optimal cardiovascular protection involves a *multifactorial strategy* that includes at least 17 different factors responsible for vascular disease.

Life Extension believes that innovative strategies for decreasing vascular risk should incorporate *thorough* cholesterol and lipoprotein testing, as well as strategic nutrient and pharmaceutical intervention, for optimal health effects and vascular support.

## THE BLOOD LIPIDS: CHOLESTEROL AND TRIGLYCERIDES

### Cholesterol

Cholesterol is a wax-like steroid molecule that plays a critical role in metabolism. It is a major component of *cellular membranes,* where its concentration varies depending on the function of the particular cell. For example, the membrane of liver cells contains fairly large fractions of cholesterol (~30%).[1]

The cholesterol in cell membranes serves 2 primary functions. First, it modulates the fluidity of membranes, allowing them to maintain their function over a wide range of temperatures. Second, it prevents leakage of ions (molecules used by the cell to interact with its environment) by acting as a cellular insulator.[2] This effect is critical for the proper function of neuronal cells, because the cholesterol-rich *myelin sheath* insulates neurons and allows them to transmit electrical impulses rapidly over distances.

Cholesterol has other important roles in human metabolism. Cholesterol serves as a *precursor to the steroid hormones,* which include the sex hormones (androgens and estrogens); mineral corticoids, which control the balance of water and minerals in the kidney; and glucocorticoids, which control protein and carbohydrate metabolism, immune suppression, and inflammation. Cholesterol is also the *precursor to vitamin D.* Finally, cholesterol provides the framework for the synthesis of bile acids, which emulsify dietary fats for absorption.

### Triglycerides

Triglycerides are *storage lipids* that have a critical role in metabolism and energy production. They are molecular complexes of glycerol (glycerin) and 3 fatty acids.

While glucose is the preferred energy source for most cells, it is a bulky molecule that contains little energy for the amount of space it occupies. Glucose is primarily stored in the liver and muscles as glycogen. Fatty acids, on the other hand, when packaged as triglycerides, are denser sources of energy than carbohydrates, which make them superior for long-term energy storage (the average human can only store enough glucose in the liver for about 12 hours worth of energy without food, but can store enough fat to power the body for significantly longer).

## LIPOPROTEINS: BLOOD LIPID TRANSPORTERS

Lipids (cholesterol and fatty acids) are unable to move independently through the bloodstream, and so must be transported throughout the body as lipid particles. The lipid particles that transport cholesterol in circulation are called *lipoproteins*. Contained within these lipoproteins are one or more proteins, called *apolipoproteins*, which act as molecular "signals" to facilitate the movement of lipid-filled lipoproteins throughout the body. Lipoproteins can also carry fat-soluble antioxidants, like CoQ10, vitamin E, and carotenoids, which protect the transported lipids from oxidative damage. This is why vitamin E and CoQ10 have performed so well in cardiovascular studies—because they prevent the oxidative modification of LDL particles, which in turn protects the blood vessel lining from damage. This will be discussed in greater detail in forthcoming sections in this protocol.

Four main classes of lipoproteins exist, and each has a different, important function:

- **Chylomicrons (CMs)** are produced in the small intestines and deliver energy-rich dietary fats to muscles (for energy) or fat cells (for storage). They also deliver dietary cholesterol from the intestines to the liver.

- **Very low-density lipoproteins (VLDLs)** take triglycerides, phospholipids, and cholesterol from the liver and transport them to fat cells.

- **Low-density lipoproteins (LDLs)** carry cholesterol from the liver to cells that require it. In aging people, LDL often transports cholesterol to the linings of their arteries where it may not be needed.

- **High-density lipoproteins (HDLs)** transport excess cholesterol (from cells, or other lipoproteins like CMs or VLDLs) back to the liver, where it can be reprocessed and/or excreted from the body as bile salts. HDL removes excess cholesterol from the arterial wall.

Among its myriad functions, the liver has a central role in the distribution of cellular fuel throughout the body. Following a meal, and after its own requirements for glucose have been satisfied, the liver converts excess glucose and fatty acids into triglycerides for storage and packages them into VLDL particles for transit to fat cells. VLDLs travel from the liver to fat cells, where they transfer triglycerides/fatty acids to the cell for storage. VLDLs carry 10–15% of the total cholesterol normally found in the blood.[3]

As VLDLs release triglycerides to fat cells, their cholesterol content becomes proportionally higher (which also causes the VLDL particle to become smaller and denser). The loss of triglycerides causes the VLDL to transition to a low-density lipoprotein (LDL). The LDL particle, which averages about 45%

cholesterol, is the primary particle for the transport of cholesterol from the liver to other cells of the body; about 60–70% of serum cholesterol is carried by LDL.[4]

During the VLDL to LDL transition, an *apolipoprotein* buried just below the surface of the VLDL called *ApoB-100*, becomes exposed. ApoB-100 identifies the lipoprotein as an LDL particle to other cells. Cells which require cholesterol recognize ApoB-100 and capture the LDL, so that the cholesterol it contains can be brought into the cell. Each LDL particle expresses exactly one ApoB-100 molecule, so measurement of ApoB-100 levels serves as a much more accurate indicator of LDL number than LDL-C (LDL cholesterol) level.

Because of the correlation between elevated blood levels of cholesterol carried in LDL and the risk of heart disease, LDL is commonly referred to as the "bad cholesterol." LDL is, however, more than just cholesterol, and its contribution to disease risk involves more than just the cholesterol it carries.

All LDL particles are not created equal. In fact, *LDL subfractions* are divided into several classes based on size (diameter) and density, and are generally represented from largest to smallest in numerical order beginning with 1. The lower numbered classes are larger and more buoyant (less dense); size gradually decreases and density increases as the numbers progress. Smaller, denser LDLs are significantly more atherogenic for 2 reasons: they are much more susceptible to oxidation,[5-7] and they pass from the blood stream into the blood vessel wall much more efficiently than large buoyant LDL particles.[8] A more comprehensive lipid test, such as the *Vertical Auto Profile (VAP) Test* or *NMR* (nuclear magnetic resonance), allows for assessment of the size and density of LDL particles, a feature that dramatically increases the prognostic value and sets these advanced tests apart from conventional lipid tests. If an individual is found to have a greater number of small dense LDLs they are said to express LDL *pattern B* and are at greater risk for heart disease than an individual with more large buoyant LDL particles, which is referred to as *pattern A*.

*HDLs* are small, dense lipoprotein particles that are assembled in the liver, and carry about 20–30% of the total serum cholesterol.[9] Cholesterol carried in the HDL particle is called "good cholesterol," in reference to the protective effect HDL particles can have on cardiovascular disease risk. HDL particles can pick up cholesterol from other tissues and transport it back to the liver for re-processing and/or disposal as bile salts. HDL can also transport cholesterol to the testes, ovaries, and adrenals to serve as precursors to steroid hormones. HDLs are identified by their apolipoproteins *ApoA-I and ApoA-II*, which allow the particles to interact with cell surface receptors and other enzymes.

The movement of cholesterol from tissues to the liver for clearance, mediated by HDLs, is called *reverse cholesterol transport*. If the reverse cholesterol transport process is not functioning efficiently, lipids can build up in tissues such as the arterial wall. Thus, reverse cholesterol transport is critical for avoiding atherosclerosis. Interestingly, a link between the male hormone testosterone and reverse cholesterol transport has been discovered—testosterone enhances reverse cholesterol transport.[10] Although it is known that testosterone decreases levels of HDL, it also improves HDL *function*. This effect is mediated by a protein in the liver called scavenger receptor B1 that acts to stimulate cholesterol uptake for processing and disposal. Testosterone beneficially increases scavenger receptor B1.[11] Testosterone also increases the activity of an enzyme called hepatic lipase, another facilitator of reverse cholesterol transport.[12]

Aging men experience a decline in testosterone levels, as well as a simultaneous increase in heart disease risk, which suggests that these phenomena may be related. Indeed, studies have shown that men with even slightly lower testosterone levels were over 3 times as likely to exhibit signs of early coronary artery disease.[13] In order to maintain optimal reverse cholesterol transport efficiency, aging men should strive to maintain a free testosterone in the youthful range of 20–25 pg/ml. Those men interested in learning more about the link between heart disease and declining testosterone levels and ways to boost testosterone naturally should read Life Extension's "Male Hormone Restoration" protocol.

## BLOOD LIPIDS AND LIPOPROTEINS AND DISEASE RISK

The initial association between cholesterol and cardiovascular disease was born out of the detection of lipid and cholesterol deposits in atherosclerotic lesions during the progression of atherosclerosis.[14] Subsequently, studies have elucidated a role of LDLs in cardiovascular disease development, particularly the role of *oxidized LDL* (ox-LDL; LDL particles that contain oxidized fatty acids) in infiltrating and damaging arterial walls, and leading to development of lesions and arterial plaques.[15,16]

Upon exposure of the fatty acid components of LDL particles to free radicals, they become oxidized and structural and functional changes occur to the entire LDL particle. The oxidized LDL (ox-LDL)

particle can damage the delicate *endothelial lining* of the inside of blood vessels.[17] Once the ox-LDL particle has disrupted the integrity of the endothelial barrier additional LDL particles flood into the arterial wall (intima). Upon recognition of the presence of the ox-LDL within the intima, immune cells (macrophages) respond by engulfing it in an effort to remove it. But, the immune cells have then become too enlarged (by engulfing multiple ox-LDL particles) to escape back through the endothelial layer and become trapped within the intima, where they continually release *cytokines*, causing oxidative and inflammatory reactions to occur, resulting in the oxidation of additional native LDL particles and recruitment of more immune cells. This accumulative cycle results in the formation of atherosclerotic plaque deposits, which cause the arterial wall to protrude and disrupt blood flow, a process referred to as *stenosis*.

The recognition that ox-LDL is an initiator of endothelial damage allows for a clearer understanding of LDL's role in the grand scheme of heart disease. Although an elevated number of native LDL particles does not directly endanger endothelial cells, it does mean that there are more LDL particles available to become oxidized (or otherwise modified), which then become more likely to damage endothelial cells.

Lowering serum cholesterol to an "optimal" range (total cholesterol 160–180; LDL-C 50–99) is one of the most frequently used strategies for reducing heart disease risk in persons without CHD.[18] This approach, however, only addresses a portion of the risk. The actual predictive power of high LDL cholesterol for cardiovascular risk is likely much more complex, and has been the subject of several investigations. (Standard therapy for those at *increased risk* for heart disease is to keep LDL <70 mg/dl.)

## THE MULTIFACTORIAL PATHOLOGY OF VASCULAR DISEASE

Analysis of the decline in CHD death rates from 1980 to 2000 by mathematical modeling highlighted the need to address multiple risk factors to protect against the end result of heart disease: mortality. In this study, cholesterol reduction accounted for only 34% of the reduction in death rate in individuals with heart disease. To put this into context, the same model estimated that reductions in systolic *blood pressure* were responsible for 53% of the death rate reduction, and smoking cessation accounted for 13%.[19] In another comprehensive review of studies of CHD risk factors, non-HDL cholesterol increased the risk of CHD less than either elevated *C-reactive protein* (CRP; a marker of systemic inflammation) levels or high systolic blood pressure.[20] In the Copenhagen Heart Study, which tracked 12 000 participants for 21 years, high cholesterol was the sixth most relevant risk factor for developing CHD in both men and women; diabetes, hypertension, smoking, physical inactivity and no daily alcohol intake (light alcohol consumption is heart-healthy) presented larger risks for the disease.[21] The controversial JUPITER trial, which examined prevention of CHD by statin drugs in persons with very low LDL-C (but elevated hs-CRP) supported the conclusion that non–LDL-C risk factors (such as inflammation) represent enough risk for CHD to warrant treatment, even if lipids are within low-risk ranges.[22]

In order to reduce risk, there must be a systematic approach and understanding of the multiple factors of cardiovascular risk and atherosclerosis. Optimal cholesterol management is important for risk reduction, but so are the multiple risk factors that Life Extension has long identified. Accordingly, efforts to lower cholesterol to mitigate cardiovascular risk will only be met with optimal success if paired with measures to reduce other risk factors such as inflammation, oxidation, hypertension, excess plasma glucose, excess body weight, fibrinogen, excess homocysteine, low vitamin K, insufficient vitamin D, hormone imbalance, and so on. Mainstream medicine is quick to point out that 10–15% of patients with coronary heart disease have no apparent major risk factors.[23]

Life Extension members are well aware of the need to address every risk factor for heart disease to improve outcome.

## HIGH BLOOD SUGAR INCREASES THE ATHEROGENICITY OF LDL

Elevated levels of blood sugar create ideal conditions for *glycation reactions* to occur. Glycation is a process by which a protein or a lipid is joined together, nonenzymatically, with a sugar. The resultant product is a highly reactive molecule that is capable of damaging tissues it comes in contact with.

Glycation of LDL particles is a well-documented phenomenon that greatly increases the atherogenicity of LDL. *Glycated LDL* has been shown to be significantly more susceptible to oxidation than native LDL,[24] and to substantially impair endothelial function.[25] In addition, glycated LDL stimulates oxidative stress and inflammation in vascular smooth muscle cells,[26] which reside in the outer layer of the arterial wall; this exacerbates plaque buildup within blood vessel walls. Glycated, oxidized LDL causes degradation of endothelial nitric oxide synthase (eNOS), a critical enzyme involved in maintaining proper vasodilatation and blood flow.[27] Moreover, once LDL has become glycated it is no longer recognized by

the LDL receptor on cell surfaces, meaning that it will remain in circulation and is more likely to contribute to the atherosclerotic process.[28]

Individuals with diabetes are known to be at substantially greater risk for developing atherosclerosis than normoglycemics; glycated LDL plays a major role in the increased cardiovascular disease prevalence in this population.[29] Because the production of glycated LDL depends on the concentrations of sugars (particularly glucose and fructose) in the blood, maintaining ideal postprandial (125 mg/dL) and fasting (70–85 mg/dL) glucose levels is an effective strategy for reducing heart disease risk.

## BLOOD LIPID MEASUREMENT

The determination of the relative levels of the blood lipids and their lipoprotein carriers is an important step for assessing cardiovascular disease, as well as determining appropriate measures for attenuating this risk. Most physicians conduct a routine, fasting blood chemistry panel during a patient's annual physical. This test includes the classic lipid panel or lipid profile, which measures total cholesterol, HDL, and triglycerides from a fasting blood sample; levels of LDL-C are calculated from these data.[30] An extended lipid profile may also include tests for non-HDL and VLDL.

The recognition of the relative risks of the different subclasses of lipoprotein particles has led to the development of advanced lipid testing, which may have an improved prognostic power over conventional lipid panels in its ability to assess additional risk factors for CHD (such as LDL particle size, VLDL remnants, *lipoprotein(a), or ApoB-100*). The *Vertical Auto Profile (VAP) Test* is a comprehensive advanced lipid test that uses advanced techniques to separate and quantify lipoproteins from a blood sample. The standard VAP can *directly measure* LDL-C levels, and *subclassify LDLs by particle size and density*, and HDL, VLDL subclasses, as well as ApoB-100.

A comparison between standard lipid tests and the VAP test is provided in the table below.

| Vertical Auto Profile (VAP) | Classic Lipid Panel |
| --- | --- |
| Directly measures LDL (more accurate assessment of LDL and therefore more prognostic of risk for heart disease) | Estimates LDL using a calculation |
| | Calculated levels lose accuracy when triglycerides are very high (>400 mg/dL) |
| Measures ApoB-100, which is a direct indication of the LDL particle number (more particles are associated with higher atherogenic risk) | Not included |
| Measures Lp(a) (some evidence suggests that Lp(a) is more atherogenic than LDL) | Not included |

| Vertical Auto Profile (VAP) | Classic Lipid Panel |
|---|---|
| Identifies LDL density pattern (a small, dense pattern is more atherogenic (pattern B); a large buoyant pattern is less atherogenic (pattern A) | Not included |
| Specifies lipoprotein subclass levels (some subclasses of lipoproteins are more atherogenic than others) | Not included |

Other lipid tests include the following:

1. A gradient gel technique developed by Berkeley HeartLab,[31] which, while not as comprehensive as the VAP test, is able to quantify all 7 LDL subclasses.

2. Nuclear magnetic resonance (NMR) spectroscopy,[32] which determines much of the same information as the other 2 techniques (VAP and Berkeley), but it is the only one test that can quantitate LDL particle number (although this is not necessarily an advantage over the VAP test, since this is functionally the same as directly quantitating ApoB-100).

# CONVENTIONAL APPROACHES TO MANAGING BLOOD LIPIDS AND LIPOPROTEINS

Reduction of total and LDL cholesterol (and/or triglycerides) by conventional medical therapies usually involves inhibiting cellular cholesterol production in the body, or preventing the absorption/reabsorption of cholesterol from the gut. By reducing the availability of cholesterol to cells, they are forced to pull cholesterol from the blood (which is contained in LDL particles). This has the net effect of lowering LDL-C. Therapies that increase the breakdown of fatty acids in the liver or lower the amount of VLDL in the blood (like fibrate drugs or high-dose niacin)[33] also result in lower serum cholesterol levels. Often, complementary strategies (such as statin to lower cholesterol production plus a bile acid sequesterant to lower cholesterol absorption) are combined to meet cholesterol-lowering goals.

Reduction of cellular cholesterol production is the most frequent strategy for reducing cardiovascular disease risk, with HMG-CoA reductase inhibitors (statins) being the most commonly prescribed cholesterol-lowering treatments. Statins inhibit the activity of the enzyme HMG-CoA reductase, a key regulatory step in cholesterol synthesis. Since cholesterol levels in cells are tightly controlled (cholesterol is critical to many cellular functions), the shutdown of cellular cholesterol synthesis causes the cell to respond by increasing the activity of the LDL receptor on the cell surface, which has the net effect of pulling LDL particles out of the bloodstream and into the cell. Statins may also reduce CHD risk by other mechanisms, such as by reducing inflammation.[34]

Statins may induce serious side effects in some individuals, the most common being muscle pain or weakness (myopathy). The prevalence of myopathy is fairly low in clinical trials (1.5–3.0%), but can be as high as 33% in community-based studies and may rise dramatically in statin users who are active (up to 75% in statin-treated athletes).[35,36] Occasionally, statins may cause an elevation of the liver enzymes aspartate aminotransferase (AST) and alanine aminotransferase (ALT). These enzymes can be monitored by doing a routine chemistry panel blood test. Additionally, by inhibiting HMG-CoA reductase (an enzyme not only required for the production of cholesterol, but other metabolites as well), statins may also reduce levels of the critically important antioxidant molecule CoQ10.

Lowering cholesterol absorption from the intestines reduces LDL-C in a different fashion; by preventing uptake of intestinal cholesterol, cells respond by making more LDL receptor, which pulls LDL particles out of the bloodstream. Ezetimibe and bile acid sequestrants (colesevelam, cholestyramine, colestipol) are 2 classes of prescription treatment that work in this fashion. Ezetimibe acts on the cells lining the intestines (enterocytes) to reduce their ability to take up cholesterol from the intestines. While ezetimibe does reduce LDL levels, the results of several major trials[37–39] failed to show the benefit of ezetimibe as part of a combination therapy for reducing risk of cardiovascular disease, and it may actually increase the risk of atherosclerosis if prescribed to patients already on statins for reasons that are not clear.[40] Bile acid sequestrants bind to bile acids in the intestine, which reduces their ability to emulsify fats and cholesterol. This has the net effect of preventing intestinal cholesterol absorption. Bile acid sequestrants may also increase HDL production in the liver, which is usually inhibited by the reabsorption of bile acids.[41]

# NUTRITIONAL APPROACHES TO MANAGING BLOOD LIPIDS AND LIPOPROTEINS

Nutritional approaches to blood lipid and lipoprotein management mirror many of the strategies of conventional therapies. Dietary modifications aim to reduce the intake and uptake of fats and cholesterol from the diet. The inclusion of specific dietary compounds with cholesterol-lowering (hypocholesterolemic) or cardio-protective properties may also reduce cardiovascular disease risk by several different mechanisms.

## Diet

**Therapeutic Lifestyle Changes (TLC) diet.** Diet is an important determinant of cardiovascular disease risk; both conventional and alternative approaches advocate dietary and lifestyle changes as the first step in meeting lipid management goals. The National Cholesterol Education Program (NCEP) developed the Therapeutic Lifestyle Changes (TLC) diet[42] for medical professionals to help patients pursue nutritional options for lowering cholesterol. The TLC diet recommends no more than 25–35% of daily calories from total fat, with up to 20% as monounsaturated, 10% as polyunsaturated, and <7% as saturated fats. This relatively high allotment of fat calories allows for increased unsaturated fat intake like omega-3 fatty acids in place of carbohydrates for patients with metabolic syndrome.

Carbohydrates and proteins should provide 50–60% and 15% of total calories, respectively. Dietary cholesterol intake should be less than 200 mg per day. Optional dietary guidelines include the addition of 10–25 g of *soluble fiber*, and 2 g of *plant sterols* per day. Total calories are adjusted to maintain body weight and prevent weight gain, and enough moderate exercise to burn at least 250 calories per day is recommended.

**Dietary Approaches to Stop Hypertension (DASH) diet.** Although not designed as a hypocholesterolemic diet, the DASH (Dietary Approaches to Stop Hypertension) eating plan encourages many of the same heart-healthy eating habits.[43] The first DASH eating plan (originally called the "combination diet") focused on fruits, vegetables, and whole grains, and was especially high in fiber (31 g/day) and potassium (4.7 g/day), and low in animal products. Ironically, the original DASH was not a low-sodium diet (allowing up to 3 g/day), but was nonetheless hypotensive.[44] The low-sodium DASH diet has demonstrated even greater hypotensive effects when limiting sodium to 1.5 g/day.[45] Recall that hypertension is a major coronary heart disease factor. Hypertension magnifies the danger posed by excess LDL by damaging the endothelial barrier, allowing increased permeability.

**Calorie restriction.** Calorie restriction (CR) is the dramatic reduction of dietary calories (by up to 40%), to a level short of malnutrition.[46] Restriction in energy intake slows down the body's growth processes, causing it to instead focus on protective repair mechanisms; the overall effect is an improvement in several measures of wellbeing. Observational studies have tracked the effects of CR on lean, healthy individuals, and have demonstrated that moderate CR (22–30% decreases in caloric intake from normal levels) improves heart function, reduces markers of inflammation (C-reactive protein, tumor necrosis factor [TNF]), reduces risk factors for cardiovascular disease (LDL-C, triglycerides, blood pressure) and reduces diabetes risk factors (fasting blood glucose and insulin levels).[47–50] Preliminary results of the Comprehensive Assessment of Long-Term Effects of Reducing Intake of Energy (CALERIE) study, a long-term multicenter trial on the effects of calorie-restricted diets in healthy, overweight volunteers[51] has shown that moderate CR can reduce several cardiovascular risk factors (LDL-C, triglycerides, and blood pressure, C-reactive protein).[52]

## REPLACING LOST HORMONES TO ACHIEVE OPTIMAL CHOLESTEROL LEVELS

Due to the role of cholesterol as a precursor to steroid hormones, some researchers have speculated that the elevation in cholesterol seen with advancing age is a compensatory effort by the body to restore levels of hormones to more youthful levels.

In a small clinical trial, Sergey Dzugan and Arnold Smith found that restoring youthful hormone levels with the use of bioidentical hormone replacement therapy (BHRT) resulted in a significant reduction in cholesterol levels in 20 individuals with high cholesterol.[53]

Hormone replacement therapy has been shown to reduce cardiovascular risk in aging women,[54] and aging men with lower testosterone levels are at significantly greater risk for heart disease.[55] Thus, aging individuals should consider optimizing their hormone levels in order to reduce cardiovascular risk. More information on this topic can be found in Life Extension's Hormone Replacement Therapy protocols for men and women.

## NUTRIENTS FOR LIPID MANAGEMENT

There are several nutrients that have been identified as potential agents for promoting a favorable lipid profile; many of them work by the same principles as conventional therapies (such as reducing cholesterol synthesis, or interfering with cholesterol absorption in the gut). Several also have additional activities (antihypertensive, inhibition of LDL oxidation, anti-inflammatory) that complement their cholesterol-lowering activity and lend to their overall reductions in fatal and nonfatal cardiovascular events.

## Inhibiting Cholesterol Synthesis

**Pantethine.** Pantethine and its metabolites appear to act on the body's fat and cholesterol metabolism pathways. Pantethine is a derivative of pantothenic acid (vitamin B5), and can serve as a source of the vitamin. One notable function of vitamin B5 is its conversion into coenzyme A, a necessary factor in the metabolism of fatty acids into cellular energy. The pantethine derivative cysteamine may also function to reduce the activity of liver enzymes that produce cholesterol and triglycerides.[56] Studies of pantethine consumption have demonstrated significant reductions in total and LDL cholesterol (up to 13.5%), triglycerides, and elevation of HDL-C in hypercholesterolemic subjects (individuals with high cholesterol)[57,58] and diabetic subjects[59] when taken at 900–1200 mg/day, although significant effects on triglycerides have been observed at dosages as low as 600 mg/day.[60]

**Red yeast rice.** Red yeast rice is a traditional preparation of rice fermented by the yeast *Monascus purpureus*. The yeast produces metabolites (monacolins) that are naturally occurring HMG-CoA reductase inhibitors (one of these, monacolin K, is chemically identical to lovastatin[61]). A comprehensive review of 93 randomized trials including nearly 10 000 patients has demonstrated that commercial preparations of red yeast rice produced reduction in total cholesterol, LDL-C, triglycerides, and an increase in HDL-cholesterol.[62] A long-term (4.5-year) multicenter study of nearly 5000 patients with a previous heart attack and high total cholesterol levels demonstrated that a commercial red yeast rice preparation reduced the incidence of major coronary events, including nonfatal heart attack and cardiovascular mortality, when compared to placebo.[63] Red yeast rice extracts have also been shown to be well tolerated and effective in lowering LDL in patients with statin intolerance.[64,65]

Due to regulations regarding their labeling in the United States, standardization of commercial red yeast rice preparations for monacolins is problematic, thus levels of monacolins can vary dramatically between red yeast rice products.[66] There are some standardized red yeast rice products that are standardized for monacolin K content.

**Garlic.** Garlic has been substantiated by several human trials, particularly its ability to support favorable blood lipid profiles. Three separate analyses of 32 blinded, controlled human trials of garlic consumption in healthy patients or patients with high cholesterol and triglycerides confirm significant reductions in total cholesterol by an average of 7.3 mg/dL, and triglycerides by an average of 4.2 mg/dL.[67–69] While the average cholesterol reductions across all human studies are modest, greater reductions in total cholesterol were realized in patients who were initially hyperlipidemic or hypertriglycemic (>11 mg/dL reduction), took the extract for over 12 weeks (11 mg/dL reduction), or took a garlic powder (as opposed to an oil or aged extract; 12 mg/dL reduction).[70]

Garlic also reduces systolic and diastolic blood pressure (SBP and DBP) in hypertensive individuals, and systolic blood pressure in persons with normal blood pressure. A recent review and analysis of 11 controlled human trials of garlic showed a mean decrease of 4.6 ± 2.8 mm Hg for SBP in the garlic group compared to placebo, while the mean decrease in the hypertensive subgroup was 8.4 mm Hg for SBP and 7.3 mm Hg for DBP.[71]

**Indian gooseberry.** Indian gooseberry (amla; *Emblica officinalis*) has been used traditionally as a nutrient-dense food in Indian regions, and in Ayurvedic medicine for treating a variety of conditions. Modern scientific inquiry has revealed considerable evidence in support of the medicinal use of this nutritional powerhouse. Analytical studies on extracts of Indian Gooseberry highlight its potent antioxidant properties[72] animal studies carry these findings forward by showing that orally administered amla extract significantly reduce levels of oxidized LDL.[73,74] In human studies, extracts of amla have been shown to attenuate elevations in LDL, total cholesterol, and triglycerides, and boost levels of protective HDL.[75] In a study examining the antioxidant activity of amla extract in subjects with metabolic abnormalities, 4 months of supplementation was shown to dramatically bolster plasma antioxidant power and suppress oxidative stress.[76]

Studies suggest that amla extract may also protect against LDL glycation by modulating blood glucose levels. In diabetic patients amla not only significantly reduced post-prandial glucose levels, but also lowered lipid and triglyceride levels over a 21-day period[77]. In an animal model of metabolic syndrome induced by a high-fructose diet, concomitant administration of amla extract reined in rising cholesterol and triglyceride levels, and also significantly repressed the expression of inflammation-related genes, which are typically elevated in metabolic syndrome models.[78] Extracts of the antioxidant-rich fruit also reduce levels of advanced glycation end products (AGEs), which are formed by the same process as glycated LDL.[79] By limiting the amount of LDL particles that become glycated, amla may help maintain proper cellular uptake of cholesterol and reduce the amount of LDL-C available to infiltrate the arterial wall.

## THE ROLE OF BILE ACIDS IN DIETARY FAT ABSORPTION

**Bile acids** are excreted from the liver into the small intestine where they facilitate the absorption of dietary fats into the bloodstream. The *absorption* of dietary fats is dependent on bile acids and the *lipase* enzyme. An intact soluble fiber binds to *bile acids* in the small intestine, thus helping to impede *absorption* of dietary fats (while simultaneously reducing serum LDL and cholesterol).

Specially processed, propolmannan is a polysaccharide fiber derived from a plant that grows only in the remote mountains of Northern Japan. Propolmannan is patented in 33 countries as a purified fiber that does not break down in the digestive tract.

Published studies reveal propolmannan's ability to not only increase the amount of bile acids in the feces, but also reduce the rate of carbohydrate absorption and the subsequent glucose/insulin spike in the blood. When propolmannan is taken before meals, consistent and significant reductions in blood triglyceride, LDL, and cholesterol are observed.[80]

**Soluble fibers.** Soluble fibers include nondigestible and fermentable carbohydrates, and their sufficient intake has been associated with lower prevalence of cardiovascular disease.[81] When included as part of a low-saturated fat/low-cholesterol diet, they can lower LDL-C by 5–10% in hypercholesterolemic and diabetic patients, and may reduce LDL-C in healthy individuals as well.[82] The cholesterol-lowering properties of soluble oat fiber, psyllium, pectin, guar gum, beta-glucans from barley, and chitosan are substantiated by dozens of controlled human clinical trials.[83–85] Soluble fibers lower cholesterol by several potential mechanisms.[86] They may directly bind bile acids or dietary cholesterol, preventing/disrupting their absorption. Their high viscosities (measure of a liquids thickness) and effects on intestinal motility may slow or limit macronutrient uptake. They can also increase satiety, which can limit overall energy intake.

**Prebiotics.** Prebiotics, a subset of soluble fiber, have gained attention in recent years in their ability to be selectively fermented by gut flora for a diversity of potential health-promoting benefits. The fermentation of prebiotic fibers into short-chain fatty acids such as acetate, butyrate, or propionate may inhibit cholesterol synthesis in the liver.[87] In human trials, the prebiotic fibers inulin and dextrin have induced reductions in serum levels of total cholesterol (–9% and –2% for inulin and dextrin, respectively), LDL-C (–1% for dextrin), and triglycerides (–21% for inulin).[88,89]

**Plant sterols.** Plant sterols (phytosterols) are steroid compounds found in plants that function similarly to cholesterol in animals (as components of plant cell membranes, and precursors to plant hormones). Like cholesterol, they can exist as free molecules or as sterol—esters. Esters of sterols have a higher activity and better fat solubility, which allows for lower effective dosages (2–3 g/day as opposed to 5–10 g/day for unesterified sterols).[90] Sterols themselves are poorly absorbed from the diet, but because of their chemical similarity to cholesterol, they are thought to compete with cholesterol for absorption in the intestines, which has the net effect of reducing LDL levels.[91] Sterols may also reduce cholesterol production in the liver, reduce the synthesis of VLDLs, increase LDL particle size, and increase LDL uptake from the blood[92,93] HDL and/or very low-density lipoproteins are generally not affected by sterol intake.[94]

There have been numerous studies of the effects of sterol esters on reducing mean total cholesterol and LDL-C cholesterol in healthy, hypercholesterolemic, and diabetic individuals. An analysis of 57 trials involving over 3600 individuals has reported an average LDL-C reduction of 9.9% at a mean intake of 2.4 g sterol esters/day.[95] Sufficient evidence of the cholesterol-lowering effects of sterols has prompted the U.S. Food and Drug Administration to permit the health claim that sterol esters may be associated with a reduced risk of coronary heart disease, when taken at sufficient levels in the context of a healthy diet, one of only 12 permissible health claims granted by this organization.[96] The NCEP[97] and American Heart Association[98] both support the use of sterols in their dietary recommendations.

**Guggul/Gum guggul.** Guggul/Gum guggul, the resin of the *Commiphora mukul* tree, has a history of traditional usage in Ayurvedic medicine and is widely used in Asia as a cholesterol-lowering agent. Guggulipid is a lipid extract of the gum that contains plant sterols (guggulsterones E and Z), the proposed bioactive compounds.[99] In an analysis of 20 human studies on guggulipid, most of the evidence support a significant reduction in serum total cholesterol, LDL, and triglycerides, as well as an elevation in HDL.[100] However, most of these studies were small, and had significant design flaws (such as lack of controls or statistical analysis). More recent studies, with better designs, have produced conflicting results. The first, a 36-week study of the effects of 25 mg of guggulsterones on 61 hypercholesterolemic patients demonstrated significant reductions of total cholesterol by 11.7%, LDL by 12.5%, and triglycerides by 15%.[101] A second study revealed an opposite effect; this larger study (103 patients) looked at low- (25 mg) and high- (50 mg) dose guggulsterones on blood lipid parameters for 8 weeks, and observed increases in LDL-C (4 and 5% for the low- and high-dose groups, respectively).[102] In the most recent study, 12-week administration of 540 mg raw guggul demonstrated modest reductions in both total cholesterol and HDL (3–6%), although the clinical significance of this outcome is not clear.[103]

**Soy protein.** Soy protein has value as an anti-hypercholesterolemic agent not only because of the potential lipid-lowering effects of its included isoflavones (which may increase the amount of LDL receptors and help to clear LDL particles from the blood), but also for its potential as an alternative to other high-fat/high-cholesterol protein sources. A 1995 meta-analysis of 38 controlled human clinical trials (30 conducted on hypercholesterolemic patients) revealed that compared to animal protein, an average intake of 47 g/day of soy protein resulted in significant improvements in blood lipid/lipoprotein parameters. Across the studies there were observable average reductions in total cholesterol (9%), LDL-C (12.9%), triglycerides (10.5%), and VLDL-C (2.6%), as well as a nonsignificant increase in HDL-C (2.4%).[104] These data were the foundation for the Food and Drug Administration (FDA) approval of the food-labeling health claim for soy protein in the prevention of CHD.[105]

More recently, a second meta-analysis of 41 soy protein studies (including 32 new studies performed after 1995) confirmed the antihypercholesterolemic properties of soy protein. The average reductions in blood lipids were smaller (5.3% for total cholesterol, 4.3% for LDL-C, 6.3% for triglycerides, and a 0.8% increase in HDL-C), but this analysis was limited to studies that used soy protein isolates (which contain no cholesterol-lowering fiber).[106] Some of this difference may also be explained by baseline lipid levels; persons with moderate to severe hypercholesterolemia showed the largest decreases in serum cholesterol when soy is added to the diet.[107]

Isoflavone-enriched soy proteins may have additional lipid-lowering benefits. In the 11 human trials that compare isoflavone-enriched soy to isoflavone-free soy, the enriched soy products (which delivered an average of 102 mg isoflavones/day) lowered total and LDL cholesterol more than isoflavone-free soy, by 1.7% and 3.5%, respectively.[108]

## Inhibiting Oxidation and Glycation of LDL

**Coenzyme Q10 (CoQ10).** The generation of chemical energy in the form of ATP by the mitochondrial electron transport chain is essential for the existence of life as we know it. Delicate endothelial cells that line the arterial walls depend on healthy mitochondrial function to control blood pressure and vascular tone. Oxidized or glycated LDL can sabotage endothelial mitochondrial function and damage the endothelial barrier, setting the stage for the atherosclerotic cascade to initiate.[109,110] CoQ10 is an integral component of mitochondrial metabolism, serving as an intermediary transporter between 2 major checkpoints along the road to ATP production. Interestingly, CoQ10 is also the only known endogenously synthesized lipid-soluble antioxidant,[111] and is thus incorporated into LDL particles, where it serves to protect against oxidation. Because of these dual roles insufficient levels of CoQ10 expedite atherogenesis from 2 angles—by limiting mitochondrial efficiency in endothelial cells and leaving LDL particles vulnerable to oxidative damage.

As noted above, statin drugs, which are typically used to treat high cholesterol, ironically also suppress levels of CoQ10 in the blood.[112] Individuals taking a statin drug should always supplement with CoQ10.

**Carotenoids.** Carotenoids are common constituents of the LDL particle. *Beta-carotene* is the second most abundant antioxidant in LDL; other common dietary carotenoids (*lycopene, lutein*) may be transported by LDL particles as well.[113] Together, these 3 carotenoids have an indispensable role in the protection of LDL particles from oxidative damage; their serum levels have been demonstrated to be the most predictive of the degree of LDL oxidation in humans.[114] Carotenoids may also possess additional lipid-lowering activities independent of their antioxidant potential. The best-studied in this respect is lycopene; an analysis of 12 human trials of *lycopene* reveals an average reduction in LDL-C of approximately 12%.[115] Potential mechanisms for this action are suppression of cholesterol synthesis by the inhibition of the HMG-CoA reductase enzyme, or an increase in the rate of LDL degradation.[116] Astaxanthin, a carotenoid found in some fish and marine oils, can increase HDL.[117]

**Vitamin E.** Natural tocopherols and tocotrienols together form *vitamin E*. These fat-soluble antioxidants have been studied for decades and are known to protect against some cardiovascular events. Vitamin E strongly inhibits the oxidation of LDL particles.[118,119]

Alpha tocopherol is the best known form of vitamin E and is found in the largest quantities in blood and tissue. It is critical, however, for anyone supplementing with vitamin E to make sure they are also getting adequate *gamma tocopherol* each day. The key benefit is gamma tocopherol's ability to dramatically reduce inflammatory threats, a major cause of virtually all degenerative diseases. One of the most important benefits of gamma tocopherol is its ability to improve *endothelial function* by increasing *nitric oxide synthase*, the enzyme responsible for producing vessel-relaxing nitric oxide.[120] One major way it produces this effect is by sponging up destructive reactive nitrogen species, such as peroxynitrite.[121] In fact, gamma tocopherol is able to "trap" a variety of reactive nitrogen species and halt their negative effects on a host of cellular processes.[122]

Supplementation in humans with 100 mg per day of gamma tocopherol resulted in a reduction in several risk factors for vascular disease such as platelet aggregation and LDL cholesterol levels.[123]

**Pomegranate.** Pomegranate is now widely viewed as a *superfruit* with a myriad of health benefits, and rightfully so; dozens of placebo controlled clinical trials have been carried out on pomegranate juice, or pomegranate extract. With respect to lipid management, the efficacy of pomegranate is rivaled by very few natural compounds. The high concentration of polyphenols (particularly punicalagins) in pomegranate makes it an ideal ingredient for suppressing LDL oxidation.[124,125]

Consumption of pomegranate polyphenols significantly lowered total and LDL cholesterol concentrations while maintaining HDL levels in subjects with elevated cholesterol profiles.[126] Pomegranate also suppresses immunoreactivity against oxidized LDL, a mechanism which would be expected to limit plaque formation in the intimia.[127] In fact, this is exactly what was shown in a long-term study of pomegranate consumption. Subjects received either pomegranate juice or placebo for 3 years; in the group receiving the placebo, carotid intima media thickness (cIMT; a measure of atherosclerosis) *increased* by 9% one year after study initiation, while in the group receiving pomegranate, cIMT was *reduced* by an astonishing 30%. Moreover, pomegranate significantly reduced oxidized LDL concentrations, and increased serum antioxidant activity, compared to placebo, while simultaneously *lowering blood pressure*. This study also showed that pomegranate nearly doubled the activity of *paraoxonase-1 (PON-1)*, an antiatherogenic enzyme

that optimizes the function of HDL and protects lipids from oxidative damage.[128] Both groups in this study continued on standard therapy that may have included statins, anti-hypertensives, etc.

**Polyphenols.** Polyphenols are a diverse set of phytonutrients that are ubiquitous in the diet. Polyphenol intake has been associate with lower risk of cardiovascular mortality, and may partially explain the health benefits of several common foods (tea, fruits, vegetables, wine, chocolate).[129] Flavonoids, the largest and best studied class of polyphenols, include catechins from green tea and chocolate, theaflavins from black tea, soy isoflavones, flavan-3-ol polymers from red wine, and anthocyanidins from grapes and berries. A systematic analysis of over 130 human studies of flavonoids revealed significant improvements in endothelial function (cocoa and black tea polyphenols) and blood pressure (anthocyanidins, isoflavones, cocoa); however, only green tea catechins exhibited significant cholesterol (LDL-C) lowering in this analysis (averaging about 9 mg/dL over 4 studies).[130] Subsequently, a study of black tea extract in 47 mildly hypercholesterolemic Japanese men and women demonstrated an 8% reduction in total cholesterol and 13% drop in LDL-C after 3 months.[131]

Other polyphenolic compounds with significant lipid modification potential based on human studies include methylated citrus flavonoids (polymethoxyflavones), which were shown to lower total-cholesterol, LDL-C, and triglycerides by 27%, 25%, and 31%, respectively, when combined with tocotrienols in a small pilot trial.[132] Additionally, the red wine polyphenol resveratrol was shown to incorporate into the LDL particles of human volunteers following ingestion of a high-resveratrol wine, potentially acting as a resident antioxidant.[133] This is consistent with resveratrol's role in the prevention of LDL oxidation observed in humans.[134]

**Curcumin.** Curcumin has a variety of protective roles in CVD, potentially reducing oxidative stress, inflammation, and the proliferations of smooth muscle cells and monocytes.[95] Small human trials have revealed the effects of curcumin on reducing lipid peroxidation[135,136] and plasma fibrinogen,[137] both factors in the progression of atherosclerosis.[138] Curcumin may also reduce serum cholesterol by increasing the production of the LDL receptor,[139,140] but despite successes in animal models, human data on the antihypercholesterolemic effects of curcumin is conflicting. A small study of 10 healthy volunteers revealed significant decreases in lipid oxidation products (–33%) and total cholesterol (–12%), with a concomitant increase in HDL-C (29%) when using

500 mg curcumin daily for 7 days.[141] In two subsequent studies, low-dose curcumin showed a nonsignificant trend toward lowering total cholesterol and LDL-C in acute coronary patients,[142] while high dose-curcumin (1–4 g/day) exhibited nonsignificant increases in total, LDL, and HDL cholesterol.[143]

## Enhancing Cholesterol Elimination

**Artichoke.** Artichoke has traditional usage as a liver protectant and choleretic (compound that stimulates bile flow). In stimulating bile flow, artichoke may aid the body in the disposal of excess cholesterol. In vitro studies suggest its antiatherosclerotic effects may also be linked to an antioxidant capacity that reduces LDL oxidation, or the ability of one of its constituents, luteolin, to indirectly inhibit HMG-CoA reductase.[144]

In addition to several uncontrolled human studies and case reports,[145] 2 randomized, controlled trials support the ability of artichoke extracts to lower total and/ or LDL cholesterol. In the first trial, artichoke extract (1800 mg/day) for 6 weeks reduced total cholesterol (–9.9%) and LDL-C (–16.6%) in 71 hypercholesterolemic patients, with no differences in HDL-C or triglycerides.[146] In the second, also in hypercholesterolemic patients, 1280 mg of artichoke extract/day for 12 weeks reduced total cholesterol by 6.1%, when compared to a control group. Changes in LDL-C, HDL-C, and triglycerides were insignificant.[147] Artichoke extract also improved parameters of endothelial function in a small human trial.[148]

## Optimizing the Lipid Profile

**Niacin/nicotinic acid.** Niacin/nicotinic acid (vitamin B3) is an essential nutrient with roles throughout human metabolism. At dosages substantially above the recommended daily intake (RDI), prescription niacin treatments can significantly raise HDL-C (by 30–35% in some cases, at dosages averaging 2.25 g/day).[149,150] Niacin can also change the distribution of LDL by increasing the amount of large buoyant LDL and reducing the amount of small dense LDL.[151] Niacin can also reduce the susceptibility of LDL to oxidation.[152]

In 2010, the results of 7 published studies on the effects of niacin therapy were combined to examine the overall effect. This *meta-analysis* is considered more powerful than an individual study because it increases the sample size. The results showed that patients taking niacin (compared with a placebo) had significant reductions in nonfatal myocardial infarction and transient ischemic attack.[153]

On May 26, 2011, the National Institutes of Health stopped a clinical trial of a prescription-strength level of niacin 1 year prior to its projected completion. The participants were 3400 patients with stable heart disease, well-controlled LDL, and elevated triglycerides. They added high-dose, extended-release niacin to their statin therapy. The level of niacin used in the study was much higher than that contained in dietary supplements. As shown in previous studies, the niacin drug successfully elevated HDL and lowered triglycerides, but failed to reduce the risk for heart attack or stroke. The findings of this trial highlight the multifactorial pathology of cardiovascular disease; Life Extension believes that had these patients been receiving antioxidants like CoQ10 to reduce LDL oxidation, pomegranate to improve endothelial function, and fish oil to regulate triglyceride levels there would have been a strong reduction in risk. Mainstream media outlets have used this study as a basis for headlines suggesting that niacin is ineffective for promoting cardiovascular health. However, the lesson that should be taken from these findings is that optimal cardiovascular protection requires a multimodal approach, and should not be limited to one or two interventions.

**Fish oil.** Fish oil is a source of omega-3 fatty acids (eicosapentaenoic acid [EPA] and docosahexaenoic acid [DHA]), which cannot be synthesized by humans but are nonetheless essential for several metabolic processes. Aside from reductions in the risk of cardiovascular mortality and nonfatal cardiovascular events (supported by studies of tens of thousands of moderate- and high-risk patients),[154] fish-oil fatty acids significantly reduce serum triglycerides. Forty-seven studies, comprising over 15 000 patients, have confirmed an average triglyceride reduction of 30 mg/dL, at an average intake of 3.35 g EPA plus DHA over 24 weeks.[155] Triglycerides were reduced in a dose-dependent manner, and were dependent on baseline levels (reductions of >40% were observed in patients with the highest starting triglyceride levels). Slight increases in LDL-C and HDL-C were also observed in these studies, although other large analyses failed to detect any significant effects of fish oil on cholesterol.[156] The mechanism by which EPA + DHA lowers triglycerides is thought to occur via slowing the release of VLDL particles into the plasma, or increasing lipid degradation and clearance of triglyceride-rich lipoproteins from the blood.[157] Lowering triglyceride levels is a known strategy for increasing the amount of large buoyant LDL and reducing the amount of small dense LDL.

Prescription fish oil uses a highly concentrated EPA+DHA fish oil ester that provides a dosage of 3.36 g of omega-3 in 4 capsules; its degree of triglyceride reduction (up to 45%) is similar to nonprescription fish oil at a similar dose (usually requiring several more capsules).[158] Nonprescription fish oil supplements sell at a fraction of the price of prescription fish oil and usually require one or more additional capsules to be taken daily to obtain the same amount of EPA/DHA.

## Life Extension Suggestions

Those with vascular disorders often manifesting as coronary artery disease should consider using a wide range of supplements, hormones, and drugs to suppress the multiple risk factors involved in atherosclerosis progression. Healthy individuals should carefully follow blood test results to ascertain which nutrients are more important.

### Inhibiting Cholesterol Synthesis
- **Pantethine:** 400–1200 mg daily
- **Red yeast rice:** 600–1200 mg daily
- **Garlic,** standardized extract: 1500–3000 mg daily
- **Amla** (Indian gooseberry), standardized extract: 500–1000 mg daily
- **Statin drug** (lowest dose needed to optimize LDL levels, ideally below 80 mg/dL)

### Inhibiting Absorption of Dietary Cholesterol
- **Dietary fiber:** 25–30 g daily
- **Propolmannan:** 2000–6000 mg daily
- **Prebiotics:** 5000–10000 mg daily
- **Plant sterols:** 600–1200 mg daily
- **Soy isoflavones:** 54–108 mg daily

### Enhancing Cholesterol Elimination
- **Artichoke leaf,** standardized extract: 500–1000 mg daily

### Inhibiting Oxidation and Glycation of LDL
- **CoQ10** (as ubiquinol): 100–300 mg daily

- **High gamma tocopherol vitamin E:** 350–700 mg daily
- **Pomegranate, standardized extract:** 500–1000 mg daily
- **Beta carotene:** 25000 IU daily
- **Lycopene:** 15–30 mg daily
- **Trans-resveratrol:** 250–500 mg daily
- **Green tea,** standardized extract: 700–1400 mg daily
- **Black tea,** standardized extract: 350–700 mg daily
- **Curcumin:** 400–800 mg daily

### Optimizing the Lipid Profile
- **Niacin:** 1000–2500 mg daily
- **Omega-3 fatty acids** (EPA and DHA): 1400 mg of EPA, 1000 mg DHA daily

### Improving Reverse Cholesterol Transport
- **Testosterone replacement** (men)

In addition, the following blood testing resources may be helpful:

- VAP™ Test
- Omega Score®
- CoQ10 (coenzyme Q10)
- Female Comprehensive Hormone Panel or Male Comprehensive Hormone Panel; or Female Panel or Male Panel
- Chemistry Panel and Complete Blood Count (CBC)

## REFERENCES

References available at: www.lef.org/dpt5/ch39

# 40

# Chronic Fatigue Syndrome

Chronic fatigue syndrome (CFS), also known as chronic fatigue and immune dysfunction syndrome, is a mysterious medical condition that affects approximately 500000 Americans.[1] The disease has no known cause and there is no test that can measure for it.

Rather, CFS is defined as a set of symptoms that include prolonged, overwhelming fatigue that begins upon awakening and lasts throughout the day. The fatigue may worsen with exercise or physical activity. Other symptoms associated with CFS include mood swings, muscle spasms, pain, headache, sleep disturbances, and loss of appetite.[2,3] There is typically no evidence of muscle weakness, joint or nerve abnormalities. Also, CFS is not considered a primary psychological disorder, although it may have psychological elements (eg, depression).[4]

Chronic fatigue syndrome primarily affects women age 25–45, but can affect anyone. While the cause of CFS is unknown, it can be triggered by a number of factors, including infectious agents, mental or physical stress, nutrient deficiencies, immune system abnormalities or allergies, hormonal abnormalities, and low blood pressure. It tends to run in families, so some researchers have hypothesized there may be a genetic predisposition. Oxidative stress may also play a role in the disease.[2,5]

Several famous clusters of cases have occurred, such as an outbreak in Los Angeles County Hospital in 1934; but no common environmental or infectious cause was ever discovered.[6] In recent years, as researchers have learned more about the disease, some clinicians have begun calling for CFS to be classified into different subgroups, depending on other factors present (eg, family history, viral status, and sociodemographic factors).[7] This thinking reflects the idea that CFS may have multiple, interlocking causes or triggers.

## CAUSES OF CFS

### Infectious Disease

To date there is no specific correlation between any infectious agent and CFS.[6] Anecdotally, many CFS sufferers believe that their condition began with a flu-like illness, although for others the disease arises spontaneously.[4]

### Immune Disorders

Many patients with CFS have impaired immune function, as indicated by increased production of cytokines, decreased natural killer cells, alterations in T-cell expression, or increased allergies or autoimmune diseases—although it is unclear whether these conditions were caused by CFS itself.[8–15]

### Dental Amalgam Toxicity

Some research shows a possible correlation between dental amalgam, metal toxicity, and CFS symptoms. In one study, 83 patients (76%) reported long-term health improvement following the removal of dental metal. This effect is believed to be related to a hypersensitive allergic response.[16]

### Oxidative Stress

Studies suggest that oxidative stress may play a role in the development of CFS.[17–19]

### Endocrine System Disorders

Stress, both physical and emotional, can lead to increased levels of cortisol and other hormones. An article in the *Journal of Affective Disorders* concluded that CFS may be associated with low cortisol levels and increased serotonin function.[20] Aluminum is increased in CFS, while DHEA and iron are reduced in female patients.[21,22]

### Low Blood Pressure

Low blood pressure is a common finding in CFS. In one study, neurally mediated low blood pressure was documented in 96% of CFS patients.[23] Medications for the treatment of neurally mediated low blood pressure resulted in improvement in two-thirds of patients.[24] Orthostatic hypotension (low blood pressure that occurs when going from a lying to a standing position) is also a common symptom in chronic fatigue patients.[25]

## DIAGNOSING CFS

Diagnosing CFS is difficult because its symptoms are vague and the disorder often mimics other syndromes or diseases, such as influenza or other viral infections.[5,26–28] Illnesses that may mimic CFS include hypoglycemia, hypothyroidism, depression, environmental illness, food allergies, eating disorders, sleep apnea, autoimmune disease, infections, mononucleosis, and cancer.

A CFS diagnosis can be made only when the patient has suffered from persistent, unexplained fatigue for at least 6 months. In addition to fatigue, 4 of the following symptoms must be present[29]:

- Unrefreshing sleep
- Cognitive impairment, especially short-term memory or concentration
- Sore throat
- Tender lymph nodes
- Aching or stiff muscles
- Multijoint pain without swelling or redness
- Headaches of a new type, pattern, or severity
- Postexertion malaise lasting more than 24 hours
- Persistent feeling of illness for at least 24 hours after exercise

A number of other symptoms have been reported by CFS patients, including abdominal pain, alcohol intolerance, bloating, chest pain, chronic cough, diarrhea, dizziness, dry eyes or mouth, earache, irregular heartbeat, jaw pain, morning stiffness, nausea, night sweats, shortness of breath, skin sensation, tingling sensations, and weight loss.[30]

Chronic fatigue syndrome tends to arise suddenly in otherwise active individuals. In a typical disease course, an otherwise ordinary flu-like illness or some other stressor will leave behind unbearable exhaustion and symptoms of CFS. This condition is frequently mistaken for a recurrence of the infection, sending the patient back to the doctor for more tests. Repeated tests will reveal no characteristic abnormalities, yet symptoms worsen, eventually resulting in sleep disturbances and depression. Many patients with CFS feel their concerns are initially dismissed by physicians, friends, and family, which may contribute to a sense of isolation.

Once diagnosed, the symptoms may fluctuate, but CFS is not a progressive disease. Instead, most patients tend to get better by degrees, and some will fully recover.[6]

There is no single laboratory test to confirm CFS. Instead, physicians should perform a wide variety of blood and cognitive testing in an effort to rule out other diseases. Recent research into CFS suggests that there may be several subclasses of the disease, based on differences in disabilities, sociodemographic factors, viral status, and other biomarkers, and thus different modes of diagnosis and treatment may be appropriate.[7]

## TREATING CFS

There are no prescription medications approved by the Food and Drug Administration (FDA) for use in treating CFS. There are, however, a number of medications used to treat the various symptoms of CFS, depending on the subclass of the disease and how it manifests itself. These medications include antidepressants, antihistamines, decongestants, central nervous system depressants (or stimulants), mineralocorticoids, and expectorants.[6,31]

One medication showing potential is Ampligen®, an experimental antiviral medication that stimulates the production of interferon. In 2 studies, CFS patients treated with Ampligen® demonstrated improvements in cognition and performance. The drug has not yet been approved by the FDA and is in various stages of approval around the world for a wide range of conditions.[32]

## WHAT YOU HAVE LEARNED SO FAR

- Chronic fatigue syndrome (CFS) is characterized by long-term fatigue, as well as sleep-related difficulties, cognitive difficulties, sore throat, tender lymph nodes, or other symptoms.
- The cause of CFS is unknown, although it can be triggered by a wide range of events. There may be multiple causes.
- It is estimated to affect about 500 000 people in the United States, although it mostly affects women age 25–45.
- The diagnosis of CFS is made by excluding other conditions that can have similar symptoms, such as depression or viral illness. A variety of blood tests and other analyses are sometimes needed to rule out other conditions and correctly diagnose CFS. It is still frequently misdiagnosed.
- There is no standard, approved treatment for CFS.

## REGAINING ENERGY THROUGH NUTRITION

In most cases, CFS symptoms gradually improve over time. Life Extension believes that the best approach to CFS is to boost energy levels and support healthy immune function. A full evaluation of hormonal status can also be considered, with blood tests measuring the levels of hormones such as DHEA, pregnenolone, estrogen, testosterone, and others. If levels are low, bioidentical hormone replacement may be helpful. For more specific information on hormone restoration, see Female Hormone Restoration and Male Hormone Restoration protocols.

Several nutrients have been suggested to be deficient in CFS patients, including B vitamins, antioxidants, vitamin C, magnesium, sodium, zinc, L-tryptophan,

L-carnitine, CoQ10, and essential fatty acids. Nutritional deficiencies influence the symptoms of the syndrome as well as the recovery process.[33–35]

## Fighting Fatigue: The Leading Candidates

Free radicals and other potent oxidants may contribute to the development of CFS. One study showed that protein oxidation was significantly elevated in the blood of CFS patients.[36]

A number of studies have looked at nutrients or hormones with immune-boosting properties and found promising results with CFS. In one study conducted at the University of Iowa, 155 patients with CFS were asked to report on their care regimens, including prescription medications, yoga, and nutrients. Three supplements in particular appeared to be beneficial.[37]

**Coenzyme Q10.** Coenzyme Q10 (CoQ10) is a potent antioxidant that aids in metabolic reactions, including the process of forming adenosine triphosphate (ATP), the molecule used by the body for energy.

In one study of 20 female patients with CFS (requiring bed rest following mild exercise), 80% were deficient in CoQ10. After 3 months of CoQ10 supplementation (100 mg/day), exercise tolerance more than doubled, 90% had reduction or disappearance of clinical symptoms, and 85% had decreased postexercise fatigue.[38]

In the University of Iowa study, CoQ10 emerged as the leading therapy for CFS, with 69% of patients reporting it was helpful.

**DHEA.** DHEA has also been singled out for its ability to help CFS patients. The DHEA levels of many CFS patients are low compared to optimal ranges.[21,39] One study speculated that DHEA deficiency might be related to CFS symptoms.[40]

Produced primarily by the adrenal glands, DHEA is a valuable hormone whose levels decline with age. DHEA has been shown to improve energy levels in chronic fatigue patients.[40]

In a study of 15 subjects with CFS, 15 subjects with major depression, and 11 healthy subjects, DHEA levels were significantly lower in the CFS subjects compared to the healthy group. The authors concluded that DHEA has a potential role both therapeutically and as a diagnostic tool in CFS.[22,39]

Another study of DHEA levels in 22 CFS patients found normal DHEA levels but a blunted serum DHEA response curve to adrenocorticotropic hormone (ACTH) injection. ACTH normally stimulates the adrenal glands to secrete DHEA. The authors concluded that endocrine abnormalities may play a role in CFS.[41] See the Stress Management protocol for more information.

## Nutrient Deficiencies

CFS patients are also frequently deficient in a number of other vital nutrients. While the research is not exhaustive, CFS-related deficiencies may be helped through supplementation.

**Vitamin B6.** Some data provide evidence of reduced functional B vitamin status, particularly of pyridoxine (vitamin B6) in CFS patients.[42]

**Folate.** An article in the journal *Neurology* described a study in which folate levels were measured in 60 patients with CFS. Researchers found that 50% of patients had values below 3.0 mcg/L.[43]

**Glutathione.** Glutathione has been shown to help prevent damage to DNA and RNA, detoxify heavy metals, boost immune function, and assist the liver in detoxification. Levels of intracellular glutathione decrease with age.

An article in the *Medical Hypotheses* journal proposed that glutathione may be depleted in CFS patients. The authors proposed that glutathione depletion also causes the muscular fatigue and myalgia associated with CFS.[33]

Cysteine is a precursor to glutathione. It has been hypothesized that glutathione and cysteine metabolism may play a role in skeletal muscle wasting and muscle fatigue. The combination of abnormally low plasma cysteine and glutathione levels, low natural killer cell activity, skeletal muscle wasting or muscle fatigue, and increased rates of urea production define a complex of abnormalities that is tentatively called "low CG syndrome." These symptoms are found in patients with HIV infection, cancer, major injuries, sepsis, Crohn's disease, ulcerative colitis, CFS, and to some extent in overtrained athletes.[44]

Supplements used to raise cellular glutathione levels include N-acetylcysteine (NAC) (with vitamin C), lipoic acid, whey protein, L-cysteine, and glutathione.

**Lipoic acid.** Lipoic acid is known as the "recycler" antioxidant because it can restore the antioxidant properties of vitamins C and E after they have been neutralized by free radicals. It also stimulates the production of the antioxidant glutathione and helps in the absorption of CoQ10.[3,45,46] The body produces glutathione in limited amounts.

**Essential fatty acids.** Essential fatty acids are the fatty acids that cannot be made by the body. Essential fatty acids are crucial for rebuilding and producing new cells, and required for normal brain development.[3]

The use of essential fatty acids for postviral CFS was examined in a double-blind, placebo-controlled study of 63 adults. The patients had been ill for 1–3 years after an apparent viral infection and had severe fatigue, myalgia, and a variety of psychiatric symptoms. Study subjects received either placebo or a preparation containing linolenic, gamma-linolenic, eicosapentaenoic (EPA), and docosahexaenoic (DHA) acids (eight 500-mg capsules daily) over a 3-month period. The treatment group showed continual improvement, compared with uneven results in the placebo group.[47] The essential fatty acid composition of the subjects' red cell membrane phospholipids was analyzed at the first and last visits. The essential fatty acid levels were abnormal at baseline and corrected by active treatment. The authors concluded that essential fatty acids provide a rational, safe, and effective treatment for patients with postviral CFS.

In a case series of CFS patients, researchers administered essential fatty acids with other treatment protocols and observed a 90% gain in improvement within 3 months among two thirds of CFS patients.[48]

### Energy Boosters

A number of nutrients have been studied for their ability to boost cellular energy—a possibly important concern among CFS patients. These include the following:

**NADH.** Reduced B-nicotinamide dinucleotide (NADH), along with CoQ10, is essential for the production of cellular energy.

A randomized, double-blind, placebo-controlled crossover study examined the use of NADH in CFS: 26 eligible patients diagnosed with CFS received either 10 mg of NADH or placebo for a 4-week period. Eight of 26 (31%) responded favorably to NADH, in contrast to 2 of 26 (8%) to placebo.[49]

**L-carnitine.** Although the research is somewhat inconsistent, several studies have found deficiencies of the amino acid L-carnitine among CFS patients. L-carnitine is known to boost energy levels. The lack of consistency in research suggests a number of other nutritional deficiencies, including carnitine, B-complex vitamins, essential fatty acids, L-tryptophan, zinc, magnesium, and others, may be related.[50]

Studies show that carnitine given as a supplement to CFS patients results in better functional capacity and lessening of disease symptoms.[51,52] Other studies have shown a dose of 1000–2000 mg daily has resulted in improvement.[50,53]

Acetyl-L-carnitine relieved mental fatigue, and propionyl-L-carnitine alleviated general fatigue in a study comparing the two in CFS patients.[54]

**Magnesium.** Magnesium participates in energy metabolism and protein synthesis. The body vigilantly protects blood magnesium levels, in part because 350 enzymatic processes depend on magnesium for activation. Magnesium is stored in tissues and bone, sharing skeletal residency with calcium and phosphorus.[55]

A randomized, double-blind, placebo-controlled study was conducted of CFS patients found to have low magnesium levels. In the clinical trial, 32 CFS patients received either placebo or intramuscular magnesium sulfate weekly for 6 weeks. Patients treated with magnesium reported improved energy levels, better emotional state, and less pain.[56]

A new magnesium compound, magnesium-L-threonate, allows for oral administration while boosting levels of magnesium in the brain.[57] However, another study found that magnesium supplementation resulted in a significant worsening of symptoms between 6 and 24 months.[37] Although some people may find magnesium supplementation helpful, if symptoms worsen, it should be discontinued.

**Glutamine.** Glutamine is a conditionally essential amino acid needed during periods of excessive stress. Glutamine is the preferred energy for enterocytes, the cells lining the gastrointestinal tract. Glutamine is also one of the 3 amino acids necessary to make glutathione, a potent scavenger of free radicals.

Supplementation with glutamine might benefit chronic fatigue patients by enhancing gut motility, improving plasma glutamine levels, and boosting glutathione.[58,59]

**Rhodiola.** Rhodiola (*Rhodiola rosea*) has been extensively studied in cell cultures, animals, and humans. It has shown antifatigue and depression, physical endurance, anticancer, immune-enhancing, and sexual stimulating effects.[60]

A study conducted at the Russian Academy of Natural Sciences demonstrated that rhodiola helps boost physical working capacity. In an animal study, an oral rhodiola extract boosted ATP content in the mitochondria of skeletal muscles, such that rhodiola-supplemented rats were able to swim 25% longer than control rats before reaching exhaustion.[61] This is consistent with research demonstrating that rhodiola helps improve exercise endurance in humans after a single dose (200 mg of *Rhodiola rosea*, containing 3% rosavin and 1% salidroside).[62]

Similar results were observed in a study that measured capacity for mental work within the context of fatigue and stress.[63] Scientists at the Centre of Sanitary and Epidemiological Inspection in Moscow gave rhodiola to 161 young cadets and measured the results using an antifatigue index. The results indicated a highly significant reduction in fatigue.

## Life Extension Suggestions

### For Immune Enhancement and General Nutrient Support
- **Comprehensive multivitamin/multinutrient formula:** per label instructions
- **Glutathione:** 250–500 mg daily
- **N-Acetyl-cysteine (NAC):** 600–1800 mg daily
- **R-lipoic acid:** 240 mg–480 mg daily
- **Fish oil (with olive polyphenols):** providing 1400 mg EPA and 1000 mg DHA daily
- **Folic acid:** 800–1000 mcg daily
- **Vitamin B6:** 100 mg daily

### For Energy Enhancement
- **Coenzyme Q10,** as ubiquinol: 100 mg 3 times daily
- **Magnesium:** 144 mg daily as magnesium L-threonate; 320 mg daily as magnesium citrate
- **DHEA:** 15–25 mg daily for women; 25–75 mg daily for men (depending on blood test results)
- **NADH:** 5 mg twice daily
- **Gamma linolenic acid (GLA):** 300–600 mg daily
- **L-carnitine:** 500–2000 mg daily, on an empty stomach
- **Rhodiola rosea, standardized extract:** 250 mg daily

### For Intestinal Tract Support
- **Glutamine:** ≥1 g daily

## REFERENCES

References available at: www.lef.org/dpt5/ch40

# 41

# *Chronic Kidney Disease*

You may be surprised to learn that until 2002; no standard definition for chronic kidney disease (CKD) existed within the medical community.[1] Before then, conflicting classifications had created a state of confusion as to how many Americans were afflicted with this progressive, life-threatening condition.

Once proper categorization of the various phases of CKD was established, the stark and daunting scale of this modern epidemic emerged.

We now know that as many as 26 million Americans currently suffer from some form of chronic kidney disease.[2,3] Aging individuals are especially vulnerable.[4]

When you consider that the risk of cardiovascular mortality in CKD sufferers is 30 times that of the general population,[5] the steady increase in kidney disease rates seen today amounts to a public health disaster. Unfortunately, public awareness of this threat remains low.

Life Extension has long emphasized the need for vigilance through routine testing (at least once a year) to monitor kidney health. In addition to the standard tests for measuring kidney function (ie, creatinine, albumin, and BUN/creatinine ratio), certain individuals should insist that their doctor test for cystatin-C, a largely overlooked blood marker providing a far more precise measure of renal function.[6] Optimal levels are below 0.91 mg/L.

Individuals should keep a record of their test results. Once any sign (such as an increase in creatinine) of disease is detected, it is imperative that immediate steps be taken to halt its progress, as kidney function can decline precipitously and kidney damage may be irreversible. Fortunately, Life Extension members are already taking a variety of nutrients that support kidney health.

In this protocol, you will discover recent scientific advances in our understanding of how CKD unfolds, the specific risk factors that contribute to its progress, and how to bring them under control.

You will also learn of safe, low-cost, natural interventions that have been shown to stop CKD in its tracks, long before end-stage renal disease (ESRD)

renders dialysis, kidney transplant, or both as the only option(s).

## PYRIDOXAMINE OR PYRIDOXAL-5-PHOSPHATE: POTENT KIDNEY DEFENSE

The formation of advanced glycation end-products (AGEs) is a well-established factor in the onset and progression of kidney disease. Nutrients that have been conclusively shown to mitigate the effects of these lethal agents constitute a front-line, low-cost intervention.

A formidable AGE antagonist is the vitamin B6 compound, pyridoxamine. A plethora of research confirms its power to halt formation of AGEs.[7–9] Evidence has also emerged that pyridoxamine drastically limits formation of equally deadly advanced lipoxidation end-products (ALEs)—another catalyst for kidney disease.[10–12]

A team of biochemists at the University of South Carolina were able to show that pyridoxamine traps the reactive molecules formed during lipid (fat) peroxidation and accompanies them harmlessly into the urine.[11,13]

Their colleagues subsequently found that neutralizing AGEs and ALEs can prevent kidney disease and lipid profile abnormalities in diabetic rats.[14] They found that rats supplemented with pyridoxamine had lower levels of albumin (protein) in their urine, lower plasma levels of the waste product creatinine, and less dramatically elevated blood lipids than the placebo-treated rats, all directly related to the reduction of AGEs/ALEs.

They subsequently examined whether similar results could be obtained in non-diabetic rats.[15] Three groups of rats were studied:

- Lean (healthy)
- Obese without treatment
- Obese treated with pyridoxamine

As expected, AGE and ALE formation underwent a 2- to 3-fold increase in obese, untreated rats as compared to lean rats. Conversely, those increases were absent in obese rats treated with pyridoxamine. Treated rats also experienced a smaller increase in plasma triglycerides, cholesterol, and creatinine levels as compared to the obese, untreated rats.[15]

In an equally compelling development, hypertension in the rats treated with pyridoxamine resolved, as did thickening of blood vessel walls. Untreated rats displayed urinary evidence of renal disease (albuminuria) that in contrast had been nearly normalized in supplemented rats. This provides powerful evidence of pyridoxamine's multitargeted protective effect against CKD.[15]

In 2004, the same research team made a landmark discovery. While studying the relative effects of pyridoxamine (along with a variety of additional natural antioxidants) on the progression of kidney disease in diabetic rats, they decided to examine how these natural compounds stacked up against enalapril, a standard pharmaceutical intervention used to prevent CKD.[10] Enalapril is an ACE inhibitor, one of a class of drugs commonly used to control blood pressure and kidney disease.

They found that pyridoxamine therapy was the most effective at preventing the progression of kidney disease, followed by vitamin E and lipoic acid. Enalapril, the prescription drug, proved to be the least effective intervention. Pyridoxamine also limited lipid profile abnormalities as well as the formation of AGEs and ALEs, offering a far broader spectrum of preventive effects than enalapril.[10]

Researchers at the University of Miami advanced these findings by treating diabetic mice with both pyridoxamine and enalapril.[16] They found that pyridoxamine alone provided substantial benefit, cutting albuminuria and damage to the glomeruli (capillaries that carry blood within the kidneys). Combining enalapril with pyridoxamine reduced kidney disease mortality in these animals as well, leading the researchers to suggest that the ACE-inhibitor (enalapril)/pyridoxamine combination might be useful.

A convincing body of research on pyridoxamine therapy in humans with CKD has emerged. In 2007, a team of researchers at Harvard University set out to determine optimal interventions to halt the progression of kidney disease in diabetics.[17] They conducted two 24-week, multicenter placebo-controlled trials in patients with known diabetic nephropathy—treatment of which is known to delay the onset of end-stage renal disease in diabetics. Doses of pyridoxamine ranged from 50 to 250 mg twice daily.

Pyridoxamine significantly inhibited the rise in blood levels of the waste product creatinine, one of the key biomarkers of kidney dysfunction and a predictor of kidney failure. Urinary levels of inflammatory cytokines were also significantly lower in the treated group compared to controls.

Pyridoxamine has been firmly established as a front-line, safe, low-cost intervention in CKD caused or exacerbated by AGEs and ALEs. Further, this natural vitamin B6 compound has been shown to significantly

improve outcomes of experimental kidney transplants and other forms of kidney disease.[18-20]

It therefore borders on criminal that in January 2009, the Food and Drug Administration (FDA) classified this potent, entirely safe CKD therapeutic as a drug, putting it out of reach for many Americans suffering from this deadly condition. No one should be forced to bear the outrageous burden of costly pharmaceuticals and their toxic side effects when a perfectly safe alternative exists.

Fortunately, there is another equally safe option available—another form of vitamin B6 known as pyridoxal-5-phosphate (P5P) that also exerts potent anti-AGE effects. It has been shown to prevent the progression of diabetic kidney disease in preclinical models.[21] In fact, as far back as 1988, P5P was used by a German research group to reduce blood lipids in humans with chronic kidney disease.[22]

# FOUR COMPLEMENTARY KIDNEY PROTECTORS

## Coenzyme Q10

Because of the tremendous blood flow and high concentration of metabolic toxins continuously circulating through the kidneys, they are the site of extraordinary oxidative stress, which is known to contribute to progressive kidney damage and its complications (ie, high LDL and increased cardiovascular disease risk).[23]

Coenzyme Q10 (CoQ10) fortifies the body's natural antioxidant capacity and reduces levels of oxygen-free radicals, indicating an important defense against CKD. As it happens, CoQ10 has been used experimentally to control hypertension and kidney disease in laboratory animals since the early 1970s.[24,25]

Human studies have shown that CoQ10 levels substantially decline, while markers of oxidation such as malondialdehyde are dramatically elevated in kidney disease patients with even mild renal dysfunction.[26] These decreased CoQ10 levels make circulating lipoproteins (such as LDL) more vulnerable to oxidative damage. This in turn increases risk for further cardiovascular damage, adding to the renal burden and substantially increasing the risk of kidney disease.[27]

In 2001, a team of European researchers published compelling evidence for how effective nutritional intervention can be in patients with established kidney disease.[28] Subjects received antioxidant therapy with vitamins C, E, and riboflavin (vitamin B2) for 1 month preceding the addition of CoQ10 therapy for 2 months. Following supplementation, CoQ10 levels in the blood increased from just one quarter to nearly 4 times the normal reference levels. The study was too brief to demonstrate any change in kidney function. However, evidence from animal trials the same year showed that increasing CoQ10 levels in tissues of diabetic rats resulted in a reversal of oxidative stress markers in the kidney, heart, and liver.[29]

By 2004, definitive evidence of the benefits of CoQ10 in human kidney disease patients was demonstrated by European researchers working with transplant recipients. Transplant recipients undergo tremendous oxidative stress and as a result, typically have marked disturbances in lipid profiles. The researchers provided their patients with 30 mg of CoQ10 3 times daily for 4 weeks, and monitored levels of oxidation factors (such as malondialdehyde), natural antioxidant enzymes in the body, and lipid profiles.[30]

Significant improvements were seen after just 4 weeks, with reduction in LDL, increase in beneficial HDL, and a decrease in presence of inflammatory cells noted. These results suggest a potentially dramatic improvement in both quality of life and survival rates for patients with early-stage kidney disease as well as those requiring dialysis or transplantation.

Animal studies have also shown that CoQ10 can protect kidney tissue from numerous nephrotoxic drugs, including gentamicin, a powerful antibiotic with a notorious propensity for causing kidney damage.[31,32] These findings are significant not only because they offer protection in patients who might be exposed to such drugs, but they teach us about CoQ10's potent ability to combat the extreme oxidant stress that the kidney faces as it deals with a variety of foreign chemicals.

## Silymarin

Silymarin is extracted from milk thistle (*Silybum marianum*), a plant rich in the following flavonolignans (natural phenols composed of flavonoid and lignin): silychristin, silydianin, silybin A, silybin B, isosilybin A, and isosilybin B—collectively known as the silymarin complex.

This safe, natural compound has a long history as a traditional therapy for liver and kidney conditions.[33,34] It has been used in Western medicine for more than a quarter of a century, owing to its potent antioxidant and nephron-protective effects, as the treatment of choice for kidney injury resulting from severe mushroom poisoning.[35] In fact, we've known since 1979 that kidney injury (via mushroom poisoning) in animals who are pretreated with silymarin can be almost

entirely preventable.[36] This makes it a natural choice for protection against drug-induced kidney damage since so many drugs can act like poisons, exerting extreme oxidant stress on kidney tissue.

Mushroom poisons (mycotoxins) are among the most deadly natural toxins known. Their kidney toxicity is surpassed only by some of the most aggressive chemotherapy agents. Physicians have therefore looked to silymarin as a potential "renoprotective" agent for patients undergoing chemotherapy.

Silymarin is also protective against several classes of nephrotoxic drugs, in particular cisplatin and Adriamycin®, two of the most potent and damaging (owing to oxidative damage and severe inflammation) chemotherapeutic drugs.[26,37,38] Researchers around the world have found that silymarin and its components reduce and often prevent the kidney damage caused by these drugs.[39–42]

Silymarin's ability to protect against the oxidative stress produced by potent drugs suggests that it may be useful in protecting against more subtle, chronic injury by free radicals—particularly those generated by chronic blood glucose elevations. German researchers, for instance, have found that silymarin could prevent injury to renal cells incubated with elevated glucose concentrations while blocking production of oxidative stress markers.[43]

Silymarin's protective power also extends to ischemia/reperfusion injury (restoration of blood supply following restriction of blood flow). Turkish researchers demonstrated that by pre-treating animals with silymarin, they could completely prevent visible and functional damage to kidney structures exposed to this kind of injury.[44,45] Studies such as these suggest that by maintaining optimal antioxidant function through supplementation, we may be able to prevent much (if not most) of the chronic oxidative damage to which our kidneys are exposed on a daily basis. As a result, they have huge implications for the general population.

## Resveratrol

The considerable advance in our understanding of the cyclical relationships between oxidative stress, endothelial dysfunction, inflammation, atherosclerosis, and chronic kidney disease points to resveratrol as an intervention in the chain of events that ultimately lead to renal failure.[46]

Italian researchers are among the leaders in resveratrol research. Early in this century, one group published research demonstrating the impact of resveratrol on preserving kidney structure and function in rats exposed to ischemia/reperfusion injury.[47,48]

Japanese and Indian urologists followed that up with reports detailing the mechanisms by which resveratrol combats oxidative damage following reperfusion, markedly reducing kidney dysfunction.[49–53] Bacterial infection (sepsis) is a common cause of kidney failure in the intensive care unit and following surgery or trauma. Turkish physiologists demonstrated that resveratrol can reduce or prevent both kidney and lung injury in septic rats.[54]

Resveratrol, due to its antioxidant and anti-inflammatory potential, has been utilized in studies to prevent drug-induced kidney damage. The following results were noted when rats, exposed to antibiotic gentamicin, were treated with resveratrol: (1) nephrotoxicity was significantly reduced, (2) more rapid healing of injured kidney tissue was attained, and (3) a dramatic reduction in markers of oxidant injury was observed.[55] A team of toxicologists in Brazil demonstrated its protective power against cisplatin, the powerful chemotherapy agent responsible for so much drug-induced kidney damage.[56] Finally, Indian pharmacologists were successful in protecting animal kidneys from damage caused by cyclosporine A (another common chemotherapy and immune-suppressant drug) by pretreating the animals with resveratrol.[53]

Since diabetes is the leading cause of kidney disease—and because the damage it inflicts is largely mediated by free radical production resulting from destructive alteration of proteins by glucose (glycation)—researchers have explored resveratrol as a preventive in diabetic kidney damage. Promising results have come from Indian pharmacologists who significantly attenuated kidney damage in rats with experimentally induced diabetes, even 4 weeks after the diabetes was induced.[57]

In the researchers' own words, "The present study reinforces the important role of oxidative stress in diabetic kidney disease and points towards the possible antioxidative mechanism being responsible for the renoprotective action of resveratrol."

## Lipoic Acid

Like resveratrol, lipoic acid is a powerful antioxidant with few known side effects.[58] Lipoic acid has been successfully employed in the laboratory to block the oxidative damage caused by ischemia/reperfusion injury, thereby opening the door to another effective treatment for this common cause of acute kidney failure.[59] In 2008; researchers showed that they could reverse all adverse effects on renal function and lab abnormalities following experimental ischemia/reperfusion injury in animals.[60]

Lipoic acid has been comprehensively studied worldwide for its power to prevent or mitigate drug-induced kidney damage. We know that lipoic acid is an effective kidney-protective agent against damage inflicted by Adriamycin®,[61,62] the immunosuppressive drug cyclosporine A,[58,63,64] and even against acute toxic doses of the pain reliever acetaminophen.[65] In studies examining the protective benefits of lipoic acid against cyclosporine toxicity, it helped to normalize blood lipid abnormalities.[64]

Nephrologists at Georgetown University examined lipoic acid in the context of diabetic kidney disease. Their results showed that it can improve renal function in diabetes by lowering sugar levels.[66]

They also demonstrated that lipoic acid lowers protein loss in urine and improves kidney structure and function by reducing oxidative stress in diabetic laboratory animals.[66]

In yet another compelling study, Korean researchers showed that they could improve kidney patients' responses to the vasodilator (blood vessel relaxer) nitric oxide (NO) by supplementing them with lipoic acid.[67] Loss of endothelial responsiveness to NO is a cause of vascular disease in diabetics. A chemical called asymmetric dimethylarginine (ADMA) is a sensitive marker and predictor of cardiovascular outcome in patients with end-stage renal disease. Fifty patients on hemodialysis were treated with 600 mg lipoic acid daily for 12 weeks. ADMA levels remained unchanged in the control group but fell significantly in the treatment group, suggesting that lipoic acid may reduce the risk of cardiovascular complications in this group of patients.

## Overcoming CKD-Related Fatigue

**L-carnitine.** L-carnitine, an amino acid–derived nutrient crucial to cellular energy management, may play a vital role in kidney disease prevention and management.[68,69] Carnitine deficiency is itself a known causative factor in the development of kidney disease. Conversely, patients with kidney disease frequently develop carnitine deficiency, especially those on dialysis. Carnitine therapy is known to lead to improvements in many kidney disease–related complications including cardiovascular disease, anemia, decreased exercise tolerance, weakness, and fatigue.[69]

As noted earlier, CKD sufferers are at very high risk for developing cardiovascular complications, including heart attacks and heart failure. This is thought to be related in part to the massive oxidative stress induced by kidney disease and in part to inadequate energy management in cardiac tissues induced by carnitine deficiency.[70] The frequent result of these interrelated factors is a massive deterioration in energy, exercise tolerance, quality of life—and perhaps, longevity.[71]

Based on patient reported outcomes, scientists in Kentucky discovered that supplementation with L-carnitine could improve general health, vitality, and physical function in people on dialysis.[72] In 2001, research by clinicians at Los Angeles Medical Center showed that L-carnitine given intravenously to dialysis patients could reduce fatigue and preserve exercise capacity.[73] A literature review by nephrologists at Vanderbilt University indicated that L-carnitine supplementation should be used to improve red blood cell count in dialysis patients whose anemia doesn't respond to therapy with the hormone erythropoietin.[74] Finally, data from Italy demonstrated that L-carnitine supplements could help suppress levels of the inflammatory marker C-reactive protein, potentially reducing cardiovascular risk in dialysis patients.[75]

### Additional Nutrients That May Benefit CKD

**Folic acid.** Folic acid is well known for its capacity to reduce levels of the metabolite homocysteine, which is strongly associated with cardiovascular disease and dramatically elevated in individuals with kidney disease or kidney failure.[76–79]

**Omega-3 fatty acids.** Omega-3 fatty acids have been shown to help improve cardiovascular risk factors,[80–82] and kidney function in patients with established kidney disease.[83,84] Research published in 2009 suggests that diets rich in omega-3s may actually prevent kidney disease.[85,86]

**Vitamins C and E.** Through its powerful antioxidant effects, vitamin E may help prevent the onset of CKD. Vitamins E and C may mitigate the development of cardiovascular and other complications in patients with chronic kidney disease.[87–92]

## SUMMARY

Chronic kidney disease (CKD) is rapidly approaching epidemic proportions, with up to 26 million Americans suffering from some form of kidney disease. Kidneys filter 200 quarts of blood daily. The high-pressure and toxin-rich environment surrounding kidneys renders these delicate, highly complex organs especially vulnerable to damage, dysfunction, and disease.

High blood pressure, elevated blood sugar, NSAIDs (such as ibuprofen), certain medications, and high-protein diets are the most common threats to kidney health. The potentially lethal insults they inflict include oxidative stress, production of advanced glycation and lipoxidation end-products (AGEs and ALEs), inflammation, and an excessive filtration burden that taxes renal function over time.

Nutrients such as pyridoxal-5-phosphate (P5P) fight AGEs and ALEs. CoQ10, silymarin, resveratrol, and lipoic acid are also clinically supported, potent interventions. Omega-3 fatty acids help quell inflammation, contributing to enhanced kidney health. A host of additional nutrients complement these actions, including folic acid (folate) and vitamins C and E.

### Life Extension Suggestions

- **Pyridoxal-5-phosphate** (P-5-P): 50–250 mg twice daily, 30 minutes before meals
- **Coenzyme Q10** (as ubiquinol): 100–300 mg daily, anytime
- **Silymarin:** 720 mg silymarin along with 270 mg silibinin daily, with meals
- **Trans-resveratrol:** 100–500 mg daily in divided doses
- **R-lipoic acid:** 200 mg once or twice daily, 30 minutes before meals
- **L-carnitine:** 500–2000 mg daily, on an empty stomach
- **Fish oil** (with olive polyphenols): At least 1400 mg/day of EPA and 1000 mg/day of DHA
- **Natural vitamin E:** 100–400 IU alpha-tocopherol and 200 mg gamma-tocopherol daily
- **Vitamin C:** Up to, but not exceeding, 3000 mg daily
- **Folic acid** (as methylfolate): 1000 mcg daily

In addition, the following blood testing resources may be helpful:

- Chemistry Panel and Complete Blood Count (CBC)
- CoQ10 (Coenzyme Q10)
- Cystatin-C

## REFERENCES

References available at: www.lef.org/dpt5/ch41

# 42

# Chronic Obstructive Pulmonary Disease (COPD)

Chronic obstructive pulmonary disease (COPD) is an underdiagnosed lung disease characterized by persistent inflammation and airflow obstruction. COPD is preventable and treatable, but not fully reversible.[1-7]

COPD is the fourth-leading cause of death in most industrialized countries and is predicted to become third by 2020.[8] This increase is due primarily to a global epidemic of tobacco smoking, a leading risk factor for COPD.[9]

COPD encompasses two main conditions[2,10,11]:

- *Emphysema*, which damages and enlarges the *alveoli*, the tiny sacs where oxygen transfer takes place in the lungs
- *Chronic bronchitis*, in which a chronic cough accompanies persistent inflammation of the airways

The goal of COPD treatment is to slow or prevent disease progression, improve exercise tolerance, improve health status, prevent and treat exacerbations, and reduce mortality. Smoking cessation is the most crucial step to prevent COPD or delay its progression.[2,12]

Conventional therapies such as inhaled corticosteroids, inhaled anticholinergics, and beta2-agonists are helpful in treating COPD.[13] However, *inhaled corticosteroids* may increase the risk of *pneumonia*,[14] and *osteoporosis*[15] and *inhaled anticholinergics* may increase the risk of *death*.[16]

After reading this protocol, you will understand what causes COPD, how therapy can relieve symptoms, and how lifestyle changes can reduce exacerbations. You will also learn about novel therapies and natural compounds that can target some key mechanisms that drive COPD progression, including *inflammation* and *oxidative stress*.

## UNDERSTANDING THE CAUSES OF COPD

COPD is a slowly progressing disease that often develops over decades as a result of chronic exposure to inhaled irritants, which trigger an inflammatory response in the lungs.[1] In a typical case, a patient will experience declining lung function for many years before being diagnosed with COPD and receiving

**Bronchitis and Emphysema**

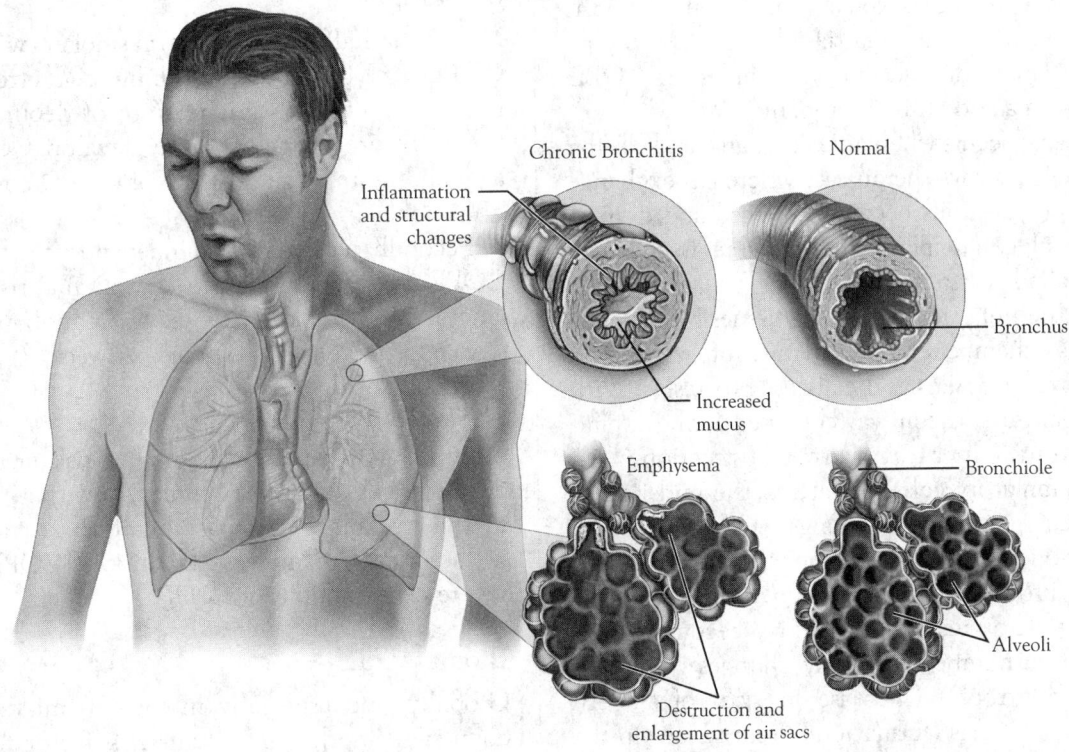

Chronic Bronchitis

Normal

Inflammation and structural changes

Increased mucus

Bronchus

Emphysema

Bronchiole

Alveoli

Destruction and enlargement of air sacs

therapy. During this time, the lungs are undergoing several changes characteristic of COPD.[17]

*Three pathologic processes* play a significant role in COPD-related lung damage: (1) oxidative stress, (2) inflammation, and (3) an imbalance in enzymes (eg, proteases) involved in cell injury and repair.[11]

The bulk of lung tissue is composed of *alveoli*—tiny air sacs where the exchange of oxygen and carbon dioxide takes place. Having a large surface area and blood supply makes the lungs susceptible to oxidative injury caused by reactive oxygen species (ROS) and free radicals either in air pollutants or released through metabolic processes. Cigarette smoke itself contains numerous oxidizing agents.[18]

As a first line of defense, the lungs produce antioxidants such as glutathione, catalases, and peroxidases to detoxify the reactive species. However, in COPD, increased oxidant burden and/or decreased antioxidant defense causes an imbalance (*oxidative stress*) between the amount of ROS and the body's ability to neutralize them.[19] Oxidative stress can cause the air sacs to become less elastic, and the extracellular matrix of the lungs to become damaged.[11,18]

The underlying cause of COPD damage is an *inflammatory response* mounted by the immune system. Chronic exposure to an irritant (eg, cigarette smoke) causes inflammatory cells (eg, neutrophils, macrophages, eosinophils) to gather in the air spaces of the lung. In response to the toxins, macrophages release inflammatory chemicals and begin to recruit more immune-system cells, which in turn release more inflammatory chemicals as well as protease enzymes that degrade the extracellular matrix.[2,11,20]

The two main disease types encompassing COPD are emphysema and chronic bronchitis.[11]

*Emphysema* occurs when alveoli enlarge and cluster. This process destroys the air sacs where gas exchange occurs. As tissue walls become damaged and disintegrate, the alveoli expand and coalesce into larger, thinner-walled air sacs (ie, blebs or bullae). As the walls lose their elasticity, the lung tissues become less efficient gas chambers. Gas exchange for oxygen and carbon dioxide worsens as the disease progresses. With weakened air sacs, the airway collapses during expiration (breathing out) causing airway obstruction.[2,17]

As inflammatory cells migrate to the midsize airways, mucus glands in the lungs become enlarged, causing more mucus production and cough. Over time, the bronchial walls thicken, airways narrow (becoming deformed), and airflow becomes more limited.[2,17] A number of airway changes occur, including hypertrophy (increase in size) of smooth muscle cells, fibrosis (formation of scar tissue) in the airway walls, and infiltration of inflammatory cells. The term for the lung damage and inflammation of the mucus membrane in the airways is *chronic bronchitis*. Chronic bronchitis is diagnosed by the presence of cough and sputum production for at least 3 months in each of 2 consecutive years.[2]

Because changes in the lungs develop incrementally, symptoms appear gradually and may be present for many years before medical treatment is initiated. Progressive and chronic coughing, sputum production, and shortness of breath (dyspnea) are the characteristic symptoms of COPD.

A majority of people with COPD also suffer from other medical conditions (eg, heart disease, osteoporosis, anemia, metabolic syndrome, diabetes, depression, respiratory infections, wasting of the skeletal muscles, and lung cancer) that can affect prognosis.[2,21] Poor lung function and poor nutrition may also exacerbate muscle weakness, abnormalities in fluid and electrolyte balance, and depression.[2,22]

## CAUSES AND RISK FACTORS

Smoking is a primary risk factor for COPD, accounting for up to 75% of all COPD cases globally. Genetics, occupational exposure to gases and fumes, and exposure to biofuel account for the remaining cases.[23,24] People exposed to more than one risk factor can develop COPD earlier, or have more severe symptoms and exacerbations.[2]

### Smoking

More than half of all long-term smokers will develop COPD.[25,26] Moreover, life-long cigarette smokers have a significantly higher rate of decline in lung function, are more likely to develop COPD with age, and more frequently die of COPD compared to nonsmokers.[27,28]

Secondhand smoke is an independent risk factor for COPD.[29,30] Evidence shows that COPD risk doubled among never-smokers exposed to secondhand tobacco smoke for more than 20 hours per week.[30]

### Occupational Exposure

Occupational exposure is another risk factor in the development of COPD. Studies show that toxic gases in the workplace, such as chemical dust and fumes in factories, can increase the risk of COPD[23,25] and severe exacerbations of COPD.[31]

### Biomass Fuel

Globally, and especially in low- to middle-income countries, another important risk factor for COPD may be exposure to air pollutants such as solid or biomass fuels (eg, coal, straw, animal dung, and wood).[23,25] Of these fuels, wood smoke, followed by mixed biomass smoke, is the most notable COPD risk factor.[32]

## Asthma (Bronchial Hyperresponsiveness)

Childhood asthma is a risk factor for the development of COPD later in life, and asthma in the elderly shares many similarities with COPD (eg, shortness of breath, wheezing, coughing, decline in lung function and treatment options).[2,29,33] Also, airway obstruction becomes more severe with long-term asthma. Therefore, it is necessary for doctors to distinguish the two conditions in order to properly diagnose and manage them.[34]

Clinically distinguishing asthma and COPD is typically straightforward among middle-aged and younger people. However, in the elderly, especially those who smoke, differentiating between the two conditions can be difficult using standard clinical lung function assessments. More comprehensive diagnostic testing, including allergy testing, CT scanning of the lungs, and advanced biomarker analyses that characterize COPD versus asthma based on the profile of inflammatory mediators in the blood, allow modern clinicians to confidently categorize most patients.[34,35]

Treatment response can also aid in the differentiation of the two conditions. For example, asthma is typically significantly reversible using bronchodilators, while COPD is only minimally reversible.[34]

## Alpha-1-Antitrypsin Deficiency

Alpha-1-antitrypsin deficiency is a rare (up to 3% of COPD patients), inherited cause of COPD, occurring primarily in individuals of northern European descent. This genetic defect causes the body to produce a decreased amount of the protein alpha-1-antitrypsin, which normally prevents neutrophil elastase from damaging the alveoli. Emphysema typically develops by early middle age in people with severe alpha-1-antitrypsin deficiency, especially in those who smoke.[13,36–38]

## DIAGNOSIS

Physicians typically consider COPD in patients with chronic cough, sputum production, shortness of breath, decreased exercise tolerance, and a history of exposure to tobacco smoke.[2]

Early in the disease, physical examination(s) may be normal. Later in the disease, however, the classic "barrel chest" may occur due to residual air trapped in the lungs, leading to their hyperinflation. In addition, the increased effort required to exhale can produce wheezing, while pursed lips or grunting respirations may signal efforts to keep the airways open by increasing pressure at the beginning of expiration.[2,17,24] Also, severe to very severe COPD commonly results in fatigue, weight loss, and anorexia.[2]

*Spirometry* is the gold standard for diagnosing and monitoring progression of COPD. This breathing test includes forced expiratory volume in one second (FEV1)—the greatest volume of air that can be breathed out in the first second of a large breath, and the forced vital capacity (FVC)—the greatest volume of air that can be breathed out in a whole large breath. In healthy people, at least 70% of the FVC comes out in the first second (ie, the FEV1/FVC ratio is >70%). In fact, the FEV1/FVC ratio <70% is a diagnostic characteristic of COPD.[2,39]

Other tests (eg, x-rays, computed tomography, and magnetic resonance imaging) may be performed if complications such as pneumonia are suspected.

The serum alpha-1-antitrypsin level may also be measured to detect alpha-1-antitrypsin deficiency. This testing may be especially considered for individuals of northern European descent with a personal history of COPD before age 50, family history of COPD or emphysema, and limited exposure to inhalants or irritants.[36,37,40]

Exacerbations of COPD often develop following a viral upper respiratory or tracheal infection. Assessment of COPD exacerbations is based on the degree of airflow limitation, duration, or worsening of new symptoms, and number of previous episodes. Clinical tests (eg, electrocardiography, blood count, and presence of infections) may also be performed to assess the severity of an exacerbation.[2]

## TREATMENT FOR COPD

There is no cure for COPD. However, both pharmacologic and lifestyle management strategies can help improve health status and physical function.[2,41]

According to the Global Initiative for Chronic Obstructive Lung Disease (GOLD), effective COPD management has the following goals[2]:

- Preventing disease progression
- Relieving symptoms
- Improving exercise tolerance and health status
- Preventing and treating complications and exacerbations
- Reducing mortality

## Pharmacologic Therapy

**Bronchodilators.**    Bronchodilators are the first-line therapy for mild COPD. Bronchodilators relax airway smooth muscles, making it easier to breathe. Treatment may begin with a rescue bronchodilator used "as needed" during mild episodes of COPD. In more severe COPD, combination bronchodilator therapy (ie, a rescue bronchodilator combined with a controller [long-acting] bronchodilator) may help relieve symptoms.[2,24]

Bronchodilators include the following:

- Short-acting *beta2-adrenergic agonists* (SABAs) (eg, albuterol and levalbuterol) are rescue medications used "as-needed" to relieve acute symptoms by relaxing airway smooth muscles.[42] The effect(s) of SABAs are immediate, but usually wear off within 4–6 hours. Long-acting beta2-adrenergic agonists (LABAs) (eg, salmeterol and indacaterol) are effective for 12 or more hours.[2] LABAs can significantly reduce exacerbations and improve respiratory health, but do not reduce hospitalization or mortality.[43] Side effects of beta-2-agonists include increased heart rate and blood pressure, trembling, and cardiac arrhythmias.[44]

- *Anticholinergics* (eg, ipratropium and tiotropium) prevent contraction of airway smooth muscle and can reduce exacerbations as well as improve symptoms and health status.[2,45,46] The main side effect of anticholinergics is dry mouth. A comprehensive review showed that tiotropium mist inhaler is associated with a *50% increased risk of death* in people with COPD.[16] Another study showed the use of anticholinergic inhalers increased risk of acute urinary retention among COPD patients with benign prostatic hyperplasia (BPH) (ie, benign enlargement of the prostate).[47]

- *Methylxanthines* (eg, theophylline) are a group of alkaloids commonly used for their effects as mild stimulants and bronchodilators.[48] They are not as well tolerated as inhaled LABAs. Side effects include headache, insomnia, nausea, heartburn, and abnormal cardiac rhythms (which have potential to be fatal in some individuals).[2]

**Corticosteroids.**    Inhaled steroid medications (eg, fluticasone and budesonide) reduce airway inflammation and frequency of exacerbation(s). They can be effective in severe COPD, especially that which co-occurs with asthma.[49,50] At low doses, regular use can improve symptoms, lung function, and quality of life. Side effects include hoarse voice, cough, and oral fungal infection.[51] Inhaled corticosteroids may also increase the risk of pneumonia and impair bone health.[14,49]

Combining inhaled corticosteroids with a LABA significantly reduces morbidity and mortality in COPD when compared to steroids alone, although much of the benefit may be due to the LABA.[49,52] Oral corticosteroids (eg, prednisone, prednisolone), due to their adverse effects (eg, muscle weakness and respiratory failure), are not recommended for long-term use in patients with COPD.[2]

## Other Treatments

**Oxygen therapy.**    Long-term oxygen therapy may be recommended for severe COPD when oxygen level during rest falls below the normal threshold twice over a 3-week period, or if there is evidence of pulmonary hypertension or failure. Stable but very severe COPD may require ventilator support to improve survival.[2]

**Surgery.**    Surgery may be a last option for very severe COPD that does not improve with medication and is accompanied by emphysema in the upper lobe of the lungs.[2] In a bullectomy procedure, larger air sacs (bullae) that have been damaged by emphysema are removed. Surgical removal of these bullae can help restore lung volume and allow the remaining healthy parts of the lung to function better. In lung volume reduction surgery (LVRS), damaged tissues of the lung(s) are removed. LVRS may improve breathing and quality of life, but can be costly. Lung transplantation may also be considered and can improve the quality of life and lung function in a select group with very severe, end-stage COPD.[2]

**Preventive vaccines.**    Because COPD increases susceptibility to lower respiratory tract infections, preventive vaccines, such as pneumococcal and influenza vaccinations, are recommended in all COPD cases.[24] Data show that long-term use of antibiotics does *not* affect the frequency of exacerbations. Unless used to treat bacterial infections, antibiotics are not recommended for long-term COPD therapy.[2]

## Lifestyle and Dietary Management

**Smoking cessation.**    Quitting smoking is the most important step to prevent or slow down the progress of COPD. Comprehensive smoking-cessation programs include counseling, organized "quit" plans, and when necessary, nicotine replacement therapy (eg, gum, skin patches, and other methods). The National Network of Tobacco Cessation Quit lines at 1-800-QUITNOW (1-800-784-8669) can provide smokers in every state access to information and support to quit smoking.[53]

Avoiding secondhand smoke and air pollutants that contribute to COPD symptoms and exacerbations of the disease are also beneficial.[2]

Although tobacco smoking cessation can help slow disease progression and prevent exacerbations in some cases of severe or very severe COPD, with cardiovascular and respiratory benefits becoming evident within one year of cessation, lung function will not be completely restored by stopping smoking.[54]

**Pulmonary rehabilitation.** Air passage obstruction in COPD causes the lungs and heart to work harder to carry oxygen throughout the body. General muscle wasting also becomes a risk as COPD progresses. *Exercise programs* can strengthen chest muscles and facilitate breathing, reduce depression and anxiety related to COPD, and improve recovery along with health status after hospitalization.[55] Multidisciplinary pulmonary rehabilitation programs provide well-monitored exercise programs.

*Breathing exercises* induce relaxation and make breathing easier. Pursed-lip breathing stimulates relaxation, increases oxygen intake and prevents shortness of breath. It has been shown to increase exercise and walking endurance, as well as shorten recovery time(s) in patients with moderate to severe COPD.[56] Breathing exercises are an important part of a COPD rehabilitation program. Respiratory therapists work closely with physicians to personalize the best regimen for each individual.

**Diet and COPD.** Progressive weight loss, muscle wasting, and malnutrition are common with moderate to severe COPD.[41,55] Nutritional support can contribute to weight gain and muscle mass restoration in COPD.[41] In a 3-year, randomized, controlled COPD trial, higher intake of antioxidant-rich foods (ie, fresh fruits and vegetables) resulted in significantly improved pulmonary function while an unrestricted diet resulted in lung function decline.[57] Further, a large study showed that a healthy diet (ie, fruits, vegetables, fish, and whole grains) was associated with lower risk of COPD.[58]

# NOVEL AND EMERGING THERAPIES

Despite use of current treatments, lung function continues to decline in long-term COPD. Therefore, new classes of drugs and/or nonpharmacologic therapies to reduce disease progression are needed.[59,60] Several novel drug therapies are being developed that may offer benefit to people with COPD.

## New Bronchodilators

*Indacaterol* (Arcapta Neohaler®), an ultra-long-acting beta2-agonist, was approved by the Food and Drug Administration (FDA) in July 2011.[61] It is a bronchodilator with rapid-onset action that remains effective for 24 hours or longer. In clinical trials, a once-daily treatment of indacaterol significantly improved shortness of breath and lung function, exercise endurance, and lung hyperinflation compared to placebo among COPD patients. Also, fewer subjects receiving indacaterol experienced COPD worsening compared to placebo.[62–64]

*Glycopyrronium bromide*, a novel anticholinergic with rapid-onset action that lasts for 24 hours, is being investigated as a new COPD treatment.[65] In a clinical trial among COPD patients, significant improvement in forced expiratory volume (FEV1) occurred 5 minutes after dosing and continued to be evident through week 26 of treatment.[66]

## Anti-Inflammatory Agents

*Phosphodiesterase-4 (PDE-4) inhibitors* can be used to reduce airway inflammation and exacerbations in severe to very severe COPD with a history of exacerbation and chronic bronchitis. A majority of clinical trials used *roflumilast* (Daxas®) and *cilomilast* (Ariflo®), second-generation, oral PDE-4 inhibitors. Roflumilast, in particular, is approved in the United States, Canada, and European Union.[67] Adverse side effects of PDE-4 inhibitors are nausea, diarrhea, weight loss, sleep problems, and headache.[68]

A safety concern with the anti-inflammatory agents under development is their ability to affect innate immunity, potentially increasing the risk of lung infection and perhaps cancer among people predisposed to COPD.[69]

## Statins

Statins, which treat cardiovascular disease by lowering cholesterol and combatting inflammation, may have potential as a therapy for COPD exacerbations.[70,71] Statins possess a variety of biological functions including modulation of the inflammatory response, as well as tissue-remodeling pathways, both of which are of potential benefit in treating COPD. Analysis of a large randomized trial on statins and cardiovascular disease found that treatment with pravastatin (Pravachol®) reduced exacerbations and death due to COPD.[72] Another randomized trial found that pravastatin use for 6 months improved exercise performance in COPD.[73] A prospective trial reported that statin treatment in the first year after hospitalization for COPD exacerbation reduced risk and severity of exacerbations and improved quality of life.[71]

# TARGETED NUTRITIONAL STRATEGIES

## Vitamin D

The mechanism by which vitamin D affects the pathogenesis of COPD is unclear. However, studies show that vitamin D can modulate the activity of various immune cells,[74] inhibit inflammatory responses,[75] and regulate airway smooth muscles.[76]

A review of molecular and animal experiments showed that vitamin D regulates airway contraction, inflammation, and remodeling in airway smooth muscles characteristic of COPD.[76] A cross-sectional study found that higher plasma levels of vitamin D are associated with increased bone mineral density and exercise capacity in people with COPD.[77] Evidence also showed that high-dose vitamin D supplementation improved respiratory muscle strength and exercise capacity in people with COPD.[78]

A study among 414 smokers with COPD showed that vitamin D deficiency is highly prevalent in this population, and correlates with disease severity. The study also found that genetic determinants for low vitamin D levels were associated with an increased risk of COPD.[79]

Other COPD intervention studies are underway to examine the effect(s) of 3000–6000 IU of vitamin D3 on rehabilitation (NCT01416701), as well as time to first upper respiratory infection and first moderate-to-severe exacerbation (NCT00977873).[80]

## Antioxidants: Vitamins A, C, and E

*Vitamin A* plays a role in proper lung development (in the embryonic stage) and repair of damaged tissue. Animal models showed that mice with low vitamin A levels were more likely to develop emphysema after 3 months of exposure to cigarette smoke compared to mice with normal vitamin A levels.[81] In one study, high dietary vitamin A intake (>2770 IU daily) was associated with a 52% reduction in risk of COPD.[82]

*Vitamin E* levels are low in smokers, increasing their susceptibility to free radical damage.[83] A 10-year, randomized, population-based trial of 38 597 healthy women reported that supplementing with 600 IU of vitamin E reduced the risk of chronic lung disease by 10%.[84]

A review of population studies reported that low levels of *vitamins E and C* were associated with more wheezing, phlegm, and dyspnea. Levels of *vitamins E and A* were significantly lower during acute exacerbations of COPD compared to stable COPD.[85] A case-control study showed that people with COPD had significantly lower serum levels of *vitamins A, C, E, and carotenoids* compared to healthy controls. The COPD group also had higher white blood cell DNA damage and consumed fewer vegetables and fruits than the healthy group.[86]

## N-Acetylcysteine (NAC)

N-acetylcysteine (NAC), a glutathione precursor, can dissolve mucus (mucolytic properties) and repair damage caused by reactive oxygen species.[87,88]

A comprehensive review of studies reported that oral NAC lowered the risk of exacerbations and improved symptoms in patients with chronic bronchitis compared to placebo.[89] NAC (600 mg) given twice daily for 2 months reduced the oxidant burden in the airways of people with stable COPD.[90] Experimental and clinical studies also showed that NAC can reduce symptoms, exacerbations, and slow declining lung function in COPD.[91]

Treating moderate-to-severe COPD with 1200 mg of oral NAC daily for 6 weeks improved performance on lung function tests after exercise. NAC treatment also reduced air trapping in the lungs compared to placebo.[92] Clinical evidence indicates that administering 1200–1800 mg of NAC daily counteracts oxidative stress among subjects with COPD.[90,93] In contrast, a large multicenter COPD trial reported no difference between NAC and placebo in the decline of lung function. However, those taking NAC who were not on corticosteroids appeared to have fewer exacerbations.[94]

A clinical trial is underway to investigate the effect of adding 1200 mg of NAC daily to standard treatment to reduce air trapping and exacerbations in stable COPD.[95]

## Ginseng

Ginseng has traditionally been used in Chinese medicine to treat a wide range of respiratory symptoms.[96] A review of 12 small randomized studies showed that ginseng may be a potential adjunct therapy in patients with COPD. Oral ginseng formula combined with pharmacotherapy improved respiratory symptoms and quality of life, and reduced exacerbation of COPD compared to placebo, nonginseng formula, or pharmacotherapy alone.[96] These results confirmed a previous study on the effects of 200 mg of ginseng extract daily on pulmonary function tests.[97] Pulmonary function and exercise capacity were significantly improved among people with moderate-to-severe COPD taking ginseng extract compared to placebo. A 2011 article reported that there is a large, multicenter, randomized, controlled study underway to evaluate the safety and efficacy of 200 mg of standardized root extract of

Panax ginseng daily for 24 weeks among people with moderate COPD.[98]

## Sulforaphane

Emerging evidence shows that sulforaphane, a compound in broccoli and other cruciferous vegetables, can potentially augment the anti-inflammatory effects of corticosteroids in COPD.[99] A study showed that histone deacetylase 2 (HDAC2), an enzyme that enables corticosteroids to reduce inflammation, was low in the lung tissue of people with COPD.[100,101] Evidence revealed that sulforaphane can restore corticosteroid sensitivity and increase the activity of HDAC2.[99] Sulforaphane can also counteract oxidative stress by activating Nrf2, a chemical pathway involved in protecting cells from oxidative stress caused by cigarette smoke and other irritants.[99,102,103]

## Coenzyme Q10

Coenzyme Q10 (CoQ10) is a powerful antioxidant.[104] Indirect evidence shows potential benefit of supplementation in people with COPD who have low CoQ10 levels.[105]

A case–control study showed that CoQ10 levels were lower and oxidative stress markers increased during exacerbation of COPD, indicating an imbalance in antioxidant defense during those periods. The authors suggest supplementation with CoQ10 may reduce COPD exacerbation.[105]

A study of the effects of CoQ10 on the exercise performance of athletes and nonathletes showed that plasma levels of CoQ10 increased after 2 weeks of supplementation. Participants who supplemented with COQ10 also experienced less fatigue and increased muscle performance compared to placebo.[106] These results support a previous study wherein CoQ10 supplementation (90 mg daily for 8 weeks) improved exercise performance in people with COPD.[107]

## Omega-3 Fatty Acids

Omega-3 fatty acids such as eicosapentaenoic acid (EPA) and docosahexaenoic acid (DHA) help protect against damaging inflammatory reactions, build healthy cell membranes, and repair tissues.[108–110] Omega-6 fatty acids, such as linoleic acid (LA) and arachidonic acid (AA), mediate pro-inflammatory activities.[109]

A study of clinically stable COPD reported that high dietary intake of omega-3 fatty acids decreased the risk of elevated blood inflammatory markers in COPD, while higher dietary intake of omega-6 fatty acids increased the risk of elevated inflammatory markers.[111]

EPA and DHA supplementation can reduce the destructive effects of chronic inflammation.[108] One study showed a significant improvement in shortness of breath and a decrease in inflammatory markers in serum and sputum in a COPD group receiving omega-3 supplementation compared with controls.[112]

*Boswellia serrate.* Cell culture and animal studies report that boswellic acids, specifically acetyl-11-keto-beta-boswellic acid (AKBA), from *Boswellia serrata* can inhibit 2 enzymes involved in inflammation: 5-lipoxygenase (5-LOX) and cathepsin G (catG).[113,114] 5-LOX stimulates the manufacture of proinflammatory leukotrienes and promotes the migration of inflammatory cells to the inflamed body area. 5-LOX has been shown to cause bronchoconstriction and promote inflammation.[113] Cathepsin is a protein-degrading enzyme that attracts T cells and other leukocytes (white blood cells) at the sites of injury.[114] Animal studies showed that synthetic cathepsin inhibitors reduced smoke-induced airway inflammation,[115] as well as airway hyperresponsiveness and inflammation.[116]

Studies in asthma suggest an anti-inflammatory role for *Boswellia serrata* in pulmonary disease. For instance, a randomized controlled trial showed that daily treatment with *Boswellia serrata* extract (BSE) increased the lung function of people with asthma compared to a control group.[117]

## Resveratrol

Resveratrol, a molecule found in red wine, grapes, and Japanese knotweed, has antioxidant and anti-inflammatory properties that may protect against COPD and asthma.[118] A cell culture study found that resveratrol inhibited the release of all measured inflammatory mediators (cytokines) from immune cells extracted from the alveoli of smokers and nonsmokers with COPD. In contrast, the corticosteroid dexamethasone did not inhibit the release of some cytokines in smokers with COPD.[119] Moreover, while resveratrol attenuated the release of inflammatory mediators in airway smooth muscle cells, it preserved signaling of a protein called vascular endothelial growth factor (VEGF), which may be protective against emphysema. Meanwhile, although corticosteroids significantly reduced inflammatory mediators, they also suppressed VEGF signaling.[120] In another study, resveratrol inhibited inflammatory cytokine release from alveolar macrophages in smokers and nonsmokers with COPD in a dose-dependent manner.[121]

## Zinc

The concentration of zinc is lower than normal in people with COPD; the level is even lower in severe cases.[122] A clinical trial showed that critically ill people with COPD spent significantly less time on mechanical ventilation after receiving an intravenous cocktail of selenium, manganese, and zinc, compared to those who did not.[123] Another study demonstrated that treatment with 22 mg of zinc picolinate for 8 weeks significantly increased the levels of an important antioxidant, superoxide dismutase, in COPD patients.[124]

## L-Carnitine

Respiratory infections increase the frequency and severity of exacerbations. L-carnitine modulates immune function, supports fatty acid and glucose metabolism, and may prevent wasting syndrome.[125–128] In one clinical trial, 2 g of L-carnitine daily improved exercise tolerance and the strength of respiratory muscles in people with COPD. Blood lactate level, which is associated with muscle fatigue, was also reduced with L-carnitine supplementation.[129,130]

## Essential Amino Acids and Whey Protein

COPD is associated with muscle wasting and weight loss (ie, sarcopenia, cachexia), especially in elderly people; and a higher degree of wasting predicts mortality in this population.[131,132] Supplementation with essential amino acids, which are central to anabolic processes that help sustain muscle mass with advancing age, may help combat wasting in aging people with COPD.[133] In a 12-week study involving 32 COPD patients aged 75 (mean) with impaired lung function, supplementation with 8 g of essential amino acids daily lead to gains of body weight and fat-free mass, as well as improved physical function and several biomarkers compared to placebo.[133] Whey protein is a good source of essential amino acids and evidence indicates that whey protein may support muscle protein synthesis even more so than its constituent essential amino acids in an aging population.[134]

## Melatonin

Poor sleep quality is prevalent among individuals with COPD, and oxidative stress is a significant contributor to lung deterioration and disease progression.[135,136] Since the hormone melatonin is both a powerful antioxidant and a regulator of the sleep–wake cycle, it has received attention within the COPD research community for its potential to target these two important aspects of the disease.[137,138] Observational data indicate that melatonin levels decline and oxidative stress increases during COPD exacerbations.[135] Clinical trials have shown that administering 3 mg of melatonin to COPD patients improves sleep quality and attenuates oxidative stress.[136,139,140]

## Life Extension Suggestions

- **Vitamin D:** 5000–8000 IU daily, depending on blood levels of 25-OH-vitamin D
- **Vitamin A:** 5000 IU
- **Vitamin C:** 1000–2000 mg daily
- **Natural vitamin E:** 100–400 IU alpha-tocopherol and 200 mg gamma-tocopherol daily
- **N-acetyl-cysteine** (NAC): 600–1800 mg daily
- **Panax ginseng:** 200 mg daily
- **Broccoli extract:** 400 mg daily for individuals weighing up to 160 lbs; 800 mg daily for individuals weighing over 160 lbs
- **Coenzyme Q10** (as ubiquinol): 100–300 mg daily
- **Fish oil** (with olive polyphenols): providing 1400 mg EPA and 1000 mg DHA daily
- **Boswellia serrata extract** (standardized to 20% AKBA): 100 mg daily
- **Resveratrol:** 250 mg daily
- **Zinc:** 30 mg daily
- **L-carnitine:** 500–2000 mg daily
- **Whey protein isolate:** 20–40 g daily
- **Melatonin:** 0.3–5 mg before bed (sometimes up to 10 mg)

In addition, the following blood test may provide helpful information:

- Coenzyme Q10

## REFERENCES

References available at: www.lef.org/dpt5/ch42

# 43

# Cirrhosis and Liver Disease

The liver is the largest organ in the body, weighing up to 2.5% of total lean body mass. Located in the upper right quadrant of the abdomen, the liver varies in size and shape, depending on each person's anatomy. Its main function is to metabolize substances in the blood in preparation for excretion, although it has many other important functions, including synthesis of most essential proteins, production of bile, and regulation of nutrients such as glucose, cholesterol, and amino acids.

The main type of liver cell is called a hepatocyte. These cells comprise about two-thirds of the liver's mass. The liver's blood supply comes from the hepatic artery, which supplies oxygen-rich blood. The liver also receives blood from the portal vein, which filters blood from the stomach, intestines, pancreas, and spleen.

The most common liver function tests are enzyme, bilirubin, albumin, and prothrombin time (PT) tests. The liver contains thousands of enzymes, only a few of which are routinely measured as indicators of liver function. These enzymes include the following.

- **Alkaline phosphatase (ALP).** Abnormal levels may indicate bile obstruction, liver injury, or some forms of cancer.
- **Alanine transaminase (ALT).** Abnormal levels may indicate hepatitis or other liver cell injury.
- **Aspartate transaminase (AST).** Abnormal levels may indicate injury to the liver, heart, muscle, or brain.
- **Gamma-glutamyl transpeptidase (GGT).** Abnormal levels may indicate organ damage, drug toxicity, alcohol abuse, or pancreatic disease.
- **Lactic dehydrogenase (LDH).** Abnormal levels may indicate damage to the liver, heart, or lung, and excessive breakdown of red blood cells.
- **5´-nucleotidase.** Abnormal levels may indicate impaired bile flow.

The other major liver tests include the serum bilirubin test, which measures bile excretion, and the albumin test, which can indicate liver damage. Finally, the PT test measures the time needed for blood to clot. Because most blood clotting factors are produced in the liver, and they have rapid turnover, this test can help measure the liver's ability to synthesize cells. Prothrombin may be elevated in hepatitis and cirrhosis as well as in disorders related to vitamin K deficiency.

Taken together, these tests provide physicians with a relatively complete picture of liver function and can help diagnose liver disease.

## FORMS OF LIVER DISEASE

The many possible liver diseases can be grouped loosely into three categories: hepatocellular diseases, cholestatic diseases, and mixed forms. In hepatocellular diseases, the liver is typically inflamed and shows signs of injury. Over time, liver cells may begin to die. Causes of hepatocellular liver disease include alcoholic cirrhosis and viral hepatitis, both of which attack liver cells directly. In cholestatic diseases, the flow of fluid through the liver is blocked by such things as gall stones, liver cancer, or biliary cirrhosis. In mixed forms of liver disease, both conditions are present.

The pattern and onset of symptoms can help physicians determine what kind of liver disease is present. Symptoms of liver disease include jaundice, fatigue, itching, pain in the upper abdomen, distention of the abdomen, and intestinal bleeding. However, many forms of liver disease have no symptoms and are diagnosed only during routine blood tests that detect abnormalities in the markers of liver function.

Cirrhosis is an end-stage liver disease. It is characterized by chronic injury to the liver cells, fibrosis (scarring) within the liver, and the formation of regenerative nodules. The causes of cirrhosis include the following.

### Alcohol Consumption

Excess alcohol consumption is a primary cause of cirrhosis. However, only 10–20% of alcoholics develop cirrhosis.[1]

Alcohol lowers the liver's levels of antioxidants, including vitamin E[2,3] and S-adenosyl-L-methionine (SAMe),[4] making the liver vulnerable. In addition, alcohol lowers glutathione, an important internal antioxidant.[5,6]

Because heavy drinkers consume a substantial number of calories as alcohol, they consume less vitamin- and mineral-rich food than they otherwise might, exacerbating alcohol-induced nutritional deficiencies. Virtually all individuals with alcoholic hepatitis suffer from malnutrition to a degree more or less proportional to the severity of their disease.[7]

Survival in alcoholics with moderate or severe hepatitis is directly proportional to how much food they consume. Mortality drops to zero in those consuming 3000 or more calories during treatment.[8] Similar results were seen with alcoholic cirrhosis patients, except for the most severely malnourished, who may have been too compromised to recover.[9–11]

In addition to antioxidant depletion, alcoholics tend to have a number of other nutritional deficiencies. These include low levels of vitamin C, riboflavin, zinc, pyridoxine (vitamin B6), and vitamin A.[12–17]

## Hepatitis

Hepatitis, another common cause of liver cirrhosis, is caused by infection with the hepatitis B or C virus. Because the symptoms of infection are mild and flu-like, viral hepatitis often goes undiagnosed. Blood donors sometimes find out they are infected when their donated blood undergoes routine screening. Viral hepatitis causes chronic liver inflammation, which results in cirrhosis in the majority of those infected.

## Nonalcoholic Fatty Liver Disease

The most common cause of fatty liver disease is alcohol consumption, but it can also be caused by a number of other conditions, including obesity, diabetes, and elevated triglyceride levels. If the condition is associated with obesity, it is sometimes called nonalcoholic fatty liver disease (NAFLD). Up to one-third of patients with NAFLD also have type 2 diabetes, high cholesterol levels, or both. NAFLD is closely associated with metabolic syndrome, a related cluster of conditions including obesity, diabetes, elevated triglycerides, and high blood pressure, which is considered a major risk factor for heart attack. Fatty liver disease is exacerbated by inflammation within the liver, which may hasten its progression to cirrhosis.

## Biliary Cirrhosis

Biliary cirrhosis results from prolonged obstruction of or injury to the biliary system. One of the liver's functions is to secrete bile, which is used in the gut in the normal breakdown and absorption of fats from the diet, among other things. Primary biliary cirrhosis, which has no known cause, is characterized by inflammation of the liver and destruction of liver bile ducts by scar tissue. It is associated with various autoimmune diseases, such as Raynaud's phenomenon.

## Cardiac Cirrhosis

Cardiac cirrhosis occurs when prolonged, severe right-sided congestive heart failure leads to chronic liver injury, inflammation, and the formation of scar tissue in the liver (fibrosis). The heart cannot handle the venous circulation, causing blood to back up in the body's major veins. Eventually, the liver becomes engorged and swollen.

## Inherited Disorders

Various inherited disorders can cause cirrhosis.

Whatever the cause of cirrhosis, it is a difficult disease to manage in its advanced stages, in part because of the complications that it causes. For example, people suffering from cirrhosis also frequently suffer from portal hypertension (ie, elevated blood pressure in the vein that drains into the liver). This, in turn, can cause complications in the stomach and esophagus, such as ascites. Portal hypertension occurs in about 60% of cirrhosis cases in the United States.[18] The treatment of portal hypertension often focuses on relieving the underlying liver disease. In serious cases, drugs such as diuretics might be prescribed to reduce blood pressure.

Cirrhosis may entail other complications:

- **Esophageal varices.** Portal hypertension can cause varicose veins in the esophagus. They can rupture, requiring emergency surgery.

- **Ascites.** The pressure created by portal hypertension can also cause the liver and intestines to exude fluid into the abdominal cavity, which can become swollen and distended, a condition known as ascites.

- **Hepatoma.** A compromised liver is more susceptible to cancer. Hepatocellular carcinoma occurs in about 10–20% of cirrhotic patients.[19] Liver cancer is relatively asymptomatic. It is usually not detected until it has progressed significantly. Consequently, the patient's prognosis is usually poor.

- **Hepatic encephalopathy.** This is a complex condition characterized by psychological and personality disturbances. Its specific cause is unknown; in serious cases, it can result in coma or death.

While cirrhosis is irreversible, it is usually the result of a chronic condition and thus takes a long time to develop. In fact, many people with developing liver disease (eg, fibrotic livers) have no symptoms, and their condition is detected only by routine blood tests. If the condition is detected early enough, the patient may have an opportunity to arrest the cirrhotic process before it goes too far.

As is the case with many other diseases, cirrhosis is characterized by inflammation (hepatitis literally means "inflammation of the liver"). This liver inflammation is often caused by a rise in free radicals within the liver. Under normal circumstances, the liver maintains a supply of internal antioxidants to neutralize the free radicals generated by the toxins processed in the liver. However, when the liver antioxidants are low, or when the liver is overwhelmed by continued toxic insults (eg, alcohol or chronic drug use), damage from free radicals increases, resulting in inflammation and the formation of scar tissue (fibrosis). Thus, it is important to maintain a healthy supply of antioxidants and make positive lifestyle changes, such as abstaining from all alcohol and avoiding environmental toxins whenever possible, to reduce the strain on the liver.

If cirrhosis is allowed to progress and the liver's function is compromised beyond repair, the only solution is a liver transplant. This is a complicated medical procedure with a significant risk of organ rejection, and even in successful cases, lifelong follow-up therapy with immunosuppressant drugs will be necessary.

## DIAGNOSIS OF LIVER DISEASE AND CIRRHOSIS

The symptoms of cirrhosis may be insidious, or there may be no symptoms at all for many years. If symptoms are present, they can include jaundice (yellowing of the eyes and skin), lethargy, bleeding from varices, and spidery veins under the skin.

While it can be difficult to diagnose liver disease by its symptoms alone, early liver damage is often apparent from blood test results. Standard blood tests of liver enzymes or bilirubin may show a suspicious elevation as well as alert the clinician to the possibility of liver dysfunction.

The deposition of fat in the liver (such as in fatty liver disease) can also be detected by diagnostic imaging techniques, such as computed tomography scanning, ultrasound, and magnetic resonance imaging.

## TREATMENT OF LIVER DISEASE

The treatment goal with regard to the liver is to prevent liver disease and, if diagnosed, to stop its progression toward cirrhosis. Cirrhosis is an end-stage disease with a poor prognosis and can require a liver transplant if liver failure occurs. Thus, lifestyle changes that support liver health, especially abstention from alcohol, are the cornerstone of treatment for liver disease. No matter the cause of cirrhosis, alcohol aggravates the condition and should be avoided.

In addition, physicians will attempt to treat the complications of cirrhosis, including portal hypertension and ascites, with various medications. In general, however, the use of medications must be approached with caution in people with liver disease because the liver metabolizes many of these substances. For example, aspirin should be avoided in patients with cirrhosis because of its effects on coagulation and the gastric mucosa.[18] The following conventional medicines are often prescribed to treat cirrhosis or fibrotic liver disease:

- **Corticosteroids.** These drugs have been shown to reduce the inflammation that characterizes liver disease. While they may be helpful to patients with alcoholic hepatitis and encephalopathy, they are less helpful to patients with alcoholic cirrhosis.[18,20,21]
- **Ursodiol.** Among people with biliary cirrhosis, this drug replaces lost biliary acids. Side effects are rare. This drug may not halt progression of the disease.[18]

### WHAT YOU HAVE LEARNED SO FAR

- The liver is the largest internal organ. It filters the blood from the digestive system, metabolizing toxins and monitoring nutrients such as glucose and cholesterol.
- Liver disease often develops over years, without obvious symptoms. Many people are diagnosed with liver disease after abnormalities are detected during routine blood tests.
- Cirrhosis occurs when the liver is inflamed and scar tissue forms. It is irreversible; thus prevention of liver disease is ideal. Cirrhosis can be caused by alcohol consumption, hepatitis, right-sided heart failure, and other conditions.
- Antioxidants, which neutralize the toxins processed by the liver, are an important element in liver health.
- Treatment of liver disease is limited because many drugs are metabolized by the liver; thus only a few drugs, including corticosteroids, which have significant side effects, are routinely used to treat liver disease.

## NUTRITIONAL AND SUPPLEMENTAL SUPPORT

Because they are often metabolized in the liver, nutritional supplements (like conventional pharmaceuticals) should be used with caution by people with liver diseases. It is important that people with liver disease work in close cooperation with a knowledgeable and qualified physician to design a program of nutritional support.

Nevertheless, there have been numerous nutritional approaches studied that can help slow the inflammation associated with advancing liver disease and support healthy liver function. For more detailed information, please see the Inflammation (Chronic) protocol. It is also critical that alcohol be strictly avoided.

The following nutrients have been shown to enhance liver function and reduce inflammation.

## Fish Oil

Omega-3 fatty acids and sesame lignans have been shown to reduce inflammation, which is a distinctive feature of liver disease and cirrhosis.[22–27]

Studies have shown that reducing the ratio of omega-6 to omega-3 fatty acids prevents liver damage induced by total parenteral (intravenous) nutrition in newborn piglets, rats, and humans.[28–31] Thus, it may be prudent for patients with cirrhosis to take fish oil supplements and lower their consumption of omega-6 fats, such as those found in corn oil.

It is important that any increase in fatty acids be accompanied by an increase in vitamin E. Without supplemental vitamin E, even fish oil can be detrimental. Diets containing 35% of calories from fish oil are likely to exacerbate liver damage due to alcohol and other toxins because fish oil's polyunsaturated bonds are so readily oxidized by free radicals.[32,33,34]

Monounsaturated oils, such as olive oil, should be the major source of fat calories for those with cirrhotic liver disease. Monounsaturated oils are preferable since saturated fats from animal sources usually contain considerable amounts of arachidonic acid, the precursor to inflammatory prostaglandins. For those whose main source of fat calories is animal fat, supplementation with eicosapentaenoic acid (EPA) may help reduce the buildup of proinflammatory arachidonic acid and reduce levels of inflammatory mediators.[22]

In addition to using olive oil instead of corn oil or animal fats, people with liver disease would most likely benefit from supplementation with a dose of fish oil high enough to inhibit inflammatory prostaglandin synthesis without providing a significant target for reactive oxygen species (ROS). While more work is needed to determine how much fish oil is too much, the nutrition studies cited above suggest that supplementation with fish oil should be limited to about 10% of total calories.[35] Also, maintaining high levels of antioxidant nutrients such as vitamin E will help limit oxidant damage from polyunsaturated fats.

## S-Adenosylmethionine (SAMe)

By increasing oxidative stress, many liver toxins (eg, alcohol and acetaminophen) deplete glutathione and other important antioxidant molecules. As a result, SAMe, a glutathione precursor, is also decreased.[36] In both rodents and nonhuman primates, depletion of antioxidants occurs at early stages of liver disease. Supplementation with SAMe restores levels of glutathione and decreases liver damage in animals; it has been recommended as an area of study for humans with early liver disease or chronic exposure to liver toxins, including alcohol.[36,37]

In one clinical trial, 123 patients with alcoholic liver cirrhosis were given either a placebo or 1200 mg daily of oral SAMe. At the end of the 2-year trial, 30% of the placebo-treated patients had died, compared with 16% of the SAMe group. When patients with the most severe disease were excluded from the calculation, these numbers became 29% in the placebo group and 12% in the SAMe group.[38] The livers of those patients with the most advanced cirrhosis may have been too damaged to respond to the SAMe.

## Polyenylphosphatidylcholine (PPC)

Phosphatidylcholine is produced in the liver through a process involving SAMe. Supplementing alcohol-treated rats or baboons with PPC during alcohol feeding prevents the depletion of SAMe.[39]

In rats, PPC treatment accelerated regression of preexisting fibrosis.[40] In a baboon study, none of the animals fed 2.8 g PPC per 1000 calories (about 2 g daily per 20 kg body weight) developed fibrosis or cirrhosis, even after 6.5 years of alcohol feeding, whereas 10 out of 12 untreated baboons developed fibrosis or cirrhosis.[41] In addition to preventing alcohol-induced oxidative stress, PPC stimulates the enzyme responsible for the breakdown of liver collagen.[41]

Among humans, 2 years of treatment of alcoholic cirrhosis patients with 4.5 g daily of PPC resulted in favorable changes in two blood parameters of liver damage, bilirubin and liver transaminases, among certain subgroups. Fibrosis, however, continued to progress, leading the authors to conclude that while PPC is effective in preventing liver damage among animals, it is less effective among humans with long histories of drinking.[42]

## Silymarin

A standardized plant extract from milk thistle, silymarin contains about 60% silibinin.[43] Silymarin appears to inhibit the formation of mediators of inflammation, such as leukotrienes.[44] In animal studies, silymarin protected the liver from carbon tetrachloride damage and slowed the accumulation of scar tissue in the biliary tract.[43,45,46] In baboons, silymarin slowed the progression of alcohol-induced liver fibrosis.[47]

Some placebo-controlled human trials have shown promising results. In one study, mortality was 39% among alcoholic cirrhosis patients treated with Legalon (a proprietary standardized product containing 70–80% silymarin) after 24–41 months. Mortality was 58% in placebo-treated patients.[48] In another clinical study, this same silymarin preparation normalized blood levels of bilirubin and other markers of liver disease after 6 months.[49] Favorable changes in blood chemistry were noticed in as little as 4 weeks.[50]

Improvements were also observed with a silymarin-phospholipid complex in patients with chronic active hepatitis.[51] Recently, an Italian firm developed a proprietary preparation of silibinin complexed with both vitamin E and phospholipids. The complex successfully protected rat livers against necrosis and inhibited collagen formation in rats after bile duct obstruction.[52]

## Antioxidants

Since cirrhosis is the result of chronic injury to the liver from free radicals, antioxidant therapy may slow the progression of the disease. Studies have found that people with cirrhosis have low levels of vitamin C and vitamin E.[53]

In one remarkable study, patients with hepatitis C were given 7 oral antioxidants, glycyrrhizin (500 mg twice daily), schisandra (500 mg 3 times daily), silymarin (250 mg 3 times daily), ascorbate (2 g 3 times daily), lipoic acid (150 mg twice daily), L-glutathione (150 mg twice daily), and alpha-tocopherol (800 IU daily) for 20 weeks. Four different intravenous antioxidant preparations, including glycyrrhizin (120 mg), ascorbic acid (10 g), L-glutathione (750 mg), and B-complex (1 mL; composition not specified), were also administered twice weekly for the first 10 weeks. No significant side effects were observed. Normalization of liver enzymes, which indicated reduced liver injury, occurred in 44% of patients. One-fourth of the patients showed viral load decreases of 90% or more. Histologic improvement was noted in 36% of patients.[54]

Consistent with these findings, an Italian study demonstrated that eating foods high in antioxidants (fruits and vegetables) decreased the progression of cirrhosis, while a high level of fatty animal products and sugar from nonfruit sources increased it.[55]

Animal products are high in arachidonic acid, a precursor to inflammatory mediators such as prostaglandins and leukotrienes, and sugars from nonfruit sources are more likely to increase insulin levels because fiber is not present to slow the absorption of sugar. High insulin levels stimulate the conversion of arachidonic acid into inflammatory prostaglandins. The resulting inflammation generates high levels of ROS. Thus, cirrhotic patients should avoid nonfruit sources of sugar or consume additional fiber when nonfruit sugars are consumed.

Selenium, a potent antioxidant, appears to protect against hepatic cancers. In a 4-year trial, selenium-enhanced table salt reduced primary liver cancer 35% in study participants compared with controls. In a study involving hepatitis B patients, one 200-mcg tablet of selenium daily reduced the incidence of primary liver cancer to zero. When selenium supplementation ceased, primary liver cancer incidence began to rise, indicating that hepatic carcinoma risk may be minimized with selenium supplementation.[56]

## N-Acetylcysteine (NAC)

NAC is a slightly modified version of the sulfur-containing amino acid cysteine. When taken internally, NAC replenishes intracellular levels of the natural antioxidant glutathione (GSH), helping to restore cells' ability to fight damage from ROS.[57]

## Schisandra and Melon Pulp Concentrate

As the body loses its natural primary antioxidant mechanisms, it accumulates lipid peroxidation products, and liver mitochondria begin to fail. Purified extract from a non-GMO *Cucumis melo* melon has been found to be rich in superoxide dismutase (SOD), the first enzyme in your body's mitochondrial oxidant protection system.[58,59] Melon-derived SOD quickly converts primary free oxygen radicals into hydrogen peroxide. That hydrogen peroxide must be rapidly converted into water to complete the mitochondrial oxidant detoxification process. That task is handled by a second liver-protective agent, an extract of the Chinese vine *Schisandra chinensis*.

Schisandra extract has been known to protect liver function for more than four decades,[60] but it is only recently that we have learned that it does so by boosting mitochondrial antioxidant function.[61] In that fashion, the extract confers powerful protection against a host of oxidative liver toxins (including mercury).[61–67]

In an open label trial of 56 patients with acute or chronic hepatitis, cirrhosis, or fatty liver (steatosis), 22.5 mg per day of schisandrins resulted in decreased serum markers of liver cell injury, even in patients with cirrhosis.[68] A placebo-controlled study of the same extract formulation in patients with chronic hepatitis (a condition that imposes extreme oxidant stress on liver tissue) resulted in significant decreases in liver damage markers after just 1 week.[68] Neither study detected any side effects of the extract.

## Branched-Chain Amino Acids

Branched-chain amino acids (BCAAs) are essential amino acids (ie, must be obtained in the diet because the human body cannot make them). BCAAs include leucine, isoleucine, and valine. Cirrhotic patients have an increased energy requirement that BCAAs seem to fill better than glucose or amino acids.[69] Supplementing the diet with these amino acids lowers hospital admission rates and improves nutritional parameters, liver function tests, and overall quality of life in patients with liver disease.[70] In addition, supplementing with BCAAs after surgery for hepatic carcinoma shortens hospital stays and improves the return of liver function.[71] Encephalopathy is also alleviated after treatment with BCAAs.[72]

## Life Extension Suggestions

- **Polyenylphosphatidylcholine (PPC):** 1800–2700 mg daily
- **Branched-chain amino acids (BCAAs):** 2400 mg daily
- **Milk thistle, standardized extract:** 750 mg daily
- **L-glutathione:** 250–500 mg daily
- **N-acetyl-cysteine (NAC):** 600–1800 mg daily

- **S-adenosylmethionine (SAMe):** 1200 mg daily
- **B-complex vitamin including:**
  - **Thiamine** (B1): 100 mg
  - **Riboflavin** (B2): 50 mg
  - **Niacin:** 200 mg
  - **Vitamin B6:** 75 mg
  - **Folate** (preferably as L-methylfolate): 800 mcg
  - **Vitamin B12:** 1000 mcg
  - **Biotin:** 600 mcg
  - **Pantothenic acid:** 1000 mg
  - **Choline:** 45 mg
  - **Inositol:** 250 mg
  - **Para-aminobenzoic acid (PABA):** 100 mg
- **Vitamin C** (ascorbic acid): 6000 mg daily
- **Vitamin E** (as high gamma tocopherol mix with sesame lignans): 359 mg daily
- **Selenium:** 200 mcg daily
- **Fish oil,** with olive polyphenols: providing 1400 mg EPA and 1000 mg DHA daily
- **Schisandra chinensis standardized extract:** 250 mg daily
- **Melon pulp concentrate:** 10 mg daily
- **Soluble fiber:** 2000–6000 mg daily

## REFERENCES

References available at: www.lef.org/dpt5/ch43

# 44

---

# *Colorectal Cancer*

---

Colorectal cancer remains the second most common cause of cancer death in the United States, although as much as 70% of cases thought to be *preventable* through moderate dietary and lifestyle modifications.[1,2]

The colorectal cancer mortality rate has consistently declined in recent decades due largely to enhanced accuracy of early detection techniques, such as colonoscopy. However, the outlook for colon cancer patients rapidly diminishes if the cancer has metastasized to other organs or lymph nodes before detection.

If the cancer is detected while still localized in the colon, it is removed surgically and adjuvant techniques may be employed postsurgery to improve the chance for sustained disease-free survival. Treatment for advanced metastatic colon cancer usually encompasses multiagent chemotherapy accompanied by palliative radiation.

Unfortunately, conventional standardized chemotherapy regimens may be ineffective for some patients due to genetic resistance against the drugs employed. Further, rarely do mainstream oncologists implement *nutritional therapeutics* or novel drug strategies to target genetic abnormalities associated with colon cancer growth, despite the fact that many peer-reviewed studies highlight the potential value of these agents.

Investigations have shown that several factors such as dietary habits, nutritional status, and *inflammation* influence the genetics involved in colon cancer development and progression, thus revealing multiple targets of interest in the prevention and management of colon cancer.

For example, a review of 9 studies found that for every 10 ng/mL *increase* in serum *vitamin D*, the relative risk of colorectal cancer *decreased 15%*.[3] Another landmark trial revealed that daily *low-dose aspirin* reduced the risk of developing colon cancer by 24% and the risk of dying from the disease by 35%.[4]

In recent years, the introduction of advanced cancer analytical technology such as *circulating tumor cell testing* and *chemosensitivity assays* has improved outlook considerably by paving the way toward individually tailored treatments based on the unique cellular characteristics of each patient's cancer.

In this protocol, you will learn about several *unappreciated* risk factors for colorectal cancer, and gain insight into several genetic and molecular mechanisms that drive the evolution from healthy cells to cancerous cells in the colon. You will also discover *evidence-based* methods for targeting these risk factors and carcinogenic mechanisms using natural compounds and novel drug strategies. Life Extension will also present resources and guidance for thoroughly analyzing the unique biological characteristics of your cancer cells, which is a critical step towards establishing an effective, personalized cancer treatment regimen.

## ABOUT THE COLON

The colon is the third-to-last section of the gastrointestinal tract in humans, followed by the rectum and anus. Food is mostly digested by the time it reaches the colon, so the role of this segment of the large bowel is to absorb water, some short chain fatty acids from plant fiber and undigested starch, sodium, and chloride, and compact waste to be eliminated during defecation. Moreover, colonic bacteria play a central role in metabolic detoxification by secreting chemicals that encourage excretion of toxins and pathogens. Beneficial bacteria in the colon (*probiotics*) also ferment dietary fiber and generate compounds, such as *butyrate*, which nourish cells in the colon wall and protect against carcinogenesis.

## CAUSES OF AND RISK FACTORS FOR COLON CANCER

Risk factors for colorectal cancer include age (90% is found in those over 50), personal history of polyps or adenomas, family history of colorectal cancer, and diagnosis of inflammatory bowel disease (IBD) (Crohn's or ulcerative colitis). Other risks include a diet high in fat or low in fruits and vegetables, physical inactivity, obesity, smoking, and excessive alcohol consumption.[5]

### Lifestyle

As mentioned in the introduction of this protocol, as much as 70% of colon cancers are thought to be *preventable* through diet and lifestyle modification.[1]

Factors such as diet, physical activity level, tobacco use, alcohol consumption, and sleep patterns are associated with increased risk of colorectal cancers.[6] Obesity and physical inactivity are known to increase biomarkers of inflammatory processes, such as fecal *calprotectin* and serum *C-reactive protein* (CRP). Elevated levels of inflammation are linked with higher rates of colorectal cancer. Simple changes such as increasing consumption of dietary fiber and vegetables effectively suppress inflammatory markers blunt colon cancer risk.[7]

A colon cancer treatment or prevention plan should start with foundational lifestyle measures that include physical activity and a diet rich in plant foods; patients should also strive to attain a healthy body weight.

## Genetics and Family History

Genetic alterations, both inherited and noninherited, are responsible for the carcinogenic process in colon cancer. About 75% of colorectal cancers are "sporadic," meaning that they arise in those without any family history of this disease, while the remaining 25% have an inherited predisposition that raises risk.[8]

Two familial disorders raise risk significantly: *familial adenomatous polyposis* (FAP) and *hereditary nonpolyposis colon cancer* (HNPCC, or Lynch syndrome). These inherited disorders are responsible for 1–2% and 3–5% of all colorectal cancers, respectively.

Familial adenomatous polyposis syndrome causes hundreds to thousands of polyps to form before age 30 and often leads to colon cancer at a young age (average age 39 years). Familial adenomatous polyposis arises from inherited mutations of the adenomatous polyposis coli (APC) gene, a gene mutation that is also present in 60–80% of sporadic colon cancers.

Hereditary nonpolyposis colon cancer does not cause the multitude of polyps, but polyps are much more likely to become cancerous in those with this disorder. Those with hereditary nonpolyposis colon cancer have mutated *mismatch repair genes* (MMR genes), which fail to make necessary corrections to errors in DNA replication, allowing mistakes in the DNA to accumulate and colon cancer to ensue.

## Metabolic Syndrome and Inactivity

Higher levels of insulin and glucose in the blood can increase the risk of developing colorectal cancers.[9] An analysis of clinical data from 1966 through 2005 found that a diagnosis of diabetes *raised* the risk of colon cancer by more than 30% in both men and women.[10]

A recent study, which looked at much of the previous data on diabetes and risk of colon cancer, concluded that diabetes is an independent risk factor for developing colon cancer.[11]

The link between elevated insulin levels and colon cancer may be mediated through the *insulin-like growth factor-1 receptor* (IGF-1R). Insulin activates IGF-1R, which in turn functions to stimulate cellular growth and proliferation. Overexpression of IGF-1R has been observed in colon cancer cells, suggesting an increased sensitivity to the growth-promoting effects of insulin.[2]

Obesity is a risk factor for developing cancers in general, and studies show that reducing weight can reduce inflammation in the colon, thereby reducing risk of colorectal cancers.[12] Adipose tissue (fat tissue) is not simply an inert storage system for excess calories—it actively produces many *adipokines*, or chemical messengers, that circulate throughout the body. One such adipokine, *leptin*, is linked specifically to the increased risk of developing colon cancer.[13]

Regular physical activity, which combats all the components of metabolic syndrome, is associated with a decreased risk for colorectal cancer as well. One study compared those who did not have a sedentary job with those that worked a sedentary job for ≥10 years; the risk of cancer arising in the left (distal) colon was doubled, and the risk of developing rectal cancer increased 44%.[14]

## Inflammation

People with chronic inflammatory conditions of the bowel, such as Crohn's disease or ulcerative colitis (UC), have up to a 6 times greater risk of developing colon cancer than those without the conditions.[15] However, the inflammatory process is involved in the development of colorectal cancer growths even in those without Crohn's or ulcerative colitis.[16,17]

**Cyclooxygenase-2.** Cyclooxygenase-2 (COX-2) is an enzyme that produces inflammatory end products by converting the omega-6 fatty acid *arachidonic acid* into *prostaglandin E2*, which promotes growth of cancerous cells; COX-2 is often overexpressed in colon cancer. Aspirin blocks COX-2 and has been shown to also lessen the development of colorectal cancers.[18]

**5-Lipoxygenase.** Lipoxygenase (5-LOX), similar to COX-2, metabolizes *arachidonic acid* into metabolites that drive development and progression of cancer. In colorectal cancer, 5-LOX expression was shown to correlate with the density of blood vessel growth within tumors.[19] Moreover, 5-LOX is overexpressed in precancerous polyps, and inhibition of 5-LOX caused a suppression of tumor growth in a murine colorectal cancer model.[20] A compound extracted from *Boswellia serrata*, called 3-O-acetyl-11-keto-β-boswellic acid (AKBA), is a powerful inhibitor of 5-LOX and may modulate the cellular properties of colorectal malignancies.[21,22]

For a complete discussion of the roles of COX-2 and 5-LOX in cancer development and progression, see the protocol "Cancer Treatment: The Critical Factors" protocol.

More recently, *nuclear factor-kappa B* (NF-κB), a proinflammatory mediator that influences more than 500 genes involved in proliferation, angiogenesis, immune evasion and metastatic spread, has been the topic of intense research. Not surprisingly, NF-κB is a target for thwarting cancer's growth and many natural agents act on NF-κB to prevent its signaling. The most notable natural agent able to suppress NF-κB signal transmission is *curcumin*.[23] High intake of curcumin, and resultant inhibition of NF-κB, may be one reason that the incidence of colon cancer in India is so much lower than in the United States or Europe.[24]

## Low Vitamin D Levels

More akin to a hormone than a vitamin, vitamin D broadly influences the genome by activating the vitamin-D receptor in the cell nucleus. Activation of the vitamin D receptor is estimated to modulate as many as 2000 genes, many of which are related to inflammation and cellular mutation—initial drivers in all cancers.[25]

As mentioned in the introduction of this protocol, a review of 9 studies found that for every 10 ng/mL increase in serum vitamin D, the relative risk of colorectal cancer decreases 15%.[3] These findings are consistent with the conclusion of a large, case–control study across 10 European countries, which also found that as vitamin D blood levels rose, the risk for colorectal cancer declined considerably. Compared with those in the lowest quintile (1/5th) (<10 ng/mL), those in the highest (>40 ng/ml) had a 40% *lower* risk of developing colorectal cancer.[26]

Individuals with colon cancer appear to have lower levels of vitamin D at the time of diagnosis as well. Serum vitamin D levels were insufficient (<29 ng/mL) in 82% of patients with stage IV colon cancer at the time of diagnosis.[27]

Low levels of vitamin D may adversely impact prognosis as well. One large study found an inverse association between serum *25-hydroxyvitamin D* at the time of diagnosis and colon cancer mortality.[28] Individuals with *25-hydroxyvitamin D* levels *over* 32 ng/mL had a 72% reduction in mortality compared to those with blood levels *less than* 20 ng/mL.

Life Extension encourages the maintenance of serum 25-hydroxyvitamin D levels between 50 and 80 ng/mL for optimal health. This typically necessitates supplementation with 5000–8000 IU of vitamin D daily, but supplemental doses should always be determined by blood test results.

## Low Folate and B-Vitamin Intake

Homocysteine is an indirect marker for folate, B6, and B12 status. Homocysteine can be high when there is a deficiency in any of these B vitamins. Folate deficiency is associated with greater risk of developing colorectal cancers. In a large pooled analysis of data from 13 prospective studies including over 725 000 subjects, the highest quintile of folate intake was associated with a 15% reduced risk of colon cancer compared to the lowest quintile of intake.[29]

## PATHOLOGY AND TUMOROGENESIS

Colorectal cancers begin with *epithelial cells* that line the surface of the colon along finger-like projections called *villi*. The spaces between the villi are called *crypts*, and at the base of each crypt are immature stem cells that give rise to ever-renewing cells that migrate up the crypt and toward the tips of the villi. This normal cellular process is strictly governed by a balance of cellular renewal (normal proliferation) and cellular death (apoptosis), as well as elegantly choreographed expression of various genes along the path from immature stem cells to mature epithelial cells.

Early in the course of colon cancer development, however, the normal renewal of cells is disturbed. Cellular maturation (differentiation) is blocked and apoptosis is impaired leading to an accumulation of immature cells in the crypts. This is called an "aberrant crypt," and it is the first step in the carcinogenic process of colorectal cancers.[30,31] These aberrant crypts almost always involve a genetic pathway that both embryos and colon cancer have in common, a pathway called *Wnt*.[32] Many natural agents exert protective action through influencing this Wnt pathway, including components of *black tea*,[33] *green tea*,[34] and *turmeric*.[35]

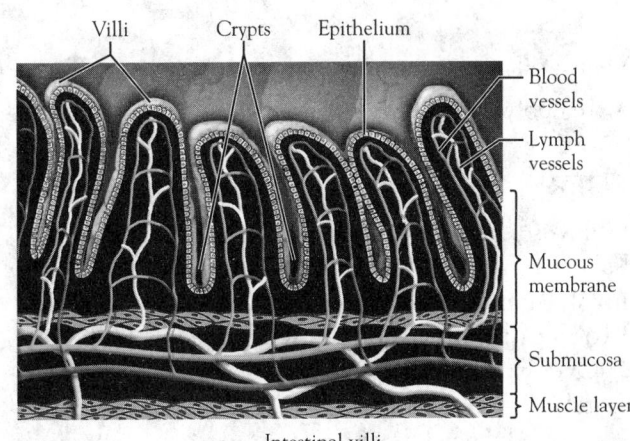

Intestinal villi

Once the aberrant crypt forms, it may go on to become a polyp, which is a growth along the lining of the colon that can be seen during a colonoscopy exam. Polyps are benign, but they can progress to adenomas, which are considered precancerous. If further mutations occur, an adenoma can then progress to cancer over years or decades. This is the primary reason that screening colonoscopies are recommended, to remove the polyps or adenomas before they have a chance to become cancer.

## Genetic Abnormalities in Colorectal Cancer

Several genes and/or genetic processes are frequently malfunctional in colon cancer cells, and therefore have become intriguing targets for treatment interventions. Some dietary compounds have been shown to influence these genes and may modulate colon cancer development and progression.

## KRAS

KRAS is a gene that orchestrates cellular receptor sensitivity to a number of growth factors. When KRAS is activated, cellular proliferation is enhanced, while deactivated KRAS slows proliferation. In several types of cancer, including colorectal cancer, KRAS is mutated in such a way that causes it to be chronically activated, leading to unabated cellular proliferation. Mutations in KRAS are present in up to 40% of colorectal cancers.[2]

While drugs that *directly* target KRAS are not yet available, the mutational status of this gene helps determine the likelihood that certain anticancer agents will be effective. For example, the anti–epidermal growth factor receptor (EGFR) antibodies cetuximab and panitumumab may be ineffective if activating mutations in KRAS are present.[36]

Several natural compounds have been shown to target the KRAS pathway, including the following:

- Perillyl alcohol, a substance extracted from citrus fruits[37,38]
- Curcumin[39]
- Fish oil[40]
- Tea polyphenols[41]

## EGFR

EGFR is a protein expressed on the surface of epithelial cells that variably regulates a number of pathways involved in cellular growth and proliferation. The KRAS pathway is among those affected by EGFR.

Overexpression of EGFR is observed in approximately 65–70% of colon cancers, and is associated with an advanced disease stage.[2]

Activation of EGFR stimulates KRAS-induced signal transduction leading to proliferation. However, in KRAS mutant (upregulation; overexpression) cancer cells, binding of EGFR is not necessary to activate KRAS. Therefore, medications sometimes used to treat colon cancer, called anti-EGFR antibodies, are only effective in patients not harboring a KRAS mutation.[42] For example, *cetuximab* is a monoclonal antibody against EGFR indicated for metastatic colorectal cancer in patients *not* carrying a KRAS mutation.

Natural compounds shown to modulate EGFR include:

- Genistein (an isoflavone from soy)[43]
- Curcumin[44]
- American ginseng[45]

**Note:** *Targeting EGFR directly may not be beneficial in a colorectal cancer patient overexpressing KRAS (constitutional activation). However, the aforementioned nutrients may also influence transcription downstream of EGFR and KRAS; thus they may be capable of inducing cell cycle arrest in KRAS mutant or wild type cancer cells. For example, curcumin was shown to act synergistically with dasatinib to reduce KRAS mutant colon cancer cell viability through alternative pathways[39]; the other nutrients likely target additional pathways as well.*

## Microsatellite Instability and Mismatch Repair Mutations

The human genome contains thousands of short, repeated base pair sequences called *microsatellites*, which vary in length from person to person, but are all the same length in an individual. DNA damage induced by factors such as oxidative stress and chemical carcinogens can cause dysfunction of genes responsible for ensuring that the microsatellites remain of consistent length; these genes are called *mismatch repair genes*. Mismatch repair gene mutations lead to microsatellite instability (MSI)–the lengthening or shortening of microsatellites. This causes dysfunction in the region of the genome containing the unstable microsatellites. If this occurs in a tumor suppressor region, the consequence can be uncontrolled cell growth, the hallmark of cancer.

MSI is found in about 15% of colorectal cancers.[46]

Ironically, MSI (versus stable microsatellites) is associated with a better prognosis in colorectal cancer,[42] likely for the same reasons that it leads to cancer in the first place–the cells are unable to repair major DNA damage and thus more readily succumb to apoptosis.

Tea polyphenols[47,48] have been shown to inhibit the proliferation of MSI colon cancer cells.

Cells with disrupted MMR function are highly sensitive to the apoptotic effects of curcumin.[49]

# SCREENING FOR COLORECTAL CANCER

## Colonoscopy

Colonoscopy is an endoscopic process using a lens that allows a physician to visualize the mucosa from the rectum to the start of the colon (ileo-cecal junction). Removal of adenomatous polyps during colonoscopy has been proven to lower the risk of colorectal cancer.[50,51]

Screening colonoscopies are recommended beginning at age 50, but those with any risk factors and/or a family history should consider screening at an earlier age.

How a colonoscopy is performed and by whom may influence whether adenomas or cancers are detected. During a 15-month period, analysis of 7882 colonoscopies performed by 12 experienced gastroenterologists found that the time it took to withdraw the colonoscope influenced detection rates. Gastroenterologists who took less than 6 minutes to withdraw the scope were much less likely to detect cancer than those who withdrew the scope more slowly (up to over 16 minutes). Even advanced cancers were more likely to be missed when the scope was withdrawn more quickly.[52]

The time of day the colonoscopy is performed may also influence its reliability. In a chart review of a total of 2087 colonoscopies at Metro Health Medical Center in Cleveland, Ohio, those done in the afternoon had a significantly higher failure rate compared to those done in the morning.[53] The "failure" of a colonoscopy means that the scope could not reach the start of the colon (the cecum). This incomplete look at the colon often necessitates repeating the scoping procedure or undergoing further imaging, such as a CT scan.

The rate of incomplete colonoscopies may be influenced by who performs the procedure. In a study designed specifically to look at factors that lead to incomplete colonoscopies, the elderly, females, and those that have had prior abdominal or pelvic surgeries are more likely to have an incomplete colonoscopic evaluation. In this same study, the researchers found that having the colonoscopy done in an office rather than hospital setting tripled the risk of new or

missed colon cancer in men and doubled it in women.[54]

## Computer Tomographic Colonoscopy

Computer tomographic colonoscopy (CTC) is sometimes referred to as a "virtual colonoscopy." It involves the use of CT imaging the colon. Preparation for CTC is much like a traditional colonoscopy with the use of laxatives to create an empty bowel. Carbon dioxide or air is infused through the rectum to create a smoother surface to assess. CTCs are useful for larger polyps but may not pick up smaller or flattened polyps as well as traditional colonoscopy. If any polyps or suspicious areas are seen on CTC, the patient must then undergo a colonoscopy to visually assess and/or remove the polyps.

CTC is limited to some extent relative to a traditional colonoscopy in that if a polyp is detected, it cannot be removed during the procedure. This is a disadvantage as the patient will then need to undergo a traditional colonoscopy following the CTC to remove the polyp. Another disadvantage of virtual colonoscopies is the high levels of radiation needed to perform the procedure.

## Fecal Occult Blood Test

Fecal occult blood test (FOBT), a simple test for detecting occult blood in the stool, is recommended as routine screening for colorectal cancers. Long before blood can be seen by the naked eye, minute quantities may signify the presence of cancer. The association of a positive FOBT with actual colorectal cancer, however, is fairly low—only 10%.[55] This is because occult blood more often comes from benign conditions, such as minor hemorrhoids; an FOBT may even detect bleeding associated with the upper gastrointestinal tract.

The FOBT is about 70% sensitive to the detection of colorectal cancer, while a colonoscopy performed by an experienced gastroenterologist is roughly 95% sensitive.[56,57]

---

# INDIRECT TESTS FOR COLON CANCER AND EMERGING TECHNIQUES

A blood-based means of detecting colon cancer may be right around the corner. Colon cancer–specific antigens (CCSAs) are nuclear matrix proteins unique to colon cancer cells. When circulating, these CCSAs serve as a "fingerprint" indicating that either colon cancer or a premalignant adenoma is likely present.[58] Circulating levels of several of the CCSAs, including CCSA-2, CCSA-3, and CCSA-4, have all been independently shown to be both sensitive and specific to colon cancer or premalignant adenomas.[59,60] While this test is not commercially available yet, ongoing research is looking at optimizing combinations of the various CCSAs to predict the likelihood of colon cancer with great accuracy. In the future, this blood test may be used to gauge the urgency for colonoscopy screening.

*Calprotectin* in the stool has been used as a marker for IBD, and is a useful tool in determining the possibility of adenoma or colorectal cancer.[61,62] Fecal calprotectin is a product of granulocyte formation, a hallmark of chronic inflammation, and as such is not specific to the cancerous process but indicates that inflammation is present. In one study, of the patients referred for colonoscopy due to abdominal symptoms, elevated calprotectin was found in 85% of those with colorectal cancer, 81% of those with IBD, and only 37% of those with normal findings.[63]

Since precancerous adenomas and colon cancer arise in the lining of the colon, the cells involved are shed with the stool on passing. With advances in technology and molecular biology, examining the stool for unique DNA changes, or *molecular markers in the stool* that signify cancer, is an area of interest.

The next generation of stool testing for colon cancer involves the *stool DNA* (sDNA) test, which was able to detect 64% of precancerous adenomas >1 cm and 85% of colon cancers, and the *fecal immunochemical test* (FIT).[64] A patented stool DNA test called PreGen-Plus(tm) is approximately 65% sensitive to the detection of colorectal cancers,[65] but the high cost of this test may limit its utility for many consumers.

These noninvasive tests remain less sensitive than a colonoscopy, and have advantages and disadvantages that should be discussed with a health care provider.[50]

## PROGNOSIS

Following diagnosis, oncologists and pathologists must analyze the extent to which the cancer has progressed and determine whether it has metastasized to other organs. This process, called "staging," is crucial in guiding treatment.

Cancer confined to the mucosa of the colon wall is classified as *stage I* and is easily removable by surgery in the great majority of cases. When the cancer has penetrated deeper into the muscle layers of the colon, or has just perforated the colon wall, it is classified as *stage II*. Stage II colon cancer also carries a fairly good prognosis. *Stage III* is defined by detection of cancer in nearby lymph nodes, tissues, or organs. *Stage IV* colorectal cancer defines metastasis to one or more distant organs, such as the lungs.

The outlook diminishes as stages advance; surgery is usually no longer a curative option for cancer not contained within the colon or isolated to nearby tissue (colon cancer with isolated liver or lung metastasis can rarely be treated effectively with

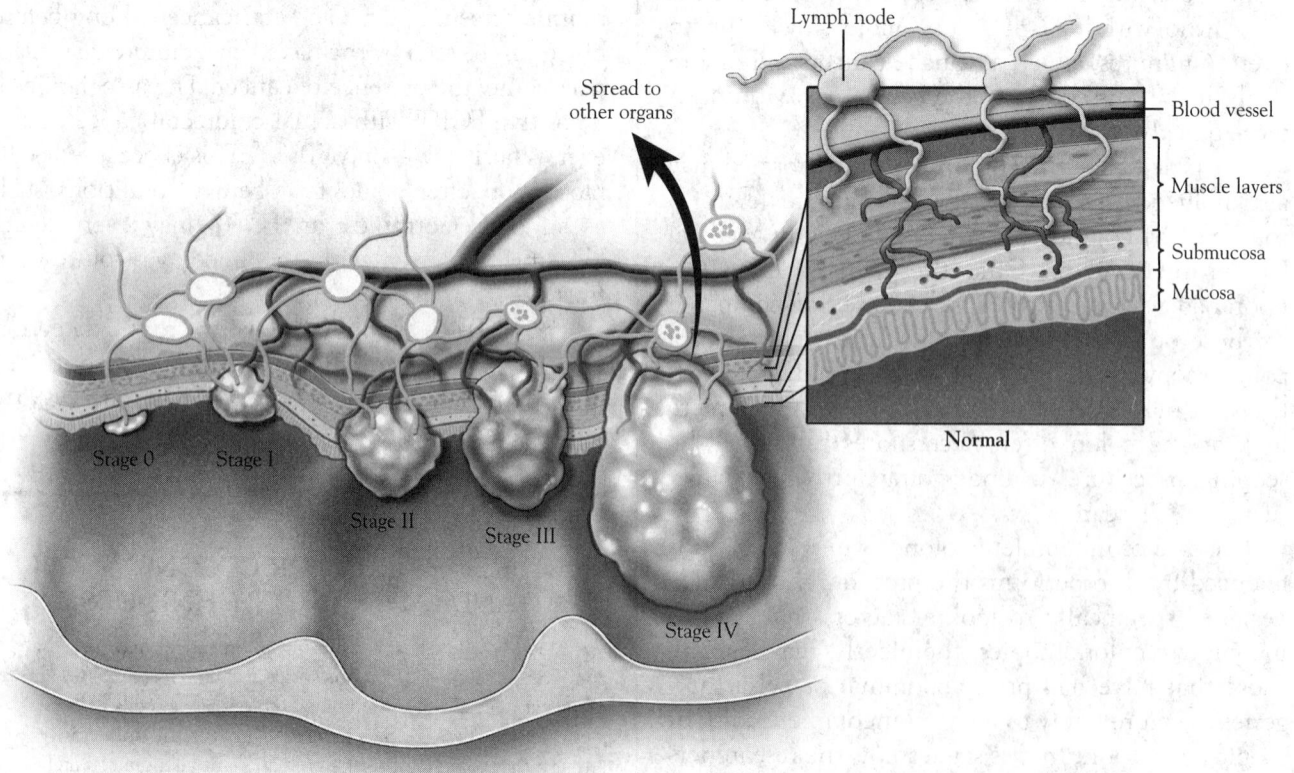

Stages of Colon Cancer

surgery). Five-year survival rates for stage I colon cancer are very good, at about 90%, while the median survival plummets to just 6 months in advanced stage IV cancer.[66]

A valuable innovation in cancer prognostic technology is *circulating tumor cell* testing. Circulating tumor cell testing involves the detection of cancer cells in the bloodstream. These circulating tumor cells are the "seeds" that break away from the primary site of cancer and spread to other parts of the body. Understanding circulating tumor cells is critically important since it is the spread of cancer to other parts of the body—and not the primary cancer—that is very often responsible for the death of a person with cancer. For a detailed discussion of circulating tumor cell testing, please refer to section 3 of the "Cancer Treatment: The Critical Factors" protocol.

# CONVENTIONAL TREATMENT OF COLORECTAL CANCER

Colorectal cancer treatment is adjusted in accordance with the characteristics of each patient's cancer. Surgery is a mainstay for treatment of stage I and most stage II cancers, while stage III and IV cancers are treated with chemotherapy and radiation. Advanced cancers are treated with an aim of reducing symptoms and improving quality of life, as they cannot be cured in most cases.

## Surgery

Surgery is the most common local treatment and usually the first-line treatment for patients diagnosed with localized colorectal cancer. Overall survival rates vary between 55% and 75%, with most recurrences of cancer seen within the first 2 years of follow-up. For patients whose cancer has not spread to the lymph nodes, survival with surgery alone varies from 75–90%. Surgery can also be performed for cancer metastases confined to the liver or lung whenever possible. Surgical removal of metastatic lesions results in long-term survival in a significant number of patients.[67]

In some cases, the patient will require a colostomy, which is an opening into the colon from outside the body that provides an exit for fecal waste. A colostomy may be temporary or, if the surgery is very extensive, may be permanent. Total colonic resection is sometimes performed as a prophylactic measure for patients with familial polyposis and multiple colon polyps.

Nutritional supplementation and dietary modification should be considered before, during, and after surgery (for more information, see the "Cancer Surgery" protocol).

## Radiofrequency Ablation

Radiofrequency ablation (RFA) uses radiofrequency energy produced by an electrode that creates temperatures above 60°C (about 140°F) within the tumor, resulting in cancer cell death. RFA is used as an alternative to surgery in patients with inoperable colorectal liver metastases.[68,69] Although RFA is unlikely to cure patients, it has a definite role in palliative therapy/relieving symptoms.[70]

## Radiation Therapy

Radiation therapy (also known as radiotherapy) uses targeted, high-energy ionizing x-rays to destroy cancer cells. It is typically used after surgery to eliminate any remaining microscopic cancer cells in the vicinity. However, it may be used prior to surgery to reduce the tumor volume, which enables the removal of tumors previously considered inoperable. Intraoperative radiation therapy (IORT) has the advantage of maximally irradiating the tumor bed while reducing damage to surrounding, normal organ tissue from the field of radiation.

For more information regarding radiation therapy and prevention of its well-known side effects, see the "Cancer Radiation Therapy" protocol.

## Adjuvant Therapy

The goal of adjuvant therapy is to eliminate any cancer cells that may have escaped the localized treatment. Adjuvant means "in addition to," and adjuvant therapy is used in combination with surgery and radiation (see "Complementary Alternative Cancer Therapies" protocol). Several types of adjuvant treatments are typically used for early-stage colorectal cancer: chemotherapy, radiotherapy, immunotherapy, nutritional supplementation, and dietary intervention.

**Chemotherapy.** Chemotherapy uses drugs that can be taken orally or injected intravenously to kill cancer cells. Chemotherapy usually begins 4–6 weeks after the final surgery, although some oncologists may initiate chemotherapy sooner than postsurgery. Typical chemotherapy for colon cancer consists of a combination of drugs that have been found to be the most effective, such as *FOLFOX4* (oxaliplatin, 5-fluorouracil (5-FU), and leucovorin) or *FOLFIRI* (folinic acid, 5-FU, and irinotecan), followed by *FOLFOX6* (folinic acid, 5-FU, and oxaliplatin).[71]

For many tumors, the potential for eradication using chemotherapy is slight.[72] However, chemotherapy using oxaliplatin may make metastatic colorectal cancer patients eligible for liver cancer removal.[73] Nevertheless, chemotherapy drugs have many side effects that can damage or destroy some healthy tissues as well. For information on natural compounds that may help to reduce such adverse effects, refer to the "Chemotherapy" protocol.

*Chemoresistance* is a major hurdle in the treatment of all cancers. This phenomenon occurs when genetic abnormalities make cancer cells resistant to chemotherapeutic drugs. Fortunately, some natural agents may combat chemoresistance.

Studies show that *curcumin* can inhibit the development of chemoresistance to FOLFOX through effects on insulin-like growth factor 1 receptor (IGF-1R) and/or EGFR.[74] When curcumin was used in combination with the targeted drug dasatinib, colon cancer cell resistance to FOLFOX was eliminated.[39] Curcumin has also been shown to sensitize colorectal cancer cells to the lethal effects of radiation therapy.[75]

**Antiangiogenic therapies.** Antiangiogenic therapies stop tumors from forming new blood vessels (eg, by inhibiting vascular endothelial growth factor [VEGF] activity) and therefore impede tumor growth. A targeted antiangiogenic agent, bevacizumab (Avastin®), which is a humanized monoclonal antibody targeting circulating VEGF, prolonged survival of metastatic colorectal cancer patients who had inoperable tumors.[76] Interestingly, in patients with metastatic colorectal cancer, the addition of Avastin® to irinotecan, fluorouracil, and leucovorin improves survival regardless of the level of VEGF expression.[77] However, side effects from Avastin® can be severe and improvements in survival seldom result in cures for advanced cases.

## NOVEL AND EMERGENT MODALITIES IN COLON CANCER PREVENTION AND MANAGEMENT

### COX-2 Inhibitor Drugs

**Aspirin.** It has long been known that aspirin may offer protection from developing a variety of cancers. Recently, a large retrospective look at data over a 20-year period showed that low-dose aspirin (75–81 mg) for >5 years reduced the risk of colon cancer by 24%, and was most effective at reducing risk of right-sided (proximal) colon cancer, a staggering 70%.[4] Importantly, not just risk of being diagnosed, but also the risk of dying from colon cancer was reduced by up to 40% in those that took aspirin (any dose) for >5 years.[18]

Aspirin's anticancer properties stem in part from its capacity to inhibit the action of *cyclooxygenase-2* (COX-2), an enzyme that plays a central role in onset and progression of most cancers, and is overactive in 50% of adenomas and 80% of colorectal cancers.[78–80] Aspirin also beneficially modulates activity of the protein complex *nuclear factor-kappa B* (NF-κB), the so-called "master switch" that stimulates the growth of a variety of cancers, including colorectal cancers.[81]

**Celecoxib.** Celecoxib is a nonsteroidal anti-inflammatory drug (NSAID) that inhibits COX-2. In one study, 1561 individuals with a history of adenomas were recruited to take either celecoxib (400 mg/day) or placebo. Follow-up colonoscopies at 3 years found that the risk of developing adenomas was halved in the celecoxib group.[82] One study suggested a synergistic effect when celecoxib is taken with *fish oil*.[83] However, while celecoxib can reduce adenoma formation, it is also well documented to raise the risk of cardiovascular events,[84,85] leaving a risk/benefit equation that should be seriously considered.

> **Note:** *Additional information about inhibiting the COX-2 enzyme can be found in step 4 of the "Cancer Treatment: The Critical Factors" protocol.*

### Metformin

Metformin is an oral antidiabetic drug that works by suppressing the production of glucose in the liver and boosting insulin sensitivity in peripheral tissues. Metformin is currently considered the treatment of choice for type 2 diabetes.

As with other malignancies, colorectal cancer risk is increased in diabetics, and there is a growing body of evidence that advanced glycation end products (AGEs), which are a consequence of elevated blood glucose, and insulin-receptor signaling, are involved in the initiation and propagation of these common tumors.[86,87]

Moreover, colorectal cancers are among malignancies most closely associated with obesity. Obese individuals are deficient in the *protective* hormone adiponectin, which activates tumor-suppressing AMP-activated protein kinase (AMPK). Metformin, by independently activating AMPK, may circumvent this deficiency and help to reduce its impact on colorectal cancer risk.[88] Naturally, these findings have piqued interest in investigating the potential role of metformin against colorectal cancer.

In 2011, researchers conducted a comprehensive review of observational data on the use of metformin and the risk of colorectal cancer in diabetic patients.[89] This review encompassed five studies including nearly 110 000 subjects. Compared to all other antidiabetic treatments, the use of metformin was associated with a 37% lower risk of colorectal cancer.

While this review provides compelling data in support of the protective role of metformin against colorectal cancer, it should be noted that the trials included were observational in nature; the protective effects of metformin must still be substantiated in clinical intervention trials.

Nonetheless, Life Extension suggests that colorectal cancer patients, especially those who are overweight or have a fasting glucose level of >85 *mg/dL*, ask their health care provider if metformin would be a positive addition to their regimen.

## Cimetidine

Cimetidine, or Tagamet®, reduces the production of stomach acid by binding with H2 receptors on the acid-secreting cells of the stomach lining. These receptors normally bind with histamine to produce stomach acid, which helps to break down food. By competing with histamine to bind with H2 receptors, cimetidine reduces the stomach's production of acid. This mechanism of action accounts for cimetidine's use in managing gastroesophageal reflux disease (GERD), a condition marked by an excess of stomach acid. Before stronger antiemetic drugs became available, cimetidine was prescribed to treat nausea associated with chemotherapy. As far back as 1988, scientists observed that colon cancer patients who had been treated with cimetidine had a notably better response to cancer therapy than those who did not receive cimetidine.[90]

Cimetidine functions via several different pathways to inhibit growth of tumors. It inhibits proliferation of cells, blocks new blood vessel growth, and interferes with cell-to-cell adhesion, a necessary process in the spread of cancer.[91] It also has positive effects on immune function.

In a 1994 study, just 7 days of cimetidine treatment (400 mg twice daily for 5 days preoperative and intravenously for 2 days postoperative) in colorectal cancer patients decreased their 3-year mortality rate from 41% to 7%. In addition, tumors in the cimetidine-treated patients had a notably higher rate of infiltration by lymphocytes, a type of white blood cell.[92] These tumor-infiltrating lymphocytes, part of the body's immune response to the tumor, serve as a good prognostic indicator.

Since cimetidine is a histamine receptor *antagonist*—that is, an agent that binds with a cell receptor without eliciting a biological response—it may help circumvent immunosuppression caused by increased histamine levels in a tumor's microenvironment.[93] While histamine appears to stimulate the growth and proliferation of certain types of cancer cells, inhibiting histamine's action may be only one mechanism by which cimetidine fights cancer.

Cimetidine inhibits cancer cell adhesion by blocking the expression of an adhesive molecule—called E-selectin—on the surface of endothelial cells that line blood vessels.[94] Cancers cells latch onto E-selectin in order to adhere to the lining of blood vessels.[95] By preventing the expression of E-selectin on endothelial cell surfaces, cimetidine significantly limits the ability of cancer cell adherence to the blood vessel walls.

Administering cimetidine may enable the immune system to mount a more effective response, possibly minimizing the risk of growth and spread from surgical resection of the tumor. Recent studies suggest that cimetidine enhances local tumor response through the production of Interleukin-18 (IL-18) by immune cells (monocytes).[96] IL-18 blocks new blood vessel growth and encourages apoptosis of cancer cells.

A report in the *British Journal of Cancer* examined findings of a collaborative colon cancer study conducted by 15 institutions in Japan. First, all participants had surgery to remove the primary colorectal tumor, followed by intravenous chemotherapy treatment. They were then divided into 2 groups: one group received 800 mg of oral cimetidine and 200 mg of fluorouracil (a cancer-fighting medication) daily for 1 year, while a control group received fluorouracil only. The patients were followed for 10 years. Cimetidine greatly improved the 10-year survival rate: 85% of the cimetidine-treated patients survived 10 years, compared to only 50% of the control group.[97] Cimetidine produced the greatest survival-enhancing benefits in those whose cancer cells showed markers associated with the tendency to metastasize.

Several other studies have corroborated cimetidine's benefits in colorectal cancer. For instance, in a Japanese study in 2006, colorectal cancer patients who received cimetidine following surgical removal of recurrent cancer had an improved prognosis compared to those treated with surgery alone.[98]

## Vaccines and Immunotherapies

An enlightened medical approach to cancer treatment involves the use of cancer vaccines. The concept is the same as using vaccines for infectious diseases, except that tumor vaccines target cancer cells instead of a virus. Another distinguishing feature of tumor vaccines is that while viral vaccines are created from a generic virus, tumor vaccines can be *autologous*, that is, they can be produced using a person's own cancer cells that have been removed during surgery. This is a critical distinction since there can be considerable genetic difference between cancers. This highly individualized cancer vaccine greatly amplifies the ability of the immune system to identify and target any residual cancer cells present in the body. Cancer vaccines provide the immune system with the specific identifying markers of the cancer that can then be used to mount a successful attack against metastatic cancer cells.

Autologous cancer vaccines have been studied extensively, with the most encouraging results noted in randomized, controlled clinical trials including >1300 colorectal cancer patients in which tumor vaccines were given after surgery. These trials reported reduced recurrence rates and improved survival.[99] Unlike chemotherapy, which can cause severe side effects and toxicity, cancer vaccines offer the hope of a "gentler" type of therapy with improved long-term safety.[100]

In a landmark study reported in 2003, a total of 567 individuals with colon cancer were randomized to receive surgery alone, or surgery combined with vaccines derived from their own cancer cells. The median survival for the cancer vaccine group was >7 years, compared to the median survival of 4.5 years for the group receiving surgery alone. The 5-year survival was 66.5% in the cancer vaccine group, which dwarfed the 45.6% 5-year survival for the group receiving surgery alone.[101] This glaring difference in 5-year survival clearly displays the power of individually tailored cancer vaccines to greatly focus a person's own immunity to target and attack residual metastatic cancer cells.

Monoclonal antibody therapies currently employed in colorectal cancer therapy include bevacizumab, which targets VEGF, and panitumumab and cetuximab, which target EGFR.

For a detailed discussion of cancer vaccines, please review the "Cancer Vaccines and Immunotherapy" protocol.

## PERSONALIZING YOUR CANCER TREATMENT REGIMEN

All cancers, including colon cancer, can have unique genetic characteristics from person to person. Gene expression profiles can highlight minute differences in the character of a cancer, and help identify which anticancer drugs will be most effective.

In one study, a 50-gene array conducted on resected colon cancers (stage I or II patients) determined that those with more "aggressive" patterns may be ideal candidates for interventions with specific preventative agents such as cox-2 inhibiting agents.[102] Such testing may be able to determine with great precision which natural or prescriptive agent to choose based on the molecular characteristics of the cancer. Specifically, tests for KRAS mutational status, EGFR expression, microsatellite instability, and other relevant tests are available currently.

Cancers have traditionally been treated as follows: if one therapy proves ineffective, then try another until a successful therapy is found or all options are exhausted. Evaluating the molecular biology of the tumor cell population helps to eliminate the need for this trial-and-error method by providing individualized information to help determine the optimal therapy before initiating treatment. This can save the patient time and money and most importantly, it may provide a better opportunity for "first-strike" eradication.

Life Extension recognizes the value that advanced cancer testing delivers to cancer patients and suggests that every cancer patient test their cancers as extensively as possible. For more information on testing the unique biological characteristics of your cancer, refer to steps 1 and 2 of the "Cancer Treatment: The Critical Factors" protocol.

## DIETARY AND LIFESTYLE CONSIDERATIONS FOR COLON CANCER

### Diet

There is a 25-fold difference among geographical areas in incidence of colorectal cancers, within North America, Australia, New Zealand, Western Europe, and select areas of Eastern Europe having the highest rates.[103] People who migrate from low-rate areas to high-rate areas see an increase in development of colorectal cancers, indicating that the cultural environment and dietary habits contribute significantly to risk.[104]

In general, Western diets contain too much red meat and not enough fruits and vegetables compared to non-Western diets. Fruits and vegetables, in addition to the vitamins, minerals, and fiber they provide, contain thousands of other compounds (phytochemicals) that have anticancer effects. Phytochemicals that lessen cancer risk are the *phenolic* compounds, including hesperdin, anthocyanins, quercetin, rutin, epigallocatechin-3-gallate (EGCG), and resveratrol, among others.[105–108]

Many cultures outside the United States also use a more diverse and greater proportion of herbs and spices in their cooking. Many spices have antiinflammatory effects and daily consumption of a variety of spices may contribute to the lower rates of colorectal cancers in non-Western cultures.[109,110]

Perhaps the most well-studied spice with a potent anti-inflammatory action is turmeric; its active ingredient is curcumin. Curcumin, through its modifying action of NF-κB, affects hundreds of molecules involved in proliferation, survival, migration, and new blood vessel development.

While there is some controversy over the precise components of the diet that influence colorectal risk, there is no real debate that whole foods, with the nutrients and fibers intact, provide protection against colorectal cancers. A recent look at data from a study using the Dietary Approaches to Stop Hypertension (DASH) diet, which is high in whole grains, fruit, and vegetables; moderate amounts of low-fat dairy; and low amounts of red or processed meats, desserts, and sweetened beverages, found that the DASH diet reduced the risk of colon cancer by nearly 20% and rectal cancers by 27%.[111]

A healthy diet not only reduces risk, but appears to favorably affect outcomes once colon cancer has been diagnosed as well. A study of patients with stage III colon cancer divided their dietary habits into 2 dietary patterns. The "Prudent" pattern was characterized by high intakes of fruits and vegetables, poultry, and fish; and the "Western" pattern was characterized by high intakes of meat, fat, refined grains, and dessert. Those with the prudent diet had less recurrence of colon cancer and were more likely to still be alive at the 5-year point.[112]

### Exercise

Population studies show that those who *exercise* have reduced risk of developing many cancers, including breast, prostate, lung, pancreatic, and colon cancer.[113] A study in the *Journal of the American Medical Association* showed that overweight survivors of cancer who took part in nutritional improvement, exercise, and modest weight loss had less functional decline than nonparticipants.[114]

Exercise may protect against the development of cancers by reducing the likelihood of obesity and/or diabetes, but there are other, more direct effects as well. Fat, or adipose tissue, releases chemical messengers called *adipokines*. These adipokines increase inflammation and create glucose dysregulation and other metabolic disturbances. Recently, *myokines* from muscle have also been discovered. These myokines, which are made when muscles contract, appear to have a cross-talk with the adipokines, and the net effect is that myokines lead to improved glucose utilization and less fat deposition.[115] Therefore, usage of muscle and reduction of adipose through exercise results in a reduction of inflammation overall.

Maintaining normal weight protects against many cancers[116] and may be one reason that diet and exercise are linked so strongly to the reduction of risk of colorectal cancer.[117]

## NUTRITIONAL SUPPORT FOR COLON CANCER

### Multivitamin

Many nutrient deficiencies can increase risk of cancer, and biochemical variations in each person's ability to utilize nutrients from food may lead to some harboring a nutrient deficiency despite eating well.[118] Multivitamin supplements vary in forms and formulations of the nutrients they contain. All multivitamins contain folate, which is often cited as the nutrient responsible for conferring protection from colon cancer. Since several other nutrients have also been shown to lower risk, it is possible that there is synergy among nutrients that lead to protection.

Several studies indicate that multivitamin use is linked with a lower risk of colon and rectal cancers.[119–121] Recently, a large pooled analysis of 13 clinical studies showed multivitamin use was associated with a 12% lower risk of colon cancer versus nonuse.[122] Moreover, an animal model revealed that experimental rats given a multivitamin in their drinking water were 84% less likely to developed chemical-induced aberrant crypt foci in their colons compared to their counterparts who received the chemical carcinogen without multivitamins.[123]

In addition, a 3-year clinical trial looked at a mixture of beta-carotene 15 mg, vitamin C 150 mg, vitamin E 75 mg, selenium 101 mcg, and calcium carbonate (1.6 g daily) versus placebo and found that the supplement group had significantly less adenoma formation.[124]

### Vitamin D

The World Cancer Research Fund conducted a systematic review of studies on colorectal cancer and vitamin D intake and 25-hydroxyvitamin D status. They confirmed that higher vitamin D intake and 25-hydroxyvitamin D status were associated with reduced colon cancer risk.[125]

The active form of vitamin D, 1,25-dihydroxycholicalciferol has been shown to directly increase the expression of tumor suppressor *cystatin D* in colon cancer.[126] This is of interest because both normal and malignant colon epithelial cells have the enzyme required to transform circulating

25-hydroxycholicalciferol to the active 1,25-dihydroxycholicalciferol, which is then used intra-cellularly to thwart the growth of the colon cancer.[127]

In one study, 1179 postmenopausal women were randomized to receive calcium (1500 mg/day), calcium with vitamin D (1500 mg and 1100 IU), or placebo. After 4 years, the incidence of cancers was less in women receiving the calcium with vitamin D, but not the calcium alone or placebo.[128] These results were in keeping with earlier data in women (46–70 years old) showing that higher vitamin-D status was associated with less risk of developing colon cancer.[129]

Precancerous lesions, or adenomas, are more likely to develop in those with lower circulating levels of vitamin D. A review of 12 studies of vitamin-D consumption and 7 studies of circulating vitamin D found that high versus low dietary intake of vitamin D reduced the risk of adenoma development by 11% and high versus low circulating levels of vitamin D reduced the risk by 30%.[130]

Higher circulating levels of 25-hydroxycholicalciferol (25[OH]D) are protective against colorectal cancer. For example, pooled data from the Physician's Health Study combined with 8 prospective trials showed the risk of developing colorectal cancer was lower for those with higher 25(OH)D status.[131]

## Vitamin E

Vitamin E is a family of eight naturally occurring compounds, four tocopherols, and four tocotrienols. All forms of vitamin E are antioxidants, able to neu-tralize free radicals directly as well as recycle other antioxidants. Over the decades, studies have been predominantly on alpha-tocopherol, although more recent evidence suggests that *gamma tocopherol* is the more active cancer preventative agent, particularly for colon cancer.[132–134] Importantly, gamma tocoph-erol was more effective at inhibiting COX-2 than alpha-tocopherol, which may result in improved protection from colon cancer.[135]

Oxidized compounds reach the epithelial cells of the colon and rectum both from dietary sources and from normal bacterial metabolism in the colon. Alpha- and gamma-tocopherol have been shown to mitigate the oxidative damage, thus lowering the carci-nogenic potential of these compounds.[136] In an animal model, a mixture of tocopherols high in gamma tocoph-erol lessened colon cancer development through anti-oxidant, anti-inflammatory, and other anticarcinogenic mechanisms.[137]

Several clinical studies suggest a benefit attributable to vitamin E. In one study, intake of supplements con-taining alpha-tocopherol (>200 IU/day) significantly reduced the risk of colon cancer development com-pared to no vitamin E intake.[119] In two other studies, those with the highest intakes of vitamin E had reduced risk of developing colorectal cancer as well.[138,139]

Tocotrienols may have their own unique anticancer mechanisms. Tocotrienols were found to increase apop-tosis in colon cancer cells through modulation of the balance between pro and antiapoptotic mediators.[140,141]

## Calcium

Higher calcium intake appears to lower the risk of developing colorectal cancer.[142,143] Calcium may pro-tect the mucosa of the colon and rectum through binding carcinogenic bile acids,[144] or through encour-aging proper maturation (differentiation) of colorectal cells. Supplemental calcium, as well as vitamin D, was shown to induce favorable cellular changes in colonic cells of patients with adenomas.[145]

A study of 92 men and women with a history of adenoma compared the effects of calcium and vita-min D alone and together on the normal cellular turnover of the colonic epithelium. Both calcium and vitamin D, alone and together, enhanced apoptosis of normal epithelial cells.[146] Interestingly, one study showed that up to 5 years after stopping the calcium supplementation, there was still less adenoma forma-tion.[147] Another study showed that vitamin D and calcium taken as a supplement was associated with reduced risk, but this benefit was not found from dietary sources alone, indicating that supplementa-tion may be necessary to attain benefit.[148] Two studies in men with previous adenomas showed a risk reduc-tion of 36% for future adenomas with supplemental calcium (1200 mg/day for 4 years in one study, and 2000 mg/day for 3 years in the other).[149]

## Selenium

Selenium deficiency has been linked to formation of many cancers, including colorectal cancer.[150] Selenium is incorporated into proteins within cells, called "sele-noproteins," involved with protecting the cells from free radical accumulation that can lead to DNA dam-age. Some of these proteins include glutathione per-oxidases (GPx), thioredoxin reductases (TrxR), and selenoprotein P (SePP). People who form adenomas are more likely to be deficient in selenium as well as the selenoproteins that protect DNA from damage. Repletion of selenium through supplementation re-stored both deficiencies, presumably leading to protec-tion from further adenoma formation.[151]

There have been a number of studies showing that selenium is lower in those with adenomas or colorectal cancer compared to controls.[152–154] Selenium may afford even more protection in current smokers and those who have quit <10 years previously.[155]

Selenium supplementation at the time of cancer surgery can increase local immune function, an effect that may reduce recurrence.[156] There may also be synergistic effects of selenium with other nutrients such as folate.[157]

A clinical trial of 200 mcg of selenium versus placebo found that the incidence of colorectal cancer was significantly less in those taking selenium.[158]

Selenium may also synergize with some cancer treatment drugs.[159] In a phase I clinical trial using high doses of *selenomethionine* alongside the chemotherapy drug irinotecan, the authors remarked "unexpected responses and disease stabilization were noted in a highly refractory population."[160] Selenium in high amounts can be toxic, and evidence suggests that doses in the 200–400 mcg range are most beneficial.[161]

## Folate

Folic acid is necessary for the synthesis of both S-adenosylmethionine (SAMe) and deoxythymidine monophosphate (dTMP). dTMP and SAMe are needed in the synthesis and function of DNA, respectively. Therefore, a deficiency of folic acid may disrupt proper DNA synthesis or function. A pooled analysis of 13 studies involving over 725 000 participants, found a 2% risk reduction for every 100 mcg/day increase of total folic acid intake.[162] In a large population study, those taking the highest amount of folate from diet and supplements (>900 mcg/day) had a 30% reduced risk of developing colon cancer versus those with the lowest consumption (<200 mcg/day).[163]

Alcohol consumption increases the risk of colon cancers, and evidence suggests this may be potentiated by polymorphisms in genes that produce enzymes involved in folate metabolism.[164] Maintaining adequate levels of folate, and its co-nutrient methionine, may offer protection from colon adenoma development, particularly in those consuming alcohol or those with genetic polymorphisms in folate metabolism.[165]

## Green Coffee and Chlorogenic Acids

Greater coffee consumption has been linked with a lower rate of a variety of cancers, including colon cancer.[166,167]

Coffee contains powerful antioxidant compounds, called *chlorogenic acids*, which have been shown to exert several potentially chemopreventive effects, including favorably modulating glucose metabolism, and quelling inflammation.[168,169] In fact, a recent study found that chlorogenic acids were able to interfere with a variety of cellular processes that drive colon cancer metastasis, including NF-κB signaling.[170]

However, the roasting process used to prepare conventional coffee beverages destroys the majority of these beneficial chlorogenic acids. Therefore, drinking coffee is an inefficient means of obtaining these bioactive compounds.

Recent scientific innovation has led to the availability *green coffee bean extract* standardized to 50% chlorogenic acids. Supplementation with green coffee bean extract is a viable option for obtaining robust quantities of bioactive chlorogenic acids.

## Garlic

Consumption of garlic has been linked with lower colon cancer risk.[171] Garlic has been shown to reduce the carcinogenic potential of compounds such as nitrosamines, as well as exert antiproliferative effects.[172,173] Components that may be responsible for the cancer-protective effects of garlic include organosulfur compounds and flavonoids.

There are many mechanisms that can explain how garlic reduces carcinogenesis in the colon and rectum.

- Inhibition of cell growth and proliferation directly
- Inhibition of new blood vessel growth
- Increased cell death (apoptosis)
- Increased detoxification of carcinogens
- Suppression of carcinogen activating enzymes
- Inhibition of cyclooxygenase-2 (thereby inhibition of inflammation)
- Antioxidant action, squelching free radicals in the bowel[174]

One clinical trial showed that supplementing with aged garlic extract reduced the formation of precancerous adenomas in patients with a history of adenomas.[175]

## Ginger

Like garlic, ginger has been a mainstay of traditional medicine for >2500 years. Ginger's multiple chemopreventive benefits have been reported in a wide range of experimental models.[176] Key compounds in ginger and its extracts limit the oxidative damage to cells caused by free radicals. They also lower levels of signaling molecules called cytokines, specifically those that provoke an inflammatory response. This dual mode of action may inhibit initiation of carcinogenesis and limit expansion of existing malignancies.[177,178] Some ginger components also increase the activity of vital enzymes that detoxify carcinogens present in the body.[179,180]

Indian researchers provided direct evidence of ginger's chemopreventive power in rats with chemically induced colon cancers in two recent studies.[181,182] After injection with a potent carcinogen, animals were either supplemented with ginger or given normal diets. In both studies the incidence of cancers and the number of individual tumors were significantly reduced in the supplemented groups. The first study also detected lower levels of oxidative agents and higher levels of natural antioxidants in supplemented animals, while the second study further showed a decrease in the activity of bacterial enzymes that release intestinal toxins and damage the colon's natural protective mucous layer.

In a recent clinical trial, 30 healthy subjects consumed 2 g of ginger or a placebo each day for 28 days. Colon biopsies were taken at baseline and at day 28 and assessed for levels of inflammatory markers. The subjects who received ginger displayed significantly lower levels of prostaglandin E-2 (PGE-2) and 5-HETE, two inflammatory fatty acid metabolites, in their tissue samples than those who received a placebo.[183] These findings are encouraging due to the role of inflammation in driving colon cancer growth.

## Modified Citrus Pectin

Modified citrus pectin (MCP) is a type of soluble dietary fiber derived from citrus fruits that has been modified by pH and heat to form smaller units of absorbable galactose residues that are able to bind to cancer cells. Specifically, MCP binds to *galectin-3*, a protein expressed by cancer cells that is involved in cell-to-cell adhesion, survival, and spread to distant organs (metastasis).[184,185] Nullifying the effects of galectin-3 by finding agents to bind to it is one means of inhibiting these procancerous mechanisms.[186,187] MCP has been shown to effectively bind galectin-3 and inhibit growth and metastasis of various cancers,[188] including colon cancer.[189]

Interfering with galectin-3 and preventing metastasis is particularly important in colorectal cancer, where spread to the liver means a much worse prognosis than limited or local disease. Galectin-3 levels appear to be increased in colon cancer, and are associated with advanced disease stage,[190,191] confirming that galectin-3 is an important molecule in the growth and spread of colon cancers.

Additional discussion on the role of MCP in combatting cancer metastasis can be found in the Life Extension Magazine article titled "Fighting Cancer Metastasis and Heavy Metal Toxicities with Modified Citrus Pectin."

## Curcumin

Curcumin is derived from the spice turmeric (*Curcuma longa*), an ancient spice used throughout Asia. Cultures in which diets high in turmeric are consumed have much lower rates of colon cancer than Western cultures.[109] Curcumin is a powerful anti-inflammatory compound that acts on NF-κB, a proinflammatory mediator that influences hundreds of genes involved in the growth and spread of cancer. In addition, curcumin regulates tumor suppressor pathways and triggers mitochondrial-mediated death in cancer cells.[192,193]

Despite aggressive surgical care and chemotherapy, nearly 50% of people with colorectal cancers develop recurrent tumors.[194] This may be due in part to the survival of dangerous colon-cancer stem cells that resist conventional chemotherapy and act as "seeds" for subsequent cancers.[195] There is evidence that combining curcumin with FOLFOX, the first-line chemotherapy drug combination of 5-fluorouricil, leukovorin, and oxaliplatin, eliminates the persistent pool of colon-cancer stem cells,[196] and potentiates the lethality of FOLFOX on cancer cells.[197]

Finally, curcumin interferes with tumor invasiveness and blocks molecules that would otherwise open pathways to penetration of tissue.[1] It also helps to starve tumors of their vital blood supply and it can oppose many of the processes that permit metastases to spread.[198] These multitargeted actions are central to curcumin's capacity to block multiple forms of cancer before they manifest.[199]

Curcumin also creates a gastrointestinal environment more favorable to optimal colon health by reducing levels of so-called secondary bile acids, natural secretions that contribute to colon cancer risk.[200] That has a direct effect, inhibiting proliferation of cancer cells and further reducing their production.[201]

A novel feature of curcumin is its ability to bind to and activate vitamin D receptors (VDRs) in colon cells.[202] Binding to VDRs elicits a host of antiproliferative and anti-inflammatory actions.

Curcumin given to patients undergoing treatment for colon cancer led to weight gain, decreased circulating inflammatory mediator tumor necrosis factor-alpha (TNF-α), and increased apoptosis.[203]

## Omega-3 Fatty Acids

There is a substantial amount of experimental, population-based studies and clinical trials showing that risk of colorectal cancer is reduced with higher intakes of omega-3 fatty acids.[204–210]

EPA (2 g/day for 3 months) reduced crypt cell proliferation and promoted proper apoptosis of colonic epithelial cells in patients with a history of colonic adenomas.[211] Separately, a large population study of physicians found that those who consumed fish oil supplements during a 10-year period had a 35% reduction in the risk of developing colon cancer.[212]

Omega-3 fatty acids may prevent colorectal cancer through supporting normal turnover of the epithelial cells by encouraging apoptosis.[208] Fish oils reduce the protumor effects of many molecules involved in the growth and spread of colon cancer, including VEGF, platelet-derived growth factor (PDGF), platelet-derived endothelial cell growth factor (PDECGF), COX-2, PG-E2), nitric oxide, NF-κB, matrix metalloproteinases, and beta-catenin.[213]

DHA, an omega-3 fatty acid found in fish oil, disrupts cell signaling in colon cancer and is synergistic with butyrate in inducing apoptosis.[214,215]

Fish oil (2.5 g/day) normalized abnormal rectal proliferation patterns in patients with a history of adenomas, and this is thought to be through reducing the availability of inflammatory omega-6 fatty acid, arachidonic acid, and modifying vitamin E availability.[216,217]

Chemotherapies induce cell death by inducing DNA damage in quickly dividing cells, tipping the death/survival pathways toward cellular self-destruction (apoptosis). Experiments have shown that EPA and DHA can make cancer cells more vulnerable to damage from chemotherapy and radiation, thus encouraging the cells to turn on cell death pathways in lieu of repair pathways.[218–220] Eventual resistance of colon cancer cells to the cytotoxic effects of chemotherapy may also be lessened with EPA/DHA.[221]

## Polysaccharide-K

Polysaccharide-K (PSK) is a mushroom polysaccharide complex used more commonly in other countries such as Japan and Australia for immune support in cancer care. Pure PSK cannot be obtained in the United States, but the mushroom *Trametes versicolor* (formerly called *Coriolus versicolor*) is high in this polysaccharide and is often substituted. Many mushrooms have some immune enhancing properties, but PSK can also suppress activation of NF-κB, therefore reducing the expression of hundreds of procancerous genes.[222]

A review of 3 clinical trials in patients who had surgery and chemotherapy for their colon cancer showed that overall survival was improved by 29% with the addition of PSK.[223]

A group of colon cancer patients were randomized to receive chemotherapy alone or chemotherapy plus PSK, which was taken for 2 years. The group receiving PSK had an exceptional 10-year survival of 82%. The group receiving chemotherapy alone had a 10-year survival of only 51%.[224] In a similar trial reported in the *British Journal of Cancer* in 2004; colon cancer patients received chemotherapy alone or combined with PSK (3 g/day) for 2 years. In the group with stage 3 colon cancer, the 5-year survival was 75% in the PSK group. This compared to a 5-year survival of only 46% in the group receiving chemotherapy alone.[225]

## Sulforaphane

Sulforaphane is a compound found in cruciferous vegetables, such as broccoli and kale. It improves the elimination of toxic substances by the liver. It also may have a more direct role in thwarting the growth of cancers, including colorectal cancer, through reactivation of tumor suppressor genes that were formerly silenced.[226,227]

Sulforaphane inhibited the formation of colon tumors in an animal model.[228] It is also able to induce apoptosis in colon cancer cells with impaired apoptosis capability.[229]

Sulforaphane appears to protect normal colon cells while encouraging self-destruction of colon cancer cells.[230] When added to oxaliplatin, sulforaphane improved the ability of the drug to kill colon cancer cells.[231]

In one study, sulforaphane was synergistic with indole-3-carbinol, another compound from cruciferous vegetables. Together the compounds resulted in greater toxicity to colon cancer cells than either compound alone.[232]

## Resveratrol

Resveratrol is a polyphenol found in grapes, peanuts, and mulberries. Resveratrol suppresses colitis and colitis associated colon cancer in mice.[233] Grape powder and resveratrol inhibited the carcinogenic Wnt pathway in normal colonic mucosa.[234,235] Resveratrol also inhibits the COX-2 enzyme, suppressing inflammation.[236] Resveratrol may synergize with butyrate in the colon as well.[237]

Resveratrol has been shown to reduce aberrant crypt formation[238,239] and adenoma formation,[240] as well as induce apoptosis of colon cancer cells.[241,242]

A small study of 20 patients scheduled for colon resection to remove malignancy showed that a dose of 0.5–1.0 g/day for 8 days prior to surgery resulted in adequate levels of resveratrol in the tumors to have biological effects. This was particularly true for tumors on the right (proximal) side.[243]

Resveratrol may also increase the sensitivity of colon cancer cells to the killing effects of chemotherapy.[244]

## Green Tea Extract

Green tea contains potent antioxidants known as catechins, the most well studied of which is epigallocatechin-3-gallate (EGCG), which has been found to inhibit carcinogenesis in various cancers, including colorectal cancers.[245–247]

Green tea extract is well established to have anti-cancer actions on growth, survival, angiogenesis, and metastatic processes of cancer cells,[248,249] and favorable effects on immune function.[250] Green tea has also been shown to reduce the carcinogenicity of nitrosamines, carcinogenic compounds from cooked meats.[251]

A meta-analysis of consumption of green tea across populations found that those consuming the highest levels of green tea had an 18% lower risk of developing colorectal cancer compared to those consuming the lowest amounts.[252] In a clinical study, green tea extract (equivalent of >10 cups/day, or about 150 mg EGCG) reduced adenoma formation, both number and severity, in those with a prior history of adenomas.[253]

## Milk Thistle

Milk thistle (*Silybum marianum*) contains silibinin and silymarin, flavonoid compounds shown to have numerous anticancer effects. Milk thistle is generally used to improve the break down and elimination of chemicals and toxins, so it is not surprising that silymarin was able to prevent chemically induced colon cancer in mice.[254] In another animal study, silymarin, along with quercitin, curcumin, and rutin, all independently reduced aberrant crypt formation, an early process in colon cancer formation.[255] Silymarin also inhibits angiogenesis,[256] a necessary process for tumor growth.

Silibinin has been shown to inhibit colorectal carcinogenesis directly.[257] Silibinin blocks proliferation, reduces new blood vessel growth, and induces cell death (apoptosis) of colorectal cancer cells.[258–261] It may achieve some of these antitumor effects through disruption of signaling pathways within cancer cells as well as by blocking activation of NF-κB.[262]

## Quercetin

Quercetin belongs to a class of potent antioxidants called flavonoids. These are what give apples their color. Onions, garlic, tea, red grapes, berries, broccoli, and leafy greens are also rich sources of quercetin.

This flavonoid is well known to nutritional scientists as a potent free radical-scavenger.[263] Quercetin also happens to possess a singular cancer-fighting feature: it can prevent cancer caused by chemicals. Its unique molecular structure enables it to *block* receptors on the cell surface that interact with carcinogenic chemical compounds. This makes it a perfect anticancer agent for the colon, where carcinogenic chemicals tend to accumulate.[263]

Researchers in Greece have also discovered that quercetin dramatically suppresses one particular cancer-causing gene in colon cells. This makes quercetin supplementation an ideal form of early prevention for individuals with a family history of colon cancer.[264]

Dutch scientists uncovered even more evidence of its cancer-preventive power at the genetic level. In an animal study, quercetin reduced "cancer gene" activity and *increased* "tumor-suppressor gene" activity in colon cells after 11 weeks.[265]

In yet another promising animal study, scientists in South Carolina were able to halt the development of aberrant crypts. Cancer-prone rats fed a diet high in quercetin[35] underwent a four-fold reduction in the number of aberrant crypts compared to a control group. Similar research has yielded additional evidence of quercetin's capacity to reduce emerging aberrant crypts—a vital first step in preventing colon cancer from developing at all.[266]

In 2006, scientists at the Cleveland Clinic evaluated patients suffering from familial adenomatous polyposis. They discovered that a combination of curcumin and quercetin could cause these growths to diminish substantially. The researchers supplemented the patients with 480 mg of curcumin and 20 mg of quercetin orally, 3 times a day for 6 months. Every single patient experienced a remarkable decrease in polyp numbers and size, with average reductions of 60% and 51%, respectively.[267]

## N-Acetylcysteine

N-acetylcysteine (NAC) is a slightly modified version of the sulfur-containing amino acid cysteine. When taken internally, NAC replenishes intracellular levels of the natural antioxidant glutathione (GSH), helping to restore cells' ability to avoid damage from reactive oxygen species. NAC suppresses the NF-κB, which in turn prevents activation of multiple inflammatory mediators.[268,269] NAC also regulates the gene for COX-2, the enzyme that produces pain- and inflammation-inducing prostaglandins in a wide array of chronic conditions.[270]

NAC (800 mg/day) reduced the rate of proliferation of the cells in the colonic crypts in patients with a history of adenomatous polyps.[271] This is in keeping with a study showing that those with a history of polyps had a 40% reduction in recurrence using 600 mg of NAC daily.[272]

## Life Extension Suggestions

Life Extension's approach includes avant-garde cancer testing technology coupled with evidenced-based regimen of natural compounds and novel drug strategies to complement conventional colon cancer treatment.

*Note:* This protocol should not be used in isolation. Individuals with colorectal cancer should also review the content in other Life Extension cancer protocols, including the following:

- Cancer Treatment: The Critical Factors
- Cancer Adjuvant Therapy
- Cancer Radiation Therapy
- Cancer Surgery
- Cancer Vaccines and Immunotherapy
- Chemotherapy
- Complementary Alternative Cancer Therapies

### Primary Supplements
- **Comprehensive multivitamin:** per label instructions
- **Vitamin D:** 5000–8000 IU daily with food. Blood levels of vitamin D3 should be regularly monitored, to achieve a blood level of 50–80 ng/mL
- **Vitamin E,** as high gamma-tocopherol blend: 359 mg daily
- **Selenium,** as Se-methylselenocysteine: 200–400 mcg daily
- **Folate,** as L-methylfolate: 1000 mcg daily

- **Modified citrus pectin:** 15 g daily
- **Curcumin,** as highly absorbed BCM-95®: 2400 mg daily
- **Fish oil:** 700–4200 mg of EPA, 500–2000 mg of DHA daily with food
- **PSK:** 3 g daily
- ***Boswellia serrata* extract,** standardized to 20% AKBA: 100–200 mg daily

### Secondary Supplements
- **Quercetin:** 250–500 mg daily
- **N-Acetylcysteine:** 600–1800 mg daily
- **Soy isoflavones:** 135–270 mg daily
- **Green coffee bean extract,** standardized to 50% chlorogenic acids: 400 mg before meals, up to 3 times daily
- **Perillyl alcohol:** 2000 mg, 4 times daily
- **Calcium:** 1200 mg daily
- **Garlic,** standardized extract: 1200–4800 mg daily
- **Ginger,** standardized extract: 150–450 mg daily
- **Milk thistle,** standardized extract: 750–1500 mg daily
- ***Trans*-resveratrol:** 250–500 mg daily
- **Green tea,** standardized extract: 725–1450 mg daily
- **R-lipoic acid:** 300 mg twice daily
- **American ginseng:** 250–500 mg daily

### Innovative Drug Strategies
- **Metformin:** 250–500 mg, 2–3 times daily before meals
- **Cimetidine:** 800 mg daily
- **Aspirin** (low dose): 81 mg daily

## REFERENCES

References available at: www.lef.org/dpt5/ch44

# 45

# Common Cold

## PREAMBLE

If you are reading this because you have developed cold symptoms, it is critical that you act quickly to halt the rapid replication of viruses occurring in your body at this very moment. Go to the nearest health food store or pharmacy and purchase:

1. **Zinc lozenges.** Start sucking on 2 zinc lozenges (13–24 mg of zinc in each lozenge) immediately and again every 2–3 hours for the first day or two. Then slowly reduce the dose until symptoms dissipate.
2. **Garlic.** Take 9000–18000 mg of a high-allicin garlic supplement each day until symptoms subside. Take with food to minimize stomach irritation.
3. **Vitamin D.** If you do not already maintain a blood level of *25-hydroxyvitamin D* over 50 ng/mL, then take 50000 IU of vitamin D the first day and continue for 3 more days and slowly reduce the dose to around 5000 IU of vitamin D each day. If you already take around 5000 IU of vitamin D every day, then you probably do not need to increase your intake.
4. **Cimetidine.** Take 800–1200 mg daily in divided doses. Cimetidine is a heartburn drug that has potent immune enhancing properties. (It is sold over the counter [OTC] in pharmacies.)
5. **Melatonin.** Take 3–50 mg at bedtime.

*Do not delay implementing the above regimen.* Once the cold virus infects too many cells, it replicates out of control and strategies like zinc lozenges will not be effective. Treatment must be initiated as soon as symptoms manifest.

## INTRODUCTION

The common cold is a viral infection of the upper respiratory tract that causes symptoms such as a runny or stuffy nose, sneezing, coughing, and sore throat.[1–3] Systemic symptoms such as mild headache, fatigue, fever, and muscle aches can occasionally occur with the common cold as well. However, if these symptoms are severe and/or accompanied by fever or significant exhaustion, they likely indicate the "flu," which is a distinct type of viral respiratory infection caused by an influenza virus.[4–6]

It has been estimated that the U.S. population contracts approximately 1 billion colds per year, and the common cold is a leading cause of medical visits and missed days at work or school.[7,8] Although most cases of the common cold are mild and self-limiting, the illness represents a major economic burden to society in terms of lost productivity and treatment expenditure.[1,9,10]

Treatment strategies for the common cold are generally aimed at relieving symptoms, shortening duration, and minimizing the risk of complications.[8,11]

Conventional cold treatments include OTC analgesics and decongestant medications.[8,12] However, these strategies are minimally effective,[13] and even when used appropriately, may be associated with significant side effects.[14]

A number of specific antiviral drugs have some degree of effectiveness against common cold viruses. One exciting candidate is Biota's *vapendavir*, which recently met key milestones for benefit in a phase IIb human rhinovirus trial in asthmatic patients in March 2012.[15] The readily available OTC drug *cimetidine*, approved for the treatment of reflux and "heartburn," has antiviral properties as well, and may be a useful common cold treatment.

Several innovative and integrative strategies such as vitamin D, garlic, zinc, *Astragalus*, beta-glucan, and probiotics have been shown in scientific studies to help manage symptom duration and intensity associated with the common cold.[9]

## DEVELOPMENT AND PROGRESSION OF THE COMMON COLD

While the common cold may be caused by over 200 distinct and continually evolving viral pathogens; rhinoviruses, coronaviruses and respiratory syncytial viruses appear to be some of the most common.[1,16–18]

Infection occurs when the cold-causing virus comes into contact with mucous membranes in the nose or eyes. Common cold infections generally result in a non-specific acute inflammatory response that stimulates the release of various inflammatory cytokines and other immune mediators. In fact, many of the symptoms associated with the common cold are a result of inflammation caused by this immune response, rather than by the virus itself.[1,2,5,19] For example, the release of a proinflammatory peptide called bradykinin is a major contributor to sore throat symptoms.[1,20] Stuffy nose symptoms result from increased pooling of blood in nasal blood vessels and increased nasal secretions. Likewise, runny nose occurs due to enhanced permeability of nasal blood vessels, which allows serum to leak into the nasal mucosa.[1]

Although infection with a virus known to cause the common cold generates an adaptive immune response that helps protect against repeated infection by the same or very similar virus, the sheer volume of distinct viruses that can cause the common cold makes developing immunity against the common cold itself very challenging.[1,2,5] However, infection by a cold virus can decrease the risk and severity of reinfection with the same virus.[1]

---

## NEW UNDERSTANDING OF THE HUMAN IMMUNE SYSTEM PAVES WAY FOR POTENTIAL COMMON COLD TREATMENT

For at least the last 100 years it has been assumed that the ability of antibodies produced by the immune system to protect against pathogens ends at the cellular membrane. In other words, scientists have thought that once a virus enters a cell it escapes the attack of antibody-mediated immunity, leaving only one option to eliminate the virus–kill the cell that harbors it. However, emergent research suggests this is not the case.

A specialized protein within cells called TRIM21 has been shown to bind to virus-bound antibodies within the cell and initiate an intracellular immune response.[21]

Researchers have proposed that delivery of exogenous TRIM21, perhaps as a nasal spray, may help up-regulate immunity against some cold-causing viral pathogens and eliminate them in as little as a few hours.[22,23]

Although more research is needed before these findings can be applied clinically, the discovery of an intracellular defense system against viruses opens the door to promising new interventions for the common cold and other viral diseases.

## COMMON COLD SYMPTOMS

The clinical symptoms of the common cold generally occur within 24–72 hours of infection, and typically begin with runny nose and a sore or "scratchy" throat. Sore throat symptoms usually subside by the second or third day of infection, after which nasal symptoms typically become the most bothersome.[1,2,5,16] Three out of every 10 people with the common cold may develop an unproductive cough, often beginning after the onset of nasal symptoms, and persisting as the cold resolves.[1,2,5,16] As a whole, these symptoms may last anywhere from 2–14 days, but most people recover within 7–10 days. Nasal symptoms lasting longer than 2 weeks may be due to seasonal allergies rather than the common cold.[24]

Occasionally, common cold infections are associated with other complications such as ear and/or sinus infection. The common cold has also been known to exacerbate certain diseases of the upper respiratory tract such as asthma, bronchitis, cystic fibrosis, and COPD. Patients who experience high fever, intense sinus pain, severely swollen glands, and/or cough that produces mucus (ie, productive cough) may have a more serious illness, and should notify their healthcare provider immediately.[2,8,24,25]

## COMMON COLD PREVENTION

Suggestions for preventing the common cold include:

- **Avoid others while you have cold symptoms and are contagious (ie, 2–7 days).** Depending on the offending virus, the common cold may be transmitted from

---

## Common Cold versus Flu: Comparison of Characteristics[4,8,128–130]

| Feature | Colds | Flu |
|---|---|---|
| Etiologic agent | >200 viral strains; rhinovirus most common | 3 strains of influenza virus: influenza A, B, and C |
| Site of infection | Upper respiratory tract | Entire respiratory system |
| Symptom onset | Gradual: 1–3 days | Sudden: within a few hours |
| Fever, chills | Occasional, low grade (<101° F) | Characteristic, higher (>101° F), lasting 2–4 days |
| Headache | Infrequent, usually mild | Characteristic, more severe |
| General aches, pains | Mild, if any | Characteristic, often severe and affecting the entire body |
| Sore throat | Common, usually mild | Sometimes present |
| Cough, chest congestion | Common; mild to moderate, with hacking, productive cough | Common; potentially severe dry, nonproductive cough |
| Runny, stuffy nose | Very common, accompanied by bouts of sneezing | Sometimes present |
| Fatigue, weakness | Mild, if any | Usual, may be severe and last 2–3 weeks |
| Extreme exhaustion | Rarely | Frequent, usually in early stages of illness |
| Season | Year-round, peaks in winter months | Most cases between November and February |
| Antibiotics helpful? | No, unless secondary bacterial infection develops | No, unless secondary bacterial infection develops |

one person to another via inhalation. This is because viral particles are small enough to be suspended in the air when an infected person coughs, sneezes, or blows their nose. Since some viruses can live for up to 3 hours on human skin, the cold can also be transmitted via direct contact with an infected person.[2,26,27]

- **Infected individuals should direct their cough or sneeze into the inner crook of their elbow, rather than into their hand(s) or directly into the air.** The contagious particles from a cough or sneeze occasionally land on environmental objects or surfaces, where rhinoviruses can also survive for up to 3 hours.[26–28]

- **Avoid touching eyes, nose, and/or mouth during cold outbreaks.** For most people this task is extremely difficult, especially since the average person touches their face approximately 16 times per hour. Given that unconscious face touching is almost unavoidable, hand washing/sanitizing and using surface disinfectants to prevent the spread of the common cold is important.[26–28]

- **Lifestyle modifications such as exercising have proven to be effective at reducing the number of common cold infections.**[29] Individuals who become infected with mild to moderate cases of the cold should continue their exercise routine, provided their symptoms are not body-wide.[30]

- **Adequate sleep quantity and quality are important for protecting against common cold.** Sleep is known to modulate the immune responses through the production of regulatory cytokines.[31,32]

- **When possible, limit your exposure to children (particularly via day-care centers) during peak cold season.** Since children are much more likely to contract a cold than adults (6–8 versus 2–4 colds per year, respectively), the adult risk of infection increases with increased contact with children, especially in close quarters.[1,10] If this cannot be avoided, you should take extra precautions to wash/sanitize your hands and disinfect surfaces that may be contaminated.[26–28]

# CONVENTIONAL TREATMENT

Although the common cold is caused by viral infection, due to the sheer volume of potential common cold viruses and treatment timing, targeted antiviral drugs are not typically beneficial.[19] In addition, *antibacterial drugs (ie, antibiotics) are of no benefit* in the treatment of the common cold,[1] except for in severe cases involving complication such as secondary bacterial sinusitis.[16] In fact, *the use of antibacterial medications for treating uncomplicated colds is likely to do more harm than good*, as they can induce adverse reactions as well as contribute to the development of drug resistant pathogens.[33]

## Over-the-Counter Cold Medicines

Nearly $3 billion worth of OTC cold medicines are purchased each year, but randomized trial evidence suggests minimal effectiveness.[1,34,35]

Following are commonly used OTC cough and cold medications along with their specific indications.[1,36,37]

**Oxymetazoline and pseudoephedrine.** These drugs are alpha-adrenergic agents. When use topically or orally, these agents may help *relieve stuffy nose symptoms* by causing blood vessels to constrict.[38] Decongestants like pseudoephedrine can increase blood pressure and should not be used by people with hypertension.[36]

**Diphenhydramine.** Diphenhydramine blocks the effects of histamine in the body, which is a proinflammatory component of the immune system. It may be beneficial for treating runny nose, sneezing, coughing, and nausea.[1,39,40] Diphenhydramine also causes sedation and may cause arrhythmia and/or tachycardia and so should be used with caution by people who have heart problems.[36]

**Dextromethorphan.** Dextromethorphan is a cough suppressant drug. It appears to reduce coughing via several actions within the brain.[41,42] Potential side effects of dextromethorphan include confusion, excitability, gastrointestinal disturbances, irritability, nervousness, and sedation.[36]

**Mild analgesics.** Acetaminophen and nonsteroidal anti-inflammatory drugs (NSAIDs) (eg, aspirin, ibuprofen, and naproxen) are drugs that provide analgesic, fever-reducing, and anti-inflammatory effects. These drugs may help alleviate painful symptoms such as a sore throat or muscle pain associated with the common cold.[1] It is important to consider that acetaminophen is an ingredient in many OTC cold medicines and can be toxic if consumed in excess. Therefore, it is imperative to read the labels of cold medicines carefully to avoid excess consumption of acetaminophen. Life Extension suggests that at least 600 mg of *N-acetyl cysteine* be taken with each dose of acetaminophen to help the liver detoxify harmful metabolic derivatives of the drug. More information is available in the Acetaminophen and NSAID Toxicity protocol.

People taking combination cough and cold medicines should be conscious of all the ingredients and doses contained within (eg, some products contain up to 5 distinct ingredients), and make sure that they are not duplicating therapy or taking more than is recommended.[43,44] Given that OTC drugs have not been demonstrated to be beneficial for the treatment of cold in young children and their potential for toxicity, these medications are not recommended for children under 4.[1]

**Cimetidine.** Cimetidine is an OTC drug that blocks certain histamine receptors (ie, histamine receptor type 2 antagonist); it is approved by the Food and Drug Administration (FDA) for inhibition of gastric acid secretion. In addition to its usefulness for treating gastric or duodenal ulcers,[45,46] cimetidine has also been shown to augment immune response against viral pathogens.[47–51]

One of cimetidine's important actions is inhibition of suppressor T-cells, which are cells of the immune system that normally "turn down" the immune response.[49,52] In other words, taking cimetidine at the first sign of a cold may allow for a more robust immune response by countering the effects of these intrinsic immune regulators.

---

## NEW DRUG SIGNIFICANTLY REDUCES COLD SYMPTOMS IN CLINICAL TRIAL

Results of a phase II clinical trial show that a new antiviral, vapendavir, reduced symptoms of rhinovirus infection among people with asthma.[15]

Vapendavir works by blocking entry of viruses into host cells, thereby preventing infection.

Compared to those who took a placebo, vapendavir recipients experienced significantly less cold symptoms during days 2 and 4 of infection, when symptoms are typically worst. Moreover, those who took the new drug experienced earlier improvement of symptoms compared to those who took a placebo (1.7 days versus 2.5 days).

More trials are needed before vapendavir becomes widely available as a common cold treatment, but these early results are encouraging.

---

# TARGETED NUTRITIONAL THERAPIES

After infection, viruses causing the common cold multiply rapidly. While most people wait until their symptoms become unbearable, then use an OTC medication, Life Extension recommends aggressive action when the viral count is still relatively low and symptoms are mild.

## Vitamin D

Evidence suggests vitamin D has a significant role in the regulation of the human immune system, and may reduce the risk of certain bacterial and viral infections.[53,54] Theoretically, vitamin D supplementation may produce a sufficient amount of *cathelicidin* (a naturally occurring antimicrobial and antiviral) to cure viral respiratory infections such as the common cold.[55,56] Furthermore, data show that higher vitamin D levels are associated with a decreased risk of contracting a seasonal viral infection.[57,58] Life Extension recommends an optimal 25-hydroxyvitamin D blood level between 50 and 80 ng/mL.

## Vitamin C

Evidence shows that vitamin C augments several aspects of the immune system and helps defend against infections (especially viral infections).[59–62] Vitamin C enhances the production and action of white blood cells; for example, it increases the ability of neutrophils (a type of white blood cell) to attack and engulf viruses.[61,63,64] Vitamin C has been shown to reduce the chances of catching a cold, and may reduce cold duration.[60,65] Upon review of clinical data from 2 studies, researchers found that using vitamin C (1000 mg) plus zinc (10 mg) during a cold could reduce runny nose symptoms by up to 27% over 5 days of treatment compared to placebo.[9]

## Zinc

Zinc helps maintain a healthy immune system, and zinc deficiency has been linked to significant immune impairment and susceptibility to infections.[8,9] Unfortunately, zinc deficiency is a common problem affecting approximately 2 billion people worldwide, even many people in Western populations. Correcting zinc deficiency through supplementation has been shown to bolster aspects of the immune system involved in fighting viral infections.[9,66,67] Zinc's antiviral properties may come from its ability to prevent the rhinovirus from attaching to cells in the nasal passages. In addition, zinc has been shown to prevent viral replication, reduce histamine release, and inhibit the production of other inflammatory mediators.[7] A comprehensive review concluded that zinc supplementation was associated with a significant reduction in the duration and severity of the common cold (when administered within 24 hours of onset of symptoms). It was also found that zinc supplementation over 5 months was helpful for preventing the common cold.[7] Clinical trials of zinc lozenges (as zinc gluconate and zinc acetate) have shown benefit in reducing the duration of colds when taken at doses of 13–23 mg every 2–3 waking hours.[7,68]

## DHEA

Dehydroepiandrosterone (DHEA) is a steroid hormone synthesized by the adrenal gland. Research has revealed that DHEA possesses powerful immune-enhancing and antiviral properties, and can enhance resistance to many different experimental infections.[8,69–71] DHEA accomplishes this in part by modulating several aspects of the immune system. For example, administering 50 mg of DHEA daily to an elderly population resulted in an increase in natural killer cell activity, a 62% increase in B-cell activity and a 40% increase in T cell activity, all of which are important for defending against infectious pathogens.[8]

DHEA supplementation is likely to be especially important among the aging and elderly, since DHEA levels decline sharply with age.[8,72]

## Melatonin

Melatonin is a hormone produced in the brain and the gut. It helps regulate the sleep-wake cycle and is a powerful antioxidant. Research indicates that melatonin helps combat many types of viral infections.[73–75] For example, melatonin appears to "prime" the immune system by interacting with specialized immune cells called "T-helper cells," allowing for a more efficient immune response against pathogens. Furthermore, melatonin administration is also associated with an increased production of antibodies.[76]

Melatonin's role as an antioxidant may be helpful during a cold as well, since most viral infections are associated with high amounts of oxidative stress.[75] This may be especially true for elderly populations, since these patients frequently experience age-related impairment of the immune system, which coincides with declining melatonin concentrations.[77]

## Astragalus Membranaceus

*Astragalus membranaceus* is a Chinese herb that contains a number of immune-stimulating ingredients such as polysaccharides, flavonoids, trace minerals, and amino acids. While it has been traditionally used to treat colds and flu as well as for increasing stamina and overall vitality, much of the research performed on *Astragalus membranaceus* is focused on its application for treating immune deficiency conditions.[8,78] In a clinical study comparing various natural products (ie, echinacea, *Astragalus membranaceus*, and licorice),

*Astragalus membranaceus* demonstrated the strongest ability to activate immune cells.[8]

## Elderberry

Elderberry, also known as *Sambucus nigra*, has been used for its medicinal properties since at least 400 BC.[8,79] The purplish-black fruits of the elderberry plant are a rich source of antioxidants, and have long been considered a folk remedy for the treatment of influenza as well as the common cold.[80,81] Even today, elderberry extracts are commonly employed as an alternative to conventional drugs for the management of a variety of viral infections and are recognized as supportive agents against common cold.[79] Researchers believe that elderberry fights colds by activating white blood cells that engulf pathogens. The German Commission E (a therapeutic guide for the safety and efficacy of herbal products) has identified the constituents of elderberry as effective for the relief of colds.[8]

## Garlic

Garlic (ie, *allium sativum*) has been traditionally used for both its culinary and therapeutic properties.[10] A clinical survey found that garlic is one of the most common herbs used for its medicinal properties including for the treatment of colds, flu, and cough.[82] When raw garlic is chopped or chewed, it releases an active organosulfur compound called allicin, which has demonstrated antiviral activity against rhinovirus and a variety of other pathogens. While studies evaluating the use of garlic/allicin for the *treatment* of the common cold are lacking, evidence suggests it may be useful for the *prevention* of such infections.[13] For example, one clinical study demonstrated that an allicin-containing garlic supplement taken once daily (over a 12-week period) was associated with 65% fewer colds than the placebo group (24 versus 65). When compared to placebo, garlic/allicin supplementation was also linked to 70% reduction in symptom duration (~ 1.5 versus 5 days).[83]

## Andrographis

*Andrographis paniculata* has been effectively used among Asian cultures for the treatment of colds for centuries.[84–88] It is reported to have anti-inflammatory, blood pressure lowering, antiviral, and immune-stimulant properties.[89] A 2009 study found that an extract of Andrographis enhanced immune function as well as reversed drug-induced immunosuppression.[90] Accumulating evidence suggests that *Andrographis paniculata* is effective as an alternative treatment option for the common cold.[91-93] For example, a 2010 study found that a standardized extract of *Andrographis paniculata* was more than twice as effective as placebo at reducing symptoms of upper respiratory tract infections.[94] Preliminary evidence suggests that *Andrographis paniculata* may be effective for the *prevention* of colds as well.[91]

## Lactoferrin

Lactoferrin is an iron-binding protein found in milk. It is a powerful immune modulator and has shown marked ability to fight bacteria, fungi, protozoa, and viruses.[8,95,96] Laboratory studies reveal lactoferrin inhibits viral infection by interfering with the ability of certain viruses to bind to cell receptor sites and prevents entry of viruses into host cells.[97,98] In addition, lactoferrin may be beneficial for alleviating the symptoms or complications of viral infections like the common cold, because it suppresses free radical-mediated damage.[8]

## Beta-Glucan

Beta-glucans are naturally occurring glucose polymers that constitute the cell walls of certain plants and pathogenic agents.[99] These polysaccharides have been shown to increase host immune defense, and are associated with enhancing macrophage and natural killer cell function.[99,100] Beta glucans also appear to mitigate the symptoms of the common cold. The Montana Center for Work Physiology and Exercise Metabolism examined beta glucans' ability to mitigate upper respiratory infections in a single blind, randomized trial in 2008; participants who consumed beta-glucans had 23% fewer upper respiratory tract infections compared to the group taking a placebo.[101]

## Probiotics

Probiotics are defined as living microorganisms (ie, bacteria and fungi) that confer a health benefit to the host when administered in adequate amounts.[102,103] Clinical studies suggest that certain probiotics may help *prevent* viral respiratory tract infections such as the common cold by enhancing the immune system. Some probiotics are associated with a reduction in severity and duration of symptoms caused by common upper respiratory tract infections.[103-108] Probiotics may be useful for managing infectious diseases because of their potential for stabilizing the micro-flora of the gut, enhancing resistance against pathogenic colonization, and modulating immune functions.[105,107,109] A 2011 clinical study found that a probiotic lactobacilli

was able to strengthen the body's immune defense against viral infections and reduce the risk of acquiring the common cold.[110] Furthermore, the consumption of yogurt fermented with *Lactobacillus* augmented natural killer cell activity and reduced the risk of catching common cold infections among the elderly.[111]

## Echinacea

Echinacea is an herb that was first utilized for its medicinal value by the Native Americans in the treatment of cough, sore throat, and tonsillitis.[112] Today, echinacea represents one of the most popular herbs used for the treatment and prevention of upper respiratory tract infections (like the common cold) in both European and American markets.[113-115] Clinical evidence shows that echinacea has beneficial effects on the common cold, including reduced severity and duration of cold symptoms, as well as increases in monocytes, neutrophils, natural killer (NK) cells, and total white blood cell count.[8] A 2010 clinical study found that a standardized extract of *E. purpurea* was able reduce the risk of common cold among athletes.[116]

## Honey

Honey has been used since ancient times as a cough and cold remedy in some countries.[117] Studies have shown that honey possesses antimicrobial properties and helps combat infection in a variety of clinical settings.[118] Clinical trials have compared the efficacy of honey to that of placebo and several conventional medicines for relieving symptoms of the common cold.[117] Evidence suggests that honey can relieve symptoms of the common cold in adults and children more effectively than some, but not all, conventional medicines.[119-122]

## Life Extension Suggestions

- **Zinc lozenges:** Start sucking on 2 zinc lozenges (13–24 mg of zinc in each lozenge) immediately and again every 2–3 hours for first day or two. Then slowly reduce the dose until symptoms dissipate.
- **Vitamin D:** If you do not already maintain a blood level of *25-hydroxyvitamin D* over 50 ng/mL, then take 50 000 IU of vitamin D the first day and continue for 3 more days and slowly reduce the dose to around 5000 IU of vitamin D each day. If you already take around 5000 IU of vitamin D every day, then you probably do not need to increase your intake.

- **Vitamin C:** 5000–20000 mg daily
- **Beta-glucan:** 100 mg daily (increase up to 600 mg as needed)
- **Andrographis paniculata extract:** 25 mg daily (increase up to 150 mg as needed)
- **Dehydroepiandrosterone (DHEA):** 200–400 mg early in the day. This is much higher than normal, but DHEA has shown some unique benefits in boosting one's ability to mount a strong immune response and also protect against dangerous inflammatory cytokine responses that sometimes occur in response to viral infections.
- **Melatonin:** 3–50 mg at bedtime. (Ordinarily, melatonin is taken at levels of just 1–3 mg per evening.) Melatonin induces a powerful immune response and this high dose can facilitate the deep sleep one often needs to fend off an infection. This dose of melatonin will make you extremely tired, so please take this only before bedtime and do not operate any machinery or vehicles after ingestion.[123]
- **Astragalus membranaceus,** standardized to 0.4% (1.8 mg) 4'-hydroxy-3'-methoxyisoflavone 7: 450 mg daily
- **Elderberry:** 2400–4800 mg daily or 1–4 tablespoons daily
- **High-allicin garlic:** 9000–18000 mg daily. This potent form of garlic will cause upper gastrointestinal upset if not ingested with food. The intake of high levels (eg, 9000 mg) may cause malodorous body odor, but saturating the body with this pungent garlic is the objective. Garlic has shown antiviral properties in a number of published studies.[124,125]

- **Aged garlic extract:** 3600 mg daily. There are unique immune-boosting compounds in aged garlic that work differently than those found in high-allicin garlic.[167]
- **Lactoferrin:** 1200 mg daily. This natural constituent of mother's milk has documented antiviral and anti-inflammatory properties that may help alleviate the symptoms of viral infections.[8,98]
- **Probiotics:** per label instructions
- **Echinacea,** standardized to 3.84% echinacosides (9.6 mg): 250–500 mg daily
- **N-acetyl cysteine:** at least 600 mg with each dose of acetaminophen

### Over-the-Counter Drug Support

**Cimetidine,** 800–1200 mg daily. This drug is sold OTC in pharmacies to combat heartburn, but its beneficial side effect is to boost immune function by reducing suppressor T cells, thereby keeping the immune system in a hyperactive state.[127] While sold OTC, it would still be wise to read the package insert in case this drug is contraindicated for you. For most people, cimetidine provides powerful immune system stimulation that is particularly effective against certain viruses.

In addition, the following *blood test* may be helpful:

- Vitamin D, 25-Hydroxy

### REFERENCES

References available at: www.lef.org/dpt5/ch45

# 46

# Complementary Alternative Cancer Therapies

Mainstream medical treatment of cancer revolves around surgery, chemotherapy, and radiation therapy, used either alone or in combination.[1,2] Chemotherapy and radiation therapy cannot discriminate between cancer cells and healthy cells; thus, they damage both types of cells and cause serious and often debilitating side effects, frequently forcing patients to abandon treatment.[3–5] Therefore, it is not surprising that many cancer patients now opt to complement conventional treatments with alternative therapies that may not only temper the adverse side effects of conventional cancer therapy, but also improve its effectiveness via independent anticancer effects.

## WHAT ARE COMPLEMENTARY ALTERNATIVE THERAPIES?

Complementary alternative medical therapies (CAM) comprises an array of remedies that lie outside what is traditionally considered conventional medical treatment for cancer. These include the use of herbal, vitamin, and nutritional supplements, as well as physical and psychological interventions such as exercise, relaxation, massage, prayer, hypnotherapy, and acupuncture.[6–8] The use of CAM as a component of integrated cancer treatment regimens may help patients reduce the side effects associated with conventional cancer treatments, alleviate symptoms, enhance immune function, and provide greater quality of (and control over) life.[9,10]

The use of CAM is popular among cancer patients undergoing conventional treatment.[7,8] Millions of patients use CAM therapies to help control their disease. In the United States, 91% of cancer patients implemented at least one form of CAM in addition to undergoing conventional cancer treatment.[11] The most popular forms of CAM were exercise, relaxation, and prayer.[11]

Although most physicians acknowledge the benefits of physical and psychological CAM therapies, the role of nutritional and mineral supplements, particularly when used in conjunction with chemotherapy and radiation therapy, is an issue of considerable controversy.

## CANCER PATIENT NUTRITION: THE USE OF DIETARY SUPPLEMENTS/ANTIOXIDANTS DURING CONVENTIONAL TREATMENT

In the following section, we summarize key findings from published studies demonstrating that dietary supplements influence clinical outcomes and long-term survival, as opposed to showing only a short-term benefit.

1. Encouraging results from a clinical study have shown that the use of antioxidants during chemotherapy treatment does not compromise the treatment. In this study of lung cancer patients, supplementation with vitamins C, E, and beta-carotene did not interfere with the effectiveness of chemotherapy.[12] In fact, recipients of chemotherapy who took antioxidants had better response rates and overall survival than those who received chemotherapy alone; however, these differences did not reach statistical significance.[12,13]

2. In a study of non–small cell lung cancer patients over 60 years of age who had undergone surgery to remove their primary tumor(s), doctors compared survival in vitamin users to nonusers and measured blood folate levels as an indicator of folic acid intake. The average survival of nonusers was 11 months compared to 41 months for vitamin users; in other words, supplement users survived almost 4 times longer than did nonusers. Patients with higher blood folate levels also had improved long-term survival.[14] The Mayo Clinic researchers who conducted this study have conducted further studies with larger patient samples, and their results consistently show improved survival and quality of life in non–small cell lung cancer patients who use vitamin and mineral supplements.[15,16]

3. Another study examined a group of transitional cell bladder cancer patients. One group was given BCG (a tuberculosis vaccine) immune-augmentation therapy plus the recommended daily allowance (RDA) of vitamins. The second BCG-treated group (the megadose group) received the RDA plus 40000 IU vitamin A, 2000 mg vitamin C, 400 IU vitamin E, 100 mg vitamin B6, and 90 mg zinc. After 5 years,

cancer recurrence rates were 91% in the low-potency RDA vitamin group versus 41% in the megadose group. In this study, large doses of vitamins resulted in a 55% reduction in cancer recurrence.[17]

4. Uveal melanoma is a rare form of melanoma that occurs in the iris of the eye.[18] Nine random high-risk patients with uveal melanoma had standard conventional therapy to eradicate their primary tumors. The patients were then put on a nutritional supplement regimen consisting of folic acid, trace minerals, amino acids, and fatty acids. After 80 months of follow-up, none of the 9 patients experienced recurrent disease compared to a similar group of patients who did not receive these supplements. Given that 100% of these high-risk patients were free of disease after almost 7 years, the results provide further evidence of the potential value of nutritional supplementation for cancer patients.[18]

5. Studies of breast cancer patients have shown that those using antioxidants are less likely to suffer a recurrence or die from their cancer.[19]

6. The effectiveness of 5-fluorouracil (5-FU), a chemotherapy agent used to treat breast cancer, was improved when it was administered in combination with folic acid.[20] 5-FU is also commonly used in colon, liver, and pancreatic cancers, but has not shown a high degree of efficacy.[21] A randomized trial of patients with metastatic colorectal carcinoma compared the effects of 5-FU administered alone and in combination with folic acid. Compared to the group receiving 5-FU alone, the patients receiving 5-FU plus folic acid experienced a 76% overall tumor reduction. Survival in the group receiving 5-FU plus folic acid was 47% greater than in the group receiving 5-FU alone. The addition of folic acid to this chemotherapy drug regimen resulted in an improved therapeutic profile and significantly prolonged survival time.[22] These results are summarized in Table 1.

**Table 1: Effect of Folic Acid on Effectiveness of 5-FU Chemotherapy**

|  | 5-FU | Folic Acid and 5-FU | Difference |
|---|---|---|---|
| Complete or partial remission | 9% | 16% | 7% |
| Arrest of tumor growth | 20% | 60% | 40% |
| Progression | 71% | 24% | 47% |

7. Advanced cancer patients exhibit a range of defects in their immune capacity that likely contribute to an increased susceptibility to infections and disease progression.[23] A study of 12 advanced colorectal cancer patients sought to determine whether supplementation with vitamin E could enhance immune function. The patients received a daily dose of 750 mg (<1200 IU) of vitamin E beginning 2 weeks prior to intervention with chemotherapy or radiation treatment. Short-term supplementation with vitamin E led to increased white blood cell (lymphocyte) counts (CD4:CD8 ratios) and enhanced the lymphocytes' ability to produce interleukin-2 and IFN-gamma, which are required for the immune system to destroy cancer cells.[24]

While all the studies mentioned above (and many others) showed the benefit of dietary supplements for cancer patients simultaneously undergoing conventional medical treatment, some studies have failed to show any benefit or have shown mixed effects from taking nutritional supplements.[25] In one study, high levels of folic acid supplementation were associated with greater reductions in neutrophils (a type of white blood cell); however, the same study showed that low neutrophil levels caused by chemotherapy could be improved by vitamin E supplements.[26] A preponderance of evidence supports the use of antioxidants with conventional cancer treatments.[27] However, cancer patients are advised to consult physicians who are experienced in both conventional cancer treatments and nutritional oncology.

## Prescription Antioxidants Versus Natural Antioxidants

Proponents of dietary supplementation for cancer patients argue that the use of supplements containing multiple high-dose antioxidants before and during conventional therapy may improve treatment efficacy by increasing tumor response and decreasing normal tissue toxicity. Conventional therapy produces toxicity during treatment that can be severe enough to cause its discontinuation. Therefore, if dietary supplements can reduce the toxicity to normal cells, or increase the response of tumor cells to conventional therapy, this would represent a significant improvement over current strategies for managing cancer.[27]

Critics argue that antioxidant supplements should not be used with conventional free-radical–generating cancer therapies because they would protect cancer cells from death due to free-radical damage.[28,29] However, synthetic antioxidants available as prescription drugs reduce toxicities associated with conventional treatments. For example, amifostine, a synthetic version of the amino acid cysteine,[30,31] is prescribed by oncologists to reduce the toxicity of conventional treatments without compromising their effectiveness.[30,32] Mesna, another synthetic antioxidant available as a prescription drug, improves the efficacy of the anticancer drug ifosfamide, which would otherwise damage the urinary system.[33] These prescribed, synthetic antioxidants have been investigated in many randomized, controlled clinical trials of cancer patients.[34,35]

Naturally occurring antioxidants and enzymes are often depleted in cancer patients undergoing aggressive therapies, leaving healthy cells defenseless against free-radical damage. Therefore, it could be argued that supplementing with antioxidants does not add something foreign to the body (unless they are synthetic), but instead replaces natural substances lost as a result of treatment.[36,37] Replenishing normal antioxidant levels reduces the adverse side effects associated with chemotherapy and radiation therapy,[30,33] and actually improves patient outcomes.[19,24,38,39] For more information on these studies, please refer to the protocols on Cancer Radiation Therapy and Chemotherapy.

# PHYSICAL AND PSYCHOLOGICAL SUPPORTIVE CAM THERAPIES

## Rehabilitation

Rehabilitation programs for cancer patients involve a combination of physical and psychological interventions that improve the patient's physical comfort and ability to function.[40,41] These are thought to alleviate the emotional distress caused by the patient's loss of mobility and need for self-care.[42,43]

## Acupuncture

Acupuncture improves cancer symptoms and treatment-related side effects such as nausea, pain, hot flashes, and breathlessness.[44] The American Cancer Society recommends the use of acupuncture in cancer patients.[44] In a study of the use of acupuncture in cancer patients, as many as 60% of patients showed an improvement in their symptoms.[45]

## Hypnosis

Hypnosis improves the symptom of hot flashes[46] and overall quality of life by reducing anxiety and insomnia in breast cancer patients.[46] Hypnosis is also recommended as an integral part of palliative care (symptom relief) for cancer patients, with a view to reducing pain and shortness of breath.[47] In addition, hypnosis improves mental health and overall well-being in cancer patients treated with radiation therapy.[48]

## Breathing Exercises

A study of cancer patients recovering from stem cell transplantation showed that following a breathing exercise program for 6 weeks reduced levels of fatigue.[49]

## Massage and Aromatherapy

Massage and aromatherapy improve the general psychological health of cancer patients; in particular, reduce anxiety levels, pain, and nausea.[50] Breast cancer sufferers receiving massage therapy have improved immune system function and feel less depressed and angry about their circumstances.[51] A combination of aromatherapy, foot soaking, and reflexology improves the fatigue often experienced by cancer patients.[52]

## Yoga Meditation

Kundalini yoga involves a variety of meditation techniques that are effective in alleviating anxiety, fear, anger, and depression.[53] This type of yoga helped breast and prostate cancer patients think positively about their cancers.[53]

## Humor

Laughing has always been recognized as a good relaxation and coping strategy. Scientific studies have now demonstrated that laughter is able to reduce anxiety and physical discomfort in cancer patients.[54] Laughter has a beneficial effect on the immune system and improves the function of natural killer cells, which play an important role in counteracting cancer.[54-57] Laughter is also known to improve the pain threshold in cancer patients and reduce levels of stress hormones.[54]

## Positive Visualization

Adoption of hope-inspiring interventions by cancer care providers is associated with an improvement in patients' ability to cope with the fear and anxiety associated with a cancer diagnosis.[58,59]

## Exercise

Various forms of exercise, including tai chi chuan, improve the quality of life of cancer patients[60,61] recovering from surgery or undergoing treatment. Exercise alleviated fatigue and improved heart and lung function as well as overall physical well-being.[62-66]

## Hydration

Many cancer patients, particularly those with terminal disease, suffer from low levels of body fluids, or dehydration.[67] Artificial hydration in these patients improves dehydration symptoms[68] and is also useful in treating chemotherapy-related diarrhea and kidney disease.[69,70] However, artificial hydration should be approached with caution and used according to each patient's medical condition, as it can aggravate symptoms associated with water retention, such as edema.[71,72]

---

### WHAT YOU HAVE LEARNED SO FAR

- Complementary and alternative therapies (CAM) represent one of the fastest-growing adjunctive cancer treatment modalities in the United States.
- The most commonly used CAM modalities include nutritional supplements, mind–body approaches, and acupuncture.
- When used properly, nutritional supplementation can enhance the effectiveness of conventional cancer treatments, boost the immune system, and improve the patient's quality of (and control over) life.
- Many cancer patients take supplemental nutrition during cancer treatment to alleviate treatment toxicities and improve well-being.
- Synthetic antioxidants (such as amifostine), available by prescription only, are widely used by both medical and radiation oncologists to control the adverse effects of cancer treatments.

---

## THE IMPORTANCE OF NUTRITION DURING CANCER TREATMENT

The nutritional status of cancer patients is often compromised by the cancer or conventional treatment(s) used.[73] A significant number of patients recovering from cancer are malnourished[74] or have suffered considerable weight loss.[75] The nutritional status of cancer patients has an impact on a variety of important factors.

Nutritional intervention as an integral part of cancer treatment can be implemented by eating healthy foods and taking supplements or by administration of enriched formulas through a feeding tube directly into the gastrointestinal tract (enteral) or injection into the veins (parenteral).[76] Enteral nutrition is always the preferred method of feeding cancer patients when the gastrointestinal tract is functional but the oral route is compromised; parenteral nutrition should be provided only to selected patients, as it is of little benefit to most cancer patients.

However, parenteral nutrition can be administered in the comfort of the patient's home and improves the long-term survival of patients with incurable advanced disease.[77] In particular, this type of artificial feeding can be useful in gynecologic and colon cancer patients who often suffer from intestinal tract obstruction.[78] In a study comparing the different types of nutritional intervention during cancer treatment, normal oral nutrition was superior to enteral and parenteral feeding only when supported by nutritional counseling from a dietitian.[76]

### Treatment Tolerance

Nutrition intervention during cancer treatment may help patients to better tolerate cancer treatment, with less frequent adverse side effects.[79–81] In particular, patients with nasopharyngeal cancer, when artificially fed through a tube before treatment, had less weight loss and superior recovery compared to patients who received nutrition intervention only after treatment.[79]

### Survival and Overall Outcome

Malnourished cancer patients are more likely to have longer periods of hospitalization, lower survival rates, and a higher frequency of medical complications.[74,75] A study of stomach cancer patients showed that nutritional status affected the patients' quality of life, and the authors recommended increasing the number of high-protein, high-calorie meals consumed each day as a way to improve nutritional status.[82]

Studies of colorectal and head and neck cancer patients have shown the beneficial effect of nutrition on survival and quality of life.[83,84] These studies have also highlighted the importance of cancer patients having access to counseling and guidance from a dietitian. In fact, these studies showed that regular foods supported by dietary counseling were more beneficial than enriched nutritional supplements taken in the absence of qualified guidance.[83,84]

### Immune Function

Impaired nutritional status in cancer patients is associated with reduced numbers of white blood cells (most often neutropenia) and low red blood cell counts, or anemia.[73] Administration of a specialized formula enriched with nutrients (including arginine and omega-3 fatty acids) to cancer patients before surgery reduced the occurrence of infections and time spent in the hospital.[85] Due to its immunomodulatory properties, arginine helps restore immune system balance in cancer patients after surgery[86];

however, further research is necessary to define its role in the nutritional care of cancer patients.

Delays in the healing of surgical wounds—or a complete failure of the wounds to heal—often complicates the rehabilitation of malnourished cancer patients after surgery.[87] Artificial nutrition of gastric cancer patients after surgery with a formula designed to boost the immune system improves wound healing and recovery.[87]

## Cancer Development and Progression

A study of patients with high levels of prostate-specific antigen (PSA), a widely accepted indicator of the risk of developing prostate cancer, showed that a diet of low fat and high soybean-protein content induced a significant, though temporary reduction in PSA levels.[88]

# NATURAL STRATEGIES FOR BOOSTING RESISTANCE TO CANCER: PREVENTION OF CANCER DEVELOPMENT AND PROGRESSION

Natural strategies known to prevent the development and progression of cancer are discussed in following sections.

## Calcium

In clinical studies involving more than 1000 colorectal cancer patients, calcium supplements reduced the risk of recurrence of colon polyps.[89] Other studies show that calcium supplements generally reduce the risk of developing colorectal cancer in the first place.[90,91] This beneficial effect of calcium was noted for calcium obtained from both dietary sources and nutritional supplements.[90]

## Carotenoids

Clinical studies have found that supplementing with lycopene, a carotenoid that is abundant in tomatoes and tomato-based products, can protect against cancers of the prostate,[92–94] colon,[95] pancreas,[96] ovaries,[97] breast,[98] and bladder.[99]

According to the *American Journal of Clinical Nutrition*, individuals seeking broad spectrum colon protection should also include foods rich in lutein (another type of carotenoid) in their diet.[100] These include spinach, broccoli, lettuce, tomatoes, oranges, carrots, celery, and greens.

## Curcumin

Curcumin, extracted from the spice turmeric, has preventive and therapeutic anticancer properties.[101,102]

Curcumin can stop the growth of cancers of the prostate,[103,104] colon,[105] and breast.[106]

In a phase 1 clinical study of colorectal cancer patients, curcumin in doses of up to 3.6 g per day improved some clinical markers and was not associated with any toxicities.[102] Clinical studies have shown that curcumin in doses of up to 10 g per day had no adverse effects in humans.[101]

## Garlic

Garlic has long been known to have anticancer properties[107,108] due to its ability to disrupt the function of cancer-causing agents.[107]

Garlic consumption lowers the risk of developing a range of cancers, including those of the stomach, colon, mammary glands, cervix,[108,109] and prostate.[110] Garlic-derived allitridum, taken in combination with selenium, protects against the development of gastric cancer.[111]

Various other garlic extracts, including aged garlic extract, allicin, and ajoene, have a range of cancer-preventive and therapeutic capabilities.[112–114]

## Green and Black Teas

Catechins and theaflavins, compounds found in green and black teas, have anticancer properties.[115]

Clinical studies have shown that consuming 5 or more cups a day of green tea reduces the risk of developing breast cancer, and may help reduce the risk of recurrence in breast cancer survivors.[116]

Consumption of green tea also significantly improves the survival of ovarian cancer patients[117] and reduces the risk of developing cancers of the lung, breast, and prostate.[118,119]

Due to the strength of data demonstrating green tea's potential in preventing cancer, Japanese researchers are trying to develop a strategy, based on green tea consumption, for delaying cancer onset in the Japanese population, as well as reducing the risk of recurrence in cancer survivors.[120]

## Folic Acid

The use of folic acid dietary supplements, or the adoption of diets rich in fruits and vegetables containing folate, is associated with a reduced risk of developing cancer, particularly colorectal[121,122] and lung cancers.[123] Sufficient intake of folic acid is also thought to protect against breast cancer[124] because folic acid guards against DNA damage and promotes gene stability.[122]

## Melatonin

The hormone melatonin, produced by the pineal gland during night-time hours, has anticancer properties.[125,126]

The use of melatonin (20 mg per night) during chemotherapy improves survival and quality of life in lung cancer patients.[127] Melatonin also reduces the growth potential of prostate and breast cancer cells.[126,128]

Further evidence supporting melatonin's role as a cancer-preventive agent comes from studies showing an elevated risk of breast cancer in night-shift workers and others who have lower levels of melatonin due to the disruption of their waking and sleeping cycles.[125] Interestingly, blind people, who generally have higher melatonin levels, have lower rates of cancer.[129,130]

## Selenium

Selenium supplements have cancer-preventive properties,[131] particularly in reducing the occurrence of lung, colorectal, esophageal, and prostate cancers.[132] Indeed, low selenium levels are associated with a four- to five-fold increase in the risk of developing prostate cancer.[133] Higher selenium levels are associated with a reduced risk of prostate cancer.[133] Because selenium levels decline with age, selenium supplements may be of particular benefit to elderly men.[133]

However, the benefits of selenium supplements in preventing cancer appear to be cancer-specific, as some clinical studies have shown supplementation to be ineffective in protecting against basal and squamous cell carcinomas of the skin.[134] Indeed, selenium supplements may increase the risk of squamous cell carcinoma.[135]

In addition to their cancer-preventive potential, selenium supplements may enhance the effectiveness of conventional chemotherapy treatment[136] and improve quality of life for patients undergoing radiation therapy.[137]

## Silymarin

Silymarin, a milk thistle extract that demonstrates anticancer properties against prostate cancer cells, may be useful in preventing and treating prostate cancer.[138,139]

## Vitamin A

Vitamin A derivatives, known as retinoids, protect against the development of various cancers, including those of the skin, breast, and lung.[140,141] Dietary supplementation with synthetic vitamin A for 12 months in liver cancer survivors prevented recurrence of this cancer.[142] In addition to preventing cancer, vitamin A derivatives have been used to cure acute promyelocytic leukemia.[140]

## Vitamin C

Long-term human studies have shown that vitamin C dietary supplements, when used in conjunction with other antioxidants, can reduce the risk of developing cancer.[143] Similar results were found for cancers of the prostate[144] and lung.[145,146]

## Vitamin D

Moderate sun exposure causes the synthesis of vitamin D in the skin. This micronutrient is known to play a role in cancer prevention.[147,148] Indeed, medical literature dating back more than 50 years affirms that regular sun exposure is associated with a substantial decrease in death rates from certain types of cancers.[149] It is estimated that moderate sun exposure without sunscreen—that is, enough to stimulate vitamin D production but not enough to damage the skin—could prevent 30 000 cancer deaths in the United States each year.[149] The sun's most damaging rays occur between 10 a.m. and 3 p.m., the hours demanding the greatest watchfulness.

Insufficient vitamin D levels are particularly associated with increased risk of developing breast, colon, and prostate cancers.[150,151] Increased vitamin D levels, obtained through sun exposure, are associated with a reduced risk of non-Hodgkin's lymphoma.[152] Vitamin D causes bones to release calcium and can thus lead to excessively high calcium levels (hypercalcemia); however, scientists are developing synthetic versions of natural vitamin D (deltanoids) that lack this adverse side effect.[153,154]

## Vitamin E

Clinical studies have shown that vitamin E can reduce the risk of prostate and lung cancers, particularly when used in combination with selenium supplements.[155,156] Regular and long-term (over 10 years) use of vitamin E reduces the risk of death from bladder cancer.[157] Similarly, use of vitamin E supplements for longer than 3 years slightly reduces the risk of recurrence among breast cancer survivors.[19]

In addition, animal studies indicate that vitamin E may have activity against colon cancer and melanoma.[158–160]

Larger clinical studies are currently underway to further assess vitamin E's protective role against prostate cancer.[161,162]

## Vitamin K

Vitamin K has been shown in laboratory and animal studies to have anticancer properties.[163] Results from a small clinical study indicate that vitamin K may protect women with viral liver cirrhosis, a known risk factor for liver cancer, from developing the disease.[164]

## PREVENTING TUMOR SPREAD (ANGIOGENESIS, INVASION, AND METASTASIS)

Natural strategies that arrest the spread of tumors include the following.

### Alpha-Tocopherol

Alpha-tocopherol supplementation, which provides the biological activity of vitamin E, reduces levels of vascular endothelial growth factor (VEGF), a tumor growth factor that plays a critical role in the formation of new blood vessels by cancer cells and subsequent tumor invasion of other organs.[165] Levels of this cancer growth factor decreased by 11% in the supplemented group, yet increased by 10% in the nonsupplemented group.[165]

### Curcumin

Curcumin is known to arrest the growth of established cancer[166] by interfering with the production of growth factors that cancer cells need to establish new blood vessels and thus invade other organs. This is a process known as angiogenesis.[166–168]

### Green Tea

Epigallocatechin in green tea has long been known to have cancer-preventive properties.[169] Epigallocatechin prevents cancer cells from forming new blood vessels and thereby spreading to other organs.[170]

### Pomegranate Extract

A laboratory study has demonstrated that extracts of the pomegranate fruit can prevent human prostate cancer cells from invading new tissues.[171]

### Soy (Genistein)

Present in soy, genistein prevents any cancer cells that persist after surgery from invading new organs and spreading.[172] This potential to arrest the spread of cancer is linked to genistein's ability to reduce production of the growth factor VEGF, a prerequisite for cancer spread and invasion.[173]

## ENHANCING THE IMMUNE SYSTEM

A range of CAM therapies have been shown to boost immune function in cancer patients. These include the following.

### Fermented Wheat Germ

Neutropenia, a condition characterized by low numbers of white blood cells known as neutrophils, is a complication of chemotherapy that leaves patients dangerously susceptible to infections.[174] Supplementing with fermented wheat germ extract during conventional treatment reduces the occurrence of neutropenia.[175]

### Garlic

Garlic supplementation boosts immune function in cancer patients[176] by improving the function of natural killer cells and lymphocytes.[176–178]

### Herbal Medicines

Herbal medicines such as echinacea, ginseng, and astragalus strengthen the immune system and may be beneficial to cancer patients.[179,180] Red ginseng boosts the immune system of gastric cancer patients undergoing chemotherapy after surgery.[180] Patients taking red ginseng had significantly higher overall survival (76%) than nonsupplementing subjects (39%) at 5 years.[180]

### Mushroom Extracts

Mushroom extracts increase the activity of natural killer cells in gynecologic cancer patients undergoing chemotherapy.[181] A *Ganoderma lucidum* polysaccharide extract known as ganopoly (1800 mg, 3 times daily before meals for 12 weeks) boosted natural killer cell numbers in advanced-stage cancer patients.[182]

In a randomized, double-blind, placebo-controlled study of 68 patients with advanced (stage 3 or 4) non–small cell lung cancer, polysaccharide peptides (PSP) isolated from the mushroom *Coriolus versicolor* (340 mg, 3 times daily for 4 weeks) significantly improved blood leukocyte and neutrophil counts, serum IgG and IgM, and percentage of body fat compared to the control group.[183]

In a case series of 8 patients with various cancers (mostly stage 2–4), a combination of maitake mushroom (*Grifola frondosa*) MD-fraction and whole maitake powder resulted in a positive response in 23 of 36 cancer patients. Cancer regression or significant symptom improvement was observed in 69% of breast cancer patients, 63% of lung cancer patients, and 58% of liver cancer patients. The study found a less than 10–20% improvement in leukemia, stomach cancer, and brain cancer patients. In addition, when maitake was taken in addition to chemotherapy, immune-competent cell activities were enhanced 1.2–1.4 times compared to chemotherapy alone.[184]

## Immunonutrition

Patients who undergo surgery to remove a tumor mass often suffer depressed immune systems following surgery, which slows their recovery and leaves them vulnerable to infection.[86] Different forms of nutrition designed to boost the immune system assist the recovery of cancer patients after surgery.[86,185,186] For example, patients administered nutrients containing fatty acids (with the aid of a feeding tube directly into the stomach) have a more rapid recovery of immune cell numbers.[86] Oral supplements enriched with arginine and omega-3 fatty acids improved immune recovery and reduced infection rates.[185,186]

## Melatonin

Melatonin is a hormone with immune regulatory activities. Most cancer patients have low levels of melatonin.[187] Melatonin supplements (10 mg per day) improve immune function in patients suffering from a variety of cancers, including gastric, renal, prostate, and bladder cancers, without any apparent adverse effects.[188] Clinical studies support melatonin's value, demonstrating that supplements of 20 mg per day can improve immune function in cancer patients, predominantly by enhancing the immunity driven by the 2 chief antitumor messengers, interleukin-2 and interleukin-12.[189,190]

## Probiotic Bacteria

When cancer patients with neutropenia (low neutrophil counts) exhibit symptoms of infection such as fever, the condition of neutropenia is referred to as febrile neutropenia.[174] The movement of bacteria through the intestinal lining is partly responsible for febrile neutropenia.[174] Interestingly, scientists have demonstrated that colonizing the intestine with friendly probiotic bacteria reduced (by virtue of competition) infection from febrile neutropenia-causing bacteria.[174]

## Relaxation Techniques

Perhaps not surprisingly, clinical studies have now shown that humor and laughter have a positive effect on the immune system, characterized by increased numbers of natural killer cells.[54–57]

Other techniques such as massage and meditation that are designed to foster relaxation also improve immune system function in cancer patients.[51,191,192] In fact, breast cancer patients participating in a massage therapy program had increased numbers of natural killer cells and lymphocytes.[51,191]

## Vitamin E

Short-term supplementation with high-dose (750 mg) vitamin E increases both the number and activity of lymphocytes in patients with advanced colorectal cancer.[24] In addition, supplementation with vitamin E during chemotherapy reduces the loss of white blood cells (neutropenia) associated with chemotherapy.[26]

# NATURAL STRATEGIES FOR ALLEVIATING CANCER SYMPTOMS

A range of complementary strategies are known to improve symptoms experienced by cancer patients.

## Anxiety, Depression, and Stress

Aromatherapy and massage are effective in alleviating depression, anxiety, and stress in cancer patients; they also have a positive effect on quality of life.[193,194] Undergoing 30-minute massage sessions 3 times per week for 5 weeks reduces hostility and anger in cancer patients.[191] In addition to massage, progressive muscle relaxation alleviates depression and anxiety in cancer patients.[51]

The use of acupuncture, hypnosis, and exercise reduces stress and anxiety.[44,48,66]

Laughter and humor are also known to improve mood and combat depression in cancer patients.[54,55,57] This improvement in mood is accompanied by quantifiable improvements in immune system and hormonal factors that influence overall well-being.[54,56,57]

Emotional support from a spouse reduces depression and improves quality of life in cancer patients.[195] Dietary supplementation with the amino acid L-carnitine in cancer patients has been effective in treating depression.[196]

## Nausea and Vomiting

Acupuncture and finger acupressure are effective in overcoming treatment-induced nausea and vomiting.[197–199] Electroacupoint stimulation and hypnotherapy also reduce the frequency and intensity of nausea in cancer patients.[9,200]

## Poor Appetite or Cachexia

Advanced cancer is often accompanied by a condition of muscle wasting referred to as cachexia or catabolic wasting.[37,201] Metabolic imbalances caused by the disease, which include the overproduction of inflammatory factors, lead to the loss of appetite and the excessive breakdown of fat and muscle.[36] This wasting condition is associated with diminished quality of life and shorter survival.[37,201]

Dietary supplementation with *fish oils* (omega-3 fatty acids) counteracts the inflammatory factors and reverses the weight loss associated with cachexia.[37,201,202] Stabilization of this condition with fish oil supplements also leads to enhanced quality of life.[202–204] For more information, refer to the Catabolic Wasting protocol.

## Lymphedema

Lymphedema, a condition characterized by excessive swelling and retention of water under the skin, often afflicts cancer patients, particularly after radiation therapy and surgery.[205,206]

Natural strategies known to be somewhat helpful in alleviating this condition include compression bandaging, which reduces the size of the swollen area, and manual massage of the draining lymph nodes, which may alleviate mild cases of lymphedema.[206,207] The use of *selenium* may improve the benefits of physical therapies such as massage and compression.[208]

## Sexual Dysfunction

Cancer patients, in particular those with prostate cancer, often experience sexual dysfunction, or impotency, usually as a complication of their treatment.[209–211] Sexual dysfunction is also associated with surgery for bladder and colorectal cancer as well as with chemotherapy agents that damage the ovaries.[210,212]

Sexual dysfunction in prostate cancer patients can be successfully managed by the use of Viagra®.[213,214] However, some alternative therapies are also effective in managing sexual dysfunction.

Clinical studies have shown that oral supplements of L-glutamine and yohimbine, a plant extract, can improve erectile dysfunction.[215] Another dietary supplement containing a combination of ginseng, ginkgo, L-arginine, multivitamins, and minerals improves erectile dysfunction.[216,217] A nutritional supplement containing barley grass, wheat grass, kelp, chlorella, cooked brown rice, and fructooligosaccharides has also been shown to improve sexual dysfunction.[218]

## Hair Loss

A mushroom extract, originally concocted for use as an immune system booster, improves alopecia (hair loss), a condition associated with the use of conventional cancer treatments.[181] Animal studies have also shown that supplementing with the antioxidant N-acetylcysteine can protect against hair loss during conventional cancer treatments.[219]

## Fatigue

In addition to relieving stress, dietary supplementation with the amino acid L-carnitine reduces fatigue, which can be a symptom of the cancer or a side effect of conventional treatment.[196] The use of L-carnitine during chemotherapy with doxorubicin has been proposed as an adjuvant therapy since 1985.[220]

Acupuncture has also demonstrated effectiveness in alleviating cancer fatigue.[221] Cancer-related fatigue responds to a combined regimen of massage, foot soaking, and reflexology.[52] In addition, breathing exercises, conducted with the help of a health care provider, improves fatigue in patients recovering from stem cell transplantation.[49]

# NATURAL STRATEGIES FOR COUNTERACTING ADVERSE EFFECTS FROM CONVENTIONAL CANCER TREATMENT

Nutritional supplements known to counteract some of the negative side effects of conventional treatments are summarized in Table 2. In addition to these nutrients, physical and psychological therapies—including acupuncture, breathing exercises, massage, and aromatherapy—can improve these negative side effects.[44,49,50] For more information, refer to the protocols on Cancer Surgery, Chemotherapy, and Cancer Radiation Therapy.

# CLINICAL TRIALS

Numerous ongoing clinical studies are assessing the merits of various CAM therapies for cancer. Cancer patients can opt to participate in these studies or simply monitor their outcomes. The specific details and findings of these studies are subject to constant change and therefore are not provided here. Up-to-date information on ongoing clinical trials can be obtained from the National Center for Complementary and Alternative Medicine (NCCAM) at the following address:

NCCAM

9000 Rockville Pike

Bethesda, MD 20892

Email: info@nccam.nih.gov

Website: http://nccam.nih.gov/research/clinicaltrials

**Table 2:   Nutritional Supplements Known to Alleviate Negative Side Effects of Conventional Cancer Treatment**

| Cancer Treatment–Related Adverse Effects | Nutritional Supplement | References |
|---|---|---|
| Diarrhea, neuropathy, heart complications, mucositis | Glutamine | Daniele et al[222], Savarese et al[223] |
| Mucositis, fibrosis, cardiovascular complications | Antioxidants | Borek[24], Wattanapitayakul et al[225] |
| Mucositis, anemia, cardiovascular complications | Melatonin | Majsterek et al[226], Ahmed et al[227], Balli et al[228] |
| Radiation-induced cell damage | Vitamin A | Levitsky et al[229], Vorotnikova et al[230] |
| Neuropathy (nerve damage) | Vitamin E | Argyriou et al[231], Pace et al[232] |
| Nausea and vomiting | Ginger | Boon et al[233], Sharma et al[234], Manusirivithaya et al[235] |
| Nephrotoxicity (kidney damage) | Silibinin | Bokemeyer et al[236] |
| Diarrhea | Herbal remedies | Mori et al[237], Taixiang et al[238] |
| Heart damage | CoQ10 | Portakal et al[239], Bandy et al[240], Iarussi et al[241] |

## FOR MORE INFORMATION

Cancer patients who suffer from the aforementioned manifestations may wish to read the following protocols and design a program that addresses the full range of their cancer concerns:

- Chemotherapy
- Cancer Radiation Therapy
- Cancer Surgery
- Cancer Vaccines and Immunotherapy
- Catabolic Wasting
- Blood Disorders (Anemia, Leukopenia, and Thrombocytopenia)
- Immune System Strengthening

## Life Extension Suggestions

Cancer patients should consult their physicians before using any complementary alternative therapies while undergoing conventional medical treatment.

Different doses of the same nutritional supplement may be required for different applications of complementary alternative cancer therapies, such as preventing cancer, inhibiting tumor spread, enhancing/suppressing the immune system, alleviating cancer symptoms, and counteracting side effects of conventional treatment. Cancer patients who wish to adopt a CAM approach should refer to the appropriate protocol or consult an integrative practitioner for definitive advice on appropriate doses of the nutritional supplements discussed in this protocol.

The blood tests discussed in this section are available through Life Extension National Diagnostics, Inc. For ordering information, call anytime toll-free at (800) 208-3444, or visit us online at www.LifeExtension.com.

## REFERENCES

References available at: www.lef.org/dpt5/ch46

# 47

# Congestive Heart Failure

Congestive heart failure (CHF) seems to be the exception when it comes to our national battle against heart disease. While other forms of heart disease, including coronary artery disease (CAD), are becoming less common, the rate of CHF continues to rise. The rate of hospitalization for CHF increased three- to four-fold between 1971 and 1999.[1,2] It is the leading cause of hospitalization among people over age 65, accounting for about 20% of hospitalizations in this group.[3]

The increase in CHF is partly due to an aging population and our success in treating other forms of heart disease. In many instances, cases of CAD and high blood pressure that would have once resulted in fatal heart attacks are successfully managed, only to have the patient later develop CHF.

CHF occurs when the heart cannot pump efficiently enough to supply the body with freshly oxygenated blood. It affects about 5 million people in the United States.[1] Hoping to prolong survival, patients with CHF are typically treated with an array of powerful medications shown to increase survival, often at a high cost. Conventional drugs used to treat CHF have significant adverse effects and, in many cases, implantation of a life-saving medical device, or even having a heart transplant, may be necessary.

Even as CHF becomes more common, it remains very dangerous. According to statistics from the multigenerational Framingham Heart Study, 80% of men and 70% of women under the age of 65 who are diagnosed with CHF will die within 8 years. Within 1 year of diagnosis, 20% of patients will die. The 5-year mortality is about 50%.[1]

## RISK FACTORS FOR CHF

A number of conditions may lead to CHF, including:

- CAD
- History of heart attack
- Advanced age
- Irregular heartbeats, or arrhythmias
- Heart valve disease

- Thyroid disease
- Diabetes
- Drug or alcohol abuse
- Cardiomyopathy
- Congenital heart defects
- Chronic high blood pressure

Unfortunately, CHF is difficult to diagnose because it often occurs in conjunction with, or as a result of, other forms of heart disease. The best hope for patients with CHF is to catch the disease early, before it has caused permanent enlargement of the heart. The symptoms of CHF include fatigue, shortness of breath, coughing, swelling, and, when severe, bluish extremities.

## CONVENTIONAL TREATMENTS FOR CHF

Once CHF has been diagnosed, physicians usually rely on a constellation of pharmaceuticals to address its symptoms and slow its progression. The exact drugs used depend on the type and severity of CHF, but some of the more common drugs include:

### Diuretics

Sometimes called "water pills," diuretics help remove excess fluid from the body. Diuretics are often the first line of treatment. A significant side effect is the loss of potassium in urine, which may result in electrolyte abnormalities.[4]

### Angiotensin-Converting Enzyme (ACE) Inhibitors

ACE inhibitors have been shown to improve survival among patients with CHF by lowering blood pressure. Side effects include dangerously low blood pressure, dizziness, coughing, and birth defects.[5]

### Beta Blockers

Beta blockers slow the heart rate by making it less sensitive to adrenaline (epinephrine). This medication may be given after a patient's condition has stabilized with ACE inhibitors. Side effects may include weight gain, tiredness, dizziness, and sensitivity to cold. Patients with a slow heart rate, elevated systolic blood pressure, peripheral vascular disease, asthma, chronic obstructive pulmonary disease, or who have had certain heart rhythm abnormalities should not take beta blockers.[6]

### Digoxin

Digoxin is used to control symptoms of some forms of CHF and control heart rate irregularities.[6] Side effects include abdominal pain, nausea or vomiting, diarrhea, and rarely, dangerous heart rhythm abnormalities.

These drugs may be prescribed in an emergency setting while the physician works to stabilize the patient's condition and in the long-term management of CHF. While these drugs are proven to extend the lives of patients with CHF, they also cause a wide range of side effects that often require more drug therapy. Despite such intensive drug therapy, the condition of most patients with CHF will eventually worsen, requiring more serious measures. A physician may recommend insertion of a pacemaker or left ventricular assist device. In extreme cases, the patient may require a heart transplant.

Vitamins and dietary supplements have also been shown to ease the symptoms of CHF—often without the debilitating side effects of more powerful pharmaceuticals.[7] Coenzyme Q10 (CoQ10) has been widely studied in CHF and found to increase heart function, while L-carnitine and taurine have been shown to improve cardiac function and lessen the heart's workload.[8,9] Other dietary supplements and nutrients, including minerals (eg, magnesium and potassium), antioxidants (eg, R-lipoic acid and vitamins C and E), and herbs (eg, hawthorn) may help ease symptoms of CHF. Each of these will be discussed in detail later in this chapter.

The hormonal system is also affected by CHF. In the early stages of CHF, studies have shown that the body tries to compensate for reduced cardiac function with a series of neurohormonal adaptations that work to maintain normal blood pressure and increase the output of the heart.[10,11] As the disease progresses, however, this hormonal response is overwhelmed, and the body's delicate hormonal balance is damaged. While there is still much to learn about the interaction of the hormonal system and CHF, hormonal therapy may offer an option for treatment.

It is important to make lifestyle changes that will slow the progression of CHF. These changes include limiting salt intake (sometimes severely), losing weight to reduce the workload on the heart, avoiding alcohol or drugs, and monitoring water intake. As always, no program of dietary supplementation and lifestyle changes should be launched without the consent of a physician.

## WHAT YOU HAVE LEARNED SO FAR

- The rate of CHF is increasing, at least partly because of our ability to treat other forms of heart disease and partly because of the aging population.

- Half of all patients with CHF die within 5 years of diagnosis.
- Most patients with CHF have other underlying forms of heart disease, especially CAD. This complicates both the diagnosis and treatment of CHF.
- CHF cannot be reversed, but its severity can be reduced. At best, conventional medicine uses a constellation of powerful drugs to slow it down. These drugs have side effects that range from mild to severe and may dramatically reduce one's quality of life.
- Besides drugs, CHF can be treated with surgical interventions such as implantation of a pacemaker or a heart transplant.
- Some nutrients and supplements—such as CoQ10, L-carnitine, and taurine—have been shown to increase the heart's function or reduce side effects of drugs used to treat CHF.
- Lifestyle changes, including dietary modifications and avoiding drugs and alcohol (which might stress the heart), are an important part of any heart-healthy program. Patients may also be advised to limit their intake of salt and water.

## CLASSES OF CHF

CHF is classified in several ways. It may be identified by the regions of the heart that are affected, severity of the disease, or area of the cardiac cycle that is compromised. The treatment program will depend on the form of CHF and its severity.

CHF severity is usually measured according to the New York Heart Association (NYHA) classification system. This model has been used by the American College of Cardiology and American Heart Association to develop treatment guidelines.[12] The CHF classes follow:

- **Class I.** No limitation and no symptoms with ordinary physical activity.

- **Class II.** Slight limitation and symptoms with ordinary physical activity. Comfortable at rest.

- **Class III.** More pronounced limitation because of symptoms, even with less than ordinary physical activity. Comfortable only at rest.

- **Class IV.** Severe to complete limitation of physical activity. Symptoms are present with any degree of physical activity and also appear at rest.

CHF is also described by the region of the heart affected. The heart has four chambers, two each on the right and left sides. Each side of the heart has a filling chamber (atria) and a pumping chamber (ventricle). A complete cardiac cycle, or heartbeat, has all of these chambers working in concert to move blood through the body.

The right side of the heart is responsible for accepting oxygen-poor blood from the body, and then

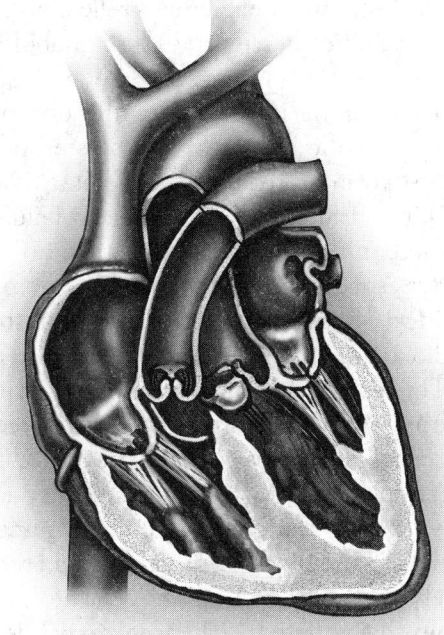

Normal Heart

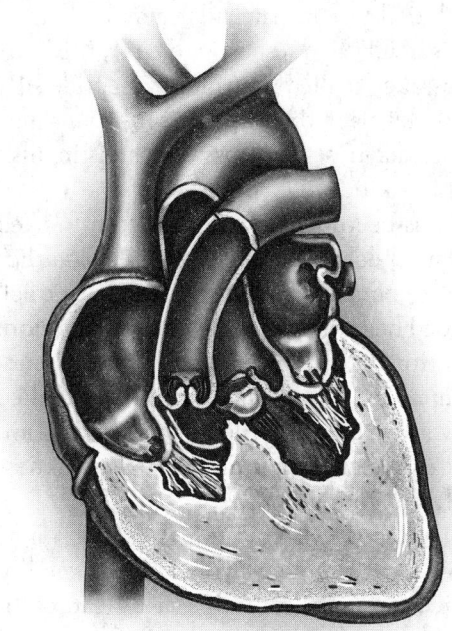

Congestive Heart

pumping it through the right ventricle, into the pulmonary arteries and into the lungs, where carbon dioxide is exchanged for oxygen. After the blood travels through the lungs, it returns to the left side of the heart through the pulmonary veins. Here, the heart's main pumping chamber (the left ventricle) pumps the freshly oxygenated blood through the aorta and out to the rest of the body.

CHF that occurs on the right side of the heart is called cor pulmonale, or right-sided heart failure. It is characterized by an expanded right ventricle. Symptoms include swelling as the blood pools in the legs and lower body.

CHF that occurs on the left side of the heart is characterized by an enlarged and weakened left ventricle. Left-sided heart failure may result in inadequate amounts of blood being pumped through the body and includes symptoms such as shortness of breath and fatigue.

CHF can also be described by the phase of the heartbeat that is affected. A normal heartbeat has 2 phases: filling and contraction. The filling phase of the heartbeat, when the ventricles are relaxed and filling with blood, is called diastole. If the lower chambers of the heart, particularly the left ventricle, cannot fill properly, it is known as diastolic heart failure.

Once the ventricles have filled with blood, they contract forcefully. This phase is called systole. If the heart cannot contract forcefully enough to expel the majority of the blood in the ventricles, it is called

systolic heart failure. Systolic heart failure is the most common form of CHF.

## DIAGNOSING CHF

Just as there is no single treatment for CHF, there is no single test used for diagnosis. Instead, physicians have traditionally relied on a patient's medical history, along with the presence of symptoms associated with CHF, and a variety of diagnostic tests.

The most common test remains the echocardiogram. This test uses sound waves to visualize the structures of the heart, allowing physicians to see the heart chambers and measure cardiac function. It also helps physicians determine how well the heart is functioning and how far the disease has progressed.

An electrocardiogram (ECG) or cardiac catheterization may also be recommended. The ECG measures electrical signals within the heart, while cardiac catheterization determines blood pressure from within the heart's chambers. In some cases, patients with CHF may have a heartbeat that is too slow (bradycardia) or too fast (tachycardia). An ECG can help physicians determine if medications to control the heart rate are necessary. Physicians may also recommend a standard exercise stress test (to evaluate an ECG reading while a patient is walking or running) or an exercise stress test (involving radionuclide scanning after injection of a radioactive substance).

While the standard test used to measure CHF is an echocardiogram (ultrasound), newer tests are showing promise. One blood test in particular may be helpful in the diagnosis of CHF. In response to CHF, the body releases a substance called natriuretic peptide. By measuring blood levels of this peptide, physicians may be able to better diagnose CHF, as well as distinguish among the various kinds of CHF.[13,14]

Once CHF has been diagnosed, it is often tracked through regular checkups and routine echocardiograms. The most common measurement used to track systolic, left-sided heart failure is the ejection fraction. Determined during an echocardiogram, ejection fraction is a measurement of how much blood is expelled from the left ventricle during the heart's contraction phase. Any measurement below 55% signals weakness in the ventricle's pumping action.

Importantly, patients with diastolic CHF who may not have severe CHF symptoms will have a normal or near-normal ejection fraction. In this case, heart catheterization may be needed to diagnose CHF.[15]

## CHF AND THE HORMONAL CONNECTION

Many people think of the heart as a simple pump that keeps blood flowing through the body. While this is true, it is also a vast oversimplification of the heart's role in the body. In fact, the heart is a highly complex organ that is responsive to all sorts of influences, including hormones. For example, when people are stressed, the body is flooded with adrenaline (epinephrine), a hormone that stimulates the heart to contract more forcefully and raise blood pressure.

Although there is much to learn, there is a clear connection between the hormonal system and cardiac health. Studies have shown that early in CHF, the body tries to compensate for reduced cardiac function with a series of neurohormonal adaptations. These changes cause certain blood vessels throughout the body to constrict (resulting in more blood flow to vital organs) and boost the output of the heart by increasing its contractile strength and heart rate.[10,11]

These changes, however, have significant drawbacks. Elevated blood pressure may lead to swelling (one of the symptoms of CHF) or congestion in the lungs that leads to coughing (another symptom). The increased force of the heartbeat may also aggravate CAD. Overall, scientists believe that the net effect of these neurohormonal adaptations is negative. The adaptations may help short term, but ultimately make the condition worse.[16]

Patients with CHF have been shown to have low levels of dehydroepiandrosterone (DHEA),[17] testosterone, and insulin-like growth factor I (IGF-I).[18] These hormonal deficiencies reflect an imbalance in the catabolic (destructive) and anabolic (constructive) hormonal systems.[19] The body's main catabolic hormone is cortisol, while one of the body's main anabolic hormones is testosterone.

A study measured blood estradiol (a dominant estrogen) in 501 men with chronic heart failure. Compared to those in the balanced estrogen quintile, men in the lowest estradiol quintile were 217% more likely to die during a 3-year follow-up, while men in the highest estradiol quintile were 133% more likely to die.[20]

The men in the balanced quintile—with the fewest deaths—had serum estradiol levels between 21.80 and 30.11 pg/mL. This is virtually the ideal range that Life Extension has long recommended its male members strive for. The men in the highest quintile who suffered a 133% increased death rate had serum estradiol levels of 37.40 pg/mL or above. The lowest estradiol group that suffered a 217% increased death rate had serum estradiol levels under 12.90 pg/mL.

The dramatic increase in mortality in men with unbalanced estrogen (ie, estradiol levels either too high or too low) is nothing short of astounding. It uncovers a gaping hole in conventional cardiology practice that is easily correctable and explains why clinical trials on aging men that fail to measure estradiol have serious shortcomings. While hormonal supplementation is somewhat controversial for heart patients, there is evidence that supportive testosterone therapy can restore testosterone levels to normal. In one study, testosterone therapy was shown to significantly improve exercise capacity and quality of life in men who had moderate to severe CHF. During the study, the men were given testosterone therapy in small doses for 12 months, enough to restore levels to within physiologic range.[21] Hormonal restoration therapy has also shown promise in lowering cholesterol levels in patients with CHF.[22] A youthful hormonal profile is closely associated with good overall health. Undoubtedly, the future will expand our understanding of the complicated interaction between hormones and CHF.

## TARGETED NUTRITIONAL STRATEGIES

### Strengthening the Heart Muscle: The Power of CoQ10

Studies have shown that nutrients and supplements can strengthen the heart muscle, with fewer side effects than the powerful pharmaceuticals often used to treat the condition. Coenzyme Q10 (CoQ10) is one of the most powerful.

The goal with nutrients and supplements, as with conventional medication, is to slow the gradual enlargement and weakening of the heart. This process, which occurs in all forms of CHF, is called cardiac remodeling. During cardiac remodeling, the heart gradually changes shape, becoming larger and thinner. Cardiac remodeling is the driving force behind the reduced quality of life experienced by patients with CHF.[23,24]

By reinforcing the heart's function, it may be possible to slow cardiac remodeling. In this regard, CoQ10 has been studied since the middle 1960s. Present in high quantities throughout the heart muscle, CoQ10 has many beneficial effects, including energy production,[25–28] an antioxidant effect,[29] and stabilizing the heart membrane.[30]

The following studies have examined CoQ10 in CHF and found that it can improve heart function.

- One meta-analysis looked at all the published studies between 1966 and 2005 of CoQ10 in CHF. It found that CoQ10 had an overall value in improving ejection fraction and diastolic volume. Although the authors called for more large studies to confirm these results, they noted that CoQ10 is generally well tolerated, with few side effects.[31]

- Researchers reviewed clinical trials involving 1000 patients with CHF and found a significant improvement in exercise tolerance as well as a lower NYHA class among those receiving CoQ10.[32]

- A study of 32 patients with NYHA class-IV CHF who were waiting for a heart transplant showed improved cardiac function and a reduction of symptoms after CoQ10 supplementation.[33]

- Among patients with CHF who had a low ejection fraction (<45%) and an elevated left ventricular diastolic volume, CoQ10 has been shown to reduce diastolic volume, which is associated with increased survival among patients undergoing coronary artery bypass surgery.[34] The degree of benefit associated with CoQ10 among these patients was shown to correlate to the severity of their CHF.[35]

Other studies have shown that withdrawing CoQ10 from patients with CHF resulted in decreased cardiac function and more severe symptoms.[36]

Previously, all supplemental CoQ10 in the world has been in its oxidized or ubiquinone form. Today, it is possible to obtain dietary supplements containing ubiquinol, the reduced form of CoQ10. The ubiquinol form of CoQ10 is more bioavailable than ubiquinone. Compared with conventional ubiquinone CoQ10,

ubiquinol was shown to absorb into the bloodstream up to 8 times better.[37–39]

In order to ascertain the effects of ubiquinol, a team of researchers identified patients with advanced CHF who had been taking 450 mg/day of ubiquinone, but whose mean total plasma CoQ10 blood level was only 1.4 µg/mL. All of these patients were then changed to 450 mg/day of ubiquinol. The results showed that ubiquinol increased mean plasma CoQ10 levels up to 4.1 µg/mL (or 2.92-fold greater than ubiquinone).[40] A review of previous studies indicates that significant clinical benefit in heart failure patients requires a plasma CoQ10 level of around 4 µg/mL.[41–43] In severe heart failure patients, the only way these higher levels can be obtained appears to be with ubiquinol— not conventional ubiquinone CoQ10 supplements.

## Increasing Energy and Blood Flow and Reducing Swelling: L-Carnitine and Taurine

Like CoQ10, the levels of L-carnitine and taurine in the heart muscle have been shown to decline among patients with CHF. By raising blood levels of both amino acids, patients with CHF have responded with fewer symptoms and improved cardiac function.

L-carnitine is essential for the transport of fatty acids into the heart muscle and mitochondria for energy production. L-carnitine is sensitive to the level of oxygen in the heart muscle. Studies have shown that patients with CHF who take L-carnitine have improved ejection fraction.[44–46] There is evidence that L-carnitine helps the heart by preventing the enlargement of the left ventricle, which is a critical step in the progression of CHF. Studies have shown that L-carnitine can help prevent left ventricular enlargement after bypass surgery in patients who have had a heart attack.[35] The same results were found among patients who have had an acute heart attack.[47] By improving ejection fraction and preventing enlargement of the left ventricle, L-carnitine addresses two of the most serious problems associated with CHF. Taurine acts by a different mechanism. Patients with CHF often have swelling caused by excessive fluid buildup in the tissues, which puts additional pressure on the heart and accelerates CHF. Diuretics, one of the standard pharmaceutical therapies in CHF, are basically designed to flush excess fluid from the body. Taurine (through well-documented pathways) has a similar effect and has been shown to help reduce fluid levels, thus reducing the workload on the heart.[9]

Taurine has a number of other positive influences as well, including minimizing the effect of the protein angiotensin II.[9] Angiotensin II causes blood vessels to constrict. This is the same protein targeted by ACE inhibitors, which are a mainstay of conventional CHF treatment. By minimizing the effect of angiotensin II, taurine may reduce cardiac remodeling.[9]

## COVERING ALL THE BASES: COMPLEMENTARY APPROACHES TO TREATING CHF

Managing CHF requires coordinating many influences and factors. The idea is to first stabilize the patient's condition (especially if the patient has acute CHF that may lead to cardiac arrest), and then develop a pharmaceutical and lifestyle program suited for the patient's metabolism. Dosages of the most popular medications often start at the lower end of their recommended range and are frequently adjusted by physicians until they get the right mix of medications to prevent symptoms, slow the disease, and keep side effects under control. A major problem with these medications is their significant side effects, which may severely reduce a patient's quality of life.

In terms of lifestyle changes, patients may be advised to limit their salt intake to 2 g per day and their water intake to 1.5–2 L per day. A heart-healthy diet—including increased intake of monosaturated oils (such as extra virgin olive oil), fruits and vegetables, fiber, and essential fatty acids—is also suggested. Finally, patients may be advised to increase their intake of garlic, onions, and celery, all of which have been shown to lower blood pressure.

A successful complementary approach uses the same principles but relies on nutrients and supplements that have far fewer side effects than conventional pharmaceuticals. The goal of complementary treatment is to:

- Restore neurohormonal and metabolic integrity
- Improve the pumping action of the heart and increase myocardial efficiency
- Decrease oxidative stress throughout the body
- Restore mineral balance (especially sodium/potassium ratios)
- Decrease vascular resistance to improve blood flow
- Lower the risk of blood clots
- Lower the risk of abnormal heart rhythms

Working with a knowledgeable physician, patients with CHF may consider adding any of these supplements to their program.

### Hawthorn

Hawthorn is a plant extract that has been shown to improve the symptoms of patients with NYHA class II or III CHF.[48] Hawthorn's benefits include relaxing blood vessels to lower blood pressure, increasing blood flow to the heart, and controlling heart rate in a way similar to digoxin.[48,49] Hawthorn helps improve exercise tolerance,[50] and has shown promise in the treatment of left ventricular dysfunction.[50–53]

### Magnesium and Potassium

Patients treated with a common diuretic (furosemide) often develop low magnesium and potassium levels, which may cause cardiac arrhythmias. Many physicians recommend that patients on furosemide also be given potassium to help prevent arrhythmias.[4] Studies have also shown that magnesium supplementation may normalize potassium and magnesium levels within the heart.[54] Blood tests can help determine whether magnesium or potassium levels are low in response to diuretic therapy.

### Antioxidant Vitamins

The dangerous effects of oxygen-free radicals on the body are well known. Elderly populations with higher blood levels of antioxidants such as vitamins C and E have been shown to have a lower incidence of heart disease.[55] Among people who have had a heart attack, supplementation with vitamins C and E has been shown to diminish the formation of free radicals and reduce damage to the heart.[56] These studies demonstrate that heart health is related to antioxidant levels. Because these antioxidants are well tolerated and slow the progression of CHF, it may be prudent to consider adding them to a CHF supplementation program.

### Lipoic Acid

Lipoic acid is an antioxidant that stimulates the creation of glutathione, another powerful antioxidant.[57] Because oxidative stress is associated with decreased cardiac function,[55] lipoic acid might be another valuable addition to the CHF antioxidant regimen.

Lipoic acid comes in two "mirror image" forms labeled "R" and "S." Research has unveiled an advanced new formulation of lipoic acid called sodium-R-lipoic acid, which reaches higher plasma levels of lipoic acid sooner than other forms.[58]

### Fish Oil

Fish oil, which is rich in omega-3 polyunsaturated fatty acids, has not been studied extensively in patients with CHF. However, there are many studies showing its value to overall cardiac health. For example, patients who take fish oil before heart surgery may avoid acute degeneration of heart tissue.[59] Fish oil has also been shown to reduce the frequency of sudden cardiac death in patients who have recently had a heart attack.[60] Researchers in the United Kingdom have launched studies to examine fish oil's ability to improve myocardial function in patients with CHF.[60]

## D-Ribose

People with CHF do not have the cardiac power to pump blood vigorously from their heart and around the body. A simple sugar molecule, D-ribose, fuels cardiac function.

Restoring the heart muscle's "tone" in patients with CHF is the goal of a host of drug treatments including diuretics, digoxin, and others. In 2003, German researchers took a natural approach—they provided daily oral D-ribose supplements or placebo for 3 weeks to 15 people with CHF.[61] The groups then reversed their treatment assignments.

During the period of D-ribose supplementation, the patients showed dramatic improvements in their heart's ability to fill and empty efficiently—changes critical to reducing fluid accumulation throughout the body and boosting energy levels as tissues gain oxygen and nutrients from the restored blood flow. Perhaps most importantly from the patients' own standpoint, they reported substantial improvements in quality of life while on the active supplement.

## Vitamin D

Abundant evidence now points to numerous cardioprotective functions of vitamin D. Vitamin D deficiency has been shown to diminish contractile function of heart muscle cells and distort heart muscle structure (triggering hypertrophy, or abnormal heart muscle growth).[62,63] Low levels of serum 25-hydroxyvitamin D have been linked with CHF.[64]

Scientists believe that elevated levels of circulating proinflammatory cytokines may contribute to heart failure, and vitamin D may offer heart-protective benefits by quelling these inflammatory mediators.[65] In a double-blind clinical trial, 123 patients with CHF were randomly assigned to receive vitamin D3 (50 mcg [2000 IU] per day) plus 500 mg of calcium or placebo plus 500 mg of calcium.[65] Over the 9-month study period, patients supplemented with vitamin D had greatly increased levels of the anti-inflammatory cytokine interleukin-10 (IL-10) and lower levels of the proinflammatory cytokine tumor necrosis factor-alpha (TNF-α). Scientists believe that by reducing the inflammatory environment in CHF patients,

vitamin D3 holds promise as an anti-inflammatory therapeutic for people suffering from heart failure.

## Pyrroloquinoline Quinone (PQQ)

In 2010, researchers released a peer-reviewed publication showing that a natural compound called PQQ promotes the formation of new mitochondria within cells.[66] The ability of PQQ to promote mitochondrial biogenesis[66] could lead to even greater improvements in cardiac output.

A study published in 2010 compared left ventricular heart muscle tissue in patients with end-stage heart failure and normal hearts. Mitochondrial DNA was decreased by 40% in failing hearts. This was accompanied by reductions of 25-80% in mitochondrial DNA-encoded proteins of failing hearts. The doctors who conducted this study concluded: "Mitochondrial biogenesis is severely impaired as evidenced by reduced mitochondrial DNA replication and depletion of mitochondrial DNA in the human failing heart . . . suggesting novel mechanisms for mitochondrial dysfunction in heart failure."[67]

## Creatine

Although creatine offers an array of benefits, most people think of it simply as a supplement that bodybuilders and other athletes use to gain strength and muscle mass. A substantial body of research has found that creatine may have a wide variety of uses.

Cardiac creatine levels are depressed in chronic heart failure, and researchers have looked at supplemental creatine to improve heart function and overall symptomology in certain forms of heart disease.

A study looked at the effects of creatine supplementation on endurance and muscle metabolism in people with CHF.[68] In particular, the researchers looked at levels of ammonia and lactate, two important indicators of fatigue and muscle performance. This study found that patients with CHF given 20 g of creatine per day had greater strength and endurance (measured as handgrip exercise at 25%, 50%, and 75% of maximum voluntary contraction or until exhaustion) and had lower levels of lactate and ammonia than the placebo group. This shows that creatine supplementation in chronic heart failure augments skeletal muscle endurance and attenuates the abnormal skeletal muscle metabolic response to exercise.

Creatine is generally taken as a "loading" phase of 15–20 g per day (generally split into doses of 5 g) for 5–7 days, followed by weeks to months of 2–5 g per day.[69]

CHF usually occurs in the presence of other forms of heart disease, especially CAD. Also, conditions such as hyperhomocysteinemia (elevated homocysteine levels) and hypercholesterolemia (high cholesterol) are associated with CHF. Patients with CHF who also have underlying cardiac disease may wish to read the following protocols and design a program that will address the full range of their cardiac problems:

- Atherosclerosis and Cardiovascular Disease
- Cholesterol Management
- Homocysteine Reduction
- High Blood Pressure

## Life Extension Suggestions

- **CoQ10 (ubiquinol):** 200–450 mg daily
- **L-carnitine:** 1–3 g daily
- **Taurine:** 2–3 g daily
- **Hawthorn:** 3000 mg daily
- **Magnesium citrate:** 160 mg (in capsule form), 1–6 times daily
- **Potassium:** 99 mg daily (or more) when instructed to do so by a healthcare professional, based on blood test results
- **Vitamin C:** 1000 mg daily
- **Vitamin E:** 800 IU daily
- **R-lipoic acid:** 240 mg daily

- **Fish oil** (with olive polyphenols and sesame lignans): providing 1400 mg EPA and 1000 mg DHA daily
- **D-ribose:** 15–30 g for advanced cardiac support in divided doses throughout the day
- **Vitamin D:** 5000–10 000 IU daily followed by vitamin D blood testing
- **Pyrroloquinoline quinone (PQQ):** 10–20 mg daily
- **Creatine:** 15–20 g daily (generally split into doses of 5 g) for 5–7 days, followed by 2–5 g daily
- **DHEA:** 25–50 mg daily (depending on blood test results)

In addition, the following blood testing resources may be helpful:

- **Omega Score®**
- **CoQ10 (Coenzyme Q10)**
- **Vitamin D, 25-Hydroxy**
- **BNP (B-Type Natriuretic Peptide)**
- **Male Panel or Female Panel**

## REFERENCES

References available at: www.lef.org/dpt5/ch47

# 48

# Constipation

Constipation is one of the most common gastrointestinal complaints in the United States, especially among elderly people. Both chronic and acute constipation can be a significant source of discomfort.

Constipation is diagnosed whenever bowel movements are difficult, hard, or painful. Contrary to popular wisdom, frequency of bowel movements is not a criterion for diagnosing constipation because of the wide range of variability among individuals. Most people have at least three bowel movements weekly, but some people have fewer and would not be diagnosed with constipation. Bowel movements should be fairly regular and pass with no straining or pain. Stool should be formed and pliable, as opposed to pebble-like and hard. It is also important to note that dramatic shifts in the frequency or manner of bowel movements (such as frequent diarrhea or the sudden onset of very painful, very difficult-to-pass bowel movements) should prompt an immediate visit to a physician to look for underlying causes.

Most individuals with constant constipation develop a variety of symptoms, ranging from abdominal pain, rectal discomfort, abdominal fullness and bloating, nausea, and loss of appetite to a general feeling of malaise. These individuals feel as if they never completely evacuate their bowels. Severe chronic constipation may be accompanied by fecal impaction.[1,2]

Most people with chronic constipation are advised to exercise and increase their intake of fiber and liquids. While these measures are effective for some people, they do not work for everybody. Many people also use fiber supplements. However, fiber supplements are not always effective. The Life Extension Foundation® has identified superior forms of fiber that may help relieve constipation when traditional fiber supplements are not adequate. If the above measures do not relieve constipation, nutritional laxatives should be considered. There are many kinds of laxatives, but using peristaltic-stimulating laxatives, which also provide health benefits, is the safest choice.

Because constipation can be caused by serious medical conditions, such as cancer, a sudden change in bowel habits among middle-aged or elderly people warrants a thorough evaluation by a physician.

## RISK FACTORS FOR CONSTIPATION

Stool is formed in the colon, which is at the lower end of the gastrointestinal tract. By the time digested food reaches the colon, most of the nutrients have been absorbed. The colon's primary job is to remove excess liquid from intestinal contents. A large number of beneficial bacteria colonize the colon and help with digestion of any remaining nutrients. Muscular peristaltic waves propel the stool (while it is in the process of being formed) toward the rectum. The stool is aided in its passage through the colon by mucus, which provides lubrication.

Bulk-forming fiber and water are essential to the healthy formation of stool. Insoluble fiber provides bulk to the stool and retains enough water to keep the stool pliable.[3] Likewise, adequate moisture is needed to keep the stool soft and prepare it for evacuation. There is, however, some disagreement among physicians about the role of fluid intake in constipation. Some studies have reported that liquid intake is not associated with constipation.[4]

For the most part, doctors usually consider the following to be risk factors for constipation.

### Lack of Exercise

Constipation has been shown to be related to inactivity.[5] Abdominal and intestinal muscles work together to move the bowels. Weak abdominal muscles can contribute to weak bowel movements.

### Some Medications

Some pain medications, especially narcotics, can cause constipation, as can some antidepressants, iron supplements, and calcium supplements.[6] Other medications that can cause constipation include calcium channel blockers, psychotropic drugs, and anticholinergics. Inadequate thyroid hormone supplementation is also thought to cause constipation.

### Certain Diseases

Tumors and some diseases may produce a rapid change in bowel movements, or even the cessation of all bowel movements.

## DIAGNOSING CONSTIPATION

During the diagnostic evaluation of constipation, physicians will attempt to determine if the condition is caused by an underlying disease, medication, or dietary cause. Constipation can be defined as the presence of two or more of the following symptoms, occurring for at least 12 weeks in the preceding

12 months (symptoms 1 through 5 must occur at least 25% of the time when defecating):[7–9]

1. Straining

2. Lumpy or hard stools

3. Sensation of incomplete evacuation

4. Sensation of anal-rectal obstruction or blockage

5. Manual maneuvers to facilitate defecation

6. Infrequent (fewer than 3) bowel movements per week

Measurement of colonic transit time (how long it takes stool to move through the colon) is sometimes used to evaluate patients with chronic constipation.[7,10]

## COMPLICATIONS OF CONSTIPATION

Complications of constipation include hemorrhoids (which are caused by straining to have a bowel movement) and anal fissures (which are tears in the skin around the anus). As a result, rectal bleeding (appearing as bright red streaks on the surface of the stool) may occur.[11–13]

Sometimes straining causes a small amount of intestinal lining to push out from the anal opening. This condition is known as rectal prolapse. Treatment requires pushing the prolapsed portion of the bowel back into the body, which can be done manually in a doctor's office. In some cases, incarcerated rectal prolapse (ie, the prolapsed portion of the bowel becomes trapped) may occur. This is an emergency that requires surgery.[14]

Constipation can contribute to a loss of bladder control by weakening the pelvic floor muscles as a result of straining. A full bowel pressing on the bladder, causing it to empty prematurely or block the outflow of urine, is not uncommon. People who have bladder control problems often do not drink enough fluids for fear of incontinence, which can also worsen constipation.[15]

## SCREENING FOR CONSTIPATION

Among middle-aged or elderly people, severe constipation or an abrupt change in bowel habits should prompt a thorough medical evaluation. Patients should be screened for thyroid hormone levels as well as electrolyte levels (such as potassium, calcium, glucose, and creatinine). Other measures should include evaluation of fecal occult blood and a white blood cell count. Colorectal screening is mandatory in patients older than 50 years who experience a change in bowel habits. Screening tests include sigmoidoscopy or colonoscopy (flexible tube or virtual) and barium enema. These tests are used to detect colorectal cancer. Of all the diagnostic tests available, flexible-tube colonoscopy is superior at detecting polyps (defined as precancerous lesions). Polyps can be removed during flexible-tube colonoscopies.

Constipation is also a relatively common complaint among children, affecting up to an estimated 10% at some point. Although constipation in children is usually caused by diet, it may be an indication of a significant organic disorder that can be determined by a thorough medical history and physical examination. Constipation that is present from birth or that begins in the neonatal period is most likely congenital in origin.

## CONVENTIONAL TREATMENTS FOR CONSTIPATION

### Fiber Therapy

The average American eats only 10–15 g of fiber daily.[16] Typical recommendations are 20–35 g of dietary fiber daily.[17] Fiber is excellent for overall intestinal health and alleviating chronic constipation. Although humans cannot digest fiber, the 5 lbs of friendly bacteria present in their digestive tract use fiber for fermentation and production of useful short-chain fatty acids that the cells of the intestine use for energy.

Most foods contain a mixture of soluble and insoluble fiber. Both are important in treating constipation. Soluble fiber is contained in oats, apples, lentils, barley, breads, and cereals. It is able to mix evenly with water, forming a soft gel. Insoluble fiber is contained in raw wheat bran, other whole grains, fruits, and vegetables. It mixes unevenly with water, forming a soft pulp. The body does not absorb soluble or insoluble fiber during digestion. Fiber contributes volume to the stool mass, making it easier for the colon to push and propel larger and softer stools out of the body. Insoluble fiber encourages contraction of the colon.

Both fiber types contribute volume to individual stool masses. A larger mass of stool is easier for the colon to push against and propel, so larger, softer stools are easier to move and pass.

The following supplements may succeed at moving the bowels when regular fiber supplements fail to correct chronic constipation:

**Chitosan.** Chitosan is a fiber composed of chitin, a component of the shell of shellfish. Chitosan has the ability to bind fat from food in the stomach and the intestines. When fat content in the bowel increases, it makes the feces soft and smooth. If you do not obtain results from other commonly used fiber sources, six 500-mg capsules of chitosan along with 1000 mg of vitamin C before each meal may help alleviate constipation. Ascorbic acid (vitamin C) helps transform chitosan in the stomach and intestine into a fat-absorbing gel. Chitosan should not be used by people who have shellfish allergies.

**Glucomannan.** Glucomannan is a water-soluble dietary fiber derived from the konjac root (*Amorphophallus konjac*). Glucomannan is considered a bulk-forming laxative that promotes a larger, bulkier stool.[18] Glucomannan generally helps produce a bowel movement within 12–24 hours.

Constipation is frequently encountered during pregnancy. A preparation of lactulose and glucomannan is effective and well-tolerated in pregnant women. Pregnant women with constipation who were treated with a preparation of 3–6 g of glucomannan and 8–16 g of lactulose twice daily for 1–3 months showed a return of normal frequency of evacuations. The formula also helped control weight gain.[19]

In one study, laxative use was significantly reduced in a long-term care facility when an interdisciplinary program was implemented based on prevention and health promotion. Specifically, increased fluid and fiber intake, timely toileting habits, and regular activity or exercise led to a 50% reduction in the number of patients receiving laxatives.[20]

## Laxatives and Other Therapies

Laxatives are considered a first-line medical therapy for constipation. Many people are concerned about the use of laxatives, believing that laxatives are addictive or that their long-term use will compromise the person's ability to have normal bowel movements.

The function of laxatives is to speed the passage of intestinal contents through the gastrointestinal tract or provide the bulk needed for normal stool formation.

Studies designed to evaluate whether laxatives and fiber therapies improve symptoms and the frequency of bowel movements in adults with chronic constipation have generally shown that fiber and laxatives decreased abdominal pain and improved stool consistency compared with placebo.

The four classes of laxatives are *bulk-forming*, *osmotic*, *stimulant*, and *emollient*.

**Bulk-forming laxatives.** Bulk-forming laxatives are the most commonly recommended initial treatments for constipation. Bulk-forming laxatives may work as quickly as 12 hours after use or take as long as 3 days to be effective. Some bulk-forming laxatives are derived from natural sources such as agar, psyllium, kelp, and plant gum. Others are synthetic cellulose compounds such as methylcellulose and carboxymethylcellulose. Natural and synthetic bulk-forming laxatives act similarly. They dissolve or swell in the intestines, lubricate and soften the stool, and make the passage of bowel movements easier and more frequent. Bulk-forming laxatives are not absorbed from the intestines into the body and are safe for long-term use. They are also safe for elderly patients to use.[21-24]

Psyllium is a bulk-forming laxative that is high in fiber. Psyllium seeds contain 10–30% mucilage. The laxative properties of psyllium are caused by the swelling of the husk when it comes in contact with water. This forms a gelatinous mass and keeps the feces hydrated and soft. The resulting bulk stimulates a reflex contraction of the walls of the bowel, causing them to empty.[25] Studies have shown that psyllium fiber is more effective than lactulose and other laxatives, and causes more frequent and bulkier bowel movements. It has also been documented to result in a lower incidence of adverse effects.[21,25]

**Osmotic laxatives.** Osmotic laxatives work by increasing the amount of water in the small intestine and colon, which increases the size and pliability of the stool. When ingested on an empty stomach, they may take only 1–2 hours to take effect. Common osmotic laxatives include milk of magnesium, sorbitol, magnesium citrate, and polyethylene glycol–based formulations. Lactulose is a prescription carbohydrate osmotic laxative that is partially broken down by bacteria in the colon into acids that cause water to accumulate in the colon. Osmotic laxatives can cause severe diarrhea and dehydration, so a physician should carefully monitor their use. In some cases, too much fluid can accumulate in the colon, causing electrolyte disorders. Polyethylene glycol does not contain electrolytes and is suggested for use in patients with heart and kidney disease.

**Stimulant laxatives.** Stimulant laxatives increase motor activity of the bowels by directly stimulating the nerve plexus in the intestinal wall, causing increased movement and the stimulation of local reflexes.[13,21,26,27] Stimulant laxatives should only be used when osmotic laxatives have been ineffective, or in preparation for rectal or bowel examinations. Results occur in 6–10 hours. Examples of stimulant laxatives include senna, bisacodyl, and dehydrocholic acid. Stimulant laxatives can cause dehydration and electrolyte problems, in addition to structural and muscular changes in the colon (such as cathartic colon) with long-term use.[28] In some products, stimulant laxatives are combined with bulk-forming laxatives. Studies have shown that these combination products may be safe to use for up to a year.[29]

**Emollient laxatives.** Emollient laxatives are generally divided into two groups: mineral oil and docusates. Mineral oil works by coating the inside of the colon with a thin layer of oil, which helps retain water in the colon and adds moisture and bulk to the stool. It is often used to prevent straining in patients for whom it would be dangerous to strain.[13,21,26] Generally, if physicians recommend mineral oil supplementation for constipation, they advise taking 5–30 mL at bedtime. However, chronic mineral oil ingestion can result in malabsorption of fat-soluble vitamins and minerals (and, in some cases, can cause inflammation of the lungs). Physicians do not recommend mineral oil for continuous treatment of constipation.

Docusates promote water retention in the fecal mass, thus softening the stool. They are generally used to prevent straining and are most beneficial when the stool is hard. However, it may be 3 days before a patient experiences results. Fecal softeners should not be used exclusively but may be useful in combination with stimulant laxatives.

**Drug therapies.** Prucalopride is a novel, selective and specific serotonin (5-HT4) receptor agonist that belongs to a new class of medications known as benzofurancarboxamides. Prucalopride may increase the frequency of bowel movements and improve colonic transit, which are key factors in the treatment of chronic constipation.[30–32] It works by operating on serotonin receptors in the gut that stimulate motility.

Tegaserod is a serotonin subtype 4 receptor partial agonist for patients who have chronic constipation. Tegaserod treatment produces significant improvements in the symptoms of chronic constipation and is safe and well-tolerated.[33–35]

**Exercise.** Exercise is an important factor in the management of constipation. Regular exercise (especially abdominal muscle exercises) and brisk walking are recommended according to the age and physical condition of the individual.

# NATURAL STRATEGIES TO REDUCE CONSTIPATION

## Supplements to Aid Elimination

Certain herbal-based formulations containing black radish, artichoke, deoxycholic acid, peppermint and wormwood extract help stimulate peristalsis, speed digestion of fats, and prevent stagnation of food in the digestive tract.

**Black radish extract.** Black radish extract has a high fiber content, which can increase peristaltic movements and add bulk to the stool.[36] It can also help increase the secretion of mucus in the colon, which aids in elimination.[37]

**Peppermint.** Peppermint, with its active ingredient menthol, is a natural antispasmodic that relaxes smooth muscle, the same type of muscle that lines the walls of the intestines. Among patients with constipation secondary to irritable bowel syndrome, peppermint oil helps to relieve symptoms and improve quality of life.[38]

## Probiotics and Prebiotics for Healthy Digestion

The colon has a robust population of beneficial bacteria that help digest any remaining nutrients. Beneficial bacteria include *Lactobacillus acidophilus* and *Bifidobacterium bifidum* (*B. bifidum*). A healthy population of beneficial bacteria is essential for proper digestion. Among elderly bed-ridden Japanese, intake of yogurt containing *B. bifidum* was reported to improve the frequency of bowel movements.[39] Another study found that commercial probiotic preparations helped increase bowel movement frequency among elderly people.[40]

People with irritable bowel syndrome suffer from alternating bouts of diarrhea and constipation, often suffering painful abdominal bloating and gas production. Bifidobacteria supplementation produced a significant reduction in abdominal distension and improved symptom scores along with faster bowel transit times (which reduces cancer risk).[41,42] Several recent studies demonstrate significant improvements in measures of gastrointestinal well-being, decreases in digestive symptom scores and bloating, and increases in health related quality of life during bifidobacteria supplementation.[43,44]

In addition, prebiotics, or fructo-oligosaccharides, have been shown to promote normal bowel movements. Fructo-oligosaccharides are sugars that are fermented by beneficial bacteria and aid in digestion.

In one study, elderly patients who were constipated benefited from taking fructooligosaccharides.[45]

## Supplements to Relieve Acute Constipation

Some cases of constipation are caused by insufficient peristalsis, which means there is not enough colon contractile activity to completely evacuate the bowels. However, there are specific nutrients that, if taken at the right time, can induce healthy colon peristaltic action without producing adverse effects.

**Vitamin C and magnesium.**   On an empty stomach, certain nutrients have been shown to induce healthy colon peristalsis. One combination is 4–8 g of vitamin C powder and 1500 mg of magnesium oxide powder taken with the juice of a freshly squeezed grapefruit. A convenient product sold by several vitamin companies is a buffered vitamin C powder that contains magnesium and potassium salts mixed with ascorbic acid. Depending on the person, a few teaspoons (or, in some cases, 1–2 tablespoons) of this buffered vitamin C powder can produce a powerful but safe laxative effect within 45 minutes. This therapy has to be individually adjusted so it will not cause day-long diarrhea.

**Vitamin B5.**   Also on an empty stomach, vitamin B5 (pantothenic acid) in a dose of 2000–3000 mg will produce a rapid evacuation of bowel contents. Vitamin B5 powder is unpalatable, but there are many health benefits attributed to it, in addition to its ability to stimulate peristalsis. Nutritional laxatives such as magnesium, ascorbic acid, and pantothenic acid are becoming more popular with people who have constipation that is resistant to fiber therapies.

## SUMMARY

Here are some steps you can take to improve your digestion and help relieve constipation.

- Increase your fiber intake. Add more fruits and vegetables, in addition to whole grains and bran, to your diet.
- Add legumes to daily meals, either as a side dish or part of a casserole. They are among the foods that offer the most fiber per serving and they encourage the growth of bacteria in the colon, adding to stool bulk.
- Cut back on low-fiber foods such as meats, cheeses, and processed foods.
- Drink plenty of water (about 8 full glasses daily). As you increase your intake of fiber, you may also need to step up your fluid intake. Caffeine-containing drinks such as coffee, tea, and colas have a mildly dehydrating effect on the body, but they do promote contractions in the bowel and can sometimes facilitate bowel movements.
- Eat on a regular schedule to give your body a chance to regulate elimination.
- Respond to your body's signals to pass stool. This will keep your bowel movements regular. Resisting the urge to move your bowels for too long can result in impaction and overflow incontinence, in which liquid stool bypasses the impacted stool and leaks out.

## Life Extension Suggestions

- **Chitosan:** 600–2400 mg daily
- **Soluble fiber:** 5–15 g daily
- **Probiotics:** per label instructions
- **Prebiotics** (as fructo-oligosaccharides and inulin): 5000–10000 mg daily
- **Magnesium** (as magnesium citrate): 160–320 mg daily
- **Multiple herbal extract formula** providing 320–640 mg of:
  - Black radish extract
  - Deoxycholic acid
  - Artichoke extract
  - Peppermint oil
  - Wormwood extract
- **Vitamin C** (ascorbic acid): 1000–4000 mg daily

## REFERENCES

References available at: www.lef.org/dpt5/ch48

# 49

---

# *Depression*

---

Depression is a state of psyche characterized by a spectrum of negative feelings ranging in scope from minor unhappiness to overwhelming despair. Although generally associated with emotional or psychological symptoms, depression can be accompanied severe pain or other physical symptoms as well; depression is capable of dramatically influencing the lives of those it affects.

Recent data estimate the overall prevalence of depression at about 11.1% of the American population, or nearly 35 million individuals,[1] and predictive models suggest that up to 50% of the population will experience at least one episode of depression during their lives.[2]

The framework underlying the pathogenesis of depression is complex and variable among individuals; both *psychological* and *biological* factors influence a person's state of mind at any given time. For example, emergent research links depression with several metabolic phenomena, including *inflammation*, *insulin resistance*, and *oxidative stress*. Intriguing preliminary data also suggest that *mitochondrial dysfunction* plays a previously unappreciated role in depression. Moreover, the role of *hormones* in depression is considerable, including stress hormones (glucocorticoids) and sex hormones (testosterone, estrogen). Many people affected by depression may be suffering from *hormonal imbalances* that significantly contribute to their symptoms.[3]

The mainstream medical establishment relies heavily upon *psychoactive drugs* that *manipulate brain chemistry* as the frontline treatment.[4] Unfortunately, the success rate of pharmacologic intervention for depression is a mere 50% *or less* and these medications are fraught with potential side effects, including a proclivity to increase suicidal ideation with some antidepressant drugs.[5]

Life Extension, on the other hand, acknowledges and appreciates the complex nature of depression and advocates a *comprehensive management strategy* that includes proactive lifestyle changes, behavioral therapy, hormone restoration, and targeted nutritional support to complement conventional antidepressant treatment and balance brain chemistry holistically.

## TYPES OF DEPRESSION AND ASSOCIATED SYMPTOMS

Although depression is a clearly defined disorder with mental and physical symptoms, unlike other disorders, doctors cannot diagnose it using a blood panel or other form of lab test. Instead, they use carefully developed clinical guidelines as defined in the *Diagnostic and Statistical Manual of Mental Disorders* (DSM).

Depression has various forms. The most common are major depressive disorder and dysthymic disorder.

### Major Depressive Disorder (Major Depression)

Major depressive disorder can be very disabling, preventing the patient from functioning normally. A combination of symptoms sabotages the patient's ability to sleep, study, work, eat, and enjoy formerly pleasurable activities. Some people may experience only a single episode, while others experience recurrent episodes.

### Dysthymic Disorder (Dysthymia)

Dysthymia, also known as chronic mild depression, lasts longer than 2 years. Symptoms are not disabling or as severe as those of major depression; however, the patient finds it difficult to function normally and does not feel well. A person with dysthymia may also experience periods of major depression.

### Psychotic Depression

Psychotic depression is a severe depressive illness that includes hallucinations, delusions, or withdrawal from reality.

### Postpartum Depression (Postnatal Depression)

Postpartum depression, also known as postnatal depression (PND), affects 10–15% of all women after giving birth. This is not to be confused with the "baby blues," which a mother may feel briefly after giving birth. The development of a major depressive episode within a few weeks of giving birth likely indicates PND. Sadly, many of these women go undiagnosed and suffer for long periods without treatment and support.

### Seasonal Affective Disorder (SAD)

The incidence of SAD increases along with the distance from the Equator. A person who develops a depressive illness during the winter months with symptoms that go away during spring or summer may have SAD. Accumulating evidence points to *vitamin D deficiency* as a contributing factor in SAD and in other forms of depression.[6]

## Bipolar Disorder (Manic-Depressive Illness)

A patient with bipolar disorder experiences (oftentimes extreme) highs (mania) and lows (depression) in mood. The frequency at which an individual reverts from mania to depression, and vice versa, determines where they lie on the *bipolar spectrum*—a diagnostic tool used to measure the severity of bipolar disorder.

# DIAGNOSING DEPRESSION

A diagnosis of clinical depression requires that the patient experience at least 5 of the 9 symptoms below, as described by the DSM, for most of the day, nearly every day, for at least 2 weeks. One of the symptoms must be either a constant feeling of sadness, anxiety, and emptiness, or loss of interest in formerly pleasurable activities.

If any of these symptoms affects your relationships and your ability to function at home or work, consult with a health care practitioner qualified to assess and treat depression.

## Emotional Symptoms

- Constant or transient feelings of sadness, anxiety, and emptiness
- Feeling restless; may experience irritability
- Feeling hopeless
- Feeling worthless or guilty for no reason; suicidal thoughts may occur
- Loss of interest in activities or hobbies once enjoyed; may lose interest in sex

## Physical Symptoms

- Disturbed sleep patterns; may sleep too little or too much
- Low energy; fatigue
- Significant weight loss or gain due to a change in eating habits; either loss of appetite or eating too much
- Difficulty concentrating, remembering details, or making decisions

# CAUSES OF DEPRESSION

Research spanning the last 20–30 years has examined a range of influences that contribute to depression. These include genetics, brain chemistry, early life trauma, negative thinking, one's personality and temperament, stress, and difficulty relating to others.[7] Moreover, emerging scientific research suggests that metabolic phenomena such as inflammation, oxidative stress, and hormonal imbalances can cause or exacerbate depression as well.[8,9]

## Impaired Stress Response

When a person experiences stress—whether it is physical or emotional, internal or external—the body copes through a complex system of adaptive reactions. This response involves the release of *glucocorticoids*, or stress hormones, which stimulate adaptive changes throughout the body.

A stress response is designed to help us confront or escape danger by redirecting blood flow to the muscles, dilating the pupils, inhibiting digestion, and releasing stored fatty acids and glucose (blood sugar) to be used by the muscles. This process is known as the *fight-or-flight response*.

The fight-or-flight response originates in the brain. When the *hypothalamus*, the brain's "control tower," perceives a threat, it sends chemical signals to the brain's *pituitary gland*, also known as the master hormone gland. The pituitary gland then sends chemical signals to the *adrenal glands*, which sit atop the kidneys. The adrenal glands then release the stress hormone *cortisol*, which triggers many of the physiologic responses to danger.

Almost all animals share the fight-or-flight response, as it is paramount for survival. Although we were designed to undergo this response on only an occasional basis, modern humans cope with relentless stress. Such things as financial worries, deadline pressures at work or school, emotional challenges, excessive caloric intake, poor diet, obesity, inactivity, and environmental toxins *chronically* activate the *hypothalamic-pituitary-adrenal axis*, keeping us in a perpetual fight-or-flight response. The result is an increased rate of cardiovascular disease, diabetes, and mood disorders such as depression and anxiety.

The relationship among chronic stress, depression, and anxiety is complex, but incredibly powerful. For instance, the chronic elevation of glucocorticoids (primarily cortisol) caused by chronic stress actually changes the *physical structure* of the brain.

Chronic exposure to glucocorticoids shifts dendrites, the branches of neurons that receive signals from other neurons, into less functional patterns. Research links this phenomenon with alterations in mood, short-term memory, and behavioral flexibility.[10] Glucocorticoids blunt the brain's sensitivity to *serotonin*, the mood-regulating neurotransmitter most often associated with depression.[11,12] Chronic stress also increases one's susceptibility to neuronal damage and impairs neurogenesis, the process by which new neurons are "born."[10]

Interestingly, emerging research suggests that drugs used to treat anxiety and depression may stabilize mood not only by acting on neurotransmitters, but also by regulating the brain's receptors for stress hormones.[13] These new findings strongly support the importance of controlling the stress response in order to alleviate mood disorders. Indeed, several genetic and epidemiologic studies have linked excessive stress, and the inability to adapt efficiently to stress, with increased rates of anxiety and depression.[14-16]

Fortunately, a number of relaxation techniques and coping styles can improve depression, further emphasizing the role of stress in depression. These approaches include mindfulness-based stress reduction,[17] meditation,[18] biofeedback,[19] progressive muscle relaxation,[20] and an integrative health approach that combines relaxation, nutrition, and exercise.[21]

Recent studies suggest that some of these techniques influence genetic activity regulating depression.[20] Brain imaging techniques show that meditation significantly affects neurotransmitter levels and the activity of various parts of the brain that facilitate relaxation.[18]

## Traumatic Events and Post-Traumatic Stress Disorder

Research establishes that trauma, such as the sudden loss of a family member, sexual abuse, or war-related traumas, contributes significantly to prolonged periods of depression. The effects are more pronounced when the trauma occurs in childhood; childhood trauma can considerably alter the structure and function of the brain, increasing susceptibility to depression and anxiety later in life.[22]

## Social Network and Personal Relationships

Lack of meaningful social contact with others has been linked to depression, while evidence increasingly shows that close personal relationships and social networks positively affect mood and health.[23] Loving relationships, social connection and support, work-related passion and recognition, and a good marriage help prevent depression.[24,25] Interestingly, it also has been shown that while a good marriage benefits both men and women, it seems to be more important for men from an overall health standpoint.

## Neurotransmitter Imbalances

Magnetic resonance imaging (MRI) shows that the areas of the brain that orchestrate thinking, sleep, mood, appetite, and behavior function abnormally in depressed patients compared to nondepressed individuals. In addition, an imaging technique called single-photon emission computed tomography (SPECT) shows changes in brain blood flow and neurotransmitter activity in the depressed person's brain.[26,27] Although imaging technology can identify neurotransmitter imbalances, it cannot reveal *why* depression has occurred.

## Comorbid Conditions

Depression is more common in those with HIV/AIDS,[28] heart disease,[29] stroke,[30] cancer,[31] diabetes,[32] Parkinson's disease,[33] and many other illnesses. Research shows a person with both depression and a serious illness is more likely to experience severe symptoms and find it harder to adapt to the medical condition. Studies also show that treating depression in this population may improve symptoms of the co-occurring illness in some instances.

Additionally, people dependent on alcohol or narcotics are significantly more likely to be depressed.[34]

## Mainstream Medicine Overlooks Factors that Contribute to Depression

The mainstream view on the cause of depression relies largely on the *monoamine hypothesis*, a theory proposing that deregulation in neurotransmitter signaling is the sole cause of depression. This has been the grounds for the primary utilization of antidepressant drugs in the management of depression for decades. However, this theory fails to take into account various other well-studied causes, and partly explains the poor success rate of antidepressant medications.

Conventional medicine overlooks several important *biological factors* that influence depression, thereby undermining the likelihood that a holistic strategy will be employed to thoroughly manage a patient's depression.

If left unchecked, aberrations among these under-appreciated factors may work together to create metabolic and neurochemical imbalances that provoke mood changes and initiate depression.

Critical omissions from conventional assessment of depression include:

- Hormonal imbalances
- Nutritional deficiencies or insufficiencies
- Oxidative stress and mitochondrial dysfunction
- Insulin resistance
- Chronic inflammation

**Hormonal imbalances.** Balanced and youthful concentrations of hormones can help control depression, and astute clinicians often find hormonal imbalances in patients with depression. Because a wide range of hormones can influence depression, it is important to discern which hormone(s) may be an underlying factor when considering depression.

For example, *thyroid function* directly affects metabolism and brain function, and low thyroid activity can contribute to depression. Conventional medicine relies on overly broad thyroid lab ranges, failing to recognize many cases of *suboptimal* thyroid function.

Overt hypothyroidism has been shown to perturb serotonin signaling in the brain, which can contribute to depression.[35] Furthermore, because the brain requires sufficient thyroid hormones to function optimally, a low thyroid hormone status can contribute to overall loss of function and degeneration in the brain, including the areas of the brain that govern mood.[36] Hashimoto's thyroiditis, an autoimmune thyroid disease, can cause a person's metabolism to swing between overly active to overly depressed. These swings can mimic the symptoms of bipolar disorder and cause misdiagnosis and inappropriate treatment.[37–40]

*Sex hormones* also influence mood and depression. Women are more susceptible to anxiety than men and also experience more depression when they are pregnant, postpartum, premenstrual, and menopausal than at other times in life. These general observations have piqued the interest of scientists and given rise to an expanding body of research linking depression with sex hormone imbalances.

By now, it is well known that most steroid hormones (eg, pregnenolone, estrogen, progesterone, testosterone, and DHEA) are neurologically active. In fact, the brain contains large numbers of receptors for DHEA, estrogen, and progesterone. These hormones affect many functions in the brain, including the regulation of mood.

Accordingly, a number of studies link hormonal imbalances to various depressive disorders.[41–44] In the *follicular phase* of menses, when estrogen levels are high, women produce more serotonin and experience an improved mood. When estrogen decreases during the premenstrual period, serotonin levels drop, contributing to the negative mood and personality shifts associated with premenstrual syndrome (PMS).[45]

Likewise, the drop in estrogen during menopause is associated with reduced serotonin production and a negative impact on mood and cognition. This is evidenced by the fact that SSRIs have been shown to improve mood and cognitive function in menopausal women.[46]

In addition, testosterone deficiency has been linked with depression in men, which is not surprising since testosterone plays an important role in brain function, including mood regulation.[47,48] In studies, select populations of men were more likely to be depressed if their total and/or free testosterone levels are low; these included those with heart disease, HIV/AIDS, and the elderly.[49,50]

Medical research acknowledges the link between hormonal imbalances and depression; however, conventional doctors rarely evaluate and address hormone status when treating depression. Instead, they frequently dismiss such imbalances as a normal part of aging, while in truth, restoring youthful hormonal status may effectively combat multiple health deficits associated with aging, including mood imbalances.

The role of hormones in treating depression will be examined more closely in the Hormone Restoration section.

**Nutritional deficiency or insufficiency.** Nutrition plays an essential role in brain function, and poor nutrition significantly increases one's risk for depression. Dietary nutrients influence nervous system function in multiple ways. Important dietary nutrients follow:

- **B-complex vitamins.** B-complex vitamins serve as *cofactors* for the production of neurotransmitters. Inadequate levels of B-vitamins, especially folate, vitamin B12, niacin, and vitamin B6, can disrupt neurotransmitter synthesis. This not only may lead to mood alterations, but also can impact overall brain function, memory, and cognition.

- **Optimal balance of omega-3 and omega-6 fatty acids.** Fatty acids are critical components of nerve cell membranes and play an important role in neuronal communication. Fatty acid imbalances can impair the transmission of messages between nerve cells, leading to cognitive deficits and mood alterations, including depression.[51]

- **Vitamin D activity.** A vitamin D insufficiency, which is very common even among dedicated supplement users,[52] is linked with seasonal depression. Recent evidence suggests that it also may contribute to general depression through its considerable influence on genetic activity, its ability to control inflammation, and other mechanisms.

It is important to remember that optimal brain function necessitates all of these nutritional aspects be addressed simultaneously.

**Oxidative stress and mitochondrial dysfunction.** Brain tissue is particularly susceptible to oxidative damage due to its high concentrations of phospholipids and the exhaustive metabolic rate among neurons. A growing body of research suggests that oxidative stress contributes to depression and other brain-related disorders.[53] This is thought to result from either an increase in damaging reactive oxygen species, a decrease in antioxidant defense mechanisms, or a combination of the two. These mechanisms become especially important with advancing age.[54]

Newer research sheds light on the critical role of mitochondria and neurotransmission and mood regulation. Mitochondria are the "powerhouses" in each cell that generate energy. In an intriguing study, researchers measured the content of mitochondrial DNA within white blood cells in aging patients who were depressed, and in an age-matched group who were not depressed. The subjects with depression had *significantly fewer mitochondria* than nondepressed controls, leading researchers to suggest that "mitochondrial dysfunction could be a mechanism of geriatric depression."[55] In a similar study, greater numbers of mitochondria in peripheral cells were associated with improved cognitive function in healthy elderly women.[56]

Preliminary research suggests that 2 nutrients, *coenzyme Q10* and *acetyl-L-carnitine*, which support mitochondrial function, may influence depression. A small study of 35 depressed patients in comparison to 22 healthy volunteer controls showed that plasma CoQ10 levels were significantly lower in the depressed patients. Levels were also lower in treatment-resistant patients, as well as those with chronic fatigue.[57]

Several studies of geriatric depression have investigated *acetyl-L-carnitine*.[58] One study compared treatment with acetyl-L-carnitine to the medication amisulpride, an antipsychotic medication commonly used to treat depression. In 204 patients with chronic depression, both acetyl-L-carnitine and the pharmaceutical drug improved symptoms.[59] Acetyl-L-carnitine also has been found to relieve depression and improve quality of life in patients with liver disease,[60] and to ease depressive symptoms significantly in patients with fibromyalgia.[61]

Another nutrient, *pyrroloquinoline quinine* (PQQ), is an enzyme involved in the *generation of new mitochondria* and the maintenance of antioxidant defense systems.[62–64] Supplemental PQQ has been shown to increase mitochondrial activity levels and to be neuroprotective in animal models.[65–67] Since fewer mitochondria have been observed in depressed patients,[55] PQQ may be supportive in this population.

**Insulin resistance.** Recent data suggest a direct link between insulin resistance and depression. In a small clinical study, treatment of depressed patients with the insulin-sensitizing drug *pioglitazone* alleviated depression while simultaneously improving their cardiometabolic risk profiles.[68] Evidence suggests that another popular glucose control agent, *metformin*, may influence psychiatric health as well.[69] Individuals who are overweight, have suboptimal glucose control, or have diabetes with concurrent depression may find that losing weight and gaining control over their glucose levels eases their depressive symptoms.

Scientific literature indicates that for *optimal health*, fasting glucose levels should fall *between 70 and 85 mg/dL*, and 2-hour postprandial (2 hours after a meal) glucose levels should not exceed *120 mg/dL*.

**Chronic inflammation.** Several studies support the role of inflammation and immune system deregulation in depression. Studies have found elevated levels of inflammatory cytokines (signaling molecules with which immune cells communicate) in patients suffering from major depression,[70] late-life depression,[71] and in patients who do not respond to SSRIs.[72] These cytokines include the interleukins IL-1beta and IL-6, as well as the cytokines INF-gamma and TNF-alpha.

Studies show an association between the systemic inflammation marker *C-reactive protein* (C-RP) and major depression.[73] C-RP levels also are associated with a number of age-related diseases, such as atherosclerosis, so C-RP levels should be kept below *1.0 mg/L* to maintain optimal health.

In prospective studies involving patients being treated with recombinant cytokines for immune-related conditions, depression is observed to develop after inflammation initiates several other undesirable metabolic cascades. This has led some researchers to identify depression as a late-stage consequence of chronic inflammation.[74]

Research innovations suggest that future antidepressant medications may be anti-inflammatory in nature.[75]

## CONVENTIONAL MEDICAL APPROACHES—CHALLENGES AND BENEFITS

As mentioned earlier, mainstream medicine typically relies on antidepressants as first-line treatment for depression.[4] However, in many cases, this first-line treatment is met with failure. The result is a diagnosis of *"treatment-resistant depression,"* and, if severe enough, more drastic measures will be undertaken in attempt to alleviate depressive symptoms. Instead of addressing the multiple other potential contributors to depression mentioned in the protocol, conventional physicians opt to appease treatment-resistant depression with procedures like *electroconvulsive therapy*, which happens to cause memory loss.

Sadly, although research has given rise to promising new modalities for relieving depression, such as *transcranial magnetic stimulation*, mainstream medicine has yet to advance past the archaic model of psychiatric medicine that has been in place for decades.

This section of the protocol will discuss typical conventional treatment options and also introduce some promising new techniques that are quickly gaining the attention of patient-minded clinicians.

## Medications Typically Used to Treat Depression

Several classes of medications may be employed to treat depression. Depending on patient symptoms and history, medications from the following 4 classes are typically utilized.

Most antidepressant medications work by altering signaling within the brain. They do so by manipulating the level of neurotransmitters in the synaptic junction, the finite space between 2 neurons in which signaling molecules are released and reabsorbed to facilitate neuronal communication.

While antidepressants may temporarily improve mood, they do so in a way that is somewhat artificial and unlikely to be effective for an extended period of time. There is disturbing evidence that some antidepressants may cause the brain to adapt to their presence, requiring increasing dosage and leading to withdrawal symptoms upon cessation.

Moreover, an under-recognized condition known as *antidepressant discontinuation syndrome* may arise in as many as 20% of patients upon abrupt discontinuation of an antidepressant medication. This phenomenon is likely the result of the brain having adapted to the medication, and now being deprived of it, malfunctions for a time until it can readapt to the lack of the drug. Symptoms of antidepressant discontinuation syndrome include flu-like symptoms, insomnia, nausea, hyperactivity, and sensory disturbances, among others.[76]

**Selective serotonin reuptake inhibitors.** Selective serotonin reuptake inhibitors (SSRIs) comprise one of the most popular classes of antidepressants. Fluoxetine (Prozac®), citalopram (Celexa®), and sertraline (Zoloft®) are all SSRIs. They tend to have the fewest side effects of antidepressant drugs. Primary side effects are decreased sexual desire and delayed orgasm. Other side effects—digestive symptoms, headaches, insomnia, and anxiousness—often decrease over time.[77]

**Serotonin and norepinephrine reuptake inhibitors.** Serotonin and norepinephrine reuptake inhibitors (SNRIs) include duloxetine (Cymbalta®), venlafaxine (Effexor®), and desvenlafaxine (Pristiq®). The side effects for these medications are similar to those of SSRIs.

**Atypical antidepressants.** Atypical antidepressants are norepinephrine and dopamine reuptake inhibitors (NDRIs) such as bupropion (Wellbutrin®), trazadone (Desyrel®), and mirtazapine (Remeron®). They have a different mechanism of action and side-effect profile than other antidepressants. For example, NDRIs generally do not cause sexual dysfunction as a side effect; however, they can increase blood pressure and risk of a seizure. Other minor effects include loss of appetite, headaches, dry mouth, nervousness, anxiety, stomach pain, constipation, insomnia, and more.

**Older antidepressants.** Older antidepressants include the tricyclic antidepressants amitriptyline, amoxapine, desipramine (Norpramin®), doxepin, imipramine (Tofranil®), nortriptyline (Pamelor®), protyptyline (Vivactil®), trimipramine (Surmontil®); and the monoamine oxidase inhibitors (MAOIs) tranylcypromine (Parnate®) and phenelzine (Nardil®). Doctors do not use these medications frequently because they tend to have more frequent and severe side effects. For example, tricyclic antidepressants can cause an abnormal heart rhythm and drowsiness. MAOIs can increase the risk of severe reactions to foods, drinks, and other medications, as well as significantly increase blood pressure, which may lead to a heart attack or stroke. Other side effects of both these classes of medication include constipation, headaches, anxiety, and dry mouth.

## Electroconvulsive Therapy

A long-standing treatment still used in conventional medicine is electroconvulsive therapy (ECT). It is most often reserved for people with suicidal ideation, psychotic depression, or those who have not responded to other treatments. It is reportedly effective in up to 90% of patients, which is why it is still available,[78] although it is important to question the extent of the benefit and how long the effects last.

ECT is associated with short-term memory loss, and it appears that some aspects of memory may be affected for an extended time.[79] Moreover, ECT may negatively influence other realms of cognition unrelated to memory. In fact, one group of reviewers stated that "clinicians should take the non-memory cognitive effects of ECT into account, and patients should be informed of their existence before they sign consent for ECT."[80]

# OTHER MEDICAL APPROACHES AND EMERGING THERAPIES

## Cognitive Behavioral Therapy

Cognitive behavioral therapy (CBT) is a nonpharmacologic means of therapy often employed to relieve depression. CBT is typically initiated if primary treatment with antidepressant medications fail, but it is sometimes used as part of first-line treatment alongside antidepressants.

CBT is centered on the belief that depression is closely linked with negative thinking (ie, thought patterns that negatively reinforce depressed mood). The goal of CBT is to help the patient recognize and replace negative thinking with more positive, constructive thoughts. CBT has been studied in various settings and has shown efficacy both independently and in combination with other conventional treatment regimens.

A recent review of studies using CBT in treatment-resistant depression found that CBT performed as well as pharmacotherapy when used in conjunction with a primary medication, or in cyclical fashion involving switching from pharmacotherapy to CBT and back again.[81] This same review also pointed out that when a patient with treatment-resistant depression switched antidepressants, greater relief was attained when the switch was accompanied by CBT. A 2010 clinical trial revealed that CBT effectively relieved depression and/or anxiety in patients with chronic obstructive pulmonary disease.[82]

CBT is also effective in young people with depression, and may be preferable over psychotropic drugs for some parents since it lacks harsh side effects. In one trial, CBT was compared to standard-of-care (pharmacotherapy) in children ages 8–15. CBT was superior to pharmacotherapy in several aspects, including patient alliance to treatment.[83] Moreover, CBT may have an overall cost advantage versus pharmacotherapy.[83]

Life Extension suggests that every patient with depression talk with a qualified health care provider about cognitive behavioral therapy as an adjuvant, or alternative to pharmacotherapy.

## Physical Activity

Research supports the use of exercise, primarily aerobic or weight training, as a preventive and adjuvant treatment (used in conjunction with medication) of mood disorders and depression. Some studies have found that exercise alone is as effective as medication for relieving depression,[84] and that exercise can reduce depression recurrence rates.[85] A recent study looked at 202 adults with major depression who participated in 4 months of exercise, took the medication sertraline, or took a placebo. A 1-year follow-up showed that exercise was as effective as the medication at relieving depression and that exercise during the follow-up period extended the benefits.[86]

## Light Therapy

Research shows morning *light therapy* from a light-therapy lamp is effective at treating seasonal affective disorder (seasonal depression), and that it is equally or possibly even more effective than antidepressants, in this type of depression.[84] A study of 98 patients with seasonal depression illustrated this. Depressed subjects were randomly assigned to 8 weeks of therapy with light in the morning (30 minutes, 10000 lux, and a placebo pill) or 30 minutes of dim light (100 lux and 20 mg of fluoxetine), with both groups experiencing a 67% response rate.[87]

Light therapy for nonseasonal depression is not well established, although results are promising; light therapy may be more helpful as an adjuvant treatment than as a stand-alone treatment.

## Transcranial Magnetic Stimulation

Interestingly, a new procedure called *transcranial magnetic stimulation* (TMS), which uses magnetic fields to stimulate nerve cells in the brain, is widely researched and showing promising results as a treatment for depression. The Food and Drug Administration has approved TMS for people who have not responded to medication, and it is often compared to the controversial ECT. It is a possible alternative to ECT, as it is more humane and causes fewer adverse effects.

A recent study of 190 patients with major depression treated with TMS showed a clinically significant improvement in symptoms.[88] In a recent review, TMS was concluded to be as effective as CBT or pharmacotherapy for relieving depression.[89]

TMS is becoming more widely available in hospitals and private practices. However, because it is relatively new, it is important to ask how long the treatment has been offered, how many patients have been treated, and what the success rates are.

# DIETARY CONSIDERATIONS FOR DEPRESSION

Dietary factors should always be addressed when managing depression, as evidence demonstrates that various aspects of diet can affect the disorder.

Individuals with depression may consume too many inflammatory omega-6 fatty acids and saturated fats, so increasing consumption of omega-3's and decreasing consumption of trans-fats, saturated fat, and excess omega-6 fatty acids is recommended.[90]

Omega-3 fatty acids[91] and folate[92] both appear to be very important in mood management. Although the role of these nutrients in the diet is important, one should augment the diet with supplements as described below for maximum benefit in addressing symptoms of depression or in trying to prevent a recurrence. As described later in this protocol, omega-3 fatty acids have been shown to decrease susceptibility to depression and may help as an adjuvant therapy. Foods high in omega-3's include deep-water fish such as salmon, mackerel, sardines, and tuna, as well as flax seeds, and some nuts (eg, walnuts).

Evidence suggests that limiting sugar intake to control blood sugar levels is another important approach to depression. This would include addressing hyperglycemia (high blood sugar), hypoglycemia (low blood sugar), or reactive hypoglycemia (low blood sugar that occurs within 4 hours of eating). Reactive hypoglycemia may be more common in people who are not overweight. To address high or low blood sugar, it is important to limit or avoid sugar and refined carbohydrates, eat small meals 4–6 times per day, eat a balance of healthy proteins, fats, and complex carbohydrates, and decrease caffeine. The nutrients magnesium and chromium and practicing relaxation techniques also help manage hypoglycemia.

Evidence also suggests that an anti-inflammatory Mediterranean diet may help prevent or manage depression.[93] A Mediterranean diet, which is rich in omega-3 fatty acids and polyphenolic antioxidants, could serve as a foundation to which targeted dietary supplements are added for maximum response. The diet generally includes good quantities of fish, vegetables, unrefined grains, beans or legumes, fruit, and olive oil. It includes moderate amounts of dairy (mostly cheese and yogurt) and red wine, and limits meats to small portions.

## Hormone Restoration Therapy

Although some physicians routinely screen for underlying hormonal disorders and/or imbalances as part of depression management and use hormonal therapy in protocols for depression, most typically do not. Instead, they may consider hormonal imbalances a normal part of aging. Also, many ascribe to the philosophy of looking at studies of averages of population data as opposed to individual cases for potentially beneficial therapeutic programs, which can cause patients who may benefit from hormone restoration to go untreated.

**Thyroid.** Thyroid dysfunction may be a significantly underappreciated cause of depressive symptoms. In one study, thyroid disorders were associated with a 22% higher likelihood of depression in women.[94]

Studies have shown that treating subjects within so-called "normal" thyroid hormone levels may still be beneficial. In one such pilot study involving 17 female patients with depression, 11 (64.7%) saw significant improvement in response to a moderate dose of l-thyroxine.[95] Similarly, in a study of 225 subjects with treatment-resistant depression, augmenting primary antidepressant therapy with thyroid hormone was found to be roughly as effective as adding a second antidepressant medication for providing relief of symptoms.[96]

Life Extension suggests maintaining a TSH (thyroid-stimulating hormone) of 1–2 μIU/mL (typical lab normal range is 0.45–4.5 μIU/mL) to avoid the consequences of subclinical thyroid dysfunction, which may include depression. To learn more about suboptimal thyroid function and how it may be impacting your life, read the Thyroid Regulation protocol.

**DHEA.** DHEA is an important steroid hormone often referred to as a neurosteroid because it serves a variety of functions in the brain. DHEA levels decrease with age and stress, and people with depression often have low levels of DHEA. In one study, blood samples from women with a history of depression contained lower levels of select neurosteroids, including DHEA, than women with no depression history.[97] Interestingly, experiments showed the women with a history of depression may metabolize progesterone differently than healthy women, reflecting an adaptive effort by the body to compensate for low neurosteroid levels.

A number of studies have examined the role of DHEA in depression, with very encouraging results. DHEA has been shown to modulate serotonin levels in the brains of laboratory animals.[98,99] DHEA has also performed well in human trials. DHEA therapy significantly benefited patients with HIV/AIDS and depression.[100] In a randomized, placebo-controlled, double-blind study, researchers studied the effects of 90 mg DHEA daily for 3 weeks and 450 mg daily for 3 weeks as a stand-alone treatment for both mild and severe depression. They found that DHEA therapy resulted in a significant improvement in symptoms compared with the placebo.[101]

**Testosterone.** Studies indicate that some depressed men have low levels of testosterone.[102,103] In addition, several clinical trials have shown that testosterone replacement therapy, usually transdermal testosterone gel, can relieve depression in men with low testosterone, metabolic syndrome, and HIV/AIDS.[50,104–106]

Aging men should maintain their *free testosterone* level in the youthful range of 20–25 pg/mL to stabilize mood and avert other age-related diseases, such as cardiovascular disease and metabolic syndrome. Men interested in restoring their hormone levels should read Life Extension's Male Hormone Restoration protocol.

**Estrogen.** Estrogen is critically important for brain function and linked to depression, especially in perimenopausal or postmenopausal women.[107] Women using estrogen replacement therapy to alleviate menopause symptoms appear to experience reduced depression.[108] In some older women being treated for depression, estrogen replacement therapy may actually improve the effects of conventional antidepressants.[109]

Estrogen is thought to prevent depression through its association with serotonin regulation in the brain.[110–112] Animal studies show that estrogen may facilitate the effects of antidepressants by modulating serotonin receptors. This suggests that an estrogen imbalance may dampen the efficacy of antidepressant medications.[113,114]

Further evidence suggests that estrogen promotes *neuroplasticity*, the process by which the brain adapts structurally and functionally to new stimuli.[110,115] Disturbances in neuroplasticity may lead to recurrent depression.[116]

Women interested in learning more about the benefits of restoring their hormone levels should read Life Extension's Female Hormone Restoration protocol.

**Melatonin.** Melatonin is a hormone produced in the pineal gland in the brain; it is involved in sleep–wake function and other circadian rhythms. Melatonin decreases with age and some studies link low levels of melatonin with symptoms of depression.

A double-blind, placebo-controlled pilot study of perimenopausal and postmenopausal women who took 3 mg of melatonin at bedtime for 6 months showed significant improvement in depressive symptoms.[117] Recently, another well-controlled preliminary study looked at 33 participants with major depression and early morning waking who took 6 mg of melatonin for 4 weeks. The results suggested improvement in sleep and depressive symptoms.[118]

Studies of the medication *agomelatine*, which acts on melatonin receptors in the brain, support melatonin's influences on depression.[119] Some studies suggest that this drug may be as effective as venlafaxine, fluoxetine, and sertraline in relieving depression.[120]

# NUTRIENTS TO BALANCE BRAIN CHEMISTRY

Depression is a *multifactorial* condition, and efficient relief requires addressing multiple neurochemical and metabolic *imbalances* that may underlie mood disturbances. The nutrients listed in the protocol are categorized according to their evidence-based mechanisms of action in brain health and mood regulation.

## Broad-Range Nervous System Effects

**Omega-3 fatty acids.** Omega-3 fatty acids are long-chain polyunsaturated fatty acids found in fish and various oils, such as flaxseed or canola oil.[121] The brain has a high concentration of polyunsaturated fatty acids, which are found mostly in cell membranes. They affect adaptability of the nervous system, nerve cell conduction and function, and neurotransmitter synthesis.[51,122] Several research models exhibit the influence of omega-3 fatty acids in depression, including dietary studies,[123] nutritional status studies showing positive effects associated with higher omega-3 to omega-6 fatty acid ratios,[124] and intervention studies that look at both eicosapentaenoic acid (EPA) and docosahexaenoic acid (DHA) taken as a stand-alone treatment and as an adjunct to medication.[91]

One investigation showed that adding the omega-3 fatty acid EPA to conventional antidepressant treatment relieved depressive symptoms.[125] Among children with depression, supplementation with omega-3 fatty acids demonstrated "highly significant" effects on symptom scores.[126] In a review article from 2006, researchers analyzed results from 6 published studies and found that omega-3 fatty acids can reduce symptoms of depression among adults as well.[127]

Because they are anti-inflammatory, omega-3 fatty acids also reduce the risk of cardiovascular disease, which is highly associated with depression.[128,129] In fact, the American Heart Association recommends fish oil for both preventing an initial heart attack and for preventing a second attack when one has already occurred.

Omega-3 fatty acids are counterbalanced with the inflammatory omega-6 fatty acids. Typically, Americans consume far too many omega-6's and not nearly enough omega-3's.

The ratio of omega-6 to omega-3 fatty acids is important. You can learn your ratio easily with the *Omega Score®* test. This test can help you assess your risk for depression, heart disease, and other age-related ailments. It can also help you evaluate whether you take enough fish oil or other omega-3 supplements. More information about the importance of maintaining an optimal omega-6 to omega-3 ratio of *less than 4:1* can be found in the *Life Extension Magazine* article titled "Optimize Your Omega-3 Status."

**Magnesium.** Magnesium, a cofactor for more than 300 enzymes in the body, is important for blood-sugar regulation and has a calming effect on the nervous system.[130] Some evidence shows a link between magnesium deficiency and depression,[131] and a recent, comprehensive review in the *Journal of Medical Hypotheses* suggests that magnesium supplementation is a viable approach for depressive symptoms.[132]

A major hurdle for supplemental magnesium historically has been delivery into the brain. This is a barrier that has limited the ability of typical magnesium supplements to target conditions that arise from within the central nervous system such as depression and anxiety. However, in a recent scientific breakthrough, researchers collaborating from Beijing, Ontario, the University of Texas, and the Massachusetts Institute of Technology have developed a highly advanced form of supplemental magnesium called *magnesium-L-threonate*.

Magnesium-L-threonate was shown in multiple animal models to not only effectively penetrate deep into the brain, but also to trigger enhancements in learning and memory by optimizing neuronal communication and reinforcing brain structure in key areas of the cortex, the most advanced aspect of the human brain.[133,134] Since magnesium-L-threonate is readily able to diffuse across the blood–brain barrier, while other forms of magnesium are not, it appears to be the ideal form of supplemental magnesium for those with depression of other mood disorders.

## Supporting Neurotransmitter Synthesis

**L-tryptophan and 5-hydroxytryptophan (5-HTP).** L-tryptophan and 5-hydroxytryptophan (5-HTP) are immediate precursors to serotonin. L-tryptophan is essential for the brain to synthesize serotonin, and several studies have shown that acute tryptophan depletion can cause depression in humans. In fact, some foreign countries license L-tryptophan as an antidepressant.[135]

In one study, healthy women given L-tryptophan for 14 days experienced increased recognition of happy faces and words, and decreased recognition of negative words. The research team concluded that L-tryptophan had improved the study participants' supply of serotonin in a manner similar to that of SSRIs.[135] In another study of the effects of acute tryptophan depletion on healthy women and on patients with bulimia nervosa,

both groups were given amino acid mixtures to decrease their plasma L-tryptophan levels. Both groups experienced an increase in depression.[136] Other studies have found L-tryptophan depletion can lead to recurrence of depression in those who are in remission from depression[137] or in those with seasonal depression.[138]

Methylation is a process in which a molecule passes a methyl group to another molecule. Methylation is essential to multiple functions in the body, including the production of neurotransmitters. One can supply raw materials to support methylation reactions by supplementing with S-adenosyl-methionine (SAMe) or by providing metabolic *cofactors* such as folate, vitamin B12, and vitamin B6. These nutrients are necessary for neurotransmitter production and have other regulating effects.

**SAMe.** SAMe, which can be found in almost every tissue in the body, assists with production of creatine, glutathione, taurine, L-carnitine, and melatonin.

Research shows that SAMe can benefit depressed patients who do not respond to SSRIs. In a well-controlled, 6-week, double-blind trial, 73 subjects with treatment-resistant depression were treated with an SSRI plus placebo, or an SSRI plus 1600 mg SAMe daily. The group receiving the SAMe experienced significantly better response rates and remission compared to the placebo control group.[139] Intriguingly, the group that received SAMe also displayed improved memory function over those receiving placebo. A smaller 6-week study revealed a response rate of 50% and a remission rate of 43% in subjects taking 800–1600 mg a day of SAMe as an adjunct to their antidepressants.[140]

**Folate.** Research shows that low blood levels of folate are associated with depression,[141] and may also be predictive of poor response to antidepressant medication.[142] Clinical trials have also demonstrated that folic acid both relieves depression on its own and enhances the effect of antidepressants. In one study, patients given 500 mcg folic acid daily in conjunction with fluoxetine experienced a significant improvement in depressive symptoms compared with patients receiving the antidepressant alone; women particularly benefited.[143] Because relapse is associated with low serum folate, it is important to maintain folate supplementation for a year following a depressive episode.[144]

The form of supplemental folate is important since a considerable portion of Americans may have a genetic polymorphism that impairs folate metabolism.[145] In fact, mutations in the gene (MTHFR) that converts folic acid into the active *5-methyltetrahydrofolate* (5-MTHF) are associated with depression.[146] Therefore, taking supplemental 5-MTHFdirectly, which can cross the blood–brain barrier, may be more effective in supporting healthy neurotransmission and decreasing potentially neurotoxic *homocysteine* levels.

**Vitamin B12.** Vitamin B12 should always be measured in the event of depression (or any other psychological problems), as a vitamin B12 deficiency can be a reversible cause of various neuropsychiatric disorders.[147] One should also consider whether a vegetarian diet or malabsorption due to celiac disease or gluten enteropathy is a factor in B12 deficiency.

Weaker digestion, reduced absorption of nutrients, and hypochlorhydria (inadequate stomach acid needed to break down proteins that contain vitamin B12) are common in the aging population and associated with B12 deficiency; B12 levels should be tested in an older person with symptoms of depression. Evidence suggests that the *methylcobalamin* form of B12 may have more beneficial metabolic effects than cyanocobalamin.[148,149]

**Vitamin B6.** Vitamin B6 is a cofactor for the production of most neurotransmitters, but it is particularly important for serotonin synthesis.[150] B6 levels are often low in women taking oral contraceptives and research has shown that B6 supplementation in these women can improve mood. For example, one study showed 22 women who had depression associated with oral contraceptive use and B6 deficiency saw significant improvement in their symptoms with B6 supplementation.[151]

A more recent study examined blood levels of *pyridoxal-5-phosphate* (P5P), a metabolically active form of B6, in the blood of 251 elderly individuals living in Massachusetts. The investigators found that deficient levels of P5P *doubled* the likelihood of depression in this population. Accordingly, when dietary composition was assessed, those with higher daily B6 intakes were less likely to be depressed.[152]

## Blood Sugar Regulation and Insulin Resistance

**Green coffee.** Recent data link increasing consumption of coffee with decreased risk of depression.[153] In fact, this relationship proved to be dose dependent, meaning that the more coffee study participants drank, the less likely depression would strike them. These findings are corroborated by a similar study conducted in 2010, which supports the link between increasing coffee consumption and decreased depression risk.[154] Interestingly, this last trial was unable to link caffeine with depression risk, suggesting that other compounds in coffee may be responsible for the mood-elevating effect.

Conventional coffee preparation, which involves roasting the green coffee beans at high temperatures to attain the desired flavor profile, dramatically lowers levels of health-promoting coffee constituents called *chlorogenic acids*.

Chlorogenic acids have been shown in several studies to aid in controlling blood sugar levels, especially those glucose spikes which occur after a high-carbohydrate meal.[155,156] In a 12-week study, consumption of chlorogenic acid–fortified instant coffee lead to a considerable reduction in body weight when compared to regular instant coffee.[157] As elevated glucose levels and excess body weight are common among depressed people, chlorogenic acids may help combat some symptoms of depression tied to insulin resistance and irregularities in glucose metabolism.

*Green coffee*, the primary source of chlorogenic acids, cannot be consumed as a beverage due to its extremely bitter taste. Consuming *green coffee extract* standardized to chlorogenic acids is an effective means of obtaining biologically active concentrations of chlorogenic acids.

The potential role of chlorogenic acids in mediating the mood boost associated with coffee consumption, and their thoroughly studied antihyperglycemic properties give rise to promising multimodal depression protection.

**Chromium.** Chromium has been studied for its role in regulating blood sugar by facilitating the uptake of glucose into cells, and some research indicates that it may be beneficial in depression as well.[158]

In one case series of 5 patients with minor depression, chromium supplementation led to remission.[159] Two other pilot studies found that chromium picolinate supplementation benefited atypical depression.[160,161] Finally, although not studied for seasonal depression, chromium may help regulate blood sugar and cravings for sugar and carbohydrates in relation to seasonal depression.

## Antioxidant Effects

**N-acetyl-cysteine (NAC).** NAC is one of the best-researched antioxidants for depression. NAC is a precursor to glutathione, one of the body's most powerful antioxidants. Research has found glutathione depletion and oxidative stress in people with bipolar depression. Two recent studies showed NAC is a safe and effective adjunctive treatment that improves depression in patients with bipolar disorder.[162]

**Lipoic acid.** Although lipoic acid has not been well studied for depression, it is one of the most effective supplemental antioxidants, since it helps recycle other antioxidants, such as vitamin C.[163] It also may benefit blood sugar regulation and neurologic function, as evidence shows it can help diabetic neuropathy.[164]

**Vitamins C, E, and selenium.** In general, antioxidants may help buffer nerve cell damage in cases of chronic or recurrent depression, although they also serve other roles in brain health. For example, the antioxidant vitamin C is an important cofactor in the synthesis of serotonin, norepinephrine, and adrenal hormones that mediate stress. Vitamin E helps protect nerve cell membranes, and low selenium levels are associated with depression[165]

## Additional Nutrients

**St. John's wort.** St. John's wort (*Hypericum perforatum*) is a medicinal herb used to treat neurologic and psychiatric disorders, including depression.[166] Compared to a placebo, *H. perforatum* extract is more effective at targeting mild to moderate depression, and reducing symptoms and recurrence rate.[167] Its effectiveness is considered comparable to antidepressant medications, but its actions are more complex.[168,169]

St. John's wort's mechanism of action on depression is not entirely understood, even though it is one of the most researched herbs for depression. St. John's wort has been shown to inhibit serotonin and norepinephrine reuptake, thus increasing their availability at the synapse.[166] Other investigators found that it influences dopamine and GABA activity. Its antidepressant qualities also can be linked to its antioxidant and anti-inflammatory properties that normalize an overactive hypothalamus-pituitary-adrenal axis and stress response.[170]

While additional research is ongoing to identify all of the antidepressant mechanisms of action, experimental models and clinical trials alike have shown that treatment with St. John's wort delivers positive response rates for mild to moderate depression.[171–173]

**Vitamin D.** Growing evidence suggests that vitamin D significantly affects depression. This is not surprising in seasonal depression, since the skin synthesizes vitamin D in response to sunlight, which is less available in the winter.[174,175] However, vitamin D has been found to play other roles in depression. For example, in a study of 7358 patients age ≥50 with a cardiovascular diagnosis and no history of depression, low vitamin D levels significantly increased the risk of developing depression.[176]

Studies also find that vitamin D3 (cholecalciferol) supplementation can improve symptoms of depression. One well-controlled study of 441 overweight and obese participants showed an association between low vitamin D levels and depression. High-dose vitamin D

supplementation (20 000–40 000 IUs/week or 2800–6000 IUs/day) for 1 year improved mood.[177] Another pilot study noted significant improvement in depression in 6 of 9 women with low levels of vitamin D upon supplementation.[175]

Vitamin D's effectiveness may be related to the high prevalence of vitamin-D deficiency in the general population, its importance in blood-sugar regulation, and its importance in overall regulation of genetic activity.

**Zinc.** Zinc is a trace element known to help regulate the nervous system,[178] and may be specifically related to depression.[179] Increasing evidence shows that decreased blood levels of zinc are associated with depression,[180–182] and, in depressed subjects, lower levels of zinc are associated with worse depression.[183] One pilot study of 20 depressed patients also showed that 25 mg of zinc per day augmented benefits of antidepressant medication.[184]

Animal studies show that antidepressants and electroconvulsive shock treatments change zinc concentrations in areas of the brain associated with depression.[185] In further animal research, zinc also was shown to enhance antidepressant effects of imipramine,[186] and influence serotonin levels and activity in several brain regions.[187]

**Inositol.** Inositol levels in the brain and cerebrospinal fluid were found to be lower in subjects with depression. One well-controlled trial showed that taking 12 g per day of inositol helped relieve symptoms in 39 patients with depression.[188]

Further research on bipolar depression suggests beneficial influences of inositol.[189] A well-controlled but small trial of 17 participants with bipolar depression showed varied responses. Four of 9 patients experienced significant improvement with inositol supplementation compared to zero of 8 who took a placebo.[190]

Inositol, a *second-messenger* precursor, has important cellular communication functions in the nervous system. Interestingly, inositol is also involved with insulin signaling and function. It therefore may have more of an effect on overweight or obese individuals, as well as those who are insulin resistant, such as those with metabolic syndrome or women with polycystic ovarian syndrome (PCOS). These findings require further research and replication.

## Life Extension Suggestions

Depression is a *multifactorial* condition, and efficient relief often requires addressing multiple neurochemical and metabolic *imbalances* that may underlie mood disturbances. The nutrients listed in this protocol are categorized according to their evidence-based mechanisms of action in brain health and mood regulation.

Many of these suggestions may serve as adjuvants to conventional therapies for depression. Always consult a qualified health care professional before combining any supplements with an antidepressant medication.

### Broad-Range Nervous System Effects
- **Fish oil** (with olive polyphenols): 1400 mg EPA and 1000 mg DHA daily
- **Magnesium L-threonate:** 2000 mg daily (supplying 144 mg elemental magnesium)

### Supporting Neurotransmitter Synthesis
- **5-hyroxytryptophan (5-HTP):** 50–200 mg daily
**OR**
- **Tryptophan:** 1000–2000 mg daily

### Supporting Methylation Reactions
- **S-Adenosylmethionine (SAMe):** 400–1200 mg daily
- **L-methylfolate:** 1000 mcg daily
- **Vitamin B12** (as methylcobalamin): 1000–8000 mcg daily
- **Vitamin B6** (as pyridoxal 5-phosphate): 100 mg daily

### Supporting Blood Sugar Regulation
- **Chromium:** 500 mcg daily
- **Green coffee bean extract,** standardized 50% to chlorogenic acid: 400 mg before each meal, up to 3 times daily

### Antioxidant Effects
- **N-acetyl-cysteine:** 600–1200 mg daily
- **R-lipoic acid:** 300–600 mg daily
- **Vitamin C:** 1000–2000 mg daily
- **Vitamin E,** as high gamma-tocopherol mix: 350 mg daily
- **Selenium,** as Se-methylselenocysteine: 200 mcg daily

### Supporting Mitochondrial Health
- **Coenzyme Q10** (as ubiquinol): 100–200 mg daily
- **Pyrroloquinoline quinine (PQQ):** 10–20 mg daily
- **Acetyl-L-carnitine:** 1000–2000 mg daily

### Hormone Restoration
Men and women with depression consider restoring their hormone concentrations to youthful levels with the use of natural bioidentical hormones. More information is available in the Male Hormone Restoration and Female Hormone Restoration protocols. A natural, over-the-counter hormone that men and women should consider optimizing follows:

- **DHEA:** 15–50 mg daily for women or 25–75 mg daily for men

In addition, thyroid hormone irregularities may contribute to depression. Therefore, those with known or suspected thyroid dysfunction should refer to the Thyroid Regulation protocol.

### Additional Nutrients
- **Vitamin D:** 5000–8000 IU daily (depending on blood test results)
- **Zinc:** 30 mg daily
- **Inositol:** 2000–10 000 mg daily
- **Comprehensive multivitamin/multinutrient formula:** per label instructions
- **St. John's wort,** standardized extract: 300–600 mg daily

In addition, the following blood testing resources may be helpful:

- Female Panel or Male Panel
- Thyroid Panel (TSH, T4, Free T4, Free T3)
- Cortisol AM/PM
- Insulin (fasting)
- Serotonin, whole blood
- Vitamin B12 and folate
- Vitamin D, 25-Hydroxy
- RBC magnesium
- Omega Score®
- Cytokine Panel

## REFERENCES

References available at: www.lef.org/dpt5/ch49

# 50

# DHEA Restoration Therapy

It is no accident that youth is associated with high levels of hormones. Produced throughout the body, sex hormones are critical to maintaining vibrancy and good health. In recent decades, scientists have begun to understand the powerful benefits of replacing hormones lost to aging. However, there are serious questions about the safety of conventional hormone replacement therapy, which relies on hormones that are synthesized from animals (eg, Premarin®) or created in a lab (eg, Provera®). Most recently, the widespread prescribing of these two hormones among menopausal women has come under scientific scrutiny because of the increased risk of stroke and heart attack.

As an alternative, *bioidentical hormone replacement therapy* may be one of the best things that aging people can do for themselves because of the wide-ranging benefits of bioidentical hormones on everything from the cardiovascular system to the aging brain and bones. What is required, however, is an approach that harnesses the wisdom of the body and relies on bioidentical hormones to replace those that decline with age.

In 1981, Life Extension introduced dehydroepiandrosterone (DHEA) in an article that described the multiple antiaging effects of this steroid hormone. At the time, DHEA replacement therapy was almost unheard of. Today, DHEA replacement therapy has been studied extensively, and decreased DHEA levels have been implicated in heart disease, high cholesterol, depression, inflammation, immune disorders, schizophrenia, Alzheimer's disease, diabetes, HIV, and osteoporosis.[1-3]

What is DHEA, and how does it work? DHEA is the most common steroid hormone in the body. It is produced mainly by the adrenal glands, and to a lesser extent, elsewhere in the body (including fat cells). DHEA is metabolized from pregnenolone, the body's "master hormone," which itself is metabolized from cholesterol. DHEA can be metabolized into other sex hormones, including testosterone, estrogens, and up to 150 individual metabolites.

Although there are still important research questions to answer, there is no question that youthful DHEA levels are closely associated with good health, and that low levels have been connected to various diseases. Unfortunately, after about age 35, DHEA begins to decline.[4,5] Women, who tend to have lower levels, lose DHEA much more quickly than men as they age. Concentrations remain roughly 30% higher in men.[6] DHEA levels also vary according to ethnicity.[6-8] By age 70, DHEA levels may be only 20% of young-adult levels.[9]

Modern hormone replacement therapy strives to recreate the youthful balance of hormones in the body—and this is where DHEA's value really stands out. Because it is metabolized into other hormones, supplementing with DHEA may allow the body to choose which hormone is needed, and then synthesize that hormone from available DHEA. This may account for the astonishing range of benefits that many researchers attribute to this hormone. DHEA's separate metabolites, including 7-Keto® DHEA, have also been shown to have individual benefits, including lowering cholesterol, burning fat, and boosting the immune system.

There are many provocative theories that may one day help explain DHEA's role in certain diseases. For instance, many elderly people suffer from high cholesterol levels, which are a risk factor for heart disease. In this age group, the rate of heart disease rises much more rapidly among women than men, partly because of the loss of hormones during menopause. Clearly, there is a link between heart disease and sex hormones, and this phenomenon raises an intriguing possibility. Because sex hormones are synthesized from cholesterol, perhaps elevated cholesterol levels represent the body's attempt to supply more of the raw materials for hormone production. Indeed, one study showed a drop in cholesterol levels after comprehensive natural hormone therapy.[10] More information on this topic can be found in Life Extension's Male Hormone Restoration and Female Hormone Restoration protocols.

As part of a comprehensive approach to fighting the diseases of aging, Life Extension suggests that people monitor their blood levels of DHEA and strive to reproduce hormone levels of a healthy 21-year-old. Fortunately, supplemental DHEA is well tolerated with only minimal side effects, even at relatively high doses.

## WHAT YOU HAVE LEARNED SO FAR

- DHEA is a hormone produced from the synthesis of pregnenolone. It may be metabolized into other sex hormones including testosterone and estrogen. DHEA is the most prevalent steroid hormone in the body.

- Low DHEA levels are clearly associated with a range of diseases, including heart disease, diabetes, inflammation, Alzheimer's, and others.
- DHEA levels drop dramatically as people age. There are pronounced differences in the average DHEA levels of men and women, with women on average having lower DHEA levels.
- DHEA replacement therapy can restore youthful DHEA levels.

# DHEA: FIGHTING INFLAMMATION

Inflammation is an insidious condition, and we are learning more every year about its association with a host of diseases. Inflammation is caused by internal chemicals called inflammatory cytokines that are released as part of the immune system response. These chemicals, including tumor necrosis factor-alpha (TNF-α), interleukin-6 (IL-6), interleukin-1 beta (IL-1β), and/or leukotriene are present in greater concentrations as we age. Reducing the concentration of inflammatory cytokines to reduce the risk of serious disease is one goal of nutrient and hormone therapy.

DHEA supplementation has been shown to improve several aspects of the immune system—cytokine production and T cell, B cell, natural killer cell, and monocyte function—in postmenopausal women and elderly men.[11] DHEA appears to be especially valuable against IL-6 and TNF, both of which are elevated in patients with inflammatory arthritis.[12–15] Systemic lupus erythematosus is another chronic inflammatory condition, affecting approximately 1 in every 700 women, usually younger women.[16] Treatment of this type of lupus with DHEA (50–200 mg daily) caused clinical improvement and decreased lupus flares by 16%.[17,18]

## DHEA IN WOMEN

Throughout their reproductive lives, women experience higher levels of estrogen produced by the ovaries. This estrogen has a cardioprotective effect, which accounts for women's lower rates of heart disease. However, around age 50, women undergo menopause, or failure of the ovaries and cessation of menstruation. This period is distinguished by a rapid drop in the level of sex hormones, including estrogen, DHEA, testosterone, pregnenolone, and progesterone. Various diseases have been connected to this rapid loss of hormonal protection, including heart disease and osteoporosis.[19] While many of the symptoms of menopause are caused by the loss of estrogen, there are also side effects associated with the drop in DHEA and testosterone among menopausal women, including the following[20]:

- Decreased libido
- Decreased strength

- Decreased muscle mass
- Decreased bone density
- Decreased energy

In menopausal women, DHEA therapy is sometimes androgenic. In other words, it tends to raise the blood levels of male sex hormones such as testosterone,[21] which accounts for the small risk among some women of increased hair growth.[22] However, there is growing evidence that a modest increase in testosterone benefits women. For example, it appears to improve bone metabolism and decrease menopausal symptoms,[23] as well as increase sexual desire.[24]

One analysis of existing studies found that DHEA had these benefits among postmenopausal women:

- A 30–50 mg daily dose improved mood, sense of well-being, and sexual appetite and activity among women with adrenal insufficiency.[25]
- A long-term trial of women over 60 reported significant increases in bone mineral density.[25]
- A study among women age 70–79 showed improvements in sexual desire, arousal, and enjoyment.[25]

## DHEA IN MEN

Studies of men have shown that DHEA replacement therapy is an important complement to testosterone therapy. Among aging men, the amount of "free" testosterone, or testosterone that is available to the body, falls more quickly than the level of total testosterone. Thus, it is important to design a hormone replacement program that raises the level of free testosterone. In a 1997 study, DHEA levels were shown to parallel the levels of free testosterone in the blood. The study authors suggested that DHEA might help raise free testosterone. If this conclusion is correct, then DHEA replacement therapy would not only raise the blood level of DHEA, but also the level of free testosterone.[26]

Still, other studies have shown that DHEA may be an effective therapy for erectile dysfunction. Although there are conflicting studies in this regard, a few have shown that among men without heart or vascular disease, DHEA has improved erectile dysfunction.[21]

## DHEA AND CANCER

In any discussion of hormone replacement therapy, the question of cancer will naturally arise. Certain cancers, especially breast and prostate cancer, may be hormone mediated. In other words, supplementation with hormones may cause cancer cells to proliferate. For this reason, men and women with histories of hormone receptor–positive cancers, or with existing tumors, are warned away from hormone therapy that might aggravate their condition.

The situation, however, is not clear-cut. In numerous studies, DHEA has shown anticancer properties.[15,27–31] According to studies using animal models and cell cultures (both animal and human), DHEA has been shown to inhibit cancer development in a number of tissues, including:

- Mammary gland[27,32]
- Skin[27]
- Colon[33–35]
- Liver and thyroid[36]

## DHEA and Breast Cancer

Because DHEA may be converted into estrogen, women with breast cancer are advised not to begin DHEA therapy, which may theoretically increase the severity of their cancer. To date, no large studies have been conducted on the use of DHEA in women with breast cancer. Healthy women taking DHEA should also monitor their blood levels of estrogen and free testosterone to make sure that DHEA is creating youthful hormone balance.

## DHEA and Prostate Cancer

Men should not begin DHEA therapy before having their prostate-specific antigen (PSA) levels tested and undergoing a digital rectal exam to measure the size and consistency of the prostate. Men with prostate cancer or severe benign prostate disease are advised to avoid DHEA because it can be converted into testosterone, which may promote cell proliferation or cause an increase in DHT (dihydrotestosterone). However, among healthy men, one study showed that DHEA did not increase PSA levels.[37] To make sure that DHEA is tolerated, men should consider having their DHEA blood levels tested every 6 or 12 months after beginning therapy, along with testing levels of free testosterone, estrogen, and DHT. The DHT form of testosterone plays an important role in the development of benign prostatic enlargement, and is believed to contribute to the progression of prostate cancer.

## DHEA AND OTHER CONDITIONS/DISEASES

Many of the studies examining DHEA have found an overall benefit among study subjects, especially the elderly. Nevertheless, it is helpful to understand some of DHEA's chemical interactions to gain insight into its many roles inside the body.

DHEA owes many of its beneficial properties to its ability to inhibit an enzyme called glucose-6-phosphate dehydrogenase (G6PD). DHEA's anticancer properties are due at least in part to its ability to inhibit G6PD.[38,39] DHEA's cardioprotective properties may also be partly due to G6PD inhibition.[40,41]

Beyond its broad benefits, a survey of studies found that DHEA was active in fighting many conditions and diseases.

## Alzheimer's Disease

Patients with Alzheimer's disease have higher levels of cortisol (the "stress" hormone),[42] and imbalanced cortisol/DHEA ratios[43] In a group of severely afflicted Alzheimer's patients, Dehydroepiandrosterone sulfate (DHEA-S) levels were significantly lower.[43] Other studies have examined the role of vascular endothelial growth factor (VEGF) among Alzheimer's patients. VEGF has been shown to protect the brain, and scientists now believe that low VEGF levels may be connected to the progression of Alzheimer's disease. DHEA-S was shown to significantly increase the bioavailability of VEGF in the brain, leading the study authors to conclude that it could be a valuable treatment for Alzheimer's and aging.[44]

## Cardiovascular Disease

There is a clear relationship between DHEA levels and cardiovascular disease. As DHEA declines, the incidence of cardiovascular disease rises in men[45–49] and in women.[50] Diabetic men with the lowest DHEA levels have a significantly greater chance of developing coronary heart disease.[51] The risk of death is higher among those with the lowest levels of DHEA in men younger than age 70.[52]

DHEA plays a protective role in the development of atherosclerosis and coronary artery disease,[53,54] especially among men. Several mechanisms are involved: inhibition of G6PD (which can modify the lipid spectrum), suppression of platelet aggregation, and reduced cell proliferation.[55] Men with lower DHEA-S are more likely to have atherosclerosis[46] and calcified deposits in the abdominal aorta.[56] Because cortisol increases the risk of heart attack and the severity of atherosclerosis in men,[57] raising DHEA levels to increase the DHEA/cortisol ratio has promise for reducing cardiovascular risk.[48] However, the same associations are lacking in women.[45]

## Myocardial Infarction

Low DHEA is related to premature heart attack in men.[58] Severely ill cardiac patients and those with acute heart attack have lower DHEA levels for as long as 3–4 months after the event.[59,60]

## Metabolic Syndrome

Metabolic syndrome is characterized by several conditions, which are all associated with elevated risk for heart disease (eg, increased insulin resistance, obesity, and abnormal cholesterol levels). In metabolic syndrome, these individual risk factors act synergistically, raising the risk of heart disease higher than their individual risk levels alone. Although research is still continuing, scientists have linked elevated cholesterol to lower DHEA levels.[61] Long-term DHEA supplementation improves insulin sensitivity by 30%, raises high-density lipoprotein (HDL) cholesterol by 12%, and lowers low-density lipoprotein (LDL) cholesterol by 11% and triglycerides by 20%.[62] The lowering of LDL by DHEA has an antioxidant effect, which could have antiatherogenic consequences.[63–66] DHEA also decreases abdominal fat, an important characteristic of metabolic syndrome.[67,68]

## Cognitive Decline

One of the most distressing elements of aging is the loss of mental "sharpness." Once again, DHEA has been shown to improve measures of cognitive function in laboratory studies.[69,70] Abnormal balances in the brain between DHEA-S and cortisol have been shown to decrease brain function.[71,72]

## Depression

DHEA has been extensively studied in depression. DHEA levels are reduced in major depressive disorders in both adolescents and adults, and an elevated cortisol/DHEA ratio predicts a delay in recovery.[73,74] Women lacking detectable DHEA have an increased occurrence of depression.[75]

DHEA has also been a useful remedy for depression.[76] A well-conducted study by the National Institute of Mental Health found DHEA to be quite effective in treating midlife, long-lasting, mild depression (dysthymia). The symptoms that improved most significantly were inability to gain pleasure from normally pleasurable experiences (anhedonia), loss of energy, lack of motivation, emotional "numbness," sadness, inability to cope, and worrying.[77] In another study, 3 months of DHEA supplementation improved self-reported physical and psychological well-being in age-advanced individuals.[78] These results were supported by a recent study that showed DHEA therapy improved depression among middle-aged people.[79]

## Diabetes

DHEA appears to increase insulin sensitivity. Insulin resistance is an early indicator of type 2 diabetes and is closely associated with obesity, which are both major risk factors for heart disease. A decrease in DHEA-S is associated with the development of type 2 diabetes.[80] Among women with deficient adrenal glands, DHEA supplementation was shown to significantly increase insulin sensitivity, and the study authors concluded that DHEA might be a valuable treatment for type 2 diabetes.[81] DHEA has also been shown to increase insulin sensitivity among obese women.[68]

## HIV/AIDS

HIV-positive men with lower DHEA levels have comparably lower CD4 cell counts,[82] and are 2.3 times more likely to progress to AIDS.[83,84] HIV-positive men have a dramatically elevated cortisol/DHEA ratio that parallels their nutritional and disease status.[83–87]

## Immune System

DHEA has been shown to enhance the immune response against a wide range of viral, bacterial, and parasitic pathogens. In one animal study, DHEA supplementation showed a significant reduction in the level of internal parasites.[88]

## Osteoporosis

Osteoporosis (bone thinning) affects millions of late-middle-aged to elderly individuals of both sexes, but is more common in women than men. In women, a major contributing factor is the loss of estrogen at menopause, which parallels the decline in DHEA. DHEA appears to exert a positive role in bone metabolism by inhibiting bone resorption and stimulating bone formation.[89,90] It also seems to aid calcium absorption.[91,92] DHEA has proved effective in clinical trials treating osteoporosis.[67] However, a correlation between DHEA and bone mineral density appears variably in women and not at all in men.[93–97]

## Stress

DHEA levels are closely tied to stress. Studies have shown that traumatic events such as burns or illnesses significantly decrease DHEA, testosterone, and androstenedione levels, while increasing the level of cortisol.[98–100] Calmness, such as that seen in individuals practicing transcendental meditation, is associated with higher levels of DHEA.[101] In one study, participants in a stress-reduction program increased DHEA by 100% and reduced stress hormone production (cortisol) by 23%.[102]

# 7-KETO® DHEA: THE PERFECT PARTNER

Among DHEA's many metabolites, one has attracted significant attention for its unique ability to lower cholesterol, burn fat, and improve the immune system. This metabolite, known as 7-Keto® DHEA, is not converted into estrogen or testosterone, so it may be safely used among people with hormone-dependent diseases, including cancer.

Scientific studies have shown that 7-Keto® can help people burn fat through a process known as "thermogenesis." This means the body's metabolic rate is accelerated, generating heat and energy that consumes calories and burns fat. 7-Keto® accomplishes this by boosting the levels of liver enzymes that stimulate fatty acid oxidation.

In one study of 30 overweight adults, study subjects received 100 mg of 7-Keto® twice daily or placebo. They also participated in a supervised exercise and diet program. At the end of the study, those taking 7-Keto® lost 6.3 pounds on average, versus 2.1 pounds for the control group.[103]

7-Keto® has also been studied for its immune-boosting and cholesterol-lowering properties. In a study on cholesterol levels, human volunteers applied a gel containing 25 mg of 7-Keto® for 5 consecutive days. At the end of the study, the subjects taking 7-Keto® experienced a rise in good HDL cholesterol and a slight reduction in harmful LDL cholesterol.[104]

Another study looking at immune function found that 4 weeks of 7-Keto® supplementation improved immune function in elderly men and women. In this study, subjects over age 65 took 100 mg of 7-Keto® twice daily or placebo. The subjects on 7-Keto® experienced a significant decrease in immune suppressor cells and an increase in immune helper cells.[105]

Because 7-Keto® is not converted into estrogen or testosterone, it may be the perfect complement to DHEA therapy, as well as providing an option for people who have hormone dependent cancers. In some women, high doses of DHEA may cause the growth of unwanted hair or acne. By adding 7-Keto® to a daily program, it may be possible to lower the dosage of DHEA.

## Life Extension Suggestions

Because of the overwhelming evidence connecting low levels of DHEA to the degenerative diseases of aging, Life Extension suggests that all people over age 40 begin DHEA therapy. For most people, the starting dose of DHEA is 15–75 mg, taken in a single daily dose. Many studies have used a daily dose of 50 mg. One recent study showed that doses <30 mg were not enough to significantly support blood levels of DHEA in young adults.[106]

Ideally, DHEA replacement therapy should begin with blood testing to establish a base range. Since almost everyone over age 35–40 has lower than optimal levels of DHEA, most people begin supplementation and test their blood DHEA levels later to make sure that they are taking the proper dose. Normal serum reference ranges and ideal ranges of DHEA-S follow:

|  | Normal (depending on age) | Ideal |
|---|---|---|
| Men | 16.2-492 µg/dL | 350-490 µg/dL |
| Women | 12-407 µg/dL | 275-400 µg/dL |

After 3–6 weeks, another test is recommended to measure serum DHEA. All individuals react differently to DHEA replacement therapy, so it is a good idea to closely monitor your blood levels and side effects. If side effects appear, it may be possible to add 7-Keto® DHEA and reduce the dose of DHEA.

Those with compromised liver health should use DHEA sublingual tablets, which bypass liver metabolism. Otherwise, capsules containing the more common micronized DHEA are quite effective in restoring DHEA to youthful ranges.

## REFERENCES

References available at: www.lef.org/dpt5/ch50

# 51

# *Diabetes*

The consequences of uncontrolled diabetes are severe blindness, kidney failure, increased risk of heart disease, and painful peripheral nerve damage. Today, most practitioners focus treatment on strict blood sugar control. While diabetes is characterized by excess blood glucose (the form of sugar used by cells as energy), this simplified approach can actually hasten the progression of the most common form of diabetes and does nothing to address the damage it causes.

A new approach to diabetes recognition and treatment is needed because the conventional wisdom has failed us. America is in the midst of a diabetes epidemic. Over the past 20 years, the number of adults diagnosed with diabetes has more than doubled, and children are being diagnosed with diabetes in alarming numbers. Diabetes has rapidly emerged as a leading culprit in the epidemic of heart disease, as well as being a leading cause of amputation and blindness among adults.

It is crucial that diabetics (and those predisposed to diabetes) understand the ways in which blood glucose causes damage and take active steps to interrupt these processes. The most notorious process is glycation (ie, sugar molecules reacting with proteins to produce nonfunctional structures in the body). Glycation compromises proteins throughout the body, and thus is a key feature of diabetes-related complications (eg, nerve damage, heart attack, and blindness).

Oxidative stress is also central to the damage caused by diabetes. Diabetics suffer from high levels of free radicals that damage arteries throughout the body. It is important that diabetics understand the need for antioxidant therapy to help reduce oxidative stress and lower the risk of diabetic complications.

## THE DIFFERENCE BETWEEN TYPE 1 AND TYPE 2 DIABETES

There are two types of diabetes: type 1 and type 2. Underlying both forms of diabetes is a disorder of insulin production, use, or both. Insulin is a hormone responsible for transporting glucose into cells. When there is excess glucose in the blood, insulin is secreted from the pancreas and signals the liver and muscles to store glucose as glycogen. Insulin also stimulates adipose tissue to store glucose as fat for long-term energy reserves. Insulin receptors are found in all cells throughout the body. In a healthy person, blood glucose levels are extremely stable.[1] Normal fasting glucose levels range between 70 and 100 mg/dL.

## Type 1 Diabetes

Type 1 diabetes, formerly known as insulin-dependent diabetes, is an autoimmune condition that occurs when the body attacks and destroys the cells (called beta-cells or β-cells) that make insulin. Type 1 diabetes accounts for about 5–10% of cases. Because type 1 diabetics can no longer make insulin, insulin replacement therapy is essential.

## Type 2 Diabetes

Type 2 diabetes, formerly known as non–insulin-dependent diabetes, occurs when the body is no longer able to use insulin effectively and gradually becomes resistant to its effects. It is a slowly progressing disease that goes through identifiable stages. In the early stages, both insulin and glucose levels are elevated (conditions called hyperinsulinemia and hyperglycemia, respectively). In the later stages, insulin levels are reduced, and blood glucose levels are very elevated. Although few people are aware of this crucial distinction, therapy for type 2 diabetes should be tailored to the stage of the disease.

Risk factors for type 2 diabetes include aging, obesity, family history, physical inactivity, ethnicity, and impaired glucose metabolism.

### Type 2 Diabetes

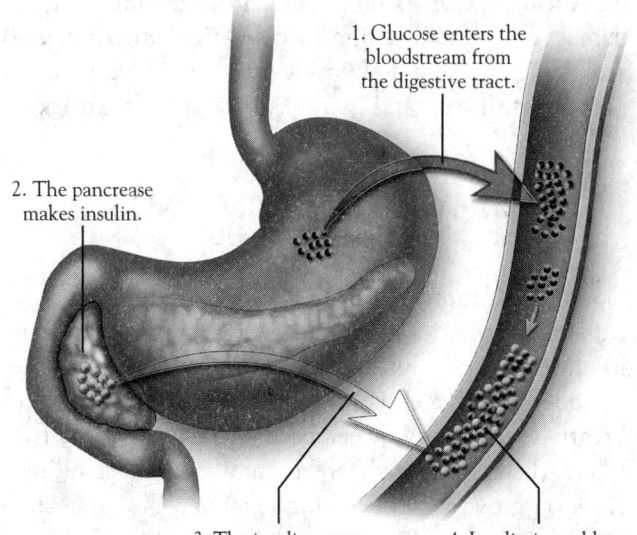

1. Glucose enters the bloodstream from the digestive tract.

2. The pancrease makes insulin.

3. The insulin enters the bloodstream.

4. Insulin is unable to facilitate cellular glucose uptake. Glucose builds up in the blood vessels.

# THE DIABETES DAMAGE CASCADE

Glycation and oxidative stress are central to the damage caused by diabetes. Unfortunately, neither of them figures into conventional treatment for diabetes, which is generally concerned only with blood sugar control.

Glycation occurs when glucose reacts with protein, resulting in sugar-damaged proteins called advanced glycation end products (AGEs).[2,3] One well-known AGE among diabetics is glycated hemoglobin (HbA1c). HbA1c is created when glucose molecules bind to hemoglobin in the blood. Measuring HbA1c in the blood can help determine the overall exposure of hemoglobin to glucose, which yields a picture of long-term blood glucose control.

Glycated proteins damage cells in numerous ways, including impairing cellular function, which induces the production of inflammatory cytokines[4] and free radicals.[5,6] In animal studies, inhibiting glycation protects against damage to the kidney, nerves, and eyes.[5,7] In a large human trial, each 1% reduction in HbA1c correlated with a 21% reduction in risk for any complication of diabetes, a 21% reduction in deaths related to diabetes, a 14% reduction in heart attack, and a 37% reduction in microvascular complications.[8]

High levels of blood glucose and glycation also produce free radicals that further damage cellular proteins[9] and reduce nitric oxide levels. Nitric oxide is a potent vasodilator that helps keep arteries relaxed and wide open. Oxidative stress in diabetes is also linked to endothelial dysfunction, the process that characterizes atherosclerotic heart disease. According to studies, diabetes encourages white blood cells to stick to the endothelium (ie, the thin layer of cells that line the inside of arteries). These white blood cells cause the local release of proinflammatory chemicals that damage the endothelium, accelerating atherosclerosis.[10] Diabetes is closely associated with severe coronary heart disease and increased risk of heart attack.

# SYMPTOMS AND DIAGNOSIS OF DIABETES

Common symptoms of diabetes include increased thirst and urination, unusual weight changes, irritability, fatigue, and blurry vision. Clinical abnormalities include hyperglycemia and glucose in the urine. The breath might smell sweet because of ketones in the blood (ketosis), which are naturally sweet smelling. Dark outgrowths of skin (skin tags) may also appear.

The most common clinical tests used to diagnose diabetes are measures of blood glucose. The fasting plasma glucose (FPG) test measures the amount of glucose in the blood after fasting. Prediabetes is diagnosed if the fasting blood glucose level is between 100 and 125 mg/dL. Diabetes is diagnosed if the fasting blood glucose level rises to ≥ 126 mg/dL.

The oral glucose tolerance test (OGTT) is used to measure insulin response to high glucose levels. During this test, patients are given glucose, and the rise in blood glucose levels is measured. Prediabetes is diagnosed if the glucose level rises to between 140 and 199 mg/dL. Diabetes is diagnosed if blood glucose levels rise to ≥200 mg/dL.

The HbA1c test is also helpful in diagnosing less severe cases of diabetes. From this test, clinicians can estimate the average blood glucose level during the preceding 2–4 months. Normally 4–6% of hemoglobin is glycosylated, which corresponds to average blood glucose between 60 and 120 mg/dL. Mild hyperglycemia increases HbA1c to 8–10% (or 180–240 mg/dL), while severe hyperglycemia increases HbA1c values up to 20%. For diabetics, a healthy HbA1c level is less than 7%, which corresponds to an average blood glucose level of ≤ 150 mg/dL.

# THE TRUTH ABOUT TYPE 2 DIABETES THERAPY

Before discussing therapy for type 2 diabetes, it is important to understand the logic behind conventional therapy and to understand why this logic is flawed. Type 2 diabetics are routinely told they need to boost their insulin levels, which will help drive blood glucose into their cells and lower their blood glucose levels. Unfortunately, this assumption defies common sense.

In the early stages of type 2 diabetes, insulin levels are already elevated (hyperinsulinemia). This is because the problem is not with insulin production, but rather a metabolic defect of insulin utilization. The delicate insulin receptors on cell membranes are less responsive to the insulin than are the receptors of people without type 2 diabetes, which means that less glucose is absorbed from the bloodstream than is normal, and glucose levels slowly rise.

This elevation in glucose upsets the body's natural balance, prompting the pancreas to discharge copious amounts of insulin to normalize glucose levels. This short-term, biological fix successfully drives glucose into cells, thereby lowering blood glucose levels, but it also hastens the progression of the disease. Eventually, the fragile insulin receptors become less sensitive (insulin resistant), which means that the pancreas must secrete even more insulin to keep clearing the blood of glucose. In later stages of the disease, the pancreas becomes "burned out" and can no longer produce adequate insulin. Insulin levels drop far below normal, allowing blood glucose to rise even higher and inflict greater damage.

Unfortunately, many early-stage diabetics are prescribed drugs (eg, sulfonylureas) designed to boost insulin levels. Considering that insulin levels are already high, this strategy is counterproductive and may actually serve to hasten the disease by further exhausting the insulin receptors on cell membranes. Also, insulin itself is a powerful hormone that, in high levels, can inflict damage. Evidence suggests that high levels of insulin may suppress growth hormone synthesis and release among obese and overweight people (who are prone to hyperinsulinemia).[11] There is also evidence that increased levels of insulin contribute to the proliferation of colorectal cells, which suggests that high levels of insulin may be a factor in the development of colorectal cancer.[12]

## A PROGRAM FOR EARLY DIABETICS

There are acute differences between early and advanced stages of diabetes. Thus, it doesn't make sense to treat all people with type 2 diabetes the same. In the early stages of the disease, people suffer from both hyperglycemia and hyperinsulinemia. Rather than take drugs that further increase the level of insulin in the blood, people with type 2 diabetes would do better to pursue therapies that increase the sensitivity of insulin receptors on the cell membranes.

One of the best defenses against mild to moderate type 2 diabetes and hyperinsulinemia is improved diet and exercise. Although the disease has a genetic component, many studies have shown that diet and exercise can prevent it.[13–16] One study also showed that while some medications delay the development of diabetes, diet and exercise work better. Just 30 minutes a day of moderate physical activity, coupled with a 5–10% reduction in body weight, produces a 58% reduction in the incidence of diabetes among people at risk.[17] The American Diabetes Association recommends a diet high in fiber and unrefined carbohydrates, and low in saturated fat.[18] Foods with a low glycemic index are especially recommended because they blunt the insulin response. For more information on glycemic index, see the Obesity and Weight Loss protocol.

The high-carbohydrate, high-plant-fiber (HCF) diet popularized by James Anderson, MD, has substantial support and validation in the scientific literature as the diet of choice in the treatment of diabetes.[19,20] The HCF diet is high in cereal grains, legumes, and root vegetables, and restricts simple sugar and fat intake.

The diet consists of 50–55% complex carbohydrates, 12–16% protein, and <30% fat, mostly unsaturated. The total fiber content is 25–50 g daily. The HCF diet produces many positive metabolic effects, including the following: lowered postmeal hyperglycemia and delayed hypoglycemia, increased tissue sensitivity to insulin, reduced low-density lipoprotein (LDL) cholesterol and triglyceride levels, increased high-density lipoprotein (HDL) cholesterol levels, and progressive weight loss.

A healthy diet for diabetics is also rich in potassium. Potassium improves insulin sensitivity, responsiveness, and secretion. A high potassium intake also reduces the risk of heart disease, atherosclerosis, and cancer. Insulin administration induces potassium loss.[21,22]

Obese people have a far greater tendency to develop type 2 diabetes than slim people. Therefore, weight loss accompanied by increased exercise and a healthy diet is effective for diabetes prevention and treatment.[23–25]

## METFORMIN: INCREASING INSULIN SENSITIVITY

In addition to diet and exercise, the prescription drug Metformin has been proven to increase insulin sensitivity in people with mild to moderate hyperglycemia. Metformin is now the most commonly prescribed oral antidiabetic drug worldwide. It works by increasing insulin sensitivity in the liver.[26] It also has a number of other beneficial effects, including weight loss, reduced cholesterol-triglyceride levels, and improved endothelial function.

Metformin is better tolerated than many other antidiabetic prescription drugs, but people with congestive heart failure, or kidney or liver disease are not candidates for metformin therapy. Neither are people who consume alcohol in excess. A benchmark assessment of kidney function, followed by an annual renal evaluation, is essential. Vitamin B12 levels should also be checked regularly because chronic use of metformin can cause a folic acid and B12 deficiency, resulting in neurologic impairment and disruption in homocysteine clearance. Also, metformin should not be used for 2 days before or after having an x-ray procedure with an injectable contrast agent because of the rare risk of lactic acidosis.

Metformin is effective on its own, but it may also be prescribed in combination with another class of insulin sensitizers called thiazolidinediones (TZDs; eg, pioglitazone or Actos®, and rosiglitazone or Avandia®). TZDs increase insulin sensitivity and stimulate release of insulin from β-cells in the pancreas. TZD treatment also improves blood pressure and relieves vascular and lipid defects.[27] However, TZDs have potentially serious side effects, including liver toxicity, which requires regular monitoring of liver function.[28,29]

In addition to these two prescription drugs, many nutrients have been shown to increase insulin sensitivity, protect vulnerable cell membranes, and reduce the damaging effects of elevated glucose (see "Nutritional Supplementation for Diabetics" section below). Ideally, a combination of improved diet, exercise, supplementation, and insulin-sensitizing prescription drugs can reverse mild to moderate hyperglycemia before stronger drugs are needed and permanent damage is done.

# DRUG THERAPY FOR ADVANCED DIABETICS

Some people, however, will not have the benefit of this knowledge before their type 2 diabetes advances to a more dangerous stage. In severe hyperglycemia, the pancreas becomes burned out after producing high levels of insulin for a long time. Insulin levels drop as a result of decreased production, and blood glucose levels are allowed to rise to very high, toxic levels. Although diet and exercise, along with supplementation, are still strongly recommended, prescription drugs might also be necessary.

Sulfonylurea drugs stimulate pancreatic secretion of insulin. Unfortunately, they are often prescribed as first-line treatment for mild to moderate type 2 diabetics, even when their use is inappropriate. By increasing levels of insulin, which are already raised, sulfonylurea drugs actually hasten the progression of early type 2 diabetes by exhausting insulin receptors faster, which causes the pancreas to burn out more quickly. Sulfonylurea drugs should really be considered a "last resort" for people with severe hyperglycemia.

Insulin replacement therapy is also a last resort for type 2 diabetics. While insulin therapy is universal and essential among type 1 diabetics, it is reserved for severe, refractory (nonresponsive to treatment) type 2 diabetics only. Proper dosing and monitoring of blood glucose are essential as too much insulin causes low blood sugar and coma, and too little insulin creates hyperglycemia. A new delivery system for insulin was recently approved by the Food and Drug Administration. This new system allows for inhaled insulin.

## WHAT YOU HAVE LEARNED SO FAR

- Diabetes is caused by abnormal metabolism of glucose, either because the body does not produce enough insulin or because the cells become desensitized to the effects of insulin.
- Type 1 diabetes is caused by an autoimmune reaction that destroys insulin-producing β-cells in the pancreas. Type 2 diabetes is caused by decreased insulin sensitivity.
- Type 2 diabetes has reached epidemic proportions in the United States. The incidence of this disease, which is caused by obesity and genetic predisposition, has increased dramatically over the past 5 years. It is more common among older people than in other segments of the population, although it is also affecting children at increasing rates.
- People with mild to moderate type 2 diabetes should avoid drugs and therapies that increase levels of insulin. Their disease is characterized by elevated levels of both insulin and glucose. Instead, therapy should focus on strategies to increase insulin sensitivity.
- Possible complications in diabetes arise from damage to enzymes and other proteins that impair their function and from resulting damage to blood vessels. The subsequent decreased blood flow, increased vulnerability to oxidant stress, and decreased antioxidant capacity all interact to produce end-organ damage to the eyes, nerve tissue, kidneys, and cardiovascular system.
- Type 1 diabetics always require insulin therapy to replace their lost insulin.

# NUTRITIONAL SUPPLEMENTATION FOR DIABETICS

Type 1 diabetics will need to be on insulin therapy for life, although the supplements mentioned in this section may help offset some of the complications caused by diabetes (eg, reduced antioxidant capacity and glycation) as well enhance glucose metabolism. Type 2 diabetics can counteract the progression of their disease by improving insulin sensitivity, enhancing glucose metabolism, and attempting to mitigate the complications of diabetes. The following supplements have been shown to improve blood sugar control or limit diabetic damage:

## Lipoic Acid

As a powerful antioxidant, lipoic acid positively affects important aspects of diabetes, including blood sugar control and the development of long-term complications such as disease of the heart, kidneys, and small blood vessels.[30-36]

Lipoic acid plays a role in preventing diabetes by reducing fat accumulation. In animal studies, lipoic acid reduced body weight, protected pancreatic β-cells from destruction, and reduced triglyceride accumulation in skeletal muscle and pancreatic islets.[35,37]

Lipoic acid has been approved for the prevention and treatment of diabetic neuropathy in Germany for nearly 30 years. Intravenous and oral lipoic acid reduces symptoms of diabetic peripheral neuropathy.[38] Animal studies have suggested that lipoic acid is more effective when taken with gamma-linolenic acid (GLA).[39,40]

Diabetes also damages deep nerves that control vital organs, such as the heart and digestive tract. In a large clinical trial, diabetics (with symptoms caused by nerve damage affecting the heart) showed significant improvement without significant side effects from 800 mg oral lipoic acid daily.[41,42]

## Biotin

Biotin enhances insulin sensitivity and increases the activity of glucokinase, the enzyme responsible for the first step in the utilization of glucose by the liver. Glucokinase concentrations in diabetics are very low. Animal studies have shown that a high biotin diet can improve glucose tolerance and enhance insulin secretion.[43,44]

## Carnitine

An extensive body of literature supports the use of carnitine in diabetes.[45] Carnitine lowers blood glucose and HbA1c levels, increases insulin sensitivity and glucose storage, and optimizes fat and carbohydrate metabolism. Carnitine deficiency is common in type 2 diabetes. In a large human trial, acetyl-L-carnitine helped prevent or slow cardiac autonomic neuropathy in people with diabetes.[46]

## Carnosine

Carnosine is a glycation inhibitor that has been shown to exhibit protective effects against diabetic nephropathy and reduce the formation of AGEs.[47,48]

Studies show that diabetics' cells have lower-than-normal carnosine levels, similar to levels in older adults.[49] Carnosine lowers elevated blood sugar levels, limits oxidant stress and elevated inflammation, and prevents protein cross-linking in diabetics and otherwise healthy aging adults.[50–54] Additionally, carnosine works "behind the scenes" to offer the following protection (for diabetics) against the physiologic destruction caused by high blood sugar:

- Carnosine reduces oxidation and glycation of low-density lipoprotein (LDL), which helps decrease the incidence of diabetes-induced atherosclerosis.[55,56]

- Carnosine reduces protein cross-linking in the lens of the eye and helps to reduce the risk of cataract (a common diabetic complication).[48,57]

- Carnosine supplementation also prevents the microscopic blood vessel damage that produces diabetic retinopathy, a major cause of blindness in diabetics.[58]

- Carnosine supplements prevent loss of sensory nerve function (neuropathy) in diabetic animals.[59]

## Chromium

Chromium is an essential trace mineral that plays a significant role in sugar metabolism. Chromium supplementation helps control blood sugar levels in type 2 diabetes and improves metabolism of carbohydrates, proteins, and lipids. Several studies have shown encouraging results from chromium supplementation:

- A controlled human study of type 2 diabetics compared two forms of chromium (brewer's yeast and chromium chloride).[60] Both forms of chromium significantly improved blood sugar control. Positive results were also seen in two smaller human trials.[61,62]

- A large human trial compared the effects of 1000 mcg chromium, 200 mcg chromium, and placebo.[63] HbA1c values improved significantly in the group receiving 1000 mcg after 2 months and in both chromium groups after 4 months. Fasting glucose was also lower in the group taking the higher dose of chromium. Chromium is a highly reactive metal ion, requiring balance through additional organic materials in order to stabilize and enhance its effects. *Amla* (Indian gooseberry) and shilajit have more recently been shown to synergistically enhance chromium's beneficial action. In a randomized clinical trial of 150 individuals with type 2 diabetes, *200 mcg* twice per day of this novel chromium compound in addition to standard medication induced a greater reduction in fasting blood glucose than placebo (*14.6%* on average) and lowered postprandial blood glucose (*14.2%*) after just 2 months.[64]

## Coenzyme Q10

Coenzyme Q10 (CoQ10) improves blood sugar control, lowers blood pressure, and prevents oxidative damage caused by disease. In a controlled human trial, type 2 diabetics given 100 mg CoQ10 twice daily experienced improved glycemic control as measured by lower HbA1c levels and blood pressure.[65] In a separate study, CoQ10 improved blood flow in type 2 diabetics, an outcome attributed to CoQ10's ability to lower vascular oxidative stress.[66] In a third study, improved blood flow correlated with decreased HbA1c.[67]

In animal studies, CoQ10 quenched free radicals, improved blood flow, lowered triglyceride levels, and raised HDL levels, suggesting a role for CoQ10 in preventing and managing complications of diabetes.[68] Animal studies have also shown that CoQ10 levels are depleted by diabetes.[69]

## Dehydroepiandrosterone

Recent studies have yielded very encouraging results supporting dehydroepiandrosterone (DHEA) supplementation in diabetics. DHEA has been shown to improve insulin sensitivity and obesity in human and animal models.[70] Although its mechanism of action is poorly understood, it is thought that DHEA improves glucose metabolism in the liver.[70]

Animal studies have also demonstrated that DHEA increases β-cells on the pancreas, which are responsible for producing insulin.[71]

In humans, DHEA levels are sensitive to elevated glucose; thus, higher glucose levels tend to be associated with decreased DHEA levels.[72] One proposed mechanism of action in humans is linked to DHEA's metabolism into testosterone. DHEA is an adrenal hormone that can be converted into either testosterone or estrogen. Studies have shown that testosterone improves insulin sensitivity in men, suggesting that DHEA's conversion into testosterone may be responsible for its beneficial effects in improving insulin sensitivity.[73]

## Essential Fatty Acids

In human experiments, omega-3 fatty acids lowered blood pressure and triglyceride levels, thereby relieving many of the complications associated with diabetes. In animals, omega-3 fatty acids cause less weight gain than other fats do; they have also been shown to have a neutral effect on LDL, while raising HDL and lowering triglycerides.[74] There are two types of essential fatty acids:

**Omega-3.** Marine oil contains omega-3 fatty acids. The research on omega-3 fatty acids stems from studies of the Inuit (Eskimo) people, who seldom suffer from heart attacks even though their diets contain an enormous amount of fat from fish, seals, and whales, presumably because these are very high in omega-3 fatty acids. Omega-3 fatty acids found in marine oil lower blood triglyceride levels, contribute to "thinning" blood, and decrease inflammation.[75] These effects partially explain many of fish oil's benefits.

**Omega-6.** Diabetic neuropathy is a gradual degeneration of peripheral nerve tissue. There is some evidence that GLA, an omega-6 fatty acid, can be helpful if given long enough to work. In one double-blind, placebo-controlled study, 111 people with mild diabetic neuropathy received either 480 mg daily of GLA or placebo. After 12 months, the group taking GLA was doing significantly better than the placebo group in 13 out of 16 measures of nerve function, with patients whose diabetes was under control doing best.[76] There is also evidence that GLA is more effective for diabetic neuropathy when combined with lipoic acid.[40]

## Fiber

Eating a diet rich in high-fiber foods prevents and reduces the harm caused by chronically elevated blood glucose. One study reported the results of diabetic individuals consuming a diet supplying 25 g of soluble fiber and 25 g of insoluble fiber (about double the amount currently recommended by the American Diabetes Association). The fiber was derived from foodstuffs, with no emphasis placed on special or unusual fiber-fortified foods or fiber supplements. A high-fiber diet reduced blood glucose levels by an average 10%.[77]

Fiber is also valuable because it produces a feeling of satiety, reducing the desire to overeat. Because high-fiber foods are digested more slowly than other foods, hunger pangs are forestalled. For the most part, fibrous foods are healthful (nutrient dense and low fat).

Fiber should be added slowly, gradually replacing low-fiber foods, for the following reasons: (1) insulin and prescription drugs may have to be adjusted to accommodate lower blood glucose levels, and (2) without a gradual introduction of the new material, intestinal distress could occur, including bloating, flatulence, and cramps.

Some individuals prefer to bolster fiber volume by adding supplemental fiber in the form of pectin, gums, and mucilages to each meal. Calculate the amount of fiber gained from foodstuffs and supplement with enough to compensate for shortfalls. Monitor blood glucose levels closely to assess gains and adjust oral or injectable hypoglycemic agents.

**Propolmannan.** Specially processed, propolmannan is a polysaccharide fiber derived from a plant (*Amorphophallus konjac*) that grows only in the remote mountains of northern Japan.

Used throughout Asia as a source of bulk in the diet, it creates a viscous barrier that impedes carbohydrate digestion, suppressing postprandial (after-meal) blood sugar surges. Propolmannan also slows "gastric emptying"—the passage of food from the stomach into the small intestine—impeding carbohydrate overexposure in the digestive tract. Propolmannan's power to safely suppress postprandial glucose surges has generated compelling results. In a group of 72 diabetics given konjac foods, postprandial glucose levels fell by an average of 84.6%.[78]

In placebo-controlled human studies, those taking propolmannan before meals lost 5.5–7.92 *pounds* after 8 weeks *without* changing their diets. The placebo groups in these studies showed no significant weight loss. The propolmannan groups also showed reductions in blood lipid/glucose levels.[79,80]

## Flavonoids

Flavonoids are antioxidants that help reduce damage associated with diabetes. In animal studies, quercetin, a potent flavonoid, decreased levels of blood glucose and oxidants. Quercetin also normalized levels of the antioxidants superoxide dismutase, vitamin C, and vitamin E. Quercetin is more effective at lower doses and ameliorates the diabetes-induced changes in oxidative stress.[81]

## Magnesium

Diabetics are often deficient in magnesium, which is depleted by medications and the disease process.[82–84] One double-blind study suggested that magnesium supplementation enhanced blood sugar control.[85]

## N-Acetylcysteine (NAC)

NAC is a powerful antioxidant that is used to treat acetaminophen overdose. Among diabetic rats, it has also demonstrated the ability to protect the heart against endothelial damage and oxidative stress that is associated with heart attacks among diabetics. In one study, NAC was able to increase the availability of nitric oxide in diabetic rats, thus improving their blood pressure as well as reducing the level of oxidative stress in their hearts.[86] In a human study examining the effects of broad-based antioxidants, NAC, in addition to vitamins C and E, was able to reduce oxidative stress after a moderate-fat meal.[87]

## Silymarin

In animal studies, silymarin was shown to improve insulin levels among induced cases of diabetes.[88] A small, controlled clinical study evaluated type 2 diabetics with alcohol-induced liver failure.[89] Those receiving 600 mg silymarin daily experienced a significant reduction in fasting blood and urine glucose levels. Fasting glucose levels rose slightly during the first month of supplementation but declined thereafter from an average of 190 mg/dL to 174 mg/dL. As daily glucose levels dropped (from an average of 202–172 mg/dL), HbA1c also substantially decreased. Throughout the course of treatment, fasting insulin levels declined by almost one-half, and daily insulin requirements decreased by about 24%. Liver function improved. A lack of hypoglycemic episodes suggests silymarin lowered as well as stabilized blood glucose levels.

## Vitamin B3

Vitamin B3 (niacin) is required for the proper function of more than 50 enzymes. Without it, the body is not able to release energy or make fats from carbohydrates. Vitamin B3 is also used to make sex hormones and other important chemical signal molecules.

In the past, the use of niacin was discouraged in diabetic individuals because it was found to increase insulin resistance and degrade glycemic control, particularly at high doses.[90] However, emerging clinical evidence shows that niacin is both safe and effective for diabetics.[91]

There is evidence that niacin reduces the risk of developing type 1 diabetes.[92,93] Niacinamide helps restore β-cells, or at least slow their destruction. Because niacin can disrupt blood sugar control in diabetics, individuals taking any form of niacin, including inositol hexaniacinate, must closely monitor blood sugar levels and discontinue treatment in the event of worsening of diabetic control. Inositol hexaniacinate has long been used in Europe to lower cholesterol levels and improve blood flow in individuals with intermittent claudication.

## Vitamin C

Several preclinical studies evaluated vitamin C's role during mild oxidative stress. The aqueous humor of the eye provides surrounding tissues with a source of vitamin C. Since animal studies have shown that glucose inhibits vitamin C uptake, this protective mechanism may be impaired in diabetes.[94] Supplementation with antioxidant vitamins C and E plays an important role in improving eye health.[95] High vitamin-C intake depresses glycation, which has important implications for slowing diabetes progression and aging.[96]

Vitamin C, through its relationship to sorbitol, also helps prevent ocular complications in diabetes. Sorbitol, a sugar-like substance that tends to accumulate in the cells of people with diabetes, tends to reduce the antioxidant capacity of the eye, with a number of possible complications. Vitamin C appears to help reduce sorbitol buildup.[97]

Vitamin C also has a role in reducing the risk of other diabetic complications. In one clinical study, vitamin C significantly increased blood flow and decreased inflammation in patients with both diabetes and coronary artery disease.[98] Three studies suggest that vitamin C, along with a combination of vitamins and minerals,[99] reduces blood pressure in people with diabetes.[100] and increases blood vessel elasticity and blood flow[101]

## Vitamin E

Vitamin E has been shown to significantly reduce the risk of developing type 2 diabetes.[102] One double-blind trial found a reduction in the risk of cardiac autonomic neuropathy, or damage to the nerves that supply the heart, which is a complication of diabetes.[103] Additional evidence documented benefits for diabetic peripheral neuropathy,[104] blood sugar control,[105–108] and cataract prevention.[106–109] In addition, vitamin E enhances sensitivity to insulin in type 2 diabetics.[106,107]

# BOTANICAL SUPPLEMENTS FOR DIABETES

Before insulin, botanical medicines were used to treat diabetes. They are remarkably safe and effective. However, because many botanical medicines function similarly to insulin, people taking oral diabetes medications or insulin should use caution to avoid hypoglycemia. Botanical medicines should be integrated into a regimen of adequate exercise, healthy eating, nutritional supplements, and medical support.

## Cinnamon

Cinnamon has been used for several thousand years in traditional Ayurvedic and Greco-European medical systems. Native to tropical southern India and Sri Lanka, the bark of this evergreen tree is used to manage conditions such as nausea, bloating, flatulence, and anorexia. It is also one of the world's most common spices, used to flavor everything from oatmeal and apple cider to cappuccino. Recent research has revealed that regular use of cinnamon can also promote healthy glucose metabolism.

A study at the U.S. Department of Agriculture's Beltsville Human Nutrition Research Center isolated insulin-enhancing complexes in cinnamon that are involved in preventing or alleviating glucose intolerance and diabetes.[19] Three water-soluble polyphenol polymers were found to have beneficial biological activity, increasing insulin-dependent glucose metabolism by roughly 20-fold in vitro.[19] The nutrients displayed significant antioxidant activity as well, as did other phytochemicals found in cinnamon, such as epicatechin, phenol, and tannin. Moreover, scientists determined that these polyphenol polymers are able to upregulate the expression of genes involved in activating the cell membrane's insulin receptors, thus increasing glucose uptake and lowering blood glucose levels.[110]

The problem with long-term cinnamon use is the presence of highly reactive aldehyde compounds.

These toxic fat-soluble compounds accumulate in the body over time. An aqueous extract of cinnamon has been identified and through a patented process, delivers cinnamon's beneficial water-soluble nutrients while *removing* deleterious fat-soluble toxins.

In a recent double-blind, placebo-controlled trial,[111] a group of individuals (average age 61) with high blood sugar taking 500 mg daily of this form of cinnamon extract experienced an average decline of 12 mg/dL in fasting blood glucose after just 2 months. It *also* produced a significant decrease in postprandial glucose spikes (by an average of 32 mg/dL) after ingesting 75 g of carbohydrates. These findings support previous clinical data on similar aqueous cinnamon extracts, in which diabetic patients saw their fasting glucose drop an average of 10.3% after 4 months.[112]

## Brown Seaweed and Bladderwrack

Another approach in managing glucose levels is to blunt the conversion of starches into their component sugars in the gastrointestinal tract. This can be accomplished safely and effectively by introducing natural enzyme inhibitors that halt carbohydrate metabolism in the gut. The most attractive targets are the sugar-producing alpha-amylase and alpha-glucosidase enzymes.

Extracts from a variety of seaweeds have inhibitory effects on these enzymes.[113–116] Animal studies have revealed that inhibiting these enzymes lowers blood sugar levels.[117,118] In a recent double-blind, placebo-controlled clinical trial, a single dose of 500 mg daily of bladderwrack and seaweed significantly increased insulin sensitivity while inducing a 48.3% decline in postprandial glucose levels in healthy individuals.[119]

## Irvingia Gabonensis

Published studies show that extract of the African mango *Irvingia gabonensis* inhibits *alpha-amylase*–mediated conversion of carbohydrates into sugar.[120]

In 2006, researchers studied the effect of Irvingia in rats who were artificially induced to develop diabetes. A single oral dose of Irvingia lowered plasma glucose 2 hours after treatment.[121]

In 1990, researchers studied the effects of Irvingia on eleven human type 2 diabetics. Compared to baseline, there were significant reductions in blood triglyceride levels (16%), total cholesterol (30%), LDL (39%), and glucose (38%), while HDL-cholesterol levels were increased by 29% after 4 weeks of supplementation. These desirable biochemical effects were accompanied by improved clinical states.[122]

Adiponectin is a hormone that plays a critical role in metabolic abnormalities associated with type 2 diabetes, obesity, and atherosclerosis.[123–133] Higher levels of adiponectin enhance insulin sensitivity; enhancing insulin sensitivity as we age is important to long-term metabolic health. Adipogenic transcriptional factors involved with adiponectin are also involved in the formation of new adipocytes, fat burning, and endothelial function.[134-136] Irvingia increases beneficial adiponectin levels and inhibits adipocyte differentiation mediated through the suppression of adipogenic transcription factors.[136]

## White Kidney Bean

Extracts from the common white kidney bean, *Phaseolus vulgaris*, are powerful blockers of the enzyme alpha-amylase.[137,138] White bean extract shows enormous potential for preventing the blood sugar and insulin spikes associated with many chronic health disorders.[139]

Amylase inhibition with white bean extract has proven particularly effective in reducing glycemia (sugar load in the blood) in studies on diabetic animals. Supplementation in diabetic rats not only substantially lowered mean blood sugar levels, but it also reduced the animals' total food and water intake (water intake is increased in untreated diabetes because of the amount lost in sugar-laden urine).[140]

White bean extract has yielded equally compelling results in human studies. It has been shown to diminish the effects of high-glycemic index foods (like white bread) that are notorious for producing sharp, potentially dangerous postprandial blood sugar spikes, helping to alleviate metabolic burden throughout the body.[141]

In one notable study, postprandial blood sugar levels were measured in a group of healthy subjects after consuming 50 g of carbohydrate in the form of wheat, rice, and other high-carbohydrate plant foods.[142] Phaseolus vulgaris inhibited the average postingestion spike in blood sugar by 67%.

## Green Coffee Extract

Coffee contains some well-studied phytochemicals such as chlorogenic acid, caffeic acid, ferulic acid, and quinic acid.[143] Some of coffee's most impressive effects can be seen in blood glucose management. Chlorogenic acid and caffeic acid are the two primary nutrients in coffee that benefit individuals with high blood sugar. Glucose-6-phosphatase is an enzyme crucial to the regulation of blood sugar. Since glucose generation from glycogen stored in the liver is often overactive in people with high blood sugar,[144] reducing the activity of the glucose-6-phosphatase enzyme leads to reduced blood sugar levels, with consequent clinical improvements.

Chlorogenic acid has been shown to inhibit the glucose-6-phosphatase enzyme in a dose-dependent manner, resulting in reduced glucose production.[145] In a trial at the Moscow Modern Medical Center, 75 healthy volunteers were given either 90 mg chlorogenic acid daily or a placebo. Blood glucose levels of the chlorogenic acid group were 15–20% lower than those of the placebo group.[146] Chlorogenic acid also has an antagonistic effect on glucose transport, decreasing the intestinal absorption rate of glucose,[147] which may help reduce blood insulin levels and minimize fat storage.

In another trial, researchers gave different dosages of green coffee bean extract, standardized for chlorogenic acid, to 56 people. Thirty-five minutes later, they gave the participants 100 g of glucose in an oral glucose challenge test. Blood sugar levels dropped by an increasingly greater amount as the test dosage of green coffee bean extract was raised (from 200 mg to 400 mg). At the 400-mg dose, there was a full 24% decrease in blood sugar—just 30 minutes after glucose ingestion.[148]

Green coffee bean extract found in unroasted coffee beans, once purified and standardized, produces high levels of chlorogenic acid and other beneficial polyphenols that can suppress excess blood glucose levels. Roasting destroys much of the coffee bean's beneficial content.

## Garlic

Allium is the active component in garlic and onions. Allium compounds are sulfur-donating compounds that help reconstitute glutathione, a major internal antioxidant. This mechanism is probably responsible for allium's positive effects. Allium has a number of positive effects that may help reduce the risk of diabetic complications, including the following:

- Reducing the risk of cardiovascular disease, including atherosclerosis[149-152]
- Decreasing oxidative stress[153]
- Promoting weight loss and insulin sensitivity in animal models of diabetes[154]
- Lowering blood pressure[155-158]
- Improving cholesterol profile[157,159-169]

## Green Tea

The compounds in these plants, including epicatechin, catechin, gallocatechin, and epigallocatechin, are powerful antioxidants, particularly against pancreas and liver toxins[170] Animal studies have shown that epigallocatechins, in particular, may have a role in preventing diabetes.[171] In studies with rats, epigallocatechins prevented cytokine-induced β-cell destruction by downregulating inducible nitric oxide synthase, which is a pro-oxidant.[172,173] This process could help slow the progression of type 1 diabetes. In vitro studies have also shown that green tea suppresses diet-induced obesity,[174] a key risk factor in developing diabetes and metabolic syndrome.[175]

## Vitamin D

Vitamin D has far-reaching implications that extend beyond promoting bone health. Over the past 40 years, research has shed light on the intersecting pathways of vitamin D and many other aspects of health.

Evidence from animal experiments and human observational studies suggests that vitamin D may help prevent type 1 diabetes, perhaps by acting as an immune system modulator.[176] Researchers demonstrated that the pancreatic β-cells of mice contain receptors for 1,25-dihydroxyvitamin D. When they administered this active form of vitamin D to mice early in life, the animals demonstrated a reduced incidence of type 1 diabetes. However, diabetes incidence was not affected when 1,25-dihydroxyvitamin D was administered to mice later in life. Vitamin D appears to limit the expression of certain cytokines, which may prevent the autoimmune attack on pancreatic cells that can lead to diabetes.[177]

Human studies likewise suggest that vitamin D may have a protective effect against type 1 diabetes. In a large-scale investigation, more than 12 000 pregnant women in Finland enrolled in a trial studying the relationship between vitamin D intake and type 1 diabetes in infants. After 1 year, children who supplemented with the suggested study dose of vitamin D[178] (2000 IU daily) had a much lower risk of type 1 diabetes than children who did not supplement.[179]

Vitamin D supplementation may reduce susceptibility to type 2 diabetes by slowing the loss of insulin sensitivity in people who show early signs of the disease. Researchers studied 314 adults without diabetes and gave them either 700 IU of vitamin D and 500 mg of calcium daily or a placebo for 3 years.[180] Among subjects who had impaired (slightly elevated) fasting glucose levels at the study's onset, those taking the active supplement had a smaller rise in glucose levels over 3 years than did the controls, as well as a smaller increase in insulin resistance. The researchers concluded that for older adults with impaired glucose levels, supplementing with vitamin D and calcium may help avert metabolic syndrome and type 2 diabetes.

## Ginkgo Biloba

Animal studies demonstrate that ginkgo improves glucose metabolism in muscle fibers and prevents atrophy.[181] Animal studies also show that ginkgo biloba extracts significantly inhibit postmeal sugar levels and act as antihyperglycemic agents.[182]

Ginkgo biloba extract has been shown to prevent diabetic retinopathy in diabetic rats, suggesting a protective effect in human diabetics.[183] In a preliminary clinical trial,[184] type 2 diabetics were given ginkgo extract orally for 3 months, which significantly reduced free radical levels, decreased fibrinogen levels, and improved blood viscosity. Ginkgo extracts also improved retinal capillary blood flow rate in type 2 diabetic patients with retinopathy.

Ginkgo has also been observed to lower blood glucose levels. It was studied in type 2 diabetics at a dose of 120 mg for 3 months. Ginkgo supplementation produced an increase in liver metabolism of insulin and oral hypoglycemic medications, which corresponded to a reduction in plasma glucose levels.[185] Type 2 diabetics with pancreatic exhaustion received the most benefit. Ginkgo does not appear to increase beta cell production; rather it enhances liver uptake of existing insulin, thereby reducing high insulin levels.

## Blueberries

Native to North America, blueberries have long been used in food preparation and for therapeutic purposes.[186] Many of the health benefits attributed to blueberries have been linked to their potent antioxidant properties. Scientists attribute these powerful antioxidant properties to polyphenols in blueberries known as anthocyanins.

In published studies, blueberries block carbohydrate metabolism in the intestine by up to 90% compared with the prescription drug acarbose.[187,188]

Additionally, blueberries have been shown to lower baseline blood sugar levels in those diagnosed with type 2 diabetes by 37%.[189–191]

In a double-blind, placebo-controlled study, 32 obese, insulin-resistant (prediabetic) adult men and women drank smoothies made with freeze-dried blueberry powder for 6 weeks. A placebo control group consumed smoothies without blueberry extracts.[192] Fasting blood samples were obtained with a clamp technique considered state of the art for precise determination of insulin sensitivity. With no changes in body weight or composition compared to controls, the blueberry group showed a statistically significant and much greater improvement in insulin sensitivity (22.2% plus or minus 5.8%) versus the placebo arm (4.9% plus or minus 4.5%).

## Vaccinium Myrtillus (Bilberry)

Studies of diabetic rats show that bilberry decreases vascular permeability.[193] Studies of diabetic mice receiving an herbal extract containing bilberry demonstrated significantly decreased blood glucose levels.[194,195]

A double-blind, placebo-controlled trial of bilberry extract in 14 people with diabetic retinopathy or hypertensive retinopathy (damage to the retina caused by diabetes or hypertension, respectively) found significant improvements in the treated group.[196] Other open clinical trials in humans also showed benefits. A preliminary study of 31 people with retinopathy documented that bilberry reduced vascular permeability and reduced hemorrhage.[197]

## Life Extension Suggestions

Under no circumstances should people suddenly stop taking diabetic drugs, especially insulin. A type 1 diabetic will never be able to stop taking insulin. However, it is possible to improve glucose metabolism, control, and tolerance with the following supplements:

- **R-lipoic acid:** 240–480 mg daily
- **L-carnitine:** 500–1000 mg twice daily
- **Carnosine:** 500 mg twice daily
- **Chromium** (Crominex™): 500 mcg daily
- **CoQ10,** in the form of ubiquinol: 100–300 mg daily
- **DHEA:** 15–75 mg early in the day, followed by blood testing after 3–6 weeks to ensure optimal levels
- **EPA/DHA:** 1400 mg EPA and 1000 mg DHA daily
- **Fiber** (guar, pectin, propolmannan, or oat bran): 20–30 g daily at least, up to 50 g daily
- **Propolmannan:** 2 g twice daily
- **GLA:** 900–1800 mg daily
- **Quercetin:** 500 mg daily
- **Magnesium:** 140 mg daily as magnesium L-threonate; 320 mg daily as magnesium citrate
- **N-acetylcysteine (NAC):** 500–1000 mg daily

- **Silymarin:** containing 750 mg *Silybum marianum*, standardized to 80% silymarin, 30% silibinin, and 8% isosilybin A and isosilybin B
- **Vitamin C:** at least 2000 mg daily
- **Vitamin E:** 400 IU daily (with 200 mg gamma tocopherol)
- **Garlic:** 1200 mg daily
- **Green tea extract:** 725 mg green tea extract (minimum 93% polyphenols)
- **Ginkgo biloba:** 120 mg daily
- **Bilberry extract:** 100 mg daily
- **B complex:** containing the entire B family, including biotin and niacin
- **Cinnamon extract:** 175 mg (*Cinnamomum cassia*) standardized to 2.5% (4.375 mg) A-type polymers 3 times daily
- **Green coffee bean extract:** 200–400 mg (standardized to contain chlorogenic acid) 3 times daily
- **Vitamin D:** 5000–10 000 IU daily
- **Brown seaweed and bladderwrack:** 100 mg 3 times daily
- *Irvingia gabonensis:* 150 mg twice daily
- **White kidney bean:** 445 mg twice daily
- **Blueberry:** standardized to contain 50 mg 3,4–caffeoylquinic (chlorogenic) acid, and 50 mg myricetin) or 22.5 g blueberry bioactive freeze-dried powder

In addition, the following blood testing resources may be helpful:

- Fasting glucose
- Postprandial glucose test
- HbA1C
- Fasting insulin
- 25-Hydroxy, Vitamin D
- CoQ10
- Omega Score®

## REFERENCES

References available at: www.lef.org/dpt5/ch51

# 52

---

# *Digestive Disorders*

---

It is estimated that some form of digestive disorder affects more than 100 million people in the United States. For some people, digestive disorders are a source of irritation and discomfort that may cause them to drastically limit their lifestyles and frequently miss work. For others, the disorders may be extremely crippling and even fatal.

## THE GASTROINTESTINAL TRACT

The gastrointestinal (GI) tract is a long muscular tube that functions as the food processor for the human body. The digestive system includes the following organs: mouth and salivary glands, stomach, small and large intestines, colon, liver, pancreas, and gallbladder.

Irritations or inflammation of the various sections of the GI tract are identified as gastritis (stomach), colitis (colon), ileitis (ileum or small intestines), hepatitis (liver), and cholecystitis (gallbladder).

The GI tract is not a passive system. Rather, it has the capability to sense and react to materials passed through it. For a healthy digestive system, every person requires different food selections that match their GI tract capacity.

## THE DIGESTIVE PROCESS

The GI tract breaks down foods by first using mechanical means (eg, chewing) and then via the application of a host of complex chemical processes (from saliva to colon microbes). Since the GI tract is the point of entry for the human body, everything eaten has an impact on the body. The food eaten and passed through the GI tract contains nutrients as well as toxins. Toxins can include, but are not limited to, food additives, pesticides, and specific foods that induce a reaction from the GI tract.

The process of digestion is accomplished via the surface of the GI tract using secretions from accessory glands. The two glands providing the majority of digestive chemicals utilized by the GI tract are the liver and the pancreas. The function of the liver is to control the food supply for the rest of the body by further processing the food molecules absorbed through the intestines. The liver does this by dispensing those food molecules in a controlled manner and filtering out toxins that may have passed through the GI tract wall.

Another very important function of the GI tract is as a sensory organ. By rejecting foods through objectionable taste, vomiting, diarrhea, or any combination of these symptoms, the sensing capacity of the GI tract can protect the body. The surface of the GI tract has a complex system of nerves and other cells of the immune system. The surface of the GI tract, or mucosa, is part of a complex sensing system called the mucosa-associated lymphatic tissue (MALT). The immune sensors in the MALT trigger responses such as nausea, vomiting, pain, and swelling. Vomiting and diarrhea are abrupt defensive responses by MALT when it senses foods with a strong allergic or toxic component. This kind of food intolerance is responsible for many digestive problems. The GI tract is "hard-wired" to the brain via hormonal, neurotransmitter-mediator chemical communication.

The GI tract is a muscular tube that contracts in a controlled rhythm to move food through the different sections (peristalsis). Strength and timing variations in contractions can cause cramping (very strong contractions) and diarrhea (very frequent contractions). When the contractions are slow and irregular, constipation may occur. Motility disorder is the general term used to describe problems with peristalsis.

Food allergy is sometimes the primary cause of GI tract problems. Chronic diseases can have their origin in food allergies. The dysfunction, discomfort, and disease associated with the GI tract can be the result of local immune responses to food selections or combinations of foods. Food selections are a result of personal tastes, social fads, ethnic culture, religion, and, to a larger degree, local or seasonal availability. Food selections made in modern affluent society are based on a developed taste for a rich diet centered on meats and dairy products loaded with fats, high concentrations of proteins, and fat-soluble toxins. Advertising and misinformation about healthy diets have overshadowed human nutritional needs.

Chewing, swallowing, and peristalsis comprise mechanical digestion, in which food is broken down into tiny particles, mixed with digestive juices, and moved through the digestive tract. Digestive enzymes break down large food molecules into small molecules that can be absorbed into the blood or lymph in the process of chemical digestion.[1]

Human evolutionary history clearly shows that we are primarily herbivores. Human saliva contains alpha-amylase, an enzyme specifically designed to break down complex carbohydrates into sugar compounds. Our teeth are designed to cut vegetable matter and grind grains.

The so-called canine teeth of humans bear no resemblance to the canines of even a domestic house cat. The human digestive system is long, and the food is processed slowly to extract all the nutrients from plant material. Conversely, carnivores have short digestive tracts that digest flesh very quickly. The digestive systems of carnivores are able to eliminate the large amount of cholesterol consumed in their diets, and carnivores do not have alpha-amylase present in their saliva.

## Dietary Shifts and Digestive Disorders

The effect of the shift in our diets during the past 100 years has resulted in 44% of Americans and Canadians being afflicted with heartburn, 5% of the population suffering from peptic ulcer disease, and 20–40% of Americans plagued with nonulcer dyspepsia. Over-the-counter medications for these ailments are a multibillion-dollar industry. Nearly every hour, there is at least one television commercial selling an antacid or similar product.

# GI SYMPTOMS

There are five basic symptoms indicating a GI tract problem. These symptoms are generally associated with dietary problems or specific food allergies. It is critical that anyone suffering from serious GI tract problems work closely with a physician to test for more developed and serious GI tract diseases. The physician should also be experienced in working with dietary factors and food allergies.

## Nausea and Vomiting

Nausea and vomiting can vary from an unsettled feeling in the stomach to the violent action of immediate vomiting. Patients with nausea and vomiting symptoms should assume the ingestion of a reactive food (ie, food containing toxins) or poisoning with a pathogen such as *Salmonella*. Vomiting immediately after eating is usually proceeded by excessive watery salivation. Some chronic low-intensity nausea can occur for a protracted time due to sustained low-level food allergies or problems with food combinations. Patients with low-level nausea usually see their symptoms disappear with dietary change(s). Nausea and vomiting are also linked with migraines caused by food allergies (see the Migraine Headache protocol).

## Bloating

Bloating can result from excessive gas in the digestive system, failure of the digestive tract to sustain youthful peristaltic contractions, or a lack of sufficient quantities of digestive enzymes and bile acids to rapidly break down food. Intestinal gas results from food fermentation and swallowing air while eating. The bloating from intestinal gas is different from that which occurs in the colon.

## Constipation

Constipation is the decreased frequency or slowing of peristalsis, resulting in harder stools. When the GI tract is slowed down, feces can accumulate in the colon with attending pain and toxic reactions. A spastic colon results when the colon contracts out of rhythm in painful spasms blocking movement of the stool. Some patients experience painful days of constipation followed by forceful diarrhea and watery stool, often accompanied by abdominal cramps.

## Diarrhea

Diarrhea is the increased frequency of bowel movements, which are also loose or watery. If diarrhea increases, the possibility of celiac disease is considered. Celiac disease is a serious disease that allows certain macromolecules to pass through the intestinal wall. If blood appears in the stool, ulcerative colitis is likely. Protracted bouts of diarrhea can result in nutritional deficiencies due to poor absorption of essential nutrients.

## Abdominal Pain

Abdominal pain appears in different patterns and with varying intensities. Cramping occurs because of muscle spasms in abdominal organs. Severe cramping pain, often called colic, usually occurs from problems with strong allergic response to food. Abdominal cramping near the navel is typically from the small intestine, and near the sides, top, and bottom of the lower abdomen, the pain is associated with the colon.

Diseases associated with central GI tract disorders include depression, migraine, asthma, sinusitis, and fibromyalgia. These diseases have been diagnosed with specific patterns of food allergy response. All of these diseases also have links to irritable bowel syndrome (IBS) (see the Irritable Bowel Syndrome [IBS] protocol for more information).

# STEPS TO A HEALTHIER DIGESTIVE SYSTEM

## Elimination Diets

Elimination diets are a good method of determining what foods cause an allergic reaction in the GI tract lining. Planning and following such diets are a safe starting point for anyone desiring to track their GI tract response to food. Interview physicians to learn who may be most qualified to assist in planning an elimination diet. A very good indicator of a healthy GI tract is regular transit time for complete food digestion. Patients who are regular are usually in optimum GI health.

## Digestive Enzymes

Aging causes many people to experience problems with digestion. It is estimated that after age 40 there is an approximate decrease of 20–30% in the body's ability to produce enzymes. The use of specific enzymes can help improve the efficiency of digestion. Enzymes can be used to enhance the proper breakdown of foods in order to more properly digest, absorb, and utilize nutrients.

Enzymes are essential to the body's absorption and utilization of food. The capacity of the living organism to make enzymes diminishes with age, and some scientists believe that humans could live longer and be healthier by guarding against the loss of our precious enzymes.

Enzymes are responsible for every activity of life. Even thinking requires enzyme activity. The two primary classes of enzymes responsible for maintaining life functions are digestive and metabolic. The primary digestive enzymes are proteases (to digest proteins), amylases (to digest carbohydrates), and lipases (to digest fats). These enzymes function as a biological catalyst to help break down food. Raw foods also provide enzymes that naturally break down food for proper absorption. Metabolic enzymes are responsible for the structuring, repairing, and remodeling of every cell, and the body is under a great daily burden to supply sufficient enzymes for optimal health. Metabolic enzymes operate in every cell, every organ, and every tissue, and they need constant replenishment.

Digestion of food takes high priority and has a high demand for enzymes. When we eat, enzymatic activity begins in the mouth, where salivary amylase, lingual lipase, and ptyalin initiate starch and fat digestion. In the stomach, hydrochloric acid activates pepsinogen to pepsin, which breaks down protein, and gastric lipase begins the hydrolysis of fats. Without proper enzyme production, the body has a difficult time digesting food, often resulting in a variety of chronic disorders.

Poor eating habits (eg, inadequate chewing and eating on the run) may result in inadequate enzyme production and, hence, malabsorption of food (which is exacerbated by aging because this is a time of decreased hydrochloric acid production) as well as a general decline in digestive enzyme secretion.

Saliva is rich in amylase, while gastric juice contains protease. The pancreas secretes digestive juices containing high concentrations of amylase and protease, as

well as a smaller concentration of lipase. It also secretes a small concentration of maltase, which reduces maltose to dextrose. Animals eating raw food often have no enzymes at all in saliva, unlike humans. However, dogs fed a high carbohydrate, heat-treated diet have been found to develop enzymes in their saliva within a week in response to enzyme-depleting foods.

One of America's pioneering biochemists and nutrition researchers, Edward Howell,[2] cites numerous animal studies showing that animals fed diets deficient in enzymes have an enlarged pancreas, as huge amounts of pancreatic enzymes are squandered in digesting foods devoid of natural enzymes. The result of this wasteful outpouring of pancreatic digestive enzymes is a decrease in the supply of crucial metabolic enzymes and impaired health.

How significant is an enzyme deficiency to overall health? For starters, organs that are overworked will enlarge in order to perform the increased workload. Those with congestive heart failure or aortic valvular disease often suffer from an enlarged heart. When the pancreas enlarges in order to produce more digestive enzymes, there results a deficiency in the production of life-sustaining metabolic enzymes, as available enzyme-producing capacity is used in digesting food instead of supporting cellular enzymatic functions. The tremendous impact that wasting pancreatic enzymes can have on health, and even life itself, has been established in animal studies. The critical question is how this applies to human health.

For much of the 20th century, European oncologists have included enzyme therapy as a natural, nontoxic therapy against cancer, and almost all leading alternative cancer specialists treating Americans prescribe both food enzymes and concentrated enzyme supplements as primary or adjuvant cancer therapies. A New York City cancer specialist, Nicholas Gonzalez, uses very high doses of supplemental pancreatic enzymes as a primary antitumor therapy. His clinical successes have led conventional drug companies to seek to duplicate these natural therapies and offer them as adjuvant drug therapies. If pancreatic enzymes are effective in treating existing cancers, one might assume that maintaining a large pool of these enzymes in the body should help prevent cancer from developing. Studies have shown that people who eat fresh fruits and vegetables (with high levels of natural enzymes) have significantly reduced levels of cancer and other diseases. It has not been proven that the high enzyme content of these foods is partially responsible for their anticancer effect, but the evidence is compelling.

The pancreas and liver are digestive organs that produce most of the body's digestive enzymes. The remainder should come from uncooked foods, such as fresh fruits and vegetables, raw sprouted grains, seeds and nuts, unpasteurized dairy products, and enzyme supplements.

Food in its natural, unprocessed state is vital to the maintenance of good health. The lack of it in the modern diet is thought to be responsible for degenerative diseases. Cooking food, particularly for long periods of time and at more than 118°F, destroys enzymes in food and leaves what is often consumed in today's enzyme-less diet. This is one reason why, by middle age, we may become metabolically depleted of enzymes. Our glands and major organs suffer most from this deficiency. The brain may shrink as a result of an overcooked, overly refined diet that is devoid of enzymes desperately needed by the body. In an effort to meet the deficiency, the pancreas may swell. Laboratory mice fed heat-processed, enzyme-less foods develop a pancreas 2–3 times heavier than that of wild mice eating an enzyme-containing natural diet of raw food.

When uncooked food is consumed, fewer digestive enzymes are required to perform the digestive function. The body will adapt to the plentiful, external supply by secreting fewer of its own enzymes, preserving them to assist in vital cellular metabolic functions. One of the worst cooking methods is frying, since frying results in much higher temperatures than boiling. Frying damages protein and destroys enzymes.

Enzymes can also be wasted by lifestyle factors. Enzymes work harder with increasing temperatures and are used up faster. A fever, for example, induces faster enzyme action and is therefore unfavorable for bacterial activity. Enzymes can be found in urine after a fever and also may be found after strenuous athletic activity.

A natural behavior of animals is to harness the power of enzymes in food by burying or covering their food, allowing enzyme activity to start predigesting the food. By this natural behavior, animals instinctively preserve their own enzyme supply. Similarly, people of some native cultures also preserve their enzyme supply and prevent disease through efficient use of enzymes. Whales have up to 6 inches of fat to keep them warm, but their arteries are not clogged. Eskimos, who frequently consume large quantities of fat, are often not obese. Both of these groups eat the fat-digesting enzyme lipase in the form of raw foods.

Studies (both in vitro and controlled in vivo) using internal and parenteral routes have examined the effectiveness of many different types and sources of plant enzymes in several conditions, including poor digestion, poor absorption, pancreatic insufficiency, steatorrhea, lactose intolerance, celiac disease, obstruction of arteries, and thrombotic disease.

Enzymes from the *Aspergillus oryzae* fungus were subjected to numerous studies, evaluating their role in supporting healthy digestion. Additionally, human studies suggest the proteolytic enzymes derived from *A. oryzae* fungus may play a role in anti-inflammatory and fibrinolytic therapies. The enzymes appear to be relatively stable in heat, and they are also active throughout a wide pH range. This is important because most enzymes are deactivated in stomach acid. These enzymes are synthesized from fungus but contain no fungal residue even though that is their derivation. Modern filtration techniques and technology enable these fungal enzymes to be well-suited for human consumption.

According to Mark Percival,[3] the oral supplementation of digestive enzymes taken just before or at mealtime can assist digestion. Even though most supplemental enzymes are labile and will deactivate when exposed to stomach acid, Percival believes some of the enzymes will remain active if they are taken with or just before a meal. Percival says, "The enzymes are physically protected" by the meal and allow some enzymatic activity to occur in the stomach. The enzymes that get through to the small intestine may help with digestion there as well. pH plays a major role in enzymatic activity, therefore, the enzymes derived from *Aspergillus* "may be highly useful as they appear to be remarkably stable, even when subjected to an acidic environment." Edward Howell[2] adds that because enzyme activity has been shown to begin even before the food is swallowed, he chews an enzyme capsule with his food in order to immediately start the digestive process.

As early as 1947, Arnold Renshaw (Manchester, England) had obtained good results with enzyme treatment of more than 700 patients with rheumatoid arthritis, osteoarthritis, or fibrositis, noting that "some intractable cases of ankylosing spondylitis and Still's disease have also responded to this therapy." He reported that of 556 people with various types of arthritis, 283 were much improved and 219 were improved to a less marked extent. Of 292 people who had rheumatoid arthritis, 264 of them showed several degrees of improvement. More time was required before improvement was seen when the duration of the disease had been long term, although most people started to show some improvement after only 2–3 months of enzyme therapy. In spite of these favorable findings, digestive enzyme therapy has been reserved for diseases that directly result in a pathologic deficiency of pancreas-derived digestive enzymes.

According to Schneider,[4] common digestive disorders may benefit from enzyme replacement. Oral intake of exocrine pancreatic enzymes is of key importance in the treatment of maldigestion in chronic pancreatitis with pancreatic insufficiency. Schneider studied the therapeutic effectiveness of a conventional and an acid-protected enzyme preparation and an acid-stable fungal enzyme preparation in the treatment of severe pancreatogenic steatorrhea. The results showed that a supplemental enzyme preparation is best for patients with chronic pancreatitis and those who underwent a Whipple procedure (a surgical procedure performed on pancreatic cancer patients), while patients with an intact upper GI tract do best with an acid-protected porcine pancreatic enzyme preparation.

Rachman[5] reported that 58% of the population has some type of digestive disorder and a lack of optimal digestive function associated with enzyme inadequacy may lead to malabsorption and other related conditions. In the elderly, the problem is often exacerbated because the elderly may have suboptimal production of gastric hydrochloric acid. "This can be a significant factor that can impact nutrient absorption along with the creation of maldigestive-type symptoms. Bacterial production of hydrogen and methane are determined after a carbohydrate challenge. Excessive levels of these gases reflect overgrowth of bacteria in the upper gut." Rachman suggests there may be improvement with enzyme replacement. He also adds that enzymes taken orally at meals may improve the digestion of dietary protein, thereby decreasing the quantity of antigenic macromolecules that leak across the intestinal wall into the bloodstream. Such leaking may trigger the body's defenses against what it perceives to be foreign protein or polypeptide invaders, producing the symptoms of allergies.

Howell[2] agrees that allergies can respond to adding enzymes to the diet. He says excessive cholesterol levels can respond to dietary enzymes as well. Howell quoted a 1962 study by three British doctors (C.W. Adams, O.B. Bayliss, and M.Z. Ibrahim), who set out to discover why cholesterol clogs arteries, ultimately manifesting in heart disease. They found that all enzymes studied became progressively weaker in the arteries as people aged and the hardening became more severe. They suggested a shortage of enzymes is part of the mechanism that allows cholesterol deposits to accumulate in the inner part of arterial walls. As early as 1958, researcher L.O. Pilgeram conducted blood tests at Stanford University and demonstrated a progressive decline of lipase in the blood of atherosclerotic patients in advancing middle and old age.

About the same time, researchers at Michael Reese Hospital in Chicago found that enzymes in the saliva, pancreas, and blood became weaker with advancing age and speculated that fat may be absorbed in the unhydrolyzed state in atherosclerosis. They also found definite improvement in the character of fat utilization following the use of enzymes.

Intravenous (IV) administration of brinase, a proteolytic enzyme prepared from A. oryzae, was found by FitzGerald[6] to be beneficial in treating chronic arterial obstruction. Patients were observed for 3 months before being given six IV infusions of either saline or brinase for more than 2 weeks. No changes were observed during the observation period. After infusion, resumed blood flow was found in 17 of 27 obstructed arterial segments. The number of patent segments increased from 11 to 27. No improvements were observed in the patients who were treated with placebos.

Pancreatin is secreted from the pancreas. It provides potent concentrations of the digestive enzymes protease, amylase, and lipase. It is sold as a drug to treat those with pancreatic insufficiency. Pancreatin efficacy was demonstrated in a study conducted on patients taking pancreatin to maintain postoperative digestion. The effects of supplementation were determined by measuring postoperative intestinal absorption and nutritional status in a randomized trial. The patients received pancreatin or a placebo. Before the trial, patients showed abnormal digestion of fats and protein. Total energy was low at baseline and at 3 weeks after surgery. Supplementation with pancreatin improved fat and protein absorption as well as improving nitrogen balance. However, patients taking a placebo had worsened absorption after surgery. These data suggest that long-term, postoperative pancreatic enzyme supplementation is both effective and necessary in surgery patients who had pancreatitis.

Considerable evidence exists in support of the beneficial effects of enzymes, both natural and supplemental. Plant enzymes have shown obvious benefit for specific conditions. Research with intact absorption of food substrates has shown that undigested food substrates enter the blood and plant enzymes break down different food substrates that would otherwise have been passed into the blood partially digested.

Youth is the time of life when our normal ability to produce enzymes is greatest. It is also a time of rapid growth and often a time with no serious illness. As people age and their food enzymes become depleted, they often begin to suffer a broad range of health complaints.

According to Howell,[2] how long we live and our state of health are determined by our enzyme potential. Howell referred to a study by Meyer and associates at Michael Reese Hospital in Chicago that reported the presence of enzymes in the saliva of young adults is 30 times higher than in people over 69 years of age.

Therefore, humans consuming an enzyme-less diet use vast quantities of their enzyme potential from pancreatic secretions and other digestive organs, perhaps resulting in shortened life span, illness, and lowered resistance to all types of stress.

In the early 1970s, G.A. Leveille, a University of Illinois researcher, discovered that enzyme activities in the tissues become weaker with age. Leveille conducted experiments on rats and found that at the age of 18 months—considered to be old for rats—when receiving enzyme-free fabricated diets, enzyme activity shrunk to less than 20% of its level at 1 month of age. Howell[2] agrees: "[T]he more lavishly a young body gives up its enzymes, the sooner the state of enzyme poverty, or old age, is reached."

The answer is to substitute raw foods for cooked foods as much as possible. Howell recommends that we eat foods with their enzymes intact and supplement cooked foods with enzyme capsules.[2] He suggests we can stop abnormal and pathological aging processes. Howell singles out raw milk, bananas, avocados, seeds, nuts, grapes, and other natural foods as rich in food enzymes. He also suggests an enzyme supplement be taken with all cooked food. Under medical supervision, Howell suggests large doses of enzyme therapy to treat certain diseases.

Few would disagree with the old adage that "we are what we eat," but it is not quite that simple. Enzymes make the digestion of food possible. This means we must make maximum use of enzyme activity, both internal enzymes and those consumed either in food or as supplements.

## Artichoke

The artichoke plant is best known for its heart, the bottom part of its spiky flower bud that many of us have learned to appreciate as both a delicacy and a nutritious vegetable. However, other parts of this tall thistle-like plant, which never reach the dinner table, have proven to be even more beneficial for our health. Clinical studies show its large basal leaves to be effective for improving digestion and liver function, as well as cholesterol levels.

Since ancient times, humans have looked to nature for help to cure diseases. Up until modern times, most remedies were derived from the plant kingdom, and even today a large percentage of our current pharmaceutical drugs are based on plant extracts from various parts of the world. Many old herbal remedies, however, have fallen into oblivion with the development of modern medicine.

Artichoke extract is one of the few phytopharmaceuticals whose experiential and clinical effects have been confirmed to a great extent by biomedical research. Its major active components have been identified, as have some of its mechanisms of action in the human body. In particular, antioxidant, liver-protective, bile-enhancing, and lipid-lowering effects have been demonstrated, which correspond well with the historical use of the plant. More research is needed to determine in detail the mechanisms of action for these effects. However, there appears to be enough evidence to suggest a potential role for artichoke extract in some areas where modern medicine does not have much to offer.

Used as a food and a medical remedy as early as 400 BCE, the artichoke plant has a long history. At the time, a pupil of Aristotle by the name of Theophrastus was one of the first to describe the plant in detail. Enjoyed as a delicacy, an appetizer, and a digestive aid by the aristocracy of the Roman Empire, it later seemed to fall into oblivion until the 1500s, when medicinal use of the artichoke for liver problems and jaundice was recorded. In 1850 a French physician successfully used extract of artichoke leaves in the treatment of a boy who had been sick with jaundice for a month and had made no improvement from the drugs used at that time. This accomplishment inspired researchers to find out more about the effects of this extract, and their research resulted in the knowledge we have today about the extract and its mechanisms of action.

Artichoke leaf extract is made from the long, deeply serrated basal leaves of the artichoke plant. This part is chosen for medicinal use because the concentration of the biologically active compounds is higher here than in the rest of the plant. The most active of these compounds have been discovered to be the flavonoids and caffeoylquinic acids. These substances belong to the polyphenol group and include chlorogenic acid, caffeoylquinic acid derivatives (cynarin is one of them), luteolin, scolymoside, and cynaroside.

Cynarin was the first constituent of the extract to be isolated in 1934. It is found only in trace amounts of fresh leaves but is formed by natural chemical changes that take place during drying and extraction of the plant material. Cynarin was originally believed to be the one active component of the extract. Today the whole complex of compounds is considered important, since it has not yet been completely clarified which component is responsible for each effect. It is claimed that neither cynarin alone, nor fresh plant material achieves the potency of the dried total extract.[7]

Chlorogenic acid, another major component of the artichoke leaf extract, has recently become known as a powerful antioxidant with exciting potential in many applications. Laboratory investigations are ongoing all over the world with promising findings for future clinical application in areas such as HIV, cancer, and diabetes.

Most of the modern research on artichoke has been done with the German artichoke extract Hepar-SL Forte, standardized to contain 3% caffeoylquinic acids. A new, even more potent extract, standardized at 15% caffeoylquinic acids—calculated as chlorogenic acid—is now available on the American market.

**Biological effects.** The original uses of artichoke (since ancient times) have been as an aid for indigestion and insufficient liver function. The mechanism of action, however, has been essentially unknown. Recent findings have provided a new foundation for our understanding and uncovered additional benefits of the extract, such as antioxidant and lipid-lowering effects.

**Effects on the GI system.** The importance of effective liver function for overall health, and proper gastrointestinal function in particular, is rarely emphasized in health discussions in the United States. One reason might be that there is neither laboratory evidence nor specific physical symptoms to reveal an overburdened liver in the beginning stages. The symptoms may be nonspecific, such as general malaise, fatigue, headache, epigastric pain, bloating, nausea, or constipation. Discomfort following meals and intolerance of fat are also notable indications of disturbances in the biliary system.

It is estimated that at least 50% of patients with dyspeptic complaints have no verifiable disease. Because of the liver's essential role in detoxification, even minor impairment of liver function can have profound effects. It is therefore important to take such chronic complaints seriously. In Germany and France, for example, physicians frequently prescribe herbal liver remedies, such as artichoke extract, with good results when presented with these chronic but nonspecific symptoms.

The proven basis for the beneficial effects of artichoke leaf extract on the gastrointestinal system is the promotion of bile flow. Bile is an extremely important digestive substance that is produced by the liver and stored in the gallbladder. The liver manufactures about 1 quart daily of bile to meet digestive requirements. It is secreted into the small intestine, where it emulsifies fats and fat-soluble vitamins and improves their absorption. Any interference with healthy bile flow can create a myriad of immediate digestive disorders, such as bloating.

Good bile flow is also essential for detoxification, which is one of the major tasks of the liver. The liver is constantly bombarded with toxic chemicals from the environment (ie, the food we eat, water we drink, and air we breathe).

Bile serves as a carrier for these toxic substances, delivering them into the intestine for further elimination from the body. This is the major route for excretion of cholesterol. Bile's promotion of intestinal peristalsis, which helps prevent constipation, is also helpful.

When the excretion of bile is inhibited (eg, due to gallstones or gallbladder disease), toxins and cholesterol stay in the liver longer with damaging effects. Other common reasons for impairment of the bile flow within the liver itself are, for example, alcohol ingestion, viral hepatitis, and certain chemicals and drugs. In the initial stages of liver dysfunctions, laboratory tests, such as serum bilirubin, alkaline phosphatase, SGOT, LDH, and GGTP, often remain normal. It is not adequate to rely on these tests alone. Symptoms that may indicate reduced liver function are general malaise, fatigue, digestive disturbances, and sometimes increasing allergies and chemical sensitivities.

Excessive alcohol consumption is by far the most common cause of impaired liver function in the United States. It stimulates fat infiltration into the liver cells, causing fatty liver. Some livers are very sensitive to even minute amounts of alcohol; others are more tolerant. Research suggests that fatty liver condition is more serious than previously believed. It may develop to more advanced liver disease, such as inflammation, fibrosis, and cirrhosis.

Because of its long historical use for liver conditions, it seemed reasonable to investigate the artichoke plant scientifically. The first clinical studies were conducted in the 1930s with encouraging results. Interest in the artichoke intensified in the 1900s, and several excellent clinical studies were conducted in recent years.

Realizing the importance of adequate bile flow for health, German researchers set out to confirm the earlier findings of bile-promoting effect of the artichoke plant in a controlled, double-blind study on healthy volunteers.[7] The participants were given a 1-time dose of artichoke extract or placebo, and their bile secretion was measured over the following hours, using special techniques. Bile secretion was found to be significantly higher in the group that received the artichoke extract.

Another clinical study showed an improvement of symptoms in 50% of patients with dyspeptic syndrome after 14 days of treatment with artichoke leaf extract. The study involved 60 patients with nonspecific symptoms such as upper abdominal pain, heartburn, bloating, constipation, diarrhea, nausea, and vomiting. In the placebo group, as a comparison, improvements of less distinct quality were noticed in 38% of the participants.[8]

Interesting results were also demonstrated in a large open-label study of 417 participants with liver or bile duct disease. Most of these patients had long-standing symptoms, some of them for many years. They suffered from upper abdominal pain, bloating, constipation, lack of appetite, and nausea. These patients were treated with artichoke leaf extract for 4 weeks. After 1 week, about 70% of the patients experienced improvement of their symptoms, and after 4 weeks, the percentage was even higher (approximately 85%).[9]

Even more remarkable improvement was shown in another open-label study,[10] where 553 outpatients with nonspecific dyspeptic complaints were treated with a standardized artichoke leaf extract. The subjective complaints declined significantly within 6 weeks of treatment. Improvements in vomiting (88%), nausea (83%), abdominal pain (76%), loss of appetite (72%), severe constipation (71%), flatulence (68%), and fat intolerance (59%) were noted. Ninety-eight percent of the patients judged the effect of the extract to be considerably better, somewhat better, or equal to that achieved during previous treatment with other drugs. The dosage used in this study was 1–2 capsules, 3 times daily of the preparation Hepar-SL Forte. One capsule contains 320 mg of dry extract of artichoke leaves, standardized to provide 3% caffeoylquinic acid.

The study by Fintelmann[10] not only confirmed the efficacy of the artichoke extract for dyspepsia, but also demonstrated a significant effect of the extract on fat (lipid) metabolism. The researchers found a significant decline in both cholesterol and triglyceride levels in the blood, which confirmed a discovery made as early as the 1930s.

Artichoke leaf extract is well tolerated and has few side effects in recommended dosages. The use of the artichoke plant as food in many countries over hundreds of years supports the safety of consumption. More important, however, is that several rigorous studies report the absence of adverse effects when using a standardized extract compared to the placebo. In a large safety study, only one out of 100 subjects reported mild side effects such as transient increases in flatulence.

Local eczematous reactions have been reported after occupational exposure and skin contact with the fresh plant or its dried parts. Such an allergy should be considered a contraindication for external use of the extract, although no reactions to orally ingested extract have been observed so far. Because of its bile-stimulating effect, the extract should not be taken by individuals with gallstones or other bile duct occlusion.

An artichoke extract is now available in the United States. While the German artichoke products, cited in most European studies, typically contain 3% caffeoylquinic acids, this artichoke extract is standardized to contain 15% caffeoylquinic acids, calculated as chlorogenic acid.

Artichoke leaf extract has proven to be a safe and natural way to maintain and improve general health because of its many applications to improve essential physiological functions. As a nutritional supplement and antioxidant, it can safely be used as an adjunct to conventional therapies.

## HOW EASTERN EUROPEANS COPE WITH DIGESTIVE DISORDERS

The difference in life expectancy between the richest and poorest European countries is more than 10 years. In the early 1990s, overall Eastern European mortality was 20–100% higher than in the West. The reasons for these differences in mortality are attributed to poor diet, excess alcohol consumption, heavy smoking, and other dangerous health behaviors.

One explanation for the decreased life span among Eastern Europeans is that their intake of antioxidants from fruits, vegetables, and nuts is much lower compared to the West. A severe deficiency of antioxidant vitamins, along with a low intake of folic acid and flavonoids, partially accounts for the high level of cardiovascular disease in Eastern Europe.

The traditional Eastern European diet consists of lots of animal fats and protein and very little in the way of fresh fruits and vegetables. This poor diet not only shortens life span, but also creates an epidemic of acute digestive disorders.

While digestive complications increase as people age, the poor health habits of Eastern Europeans exacerbate common problems such as heartburn, bloating, gas, constipation, nausea, cramps, diarrhea, and IBS.

In the United States, over-the-counter and prescription medications for digestive ailments are a multibillion-dollar industry. Most Eastern Europeans cannot afford the high-priced synthetic products sold by Western drug companies and instead rely on a natural herbal remedy that contains cholic acid, extracts from black radish, artichoke, and peppermint. Rather than masking symptoms, this herbal preparation attacks the underlying cause of many forms of digestive disorders. Considering the magnitude of digestive disorders caused by the poor health behaviors of Eastern Europeans, the fact that this herbal remedy has such a strong track record makes it a fascinating potential solution for Americans.

This herbal remedy was introduced in Europe more than 45 years ago. Today, more than 100 million doses of the formula are sold annually in Europe.

The mechanism of action of the formula is to stimulate peristalsis of the intestines, speed digestion of fats, and prevent stagnation of food in the digestive tract. Benefits to the user are a reduction in esophageal acid reflux, alleviation of the feeling of fullness and bloating after eating, decreased digestive tract tension, alkalization of the gastric content, constipation relief, and normalized elimination.

## Black Radish Juice

Black radish juice extract is the primary active ingredient in this herbal blend. Virtually unknown in the United States, the radish contains a variety of chemicals that increases the flow of digestive juices. The most important function of black radish extract is that it encourages the liver to produce fat- and protein-digesting bile and lowers the tension of the bile ducts. It also improves peristaltic movement. Constipation is another problem that is improved or eliminated from radish consumption. Rich in fiber and digestive stimulants, a regular consumption of radishes helps regulate the bowels. Since dehydration is a major cause of constipation, radishes help hydrate and lubricate the intestines and encourage relaxed bowel movements. The root juice extract of the black radish used in this European digestive aid is the most potent part of the plant.

A bonus is the radish's ability to assist the immune system, as it contains a variety of chemicals that possess natural antimicrobial actions. Regular consumption may lead to a significant improvement in the resistance against common microbial infections, such as colds, sore throats, ear infections, and the flu.

Prahaveanu[11] described a study in which liquid radish extract was administered to mice before they were inoculated with an influenza virus. There was a significant decrease in the mortality rate and a significant increase in the rate of survival as compared to the untreated controls. Another study by[12] found it to be protective against *E. coli*—more so than penicillin G.

A second ingredient of this digestive aid is artichoke, which further increases production of bile and causes it to flow through bile ducts. Peppermint is also present, which increases secretion functions of the stomach and liver and the production of enzymes.

## Cholic Acid

Cholic acid, or pure processed ox bile, is a liver enzyme used for digestion. It is particularly helpful in digesting fats and meat protein. This popular blend also contains calcium phosphate, which neutralizes stomach acid.

This formula uses a layered delivery system to ensure that the various herbal extracts perform their intended function in the right part of the digestive tract. The ingredients are cultivated in Europe in a pesticide-free environment and are standardized to ensure uniform potency. The safety profile and demonstrated efficacy of herbs such as artichoke, black radish, and peppermint, particularly in standardized extract form, suggest that this formula may be the answer to the digestive problems of millions of Americans.

Used extensively in Europe and hailed as a huge success, this formulation simultaneously relieves digestive disorders while strengthening the digestive system. While there are numerous products that work on individual symptoms of poor digestion and elimination, this formula stands out because it relieves more than one symptom at the same time. It also helps the liver function properly by enabling the organ to release toxins and encouraging it to produce the correct amount of bile.

## The Science Behind Europe's Most Popular Digestive Aid

Immunologist Mark Pasula, president and research director of Signet Diagnostic Corporation at Oxford Nutritional Center in Florida, believes this herbal formula works because of its two-pronged approach that relieves most digestive disorders while helping build a healthy digestive system.

In short, this digestive aid has the capacity to rapidly relieve symptoms in the short-term, while healing the source of the problems in the long run. It is the formula of choice for patients with digestive complaints who have not responded to food elimination therapy. Within a short time of regularly using the formula, their digestive problems disappear and their digestive system actually strengthens.

Independent clinical research was conducted on this patented formula to analyze the therapeutic effectiveness of the formula among patients with chronic digestive problems. Results showed statistically significant improvement in symptoms during treatment. The unique blend was most successful in eliminating the most frequently occurring symptom, gas, in more than 95% of the cases. Symptoms such as constipation, intestinal pains and cramps, heartburn (reflux), and stomach pains and cramps decreased or were completely eliminated in more than 90% of the cases. Bloating ceased in more than 80%, diarrhea in about 75%, and nausea and vomiting in approximately 65% of the cases.

This digestive aid was found to minimize the assimilation of undigested toxic products that often stay in the gut for prolonged periods of time. Because of its cholepoietic and cholagogic abilities, it was particularly effective in preventing the stagnation of food and bloating in patients whose diet was rich in animal protein and fat. Because there are no specific contraindications, this herbal formula can be taken together with any medication and can be taken by patients with different respiratory, cardiovascular, and musculoskeletal disorders. The only people who should avoid this formula are those with biliary tract obstruction or gallbladder disease because of the bile-stimulating effects of the black radish and artichoke extracts. It is not known how this formula would affect those who have had their gallbladder removed.

# CONVENTIONAL TREATMENT

Some of the most popular drugs prescribed to treat digestive complaints are Prilosec or Prevacid. These drugs are known as gastric acid-pump inhibitors because of the unique way in which they block the final metabolic step in the production of stomach acid. These drugs are quite expensive but are more effective in suppressing disorders associated with excess stomach acid production than the older class of histamine-2 receptor antagonist drugs sold under the trade names Tagamet®, Zantac®, Pepcid®, and Axid®. Drugs such as Tagamet® inhibit stomach acid secretion whereas Prilosec and Prevacid® suppress virtually all stomach acid secretion.

## If You Suffer from Ulcers

Most stomach ulcers are now considered to be caused by the *Helicobacter pylori* (*H. pylori*) bacteria. Blood tests can reveal the presence of the *H. pylori* antibody.

Special antibiotic regimens are now the therapy of choice in treating ulcers. In fact, special antibiotic combinations can be used to eliminate *H. pylori* bacteria from the stomach within a matter of weeks. Drugs that reduce stomach acid are therefore more frequently prescribed to treat esophageal reflux, where stomach acid regurgitates into the esophagus to cause heartburn. If left untreated, chronic esophageal exposure to stomach acid can cause esophagitis and esophageal cancer. Also, those who fail to eradicate *H. pylori* are at a far greater risk for contracting stomach cancer.

Some people with mild esophageal reflux may be able to use natural therapies to promote youthful peristaltic action and push food more rapidly out of the stomach, thereby alleviating reflux back into the esophagus.

# NATURAL THERAPIES TO IMPROVE DIGESTIVE DISORDERS

## Phosphatidylcholine

Extracellular phospholipids, synthesized on gastric mucosa, assist in the hydrophobic (nonwettable) characteristics of the epithelium, yielding protection from stomach acid and injurious materials. The nonwettable status of the epithelium is extremely important to the health of the GI tract. This valuable protection is, however, vulnerable and can be transformed by aspirin or NSAIDs from a non-wettable (resistant to harmful substances) to a wettable (mucosa is susceptible to injury from caustic substances) state.

Once the gastric mucosa has been disturbed, ulcers loom as an ongoing threat. Polyunsaturated phosphatidylcholine (PPC) has been shown to reduce the incidence of gastric ulcers, even after aggressive experimental ulcer inducement. Individuals at high risk for gastric ulcers, such as those taking high doses of either aspirin or NSAIDs, have lessened the injurious nature of the drugs when phospholipids are bound to the anti-inflammatory drugs.[13]

As noted earlier, the basic cause of many ulcers is the spiral-shaped bacterium *H. pylori*.[14] To investigate the effect of *H. pylori* infection on the gastric mucosal barrier, phospholipid and fatty acid composition of the gastric mucosa were analyzed in healthy volunteers with and without *H. pylori* infection. The gastric PPC content of *H. pylori*-positive healthy volunteers was less than that of *H. pylori*–negative healthy volunteers ($p < 0.05$).[15] These findings suggest that *H. pylori* infection results in changes in the gastric mucosal phospholipid contents and their fatty acid composition, causing the gastric mucosa to be weakened. Attempts to increase the worthiness of the gastric mucosa appears indicated, particularly in individuals with a history of gastric ulcers or those on medicinal protocols known to impact the reliability of the mucosa.

Beyond the functions of gastric protection, polyunsaturated PPC assists in the digestion of fat. The presence of luminal PPC is important for normal lymphatic transport of absorbed digestion products of triglyceride, the major dietary fat.[16,17] Assisting in the metabolism and transport of fat may explain why some individuals find value in using lecithin in conditions of hypercholesterolemia.

PPC stimulates collagen breakdown in experimental models of liver cirrhosis. As important as this finding is relative to liver health, it also has pertinent implications regarding the integrity and maintenance of the GI tract. Bowel strictures (abnormal, temporary or permanent narrowing of the bowel) are characterized by excess deposition of collagen in the intestinal wall. A study was conducted to determine the effect of PPC in the prevention of bowel strictures. Three groups of rats were assessed: a control group, a confirmed colitis group, and a group of rats diagnosed with colitis, but receiving PPC. In conjunction with the study, collagen deposition and collagenase activity in colonic tissue were measured in all of the groups. None of the control rats, but 12 of 16 rats with colitis, developed colonic strictures.

In contrast, only 2 of 15 PPC-fed rats with colitis developed strictures. Collagen content was much higher in the rats with colitis than the PPC-fed rats with colitis and the control rats. Collagenase activity in colonic tissue was also much higher in the PPC-fed rats.[18] PPC appears to enhance collagen catabolism, restricting collagen buildup in inflamed intestinal tissue and the resulting stricture formation.

Individuals wishing to enhance the integrity of their GI tract or gain assistance in fat metabolism may wish to consider the use of unsaturated PPC. Unsaturated PPC is deemed well tolerated and without major risk factors.

## Zinc-Carnosine

Zinc is a micronutrient mineral that has multiple functions in human biology, chiefly acting as a coenzyme in many enzyme systems that defend against free radical damage.[19–22] Recognizing that H. pylori infection causes increased oxidative stress, a group of Ecuadorian scientists investigated whether zinc deficiency might cause increased inflammation in the stomachs of people infected with the organism.[23] They studied 352 patients

with dyspepsia (stomach pain and dysfunction) who had biopsy samples taken during endoscopy. Patients with H. pylori infections had significantly lower zinc concentrations in their tissue samples than uninfected patients. Indeed, the more severe the inflammation, the lower the zinc levels in the infected subjects.[23] These results and others have led some researchers to consider zinc to be a "gastric cytoprotective" (cell-saving) nutrient.[24]

Zinc also has direct anti-inflammatory effects, helping to stabilize the membranes of mast cells. Mast cells release bursts of inflammatory cytokines when stimulated by injury or allergy.[25,26] Further, zinc is an immune modulator that can reduce the recurrence rate of certain inflammation-sensitive cancers.[27]

Another essential nutrient called carnosine can boost those effects even further. Japanese scientists have led the way in developing this zinc-carnosine compound. Until quite recently, gastric cancer (the result of gastritis and ulcer disease) was the top killer cancer in Japan; the dramatic decline in gastric cancer has been attributed in large part to dietary education of the Japanese people.[28] In fact, the zinc-carnosine compound, sold as polaprezinc, is a regulated prescription antiulcer drug in Japan.[29] Fortunately, this simple nutrient compound is available in the United States as a nonprescription supplement that is safe for long-term use.

Zinc-carnosine also speeds the eradication of infection with H. pylori itself, as shown by another Japanese team in 1999.[30] The group enrolled 66 patients with known H. pylori infections and symptoms, randomly assigning them to zinc-carnosine or placebo. All patients also received a cocktail of two potent antibiotics (aimed at curbing the infections) plus a proton pump inhibitor (aimed at promoting gastric healing). Only 86% of the antibiotic-proton pump inhibitor group achieved complete cure (eradication of detectable organisms), while 100% of those receiving zinc-carnosine were cured.

In early 2007, Western scientists began to examine zinc-carnosine's mode of action and effectiveness. A British team, using a laboratory model of gut injury and repair, also conducted a clinical trial.[31] In the first study, they examined the effects of zinc-carnosine on cells lining animal digestive tracts after exposure to indomethacin (a potent NSAID notorious for its gastritis-producing tendencies) or stress. The nutrient combination reduced stomach injury by 75% and small intestinal injury by 50%. It also stimulated migration and growth of cells in and near the sites of injury, hastening the healing process nearly threefold. In the clinical trial, 10 healthy volunteers took indomethacin (50 mg) 3 times daily with either placebo or zinc-carnosine. Indomethacin increased gut permeability (impaired barrier function of the gut's lining that allows inflammation to get its start) by a factor of 3 in the placebo group, whereas there was no increase in permeability in the supplemented group. The researchers concluded that zinc-carnosine stabilized the mucosal lining cells of the stomach and small intestine.

## Cranberries

There is mounting clinical evidence of how effective cranberries and their extracts can be in mitigating *H. pylori* and other stomach ailments. Chinese researchers gave cranberry juice or a placebo drink (about 2 cups per day) to 189 adults with *H. pylori* infection.[32] They checked for chemical evidence of continued infection at days 35 and 90 of treatment. More than 14% of the juice-supplemented group versus 5% of the placebo group showed complete eradication of the organism.

A large systematic review by nutritional experts has now concluded that regular intake of cranberry juice and other dietary products "might constitute a low-cost, large-scale alternative solution applicable for populations at risk for *H. pylori* colonization".[33] It seems clear that cranberries and their extracts can take their place alongside zinc-carnosine as important components of an effective stomach health regimen.

## Licorice

Long recognized for their multiple health benefits,[21,34] licorice extracts (with the potentially blood pressure-elevating glycyrrhizin molecule removed) provide yet another nutritional weapon in fighting *H. pylori* infection.[35] Various laboratory studies have shown that these extracts have potent anti-inflammatory activities, reducing cytokine production while increasing production of protective stomach mucus.[36,37] Licorice extracts can also kill *H. pylori* in stomach tissue,[38] even antibiotic-resistant strains of the organism.[39,40] Indeed, in one laboratory head-to-head comparison, licorice extracts were as effective as famotidine in preventing ulcers,[41] and animal studies have shown a potent effect on speeding the healing of existing ulcers.[42] These characteristics of licorice neatly complement those of zinc-carnosine and cranberry extracts.

## Picrorhiza

News about another natural remedy called picrorhiza (*Picrorhiza kurroa*) is now generating intense excitement in the medical community.[43,44] Well-known to practitioners of Ayurvedic medicine, picrorhiza is a perennial herb found high in the Himalayas. Its extracts are now being found to have potent antioxidant,[45-47] immune-stimulating,[48-52] and anti-inflammatory,[53-55] properties—activities that clearly have a role in gastric protection. Since picrorhiza so dramatically combats the very changes caused by *H. pylori* (ie, infection, inflammation, oxidant stress, and tissue injury), it is no wonder that this ancient herb is now at the forefront of research on stomach health.

Already used to speed healing in other infectious gastrointestinal conditions such as hepatitis A,[48,56] picrorhiza extracts also demonstrate unique wound-healing properties, stimulating tissue growth, nerve cell recovery, and blood vessel formation that may promote recovery from tissue damage.[57-59] In a dramatic illustration of the extract's ability to combat stomach ulcers, Indian scientists administered it to rats with ulcers induced by the potent NSAID indomethacin.[60] Compared with an untreated group of animals, the supplemented group had much faster rates of ulcer healing, accompanied by a profound drop in levels of oxidized tissue components. And while antioxidant enzyme activity was decreased in the untreated animals, those treated with picrorhiza had elevated antioxidant activity.

## Life Extension Suggestions

- **Digestive enzymes:** with meals
  - Pancreatin 8x blend: 400–1200 mg daily
  - Digestive enzyme blend (protease, amylase, lactase, cellulose, lipase): 290–870 mg daily
  - Whole papaya: 200–600 mg daily
- **Herbal digestive blend:** 320–640 mg daily
  - Black radish extract
  - Deoxycholic acid
  - Artichoke extract
  - Peppermint oil
  - Wormwood extract
- **Zinc (as zinc L-carnosine):** 11 mg daily
- **Deglycyrrhizinated licorice extract (DGL):** 500 mg daily
- **Cranberry extract:** 750 mg daily
- ***Picrorhiza kurroa* extract:** 100 mg daily
- **Artichoke extract blend:** 500–1000 mg daily

## REFERENCES

References available at: www.lef.org/dpt5/ch52

# 53

# *Endometriosis*

Endometriosis is caused by the growth of endometrial tissue outside the uterus. These collections of endometrial tissue cause lower abdominal pain and may cause infertility and gastrointestinal complications. Approximately 5 million American women, mostly between the ages of 25 and 44, suffer from endometriosis, and the disease affects about 30–45% of women with infertility.[1]

The cause of endometriosis is unknown. According to the most prevalent theory, endometrial tissue refluxes into the abdominal cavity, where it becomes established. An established colony of endometrial tissue continues to act like normal endometrial tissue even though it is outside the uterus. The tissue responds to normal hormonal fluctuations in a woman's monthly cycle. During the first part of the cycle, the tissue colony thickens and grows in response to estrogen. In the latter part of the cycle, tissue degenerates and bleeds, sloughs off excess cells, and causes inflammation as well as damage to adjacent tissue.

Women with endometriosis have elevated levels of inflammatory chemicals, providing a therapeutic target for anti-inflammatory dietary supplements. In addition, Life Extension has identified novel approaches to nutritional estrogen modulation that may help reduce the severity of the disease and the risk of hormone-dependent cancers, including breast and ovarian cancer.

In about two-thirds of cases, the ovaries are colonized by endometrial tissue. Other common sites for tissue to implant include the fallopian tubes, lining of the pelvic cavity, uterine ligaments, and the outside lining of the uterus, cervix, colon, appendix, and vagina. In severe cases, adhesions of endometrial tissue are found on the vulva, bladder, kidney, arms, legs, lungs, nasal mucosa, spinal column, and sites of previous surgical incision(s).[1]

While endometrial reflux is the most common theory, it does not fully explain the disease. At least some degree of menstrual reflux occurs in 75–90% of women, yet the rate of endometriosis is much lower. Obviously, an additional mechanism must be at work.

One theory that might help explain why some women suffer from endometriosis is the autoimmune theory. According to this theory, macrophages, which would normally be expected to destroy the endometrial cells, actually contribute to their colonization. In addition, numbers of T cells and natural killer cells, which are elements of the immune system, are reduced. There is also evidence that the misplaced endometrial cells are resistant to removal by immune cells.

The autoimmune theory of endometriosis is supported by frequent finding of autoantibodies in women with endometriosis and by the high rate of other autoimmune conditions among women with endometriosis, including rheumatoid arthritis, multiple sclerosis, and systemic lupus erythematosus.[2] Women who have had recurrent immune-mediated miscarriages may be prone to endometriosis.[3]

Genetics factor into the development of endometriosis. Women who have a first-degree relative with endometriosis have a 10-fold increased risk of developing the disease.[4] Also, women with a family history of endometriosis are more likely to have earlier onset and increased disease severity than women without a family history.[5]

## HOW ENVIRONMENTAL TOXINS MAY CAUSE ENDOMETRIOSIS

An association between endometriosis and exposure to chlorinated hydrocarbons, such as polychlorinated biphenols (PCBs) and dioxin, has been demonstrated in laboratory animals[6,7]; some human data support the association. These toxic chemicals can affect hormones and disrupt immune function.

Dioxin has been shown to alter hormonal response(s) and immune system function.[8–11] One study showed a direct link between exposure to dioxin and the incidence of endometriosis in monkeys. Severity of disease was directly correlated with the dose of dioxin. The monkeys showed abnormalities in their immune systems similar to changes seen in women with endometriosis.[12,13]

Human exposure to dioxin and dioxin-like PCBs is primarily through food and pesticides. Dioxin and dioxin-like PCBs have been shown to increase the risk of multiple cancers, diabetes, and cardiovascular disease; impair prostate development and reproductive capabilities; reduce memory function; and suppress the immune system.[14–18]

## ENDOMETRIOSIS AND OTHER DISEASES

Endometriosis has been associated with an increased risk of conditions associated with abnormal immune responses: systemic lupus erythematosus, rheumatoid arthritis, multiple sclerosis, and Sjögren's syndrome.[2] Allergies, eczema, and asthma caused by a hypersensitivity reaction of the immune system are also increased in women with endometriosis. Fibromyalgia, chronic fatigue syndrome, and hypothyroidism are significantly more common in individuals with hypersensitivity reactions than in the general U.S. population.[2]

A survey revealed that 42% of women with endometriosis have underactive thyroid glands (hypothyroidism). Women with endometriosis have a higher incidence of hypothyroidism than most women in the United States.[2]

Endometriosis is also correlated with an increased risk of ovarian cancer and non-Hodgkin's lymphoma.[19,20]

# DIAGNOSIS

The many presentations of endometriosis often make diagnosis difficult. The most common symptoms of endometriosis are abnormal pelvic pain and pain during intercourse. Abnormal pelvic pain often begins 1–2 days before menstruation and may last for days or throughout the menstrual flow. Other possible symptoms include abnormal vaginal bleeding, constipation, diarrhea, frequent urination, and blood in the urine or stool. Nausea, vomiting, and fainting spells may also be present. The severity of symptoms does not correlate with the extent of the disease. Symptom severity has been proposed to correlate with the depth and location of adhesions in proximity to nerve endings.[21]

In about one-third of cases, however, endometriosis has no symptoms. In this instance, women are often diagnosed during a workup for infertility.

During a pelvic examination, doctors may identify findings characteristic of women with endometriosis. A retroverted uterus (a uterus that tilts toward the back rather than the front) may make endometriosis more likely, and tenderness during the examination, in the absence of findings that suggest infection, may also raise suspicion. Doctors may be able to feel nodules along various parts of a woman's internal anatomy that correspond to collections of endometrial tissue.

Definitive diagnosis of endometriosis requires a biopsy during explorative surgery. Surgical procedures such as laparoscopy involve a scope that is inserted through a small incision in the umbilicus (navel). The scope is used to visualize and biopsy tissue. Often ectopic tissue (tissue that is in the wrong place) is removed or destroyed at the time of the procedure. Laparotomy is a more invasive surgical procedure, usually reserved for women with extensive disease.[22]

Less-direct diagnostic techniques include measuring levels of cancer antigen 125 (CA-125) and imaging.

## Imaging

Although laparoscopy and surgery remain gold-standard diagnostic tools, some less-invasive techniques can be helpful in establishing the diagnosis of endometriosis. Unfortunately, these techniques (eg, magnetic resonance imaging and ultrasound) are likely to miss many smaller or less-active lesions. Transvaginal ultrasound (an ultrasound scan done with a probe placed in the vagina) can efficiently detect lesions larger than roughly three-quarters of an inch in diameter.[23,24]

## CA-125

CA-125 is a protein made by certain cells in the body, including those of the uterine tubes, uterus, cervix, and lining of the abdominal and chest cavities (peritoneum and pleura, respectively). CA-125 is elevated among women with endometriosis, and levels drop following surgery. However, CA-125 levels can also be elevated in a number of unrelated conditions, so it cannot be used reliably as a diagnostic or screening tool. It has value, however, in following the progression of the disease during or after treatment.

# CONVENTIONAL TREATMENT OPTIONS

Conventional medical treatment focuses on pain management, reduction of estrogen stimulation, and preservation of fertility. Treatment often begins at diagnosis with laparoscopy, when visible lesions are removed or destroyed. The following medications may be used to treat endometriosis.

## Oral Contraceptives

Estrogen and progesterone combinations are commonly prescribed to manage endometriosis. Oral contraceptives are often prescribed continuously to help maintain endometrial tissue, preventing the eventual sloughing and bleeding associated with pain, as well as tissue damage and scarring. Studies have shown that 80–100% of women taking hormone-based therapies experience effective relief.[25]

## Analgesics

Nonsteroidal anti-inflammatory drugs (NSAIDs) are commonly prescribed to manage pelvic pain. NSAID treatment may be beneficial for mild pain relief but is often ineffective for severe symptoms. Side effects of NSAIDs include gastrointestinal pain and ulcers.

## Danazol

Danazol is a synthetic form of testosterone used to thin the endometrial lining and reduce levels of estrogen. Danazol has been shown to have some immune-modulating effects as well. In one study, 89% of participants on danazol reported symptomatic improvement; 94% had improvement based on repeat laparoscopy or laparotomy.[26] Danazol's side effects include deepening of the voice and unwanted hair growth, in addition to sensitivity to sunlight.

## Gonadotrophin-Releasing Hormone Agonists

Gonadotrophin-releasing hormone agonists are used to induce a menopause-like state. Their long-term use will inhibit the release of luteinizing hormone and follicle-stimulating hormone from the pituitary, resulting in very low levels of estrogens and androgens, which will inhibit ovulation and menstruation. These drugs do not have the same effects on sex-hormone binding globulin as danazol and thus do not cause a rise in free testosterone, which translates into fewer testosterone-related side effects.

## Progestins

Progestins are synthetic progesterone derivatives prescribed when estrogen therapy is contraindicated or poorly tolerated. Progestins function similarly to other hormone therapies by inhibiting ovulation and menstruation. Ovulation often does not return promptly upon discontinuation of treatment.

---

## NATURAL PROGESTERONE (BIOIDENTICAL) VERSUS SYNTHETIC PROGESTINS (NONBIOIDENTICAL)

### What Is Natural Progesterone?

*Bioidentical natural progesterone* is made in the body or made (not extracted) in the laboratory from either soybeans or the Mexican wild yam (*Dioscorea villosa*). The process was discovered in the 1930s by Pennsylvania State University professor Russell Marker, who transformed *diosgenin* from wild yams into natural progesterone.[27] Natural progesterone refers to bioidentical hormone products that have a molecular structure identical to the hormones our bodies manufacture naturally. One of the most effective forms of bioidentical progesterone is called *micronized* progesterone. The process of micronization allows for steady and even absorption of the medication.[28] Accordingly, both the micronized progesterone and other commercially available progesterone creams contain *bioidentical* progesterone.

### What Are Synthetic Progestins?

Unlike natural *progesterone*, nonbioidentical synthetic progestins are *not* molecularly identical to the hormones found naturally in

the body. Synthetic progestins were first developed for use as contraceptive agents. Because the half-life of natural progesterone is very short, researchers sought an agent that would produce longer-lasting, more potent effects than natural progesterone. Birth control pills usually contain a synthetic progestin and a synthetic estrogen. Synthetic progestins are very potent, with just a small dose preventing ovulation and thus functioning as birth control. A slight change in the chemical structure of progesterone has allowed pharmaceutical companies to create patentable and highly profitable birth control products.

One of the most common progestins, *medroxyprogesterone acetate* (Provera®), has been linked to blood clots, fluid retention, acne, rashes, weight gain, depression, certain cancers, and other disorders.[29,30] Nonbioidentical progestins are also able to bind to glucocorticoid, androgen, and mineralocorticoid receptors, which may explain the wide range of adverse side effects many women experience while taking synthetic progestins.[31,32] The vast majority of research studies have been conducted using progestins rather than natural progesterone, which helps explain the disparity and negativity of the results.

The Food and Drug Administration has also approved a drug called Prometrium®, an oral pill containing 200 mg of natural micronized progesterone taken daily. Because orally administered progesterone is metabolized by the liver, it may be contraindicated in patients with certain liver conditions. Initial liver metabolism of progesterone (called "first-pass" metabolism) also creates higher levels of certain metabolites of progesterone than transdermal or transmucosally administered progesterone.[33]

### How to Best Administer Natural Progesterone

Natural progesterone cream may be more efficiently used, since lipophilic (fat-soluble) molecules allow it to be better absorbed through the skin. This is called "transdermal" administration. Even better absorption is obtained if the progesterone is rubbed into a mucous membrane surface (inner aspects of labia or intravaginally), called "transmucosal" administration. Another advantage of topical natural progesterone cream is that individualized dosing can be easily facilitated by varying the amount of cream applied.[34–36]

As one can readily discern from the peer-reviewed published literature, adverse side effects are clearly associated with nonbioidentical *progestins*, whereas several health benefits have been observed with the use of bioidentical *progesterone*.

---

Other drugs that have been studied for endometriosis include aromatase inhibitors (agents that interfere with estrogen and progesterone synthesis), selective estrogen receptor modulators (agents that prevent estrogen from binding to its receptors and exerting its full biological effect), and immunomodulators, including interferon.

## NUTRITIONAL AND SUPPLEMENT THERAPY

### Essential Fatty Acids

Supplementation with essential fatty acids can reduce the inflammation associated with endometriosis by interfering with the production of prostaglandins or cytokines that mediate the pain and many other symptoms seen with endometriosis.

**Docosahexaenoic acid and eicosapentaenoic acid.** Docosahexaenoic acid (DHA) and eicosapentaenoic acid (EPA) are omega-3, long-chain polyunsaturated fatty acids found primarily in the oils of fatty fish such as salmon, mackerel, sardines, herring, trout, cod, kipper, pilchard, and menhaden. DHA and EPA compete with arachidonic acid in the production of prostaglandins, thereby reducing inflammation.[37–39] Fish oils also reduce the production of cytokines, such as interleukin-1, interleukin-2, and tumor necrosis factor (TNF), all of which are involved in producing and maintaining the inflammation associated with endometriosis. DHA and EPA have also been shown to down-regulate activity of immune system inflammatory cells and production of antibodies involved in the symptoms of endometriosis.[40–42]

**Gamma-linolenic acid.** Gamma-linolenic acid (GLA) is an omega-6 fatty acid found in borage seed oil, evening primrose oil, and black currant oil. GLA is metabolized in the body to series 1 prostaglandins, which decrease the inflammatory response and inhibit arachidonic acid from forming inflammatory leukotrienes.[43] Precursors to GLA can also be taken to stimulate this anti-inflammatory biochemical pathway. Linoleic acid is an omega-6 fatty acid commonly found in corn, safflower, sesame, soybean, sunflower, walnut, and grape seed oils. Alpha-linolenic acid is an omega-3 fatty acid found in flax, canola, soybeans, walnuts, pumpkin seeds, and perilla seeds. The enzyme delta-6 desaturase requires magnesium, vitamin B6, and zinc to convert linoleic acid and alpha-linolenic acid to GLA.

## Vitamin E

Vitamin E is a fat-soluble vitamin that acts as a free-radical scavenger of lipids and fats. It protects cell membranes and prevents damage to membrane-associated enzymes. The most common form of vitamin E in American diets is gamma-tocopherol, which has been shown to decrease TNF-alpha (elevated in individuals with endometriosis).[44] Vitamin E succinate and vitamin A were found to reduce indicators of toxicity and damage in laboratory mice from dioxin exposure.[45] In addition, one study suggested that women with endometriosis are under oxidative stress, which suggests a role for vitamin E as an antioxidant.[46] Another lab study indicated that vitamin E inhibited the proliferation of endometrial stromal cells.[47]

## Vitamin C

Vitamin C (ascorbic acid) is found in many fruits and vegetables, especially citrus fruit. As an antioxidant, ascorbic acid can protect cells from reactive oxygen species known to cause tissue damage and disease. Estrogen, oral contraceptives, and smoking (along with other forms of nicotine) increase vitamin C excretion, resulting in measurably lower plasma levels of vitamin C.[48,49]

## Beta-Carotene

Beta-carotene, a precursor to vitamin A, is a carotenoid found readily in fruits, vegetables, grains, and oils. It has antioxidant activity, prevents lipid peroxidation, and may reduce free radical DNA damage.[50,51] Beta-carotene and other carotenoids provide approximately 50% of the vitamin A needed in the American diet.[52] Vitamin A helps protect against damage from dioxin exposure, which has been implicated as a cause of endometriosis.[45] In animal studies, beta-carotene has shown the ability to suppress the angiogenesis necessary for maintaining growth of ectopic endometrial tissue.[53]

## Milk Thistle

Milk thistle (*Silybum marianum*) is a member of the Compositae family. Seeds are often used medicinally for liver disease. The main active constituent is silymarin, which has been shown to inhibit TNF.[54] Studies have found that TNF is elevated in women with endometriosis. Constituents of milk thistle have demonstrated antioxidant and free-radical-scavenging functions and inhibited lipid peroxidation.[55] Silymarin may increase estrogen clearance by means of its ability to inhibit the enzyme beta-glucuronidase.[56]

## Calcium D-Glucarate

Calcium D-glucarate is the calcium salt of D-glucaric acid, a natural substance found in many fruits and vegetables. Calcium D-glucarate has been shown to inhibit beta-glucuronidase, an enzyme found in certain bacteria that reside in the gut. One of the key ways in which the body eliminates toxic chemicals as well as hormones (eg, estrogen) is by attaching glucuronic acid to them in the liver and then excreting this complex in the bile. Beta-glucuronidase is a bacterial enzyme that uncouples (breaks) the bond between the excreted compound and glucuronic acid. When beta-glucuronidase breaks the bond, the hormone or toxic chemical released is available to be reabsorbed into the body instead of excreted. Elevated beta-glucuronidase activity is associated with an increased risk of various cancers, particularly hormone-dependent cancers like breast, prostate, and colon cancer.

## Natural Progesterone

Natural progesterone is structurally identical to endogenous progesterone. It is synthesized from diosgenin, which is isolated from wild yam or soy and then converted in a laboratory to pregnenolone and progesterone. Progesterone has been shown to reduce inflammation in endometriosis and limit the growth of uterine tissue.[57]

## Nutritional Modulation of Estrogen

One strategy that may be helpful with endometriosis is to modulate estrogen through nutritional means. Estrogen has many different metabolites, and research has shown that some metabolites are stronger and more dangerous than others. Certain nutrients, such as *indole-3-carbinol*, may help increase weaker estrogens while decreasing stronger estrogens. This finding may have two benefits for endometriosis patients. First, it would reduce the stimulatory effect of estrogen on endometrial tissue, which may reduce the buildup of blood during the early part of the menstrual phase. Second, favorably altering the ratio of weaker to stronger estrogens may reduce the risk of breast and ovarian cancer.

Specifically, indole-3-carbinol has been documented to increase the ratio of weaker 2-hydroxyestrone to the stronger and carcinogenic 16-alpha hydroxyestrone.[58] It accomplishes this by encouraging synthesis of additional 2-hydroxyestrone.[59]

A related natural approach to estrogen modulation may be found in a compound called *diindolylmethane* (DIM), a byproduct of indole-3-carbinol that has shown many cancer-fighting effects.

---

### HOW DIM COMPLEMENTS I3C

Many scientists believe that I3C's beneficial effects are partly driven by one of its principal byproducts, DIM.[60,61] For instance, DIM has recently been shown to promote production of beneficial interferon gamma by breast cancer cells. According to scientists at the University of California, Berkeley, "This novel effect may provide important clues to explain the anticancer effects of DIM because it is well known that [interferon gamma] plays an important role in preventing the development of primary and transplanted tumors."[62] Recently, scientists working with cell cultures also showed that DIM activates cellular stress response pathways in breast, prostate, and cervical cancer cells. This response mimics the reaction of cells deprived of adequate nutrition, further enhancing cell susceptibility to destruction.[63] In other studies, researchers have shown that both DIM and I3C induce cell death in prostate cancer cells.[64,65]

Scientists at Wayne State University School of Medicine recently noted that "I3C and DIM affected the expression of a large number of genes that are related to the control of carcinogenesis, cell survival, and physiologic behaviors."[64]

Like I3C, DIM also stops the growth of new blood vessels that tumors require for their survival and metastasis. This newly discovered anticancer activity (antiangiogenesis) is significant. In research at the University of California, Berkeley, in both cell culture assays and live animal models of cancer, small amounts of DIM dramatically reduced biochemical markers of angiogenesis and significantly impeded the rate of new vessel growth. "This is the first study," the scientists noted, "to show that DIM can strongly inhibit the development of human breast tumor in [an animal] model and to provide evidence for the antiangiogenic properties of this dietary indole."[66]

---

## Life Extension Suggestions

Endometriosis is one of the most common causes of pelvic pain in women. It is caused by growth of endometrial tissue in inappropriate places. Because endometrial tissue is sensitive to estrogen, which causes it to grow, women with endometriosis are discouraged from eating phytoestrogens (plant-based estrogens) found in soy products. Phytoestrogens have been shown to encourage endometrial tissue growth.[67]

The following nutrients have been shown to reduce the inflammation associated with endometriosis and reduce endometrial tissue growth.

- **Omega 3 fatty acids from fish oil:** 1400 mg EPA and 1000 mg of DHA daily
- **Gamma-linolenic acid (GLA):** 1300 mg daily
- **Vitamin E:** 400 IU daily with at least 200 mg gamma-tocopherol daily
- **Vitamin C:** 1–3 g daily
- **Beta-carotene:** 25 000 IU daily
- **Milk thistle extract (*Silybum marianum*),** standardized to 80% silymarin and 30% silibinins: 750 mg daily, with or without meals
- **Natural progesterone:** 1/4–1/2 teaspoon of cream twice daily on days 15–28 of the menstrual cycle
- **Indole-3-carbinol (I3C):** 80–160 mg daily
- **3,3'-diindolylmethane (DIM):** 14–28 mg daily
- **Calcium D-glucarate:** 200 mg daily, with or without food

In addition, the following *blood tests* may provide helpful information:

- Cancer Antigen 125 (CA-125)
- Female Comprehensive Hormone Panel

---

### REFERENCES

References available at: www.lef.org/dpt5/ch53

# 54

# *Epilepsy*

*Seizures*, which are characterized by transient behavioral changes, are due to abnormal electrical activity within the brain. *Epilepsy* is a neurologic disorder denoted by the periodic occurrence of seizures; numerous types of epilepsy have been described.

Approximately 3 million people experience epilepsy in the United States and there are 200 000 cases diagnosed each year. Epilepsy most commonly begins in children under the age of 2 or adults over the age of 65. Roughly 3% of the general population will experience epilepsy by age 75.[1]

Conventional treatment for epilepsy is primarily based on antiepileptic drugs (AEDs), and often, epilepsy patients must endure significant clinical experimentation to find a regimen that works for them. Most importantly, not all patients will respond well to AEDs, either due to a lack of effectiveness or due to side effects.

Research has shed light on aspects of epilepsy that remain underappreciated by the conventional establishment. For example, special dietary regimens, such as the *ketogenic diet*, have the capacity to provide benefit for epilepsy patients and represent a potential adjuvant to mainstream therapies.

Moreover, *magnesium* is a well-known anticonvulsive agent, and studies show that magnesium deficiency is associated with epilepsy; intravenous magnesium can effectively control different types of seizures as well.[2-4] However, the efficacy of supplemental magnesium has historically been limited in the context of conditions involving the central nervous system due to the inability of most types of magnesium to efficiently cross the *blood–brain barrier*. Recently, though, scientists at the Massachusetts Institute of Technology have develop a groundbreaking new form of supplemental magnesium, called *magnesium-L-threonate*, that elevates brain magnesium levels more than conventional types of magnesium.[5]

Other important contributors to epilepsy include *oxidative stress* and *mitochondrial dysfunction*.[6] Recent evidence indicates that supplementation with mitochondrial protectants like *ubiquinol (CoQ10)* and *pyrroloquinoline quinone (PQQ)* can target these

underlying pathologic features of epilepsy and may complement the effects of conventional AEDs.[7,8]

In this protocol, you will learn how irregular electrical activity in the brain causes seizures, and how several variables influence neuronal excitability. You will also read about several novel and underutilized treatment strategies and scientifically studied natural compounds with the potential to modulate the overactive neural network of the epileptic brain.

## EPILEPSY BACKGROUND

Epileptic seizures range in severity from mild sensory disruption to a short period of staring or unconsciousness to convulsions. Seizures can manifest in a variety of symptoms, including repetitive motions, changes in breathing rate, flushing, sudden lapses in consciousness, hallucinations, rhythmic twitching of muscles or a generalized loss of muscle control.[9]

People with epilepsy have a substantially higher mortality rate than the general population. This is attributable to a phenomenon known as *sudden unexplained death in epilepsy patients* (SUDEP). SUDEP is unexpected and nontraumatic and occurs in approximately 1% of epileptics.[10] It has no clear anatomic or toxicologic cause, although it may be due to cardiac arrhythmias sometimes triggered by epileptic electrical activity. In the United States, SUDEP may account for 8–17% of all deaths in individuals with epilepsy, with greater incidence in younger individuals. Major risk factors for SUDEP include epilepsy occurring earlier in life, lying in bed in a face-down position, having poorly controlled epilepsy, and being male. In fact, the male-to-female ratio can be as high as 1.75:1.[11] One of the most important things that epileptics can do to lower their risk of SUDEP is to improve control of their disease, which for many patients can be achieved by changing their diet and taking supplements in addition to taking their AEDs. Sleeping on your back may also lower your risk of SUDEP.[12]

## NEUROBIOLOGY OF EPILEPSY

The brain contains billions of neurons, which are in constant communication with one another. During nerve cell signaling, or "firing," chemicals called *neurotransmitters* are released into the space between neurons (*synapse*) to carry the signal. Neurotransmitters influence the action of neurons, either by triggering (exciting) or discouraging (inhibiting) a neuron's firing. The firing of neurons is mediated by electrical signals; as a result, abnormal electrical activity can cause uncontrolled neuron firing, leading to seizures.

Epileptic seizures are caused by a disruption in electrical activity among neurons in the *cerebral cortex*, the most highly developed part of the human brain. Comprising about two-thirds of the brain's mass, the cortex is responsible for thinking, perception and the production and understanding of language. The cortex is also responsible for processing and interpreting the 5 senses.

The nervous system has 2 major divisions: the central nervous system and the peripheral nervous system. The central nervous system consists of the brain and the spinal cord. The peripheral nervous system also has 2 parts: the *somatic nervous system* and the *autonomic nervous system* (which is further divided into 3 parts: sympathetic, parasympathetic, and enteric). The autonomic nervous system exercises control over automatic or involuntary functions in the body, such as heart rate and respiration, among others. Although seizures emanate from the brain, there is a complex interaction between the autonomic nervous system and the central nervous system with regard to seizures.

Some seizures have a preliminary phase, known as an *aura*. An aura is a brief electrical discharge in the brain that can alert a person with epilepsy that a larger seizure is imminent. Epilepsy auras can range from a nonspecific strange or peculiar sensation to feelings of extreme fear or euphoria to the experience of strange lights or strange sounds. (Epilepsy auras are different from migraine headache auras.) The auras are actually small focal seizures that do not affect consciousness. Researchers have also developed techniques that allow them to identify the type of brain activity that occurs in auras in the hopes of learning more about how these focal electrical disturbances contribute to more generalized seizure activity.[13]

# CAUSES OF EPILEPSY AND COMMON SEIZURE TRIGGERS

There are multiple different health problems that can cause epilepsy. For example, brain tumors, either benign or malignant, brain trauma, autoimmune irregularities, and neurologic diseases such as stroke and Alzheimer's can lead to seizures.[14] These represent forms of epilepsy that are acquired and have a distinct cause.

*Idiopathic epilepsy* describes epilepsies with no identifiable cause. Genetics are thought to play a role in many cases of idiopathic epilepsy, as close relatives of an epileptic are 5 times as likely to develop epilepsy themselves.[15]

In susceptible individuals, seizures can be precipitated by the presence of certain factors referred to as triggers, which include low blood sugar (hypoglycemia), dehydration, fatigue, lack of sleep, stress, extreme heat or cold, depression, and flashing or flickering lights. Food and environmental sensitivities may trigger seizures in some people.

## Electrolyte Imbalances

Electrolytes are minerals, such as sodium and potassium, which have an electrical charge when dissolved in the body's fluids. The human brain relies on these minerals to generate the electrical currents needed for neurons to function and communicate. Consequently, alterations in the levels of these electrolytes can severely affect the electrical activity in the brain and trigger seizures in epileptics. Diminished sodium levels (hyponatremia) were associated with increased frequency of seizures in a cross-sectional study of 363 patients in a county hospital.[16] New onset epileptic seizures in a 54-year-old woman who consumed a large amount of a soft drink were described in a case report; her seizures were attributed to a sudden drop in sodium levels due to excessive fluid consumption.[17] Magnesium and calcium deficiencies can also trigger or exacerbate seizures in epileptics.[18]

## Caffeine and Methylxanthines

Methylxanthines, including caffeine, are a family of natural stimulants that can be found in many foods and beverages, including coffee, tea, and chocolate. Methylxanthines increase activity in the central nervous system and can increase the excitability of neurons. There have been case reports of increasing seizure frequency, even in patients with formerly well-controlled epilepsy, following heavy coffee consumption. In one case, 4 cups of coffee a day was associated with an increase in seizure frequency from 2 per month to several per week, and in another, 5–6 cups daily caused 2 seizures in a month in a young epileptic with well-controlled epilepsy.[19–21] Experimental models indicate that caffeine lowers the seizure threshold, thus making AEDs less effective.[22] After thoroughly reviewing the available evidence and conducting some animal model experiments, one group of investigators said that "the existing clinical data confirm the experimental results in that caffeine intake in epileptic patients results in increased seizure frequency. It may be concluded that epileptic patients should limit their daily intake of caffeine."[23]

## Stress

A 2003 study revealed that emotional stress exacerbated seizures in 64% of epileptics.[24] Other studies have corroborated these findings.[25,26] Similarly, fatigue and a lack of sleep can also trigger seizures.[27,28]

## Reactive Oxygen Species

Free radicals may play a role in epilepsy.[29,30] These compounds have the ability to damage proteins, DNA, and the membranes of cells, potentially causing neurons to fire erratically leading to a seizure. Many factors can induce production of free radicals, including head trauma and neurodegenerative diseases as well as normal cellular metabolism.[31] *Mitochondria*, the cellular energy cores in which adenosine triphosphate (ATP) production takes place, are the primary source of free radicals within the body. As we age, the efficiency and integrity of these vital organelles begins to falter, leading to increasing oxidative stress and cellular deterioration. With regard to epilepsy, a relevant consequence of age-related mitochondrial dysfunction is cellular membrane damage, which can impair cellular communication, potentially leading to seizures. Indeed, experimental models indicate that animals genetically prone to a poor ability to quench mitochondrial free radicals are more likely to have seizures than normal animals.[32] Moreover, in humans, heritable defects in the mitochondrial genome cause a subclass of epilepsy called mitochondrial epilepsy.[6]

Mitochondrial energy metabolism can be targeted with some natural compounds; in particular, *coenzyme Q10* (CoQ10) and *pyrroloquinoline quinone* (PQQ). Studies indicate that both of these nutrients quell mitochondrial oxidative stress and promote overall mitochondrial vigor; PQQ even stimulates the growth of new mitochondria via a process called mitochondrial biogenesis.[8,33] In a well-designed animal model, researchers recently showed that CoQ10 reduced the severity of seizures and quelled the seizure-induced increase in oxidative stress that is responsible for epilepsy-related neuronal damage.[7] Most important, CoQ10 augmented the effects of phenytoin, a conventional AED, and spared cognitive function in rats that had seizures.[7] In other words, when seizure-prone animals were given CoQ10 plus phenytoin, their seizures were less severe than in animals receiving the AED alone.

## Aspartame

Phenylalanine, a metabolite of aspartame, can be neurotoxic at high concentrations. Therefore, it is plausible that very high doses of aspartame may trigger seizures, though this has not been observed in controlled clinical studies. In a study of people who anecdotally reported that aspartame triggered their seizures, no seizures were produced under controlled conditions of aspartame exposure.[34] Another study of children with a particular type of seizure called petit mal seizures, however, did demonstrate changes in brain electrical activity after very high oral doses of aspartame, though none of the subjects had an actual seizure.[35] In this study, the dose administered was 40 mg/kg, or about 2800 mg for a 70-kg (154-lb) human. For perspective, a can of diet soda typically contains about 180 mg of aspartame; therefore, the dose of aspartame administered to the children in the study was equivalent to over 15 cans of diet soda for an adult. In contrast, an intensive review published in 2002 found that there was no conclusive scientific evidence linking aspartame to epilepsy.[36]

Similarly, the food additive *monosodium glutamate* (MSG) has been alleged to cause seizures. However, evidence implicating the amounts of MSG commonly encountered in food in the pathology of seizures is primarily, although not exclusively, anecdotal in nature. Monosodium glutamate can indeed induce seizures in animal models, but the dose required is equivalent to several thousand grams of MSG for a grown human—a dose highly unlikely to be attainable through dietary means alone. Nonetheless, some older reports suggest that MSG might lower seizure threshold in sensitive children.[37]

Even though peer-reviewed evidence that directly implicates these dietary excitotoxins in necessarily triggering seizures among adult humans is lacking, some innovative doctors have noted substantial, although anecdotal, benefit when their seizure patients have been advised to carefully avoid food containing MSG. Therefore, it may be prudent for seizure patients, especially children, to avoid ingestion of aspartame and MSG.

## Environmental Toxins

Many environmental toxins, including some pesticides and heavy metals, are known to trigger seizures. For instance, mercury and lead are associated with seizures.[38–40] For more information on the health impact of heavy metals, see the Heavy Metal Detoxification protocol. Also, insecticides known as organophosphates increase brain activity and can cause seizures.[41,42] Additional information is available in the Metabolic Detoxification protocol.

# DIAGNOSING EPILEPSY

Epilepsy is usually diagnosed on the basis of a combination of clinical findings, including patient history, physical examination, and laboratory testing. During an office visit, a patient will typically undergo a standard neurologic examination, which includes evaluation of orientation, reflexes, motor control, nerve function, coordination, and sensory perception. It is often helpful for a physician to examine the person as soon after seizure activity as possible.

The most common diagnostic test to detect epilepsy is the *electroencephalogram* (EEG), which monitors electrical activity in the brain. However, brain activity may be normal between seizures, so a normal EEG does not rule out a diagnosis of epilepsy. Other brain imaging studies, including magnetic resonance imaging (MRI) and computed tomography (CT) scanning, are sometimes used to identify physical causes of seizures, such as tumors or malformations in the brain's vasculature (aneurysms).

# CONVENTIONAL TREATMENTS FOR EPILEPSY

## Anti-Epileptic Drugs (AEDs)

Standard conventional treatments for epilepsy often rely on AEDs, which may need to be taken for many years. AEDs are grouped by their mechanism of action (many of the drugs listed below have multiple mechanisms of action):

- **Sodium channel blockers** (carbamazepine [Tegretol®, Carbatrol®], lamotrigine [Lamictal®], phenytoin [Dilantin®])

- **Calcium current inhibitors** (valproic acid [Depakene®, Depakote®])

- **Gamma-aminobutyric acid enhancers** (vigabatrin [Sabril®], benzodiazepines, barbituates)

- **Glutamate blockers** (topiramate [Topamax®]), also targets sodium channels

- **Carbonic anhydrase inhibitors** (acetazolamide [Diamox®])

- **Those with unknown mechanisms** (levetiracetam [Keppra®])

Drug selection is based on clinical diagnosis as well as characteristics of the AED and its side effects. The choice of drug also depends on the personal preferences and experiences of the treating physician as well as the clinical context (eg, in an emergency room, intravenous administration would be a typical approach). Sometimes the type of epilepsy can also guide the choice of drug. For example, the medication valproic acid is often more effective in treating generalized epilepsy than other AEDs.[43] On the other hand, ethosuximide, another AED, is sometimes more effective for absence seizures. In an outpatient setting, many choices are available.

The optimal treatment outcome is complete cessation of seizures with one AED, also known as monotherapy. In general, almost 50% of adult patients and 66% of pediatric patients will become seizure free with the first drug that they try.[44,45] If the first AED fails or causes intolerable side effects, another one can be selected; many physicians will opt for an AED with a different mechanism of action. If the first AED fails because of intolerable side effects, a second trial of AEDs will be successful in approximately 50% of patients; however, in patients for whom the first drug was not effective, a second AED will be effective less than 15% of the time.[46]

When successful seizure control with monotherapy cannot be achieved, other AEDs are added to the treatment regimen. Polypharmacy (the use of multiple AEDs for epilepsy) is based on a combination of the various known mechanisms of action.[47] Each medication should be titrated upward in dosage until either seizures are eradicated or side effects become intolerable. Certain individuals with intractable seizures can be treated with as many as 4 different AEDs concomitantly.

Most AEDs have some side effects that can be intolerable for patients. As a result, although AED therapy is one of the mainstays of epilepsy treatment, other options may provide significant relief with fewer or milder side effects. In most instances, careful blood monitoring must be performed to determine the blood levels of each AED especially when a patient is taking multiple AEDs or other pharmaceuticals that alter metabolism.

## Surgical Intervention

Surgery for epilepsy is a very highly specialized operation and is typically reserved for patients who do not respond well to AEDs. It should be performed only by the most experienced teams of neurosurgeons, epileptologists (neurologists specializing in epilepsy), and other physicians in major academic centers. Successful surgery for epilepsy is dependent on finding a "focal lesion," an abnormality that can be seen on a radiological imaging scan. Common examples of focal lesions include masses; less common focal lesions include scars or fibrosis. The best surgical outcomes occur in individuals who have a diagnosis of temporal lobe epilepsy, a well-circumscribed focal lesion, or abnormal EEG data that are focal in nature to match the imaging abnormality.

In these cases, the success rate, defined as patients that become seizure-free, ranges from 80–90%. For individuals who do not have matching lesions on EEG and imaging, the success rate falls to about 50% (still considered favorable). Complications are few and insignificant compared to the improved quality of life as a result of seizure reduction.[48] However, surgery is not the only procedure that can provide significant relief for epileptics.

## Other Neurologic Procedures

**Vagal nerve stimulation.** The vagus nerve, which relays information to and from the brain, has many connections to neurologic areas that are instrumental in seizures. Vagal nerve stimulation (VNS) is the only form of electrical treatment for epilepsy approved by the Food and Drug Administration (FDA). Vagal nerve stimulation was approved by the FDA in July 1997 as an adjunctive treatment for partial-type seizures in adults and adolescents older than 12 who did not respond well to AEDs. In vagal nerve stimulation, a small electrical device, about the size of a pocket watch, is implanted under the skin along with a connecting wire in the left upper chest area. Small leads are attached to the vagus nerve on the left side of the neck. The implantation takes about 2 hours. After implantation, the stimulator device is programmed to deliver electrical stimulation automatically 24 hours a day (usually every few minutes).[49]

Not only can vagal nerve stimulation reduce the severity and frequency of seizures, but it can also abort a seizure after it starts. Although the mechanism of vagal nerve stimulation therapy is still unclear, researchers think that it is able to increase inhibitory signals in the brain, helping to prevent the electrical activity that leads to seizures. Vagal nerve stimulation has been found to be safe and effective. Patients that have their seizure frequency reduced by 50% or more are classified as "responders." With long-term use, 50–80% of patients who receive vagal nerve stimulation treatment will become responders, depending on the seizure type.[50–54] Reduction of AED use was reported in 43% of patients following vagal nerve stimulation for intractable epilepsy, and subjective improvement in quality of life occurred in 84%.[55]

**Deep brain stimulation (DBS).** DBS is another novel therapy that may provide significant benefits for epileptics. This treatment involves the placement of electrodes in the brain using minimally invasive surgery that can then be used to send mild electrical currents to particular regions of the brain, such as the thalamus, the cerebellum, and other deep regions in the brain. This technique was initially developed in the 1980s as a way to reduce

tremors in patients with Parkinson's disease and has gained support for treating other movement disorders, such as dyskinesia. Its effects on these other neurologic issues have spurred interest using deep brain stimulation to treat epilepsy.[56–58]

Early clinical studies on deep brain stimulation have found that it is generally safe, with the adverse effects being transient and mild. Some patients have experienced side effects such as episodic nystagmus (uncontrollable eye movements), auditory hallucinations, and lethargy.[57] However, one of the advantages of deep brain stimulation is that it can be switched off if side effects appear and the entire procedure is reversible. Early results from multiple clinical trials of deep brain stimulation have found that it can reduce seizures in a significant portion of patients, depending on its placement.[59]

**Transcranial magnetic stimulation.** Transcranial magnetic stimulation is a noninvasive technique that uses electromagnetic currents to alter the electrical activity in the brain. This therapy has shown great promise for reducing seizures in epileptics by reducing neuronal excitability. Some of the earliest studies found that transcranial magnetic stimulation can induce a prolonged period of protection from the types of electrical activity that cause seizures.[60] Case studies have found that this technique can reduce seizure frequency by over 60% in patients.[61] The most serious side effect associated with transcranial magnetic stimulation is a headache, although there is a small risk of seizure during this treatment.[62] However, this risk is low and this technique is considered to be safe; in addition, as transcranial magnetic stimulation technology advances and is combined with EEGs, this therapy can be used in a more targeted and safer way.[63]

## NOVEL AND EMERGING DRUG STRATEGIES

The pharmaceutical industry continues to make new AEDs to provide additional options for controlling epilepsy while also minimizing side effects. One new AED, known as *levetiracetam*, has recently been approved for monotherapy. Although the specific mechanisms are unclear, levitiracetam works by inhibiting synaptic conductance in ways different than traditional AEDs, so it may be effective for the treatment of epilepsies that have not responded well to other medications.[64] Other novel AEDs are only approved for adjunctive treatment, which means they can be added onto already existing drug regimens. Three of the newest AEDs that are approved for adjunctive therapy are *eslicarabzepine acetate*, *lacosamide*, and *retigabine*.

Eslicarbazepine acetate works using a similar mechanism to an already established AED, carbamazepine, but it has less neurotoxicity.[65,66] Eslicarbazepine also has fewer reported side effects than a similar AED, oxcarbazepine and can be taken once per day. As a result, eslicarbazepine acetate is being used as an additional AED for patients who do not have adequate control of their epilepsy with other medications[67] Another recently developed AED is lacosamide.[45] This drug has been shown to reduce electrical seizure activity in the brain without affecting other aspects of brain function.[68] Lacosamide works on a different part of neurons than other AEDs, so its novel mechanism may allow it to be more effective in patients that have not responded well to other AEDs.[69,70] Similarly, the new medication retigabine also has a different mechanism than other AEDs and so it can be added onto the treatment regimens of epileptics who are still having frequent seizures with less concern about impaired effectiveness.[71]

Together, these new medications, as well as other new drugs like *stiripentol* (Diacomit®) and *rufinamide* (Banzel®), have the potential to treat previously intractable cases of epilepsy or to reduce side effects. Some researchers have also noted that diuretics, such as *furosemide* and *bumetanide*, may also be able to reduce seizures by affecting the levels of water and ions in the brain.[72] Although there have not been any recent clinical studies of the effects of diuretics on epilepsy, studies examining the effects of these medications in tissue and animal models of epilepsy have been promising, and one small clinical study published in 1976 found that diuretics were able to significantly reduce seizure frequency in some patients.[73]

## HORMONE IMBALANCE

Hormone imbalances may play a role in epilepsy. Female epileptics often have an exacerbation of their condition at specific points during their menstrual cycle, which is sometimes called *catamenial epilepsy*. Seizures in women often increase during periods of low progesterone.[74] Research has found that estrogen *increases* neuronal excitability and progesterone *reduces* neuronal activity, which suggests that an imbalance between estrogen and progesterone could increase seizure frequency.[75] Lower progesterone levels are also associated with more frequent seizures in women, and elevated estrogen levels during perimenopause also appear to exacerbate epilepsy.[76,77]

Progesterone restoration therapy has been studied as a possible treatment of epilepsy and initial results have been promising.[78] The effects of hormones on epilepsy still needs to be better elucidated, as some studies have suggested that estrogen can have proepileptic and antiepileptic properties, depending on its levels.[79] Women are not the only patients that can have their epilepsy affected by sex hormone levels; testosterone and its metabolites also have antiseizure effects.[80,81] Indeed, in a case report of a man with posttraumatic seizures, testosterone therapy caused his seizures to lessen and nearly disappear.[82] These findings suggest that maintaining optimal testosterone levels may ameliorate seizure disorders in men. Free testosterone is a good indicator of testosterone activity; optimal levels are 20–25 pg/mL.

For more information about hormone testing and hormone replacement, refer to the Male and Female Hormone Restoration protocols.

## DIETARY MANAGEMENT: THE KETOGENIC DIET AND OTHERS

The idea that diet can affect epilepsy was first postulated by Hippocrates, who noticed that fasting could prevent convulsions.[83] Currently there are 4 different dietary treatments that can be used for epilepsy: the ketogenic, medium-chain triglyceride, modified Atkins, and low-glycemic index diets.

The most widely used dietary treatment for epilepsy is the *ketogenic diet*. The ketogenic consists of high intake of fats (80%) and low intake of protein and carbohydrates; it was developed in the 1920s.[84,85] The ketogenic diet requires patients to be very careful about what they eat for it to be effective.[86,87]

The ketogenic diet is carefully designed so that fats, primarily in the form of long-chain fatty acids, provide the main source of calories in the diet. Typically patients need to consume 3–4 times as much fat by weight compared to carbohydrates and proteins; this means that with this diet, over 90% of the calories come from fat. This high-fat diet changes the body's metabolism, causing it to generate chemicals known as ketones, which can then be burned for energy. This diet is also designed to provide approximately 1 g of protein for every kg of body weight to ensure adequate protein intake. The ketogenic diet typically begins with a brief fasting period, although this is not necessary and is often based on the clinician's preferences.[88]

The way that the ketogenic diet prevents seizure is still under investigation. One of the prevailing theories is that the *ketones* produced by the diet are able to enter into the brain. From there, the ketones are able to increase the levels of chemicals that decrease neuron activity, reduce levels of reactive oxygen species and make the brain use energy more efficiently, resulting in fewer seizures.[88,89]

The ketogenic diet has consistently been proven to be an effective treatment for epilepsy. Reviews have found that over 50% of children undergoing the ketogenic diet have a greater than 50% reduction in their seizure frequency, with over 30% experiencing a decrease in seizure frequency of over 90% and more than 15% becoming completely seizure free.[90] These numbers are even greater for children that maintain the ketogenic diet for 3 months: over half of the children have their seizures reduced by 90% or more and over 30% become completely seizure free.[91] The benefits of the ketogenic diet have also been confirmed by the randomized control trial, which is the most rigorous of clinical trials.[92]

Although the ketogenic diet has traditionally been recommended for children, it may also be used with great success in adolescents and adults. Clinical studies examining the effects of the ketogenic diet on older patients have shown that the diet can produce a significant reduction in seizure frequency in this population as well.[93–95] One of the main obstacles for adolescents and adults trying the ketogenic diet is patient compliance, because the diet can be so restrictive. As a result, multiple similar diets have also been designed to try to take advantage of the concept behind the ketogenic diet without significantly reducing its effectiveness. The *medium-chain triglyceride diet* is based on the idea that shorter fat molecules, such as medium-chain triglycerides, produce more ketones and thus allow for more protein and carbohydrate in the diet. Other diet plans, including the *modified Atkins diet* and the *low-glycemic index treatment*, have also been developed to allow more flexibility. The modified Atkins diet allows for 10–30 g carbohydrates each day and has no restrictions on protein or caloric intake. The low-glycemic index treatment allows a higher amount of carbohydrates (40–60 g/day) as long as they have a glycemic index of <50. Both of these modified ketogenic diets have also proven beneficial in the treatment of epilepsy.[96]

The ketogenic diet and related metabolic treatments for epilepsy can cause some side effects and nutritional deficiencies. The most common side effects are gastrointestinal issues, such as diarrhea, constipation, nausea, vomiting, and increases acid reflux.

This diet can also raise the levels of cholesterol and other lipids in the blood. Patients undergoing the ketogenic diet may also have an increased risk of a vitamin D deficiency, leading to reduced bone strength, as well as kidney stones, selenium deficiency, and increased bruising. As a result, vitamin supplementation and careful monitoring may be needed during the ketogenic diet.[97–101]

## LIFESTYLE MODIFICATIONS

### Seizure Interruptions

Although auras do not occur in all individuals with seizure disorders, some people are aware of a change in their sensory perception (whether auditory, olfactory, sensory, visual, or gustatory, sometimes involving malaise, vertigo, or the sense of deja vu) that signals the onset of a seizure. Anecdotal reports indicate that some people have learned to interrupt their seizure process by replacing the aura-induced perception with another. In these individuals, the aura is a known signal of seizure onset. For example, if the aura is a smell or unpleasant odor, these individuals can often interrupt the seizure by immediately smelling something else (in general, something with a more pleasing smell than the aura).

Some people are able to take the interruption technique a step further. By simply relying on mental imagery (eg, remembering a pleasant, positive smell), they can arrest a seizure. Some find that anger can effectively interrupt a seizure; they are able to arrest their seizures by yelling at them. Other individuals who have seizures with an observable onset pattern enlist a support person to shout at them or give them a quick shake when the pattern commences. The techniques that successfully "interrupt" an aura vary from patient to patient and must be performed at a specific time to stop the seizure[102] However, the use of aura interruption may be able to help reduce or eliminate seizures.[103]

### Stress Reduction

Getting a good night's sleep on a regular basis is a very important component of seizure prevention. Some scientists hypothesize that one major function of REM sleep is to reduce the brain's susceptibility to epileptogenic influences.[104] Stress reduction and relaxation techniques such as meditation may also aid in reducing seizures.[105]

Physical exercise can also be an important way to relieve stress that may be particularly beneficial for epileptics. Not only can exercise reduce stress, improve social integration and improve quality of life, regular physical exercise may directly help reduce seizure frequency.[106] Physical exercise may "desensitize" neurons to emotional stress, helping avert seizures brought on by other triggers.[107]

## Biofeedback

Biofeedback, another relaxation technique, can also be helpful. When the autonomic nervous system (or the involuntary nervous system) is in a state of over-arousal, the likelihood of seizure activity can increase. Biofeedback is a technique that uses displays of some form of biological monitoring, such as an EEG, to help patients identify how their body responds to certain situations. By observing changes in EEG readings, patients are able to learn how to partially control the electrical activity in their brains and can develop the ability to reduce their risk of having seizures. Although most clinical trials involving biofeedback have been small,[108–110] a comprehensive review of many studies found that biofeedback can provide significant relief for epileptics, particularly those that have not had success with AEDs.[111] On average, almost 75% of people who try EEG biofeedback for epilepsy will experience fewer seizures. Biofeedback using other biologic responses, such as slow cortical potential feedback and galvanic skin response has also been promising.[112]

Other behavioral interventions may reduce seizure frequency as well. *Yoga* can improve quality of life and result in fewer seizures.[113,114] *Acupuncture* may also be helpful in seizure prevention. A thorough review of published trials found that acupuncture may be beneficial, but that more and better-designed studies need to be done.[115] Studies of the benefits of other relaxation techniques and *cognitive behavioral therapy* have also found a possible benefit.[116]

## NATURAL AND COMPLEMENTARY THERAPIES

Many natural compounds also affect the brain and may be able to influence epilepsy; natural compounds will likely be most beneficial as adjuvants to conventional therapies.

## Vitamins and Minerals

Epilepsy patients should also be aware that long-term use of AEDs can negatively affect their vitamin and mineral status. For instance, patients taking AEDs have significantly lower levels of *vitamin D* in their blood.[117–121] This is because many AEDs increase the activity of a liver enzyme known as cytochrome P450, which also breaks down vitamin D. Vitamin D is essential for the absorption of *calcium*; consequently, patients taking AEDS absorb less calcium in their

diet, which increases their risk of developing osteoporosis. Patients who are taking AEDs may need to take vitamin D and calcium supplements.[122]

AEDs have also been shown to reduce levels of several B vitamins, including folate and vitamins B6 and B12.[123,124] These vitamins are critical for controlling metabolism in the body; low levels of these vitamins can also lead to low red blood cell levels, causing fatigue and pallor. One of the most serious consequences of the low folate levels caused by AEDs is high levels of the compound *homocysteine*, a risk factor for heart disease[123,125,126] Elevated levels of homocysteine have been implicated in the increased risk of heart disease seen in epileptics. Moreover, some studies have indicated that elevated homocysteine may contribute to AED resistance or increase seizures in epileptics.[127] Based on these findings, some researchers call for routine supplementation with the B vitamins, especially the metabolically active form of folic acid, *L-methylfolate*, to reduce homocysteine levels.[128] Folate deficiencies can also lead to seizures, particularly in infants. Impaired folate transport in the body can be a cause of seizures that do not respond well to typical treatments.[129] In addition, epileptics often have reduced folic acid levels, possibly due to the use of AEDs.[130] Doctors of epileptics should routinely monitor folic acid, vitamin B12 and homocysteine levels in patients to help prevent an increased risk of cardiovascular disease that could otherwise be treated.

Some forms of epilepsy are directly linked to vitamin B6 deficiencies; these convulsions, known as pyridoxine-dependent seizures, can only be treated with high doses of vitamin B6.[131] Low vitamin B6 levels are also associated with general epilepsy. Even in patients without pyridoxine-dependent seizures, low levels of pyridoxine might increase seizure sensitivity, although more research needs to be done to determine if pyridoxine can treat seizures.[132] Some types of seizures cannot be treated with pyridoxine, but they can be effectively managed with *pyridoxal-5-phosphate*, the biologically active form of vitamin B6.[133–135]

Antioxidants, such as *vitamin E*, *vitamin C*, and *selenium* are able to mitigate mitochondrial oxidative stress in the brain and other tissues, lowering seizure frequency in various types of epilepsy.[136–142] Animal models have shown that *alpha-tocopherol* alone is able to prevent several types of seizures.[143,144] Epileptics are also more likely to have low vitamin E levels, though this may be a result of taking AEDs.[145]

## Magnesium

Magnesium helps maintain connections between neurons. It has been shown to suppress EEG activity and limit seizure severity in animal models, and magnesium deficiency is associated with seizures in humans.[146-148] Within the body, ionic magnesium acts as a natural calcium channel blocker, offsetting the excitatory influence of ionic calcium in a manner similar to the calcium channel blocker class of conventional AEDs.[149] Moreover, magnesium levels decline sharply following seizures in patients with idiopathic epilepsy.[150] In fact, intravenous or intramuscular magnesium is often administered to women to safely prevent eclampsia, a pregnancy-associated disorder characterized by seizures.[151]

A recently developed form of magnesium, known as *magnesium-L-threonate*, may be particularly effective in epilepsy and other neurologic disorders. This form of magnesium appears to be better at penetrating the *blood–brain barrier* and thus is more efficiently delivered to brain cells.[152,153] In fact, in an animal model, magnesium-L-threonate boosted magnesium levels in spinal fluid by an impressive 15% compared to virtually no increase with conventional magnesium. Moreover, oral magnesium-L-threonate was able to modulate learning and memory, indicating that it does indeed impact the central nervous system.[154]

Thiamine, manganese and biotin are often low in epileptics as well.[155]

## Melatonin

Melatonin plays an important role in the brain, particularly in regulating the brain's sleep–wake cycle. It also exerts a calming effect at the neuronal level by reducing glutaminergic (excitatory) signaling and augmenting GABAergic (inhibitory) signaling.[156] Melatonin is widely used as a sleep aid and to treat jet lag; the side effects of taking melatonin are mild, and it is one of the most commonly used supplements in the United States. Animal models have shown that melatonin can be effective in reducing epileptic seizures.[157,158] Melatonin has also been beneficial in humans with epilepsy, and is particularly effective in the treatment of cases of juvenile epilepsy that do not respond well to AEDs.[156] Due to its widespread use and minimal side effects, melatonin has potential to improve control of epilepsy.[159]

## Polyunsaturated Fatty Acids

Polyunsaturated fatty acids (PUFAs), such as omega-3 fatty acids, are a type of essential fat that play an important role in maintaining central nervous system health. Animal studies have suggested that PUFAs, including omega-3 and some omega-6 fatty acids, may be able to modulate neuronal excitability.[160,161] This is further supported by the fact that children on the ketogenic diet often have higher levels of PUFAs in their cerebrospinal fluid, which suggests that increased PUFA levels is one of the ways that the ketogenic diet prevents seizures.[162,163] Clinical trials in adults have yielded mixed results. In one such study, 57 epileptic patients were given 1 g EPA and 0.7 g DHA daily. Seizure activity was reduced over the first 6 weeks, although the effect was temporary. The researchers called for more in-depth studies, with larger doses and larger observational groups.[164] However, a randomized controlled trial did not find that fish oil reduced seizure frequency; although, the study did find, that PUFAs reduced seizures when administered in an open-label format, meaning when subjects knew that they were not receiving a placebo.[165] An ongoing National Institutes of Health-sponsored trial is examining the effects of fish oil on cardiac health in epileptics.[166]

Life Extension suggests that the omega-6 to omega-3 ratio should be kept below 4 to 1 for optimal health. More information on testing and optimizing your omega-6 to omega-3 ratio can be found in the *Life Extension Magazine* article titled "Optimize Your Omega-3 Status."

## Resveratrol

Resveratrol, derived from red grapes and Japanese knotweed (*Polygonum cuspidatum*), and the plant *Bacopa monnieri* both appear to be promising in the management of seizure-related neurotoxicity. Resveratrol and bacopa-derived compounds have been extensively studied in experimental settings and consistently shown to guard against neuronal damage.[167-170] In the context of epilepsy, numerous mechanisms by which resveratrol might prevent seizures have been proposed,[171] and, indeed, in an animal model resveratrol prevented chemical-induced seizures,[172] though studies on epileptic humans have yet to be performed. Likewise, bacopa has been the subject of several animal model experiments, many of which have revealed a clear benefit relating to seizure frequency and postseizure brain cell damage.[173-175] Nonetheless, bacopa also has yet to be studied in a controlled manner in a population of epileptic humans.

## Phytocannabinoids

Phytocannabinoids (pCBs), which are compounds found in marijuana that closely resemble chemicals the body produces naturally called *endocannabinoids*, have shown great potential in the treatment of epilepsy. Phytocannabinoids can affect both the central and peripheral nervous system because neurons have receptors that respond directly to binding by cannabinoids. One of the major effects of pCBs is to reduce neuronal excitability by modulating electrical activity around synapses; as a result, these chemicals are sometimes referred to as potential "circuit breakers" for neurologic disorders, including epilepsy.[176,177] Therefore, researchers have been studying the effects of tetrahydrocannabinol (THC) and other phytocannabinoids on the brain to try to develop new mechanisms for treating epilepsy.[178,179] One small clinical trial found that the phytocannabinoid, cannabidiol, did reduce seizures in epileptics who were already taking AEDs.[180] Another study that was largely based on epidemiology found an association between marijuana use and decreased risk of seizure.[181] Moreover, it has been reported that patients treated for epilepsy subjectively feel that marijuana use helps eases their epilepsy.[182] More research is needed to determine the efficacy and safety of natural and synthetic cannabinoids for the treatment of seizures. A comprehensive review of studies examining the effects of cannabinoids on seizure frequency in humans is currently being carried out by the Cochrane Epilepsy Group.[183] Marijuana is illegal except as a prescribed treatment for medical problems in certain states; Life Extension does not recommend consuming illegal drugs as a treatment for epilepsy. However, the benefits of these phytocannabinoids do suggest that marijuana-derived compounds may soon become an accepted form of therapy for epilepsy and other neurologic disorders.

## Life Extension Suggestions

Most patients with epilepsy will take AEDs. These drugs can affect vitamin status and raise homocysteine levels. Patients taking AEDs are advised to supplement with calcium and vitamin D to help prevent AED-induced osteoporosis and to regularly monitor their homocysteine levels. If homocysteine levels are elevated, patients should take steps to reduce homocysteine by using B vitamins, including L-methylfolate, vitamin B12, and vitamin B6. For more information, see the Homocysteine Reduction protocol.

Patients on a ketogenic diet are advised to take a high-potency multivitamin to ensure adequate availability of nutrients. In addition, a high fiber intake (>20 g daily) is recommended to reduce fluctuations in blood sugar levels.

The following nutrients may help modulate neuronal excitability:

- **B-complex vitamin**
  - Thiamine (B1): 75–125 mg daily
  - Riboflavin (B2): 50 mg daily
  - Niacin (B3): 50–190 mg daily
  - Folate, preferably as L-methylfolate: 400–1000 mcg daily
  - Vitamin B6, preferably as pyridoxal-5-phosphate: 75–105 mg daily
  - Vitamin B12: 300–600 mcg daily
  - Biotin: 300–3000 mcg daily
  - Pantothenic acid: 100–600 mg daily
- **Melatonin:** 0.3–5 mg before bed (sometimes up to 10 mg)
- **Vitamin D:** 5000–8000 IU daily, based on blood test results
- **Natural vitamin E:** 100–400 IU alpha-tocopherol and 200 mg gamma-tocopherol daily
- **Vitamin C:** 1000–2000 mg daily
- **Selenium:** 200 mcg daily
- **Magnesium-L-threonate:** 2000–4000 mg (providing 140–280 mg of elemental magnesium)
- **Manganese:** 1–2 mg daily
- **Calcium:** 200–1200 mg daily
- **Fish oil** (with olive polyphenols): providing 1400 mg EPA and 1000 mg DHA daily
- **CoQ10** (as ubiquinol): 100–200 mg daily
- **Pyrroloquinoline quinone** (PQQ): 10–20 mg daily
- **Trans-resveratrol:** 100–500 mg daily
- **Bacopa extract:** 100–450 mg daily
- **Bioidentical hormone replacement therapy:** see Life Extension's Male Hormone Restoration or Female Hormone Restoration protocol

In addition, the following *blood tests* can provide relevant information for epileptic patients:

- Male or Female Panel (includes glucose, C-reactive protein, LDL, homocysteine, sex hormones, and many other important tests)
- Vitamin D, 25-Hydroxy
- RBC magnesium
- Omega Score®

## REFERENCES

References available at: www.lef.org/dpt5/ch54

# 55

# *Erectile Dysfunction*

Erectile dysfunction is the inability to achieve or sustain a penile erection sufficient for satisfactory male sexual performance.[1,2] The condition affects up to 30 million American men, and is typically age-dependent.[3–5] Erectile dysfunction can cause substantial emotional distress by negatively impacting intimate relationships, self-esteem, and overall quality of life.[1,6,7]

Several pharmacologic treatments for erectile dysfunction are available (eg, Viagra® and Cialis®), but these medications provide only temporary benefits and may cause minor to severe side effects such as headache, indigestion, visual disturbances, and even blindness.[8–11]

The underlying physiology of erectile function is tied very closely to *cardiovascular health*. Therefore, men who wish to perform at their sexual peak must take steps to optimize their blood vessel health.[12–14] Studies show that improving cardiovascular risk factors via healthy lifestyle modifications and pharmacologic treatment can significantly improve male sexual function.[15]

This protocol describes the biology of penile erection and highlights the link between cardiovascular disease and sexual function in men. Medications to temporarily improve erectile function will be discussed, as will integrative strategies for reducing cardiovascular risk and improving overall male sexual function through healthy lifestyle choices, pharmaceutical drugs, and the use of scientifically studied natural compounds.

## UNDERSTANDING ERECTION PHYSIOLOGY

An erection is triggered by a complex interplay between the sympathetic and parasympathetic nervous system, with local sensory stimulation of the genital area and/or central psychogenic stimulation resulting from visual, tactile, auditory, olfactory, and/or imaginative input.[5,6] The *endothelial cells* that line the blood vessels of the penis produce vasoactive factors that dilate blood vessels, one of the most important being *nitric oxide*.

Nitric oxide, by initiating production of another chemical messenger called *cyclic guanosine monophosphate*

(*cGMP*), triggers a biochemical cascade leading to expansion (vasodilatation) of penile blood vessels and allows for increased blood flow into the *corpus cavernosum*, the two columns of spongy tissue that run along the top length of the penis.[1,5,6,16] As the corpus cavernosum fills with blood it stretches, compressing the primary site where blood exits the penis, called the subtunical venules. This compression causes resistance to blood flow out of the penis, producing and maintaining an erection.[1,5,6,17]

## CAUSES OF ERECTILE DYSFUNCTION

Achieving an erection requires coordination between many body systems, so there are several ways the process can go wrong.[18] The cause of erectile dysfunction can be biological, psychological, or both.[1]

### Biological Causes

Biological causes of erectile dysfunction include vascular, hormonal, and neurologic disorders.[2]

**Cardiovascular disease.** Cardiovascular disease accounts for up to 80% of erectile dysfunction cases.[19] *Atherosclerosis*, the most common vascular disease, impedes blood flow to the penis.[20] Cardiovascular disease and *high blood pressure* contribute to *endothelial dysfunction*, which is the most common contributing mechanism to erectile dysfunction overall.[5,6]

**Age-related decline in hormone levels.** Age-related decline in hormone levels (eg, *testosterone* and *dehydroepiandrosterone [DHEA]*) is associated with erectile dysfunction.[6,21,22] (See section titled Erectile Dysfunction and Hormones)

**Diabetes.** Diabetes can interfere with penile blood flow and damage nerves in the penis, leading to erectile dysfunction.[20]

**Age-related decline in penile elastic fibers.** Age-related decline in penile elastic fibers also contributes to erectile dysfunction.[5]

**Medication-induced erectile dysfunction.** Medication-induced erectile dysfunction can occur from several drugs including antihistamines, benzodiazepines, tricyclic antidepressants, and others.[1,23]

### Psychological Causes

Psychological causes such as depression, anxiety, stress, low self-esteem, and various other conditions can contribute to erectile dysfunction as well.[17,20] Psychological problems are often to blame for intermittent erectile dysfunction among young men, while older men with erectile dysfunction frequently have a mixture of both psychological and biological causes.[5]

# THE LINK BETWEEN ERECTILE DYSFUNCTION AND CARDIOVASCULAR DISEASE

It is important for men suffering from erectile dysfunction to discuss their symptoms with their physician.[24] In addition to recommending an effective treatment for the primary complaint of erectile dysfunction, physicians should also screen for cardiovascular disease (CVD).[5,17,25] This is because erectile dysfunction and CVD share similar risk factors, including aging, hypertension, obesity, and a sedentary lifestyle.[14,26,27] Furthermore, erectile dysfunction itself has been shown to independently increase the risk of CVD, stroke, and all-cause death.[1,6]

Since erectile dysfunction often precedes some cardiovascular events by 2–5 years,[25] erectile dysfunction is viewed as a potential early warning sign for CVD.[28] Early detection is critical since CVD is a major cause of disability and death.[14]

The abbreviation ED can help make this issue easy to understand and remember. For instance, ED stands not only for *erectile dysfunction*, but also *endothelial dysfunction*, *exercise and diet* (for prevention), and *early detection* of risk factors, which can help avoid *early death* due to CVD.[29]

# ERECTILE DYSFUNCTION AND HORMONES

## Testosterone

Many facets of male sexual function depend on male hormones (androgens) such as testosterone.[21] Testosterone helps support the production of nitric oxide,[6] but also helps maintain libido.[21] As men age, their androgen levels decline. Low androgen levels are observed in as many as one-third of men with erectile dysfunction.[10]

Androgen deficiency can directly contribute to erectile dysfunction by negatively impacting penile blood flow and increasing breakdown of cGMP.[1,30] Low testosterone is the most common reason for failure to respond to phosphodiesterase-5 (PDE5) inhibitors (eg, Viagra® and Cialis®), which are drugs that slow the breakdown of cGMP.[31]

Clinical guidelines recommend hormone level testing for aging men who suffer from sexual dysfunction. Maintaining optimal testosterone levels is not only important for sexual function, but also for cardiovascular health.[32] Moreover, low androgen levels are associated with depression, osteoporosis, insulin resistance, increased fat mass, decreased lean body mass, and cognitive dysfunction.[6,21] Life Extension recommends that ageing men target optimal *free*

*testosterone* blood levels of *20–25 pg/mL* and *total testosterone* levels of *770–1197 ng/dL*.

*Testosterone* restoration can lead to improved erectile function and libido in men with low androgen levels.[1] In fact, when PDE5 inhibitors fail, the addition of testosterone therapy is associated with substantial improvement in erectile function among men with low testosterone and may eliminate the need for PDE5 inhibitors altogether.[1,6,21,31] Refer to Life Extension's Male Hormone Restoration protocol for more information.

## DHEA

Dehydroepiandrosterone (DHEA) is a precursor to testosterone.[33,34] As with testosterone, aging is associated with decreased levels of DHEA. Circulating levels of DHEA can decline by up to 80% from age 25–80.[34] Low DHEA levels have been linked to erectile dysfunction.[22,35] Studies have shown that oral DHEA supplementation may improve sexual performance, as measured by erectile function, orgasmic function, sexual desire, intercourse satisfaction, and overall satisfaction in some men.[36,37] Life Extension recommends an optimal target blood level for DHEA-sulfate of 350–490 μg/dL.

# AROMATASE INHIBITORS, TESTOSTERONE RESTORATION, AND TESTOSTERONE/ESTROGEN BALANCE

Physicians versed in male hormone restoration know that exogenous administration of testosterone may increase estrogen (estradiol) levels in aging men, in particular aging men with significant amounts of visceral fat. The conversion of testosterone into estrogen is called *aromatization* and is mediated by an enzyme called *aromatase*.[38] Aromatase inhibitors (eg, anastrozole [Arimidex®]) are drugs that inhibit the activity of the aromatase enzyme, thereby reducing the amount of testosterone converted into estradiol.

When used concurrently with testosterone supplementation, aromatase inhibitors allow testosterone levels to rise without being converted into excess estrogen. Reports suggest that aromatase inhibitor therapy can improve sexual function in men.[38]

Maintaining healthy testosterone/estrogen balance has other important implications for aging males. For example, in a study among men with heart failure, both low and high estradiol levels were associated with significantly increased chances of death compared to "balanced" levels.[39] More about estrogen/testosterone balance in men is available in the *Life Extension Magazine* article titled, "Why Estrogen Balance Is Critical to Aging Men."

Life Extension suggests an optimal estrogen level (measured as estradiol) of 20–30 pg/mL for men.

# CONVENTIONAL TREATMENT OF ERECTILE DYSFUNCTION

## Phosphodiesterase-5 (PDE5) Inhibitors

The signaling molecule *cyclic guanosine monophosphate* (*cGMP*) is an important mediator of vasodilatation, penile blood flow, and therefore erection. The natural destruction of cGMP by the *phosphodiesterase-5 (PDE5) enzyme* effectively shuts down the erection process, returning the penis to its nonerect (flaccid) state.[6]

Medications used to treat erectile dysfunction, such as sildenafil (Viagra®), vardenafil (Levitra®), and tadalafil (Cialis®), improve erectile function by inhibiting the PDE5 enzyme, allowing an erection to persist.[6] However, approximately one-third of men with erectile dysfunction do not respond to PDE5 inhibitors.[1] Men whose erectile dysfunction is not improved by PDE5 inhibitors may have low testosterone levels and should have a testosterone blood test.[25]

Although PDE5 inhibitors are generally well tolerated, they can cause a number of side effects including headache, indigestion, visual disturbances, priapism (ie, painful, prolonged erection lasting more than 6 hours), and even blindness.[8–11] Furthermore, the use of PDE5 inhibitors is limited in some men by contraindications such as cardiovascular disease. These drugs can also interact with other medications (eg, nitrates) and cause negative reactions.[1,9–11] PDE5 inhibitors only improve erectile function, not overall sexual function.[1]

## Intracavernosal Medications

In men who are not good candidates for or do not respond well to PDE5 inhibitors, intracavernosal vasodilating medications are a second-line treatment option. These treatments are delivered via self-injection into the cavernosum. Adverse effects may include pain, prolonged erection, and fibrosis.[40–42]

**Alprostadil.** Alprostadil is synthetic prostaglandin E1, which is a biochemical signaling molecule with vasodilatory properties.[43,44] Studies show alprostadil to be effective in about 70% of men with erectile dysfunction.[43] Alprostadil can now be delivered via topical cream as well, which has demonstrated a success rate similar to injectable forms.[45,46]

**Papaverine.** Papaverine, a compound derived from the poppy plant, nonspecifically inhibits phosphodiesterase enzymes and modulates calcium signaling. It does not possess opiate properties like some other poppy derivatives such as morphine. Studies suggest a patient satisfaction rate of about 44%. Papaverine use may increase liver function tests with the potential for hepatotoxicity.[47]

**Phentolamine.** Phentolamine blocks alpha-1 and -2 adrenergic receptors. This helps facilitate erection by impairing muscle constriction. Phentolamine alone is not sufficient to trigger and sustain rigid erection, so it is used in combination with other intracavernosal agents for an additive effect. Because phentolamine is expensive and needs to be refrigerated, it may be less convenient.[47]

## Vacuum Erection Devices (VEDs)

Another alternative is utilizing a vacuum device to artificially increase penile blood flow. These devices consist of plastic cylinders that are placed over the penis and vacuumed by a pump to negative pressure to allow cavernosal expansion and erection. Constriction rings are then placed at the base of the penis to retain blood. Vacuum erection devices provide a relatively safe and efficacious alternative for those unresponsive to or unable to take oral medications. Disadvantages include lack of penile stability, which may interfere with sexual performance, and inhibited ejaculation.[47]

## Behavioral Interventions

Erectile function and overall sexual satisfaction can be considerably impacted by psychological and interpersonal factors. Evidence suggests a psychogenic contribution to as many as 40% of erectile dysfunction cases. Psychosocial variables such as anxiety about seeking erectile dysfunction treatment undermine availability of effective treatment options as well. A comprehensive review conducted in 2008 showed that group psychotherapy can significantly improve erectile dysfunction and complement pharmacologic treatment strategies.[48]

## Shock Wave Therapy

Extracorporeal ultrasound shock wave therapy is used to treat some penile disorders such as Peyronie's disease.[49,50] Application of low-intensity ultrasound shock waves to the penis is emerging as a treatment for erectile dysfunction among men without other penile disorders. In a pioneering, randomized, double-blind, sham-controlled study on 67 men, researchers showed that shock wave therapy significantly improved erectile function and penile blood flow among previous responders to PDE-5 inhibitors. Treatment was well tolerated with none of the subjects reporting discomfort or adverse events.[51] Another study showed that shock wave therapy improved erectile function in 29 men who responded poorly to PDE5 inhibitors.[52]

# LIFESTYLE AND ERECTILE DYSFUNCTION

Certain modifiable conditions and behaviors increase the chances of developing erectile dysfunction. These include lack of physical activity and obesity, as well as alcohol, tobacco, and illicit drug use.[5,23,28] Eating an unhealthy diet low in antioxidants is also linked to erectile dysfunction.[28,53]

The following lifestyle modifications may improve erectile function.[1]

## Regular Physical Exercise

Studies have shown that exercise can improve erectile function, sexual response, and overall cardiovascular health.[28,54]

## Weight Control and Diet

Obesity nearly doubles the risk of erectile dysfunction.[1] Weight control and adoption of a healthier diet (such as the *Mediterranean diet*) may reduce this risk. The principles of a Mediterranean diet include high intake of fruits, vegetables, nuts, whole grains, and fish, with low intake of refined grains as well as red and processed meats. In combination with physical activity, a Mediterranean diet may be especially beneficial for men with erectile dysfunction who also have metabolic syndrome or diabetes.[28,54-57] Furthermore, diets rich in antioxidants have been shown to improve penile blood flow, erectile activity, smooth muscle relaxation, and fibrosis.[28,58]

# TARGETED NATURAL INTERVENTIONS

A variety of natural modalities may improve erectile function and male sexual health.[10,59-61]

## L-Arginine

L-arginine is an essential amino acid with numerous metabolic actions.[62,63] It plays a significant role in erectile function by contributing to the formation of the vasodilator nitric oxide.[19,64-66]

Supplementation with L-arginine has been shown to restore erectile quality and increase sexual satisfaction by boosting nitric oxide bioactivity and improving penile blood flow.[53,67-69] The efficacy of L-arginine, combined with Pycnogenol®, a bioactive compound derived from French maritime bark with vasodilatory properties, has been tested in five independent clinical studies and been shown to improve male sexual function.[70-74] This combination is called Prelox®. The first clinical trial to report successful treatment of erectile dysfunction with Pycnogenol® and L-arginine aspartate involved 40 men aged 25–45 years suffering from mild erectile dysfunction. A regimen of 80 mg of Pycnogenol® and 1.7 g of L-arginine daily yielded significant improvement, with 32 patients (80%) enjoying normal erections. L-arginine, together with an increased amount of Pycnogenol® (120 mg daily), further increased the number of patients with restored normal erectile function. At the end of the 3-month trial, 37 patients, equivalent to 92.5% of all participants, achieved normal erectile function.[70]

L-arginine supplementation has also been shown to attenuate endothelial dysfunction associated with high cholesterol and coronary heart disease.[75] Since endothelial dysfunction diminishes the effects of PDE-5 inhibitors, L-arginine supplementation may be a useful add-on therapy for men who do not respond to these drugs.[63,75,76]

## Epimedium

*Epimedium* is a genus of over 50 distinct species of plants. It is colloquially referred to as *horny goat weed* because it was observed that goats who ate it subsequently engaged in intense sexual activity. *Epimedium* has been used in traditional Chinese medicine for centuries as a natural aphrodisiac and for the treatment of erectile dysfunction.[77-79]

Research has shown that *icariin*, a bioactive component derived from the aerial portion of the *Epimedium* plant, improves erectile and sexual function when administered orally.[79,80] Laboratory data show that icariin can inhibit PDE5, improve penile blood flow, and support endothelial integrity. Icariin also has testosterone-like properties and is associated with increased intracavernosal pressure and nitric oxide levels.[78,79,81-83]

## Yohimbine

Yohimbine, a compound derived from the bark of the Yohimbe tree, has been utilized in the treatment of erectile dysfunction for over 70 years.[84] Yohimbine's mechanism of action is thought to be its ability to enhance smooth muscle relaxation, thereby promoting penile erection. It is thought to accomplish this by blocking the effects of neurotransmitter receptors called *alpha-2 adrenergic receptors*, which promote smooth muscle contraction when activated.[85]

Clinical studies of yohimbine, alone or in combination with L-arginine, have shown improved erectile function.[59,86,87] In one clinical trial, yohimbine was effective for up to 84% of male volunteers, depending on the type of erectile dysfunction.[88] Compared to placebo, yohimbine was more effective at improving self-reported sexual function and penile rigidity.[89,90] Another study found that yohimbine improved erectile function in 42% of men with erectile dysfunction, compared to 27% of subjects taking placebo.[91] Additionally, yohimbine may be particularly effective among type 2 diabetics and those with nonbiological causes of erectile dysfunction.[84,92]

Yohimbine may cause some side effects including heart palpitations, anxiety, fine tremor, and high blood pressure. These occur infrequently and are usually reversible.[84,89,93]

## Ginseng

Ginseng belongs to the genus *Panax*, which is a group of slow-growing perennial plants with distinctively fleshy roots.[94] Five thousand years after it was first used for the treatment of erectile dysfunction in ancient China, ginseng continues to be a popular natural aphrodisiac.[95] An estimated 6 million Americans have used ginseng for the improvement of sexual dysfunction.[61,96]

Ginsenosides, the principal active constituents in ginseng, have cardioprotective, immune-stimulatory, antifatigue, hepatoprotective, and antioxidant effects. In addition, they also increase the synthesis of nitric oxide.[97] In animal studies, ginsenosides have been shown to relax penile smooth muscle tissue (through the release of nitric oxide) and potentially affect chemical pathways involving cGMP and testosterone.[98,99]

A 2009 clinical study showed that 1000 mg of Panax ginseng twice daily improved erectile function and overall sexual satisfaction among men with erectile dysfunction. The study also found that ginseng potentially increased testosterone levels. The authors concluded that ginseng could be effective for improving erectile function regardless of age and severity of dysfunction.[97] Another study showed that ginseng significantly improved penile rigidity, libido, and satisfaction among men with erectile dysfunction.[61]

## Maca

Maca (*Lepidium meyenii*) is a root vegetable belonging to the mustard (ie, *Brassica*) family.[22,100] Ancient Peruvians have cultivated maca for millennia and taken advantage of its aphrodisiac properties.[22,101] The dried root of the maca plant is a rich source of amino acids, iodine, iron, and magnesium.[100,102]

Scientific studies support the aphrodisiac activity of maca, and show that it stimulates metabolism, helps control body weight, increases energy, improves memory, and reduces stress and depression.[101,103] It also shows androgen-like effects in animals.[102] Human clinical studies suggest that maca enhances the production of sex hormones, increases libido, and improves well-being.[100–102,104] The aphrodisiac activity of maca may be due to local effects on erectile function and/or central nervous system effects.[100]

## Ginkgo Biloba

Extracts of leaves from the Ginkgo biloba tree have been used for centuries in the treatment of asthma, fatigue, circulatory problems, and vertigo.[105] It has more recently been associated with enhanced sexual desire, excitement, orgasm, and resolution, as well as neuroprotective properties.[105,106] The sexual benefits of ginkgo were discovered serendipitously when male geriatric patients taking Ginkgo biloba for memory enhancement reported improved erections.[22]

In addition to experimental data showing that Ginkgo biloba can enhance sexual behavior in rats,[107] clinical studies have revealed that it can increase penile blood supply and improve erectile function in humans.[106] Ginkgo contributes to increased blood flow by increasing nitric oxide bioavailability to vascular smooth muscles of the penis.[22,108] In one study, 120–240 mg of Ginkgo biloba extract was associated with a 76% improvement in sexual dysfunction among men being treated with antidepressants.[109]

## Muira Puama

Muira Puama (*Ptychopetalum olacoides*), also known as *potency wood*, is an herb that comes from a small bush in the rainforests of Brazil. It has been associated with enhanced erectile function and orgasm in aging men suffering the effects of fatigue or age-related complaints. In one study of 262 men suffering from poor sexual desire, more than 60% reported improvements with Muira Puama supplementation. In addition, more than half of the men with erectile dysfunction reported that Muira Puama was beneficial. While Muira Puama's mechanism of action remains unknown, its actions may be related to its plant sterol content. Plant sterols may contribute to increased synthesis of testosterone.[108]

## Chrysin

The bioflavonoid chrysin is a natural aromatase inhibitor that helps minimize the conversion of testosterone to estrogen.[110] Although chrysin has low oral bioavailability,[111] its bioavailability may be improved by co-administration with the black pepper extract piperine, thus enhancing its actions as an aromatase inhibitor.[112]

## Carnitines

Carnitine (including acetyl-L-carnitine [ALC] and propionyl-L-carnitine [PLC]) are natural amino acid compounds. Studies have linked carnitines to a variety of positive effects among men with low testosterone, including improved erection quality/function, orgasm, and general sexual well-being.[75,113] Carnitines may have testosterone-like effects in the body.[114] A 2012 study showed that 250 mg of PLC daily for 3 months (in combination with 2500 mg of L-arginine and 20 mg of niacin) successfully improved erections in 40% of men with erectile dysfunction, while nearly 77% of men reported a partial response.[75]

Carnitines may improve endothelial function by acting as antioxidants in these cells.[75] For this reason, carnitine supplementation may be generally beneficial for cardiovascular health.[113,115] Carnitine may also have a place as a combination therapy with PDE5 inhibitors, especially among patients whose erectile dysfunction is caused by underlying endothelial disorders, such as diabetes.[116]

## Vitamin D

Vitamin D insufficiency (as defined by serum levels <30 ng/mL) affects over 75% of the U.S. population. Vitamin D deficiency may be a risk factor for erectile dysfunction, since it contributes to arterial stiffness and vascular dysfunction. In a 2012 paper, researchers theorized that optimizing vitamin D levels could reduce certain risk factors for erectile dysfunction, such as arterial stiffness, diabetes mellitus, hypertension, and inflammation of the endothelium. Vitamin D has also been shown to stimulate the production of nitric oxide.[117]

## B Vitamins

Inadequate intake of B vitamins, especially folate, B6, and B12, can contribute to elevated levels of *homocysteine*. Homocysteine is a metabolic amino acid derivative that can damage endothelial cells and contribute to cardiovascular disease.[118,119] In one study, homocysteine impaired cavernosal smooth muscle relaxation. The authors proposed homocysteine as a risk factor for erectile dysfunction.[120] B vitamin supplementation can help keep homocysteine levels in a healthy range; therefore, may mitigate erectile dysfunction.[118,119,121] Life Extension

recommends that homocysteine levels be kept *below 8 μmol/L* for optimal health.

## Vitamin E

Erectile dysfunction is often associated with oxidative stress, which impairs endothelial function and reduces nitric oxide bioavailability.[122,123] Both experimental and clinical data has shown that vitamin E may be beneficial for erectile dysfunction, since it enhances endothelial cell function, scavenges free radicals, improves nitric oxide–mediated relaxation, preserves nerve function, and increases intracavernosal pressure.[123,124] Through these various actions, vitamin E has shown promising results in experimental models of erectile dysfunction caused by aging and hypertension.[123,125] Vitamin E may also be beneficial when added to PDE5 inhibitor treatment, especially if treatment with a PDE5 inhibitor alone has not been successful in the past.[124]

---

## ADULTERATED SEXUAL HEALTH SUPPLEMENTS

A number of unscrupulous marketers have attempted to take advantage of consumers by adulterating "natural" sexual health products with drug analogs.[126,127] For instance, a 2011 study identified an illegal Viagra-like compound (mutaprodenafil) in a "male enhancement" product.[128] Likewise, a 2012 analysis of nine supplements intended for enhancing male sexual performance found that only one contained a true natural product. The other supplements were found to have untested and unapproved synthetic drug analogs, which may cause significant side effects.[126,127,129] Supplements marketed for boosting testosterone, increasing libido, and/or enhancing male sexual performance are prone to contamination or spiking by profiteers.[129,130]

Insist on purchasing only the highest-quality dietary supplements from trusted, research-focused firms. Choose a brand that uses advanced analytical methods, such as high-performance liquid chromatography, gas chromatography, and mass spectrometry to ensure that products meet label claims for potency and purity, and do not contain illegal drug analogs.[127] Furthermore, be sure to choose a dietary supplement company that tests its raw materials using U.S. Pharmacopeia and other exacting pharmaceutical assay standards.

---

## Life Extension Suggestions

- **French maritime bark extract (Pycnogenol®):** 60–200 mg daily
- **L-arginine:** 700–10 000 mg daily
- **Icariin,** from *Epimedium sagittatum* extract: 60–120 mg daily
- **DHEA:** 25–75 mg daily (depending on blood test results)

- **Muira puama extract:** 425–850 mg daily
- **Maca root:** 160–320 mg daily
- **Chrysin:** 750–1500 mg daily (with black pepper extract piperine to enhance absorption)
- **Acetyl-L-carnitine:** 1000–2000 mg daily
- **Propionyl-L-carnitine:** 300–600 mg daily
- **Vitamin D:** 5000–8000 IU daily, depending on blood levels of 25-hydroxy vitamin D
- **Vitamin B6,** as pyridoxal 5'-phosphate: 100 mg daily
- **Vitamin B12:** 1000–5000 mcg daily
  **Yohimbine:** 135–450 mg daily
  **Vitamin E:** 400 IU daily with at least 200 mg gamma tocopherol
  **Ginkgo biloba,** standardized extract: 120 mg daily

**Ginseng,** standard to 15% ginsenosides: 250–1000 mg daily

In addition, the following *blood test* may be helpful:

- **Male panel** (includes Total and Free Testosterone, Estradiol, Homocysteine, DHEA-S, and Vitamin D, 25-Hydroxy)

## REFERENCES

References available at: www.lef.org/dpt5/ch55

# 56

# *Exercise Enhancement*

Exercise is a proven life extender. Thousands of clinical trials have documented the benefits of a regular exercise program. It has been shown to reduce the risk of many diseases, including heart disease, the leading killer in the United States. Exercise is effective in preventing obesity and depression, and helps people of all ages maintain flexibility, strength, and independence.

Many people who exercise regularly are not getting all the benefits possible from their exercise program. Although any sustained exercise is helpful, results are about more than the time spent exercising. Nutrition is a critical component of any exercise program, and there are proven ways to maximize an exercise program that might not be learned from a family physician or government program.

## PROVEN BENEFITS OF EXERCISE

Exercise has been shown to increase life span by an average of 1–4 years for people engaging in moderate to difficult exercise routines.[1,2] Better yet, those additional years will be healthful because exercise benefits the heart, lungs, and muscles. Even moderate levels of exercise have been documented to stave off many dreaded diseases of aging. Walking briskly for 3 hours per week reduces one's chances of developing many chronic health problems.[3] Exercise may also alleviate depression as well as enhance self-image and quality of life.[4,5]

Exercise has been shown to improve the quality of life in people with diabetes, muscular dystrophy, stroke, multiple sclerosis, myasthenia gravis, and chronic obstructive pulmonary disease.[6,7] Regular exercise can improve blood glucose control, delay or prevent type 2 diabetes, offset age-associated increases in inflammatory cytokines, and reduce cardiovascular risk, diabetes-related mortality, and depression.[8–15]

Routine exercise contributes to thicker and stronger bones.[16] Studies of postmenopausal women have shown that exercise produces increased mineral density of bone at the hip and femoral sites, areas with particularly high fracture rates in older people.[17,18] Older adults with knee osteoarthritis

showed improved balance following an exercise regimen of weight training and aerobics.[19]

Regular exercise in childhood and teen years can help ensure healthy bones late in life. Also, pregnant women can positively influence the size of their infants through exercise.[20]

## METABOLISM–GETTING THE ENERGY WE NEED

To make the most of an exercise program, it is important to understand how exercise affects the metabolic process as well as how it can be enhanced through diet and nutrition.

After food is consumed, it is broken down into components used for energy. Organic molecules, including amino acids, lipids, and simple sugars, are broken down by a process called catabolism. Simple sugars, mainly glucose, are the body's primary source of energy, followed by fats. Only when these two energy sources are depleted is protein, or muscle mass, used for energy. In general, metabolizing protein for energy is not desirable. More energy is needed to metabolize protein than carbohydrates or lipids. Also, protein catabolism (breakdown) produces ammonia as a byproduct, which is harmful to cells. Continued catabolism of protein will damage cells and body systems as well as reduce the effectiveness of any exercise program.

Ultimately, catabolism ends in the production of adenosine triphosphate (ATP) (ie, the body's main energy molecule) in the mitochondria. ATP is necessary for virtually every energy-requiring process in the body. Furthermore, ATP is essential for anabolism, or the synthesis of new organic molecules used to perform repairs, support growth, and produce secretions. When living cells use ATP to create new molecules, a high-energy phosphate bond is broken to release the energy, thereby creating adenosine diphosphate (ADP).

### Muscle Activity During Exercise

The goal of a nutritionally sound exercise program is to support healthy muscle function by providing enough energy for the exercise and recovery period. To design a healthy exercise program, it is valuable to know how energy is consumed by working muscles.

The first energy source to be used by a muscle is ATP, which is stored in the muscles in very limited quantities—enough for only one contraction. When exercise begins, more ATP must immediately be synthesized from creatine phosphate, which is also stored in muscle tissue. Like ATP, creatine phosphate stores are consumed quickly.

ATP and creatine phosphate are supported and replenished through the metabolism of glucose. Almost as soon as the muscle goes to work, glucose is released from glycogen reserves in the muscles in a process known as glycogenolysis. When adequate oxygen is available, glucose is burned through oxidative (aerobic) metabolism, with a high yield of ATP. When adequate oxygen is not available (as in sudden bursts of activity), anaerobic metabolism occurs. A byproduct of anaerobic metabolism is lactic acid. When lactic acid builds up, it creates the "burn" that is familiar to weight lifters and others who get a lot of anaerobic exercise.

As glycogen stores are depleted, the body turns to fat and then protein for energy. After a workout, during recovery, oxygen demand is high while muscles restore ATP, creatine phosphate, and glycogen.

Muscle performance and energy metabolism are determined by physical conditioning and the type of muscle fibers being used. Anaerobic activity is characterized by brief, intense workouts (eg, 50-m dashes or weight lifting). Strength training, which usually relies on short bursts of activity with relatively heavy weights,[21] builds muscle mass.

Aerobic endurance training (eg, jogging and distance swimming) involves sustained, low-level muscle activity. Increased aerobic function is used to produce weight loss (providing fewer calories are consumed than expended) as well as improved respiration and cardiovascular function. Since aerobic activity does not result in increased muscle mass, a combination of aerobic and anaerobic activities (interval training), along with reduced caloric intake and other factors (eg, nutritional status and body type) will result in both weight loss and increased muscle mass.[16]

## MUSCLES AND AGING

As humans age, our muscles atrophy and weaken (ie, sarcopenia), regardless of exercise regimen or lifestyle.[22] The muscles become smaller and less elastic, and muscle injuries become more common.[22,23] The ability to recover from injuries also decreases, as does tolerance for exercise.

Our senior years are a good time to exercise, as it improves quality of life. Sarcopenia, even in severe cases, can be reversed through strength training.[21,24] Exercise has also been shown to control body weight (very important in preventing diabetes, cardiovascular disease, and hypertension) and strengthen bones. It is important for older people to engage in regular, low to moderate exercise rather than strenuous activity.[16]

## WHAT YOU HAVE LEARNED SO FAR

- Exercise results in weight reduction, enhanced physical and mental status, reduced risk of illnesses, and extended life.
- Metabolism is the process of breaking down food for use as energy.
- During muscle contraction, ATP is used for energy. ATP stores are replenished by creatine phosphate, while glucose continues to generate new ATP from both aerobic and anaerobic metabolism.
- Aerobic activity improves cardiovascular function and results in weight loss. Strength training (resistance training) uses weights to build muscle from repeated, increased resistance.

## TESTOSTERONE REPLACEMENT

Testosterone, the male sex hormone that determines secondary sex characteristics in men, is important to capacity and endurance when exercising. As men age, they gradually lose testosterone in a process called andropause, which is somewhat similar to menopause among women. By age 70, as many as 40–50% of men have low testosterone levels.[25] Symptoms of andropause include the loss of bone and muscle mass, depression, loss of sexual function, and heart disease. At the same time that testosterone is declining, growth hormone levels are dropping.[26]

While it might seem that testosterone and growth hormone supplementation would enhance exercise, study results have been conflicting and incomplete. A few small-scale studies have shown it is possible to temporarily boost growth hormone levels by taking supplements that naturally increase growth hormone and testosterone levels; however, there is not yet enough data to recommend hormone replacement in the context of increased exercise endurance and capacity.[25] Considering that some cancers are hormone dependent, testosterone supplementation should be approached with caution by aging men who want to boost their exercise capacity and endurance. Hormone replacement therapy should be done only under the supervision of a qualified physician and after comprehensive blood testing.

## EXERCISE-ENHANCING SUPPLEMENTS

The following supplements have been shown to promote strength by supporting muscle function.

# Carnitine

Carnitine is an amino acid that helps transport fat into mitochondria, where it is metabolized. Exercise capacity is increased among people with arterial disease following carnitine supplementation.[27] In addition, studies show that carnitine supplementation increases muscle function and exercise capacity in people with kidney disease.[28]

# Carnosine

Carnosine is found in high amounts in skeletal muscle; muscle levels of carnosine are elevated during peak activity.[29] Among other reported advantages, carnosine scavenges free radicals, which is important because exercise produces abundant free radical activity.[30–33] Additionally, carnosine protects against cross-linking and advanced glycation end product formation, both of which damage protein.[34,35] Carnosine also acts as a pH buffer, protecting muscles from oxidation during strenuous exercise.[36]

# Coenzyme Q10

Coenzyme Q10 (CoQ10) is a critical component in the conversion of food and oxygen to ATP (the body's universal energy source). ATP acts as a short-term reserve to power everything from muscle activity to brain work. Over time, mitochondrial oxidant damage depletes CoQ10 stores.[37–39] Depleted CoQ10 and related mitochondrial dysfunction are major contributors to age-related diseases as well as aging itself.[40] Aged and damaged mitochondria with insufficient CoQ10 operate inefficiently, producing less energy and more reactive oxygen species.[41] This produces more mitochondrial oxidant damage, driving a vicious cycle.[42]

# Shilajit

Long known to Ayurvedic practitioners for its healing power, *shilajit* is an organic substance harvested from biomass high in the Himalayas.[43,44] It acts as a powerful *adaptogen*, providing broad systemic defense against stress and illness. Cutting-edge scientific analysis has isolated *humic substances* as the principal active ingredients that enhance mitochondrial energy flow.[45]

In 2009, a series of landmark studies detailed for the first time how shilajit works on energy metabolism.

Mice subjected to strenuous exercise experienced ATP declines in muscle, blood, and brain tissue. When supplemented with shilajit, ATP loss was sharply reduced,[46] and other biochemical markers of energy status dramatically improved. CoQ10, in particular, fell twice as fast in control mice as in supplemented mice. When given in combination, CoQ10 and shilajit displayed a more powerful *synergistic effect* than either alone.

Further analysis brought some of its key mechanisms of action to light. Shilajit contains two primary components, *fulvic acid* and *dibenzo-a-pyrones* (*DBPs*). Fulvic acid independently stimulates mitochondrial energy metabolism, protects mitochondrial membranes from oxidative damage, and helps channel electron-rich DBPs into the mitochondria to support the electron transfer chain (ie, a series of reactions coupled to the formation of ATP).[47,48] Fulvic acid works as an electron "shuttle," augmenting CoQ10 to speed electron flow within mitochondria.[49–51]

When laboratory mice were supplemented with oral CoQ10 alone, CoQ10 levels increased in heart, liver, and kidney tissue.[52] When DBPs from shilajit were added to the supplement, CoQ10 levels increased further—as much as 29% in the liver.[52]

A recent study suggests that DBPs from shilajit preserve CoQ10 in its superior *ubiquinol* form.[52]

Preliminary findings suggest that shilajit protects human tissue from lost energy in the form of ATP, while maximizing benefits from CoQ10, with dramatic improvement in exercise performance.[53] In an unpublished study, people who took shilajit *200 mg* once daily for 15 days registered *14%* higher post-exercise ATP levels in the blood—equivalent to levels in people who had not exercised at all. The average number of steps taken on a standardized dynamic exercise test rose significantly, and mean fitness scores increased by *15%*—without any intervening exercise training.

# Creatine

Studies show that creatine supplementation effectively increases lean muscle mass and strength.[54–56] Creatine donates a phosphate molecule to adenosine diphosphate (ADP) to produce more ATP for energy demands. Lactic acid buildup may also be delayed after creatine supplementation.

Studies support the use of creatine to increase strength in older people.[56,57] Other studies demonstrate that creatine can help those with degenerative neurologic disorders and enhance memory in older adults.[58–67]

# Branched-Chain Amino Acids

Amino acids are the building blocks of protein. Essential amino acids, (ie, those not synthesized by the human body) must be obtained from outside sources. The essential branched-chain amino acids (isoleucine, leucine, and valine) improve performance and prevent muscle metabolism during endurance exercise.[68–70] In a study comparing amino acid and carbohydrate supplements, amino acid supplements improved walking and isometric muscle strength in older participants.[71]

## Glutamine

Although the most abundant amino acid in the body, at times the body cannot produce all the glutamine it needs due to extreme stress caused by surgery, prolonged exercise, or infection.[68,72–74]

Various studies have shown the beneficial properties of glutamine during exercise. Athletes who engage in strenuous activity are at elevated risk of developing an upper respiratory infection. This heightened risk could be due to decreased glutamine as a result of intense exercise.[75,76] Glutamine supplementation resulted in a reduction of respiratory infection in a study of marathon runners.[77]

Glutamine, in conjunction with L-cysteine and glycine, helps promote the synthesis of glutathione (a powerful antioxidant) and regulate muscle metabolism.[78] Glutamine helps build and maintain lean muscle tissue.[68] If levels are low, the body may break down muscle to obtain glutamine, resulting in low muscle mass. Supplemental glutamine may prevent muscle breakdown as well as promote greater protein synthesis.[79,80]

## Metabolic Whey Protein

Protein supplementation has been used by fitness enthusiasts and athletes for many years. After exercise, when the body is in a catabolic state, protein supplementation can help protect the body's muscles from being metabolized for energy. Whey protein, in particular, is easily digestible and immediately available to the body. In a study comparing protein and carbohydrate supplements, participants in the protein group showed greater mechanical muscle function during resistance training than participants in the carbohydrate group.[81]

## Plant Protein

In addition to being a source of protein suitable for vegetarians, research has shown that consumption of high-quality vegetable protein exerts numerous beneficial effects in aging humans. Pea protein contains more glutamine than whey or egg protein, with comparable BCAA values to whey, egg, and casein. It also contains more arginine than these 'gold standard' animal proteins. Arginine is essential for *nitric oxide synthesis,* which promotes healthy *endothelial function* and blood vessel dilation and relaxation.[82]

## Polyenylphosphatidylcholine

Polyenylphosphatidylcholine (PPC) is a phospholipid that contains polyunsaturated fatty acids, including linoleic and linolenic acid. In addition to providing flexibility to the cell membrane, PPC can help maintain plasma choline levels during exercise. Choline, which is depleted during exercise, assists in acetylcholine formation. Acetylcholine is involved in the relay of muscle contraction signals across nerve synapses.[83]

## Vitamin D

While scientists have long known that vitamin D plays an important role in bone health, recent studies suggest that it is also essential for maintaining muscle mass in the aging population. Vitamin D helps preserve Type II muscle fibers that are prone to atrophy in the elderly. Scientists noted that vitamin D helps support both muscle and bone tissue, and low vitamin D levels seen in older adults may be associated with poor bone formation and muscle function. Thus, ensuring adequate vitamin D intake may help reduce the incidence of both osteoporosis and sarcopenia in the aging population.[84]

## D-Ribose

D-ribose, a carbohydrate molecule found in every living organism, facilitates the production of ATP.[85]

One study found that exercise-induced physical fatigue was the most important reason people stopped their workouts.[86] Vigorous exercise can drop muscle ATP levels by up to 20%, with up to a 72-hour recovery period for muscles that have been worked hard.[87,88]

The "wiped-out" feeling many of us experience after exercise is also caused by the leakage of ATP breakdown products from muscles into the bloodstream.[89] Once again, D-ribose is vital to keeping muscle ATP-based energy stores at peak capacity,[90,91] which can mean less "afterburn" and more enthusiasm for the next workout.

Exercise physiologists showed that supplementing muscles with D-ribose resulted in an up to 400% increase in the total amount of ATP produced, providing a substantial "bank" of energy to be called upon for use when needed.[92] When physiologists provided D-ribose to working muscles, they demonstrated up to a 600% rise in the rate at which ATP components were recycled for use (recycling ATP is much faster and more efficient than building it from scratch).[91,93]

Sport and exercise physiologists showed that human muscle lost ATP after extreme exercise (mimicking experimental models) and also noted that exhausted muscles took longer to replenish ATP levels than rested muscles.[87] That led them to speculate that supplementing human sprinters with D-ribose might speed the recovery of their muscle ATP levels.

In 2004, a landmark paper showed that 3 times daily supplementation with D-ribose for 3 days following extreme sprint training caused ATP levels to return to normal within 72 hours, while ATP levels remained depressed in placebo recipients.[94]

## FOR MORE INFORMATION

The following chapters may also be of interest:

- Obesity and Weight Loss
- Trauma and Wound Healing
- Male Hormone Restoration
- Female Hormone Restoration

## Life Extension Suggestions

- **Creatine:** 2–5 g daily
- **Carnitine:** 1000–2000 mg daily
- **Carnosine:** 1500–3000 mg daily
- **CoQ10,** as ubiquinol: 100–300 mg daily
- **Shilajit:** 100–200 mg daily
- **Branched-chain amino acids:** containing at least 1200 mg L-leucine, 600 mg L-isoleucine, and 600 mg L-valine

- **Glutamine:** 500–1000 mg daily
- **Whey protein:** 20–80 g whey protein daily. It is most important to consume whey protein before and immediately after your exercise session to make sure adequate protein is available to depleted muscles.
- **Plant protein:** 18 g protein from a blend of plants including pea
- **Polyenylphosphatidylcholine (PPC):** 900–1800 mg
- **Vitamin D:** 5000–8000 IU daily; depending upon blood levels of 25-OH-vitamin D
- **D-ribose:** 5 g, 1–3 times daily with food

Also, the following *blood tests* may provide helpful information.

- Vitamin D, 25-Hydroxy
- Female Comprehensive Hormone Panel or Male Comprehensive Hormone Panel
- Creatine kinase

## REFERENCES

References available at: www.lef.org/dpt5/ch56

# 57

# Eye Health

Healthy vision is accomplished through healthy eyes—and good nutrition is vital to healthy eyes. The eye is made of various structures working in concert to focus light rays from objects into images and send them to the brain via electrical impulses. The eye itself is protected in a bony orbit (socket). The socket provides protection against trauma, but cannot protect the eye from internal injuries.

The front of each eye is covered by an eyelid, which blinks periodically to spread tears over the eye surface and remove unwanted material. The eyelids also have glands that secrete oil onto the cornea, forming a portion of the tear film of the eye.

The cornea is the transparent covering through which light travels. On all sides of the cornea (covering and shaping the rest of the eyeball) lies the sclera, which is made of tough connective tissue. This sclera is the "white" of the eye, while the cornea covers the pupil and the iris (the dark hole and colored portions, respectively). The conjunctiva (a delicate, thin layer of tissue) covers the entire surface of the eyeball and lines the inner surfaces of the lids.

Beyond the cornea lies the iris, which gives the eye its color. The iris is a sphincter made of smooth muscle that contracts and expands in response to light levels. The open area in the middle of the iris is the pupil. When the iris contracts, the pupil gets smaller, thus allowing less light to enter the eye. Conversely, when the iris sphincter muscle relaxes, the pupil dilates, allowing more light into the eye.

The area between the cornea and the iris is the anterior chamber; it is filled with a fluid called aqueous humor. The aqueous humor bathes several structures in the eye. Directly behind the iris is the lens, which is held in place by small, string-like structures called *zonules*. The lens and the cornea together focus all images coming into the eye.

Behind the lens, the eye is filled with vitreous humor, a clear substance with the consistency of firm jelly. Vitreous humor fills the bulk of the eyeball and gives it the round shape needed for proper image production. The inner back surface of the eye is lined with light-sensitive nerve tissue called the retina. An easy analogy is to compare the retina of the eye to the film of a camera: both capture images. The retina consists of photoreceptors (light-detecting cells), nerve fibers, and blood vessels. There are two kinds of photoreceptors: rods and cones. Rods are extremely light sensitive but detect only black and white. Cones detect colors but require more light than rods. This explains why objects in dim light often appear in shades of grey, black, or white. Together, rods and cones capture the image and send it to the brain via the optic nerve.

The most important part of the retina is the macula. This area has a very high concentration of photoreceptors and is responsible for one's central vision. The nerve fibers in the macula and other parts of the retina coalesce to form the optic nerve, which is a sort of cable that connects the eye to the brain.

Eye health is highly dependent on healthy neurologic and cardiovascular systems. Images obtained by the eye are transferred via electrical impulses to the brain, where they are processed and in turn transformed into the mental images we "see." Thus, maintaining optimum neurological health and capacity contributes to visual functioning. Similarly, the cardiovascular system supplies the eye with oxygen-rich blood and removes waste products produced in the eye's structures. The retina and surrounding structures are especially rich in blood vessels and rely on a healthy cardiovascular system. Many nutrients have the potential to maintain or improve the eye and its function by acting on the cardiovascular and brain systems.

## HOW THE EYE SEES

When a person looks at an object, light rays bouncing off that object hit the cornea, which bends them toward the center of the retina by a process known as refraction. These bent light rays then go through the pupil and are adjusted by the lens. If the eye is focusing properly, the rays then fall onto the retina (mostly on the macula) as a clear, upside-down image. This image is captured by the photoreceptors and then transferred via the nerve fiber layer of the retina to the optic nerve, which connects to the brain, where the image is interpreted and inverted so the world appears right side up.

When the eye does not properly focus light rays from the image, the result is a refractive error. There are two types of refractive errors:

- **Spherical aberration.** Spherical aberration occurs when the focused image falls either in front of the retina (near-sightedness, or myopia) or "behind" the retina (far-sightedness, or hyperopia).

- **Astigmatism.** Astigmatism occurs when light waves interfere with each other as their distance from the central axis increases so that the image becomes blurry anywhere except in the middle. Astigmatism is usually caused by an irregularly shaped cornea. It can occur alone or in conjunction with myopia or hyperopia.

Myopia, hyperopia, and astigmatism can all usually be corrected with eyeglasses, contact lenses, or refractive surgery such as LASIK.

Besides refractive errors, most people develop presbyopia at around age 40. This disease occurs when the lens of the eye can no longer focus on near images because of age-related stiffness. For people who never wore glasses, reading glasses are usually necessary starting at around age 40. For those who already wear glasses, bifocals or another form of dual correction is often needed. Presbyopia is an irreversible condition.

## DISEASES OF THE EYE

Besides refractive and other focusing errors that cause decreased vision, many diseases can temporarily or permanently affect sight.

Since the eyelids, and the rest of the facial skin, have more lifetime sun exposure than other parts of the body, they are at increased risk of developing cancer. Skin cancer can often be treated by removing the lesion surgically.

The conjunctiva can become inflamed or infected from numerous diseases. This condition is called conjunctivitis. The most common causes of conjunctivitis include allergies, dry eyes, and viral infection (pinkeye). Bacterial and other types of infections can also cause pinkeye. Allergic reactions, dry eye, and chemical exposure can lead to inflamed conjunctiva.

Since the cornea helps focus images into the eye, maintaining clarity is essential. Both infection and injury can produce scars that leave the cornea cloudy. Clouded corneas reduce the amount of light that enters the eye, resulting in decreasing stimulation of the photoreceptors and dim vision. Scarring can also affect the shape of the cornea, producing astigmatism. Severe corneal scarring, or keratoconus, is one of the reasons for a corneal transplant operation.

If the tear system is not functioning properly, dry eye may develop. In some instances, it can be

debilitating. Dry eye can be caused by numerous rheumatologic and auto-immune diseases, such as Sjögren's syndrome, rheumatoid arthritis, and systemic lupus erythematosus. It has also been linked to many medications. Dry eye can even occur without an obvious cause. Rarely, ocular dryness is severe enough to cause permanent damage to the cornea. Dry eyes can be treated with artificial tear drops or prescription medications such as Restasis® or by unplugging of the tear drainage system.

The first internal structure in the eye is the anterior chamber, where aqueous humor bathes the back side of the cornea, the iris, and the front of the lens. If the aqueous humor is either produced too quickly or drained too slowly, pressure inside the eye can become elevated. This is one usual component of a disease process called glaucoma, which can cause irreversible vision loss. In glaucoma, the elevated pressure presses on the optic nerve fibers, reducing their blood flow, which may lead to cell damage or death. Because of the arrangements of nerve fibers in the optic nerve, glaucoma primarily produces loss of peripheral (side) vision. In advanced cases, it can also impair central vision. Vision loss due to glaucoma is permanent. Treatment includes prescription medications, laser treatments, and surgery. Animal research suggests that Ginkgo biloba supplementation may be helpful in glaucoma prevention and treatment.[1] Research has also implicated oxidative stress as a causal factor in glaucoma. Evidence now suggests that increased concentrations of reactive oxygen species play an important role in the development of glaucoma.[2]

Oxidative stress has also been implicated in the development of cataracts.[3] A cataract occurs when the lens becomes cloudy as a result of normal aging. The only cure for cataracts is surgery, although one study has suggested that antioxidant therapy may help reduce the risk of developing them.[3] Cataract surgery is very common and typically restores excellent vision in most people.

Behind the lens is the vitreous cavity. The vitreous humor can pull away from the back of the eye and form floaters, which are small condensations that appear as black spots or cobwebs in one's vision. The vitreous humor can also form a retinal hole or tear when it pulls away from the back of the eye. Either of these conditions can lead to retinal detachment, in which the retina falls away from the back of the eye. Retinal detachments are medical emergencies. A sensation of a curtain being pulled across the field of vision is a danger sign for retinal detachment. Retinal detachments are usually repaired with surgery, although the surgery is not always successful. Retinal holes or tears can often be treated with a laser to help prevent retinal detachment from worsening. Successful treatment of retinal detachment depends on early detection.

Many diseases, both exclusive to the eye and systemic, can cause serious damage to the retina. Macular degeneration is probably the most feared of all ophthalmic diseases. It occurs when the macula (which is responsible for central vision) becomes diseased, distorting central vision. Macular degeneration is a significant cause of blindness.[4]

Treatments for macular degeneration include laser treatments, surgery, and injection of prescription medications into the eye. One of the greatest nutritional breakthroughs in the treatment of macular degeneration was the release of the Age-Related Eye Disease Study, in which researchers found that vitamins C and E, beta-carotene, and zinc (plus copper) can reduce progression in certain types of macular degeneration.[5] Newer research has also implicated oxidative stress in macular degeneration. It is believed that age-related elevations in oxidative products in the eye may contribute to the development of macular degeneration.[6,7] Inflammation has also been identified as a possible aggravating factor in the development of macular degeneration.

The health of the eye is also affected by systemic disease (eg, diabetes, atherosclerosis, and hypertension), which can cause significant damage to the retina. In diabetic retinopathy, the small blood vessels of the retina become diseased and can leak blood products. Also, they do not carry enough oxygen, so some areas of the retina may become oxygen deficient. The eye may respond by forming more blood vessels (neovascularization), which are very fragile. In many cases, the blood vessels can bleed directly into the back of the eye. In people with high blood pressure, the retinal blood vessels can change shape and become unhealthy. Atherosclerotic disease can affect the small blood vessels of the eye and cause reduced blood flow.

## FOR MORE INFORMATION

Additional protocols that might be of interest include the following:

- Cataracts
- Glaucoma
- Age-Related Macular Degeneration
- Retinopathy

## HEALTHY EYES: THE BASICS

You can take several steps to protect healthy vision:

- Stop smoking. Smoking can increase one's risk of developing cataracts, macular degeneration, and many other diseases by increasing oxidative stress, narrowing blood vessels, and reducing blood flow to the eye.[8,9]

- Wear a hat and sunglasses with ultraviolet (UV) protection whenever you are outdoors. The sun's UV rays can increase the risk of developing skin cancer, cataracts, and macular degeneration.[10]

- Get regular, comprehensive eye examinations. Many eye diseases have no symptoms until late in the disease. Thus, many eye diseases are not apparent until diagnosed during a comprehensive eye examination. The American Academy of Ophthalmology currently recommends the schedule below for comprehensive medical eye examinations in healthy people with no family history, personal history, or risk factors for eye disease. Since everyone is different, consult your doctor as to how often you should get a comprehensive eye examination.[11]

  - Age 20–29: at least once
  - Age 30–39: at least twice
  - Age 40–64: every 2–4 years
  - Age ≥65: every 1–2 years

- Maintain a healthy diet and adequate nutritional intake. Your eyes rely on the nutrients you consume. This may be especially important in light of research implicating oxidative stress in major eye diseases. It is very important that all aging people maintain adequate antioxidant supplies to protect their eyes.

Some of the nutrients that benefit healthy vision work by directly supporting eye function, while others enhance blood flow to the eye by supporting the cardiovascular system. It is important that people with heart disease, such as coronary artery disease, visit their ophthalmologist and carefully follow their dietary program.

## TARGETED NATURAL THERAPIES

### Omega-3 Fatty Acids

One group of dietary supplements that affects both the eye and the cardiovascular system is omega-3 fatty acids. These essential fatty acids help prevent hardening of the arteries in both the heart and the eye by reducing inflammation. Arteriosclerosis is a pervasive and quiet enemy of the eye. The result of arteriosclerosis is a decrease in nutrients to the eye and a reduction in the removal of waste products. An added benefit of omega-3 fatty acids is an apparent lower risk of dry eye syndrome, particularly in women.[12]

## Lipoic Acid

Lipoic acid is a very powerful antioxidant that prevents free radical damage, thus reducing oxidative stress and possibly reducing the risk of degenerative eye disease. It has shown promise as a nutrient to protect rabbits' eyes from ultraviolet damage.[13]

## N-Acetyl-L-Carnosine

When administered topically, N-acetyl-L-carnosine can move easily into both the water-soluble and lipid-containing parts of the eye. Once there, it helps prevent DNA strand breaks induced by UV radiation and enhances DNA repair.[14] In the lipid areas of the eye, N-acetyl-L-carnosine partially breaks down and becomes L-carnosine. In a 1999 study of 96 patients aged ≥60 years with cataracts, 1–2 drops of a carnosine-containing solution was administered 3–4 times daily for 3–6 months. At the end of the study, the level of eyesight improved, and the lens became more transparent. For primary senile cataracts, the effective rate was 100%; for mature senile cataracts, the effective rate was 80%.[15]

## Vitamin C

Intraocular pressure can be lowered by high doses of vitamin C. The osmotic changes are thought to impact either the outflow or secretion mechanism to reduce the pressure. Vitamin C may slow the progression of glaucoma.[16,17]

## B Vitamins

A decrease in B vitamins has been linked to heart disease. Because B vitamins are poorly stored by the human body, they must be ingested on a regular basis. Low levels of B vitamins, including vitamin B12, folic acid, and niacin, have been seen in glaucoma, diabetic retinopathy, and age-related macular degeneration.[16]

While diabetes threatens whole-body health, the eyes are particularly vulnerable to damage. Damage to small blood vessels caused by diabetes can result in retinopathy (a disease of the eye's retina, which collects visual information) and even blindness.

Scientists in Germany discovered that administration of benfotiamine (a fat-soluble form of vitamin B1) helped prevent retinopathy in test subjects with diabetes. Study subjects who received benfotiamine for 36 weeks demonstrated completely normalized levels of damaging advanced-glycation end products (AGEs) in the retina, leading the research team to conclude that benfotiamine may help prevent or delay the onset and progression of diabetic retinopathy.[18]

An exciting development in *prevention* of macular degeneration came from Harvard researchers.[19]

Using 5205 women (≥40 years) known to have pre-existing cardiovascular disease or three or more cardiovascular risk factors (but who did not have macular degeneration at the start of the study), researchers conducted a large, randomized, placebo-controlled trial. Subjects were randomly assigned to receive either a combination of folic acid, pyridoxine (vitamin B6), and vitamin B12, or a placebo, and they were followed over an extended time period.

After an average of 7.3 years, researchers identified 55 cases of macular degeneration in the treatment group and 82 in the placebo group—this came out to a risk reduction of 34% in the vitamin supplemented group. That protection level rose to 41% for macular degeneration that was causing visual problems.

This was a truly stunning result, particularly since all subjects already had evidence of cardiovascular disease or increased risk, and the levels of supplementation were fairly modest—2.5 mg (2500 mcg) daily of folate, 50 mg daily of B6, and 1 mg (1000 mcg) daily of B12. Based on the study results, the author noted that "daily supplementation with folic acid, pyridoxine, and cyanocobalamin may reduce the risk of age-related macular degeneration."

While further studies are needed to determine whether B vitamins protect other populations against macular degeneration, this study provides hope that B vitamins may offer an accessible and low-cost preventive strategy against a leading cause of blindness in older adults.

## Bilberry

Studies have shown the herb bilberry to be effective in vascular disorders. Bilberry contains flavonoids and antioxidants that increase microcirculation and support retinal function.

This nutrient may be especially beneficial for individuals with macular degeneration, cataracts, diabetic retinopathy, and night blindness.[20]

Many studies have demonstrated the superior and efficient antioxidant and free radical-scavenging activity of bilberry and other related berry fruits, along with genetic signaling abilities that favor their use in health promotion and disease prevention.[21] Bilberry has also shown its strength in bolstering defense systems against harmful oxidative stress. In research involving tissue from the pigmented layer of the retina, bilberry proved a potent influence on beneficial gene pathways involved in the antioxidant response effort.[22] In addition to a huge body of research showing bilberry's benefits in vascular models of disease and atherosclerosis,[23] bilberry has also shown its protective effects in other models of inflammatory eye diseases such as uveitis, with greater protection afforded by increasing extract dosage, or the so-called dose–response.[24]

## French Maritime Bark Extract

French maritime pine bark is a powerful antioxidant rich in proanthocyanidins, which are known for their ability to scavenge and neutralize harmful free radicals. The biologic effects of French maritime pine bark also extend to the natural agent's abilities to help regulate the cell's antioxidant network and associated genes, as well as dampen gene expression related to nuclear factor-kappaB (NF-κB)–dependent pathways inside cells, which have been shown to result in anti-inflammatory effects.[25,26]

Human studies have also shown the ability of French maritime pine bark to improve vascular endothelial function,[27] which involves the delicate layer of critical lining cells inside blood vessels that possess wide-ranging effects on vessel tone, integrity, inflammation, antioxidant protection, and repair. Disorders of endothelial function have also been cited as contributing factors to the development or progression of glaucoma,[28] which lends further support to the use of French maritime pine bark.

Interest in the benefits of French maritime pine bark grew with people's understanding of the damage caused by free radicals. Mitochondrial-associated oxidative damage affects the eyes' drainage system, whose tissue integrity is essential to maintaining normal eye fluid outflow and pressure.[29] This understanding of the role played by faulty mitochondrial function in the development of glaucoma pointed investigators toward possible dietary solutions.

## Cyanidin-3-Glucoside

Anthocyanins are pigmentary compounds that lend fruits like grapes, blueberries, and black currants their dark color.

Scientists are increasingly focusing on the benefits of one anthocyanin in particular: *cyanidin-3-glucoside* or C3G.[30] Scores of studies in the past 2 years have established its potent combination of antioxidant, anti-inflammatory, DNA-protective, and gene-regulating effects.

C3G plays a unique role in protecting retinal tissue from damage. It works by multiple mechanisms at several sites in the retina. Most importantly, C3G stimulates regeneration of the retinal pigment *rhodopsin*.[31] Rhodopsin is vital to vision in dim light. When depleted, rhodopsin takes longer to return to its normal, light-sensitive state. C3G increases restoration of rhodopsin levels.[32,33]

C3G also serves to protect retinal cells against the harmful oxidation triggered by light.[34] It accomplishes this by reducing the accumulation of a fluorescent pigment called A2E that amasses with age and interferes with normal retinal function. C3G's ability to quench oxygen free radicals is credited with this effect.[34]

Retinal cells are nerve cells capable of transmitting electrical signals. C3G and other cyanidin components of berries have neuroprotective effects on retinal cells.[35]

## Carotenoids

**Beta-carotene.** This carotenoid functions as an antioxidant by disabling free radicals. Low intake of beta-carotene is associated with increased free radical damage, which increases the risk of cataracts and macular degeneration.[36]

**Zeaxanthin and lutein.** Carotenoids are found in vegetables (red, yellow, green, and orange) and fruits. Carotenoids like zeaxanthin and lutein have highly antioxidative characteristics and help prevent destructive vascular changes in the macula, decreasing the risk of age-related macular degeneration. Studies indicate that high levels of lutein may decrease the incidence of posterior subcapsular cataracts, diminish complaints of glare, and provide better color vision and more critical acuity.[37]

**Meso-zeaxanthin.** Meso-zeaxanthin, a nutritional cousin of lutein and zeaxanthin, is attracting attention for its application in eye health.[38–40] Although not present in the typical diet, meso-zeaxanthin is produced from lutein in the retina.[38,40] Together with lutein and zeaxanthin, meso-zeaxanthin helps comprise macular pigment, the region of the eye's retina that is crucial to detailed vision.[38] Like many other biochemical processes, however, the conversion of lutein to meso-zeaxanthin is reduced by aging. A deficiency in meso-zeaxanthin can therefore result in a reduction in macular pigment density. Furthermore, a lack of ingested lutein or difficulty in synthesizing meso-zeaxanthin from lutein can further reduce levels.

A study showed that when individuals were supplemented with meso-zeaxanthin, their macular pigment density increased.[39] Since optimal macular pigment density is crucial to visual health, this suggests that supplementing with meso-zeaxanthin—in addition to consuming abundant lutein and zeaxanthin—may help fend off the onset of macular degeneration.[38]

**Astaxanthin.** Astaxanthin is a carotenoid xanthophyll, found naturally in the alga *H. pluvialis*, which gives lobster and other marine life consuming it a reddish hue.

In a double-blind study, 26 individuals whose work required staring at a visual display terminal were randomly assigned to receive 5 mg astaxanthin or placebo daily for 1 month. Those who received astaxanthin had a 54% reduction of eye fatigue complaints and objective improvements in accommodation ability.[41]

Only the astaxanthin group showed significant reduction of subjective symptoms. After 4 weeks of treatment with astaxanthin, the power of accommodation was significantly improved. On the other hand, placebo did not show any significant difference.

Research into the activity of astaxanthin has shown that its antioxidant mechanism may be complementary to that of vitamin E, which is also important in eye health and may help protect against age-related macular degeneration.[42] Free radical damage by UV light or other types of injury involves spreading of subatomic, negatively charged particles known as electrons. Astaxanthin is a chemical compound that can accept electrons easily, absorbing free radicals and stopping the chain reaction of tissue damage.[43]

## Selenium

Selenium is an essential trace mineral with antioxidant properties that works in partnership with vitamin E to protect cellular integrity and cell membranes. It protects the cell membranes from free radical damage, decreasing the risk of macular degeneration, cataracts, and glaucoma. Numerous plants, including grains and garlic, contain selenium, but the concentration is highly dependent on soil content.[44]

## Taurine

High concentrations of taurine are needed within the eye to maintain optimal function and structure. It has been found to protect the lens against free radical damage.[45,46] In a series of studies performed by researchers at the University of Maryland,[45] rat lenses were cultured with a potent oxidant called menadione. The addition of physiologic amounts of taurine—enough to create a concentration roughly equivalent to that which would exist in healthy lenses—attenuated the harmful effects of the oxidant. Another study found that the lenses of diabetic rats were protected against cataract by physiological levels of taurine.[47]

## Coenzyme Q10

This nutrient has been studied in the context of age-related macular degeneration. In a randomized, double-blind, placebo-controlled trial examining the effects of coenzyme Q10 (CoQ10) combined with acetyl-L-carnitine and omega-3 fatty acids, researchers found that the nutrient mix improved and stabilized visual functions in patients with early age-related macular degeneration.[48] In an animal study, CoQ10 and vitamin E, applied topically, were found to help reduce the risk of complications after laser cornea surgery.[49]

## Vitamin A

Vitamin A, retinol, and retinyl palmitate are multifunctional and essential in virtually all tissues. Vitamin A is required by the photoreceptors of the retina for proper function. Vitamin A, as an antioxidant, has been shown to decrease lipid levels in coronary heart disease; therefore, it may protect the ocular vascular system.[44,50]

## Zinc

This mineral is required to maintain the integrity of the immune system and of carbohydrate and protein metabolism. The retina has the highest concentration of zinc of any organ system.[51] Previous studies suggest zinc may play a role in reducing the risk of age-related macular degeneration. However, other studies have presented a complex picture. At lower doses, zinc does have a protective effect against macular degeneration by supporting epithelial cells in the retina. However, at higher doses, zinc has the opposite effect.[52] Fortunately, this dangerous effect of zinc is attenuated by antioxidants, such as vitamin E, taken at the same time as zinc. Therefore, for anyone consuming zinc to help prevent age-related macular degeneration, antioxidants are recommended.[52]

## Life Extension Suggestions

- **Fish oil,** with olive polyphenols and sesame lignans: providing 1400 mg EPA and 1000 mg DHA daily
- **Lipoic acid:** 240–480 mg daily
- **Vitamin C:** 1–3 g daily
- **B-complex vitamins:**
  - Thiamine (B1): 100 mg
  - Riboflavin (B2): 50 mg
  - Niacin: 200 mg
  - Vitamin B6: 75 mg
  - Folate (preferably as L-methylfolate): 800 mcg

- • Vitamin B12: 1000 mcg
- • Biotin: 600 mcg
- • Pantothenic acid: 1000 mg
- • Choline: 45 mg
- • Inositol: 250 mg
- • Para-aminobenzoic acid (PABA): 100 mg
- **Benfotiamine:** 100–250 mg daily
- **Beta-carotene:** 5000 IU daily
- **Vitamin A:** 2500 IU daily
- **Vitamin E:** 400 IU daily (with at least 200 mg gamma tocopherol)
- **Bilberry:** 100 mg daily
- **French maritime pine bark:** 40–200 mg daily
- **Zeaxanthin:** 2.75 mg daily
- **Lutein:** at least 10 mg free lutein daily
- **Astaxanthin:** 6 mg daily

- **Mesozeaxanthin:** 1 mg daily
- **C3G (cyanidin-3-glucoside):** 2.2 mg daily
- **Selenium:** 200–400 mcg daily
- **Taurine:** 1–4 g daily
- **Zinc:** 15–30 mg daily
- **Coenzyme Q10,** as ubiquinol: 100–300 mg daily
- **Eye drops containing N-acetyl-L-carnosine:** may be applied 3–4 times daily
- **UV-blocking sunglasses**

## REFERENCES

References available at: www.lef.org/dpt5/ch57

# 58

# *Female Hormone Restoration*

U ntil 2002, mainstream physicians routinely prescribed conventional hormone replacement therapy (HRT) in order to alleviate menopausal symptoms such as hot flashes, mood swings, decreased sexual desire, vaginal dryness, and difficulty sleeping, as well as to prevent heart disease and osteoporosis. In 2002, however, the results of a landmark study, the Women's Health Initiative (WHI), identified dangers associated with conventional hormone replacement therapy in women. More than 160 000 women participated in this observational study. Conventional HRT side effects included a 26% increased risk of breast cancer, 29% increased risk of heart attack, 41% increase in risk for strokes, and a doubling in risk for blood clots relative to the untreated group. Moreover, women receiving conjugated equine (horse-derived) estrogen experienced a six-fold increased risk for uterine cancer. Only those women under 60 years of age who had undergone a hysterectomy (surgical removal of the uterus) experienced a reduction in breast cancer risk when using estrogen *without* medroxyprogesterone acetate (MPA), a synthetic progestogen.[1–6]

Given the substantial risks associated with conventional HRT, many women began to seek alternatives. Up to 70% of women taking HRT stopped, and overall, women's trust in the mainstream medical establishment declined significantly.[7,8] Data from the study also resulted in many physicians discouraging the use of conventional HRT for the prevention of osteoporosis and cardiovascular disease in aging women.[4,9]

Life Extension was not surprised by the results of the WHI study. The hormones being utilized consisted of oral *equine* (horse) estrogen and a *synthetic progestogen*, both of which differ in chemical structure from the natural hormones produced in a woman's body. Life Extension has discouraged the use of conventional HRT for many years and instead has recognized the value of *bioidentical HRT*, which uses hormones that are identical to those naturally produced in women. Conventional HRT makes use of *non-bioidentical* hormones that differ chemically from those naturally produced by a woman's body. Furthermore, the relative levels of the female hormones administered in conventional HRT are different.[10,11]

Bioidentical HRT is associated with far fewer side effects than conventional HRT and there is intriguing evidence that it may reduce the risk of certain cancers.[12]

Moreover, supplementation with scientifically studied vitamins and natural plant extracts can help promote healthy metabolism of female hormones and complement the actions of bioidentical HRT.

## UNDERSTANDING CONVENTIONAL HRT

The rationale for conventional HRT is that women's hormone levels decline with age. Replacement, therefore, should reverse troubling menopausal consequences, which include increased risk of heart attack and cancer.[13–15] While the original understanding of menopause and logic behind HRT were theoretically correct, modern science is showing that the true story of HRT is much more complex.[16]

It is impossible to isolate estrogen and progesterone from other hormones. All steroid hormones are created from cholesterol in a hormonal cascade. The first in the cascade is *pregnenolone*, which is subsequently converted into other hormones including *dehydroepiandrosterone* (DHEA), progesterone, testosterone, and various forms of estrogen. These hormones are interrelated, yet each performs unique physiologic functions. Biologically sound hormone replacement should focus on a woman's total hormone balance, not only on estrogen and progesterone.

Mainstream physicians are just now beginning to recognize *estrogen dominance*,[10] a term used to characterize the relative imbalance between excess estrogen and insufficient progesterone. Estrogen dominance helps explain many of the conditions that confront modern women in Western civilization, such as fibrocystic breast disease[17] and cancer.[18–20] Estrogen dominance can occur in any woman. However, perimenopausal women, who typically experience a more rapid decline in progesterone relative to estrogen, are especially at risk.[21]

*Conjugated equine estrogen* (CEE) is obtained from the urine of pregnant mares (horses).[22] CEE is usually given in combination with progestin, a chemical compound modified for the purpose of appearing structurally *similar* to natural, bioidentical progesterone. However, it is not the same. The structural differences between conjugated equine estrogen and chemical progestin as well as natural hormones are responsible for many of the adverse effects resulting from conventional HRT.

Another major problem with conventional HRT is the estrogen ratio. For example, the ratio in medications such as Premarin® is considerably different than the ratio observed naturally in a woman's body.[23]

## CAUSES OF ESTROGEN DOMINANCE

Beginning in perimenopause and continuing throughout menopause, the production of progesterone tends to decline more rapidly than that of estrogen. If the progesterone to estrogen ratio is unbalanced, favoring excess estrogen, a woman may become susceptible to an increased risk of fibrocystic breast disease and other health problems.[17,24]

Factors contributing to estrogen dominance include:

- Exposure to estrogen-mimicking chemicals found in herbicides, pesticides, petrochemicals (eg, BPA, bisphenol A) and PCBs (polychlorinated biphenyls) used in some cosmetics, glue, plastic, and other modern materials.[25]

- Obesity as well as increased intake of excess calories from simple sugars, fiber-deficient refined grains, and *trans*-fat from partially hydrogenated vegetable oil.

Many practitioners report that estrogen dominance is often associated with symptoms such as food cravings, bloating, weight gain, fatigue, mood swings, depression, cyclical migraine headaches, decreased sexual desire, menstrual cramps, short cycles, heavy menstrual bleeding, hair loss, fibroids, and endometriosis.

### Is Cancer Risk a Reason to Deprive Aging Women of Natural Hormones?

Concern about cancer is an important reason why more aging women do not restore their hormones to youthful levels. Hormones like estrogen and testosterone affect cell growth and proliferation. Does that mean aging women should simply accept hormone deficiency as a part of "normal" aging?

If estrogen caused breast cancer, then we would expect to see very high rates in young women of childbearing age, with a dramatic decline after menopause. This has not been observed. To demonstrate the risk of developing breast cancer as women age, we have reprinted the following statistics[26]:

| | | | |
|---|---|---|---|
| By age 25: | 1 in 19 608 | By age 60: | 1 in 24 |
| By age 30: | 1 in 2525 | By age 65: | 1 in 17 |
| By age 40: | 1 in 217 | By age 70: | 1 in 14 |
| By age 45: | 1 in 93 | By age 75: | 1 in 11 |
| By age 50: | 1 in 50 | By age 80: | 1 in 10 |
| By age 55: | 1 in 33 | By age 85: | 1 in 9 |

The genes that help regulate healthy cell growth can *mutate*. In fact, mutations in cells' regulatory genes are an underlying cause of cancer.[27] Breast cells with mutated genes may be more vulnerable to estrogen's growth-stimulating effects.

## ESTROGEN EXPLAINED

To fully appreciate the complexity of HRT, it is important to understand the various forms of estrogen and their physiologic effects. More than 15 forms of natural estrogen have been identified,[28] including estrone, estradiol, and estriol.

Each of these estrogens has particular functions. Estradiol (E2) (the predominant form in nonpregnant, reproductive females) primarily aids in the cyclic release of eggs from the ovaries (ie, ovulation). E2 has beneficial effects on the heart, bone, brain, and colon. Reduction in the level of E2 causes common menopausal symptoms such as hot flashes and night sweats. Estrone (E1), produced in the ovaries and fat cells, is the dominant estrogen in postmenopausal women. Estriol (E3) is secreted in large quantities by the placenta during pregnancy. However, it is a comparatively weak estrogen, and the form of estrogen least associated with hormone-related cancers. In Europe and Japan, E3 is frequently used for HRT.[5,12,29,30]

The three types of estrogen convert into many metabolites. E1, for example, may convert into three different forms:

- 2-hydroxyestrone
- 4-hydroxyestrone
- 16-alpha-hydroxyestrone

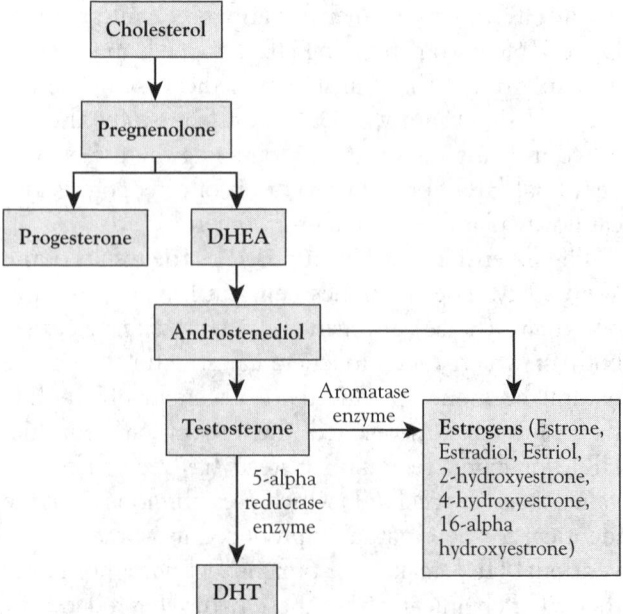

**Simplified Hormone Cascade**

Scientists have identified 2-hydroxyestrone as a "good" or chemoprotective estrogen, while 16-alpha-hydroxyestrone and 4-hydroxyestrone have been associated with the development of cancer.[31,32] The relationship between 2-hydroxyestrone and 16-alpha-hydroxyestrone is sometimes expressed as the 2:16 ratio.[28]

By increasing the ratio of 2-hydroxyestrone to 16-alpha-hydroxyestrone, it may be possible to reduce the risk of estrogen-related cancers.[28,31]

3,3'-diindolylmethane (DIM) and indole-3-carbinole (I3C) (found in cruciferous vegetables) favorably affect estrogen metabolism and help to optimize the 2:16 ratio. A placebo-controlled, double-blind study of women at increased risk for breast cancer found that 4 weeks of supplementation with I3C promoted favorable changes in the urinary estrogen 2:16 ratio.[33,34]

## Estrogen Receptors and a Closer Look at Estriol

As mentioned previously, estriol (E3) is the form of estrogen least associated with cancer. E3's protective effects become apparent when examining the differing actions that each of the three primary estrogens exerts on the estrogen receptors. In breast cells there are two distinct *classical* estrogen receptors that bind estrogens, estrogen receptor *alpha* (ER-α) and estrogen receptor *beta* (ER-β). In addition, there is one *non-classical* estrogen receptor, GPR30.[35–39] The binding of estrogen hormones to ER-α promotes breast cell proliferation, which can exacerbate the spread of existing breast cancer. Conversely, the binding and activation of ER-β attenuate breast cell proliferation and thus may slow the development of a cancerous tumor.[40–43]

Estrone (E1) and estradiol (E2) preferentially bind to and activate ER-α, thereby explaining the proliferative effects of these two hormones.[44,45] E3, on the other hand, binds to and activates ER-β.[44,45] This helps to explain E3's "antiestrogenic" activity and led a noted researcher in HRT to state the following: *"This unique property of estriol, in contrast to the selective ER [estrogen receptor] alpha binding by other estrogens, imparts to estriol a potential for breast cancer prevention, while other estrogens [estrone and estradiol], would be expected to promote breast cancer . . . Because of its differing effects on ER alpha and ER beta, we would expect that estriol would be less likely to induce proliferative [potential cancerous growth] changes in breast tissue and to be associated with a reduced risk of breast cancer."*[12]

Moreover, groundbreaking research has revealed that GPR30 mediates proliferation of breast cancer cells independently of ER-α and ER-β. E2 strongly binds to and activates GPR30, driving proliferation. E3, on the other hand, acts as an antagonist of GPR30, though it has a much lower affinity for GPR30 than E2.[39,46] Many carcinogenic toxins, including bisphenol A (BPA) and polychlorinated biphenyls (PCBs), promote the growth of breast cancer cells by functioning as agonists of GPR30.[39]

The traditional breast cancer drug tamoxifen, which blocks the activity of ER-α and ER-β, fails to suppress the cancer-promoting effects of GPR30. It is by this mechanism that some estrogen receptor-positive (ER-positive) breast cancers become drug-resistant. In fact, tamoxifen has been shown to *stimulate* the growth of drug-resistant breast cancer cells via activation of GPR30.[47]

E3, through its estrogen receptor modulatory capacity, combats the proliferative effects of E1 and E2.[39,48] These scientific findings highlight the importance of emphasizing E3 in any bioidentical hormone replacement regimen intended to restore youthful hormone balance and guard against breast cancer development.

# THE DANGERS OF AGE-RELATED HORMONE DECLINE

By the time a woman enters menopause, she may have already experienced two decades of hormonal imbalance. During the postmenopausal period, when sex hormone levels decrease significantly, aging women are at increased risk of the following diseases: heart disease, osteoporosis, Alzheimer's, and dementia, among others.

**Heart Disease.** According to the Centers for Disease Control and Prevention (CDC), heart disease is the leading killer of American women.[49] The risk for postmenopausal women is equal to that seen in men. Menopause can cause elevations in blood pressure, low-density lipoprotein (LDL) cholesterol, total cholesterol, triglycerides, as well as homocysteine levels, C-reactive protein, and interleukin-6 (an inflammatory cytokine), which are all associated with estrogen deficiency.[50–52] At the same time, high-density lipoprotein (HDL) cholesterol levels drop significantly. Estrogenic activities are vital for maintaining the integrity of the vascular endothelium, where atherosclerotic changes begin.[53] Finally, lack of estrogen replacement in the postmenopausal state may predispose women to forms of cardiac muscle disease that are only now beginning to be understood.[54]

**Osteoporosis.** Hormone deficiencies (beginning as early as age 30) are clearly associated with bone loss and osteoporosis. By the time women reach age 50, they are at a significantly increased risk of an osteoporotic bone fracture. Estrogen deficiency results in increased production of proinflammatory cytokines, which cause increased bone breakdown and inflammation.[55] Combined estrogen and androgen (ie, natural or synthetic) therapy has been shown to increase BMD more than estrogen therapy alone.[56]

**Alzheimer's and dementia.** Hormone loss is associated with neuronal degeneration and increased risk of dementia, Alzheimer's disease, and Parkinson's disease.[57,58] Estrogen stimulates degradation of beta-amyloid protein (noted to accumulate in the brain of Alzheimer's disease patients) by upregulating production of protective proteins.[59] Deficiencies in pregnenolone and DHEA, which are both neuroprotective hormones, are also linked to reduced memory and brain cell death associated with Alzheimer's disease.[60,61] These two hormones play an important role in regulating neurotransmitter systems that are involved in learning, stress, depression, addiction, and many other vital functions.[60]

## Progesterone's Balancing Act

In a healthy young woman, progesterone serves as a counterweight to estrogen during the menstrual cycle. Estrogen levels rise during the first half of the cycle and progesterone levels rise in the middle. Progesterone's job is two-fold: (1) to prepare the uterus for implantation with a healthy fertilized egg, and (2) to support the early stage of pregnancy. If no implantation occurs, progesterone levels drop until another cycle begins.

Studies have shown that progesterone has antiproliferative effects on breast cancer and leukemia cells.[62–64] Breast cancer is 5.4 times more common in premenopausal women with low progesterone levels than with favorable levels.[65] Data suggest that while bioidentical (ie, natural) progesterone does not increase risk of breast cancer, synthetic progestins used in conventional HRT do.[66]

Natural progesterone has also demonstrated neuroprotective properties. One study called for more attention to progesterone as a *"potent neurotrophic agent that may play an important role in reducing or preventing motor, cognitive, and sensory impairments [in both men and women]."*[67]

## BIOIDENTICAL HORMONE REPLACEMENT THERAPY

Bioidentical hormone formulations in measured doses (ie, tailored to individual patients) can be obtained from a compounding pharmacy with a physician's prescription. Bioidentical estrogen therapy has been utilized extensively in Europe and Japan for several years.[30]

**Estriol.** Estriol (E3) has shown beneficial effects in women at risk for cardiovascular disease. Japanese scientists found that a group of menopausal women treated with E3 for 12 months had a significant decrease in both systolic and diastolic blood pressure.[68] Another placebo-controlled study demonstrated that E3 replacement for 30 weeks improved flow-mediated dilation (a measure of arterial relaxation).[69] E3 accomplishes these effects by strongly activating nitric oxide signaling systems and stabilizing atherosclerotic plaques.[30]

E3 may further reduce cardiovascular risk through its beneficial effects on lipid profiles. One Japanese study found that E3 prevented a postmenopausal rise in total cholesterol while not inducing elevated triglyceride levels, a side effect frequently seen after treatment with conventional estrogen therapy.[70] E3, in combination with a statin drug, can reduce carotid artery intima-media thickness (a measure of atherosclerosis) in postmenopausal women with elevated blood lipids.[71]

E3 also increases bone mineral density, a vital parameter in post-menopausal women at risk for osteoporosis. In one study, women treated with E3 exhibited an increase in bone mineral density and improved climacteric (ie, menopausal) symptoms with no increased risk of endometrial hyperplasia.[72] In a second study, researchers treated postmenopausal and elderly women with either a combination of E3 and 1000 mg/day of calcium lactate or 1000 mg/day of calcium lactate alone. Bone mineral density significantly increased in women receiving E3 versus a decrease in those not receiving E3.[73] In a summary statement, the researchers wrote: *"[T]he acceleration of bone turnover usually observed after menopause was prevented by treatment with E3 [estriol]."*[74]

E3 also supports sexual and urinary health. For example, one study showed that E3-treated women reported a 68% reduction in symptoms of incontinence compared to 16% in the placebo group.[75] Women with recurrent urinary tract infections experienced a 91% reduction in infections following treatment with an intravaginal estriol cream compared to the placebo group.[76] Another study demonstrated that locally administered E3 therapy significantly increased the number of blood vessels surrounding the urethra, thereby improving its ability to maintain urine in the bladder until the desire to void the bladder is reached.[77] The addition of E3 to standard therapy for prevention of urinary tract infections reduced the number of recurrences 11-fold, and the days of antibiotic therapy more than 12-fold in another study.[78]

Stress incontinence refers to intermittent loss of urine with pelvic floor stress from laughing, coughing, and so on. Pelvic floor muscle exercises are effective in reducing stress incontinence, and studies suggest that E3 adds substantially to the beneficial effect(s).[79]

E3 can offer relief for women suffering from atrophic vaginitis, the symptoms of which include vaginal dryness, vaginal burning, and painful intercourse. After 4 weeks of treatment with an intravaginal estriol cream, researchers noted that *"atrophy of vaginal epithelium and chronic vaginitis stopped or significantly decreased. . . . The subjective complaints relating to the estrogen deficiency (vaginal burning and dryness, itching, dyspareunia [painful sex] and urinary dysfunctions) ceased. Side-effects and complications during the treatment were not found."*[80] More objective improvements to vaginal dryness and acidity have been demonstrated in recent studies.[81]

Topical estriol creams applied to the face and neck can reduce many symptoms of aging skin (eg, dryness and wrinkling). Animal studies demonstrate that estriol cream promotes collagen production and enhances skin's elasticity.[82]

Studies have also shown E3 to be effective in the treatment of menopausal symptoms. In one study, women being treated with varying doses of E3 for 6 months had decreased vasomotor symptoms of menopause (eg, hot flashes). The improvements were found to be dose-dependent. There were no detrimental effects on uterine or breast tissue.[83] Other studies have shown similar results with up to 71% of patients reporting elimination of hot flashes and sweating and 21% reporting a substantial reduction.[84]

**Progesterone.** Progesterone complements and balances the impact of estrogen in aging women. Combined with estrogen, progesterone substantially improved the amount of time that women with a history of heart attack or coronary artery disease could work out on a treadmill before reducing blood flow to the heart. Use of non-bioidentical progesterone produced no effect.[85] Another mechanism by which progesterone enhances cardiovascular health is its ability to maintain or even increase HDL levels in women receiving estrogen replacement therapy.[86–88]

Progesterone has a major role in relieving menopausal symptoms as well. Four head-to-head studies comparing progesterone to non-bioidentical synthetic progestogen (progestin) reported that women experienced greater satisfaction, improved quality of life, and fewer side effects when switched from progestin to progesterone.[89–92] The beneficial effects of progesterone compared to non-bioidentical progestin included a 30% reduction in sleep problems, 50% reduction in anxiety, 60% reduction in depression, 25% reduction in menstrual bleeding, 40% reduction in cognitive difficulties, and 30% improvement in sexual function. In the study, 80% of women reported overall satisfaction with the bioidentical progesterone formulation.[93]

---

## WHAT YOU NEED TO KNOW: BIOIDENTICAL HORMONES

- Non-bioidentical hormones are chemically different than natural hormones produced within the body. The use of non-bioidentical estrogen and synthetic progestin in the WHI trial was associated with an increased risk of breast cancer, heart attack, venous blood clot, and stroke.
- Non-bioidentical, oral conventional hormone replacement therapy is associated with an increased risk of uterine cancer.
- Bioidentical hormones have the same molecular structure as the hormones produced naturally within the body. The body does not distinguish between supplemental bioidentical hormones and the hormones produced within the body. As a result, bioidentical hormones are properly utilized, and are able to be naturally metabolized and excreted from the body.
- Current literature suggests that bioidentical progesterone is associated with a decreased risk of breast cancer.
- A scientific literature review suggests that bioidentical progesterone may be superior to progestins in treating menopausal symptoms. Estriol is also highly effective in the treatment of menopausal symptoms.
- Research on bioidentical progesterone has shown beneficial effects (eg, decreasing the risk of blood clots, protecting against atherosclerosis, and maintaining healthy HDL levels) on cardiovascular health.
- Three major types of estrogen are produced naturally in a woman's body: estrone (E1), estradiol (E2), and estriol (E3).
- Estriol has been shown to improve bone density, promote youthful skin, enhance urinary health, and improve sexual function.

---

## BEYOND ESTROGEN AND PROGESTERONE: THE COMPLETE HORMONAL PICTURE

In addition to estrogen and progesterone, it is important to monitor levels of the hormones pregnenolone, DHEA, and testosterone. Ideal bioidentical HRT goes beyond the mere suppression of symptoms caused by declining ovarian hormone levels. The real goal of Life Extension's approach to female hormone restoration is to restore hormones to youthful levels. Such an approach has wide-ranging benefits throughout the body and significantly enhances physical and psychological well-being.

**DHEA.** DHEA is a natural steroidal hormone secreted by the adrenal gland, gonads, and brain.[94] Although women usually have less DHEA than men, both sexes lose DHEA over time, suggesting an age-related decline.[95] Peak levels are typically reached when women are in their 30s, after which they begin to lose approximately 2% per year. Decreased levels of DHEA are associated with cancer, diabetes, lupus, psychiatric illness,[96] insomnia, pain, and disability.[97]

DHEA has been shown to improve mood, neurologic function, immune function, energy, feelings of well-being, and the maintenance of muscle and bone mass.[98,99] A combination of DHEA and pregnenolone has been shown to improve memory.[100] DHEA may also improve insulin sensitivity and triglyceride levels.[96,101]

Life Extension suggests that maturing women strive to keep their DHEA-sulfate (DHEA-S) levels in a range of 275–400 µg/dL to promote optimal health and vitality.

**Testosterone.** Like DHEA, testosterone levels in women gradually decrease with age.[102] Loss of testosterone affects libido, bone and muscle mass, vasomotor symptoms, cardiovascular health, mood, and well-being.[103,104] Testosterone in conjunction with estrogen has been shown to improve quality of life, vigor, mood, concentration, bone mineralization, libido, and sexual satisfaction.[103,105-107] The combination has also been shown to reduce hot flashes, sleep disturbances, night sweats, and vaginal dryness.[108] Because DHEA converts into testosterone, it is possible to raise testosterone levels with DHEA.[102,107]

Studies also suggest that testosterone, in the context of hormone restoration, may prevent or reduce estrogenic cancer risk in the treatment of women with ovarian failure.[109,110] In addition, testosterone is effective in the treatment of low libido in women.[108]

Life Extension encourages women to maintain a total testosterone level of 35–45 ng/dL and a free testosterone level of 1–2.2 pg/mL.

**Pregnenolone.** As is the case with other hormones, a significant reduction of pregnenolone begins when women reach their early 30s.[111] As the initial

hormone in the overall steroid hormone cascade, pregnenolone is derived from cholesterol. Pregnenolone deficiencies have been associated with diminished brain function and dementia.[112]

Aging women should maintain a pregnenolone blood level of 130–180 ng/dL for optimal performance.

It is very important that women have their hormone levels checked before beginning bioidentical hormone restoration therapy. To ensure safe and adequate levels, testing should occur 1 month after commencing HRT and then again 2 months later. Those women who wish to enhance their sexual desire and have already tried DHEA and pregnenolone therapy should consult with their physician about alternative options (eg, small amounts of testosterone). Women should always consult a physician before beginning HRT, especially if they have had or are at high risk (eg, first-degree relative with a diagnosis) of having hormone-responsive cancer (eg, breast or endometrial).

## MOVING FORWARD WITH BIOIDENTICAL HRT

Given the wealth of data demonstrating the superiority of bioidentical HRT, a noted researcher in hormone replacement therapy proclaimed, "*Physiological data and clinical outcomes demonstrate that bioidentical hormones are associated with lower risks, including the risk of breast cancer and cardiovascular disease, and are more efficacious than their . . . animal-derived [nonbioidentical] counterparts. Until evidence is found to the contrary, bioidentical hormones remain the preferred method of HRT.*"[12]

Compounded prescription bioidentical estrogen formulas include *Bi-Est* and *Tri-Est*. Bi-Est consists of 20% estradiol (E2) and 80% estriol (E3). Tri-Est contains 10% E2, 10% estrone (E1), and 80% E3.[113] In some situations these ratios do not meet individual needs. In one study, the amounts observed naturally in reproductive-age women were 90% E3, 7% E2, and 3% E1.[114] In this case, a prescription (based on the results of hormone tests and assessment of symptoms) is tailored to the needs of the patient by an experienced physician. A comprehensive hormone restoration program should also include progesterone, DHEA, pregnenolone, and perhaps testosterone.

There are two different philosophies regarding the dosing of hormones. The first encourages using the lowest possible dose that will ameliorate the symptoms. This more conservative approach is unlikely to cause a menstrual cycle in menopausal woman. However, it is also unlikely to bring hormones back to what Life Extension considers optimal levels.

The second approach involves significantly higher hormone dosages. The idea here is to "trick" a woman's brain into thinking she is still of reproductive age. The goal is to achieve levels that mimic the hormonal fluctuations of a menstruating woman, thereby restoring the menstrual cycle.

Utilizing the results of hormone testing and clinical evaluation(s), physicians with experience in bioidentical hormone replacement can help women find an optimal dosing strategy. Most women find that they respond desirably to bioidentical HRT when based on this combined approach. To obtain contact information for physicians in your area who are knowledgeable about bioidentical hormone replacement therapy, or to request information about Life Extension's Female Comprehensive Hormone Profile blood test, call 1-800-226-2370 or visit www.lef.org/blood.

Women taking any kind of estrogen replacement therapy (including bioidentical) should refer to the Breast Cancer Prevention protocol in order to understand the importance of making healthy lifestyle choices that could reduce the risk of breast cancer.

## How Bioidentical Estrogen-Progesterone Is Prescribed

The commercial availability of individually tailored bioidentical hormone products is limited. As a result, many physicians utilize compounding pharmacies to prepare and dispense bioidentical hormone prescriptions to their patients. To obtain the phone number of a compounding pharmacist in your area, call 1-800-226-2370.

In order to gauge the initial dose of bioidentical estrogen, the estradiol (E2) and/or total estrogen blood levels should be considered in conjunction with other hormones levels (eg, progesterone).

A menopausal woman typically has an E2 blood level of 0-19 pg/mL. With the use of bioidentical estrogen cream (eg, compounded E3 and E2), the blood E2 level may increase to 100 pg/mL or higher, which would indicate to the prescribing doctor that the formula is being *absorbed* and has increased the patient's E2 to a more youthful level.

If the patient reports that her menopausal symptoms have been resolved, most practitioners will continue the current dosage and conduct periodic follow-ups.

If, however, the patient is still having symptoms, the dose of bioidentical estrogen cream can be increased. In addition, a urinary hormone profile might be ordered to assess other estrogens and their associated metabolites. Based on the results of these tests, a more precise dose of E3, E2, progesterone, and occasionally, testosterone can be prescribed. A typical starting dose for bioidentical estrogen cream might read as follows:

---

Your Doctor's Name _____ DEA# _____

Your Doctor's Address _____

Your Doctor's Phone Number _____

Patient's Name _____ Age _____

Address _____ Date _____

*BI-EST cream:*
*0.5 mg estradiol/2.0 mg estriol per mL*
*Apply 1 mL topically every day. #60 mL*

Refill _____ times _____
(Signature)

---

Please note that this is a general suggestion for an initial prescription. A physician experienced in bioidentical hormone replacement will tailor the prescription to the individual woman's needs. The dose can be increased when severe symptoms of estrogen deficiency are present.

Women on an estrogen replacement regimen should also be prescribed *natural progesterone* (in contrast to synthetic progestin drugs like Provera®) in a dose that achieves a youthful balance. Natural progesterone produces many benefits when properly balanced with estrogen. The typical dose for topical progesterone cream may vary between 50 and 200 mg, depending on a woman's individual biochemical needs.

Typically, progesterone cream should be applied twice daily to different parts of the body. Specific dosing instructions are as follows:

- Premenstrual and perimenopausal women: 1/4 tsp. of a 2.5% progesterone topical cream (approximately 30 mg natural progesterone) twice daily, starting on day 12 of the menstrual cycle and continuing up to day 28.

- Menopausal women: 1/4 tsp. twice daily for 21 days, followed by 7 days off.

The dose can be adjusted up or down depending on a woman's symptoms and her response to treatment. If using natural progesterone cream from a pharmacy, a prescription for a postmenopausal woman might be written as follows:

```
┌─ ─ ─ ─ ─ ─ ─ ─ ─ ─ ─ ─ ─ ┐
|                                              |
|  Your Doctor's Name _____ DEA# _____   |
|  Your Doctor's Address _____     |
|  Your Doctor's Phone Number _____    |
|  Patient's Name _____ Age _____      |
|  Address _____ Date _____      |
|    PROGESTERONE cream 50 mg/mL               |
|  Directions: Apply 1 mL (pump) topically twice |
|    daily or at bedtime) days 1–25            |
|    Dispense: 1 or 2 month supply             |
|                                              |
|  Refill _____ times _____    |
|                          (Signature)         |
└─ ─ ─ ─ ─ ─ ─ ─ ─ ─ ─ ─ ─ ┘
```

A prescription for a premenopausal woman might read as follows:

```
┌─ ─ ─ ─ ─ ─ ─ ─ ─ ─ ─ ─ ─ ┐
|                                              |
|  Your Doctor's Name _____ DEA# _____   |
|  Your Doctor's Address _____     |
|  Your Doctor's Phone Number _____    |
|  Patient's Name _____ Age _____      |
|  Address _____ Date _____      |
|    PROGESTERONE cream 25 mg/0.1 cc           |
|  Directions: Apply 0.1 cc to the labia or intravagi- |
|    nally daily on days 10–25 of a 28 day cycle |
|    Dispense: 1 or 2 month supply             |
|                                              |
|  Refill _____ times _____    |
|                          (Signature)         |
└─ ─ ─ ─ ─ ─ ─ ─ ─ ─ ─ ─ ─ ┘
```

Some physicians prescribe topical progesterone similarly to estrogen, ie, in milligrams per fraction of a cubic centimeter (cc). These are applied via a syringe onto the skin, and have the dual advantage of more precise dosage adjustment and smaller volume of cream (which is less likely to make a mess on clothing).

The blood level targets in aging women might be:

- Estradiol: 90–211 pg/mL
- Progesterone: 2.0–6.0 ng/mL
- Free testosterone: 1.0–2.2 pg/mL

Before a prescription for bioidentical hormones can be written, it is important to have a baseline blood test to determine the doses of bioidenticals that might be needed. To order a comprehensive Female Panel that includes estradiol, progesterone, and free testosterone, call 1-800-226-2370.

In order to achieve optimal hormonal balance, it is important to also address testosterone levels. Although testosterone is thought of as a male hormone, it plays an important role in women's health. Testosterone levels decrease in women as they age. Low testosterone in postmenopausal women can have a negative impact on sex drive, mood, psychological well-being, bone and muscle mass, and cardiovascular health.[115-118] A physician experienced in bioidentical hormone therapy will measure testosterone levels in women and prescribe bioidentical testosterone if needed. Correcting low testosterone in women usually requires a 150–300 mcg patch or an individually prescribed testosterone cream.[119]

Since DHEA (dehydroepiandrosterone) can convert to testosterone in a woman's body (ie, naturally), a woman with low testosterone might be able to increase her level by taking 15–25 mg daily of DHEA, which is available as a low-cost dietary supplement.[120]

## Pros and Cons of Various Hormone Testing Methods

There is continuing debate regarding the best testing methods for hormones. Hormones can be analyzed in the blood, urine, or saliva. There are benefits and drawbacks to each of these methods. Life Extension currently offers blood and 24-hour urinary testing.

### Saliva Testing

**Pros**—This easy, at-home collection process is a measurement of bioavailable hormone levels.
**Cons**—Accuracy and testing variability are issues to consider. Hormone levels in saliva are significantly less than in blood, which can affect the accuracy of the test. In addition, saliva flow rate as well as gum disease (even if subclinical) will alter the results of the test. There are limited laboratories available for this type of testing.

Note: Although Life Extension does not utilize saliva testing at this time, some experienced physicians use this type of testing, in conjunction with clinical symptoms, to successfully evaluate and treat hormone deficiencies.

### Urine Testing

**Pros**—This method provides a 24-hour picture of hormone levels rather than a snapshot in time. It allows for testing of not only the three main estrogens—estrone, estradiol, and estriol—but also metabolites like 2- and 16-hydroxyestrone.

**Cons**—Inconvenient and more costly for a full hormone profile.

### Blood Testing

**Pros**—This method has been used consistently for decades. There is typically good correlation with symptoms. The testing is inexpensive, routine, and readily available through blood draw centers.

**Cons**—Blood draw involves a needle stick. Estrone and estradiol can be evaluated. This test, however, is not sensitive enough to assess estriol levels in menopausal women because the estriol test used by traditional laboratories is for the purposes of evaluating fetal growth in pregnancy, during which time levels of this hormone are much higher. Finally, there is no blood estrogen metabolite testing available.

## PHYTOESTROGENS AND NUTRITIONAL SUPPORT

Phytoestrogens are natural compounds found in some plants. They exert estrogen-like activity in the body and may be an effective alternative to bioidentical HRT for some women.

Some of the best evidence to support the use of phytoestrogens comes from Asia, where women do not typically experience many of the diseases and menopausal symptoms associated with the loss of estrogen. One explanation for this may be the phytoestrogens found in soy and other plant products consumed in Asian diets.[121–123]

Phytoestrogens bind to estrogen receptors and help modulate estrogen activity.[124] When estrogen levels are too low, their very mild estrogenic effect raises total estrogenic activity. Alternatively, when estrogen levels are too high, they compete with estrogen at cellular receptor sites, thus reducing endogenous estrogenic impact. By competing with endogenous estrogen for estrogen receptors, phytoestrogens may help prevent the growth and spread of several hormone-dependent cancers.[125] They have also been shown to decrease the risk of some degenerative diseases, including cardiovascular disease, osteoporosis, and breast and uterine cancer.[122,126–129]

Dietary and supplemental phytoestrogens present a way for women to obtain limited hormonal support without the use of hormone therapy.

**Cardiovascular Benefits:** Unlike conventional HRT, which has been shown to raise the risk of heart attack among postmenopausal women, phytoestrogens have a positive effect on the heart. In 1999, the Food and Drug Administration authorized the use of health claims on food labels that link increased soy consumption with a reduced risk of coronary artery disease.[130] One study of more than 400 women demonstrated that phytoestrogens, through their effect on the arterial walls (particularly in older women), protect against arterial degeneration and atherosclerosis.[131]

A scientific review of studies on phytoestrogens found they offer the following cardiovascular benefits:

- Improvements in lipid disturbances as a result of activating beneficial estrogen receptor subtypes[132]

- Decreased blood pressure, LDL cholesterol, total cholesterol, and triglycerides[133]

- Increased HDL cholesterol and improved cardiovascular profile[133,134]

- Lowering the overall rate of cardiovascular disease among people with higher consumption of phytoestrogens[135]

- Lowering of lipids in people with high cholesterol via genistein and daidzein, two of the most extensively studied phytoestrogens[124,136]

- Reduction in the risk of atherosclerosis due to increased levels of daidzein and genistein, which inhibit LDL oxidation[137]

In addition, a 6-month study of more than 180 women confirmed that a soy-rich diet is as effective as conventional HRT for lowering lipid levels.[138]

Furthermore, phytoestrogens have almost 3 times the radical scavenging activity as vitamins C and E, as well as help protect arterial walls.[131,139]

**Brain Protection:** Estrogen and estrogen-like compounds protect brain cells from degenerative changes due to aging and oxidative stress.[22,140]

- The phytoestrogen genistein protects animal subjects from the effects of brain ischemia, the kind of injury seen in stroke.[141–143]

- Genistein has antiapoptotic activity, protecting cultured brain cells from self-destructing over time.[144]

**Osteoporosis and Bone Health:** Studies have shown that postmenopausal women with a habitually high intake of phytoestrogens have high bone mineral density of the spine and hip.[127,145] A number of studies have been conducted on phytoestrogens and bone health, and their conclusions are as follows:

- Genistein and daidzein increase bone mineralization.[146–148]

- Genistein and daidzein decrease bone resorption and inflammatory factors while increasing osteogenic (bone-forming) proteins.[149–153]

- An isoflavone mixture of daidzein and genistein demonstrated significant increases in bone mineral density after 6 months of treatment. Women who ingested 57 mg daily of isoflavones had a 4% increase in bone mineral density.[147]

- A phytoestrogen preparation containing daidzein and genistein demonstrated protective effects on the lumbar spine.[154]

- Dietary supplementation with 54 mg daily of genistein *"may be as effective as hormone replacement therapy in attenuating menopause-related bone loss without causing the associated side effects."*[155]

**Cancer Protection:** Studies demonstrate a significantly lower incidence of sex hormone–related cancer in Asian countries.[123,156] These studies, which attribute this result to the traditionally high intake of soy isoflavones in the Asian diet, have concluded the following:

- Daily soy isoflavone consumption is associated with decreased breast cancer risk.[157] A diet containing 113–202 mg daily (depending on body size) of genistein and daidzein can increase the production of the protective 2-hydroxylated estrogen, decrease estradiol and its harmful metabolites, and lower the long-term risk of breast cancer.[158]

- Genistein and daidzein have an inhibitory effect on uterine cancer.[159]

- Genistein intake is linked with lower rates of stomach cancer.[160]

**Menopause Symptoms:** Several studies have demonstrated that natural estrogen significantly decreases hot flashes and vaginal atrophy.[161,162] Treatment with 54 mg daily of genistein safely decreased hot flashes up to 30% and should be considered as an alternative treatment for postmenopausal conditions.[163] Subsequent studies showed a decrease in hot flushes of more than 56%.[164] Another study concluded that *"genistein can be used for the management of hot flushes in postmenopausal women not treated with hormone replacement*

*therapy due to their superior efficacy to placebo and very good safety profile."*[165]

## Additional Natural Ingredients to Target the Symptoms of Menopause

**Black Cohosh.** Black cohosh has been used in the treatment of climacteric symptoms such as hot flashes, mood disturbances, diaphoresis, palpitations, and vaginal dryness.[166–168] Additionally, black cohosh conveys antiproliferative effects on breast cancer cells.[169–171] Data suggest that it is comparable to some pharmaceutical prescription medications for preventing bone loss.[172]

**Dong Quai.** Dong quai, based on its use in Chinese medicine for gynecologic disorders (ie, painful menstruation or pelvic pain, recovery from childbirth or illness, and fatigue/low vitality), is referred to as "female ginseng."[173,174] It is an effective remedy for alleviating menopausal symptoms without proliferative changes in the uterus or vagina.[175] A study demonstrated that a preparation of soy isoflavones, black cohosh, and dong quai reduced menstruation-related migraine headaches.[176]

**Licorice Root.** Licorice root exerts estrogen-like effects and has been shown to reduce body fat, positively impact testosterone metabolism,[177–179] and decrease serotonin reuptake by up to 60%, which may help alleviate menopausal depression.[180] Licorice root also assists with repair of blood vessel walls and supports arterial health, thus reducing the risk of cardiovascular disease.[181]

**Vitex Agnus-Castus.** Extracts from the fruit and leaves of vitex agnus-castus (vitex), also known as chasteberry, contain chemicals with diverse beneficial effects for the treatment of premenstrual symptoms.[182] In one study, menopausal women reported excellent symptomatic relief after using two essential oils from vitex.[183]

## Nutrients to Complement Bioidentical HRT

**Vitamin D.** Vitamin D confers significant protective effects against breast cancer. In a study, women with higher vitamin D levels had a nearly 70% reduction in their risk of breast cancer compared to women with the lowest levels.[184] Laboratory studies have shown that vitamin D suppresses growth of breast cancer by:

- Blocking signals that stimulate cancer cell growth

- Enhancing signals that inhibit cancer cell growth

- Favorably altering genetic regulators of the cell cycle[185–188]

Vitamin D helps prevent mutated cells from becoming malignant and even induces cancer cell death (apoptosis). Human studies show that doses of 1100 IU vitamin D daily plus calcium result in a 60% risk reduction for developing any cancer, compared with placebo.[189]

**Cruciferous Vegetables.** Cruciferous vegetables such as broccoli, cauliflower, cabbage, kale, and Brussels sprouts can help detoxify dangerous estrogen breakdown products that promote cancer growth.[190,191] When estrogens are metabolized via certain biochemical pathways, they become more likely to trigger cancer.[192,193] Aging adults suffer from a high prevalence of cancers associated with an imbalance in estrogen metabolism.[192,193] Cruciferous vegetables contain compounds that promote a healthier pathway for the breakdown of estrogens in the body, thus protecting against cancer.[34,194–198]

A chief component of cruciferous vegetables, indole-3-carbinol (I3C), prevents the conversion of estrogen to its breast cancer promoting *16-alpha-hydroxyestrone* form, while increasing conversion to its cancer-fighting *2-hydroxyestrone* form.[32,199,200]

**Lignans.** Lignans can slow the growth of breast cancer in women. Thirty-two women awaiting surgery for breast cancer were randomized to receive a muffin either with or without (control group) 25 g of flaxseeds. Analysis of the cancerous tissue after surgery revealed that markers of tumor growth were reduced by 30–71% in the flaxseed group, with no change noted in the control group.[201]

A recently published study found that a combination of lignans, I3C, and calcium-d-glucarate along with other supportive herbs favorably altered the 2/16-hydroxyestrone ratio in pre- and postmenopausal women. The researchers remarked, *"Supplementation with a mixture of indole-3-carbinol and . . . lignan in women significantly increased estrogen C-2 hydroxylation. This may constitute a mechanism for the reduction of breast cancer risk as well as risk for other estrogen-related cancers."*[202]

A comprehensive review of 21 studies found that postmenopausal women with higher lignan intake were significantly less likely to get breast cancer. The investigators concluded that *"high lignan exposure may be associated with a reduced breast cancer risk in postmenopausal women."*[203]

**Fish Oil.** Fish oil, with its high omega-3 fatty acid content, reduces cancer risk by a number of mechanisms. Fish oil reduces oxidative stress and suppresses production of many inflammatory mediators that contribute to cancer development.[204] It can sensitize tumor cells to chemotherapy effects (even when metastases are present), potentially reducing the doses of chemotherapy required for treatment.[205]

A study revealed that fish oil, through its effect on oxidative stress and induction of apoptosis, can prevent the progression of colon cancer.[206] In an animal model of breast cancer, fish oil supplementation was shown to reduce bone metastasis by blunting the expression of a protein called CD44, which drives cancer cell migration.[207]

**Green Tea.** Green tea polyphenols, particularly one called epigallocatechin gallate (EGCG), suppress the growth and reproduction of human breast cancer cells. They have reduced the number of breast cancer tumors in animal models of the disease.[208–210] Green tea also reduces the production of vascular endothelial growth factor (VEGF), helping to starve tumors of their blood supply while down-regulating cancer-promoting estrogen receptors and increasing apoptosis.[210–213]

**Pomegranate.** Pomegranate has been extensively studied for its antioxidant properties as well as its cancer-fighting capacity. With respect to breast cancer, pomegranate is an especially promising phyto agent due to its ability to both inhibit the cancer-promoting enzyme aromatase and suppress angiogenesis, which is the process by which tumors gain new blood vessels.[214,215]

## SUMMARY

Equine estrogens and synthetic progestins remained the staple of menopausal care until 2002, when the Women's Health Initiative (WHI) revealed the dangers associated with these *unnatural* hormone replacement methods. As women learned that conventional hormone replacement therapy was closely tied to an increased risk of certain cancers, many abandoned their trust in mainstream medicine and turned to natural bioidentical hormones as well as scientifically validated phytoestrogens for menopausal symptom relief.

Emerging science continues to undermine conventional hormone replacement therapy in favor of bioidentical hormone replacement. Studies confirming the estrogen receptor modulating abilities of the natural estrogen *estriol* provide reassurance for women who seek relief from the ravages of age-related hormone loss without the fear of increased cancer risk.

By coupling healthy diet and lifestyle habits with regular blood testing and bioidentical hormone replacement therapy, women today have a means to look and feel their best at any age.

Given the preponderance of evidence, women should feel confident that bioidentical hormone replacement, when appropriately prescribed, offers a safer and potentially more effective alternative to conventional HRT to help relieve menopausal symptoms and optimize long-term health. The addition of several proven nutrients to a bioidentical hormone regimen may help optimize estrogen metabolism and reduce cancer risk even further, offering an optimal, balanced approach to health maintenance.

## Life Extension Suggestions

A hormone replacement regimen should start with a comprehensive female hormone profile blood test and a consultation with a qualified, knowledgeable physician. Once a baseline hormone profile is established, periodic blood testing is recommended to monitor hormone levels. Women interested in hormone blood testing can call 1-800-226-2370 or visit Life Extension's Blood Testing and Laboratory Services online.

Life Extension recommends that women strive for the following optimal hormone levels.

| Hormone | Optimal Range |
| --- | --- |
| DHEA | 275–400 µg/dL |
| Total estrogen | Day 01–10: 61–394 pg/mL |
| | Day 11–20: 122–437 pg/mL |
| | Day 21–30: 156–350 pg/mL |
| | Menopause and post-menopausal: 75–200 pg/mL |
| Estradiol | Lowest dose to ameliorate symptoms: 30–50 pg/mL |
| | Typical replacement such as with a Bi-Est cream/gel: 80–100 pg/mL |
| | Higher end replacement/ restoration of menstrual cycle: 90–211 pg/mL |
| Progesterone | 18–27 ng/mL (premenopause) |
| | 2–6 ng/mL, but up to 15 for some women, especially if they are treated with higher doses of estrogen replacement (menopause and postmenopause) |
| Total testosterone | 35–45 ng/dL |
| Free testosterone | 1–2.2 pg/mL |

## Nutrients to Support Hormonal Balance and Healthy Hormonal Metabolism

- **Genistein**: 25–75 mg daily
- **Daidzein**: 20–50 mg daily
- **Black cohosh**, standardized extract: 40–80 mg daily
- **Pomegranate**, standardized extract: 400–800 mg daily
- **Green tea**, standardized extract: 725–1450 mg daily
- **Vitex**, standardized extract: 20–40 mg daily
- **Broccoli**, standardized extract: 400–800 mg daily
- **Indole-3-carbinol (I3C)**: 80–160 mg daily
- **3,3'-diindolylmethane (DIM)**: 14–28 mg daily
- **Licorice root extract**: 25–50 mg daily
- **Lignan extract** (flax or Norway spruce): 25–50 mg daily
- **Vitamin D3**: 5000–8000 IU daily
- **Omega-3 fatty acids** (from fish): 2000–6000 mg daily
- **Calcium D-glucarate**: 200–600 mg daily
- **DHEA**: 25–50 mg daily (depending on blood test results)
- **Pregnenolone**: 50–100 mg daily (depending on blood test results)
- **Progesterone cream**: per label directions

In addition, the following *blood testing* resources may be helpful:

- Female Comprehensive Hormone Panel
- Female Basic Hormone Panel
- Urinary Hormone Profile (24 hour)

## REFERENCES

References available at: www.lef.org/dpt5/ch58

# 59

# Fibrocystic Breast Disease

Breast nodules are a frequently presented gynecologic complaint. These nodules have two chief causes: benign breast disease and cancer. However, benign breast disease is the most common cause of nodules and can stem from cyst formation, obstructed ducts, inflammation, or infection. Although benign breast nodules have several causes and manifest themselves differently, for purposes of this discussion, all fibrous nodules or lumps will be referred to as fibrocystic breast disease (FBD).

According to the National Cancer Institute/ National Institutes of Health,[1,2] FBD is a common condition that affects many women at some time in their lives. FBD is most common between ages 30 and 50,[3] but younger women as well as menopausal women taking hormone replacement therapy (HRT) may also experience FBD.[4] More recently, some physicians have preferred to call FBD, fibrocystic breast "condition" or "change" (FBC).

The symptoms of FBD can vary significantly. Some women experience severe breast tenderness and pain with multiple lumps in both breasts. Other women have only mild tenderness with no detectable lumps. In some women the symptoms are relatively constant, while in others the symptoms come and go either monthly or over several months. According to the National Cancer Institute,[1] the chances of developing FBD are greater in women who have never had children, have irregular menstrual cycles, or have a family history of FBD or breast cancer.

FBD is a condition generally characterized by lumps that move freely in the breast tissue and vary in texture and size.[5] However, because the clinical signs of breast cancer are not easily distinguished from benign breast conditions, all breast lumps should be examined by a physician and not be assumed to be benign. Only a physician can determine the nature of breast lumps or changes.[1]

Because FBD is a benign condition, it usually does not lead to breast cancer.[2,6] Fortunately, only about 5% of FBD cases involve the type of changes that would be considered a risk factor for developing breast cancer. However, benign conditions may eventually result in calcifications.[7] Calcifications are quite small—sometimes as small as a grain of salt—and cannot be detected during a routine exam; however, calcifications may be detected by routine mammography. Since calcifications may be associated with some types of premalignant lesions, it is important to follow your physician's recommendations concerning the frequency of mammography.[3]

## NORMAL BREAST TISSUE

The breast is composed of 15–20 lobes of milk-secreting glands that are embedded in fatty tissue. Ducts link the lobes of these glands and have an outlet through the nipple. The area between the lobules and ducts is filled with fatty tissue. Breast tissue itself contains no muscles; however, there are small, very fine ligaments throughout the breast that attach to the skin and determine the shape of the breast. There are no muscles in the breast itself, although pectoral muscles lie just under each breast and over the ribs.[3]

The breasts undergo changes each month when a female begins to have menstrual periods. Hormones that are implicated in development of breast mammary glands and worsening premenstrual breast symptoms are estrogen and progesterone, the main female hormones, and prolactin, the milk release hormone secreted by the pituitary gland.[5] An increase in prolactin may also be responsible for some FBC changes because higher levels of prolactin seem to be connected with a higher occurrence of FBC (prolactin levels of >100 ng/mL may be a causative factor). Often the painful symptoms of FBD will decrease once menstruation begins. In some women, however, the repeated cycles of hormonal stimulation result in chronic inflammation and development of fibrous tissue. When fibrous tissue makes it more difficult for the fluid in breast cysts to escape and be normally absorbed by a woman's body, the cysts become denser, which can cause pain and pressure on surrounding tissues.[5] This fibrous tissue is similar to the type of tissue in ligaments and scars and feels firm, thick, rubbery, and ridge-like. It may also feel like small or large beads scattered throughout the breast.

In addition to naturally occurring hormones (ie, estrogen, progesterone, and prolactin), many other natural hormones (hypothalamic, other pituitary hormones, thyroid, parathyroid, adrenal, pineal, pancreas, ovarian, and duodenal hormones) can contribute to FBD.[3,8] Environmental estrogens, called xenoestrogens, may also contribute to human hormone levels. Xenoestrogens come from phytoestrogens (produced by plants), dietary estrogens from meat and dairy products, and many other chemicals such as pesticides, fertilizers, alkylphenols (used in detergents), and plastics (food packaging).[9] Additionally, as women approach menopause, they have an additional complicated decision to make concerning the use of synthetic hormone replacement therapy (HRT).[10–12]

# BREAST NODULES

As stated earlier, because breast tissue is naturally a glandular type of tissue, almost all women develop nodules or lumps in their breasts at some time or another. Lumps, also called "dominant lumps," feel different from surrounding tissue.[3] Some may be quite large, while others are small and even diffuse over time.[6] Fibrous tissue in the breast may even be mistaken for a lump. Breast nodules or lumps are the result of several medical causes, including cysts, fibroadenomas, areolar gland abscesses, breast abscesses, intraductal papillomas, mammary duct ectasia, mastitis, Paget's disease, and cancer.[13]

## Benign Nodules

**Cysts.**   Cysts are the most common cause of nodules or breast lumps. Cysts are usually smooth, round, fluid-filled, and slightly elastic. Although the fluid that comes from a cyst is often discolored, the color of the fluid is of little cause for concern unless it is bloody. Cysts occur as an isolated lump, in clusters, or widespread with well-defined lumps of various sizes. Cystic lumps are mobile and do not attach themselves to underlying breast tissue; therefore, cysts do not produce tissue deviation or dimpling. Mobility is one major characteristic that differentiates cysts from malignant nodules. However, cysts are sometimes accompanied by thickened adjacent tissue that is palpable and not so mobile. Breast cysts may also produce a discharge from the nipple that varies from clear and watery to sticky.[3]

Cysts frequently occur in the upper outer quadrant and the underside of the breast. Symptoms range from a feeling of fullness or heaviness to a dull ache, extreme sensitivity, or a burning sensation. For some women, these symptoms may be severe, making exercising or sleeping on their stomachs painful.

Cysts also often increase in size and tenderness in response to the monthly menstrual cycle because breast tissue undergoes changes related to the normal rise and fall of hormone levels.[5] After menstruation, the changes and symptoms sometimes abate. Physicians recommend that the best time for breast examination is about 7–10 days after the start of menstruation when breast tissue is more likely to be at its most normal state. Sometimes, after menopause, FBD symptoms completely disappear or become less noticeable (without HRT).[4]

The occurrence of multiple cysts in one or both breasts is also common in FBD (also called fibroadenosis or chronic cystic mastitis).[13] If a mass is determined to be a cyst, the next step is to determine if it is a simple cyst (one compartment) or a complex cyst (more than one compartment within the cyst). Simple cysts are very unlikely to be malignant.

**Sclerosing adenosis.**   Sclerosing adenosis is a benign condition with excessive tissue growth in the lobules of the breast.[2] The condition frequently causes breast pain. Sclerosing adenosis may produce lumps and appears on a mammogram as a calcification (a small deposit of calcium) in breast tissue.

**Intraductal papillomas.**   Small, wart-like, benign growths that project into the breast ducts near the nipple are intraductal papillomas.[2] They usually occur singly, but can also appear as multiple lesions. The smaller nodules are difficult to palpate. The primary sign of intraductal papilloma is nipple discharge, either clear or bloody. Breast pain and tenderness may occur.

## Nodules with Potential for Cancer

**Complex cysts.**   Complex cysts have more than one compartment within the cyst. Ultrasonography is valuable in differentiating simple cysts from complex cysts or solid masses.[14] Complex cysts are somewhat more likely to be cancerous, so doctors will often order further tests, beginning with fine needle aspiration and perhaps a biopsy, to be certain the cyst is not cancerous or pre-cancerous.

**Fibroadenomas.**   Fibroadenomas (sometimes called adenofibromas) are smooth, firm, benign tumors that are extremely mobile, feel slippery, and move around easily in the breast. They consist of structural (fibro) and glandular (adenoma) tissue.[2,13] Fibroadenomas feel round with well-defined margins and vary from pinhead in size to very large. They grow rapidly and usually occur near the nipple or on the outside of the upper quadrant. Fibroadenomas occur most often in women in their 20s and 30s and occur twice as often in African-American women as in other American women.[2] When aspirated, if there is no fluid in the lump, it is most likely a fibroadenoma. Fibroadenomas do not cause pain or tenderness. A "complex" fibroadenoma contains abnormal growths or exhibits abnormal cell changes. Although fibroadenomas themselves do not become cancerous,[2] they can act as markers for the disease. Women with a family history of breast cancer who also develop complex fibroadenomas might be at a higher risk for developing cancer than other women. Fibroadenomas are not difficult to remove and rarely recur.

**Paget's disease.** Paget's disease is a slow-growing intraductal carcinoma that begins as a scaling, eczema-like lesion on the nipple.[13] The nipple becomes red and irritated and the lesion extends along the skin and into the ducts. The lesion can progress to a mass located deep in the breast.

**Phyllodes tumor.** Phyllodes tumor is a breast tumor that might be malignant.[15] Phyllodes tumor is a rare type of breast tumor, similar to a fibroadenoma, but is composed of an overgrowth of fibrous connective breast tissue that can become quite large. Although rare, if malignancy is discovered via biopsy, the tumor and a margin of normal breast tissue are removed surgically.

# FACTORS AFFECTING INCREASED RISK OF BREAST CANCER

When a woman finds a breast nodule, the first concern is that it might be cancerous. Most of the time, breast nodules are not cancerous (benign). According to Hurley,[16] there are three basic, agreed-upon classifications of benign breast disease: nonproliferative, proliferative without atypia, and atypical hyperplasia. However, there can be an association with benign changes in the breast in young women and an increased risk of breast cancer with age, particularly later in life. Therefore, pathologists sometimes add comments to the pathology report indicating whether or not benign changes are relevant to an increased risk of cancer. One study followed 644 women with breast nodules between 1976 and 1982; the researchers found a relationship between subsequent cancer in women with multiple cysts and in 15 of the women whose cysts had been aspirated. The authors concluded that women with multiple breast cysts that have been aspirated have an increased risk of breast cancer. These women should perform more breast self-examinations and have follow-ups accordingly.[17]

Benign breast conditions are more often found in premenopausal women.[18,19] Breast cancer occurs more often in postmenopausal women (75% of cases).[20] Estimating the risk for future breast cancer from a benign condition is difficult; the extent of mammography screening differs in the population and often, significant time passes between diagnosis of benign disease in a younger woman and the increased risk

for breast cancer development in older women. Because benign breast disease is difficult to distinguish from malignant disease, diagnostic biopsy is required for a definitive diagnosis.[20]

Women diagnosed with benign disease do appear to have an overall modest increase in risk for subsequent development of breast cancer, particularly for more hyperplastic or epithelial (the covering or lining) proliferative forms. However, the evidence regarding the risk of breast cancer for nonproliferative conditions is conflicting. Some research found that the risk of breast cancer for women with nonproliferative disease is about double that of women without benign disease,[21] while others find that lesions with no proliferative changes were not associated with an increased risk.[20,22,23] According to Hurley,[16] atypical hyperplasia is a risk factor, but is not with certainty followed by breast cancer; risk applies to both breasts, with greater risk on the affected side. There is no means to predict which women will go on to develop breast cancer and the effectiveness of current screening and management methods is unknown. Further complicating a physician's ability to predict a woman's risk for breast cancer is that most women do not have a history of biopsy for a benign lesion.[20,24]

## Hormone Replacement and Breast Cancer

In the July 17, 2002 edition of the *Journal of the American Medical Association*, after decades of accumulated observational evidence, the Women's Health Initiative Investigators group raised concerns about the balance of risks and benefits for hormone use in healthy postmenopausal women. The concerns resulted from a randomized controlled primary prevention trial. The trial recruited 16 608 postmenopausal women (50–79 years of age) with an intact uterus at age 40 to U.S. clinical centers from 1993 to 1998. The study was designed to last 8.5 years. Participants in the study received placebo (8102 subjects) or conjugated equine estrogen (0.625 mg daily) plus medroxyprogesterone acetate (2.5 mg daily) in a single tablet (8506 subjects), commonly known as Prempro®. The study monitored coronary heart disease, invasive breast cancer, stroke, pulmonary embolism, endometrial cancer, colorectal cancer, hip fracture, and death due to other causes.

After 5.2 years, the data and safety monitoring board recommended stopping the trial because one statistic (for invasive breast cancer) had exceeded the stopping boundary for an adverse effect and the global index statistic supported risks exceeding benefits. Although the absolute risk was still low, investigators stopped the estrogen plus progestin part of the study.

They concluded: "Overall health risks exceeded benefits from use of combined estrogen plus progestin for an average 5.2-year follow-up among healthy postmenopausal U.S. women." Women in the other groups in the study (women taking estrogen alone, on a low-fat diet, taking calcium and vitamin D supplements, and women in the observation-only group) were advised to continue with their assigned treatment regime. However, prescribing the combination of estrogen and progestin was not recommended for long-term use or for prevention of chronic diseases.[12] Theories abound about why there appear to be complications with combination HRT, with one being that the progestin part of the therapy may have an antagonistic action on the estrogen part. Other co-factors include obesity, diabetes, and influence of family health history.

Another much smaller study of 158 women (58 using HRT with Prempro® [0.625 mg conjugated equine estrogen plus 5 mg medroxyprogesterone acetate], 51 using low-dose oral estrogen alone [estriol] 2 mg daily, and 55 using transdermal estrogen via a patch with estradiol, 50 mcg each 24 hours) evaluated the impact of different HRT regimens on mammographic breast density. Independent radiologists were unaware of the HRT and analyzed coded mammography films. The research indicated that an increase in mammographic density was more common in women taking continuous combined HRT (40%) than in those using oral low-dose estrogen (6%) or transdermal (2%) treatment. The researchers reported that increased density was already apparent at the first visit after beginning HRT. During long-term follow-up, there was very little change in mammographic status, leading to the conclusion that there was an "urgent need to clarify the biological nature and significance of a change in mammographic density during treatment and, in particular, its relation to symptoms and breast cancer risk."[10]

Scientists, environmentalists, physicians, and governmental agencies have all produced reports in support of their particular stance on hormones—whether they are safe and whether they should be used. Therefore, in light of continuing concerns about the safety of using HRT, particularly HRT containing estrogen plus a progestin component, decisions concerning hormone use and modulation are personal ones related to each woman's particular risk factors and her reasons to consider using HRT. It is more important than ever to consult a physician for guidance concerning the decision to use any hormone therapy. (For more information, see Life Extension's Female Hormone Restoration protocol.)

## Other Causes of Breast Nodules

**Mastitis.** Mastitis or postpartum mastitis is an infection in women who are breastfeeding in which a milk duct becomes blocked, causing milk to pool, permitting a bacterial infection, and resulting in inflammation.[3] The breast appears red, feels warm, and may be tender. Mastitis can be accompanied by chills, fever, and cracking of the nipple.

**Mammary duct ectasia.** Mammary duct ectasia causes ducts beneath the nipple to become clogged and inflamed, particularly in women nearing menopause or in postmenopausal women.[2] The condition can be itchy and tender, with transient pain, and may produce a thick, sticky multicolored discharge. The skin over the nodule may be a blue-green color. Nearby lymph nodes can also be inflamed.

**Pseudolumps.** Pseudolumps are normal lumpy areas of breast tissue. This type of lumpiness will often disappear or vary with cyclic hormonal levels. Pseudolumps also result from silicone injections (to enlarge the breasts) or as a consequence of breast surgery or radiation therapy.

**Fat necrosis.** Fat necrosis produces painless, round, firm lumps that form from damaged and disintegrating fatty tissue.[2] Fat necrosis is more likely to occur in obese women with large breasts. It may also develop in response to a bruise or blow to the breast. Sometimes the skin around these lumps looks red or bruised.

**Breast pain.** Mastalgia refers to breast pain that is severe enough to cause a woman to seek medical treatment. Mastalgia can occur at rest or during movement, intermittently, cyclically, or constantly and can be sharp or dull and radiate to the back, arms, or neck. Pain can be aggravated by palpation (such as during physical examination). However, mastalgia is an unreliable indicator of a serious condition such as cancer.[13] Although many women experience uncomfortable tenderness and swelling, pain characterized as severe occurs only about 15% of the time.

Breast pain not related to the menstrual cycle is called noncyclical breast pain. Noncyclical breast pain is rare and much more difficult to treat. Noncyclical breast pain can be caused by old trauma to the breast (such as a blow to the breast, biopsy, or surgery), infection, or some other condition completely unrelated to the breast.[13] Arthritis is a possible cause of breast pain. Arthritis pain is usually felt in the breastbone, at the center of the chest. Women with arthritic breast pain also may experience increased discomfort when they breathe deeply.

An early study showed that there were significant abnormalities in pituitary function (via prolactin mechanisms) seen in severe cyclical mastalgia and nodular breast disease, but not in women with non-cyclical mastalgia.[25]

## SIGNS OF BREAST CANCER

Nodules that are hard, poorly delineated, and fixed to the skin or to underlying tissue are suggestive of breast cancer. Cancerous nodules can cause dimpling, nipple deviation, or nipple retraction. They usually occur singly and are often not painful. There may be nipple discharge that is clear or bloody. Bloody discharge is more suggestive of breast cancer. Ulceration may occur in later stages.[15] (Further discussion of breast cancer is beyond the scope of this protocol. See Life Extension's Breast Cancer protocol for a discussion of additional information.)

## DIAGNOSING FIBROCYSTIC BREAST DISEASE

A health care provider experienced in diagnosing breast conditions should examine any new breast mass or lump. Additionally, if there is any skin irritation, dimpling, nipple pain or retraction, redness or scaling of the nipple or breast skin, or nipple discharge other than breast milk in lactating women, see a physician for an evaluation. Breast conditions usually can be diagnosed by an examination by a physician. It is not unusual for a physician to recommend a mammogram, ultrasound, or biopsy procedure to assist or confirm the diagnosis.[26]

A mammogram, the most frequently used diagnostic tool for breast lumps, is a type of x-ray examination. If the mammogram suggests that abnormal tissue is benign, follow the physician's recommendations and recheck the lump (in perhaps 4–6 months).[26] If the mammogram is inconclusive or indicates the need for further examination, your physician may recommend a computer-aided diagnostic procedure using ultrasound. This additional diagnostic procedure is designed to improve identification of a potentially malignant lesion.

Ultrasound uses high-frequency waves to outline a part of the body and is useful to further evaluate possible abnormalities found during mammograms or physical examinations. Besides aspiration, ultrasound is the only way to determine if the lump is a fluid-filled cyst. Fluid-filled cysts have a distinctive appearance on an ultrasound screen.

Fine-needle aspiration biopsy (FNAB) is used if the physician is almost certain that the lump is a cyst.

Aspiration is also used to extract material from a lump for further analysis.[2] A very thin needle is inserted into the breast tissue as the doctor palpates the lump. The procedure is essentially painless because nerves are located primarily in the skin, not in the breast tissue itself. Ultrasound is used to guide the needle when a lump is either difficult to palpate or very small. FNAB has decreased the need for surgical biopsy.

Core-needle biopsy uses a needle larger than the type employed with FNAB. The procedure is performed in a physician's office with local anesthesia of the breast area to be biopsied. Core-needle biopsy removes a small cylinder of tissue for examination.

Stereotactic biopsy is a newer approach that relies on a three-dimensional x-ray to guide the needle biopsy of nonpalpable mass.[2] The breast is x-rayed from two different angles and a computer plots the position of the suspicious area. Once the area is precisely identified, the radiologist uses a needle to biopsy the lesion.

Surgical biopsy may also be necessary to remove all or part of a lump for examination.[2] This procedure is done either in a physician's office or an outpatient hospital facility under intravenous sedation or local anesthesia.

There are newer methods, such as vacuum-assisted biopsy, which remove even more tissue, but so far there is no universal agreement about when these procedures should be used, even though current studies show consistent reliable results.[27–31]

## CONVENTIONAL TREATMENTS FOR FIBROCYSTIC BREAST DISEASE

Although some physicians consider FBD to be more correctly termed a condition, its symptoms cause significant pain and discomfort for many women. Women who have FBD may find relief from any of several conventional and natural treatments. Some procedures (eg, FNAB) for the conventional treatment of FBD can often be performed in a physician's office. Other procedures (eg, biopsy) are usually performed in an ambulatory or hospital surgical facility.

### Breast Cysts

Breast cysts are relatively simple to treat. Simple breast cysts are aspirated by a physician with a needle and syringe.[2] A biopsy is often not necessary. Fluid aspirated from a cyst is rarely tested unless it is bloody or the woman is older than 55 years of age. Gross, benign breast cysts disappear after aspiration. However, a cancerous lump remains even after fluid is withdrawn. Following imaging by mammography and ultrasonography, complex cysts require laboratory investigation usually beginning with fine needle aspiration and perhaps biopsy.

## Intraductal Papilloma

In intraductal papilloma, the diseased ducts can be removed surgically if discharge becomes bothersome.[1,2] The appearance of the breast is usually unchanged.

## Mastitis

Mastitis or postpartum mastitis is an infection that is treated with antibiotics.[7] Pus-filled abscesses may need to be drained or removed. Lactating women with mastitis should use a breast pump to prevent additional pooling of breast milk and discard the milk. Breast milk should not be used until the infection has responded to antibiotic treatment.

## Mammary Duct Ectasia

Mammary duct ectasia is treated with antibiotics, warm compresses, and sometimes surgery.[2]

## Hormone and Drug Therapy

The anterior pituitary gland secretes follicle-stimulating hormone (FSH), which in turn causes follicle cells in the ovaries to secrete estrogens. The anterior pituitary also secretes luteinizing hormone (LH), which causes the corpus luteum to secrete progesterone and a small amount of estrogens, including estradiol (E2). LH and FSH work together to bring about ovulation and menstruation. The corpus luteum produces progesterone for about 11 days (the luteal phase) after ovulation. About 3 days later, when levels of estrogen and progesterone are at their lowest, menstruation begins.

In an early study comparing women with normal breast tissue to women with benign breast disease, there was a significant imbalance of progesterone over estradiol during the luteal phase in women with benign breast disease.[32] When the women were grouped according to type of breast lesion, there was elevated or normal estradiol in women with adenosis tumors and increased nodularity of both breasts. Plasma progesterone was also consistently lower in all groups as compared to women with normal breast tissue. The authors concluded: "From these results it may be postulated that an imbalance in the secretion of E2 and progesterone by the corpus luteum is a constant finding in women with benign breast disease."[32]

**Oral contraceptives.** Sometimes physicians treat breast pain and swelling associated with FBD by prescribing oral contraceptives which tend to stabilize (or level out) hormone levels. Results of studies indicate that oral contraceptives have positive benefits by decreasing the symptoms of FBD, particularly in younger women.[33–35]

**Hormone replacement therapy.** Hormone replacement therapy (HRT), often recommended to postmenopausal women, may actually increase the symptoms of FBD depending on the hormone combination used. As with any type of hormone administration, however, the results and effects differed widely among women studied. When on HRT, it is important to monitor any changes in breast tissue and evaluate these changes with your physician as they relate to the positive benefits (cardiovascular, bone density) versus the risks (increased density of breast nodules) of continuing HRT.[10,36] (See Life Extension's Female Hormone Restoration protocol.)

In a 1997 study, doctors treated women with painful FBD by giving them estroprogestins (estrogen-progesterone compounds) for 3 months. They found that 60% of the women reported reduced or improved symptoms.[37] However, like HRT, estrogen replacement therapy (ERT) has also been linked to higher rates of FBD among postmenopausal women; in fact, they are twice as likely to develop FBD as women who have not used ERT.[38] Women on ERT also experience more fibroadenomas. The risk seems to increase the longer the therapy is employed.

Powerful drugs (eg, tamoxifen and Danazol) with hormonal effects are also available and are prescribed with caution when pain from FBD is severe. However, physicians are hesitant to use them because of potential side effects and interactions with other drugs or conditions.

**Tamoxifen.** Tamoxifen, a medicine that blocks the effects of estrogen hormone in the body, is primarily used to treat breast cancer that is estrogen receptor positive.[39] It has also been used in some women who do not have breast cancer, but are at high risk to develop it. Tamoxifen has been used to relieve significant breast pain associated with FBD. An early double-blind, controlled study was done with tamoxifen in 60 patients who had severe mastalgia lasting more than 6 months. The patients were treated with a placebo or 20 mg of tamoxifen for 3 months. There was relief of pain in 71% of patients receiving tamoxifen, demonstrating that tamoxifen was valuable in the treatment of severe cyclical and noncyclical mastalgia and that treatment can be achieved with few side effects.[40] How tamoxifen works and its long-term effects are not precisely known. However, the use of tamoxifen requires careful monitoring by a physician to assess side effects, blood levels, and so forth.

*Indole-3-carbinol (I3C)* (a phytonutrient with similar properties to tamoxifen) partially inactivates estrogen,[41] fights free radicals,[42] and interferes with tumor cell production.[43] See the detailed description below on I3C and how it may be used as an adjunct or alternative to tamoxifen.

**Danazol.** Danazol is a synthetic steroid prescribed for pain and infertility (caused by endometriosis) and for the pain and tenderness of FBD. When prescribed for FBD, Danazol may produce partial or complete disappearance of nodules and relief from pain and tenderness.[44-46] However, Danazol has undesirable side effects such as allergic reactions (particularly for persons who are allergic to preservatives or anabolic steroids) and drug interactions. For example, Danazol may increase the anticoagulant effect of warfarin (a drug frequently prescribed as a blood-thinning agent), increase blood sugar levels in diabetes mellitus, and increase the occurrence of migraine headaches.[47] Additionally, this synthetic testosterone derivative may cause women to develop male sexual characteristics such as facial hair.[48] Danazol is not recommended for pregnant women or women who are breast feeding because of undesirable effects to the infant. However, Danazol does help alleviate breast pain. As early as 1985, a study found that the drug eased pain in 70% of women with cyclical pain and in 31% of women with noncyclical pain.[49] Symptoms often recur after treatment with Danazol is stopped.

**Bromocriptine.** Bromocriptine helped 20% of women with noncyclical pain and 47% of women with cyclical pain.[49] Bromocriptine is a drug that affects the pituitary gland (blocks the release of the hormone prolactin) and is prescribed for menstrual problems and to stop milk production in some women. It is also used to treat other conditions such as infertility, Parkinson's disease, and acromegaly (overproduction of growth hormone). Bromocriptine has side effects, including significant nausea, allergic reactions, and interactions with drugs taken for other conditions (hypertension, mental illness, and liver conditions).

**Lisuride.** Lisuride (used in Parkinson's disease), a drug with endocrine effects similar to those of bromocriptine, reduced FBD symptoms in 63% of women studied. Estrogen levels in those patients were reduced and progesterone levels were increased.[50]

**Dehydroepiandrosterone.** Dehydroepiandrosterone (DHEA) is a steroid hormone chemically related to testosterone and estrogen. It is made by the adrenal glands from cholesterol. DHEA levels in the human body peak in the mid-20s and steadily decline beginning about the mid-30s.[51] Researchers have studied the actions of DHEA for over 20 years and have found that it may have beneficial implications in many areas, such as improving immunity; reducing menopausal symptoms; preventing cancer, heart disease, Alzheimer's disease, and chronic inflammation; improving longevity; and aiding weight loss.[51-59] DHEA should only be taken under the supervision of a physician who can monitor blood levels of steroids and cholesterol and existing health conditions.[60-62] DHEA is contraindicated in both men and women who have hormone-related cancer. (See Life Extension's DHEA Restoration Therapy protocol. Life Extension suggests specific dosing and blood testing schedules for all persons desiring to take DHEA safely.)

# NATURAL TREATMENTS FOR FIBROCYSTIC BREAST DISEASE

There are a number of natural treatments that may help women with FBD. These therapies may be employed alone or in combination with conventional treatments.

Nutritionists make several general recommendations concerning FBD and diet:

- Reduce fat to less than 20% of your diet, particularly saturated fats (animal products).
- Include more foods that are high in fiber. (Fiber is important in aiding bowel transit time.)
- Limit eggs, chicken, and dairy products.
- Include soy protein products (eg, tofu).
- Reduce caffeine intake or consider avoiding caffeine or other stimulants (eg, coffee, tea, soft drinks, and chocolate) altogether.
- Reduce or eliminate sugar, white flour, and refined foods.
- Take vitamins (beta-carotene, vitamin C, vitamin E, vitamin B-complex, vitamin B6).
- Take minerals (selenium, zinc, copper, calcium, magnesium, iodine).
- Consume omega-3 fatty acids from cold-water fish, fish oil supplements, or Perilla-seed oil supplements.

In addition, some form of daily exercise (walking, bicycle riding, yoga, weight training) and not smoking are strongly recommended.

Therefore, many choices concerning type of diet or foods to include and/or avoid will be personal ones based on each individual's particular circumstance and experience. Consult your physician with any concerns before making nutritional changes to control or treat FBD.

## Dietary Fat

Beginning as early as 1980, numerous studies have examined the relationship between FBD and dietary fat. Obesity tends to increase estrogens, free fatty acids, and triglycerides.[63–75] The typical Western diet provides about 40% of its calories from fat. However, nutritionists recommend that a healthy diet should include 30% of calories from fat with only 10% of these calories coming from saturated fat. Some researchers suggest that additional lowering of dietary fat levels (to 15%) may help stabilize hormonal imbalances that can lead to FBD.[76] In an early two-part study, investigators put 16 women on a diet with fat comprising 20% of total calories. After 3 months, the investigators found significant reductions in circulating estrogens, while levels of serum progesterone remained stable.[77,78]

In another early trial, researchers studied women who had severe cyclical FBD for at least 5 years. These women were advised to limit their dietary fat to 15% of calories consumed, while increasing complex carbohydrate consumption. After 6 months, the women reported significant reduction in the severity of premenstrual breast tenderness and swelling.[79] In a follow-up study in 1997, 817 women were randomly assigned to two groups (an intervention group to reduce intake of dietary fat and increase carbohydrates and a control group) and followed for 2 years. In all subjects, baseline mammography images were taken and compared with images that were taken 2 years later. After 2 years, there was a reduction in breast mass, leading the authors to conclude that "a low-fat high-carbohydrate diet reduced the area of mammographic density, a radiographic feature of the breast that is a risk factor for breast cancer." The authors suggested that longer follow-up of a larger number of subjects is required to determine if these effects are associated with changes in the risk for breast cancer.[80]

A study conducted at Harvard University followed more than 300 000 women.[81] These data suggested that "greater waist circumference increases risk of breast cancer, especially among women who are otherwise at lower risk because of never having used estrogen replacement hormones."

Conversely, mounting evidence also suggests that some dietary fat is desirable and provides protection for the breast.[82–84] Women experienced better breast health if their diet included moderate levels of fat. However, women desiring to add some dietary fat should not do so by merely increasing their consumption of meat, dairy products, and products with vegetable oils that contain saturated fat (palm and coconut oil). Better sources of dietary fat come from unsaturated fats such as fish, olive, peanut, and sunflower oils; olives, and avocados.

## Fatty Acids

Beneficial or essential fatty acids (EFAs), just like other vitamins and minerals, are vital for good health. EFAs are polyunsaturated fats ("good" fats) and contribute to healthy functioning of cell membranes, the skin, immune system, and cardiovascular system. Although fatty acids are essential for overall health, the body does not manufacture them; we need to obtain them through diet.

**Conjugated linoleic acid.** Conjugated linoleic acid (CLA) is a source of natural dietary fat. CLA is an essential fatty acid occurring in dairy and other products such as whole milk, cheese, and red meats from ruminant animals. CLA is considered to be "a healthy fat" because it is polyunsaturated (liquid at room temperature). Because CLA content in dairy products is directly related to the fat content, CLA levels are greatest in higher fat (rather than lower fat) products. Good dietary sources of CLA are homogenized milk, butter, plain yogurt, cheese, and ground beef. Interestingly, the CLA content of milk and other dairy products is highest in pasture- or range-fed cows.[85] Skim milk does not contain CLA.[86] As stated earlier, CLA is found in dairy products; however, it occurs at relatively low levels in these dietary sources. Therefore, we probably cannot get adequate CLA from food alone.

Animal studies have documented a number of potential health benefits of CLA: an anticarcinogenic effect, lowered total and LDL cholesterol, a reduction of body fat, increased rate of bone formation, and improved glucose utilization.[85] Although FBD is often a benign condition, there are important tumor-modulating, anticancer, and anti-inflammatory effects associated with CLA that are beneficial and perhaps preventive. In studies conducted using laboratory rats, CLA was found to confer lifelong protection against mammary cancer and reduce the density of mammary glands.

Researchers suggested that CLA fed during mammary gland development resulted in diminished mammary epithelial branching, which might possibly result in reduced mammary cancer risk. Data showed a "graded and parallel reduction of terminal end bud density and mammary tumor yield produced by 0.5 and 1% CLA. No further decrease in either parameter was observed when CLA in the diet was raised to 1.5–2%." Researchers concluded: "Optimal CLA nutrition during pubescence could conceivably control the population of cancer-sensitive target sites in the mammary gland."[87] Researchers also conducted studies in laboratory rats to investigate the role of CLA in inhibiting mammary carcinogenesis. They found that CLA "can act directly to inhibit growth and induce apoptosis of normal mammary epithelial cell organoids and may thus prevent breast cancer by its ability to reduce mammary epithelial density."[88,89] Apoptosis is the normal, healthy programmed death of cells. CLA is therefore suggested because of its antitumor effects.

**Omega-3 and omega-6 fatty acids.** Omega-3 and omega-6 fatty acids are important members of the EFA family.

Omega-6 fatty acids are generally available in adequate amounts from grains and vegetable oils commonly present in processed foods unless lifestyle (consumption of alcohol, excessive sugar, and saturated fats) or health conditions are a factor. Dried beans, including inexpensive northern beans and soybeans, are an excellent source of omega-6 fatty acids. Omega-6 fatty acids are also found in linoleic acid from safflower, sunflower, corn, and soybean oils.

Greater effort is often required to ensure that adequate omega-3 EFAs are available from daily nutrition. Omega-3 fatty acids are abundant in fish oils from mackerel, salmon, halibut, and herring. Flax seeds and green leafy vegetables also contain omega-3 fatty acids.

Women with severe mastalgia and FBD appear to have abnormal fatty-acid levels that may lead to endocrinologic hypersensitivity (imbalance of proper hormonal ratios and the resultant effect on other systems).[8,90] FBD seems to be associated with exaggerated estrogen–progesterone ratios and increased levels of prolactin.[91,92] Thus, increasing omega-6 fatty acids may reduce FBD symptoms.[93] The correct balance of omega-6 and omega-3 fatty acids will also help inhibit the inflammatory cascade that may precede the onset of fibrous tissue.

**Gamma linolenic acid.** Gamma linolenic acid (GLA), a plant-derived omega-6, is most abundant in seeds of a flower known as borage.[94–96] Although a member of the omega-6 family, it is metabolized differently than other omega-6s. Aging results in defects occurring in human enzymes responsible for producing anti-inflammatory molecules from dietary fats. The result is an increased risk for inflammatory conditions of all kinds. Supplemental GLA can counteract this acquired enzyme defect, supplying vital biochemical precursors with powerful anti-inflammatory effects.

GLA plays an important role in modulating inflammation throughout the body, especially when incorporated into the membranes of immune system cells.[97,98] In early 2010, a team of Taiwanese researchers discovered that GLA regulates the inflammatory "master

molecule" nuclear factor-kappa B or NF-κB, preventing it from switching on genes for inflammatory cytokines in cell nuclei.[99]

**Evening primrose oil.** Several European studies support using evening primrose oil to treat breast pain and cysts.[49,100–105] Evening primrose oil is a good source of beneficial gamma-linolenic acid and linoleic acid. In a 1990 survey, as many as 13% of surgeons and 30% of breast surgeons in Great Britain recommended evening primrose oil, particularly for cyclic mastalgia.[92,106] Evening primrose oil significantly improved the fatty-acid profiles of women with FBD[107] and improved pain symptoms.

**Borage and flax seed oils.** These two oils modulate inflammatory prostaglandins.[94,108] This is mainly due to the GLA-rich content in both oils. It may take 4–6 weeks before there is noticeable improvement. Nonetheless, treatment should be continued for 4–8 months.

## Fruits, Vegetables, and Dietary Fiber

A diet emphasizing fruits and vegetables benefits women with FBD. Natural, beneficial chemicals present in fruits and vegetables assist enzymes in the body to detoxify potentially harmful compounds (called carcinogens).[109] In fact, women who maintain a vegetarian diet are actually able to excrete 2–3 times more estrogen than omnivorous women. This could partially explain why vegetarian women have a lower incidence of breast cancer.[110,111]

In addition, some chemical components of fruits and vegetables benefit the function of (switch on) the parasympathetic nervous system, thus minimizing development of tumors and cysts. Increasing fiber consumption appears to be a component in reducing the symptoms of FBD in some women. Fiber assists elimination of waste from the system, decreasing levels of circulating estrogens.[109] Obtain plenty of fiber from your diet. Good sources of dietary fiber are legumes (kidney and pinto beans, peas, and lentils), vegetables (Brussels sprouts, broccoli, and carrots), raw fruits (apples, oranges, and bananas), and grains (particularly bran and oats).[112,113] Additional fiber may be obtained from dietary supplements in the form of powders or capsules.

## Indole-3-Carbinol and Diindolylmethane

Indole-3-carbinol (I3C) is a naturally occurring dietary compound (a phytochemical) found in some fruits and the cruciferous vegetables such as broccoli, cauliflower, Brussels sprouts, cabbage, turnips, kohlrabi, bok choy, and radishes. Phytochemicals are also natural anticancer compounds. I3C appears to work by partially inactivating estrogen,[41,114,115] fighting free radicals,[42] and directly interfering with tumor cell reproduction.[43] Many scientists believe that I3C's beneficial effects are partly driven by one of its principal byproducts, diindolylmethane (DIM).[116,117] Perhaps the single most important mechanism of action of I3C and DIM is modulating estrogen metabolism. Epidemiologic, laboratory, and animal studies indicate that dietary intake of I3C prevents the development of estrogen-enhanced cancers, including breast, endometrial, and cervical cancers. While estrogen increases the growth and survival of tumors, I3C has been found to arrest growth and increase apoptosis (programmed cell death).[117]

Indole-3-carbinol triggers the release of enzymes that help break down estrogen precursors into a harmless form rather than the form linked to breast cancer.[114,118–120] Cabbage and broccoli also contain sulforaphane, another phytonutrient shown to stimulate the release of enzymes that attach to cancer-causing substances and transport them from the body.[121]

The National Cancer Institute and U.S. Department of Agriculture have said that by eating 5 servings of vegetables and fruit daily, a person can cut the risk of cancer by more than 50%. Most people do not come close to meeting this guideline, particularly the recommendation for vegetables, because they either do not like cruciferous vegetables, the vegetables are not readily available, or they cannot eat the quantity required daily to meet recommended dietary guidelines for phytonutrients. Sometimes raw vegetables are not easy for the system to digest. Storage and processing by the supplier or overcooking in the home contributes to loss of phytonutrients. Often, only half the phytonutrients in any serving of raw vegetables ultimately becomes available for absorption—the other half is quickly eliminated from the body. Concentrated vegetables (particularly those with the water content removed and which are ground to the consistency of powdered sugar) are more digestible. In this form, it is estimated that 90–100% of phytonutrients, and all of their cancer-fighting properties, become available for absorption by the body.[121]

Animal studies indicate that I3C is safe at recommended doses.[122] Human trials have also found no significant side effects.[115] A study found that the naturally occurring chemical I3C found in vegetables of the Brassica genus is "a promising anticancer agent that we have shown previously to induce a G1 cycle arrest of human breast cancer cell lines, independent of estrogen receptor signaling." It was noted that a combination of I3C and antiestrogen tamoxifen cooperated to inhibit growth of the estrogen-dependent human MCF-7 breast cancer cell line more effectively than either agent used alone. Authors suggested that "I3C works through a mechanism distinct from tamoxifen." It was concluded that "these results demonstrate that I3C and tamoxifen work through different signal pathways to suppress the growth of human breast cancer cells and may represent a potential combinatorial therapy for estrogen-responsive breast cancer."[123]

**Note:** *See Life Extension's Breast Cancer protocol for more information.*

## Soy

Soy has been the subject of research for overall breast health. Some studies indicate that soy foods containing phytoestrogens (natural estrogens from plants) may offer some protective benefit. Researchers also believe that soy may play a role in balancing hormone levels in premenopausal women and perhaps in relieving premenstrual syndrome and menopausal symptoms.[124] Good dietary sources of soy are canned soybeans, tofu, soy protein bars, and tempeh.

Researchers speculate that some of the antitumor activity of soy compounds may result from production of enzymes that attack free radicals.[125] However, as with other nutrients, agreement is impossible and many authorities are reluctant to give soy universal endorsement. Others suggest that soy can modulate hormonal activity and even act as an antioxidant. If using soy, carefully monitor your breasts to assess the response of breast tissue to soy products.

## Simple and Complex Carbohydrates

Carbohydrates, whether simple or complex, might be an even greater concern in FBD than fat. Italian researchers found that heavy consumption of starchy foods, including pasta and white bread, increased breast cancer risk.[83,126] Both simple and complex carbohydrates are composed of sugar units. Simple carbohydrates are composed of 1 or 2 sugar units. Simple carbohydrates are found in fruit and vegetable juices, candy, soft drinks, and foods with added sugar. The problem with simple carbohydrates is that they induce an insulin spike upon ingestion. Insulin can promote cancer cell division, which is why consumption of starchy foods might increase cancer risk. Complex carbohydrates are made from many sugar units that structurally look like beads in a bracelet. Good sources of complex carbohydrates such as whole-grain products, fruits, vegetables, and legumes (dried beans and peas) do not induce a sharp insulin spike because they release sugar more slowly into the bloodstream. Both simple and complex carbohydrates are converted to blood sugar by the body to use as energy or fat storage. However, complex carbohydrates are better because they include vitamins, minerals, and fiber.[127]

## Vitamins

**Vitamin E.** Since 1965, using vitamin E has been recommended by some researchers for treatment of FBD.[128] However, researchers are not unified concerning the use of vitamin E to successfully treat or manage FBD and evidence has been inconclusive. Vitamin E in the form of alpha tocopherol has corrected abnormal estrogen–progesterone ratios in some patients with mammary dysplasia.[129] Results of that study, however, were not replicated in 1985.[130] Another study of 105 women with FBD found that 600 mg of vitamin E for 3 months had no effect on symptoms.[131]

**Folic acid.** Many physicians recommend taking folic acid along with vitamin E. In some women, combining the two seems to have a more beneficial effect than either alone. Folic acid, abundant in green, leafy vegetables is often deficient in the standard American diet. Women of child-bearing age are particularly encouraged to include folic acid in their diet. The more biologically-active form of folic acid, 5-methyltetrahydrofolate (5-MTHF), or L-methylfolate, is suggested for supplemental use.

**Vitamin A.** Studies have shown that vitamin A has been able to inhibit the growth of breast cancer cells.[132–135] Therefore, there is some justification for women with FBD to take vitamin A. In one of only a few studies,[136] 12 women with FBD were given 150 000 IUs of vitamin A daily for 3 months. Nine of the women reported marked pain reduction.

However, large doses of vitamin A can also be toxic. Therefore, beta-carotene may be a more practical treatment. In one study, 25 women with moderate to severe pain before their menstrual periods were given daily supplements of beta-carotene and retinol. After 6 months, most of the women reported marked reduction in breast pain with no side effects.[137] A diet high in yellow and orange fruits and vegetables will raise beta-carotene levels. You may also wish to use a beta-carotene supplement.

**Vitamin C.** The immune system requires vitamin C for proper function, tissue repair, diuretic action, anti-inflammatory responses, and adrenal hormone balance.

## Supporting Detoxification Systems

The liver supports many mechanisms including providing a detoxifying and filtering system for all body wastes as well as binding and eliminating extra hormones (including estrogen clearance). If the liver does not adequately perform its detoxifying and binding functions, estrogen stores may increase. As noted earlier, increased fiber in the diet improves removal of toxins and waste from the system. Nutrients that support the liver include *choline, S-adenosyl-methionine (SAMe), green tea,* and *N-acetyl-cysteine (NAC).* If you have FBD, consider using these supplements daily.

Herbs that support detoxification include *echinacea (Echinacea purpurea)* and *goldenseal (Hydrastis canadensis).* These herbs should be started about a week before menstruation begins, used for 7–10 days, and then discontinued for 4–7 days. Goldenseal should be followed by a probiotic that contains *acidophilus* and *Bifido* bacteria to replace good bacteria in the gut.

## Supplements and Herbs to Relieve Cyclical Pain and Reduce Inflammation

**Dandelion (*Taraxacum officinale*) and milk thistle (*Silibinin marianum*).** Dandelion and milk thistle will help to detoxify the system.[138–142] Dandelion has also been used to treat painful breasts and relieve impacted milk glands. Drink up to 2 cups of dandelion tea daily.

As the body's primary detoxifier, the liver serves as the frontline defense against chemical agents. Extracts from the milk thistle plant are among the most potent defenders of liver function. They are capable of halting and even reversing externally induced liver damage. Silymarin, silibinin, and other milk thistle components protect against these and other chemical insults. They have been conclusively shown to counteract toxicity from a wide variety of toxic substances, including ethanol,[143] organic solvents,[144] and pharmaceuticals.[145,146]

**Saw palmetto.** Saw palmetto (*Serenoa repens*) is used to treat prostate problems, but its antiestrogenic characteristics also make it useful as a treatment for hormonal disturbances. Saw palmetto should be standardized to contain 85–95% fatty acids and sterols.

*Chasteberry.* Chasteberry (*Vitex agnus-castus*) has been used to relieve FBD. Chasteberry may decrease prolactin, leading to increased progesterone production during the menstrual cycle. Also, it seems to result in a shift in estrogen-progesterone balance, regulating hormones and inhibiting release of FSH and LH. This results in less estrogen to stimulate breast tissue. Eat the equivalent of 20–40 mg of fresh chasteberry berries daily or consume a chasteberry extract standardized to 0.5% agnuside.

# OTHER CONSIDERATIONS

## Caffeine

Some women find that reducing or even eliminating caffeine intake by avoiding coffee, tea, chocolate, and soft drinks significantly decreases breast discomfort.[149] However, the topic is controversial because studies results linking caffeine and FBD have been inconsistent or inconclusive.[4,148–150]

An early study by Minton[151] was widely publicized because it claimed that abstaining totally from caffeine lessened symptoms and resolved FBD completely. According to Minton, abstinence from consuming methylxanthine (a chemical present in foods and beverages that contain caffeine) decreased the need for major breast surgery and breast biopsies because of benign disease.[151–153] A literature review on causes of breast pain found that some investigations did find an association between caffeine intake and FBD and breast pain.[105] However, other studies over the past 20 years examining the relationship of caffeine to breast conditions reported inconclusive or even the opposite conclusions.[150,154–156] One study of more than 2000 women concluded that coffee consumption was not associated with an increase of breast cancer among women with a history of FBD.[156] Another study even found "slight" evidence that the more coffee a woman consumed, the less likely she was to have breast cancer.[157]

Even though the evidence of a direct link between caffeine and FBD is inconclusive, many clinicians do recommend low caffeine intake in women with FBD. Some women report significant relief from FBD symptoms after eliminating caffeine from their diets. If you suspect caffeine might have a role in your FBD symptoms, eliminate sources of caffeine (chocolate, coffee, tea, soft drinks) from your diet for 3 months to see if your symptoms improve.

As noted above, methylxanthine is a chemical present in foods and beverages that contain caffeine. Methylxanthines increase circulating catecholamines (chemicals present in response to stress). There is some evidence that women with FBD have an increased sensitivity to catecholamines. However, as with caffeine, the studies are inconclusive.[158]

## Iodine

According to some alternative-care practitioners, a malfunctioning thyroid gland may be a precursor to many disorders in females. With hypothyroidism, hormones such as LH, FSH, and prolactin may be overly stimulated. Researchers have linked breast abnormalities, including FBD, to repeated hormonal arousal.[5] An early study of 19 women with breast pain (mastodynia) and nodularity caused by FBD reported that almost half (47%) the women had total relief after daily treatment with 0.1 mg of levothyroxine (Synthroid®). Three patients had elevated serum prolactin levels. Their prolactin levels became normal and they experienced dramatic pain relief after treatment with levothyroxine.[159]

Iodine deficiency interferes with optimum breast health, and intake of levels far higher than the recommended dietary allowance of 150 mcg may be required to achieve benefits. Daily amounts of 3000–6000 mcg may help relieve the symptoms of FBD.[160]

Iodine plays an important role in the health of women's breast tissue.[161] In the presence of chemicals and enzymes found in breast tissue, iodine has been shown to exert a powerful antioxidant effect equivalent to vitamin C.[160,162] Iodine-deficient breast tissue exhibits chemical markers of elevated lipid peroxidation, one of the earliest factors in cancer development.[160,163–166] Animal studies have shown that FBD can be induced by depriving breast tissue of iodine.[161,167,168] These changes can be reversed by iodine doses equivalent to 5000 mcg daily in humans.[160,169]

Women with FBD obtain substantial relief from oral administration of iodine at doses of 3000–6000 mcg, with 65% achieving improvements according to their own and their physicians' assessments.[170] In those studies, only 33% of placebo recipients reported any benefit. No side effects were detected at any of the doses used.[160]

Iodine also helps regulate levels of the stress hormone cortisol and contributes to normal immune function.[173,174] Abnormal cortisol levels and deficient immune function are significant contributors to the risk of breast cancer; women with FBD may also suffer from elevated cortisol levels.[173–176]

A review of three clinical studies using sodium iodide, protein-bound iodide, and molecular iodine showed clinical improvements in FBD of 70%, 40%, and 72%, respectively.[170] The review concluded that molecular iodine was nonthyrotropic (did not alter) and the most beneficial. Thus, some suggest that treating thyroid problems might reduce the risk or incidence as well as improve the symptoms of FBD.[170]

Another study looked at thyroid hormones and FBD. The data suggested that free T3 had an important role in the physiology of FBD.[177] To further examine this theory, a study looked at the levels of triiodothyronine (T3), thyroxin (T4), thyroid-stimulating hormone (TSH), and prolactin (Prl) in FBD. The authors found that T4 levels were significantly lower in women with FBD than in controls. They concluded that there seemed to be a connection between FBD and thyroid function.[178] Taking daily iodine will help support a healthy thyroid. Kelp may also be beneficial. However, be certain the seaweed is harvested from clean water. A simple, convenient source of iodine is table salt containing iodine.

## Proteolytic Enzymes

According to researchers from Germany, pancreatic enzymes may reduce tumors and cysts, inflammation, and soreness. In a study of 96 patients, cyst size was reduced significantly after women took an enzyme preparation for 6 weeks. Additionally, the women reported significant improvement and less pain. A preparation containing lipase, protease, and amylase was recommended.[179] Another proteolytic enzyme, serratiopeptidase, has been researched as a treatment option for those diagnosed with FBD. In one double-blind study published in the *Singapore Medical Journal*, 70 women with breast engorgement were randomly divided into a treatment and placebo group. There was more reduction of breast pain and swelling in the women receiving serratiopeptidase than in women not receiving the supplement. No adverse reactions were reported.[180]

## Life Extension Suggestions

- **Comprehensive multivitamin:** per label instructions
- **Soybean extract:** 3125 mg daily
- **DHEA:** 15–50 mg daily
- **Vitamin A,** as beta-carotene: 25 000 IU daily
- **Vitamin C:** 2–6 g daily
- **Folate,** as folic acid: 800 mcg daily
- **L-methylfolate:** 1000 mcg daily
- **Vitamin B12:** 300 mcg daily
- **Vitamin E,** as high gamma tocopherol mix with sesame lignans: 359 mg daily
- **Fish oil,** with olive polyphenols and sesame lignans: 1400 mg EPA and 1000 mg DHA daily
- **Conjugated linoleic acid (CLA):** 2340 mg daily
- **Gamma linolenic acid (GLA):** 299–1495 mg daily
- **Dietary fiber:** 25–30 g daily
- **Probiotics:** per label instructions
- **Iodine:** 1000–6000 mcg daily
- **Milk thistle extract:** 750 mg daily
- **Saw palmetto:** 320 mg daily
- **Pancreatin 8x blend:** 400–1200 mg daily
- **Digestive enzyme blend** (protease, amylase, lactase, cellulose, lipase): 290–870 mg daily
- **Serratiopeptidase:** 5–20 mg daily
- **Indole-3-carbinol:** 80–160 mg daily
- **Progesterone cream:** per label instructions
- **Dandelion root extract:** 1040–4160 mg daily
- **Goldenseal:** 250 mg daily
- **Castor oil:** per label instructions

In addition, the following *blood tests* may provide helpful information.

- Female Comprehensive Hormone Panel (includes sex hormones, TSH, free T3, DHEA-S, and many other important tests)
- Prolactin
- FSH and LH

## REFERENCES

References available at: www.lef.org/dpt5/ch59

# 60

# *Fibromyalgia*

Typically presenting in young or middle-aged women, fibromyalgia is a condition of soft tissue pain, muscular stiffness, unremitting fatigue, disturbed sleep, and cognitive "slowing", often associated with a variety of additional unexplained symptoms, psychological depression, and impairment of activities of daily living.

Of note, fibromyalgia was once often dismissed by the mainstream medical community as a psychological disorder without underlying medical causation because of the lack of objective medical findings on screening laboratory tests and medical imaging procedures. However, recent research has helped identify the underlying nervous system pathology for fibromyalgia, which is currently believed to be a central sensitivity syndrome.[1,2]

Fibromyalgia is currently identified as a *neurosensory disorder* characterized by disturbances in the way the central nervous system interprets and evaluates stimuli.[3]

Fibromyalgia typically is associated with other regional pain syndromes, as well as mood and anxiety disorders. In fact, significant data support the idea that fibromyalgia, chronic fatigue syndrome, regional chronic pain syndromes, and some emotional disorders all involve *abnormal perturbations of the stress response system*.[4,5] In these disorders, stress functions to cause alterations in corticotropin-releasing hormone, with associated effects on the neuroendocrine axis.

In addition, fibromyalgia often is observed in other co-morbid disease characterized by *chronic, systemic inflammation*, such as rheumatoid arthritis, systemic lupus erythematosus, and chronic hepatitis C infection.[6-8] In such cases, associated disorders of systemic inflammation, chronic stress, anxiety and depression, hormone imbalances, and impaired sleep must be treated for optimum outcome in fibromyalgia.

This protocol will summarize several potential triggers of fibromyalgia symptoms as well as outline steps that can be taken to identify and address them. Using convenient blood tests to uncover potential imbalances or deficiencies and targeting them with scientifically studied natural therapies may improve the quality of life for those with fibromyalgia.

## SYMPTOMS OF FIBROMYALGIA

The primary symptom of fibromyalgia is widespread chronic pain that persists for at least 3 months and may be accentuated at tender points. This is often accompanied by chronic fatigue and frequent sleep disturbances.[9] In addition to this triad of symptoms, other common indicators of fibromyalgia include tenderness, stiffness, mood disturbances (eg, depression and/or anxiety), and cognitive difficulties (eg, trouble concentrating, forgetfulness, and disorganized thinking).[10] Migraine and tension headaches are also present in more than half of individuals with fibromyalgia.[11] Many of those suffering from this chronic condition experience a variety of other unexplained symptoms such as:[12-14]

- Irritable bowel sensations
- Headache
- Pelvic and urinary problems
- Weight fluctuations
- Sexual dysfunction
- Cognitive dysfunction

Although these symptoms often come and go spontaneously, they are usually intense enough to impair daily function.[15]

Since each individual diagnosed with fibromyalgia is affected differently, their experience(s) will vary. For example, fibromyalgia pain has been described as deep muscular aching, soreness, stiffness, burning, or throbbing. People with fibromyalgia may also experience numbness, tingling, or strange "crawling" sensations in their arms and legs.[16] These painful sensations are typically described as "widespread"—meaning they originate above and below the waist, on both sides of the body, as well as in the spine and lower back.[17]

## POSSIBLE CAUSES OF FIBROMYALGIA

Because many fibromyalgia patients appear well upon physical examination, the diagnosis of fibromyalgia was historically considered controversial and, unfortunately, written off by many conventional physicians as a psychosomatic condition.[16,18]

### Pain Hypersensitivity

Evidence from functional magnetic resonance imaging (fMRI) studies of the brain has demonstrated that patients with fibromyalgia are more sensitive to pain than their healthy counterparts.[3] Therefore, fibromyalgia is thought to be a result of some type of *neurosensory disorder* that perturbs the central nervous system's ability to process painful stimuli.[19,20] This dysfunction appears to be a result of neurochemical imbalances that cause the brain to amplify pain through two different mechanisms: (1) *allodynia* (ie, a heightened sensitivity to stimuli that are not normally painful); and (2) *hyperalgesia* (an increased response to painful stimuli).[21] Although no one knows exactly how or why this central sensitization develops, researchers have identified several possible theories.

## Hormonal Influences and Stress

Although a causal link has yet to be established, some evidence suggests a role for sex hormones in the etiology of fibromyalgia. For example, fibromyalgia predominantly affects middle-aged women; a population whose hormones have begun to decline or fall out of youthful balance.[22,23] Furthermore, the fluctuating hormone levels caused by endocrine dysfunction commonly produce symptoms that are similar to those of fibromyalgia (eg, muscle pain/tenderness, exhaustion, and reduced exercise capacity).[24] In one clinical trial, taking the selective estrogen receptor modulator (SERM) raloxifene every other day for 16 weeks lead to significant improvements in pain and fatigue scores, reduced tender points and sleep disturbances, and greater recovery of usual activities compared to placebo among 49 women.[25] These findings implicate estrogen signaling in fibromyalgia etiology.

Likewise, perturbations in the hypothalamic-pituitary-adrenal (HPA) axis have been demonstrated in fibromyalgia patients, implicating a possible therapeutic role for dehydroepiandrosterone (DHEA) supplementation and stress management strategies.[26] It is thought that stress functions to cause alterations in corticotropin-releasing hormone (CRH), with associated effects on the neuroendocrine axis. More information is available in the Stress Management protocol.

This evidence is convergent with recent data indicating a relatively high prevalence of growth hormone deficiency among patients with severe fibromyalgia. This deficiency is linked to increased levels of blood cytokines and pain severity.[27,28] Therefore, fibromyalgia patients may benefit from hormone level testing in order to identify, and subsequently treat any underlying imbalances or insufficiencies.[27] In the case of growth hormone (GH)–deficient fibromyalgia patients, GH replacement therapy has been associated with significant improvements in symptoms and quality of life.[29]

For more information on hormone testing and natural hormone replacement, refer to the Female Hormone Restoration protocol.

## Neurotransmitter Imbalances

Symptoms of fibromyalgia might be caused by a disruption in the communication between nerves and the brain. This theory is supported by evidence indicating that fibromyalgia patients often have lower-than-normal amounts of neurotransmitters (ie, serotonin, norepinephrine, and dopamine),[30] and frequently suffer from mood disorders like depression and anxiety. A low level of serotonin is particularly significant to fibromyalgia patients as an imbalance can contribute to pain sensitivity, sleep disturbances, and mood alterations. This supports the use of antidepressants for treating fibromyalgia, since antidepressants often increase the circulating amounts of these important neurotransmitters. The problem with antidepressants is that they often come with undesirable side effects, and thus are not a very attractive option for many patients. Fortunately, supplementation with a natural building block of serotonin called 5-hydroxytryptophan (5-HTP) may improve the fibromyalgia symptoms of pain, depression, anxiety, and insomnia.[31] 5-HTP supplementation is well tolerated, and generally starts to take effect within the first 30 days of use.[26]

## Inflammation

Although fibromyalgia is not generally believed to be an inflammatory condition,[16] there is evidence suggesting that some type of inflammatory process may be contributing to its onset and/or progression.[32] While classic inflammatory processes are not observed in fibromyalgia patients, these individuals do exhibit some inflammation-related abnormalities.[33] For instance, the cerebrospinal fluid (CSF) of fibromyalgia patients commonly contains higher-than-normal levels of the inflammatory mediators *substance P* and *corticotropin-releasing hormone (CRH)*. Likewise, the serum of fibromyalgia patients commonly contains higher-than-normal levels of the proinflammatory cytokines *interleukin-6 (IL-6)*, *interleukin-8 (IL-8)*, and *substance P*, while the skin of fibromyalgia patients commonly contains higher-than-normal amounts of *mast cells*, which can produce IL-6 and IL-8.

In addition, fibromyalgia often occurs simultaneously with other chronic inflammatory conditions, such as arthritis, systemic lupus erythematosus, or chronic hepatitis C infection.[6-8] It is possible that inflammation arising from co-occurring medical conditions could play a role in the pathology of fibromyalgia. Therefore, some individuals with fibromyalgia, especially those who have been diagnosed with other medical conditions, may respond to supplementation with natural anti-inflammatory agents such as omega-3 fatty acids, curcumin, and boswellia serrata.[34–36]

## Sleep Dysfunction

Although sleep disturbance is an obvious consequence/symptom of fibromyalgia, some researchers believe that nonrestorative sleep (NRS) may actually cause and/or contribute to fibromyalgia-related pain.[37] This bidirectional relationship is further supported by studies of fibromyalgia patients showing that improvement in sleep quality is linked to significant reductions in fibromyalgia symptom intensity.[38] Since serotonin is involved in pain signaling and sleep regulation, some researchers have suggested that abnormally low serotonin levels (common among fibromyalgia patients) may be one possible explanation for this connection.[39] Clinical studies have also found that fibromyalgia patients may have low circulating levels of melatonin, which can lead to disruptions in sleep cycles.[40] Among these patients, melatonin supplementation has been shown to improve sleep and fatigue-related symptoms.[41]

As with pain, fibromyalgia-related sleep dysfunction should be managed in a step-wise fashion, starting with the least risky treatment. For many of those with fibromyalgia, improving sleep hygiene is enough to make a significant difference.[42] The sleep environment should be dark, cool, and quiet, and external distractions should be minimized. The sleep cycle should be normal (eg, consistent bedtime and morning awakening time), and healthy lifestyle considerations (eg, adequate exercise, smoking cessation, and avoiding nighttime alcohol use) may also help improve sleep quality.[43]

Patients who continue to have problems sleeping may require pharmacotherapy with agents such as zolpidem (Ambien®) and eszopiclone (Lunesta®). However, these medications can be habit forming and are not associated with subsequent pain relief.[42] On the other hand, natural supplements such as 5-HTP and melatonin are not only associated with improvements in sleep quality and pain score, but are also less likely to produce negative side effects.[26,41]

## Mitochondrial Dysfunction

Mitochondria are cellular components responsible for the generation of the energy necessary for proper cellular function. Evidence indicates that fibromyalgia symptoms may arise as a result of mitochondrial dysfunction.[44–46] For example, case reports of 2 patients with fibromyalgia revealed impaired mitochondrial function and deficiency in coenzyme Q10 (a critical compound necessary for proper mitochondrial function) in blood and skin cells.[47] Similarly, in another case report, a 41-year-old woman diagnosed with fibromyalgia, but who had been unresponsive to a variety of conventional treatments, was later found to have significant mitochondrial dysfunction.[48] Her symptoms improved dramatically when treated 4 times daily with a cocktail of mitochondrial nutrients including coenzyme Q10 (200 mg), creatine (1000 mg), L-carnitine (200 mg), and folic acid (1000 mcg). Moreover, dysfunctional mitochondria contribute to increased oxidative stress. In a study involving 20 fibromyalgia patients and 10 healthy controls, the fibromyalgia patients had greater levels of a mitochondria-derived free radical (superoxide) in their blood cells and increased lipid peroxidation compared to the healthy subjects.[49]

---

## FIBROMYALGIA AND OBESITY

While the relationship between obesity and chronic pain has been common knowledge for decades, more recent evidence suggests that this association is particularly true for fibromyalgia patients. For example:

- In 2008, researchers demonstrated significant improvement in pain scores and tender point frequency among fibromyalgia patients who underwent gastric bypass surgery.[50] This suggests that *weight loss should be an important treatment goal for obese patients diagnosed with fibromyalgia.*

- In 2009, researchers reported that 71% of fibromyalgia patients enrolled in their study were either overweight or obese and exhibited common laboratory findings associated with obesity such as elevated levels of IL-6, catecholamines, cortisol, and CRP.[51] The authors also pointed out that both obese patients and those with fibromyalgia presented with reduced sleep duration and quality, concluding that excess weight and obesity may play a significant role in fibromyalgia and its related dysfunction(s).

- In 2010, a study of 215 fibromyalgia patients reported that nearly 80% of participants were either overweight or obese. These same patients exhibited greater tender point sensitivity, reduced physical strength, reduced lower-body flexibility, shorter sleep duration, and greater restlessness during sleep.[52]

- A 2011 review article concluded that fibromyalgia patients are 40% more likely to be obese and 30% more likely to be overweight.[53] In addition to concluding that obesity is highly prevalent among fibromyalgia patients, the authors also proposed the following possible mechanisms that might explain this link:

- Alterations in the endogenous opioid system (painkilling mechanisms naturally occurring in the body)
- Endocrine system dysfunction (eg, thyroid and sex hormone imbalances)
- Systemic inflammation (eg, cytokine imbalance)
- Too little physical activity
- Cognitive and sleep disturbances
- Psychiatric conditions (eg, depression)
- Dysfunction of the growth hormone (GH)/insulin-like growth factor-1 (IGF-1) axis

# DIAGNOSING FIBROMYALGIA

Most doctors diagnose fibromyalgia on the basis of widespread pain lasting ≥ 3 months that is not attributable to any other medical condition. However, in-depth criteria for the diagnosis of fibromyalgia have been developed by the American College of Rheumatology (ACR),[17] but many physicians don't strictly adhere to these criteria.

Doctors have trouble diagnosing fibromyalgia for a variety of reasons. First, fibromyalgia patients typically do not exhibit any obvious abnormalities upon physical examination, laboratory analysis, and/or radiologic imaging. Also, fibromyalgia patients are often affected by at least one of the following disorders: chronic fatigue syndrome (CFS), irritable bowel syndrome (IBS), interstitial cystitis (IC), and temporomandibular disorder (TMD).[54]

Therefore, distinguishing the symptoms associated with fibromyalgia from the aforementioned conditions can be fairly confusing, even for experienced physicians.[55] For these reasons, fibromyalgia is primarily a diagnosis of exclusion, which means that other diseases and disorders must first be ruled out.

# CONVENTIONAL TREATMENT

Most experts in the field of fibromyalgia recommend a multifaceted, tailored treatment program incorporating both pharmacologic and nonpharmacologic therapy (ie, education, physical therapy, and cognitive behavioral therapy).[13,56] Since the experience of fibromyalgia and the reaction to therapy is largely shaped by a complex interaction of physical, psychological, and social factors, most experts suggest a multidisciplinary approach, which involves a team of clinicians from a variety of medical disciplines (eg, family practice, physical therapist, and mental health specialists).[57,58] An appropriate fibromyalgia management program should be aimed at symptomatic treatment of pain, fatigue, and sleep quality,

as well as improving physical capacity and emotional balance.[59]

## Conventional Pharmacologic Therapy

Traditional pharmacotherapy for fibromyalgia includes the wide variety of medications listed below:[60]

- Pain relievers (eg, opioids, nonopioid analgesics, local anesthetics)
- Sleep aids
- Anti-inflammatories (eg, nonsteroidal anti-inflammatory drugs [NSAIDs])
- Antidepressants
- Botulinum toxin (Botox®)
- Muscle relaxants
- Anticonvulsants

While all of the above medications are commonly used to treat fibromyalgia, the Food and Drug Administration (FDA) has only approved 3 specific drugs for this indication. In June 2007, pregabalin (Lyrica®), an anticonvulsant drug, became the first to be approved. A year later, duloxetine (Cymbalta®), an antidepressant, became the second. The most recent addition to this list is the antidepressant milnacipran (Savella®), which was FDA approved in January 2009.

Unfortunately, none of these medications are effective for the entire scope of symptoms and disabilities associated with fibromyalgia.[61] Furthermore, many patients either fail to respond or develop significant side effects to these drugs, especially since they are required to be on them long term.[20]

Pharmacotherapy is typically initiated only after less invasive strategies have failed. Since fibromyalgia patients often present with dissimilar symptoms and different symptom severities, there is no universally applicable drug treatment algorithm available. Therefore, physicians generally direct treatment at the most bothersome symptoms, organize potential therapies by mechanism of action, and start with drugs that carry the lowest side effect profile.[60]

## Conventional Nonpharmacologic Therapy

Education concerning the diagnosis and treatment of fibromyalgia is not only effective, but also one of the cheapest and least invasive interventions.[62] Educational interventions are particularly beneficial for fibromyalgia patients that have lived with the syndrome for many years, all the while believing that the symptoms were completely psychological.[13] This not only leaves individuals with fibromyalgia feeling rejected by the medical community, but also induces significant stress, potentially worsening symptoms. Therefore, becoming informed about the disorder can not only ease the fear of the unknown, but produce a significant therapeutic effect as well.[63]

Cognitive behavioral therapy (CBT) and relaxation techniques have been shown to reduce pain and improve sleep.[64] Lifestyle modifications such as exercising regularly, eliminating tobacco use, and reducing excess alcohol consumption should also be considered, as they are strongly associated with decreased pain and fatigue. Although regular aerobic fitness and strength training are significantly beneficial interventions, numerous patients are unwilling or unable to adhere to these regimens (due to pain).[65]

# DIETARY CONSIDERATIONS AND ALTERNATIVE PHYSICAL MODALITIES

## Diet

Given the known association between obesity and fibromyalgia, it is not surprising that adherence to a healthy diet can have significant benefits. According to recent evidence, vegetarian diets are particularly beneficial for decreasing the pain associated with fibromyalgia; not only because they can induce weight loss, but also because they are rich in antioxidants.[66] This is recommended based on evidence that oxidative damage (ie, free radicals) plays an important role in the development of fibromyalgia.[67,68] However, adherence to a specific dietary pattern may not be necessary if antioxidant-rich foods are consumed regularly as part of a healthy diet.[69,70]

## Complementary and Alternative Physical Modalities

In the case of *acupuncture*, some data suggests it produces short-term pain relief, but these benefits do not appear to be long-term.[28] Other promising alternative interventions include movement-based therapies such as *yoga, tai chi, mindfulness meditation,* and *hydrotherapy* (in which the patient undergoes physical therapy while in the water or simply bathes to relieve symptoms).[23,71–73]

# TARGETED NUTRITIONAL THERAPIES

Although no individual dietary supplement has been proven to be effective for relieving *all* the common symptoms of fibromyalgia, the following have either been linked to symptom improvements or recommended by experts to overcome deficits that are common among fibromyalgia patients:

## Magnesium

Research has revealed that low circulating levels of magnesium may be implicated in the development of fibromyalgia in some individuals.[74,75] Magnesium supplementation has been shown to reduce symptoms of fibromyalgia, thus making it a frequently recommended supplement.[76,77]

In one clinical trial involving 80 women (60 with fibromyalgia and 20 healthy controls), a diagnosis of fibromyalgia was associated with significantly lower red blood cell and serum magnesium levels. Furthermore, lower magnesium levels were associated with more severe fibromyalgia symptoms.[75] The trial went on to assess the effect of 8 weeks of supplementation with magnesium citrate (300 mg daily) alone or in combination with amitriptyline (10 mg daily) upon several measures of fibromyalgia severity. While both magnesium and amitriptyline alone effectively improved many of the assessed parameters, the combination of the two was more effective than either alone and significantly improved pain, tender points, depression and anxiety scores, as well as sleep disorders and irritability.

Patients with fibromyalgia should consider having a *red blood cell magnesium test* to ensure that they are not deficient in this important nutrient.

## Melatonin

Melatonin is a hormone that helps regulate the sleep–wake cycle. Clinical studies have found that some fibromyalgia patients often have low circulating levels of melatonin, which can lead to disruptions in the sleep cycle.[40] In addition, fibromyalgia patients appear to secrete less melatonin during the night than healthy controls.[78] Among these patients, melatonin supplementation has been shown to decrease symptoms of fibromyalgia.[40,41]

## S-Adenosyl-L-Methionine (SAMe)

SAMe is a natural compound made from methionine (an amino acid) and adenosine triphosphate (ATP). Supplementation with SAMe has been linked to improvements in morning stiffness, fatigue, quality of sleep, and clinical disease activity among fibromyalgia patients.[79] In addition, other studies have shown that SAMe provides relief from depression, which sometimes occurs in people with fibromyalgia.[80,81]

## D-Ribose

D-ribose is a sugar that helps increase cellular energy synthesis in muscle cells. One trial involving 41 fibromyalgia patients found that 5 g of D-ribose 3 times daily significantly improved energy, sleep, mental clarity, pain intensity, and general well-being.[82] Another small trial found that 3 g of D-ribose twice daily improved exercise capacity, vitality, and mental outlook in adults 50 and older.[83] Similarly, a case-report of a 37-year-old woman with fibromyalgia indicated that 5 g of D-ribose twice daily improved her symptoms.[84]

## Chlorella

Chlorella is a genus of single-cell green algae. It grows in fresh water and contains high concentrations of important vitamins, minerals, dietary fiber, nucleic acids, amino acids, enzymes, and other substances. Chlorella has been shown to relieve symptoms of fibromyalgia when used as a supplement.[26] In a small pilot trial, 18 patients with fibromyalgia experienced an average 22% decrease in pain intensity after taking chlorella daily for 2 months.[85]

## 5-Hydroxytryptophan (5-HTP)

5-HTP is an endogenous precursor to serotonin. It can be derived from the seeds of an African plant (*Griffonia simplificolia*). The potential utility of 5-HTP—a more direct precursor to serotonin than L-tryptophan—in fibromyalgia is supported by data indicating impaired tryptophan metabolism in fibromyalgia patients.[86] Clinical trials have shown that 5-HTP supplementation in fibromyalgia patients is associated with considerable improvements in anxiety, pain intensity, quality of sleep, fatigue, and the number of tender points.[87,88]

## Coenzyme Q10 (CoQ10)

CoQ10 is an essential component of healthy mitochondrial function, as well as a powerful antioxidant.[89] CoQ10 has demonstrated anti-inflammatory and analgesic properties in animals.[90] Researchers believe that low CoQ10 levels may play a role in the development of fibromyalgia symptoms because (1) CoQ10 has been found lacking within the blood cells of many fibromyalgia patients, and (2) subsequent CoQ10 supplementation (300 mg daily for 9 months) has been linked to a significant improvement in symptoms in a small preliminary trial.[91] Other data from case reports (see "Mitochondrial Dysfunction" section above) also suggest a role for CoQ10 in relieving fibromyalgia symptoms.

## Acetyl-L-Carnitine

Acetyl-L-carnitine is an acetylated version of the amino acid L-carnitine, which is a mitochondrial membrane compound that aids in the generation of metabolic energy and guards against oxidative damage.[92] It has been suggested that fibromyalgia syndrome may be associated with metabolic alterations including a deficit of carnitine.[93] In one double-blind, randomized, placebo-controlled trial involving 102 fibromyalgia patients, 1000 mg (oral) and 500 mg (intramuscular injection) of acetyl-L-carnitine daily significantly improved pain and cognitive symptoms more than placebo.[93] The treatment was well tolerated.

## Omega-3 Fatty Acids

Omega-3 fatty acids can only be synthesized to a limited extent by the human body, but are vital for normal metabolism. Omega-3s modulate several cellular properties and have been shown to reduce inflammation.[34] Among fibromyalgia patients, omega-3 fatty acid supplementation has been linked to significant improvements in pain severity, tender point counts, fatigue, and depression.[94] Another case report indicates that supplementation with fish oil (providing 2400–7200 mg of EPA/DHA daily) eased neuropathic pain in a small number of subjects with fibromyalgia and/or related neuropathic pain.[95] Life Extension suggests that the omega-6 to omega-3 ratio be kept at or below 4:1 for optimal health. A convenient blood test called the OmegaScore™ test measures the balance between pro-inflammatory omega-6s and anti-inflammatory omega-3s.

## Vitamin D

Patients with fibromyalgia syndrome have impaired mobility and therefore get less exposure to sunlight. This contributes to the vitamin-D deficiency frequently observed in this population.[96,97] In one trial involving 100 women with fibromyalgia, 61% were found to be vitamin-D deficient (blood levels of 25-hydroxyvitamin D <30 ng/mL).[98] Upon supplementation with vitamin D, 42 (69%) of those women reported significantly improved symptoms when their vitamin D levels reached ≥ 30 ng/mL; the improvement became more significant when their vitamin D levels exceeded 50 ng/mL. Fibromyalgia patient should have their vitamin D levels checked regularly.[98] Life Extension suggests that a 25-hydroxyvitamin D level of 50–80 ng/mL should be targeted for optimal health among most aging individuals.

## General Support

The following nutrients may render additional benefits by providing antioxidant protection and mitochondrial support:

**Superoxide dismutase (SOD).** SOD is an endogenous antioxidant found in decreased amounts among fibromyalgia patients.[68] Superoxide dismutase occurs in plants and can thus be extracted from them. In one double blind trial, supplementation with 1000 mg/day of a plant superoxide dismutase extract (GliSODin®) significantly boosted SOD activity and decreased CRP levels in athletes compared to placebo.[99]

**Vitamins A, C, E, and the mineral zinc.** Vitamins A, C, E, and the mineral zinc all provide antioxidant protection. In one study, fibromyalgia patients had lower blood levels of vitamins A and E, as well as increased lipid peroxidation when compared to healthy controls.[100] Another study found that fibromyalgia patients had lower zinc and magnesium levels than healthy controls.[74] In a survey of over 300 fibromyalgia patients, 35% reported using vitamin C[101]; and vitamin C combined with vitamin E has been shown to boost antioxidant activity in conditions related to oxidative stress.[102] All of these nutrients are available in a *comprehensive multivitamin*.

**B vitamins.** B vitamins are important cofactors in a variety of metabolic events. They were reported in a survey to be used by a quarter of fibromyalgia patients.[101] Homocysteine is a damaging metabolic by-product whose levels are kept in check by adequate B-vitamin intake. In one study, women with fibromyalgia were shown to have higher levels of homocysteine in their cerebrospinal fluid than healthy controls.[103] Other evidence indicates that a Myers' cocktail, which consists of an intravenous infusion of several vitamins (ie, B-complex vitamins), may be useful in fibromyalgia.[104,105] Moreover, B vitamins are essential for maintaining optimal mitochondrial function.[106]

**NADH.** Nicotinamide adenine dinucleotide (NADH) is a coenzyme that supports numerous metabolic reactions critical for optimal cellular function. For example, NADH helps recycle CoQ10, thereby aiding in cellular energy production. It also possesses considerable antioxidant potential.

    Supplementation with NADH has been shown to improve energy in people with chronic fatigue syndrome.[107] Similarly, NADH supplementation relieved sleepiness and cognitive deficits in people

suffering from jet lag.[108] In other trials, NADH improved cognitive function among people with Alzheimer's disease,[109] and relieved Parkinson's disease symptoms.[110] While NADH has yet to be studied in people with fibromyalgia, these findings are encouraging since fibromyalgia sufferers often experience fatigue and suboptimal cognition.

## Life Extension Suggestions

- **Comprehensive multivitamin:** per label instructions
- **Magnesium,** 140 mg daily as magnesium-L-threonate *and* 320 mg daily as magnesium citrate
- **Melatonin:** 0.3–5 mg before bed (sometimes up to 10 mg)
- **Coenzyme Q10** (as ubiquinol): 100–300 mg daily
- **Acetyl-L-carnitine:** 1000–2000 mg daily
- **B-complex vitamins** (many of these should be included in high potency multivitamin supplements):
  - **Thiamine** (B1): 75–125 mg daily
  - **Riboflavin** (B2): 50 mg daily
  - **Niacin** (B3): 50–190 mg daily
  - **Folate,** preferably as L-methylfolate: 400–1000 mcg daily
  - **Vitamin B6,** preferably as pyridoxal-5-phosphate: 75–105 mg daily
  - **Vitamin B12:** 300–600 mcg daily
  - **Biotin:** 300–3000 mcg daily
  - **Pantothenic acid:** 100–600 mg daily
- **Fish oil** (with olive polyphenols): at least 1400 mg/day of EPA and 1000 mg/day of DHA
- **5-hydroxytryptophan** (5-HTP): 50–200 mg daily
- **S-adenosyl-methionine** (SAMe): 400–1200 mg daily in divided doses with food
- **Vitamin D:** 5000–8000 IU daily, depending on blood test results
- **Creatine:** 1.25 g daily
- **Zinc:** 30 mg daily
- **DHEA:** 15–25 mg daily for women; 25–75 mg daily for men (depending on blood test results)
- **D-ribose:** 5 g, 1–3 times daily with food
- **Probiotics:** per label instructions
- **Chlorella:** 1–3 g daily
- **Plant-derived SOD blend** (including SODzyme® and GliSODin®): 2100 mg daily
- **NADH:** 5–20 mg daily in divided doses on an empty stomach
- **Curcumin** (as highly absorbed BCM95®): 400–800 mg daily
- **Boswellia serrata** (as highly absorbed Apres-Flex™): 100 mg daily

In addition, the following blood tests may provide helpful information.

- Vitamin D, 25-Hydroxy
- Omega Score®
- Red blood cell (RBC) magnesium
- Female Panel or Male Panel
- DHEA (available in the Female or Male Panel)

## REFERENCES

References available at: www.lef.org/dpt5/ch60

# 61

# *Fungal Infections (Candida)*

Fungal infections are estimated to occur in over a billion people each year, and recent evidence suggests the rate is increasing.[1-4] Fungi can infect almost any part of the body including skin, nails, respiratory tract, urogenital tract, alimentary tract, or can be systemic.[5,6] Anyone can acquire a fungal infection, but the elderly, critically ill, and individuals with weakened immunity, due to diseases such as HIV/AIDS or use of immunosuppressive medications, have a higher risk.[1,7]

Although several species of fungi are potentially pathogenic in humans, *Candida* (especially *Candida albicans*) is the organism responsible for most fungal infections. *Candida*, which is normally present within the human body, is usually harmless. However, it can cause symptoms when a weakened immune system or other factors allow it to grow unabated.[8-10]

Increased use of antibiotics and immunosuppressive drugs such as corticosteroids are major factors contributing to higher frequency of fungal infections. Antibiotics and immunosuppressive drugs, by disrupting normal bacterial colonization and suppressing the immune system, create an environment within the body in which fungi can thrive.[1,11]

Fungal infections can range in severity from superficial to life-threatening. For example, fungal infections affecting only the top layers of the skin are readily treatable and have a relatively limited impact on quality of life. However, if a fungal infection enters systemic circulation, consequences can be deadly.[12,13]

Many integrative medical practitioners believe that chronic, low-level *Candida* infestation can cause a variety of nonspecific symptoms that may resemble chronic fatigue syndrome, depression, anxiety, or fibromyalgia. This phenomenon is sometimes referred to as "*Candida*-related complex." Conventional medical practitioners do not recognize *Candida*-related complex as a disease. However, many innovative health care practitioners report improvements in patient quality of life upon treatment.[14]

Upon reading this protocol, you will have a better understanding of the various ways that fungi can infect a human host, and how conventional medicine treats these infections. In addition, you will discover several natural compounds that have antifungal activity and may complement conventional treatments for fungal infections.

## UNDERSTANDING *CANDIDA* FUNGAL INFECTIONS

*Candida albicans* is the most common fungal microorganism in healthy individuals, as well as the most common fungal pathogen causing lethal infections (particularly in high-risk groups such as immunocompromised patients).[9,10] It can be found in up to 70% of healthy individuals at any given time.[9,15,16]

*Candida* is considered an opportunistic pathogen because it can harmlessly colonize the human digestive tract, mouth, skin, and genitourinary tract.[17,18] However, when the balance of normal bacteria is upset (eg, after antibiotic treatment) or the immune system of the host is weakened (eg, treatment with systemic corticosteroids), *Candida* can proliferate.[19]

Several areas of the body may be affected by fungal infection, including those discussed in the following sections.

### Urogenital Tract

Although *Candida* is often found in the lower female urogenital tract in asymptomatic women, proliferation and subsequent infestation of this fungal species accounts for approximately one-third of all infections in the vulva and/or vagina (ie, vaginitis).[20] Also known as vulvovaginal candidiasis (VVC) or "yeast infection,"[21] this fungal infection represents the second most common cause of vaginitis in the United States (after bacterial vaginosis), and is diagnosed in up to 40% of women who present to their primary care provider with vaginal complaints.[22] Approximately 75% of women report having had at least one episode of VVC, and between 40–45% will suffer from at least 2 or more episodes within their lifetime.[23]

The most common symptoms of VVC include unrelenting itch, painful intercourse, malodorous vaginal discharge, and painful urination.[23] Although the vast majority (up to 92%) of VVC cases are caused by *Candida albicans*, other *Candida* species can also be responsible (eg, *Candida glabrata* and *Candida parapsilosis*). However, the various *Candida* species tend to produce similar vulvovaginal symptoms. Recently, researchers have reported an increased frequency of VVC caused by non-*albicans* species.[20] This trend may be attributed to selective pressure from the widespread use of over-the-counter and prescription antifungal drugs,[20] especially since some non-*albicans* species are less susceptible to many of these medications.[24]

Some evidence suggests that hormones influence the infectious process of VVC.[25] This conclusion is supported by data indicating that a majority of VVC cases occur during the reproductive years. For example, 75% of women of childbearing age are affected by VVC,[20,26,27] while only sporadic episodes of VVC are reported among premenstrual girls and postmenopausal women.[20,27] Further research reveals that fluctuating hormone levels resulting from menstruation and pregnancy, as well as the use of oral contraceptives and hormone replacement (ie, estrogen therapy), may predispose females to VVC.[28,29]

Researchers have identified several factors that may increase susceptibility to fungal infections including[20]:

- Diabetes (with poor glycemic control)
- Exposure to antibiotics (both during and after therapy)
- High levels of estrogen (eg, oral contraceptives or estrogen therapy)
- Weakened immune system from drugs (eg, corticosteroids) or disease (eg, HIV/AIDS)
- Contraceptive device utilization (eg, vaginal sponges, diaphragms, and intrauterine devices)

Although less common, men can get genital fungal infections as well.[30] Therefore, it is important that both members of a relationship receive treatment for fungal infections, even if symptoms are only evident in one person. If antifungal treatment is not initiated in both people in a relationship, the partners may continue to repeatedly infect one another.[31]

## Skin

Fungal infections of the skin (ie, cutaneous fungal infections) are a common phenomenon, affecting millions of people worldwide. While cutaneous fungal infection is not normally life threatening, it can be very uncomfortable and associated with a significant decrease in quality of life.[32,33] *Candida* is just one of a variety of microorganisms commonly found on human skin.[34] In healthy individuals, the overgrowth of *Candida* is inhibited by resident skin microorganisms (normal bacterial skin flora). However, when there is an imbalance of this normal skin flora, *Candida* can begin to reproduce in sufficient amounts to cause infection (ie, candidiasis).[35] Due to an increase in the number of immunocompromised individuals, the rate of candidiasis of the skin (ie, cutaneous candidiasis) is currently on the rise.[36]

Candidiasis can be broadly classified into 2 forms based on the degree of fungal invasion: superficial/mucosal candidiasis and deep-seated/systemic candidiasis.[33] However, superficial candidiasis of the skin and mucous membrane is much more common than deep-seated/systemic infection.[33] Among the different species of *Candida* that can be found on the skin, *Candida albicans* is by far the most common.[35] While cutaneous candidiasis can affect virtually any part of the human body (eg, finger nails, external ear, in between fingers and toes), it most often occurs in warm, moist, creased areas such as the armpit or groin.[33,34,37–39] Major symptoms of cutaneous candidiasis include itch (unrelenting and often intense) and an enlarging skin rash. Occasionally, the rash will be surrounded by smaller rashes appearing along the outer edge of the main rash.[34] These types of fungal rashes may occur on skin that is exposed to feces (eg, perineal skin), since this area is at a higher risk of becoming infected with *Candida* fungus.[35]

Individuals whose hands and/or feet remain wet for prolonged periods of time may be prone to fungal infection around or under their finger and toe nails. In these cases, the nail area commonly becomes red and swollen. The nails themselves will become thick and brittle, ultimately becoming destroyed and detached.[38–41] Although anyone's nails can become infected by fungus, these types of infections are more common among adults >60 years, and among individuals with diabetes or poor circulation.[42]

## Mouth and Throat

*Candida* infections of the mouth (ie, oral candidiasis) are widespread among humans.[43] In addition to the general factors that predispose an individual to *Candida* infection (eg, immunosuppressive drugs and antibiotics), oral candidiasis may also be caused by chronic dry mouth and oral prosthesis (dentures).[44] Although oral infection can be caused by a variety of *Candida* species, *Candida albicans* is the most common causative agent.[45]

Oral candidiasis (thrush) is characterized by whitish, velvety sores or patches appearing on the mucous membranes lining the inside of the mouth (eg, roof of the mouth and inside the lips and cheeks), as well as the throat and tongue.[46,47] These whitish sores may slowly increase in size, quantity, and may bleed easily.[47] Occasionally, oral *Candida* infections can manifest as subjective feelings of pain or taste abnormalities.[48]

In addition to infections inside the mouth, *Candida* can also take the form of perlèche (angular cheilitis),[49,50] which is commonly identified by reddish lesions and crusting at the corners of the mouth.[51] Perlèche can be associated with long-term use of ill-fitting dentures and incorrect use of dental floss (resulting in cuts at the corners of the mouth).[50]

## Systemic Infection

Although *Candida* species are normal residents of the gastrointestinal (GI) and genitourinary tracts of humans, they occasionally cause a deep-seated or systemic (disseminated) infection.[52] These serious fungal infections usually indicate the host has a weakened immune system, and can occur as a result of a superficial skin infection that invades deeper tissues, eventually reaching the bloodstream (ie, candidemia). Once the fungus is circulating throughout the body, it has the capacity to reach vital organs such as the brain, heart, and kidneys. While this form of candidiasis is rare, it is the most severe.[33] These types of fungal infections can be fatal and require prompt diagnosis and aggressive treatment in order to achieve a favorable outcome.[53]

Since the clinical symptoms of a systemic *Candida* infection can vary, and are often very similar to that of a bacterial infection, the gold standard for its proper diagnosis is a positive blood culture.[54] Advancements in blood culturing technology now allow for the rapid identification of a variety of *Candida* species in as little as 90 minutes. This reduction in laboratory turnaround time enables clinicians to optimize antifungal drug selection much faster, and ultimately improve care.[55,56]

## Intestinal Candidiasis

*Candida* organisms are a common part of the normal GI flora,[57] and are present in the gut of approximately 70% of healthy adults.[16] However, high levels of *Candida* colonization in the GI tract may be an urgent problem,[58] especially since it is associated with several GI diseases (eg, irritable bowel syndrome) and certain allergic reactions.[16,57] Furthermore, *Candida* colonization in the gut can also promote inflammation, which in turn promotes further fungal colonization in a vicious cycle.[57]

Intestinal *Candida* colonization can also lead to superficial and systemic candidiasis if the innate host barriers (ie, mucosa, immune system, intestinal microflora) are not stable.[16] Benign strains of intestinal *Candida* can also become more virulent when their gene expression is altered in such a way that they are able to form biofilms, destroy tissues, and escape host immune system defenses.[16,57] While antimycotics (eg, nystatin) are available for the treatment of intestinal *Candida* overgrowth, probiotics (having demonstrated positive results in controlled clinical trials) may also be beneficial. Probiotics may exert this effect by rebalancing the normal flora of the gut, thereby suppressing local *Candida* colonization.

Some research questions the clinical significance of yeast infestation of the intestinal mucosa, and suggests that clinical action may not always be necessary.[16]

## Fungal Sinusitis

Overgrowth of fungus in the nasal cavity (ie, fungal sinusitis or fungal rhinosinusitis) and the subsequent human immune response (eg, allergic fungal sinusitis) is currently believed to be responsible for some cases of chronic sinusitis.[59] This condition can be classified as either invasive or noninvasive, depending on the extent of fungal infection. Invasive forms of fungal sinusitis are largely limited to immunocompromised populations,[60] and are characterized by infection of the submucosal tissue, which often causes tissue necrosis and destruction.[61]

Although optimal treatment options for fungal sinusitis are still debated,[62] they typically include systemic antifungal therapy as well as surgical debridement and evacuation of infected tissue.[60] In addition to these conventional treatment options, some experts believe fungal sinusitis may also respond to probiotics as well as an antifungal diet. An antifungal diet calls for avoidance of sugar and concentrated sweets, and consists primarily of protein and fresh vegetables, along with a small amount of fruit, complex carbohydrates, and fat-containing foods.[59]

---

### CANDIDA-RELATED COMPLEX (CRC)

While overt *Candida* infection is a well-documented phenomenon, the idea that chronic low-grade *Candida* infestation (primarily in the gut and urogenital tract) can cause various, seemingly unrelated symptoms is viewed with skepticism among conventional infectious disease experts. As a result, the conventional medical community is often at odds with some innovative health care practitioners as to the treatment strategy of *Candida* infestation in chronic health conditions.

With his publication of *The Yeast Connection* in 1986, William Crook introduced the public to the concept that yeast overgrowth could potentially underlie numerous chronic symptoms.[63] Seminal scientific research published by C. Orian Truss in 1977 contributed to the development of Crook's theory.[64] The concepts and treatments described in these publications continue to be utilized in the practices of innovative health care practitioners worldwide.

The mechanism(s) by which *Candida* overgrowth might cause otherwise unexplainable symptoms are unclear. However, suppression of the immune system, with subsequent reactivation of dormant viruses like Epstein-Barr virus and herpes virus, is one hypothesis.[65] Other theories posit that

*Candida* colonization within the GI tract may contribute to "leaky gut," in which foreign particles "leak" through the intestinal barrier and contribute to systemic reactions.[16,66,67]

Although published, peer-reviewed research on the role of yeast overgrowth in chronic disease is limited, some innovative health care practitioners, including Crook, have detailed reports of improved quality of life upon treatment for suspected yeast overgrowth.[14,63] Strategies often employed to treat "chronic *Candida* infection" include use of graded doses of antimycotic medications such as nystatin, as well as strict adherence to a sugar- and starch-free diet.

# CONVENTIONAL TREATMENT

Although most cases of *Candida* infection are treated with some type of antifungal agent, the formulation of the medication (eg, pills, ointment, suppositories, or powder) will largely depend on the location and clinical presentation of the infection.[68,69]

## Mild Oral Candidiasis

Mild oral candidiasis can be treated with either clotrimazole lozenges or a nystatin swish-and-swallow suspension, but may require oral fluconazole for moderate to severe and recurrent cases.[70] An emerging treatment for oral candidiasis involves the use of mouthwash containing silver nanoparticles (SN). Although this approach requires more investigation to include safety and efficacy, it may hold therapeutic potential in the near future.[71]

## Candidiasis of the Skin

Candidiasis of the skin is most often managed with topical antifungal agents of the azole class (eg, bifonazole or ketoconazole).[72] People with candidiasis of the skin should also keep the skin as dry as possible and, if appropriate, use antifungal mouth rinses or shampoos.

## Fungal Infections of the Finger/Toe Nail Plate

Fungal infections of the finger/toe nail plate (eg, onychomycosis) are typically treated with both topical and systemic antifungals. However, long-term cure and recurrence rates, as well as costs associated with these treatments, are often unsatisfactory. For this reason, researchers have studied the effects of laser therapy for the treatment of onychomycosis; they found that this technology is capable of inhibiting the growth of the fungus on nail samples.[73] In severe cases that do not respond to drug therapy, surgical removal of all or part of the nail plate may be considered.[74]

## Vaginal *Candida*

Vaginal *Candida* infections can be treated with topical or oral antifungal drugs such as fluconazole or nystatin.[20] The species of *Candida* that a woman is infected with can influence treatment response. For example, fluconazole and nystatin are both effective for the treatment of *Candida albicans*, but in women with non-*albicans* species, only fluconazole is highly effective.[75]

## Invasive/Systemic Candidiasis

Treatment for invasive/systemic candidiasis depends on a variety of factors, but will most likely involve intravenous or oral therapy with any one of the following drug classes: polyenes, azoles, and echinocandins.[76] The polyene drug amphotericin B is a very common treatment, but is hindered by considerable kidney toxicity. Therefore, newer, less toxic derivatives of the drug (eg, liposomal amphotericin B) are a better option. The high cost of these formulations, however, can be burdensome in some circumstances.[77,78]

The side effects of most systemic antifungal drugs are comparable and include headache, GI symptoms (eg, nausea and vomiting), hepatitis, kidney toxicity, and lupus-like syndromes, among others.[78–80]

# NUTRITIONAL THERAPY FOR *CANDIDA* INFECTIONS

Given the rise in *Candida* infections,[1] and their increasing resistance against commonly used antifungal drugs,[81] novel therapies for the prevention and management of these infections are needed.[82]

## Dietary Modifications

Dietary modifications, such as limiting intake of refined carbohydrates (eg, pasta, bread, sweets, soft drinks, etc.), may be helpful for people with *Candida* infections. Higher dietary sugar is associated with vulvovaginal candidiasis, and abnormal glucose metabolism is associated with recurring vulvovaginal infections.[83] Diets rich in carbohydrates are also associated with *Candida* overgrowth in the GI tract and may contribute to mucosal invasion.[84,85] Laboratory studies indicate that excess glucose weakens the immune system's response to *Candida* as well as the azole class of antifungal drugs.[86] Candidiasis patients should maintain a healthy, well-balanced diet, as poor nutrition is a commonly overlooked risk factor for bacterial and fungal infections.[87] More information about blood sugar control is available in the Diabetes protocol.

## Probiotics

Data suggest that probiotics such as lactobacillus are beneficial against mucosal *Candida* infections,[82] and should be especially considered for women who suffer from more than 3 yeast infections per year.[88] Research shows that probiotics exert their beneficial actions by suppressing the growth of *Candida* (in various regions of the body) and inhibiting *Candida*'s ability to adhere to cell surfaces.[89]

Dietary products containing probiotic bacteria (eg, certain cheeses and yogurts) can help control *Candida* growth in the human body.[90,91] In a study, yogurt containing lactobacillus was associated with a decreased amount of vaginal yeast (detected by culture), as well as a reduced rate of vaginal discharge associated with yeast infections.[92]

While yogurt has long been considered a favorite natural remedy for vaginal candidiasis, and has been shown to suppress *Candida albicans* growth,[91,93] women must carefully choose yogurt products that are low in sugar. Supplemental probiotics containing lactobacillus, administered either orally or vaginally, can also help resolve urogenital infections (including yeast infections).[94,95] In particular, the lactobacillus species rhamnosus and reuteri have been studied for repopulating vaginal flora and reducing yeast populations.[96,97]

Probiotics may also be useful after a course of antibiotics. Antibiotics used to kill pathogenic bacteria also destroy the beneficial bacterial flora of the vagina, putting women at risk to develop yeast infections.[83] Probiotics also help rebalance gut bacteria, and thus may help avoid symptoms of leaky gut syndrome.[66]

## Resveratrol

Resveratrol, a compound found in the skin of grapes, may contribute to the anti-inflammatory characteristics of red wine. In 2007, researchers investigated (in a laboratory) the fungicidal activity of resveratrol against *Candida albicans*. They concluded that resveratrol demonstrated potent antifungal properties, and appears to be safer than conventional antifungal drugs such as amphotericin B.[98] In 2010, further research revealed that resveratrol impairs the ability of *Candida albicans* to convert into its more infectious form, and thus may be a useful agent against *Candida* infections. In fact, resveratrol's chemical structure may form the foundation of an entirely new class of antifungal drugs.[99]

## Goldenseal

Goldenseal (*Hydrastis canadensis L.*) is a botanical that has been used to fight inflammation and infection. An active ingredient in goldenseal is berberine,[100] which has been shown to have strong antifungal effects against *Candida* in a laboratory setting.[101] Berberine has also demonstrated synergistic effects against *Candida albicans* when used in combination with commonly used antifungal drugs (eg, fluconazole) in laboratory studies.[102–104] Berberine may combat *Candida* growth by interfering with the ability of the fungus to penetrate and adhere to host cells.[105] Study outcomes have been so positive that, similar to the case with resveratrol, synthetic analogs of berberine are being developed that may represent a new class of antifungal medications.[106,107]

## Lactoferrin

Lactoferrin, a protein found in mucosal secretions (eg, human colostrum/milk, tears, saliva, and seminal fluid),[108–110] possesses broad-spectrum antimicrobial activity against bacteria, fungi, viruses, and protozoa.[111] Lactoferrin demonstrates a significant antifungal effect against a variety of pathogenic *Candida* species (ie, *Candida albicans*, *Candida krusei* and *Candida tropicalis*).[112] In addition to lactoferrin's ability to interfere with *Candida* growth on its own, it also displays potent synergism with common antifungal drugs; it has been shown to enhance the antifungal activity of fluconazole against *Candida*.[111] Although lactoferrin's antifungal activity against *Candida albicans* has been well established, the mechanism by which it achieves this effect is not as clear.[109] Lactoferrin's ability to bind to iron may contribute to its antifungal activity,[113] especially since iron appears to enhance the proliferation of *Candida* species.[112]

Lactoferrin derived from both bovine and human sources inhibits growth of oral *Candida*.[110] However, bovine-derived lactoferrin has been specifically identified as a promising treatment option for oropharyngeal candidiasis.[114]

## Tea Tree Oil

Tea tree oil is an essential oil derived from leaves of the native Australian plant *Melaleuca alternifolia* (*M. alternifolia*). It is well known for its medicinal value and has been used by Australian Aborigines to treat colds, sore throats, skin infections, and insect bites.[115,116] Tea tree oil has a variety of therapeutic properties (eg, anti-inflammatory and antiseptic) and is a popular ingredient in a number of natural cosmetic products (eg, shampoo, massage oil, and skin/nail cream).[115,117,118] Tea tree oil, capable of eliminating a large number of microorganisms,[117] shows promise as a treatment for *Candida* infections.[119] Animal studies indicate that one of the active compounds in tea tree oil, terpinen-4-ol, may be especially promising for treating drug-resistant forms of vaginal candidiasis.[118] Furthermore, tea tree oil may have beneficial effects against fluconazole-resistant oropharyngeal candidiasis.[119]

Laboratory research indicates that tea tree oil may exert its yeast-killing effect by inhibiting *Candida*'s ability to replicate. It also appears to interfere with membrane properties/functions of *Candida*.[117] In addition, research has demonstrated that tea tree oil reduces *Candida*'s ability to adhere to human cell surfaces.[120]

Although tea tree oil is occasionally associated with contact dermatitis (when used topically), it is generally considered to be safe. However, it can be toxic when ingested orally, producing a variety of negative effects (eg, vomiting, diarrhea, and hallucinations).[115] Therefore, it is typically used topically and should be kept out of the reach of young children.

## Other Essential Oils

Essential oils (ie, volatile oils) refer to the compounds found within aromatic plants that give them a particular odor or scent.[121] Most essential oils are a mixture of various chemicals, which are of clinical interest due to their large spectrum of biological activities.[122]

Although tea tree oil is considered one of the most important essential oils for biological activity against *Candida*,[118] a wide variety of essential oils possess anti-*Candida* properties (eg, carvacrol, 1,8-cineole, geraniol, germacrene-D, limonene, linalool, menthol, and thymol).[123] Experimental models involving geranium oil (or its main component geraniol) show that it suppressed *Candida* cell growth.[124] In addition, clove oil and its major constituent eugenol have shown particularly potent effects against *Candida*,[125] and may be effective against multi-drug resistant forms of *Candida albicans* alone or in combination with other common antifungal drugs (eg, fluconazole or amphotericin B).[80] A laboratory study demonstrated that essential oil from Moroccan thyme may act synergistically with common antifungal drugs, potentially reducing the need for high doses, which may in turn minimize associated side effects and treatment expenses.[126] Research has also identified the essential oil of lemon verbena (*Aloysia triphylla*) as a promising alternative for the treatment of candidiasis.[127] Compounds isolated from the essential oil of oregano possess antifungal activity as well.[128]

## Garlic

For centuries, the garlic plant *Allium sativum* has been used as a popular food, spice, and herbal remedy.[129,130] Garlic has been noted to possess cardiovascular,[131] anticancer, antioxidant, and antimicrobial benefits.[130] Garlic (and its constituent allicin) can cause potent growth inhibition in yeast and be effective against mucosal and systemic/invasive candidiasis.[132,133] Research suggests that allicin, due to its effect on reducing the growth of biofilm (a component of *Candida* allowing it to become resistant to certain antifungal agents), may reduce *Candida*'s ability to become resistant to common antifungal drugs. Allicin may also decrease the production of *Candida* by disrupting its membrane.[134] A clinical trial found that the topical administration of a garlic paste was as effective at suppressing the symptoms of oral candidiasis as clotrimazole solution (the conventional antifungal treatment for this indication).[135] Likewise, a clinical study of *Candida* vaginitis concluded that there was no difference in treatment response between a vaginal cream containing garlic and thyme, and a vaginal cream containing clotrimazole.[136]

## Additional Alternative Therapies

**AHCC.** Active hexose correlated compound (AHCC) is an extract derived from fungi of the Basidiomycetes family. AHCC has demonstrated biological activity against a variety of disorders.[137] Experimental research has shown that AHCC appears to have a protective effect against *Candida* infections, especially among the immunocompromised.[138] Likewise, a 2008 experimental study suggested that supplementation with AHCC may increase the survival of hosts acutely infected with a variety of pathogens such as *Candida albicans*.[139] Additional therapies to support a healthy immune system can be found in the Immune System Strengthening protocol.

**Caprylic acid.** Caprylic acid (ie, octanoic acid) is commonly available as a nonprescription agent that is well known for its antibacterial and antifungal properties.[140]

**Boric acid.** Boric acid (ie, boracic acid or orthoboric acid) is the most common form of the mineral boron, which is often used as a supplement for building strong bones and muscles as well as supporting cognitive function and muscle coordination.[24,141] Boric acid has also been shown to inhibit the growth and reproduction of fungi (ie, fungistatic action),[24] and is used intravaginally to treat yeast infections.[141,142] In fact, a 2011 review article concluded that boric acid may be recommended as a safe, effective, and relatively cheap treatment for recurrent yeast infections.[24] Boric acid has also been proven to be efficient for the treatment of most yeast infections that are resistant to conventional therapies,[83] and thus may be considered a second-line alternative treatment option for this indication.[26]

## Life Extension Suggestions

- **Trans-resveratrol:** 250 mg daily
- **Goldenseal:** 250–550 mg daily
- **Apolactoferrin:** 285 mg daily
- **Garlic extract,** standardized to 10 000 ppm allicin potential [12 mg]: 1200–4800 mg daily
- **Probiotics:** per label instructions
- **Caprylic acid:** 60 mg daily
- **Boric acid suppository:** per label instructions

- **Oil of oregano extract:** 45–450 mg daily
- **Active hexose correlated compound (AHCC):** 1–3 g daily

---

## REFERENCES

References available at: www.lef.org/dpt5/ch61

# 62

# Gastroesophageal Reflux Disease (GERD)

Gastroesophageal reflux disease (GERD) is a chronic condition in which contents of the stomach flow back ("reflux") into the esophagus potentially causing symptoms (eg, heartburn) and injury to esophageal tissue.[1,2] GERD is one of the most common health conditions of the gastrointestinal tract, and close to 20% of Americans experience heartburn weekly.[3,4]

Pharmaceutical behemoths rake in nearly $14 billion annually from the sale of proton pump inhibitors (PPIs) in the United States alone.[5] However, long-term use of acid-blocking drugs can *impair nutrient absorption* and may lead to *deficiencies* with dangerous consequences. For example, chronic, high-dose therapy with *proton pump inhibitors* and *histamine-2 receptor blockers* can significantly increase the risk of *hip fracture*.[6]

In addition to *robbing* your body of critical nutrients like *calcium, magnesium,* and *vitamin B12,* PPIs can also cause a *rebound effect* when they are discontinued, potentially exacerbating GERD symptoms.[7–9]

Furthermore, conventional treatment strategies call for increasing the dosage or adding *another* acid-blocking drug when PPIs fail to relieve GERD symptoms, which occurs in up to 33% of cases.[10] Worse yet, as much as 69% of prescriptions for PPIs are written for *inappropriate indications.*[5]

In this protocol, you will learn about the causes of GERD, as well as evidence-based treatment strategies with scientifically studied *natural compounds,* and specific steps to take to avoid the potential dangers associated with the chronic use of pharmaceutical acid-blocking therapies.

## THE ESOPHAGUS AND DIGESTIVE TRACT

The esophagus conveys ingested material from the mouth to the stomach. It is one of the simpler regions of the gastrointestinal (GI) tract; a roughly

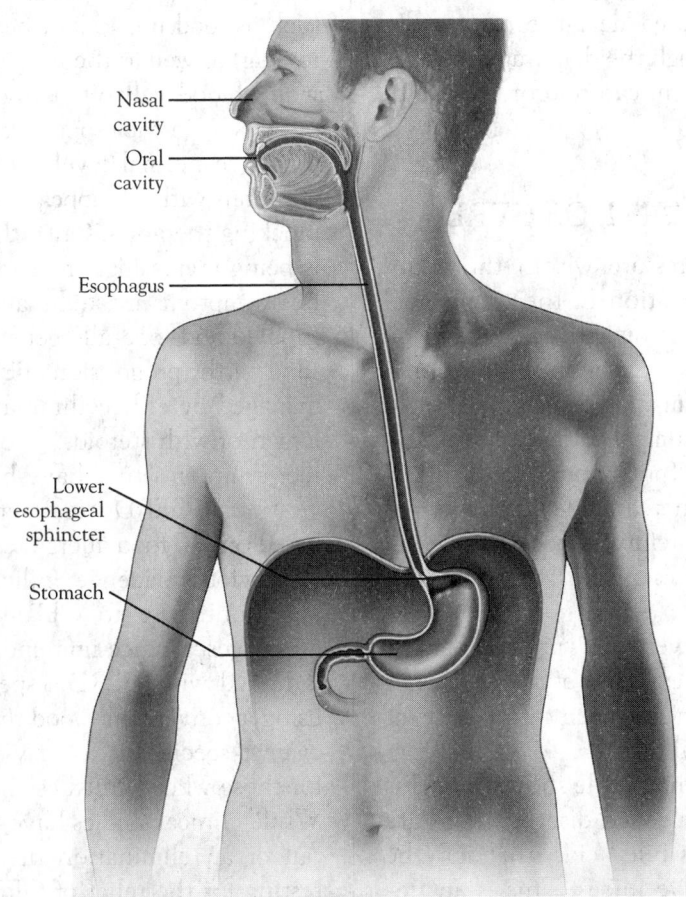

Basic anatomy of the upper digestive tract

8- to 10-inch muscular tube that runs from the back of the oral cavity (ie, pharynx), through the chest cavity, and into the abdomen where it joins with the opening of the stomach (ie, cardia). After ingested materials have traveled down the esophagus, they are emptied into the acidic environment of the stomach for chemical and mechanical digestion.

While the thick cellular layer of the stomach is a suitable barrier against stomach acid, the thinner mucus membrane of the esophagus was not designed to withstand such harsh conditions. To protect the esophagus from the potential back-flow of stomach contents (reflux), a sphincter is located at the junction between the esophagus and stomach, called the gastroesophageal or *lower esophageal sphincter* (LES). This sphincter, a circular band of thickened muscle, surrounds the lower esophagus and pinches it closed. The LES is usually closed. It opens to allow the passage of swallowed food or drink, a reflex that is triggered by the act of swallowing.

Aiding the closure of the LES is the diaphragm (a wide, flat muscle that helps to expand the lungs during respiration). Internally, the diaphragm separates the chest cavity from the abdomen, and the esophagus passes through a hole in the diaphragm (called the hiatus) on its way from the mouth to the stomach. The LES is situated near the part of the esophagus that passes through the diaphragm, so that contraction of the diaphragm can reinforce the closure of the sphincter.[11]

## THE DEVELOPMENT OF GERD

Occasionally, increased pressure within the abdomen or a momentary relaxation of the esophageal sphincter can force some stomach contents back into the esophagus. Everyone experiences occasional reflux, which can result from a large meal or physical activity or reclining after a meal. Other physiologic conditions, both normal (pregnancy) and pathologic (obesity) can also increase the likelihood of reflux. As long as gastric reflux is occasional, and promptly cleared from the esophagus, there is little risk of damage.[11]

Prolonged reflux, however, can present serious health concerns. Repeated exposure of the esophagus to the harsh chemistry of the stomach can have deleterious effects on esophageal tissue.[12]

It is important to note that while stomach acid is most often associated with reflux disease, there are other compounds, such as bile acids, that may be present in refluxed digestive juices. This is an important consideration in the diagnosis and treatment of GERD, especially when the disease is resistant to acid-suppression therapy. Many patients with treatment-resistant GERD (despite use of acid-blocking pharmaceutical therapy) may have bile in their reflux.[13,14] In one study, over half of the patients with reflux symptoms had 24-hour esophageal pH measurements within normal limits.[15,16] In some cases, stomach acid may partially neutralize damaging alkaline reflux from lower parts of the digestive tract, thus protecting the esophagus. In an animal model of small intestinal reflux, rats on acid-blocking therapy demonstrated more esophageal damage and Barrett's esophagus than control animals, a finding consistent with some human observational studies.[17]

A functional (transient LES relaxation) or mechanical (hypotensive LES) problem of the LES are the most common causes of GERD. Transient relaxation of the LES can be caused by foods (coffee, alcohol, chocolate, fatty meals), medications (beta-agonists, nitrates, calcium channel blockers, anticholinergic drugs), hormones (eg, progestins), and nicotine.[18]

*Allergy is not a risk for progression to GERD, but it can increase the incidence of a related condition—eosinophilic esophagitis* (EE). EE is characterized by upper gastrointestinal symptoms (some of which resemble GERD such as food impaction, heartburn, or difficulty swallowing) as well as the presence of *eosinophils* (a type of white blood cell often involved in allergic immune responses) in the esophagus.[19] Individuals with EE often have normal levels of acidity in the esophagus. Children with EE appear to be unresponsive to acid-blocking therapies. Once thought a rare condition, it is being increasingly recognized as a cause of GERD-like symptoms in adults and, especially children.[20,21] Inhaled and food allergens are thought to be responsible for the progression of EE. As such, it is commonly managed by either eliminating the source of the allergen or with steroids.[19] For individuals with GERD-like symptoms that have been unresponsive to conventional GERD treatments, an elimination diet based on IgE food allergy testing may be useful.[22]

Previous evidence indicates that *food sensitivities* may contribute to GERD-related irritation of the esophagus.[23] Since immunoreactivity to certain foods is linked with GERD, especially in children,[24] then using a convenient blood test to assess IgG antibodies against specific foods may prove to be a useful tool for those whose GERD symptoms fluctuate with diet. While clinical studies have yet to evaluate the potential of an elimination diet based on IgG antibody testing for the relief of GERD symptoms, similar approaches have been successful.[25]

For more information about food allergy and/or sensitivity testing, refer to the Allergies protocol.

**H. pylori Infection.** Infection with the bacteria *Helicobacter pylori*, which resides in the stomach and is associated with ulcers of the gastric lining, has been observed in up to 40% of GERD cases; though it is unclear whether *H. pylori* infection causes GERD.[26,27] Until recently some experts believed that *H. pylori* infection possibly conferred some protection against development of GERD.[28] However, more recent research suggests that this is likely not the case.[29,30] Furthermore, upon conducting a review of randomized controlled trials, Saad[29] and colleagues uncovered a significantly lower incidence of GERD symptoms in patients who had undergone *H. pylori* eradication compared to those who had not.

## AN ALTERNATIVE THEORY ON THE CAUSE OF GERD

*Hypochlorhydria.* Some high-profile alternative medical practitioners suggest that rather than *too much* stomach acid, it may be *too little* that causes GERD.[31] The proposed etiology involving *hypochlorhydria* attributes GERD symptoms to refluxed acid, and argues that just because acid is being refluxed does not necessarily mean that there is too much in the stomach to begin with. Proponents of the hypochlorhydria theory believe that inadequate stomach acid reduces lower esophageal sphincter tone, thereby allowing stomach contents to be refluxed giving rise to GERD symptoms.

*Hydrochloric acid (HCl)* in the stomach activates enzymes that help break down proteins and stimulates other digestive processes. The hypochlorhydria theory of GERD proposes *increasing* stomach acidity to alleviate symptoms, as opposed to lowering it, which is the conventional approach. To do this, alternative practitioners often administer betaine HCl, which delivers additional hydrochloric acid to the stomach. This therapy is sometimes preceded by the Heidelberg test to measure the pH of the stomach.

Although the hypochlorhydria theory lacks support in modern published, peer-reviewed scientific literature, detailed reports of using orally administered hydrochloric acid to improve gastric function are available in early articles.[32] Also, some innovative modern-day practitioners have noted clinical improvement in GERD patients using this method.[31]

## GERD SYMPTOMS AND COMPLICATIONS

Aside from heartburn, there are several other symptoms associated with GERD that reduce quality of life. These include nausea, hypersalivation (increased saliva production), globus (the sensation of a constant lump in the throat), trouble swallowing, bad breath, and dental erosion.[32] Sleep disturbances and nocturnal choking are also possible.[33] Because of the close proximity of the larynx (the opening of the windpipe) and esophagus, GERD can manifest respiratory symptoms (eg, including chronic hoarseness, cough, and laryngitis) as well. GERD can be associated with inflammation of lung tissue (pneumonitis), sinusitis, asthma, and middle ear infection (otitis media).[34,35] Recent evidence suggests that GERD may also be associated with idiopathic pulmonary fibrosis (IPF), an incurable lung disease resulting from the deposit of fibrous tissue on the lung surface. The incidence of GERD is high in IPF patients, which places them at risk for aspiration (reflux) of material into the lungs and subsequent damage.[36,37]

Prolonged exposure of the esophagus to gastric reflux can result in dramatic alterations to its function. Serious complications of GERD include:

**Peptic Stricture.** In people with long-term GERD, healing of ulcerations can lead to the deposit of fibrous scar tissue as well as a stricture (ie, narrowing) of the esophagus.[38] Segments of the esophagus with stricture are usually thickened, stiff, and may be shortened. As the esophagus shortens, it can pull the stomach up through the esophageal hiatus, resulting in hiatal hernia.[39] The prevalence of peptic stricture among patients with GERD is about 10–25%.[40] Treatment of severe peptic stricture involves the mechanical dilation of the narrowed region by a stent or balloon combined with acid suppression therapy.[33]

**Barrett's Esophagus.** Barrett's esophagus is a change in the cellular makeup of the mucus membrane of the esophagus. A normal esophagus is lined with a layer of flattened cells (squamous epithelial cells). In Barrett's esophagus, these cells are replaced by a layer of thicker, taller cells (columnar epithelial cells) similar to those found on the inner surface of the stomach or intestines.[41] This *reversible* replacement of one differentiated cell type with another mature differentiated cell type is called metaplasia, and is distinct from the cellular transformation that occurs during cancer progression. The main cause of Barrett's esophagus is thought to be an adaptation to chronic acid exposure from reflux esophagitis.[42,43] Barrett's esophagus can increase the risk of esophageal cancer. Although endoscopic examination of the esophagus can identify potential tissue changes that are indicative of Barrett's esophagus, a confirmed diagnosis requires a biopsy of the esophageal mucus membrane.[44]

**Esophageal Cancer.** The two major types of esophageal cancer are esophageal squamous cell carcinoma and esophageal adenocarcinoma. Esophageal adenocarcinoma (EAC) arises from metaplasia of tissue in the lower part of the esophagus, and is thought to develop as a result of long-term GERD and Barrett's esophagus.[45] Two large studies of Barrett's esophagus patients estimate the risk of progression to esophageal adenocarcinoma at approximately 0.27–0.4% per person per year.[46,47] The risk is highest in men and increases with age, aspirin/NSAID use, smoking, and incidence of hiatal hernia or esophageal dysplasia.[46]

# DIAGNOSIS

In patients with symptoms that suggest uncomplicated GERD (heartburn and/or regurgitation often occurring after meals and aggravated by lying down or bending over, with relief obtained from antacids), the recommended course of action is treatment for GERD with a trial of acid-suppression therapy. If the patient responds to this initial therapy, then it is reasonable to assume GERD.[48]

Self-assessments can be useful in diagnosing uncomplicated GERD. The GERD questionnaire (GerdQ) is a simple, easily interpreted six question assessment of GERD symptom frequency. In one study of 300 patients, GerdQ had 65% sensitivity, a result similar to the diagnostic accuracy achieved by gastroenterologists.[49] Using GerdQ as a patient-tailored diagnostic and therapeutic evaluation tool is beneficial compared with standard approaches to GERD management.[50]

Further diagnostic testing is only recommended if the patient does not respond to acid-suppression therapy, presents symptoms suggestive of complicated GERD (eg, dysphagia), or has been symptomatic long enough to put them at risk for Barrett's esophagus.[48]

Tests for GERD may include:

**Barium Esophagram.** Viewing the esophagus via x-ray radiography after swallowing a barium contrast solution can give insight into esophageal motility as well as detect esophageal strictures, ulcers, or severe esophagitis. It is not as sensitive or accurate at diagnosing mild esophagitis or reflux. Compared to newer techniques, it may not be as suitable for the routine diagnosis of GERD.[48]

**Upper GI Endoscopy.** Direct viewing of the esophagus via flexible esophagoscope can identify mucosal breaks, areas of sloughed cells, ulceration, or redness that is distinct from areas of normal mucus membranes. Mucosal breaks are the minimum reliable indicator of GERD.[12] Esophageal changes indicative of Barrett's esophagus can also be seen with an endoscope. However, a biopsy is required before a definitive diagnosis can be made.[51]

**Esophageal pH Monitoring.** Esophageal pH monitoring is the current gold standard for diagnosing GERD. While a person is upright and mobile, esophageal pH is monitored using a flexible catheter with pH sensor (inserted through the nose and positioned in the lower esophagus), or more recently, a wireless pH capsule attached to the lower esophagus.[52] Measurements of pH are logged over a 24-hour period.[53] Normal esophageal pH is close to 7.0, while a reflux event is recorded as a sudden (>30-second) drop in pH to below 4.0. One method measures six parameters over the study period including the percentage of time that the esophageal pH is >4 (while upright, reclined, and total), the number of reflux episodes (both total episodes and those >5 minutes), and the duration of the longest reflux episode. These parameters are then assembled into a composite score (DeMeester score) where less than 14.7 is normal.[54] Unlike endoscopy, esophageal pH monitoring provides direct physiologic measurement of acid in the *esophagus* and is the most objective method to document reflux disease, assess the severity of the disease, and monitor the response of the disease to medical or surgical treatment.

**Bilitec.** The Bilitec system uses a fiberoptic sensor to detect the presence of bile in reflux. Bile has been implicated in symptomatic reflux that is difficult to manage by conventional acid-suppression therapy.[55]

**Esophageal Manometry.** Esophageal manometry assesses esophageal and LES function by measuring pressure changes in the esophagus induced by swallowing and peristalsis. A physician passes a pressure-sensing catheter through the nose and esophagus into the stomach. The patient performs a series of 5 mL water swallows, and pressure measurements are made of the peristaltic activity of the esophagus and LES. Since manometry measures esophageal function, it is more suited for diagnosing dysphagia, or abnormal relaxation of the lower esophageal sphincter.[56]

# CONVENTIONAL PHARMACEUTICAL TREATMENT

Acid suppression therapies are the mainstay of pharmaceutical GERD treatment. Acid suppression therapy neutralizes stomach acid or reduces its secretion, minimizing the potential for damage during reflux episodes. Acid suppression therapies include antacids, histamine-2 receptor blockers, and proton pump inhibitors.

**Antacids.** Antacids that neutralize stomach acid are the first medication(s) commonly used to provide quick relief for the reflux symptoms of GERD, and are often effective for mild symptoms. Typical antacids include aluminum hydroxide or magnesium hydroxide, calcium carbonate (Tums®), and sodium or potassium bicarbonate.

**Histamine-2 Receptor Blockers (H2 Blockers).** H2 blockers prevent secretion of stomach acid by inhibiting the action of histamine, which is a stimulus for acid secretion. Examples of H2 blockers include cimetidine (Tagamet®), ranitidine (Zantac®), and famotidine (Pepcid®). H2 receptor blockers are effective for healing only mild esophagitis in 70–80% of patients with GERD and for providing maintenance therapy to prevent relapse. Tachyphylaxis has been observed, suggesting that pharmacologic tolerance can reduce the long-term efficacy of these drugs. Therefore, patients are more likely to develop resistance to the drug, limiting its long-term efficacy.[57] Still, for mild GERD symptoms, H2 blockers can be an effective treatment.

**Proton Pump Inhibitors.** Proton pump inhibitors (PPIs) (eg, omeprazole, lansoprazole, rabeprazole, pantoprazole, esomeprazole) inhibit stomach acid by preventing the secretion of protons (acid) from acid-producing cells of the stomach. Proton pump inhibitors have been found especially useful when GERD is not well controlled by H2 blockers.[58] They are the drug of choice for conventional GERD management.[59]

Acid suppression therapies can interfere with the absorption of nutrients that require stomach acid for proper digestion such as nonsupplemental iron,[60] vitamin B12,[61,62] and dietary calcium.[63]

Acid-suppression-related nutrient deficiencies carry their own health risks. Based on a study survey, the incidence of iron deficiency anemia secondary to chronic PPI usage has increased up to five-fold.[64] Elevated homocysteine (a risk factor for cardiovascular disease) has been associated with vitamin B12 deficiency induced by PPIs.[61] Chronic high-dose PPI or H2 blocker usage can more than double the risk of potentially deadly hip fracture[6,65] by impairing calcium absorption and bone metabolism. Impaired calcium absorption can also disrupt calcium balance and contribute to cardiac conduction problems. Individuals on long-term PPI therapy should monitor their iron and B12 status using convenient blood tests to identify possible drug-induced nutrient deficiencies. Homocysteine levels should be assessed as well. Long-term use of acid suppression therapy (drugs) may also be a risk factor for food allergies.[66] In one study, more than 27% of GERD patients tested positive for food allergies; avoiding allergenic foods resulted in significant improvement of GERD symptoms.[67]

One of the roles of stomach acid is to provide defense against ingested pathogens. Therefore, reductions in stomach acid due to PPI usage can lower resistance 2- to 4-fold to intestinal infections from *Salmonella*, *Campylobacter*, and *Clostridium difficile*.[68,69] Probiotics may prove a useful adjunct to PPI therapy. *Saccharomyces boulardii* (ie, probiotic yeast) was effective in reducing side effects associated with PPI usage in one study.[70] However, more investigation is needed, as a large 2012 study failed to link PPI therapy to small intestinal bacterial overgrowth.[71]

Another major problem with PPI drugs is that they are often taken for much longer periods than recommended, which could compound their potential for causing side effects. PPIs are approved for use for 14-day intervals, no more than three times yearly, but many patients take these drugs semi-permanently.[72,73] Use of PPIs for not more than 14 days at a time and not more than 3 times yearly may reduce the negative side effects of these drugs.

**Surgery.** The goal of antireflux surgery is the reconstruction of the LES mechanism. This is commonly performed by laparoscopic fundoplication, a minimally invasive technique in which a portion of the stomach (fundus) is wrapped (fully or partially) around the base of the esophagus and sutured into place. The lower portion of the esophagus passes through a small tunnel of stomach muscle,[38] thus reinforcing the closure of the LES. Additionally, as the stomach contracts, it constricts the lower esophagus (pinching it shut) instead of forcing acid into the esophagus. There are several surgical techniques for different applications. For example, patients prone to dysphagia (difficulty swallowing) may benefit more from a laparoscopic fundoplication that only partially wraps the esophagus.[74] In some cases, these surgeries can be performed as an outpatient procedure.[75]

## DIETARY AND LIFESTYLE APPROACHES TO GERD MANAGEMENT

Up to 50% of patients with GERD experience persistent symptoms, despite taking PPIs regularly.[76] Diet and lifestyle interventions are therefore an important adjunct to standard drug therapy. Education on managing stress, proper diet, physical activity, and understanding the causes and progression of GERD have shown to promote significant improvement in patient perception of their illness and well-being.[76]

Some diet and lifestyle modifications commonly suggested for GERD patients include:

**Avoid Foods and Beverages Associated with GERD Symptoms.** Several common dietary components have been associated with increases in GERD symptoms, including:

- Coffee[77]
- Chocolate[78]
- Spicy foods[79]
- Carbonated beverages[80]
- Alcohol[80,81]

Additional foods that may cause symptoms include tomatoes (cooked and raw), milk, cheese, citrus foods, cakes, and pastries.[76]

**Quit Smoking.** Smoking increases GERD symptoms by reducing (1) the ability of the LES to remain closed against increases in gastric pressure, and (2) the clearance of reflux from the esophagus.[82] The incidence of GERD increases with the duration of smoking. Based on data from a large population study, long-term (>20 years) daily smoking resulted in a 70% increase in the occurrence of reflux episodes compared to those who have smoked for >1 year.[83]

**Lose Weight.** Increased body mass and abdominal adiposity increases pressure on the stomach and lower esophagus. This can stress the lower esophageal valve, hampering its ability to maintain a seal against gastric reflux. Sustained abdominal pressure can also increase the risk of hiatal hernia.[84] Based on a survey of seven studies, overweight individuals averaged a 43% increase and obese individuals a 94% increase in GERD symptoms over individuals with a normal body mass.[85] Esophageal adenocarcinoma incidence was more frequent in overweight individuals in most of these studies.

**Monitor Meal Size and Macronutrient Composition.** Dietary fat delays gastric emptying, which may increase the probability of reflux in susceptible patients. High-fat meals are also associated with increased risk of esophageal cancer.[86] Whereas high-calorie, high-fat meals appear to elicit GERD,[87,88] reducing fat content in meals has had beneficial effects in some studies.[89,90] Low carbohydrate (>20 g) meals reduced some reflux symptoms in a small trial in obese subjects.[91] Aside from their direct effects on GERD, limitation of fat, carbohydrate, and total calorie intake are effective methods for weight reduction, which itself is an effective antireflux strategy. Weight reduction is also an effective way to positively impact many additional aspects of health and potentially enhance longevity. More information is available in the Caloric Restriction and Obesity and Weight Loss protocols.

**Avoid Eating Close to Bedtime.** GERD patients have long been advised to avoid eating close to bedtime in order to give the stomach adequate time to empty before lying down.[92] Clinical studies, however, have had mixed results regarding the minimization of GERD symptoms.[93-95]

**Elevate the Head of the Bed While Sleeping.** Several studies have suggested that raising the head of the bed 8–11 inches, or sleeping on a "wedge," can reduce the number and duration of reflux episodes.[82] This approach uses gravity to help keep stomach contents out of the esophagus. Left lateral recumbency (sleeping on one's left side) may also reduce GERD symptoms by potentially keeping the LES above the level of the stomach and reducing pressure on the valve.[82]

**Limit Aspirin and Other Nonsteroidal Antiinflammatory Drugs (NSAIDs).** Some evidence suggests that NSAID use is associated with GERD.[96] NSAIDs exert their anti-inflammatory activity by inhibiting the activity of proinflammatory cyclooxygenase (COX) enzymes. However, the COX-1 enzyme is also important for promoting the formation of the protective mucus lining of the stomach.

# TARGETED NUTRITIONAL INTERVENTIONS

**Raft-Forming Agents.** Raft-forming reflux suppressants have been used to treat GERD for more than 30 years.[97] Raft formers are combinations of a gel-forming fiber (eg, alginate or pectin) with an antacid buffer (commonly sodium or potassium bicarbonate). When the combination reaches the stomach, chemical reactions cause the release of carbon dioxide bubbles. These bubbles become trapped in the gelled fiber, converting it into a foam that floats on the surface of the stomach contents (hence "raft-forming" agent). Several studies have demonstrated that rafts reduce GERD symptoms by mechanisms independent of acid reduction. They can either move into the esophagus ahead of the stomach contents during reflux (protecting it from exposure) or may act as a barrier to reflux episodes.[98] A recent multicenter study of patients with mild to moderate GERD symptoms demonstrated that an alginate-based raft-forming agent was as effective as the PPI omeprazole at reaching an initial heartburn-free period and reducing reflux pain.[99]

The properties of raft-forming agents can be modified by adding calcium salts, which can cross-link fibers and form stiffer gels.[98] Raft formers are most effective when taken 30 minutes to 1 hour after a meal. If taken with a meal, they can mix with stomach contents and fail to form a "raft."[98]

**Melatonin.** Melatonin is a hormone most often associated with the sleep cycle, but is found at levels hundreds of times higher in the gut than in the brain.[100] Animal trials of melatonin for GERD symptoms have found it to be not only effective in preventing acid-induced esophageal damage, but also damage caused by digestive enzymes and bile.[101] Two human trials have investigated supplemental melatonin on GERD symptoms. In the first, 176 patients on a 6-mg melatonin/multinutrient combination were compared to 175 patients on a PPI (20 mg omeprazole). The effects were measured by the length of time it took for the patients to become asymptomatic (defined as no heartburn or regurgitation) for 24 hours. All patients in the melatonin group reported improvement in GERD symptoms compared to two-thirds in the PPI group. Relief was reached faster in the melatonin (7 days) versus PPI (9 days) group, with a much lower incidence of side effects.[102] A second study compared 3 groups of 9 GERD patients, each on a different regimen (3 mg melatonin, 20 mg omeprazole, or both) to a group of healthy control subjects. Heartburn and gastric pain were decreased after 4 weeks and completely resolved after 8 weeks in all treatment groups. However, only the two melatonin groups had significant improvements in LES function.[103]

**D-Limonene.** D-Limonene is a component of the essential oil of citrus fruits. In a small, unpublished study of 19 patients with GERD or chronic heartburn, 1000 mg d-limonene daily or every other day for 14 days led to the remission of symptoms in 89% of the patients. In a small follow-up investigation, 22 participants with GERD or chronic heartburn were randomized to receive 1000 mg d-limonene either once daily, every other day, or placebo. By day 4, 29% of participants on treatment experienced significant relief, which rose to 83% by day 14 compared to 30% on placebo. The mechanism of d-limonene activity in GERD is not clear; in vitro research suggests mucosal protection and increased peristalsis.[104]

**Deglycyrrhizinated Licorice (DGL).** Licorice extracts have been shown to support the health of the stomach lining and combat *H. pylori* bacteria that can cause ulcers.[105] This may convey benefits to those suffering from GERD, since recent evidence indicates that *H. pylori* eradication appears to improve GERD symptoms.[29] Unlike whole licorice, deglycyrrhizinated licorice (DGL) extracts provide beneficial licorice compounds without glycyrrhizin (a component of whole licorice that has been shown to cause side effects).

While published, peer-reviewed literature supporting the use of DGL in GERD is lacking, some innovative doctors employ DGL with positive results.[106]

## PROTECTING AGAINST BARRETT'S ESOPHAGUS AND ESOPHAGEAL CANCER

GERD increases the risk of metaplastic (ie, transformation of tissue) events that lead to Barrett's esophagus, which in turn significantly increases the risk of esophageal cancer. Therefore, the most effective way to reduce the risk of these two serious conditions is to control the symptoms of GERD. However, the following additional considerations may be beneficial as well.

Several observational studies have examined the effects of dietary patterns on the incidence of Barrett's esophagus or esophageal cancer (independently of GERD). Some foods and supplements appear to reduce cancer and metaplasia risk.

Total fruit and vegetable intake has been associated with reductions in the risk of esophageal adenocarcinoma in some studies.[107–109] It has been noted that risk reductions associated with citrus fruits as well as yellow, brassica, or raw vegetables were consistently positive.[107,110,111] Strawberries, due to their powerful antioxidants, have also piqued the interest of researchers looking for compounds able to protect esophageal tissue. In order to test the hypothesis that strawberries might protect against esophageal cancer, scientists administered freeze-dried strawberry powder to 75 patients with precancerous esophageal lesions for 6 months. At a dose of 60 g daily, freeze-dried strawberry powder improved the appearance of the esophageal tissue under microscopic examination. Moreover, several inflammatory markers were reduced, including a 63% reduction in cyclooxygenase-2 (COX-2) activity and a 62% reduction in NF-κB activity. The investigators remarked, "*Our present results indicate the potential of freeze-dried strawberry powder for preventing human esophageal cancer.*"[112]

Fiber from cereal or whole grain was generally associated with reduced risk of esophageal cancer.[107,108,113,114] On the other hand, increased consumption of animal protein, saturated fat, and dietary cholesterol consistently led to increased risk of esophageal cancer.[108,113]

Vitamins C and E, beta carotene,[113,115–117] and dietary folate[113,115,118] appear to confer a reduction in esophageal cancer risk in the majority of studies. Likewise, general supplement (ie, multivitamin) usage was associated with risk reduction in one population study.[119]

Several fruits and vegetables contain a powerful polyphenol (antioxidant) called ellagic acid. It exerts cellular protection in a variety of settings and is well documented in animal studies as an inhibitor of esophageal cancer as well as aiding in ulcer healing.[120,121]

Various other dietary constituents have been investigated in cell culture or animal models of esophageal cancer with positive results. These include sulforaphane (from broccoli),[122] vitamin E with N-acetyl cysteine,[123] proanthocyanidins (from apples), and cranberries. Betaine (trimethylglycine) intake was associated with a reduction in Barrett's esophagus in one study.[118]

## Life Extension Suggestions

The following ingredients may promote a healthy chemical environment within the esophagus:

- **Raft-forming alginate**: per label instructions
- **D-limonene**: 1000 mg daily, every other day for 20 days, 30 minutes before or 1 hour after meals
- **Melatonin**: 0.3–5 mg before bed (sometimes up to 10 mg)
- **Deglycyrrhizinated licorice (DGL)**: 760 mg as chewable tablets before each meal

The following ingredients may combat side effects of conventional treatments:

- **Probiotics**: per label instructions
- **Comprehensive multivitamin** (containing B-complex vitamins): per label instructions
- **Vitamin B12**: 1000–5000 mcg daily
- **Iron**: as needed per blood testing
- **Calcium**: 200–1200 mg daily
- **Magnesium:** 140 mg daily as magnesium-L-threonate; 320 mg daily as magnesium citrate

The following ingredients may promote healthy cellular division within the esophagus:

- **N-acetyl-cysteine (NAC)**: 600–1800 mg daily
- **Broccoli extract** (standardized to 4% glucosinolates): 400–800 mg daily
- **Apple extract** (standardized to 50% polyphenols): 600–2400 mg daily
- **Trimethylglycine** (TMG): 500–1000 mg daily

In addition, the following *blood tests* may provide helpful information:

- Vitamin B12 and Folate
- Ferritin
- Homocysteine
- *Helicobacter pylori* IgG ANTIBODIES
- Food Safe™ Allergy Test

## REFERENCES

References available at: www.lef.org/dpt5/ch62

# 63

# Gingivitis

Gingivitis is the most common and mild form of oral/dental disease. According to the Food and Drug Administration (FDA), approximately 15% of adults aged 21–50 years, and 30% of adults over 50 have gum disease.[1] Gingivitis is characterized by inflammation and bleeding of the gums. Because gingivitis is rarely painful in its early stages, it often goes unnoticed until severe irritation or receding gums occur.

The main cause of gingivitis is plaque (or biofilm), a soft, sticky film that forms on the teeth when starches and sugars react with bacteria that is naturally present in the mouth. Plaque buildup occurs between the teeth and gums, in faulty fillings, and near poorly cleaned partial dentures, bridges, and braces. If not removed within 72 hours, plaque will harden into tartar that cannot be removed by brushing or flossing.

The best defense against gingivitis is brushing and flossing after meals, as well as professional cleaning by a dental hygienist every 3–4 months.

If left untreated, gingivitis may lead to a more serious condition called periodontitis, in which the inner gum and bone pull away from teeth and form pockets. These pockets can collect bacteria and debris, and become infected or abscessed. Bacterial toxins eventually break down the underlying bone and connective tissue that hold teeth in place. The ultimate outcome is tooth loss. For more information, see Life Extension's Periodontitis and Cavities protocol.

## RISK FACTORS FOR GINGIVITIS

Several studies suggest that gum disease may be passed from parents to children as well as between couples.[2,3] Based on these findings, the American Academy of Periodontology (AAP) recommends that treatment of gum disease may involve entire families and that if one family member has periodontal disease, all family members should see a dental professional for a periodontal disease screening.

Other conditions that may contribute to gingivitis include the following.

## Medications

Certain prescription and over-the-counter drugs can create a favorable environment for plaque buildup. Cold remedies and tricyclic antidepressant drugs decrease salivation, which allows plaque and tartar to form more easily.[4] Oral contraceptives can increase microbial flora that contribute to gingivitis.[5]

Other drugs—particularly antiseizure medications such as phenytoin (Dilantin®), calcium channel blockers, antihypertension drugs, and medications that suppress the immune system—can sometimes cause an overgrowth of gum tissue.[6,7] This condition, called gingival hyperplasia, can make plaque much more difficult to remove and provide more surface for bacteria to develop.

## Infections

Viral and fungal infections can also adversely affect gum health. The herpes virus, for example, can lead to acute herpetic gingivostomatitis, a condition characterized by swollen gums and small, painful sores in the mouth.[8] Oral thrush is caused by overgrowth of the yeast known as *Candida albicans* that is normally found in the mouth. Thrush can produce white lesions on the inner cheeks and tongue that can spread to the gums.

## Disease

Certain health conditions that may not be directly associated with the mouth can affect gum health. For example, leukemia patients may develop gingivitis if leukemia cells invade the gum tissue.[8] Fanconi anemia is a rare genetic disorder that attacks bone marrow and reduces white blood cell production, leaving the patient predisposed to infections and more susceptible to gum disease.[9]

## Hormonal Changes

During periods of hormonal fluctuation (eg, pregnancy and menopause), women may become more susceptible to gingivitis due to decreased salivation and blood supply to the gums. It is also thought that increased hormone levels cause the gums to respond aggressively to bacteria-producing irritation. However, while it is clear that hormone levels play a role in the progression of periodontal disease, hormones do not specifically cause gingivitis.[10] Of particular importance to women is that several recent studies indicate that pregnant women with periodontal disease may be more likely to deliver a pre-term, low-birth-weight infant.[11]

## Poor Nutrition

A diet lacking in adequate amounts of calcium, vitamin C, and B vitamins can increase the risk of developing periodontal disease.[8,12,13]

## Smoking

Tobacco use may be one of the largest preventable risk factors for periodontal disease. According to one study, smoking may be responsible for more than half of adult cases of periodontal disease in the United States. The same study also found that smokers are 4 times more likely to develop advanced periodontal disease than people who have never smoked.[14] Smoking diminishes oxygen and nutrient delivery to gum tissue and interferes with the synthesis of cytokines that regulate immunity and inflammation. Smoking also poses a risk of periodontal therapy failure, treatment complications, and increased time to treat the disease.[15]

## Stress and Depression

Stress has been linked to an increased risk of periodontal disease, possibly because it may trigger an increase in behaviors such as smoking and poor oral hygiene. Sustained levels of financial stress and poor coping abilities, which can trigger habits such as poor diet or smoking, double the risk of developing periodontal disease.[16] Researchers have also found that clinically depressed patients are only half as likely to benefit from periodontal treatment as nondepressed patients.[17]

# GINGIVITIS AND HEART DISEASE

There is a clear association between gum disease and heart disease. A 2004 study found that 91% of patients with cardiovascular disease also suffered from moderate to severe periodontal disease.[18] While people with gum disease have a 25% greater risk of heart disease than those with healthy gums, researchers have only recently begun to uncover possible causes for this link. Researchers now believe that gum disease, which is inflammatory, causes the release of proinflammatory chemicals into the bloodstream, which triggers a systemic inflammatory response. Atherosclerosis is also an inflammatory disease, and many of the same factors that increase risk for heart disease also increase risk for gum disease, including C-reactive protein (CRP), fibrinogen, and cholesterol.[19]

This theory was supported by a recent study involving 5000 participants, which showed that oral inflammatory markers entering the bloodstream encouraged systemic inflammation.[20] This large study also confirmed that periodontal disease and body mass index are jointly associated with increased levels of CRP in assessing the risk of heart disease.

# CONVENTIONAL TREATMENT

Treatment of gum disease begins with regular brushing and flossing. It is also important to make regular trips to the dentist for cleaning and monitoring. Most dentists recommend yearly full-mouth x-rays to assess the progression of bone loss in the jaws. Life Extension, however, has long been concerned about the radiation exposure that results from undergoing medical x-rays. Even x-rays that emit low levels of radiation damage DNA, which can lead to cancer. While some dental x-rays are necessary, annual x-rays are not advisable.

A full periodontal probe with a tiny, ruler-like instrument is also performed to measure the pockets surrounding the teeth. In healthy gums, the pockets measure less than 3 millimeters (one-eighth of an inch). Pockets measuring 3–5 millimeters indicate signs of gingivitis. Pockets measuring more than 5 millimeters signify the development of periodontitis. For more information, see Life Extension's Periodontitis and Cavities protocol.

A professional cleaning to remove plaque and tartar buildup should be performed at least twice a year. Some people need to have cleanings done more frequently. Nonsurgical deep cleaning involves two procedures known as scaling and root planing, which are sometimes performed in sections of the mouth at different times, especially if there is considerable soreness and bleeding from the gums. Scaling removes plaque and tartar above and below the gum line. Root planing smoothes out the tooth root to remove bacteria buildup and encourage the gums to reattach to the teeth.

## Mouth Rinses

Mouth rinses are frequently used to help prevent gingivitis. Medicated mouth rinses containing a 0.1% solution of folic acid have effectively reduced gum inflammation and bleeding in double-blind trials.[21,22] Prescription antibacterial mouthwashes containing the ingredient chlorhexidine (Peridex®, PerioGard®) are also frequently used to treat gum inflammation.

## Decapinol®

Decapinol®, a prescription oral rinse, reduces the adherence of bacterial plaque to oral surfaces. This reduces the formation of new plaque as well as breaks up existing plaque, making it easier to remove with normal brushing. Reducing the presence of plaque also reduces the amount of bacterial toxins released into the gums. The result is a reduction in plaque and gingivitis. Decapinol® is only mildly antibacterial, so it does not upset the oral bacterial flora.

## Toothpaste

The natural and synthetic antibacterial agents in many brands of toothpaste can help keep gums healthy. Natural toothpastes contain botanical oils that have antibacterial properties, while commercial formulas offer the benefit of fluoride to help prevent cavities. The brand Colgate Total®—the only FDA-approved toothpaste for fighting gingivitis—contains triclosan, a mild antimicrobial proven to reduce plaque and pocket depths associated with gingivitis.[23,24]

## Antibiotic Therapy

Antibiotic therapy used alone or in combination with other treatments may also be recommended to treat gingivitis. Atridox® (doxycycline hyclate), PerioChip® (chlorhexidine gluconate), and Arestin® (minocycline hydrochloride) are antibiotics applied in sustained-release doses directly into the periodontal pocket. A relatively new drug called Periostat® (doxycycline hyclate) was approved by the FDA in 1998 for use in combination with scaling and root planing. Taken orally, Periostat® suppresses the action of collagenase, an enzyme that causes destruction of the teeth and gums.[25,26]

## Surgery

If a diligent regimen of proper brushing, flossing, and regular dental cleanings is followed, nearly all cases of gingivitis can be reversed in a short time. However, in advanced gingivitis, or conditions that make treatment difficult, the following surgical treatments can help.

**Curettage.**   A procedure in which diseased gum tissue in the infected pocket is scraped away, allowing the infected area to heal.

**Flap surgery.**   Involves pulling back the gums to remove tartar buildup. The gums are then sewn back in place so that the tissue fits snugly around the tooth, thereby reducing pocket depth.

**Guided tissue regeneration.**   Stimulates bone and gum tissue growth, and is often performed in combination with flap surgery. In this procedure, a small piece of mesh-like fabric is inserted between the bone and gum tissue. This keeps the gum tissue from growing into the area where the bone should be, allowing the bone and connective tissue to reattach.

**Soft tissue grafts.**   Reinforces thin gums or replace tissue where the gums have receded. The grafted tissue, usually taken from the roof of the mouth, is sewn in place over the affected area.

## Hydrogen Peroxide

Hydrogen peroxide, which is included in many toothpastes, is valuable for its ability to reach bacteria hiding among gingival folds and gaps. Hydrogen peroxide is also added to some mouthwashes to reduce gingivitis and whiten teeth.[27] Hydrogen peroxide has been used effectively for years in dentistry.

# NUTRITIONAL APPROACHES FOR HEALTHY GUMS

In addition to brushing with a good toothpaste and making regular visits to the dentist, a number of nutrients have been shown to improve gum health.

## Coenzyme Q10

Coenzyme Q10 (CoQ10), a vital nutrient needed by every cell in the body to make energy, is beneficial for a variety of diseases and disorders, including periodontal disease. In addition to energy production, CoQ10 plays a vital role as an antioxidant at the cellular level by neutralizing free radicals. As early as the 1970s, researchers found that gum tissue in people with periodontal disease was often deficient in CoQ10.[28,29] Subsequent studies have shown that CoQ10 doses of 50–75 mg daily can halt deterioration of the gums and allow healing to occur, sometimes within days of starting therapy. In one double-blind trial, 50 mg daily of CoQ10 was significantly more effective than placebo in reducing symptoms of gingivitis after 3 weeks of treatment.[30]

Stephen T. Sinatra, clinical cardiologist and author, reports that many of his patients see improvement in their gum health after beginning CoQ10 supplementation for heart disease. According to research by Sinatra, CoQ10's supportive effects on the immune system in general account for its ability to promote healing of diseased gums. Victor Zeines, a holistic dentist and author, recommends 100 mg of CoQ10 daily in combination with other supplements to help reverse gum disease naturally.

## Calcium

A study found that people who do not consume adequate amounts of calcium each day are at significantly higher risk for periodontal disease.[13] According to the American Dietetic Association, 3 of 4 people do not fulfill their daily calcium requirement. The study showed that men and women who had low calcium intakes (below the recommended dietary allowance) were almost twice as likely to have periodontal disease, as measured by the loss of attachment of the gums to the teeth.

## Vitamin D

According to a recent report from the *American Journal of Clinical Nutrition*, high blood levels of a vitamin D metabolite are associated with a decreased risk of gingivitis. Researchers at Boston University analyzed data from 6700 nonsmokers, aged 13–90+, from the National Health and Nutrition Examination Survey. The investigators analyzed blood levels of 25-hydroxyvitamin D and assessed the participants' gums for the presence of gingivitis. Participants with the highest blood levels of 25-hydroxyvitamin D were the least likely to display signs of gingivitis. The scientists noted that vitamin D may reduce susceptibility to gingivitis by exerting anti-inflammatory effects, and postulated that gingivitis may provide a useful clinical model for further investigation into the anti-inflammatory effects of vitamin D.[31]

## Folic Acid

Studies have demonstrated that folic acid is very effective in preserving gum tissue and reducing the risk of gingivitis and periodontitis.[32] Although the benefits of oral folic acid in protecting against heart disease and birth defects are well documented, new evidence suggests that using folic acid topically (as a mouthwash) can also strengthen one's oral defenses. Studies have demonstrated folic acid's ability to improve gingivitis symptoms, reduce gum tissue's inflammatory response, and make gum tissue more resilient to irritants such as bacteria and plaque.[21,33]

Folic acid has been clinically tested in mouthwash solutions to assess its benefit in treating gingivitis. One study showed significant improvement after 4 weeks of using a folic acid mouthwash. In this double-blind, placebo-controlled study of 60 patients, dietary folic acid intake did not correlate with treatment results, suggesting the importance of applying folic acid topically to the gums.[21]

A double-blind study of 30 pregnant women evaluated the effects of folic acid mouthwash and folic acid tablets versus placebo. After 28 days, folate serum levels increased significantly in both groups receiving folic acid, but only the group receiving folic acid mouthwash showed a highly significant improvement in a gingival index.[33]

Another study evaluated 30 patients with normal blood folate levels in a clinical setting. One group rinsed their mouths daily with a folate solution, and the other used a placebo mouth rinse. After 60 days, the group receiving the folic acid rinse showed significant improvement in gingival health compared to the placebo group.[34]

A double-blind study of 30 patients compared supplementation with 4000 mcg of ingested folic acid to placebo. After 1 month, plaque and gingival indices showed that folic acid supplementation appeared to increase the resistance of the gingiva to local irritants, leading to a reduction in inflammation.[35]

## Green Tea

Green tea extract is rich in a class of antioxidants called catechins. Two in particular, epigallocatechin gallate (EGCG) and epicatechin gallate (ECG), combat oral plaque and bacteria.[36–38] These green tea polyphenols work as antiplaque agents by suppressing glucosyl transferase, which oral bacteria use to feed on sugar. Other research has demonstrated that green tea extract can kill oral bacteria and inhibit collagenase activity. Collagenase, a natural enzyme that becomes overactive in the presence of bacterial overgrowth, can destroy healthy collagen in gum tissue.

Green tea extract applied topically inhibits *Streptococcus mutans* (S. mutans) bacteria, which have been implicated in the development of dental caries (the decay and breakdown of teeth and their bone support). Scientists suggested that certain extracts from green tea might be especially helpful in preventing tooth decay by preventing the development of bacterial plaque.[39] In a Chinese study, green tea extract was used to rinse and brush the teeth. The study demonstrated that S. mutans could be inhibited completely after contact with green tea extract for 5 minutes. There was no drug resistance after repeat cultures.[40] The scientists concluded that green tea extract is effective in preventing dental caries.[40] Other studies have shown that the plaque index and gingival index decreased significantly after green tea extract was used.[41]

More recent studies confirm the benefits of green tea in fighting gum disease, especially when combined with conventional treatments. In a pilot study, hydroxypropyl cellulose strips containing green tea catechins as a slow-release local delivery system were applied once a week for 8 weeks to the pockets in periodontal patients. The green tea catechins inhibited the bacteria *P. gingivalis* and *Prevotella spp.*, and a reduction in pocket depth was observed.[42]

## Hyperimmune Egg Extract

Agricultural scientists discovered long ago that they could immunize hens against germs that threaten humans. This immunity was then passed on by the hen to her egg.[43–45] Scientists have now been able to customize eggs to provide different types of immunity. At least 24 different organisms have been used to immunize a single hen, which then lays eggs that offer passive immunity to all of the organisms.[44]

Hyperimmune egg extract has been shown to reduce the volume of dental plaque, which in turn cuts down on the total load of inflammation in the mouth.[46] Animals supplemented with hyperimmune egg against the leading bacterial cause of dental caries developed significantly lower dental caries scores than did control animals.[47,48] Oral hyperimmune egg rinses have also been used successfully in humans to reduce disease-causing bacteria; the extracts remain active and present in the mouth at least overnight, offering long-standing protection.[49–51]

## Pomegranate

Researchers are finding important applications for pomegranate in the field of dental health. Clinical studies have shown that this popular antioxidant attacks the causes of tooth decay at the biochemical level with remarkable vigor.[52–56] Pomegranate literally attacks bacteria where they live. Research shows that by interfering with production of the chemicals the bacteria use as "glue," pomegranate extract suppresses bacteria's ability to adhere to the surface of the tooth.[57,58]

A study conducted in 2007 examined the effects of a mouthwash containing pomegranate extract on the risk of gingivitis.[59] Investigators noted that pomegranate's active components, including polyphenolic flavonoids (eg, punicalagins and ellagic acid), are believed to prevent gingivitis through a number of mechanisms including reduction of oxidative stress in the oral cavity, direct antioxidant activity,[60–62] anti-inflammatory effects, antibacterial activity,[63,64] and direct removal of plaque from the teeth.[54] Saliva samples were evaluated for a variety of indicators related to gingivitis and periodontitis. Subjects rinsing with pomegranate solution experienced a reduction in saliva total protein content,[59] which is normally higher among people with gingivitis,[65] and may correlate with plaque-forming bacterial content.[66]

## Xylitol

Pure xylitol is a white crystalline substance that resembles and tastes like sugar. It is found naturally in fruits such as plums, strawberries, and raspberries. Xylitol is used commercially to sweeten sugarless gum and candies.

Xylitol has been shown to inhibit the formation of plaque. In a double-blind and controlled study, Swedish researchers had 128 children chew gum containing either xylitol or the sweeteners sorbitol and maltitol, 3 times daily for 4 weeks. While both were effective against the buildup of dental plaque, only the xylitol-sweetened gum eliminated microbes found in saliva, particularly a strain of bacteria implicated in tooth decay.[67] Xylitol could thus be an essential ingredient in a targeted strategy to avert dental disease.

A double-blind, placebo-controlled study of 2630 children compared a standard fluoride toothpaste with one containing 10% xylitol. Over a 3-year period, children given the xylitol-enriched toothpaste developed notably fewer cavities than those using the fluoride-only toothpaste.[68]

## Probiotics

Probiotics have been defined as "living microorganisms which upon ingestion in certain numbers exert health benefits beyond inherent general nutrition."[69] Scientists have been interested in the makeup of the microbes that live in the mouth (the "oral flora") for decades, seeking to identify factors that promote the growth of healthy organisms and reduce the growth of those implicated in disease and inflammation.[70–73]

Probiotics not only improve oral health but can help change the stubborn composition of dental biofilm and plaque.[74,75] Reducing the total amount of plaque through teeth brushing is always a desirable goal; however, its complete elimination is not possible. Therefore, changing the actual composition of plaque from an inflammatory cytokine-rich environment to a more benign environment (dominated by neutral or even helpful organisms) can contribute to overall systemic health.[76–78]

In laboratory studies, the probiotic *Streptococcus salivarius* (*S. salivarius*) helped inhibit the formation of the sticky biofilm that can contribute to oral disease.[79] Building on these results, an animal study showed that the *S. salivarius* probiotic helped displace biofilm from the teeth, displacing cavity-causing bacteria and inhibiting tooth decay.[80] Another in vitro experiment demonstrated how effectively a second oral probiotic protects oral health.[81] In this experiment, a form of *Bacillus coagulans* (known as GanedenBC30®) was shown to competitively inhibit the cariogenic (cavity-inducing) bacterium *S. mutans*, which contributes to significant tooth decay.

## Lactoferrin

Lactoferrin, a naturally occurring antimicrobial agent, is found in saliva and gingival fluid, breast milk, tears, and other bodily fluids.

This protein is a well-known immune system booster involved in the body's responses to infection, trauma, and injury.[82]

Lactoferrin may bind to and slow the growth of periodontitis-associated bacteria.[83] In an animal study, locally applied lactoferrin powder appeared to support the healing of oral lesions.[84]

## Vitamin C

People deficient in vitamin C may be at risk of developing gingivitis.[85] In one study, a group of subjects with periodontal disease who normally consumed only 25–30 mg of vitamin C daily were supplemented with an additional 70 mg. They experienced marked improvement in gum tissue after only 6 weeks.[86] Although it is established that smoking contributes to gum disease, tobacco users may especially benefit from vitamin C supplementation, as smoking depletes the body of vitamin C.[12]

## Herbal Protection

Tea tree oil, used as an oral rinse, has been proven to kill bacteria.[87] In fact, research has shown that a tea tree oil concentration of 0.6% inhibited 14 of 15 oral types of bacteria. In one study, 49 subjects aged 18–60 with severe, chronic gingivitis were divided into groups, one of which was given a gel containing tea tree oil to apply with a toothbrush twice daily. The tea tree oil group had improved gingival index and papillary bleeding index scores attributed to the herb's anti-inflammatory properties.[88]

Camu-camu, a shrub from the Amazon rainforest, is revered for its rich supply of vitamin C, which aids in circulation, fortifying blood vessel walls, and regenerating tissue. Moreover, camu-camu has astringent, antioxidant, and anti-inflammatory properties.[89,90]

Both gotu kola and vitamin E help to heal wounds, promote connective tissue growth, and fight free radicals. Goldenseal is a medicinal plant that boosts immune function.[91]

Chamomile and red thyme oil are mild antimicrobials.[92] Finally, herbs such as parsley, spearmint, menthol, and eucalyptus are stimulating to the gums, as well as refreshing and cooling for the mouth in general.[93]

## Reducing Gum-Related Inflammation

**Fish oil and borage oil.** Because of the association between gum disease and systemic inflammation, researchers have begun looking at anti-inflammatory nutrients in the context of gum disease. In one study, 30 adults with gum disease were given a variety of polyunsaturated fatty acids, including omega-3 fatty acids from fish oil (up to 3000 mg daily) and omega-6 fatty acids from borage oil (up to 3000 mg daily). At the end of the study, clinically significant improvements were measured in both gingival inflammation and the depth of gum pockets.[94] Another preliminary human study found that omega-3 fatty acids tended to reduce inflammation, but called for more thorough research.[95] However, in light of the established connection between omega-3 and omega-6 fatty acids and inflammation, as well as fatty acids' lack of side effects, it is reasonable for people with gum disease to consider using these supplements. Other anti-inflammatory supplements include ginger and curcumin, though

neither of these has been studied in the context of inflammatory gum disease.

## Life Extension Suggestions

Healthy teeth and gums depend on regular brushing and flossing, as well as trips to a dentist every 3–4 months for cleaning and monitoring. It is also important to make lifestyle changes to protect your gums, including:

- Stopping smoking
- Consuming a diet low in fat and high in fresh fruit and vegetables
- Reducing intake of sugar, which reacts with bacteria to form plaque

Your choice of toothpaste is important. Today, the market is flooded with very strong toothpastes that contain whitening agents (usually hydrogen peroxide or carbamide peroxide). A toothpaste is now available that has been fortified with coenzyme Q10, folic acid, xylitol, green tea, lactoferrin, and other nutrients that are directly delivered to the gums every time one brushes. This novel toothpaste also contains a mild solution of 0.2% hydrogen peroxide.

A mouthwash containing tea tree oil, peppermint, eucalyptus, and other soothing nutrients may also be helpful. In addition, a mouth spray containing CoQ10, vitamin E, camu-camu, hydrogen peroxide, xylitol, peelu, tea tree oil, vitamin K1, gotu kola extract, propolis extract, and many other herbal ingredients may be very beneficial. The suggested daily usage is to spray this along the gum lines and swish it through the mouth and teeth several times.

In addition, a number of nutrients have been shown to improve the health of the gums, including:

- **Coenzyme Q10:** 100 mg daily
- **Calcium:** 200–1200 mg daily
- **Folic acid:** 800 mcg daily, taken with 300 mcg of vitamin B12 daily to prevent a vitamin B12 deficiency
- **Green tea extract**, standardized to 98% polyphenols: 725–1450 mg daily
- **Vitamin C:** 2–4 g daily (taken as 500 mg every few hours)
- **B-complex vitamins:**
  - Thiamine (B1): 100 mg
  - Riboflavin (B2): 50 mg
  - Niacin: 200 mg
  - Vitamin B6: 75 mg

- Folate, preferably as L-methylfolate: 800 mcg
- Vitamin B12: 1000 mcg
- Biotin: 600 mcg
- Pantothenic acid: 1000 mg
- Choline: 45 mg
- Inositol: 250 mg
- Para-aminobenzoic acid (PABA): 100 mg
- **Fish oil,** with olive polyphenols and sesame lignans: providing 1400 mg EPA and 1000 mg DHA daily
- **Omega-6 fatty acids:** up to 3000 mg daily of GLA
- **Vitamin D:** 5000–10 000 IU daily
- **Hyperimmune egg extract:** 3–6 tablets chewed daily on an empty stomach
- **Probiotic lozenge**, containing GanedenBC30® (*Bacillus coagulans*) and *Streptococcus salivarius* K12: per label instructions
- **Mouthwash** including ingredients such as pomegranate, green tea, and xylitol

- **Toothpaste** containing hydrogen peroxide, CoQ10, green tea, xylitol, lactoferrin, and folic acid
- **Mouth spray** with ingredients such as tea tree oil, camu-camu, gotu kola, goldenseal, chamomile, thyme, parsley, spearmint, menthol, and eucalyptus

The following *blood test* may provide helpful information:

- **Vitamin D, 25-Hydroxy**

## REFERENCES

References available at: www.lef.org/dpt5/ch63

# 64

# Glaucoma

Glaucoma is the second leading cause of irreversible blindness worldwide. The disease affects about 5 million Americans, mostly over age 40. Distressingly, many of these individuals are unaware of their affliction until long after the optic nerve has already been permanently damaged.

The term "glaucoma" refers to a group of similar conditions that damage the retina and optic nerve, leading to visual impairment. Glaucoma is sometimes called a "silent thief" because it slowly robs its victims of peripheral vision, which can go unnoticed until the loss becomes significant enough to interfere with everyday life.

Although glaucoma-related vision loss is not reversible, the progression of the disease can nearly always be slowed or halted. When diagnosed and treated early, it seldom leads to blindness.

Prescription medications and surgery can control the clinical manifestations, but the most commonly prescribed drugs carry unpleasant side effects, while there are risks associated with surgery.

Fortunately, recent scientific studies have illuminated *natural* strategies to help attenuate the progression of glaucoma. Investigations have shown that a combination of plant-based interventions derived from *French maritime pine bark* and *bilberry* target one of the most common underlying problems with glaucoma: increased pressure in the front of the eye, a condition known as elevated *intraocular pressure* (IOP).

Human studies reveal that these natural compounds complement conventional glaucoma medications as well, acting synergistically to optimize intraocular pressure.[1]

Moreover, conventional therapies do little to address a major contributor to visual impairment in glaucoma—*mitochondrial dysfunction*.[2,3] *Coenzyme Q10* and *pyrroloquinoline quinone* (PQQ) are two powerful mitochondrial protectants that may play a considerable, yet unappreciated role in maintaining visual acuity for glaucoma patients.

After reading this Life Extension protocol, you will understand how glaucoma emerges and discover that making lifestyle changes to control risk factors can lessen the risk of glaucoma development and progression. You also will learn about exciting findings related to a number of natural compounds with the ability to target multiple mechanisms underlying the progression of glaucoma.

## STRUCTURES OF THE EYE

### Back of the Eye

The eye is a spherical structure. It is connected at its rear pole to the brain via the *optic nerve*. The optic nerve is a fibrous tube containing over one million horizontally running nerve fibers (axons), each one originating from a type of retinal cell called a *ganglion cell*. The retina and optic nerve are pictured in Figure 1.

The *retina* is composed of a thin sheet of cells (and related structures) that form the back wall of the eye. Its primary role is to capture light and transform it into electrical signals. The signals are transmitted to the brain by the optic nerve, where they are interpreted as the objects we "see."

*Ganglion cell* axons are responsible for transmitting these electrical signals. The axons spread out across the retina to converge at the *optic disc*, the point of origin of the optic nerve. The optic disc is where damage from glaucoma is typically detected by an eye exam.

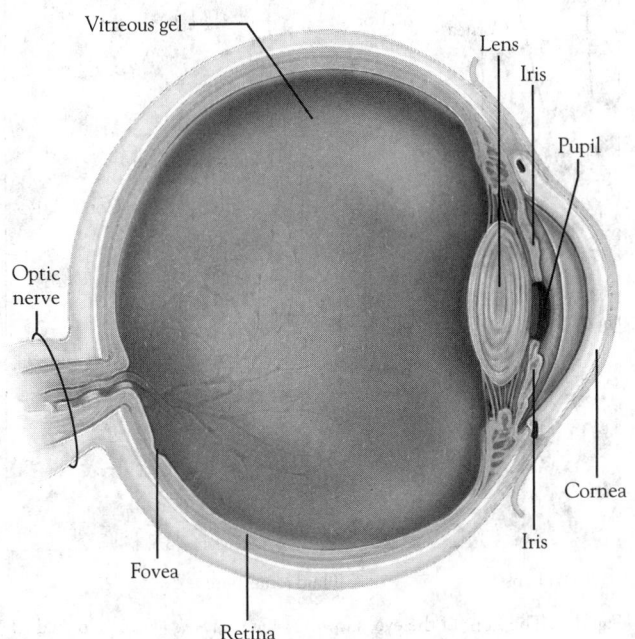

Figure 1. Structures of the eye

## Front of the Eye

When we look at our eyes in the mirror, we see four main features of the front of the eyeball: the white *sclera*, the black *pupil*, the colored *iris*, and the dome-shaped *cornea* overlaying the iris and pupil. In most cases of glaucoma, the trouble lies immediately behind the cornea in the outflow of a fluid called *aqueous humor* (or aqueous fluid). Normally, aqueous humor flows from behind the iris (posterior chamber), where it is formed, to the front of the iris (anterior chamber) where it drains through the *trabecular meshwork* into *Schlemm's canal* and ultimately into the blood circulation (Figure 2). Aqueous humor should not be confused with tears, which are formed outside the eye.

## TYPES OF GLAUCOMA

There are two major forms of glaucoma: *open-angle glaucoma* and *angle-closure glaucoma*. About 90% of cases of glaucoma are primary open-angle glaucoma (POAG). The majority of others are angle-closure glaucoma.

Less common forms of glaucoma include congenital glaucoma, which tends to run in families and is present at birth, normal tension glaucoma, pigmentary glaucoma, pseudoexfoliative glaucoma, traumatic

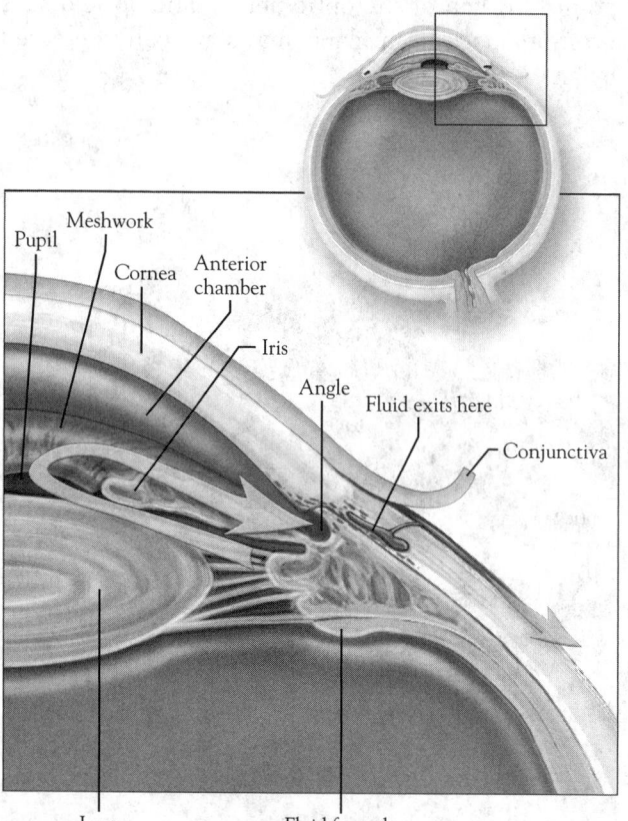

Figure 2. The front of the eye, showing where *aqueous humor* is formed behind the iris. The fluid travels to the anterior chamber and out through the trabecular meshwork and Schlemm's canal.

glaucoma, neovascular glaucoma, and iridocorneal endothelial syndrome.

In the last several years, glaucoma has come to be described as a "neurodegenerative disease" because it shares features with several brain disorders including Alzheimer's disease, amyotrophic lateral sclerosis (Lou Gehrig's disease), and Parkinson's disease.[4]

## SIGNS AND SYMPTOMS OF GLAUCOMA

Signs and symptoms of glaucoma differ depending upon the type of glaucoma. Most patients do not have any symptoms in the disease's early stages. Others may experience severe pain and rapidly compromised vision. Even without symptoms, people with glaucoma are vulnerable to a loss of peripheral vision, followed by reductions in central vision and blindness. (Symptoms should always be reported to the examining ophthalmologist or optometrist.)

- Most people with open-angle glaucoma have no symptoms until they notice a loss of peripheral vision. The vision loss can be slowly progressive, leading to tunnel vision and finally blindness.

- Closed-angle glaucoma is an acute condition (meaning it comes on quickly with a rapid rise in IOP) and is often associated with severe eye pain. Angle-closure glaucoma is a medical emergency and must be treated quickly to prevent vision loss. Symptoms may include extreme eye pain, headaches, blurred vision, red eyes, halos around lights, tender and firm eyes, and nausea and vomiting. An eye exam usually shows a shallow anterior chamber and mildly dilated pupils, sometimes drug related.

- Congenital glaucoma can be marked by excess tearing of the eyes (usually associated with a malformed tear duct drainage system), iris abnormalities, extreme sensitivity to light, and a large and hazy cornea.

## RISK FACTORS FOR GLAUCOMA

There are many risk factors for glaucoma, ranging from factors you cannot control (genetic abnormalities and age) to lifestyle factors. Some of the known risk factors for glaucoma include:

- **Intraocular pressure.** Normal intraocular pressure is between 10 millimeters mercury (mmHG) and 20 mmHg. Higher-than-normal IOP is perhaps the most significant risk factor for glaucoma. It is important to distinguish between *intraocular pressure* and *blood pressure*—they are not synonymous.

Intraocular pressure refers to the pressure caused by the aqueous humor secreted by the ciliary body, while blood pressure refers to the pressure exerted by the blood on the blood vessel (artery) wall.

- **Age.** People older than 60 are more likely to develop glaucoma. For some ethnic groups, risk begins at an earlier age.

- **Ethnicity.** African Americans have the highest risk for glaucoma in the United States (12%). Among Asian Americans and U.S. Hispanics, the glaucoma risk is 6.5%.[5]

- **Medical Conditions.** Glaucoma is especially closely related to diabetes and high blood pressure. In a 2011 study, researchers examined medical records of over 2 million people older than 40 who were enrolled in a U.S. managed care network. The records revealed a 35% increased risk in people with diabetes of developing open-angle glaucoma and a 17% increased risk in those with hypertension. Both conditions together raised the risk to 48%.[6]

  An association has also been drawn between thyroid disease and glaucoma, according to a study of 12 376 participants from the Centers for Disease Control and Prevention's 2002 National Health Interview Survey. Researchers found that the prevalence of glaucoma was almost double in people with thyroid problems versus those without thyroid problems.[7]

- **Other Eye Conditions.** Based on a study of 2650 patients where 579 patients (21.84%) had secondary glaucoma, eye-related causes, in order of frequency, were postvitrectomy surgery, eye trauma, corneal pathology, aphakia, neovascular glaucoma, pseudophakia, and uveitis. There were also cases secondary to tumor, myopia, pseudoexfoliation syndrome, retinopathy of prematurity, aniridia, iridocorneal endothelial syndrome, and chemical injury to the eye.[8]

- **Corticosteroids.** Glaucoma risk is raised by prolonged use of corticosteroids, including corticosteroid-containing eye drops for reducing eye inflammation and inhalers for treating asthma.

- **Physical Activity.** Research suggests an association between low levels of physical activity and low ocular perfusion pressure (OPP), a risk factor for glaucoma. OPP is a calculation derived from intraocular pressure (IOP) and blood pressure.[9]

Having a *family history* of glaucoma is a well-established risk factor, and the role of *genetics* in glaucoma continues to receive scientific scrutiny. In the late 1990s, researchers began identifying glaucoma gene mutations, including several in a gene that encodes for the protein TIGR found in the trabecular meshwork. They discovered the mutations by studying families with POAG. The mutation occurred in 4.4% of these patients, compared to 0.3% of the general population.[10]

Since then, several other genes (eg, *MYOC, OPTN*) have been associated with POAG. Among the most recently noted is *ADAMTS10*, which was discovered in a unique population of beagles with glaucoma.[11]

Another gene linked to glaucoma is *CYP1B1*. In some populations, *CYP1B1* mutations are found in over half of all cases of congenital glaucoma.[12]

Researchers expect to find many more genes and other events involved in the initiation and progression of glaucoma. An important aspect will be to identify people with genetic and other risk factors and to counsel them about ways to reduce the likelihood of developing glaucoma.

Lastly, other drugs besides steroids can raise the risk of glaucoma, especially of angle-closure glaucoma. Categories of drugs known as anticholinergics and adrenergics are the most common. Sulfa drugs, antihistamines, and decongestants can also cause problems. And several anticancer drugs can increase the risk of open-angle glaucoma. Because the cause of the glaucoma is linked to the particular drug usage, the first line of treatment is to discontinue the drug.

**Note:** *If you have glaucoma, make sure to inform your health care provider and pharmacist. They should know what drugs to avoid.*

## PATHOPHYSIOLOGY OF GLAUCOMA

In the past, doctors thought of glaucoma as a disease with only one major feature: increased intraocular pressure (IOP), or essentially raised pressure in the eye. Although we now know that glaucoma can occur even in people with normal IOP, this is still the most common underlying symptom of the disease. In the most common form of glaucoma—open-angle glaucoma—IOP can be subtly raised long before symptoms become discernible to the patient. This provides a critical window of time during which aggressive measures can be taken to reduce IOP and head off symptoms before they develop; hence the importance of regular eye check-ups, even if you do not have any symptoms. Once symptoms manifest and glaucoma is detected, it is important to take immediate and aggressive action to protect your eyesight.

Elevated IOP is caused by abnormal drainage of aqueous humor from the front chamber of the eye. In a healthy eye, fluid from the front chamber drains into a region known as the trabecular meshwork through an acute angle formed by the intersection of the cornea and iris. If the fluid cannot drain through this angle, it backs up into the eye itself, causing elevated IOP. There are two main reasons for a blockage at this angle: either the angle remains open and the fluid has complete access to the trabecular meshwork but for some reason its outflow is impeded (open-angle glaucoma), or there is a physical barrier in the angle, sometimes caused by deformity in the iris, that causes reduced flow (closed-angle glaucoma).

## Open-Angle Glaucoma

Open-angle glaucoma occurs even though there is no obstruction to the flow of aqueous humor. It may be caused by a mutation in the GLC1A gene, which is responsible for the production of a protein called myocilin that is normally present in the trabecular network. This condition is known as primary open-angle glaucoma (POAG). Secondary open-angle glaucoma can be caused when particulate matter, such as clumps of protein and shedded portions of surrounding cells and fibers, clog the outflow channels.

Importantly, the events leading to impaired trabecular meshwork drainage in non-genetic open-angle glaucoma share several pathological characteristics with *atherosclerosis*, such as *endothelial dysfunction*.[13–15] Therefore, individuals who wish to preserve the integrity of their trabecular meshwork should consider the suggestions in Life Extension's Atherosclerosis and Cardiovascular Disease protocol as well.

## Closed-Angle Glaucoma

Primary angle-closure glaucoma is most common in eyes with a shallow (flatter) front chamber. Secondary angle closure glaucoma is usually related to abnormal biological events in the eye, such as displacement of the iris against the cornea, which inhibits the aqueous humor from reaching the trabecular meshwork. Surgery or trauma to the eye can also lead to scar tissue that interferes with drainage. In addition, tumors can grow in the aqueous production and outflow system and interfere with the trabecular meshwork.

## Congenital Glaucoma

Congenital glaucoma is present at birth. It is related to improper formation of the aqueous fluid outflow system during fetal development. Several gene mutations

have been associated with congenital glaucoma. Congenital glaucoma is usually diagnosed at birth or within the first year of life.[16]

## Normal Tension Glaucoma

Not all people with glaucoma have elevated IOP. When IOP is normal but the person still has typical symptoms of glaucoma, the condition is called normal tension glaucoma.

## Pseudoexfoliative Glaucoma

Pseudoexfoliative glaucoma (PEX) is distinguished by clumps of amyloid protein that accumulate in the eye and ultimately end up blocking the outflow of aqueous humor by clogging the trabecular network. The cause is unknown, although a mutation in the LOXL1 gene may play a role. PEX is more common in women and in people of Northern European dissent.

## Anatomic Changes in Glaucoma

In glaucoma, the retina and optic nerve at the back of the eye grow thinner as ganglion cells and axons die. This thinning can be seen by a doctor during an ophthalmic exam. Eye doctors refer to the visible changes as "cupping."

A relatively new technology called *optical coherence tomography* (OCT) allows physicians to measure the progressive thinning of the retina and the cupping of the optic nerve and correlate the changes with visual field loss. Researchers have proposed that OCT be used for studying the effect of new drugs and devices being developed for treating glaucoma.[17] Other common tests that provide similar diagnostic information include Heidelberg retina tomography (HRT) and the GDxTM nerve fiber analyzer (GDx).

Beyond the visual symptoms of cupping, glaucoma's damage extends deep into the cells of the eye. Like all human cells, the cells of your eyes are full of structures called *mitochondria* that produce energy for the cell to function. In glaucoma, researchers are learning that the mitochondria in the retinal ganglion cell become damaged. Without healthy mitochondria, cells are unable to engage in a natural repair processes following normal wear and tear, oxidative stress, and injury. As a result, the retinal ganglion cells become susceptible to a process called apoptosis, or cell death.[18]

In the eye, it appears that *oxidative stress* is a major feature of mitochondrial damage. Free radical attack in the sensitive retinal ganglion cells causes mitochondrial damage, which in turn causes cell death. Excessive calcium within the cells is also implicated in retinal ganglion cell death.[19] Life Extension has long been at the forefront of identifying novel, natural ways to boost mitochondrial health.

Researchers have also uncovered another possible contributor to retinal ganglion cell death: excessive *glutamate*. Glutamate is the body's main excitatory neurotransmitter. Although it is vitally important to a healthy brain and nervous system, too much glutamate is toxic because it causes overstimulation of nerve cells. Normally, glutamate is cleared quickly. In glaucoma, however, it appears that high levels of glutamate in the retinal ganglion overstimulate cells, resulting in cell death. Researchers are looking at ways to reduce glutamate signaling in the eye, thus protecting the retinal ganglion cells from its toxic effects. This could be especially important for patients whose glaucoma does not respond to IOP-lowering treatment.[20]

## SUPPORTING MITOCHONDRIAL HEALTH TO PROTECT RETINAL GANGLION CELLS

As mentioned previously, oxidative stress plays a central role in the deterioration of ganglion cells that eventually leads to blindness in glaucoma.

As intraocular pressure increases, ocular blood flow is disrupted, causing, among other detriments, impaired oxygen delivery to the cells in the eye. Secondarily to poor oxygen delivery, mitochondrial function begins to decline. Suboptimally nourished mitochondria then begin to generate excessive amounts of free radicals, which destroy neighboring cellular structures, ultimately causing the cell to initiate apoptosis, or programmed cell death.

Supporting mitochondrial function with scientifically studied nutrients may mitigate the production of tissue-destroying free radicals and represent an unappreciated modality for preserving vision in glaucoma patients.

*Coenzyme CoQ10* and *pyrroloquinoline quinone* (PQQ) are two chief mitochondrial-supporting natural compounds available in the form of dietary supplements. Both of these compounds have been shown to protect mitochondrial function in a variety of disease states, and may help sustain ganglion cell mitochondrial health in individuals with glaucoma.[21,22]

## TESTS AND DIAGNOSIS

The simplest and most common test for glaucoma is an intraocular pressure reading, though increased IOP does not necessarily mean that glaucoma is the cause, and no single test alone can be used to establish a diagnosis of glaucoma. To get an IOP reading, a doctor or technician typically touches the front of the eye with a small instrument called a tonometer. Many doctors will also do a dilated eye exam. The purpose of dilating the pupil is to look directly at the inside back of the eye to check for retinal and optic nerve damage.

The doctor will probably take pictures and measurements to establish a baseline for comparing to future eye exams. A patient with glaucoma is also likely to have a visual field test to measure losses in peripheral vision and a visual acuity test to check for visual sharpness (acuity). The doctor may also use a technique called gonioscopy to study the angle of the drainage system and tonography to study the rate of fluid drainage.

Additional testing to establish a diagnosis of glaucoma often includes pachymetry (measures central cornea thickness), visual field testing, gonioscopy, and possibly nerve fiber layer scanning technology.

## TREATMENTS

Acute closed-angle glaucoma is a medical emergency that must be treated immediately. However, the more common type of glaucoma—open-angle glaucoma—can be an insidious disease with no symptoms, even as serious damage is being done to your retina and optic disk. The best approach to glaucoma is regular eye check-ups to make sure IOP is not rising, and if it is, to take aggressive measures to lower IOP.

A combination of natural therapies and conventional treatments can be used. The goal for both conventional and natural therapies is to lower IOP as much as possible and slow or halt the progression of symptoms.

### Conventional Treatment

Medications for glaucoma work by decreasing production and/or increasing drainage of aqueous fluid. Most glaucoma medications are topical—that is, in the form of eye drops. Categories of glaucoma medications are *alpha agonists*, *beta blockers*, *carbonic anhydrase inhibitors*, and *prostaglandin analogs*. A doctor may recommend a combination of glaucoma medications.

- **Alpha agonists** decrease fluid production and increase drainage. Two such drugs are apraclonidine HCl (Iopidine®) and brimonidine tartrate (Alphagan®). Dryness of mucous membranes is among the side effects caused by alpha antagonists.

- **Beta blockers** decrease production of aqueous fluid. They include timolol maleate (Istalol®, Timoptic XE®), betaxolol (Betoptic®), levobunolol HCl (Betagan®), metipranolol (OptiPranolol®), and timolol hemihydrate (Betimol®). Side effects of beta blockers include lowering of blood pressure and decreased heart rate.

- **Carbonic anhydrase inhibitors** work by decreasing aqueous fluid production. They include brinzolamide

(Azopt™), dorzolamide HCl (Trusopt®), and acetazolamide (Diamox®, Sequels®). These are available in pill and eye drop form. Systemic carbonic anhydrase inhibitor therapy may cause kidney dysfunction.

- **Cholinergic medications** lower IOP by constricting the pupil. This increases the volume of the eye's anterior chamber and improves access of aqueous fluid to the trabecular meshwork drainage system. Cholinergic medications are sometimes prescribed in combination with other glaucoma medications to help balance fluid production and drainage. Several cholinergic medications are pilocarpine HCl (Isopto® Carpine, Pilopine HS®) and carbachol (Isopto® Carbachol). Constriction of the pupil can cause poor night vision.

- Some medications contain several active ingredients. One called Combigan™ is a beta blocker and alpha agonist. It combines brimonidine tartrate and timolol maleate. Another, Cosopt®, is a beta blocker and carbonic anhydrase inhibitor. It combines dorzolamide HCl and timolol maleate. Both decrease production of aqueous fluid. An advantage is that patients get the benefit of both types of compounds in a single eye drop. A downside is the risk of side effects unique to each medicine.

- **Prostaglandin analogs** increase aqueous fluid drainage. Due to their ability to efficiently reduce IOP, prostaglandin analogs are becoming widely employed in clinical settings. Available medications are travoprost (Travatan®), bimatoprost (Lumigan®), and latanoprost (Xalatan®). Side effects of these compounds are a change in eye color and lengthening of eyelashes; the skin surrounding the eye may darken as well.

## Surgery

Most eye doctors in the United States start glaucoma treatment by prescribing a regimen of medicinal eye drops. As glaucoma progresses, patients are instructed to use higher doses or a combination of different types of eye drops. Surgery may be recommended for patients whose IOP is not responsive to medicines, whose glaucoma continues to worsen, or who experience uncomfortable side effects from glaucoma medications.

*Laser surgery* and *filtering surgery* are two common forms of surgery for POAG. Most are performed in a medical office or outpatient facility. The eye is temporarily numbed to keep the patient comfortable.

Laser surgery uses a high-energy laser beam to open obstructed trabecular drainage channels and to allow aqueous fluid to flow more freely from the anterior chamber of the eye. Many people who have this surgery, called laser trabeculoplasty, continue with glaucoma medication, although usually at a lower dose. Types of laser surgery for open-angle glaucoma include argon laser trabeculoplasty (ALT) and selective laser trabeculoplasty (SLT). SLT is a newer and more selective procedure that targets individual cells of the trabecular meshwork.

Another laser treatment called laser *cyclophotocoagulation* works differently from ALT and SLT. Instead of increasing drainage, it reduces fluid production. It does so by destroying part of the ciliary body of the eye where aqueous fluid is formed.

For patients in whom laser surgery is not ideal, there is also filtering surgery. Here the eye surgeon manually makes a small opening in the white of the eye (sclera) and removes a small part of the trabecular meshwork and nearby structures. This procedure, called a *trabeculectomy*, gives the aqueous fluid an additional outflow route. The surgeon covers the scleral opening with a natural membrane to protect the inner eye and to capture the fluid against the sclera, where it is absorbed.

An alternative to natural drainage through the opening in a trabeculectomy is drainage through a surgically implanted valve. The valve allows aqueous fluid to bypass the trabecular meshwork altogether. Aqueous fluid drains through a small tube from the anterior chamber onto the outside surface of the eye. A drainage valve is sometimes used when a trabeculectomy fails. It can also be used for treating juvenile glaucoma or glaucoma that is caused by trauma or severe eye inflammation.

Some patients may be better candidates for one or the other type of treatment (trabeculectomy or ALT/SLT). For example, ALT is generally preferred for patients older than 50. Further, a major study, called the Advanced Glaucoma Intervention Study (AGIS), supported by the National Eye Institute of the National Institutes of Health, showed a difference in treatment outcomes based on race. Caucasians had better outcomes than African Americans when medical therapy was followed initially by trabeculectomy, for unknown reasons.[23] Research comparing outcomes in Latinos and Caucasians showed no differences.[24]

Emergency glaucoma surgery for acute angle-closure glaucoma takes a different approach. A surgeon might create holes in the iris rather than the sclera. This treatment, performed using laser or conventional surgical techniques, rapidly decreases IOP by opening up the angle formed by the iris and drainage channels.

Fortunately, the risk that a patient will develop angle-closure glaucoma is predictable based on the results of routine eye exams. Therefore, regular check-ups can help avoid an acute angle closure crisis altogether because, upon detection of ocular anatomy favoring development of angle-closure glaucoma, a clinician can employ preventive procedures.

# NUTRIENTS FOR GLAUCOMA

The key with glaucoma is to detect increased IOP as soon as possible and immediately act to counter it, before stronger prescription drugs or invasive surgery become necessary. Researchers have recently discovered a pair of nutrients that target underlying mechanisms of glaucoma.

If clinical signs like increased IOP have already developed, but there are still no noticeable symptoms, it is even more important to act quickly to prevent disease progression. In this case, natural therapies, when combined with standard glaucoma medicines, may act synergistically to lower IOP; natural ingredients may also counteract the underlying damage caused by glaucoma.

## French Maritime Pine Bark and Bilberry

Human studies have shown a powerful effect of French maritime pine bark and bilberry extract on the underlying symptoms of glaucoma. These two nutrients are rich in proanthocyanidins, powerful antioxidants known for their ability to neutralize harmful free radicals. Proanthocyanidins have also been shown to support cardiovascular health.[25]

In a 2010 study combining treatment with French maritime pine bark and bilberry with the traditional glaucoma drug Latanoprost—a prostaglandin analog that increases aqueous fluid drainage—researchers found a clear benefit of the combination treatment.[1]

Pine bark and bilberry may act on a molecular level to decrease the production of aqueous humor, improve blood vessels structure and function, and decrease the resistance to fluid drainage.

Latanoprost causes smooth muscle cells, such as those in blood vessels and the eyes, to relax or contract. However, in part due to risk of side effects associated with its use, latanoprost eye drops may not be ideal for people with elevated IOP without symptoms. By contrast, the natural intervention of French maritime pine bark and bilberry is not associated with the side effects of latanoprost, which include ocular cysts, swelling, and inflammation.[26]

In this encouraging study, researchers studied 79 patients who had elevated IOP but no signs of glaucoma. Patients were randomized to receive either (1) an oral nutrient compound containing standardized French maritime pine bark extract and a phenolic bilberry (*Vaccinium myrtillus*) extract, (2) standard medical therapy with latanoprost eye drops alone, or (3) the nutrient compound and latanoprost drops, for 24 weeks.

IOP improved in patients in all treatment groups. The most rapid drop in pressure (28%) was seen in the latanoprost-only group, beginning 4 weeks after treatment began. In group 1, significant improvement began at 6 weeks. IOP reduction was 24% at week 16 and was maintained throughout the study. The most exciting results, however, were in the group receiving latanoprost *in combination* with pine bark and bilberry, those receiving the combination therapy. Patients in this group showed a 28% reduction in pressure at 4 weeks. Their reduction soared to 40% at 24 weeks. These results show the natural intervention amplifying the effect of the conventional intervention.

## Antioxidants

Pine bark and bilberry are among the newest nutrients used to fight glaucoma, but research has long supported the use of antioxidants to counter the oxidative damage caused by glaucoma. Dietary antioxidants have been shown to protect retinal ganglion cells against damage. Antioxidants include glutathione, lutein, zeaxanthin, zinc, vitamin A, vitamin C, vitamin E, beta-carotene, bioflavonoids, EGCG from green tea, and curcumin, among others.

Laboratory studies show that antioxidant treatment helps mitigate risk factors for glaucoma.[27] Research into epigallocatechin-gallate (EGCG), a powerful antioxidant found in green tea, for example, shows a potential impact on the physiology of retinal cells in patients with glaucoma.[28] The researchers used electrical measurements of retinal activity to show the effect.

Most scientists agree that more research is needed to understand the role of antioxidants in preventing or treating glaucoma and to determine effects of different doses and combinations of antioxidants in food and food supplements. Vitamin C and bioflavonoids in combination, for example, are thought to preserve the structure and function of blood vessels, which may improve blood flow to the retina and optic nerve to prevent glaucoma or slow decline in vision.

**Vitamin C** is also used in the formation of collagen, which gives strength and structure to tissues in the body. In the eye, collagen helps maintain the integrity of blood vessels and the trabecular meshwork. A recent study found that vitamin C serum levels were significantly lower in normal-tension glaucoma patients than in healthy controls.[29]

**Vitamin A** is necessary for the formation of *rhodopsin*, a pigmented compound in specialized retinal cells that allow the eye to see in low light. The eyes are strong indicators of vitamin A deficiency, becoming dry, itchy, or inflamed, and experiencing night blindness when levels are insufficient.[30] Most anyone taking a multivitamin supplement will not be deficient in vitamin A.

Vitamin A can be obtained through food (green leafy vegetables, liver, kidney, egg yolks, butter, fortified dairy products, cold-liver oil, and orange-colored foods, for example) or supplemental beta-carotene. Beta carotene is a pro-vitamin of vitamin A. It is converted, as needed, into vitamin A in the liver or during intestinal absorption.

**Ginkgo biloba** extract has been studied as a neuroprotector of retinal ganglion cells in glaucoma due to its ability to open (dilate) blood vessels and its antioxidant effect. Along with oxidative stress and high IOP, blood vessel inadequacy has also been proposed as a contributor to glaucoma, especially in normal tension glaucoma.

Ginkgo biloba has been shown to increase blood volume and velocity of blood flow in the eyes of healthy people.[31] In patients with normal tension glaucoma, studies show that it improves visual field loss.[32,33] These encouraging findings will hopefully lead to more research.

**Coleus forskohlii** is one of 200 varieties of the plant Coleus (*Solenostemnon*) found around the world. The therapeutic ingredient in *Coleus forskohlii* is found in its root, which was used originally in a paste form for treating a variety of disorders including cardiovascular conditions because of its vasodilating effect. *In vitro* studies show its significant antioxidant properties.[34] In clinical studies involving both animals and humans, a special preparation of *Coleus forskohlii*, applied directly to the eye, was shown to reduce IOP by increasing intraocular circulation and decreasing aqueous humor inflow into the posterior cavity.[35,36] Benefits were observed about an hour after application and remained significant for at least 5 hours.

*Coleus forskohlii* has also been used in the treatment of hypothyroidism as well, a condition in which the thyroid gland underperforms. Interestingly, hypothyroidism is a proven risk factor for glaucoma.[7]

## The Value of Minerals

*Magnesium* has long been recognized as nature's calcium balancer. Previous studies have demonstrated that calcium channel-blocking drugs offer benefits for some glaucoma patients. Armed with this revelation, researchers at the University Eye Clinic in Basel, Switzerland, evaluated the effect of supplemental magnesium on glaucoma patients. Magnesium (121.5 mg twice daily) was administered to 10 glaucoma patients for 1 month. At the conclusion of the study, results substantiated that magnesium supplementation improved the peripheral circulation, with an accompanying beneficial effect on the visual field in patients with glaucoma.[37]

Magnesium also has the ability to suppress the sympathetic nervous system. This is a reputation that earned magnesium credit in cardiology,[38] acting as an anti-adrenergic, meaning that it can block the "fight-or-flight" reaction, which causes the pupil to dilate and put added pressure on the drainage angle in the anterior chamber of the eye.

The trace mineral *chromium* has won credit beyond stabilization of blood glucose levels by improving focusing of the eye and lowering IOP.[39] *Selenium* has also been associated with glaucoma[40] and *zinc* with other vision disorders including age-related macular degeneration.[41]

## Melatonin

Small amounts of the pineal hormone melatonin are synthesized in the retina of humans and most other animals. Melatonin is a powerful antioxidant that may help reduce oxidative damage in the eye. In studies of animals with induced glaucoma, researchers found that placing melatonin in the anterior chamber of the eye reversed the negative effect of ocular hypertension on retinal function and diminished the impact of ocular hypertension on retinal ganglion cells. These results indicate that melatonin could be a valuable resource for treating glaucoma.[42]

## Others

Rutin, a bioflavonoid from the citrus family, has demonstrated the ability to lower IOP when used in conjunction with standard drugs. Moreover, experiments have revealed that orally ingested rutin is capable of reaching the eyes.[43]

---

## MARIJUANA FOR GLAUCOMA

It is well documented that active ingredients in marijuana lower IOP in people with and without glaucoma. Marijuana has been tested as a glaucoma treatment in its smokable form and as pills[44] and eye drops (as synthetic cannabinoids). Patients and doctors see potential advantages of all formulations but with some caveats.

Doctors are quick to point out the negative impact of frequent smoking on lung health (the IOP-lowering effect lasts only 3–4 hours) and the mood-altering effect of marijuana on cognition and motor skills, which could interfere with carrying out activities of daily living.

The pills and eye drops contain the active ingredient in marijuana, *tetrahydrocannabinol* (THC). This is effective in some people, but others find the side effects of THC uncomfortable. As for eye drops, it has not been possible to develop a compound that provides a sufficient dose of THC to the inside of the eye.

Another effect of marijuana—it lowers blood pressure—could also be a problem in glaucoma. As mentioned earlier, there is growing evidence that poor blood supply to the optic nerve could contribute to glaucoma. Therefore, marijuana's effect on blood supply to the eye might cancel out any improvement from IOP lowering treatments. More research is planned to study THC as a potential therapy for glaucoma.[28]

# LIFESTYLE TIPS FOR CONTROLLING IOP

## Exercise

Research findings show that physical activity can have a long-term beneficial effect on ocular perfusion pressure (OPP) (OPP is a measurement derived from IOP and blood pressure), which reflects the status of blood vessels at the optic disc.[9] This is an important finding given that low OPP is a risk factor for glaucoma.

The benefit appears to be related to cardiovascular fitness. In a study of over 5500 men and women, researchers questioned participants about rates of earlier physical activity (15 years previously) and then tested them for intraocular pressure (IOP) and blood pressure. They found an association between higher levels of activity and a 25% reduced risk of low OPP.

## Caffeine and Glaucoma

Older research shows that caffeine can cause a temporary increase of IOP.[45] The increase lasts for about 2 hours. Researchers looked at dietary histories of nearly 80 000 women in the Nurses' Health Study (NHS) and over 42 000 men in the Health Professionals Follow-up Study (HPFS) to determine whether repeated caffeine intake throughout the day would sustain IOP elevation and increase the risk of developing primary open-angle glaucoma. They found no such association between overall caffeine intake and increased risk of primary open-angle glaucoma.[46]

## Could Coffee Be Protective against Glaucoma?

Green coffee beans and brewed coffee contain antioxidant compounds that have neuroprotective actions.[47]

The antioxidant properties of green coffee come largely from the phenol *chlorogenic acid*. Other antioxidants in coffee include caffeic acid, quinic acid, and ferulic acid. Researchers report that green coffee has the strongest antioxidant properties, followed by instant coffee. Antioxidant activity decreases during roasting by 50–90%.[48,49] The antioxidant properties of instant coffee are partially related to the production during roasting of the free radical scavenger ApV, which is a zinc-chelating substance formed from chlorogenic acid, sugar, and proteins.

The neuroprotective effect of chlorogenic acid has been demonstrated in cell cultures of rat retinal ganglion cells where researchers found that chlorogenic acid produced a concentration-based inhibition on oxidative stress-induced neurotoxicity.[50]

## Emotional Stress and Glaucoma

As described earlier, closed-angle glaucoma can be related to a structural abnormality in the eye where a narrow angle between the iris and cornea impedes the outflow of aqueous fluid. Acute stress (the flight-or-fright reaction) can narrow the angle even further (by dilating the pupil) and cause an acute glaucomatous event.

## Smoking and Glaucoma

Cigarette smoking has been linked to several age-related eye diseases, including age-related macular degeneration, cataract, and severity of diabetic eye disease.[51] Although some findings have suggested a role for smoking in glaucoma,[52] others, including a systematic review of 11 earlier research studies, show little evidence that cigarette smoking causes primary open-angle glaucoma.[53] However, the authors of the review article question the quality of several of the studies that showed no influence of cigarette smoking on glaucoma and, given the clear link between smoking and other eye diseases, believe that further research is needed to confirm their findings.

## Sunglasses and Glaucoma

Although exposure to bright light and sun does not appear to be a risk factor for glaucoma, many people with glaucoma experience a sensitivity to light and glare. The problem can be solved by wearing sunglasses that block at least 99% of UVB rays and 95% of UVA rays.

# SUMMARY

Glaucoma is a common cause of blindness worldwide. It occurs more often in African Americans, Latinos, and Asians than in Caucasians. The most common event associated with glaucoma is an increase in intraocular pressure. Many therapies are designed to lower IOP in order to decrease pressure on the retina and optic nerve. Uncontrolled pressure damages retinal ganglion cells and their axons and causes the loss of peripheral vision and, if untreated, can lead to complete blindness. Glaucoma is a multifactorial condition. Genetic defects and nutritional deficiencies are risk factors for glaucoma. Certain behaviors influence IOP and may impact the development and/or progression of glaucoma.

New natural interventions, including a combination of pine bark and bilberry, show great promise in reducing the underlying symptoms of glaucoma, especially when used in combination with traditional glaucoma medications. Antioxidants are also valuable to reduce oxidative damage to the eyes, while minerals are important for general eye health.

In the future, more research is needed to understand the multiple underlying factors that contribute to glaucoma and develop conventional and natural interventions that will help prevent and reverse this major cause of blindness.

## Life Extension Suggestions

- **Blend of French maritime pine bark extract and bilberry extract**: 120–240 mg daily
- **Zeaxanthin and meso-zeaxanthin blend**: 3.75 mg daily
- **Lutein**: 10 mg daily

- **Green tea**, standardized extract: 725–1450 mg daily
- **Coenzyme Q10** (as ubiquinol): 100–200 mg daily
- **Pyrroloquinoline quinone** (PQQ): 10–20 mg daily
- **Curcumin** (as highly absorbed BCM-95®): 400–800 mg daily
- **Vitamin A**: 500 IU acetate and 4500 IU beta-carotene daily
- **Natural Vitamin E**: 100–400 IU alpha-tocopherol and 200 mg gamma-tocopherol daily
- **Vitamin C**: 1000–2000 mg daily
- **Selenium**: 200 mcg daily
- **Zinc**: 30–50 mg daily
- **Chromium** (Crominex™): 500 mcg daily
- **Green coffee**, standardized extract: 200–400 mg before each meal up to 3 times daily
- **Ginkgo biloba**, standardized extract: 120 mg daily
- **Coleus forskohlii,** standardized extract: 100 mg daily
- **Magnesium**: 140–500 elemental mg of highly absorbable magnesium
- **Melatonin**: 0.3–3 mg 30–60 minutes before bed

## REFERENCES

References available at: www.lef.org/dpt5/ch64

# 65

# Gout and Hyperuricemia

Gout is one of the oldest known and most common forms of *arthritis*; it is a crystal deposition disease in which crystals of *monosodium urate* form in joints and other tissues. Gout attacks cause a characteristic painful inflammation of one or more joints of the extremities, or nodules in soft tissues called *tophi*. An acute attack of gout, although brief and usually subsiding spontaneously, can be temporarily debilitating, and predisposes an individual to subsequent attacks.

Once a disease of only the affluent (who could afford the purine-rich foods and drink linked to gout risk), this "disease of kings" has rapidly become a disease of everyman. The prevalence of gout among United States adults, according to the National Health and Nutrition Examination Survey (2007–2008) is estimated at 3.9% (8.3 million people), favoring men over women by almost 3:1.[1] This represents a significant 44% increase in gout frequency from previous estimates just a decade earlier.[2]

The primary risk factor for gout is elevated levels of a metabolic byproduct called *uric acid* in the blood; this condition is known as *hyperuricemia*. Hyperuricemia is estimated to affect over 21% of the United States population, and doubles in frequency between ages 20 and 80 years.[1]

Hyperuricemia increases the risk of not only gout, but other diseases as well, including *hypertension*, *kidney disease*, and *metabolic syndrome*. Even during the asymptomatic periods between gout attacks, the body is exposed to periods of low-grade *chronic inflammation*. The propensity for excessive blood uric acid and gout is also increased by other disease states; therefore, a gout or hyperuricemic patient should consider Life Extension's suggestions and protocols for Obesity and Weight Loss, Inflammation (Chronic), Atherosclerosis and Cardiovascular Disease, High Blood Pressure, and Kidney Health as well.

## URIC ACID METABOLISM

Uric acid is the final product of *purine* metabolism in humans. Purines are components of nucleosides, the building blocks of DNA and RNA. Purine nucleosides (*adenosine* and *guanine*) are used in the creation of other metabolically important factors as well, such as *adenosine* triphosphate (ATP; the energy-carrying molecule), S-*adenosyl*methionine (SAMe; the methyl donor), and nicotinamide *adenine* dinucleotide (NADH; an important cofactor in energy production and antioxidation). Given the importance of purine-containing molecules for survival, vertebrates, including humans, have developed robust systems for synthesizing sufficient purine nucleosides for their metabolism using readily available materials (such as glucose, glycine, and glutamine), as well as recycling purine nucleosides from throughout the body or from the diet.

In mammals, excess purine nucleosides are removed from the body by breakdown in the liver and excretion from the kidneys. For most mammals, the purines are first converted into the intermediate uric acid, which is then metabolized by the enzyme *uricase* into the compound *allantoin*. Allantoin is a very soluble compound that can easily travel through the bloodstream, become filtered by the kidneys, and be excreted from the body. In contrast to other mammals, humans and other primates lack a functional uricase enzyme, and can only break purines down into uric acid.

The levels of uric acid in the blood depend on two factors. The first is the rate of uric acid synthesis in the liver. Since uric acid results from purine degradation, its levels are influenced by both the amount of purines synthesized in the body, as well as the amounts of purines absorbed from the diet.[3] The second determinant of blood uric acid levels is the rate of uric acid excretion from the kidneys. Excretion has the greatest effect on blood uric acid levels, with about 90% of hyperuricemia cases attributed to impaired renal excretion.[4] Impaired excretion is most often due to abnormalities in the kidney urate transporter (called URAT1) or organic ion transporter (OAT), both of which control the movement of uric acid out of proximal kidney tubules and into urine.[5]

One of the most intriguing aspects of uric acid is that although it appears to be a "waste product" of purine metabolism, only about 10% of the uric acid that enters a normal human kidney is excreted from the body.[3] In other words, rather than eliminating uric acid, a healthy kidney returns up to 90% of it to the bloodstream. The reason for this is likely due to the role of uric acid as one of the most important antioxidants in body fluids, responsible for the neutralization of over 50% of the free radicals in the bloodstream.[6]

The ability of humans and primates to preserve blood levels of uric acid (due to slow kidney filtration and lack of a uricase enzyme) was probably advantageous to our evolution, by increasing antioxidant capacity of the blood.[7]

Humans and primates are among the few mammals that cannot produce their own vitamin C, and may have evolved the ability to preserve uric acid to compensate for this.[8] For example, blood uric acid levels in humans are normally about 6 times that of vitamin C, and about 10 times the levels in other mammals.[9] Like vitamin C, uric acid has a principal role in protecting high-oxygen tissues (like the brain) from damage, and low blood uric acid levels have been associated with the progression or increased risk of several neurologic disorders, including amyotrophic lateral sclerosis (ALS)[10] and multiple sclerosis (MS),[11] and Huntington's,[12] Parkinson's,[13] and Alzheimer's diseases.[14]

## HYPERURICEMIA AND THE DEVELOPMENT OF GOUT

Uric acid is a metabolic "waste product" with poor solubility in body fluids, yet its potential role as a primary antioxidant in body fluids suggests that it should be kept at sufficient levels in the blood. Clearly, these diametric properties of uric acid define a range for normal blood uric acid levels. Commonly, the upper limit of this range is taken as 8.6 mg/dL in men and 7.1 mg/dL in women (although some laboratories and research groups use different limits).[15–17] Uric acid levels above this limit are considered hyperuricemic.

**Anatomy of gout**

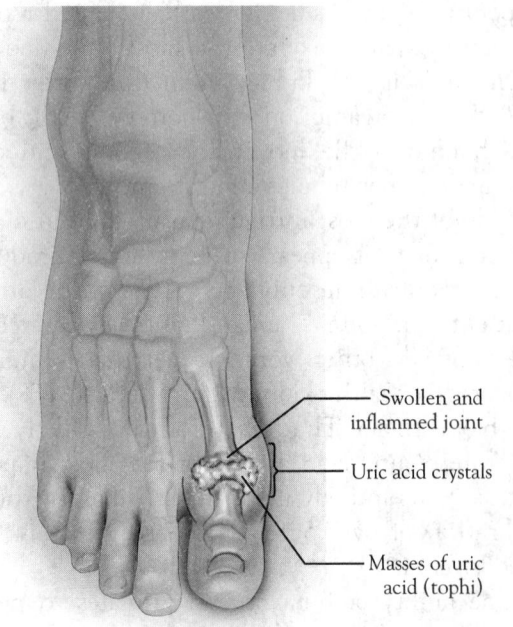

- Swollen and inflamed joint
- Uric acid crystals
- Masses of uric acid (tophi)

Hyperuricemia is a primary risk factor for the development of gout, although it is likely that many hyperuricemic individuals will not develop symptoms.[7] While the risk of a gout attack increases with blood uric acid, the annual occurrence of inflammatory gout is fairly low; persons with blood uric acid levels between 7 and 8.9 mg/dL have a 0.5–3% change of developing the disease, which rises to 4.5% at levels over 9 mg/dL.[18]

Hyperuricemia without symptoms (asymptomatic hyperuricemia) is also a risk factor for other diseases. Although patients with asymptomatic hyperuricemic may never experience the symptoms of a gout attack, ultrasound studies have revealed that up to one-third may have urate deposits and evidence of inflammation in their joints and surrounding soft tissues.[19]

As local serum uric acid concentrations rise above their limit of solubility, monosodium urate can begin to precipitate out of the blood, forming needle-like crystals preferentially in cartilage and fibrous tissues. Here, the crystals may reside for years without causing problems.[20] Urate crystals within tissues have two fates—they can redissolve in body fluids and reenter circulation, or may be "shed" from the tissue. Shed monosodium urate crystals can enter nearby joint spaces or bursa (the fluid-filled sacs that provide cushioning between tendons and bones around a joint) where they are quickly engulfed by immune cells. This activates a localized inflammatory response, leading to the characteristic arthritis of gout.[21]

Gout is commonly divided into distinct "phases" of recurrent attacks of acute gout interspersed with symptom-free periods, with cumulative crystal deposition gradually contributing to a chronic condition (chronic tophaceous gout).

An attack of acute gout usually appears as a sudden inflammatory arthritis of a single joint in the lower extremities, most often the *metatarsophalangeal joint* of the big toe (the "ball" of the foot). At this joint, gout is called *podagra*. Other joints that are frequently affected include the mid-foot, ankle, knee, wrists, and finger joints. The skin may be red and shiny above the affected area. Attacks often begin in the early morning and peak in 6–24 hours. The pain is severe, and patients often cannot wear socks or touch bedsheets during flare-ups.[22] Even without treatment, the attacks typically subside spontaneously within several days to 2 weeks. Acute gout attacks can also be accompanied by high fever and leukocytosis (elevated white blood cell count).[20]

Gout attacks can be triggered by a variety of factors, many of which reduce the solubility of urate in the blood. The factors include infection, trauma to the joint, rapid weight loss, dehydration, acidosis, and lower body temperature (which explains the timing of gout attacks and why they most frequently occur in the extremities).[22]

Following resolution of an acute attack, a patient can enter an "intercritical period," or a period without symptoms. Although the patient may be asymptomatic, monosodium urate crystals and low-grade inflammation can persist in the joint during this period.[23] Once an initial acute gout attack has occurred, further attacks are likely to follow. Recurrent attacks of acute gout often lead to chronic tophaceous gout, in which monosodium urate deposits (tophi) form in the soft tissues, usually along the rim of the ear, over the elbow joint, and in the joints of the fingers and toes. Tophi reduce the growth and viability of bone cells (osteoblasts),[24] and if left untreated, tophaceous gout can lead to significant joint erosion and loss of function.[22]

## THE ROLE OF HYPERURICEMIA IN OTHER CONDITIONS

Although hyperuricemia is most often associated with gout, elevated blood levels of uric acid have also been associated with other diseases. Hyperuricemia and gout are both risk factors for kidney or bladder stones (urolithiasis). Both conditions increase the risk of forming not only uric acid stones, but also the more common calcium oxalate stones. The presence of calcium oxalate stones is 10–30 times higher in gout patients than those without gout.[25] Deposits of monosodium urate crystals in kidney tissues can result in kidney damage (nephropathy), either acutely by formation of crystals within the tubules of the kidney, or through a chronic inflammatory response to urate deposits in other tissues of the kidney.[26] Prior to the development of uric acid-lowering treatments, kidney disease occurred in up to 40% of gout patients; renal failure was the usual cause of death in 18–25% of these patients.[27]

Hyperuricemia is a risk factor for cardiovascular diseases in high-risk groups, and has been associated with small increases in the risk of coronary events,[28] heart failure,[29] and stroke.[30] It is often seen in patients with hypertension; high blood pressure has long been thought to contribute to elevated blood uric acid, possibly due to reduced blood flow to the kidneys and lower urate excretion.[31] However, recent experimental and epidemiologic data suggest that the opposite may be true: a comprehensive review of 18 observational studies revealed that for each 1 mg/dL increase in blood uric acid, the risk of hypertension increased by 13%.[32] This effect was more pronounced in women and young adults. Lowering of uric acid levels in hyperuricemic, hypertensive adolescents reduced their blood pressure as well.[33] Ironically, the increased risk of cardiovascular diseases associated with hyperuricemia may be due to increases in oxidative stress: xanthine oxidase,

the enzyme that synthesizes uric acid, also produces free radicals in the process.[6]

Hyperuricemia is an integral part of metabolic syndrome,[20] and epidemiologic studies have demonstrated that elevated uric acid levels substantially increase metabolic syndrome risk (and vice versa).[34,35] Data from the Multiple Risk Factor Intervention Trial (MRFIT) showed that hyperuricemia was associated with increased risk of type 2 diabetes, and that male patients with gout had a 41% increased risk for the disease.[36]

## RISK FACTORS FOR GOUT

Hyperuricemia is the primary risk factor for gout, and is required, although not sufficient, for the progression of the disease. The risk of gout increases with age and is more common in men; increased risk is also associated with other medical conditions including hypertension, obesity, renal insufficiency, early menopause (hormone therapy can reduce this risk), hypercholesterolemia, and surgery. Some medications increase gout risk (which is reversible upon discontinuation), particularly loop and thiazide diuretics, but also antituberculosis drugs, cyclosporin, and levodopa.[20,37–39] Aspirin has a dual effect on uric acid levels; low doses inhibit excretion and increase blood levels, while very high doses (>3000 mg/day) reduce levels.[20] At 75 mg/day in elderly patients, the increase in blood uric acid is about 6%.[40]

Uric acid levels are very sensitive to dietary influences. High-purine foods, particularly red meat, fish, and shellfish, have long been known to increase hyperuricemia and gout risk. Data from the Health Professionals Follow-up Study, which followed over 47 000 health professionals for 12 years, revealed that individuals with the highest intakes of beef, pork, or lamb (>1.9 servings/day) and seafood (>0.6 servings/day) increased their risk of gout by 77% and 53%, respectively.[41] There were no associations between total protein intake, total animal protein (including dairy protein, poultry, and eggs) intake, or purine-rich vegetable intake and the incidence of gout.

Alcoholic beverages increase blood uric acid and gout risk.[42,43] In one study, individuals who consumed one beer or one serving of spirits per day had 1.75 and 1.22 times the incidence of gout, respectively, than individuals who consumed less than one drink a month. Drinking over two beers/day increased gout risk 2.5-fold.[42] Wine does not appear to affect gout risk. Alcohol metabolism to acetate accelerates the breakdown of purine-containing nucleotides (like ATP) and raises blood uric acid.[44] Alcohol can also lower body temperature in the extremities which may precipitate an acute attack independent of blood uric acid concentration (gout attacks can occur in alcoholics at lower blood urate levels than in nonalcoholics).[45] Beer, despite having less alcohol per serving than the other beverages, is more hyperuricemic due to its high purine content.[46]

Fructose has been positively associated with both gout and hyperuricemia risk in some studies, but has had no significant effect in others. In the third National Health and Nutritional Examination Survey of 14761 individuals over 20 years old (NHANES III), individuals who consumed one or more sweetened soft drinks per day had levels of blood uric acid that averaged 0.5 mg/dL higher than nondrinkers.[47] By comparison, persons who consumed an equivalent amount of orange juice had blood uric acid levels that averaged only about 0.15mg/dL higher than non-juice drinkers. An analysis of more recent NHANES data,[17] however, failed to find any significant association between total fructose consumption and hyperuricemia risk. These results, in addition to the conflicting results of several metabolic studies of fructose in human volunteers, suggest that the relationship between fructose and hyperuricemia may be sensitive to factors aside from just the amount of ingested sugar.[17]

## DIAGNOSIS OF GOUT

Gout usually presents with characteristic inflamed, painful joints in the extremities, but these symptoms are also common to other conditions, particularly *pseudogout* (a related condition caused by the accumulation of calcium pyrophosphate crystals in the joint) or septic arthritis (caused by joint infection). Blood tests can determine whether the patient is hyperuricemic (typically a serum concentration above 7 mg/dL in males and above 6 mg/dL in females). While hyperuricemia is the most important risk factor for gout, its diagnostic power may be limited; as some hyperuricemic patients may never develop the disease, and blood urate levels may be normal during an acute attack (in one study, 14% of patients had blood uric acid levels of <6 mg/dL during their gout attacks).[48]

The European League against Rheumatism (EULAR) recently published guidelines for gout diagnostic criteria, based on accumulated studies of gout diagnoses. According to their analysis, the most definitive feature in the diagnosis of gout is the identification of monosodium urate crystals in synovial (joint) fluid or aspirates of tophi.[15] This involves the insertion of a fine needle into the joint or tophus and withdrawing a fluid sample, which is subsequently examined under a microscope.[49] The presence of large needle-shaped crystals confirms the presence of monosodium urate, and can be used to differentiate gout from pseudogout or septic arthritis.

The presence of urate crystals in the joints of asymptomatic patients can be used to identify intercritical periods in patients with recurrent gout, or can be used to screen patients who may benefit from urate-lowering therapy prior to their first acute gout attack. Screening of the joints of the extremities using ultrasound is being explored as a noninvasive method to improve the detection of urate crystals in asymptomatic patients. In a pilot study, ultrasound correctly identified urate crystals in the joints of asymptomatic, hyperuricemic volunteers with an accuracy of 81%.[50]

## CONVENTIONAL TREATMENT OF GOUT

Treatments for acute gout attacks typically manage pain and inflammation, and include nonsteroidal anti-inflammatory drugs (NSAIDs), corticosteroids, and colchicine. While treatments for acute gout are typically short term, there are risks of significant gastrointestinal side effects for NSAIDs and colchicine in some individuals. Moreover, although colchicine is approved by the Food and Drug Administration (FDA) to treat acute gout flares, it has a low therapeutic index, meaning that the dose required to exert a beneficial effect is near that which is potentially toxic. Aspiration of affected joints to relieve pressure and injection of long-acting steroids are commonly used treatments in practice, although they have not been investigated in controlled trials.[51]

After the initial attack has subsided, patients are usually encouraged to adopt lifestyle changes that may reduce hyperuricemia and gout risk (such as lower purine diets, weight loss, or exercise). Many will be placed on longer-term, uric acid-reduction therapy. Recall that uric acid levels are controlled by the rate of uric acid production and the rate of uric acid excretion; current therapies address one or the other of these two aspects.

### Xanthine Oxidase Inhibitors

Xanthine oxidase inhibitors reduce the activity of xanthine oxidase, the final step in uric acid synthesis. This has the effect of lowering uric acid production. Allopurinol (Zyloprim) has a long history of usage as a xanthine oxidase inhibitor; recently febuxostat (Uloric) has been approved for treatment of hyperuricemia in the United States. Febuxostat exhibits greater uric acid-lowering effects than allopurinol, although the incidence of gout flares is similar between the two drugs.[52]

## Uricosuric Drugs

Uricosuric drugs increase the excretion of uric acid from the kidneys, primarily by reducing the absorption of uric acid from the kidneys back into the blood. Probenecid (Benemid) and sulfinpyrazone (Anturane) are two examples. These drugs tend to increase urinary uric acid levels, which can cause kidney stones.

## Surgical Removal

The tophi of chronic gout, if severe enough to cause joint dysfunction or deformity, can also be treated by surgical removal.[53,54]

---

## INNOVATIVE NEW DRUGS FOR THE MANAGEMENT OF CHRONIC GOUT

As mentioned earlier in this protocol, in most mammals uric acid is converted into the more soluble compound *allantoin* by an enzyme called *uricase*. This conversion allows for the urinary excretion of allantoin, thereby reducing uric acid blood levels. However, humans are unable to facilitate this conversion due to an evolutionary loss of the uricase enzyme.

Recently, scientists have recreated the mammalian uricase enzyme in the laboratory and generated injectable medications that deliver the *recombinant* enzyme into the blood. Once in the bloodstream, the recombinant uricase enzyme breaks down uric acid into allantoin, which is then easily excreted through the human kidneys.

By injecting this enzyme otherwise not present in higher primates, the rate of uric acid excretion can be expedited.

Two such medications are available—*rasburicase* (Elitek®), and a chemically modified version of this same drug, called *pegloticase* (Krystexxa®). Pegloticase is FDA approved to lower uric acid levels in patients with chronic gout.[55]

In two concurrent randomized, double-blind, placebo-controlled trials, pegloticase, administered at a dose of 8 mg either every 2 weeks or every 4 weeks, efficiently lowered uric acid levels.[56] The participants in these studies consisted of patients with chronic gout, which had not been relieved by allopurinol, and blood uric acid levels above 8.0 mg/dL at baseline. Reduction of uric acid levels to ≤6.0 mg/dL was the primary endpoint, and was achieved in 38% of patients receiving biweekly injections, and in 49% of those receiving monthly injections.

However, pegloticase may cause some side effects. In the studies mentioned above, between a quarter and a half of subjects experienced an injection site reaction, of which 6.5% were considered to be anaphylaxis. This means that physicians may opt to administer corticosteroids before pegloticase in order to suppress the immune system in hopes of avoiding an inflammatory response. The long-term effects of corticosteroids in combination with pegloticase have not been studied as of yet, so the side effects in gout patients remain unknown.[57]

Many physicians may not be aware of the availability of pegloticase for lowering uric acid levels in gout patients due to its recent FDA approval. Individuals with chronic gout that has not improved after the use of conventional gout medications should consider asking their health care professional if pegloticase is right for them.

---

## DIETARY APPROACHES TO CONTROL HYPERURICEMIA AND REDUCE GOUT RISK

Lifestyle can have a significant influence on the development of hyperuricemia and gout. Accumulated data from several large epidemiologic studies suggest several possible modifications for significant reductions in gout risk[58]:

### Exercise Daily and Reduce Weight

Increased adiposity is associated with increased uric acid levels and gout risk.

### Limit Red Meat Intake

Beef, pork, and lamb are high-purine foods that can significantly increase gout risk.

### Adjust Fish Intake to Individual Needs

Carefully balance the benefits of omega-3 fatty acids with the increased gout risk, or consider taking an omega-3 supplement. High quality fish oil supplements are highly purified and the purine content in these oils is either undetectable or present in trace amounts that pose no risk of raising gout levels.

### Drink Skim Milk or Consume Other Low-Fat Dairy Products, up to 2 Servings/Day

Dairy consumption is inversely associated with gout risk.

### Consume Vegetable Protein, Nuts, and Legumes

Nuts and legumes are good sources of non-uricemic protein; legumes and vegetables (even those high in purines) are not associated with gout risk.

### Reduce Alcohol Intake

Moderate alcohol consumption has cardiovascular benefits, but beer and spirits significantly increase gout risk. Red wine, on the other hand, appears not to increase gout risk.

### Limit Intake of Sugar-Sweetened Beverages

Fructose in these beverages might increase hyperuricemia and gout risk. Although fruits also contain fructose, it is usually present at lower levels and most have health benefits that justify their consumption.

# TARGETED NATURAL INTERVENTIONS

In addition to diet and lifestyle changes, several individual dietary factors may reduce hyperuricemia or gout risk.

## Vitamin C

Vitamin C is an essential water-soluble antioxidant vitamin in humans, which has been shown in laboratory tests to exert a uric acid-lowering effect by inhibiting the enzyme xanthine oxidase.[59] In a comprehensive review of 13 randomized controlled trials of vitamin C supplementation in a total of 556 adults with normal kidney function, an average reduction in blood uric acid of 0.35mg/dL was observed for an average dose of 500 mg/day for a median duration of 30 days.[60] The most significant reductions were observed in persons with higher initial baseline uric acid concentrations (patients with a blood uric acid level of >4.85 mg/dL saw a 0.78 mg/dL reduction). In a large study (184 healthy subjects), vitamin C also increased the glomerular filtration rate (the rate at which blood is filtered in the kidney and a measurement of kidney function) when compared to the control group.[61] Future trials are necessary to determine whether vitamin C intervention can prevent the incidence and recurrence of gout. Plasma levels of vitamin C are also inversely associated with blood pressure,[62,63] which may be an independent risk factor for gout.

## Cherries

Cherries are a traditional gout treatment rich in polyphenol antioxidants,[64,65] and a small set of clinical cases in the 1950s documented decreased duration and severity of gout attacks in 3 people on cherry-supplemented diets.[66] Two more recent investigations have demonstrated a potential role of cherries in the management of gout, although they present conflicting mechanisms for this action. After a single dose of 280 g cherries, the blood urate levels in 10 healthy women dropped by 14% after 5 hours, while urinary urate levels increased.[64] Markers of inflammation (CRP) also decreased slightly. A second study of 100 patients with recurrent gout taking 15mL/day of cherry juice concentrate for 4–6 months also revealed decreases in markers of inflammation, as well as a >50% reduction in the number of acute gout attacks for 92% of treated patients.[67] However, uric acid levels were not lowered in this group, and averaged 7.8 mg/dL. Cherry consumption has also been observed to increase in blood uric acid.[68] Although it appears that cherries may reduce the frequency of gout attacks, the mechanism for this action clearly does not depend solely on lowering blood uric acid levels.

## Coffee

More than 50% of Americans drink coffee, and the average per capita intake is 2 cups per day.[69] Coffee contains both caffeine and polyphenolic antioxidants that may have independent roles in the reduction of gout risk. The relationship between coffee consumption and the risk of gout has been examined in two large observational studies. In the Nurse's Health Study, 89 433 women were tracked over 26 years for their consumption of coffee—those who consumed more coffee had a lower risk of gout.[70] The largest reductions in risk were observed in women who consumed over 4 cups of caffeinated coffee per day (–63%), although modest consumption of decaffeinated coffee (>1 cup/day) reduced gout risk by 23%. In the same population, tea had no effect. A similar study of 45 869 men for 12 years demonstrated a similar effect for both caffeinated and decaffeinated coffees, which was significant at coffee intakes over 4 cups a day (–40% risk).[71]

Much of the protective effect of coffee against acute gout can be attributed to caffeine in the above studies; caffeine (1,3,7-trimethyl-xanthine) is a competitive inhibitor of xanthine oxidase.[72] The protective effect of decaffeinated coffee suggests other compounds may also important. For example, some evidence suggests that iron overload may contribute to the development of gout, and *chlorogenic acids* from coffee have been shown to reduce iron absorption.[73] Conventional coffee, due to the roasting process, contains very little chlorogenic acids. However, recent innovations have led to the availability of a *green coffee extract high in chlorogenic acids*, which can be taken in the form of a supplement. Green coffee extract supplements are a superior source of chlorogenic acids and other healthful coffee compounds as compared to conventionally roasted coffee beans used to make coffee beverages.[74,75]

## Fiber

An analysis of fiber intake data in 9384 adults without cancer, diabetes, or heart disease from the National Health and Nutrition Examination Survey (NHANES) 1999–2004 revealed a significant association between higher fiber intake and lower hyperuricemia risk. The study, which used a higher blood uric acid limit for the definition of hyperuricemia (8.4 mg/dL for men and

7.4 mg/dL for women), demonstrated a 55% reduction in hyperuricemia risk between the highest fiber consumption (9.5 g fiber/1000 kcal of total food intake, or 19 g fiber/day for the average 2000-kcal diet) and the lowest (<4.6 g/1000 kcal; <9.2 g fiber/day).[17] A smaller case-controlled study of 92 gout patients and 92 gout-free controls demonstrated a statistically significant reduction in the risk of gout among persons with the highest intake of total and soluble fiber.[76] While these mechanisms for this reduction is unknown, dietary fiber may inhibit purine or adenine absorption in the digestive system.[77] Fiber has also been shown to reduce other independent risk factors for gout, including hypertension[78,79] and high cholesterol.[80]

## Folate

A small case-controlled study of 92 gout patients and 92 gout-free controls demonstrated a statistically significant reduction in the risk of gout among persons who consumed over 51.5 mcg/day of folate from food sources (a 70% reduction compared to those who consumed less than this value).[76] No significant effects on gout risk were observed for vitamins A, E, or the other B vitamins in this study.

## Chinese Herbs

Several Chinese medicinal plants have been tested for xanthine oxidase inhibitory activity. The most active was the methanol extract of Chinese cinnamon (*Cinnamomum cassia*), followed by *Chrysanthemum indicum* and *Lycopus europaeus*. Among water extracts, the strongest inhibition was observed with *Polygonum cuspidatum*, which is an excellent source of the polyphenol *resveratrol*.[81] These herbs have been used in China to suppress gout.[81] Extracts from two traditional Chinese antigout treatments (*Paederia scandens* and *Smilax china*) both decreased blood uric acid concentration in rats with experimentally induced hyperuricemia.[82,83]

## Flavonoids

Flavonoids may lower blood uric acid through their ability to inhibit the enzyme xanthine oxidase; olive leaf constituents, milk thistle constituents, apigenin, myricetin, luteolin, and genistein have all shown this ability in laboratory experiments; apigenin had an inhibitory activity comparable to the synthetic xanthine oxidase inhibitor allopurinol.[84–87] In fructose-induced hyperuricemic rodents, quercetin, rutin, kaempferol, myricetin, and puerarin all significantly reduced blood uric acid to levels equivalent

to healthy control animals.[88,89] Grape seed procyanidins were found to have uric acid-lowering effects in rats with hyperuricemia. The procyanidin-treated animals exhibited normal growth compared to animals treated with allopurinol, which exhibited some retarded growth.[90]

---

## ANTI-INFLAMMATORY NUTRIENTS: A POTENTIAL ROLE IN CHRONIC GOUT?

While hyperuricemia and urate crystal formation are requirements for an acute gout attack and a contributing factor for chronic gout, inflammation is clearly central to the disease. Several labs have investigated the chemical cascades that mediate this process. Under certain conditions, cells of the innate immune system (the *macrophages* or "big-eaters") that reside within tissues recognize the presence of urate crystals. Through a process that is still not fully elucidated, these cells are stimulated to produce proinflammatory cytokines (particularly IL-1β), which recruit inflammatory white blood cells (*neutrophils*) to the site of crystal deposition.[91,92] The circumstances surrounding the cessation of inflammation in acute gout are equally puzzling. Data suggest a yet-unidentified gout promoting "factor" that must be present with the urate crystals in order for an acute attack to occur.[93]

Although it seems a reasonable assumption that anti-inflammatory nutrients may have a role in mitigating gout attacks, research in this specific area is lacking. The quick progression and resolution of acute gout may make it less amenable to nutrient "interventions" (many of which have only been tested for their long-term effects on inflammation). However, the intercritical periods between attacks have been associated with sustained low-level inflammation,[94] a situation more readily addressed by dietary modification. Nutrients that have been shown to attenuate joint inflammation and reduce proinflammatory cytokines (including IL-1β), such as *curcumin*,[95,96] *omega-3 fatty acids*,[97] and *resveratrol*[98] may be especially suited for this purpose. Experimental diets high in the omega-3 fatty acid EPA and the healthy omega-6 fatty acid GLA were shown to reduce urate crystal-induced inflammation in a rat model.[99] Omega-3 supplements may be more suitable for hyperuricemic patients who are limiting fish intake.[70]

---

## Life Extension Suggestions

- **Vitamin C:** 1000–2000 mg daily
- **Cherry extract:** 1000–3000 mg daily
- **Green coffee extract** (standardized to 50% chlorogenic acid): 400–1200 mg daily
- **L-methylfolate:** 1000 mcg daily
- **Quercetin:** 250–500 mg daily
- **Grape seed,** standardized extract: 100–200 mg daily

- **Olive leaf,** standardized extract: 500–1000 mg daily
- **Milk thistle,** standardized extract: 750 mg daily
- **Fiber:** ingest 30–40 g of fiber daily from food and supplemental sources
- **Fish oil** (with olive polyphenols): 1400 mg EPA and 1000 mg DHA daily
- **Curcumin** (as highly absorbed BCM-95®): 400–800 mg daily
- *Trans*-**resveratrol:** 250–500 mg daily

In addition, the following blood testing resources may be helpful:

- Chemistry Panel and Complete Blood Count (CBC)
- Omega Score®

## REFERENCES

References available at: www.lef.org/dpt5/ch65

# 66

# *Hangover Prevention*

Aging makes us increasingly vulnerable to alcohol-induced hangover, liver injury, and damage to the central nervous system. Because alcohol consumption produces toxic compounds and causes vitamin deficiencies, in the best of all possible worlds it would be better not to drink alcohol at all. For those who still want to drink, it is possible to do so more safely. The first suggestion would be to drink only moderately and follow the preventive measures outlined in this protocol.

*Warning:* What follows is for those who choose to drink moderately. These suggestions are not for those who suffer from alcoholism. Simply put, an alcoholic has "lost the power of choice in drink" and is "without defense against the first drink." In short, an alcoholic cannot drink safely. The Foundation is all too aware that an alcoholic may easily misinterpret the following information as a license to drink. It is not. It is only for those who drink by choice and do so in moderation.

The consumption of alcohol results in the formation of two very toxic compounds, acetaldehyde and malondialdehyde. These compounds generate massive free-radical damage to cells throughout the body. The free-radical damage generated by these alcohol metabolites creates an effect in the body similar to that caused by radiation poisoning. That is the reason why people feel so sick the day after consuming too much alcohol. If the proper combination of antioxidants is taken at the time alcohol is consumed or before the inebriated individual goes to bed, the hangover and much of the cellular damage caused by alcohol may be prevented.

## THE ASTRONOMICAL COST OF HANGOVERS

A study in *Annals of Internal Medicine* compiled the enormous cost of lost productivity induced by hangovers.[1] An excerpt from this study follows:

"The alcohol hangover is characterized by headache, tremulousness, nausea, diarrhea, and fatigue combined with decreased occupational, cognitive, or visual-spatial skill performance. In the United States,

related absenteeism and poor job performance cost $148 billion annually (average annual cost per working adult, $2000). Although hangover is associated with alcoholism, most of its cost is incurred by the light-to-moderate drinker. Patients with hangover may pose substantial risk to themselves and others despite having a normal blood alcohol level. Hangover may also be an independent risk factor for cardiac death."

Based on these statistics, hangover causes a significant economic loss in the United States. The staggering cost of alcoholic hangover could be significantly mitigated if drinkers took the right antioxidants before going to bed.

## PROTECTING AGAINST HANGOVER AND CELLULAR DAMAGE

Nutrients that neutralize alcohol byproducts and protect cells against the damaging effects of alcohol include vitamin C, vitamin B1, S-allyl-cysteine (antioxidant found in garlic), glutathione, vitamin E, and selenium.[2-6] These nutrients can be taken at the time the alcohol is consumed or before bedtime to help prevent a hangover.

### Vitamin C

Vitamin C is one of the essential nutrients depleted by alcohol consumption.[7] Because it is the body's primary water-soluble dietary antioxidant, this depletion results in severe oxidative stress in daily drinkers.[8] Vitamin C is also an essential cofactor for many enzymes, and its depletion lowers levels of internally produced antioxidant enzymes such as superoxide dismutase (SOD), catalase, and glutathione peroxidase.[9] Low levels of these antioxidants may be associated with increased rates of cancers in humans, whether or not they consume alcohol.[10]

### Vitamin B1

Thiamine (vitamin B1) is an essential water-soluble vitamin. Thiamine deficiency can cause lethargy, fatigue, apathy, impaired awareness, loss of equilibrium, disorientation, memory loss, anorexia, muscular weakness, and eventually death.[11] Alcohol consumption depletes thiamine and produces the same symptoms as nonalcoholic thiamine deficiency.[12] Thiamine deficiency damages brain cells and other nerve cells throughout the body. Thiamine deficiency—rather than the toxic effects of ethanol—has been proposed as the primary cause of cerebellar degeneration in alcoholics.[13]

## Garlic Extract (S-allyl-cysteine)

Because the heavy consumption of alcohol produces many deleterious effects within the body, including an increased risk of cancer, liver disease, and neurologic disease, it is suggested that hangover-prevention ingredients such as garlic be taken any time alcohol is consumed. Garlic contains S-allyl-cysteine, a neutralizer of acetaldehyde.

S-allyl-cysteine scavenges free radicals and reduces oxidative stress.[14,15] In experimental animal models, S-allyl-cysteine helped protect the nervous system from neurotoxins and the kidneys against damage from reactive oxygen species.[14,15]

## Vitamin E

Brain and liver cells contain the lion's share of lipids among the body's organs, and lipid peroxidation rates are highest in the brain and liver due to their fat content. Accordingly, vitamin E content is also highest in these organs.

Nature has tailored vitamin E to block the peroxidation process, thus explaining its concentration in these two organs and its depletion by alcoholism and cirrhosis.[9,16,17] Vitamin E is an essential nutrient that may prevent damage caused by alcohol in the brain and liver.[18,19] As such, it is a supplement that should always be taken by those who consume alcohol.

## Selenium

In humans, low selenium status is associated with increased risk of colon cancer.[20] Selenium levels tend to be reduced in people who drink alcohol regularly.[21] That is especially concerning because selenium deficiency is a major risk factor for liver cancer; conversely, people with the highest levels of selenium in their tissues have a 50% reduction in risk for this cancer.[22]

## Glutathione

Oxidative stress combined with acetaldehyde causes a profound impairment of the body's natural antioxidant systems, by depleting stores of a compound called glutathione.[23] Restoring cellular healthy glutathione levels, therefore, seems to be a natural strategy to prevent alcohol-related cancers.

Glutathione, one of the body's most important natural antioxidants, plays a key role in alcohol detoxification. In the liver, glutathione binds to toxins and transforms them into compounds that can be excreted in the bile or urine. The liver's supply of glutathione may be exhausted by binding to carcinogens produced during alcohol detoxification by the liver. The direct conjugation of acetaldehyde and glutathione has been observed in acute models of alcohol ingestion. When depleted by chronic alcohol ingestion, glutathione becomes unavailable for ordinary regulatory processes.

These findings should not surprise anyone who understands that the ingestion of alcohol inflicts massive free-radical damage throughout the body. When a person is exposed to a known toxic substance (such as alcohol), it makes sense to take an antidote (antioxidants) to provide at least partial protection against the short-term (hangover) and long-term (degenerative disease) effects.

## Additional Support

**N-acetyl cysteine.** N-acetyl cysteine (NAC) powerfully replenishes glutathione levels in tissues, helping to fend off the consequences of acute oxidative stress.[24,25] Rats supplemented with NAC prior to treatment with acetaldehyde are potently protected against toxicity and death; the effect is even more powerful when combined with vitamin C and thiamine.[25] Independently, NAC binds acetaldehyde directly, further preventing its damaging effects.[26]

**Chlorophyllin.** Chlorophyllin is a water-soluble form of the green plant pigment chlorophyll.[27,28] It has been evaluated as a chemopreventive agent in populations at high risk for liver cancer, one of the most common tumors known, and one that is frequently caused by ingested toxins.[27–29] Chlorophyllin is a large molecule thought to bind to many carcinogens and toxins, enhancing their excretion from the body before they damage DNA.[29,30] Binding to toxins in the intestine prevents their uptake, further reducing their cancer-producing effects.[29] Chlorophyllin also induces important enzymes that protect against oxidants arising from toxins such as acetaldehyde, while also reducing expression of inflammatory mediators.[31,32]

**Grape seed extract.** Extracts of grape seeds are known to be powerful antioxidants with health benefits for many tissues. In both animal and human studies, these extracts reduce markers of oxidative damage and enhance natural antioxidant mechanisms to protect cells and DNA from injury.[33–37] Grape seed extracts have been shown to prevent alcohol-induced oxidative damage in all tissues examined in animal studies.[38,39] These extracts are highly bioavailable in humans, making them especially appealing in combating the cancer-causing effects of alcohol.[40,41]

**L-theanine.** L-theanine is a nonprotein amino acid found exclusively in green tea.[42,43] It contributes significantly to the favorable taste of green tea and has numerous health-promoting benefits.[42] Research from Japan shows that theanine is a powerful antidote to the effects of alcohol. If theanine is given to mice before or after they drink alcohol, it significantly lowers blood levels of alcohol.[44] It works by modulating alcohol chemistry.

Theanine accelerates the breakdown of acetaldehyde and blocks toxic radicals.[44] The remarkable powers of theanine to intercept free radicals were demonstrated in the same study. It blocked radicals caused by alcohol and suppressed levels to below normal for 5 hours. Theanine also helps to counteract the alcohol-induced loss of glutathione.[44]

**S-adenosylmethionine (SAMe).**   As already discussed, supplementing with the right antioxidants while consuming ethanol significantly reduces consequences of these free radicals throughout the body. SAMe has additional value because, like NAC, it helps restore depleted glutathione in alcohol-damaged cells, providing additional antioxidant protection.[45,46]

Ethanol also depresses an enzyme required to convert methionine into S-adenosylmethionine (SAMe),[47] resulting in a deficiency of SAMe. Alcohol-induced depletion of SAMe can be overcome by SAMe supplementation, which restores hepatic SAMe levels.[48–51]

Supplementation with SAMe may help support healthy liver function. For those who cannot afford SAMe, supplementation with trimethylglycine (TMG, also known as glycine betaine), folic acid, and vitamin B12 could help the liver to synthesize SAMe.

**Probiotics.**   One reason that 30% of alcoholics develop cirrhosis may be a leaky gastrointestinal system. According to research,[52] another factor might be a gut-derived endotoxin. This would suggest that the use of probiotic substances might aid in the prevention of cirrhosis or other liver damage. Probiotics are beneficial bacteria that help to recolonize the intestinal tract. Intestinal flora (bacteria) help our digestive system absorb nutrients and act as a protective barrier in keeping toxins out. Along with taking a probiotic formula, a supplement to nourish intestinal flora such as fructo-oligosaccharides (FOSs) is suggested. FOSs help reduce the formation of toxic liver metabolites and therefore is beneficial to people with chronic liver problems.

**Magnesium.**   Chronic alcohol consumption can constrict arteries in the brain and lead to neurologic deficit.[53] Daily supplementation could help keep cerebral blood vessels open by blocking excess infiltration of calcium into endothelial cells.

**Milk thistle extracts—silymarin and silibinin.** Silymarin is a compound extracted from the milk thistle plant. It has long been used to improve liver health and enhance excretion of toxins, particularly those that are related to alcohol toxicity. Silymarin is a powerful antioxidant and protects DNA from cancer-inducing damage, especially in alcohol-induced liver disease.[54,55] It inhibits conversion of ethanol to acetaldehyde and reduces cell proliferation in laboratory models of liver cancer.[56]

Those who drink routinely might consider taking a special milk thistle extract called silibinin, which may have a protective effect on the liver.[57] Clinical evidence supports silibinin for alcohol-induced cirrhosis.[58,59] Silibinin is the most active constituent of silymarin. In Germany, silibinin is sold as a drug to treat liver diseases.

**Picrorhiza.**   *Picrorhiza kurroa* is a member of the figwort family, with a long history of use in traditional south Asian medical systems.[60] *Picrorhiza* extracts given to laboratory animals following chronic alcohol ingestion reverse most of the deleterious biochemical changes induced by alcohol.[61,62] A powerful antioxidant,[60] *Picrorhiza* also has specific anticancer effects, inhibiting toxin-induced cancer generation and increasing life span of tumor-afflicted animals.[63,64]

**Polyenylphosphatidylcholine (PPC).**   PPC is a fat-soluble nutrient with many health-promoting benefits. These include protecting the liver, sustaining cardiovascular health, and supporting nervous system and gastrointestinal function. Dietary sources of PPC include soybeans, liver, oatmeal, cabbage, cauliflower, egg yolk, meat, and vegetables.

For those who consume large amounts of alcohol (ie, binge drinkers), PPC supplementation is recommended prior to alcohol consumption. The administration of PPC has been shown to provide significant protection against certain forms of alcohol-induced liver injury in animals via several unique mechanisms.[48–51,65] PPC also reduces gastric irritation.[66]

In a study in mice, alcohol administration induced numerous changes, depleting the liver-supportive nutrients SAMe and glutathione, as well as increasing lipid peroxidation. PPC protected against these effects, restoring levels of SAMe and glutathione, and relieving oxidative stress in the liver.[67]

In a study of baboons, PPC helped to prevent alcohol-induced cirrhosis. PPC also helped to prevent two common detrimental effects of alcohol: the formation of fatty liver and the elevation of blood lipid levels.[68] In a human study, investigators examined the effects of PPC on heavy alcohol drinkers. While PPC treatment for 2 years did not affect the progression of liver fibrosis, it did promote favorable changes in blood levels of bilirubin (a liver-produced waste product) and liver transaminases (enzymes that are elevated by liver damage).[69]

**European medications.** European medications such as Picamilon (50 mg, 3 times/day) and Pyritinol (200 mg, 3 times/day) could help prevent and restore neurologic function lost due to chronic ethanol intake. An expensive prescription drug called Nimotop® (nimodipine), at the dosage of 30 mg 3–4 times per day, can slowly repair central nervous system damage caused by excess alcohol intake.

## Life Extension Suggestions

Take the following supplements prior to alcohol consumption or before going to bed:

- **Glutathione** (reduced): 50 mg
- **N-acetyl-L-cysteine** (NAC): 1200 mg
- **Vitamin C:** 3000 mg
- **Vitamin E:** 50 IU
- **Thiamine** (vitamin B1): 100 mg
- **Selenium:** 25 mcg
- **Chlorophyllin:** 20 mg
- **Grape seed extract** (standardized to proanthocyanidins): 20 mg
- **Silymarin** (milk thistle extract): 20 mg

- *Picrorhiza kurroa* **extract** (root standardized to kutkin): 15 mg
- **Garlic extract:** 400–800 mg
- **Polyenylphosphatidylcholine** (PPC): 1800–3600 mg
- **L-theanine:** per label instructions

These supplements can be taken regularly:

- **Milk thistle extract:** standardized to contain 600 mg silymarin and 225 mg silibinin daily
- **Probiotic:** per label instructions
- **Fructo-oligosaccharide** (FOS): per label instructions
- **Magnesium:** 500–1500 mg daily
- **S-adenosylmethionine** (SAMe): 400–1200 mg daily, or an alternative to raise SAMe levels in the liver includes the following:
  - **Trimethylglycine** (TMG): 500 mg daily
  - **Folic acid:** 800 mcg daily
  - **Vitamin B12:** 500 mcg twice daily

**Note:** *Alcohol depletes many vitamins and minerals from the body, so taking high-potency vitamin-mineral supplements throughout the day is very important. For protecting and restoring liver function lost because of alcohol damage, see the "Cirrhosis and Liver Disease" protocol.*

## REFERENCES

References available at: www.lef.org/dpt5/ch66

# 67

# Hearing Loss and Tinnitus

Hearing loss is one of the most common chronic conditions in older adults, with an estimated 36 million Americans reporting some degree of hearing impairment.[1,2] Next to arthritis, it is the second most common handicapping condition.[3,4] Although hearing loss is more common with age, approximately 8.5% of American adults aged 20–29 have significant hearing loss, a number that appears to be rising.[5]

Hearing loss and a related condition, *tinnitus* or "ringing in the ears," can become severe obstacles in communicating and interacting with others, contributing to poor quality of life. Moreover, hearing loss can lead to reduced neurologic activity in the parts of the brain that process speech, and atrophy in the parts that process sound in general.[6–8]

## UNDERSTANDING HEARING LOSS AND TINNITUS

Hearing loss can be *conductive*, *sensorineural*, or *mixed*, which is a combination of conductive and sensorineural. The type of hearing loss is correlated with the anatomic part of the ear affected (outer, middle, or inner ear). Generally, damage to the outer and middle ear causes conductive hearing loss, whereas inner ear damage results in sensorineural hearing loss.[9]

### Conductive Hearing Loss

Outer and middle ear conductive hearing loss could be caused by infections, trauma, congenital malformations, or tumors in the outer ear. Otitis media, a common childhood disease that can also affect adults, is one of the most common types of ear infections to cause hearing loss; similarly, viral infections of the upper respiratory tract can affect the ear and cause temporary hearing loss. Trauma to the tympanic membrane, one of the middle ear structures that help translate sound waves into interpretable neurologic signals, can also result in conductive hearing loss. The tympanic membrane can become damaged by direct trauma, which can be caused by a foreign body such as a cotton swab (eg, Q-tip®),

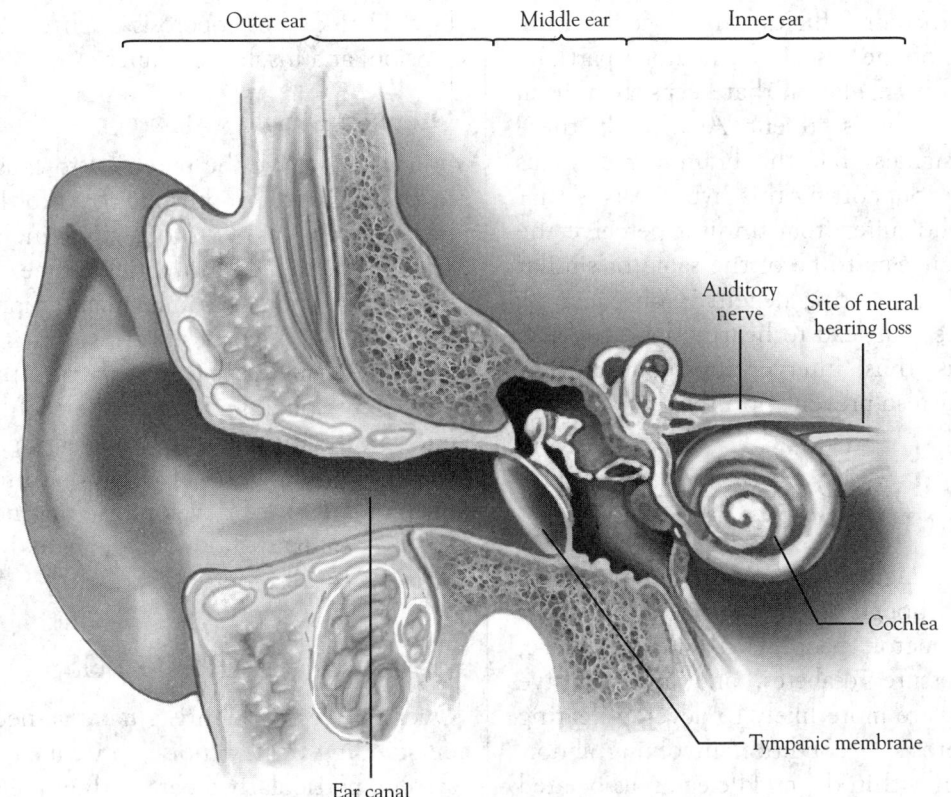

Outer ear     Middle ear     Inner ear

Auditory nerve

Site of neural hearing loss

Cochlea

Tympanic membrane

Ear canal

Anatomy of the Ear

infection, and sudden changes in air pressure (middle ear barotrauma).[10]

## Sensorineural Hearing Loss

Damage to the inner ear is usually responsible for hearing loss that progresses over time. *Presbycusis*, or age-related deterioration of hearing ability, is marked by the gradual loss of high-frequency hearing on both sides in elderly individuals.[11] Presbycusis is also associated with tinnitus. Excessive noise can also cause sensorineural hearing loss that can gradually increase over time. Loud noise damages the delicate structures in the ear both due to trauma and accumulation of free radicals and excess glutamate, as well as altering intracellular magnesium and calcium levels.[12] Infections and a condition called Ménière's disease can also lead to inner ear damage and sensorineural hearing loss.[10,13]

## Tinnitus

Closely linked to hearing loss is a condition known as *tinnitus*, characterized by a persistent ringing sensation in the ears. Although tinnitus can be triggered by a variety of causes, the majority of cases are associated with hearing loss.[14] Researchers are still working to understand the process behind tinnitus. One popular hypothesis is when the hair cells (specialized nerve cells that help translate sound waves into interpretable signals for the brain, not to be confused with hair follicles) in the cochlea are damaged, some of the associated neurons partially lose the inhibitory regulation that keeps them from firing when no sound is present. As a result, these neurons send signals that the brain perceives as persistent noise. Supporting this hypothesis is that many people who suffer from tinnitus perceive the "ringing" in their ears to be of the same or similar frequency to their hearing deficits. Consequently, similar processes that lead to hearing loss may also lead to tinnitus; thus, interventions that prevent hearing loss may also prevent tinnitus.[14]

## CAUSES OF AND RISK FACTORS FOR HEARING LOSS

A number of risk factors can predispose a person to hearing loss. Although advancing age is the most important risk factor, people with heart disease, high blood pressure, diabetes, and an extensive smoking history are more likely to develop hearing loss.[3,15] Otosclerosis, a condition involving abnormal bone growth within the middle ear, is associated with both conductive and sensorineural hearing

loss.[16–19] In addition, hearing loss is more common in men.[5]

## Noise Exposure

Repeated exposure to loud noises from occupational sources, recreational activities, or firearms strongly correlates with an increased risk of unilateral (hearing loss in one ear), bilateral (hearing loss in both ears), and high-frequency hearing loss.[5] According to a 2007 report, approximately 30 million Americans are exposed to dangerous levels of noise every day, with 10 million adults and 5.2 million children affected by irreversible hearing loss due to excessive noise exposure.[20] In addition, noise-induced hearing loss is the largest single category of compensated occupational disease in Europe.[21]

The National Institute of Occupational Safety and Health considers noise levels above 85 decibels to be harmful.[22] Although sustained levels of loud noise are dangerous, impulse noise (ie, large bursts of loud noise) can also damage hearing. In fact, research suggests that short exposure to very loud noise, such as that experienced by soldiers, can be more damaging to the auditory system than continuous noise.[23]

Not only does excessive noise damage hearing, it may also increase blood pressure and heart rate, increase physiologic stress, and raise cortisol levels.[20] Elevated cortisol levels are associated with an increased risk of osteoporosis, high cholesterol, hypertension, and insulin resistance.[24]

## Ototoxic Drugs

Some drugs have the potential to cause hearing loss or tinnitus because they are toxic to the ear or "ototoxic." Examples of ototoxic drugs include high doses of aspirin, some antibiotics, some chemotherapy drugs, and some anti-inflammatory medications.[25–29] For example, high doses of aspirin in the range of 2000–4000 mg daily can cause tinnitus and hearing loss via peripheral effects on the cochlea and central effects on nerves involved in hearing. These effects usually subside within 1–3 days of discontinuing aspirin.[30–33] Risk of developing drug-induced hearing loss is greater in those with impaired kidney health or inner ear disorders.[26]

## HOW HEARING LOSS OCCURS

Over the years, scientists have gained a better understanding of how noise can damage the auditory system, particularly a part of the inner ear known as the cochlea. The cochlea contains specialized nerve cells, known as hair cells, which help translate sound waves into interpretable signals for the brain. Loud sounds damage hair cells through direct mechanical trauma and secondary metabolic damage. Direct mechanical trauma typically causes immediate structural damage to cochlear hair cells and can potentially cause immediately detectable hearing loss. The metabolic effects of loud noise, however, can accumulate for days or even weeks after initial sound exposure.[34]

Loud noise affects metabolism in hair cells by decreasing oxygen supply and increasing energy demands. Loud noise can disrupt the flow in blood vessels that supply oxygen to hair cells, depriving these cells of nutrients needed to function and leading to cell damage through a process known as ischemia. At the same time, the increased stimulation due to noise forces the hair cells to be metabolically more active. The end result is that, during this period of intense stimulation, these hair cells burn through their energy reserves, resulting in the formation of reactive oxygen species (ROS). These ROS have the ability to damage proteins and lipids and can ultimately lead to death of the hair cells.[35]

Hair cells may also be damaged by inflammatory mediators known as cytokines. Animal studies have found an increase in certain proinflammatory cytokines in response to loud noise. These cytokines include interleukin-6 (IL-6) and tumor necrosis factor-alpha (TNF-α), two compounds that can be toxic to nerve cells at high levels.[36] In addition, overstimulation of hair cells can cause them to release large amounts of the neurotransmitter glutamate. Although glutamate release is needed to help translate sounds into neurological signals, too much glutamate can result in significant "excitotoxicity," in which excessive stimulation damages nerve cells.[37]

## THERAPIES FOR HEARING LOSS AND TINNITUS

### Hearing Loss

**Hearing aids.** One of the most common treatments for hearing loss is the use of hearing aids. Hearing aids are devices that amplify sound waves, making it easier to hear sounds. There are a variety of hearing aids available, and people who are hard of hearing typically need to go to a trained specialist to determine exactly what type of hearing aid is appropriate.[38] Studies estimate, however, that only about 15–20% of people who could benefit from hearing aids use them. This may be due to cost or because people often consider mild

hearing loss inconsequential, and therefore do not seek treatment.[39,40]

## HORMONE REPLACEMENT THERAPY FOR HEARING LOSS

One interesting development in the field of hearing loss research is the potential link between *aldosterone* levels and hearing loss. Aldosterone is a hormone that helps to regulate blood pressure and electrolyte levels. Research has found that higher aldosterone levels may help protect the cochlea from age-related hearing loss.[41] A case study has also been published detailing a child with genetically low aldosterone levels and otherwise unexplained sensorineural hearing loss.[42] Currently, the Tahoma Clinic in Seattle is recruiting volunteers for a study examining the effects of aldosterone supplementation on hearing loss.[43]

### Tinnitus

**Behavioral therapies.** Treatment for tinnitus includes behavioral therapies (ie, therapeutic behavior modification). One specialized therapy, known as tinnitus retraining therapy, aims to train the brain to ignore symptoms of tinnitus unless specifically focusing on ringing in the ears. Cognitive-behavioral therapy and biofeedback can also be used to help learn to manage responses of the mind and body to tinnitus, thus allowing people to minimize its effects on their daily lives.[44-46]

**Masking and electrical stimulation.** Sound-masking devices are commonly used to treat tinnitus. These devices emit low levels of noise designed to help reduce the perception of tinnitus.[47] However, it has been seen that masking by itself is not as effective in reducing the severity of tinnitus as certain other treatment options, such as relaxation techniques, counseling, and tinnitus retraining.[48]

Electrical stimulation of the cochlea, via electrodes placed on parts of the ear, can also provide relief from tinnitus in people who also have hearing loss.[45,49]

**Neuromodulation.** One emerging treatment for tinnitus is neuromodulation, a process that helps correct the "misfiring" or continuous "firing" of neurons in the brain leading to tinnitus. Various methods and devices for this purpose are being researched.[50] One of them, called repetitive transcranial magnetic stimulation (rTMS), uses magnetic pulses to modulate brain activity; preliminary results show that it is effective for reducing tinnitus symptoms.[51] Deep brain stimulation, a technique in which electrodes are carefully placed in certain areas of the brain in order to deliver therapeutic electrical signals, has also been researched as a potential treatment for tinnitus.[52] One of the most novel therapies to treat tinnitus is acoustic stimulation. A device used for this treatment has been found to be both safe and effective,[53] and has the added advantage of being relatively small and portable.[50]

**Medications.** Some drugs have been shown to partially relieve tinnitus or ease emotional distress associated with tinnitus or hearing loss; these include antidepressants, sleep aids, and antipsychotics.[54,55] However, efficacy has proven inconsistent in trials and more evidence is needed before the best drug strategy can be determined.[56,57]

# TARGETED NUTRITIONAL THERAPIES

## Antioxidants

Antioxidants are compounds that have the ability to neutralize damaging ROS. Since ROS are involved in the development and progression of tinnitus and hearing loss, antioxidants represent a promising therapeutic strategy.[58–60]

**N-acetyl cysteine.** N-acetyl cysteine (NAC) is a naturally occurring antioxidant that has been used for years to treat acetaminophen overdose and break up mucus; it also increases the production of glutathione, one of the most prevalent antioxidants in the body.[61] NAC has been studied as a potential therapeutic agent to protect hair cells from damage due to excessive noise as well. A 2011 study on military recruits found that NAC was able to protect the cochlea from damage due to noise from firing a gun in an enclosed space.[62] Animal studies have also found that NAC has a protective effect against continuous loud noises[63,64] as well as impulse noise.[65] Another animal study showed that NAC may reduce noise-induced hearing loss even when administered after exposure to dangerous levels of noise.[66] NAC has generated interest in the field of hearing loss because it is safe for human consumption and has already been approved for some uses in humans (eg, treatment of acetaminophen toxicity).[61]

**Acetyl-L-carnitine.** Mitochondria are the energy power plants of the cell. They are also the site of ROS production, especially when the cell is under stress. In cochlear hair cells, mutations in mitochondrial DNA and declining function of the mitochondria have been found to cause age-induced hearing loss.[67] As a result, compounds that help maintain mitochondrial health, such as acetyl-L-carnitine,

may help protect cells from damage. Animal studies have found that acetyl-L-carnitine is able to protect the cochlea from both continuous and impulse noise damage as well as prevent loss of hair cells.[65,68] Acetyl-L-carnitine was also found to reduce mutations in mitochondrial DNA, suggesting that it could prevent not only noise-induced hearing loss, but also age-related hearing loss.[69] Much like NAC, acetyl-L-carnitine appears to be effective even when administered after exposure to loud noise(s).[66,70] In one animal study, acetyl-L-carnitine was shown to protect against ototoxicity induced by the chemotherapeutic drug cisplatin.[71]

**Lipoic acid.** Lipoic acid has been found to reduce age-related hearing loss.[69] Preliminary animal studies have also found that lipoic acid can help protect against noise-induced hearing loss and preserve inner-ear mitochondrial function.[72,73] This may be partly due to the effect it has on glutathione (ie, a naturally occurring antioxidant in the body). Studies have found that increasing glutathione levels help protect the cochlea from damage due to loud noises.[74] In one laboratory study, lipoic acid was shown to increase glutathione levels in nerve cells, protecting them from damage.[75] Lipoic acid may also be able to counteract the action of toxins (eg, carbon monoxide) that aggravate the effects of noise and make normally safe levels of volume harmful to the ear.[76] In a clinical trial among 46 elderly subjects with hearing loss, 8 weeks of treatment with lipoic acid (60 mg/day) combined with 2 other free radical scavengers (vitamin C 600 mg/day and rebamipide 300 mg/day) significantly improved hearing at all frequencies tested.[77]

**Vitamins.** Dietary supplementation with vitamins that have antioxidant capabilities can help protect the hair cells of the cochlea. One animal study showed that a 35-day pretreatment regimen of vitamin C may be able to protect against noise-induced hearing loss.[78] Similarly, supplementing animals with certain forms of vitamins A and E have shown significant protective effects.[79,80] The length of time that vitamins need to be taken prior to noise exposure may vary depending on the vitamin. For example, vitamin E appears to be effective with 3 days of pretreatment, vitamin A may only require 2 days to be effective, and vitamin C may require a longer pretreatment period. In addition, taking vitamins in combination may be more effective than any one of them alone.[74] For example, a combination of B vitamins, vitamins C and E, and L-carnitine protected rodents from cisplatin ototoxicity.[81]

**Folate and vitamin B12.** Folate and vitamin B12 are important for the functioning of many cells in the body, including nerve cells. They also help reduce levels of homocysteine, a potentially toxic compound found in the body. Elevated homocysteine levels are linked to an increased risk of hearing problems.[82,83] Vitamin B12 injections (1 mg for 7 days followed by 5 mg on day 8) protected against noise-induced hearing loss in healthy volunteers aged 20–30 years.[84] Researchers have found that patients with low levels of folate in their blood are more likely to develop hearing loss,[82,83,85] and that low vitamin B12 levels are associated with hearing loss[82] and tinnitus.[86]

**Magnesium.** Because loud noise impairs blood flow to the cochlea, researchers have also examined compounds that could help improve circulation to the hair cells and prevent their death. Magnesium is known to help expand blood vessels and improve circulation; it also helps control the release of glutamate, one of the major contributors to noise-induced hearing loss.[87] Animal studies have found that magnesium deficiency increases the risk of noise-induced hearing loss.[88,89] A combination of magnesium and other antioxidants may synergistically prevent hearing loss, potentially because magnesium's ability to increase blood flow also helps transport the protective antioxidants.[87] Other animal studies have determined that magnesium can protect against impulse noise damage.[90,91] Magnesium's benefits have been demonstrated in human trials as well; magnesium supplementation (122 mg daily for 10 days) reduced noise-induced hearing loss in men aged 16–37 years.[92] Studies have also found that both intravenous magnesium and oral magnesium supplementation may be beneficial for other types of hearing loss, such as sudden sensorineural hearing loss.[93,94]

**Melatonin.** Melatonin, a hormone critical for healthy sleep,[95] has powerful antioxidant properties. Animal studies have found that it is effective at preventing hearing damage after exposure to loud noises.[96,97] It is also effective at treating other types of hearing loss caused by ROS, such as due to the chemotherapy drug cisplatin.[98] Researchers have discussed the potential for melatonin to act as a protectant against age-related hearing loss.[99] For example, it was noted in a study that low plasma levels of melatonin were associated with significant high-frequency hearing loss among elderly subjects.[100]

Additionally, melatonin has been tested as a treatment for tinnitus, both in combination with the medication sulpiride (an atypical antipsychotic) and on its own. On its own, melatonin provides relief from tinnitus, especially in people with significant sleep problems.[101-103] When combined with sulpiride, melatonin reduces the perception of tinnitus by diminishing the activity of dopamine, a chemical in the brain. In one study, sulpiride alone relieved tinnitus in 56% of subjects while melatonin alone reduced tinnitus in 40%. However, when used together, 81% of subjects reported relief from their tinnitus symptoms.[104]

**Ginkgo biloba.** Ginkgo biloba, a commonly used herbal supplement, has attracted interest as a means of protecting against hearing loss as well as a treatment for tinnitus. Early animal studies found that when a standardized preparation of Ginkgo biloba extract was given as a supplement to animals, it reduced behavioral manifestations of tinnitus.[105] This extract, at a dose of 160 mg daily over a 12-week period, was also effective at reducing symptoms in humans.[106] However, other studies have found negligible or no effect[107,108]; therefore, more research is needed in this area. Ginkgo biloba may also be effective at preventing hearing loss that causes tinnitus; an animal study found that a Gingko biloba extract was able to reduce drug-induced oxidative damage to hair cells in the cochlea.[109]

**Coenzyme Q10.** Coenzyme Q10 (CoQ10) supports mitochondrial function and has significant antioxidant properties.[110] Animal studies have found that supplementation with CoQ10 reduced noise-induced hearing loss and the death of hair cells.[111-113] Human studies have also yielded promising results, as 160–600 mg of CoQ10 daily was found to reduce hearing loss in people with sudden sensorineural hearing loss and presbycusis.[114-116] Also, a small preliminary trial found that CoQ10 supplementation alleviated tinnitus in those whose CoQ10 blood levels were initially low.[117] Another small trial found that CoQ10 may slow progression of hearing loss associated with a mitochondrial genetic mutation.[118]

**Zinc.** Zinc, a mineral involved in many physiologic processes (including nervous system function), has antioxidant and anti-inflammatory properties.[119,120] Evidence suggests that inadequate zinc intake may be associated with impaired hearing.[121] Researchers have found that zinc supplementation may be helpful in treating some forms of hearing loss.[122] In addition, low levels of zinc correlate with perceived loudness of tinnitus in afflicted individuals.[123]

**Omega-3 fatty acids.** Long-chain omega-3 (n-3) polyunsaturated fatty acids (PUFAs), long recognized as important for health, may also affect hearing loss; a preliminary study found that participants with the highest blood levels of these beneficial fats suffered the least amount of hearing loss over time.[124] In another study, greater fish or fish oil consumption was associated with less hearing loss among nearly 3000 subjects over 50 years of age. The authors remarked that "*dietary intervention with n-3 PUFAs could prevent or delay the development of age-related hearing loss.*"[125]

## Life Extension Suggestions

- **N-acetyl-cysteine** (NAC): 600–1800 mg daily
- **Acetyl-L-carnitine:** 1000–2000 mg daily
- **R-lipoic acid:** 240–480 mg daily
- **Vitamin C:** 1000–2000 mg daily
- **Vitamin A:** 5000 IU (as 90% beta-carotene and 10% acetate) daily in divided doses
- **Vitamin E:** 100–400 IU alpha-tocopherol and 200 mg gamma-tocopherol daily
- **Zinc:** 30 mg daily
- **Coenzyme Q10,** as ubiquinol: 100–300 mg daily

- **Fish oil (with olive polyphenols):** providing 1400 mg EPA and 1000 mg DHA daily
- **Ginkgo biloba**, standardized extract: 120 mg daily
- **Magnesium:** 140 mg daily as magnesium-L-threonate, 320 mg daily as magnesium citrate
- **Melatonin:** 0.3–5 mg before bed (sometimes up to 10 mg)
- **Folate:** 400 mcg–1000 mcg daily
- **Vitamin B12:** 300 mcg–5000 mcg daily
- **Earplugs:** per label instructions

In addition, the following *blood tests* may be helpful:

- Omega Score®
- Coenzyme Q10 (CoQ10)

## REFERENCES

References available at: www.lef.org/dpt5/ch67

# 68

# *Heavy Metal Detoxification*

There are 35 metals that concern us because of occupational or residential exposure; 23 of these are the heavy elements or "heavy metals": antimony, arsenic, bismuth, cadmium, cerium, chromium, cobalt, copper, gallium, gold, iron, lead, manganese, mercury, nickel, platinum, silver, tellurium, thallium, tin, uranium, vanadium, and zinc.[1] Small amounts of these elements are common in our environment and diet and are actually necessary for good health, but large amounts of any of them may cause acute or chronic toxicity (poisoning). Heavy metal toxicity can result in damaged or reduced mental and central nervous function, lower energy levels, and damage to blood composition, lungs, kidneys, liver, and other vital organs. Long-term exposure may result in slowly progressing physical, muscular, and neurologic degenerative processes that mimic Alzheimer's disease, Parkinson's disease, muscular dystrophy, and multiple sclerosis. Allergies are not uncommon, and repeated long-term contact with some metals (or their compounds) may cause cancer.[2]

For some heavy metals, toxic levels can be just above the background concentrations naturally found in nature. Therefore, it is important to learn about heavy metals and take protective measures against excessive exposure. In most parts of the United States, heavy metal toxicity is an uncommon medical condition; however, it is a clinically significant condition when it does occur. If unrecognized or inappropriately treated, toxicity can result in significant illness and reduced quality of life.[3] For persons who suspect that they or someone in their household might have heavy metal toxicity, testing is essential. Appropriate conventional and natural medical procedures may need to be pursued.[4]

The association of symptoms indicative of acute toxicity is not difficult to recognize because they are usually severe, rapid in onset, and associated with a known exposure or ingestion.[3] Symptoms include: cramping, nausea, and vomiting; pain; sweating; headache; difficulty breathing; impaired cognitive, motor, and language skills; mania; and convulsions. Symptoms of chronic exposure (impaired cognitive, motor, and language skills; learning difficulties; nervousness and emotional instability; and insomnia, nausea, lethargy, and feeling ill) are also easily recognized; however, they are much more difficult to associate with their cause. Symptoms resulting from chronic exposure are very similar to symptoms of other health conditions and often develop slowly over months or even years. Sometimes symptoms of chronic exposure subside; thinking the symptoms are related to something else, people postpone seeking treatment.

## Definition of a Heavy Metal

"Heavy metals" are chemical elements with a specific gravity at least 5 times that of water. The specific gravity of water is 1 at 4 °C (39 °F). Specific gravity is a measure of density of a given amount of a solid substance when it is compared to an equal amount of water. Some well-known toxic metals with a specific gravity 5 or more times that of water are arsenic (5.7), cadmium (8.65), iron (7.9), lead (11.34), and mercury (13.546).[5]

## Beneficial Heavy Metals

In small quantities, certain heavy metals are nutritionally essential for a healthy life. Some of these are trace elements (eg, iron, copper, manganese, and zinc). These elements, or some form of them, are commonly found naturally in foodstuffs, fruits and vegetables, and in commercially available multivitamin products.[2] Diagnostic medical applications include direct injection of gallium during radiologic procedures, dosing with chromium in parenteral nutrition mixtures, and using lead as a radiation shield around x-ray equipment.[6] Heavy metals are also common in industrial applications such as the manufacture of pesticides, batteries, alloys, electroplated metal parts, textile dyes, steel, and so forth.[2] Many of these products are in our homes and add to quality of life when properly used.

## Toxic Heavy Metals

Heavy metals become toxic when they are not metabolized by the body and accumulate in the soft tissues. Heavy metals may enter the human body via food, water, air, or absorption through the skin in agriculture, manufacturing, pharmaceutical, industrial, or residential settings. Industrial exposure is common in adults. Ingestion is the most common route in children.[6] Children may develop toxic levels from normal hand-to-mouth activity (ie, coming in contact with contaminated soil or eating non-food objects [eg, dirt or paint chips]).[4] Less common routes of exposure include a radiologic procedure, inappropriate dosing or monitoring during intravenous (parenteral) nutrition, a broken thermometer,[7] or a suicide or homicide attempt.[8]

As a rule, acute poisoning is more likely to result from inhalation or contact with dust, fumes or vapors, or materials in the workplace. However, lesser levels of contamination may occur in residential settings, particularly in older homes with lead paint or old plumbing.[2] The Agency for Toxic Substances and Disease Registry (ATSDR) in Atlanta, Georgia (a part of the U.S. Department of Health and Human Services) was established by congressional mandate to perform specific functions concerning adverse human health effects and diminished quality of life associated with exposure to hazardous substances. The ATSDR is responsible for assessment of waste sites and providing health information concerning hazardous substances, response to emergency release situations, and education and training concerning hazardous substances.[9] In cooperation with the U.S. Environmental Protection Agency, the ATSDR has compiled a Priority List for 2001 called the "Top 20 Hazardous Substances." The heavy metals arsenic (1), lead (2), mercury (3), and cadmium (7) appear on this list.

Note: *The ATSDR provides comprehensive protocols called Medical Management Guidelines for Acute Chemical Exposures in Volume III of the Managing Hazardous Material Incidents Series. These protocols have a Chemical Abstracts Service (CAS) number and give a description of toxic substances, routes of exposure, health effects, prehospital, triage, and emergency medical department care, antidotes and treatment, disposition and follow-up, and reporting instructions. The series may be viewed or downloaded from the ATSDR website at no cost.*

# COMMONLY ENCOUNTERED TOXIC HEAVY METALS

As noted earlier, there are 35 metals of concern, 23 of them heavy metals. Toxicity can result from any of these metals. This protocol will address the metals most likely encountered in our daily environment. Four metals included in the ATSDR's Top 20 Hazardous Substances list will be covered in this protocol. Iron and aluminum, which do not appear on the ATSDR's list, will also be discussed.

## Arsenic

Arsenic, number 1 on the ATSDR's top 20 list, is the most common cause of acute heavy metal poisoning in adults. Arsenic is released into the environment by the smelting process of copper, zinc, and lead, as well as the manufacturing of chemicals and glasses. Arsine gas is a common byproduct produced by the manufacturing of pesticides that contain arsenic. Arsenic may be also be found in water supplies worldwide, leading to exposure of shellfish, cod, and haddock. Other sources are paints, rat poisoning, fungicides, and wood preservatives. Target organs are the blood, kidneys, and central nervous, digestive, and skin systems.[6,10]

## Lead

Lead is number 2 on the ATSDR's top 20 list. Lead accounts for most cases of pediatric heavy metal poisoning.[6] It is a very soft metal and was used in pipes, drains, and soldering materials for many years. Millions of homes built before 1940 still contain lead (eg, in painted surfaces), leading to chronic exposure from weathering, flaking, chalking, and dust. Every year, industry produces about 2.5 million tons of lead throughout the world. Most of this lead is used for batteries. The remainder is used for cable coverings, plumbing, ammunition, and fuel additives. Other uses include paint pigments and in PVC plastics, x-ray shielding, crystal glass production, and pesticides. Lead targets the bones, brain, blood, kidneys, and thyroid gland.[2,11]

## Mercury

Number 3 on ATSDR's top 20 list is mercury. Mercury is generated naturally in the environment from degassing of the earth's crust, from volcanic emissions. It exists in 3 forms: elemental mercury, organic and inorganic mercury. Mining operations, chloralkali plants, and paper industries are significant producers of mercury.[12] Atmospheric mercury is dispersed across the globe by wind and returns to the earth in rainfall, accumulating in aquatic food chains and lake fish.[13] Mercury compounds were added to paint as a fungicide until 1990. These compounds are now banned; however, old paint supplies and surfaces painted with these old supplies still exist. Mercury continues to be used in thermometers, thermostats, and dental amalgam. (Many researchers suspect dental amalgam to be a possible source of mercury toxicity.[14,15]) Medicines, such as mercurochrome and merthiolate, are still available. Algaecides and childhood vaccines are also potential sources. Inhalation is the most frequent cause of exposure to mercury. The organic form is readily absorbed in the gastrointestinal tract (90–100%); lesser, but still significant amounts of inorganic mercury are absorbed in the gastrointestinal tract (7–15%). Mercury targets the brain and kidneys.[6,16]

## Cadmium

Cadmium, number 7 on ATSDR's top 20 list, is a by-product of the mining and smelting of lead and zinc. It is used in nickel-cadmium batteries, PVC plastics, and paint pigments. It can be found in soils because insecticides, fungicides, sludge, and commercial fertilizers that use cadmium are used in agriculture. Cadmium may be found in reservoirs containing shellfish. Cigarettes also contain cadmium. Lesser-known sources of exposure are dental alloys, electroplating, motor oil, and exhaust. Inhalation accounts for 15–50% of absorption through the respiratory system; 2–7% of ingested cadmium is absorbed in the gastrointestinal system. Cadmium targets the liver, placenta, kidneys, lungs, brain, and bones.[6,17]

## Iron

Discussion of iron toxicity in this protocol is limited to ingested or environmental exposure. Iron overload disease (hemochromatosis), an inherited disorder, is discussed in a separate protocol. Iron does not appear on the ATSDR's top 20 list, but it is a heavy metal of concern, particularly because ingesting dietary iron supplements may acutely poison young children (eg, as few as five to nine 30-mg iron tablets for a 30-lb child).

Ingestion accounts for most of the toxic effects of iron because iron is absorbed rapidly in the gastrointestinal tract. The corrosive nature of iron seems to further increase the absorption. Most overdoses appear to be the result of children mistaking red-coated ferrous sulfate tablets or adult multivitamin preparations for candy. Fatalities from overdoses have decreased significantly with the introduction of child-proof packaging. In recent years, blister packaging and the requirement that containers with 250 mg or more of iron have child-proof bottle caps have helped reduce accidental ingestion and overdose of iron tablets by children. Other sources of iron include drinking water, iron pipes, and cookware. Iron targets the liver, cardiovascular system, and kidneys.[6]

## Aluminum

Although aluminum is not a heavy metal (specific gravity of 2.55–2.80), it makes up about 8% of the Earth's surface and is the third most abundant element.[18] It is readily available for human ingestion through the following sources: food additives, antacids, buffered aspirin, drinking water, automobile exhaust, tobacco smoke, and use of nasal sprays, astringents, antiperspirants, aluminum foil, aluminum cookware, cans, ceramics, and fireworks.[18]

About 20 years ago, researchers began to find what they considered to be significant amounts of aluminum in the brain tissue of Alzheimer's patients. Although aluminum was also found in the brain tissue of people without Alzheimer's disease, recommendations to avoid sources of aluminum received widespread public attention. As a result, many organizations and individuals began to dispose of all their aluminum cookware and storage containers, and become wary of other possible sources of aluminum (eg, soda cans, personal care products, and drinking water).[19]

However, although there were studies that demonstrate a positive relationship between aluminum in drinking water and Alzheimer's disease, the World Health Organization (WHO) had reservations about a causal relationship because the studies did not account for total aluminum intake from all possible sources.[20] Although there is no conclusive evidence for or against aluminum as a primary cause for Alzheimer's disease, most researchers agree it is an important factor in dementia and deserves continuing research. Reducing exposure to aluminum is a personal decision. Workers in the automobile manufacturing industry also have concerns about long-term exposure to aluminum (contained in metalworking fluids) and the development of degenerative muscular conditions as well as cancer.[21,22] The ATSDR has compiled a ToxFAQs to answer the most frequently asked health questions about aluminum. Aluminum targets the central nervous system, kidney, and digestive system.

## SYMPTOMS OF EXPOSURE AND TOXICITY

Exposure to toxic heavy metals is generally classified as acute, 14 days or less; intermediate, 15–354 days; and chronic, more than 365 days (ATSDR). Additionally, acute toxicity is usually from sudden or unexpected exposure to a high level of the heavy metal (eg, careless handling, inadequate safety precautions, or accidental spill or release of toxic material often in a laboratory, industrial, or transportation setting). Chronic toxicity results from repeated or continuous exposure, leading to an accumulation of the toxic substance in the body. Chronic exposure may result from contaminated food, air, water, or dust; living near a hazardous waste site; spending time in areas with deteriorating lead paint; maternal transfer in the womb; or participating in hobbies that use lead paint or solder. Chronic exposure may occur in either the home or workplace. Symptoms of chronic toxicity, often similar to many common conditions, may not be easily recognized. Routes of exposure include inhalation, skin or eye contact, and ingestion.[2-4,6,19,20,23]

## Arsenic

Exposure to arsenic occurs mostly in the workplace, near hazardous waste sites, or in areas with high natural levels. Symptoms of acute arsenic poisoning are sore throat from breathing, red skin at contact point, or severe abdominal pain, vomiting, and diarrhea, often within 1 hour after ingestion. Other symptoms are anorexia, fever, mucosal irritation, and arrhythmia. Cardiovascular changes are often subtle in the early stages, but can progress to cardiovascular collapse.

Chronic or lower levels of exposure can lead to progressive peripheral and central nervous changes, such as sensory changes, numbness and tingling, and muscle tenderness. A typical symptom is a burning sensation ("pins and needles") in hands and feet. Neuropathy (inflammation and wasting of the nerves) is usually gradual and occurs over several years. There may also be excessive darkening of the skin (hyperpigmentation) in areas not exposed to sunlight, excessive formation of skin on the palms and soles (hyperkeratosis), or white bands of arsenic deposits across the bed of the fingernails (usually 4–6 weeks after exposure). Birth defects, liver injury, and malignancy are possible. Arsenic has also been used in homicides and suicides.

## Lead

Acute lead exposure is also more likely to occur in the workplace, particularly in manufacturing processes that include the use of lead (eg, where batteries are manufactured or lead is recycled). Even printing ink, gasoline, and fertilizer contain lead. Symptoms include abdominal pain, convulsions, hypertension, kidney dysfunction, loss of appetite, fatigue, and sleeplessness. Other symptoms are hallucinations, headache, numbness, arthritis, and vertigo.

Chronic exposure to lead may result in birth defects, mental retardation, autism, psychosis, allergies, dyslexia, hyperactivity, weight loss, shaky hands, muscular weakness, and paralysis (beginning in the forearms). Children, who are particularly sensitive to lead (absorbing as much as 50% of the ingested dose), are prone to ingesting it because they chew on painted surfaces and eat products not intended for human consumption (eg, hobby paints, cosmetics, hair colorings with lead-based pigments, and playground dirt). In addition to symptoms found in acute lead exposure, symptoms of chronic lead exposure could include allergies, arthritis, autism, colic, hyperactivity, mood swings, nausea, numbness, lack of concentration, seizures, and weight loss.

## Mercury

Acute mercury exposure may occur in the mining industry and the manufacturing of fungicides, thermometers, and thermostats. Liquid mercury, because of its beautiful silver color and unique behavior when spilled, is particularly attractive to children. Children are more likely to undergo acute exposure in the home from ingesting mercury either from a broken thermometer or drinking medicine that contains mercury. Because mercury vapors concentrate at floor level, crawling children are subject to a significant hazard when the mercury is sprinkled throughout the house during religious ceremonies or an accidental spill.[24] Mercury spills are difficult to clean up, and mercury may remain undetected in carpeting for some time. Symptoms of acute exposure are cough, sore throat, shortness of breath, abdominal pain, nausea, vomiting, diarrhea, headache, weakness, visual disturbances, tachycardia, hypertension, and a metallic taste in the mouth.

Chronic exposure to mercury may result in permanent damage to the central nervous system[25] and kidneys. Mercury can also cross the placenta from mother to fetus (levels in the fetus are often double those in the mother) and accumulate, resulting in mental retardation, brain damage, cerebral palsy, blindness, seizures, and inability to speak.

Dental amalgam is also suspected as being a possible source of mercury toxicity from chronic exposure. Some physicians suggest that amalgam fillings could be part of the explanation for the explosion of learning problems and autism in children since World War II, a time period corresponding with the introduction and widespread use of mercury amalgam.[15] Studies in both animals and humans have confirmed the presence of mercury from amalgam fillings in tissue specimens, blood, amniotic fluid, and urine.[14,26-30] However, according to Robert M. Anderton of the American Dental Association, "There is no sound scientific evidence supporting a link between amalgam fillings and systemic diseases or chronic illness."[31]

The American Dental Association (ADA) does acknowledge that amalgam contains mercury and reacts with others substances. However, the ADA concludes that amalgam continues to be a safe material.[32] Researchers reported finding "no significant association of Alzheimer's disease with the number, surface area, or history of having dental amalgam restoration" and "no statistical significant differences in brain mercury levels between subjects with Alzheimer's disease and control subjects."[33]

The metallic mercury used by dentists to manufacture dental amalgam is shipped as a hazardous material to dental offices. Although the ADA does not advise removing existing amalgam fillings from teeth, it does support ongoing research to develop new materials that will prove to be as safe as dental amalgam.[31] Symptoms of chronic exposure in adults and children could include tremors, anxiety, forgetfulness, emotional instability, insomnia, fatigue, weakness, anorexia, cognitive and motor dysfunction, and kidney damage. People who consume fish more than twice weekly show very high serum levels of mercury.

## Cadmium

Acute exposure to cadmium generally occurs in the workplace, particularly in the manufacturing of batteries and color pigments used in paint and plastics, as well as in electroplating and galvanizing processes. Symptoms of acute cadmium exposure are nausea, vomiting, abdominal pain, and difficulty breathing.

Chronic exposure to cadmium can result in chronic obstructive lung disease, kidney disease, and fragile bones. Protect children by carefully storing products containing cadmium, especially nickel-cadmium batteries. Symptoms of chronic exposure could include alopecia, anemia, arthritis, learning disorders, migraines, growth impairment, emphysema, osteoporosis, loss of taste and smell, poor appetite, and cardiovascular disease.

## Aluminum

Although aluminum is not a heavy metal, environmental exposure is frequent, leading to concerns about cumulative effects and a possible connection with Alzheimer's disease.[18] Acute exposure is more likely in the workplace (eg, unintentional breathing of aluminum-laden dust from manufacturing or metal-finishing processes).

Chronic exposure may occur in the workplace from accumulated exposure to low levels of airborne aluminum dust and handling aluminum parts during assembly processes over many years. In the home, we are in constant contact with aluminum in foods and water, cookware and soda cans, and other items with high levels of aluminum (eg, antacids, buffered aspirin, treated drinking water, nasal sprays, toothpaste, and antiperspirants).[18,19] Citric acid (eg, in orange juice) may increase aluminum levels by its leaching activity.

Aluminum-based coagulants are used in the purification of water. However, the beneficial effects of using aluminum to treat water have been balanced against potential health concerns. Water purification facilities follow a number of approaches to minimize the level in "finished" water.[20] Symptoms of aluminum toxicity include memory loss, learning difficulty, loss of coordination, disorientation, mental confusion, colic, heartburn, flatulence, and headache.

## LABORATORY TESTING AND DIAGNOSIS FOR THE PRESENCE OF HEAVY METALS

Diagnosing heavy metal toxicity requires observation of presenting symptoms, obtaining a thorough history of potential exposure, and laboratory tests. Routine laboratory tests include blood tests, liver and renal function tests, urinalysis, fecal tests, x-rays, and hair and fingernail analysis. Many of these tests are not routinely performed in a doctor's office. However, your physician can take blood samples and send them to the appropriate testing laboratory. Chest x-rays are recommended for persons with respiratory symptoms, and abdominal x-rays can detect ingested metals (refer to the ATSDR ToxFAQs for specific information).

## Arsenic

Arsenic levels can be measured in blood, urine, hair, and fingernails. Because arsenic clears fairly rapidly from blood, blood tests are not always useful.[4] Urine tests are the most reliable for arsenic exposure within the past few days; hair and fingernail tests are used to measure exposure over the past several months.[10] Abdominal x-rays can reveal metallic fragments.[3]

> **Note:** *Hair treatments (including hair dyes) can contaminate hair samples. When testing for any heavy metal, the most accurate results are obtained from hair that has not been chemically treated for at least 2 months.*

## Lead

When symptoms of lead toxicity are present, blood testing is done. Blood lead levels in children higher than 10 µg/dL are considered to be of concern.[3,11] Symptoms in adults may not appear until blood lead levels exceed 80 µg/dL.[4] However, medical treatment is usually necessary in children with levels of 45 µg/dL. Significantly lower levels of 30 µg/dL in children can cause mental retardation or cognitive and behavioral problems.[11] A complete blood count (CBC) is also done to check for abnormalities on red blood cells (basophilic stippling). In children, long-bone x-rays may reveal bands called "lead lines" that indicate failure of the bone to rebuild. These bands are not actual lead concentrations, but bone abnormalities. Adults do not have lead lines. X-rays of the abdomen can reveal swallowed objects, such as paint chips, fishing sinkers, curtain weights, or bullets.[3] A less common test is measurement of lead in teeth.[11] All children with brain-related symptoms should be considered for lead toxicity.[3]

## Mercury

A 24-hour urine specimen is collected for measurement of mercury levels. Chest x-rays can reveal a collection of mercury from exposure to elemental mercury or a pulmonary embolism containing mercury.[3] Abdominal x-rays can reveal swallowed mercury as it moves through the gastrointestinal tract. Blood and urine samples are used to determine recent exposure, as well as exposure to elemental and inorganic forms of mercury. Scalp hair is used to test for exposure to methylmercury. Liver and kidney function tests are also important in severely exposed persons. Blood mercury levels should not exceed 50 µg/L (see the ATSDR Medical Management Guidelines).

## Cadmium

Laboratory testing procedures for cadmium toxicity include collection of a 24-hour urine specimen, CBC, and hair and fingernail clippings. Blood levels show recent exposure; urine levels show both recent and earlier exposure (ATSDR). Blood levels of cadmium above 5 µg/dL and creatinine in urine above 10 µg/dL suggest cadmium toxicity.[4]

**Note:** *The ATSDR is unsure of the reliability of tests for cadmium levels.*

## Aluminum

Testing procedures measure aluminum levels in blood, urine, hair, fingernails, and feces.[18] According to a spokesperson at the ATSDR in spring 2002, average aluminum levels are recognized as less than 0.01 mg/L. However, blood testing might underestimate the total body level of aluminum; postmortem brain, lung, and bone measurements reveal much higher levels of aluminum than blood tests.

# SIGNIFICANCE OF INDIVIDUALIZED TREATMENT REGIMENS

Treatment regimens vary significantly and are tailored to each individual's medical condition and circumstance(s) of exposure. Providing a complete history, including occupation, hobbies, recreational activities, and environment, is critical in diagnosing heavy metal toxicity. A possible history of ingestion often facilitates a diagnosis, particularly in children. Physical examination findings vary with age, health status, amount or form of the substance, and time since exposure (absorption rate).[3]

Allopathic (conventional), alternative, and naturopathic (to a lesser extent) practitioners treat heavy metal toxicity. Once toxicity is confirmed, all cases (even suspected) should be brought to the attention of a professional experienced in diagnosing and treating poisoning. Professionals often consult with regional poison control centers or medical toxicologists for added expertise. Emergency room personnel and first responders are trained in recognizing symptoms and in the proper handling, decontamination, and treatment techniques for acute exposure cases (see the ATSDR Medical Management Guidelines).

Conventional and alternative medical treatment includes chelation therapy, supportive care (intravenous fluids, cardiac stabilization, exchange transfusion, dialysis), and decontamination (charcoal, cathartics, emesis, gastric lavage, surgery). These procedures typically require hospitalization or treatment in a health care or clinical setting.[34] Follow-up laboratory testing is required until reference levels are within and remain in normal range(s), particularly with acute exposure or if symptoms continue after treatment.[35,36] Additionally, if homicide or suicide is suspected, proper medical and legal resources should be involved.[3] Medical personnel should report exposure(s) to the appropriate agency to prevent additional public health risks either in the workplace or at home.[2-4,6,18,19,35,37-40]

Therapies to remove heavy metals from humans include chelation and decontamination procedures, as well as supportive measures, often used in combination. Therapies can be very complex and highly individualized, tailored to the specific needs of each individual and requiring the expertise of trained and experienced professionals, sometimes a team of professionals. Self-diagnosis and treatment are not appropriate.

## Chelation Therapy

Chelation is a chemical process with applications in many areas, including medical treatment, environmental site rehabilitation, water purification, and so on. In the medical environment, chelation is used to treat cardiovascular disease, heavy metal toxicity, and remove metals that accumulate in body tissues due to genetic disorders (hemochromatosis). This section will address the use of chelation therapy for the removal of heavy metals as a result of ingested or environmental exposure.

Chelation therapy, simply defined, is the process by which a molecule encircles and binds (attaches) to the metal and removes it from tissue.[34] Depending on the drug used, chelating agents specific to the metal are given orally, intramuscularly, or intravenously. Once the bound metal leaves the tissue, it enters the bloodstream, is filtered from the blood in the kidneys, and then eliminated in the urine.[4] The decision to chelate should be made only by professionals with experience using chelation therapy, preferably in consultation with a poison control center or medical toxicologist.

Typically, a patient receives a programmed series of intravenous infusions, intramuscular injections, or oral administration of a chelating agent (possibly a combination of the three). Therapy is often lengthy (from a few hours in an emergency room to several days of in-patient treatment in a hospital). Repeated courses of treatment are sometimes required.[36] Chelation may be uncomfortable due to the side effects of the medicine itself or route of administration (eg, pain in the area surrounding an injection site).[3] Frequent follow-up testing is required to determine the amount of the metal removed. Sometimes, as in the case of lead, testing may show a rapid decline initially, then a leveling off over time. In the case of lead, this leveling off is caused by lead continuing to enter the blood from the bones where it has been stored ("rebound effect"). The leveling off effect is used as a guide for determining how long chelation therapy should be continued.[36] As time passes following exposure, chelation therapy is less effective in reducing the severity of poisoning and risk of serious delayed effects (see the ATSDR Medical Management Guidelines). It cannot reverse neurologic damage already sustained.

Acutely poisoned symptomatic persons or persons with a clear history of exposure to a toxic heavy metal may require chelation therapy to start before confirmation can be obtained from a laboratory (see the ATSDR Medical Management Guidelines). However, asymptomatic patients are not usually treated with chelation therapy until after test results reveal levels that require treatment. There is growing interest in removing toxic metals from asymptomatic persons known to have received low levels of environmental exposure to heavy metals.[12]

This interest has been generated due to the toxic effects (or damage) that may occur at levels previously thought to be safe. According to Goyer, "It is clear that the margin between the levels of exposure for persons living in the industrialized nations of the world and levels of exposure currently recognized as producing the lowest adverse effect is small." Goyer listed low-level exposure to lead as possibly causing impaired cognitive and behavioral development in children, accumulation of cadmium being associated with renal tube dysfunction, and allegations that mercury vapor from dental amalgam may be a possible cause of chronic health problems.[12] Mercury vapor is released from amalgam in new fillings when old amalgam fillings are replaced[14] and when amalgam is scraped during cleaning.

Chelation is effective in treating arsenic, lead, iron, mercury, and aluminum poisoning. However, chelation is not considered to be particularly effective in treating cadmium poisoning; although it may be used to prevent further absorption in the gastrointestinal tract. There is no effective treatment for cadmium poisoning.[17,34,36]

**Chelating agents.** Dimercaprol (also known as BAL or British anti-Lewisite) is an agent frequently used in chelation therapy. Oral chelating agents used as alternatives to BAL are 2,3-demercaptosuccinic acid (DMSA), dimercaptopropanesulfonate (DMPS), and D-penicillamine (ATSDR MMG). Another agent, deferoxamine, is often used to chelate iron. Ethylenediaminetetraacetic acid (ETDA), one of the first chelators developed, also has an affinity for lead.

- **Dimercaprol.** BAL is a chelating agent administered by injection in the treatment of acute poisoning by certain heavy metals (eg, arsenic, lead, mercury, gold, bismuth, and antimony). Contraindications to using BAL are preexisting kidney disease, pregnancy, hypertension, and current use of medicinal iron. BAL has significant side effects that are frequent and include pain at the injection site, hypertension, tachycardia, abdominal pain, nausea, vomiting, headache, burning sensation of the lips, excessive salivation, rhinorrhea, tearing, fever, muscle pain, muscle spasms, profuse sweating, and a feeling of chest constriction. BAL is considered to be the most toxic of the chelating agents.[36] However, side effects can be medically managed and are seldom severe enough to end treatment.[41]

- **Dimercaptosuccinic acid.** DMSA, an oral chelating agent, is an analogue of (similar to) BAL. DMSA is used in conjunction with or as an alternative to BAL for lead and mercury toxicity. DMSA is less toxic than BAL, and it is sometimes substituted for BAL when the patient's condition improves. DMSA is also used when intolerance to BAL develops. Although DMSA is similar to BAL, it has fewer and milder side effects (eg, nausea, vomiting, diarrhea, rhinitis, cough, and rash) (see the ATSDR Medical Management Guidelines). An interesting study on thiol-chelating substances showed that DMSA was more effective than DMPS and SAMe (S-adenosylmethionine) in protecting mice from acute hepatic or renal toxicity caused by arsenic; also, all 3 substances were nontoxic to the liver or kidneys of mice.[42] Contraindications to using DMSA are preexisting kidney or liver disease and pregnancy. Hydration is essential. DMSA is not used in conjunction with ETDA or D-penicillamine.[38]

- **Dimercaptopropanesulfonate.** DMPS is another analogue of BAL. It has been shown to be less effective and have more side effects than DMSA.[43] DMPS is the drug of choice in Europe and Asia; however, the Food and Drug Administration (FDA) has not approved DMPS for chelating purposes in the United States. It does, however, appear on the FDA list of drugs that appear to be safe. In the United States, DMPS is distributed to pharmacists in bulk for compounding and dispensing in oral and injectable forms.[44,45]

- **D-Penicillamine.** D-penicillamine is an oral chelating agent used to treat heavy metal toxicity, particularly arsenic and mercury. Side effects are gastrointestinal intolerance, nausea, vomiting, and itchy skin (wheals). Contraindications are allergy to penicillin, possible interaction with other drugs (immunosuppressants, digoxin), severe blood disorders, kidney insufficiency, and pregnancy.[40]

- **Deferoxamine.** Deferoxamine is used to chelate iron, especially acute iron poisoning in small children. It is also used to chelate aluminum. Deferoxamine is administered by injection or intravenously. Common side effects are blurred vision, wheezing, rapid heartbeat, seizures, itching, skin rash, bluish skin, and redness and pain at the injection site. Gastrointestinal discomfort, fever, cramping, and bruising are less common. Contraindications are allergies to certain foods or dyes, other medicines currently being taken, pregnancy or breast feeding, and kidney disease.[37]

- **Ethylenediaminetetraacetic acid, edetate disodium.** Ethylenediaminetetraacetic acid, edetate disodium (EDTA), one of the oldest chelating agents, came into prominence in the 1950s. EDTA has an affinity for lead. It is often used intravenously as a second-line treatment in combination with BAL. Common side effects are gastrointestinal upset and headache. More serious side effects can include seizures, numbness or tingling in the hands and feet, irregular heartbeat, skin rash, fever or chills, and blood in the urine.[3] EDTA is contraindicated with pregnancy and kidney disease. It can also interact with insulin and heart medicines.[39]

Table 1 summarizes chelating agents, heavy metals they are used to treat, route of administration, and brand name(s).

## Gastrointestinal Decontamination

In addition to chelation therapy, the following decontamination procedures are often required: gastric lavage, whole bowel irrigation, emesis, charcoal, or cathartics.

**Gastric lavage.** Gastric lavage is washing out of the stomach with sterile water or a salt solution to remove swallowed irritants or poisons.[34] Gastric lavage is accomplished by placing a plastic tube into the stomach via the mouth and esophagus. Normal saline, water, or a combination is introduced into the stomach via the tube. Gastric lavage is not indicated if the substance ingested is an alkaline corrosive. It is done in a health care environment or hospital and is most effective within the first hour of ingestion. Gastric lavage is not effective in removing large tablets, large clumps of

## Table 1:  Chelating Agents[3,6,36,37–40,45,48,91,141]

| Chelating Agent | Heavy Metal | Route[b] | Brand Name(s) |
|---|---|---|---|
| Dimercaprol (BAL) | Arsenic<br>Lead<br>Mercury (inorganic)[a] | IM | Dimercaprol<br>Injection B.P.<br>BAL in Oil |
| Dimercaptosuccinic acid (DMSA)<br>(succimer) | Arsenic<br>Lead<br>Mercury | PO | Chemet |
| Dimercaptopropane-sulfonate (DMPS) | Arsenic | PO<br>IM | Bulk form (for compounding<br>by pharmacists) |
| D-penicillamine | Arsenic<br>Mercury<br>Lead | PO | Metalcaptase<br>Penicillamine<br>Cuprimine<br>Depen |
| Ethylenediaminetetra-acetic acid (EDTA)<br>(edetate disodium) | Lead | IV | Chealamide Versenate |

[a] *Not methylmercury poisoning.*

[b] *Under supervision of a physician. IM, intramuscular; PO, per oral or by mouth; IV, intravenous.*

tablets, or other material,[46] but it is indicated for arsenic.[3] Insertion of the tube may injure the esophagus. Gastric lavage is more effective in adults than children because a larger tube can be used.[46,47]

**Whole bowel irrigation.** Bowel irrigation is emptying of the bowel with large volumes of solutions (eg, Golightly, Colyte, sterile water) used to remove swallowed irritants or poisons (eg, arsenic and lead) from the bowel.[3,47] The fluid may be administered orally or via gastric tube until the bowel fluid has the same appearance as the solution administered.[46,47] Whole bowel irrigation is indicated if some time has elapsed since ingestion of the toxin and the toxin will not be effectively bound by charcoal. It can take several hours. The side effects include nausea, vomiting, diarrhea, and cramping. Whole bowel irrigation is not indicated if mental status is impaired or bowel sounds are decreased.[48]

**Emesis.** Emesis (ie, forceful emptying [vomiting] of the stomach) is most effective for recent oral ingestion of noncorrosive substances. Ipecac syrup USP, considered an essential emesis agent in many homes with young children, has been the cornerstone of poison management.[48] If instructed by a physician, ipecac may be given in the home prior to arrival of emergency personnel or treatment in an emergency department, often preventing significant absorption from stomach contents.[46] However, use of ipecac is only effective when administered within the first 5–20 minutes after ingestion of a toxin. After a toxin has left the stomach, inducing emesis with ipecac is useless. Administering it after the first few minutes may actually delay further medical treatment.[48] Ipecac may take 20 minutes to produce forceful vomiting,[47] and the vomiting may last for some time (2–4 hours). Emesis should not be induced if the patient is having difficulty maintaining consciousness, the toxin is caustic or might cause choking (eg, a clump of pills), or the person has gastrointestinal bleeding.[48] When appropriate, emesis is induced in cases of acute arsenic or mercury poisoning.[34]

Contact a physician, emergency department, or poison center before using emesis.

**Charcoal.** Charcoal is administered in single- or multiple-dose regimens, either intravenously or orally. Single doses are most effective if administered within the first hour after ingestion. Multiple-dose regimens are often used in complicated cases and children because smaller doses (half a single dose) appear to be better tolerated than the larger single dose.[48] Charcoal should not be administered for caustic or corrosive material, and bowel sounds must be present. Its

usefulness is limited in certain pesticides and compounds that are poorly water soluble (eg, iron and elemental metals).[48] Gastrointestinal decontamination with activated charcoal is indicated to aid in removal of mercury.[3]

**Cathartics.** Cathartics are used to aid moving toxic material through the gastrointestinal tract, remove and reduce concentrations, or decrease absorption of toxic materials.[47,48] A cathartic agent increases intestinal action, increases the bulk of feces, makes feces soft, or adds water to the intestinal wall, the term implying fluid bowel materials.[1] Cathartics are often used in conjunction with charcoal in adults, particularly to prevent impaction or formation of charcoal "briquettes." Cathartics are not recommended for children under 1 year and should be used with caution in children under 3 years of age. Cathartics can produce significant diarrhea and electrolyte imbalance. They are not indicated if bowel sounds are absent.[48]

**Supportive measures.** IV fluids, dialysis, and drugs to treat complications resulting from heavy metal toxicity and treatments (eg, shock, anemia, kidney failure, breathing difficulties, cardiac irregularities, infections) may be required. Close monitoring of symptoms by medical personnel and immediate response to them are also required.[34,35,47,48]

## Treatment Regimes for Selected Heavy Metals

**Arsenic.** Chelation therapy shortens the distribution of arsenic in the blood and reduces the body burden. It can reduce the risks of serious delayed effects, but chelation does not reverse damage from delayed effects of acute arsenic poisoning (see the ATSDR Medical Management Guidelines). BAL, DMSA, and D-penicillamine are the primary drugs used to removew arsenic. Chelation therapy with injectable BAL is the primary form of treatment for acute arsenic toxicity. The oral chelating agent DMSA is also an effective treatment choice.

Supportive care with abundant fluids to increase elimination of arsenic may be required. Exchange transfusion and hemodialysis may also be necessary in the event of kidney failure. However, these treatments are supportive and do not remove arsenic.[6] Decontamination of the gastrointestinal system with gastric lavage aids in reducing continued absorption of arsenic. Whole bowel irrigation may also be necessary. Use supportive measures, such as correcting heart rhythm irregularities and hypotension.[3]

**Mercury.** Chelation therapy is the usual treatment method for mercury poisoning, using BAL, DMSA, or D-penicillamine.[3] BAL is widely used for inorganic mercury poisoning,[6] with D-penicillamine used as an alternative. Other treatments are activated charcoal for gastrointestinal decontamination (unless there is evidence of corrosive damage in the gastrointestinal tract),[3] gastric and whole bowel lavage, and supportive measures. However, charcoal is not usually given when elemental mercury is ingested because elemental mercury is poorly absorbed in the gastrointestinal tract (see the ATSDR Medical Management Guidelines; and *Life Extension Magazine*, May 2001, "Mercury Amalgam Toxicity: Your Next Visit to the Dentist May Not Be as Innocent as You Think" for a detoxification protocol to be used in conjunction with the removal of mercury amalgams).

**Iron.** Chelation with the drug deferoxamine is commonly used with blood serum levels greater than 500 µg/dL. This level is only a guide. Much lower levels are known to produce cardiovascular difficulties, and some persons with higher levels exhibit no symptoms. Deferoxamine binds to absorbed iron very well and is eliminated in urine. Deferoxamine may be administered via injection or intravenously; however, intravenous administration is less painful and more efficient. Supportive care with special attention to fluid balance and cardiovascular stabilization are essential in iron poisoning.[6]

Blood levels are used as a guide to therapy, but the estimated ingested amount is often used to determine initial course of action. If the person is symptomatic, however, or if the amount ingested exceeds 20 mg/kg (or as few as five to nine 30-mg tablets for a 30-lb child), gastrointestinal decontamination is recommended. Inducing emesis is an option within the first hour after ingestion. Gastric lavage may also remove fragments of tablets.[6]

*Note: BAL chelation is contraindicated for iron toxicity because it can combine with medicinal iron to become very toxic (see the ATSDR Medical Management Guidelines).*

**Lead.** In 1991, chelation therapy with DMSA received FDA approval for children with blood lead levels >45 µg/dL.[36] A major advantage of DMSA is that it can be given orally, which leads to better compliance by the patient. DMSA is relatively safe and significantly reduces blood levels of iron.[49] BAL, D-penicillamine, and EDTA are also used.[36] Whole bowel irrigation is used if x-rays indicate the presence

of lead.[3] Follow-up blood testing is required because stored lead in bones may continue to be released with long-term lead exposure.[36]

**Aluminum.** Although deferoxamine has not been approved by the FDA for aluminum chelation, it has been used since 1980 as a first-line treatment in cases of aluminum toxicity. It is important to remember that deferoxamine is used to chelate iron. Therefore, during chelation treatment for aluminum, iron would also be chelated. EDTA may also be used.[36]

**Cadmium.** There is no medical chelating method known to be effective for the treatment of cadmium toxicity; however, DMSA may be used in cases of acute oral cadmium poisoning to help prevent additional absorption of cadmium in the gastrointestinal tract.[36] Eliminating exposure to cadmium is the only known method for preventing cadmium toxicity.[17]

# PREVENTING HEAVY METAL POISONING

Occupational exposure can be reduced by engineering solutions that address the manufacturing process, collecting and removing fumes, reducing dust, and substituting other materials when possible. In recent years, the pottery industry has replaced certain lead compounds in their products used as dishes or food containers. In most countries, laws have been passed to protect workers by setting limits of exposure, requiring monitoring in the workplace and medical surveillance of workers, and making the following recommendations[2]:

- No smoking, eating, or drinking in work areas.
- Provide appropriate protective clothing that will remain at the facility.
- Provide showering facilities as needed.
- Work clothes and street clothes will not be kept in the same area.

Three agencies in the United States that provide information and guidance are the Occupational Safety and Health Administration (OSHA), National Institute for Occupational Safety and Health (NIOSH), and Agency for Toxic Substances and Disease Registry (ATSDR). Local health departments, regional poison control centers, and clinics that specialize in occupational and environmental health conditions can also provide valuable resources and guidance.

In the home, practical measures include raising awareness of possible sources of exposure and reducing the threat of exposure. Think carefully about the necessity of having products containing toxic metals around the house or in the garage (eg, fertilizers, fungicides, insect or rodent poisons, lead-based paint, refinishing chemicals, household cleaning agents, hobby supplies, photographic chemicals, batteries, etc.). Use alternatives when possible. When these products are necessary, store them carefully and dispose of them properly. Medicines and personal health care products should be stored so they are in a location well out of the reach of children. Emphasize safety rules with children. If appropriate, before leaving the workplace, follow decontamination procedures to remove toxic materials from clothing, shoes, skin, and hair. Consider cumulative exposures, such as from cookware, storage containers, medicines, water, foodstuffs, and the environment.[50]

1. Use the least harmful product possible.

2. Buy only as much as needed.

3. Read labels. Know potential hazards of products.

4. Store products in their original container. Read the label every time a product is used. Refer to the label in case of an accidental spill or ingestion. Never store household chemicals in a food container, even if the container has been relabeled.

5. Support and use established disposal programs and facilities.

6. Become familiar with symptoms of and first aid procedures for ingestion of substances containing toxic metals.

## NATURAL THERAPIES TO PROMOTE CHELATION, DETOXIFICATION, AND PROTECTION

There is no substitute for prompt and professional medical attention in cases of heavy metal toxicity. However, many herbs and supplements have natural chelating characteristics and properties that help detoxify the body. Important supplements to consider are antioxidants, herbs, minerals, essential amino acids, phytoextracts, detoxifying agents, protective agents, and fiber (see also Life Extension's Immune System Strengthening protocol).

### Antioxidants

Vitamins C, E, and A, alpha-lipoic acid, glutathione, lactoferrin, selenium, and zinc are important antioxidants that aid overall health by increasing protection from oxidative stress.

**Vitamin C.** Vitamin C has long been recognized as having positive effects for the prevention of heart disease and some forms of cancer, improving immune function, maintaining healthy skin and blood vessels,

accelerating healing, and reducing allergic reactions. A steady supply of vitamin C is vital to overall health. Because the human body cannot manufacture or store vitamin C, requirements must be met from dietary sources, such as citrus fruit, vegetables, and supplements. Vitamin C is particularly beneficial as an antioxidant to protect the lungs. It has been shown to protect the airways from inhaled (environmental) oxidants.[51] Additionally, researchers have shown that vitamin C can help reduce harmful effects of lead, aluminum, copper, silica, and radiation.[51-56]

**Vitamin E.** Some benefits of vitamin E include synergy with vitamin A, reducing cellular aging, reducing risk of Alzheimer's disease, protecting the nervous system, preventing abnormal blood clotting, lowering risk of heart disease,[57] protecting immune function, lowering risk of certain cancers, and protecting lungs from toxins and pollutants.[54]

As early as 1981, studies using 3 different feeding experiments revealed that when animals received silver, copper, cobalt, tellurium, cadmium, and zinc, they frequently developed lesions characteristic of selenium and vitamin E deficiency, such as necrosis (local destruction of tissue due to disease or injury) of cardiac and skeletal muscle as well as smooth muscle of the intestine and gizzard. In another study, vitamin E and selenium rendered complete protection from muscle lesions produced by copper, cobalt, tellurium, cadmium, and zinc. Vitamin E also produced protection against lesions caused by silver. There was partial protection using selenium.[58] Ten years later, in yet another animal study, researchers found that cadmium caused a negative change in kidney, liver, and blood biochemical markers. When administered along with vitamin E, both cadmium-induced biochemical alterations and accumulation of cadmium in the kidneys, liver, and blood were reduced. Researchers concluded the antioxidant properties of vitamin E seemed to be responsible for protection from cadmium toxicity.[59]

Another study examined lipid peroxidation (oxidative damage) and cell death on liver cells caused by iron (ferrous sulfate) in animals. Researchers found that vitamin E reduced lipid peroxidation by 39% and increased cell viability by 12%. However, the greatest protective effect against iron-induced lipid peroxidation occurred when vitamin E, glutathione (GSH), and N-acetyl-cysteine (NAC) were combined. The combination reduced lipid peroxidation by 94% in iron-treated cells.[60]

**Vitamin A.** Vitamin A (retinol) is essential for normal cell growth and protection from various diseases. Vitamin A has also been shown to help inhibit cancer cell proliferation (particularly against leukemia) and aid in a return to normal cell growth patterns. Vitamin A has shown protective effects against tumor growth as well.[61] Beta-carotene, a potent source of vitamin A (via the liver), is another important antioxidant. However, continuous, high doses of vitamin A or beta-carotene are not recommended. Pregnant women should not take vitamin A.

**Alpha-lipoic acid.** Alpha-lipoic acid, a potent free radical scavenger, has the ability to detoxify metals and regenerate other antioxidants (eg, vitamins C and E, coenzyme Q10, and glutathione). Alpha-lipoic acid has also been used in the treatment of heart disease, diabetes, and other oxidant-related diseases. In a study, lipoic acid improved the thiol capacity of cells by increasing glutathione levels and reducing malondial-dehyde levels in lead-exposed cells.[62]

*Note: Thiols participate in detoxification activity in the body. Malondialdehyde occurs in the bloodstream as a product of lipid peroxidation. It also occurs naturally in a variety of foods, depending on source and method of preparation.*

Another study used 2 different lipoic acid protocols on exposure to mercury and neurotoxicity. Authors concluded that "the ameliorating effect of lipoic acid and its therapeutic efficacy during various modes of therapy on the antioxidant status were established in the nervous tissues."[63] Other toxic substances such as cyanide, glutamate, or iron ions have been shown to be neurotoxic. Prolonged pretreatment with lipoic acid provided protection for the cells.[64] Alpha-lipoic acid also appears to have positive effects for cadmium toxicity, providing a protective effect for cadmium-induced cell dysfunction and membrane damage in hepatocytes (the most basic liver cells that perform all functions of the liver).[65,66]

**Glutathione.** Glutathione is a tripeptide (chain of amino acids) that functions as a modulator of cellular homeostasis (the orderly status of cell life), including detoxification of oxyradicals and carcinogens. If glutathione is depleted, an organism can be predisposed to incur stress from pollutants.[67] Glutathione and gluta-thione-related enzymes are important antioxidants. These enzymes appear to play an important role in detoxifying carcinogens.[68–70]

Glutathione status has also been shown to have an impact on the ability of the body to handle heavy metals such as cadmium, lead,[71,72] iron, and mercury. The prooxidative effects of heavy metals are compounded by the fact that they also inhibit antioxidative enzymes

and deplete intracellular glutathione. Heavy metals also have the potential to disrupt the metabolism and biological activities of many proteins because of their high affinity for free sulfhydryl groups. When glutathi-one status is elevated or increased by supplementation and there is exposure to cadmium, lead, iron, or mercury (either independently or along with nutrients such as zinc or selenium), exposed tissues were able to stop damage by the lipid peroxides created by exposure to the metals.[73–78] In a study in rats, researchers concluded their results indicated increases in renal gluta-thione (glutathione S-transferase or GST) "occur at levels of lead that are environmentally significant and that these changes precede cellular damage." They suggested that GST "may serve as a tissue biomarker of lead exposure."[72]

Additionally, glutathione appears to play a major role in arsenic toxicity.[68–70] It is the most abundant cellular thiol in the body.[68] Arsenic toxicity appears to be a result of the ability of arsenite to bind to protein thiols, causing the thiols to be unavailable for detoxi-fication activity. Researchers examined the effect of arsenic on the activity of a variety of glutathione en-zymes; they concluded that many more studies are needed to understand the relationship between gluta-thione-related enzymes and the products of arsenic metabolism in the role of arsenic toxicity and carcino-genesis.[68] It was noted that "these observations further demonstrate that glutathione is an important compo-nent of MRP1-mediated cellular resistance to arsenite and antimony."[69]

Glutathione is also closely tied to immunity, pro-tecting cells, and assisting the liver in detoxifying harmful compounds and toxins. When taking glutathi-one, vitamin C is also recommended because it assists glutathione in maintaining its powerful free radical-suppressing effects.

**Lactoferrin.** Lactoferrin, a natural component of cow and human milk, is a subfraction of whey with well-documented antiviral, antimicrobial, anticancer, and immune modulating and enhancing effects. How-ever, lactoferrin's best-known role is as an iron-binding protein. Lactoferrin acts as an antioxidant, scavenging free iron and helping prevent uncontrolled iron-based free radical reactions. Although lactoferrin is both an iron scavenger and donor (depending on the cellular environment), it has been found to scavenge or donate iron appropriately depending on what the body needs at any given time. At normal physiologic pH, lactofer-rin binds tightly to iron, diminishing oxidative stress to tissues.[79] Researchers examining the role of whey pro-teins, multifermented whey proteins, and lactoferrin in oxidative stress concluded that "whey protein, lactoferrin and multifermented whey are good candidates as dietary inhibitors of oxidative stress and should be considered as potential medicinal foods in various pathologies as HIV infection and cancer."[80]

**Selenium and zinc.** Deficiency of selenium and zinc, important antioxidant micronutrients, contributes to compromised immunity[81] and lowered defense against free radicals.[82,83] Selenium and zinc act as cofactors of antioxidant enzymes to protect against oxygen free radicals produced during oxidative stress.[84] Selenium is often found to be deficient in persons who suffered physical trauma. It was concluded that patients who experienced severe trauma had fewer infections and less organ dysfunction when they received selenium supplementation.[82] Studies on the protective benefits of selenium have implications in the management of persons receiving chemotherapy, enhancing mediation of oxygen free-radical damage to normal tissue and decreasing side effects (eg, nausea, emesis, vertigo, unsteady gait, and seizures caused by chemicals and drugs used in chemotherapy).[85] This is a possible characteristic of persons with brain tumors who frequently have low blood levels of selenium.[83,85]

## Herbs

Herbs and herbal extracts have been used and studied for years, particularly in Europe and China.[86] Many modern-day drugs have been derived either directly or indirectly from herbal origin. Herbs are often complexed (combined) to assist in blood purification and detoxification (eg, dandelion root, yellow dock root, sarsaparilla root, echinacea, and licorice root).

**Cilantro.** *Coriandrum sativum* is a European herb in the parsley family. The leaves are cilantro (also Chinese parsley) and the fruit is coriander. Cilantro leaves are commonly used as a seasoning herb. However, dried coriander seeds, which are used as a spice, have an entirely different flavor than the leaves. Coriander stimulates appetite, helps increase secretion of gastric juices, and aids the digestive system. Essential oils of cilantro are considered to have antifungal and antibacterial properties.[14,87]

Studies found that antibiotics used to treat infection were not effective in the presence of heavy metals such as mercury and lead. These metals appeared to coexist with infections such as *Chlamydia trachomatis* and *Herpes simplex*, as well as with cytomegalovirus and other microorganisms, including viruses responsible for cancer. Even with rigorous treatment and taking precautions to guard against reinfection, patients often had a recurrence of infection within several months after completing treatment. However, after eating soup containing cilantro (by chance) along with an experience following a cardiac thallium study, it was noted that cilantro successfully eliminated mercury deposits (mercury resulted as a decay product of thallium).[14,87] Researchers then gave subjects a course of either antibiotics or antiviral drugs along with cilantro. The amount of cilantro varied among subjects because some did not like either cooked or raw cilantro. Researchers found that cilantro worked synergistically with antibiotic drugs and rapidly reduced symptoms and infection. They also found that cilantro accelerated the elimination of mercury, lead, and aluminum through the urine. They hypothesized that certain infectious organisms somehow use mercury or lead to protect themselves from antibiotics or deposits of heavy metals somehow make antibiotics ineffective.[87]

The same researchers investigated the potential health hazard of mercury in dental amalgam. In this case study, they monitored a patient having amalgam fillings removed. Even though considerable care was used so the patient would not swallow minute particles of amalgam during the removal process (drilling), significant deposits of mercury were still found in the patient's lungs, kidneys, liver, and heart. These deposits were not present prior to the amalgam removal. However, the mercury deposits were eliminated by taking oral cilantro 4 times a day. Cilantro detoxification treatment was initiated before the removal procedure and continued for about 2–3 weeks afterward.[14]

**Garlic.** Garlic has been valued for centuries for its medicinal properties. Research has shown that garlic can protect against various pollutants and heavy metals.[88] Garlic is also important for its ability to prevent certain kinds of cancer, prompting the National Cancer Institute to develop a $20.5 million program to study plant-derived compounds in common foods that may have cancer-prevention effects. Some scientists speculate that garlic may protect against cancer by its ability to help the body inactivate and eliminate cancer-causing substances without damage. Depending on personal requirements or preferences, garlic supplements are available in a wide range of potencies. The aged form of garlic is organically grown then harvested and aged to produce a mild, odor-free garlic extract.

**Green tea.** Green tea is a powerful antioxidant that may protect cells from mutation caused by cancer-causing agents and damage caused by free radicals.[89] For years, studies conducted in Japan demonstrated that persons who consumed green tea had a lower incidence of several types of cancer (stomach, liver, pancreas, breast, lung, esophagus, and skin).

## Minerals

In addition to the vitally important function of maintaining healthy bones and helping restore bone density if lost, calcium is required for proper liver function. Kidneys assist in processing body waste; however, the liver is the organ with the primary function of processing body waste. Additionally, through complex chemical processes, the liver is also responsible for providing building and maintenance materials for all other organs and tissues, providing vital digestive enzymes, and storing glucose not immediately needed by cells.[90] Adequate absorption of calcium can be compromised by an existing condition of the liver or intestinal tract. To aid optimized liver function, ensure that adequate dietary calcium is provided.

## Essential Amino Acids

Amino acids, the basic chemical "building blocks" of life, are derived from dietary protein that is broken down into individual amino acids by the body. The body then reassembles the amino acids into new and vital structures essential to produce protein structures for genes, enzymes, hormones, body fluids, and neurotransmitters.[91] A deficiency in essential amino acids can negatively affect protein synthesis. Exposure to pollution, chemicals, and agricultural pesticides contribute to amino acid deficiency. L-cysteine and the acetylated form, N-acetyl-cysteine (NAC), act as antioxidants and liver protectants. Taking vitamin C along with either L-cysteine or NAC will help maintain their powerful free radical-suppressing effects.

**Cysteine and N-acetyl cysteine (NAC).** L-cysteine is a conditionally essential amino acid, one of 3 sulfur-containing amino acids. The other two are taurine (produced from L-cysteine) and L-methionine. L-cysteine can be produced from L-methionine in the body by a complex multistep process. L-cysteine acts as an antioxidant and has a pivotal role in inducible, endogenous (internal) detoxification mechanisms in the body. Exposure to metal(s) impacts our supply of cysteine.[92]

NAC is the acetylated (or combined) form of L-cysteine, which is more efficiently absorbed and used. NAC works in the extracellular environment and is a precursor of intracellular cysteine and glutathione. NAC has been used as a liver protectant, as well as to break up pulmonary and bronchial mucus. For decades, NAC has proven to be a safe and effective prophylaxis (prevention agent) and therapy for a variety of conditions, even in very high doses, mostly involving glutathione depletion and alterations of the redox status.[93]

**Note:** Redox = red(uction) + ox(idation)

NAC has an impressive list of protective effects including antioxidant activity, decrease of the biologically effective dose of carcinogens, anti-inflammatory activity, immunologic effects, inhibiting progression to malignancy, inhibiting metastasis, and protection from adverse effects of chemopreventive and chemotherapeutic agents. Although their studies were primarily directed at chemoprevention treatment and complementary approaches in high-risk individuals (eg, smokers or ex-smokers), authors noted "there is overwhelming evidence that NAC has the ability to modulate a variety of DNA damage and cancer-related end-points."[93]

**Glycine.** Glycine is another conditionally essential amino acid found in plant and animal protein. Chemically, glycine is the most simple and ubiquitous (seemingly present everywhere) of all the amino acids. It combines with many toxic substances and converts them to harmless forms, which are then excreted from the body. Glycine has a calming effect on the brain. It may also be a growth hormone releaser. Along with cysteine and glutamic acid, glycine is also a component of glutathione. In a study of Stronger Neo-Minophagen C, a Japanese drug containing glycine, glycyrrhizin, and cysteine, which is said to be protective against chronic cadmium toxicity, authors concluded that the reported beneficial effects were from glycine. Glycine appeared to reduce the oxidative stress of chronic cadmium toxicity.[94]

**Carnosine.** Carnosine chelates (binds to) ions of copper, zinc, and iron, which in excess are known to induce production of amyloid beta and other proteins found in Alzheimer's and Parkinson's diseases.[95-98]

**L-carnitine.** L-propionyl carnitine, a form of carnitine, is known to improve heart muscle recovery after a heart attack. It acts as an energy source for heart muscles and an anti-free radical agent in damaged heart tissue; the latter effect a result of iron chelation.[99] Another form, acetyl-L-carnitine, exhibits powerful antioxidant effects that reverse the impact of iron-induced oxidative stress in human cells.[100]

## Detoxifying/Chelating Agents

**Alfalfa.** Although most people consider alfalfa to be a plant primarily grown for animal feeds, and it has been widely studied for that purpose, alfalfa (also called buffalo herb, buffalo grass, Chilean clover, lucerne, and purple medic) is an excellent source of protein for humans. Alfalfa is high in vitamins A, D, E, B6, and K, calcium, magnesium, chlorophyll, phosphorus, iron, potassium, trace minerals, and several digestive enzymes. Alfalfa is also a high-fiber substance (21% crude fiber, 42% dietary fiber). High-fiber diets are generally recommended for reducing cholesterol, improving diabetes, and protecting against colon cancer. Researchers found that because of its high-fiber content, alfalfa has properties to bind to material in the colon and aid in its removal.[101] More studies are required, however, to determine whether alfalfa can induce activity in a complex cellular system to inactivate dietary chemical carcinogens in the liver and small intestine and remove them before causing harm to the body.

Alfalfa should not be taken by individuals with toxic or chronic iron overload.

**Chlorella.** Chlorella is a single-cell, fresh water algae that is rich in protein, vitamins, minerals, chlorella growth factor, and other beneficial substances. It is about the size of a human erythrocyte (red blood cell) (ie, about 2–8 microns in diameter). Chlorella is high in chlorophyll, giving it a rich green color. For many years, chlorella has been accepted as a detoxifier, and is commonly used in colon cleansing regimes. Chlorella appears to bind to heavy metals as well as other toxic substances in the bowel and help with the detoxification process. Chlorella also increases serum albumin levels necessary for optimum health.

Many reports have come from Japanese research studies that followed the nuclear catastrophe resulting from atomic bombs being dropped on Hiroshima and Nagasaki in 1945. In a report on animals, authors noted that chlorella (8 g daily) increased elimination of cadmium 3-fold in feces and 7-fold in urine.[102] Other researchers from Japan showed that chlorella helped detoxify uranium and lead.[103] Chlorella has detoxification potential for similar compounds, such as dioxin and polychlorinated biphenyls (PCBs) (ie, chemical compounds used in plastics, insulation, and flame retardants, with potential to cause cancer and liver damage). Other research indicates that chlorella is useful in detoxification of high levels of mercury in the body caused by removal of mercury amalgam. Some dentists recommend chlorella to patients having mercury amalgams replaced (as well as to themselves and staff who can incur accidental exposure from day-to-day exposure to amalgam filling procedures).[15]

**Methylsulfonylmethane (MSM).** Methylsulfonylmethane or dimethyl sulfone (MSM) is a naturally occurring sulfur compound. Dimethylsulfoxide (DMSO) and dimethylsulfide (DMS) are closely related compounds. In its purified form, MSM has no odor and is a slightly bitter tasting, water-soluble, white crystalline powder that contains 34% elemental sulfur (chemical formula of [CH3]2SO2). The origins of MSM begin with phytoplankton in the ocean. DMS is produced through a complex process occurring in the ocean. DMS escapes as gas and rises into the upper atmosphere. Some atmospheric chemists suggest that MSM and its related compounds, DMSO and DMS, are the source of 85% of sulfur compounds in all living organisms. In the atmosphere, DMS is oxidized by ozone and ultraviolet light into its chemical cousins, DMSO and MSM. DMSO and MSM return to the earth in rain, where they are absorbed by the soil. Plants rapidly take up and concentrate the two compounds. Next, animals eat the plants, which completes the cycle.[104]

As a result of the cycle that began with phytoplankton, MSM occurs naturally in the human body as a result of the food we eat. MSM is a normal component of fresh fruits, vegetables, seafood, and meat; it can also be found in tea, coffee, and chocolate. MSM can be detected in the circulatory system (about 0.2 ppm in a normal adult male) and in human urine. Normal adult humans excrete from 4–11 mg of MSM daily in urine. The concentration of MSM decreases with age in vertebrates. Therefore, some research suggests a minimum concentration of MSM must be maintained in the body to preserve normal function and structure.[104]

Chelation involves a sulfur donor. Because MSM is a compound that contains sulfur, it could theoretically be beneficial as part of a detoxification protocol for heavy metals (eg, there is a sulfur component in glutathione, methionine, cysteine, and NAC). After administering cadmium to rats, cysteine and methionine were given in combination. Researchers found that cadmium was removed from the circulatory system, preventing its deleterious effects.[105] In addition to its detoxifying potential, MSM has potential for allergy response reduction, control of hyperactivity, constipation relief, cancer prevention, and inflammatory conditions (eg, rheumatoid and degenerative arthritis).[104]

**Rutin.** Rutin is a phytoextract (plant extract) found in many plants, particularly buckwheat. Other rich sources of rutin are black tea and apple peel. Rutin is thought to have antioxidant, anti-inflammatory, anticarcinogenic, and cytoprotective activities.[106–110] Studies in animals demonstrated that rutin has anti-inflammatory potential in colitis, reducing tissue damage.[109,110] Researchers reported free-radical scavenging and iron-chelating ability that significantly protected against cellular damage.[111]

**Modified citrus pectin.** In some instances, chelation therapy involves the infusion of compounds via a catheter placed in an arm vein. This procedure must be done in a clinical setting over a specified course of treatments. In contrast, chelation therapy using modified citrus pectin (MCP) is done via the oral route and can be administered to the patient in almost any clinical setting, since the supplement can be ingested anywhere.

A pilot trial evaluating MCP's chelating effects provided evidence that orally administered MCP significantly increases urinary excretion of toxic metals. In a study published in 2006, 8 healthy individuals were given 15 g of MCP daily for 5 days and 20 g of MCP on day 6. Twenty-four-hour urine samples were collected on days 1 and 6 and analyzed for toxic and essential elements. The investigators reported that significant urinary excretion of arsenic, mercury, cadmium, and lead increased within 1–6 days of MCP treatment. There was a 150% increase in cadmium excretion and 560% increase in lead excretion on day 6.[112] Essential minerals such as calcium, zinc, and magnesium were not noted to increase in the urinary analysis, indicating that MCP treatment did not deplete these nutrients.

In a case study report, 5 patients with different illnesses were given either MCP alone or in combination with alginate (MCP/alginate complex) for up to 7 months. Each one had a gradual decrease of total heavy metal burden, which is believed to have played an important role in the patients' recovery and health maintenance. The patients had a 74% average decrease in toxic heavy metals after treatment. This is the "first known documentation of evidence" of a possible correlation between positive clinical outcomes and a reduction of toxic heavy metal load using MCP alone or as an MCP/alginate complex. Authors recommended "further studies be performed to confirm the effectiveness of this gentle nontoxic chelating system as an alternative to harsher chelators in the treatment of patients with a heavy metal body burden."[113]

**Quercetin.** Quercetin, a flavonoid found in berries and other plants, chelates iron atoms as powerfully as prescription drugs used in managing severe cases of iron overdose.[114,115] Quercetin's antioxidant effects are likely to be closely related to its strong iron-chelating capacity, and account for its ability to prevent the DNA strand damage that precedes cancer development.[116,117]

Studies of quercetin reveal it can prevent kidney damage associated with acute iron overload from muscle breakdown, one of the leading causes of acute renal failure.[118] Similarly, liver injury from long-term exposure to iron is prevented in laboratory animals supplemented with quercetin.[119,120]

**Cranberry and pomegranate.** Dark-colored and red fruits are known to have many health benefits, in large part because of their high polyphenol content. Cranberry and pomegranate extracts rich in polyphenols have now been shown to have potent iron-chelating capabilities, in some cases completely suppressing iron-catalyzed oxidant reactions.[114,121]

**Curcumin.** The unexpected discovery that curcumin is also a powerful iron chelator has given us new insight into its multimodal mechanisms of action in gaining control of age-related iron accumulations in the brain, heart, and liver.[122–125]

Iron chelation by curcumin is now recognized as one of the mechanisms that prevents cognitive deficits and pathologic tissue changes in animal models of Alzheimer's disease.[126] In addition, curcumin induces increased genetic expression of ferritin (ie, the body's natural iron-binding and transport protein), further sequestering iron away from vulnerable tissues.[122] These multiple capabilities lead directly to a reduction in iron levels within iron-overloaded organs.[122,125,127,128]

**Dietary fiber.** Choosing foods with high fiber content and supplementing the diet with additional fiber (eg, psyllium, acacia, apple pectin, and oat and wheat bran) aid the body in ridding itself of toxins. When adding dietary fiber, use small amounts at first so the digestive system can adjust. If gas or bloating occurs, reduce the amount until tolerance is achieved.

## Protective Agents

**S-Adenosylmethionine.** S-adenosylmethionine (SAMe) (also known as SAM or AdoMet) has been called "the liver's super-nutrient." Nothing else comes close to SAMe for providing a spectrum of health benefits for the liver. As a preventive agent, SAMe can reverse the destructive effects of chemicals and alcohol as they occur. It also has a central role in liver biochemistry. SAMe performs 2 crucial functions: methylation and trans-sulfuration. One result of trans-sulfuration is a transformation into glutathione, the liver's most vital substance. Glutathione, a natural antioxidant for the liver, is crucial for liver function. Because the liver also contains the third highest amount of SAMe in the body (after the adrenal and pineal glands) and it is so important for liver function, SAMe can be considered an essential nutrient for the liver.

The principal function of the liver is to break down damaging substances encountered by the body (drugs, alcohol, infections, or even our own body products). Therefore, poor liver function is invariably accompanied by glutathione depletion. In addition to its many other functions, SAMe also plays a leading role in liver regeneration. Anyone concerned with the effects of drugs, toxic chemicals, alcohol, and aging on the liver should consider taking SAMe for its protective benefits.

Several studies were conducted to investigate the role of SAMe in arsenic toxicity.[42,129,130] A study demonstrated that arsenic interferes with DNA methyltransferases, causing tumor suppressor genes to be inactivated. The study suggests that arsenic-induced malignant transformation is linked to DNA hypomethylation subsequent to depletion of SAMe, potentially resulting in aberrant gene activation, including cancer genes.[130]

**Note:** *In methylation, a compound is derived from ethanol in which hydroxyl hydrogen is replaced by a metal.*

Researchers conducted a study in mice to determine SAMe's role in increasing removal of cadmium from target organs by diethylenetriamine penta acetic acid (DTPA). Results indicated significant removal of cadmium concentration from the blood in DTPA-plus-SAMe-treated animals compared to either one of the substances alone. They also found that treatment with SAMe alone was effective in correcting zinc and glutathione concentrations.[131]

Research was done in mice to investigate the beneficial effects of SAMe on acute and chronic lead exposure.[132] Mice were treated with subcutaneous SAMe for 20–22 days. In all test subjects, there was significant recovery of erythrocytic (red blood cell) ALA-D following SAMe therapy. There was also decreased lead content in blood, liver, and kidneys, with near normal levels attained in 2 weeks. Diminished glutathione (GSH) concentration in the blood and liver also reached normal levels following SAMe administration.

**Silibinin.** Silibinin (also known as silybin) is the most biologically active ingredient in silymarin. Silymarin is an extract derived from the herb milk thistle (a member of the *Compositae* or daisy family). Silymarin and its main active ingredient, silibinin, help prevent toxic liver damage. Standardized milk thistle extract usually consists of a minimum of 35% silybin (by HPLC analysis).

A study compared the effectiveness of silymarin with silibinin to inhibit copper-induced oxidation of low-density lipoproteins *in vitro*. Silymarin and silibinin were found to be equally effective in prolonging the initial "lag phase" (the slow stage of the oxidation process). As a result, authors concluded that "silybin is the most important compound of silymarin in protecting LDL from oxidation."[133]

There have been a few studies to investigate the activity of silibinin on heavy metals. This research supports the use of silibinin as an adjunct for liver, kidney, pancreatic, and other organ support in any heavy metal detoxification program. Silibinin is important for heavy metal detoxification due to its ability to aid liver function and regeneration,[134,135] elevate glutathione enzyme levels,[136] reduce oxidation,[133,134] and improve cellular thiol status.[137]

If the liver has already been damaged by toxic substances, silymarin and silibinin can help speed up liver regeneration by accelerating the rate of protein synthesis in the liver, leading to faster cell regeneration.[138,139] German researchers discovered that silibinin also protected the kidneys from toxic injury and produced accelerated kidney regeneration after toxic damage (eg, from agents such as chemotherapy drugs).[140] Because kidneys can be damaged by analgesics, chemotherapy drugs, and other toxic substances, the finding that silibinin has protective benefits and even stimulates regeneration has tremendous clinical interest.

## CONCLUSION

For most people, acute heavy metal toxicity will rarely be a concern or pose a problem. However, certain groups are at a higher risk:

- Those living in homes that contain lead pipes and lead-based paint or in areas having high environmental levels of elemental mercury, iron, or aluminum
- Those working in industries that manufacture batteries, pesticides, and fertilizers
- Those working in industries involved in metal finishing
- Those handling chemicals in scientific or laboratory settings

Heavy metal exposure can be considered acute (from an accident) or chronic (from long-term exposure). Unrecognized or untreated toxicity will likely result in illness and reduced quality of life. Testing is essential if you or someone in your household might have heavy metal toxicity. If test results are positive, initiation of appropriate conventional and natural medical procedures described earlier in the protocol might be required. However, there are many natural chelating, detoxifying, anti-inflammatory, and antioxidant products that can aid your vital organs in performing at their best.

# SUMMARY

If you suspect you have heavy metal toxicity, consult your physician. If you have a specific medical condition or are taking prescription medication, consult your physician about possible contraindications before using any suggested product. More aggressive treatment approaches for chelation therapy require supervision and monitoring by a qualified medical health professional.

Observe workplace safety rules and follow procedures to protect yourself in the workplace. When leaving the workplace, follow decontamination procedures to avoid wearing contaminated clothing that could potentially expose other persons, particularly children in the home. At home, raise your awareness of potential sources of exposure to toxic materials. Take measures to limit access to toxic products. Whenever possible, replace toxic products with less dangerous alternatives. Properly dispose of those no longer needed. Learn to recognize symptoms of ingested toxic substances. Learn first aid procedures. Display emergency contact numbers by the telephone.

Strive to achieve proper, balanced nutrition by choosing fresh (organic when possible) fruits, vegetables, grains, lean meat, and cold-water fish.

Consider taking supplemental antioxidants, herbs, minerals, amino acids, phytoextracts, detoxifying agents, protective agents, and fiber as adjuncts to a healthy diet to enhance vital organ functioning and aid in the body's natural detoxifying actions. The dosage recommendations listed below are for healthy persons.

## Life Extension Suggestions

- **Comprehensive multivitamin:** per label instructions
- **Selenium:** 200–400 mcg daily
- **Vitamin E:** 400 IU daily (with 200 mg gamma tocopherol)
- **Vitamin C:** 2000–6000 mg daily
- **Vitamin A**, as beta-carotene: 25 000 IU daily
- **Glutathione:** 250 mg daily
- **Zinc:** 30 mg daily
- **Lactoferrin**, providing 95% of apolactoferrin: 300 mg daily
- **Aged garlic extract:** 600–1200 mg daily
- **Cilantro oil:** Steep 1–15 drops in hot water 2 times daily (5 days on, 2 days off). During mercury chelation therapy, stop using cilantro after 2 weeks or on the day therapy begins during the third week.
- **Green tea**, standardized extract: 725 mg once to twice daily
- **Calcium:** 200–1200 mg daily
- **N-acetyl-cysteine (NAC):** 600–1200 mg daily
- **Alfalfa sprouts:** Available as a food product in most health-food stores, and may be added to salads or blended into a juice. Dried herbs from alfalfa leaves and sprouts may be brewed into a tea—1 oz steeped in 1 pint of water for 20 minutes—2 cups daily. Dried powder capsules may also be taken at a dose of 4–6 capsules daily. Due to its high iron content, alfalfa should not be taken by individuals with toxic or chronic iron overload.
- **Rutin:** Include citrus fruit and foods containing buckwheat flour in your diet as natural sources of rutin. A convenient source of supplemental rutin is 1/4 tsp of rutin powder taken 2–3 times daily with a beverage.
- **Methylsulfonylmethane (MSM):** 3000 mg daily
- **R-lipoic acid:** 240 mg once or twice daily, 30 minutes before meals
- **Glycine:** 3000 mg on an empty stomach
- **Chlorella:** 1000 mg, 2–3 times daily
- **Propolmannan:** 2000 mg twice daily with 8–16 oz of water 30 minutes before the heaviest meals
- **S-adenosylmethionine (SAMe):** 400 mg, 2–3 times daily in divided doses on an empty stomach. Take with co-factors vitamins B12, B6, and folic acid.
- **Milk thistle extract (*Silybum marianum*)**, standardized to 80% silymarin and 30% silibinin: 750 mg daily, with or without meals
- **Modified citrus pectin:** 1500 mg twice daily on an empty stomach
- **Modified alginate complex:** 750 mg twice daily on an empty stomach
- **Quercetin**, as quercetin glycoside derivatives and free quercetin: 250 mg, 1–2 times daily with or without food
- **Carnosine:** 1000–1500 mg daily with or without food
- **Cranberry extract:** 500 mg daily
- **Standardized pomegranate extract:** 500–1500 mg daily
- **Curcumin**, as highly absorbed BCM-95®: 400 mg daily
- **Acetyl L-carnitine and propionyl L-carnitine:** 1400 mg daily

In addition, the following *blood tests* may provide helpful information:

- Female panel or Male panel
- Heavy Metals panel
- Ferritin
- Serum Iron

- Transferrin
- Copper

## REFERENCES

References available at: www.lef.org/dpt5/ch68

# 69

# *Hemochromatosis*

Iron is an essential micronutrient. However, free iron rapidly catalyzes the generation of damaging free radicals and subsequent oxidant stress. In fact, excess iron can damage cells and tissues, and iron overload is associated with increased risk of cancer and heart disease along with neurologic, endocrine, and musculoskeletal disorders.[1–5]

Iron is unusual among dietary nutrients in that both iron deficiency and iron excess are relatively common health concerns; however, little understood or recognized is that the difference between iron deficiency or overload is often a question of a scant few milligrams of iron.[6–8]

Conditions that predispose to accumulation of excess iron can be hereditary (eg, hemochromatosis) or acquired (eg, excess iron ingestion, chronic liver disease). Poorly appreciated by mainstream medicine is the fact that iron has a tendency to accumulate within cells during the aging process,[9,10] further exacerbating the detrimental impact of aging in the body.

Iron overload is not typically detected until 40–60 years of age.[11] However, recent advances in the understanding of the genetic basis of hereditary iron overload disorders, availability of blood markers, and development of noninvasive techniques to assess tissue iron stores have facilitated early detection and faster treatment of iron overload disorders.[12–15]

This protocol will present an overview of iron overload disorders (acquired and hereditary), and will highlight state-of-the-art methods in diagnosing and treating excess iron stores. Additionally, advances in dietary approaches to managing iron intake will be reviewed.

## BIOLOGY AND PATHOPHYSIOLOGY

The body absorbs 10% (1–2 mg) of the iron encountered in dietary sources each day, but has no efficient means of rapidly eliminating excess iron, other than loss of blood. Iron absorption is regulated in the gastrointestinal (GI) tract at the initial part of the small intestine called the duodenum, which lies just beyond the stomach in the digestive tract.[6,16,17]

Following absorption, iron is normally bound to specific storage or transport proteins when not in use; this limits the possibility of excess free iron catalyzing generation of damaging free radicals. Iron travels through the bloodstream bound to transferrin (an iron transport protein).

Cells that require iron (eg, red blood cells) express a transferrin receptor on their surface, which captures circulating transferrin and pulls it into the cell, causing it to release the bound iron.

Iron, in excess of what is needed to satisfy metabolic demand, is stored bound to the iron storage protein ferritin.[17,18] Both ferritin and transferrin are used as blood markers to monitor iron load (see Diagnosis section). Iron overload results from an elevated total body iron pool. There are primary (inherited) and secondary (acquired) causes of iron overload; many involve dysregulation of iron absorption from the gut. However, iron overload secondary to repeated blood transfusions can occur in patients with certain types of anemia.[6,19]

Despite its many important metabolic roles, iron is a potent free radical generator. Damaging reactive oxygen species are constantly produced during cellular energy generation. Antioxidant enzymes (eg, superoxide dismutase and catalase) normally eliminate these pro-oxidant compounds, sparing cells from oxidative damage. Iron, however, can readily convert these reactive oxygen species into damaging hydroxyl radicals that are not cleared by antioxidant enzymes. Hydroxyl radicals can damage DNA and cellular proteins, as well as decrease the integrity of cellular membranes.[6,20,21] *Iron balance* (homeostasis) in humans is predominantly controlled by limiting intestinal absorption, as well as efficient recycling of the body pool because virtually no iron is excreted.[6]

Iron balance is regulated by the peptide hormone hepcidin.[22] Hepcidin, produced by the liver in response to high iron stores or inflammation, travels through the bloodstream to the intestines where it reduces iron absorption. It is thought that both genetic and acquired causes of iron overload may share a common mechanism of low hepcidin production.[4]

Normal iron absorption (1–2 mg/day) and dysregulated iron absorption differ by only a few milligrams each day, yet this is sufficient to outpace iron loss— approximately 1 mg/day in adult men—which occurs very slowly through the sloughing of GI and skin cells.[6,16]

As the total body iron pool rises, its levels exceed the capacity of iron storage and transport proteins (ferritin and transferrin, respectively) to keep it safely bound.[23] Increased levels of non–transferrin-bound iron in the blood can enter cells, thus increasing free cellular iron levels. It is this free iron that is available for generating free radicals within cells, and is responsible for the cellular and tissue toxicities characteristic of iron overload.[23]

# CAUSES AND RISK FACTORS

## Primary Iron Overload

Primary iron overload results from inherited defects in genes involved in iron absorption, transport, or regulation.

**Hemochromatosis.** Hemochromatosis, the most common disease of primary iron overload, can be partitioned into four types. The most common is classic (type I) or HFE hemochromatosis. HFE hemochromatosis results from the inheritance of 2 mutant copies of the HFE or high Fe (iron) gene (C282Y and H63D).[11,24] These defective genes are thought to increase iron absorption by lowering production of hepcidin, and increasing iron uptake from intestinal cells.

The other 3 types of hemochromatosis are much more rare: type II is a more severe iron overload due to defective production of hepcidin; type III is a defect in the transferrin receptor (unable to uptake iron from the blood); and type IV results in defects in the removal of iron from certain cells (liver macrophages). Type IV may also cause the intestines to become insensitive to hepcidin, resulting in uncontrolled iron absorption.[19]

**Additional disorders.** Other hereditary iron overload disorders are extremely rare. They include atransferrinemia (lack of the transferrin iron transporter), mutation in the ferritin gene, and neurodegeneration with brain iron accumulation (NBIA).[19,25]

## Secondary Iron Overload

Secondary iron overload can result from a variety of conditions.

**Repeated blood transfusions to treat certain types of anemia.** Additional iron is introduced with each transfusion, and since humans have no mechanism for its excretion, iron overload becomes possible. Iron overload in transfusion patients presents additional treatment challenges, as phlebotomy, the gold standard for iron overload treatment in hereditary hemochromatosis, is usually not feasible in anemic patients.[26]

**Chronic liver disease.** Chronic liver disease, caused by, for example, alcoholic fatty liver and the hepatitis C virus, can compromise the liver's ability to produce the iron regulatory hormone hepcidin and the iron transport protein transferrin.[4,23]

**Additional sources.** Other sources of secondary iron overload include *excessive dietary intake*, *parenteral iron* (such as intravenous iron for anemia management), and *long-term hemodialysis*.[13,19]

# SIGNS, SYMPTOMS, AND CONSEQUENCES OF IRON OVERLOAD

The classic symptom of iron overload is *skin hyperpigmentation* (to a bronze or grey color), due to deposits of iron and melanin complexes in the skin. The *liver*, as a primary source of iron storage, is particularly susceptible to iron overload and related damage, which may range from enlargement (hepatomegaly) and elevated serum liver enzymes, to fibrosis or cirrhosis.[4]

Long-term iron overload can result in *liver cancer*.[2] High-serum iron (measured as greater than 60% transferrin saturation) increases the 10-year absolute risk of liver cancer almost 6-fold and risk of any cancer over 3-fold.[27]

Iron accumulation in *endocrine organs* has been associated with *diabetes*, *hypogonadism* (decreased production of sex hormones), and less commonly *hyper- or hypo-thyroidism*; some of these may be reversed by bringing iron levels back into a healthy range.[4,28]

*Osteoporosis* is possible with severe iron overload, and may be due to hypogonadism.[4,29]

*Arthropathy* (joint disease with or without inflammation) is common with iron overload, causing pain with minimal inflammation in the joints of the hands, wrists, elbows, shoulders, and hips.[4]

Iron deposition in the *heart* can cause *cardiomyopathy*, *arrhythmia*, *heart failure*, and *sudden cardiac death*.[30,31] It can also increase vascular damage and *atherosclerosis* risk.[32]

The *brain* is another potential site of excess iron accumulation, as it requires iron for several neuron-specific reactions, such as the synthesis of myelin, which sheaths neuronal axons, and the production of neurotransmitters.[33] Excess iron can form complexes with melanin in the substantia nigra of the brain in much the same way it does in skin; this has been observed in the brains of *Parkinson's disease* patients, and may be related to progression of the disease.[1,3,34] Iron deposits in the amyloid plaques of *Alzheimer's disease* patients may contribute to neurodegeneration through free radical toxicity.[35] Abnormal brain iron deposition has also been observed in *multiple sclerosis* as well as other neurodegenerative movement disorders.[25,33]

*Bacteria* require iron for many of the same reactions as humans; excess iron in the blood or tissues can *stimulate the growth of invading pathogens.*[19]

## IRON OVERLOAD AND ENDOCRINE DYSFUNCTION

*Hormonal imbalance* is a significant problem among individuals with primary or secondary iron overload.[36–38]

Excess iron accumulates in the *pituitary gland* and disrupts synthesis of gonadotropin-releasing hormone (GnRH), which is responsible for stimulating the production of sex hormones from the gonads (ie, testes and ovaries). The consequence of this disruption is abnormally low levels of important sex hormones like testosterone and estrogen.[37,38]

However, pituitary dysfunction alone does not account for all the hormonal perturbations observed in all iron overload cases.[39] This can be partly explained by another phenomenon observed among some iron overload patients—elevated *sex hormone–binding globulin (SHBG)* levels—although the mechanism for this elevation is not entirely clear.[40]

SHBG is a transport protein that carriers sex hormones through circulation. The problem, however, is that when hormones are bound to SHBG, their ability to bind and activate their receptors is greatly hindered. So, when SHBG levels are elevated due to iron accumulation in the liver, hormonal signaling may be disrupted.[41]

Thus, iron accumulation in the brain and the liver among those with iron overload may precipitate considerable hormonal irregularities, which can lead to a barrage of complications ranging from *diabetes* to *cardiovascular problems* and *loss of libido* to *osteoporosis.*[42–45]

An unfortunate reality is that many conventional physicians may not appreciate the role of iron overload in hormone-related complications.[46,47] Therefore, it is likely that many patients whose hormone-related ailments may be attributable to excess iron levels are not properly diagnosed and treated.

Life Extension suggests that individuals with known or suspected hormonal imbalances consider *blood tests for iron overload*. Likewise, individuals with iron overload should consider *blood tests for hormone imbalances*. Identification and treatment of these commonly concurrent conditions may improve quality of life for many people.

## DIAGNOSIS

Given the potential involvement of elevated tissue iron in the progression of several seemingly unrelated diseases, surveillance of total body iron content may present an important measure of disease prevention. Historically, excessive iron has been diagnosed only after sufficient damage has occurred to reveal characteristic symptoms (hyperpigmentation, liver enlargement, and joint problems); however, there are several tests that can monitor iron status before signs and symptoms of frank iron overload occur. Annual blood testing for iron load can allow early detection of subclinical elevations that can be addressed by diet, lifestyle changes, and/or conventional therapies.[6,13,14]

*Serum ferritin* and *transferrin saturation* are blood tests that can detect iron overload, even before symptoms appear.[6,13,14] Other important tests for diagnosing iron overload include serum iron, total iron binding capacity (TIBC), HFE test, liver biopsy, and magnetic resonance imaging (MRI).

**Serum ferritin.** This test measures the iron storage protein ferritin in the blood serum. While typically an intracellular storage protein, blood levels of ferritin increase proportionally to body stores (1 ng/ml of serum ferritin represents approximately 8 mg of stored iron).[13] Infection, inflammation, or liver disease can elevate serum ferritin levels, complicating measurements in individuals with these conditions; a high-sensitivity C-reactive protein (hs-CRP) test can be used to rule out inflammation.[6]

**Transferrin saturation.** Transferrin saturation (TSAT) measures the ratio of serum iron and total iron-binding capacity of transferrin multiplied by 100.[13] Elevated TSAT is seen in several genetic causes of iron overload.[14]

**Serum iron.** Serum iron measures the total iron in blood serum.[13]

**TIBC.** TIBC measures total binding capacity of transferrin (the iron transport protein) in the serum (an indirect measurement of transferrin).[13]

**HFE test.** An HFE test is a genetic test for the presence of either of the 2 main mutations (C282Y and H63D) of the HFE gene. These mutations are the most common causes of hereditary hemochromatosis. An individual with type I hemochromatosis generally carries 2 copies of the C282Y gene, or one copy of each mutant gene.[15] Positive HFE analysis confirms the clinical diagnosis of hemochromatosis in asymptomatic individuals with blood tests showing increased iron stores; it is also predictive of risk in individuals with a family history of hemochromatosis.[19]

**Liver biopsy.** Liver biopsy can be used as a direct measure of nonheme iron and for the diagnosis of non-HFE hemochromatosis. Liver iron concentrations of >15 mg/g dry weight increase the risk of iron-associated cardiovascular disease and early death. The threshold for liver injury and fibrosis is about 22 mg/g.[13]

**MRI.** The development of MRI of the liver and heart now offers a noninvasive method for assessing iron stores in these organs. *R2-MRI* (also known as

*FerriScan*) is now specifically recommended as a method to measure liver iron concentrations in clinical practice guidelines. It is also used for monitoring the efficacy of iron chelation therapy.[12,13,48]

# CONVENTIONAL TREATMENT

## Phlebotomy

The standard treatment for patients with iron overload is bloodletting (phlebotomy or venesection) in the absence of anemia and chelation in the iron-loading anemias.[14,19] One unit (about 450 ml) of blood contains approximately 200–250 mg of iron, depending on the hemoglobin concentration; it is often recommended to remove one unit per week (as tolerated). In patients who have very high total body iron stores >30 g, therapeutic phlebotomy (ie, removal of blood) may take up to 1–2 years to adequately reduce iron stores, until serum ferritin levels and transferrin saturation values fall within normal ranges. Ferritin levels are then typically maintained by removal of 2–4 units of blood per year.[19]

A potential drawback of phlebotomy is a decrease in hepcidin levels and excess iron absorption.[14] Removal of blood initiates the compensatory synthesis of new red blood cells in bone marrow. These new red blood cells have increased iron requirements through enhanced production of the oxygen-carrying protein hemoglobin. Thus, hepcidin levels may be further decreased so that additional iron can be absorbed to meet increased demand.[49]

In one study among patients with hereditary hemochromatosis, phlebotomy was associated with decreased hepcidin levels; although subjects' hepcidin levels were low initially.[49,50] Targeting a serum ferritin level slightly above the recommended range during maintenance phlebotomy may help some patients avoid increased iron absorption caused by low hepcidin levels.[49]

## Iron Chelation

For patients refractory to phlebotomy treatment, or for those in which blood removal is not feasible (eg, iron-loading anemia patients), iron chelation is the standard therapy.

Currently, there are three Food and Drug Administration (FDA)–approved iron chelating agents. Deferoxamine mesylate (Desferal®) is an injectable iron chelator that has been in use since the 1960s. It can bind and remove iron from ferritin stores or abnormal tissue deposits, but not from sites of active metabolic iron usage (such as transferrin or hemoglobin). Deferoxamine has considerable drawbacks; it can elicit hypersensitivity and systemic allergic reactions,

and its short half-life requires treatment via a slow injection over a period of 4–12 hours.[6]

The development of oral iron chelators has enabled more convenient dosing and improved patient compliance. Deferiprone (Ferriprox®) is a synthetic analog of mimosine (a naturally occurring iron chelating compound, originally derived from the *Mimosa pudica* plant).[6,51] Its rapid metabolism by the liver requires that it be taken in high doses for efficacy. Side effects of deferiprone include GI discomfort and skin rash. Deferasirox (Exjade®), an orally bioavailable chelator with a longer half-life and smaller effective dose than deferiprone, has been approved in the United States for treatment of secondary iron overload due to ineffective erythropoiesis since 2005. It exhibits some of the same side effects as deferiprone, with the possibility of more serious side effects (eg, liver failure and renal dysfunction). It is also very expensive. Due to its small molecular size (compared to deferoxaminedeferoxamine), deferasirox is able to move throughout the body, removing iron from the active sites of several critical iron-containing enzymes.[6,52]

# EMERGING THERAPIES

The evolution of the therapeutic treatment for iron overload has been slow. Almost a hundred years passed between the first description of hemochromatosis in 1889 and the establishment of phlebotomy as a treatment; only recently have more precise metabolic and genetic mechanisms of iron overload been elucidated.[19]

## Iron Chelators

There appears to be increasing interest in the development of safer iron chelators with enhanced iron-clearing activity.[53] High-molecular-weight derivatives of deferoxamine, attached to natural or synthetic fibers, retain the iron-binding activity of the classic drug, while offering reduced toxicity and longer time in circulation, thus overcoming some of the shortcomings of deferoxamine alone.[53] A new oral chelator (FBS0701) is currently in clinical trials. It has an activity similar to the FDA-approved deferasirox, but with a significantly better safety profile (especially for kidney function).[54] Restoring iron regulatory function through the administration of transferrin, hepcidin, or modified hepcidin molecules (minihepcidin) is also being explored as a potential therapy.[14,55]

## Erythrocytapheresis

Erythrocytapheresis, selective removal of red blood cells from blood while preserving blood volume, has been investigated as an alternative to conventional phlebotomy.[56] Erythrocytapheresis can remove more red blood cells per procedure (achieving desired reductions in serum ferritin in fewer procedures), with no significant differences in cost, quality of life, or frequency of adverse events.[56] However, it may demonstrate some of the same drawbacks as phlebotomy (eg, lowering hepcidin levels).

## Bone Marrow Transplantation and Novel Stem Cell Therapies

Understanding genetic iron regulatory mechanisms may allow practitioners another therapeutic direction to address iron overload. Restoration of functional iron regulatory genes in patients with hereditary iron dysregulation may prove a viable treatment. Bone marrow transplantation has already proven to be an effective approach for treating young patients with β-thalassemia. In a survey of 115 transplant procedure patients between 1983 and 2006, 89% (103) survived to an average 15-year follow-up, with 96% (99) of those survivors no longer requiring blood transfusions.[57] Stem cells from bone marrow may also be used to reconstitute iron regulation elsewhere in the body. When type I hemochromatotic mice (containing two mutant copies of the HFE gene) were transplanted with bone marrow from healthy donor mice, donor stem cells were detected in the liver (constituting 11% of total liver cells) and intestine after 6 months. In both cases, the stem cells had transformed (differentiated) into cell types appropriate for those organs (liver hepatocytes and intestinal myofibroblasts), partially restored the expression of iron regulatory genes (including HFE), and reduced iron content in these tissues compared to control animals.[58]

## DIETARY AND LIFESTYLE CONSIDERATIONS

Population studies suggest *limiting dietary iron intake* may lower serum iron burden. In one study of men and women with a high incidence of HFE mutations (approximately 40% of the test group had at least one mutation in the HFE gene), the frequency of red meat and alcohol consumption was associated with higher serum ferritin levels, and noncitrus fruits with lower serum ferritin levels in men.[59] Similarly, a study of women saw modest associations between the intake of alcohol, red meat, and heme iron as well as serum ferritin.[60] In addition to the heme form of iron found in meats, nonheme iron can be found in plant-based foods (eg, leafy greens, legumes, and fortified breads and cereals).[61] The

contribution of nonheme iron to iron overload is unclear; neither of the above studies reported significant increases in serum ferritin levels associated with nonheme iron consumption.[59,60] The long-term effects of low-iron diets on disease progression are unknown, and clinical studies of dietary iron restriction are lacking.

Foods high in ascorbic (vitamin C) and citric acid (eg, citrus fruits) may enhance the absorption of nonheme iron.[62] Supplemental vitamin C >500 mg/day should be avoided in patients with iron overload,[63] especially at mealtimes.

Yearly blood donation may also help to maintain iron levels. Blood donors had an average 33% decrease in serum ferritin levels compared to nondonors in one study.[60]

Life Extension advises against taking supplemental iron unless needed (ie, due to a deficiency). Iron needs should be determined with yearly blood testing. Because excessive iron intake may be associated with, or increase the risk of several degenerative diseases, Life Extension multivitamins are formulated without iron. Pregnant women, due to increased iron requirements, should consult their physician to determine if iron supplementation is appropriate.

## TARGETED NUTRITIONAL STRATEGIES

Several dietary constituents have been investigated for their ability to treat iron overload. They work by either reducing or inhibiting iron absorption from the gut, or binding excess iron in the blood and tissues to help draw it out of the body. Additionally, the significant contribution of free radical damage to the progression of iron-overload associated diseases suggests a role for increasing antioxidant consumption.

### Lactoferrin

Lactoferrin is an iron-binding protein analogous to the iron transporter transferrin; it binds and sequesters iron in areas outside of the bloodstream such as the mucous membranes, GI tract, and reproductive tissues.[64] It is present at high concentrations in milk, and is secreted by immune cells (neutrophils) as an antibacterial compound at sites of infection or inflammation.[65,66]

The antimicrobial effects of lactoferrin are attributed to its ability to deprive pathogenic microorganisms of the iron needed for growth.[66] Experiments also suggest lactoferrin may have antioxidant and anti-inflammatory properties, and may influence the expression of inflammatory genes.[65,67,68] Evidence suggests that low-iron *apolactoferrin* may be protective against iron-mediated, free radical damage; it reduced iron-catalyzed formation of hydroxyl radicals in vitro.[69]

## Polyphenols

Polyphenols such as chlorogenic acid,[70] quercetin, rutin, chrysin,[71] punicalagins (from pomegranate),[72] and proanthocyanidins (from cranberry) have been shown to bind iron in vitro.[73] In an in-vitro binding study of 26 flavonoids (a type of polyphenol) isolated from a variety of sources (including tea catechins, hesperidin, naringenin, and diosmin), several were nearly as effective as deferoxamine at chelating ferrous iron when supplied at a 10:1 flavonoid/iron ratio. When supplied at a 1:1 ratio, quercetin, myricetin, and baicalein (a flavonoid from skullcap) continued to chelate iron with the same efficiency as deferoxamine.[74] As antioxidants, polyphenols may also reduce iron-catalyzed free radical generation.[75]

In a mouse model of iron overload (>2000 mg iron/g of liver weight), both quercetin and baicalin (fed as 1% of water, which is roughly equivalent to 15 g for a 70-kg human) reduced iron-induced lipid peroxidation and protein oxidation in the liver, decreased liver iron stores as well as serum ferritin, and increased fecal excretion of iron.[76] Clinical studies are necessary to confirm polyphenol's effect(s) in humans.

## Pectin

Pectin is an indigestible fiber that binds tightly to nonheme iron, thus interfering with its absorption. In a small study of 13 patients with idiopathic hemochromatosis (conducted before the genetics of hemochromatosis had been discovered), iron absorption decreased by nearly half following a loading dose of 9 g/m² of pectin (about 15 g for the average adult). Cellulose fiber had no effect on iron binding.[77]

## Milk Thistle

Milk thistle and its flavonoid constituent (ie, silymarin) have iron chelation and hydroxyl radial quenching properties.[78,79] In HFE hemochromatosis patients, 140 mg of silybin (the main component of silymarin) taken with a test meal containing about 14 mg of nonheme iron reduced iron absorption by over 40%.[80] When combined with soy phosphatidylcholine, silybin treatment for 12 weeks demonstrated a modest (13%) reduction in serum ferritin (indicative of reduced total body iron stores) in patients with chronic hepatitis C.[81] When combined with the injectable iron chelator

deferoxamine, silymarin resulted in more effective reductions in serum ferritin than deferoxamine alone in patients with β-thalassemia.[82]

## Curcumin

Curcuminoids, which are derived from the spice turmeric, are antioxidants and iron chelators. In experimental models, they have been shown to reduce iron-catalyzed oxidative damage of DNA,[83] liver damage associated with iron-associated lipid peroxidation,[84] and free radical damage due to iron in amyloid plaques characteristic of Alzheimer's disease.[85] In β-thalassemic mice, curcumin bound iron in the blood reduced cardiac iron deposits in mice fed a high-iron diet,[86] and reduced iron-associated lipid peroxidation when combined with the IV chelator deferiprone.[87] The iron chelation effects of curcumin in the liver depend on total iron intake. At low dietary iron concentrations, curcumin demonstrated a significant reduction in transferrin saturation and plasma iron in mice given curcumin as 2% of their diet.[88] Mice on high iron diets, however, saw significant decreases in liver ferritin (indicative of a decrease in iron storage capacity), but no changes in total plasma iron or transferrin saturation when given curcumin as 2% of their diet.[88,89]

## Green Tea

Green tea catechins are potent antioxidants that demonstrate an iron-chelating activity similar to the injectable chelator deferoxamine in test tube studies.[90] The addition of green tea extract with a high epigallocatechin gallate (EGCG) content to blood samples from β-thalassemia patients rapidly chelated non–transferrin-bound iron, and modestly reduced markers of lipid peroxidation.[91] The ability of green tea catechins to cross the blood–brain barrier implicates them as possible agents for the chelation of abnormal iron deposits characteristic of several neurodegenerative disorders.[90] Studies examining the effect(s) of green tea consumption on iron status in humans are conflicting. Several studies have shown no association between tea consumption and iron absorption, serum ferritin, or hemoglobin levels in individuals with adequate iron intake.[92–94] However, 2 studies did show reductions in serum ferritin and iron absorption with high consumption levels of green tea[95] and green tea extract,[96] respectively.

## Alpha Lipoic Acid

Alpha lipoic acid is an important antioxidant and enzyme co-factor. In cell culture, alpha-lipoic acid (in its reduced form, dihydrolipoic acid) protects neurons against oxidative damage catalyzed by iron or Alzheimer's beta amyloid[97] In a preclinical trial, R-alpha-lipoic acid (R-LA) was fed to older rats with age-related accumulation of iron in the cerebral cortex. Following 2 weeks of R-LA supplementation, iron levels dropped to those indicative of younger rats.[98]

## Carnitine

Carnitine is an internal shuttle that helps move fatty acids into the mitochondria for conversion into energy. Carnitine esters (acetyl-L-carnitine and propionyl-L-carnitine) are derivatives that may have additional antioxidant activities that confer advantages over carnitine alone.[99] When combined with alpha lipoic acid, acetyl-L-carnitine attenuated the production of free radicals in cultures of iron-overloaded human fibroblasts.[100] In test tube studies, propionyl-L-carnitine inhibits superoxide radicals, and reduces lipid peroxidation catalyzed by hydrogen peroxide.[101] It is also proposed that propionyl-L-carnitine can reduce the production of hydroxyl radicals generated by iron, because of its iron-chelating activity.[102]

## Life Extension Suggestions

- **Green tea extract**, standardized to 98% polyphenols: 725–1450 mg daily
- **Curcumin**, as highly absorbed BCM-95®: 400–800 mg daily
- **Milk thistle**, standardized extract: 750 mg daily
- **Lactoferrin** (apoloactoferrin): 300 mg daily
- **R-lipoic acid:** 300–600 mg daily
- **L-carnitine**, as acetyl L-carnitine and propionyl L-carnitine: 1400 mg daily
- **Diosmin:** 600 mg daily
- **Quercetin,** as quercetin glycoside derivatives and free quercetin: 250–500 mg daily
- **Grape extract complex:** 150 mg daily
- **Modified citrus pectin**, with alginate complex: 1.5–3 g daily

In addition, the following *blood tests* may provide helpful information:

- Male or Female Panel
- Ferritin
- Serum iron
- Transferrin

## REFERENCES

References available at: www.lef.org/dpt5/ch69

# 70

# *Hepatitis B*

Hepatitis B is an infectious liver disease caused by the *hepatitis B virus (HBV)*.[1–3] While most adults infected with HBV recover, a portion can develop *chronic hepatitis B*, risking serious illness or death from cirrhosis, hepatocellular carcinoma (liver cancer), or liver failure.[4–7]

According to 2009 World Health Organization estimates, more than 2 billion people have been exposed to the hepatitis B virus and 360 million are chronically infected worldwide.[6] It has been estimated that 12 million people in the United States have been exposed to HBV, with roughly 700 000 being chronically infected.[8]

Chronic HBV infection often does not cause symptoms in its early stages, so only about 33% of adults with chronic hepatitis are aware they are infected. Of those eligible for treatment for chronic HBV, only about 12.5% are receiving it.[9]

While the availability of HBV vaccination has decreased the incidence of HBV infection in the United States, about 43 000 cases of acute hepatitis B still occur each year.[10] Rates of vaccination are relatively low among high-risk populations (eg, illicit IV drug users, individuals with HIV, and hemophiliacs); according to a 2007 Centers for Disease Control and Prevention survey, over 51% of high-risk adults remained unvaccinated in the United States.[11]

Standard therapies for chronic HBV infection and hepatitis are limited, and are not effective in all cases.[9,12] Additionally, the unique life cycle of the HBV allows it to evolve and develop resistance to antiviral drugs.[13]

Overlooked is an abundance of published research documenting potent *antiviral* and *liver-protecting* properties of easy-to-obtain nutrients.

Fortunately, minimization of risk factors for HBV can reduce transmission of the virus, while new diagnostics and emerging treatments continue to advance the ability to combat this disease. This protocol will review these conventional treatments, as well as discuss nutritional approaches for addressing HBV infection and chronic liver disease progression.

# DEVELOPMENT AND PROGRESSION OF HBV INFECTION

## HBV Biology

The hepatitis B virus infects humans and higher primates, entering and replicating within liver cells (hepatocytes), and secreting new virus particles into circulation.[6,14] HBV is extremely effective at targeting hepatocytes; less than 10 individual virus particles are sufficient to establish an infection.[15] Upon infection, HBV DNA enters the nucleus of the hepatocyte, where it serves as the reservoir for formation of virus particles for the lifetime of the cell and makes treatment of HBV challenging.[5,16] Replication of HBV requires the activity of a viral reverse transcriptase enzyme, which is prone to introducing mutations into the viral genome and potentially allowing the virus to become resistant to some treatments.[5,17]

Following an incubation period of 1–4 months, acute symptomatic hepatitis occurs in about one-third of infected adults, 10% of young children, and rarely in infants.[5] Acute hepatitis B resolves on its own in over 95% of adult cases.[17] The acute infection is considered resolved when *hepatitis B surface antigen* (HBsAg) can no longer be detected in the blood within 6 months of infection.[5] HBsAg, a lipoprotein that forms part of the protective coating of the virus particle, is a marker for disease progression. Many individuals with HBV infection (7–40%) who are HBsAg-positive may also carry the hepatitis B e-antigen (HBeAg), a viral protein associated with high infectivity.[6] After resolution of an acute infection, an individual generally develops lifelong immunity against HBV-associated hepatitis, although the virus itself is not cleared from the liver.[5] Small amounts of viral DNA can be detected in blood years after recovery from acute hepatitis B.[17] Thus, immunosuppression (eg, corticosteroid therapy) has the potential to reactivate an HBV infection.

There are several genetic strains of HBV (genotypes A–H), which vary in geographic distribution, response to treatment, and risk of progression to advanced liver disease.[17,18] In the United States, HBV genotypes A and D are more common in African Americans and Caucasians, whereas HBV genotypes B and C are more common among persons of Asian ancestry.[4] Severe liver disease and hepatocellular carcinoma is more likely from infection with genotypes C and D. Response to interferon treatment (a conventional therapy) is greater in genotypes A and B (than C or D), and thymosin treatment is twice as effective in genotype B than C.[18,19] Although not yet standard for HBV treatment, genotyping could enable clinicians to identify and provide appropriate therapy for those at increased risk of disease progression.[18]

## Transmission and Infectivity

HBV is transmitted through the skin (eg, injection) or via mucosal exposure to infected blood or other body fluids, mainly semen or vaginal fluid.[6] In geographic areas with low HBV prevalence (such as the United States), sexual transmission and use of contaminated needles by illicit drug users are major risk factors for infection.[20]

In areas of high HBV prevalence (such as the Asia Pacific region), the virus is most commonly spread from infected mother to child at birth or child to child during early childhood. About 90% of mothers with high viral load will infect their babies with HBV.[17] HBV can also infect sperm, enabling possible transmission from infected father to embryo during conception.[21] The likelihood of parent-to-child transmission can be reduced by vaccination.[22]

Individuals with acute or chronic HBV infection should be considered infectious any time HBsAg is present in the blood. HBsAg can be found in blood and bodily fluids for 1–2 months before and after the onset of symptoms. HBsAg can be identified in serum 30–60 days after exposure to HBV. Other markers of infectivity include *HBeAg* and *HBV DNA*. HBeAg is a viral protein that indicates ongoing viral replication and increased infectivity. HBV DNA is a marker of viral replication; higher viral loads correlate with greater infectivity[6,23,24]

# OUTCOMES OF HBV INFECTION

## Asymptomatic or Acute HBV Infection

Acute HBV infection is asymptomatic in most individuals (symptomatic acute hepatitis B occurs in only about one-third of infected adults, 10% of children, and rarely in infants).[5] Symptoms are similar to those of other types of viral hepatitis, and include loss of appetite, fatigue, nausea, vomiting, abdominal pain, joint pain, mild fever, dark urine, and jaundice (yellowing of the skin and eyes due to accumulation of bilirubin secondary to liver dysfunction).[2] The majority of acute hepatitis cases resolve, and the infected person eventually develops immunity to the virus.[5,17]

## Chronic HBV Infection

Some acutely infected individuals will progress to chronic HBV infection. Chronic HBV carriers are identified by the presence of *hepatitis B surface antigen (HBsAg)* in their blood for over 6 months, a HBV DNA blood level of 2000–20000 IU/mL, and persistent or intermittent increases in liver enzymes. People with viral DNA loads of less than 2000 IU/mL are considered inactive carriers.[25]

Age of infection has a significant effect on persistence of HBV[5,6]; 90% of children infected at birth will develop chronic HBV, compared to 20–30% of children aged 1–5 and 1–5% of adults.[5] Chronic HBV infection increases the risk of serious liver disease, including cirrhosis and hepatocellular carcinoma.[4] Dysbiosis (detrimental changes in intestinal flora) is also possible.[26]

## Cirrhosis

Cirrhosis, the end stage of any chronic liver disease,[27] involves functional liver tissue being replaced by fibrous tissue and scarring. Ascites (buildup of fluid in the abdomen), hepatic encephalopathy (depressed brain function due to accumulation of toxins in the brain), bacterial infection of the abdomen, and cancer are complications of cirrhosis.[27,28] Cirrhosis is generally irreversible, although studies suggest that some HBV-mediated cirrhosis may be reversible with treatment.[9]

## Hepatocellular Carcinoma

Liver cancer is the fifth most common cancer in men and seventh most common in women worldwide. Hepatocellular carcinoma (HCC) is the most common form of liver cancer. Approximately 80% of HCC cases are associated with chronic HBV or hepatitis C virus (HCV) infection.[4] HCC risk increases with viral load. In the REVEAL-HBV study of liver disease in chronic HBV patients, individuals with the highest viral loads at study entry (over 1 million copies of HBV DNA per ml in blood) had almost 11 times the risk of HCC than those with viral loads of less than 10000 copies/ml of blood.[29]

## Fulminant Hepatitis

Fulminant hepatitis is an acute hepatitis leading to acute liver failure and hepatic encephalopathy within a rapid period of time (<8 weeks after the onset of jaundice).[30] From 7–33.7% of fulminant hepatitis cases stem from HBV infection.[30] Fulminant hepatitis is rare in HBV-infected children, and develops in 0.1–0.6% of acute hepatitis cases in adults.[5] HBV-mediated fulminant hepatitis has a mortality rate of about 70%.[6]

# CAUSES AND RISK FACTORS FOR HEPATITIS B AND HBV INFECTION

Risk factors for HBV transmission or the progression of HBV disease include the following.

## Gender

Chronic hepatitis B progresses more rapidly in males than females; cirrhosis and HCC predominate in men and postmenopausal women.[4,31] High serum levels of testosterone have been associated with increased HCC risk in HBV carriers.[32] Additionally, among 42 men who underwent liver resection for HCC between 1995 and 1999, those whose preoperative testosterone levels were in the upper half of the distribution had greater disease recurrence and poorer survival rates over a 5-year follow-up.[33] In contrast, premenopausal women have lower liver iron stores and reduced production of proinflammatory cytokines, both reducing risk of liver disease; this also suggests a potential protective role of estrogens.[31]

## HIV Infection

An estimated 10% of the 40 million people infected with HIV worldwide are also infected with HBV. HIV infection significantly increases the risk of developing cirrhosis and HCC in individuals carrying both viruses,[6] and HBV increases the rate of mortality in HIV patients on antiretroviral therapy.[34]

## Alcohol Use

A few studies investigating the association between alcohol intake, HBV infection, and the progression of liver disease found a 1.2–3 times increased risk of HCC among heavy alcohol users.[4]

## Sexual Behavior

Hepatitis B is considered a sexually transmitted disease (STD), and in areas with low HBV incidence such as the United States, sexual transmission represents a major route of infection. While homosexual men have the highest risk of infection (70% infected after 5 years of activity), heterosexual transmission has been increasing in frequency. In heterosexuals, multiple or high-risk partners (such as HBV carriers or illicit IV drug users), history of STD, and long duration of sexual activity all increase risk of transmission.[35]

## Intravenous (IV) Illicit Drug Use

Injection of illicit IV drugs is a major route of HBV infection in areas of low HBV incidence. In the United States and Western Europe, 23% of hepatitis B patients were infected by needles.[35]

## Contact with Infected Fluids

Individuals in frequent contact with potentially contaminated blood products or bodily fluids (eg, health care workers, lab technicians, police, firefighters, and patients requiring frequent transfusions or hemodialysis) are at increased risk of HBV infection.

Contaminated instruments (eg, those used for surgery, body piercing, acupuncture, or tattooing) also represent possible sources of infection.[35]

## Parent-to-Child Transfer

As mentioned earlier, mother-to-child transfer is a significant source of viral transmission in both high-prevalence and low-prevalence geographic areas. In contrast to transmission by sexual contact, drug use, or contact with infected blood (which all have a <5% risk of chronic infectivity), infection at birth carries a 90% risk of chronicity.[5,35]

# DIAGNOSIS

There are several tests for diagnosing HBV infection; the tests monitor either viral load or liver function.

## Tests for HBV Viral Load

Quantification of HBV DNA in the blood by polymerase chain reaction (PCR) or newer real-time PCR tests are indicative of the activity of HBV replication. Levels above 2000 IU/ml indicate active or chronic infection, while levels below this indicate inactive carriage of the virus.[25]

Serum HBsAg level is also a marker of infected liver mass and the amount of HBV DNA in infected hepatocytes. When combined with PCR testing, a blood test for HBsAg levels can be used to monitor progression of chronic HBV infection or identify inactive carriers.[25]

Other serologic tests for viral load include quantification of HBeAg, a marker for high-infectivity HBV, as well as the detection of antibodies to HBV antigens (anti-HBs, anti-HBe, and anti-HBc, an antibody to the HBV core antigen), which can indicate a prior or chronic infection.[6,25] Testing for anti-HBc IgM antibody can identify acute HBV infection.[36]

## Liver Function Tests

There are several blood tests that are not specific to HBV and nonspecifically assess liver function, but are important in the diagnosis of infection; these include alanine aminotransferase (or ALT, a marker of liver cell damage), bilirubin (an indicator of liver excretion function), and albumin levels and prothrombin time (indicators of liver synthesis function).[17] Most of these markers can be measured in routine blood tests. Fibrometers (ie, liver-fibrosis–specific blood panels), which combine some of these markers with other liver-specific markers, are also available.[37]

## Liver Biopsy

Liver biopsy is an important, but invasive technique for grading liver damage. Newer noninvasive methods use imaging techniques to assess liver stiffness (a direct physical property of the liver that increases as the liver is filled with connective tissue during fibrosis). These include transient elastography (an ultrasound technique) and magnetic resonance elastography.[37]

# CONVENTIONAL TREATMENT FOR HEPATITIS B

Acute hepatitis B typically resolves on its own and may not require treatment.[17] The goal of chronic hepatitis B treatment is to suppress HBV viral replication, which may limit hepatitis progression and may lower the risk of some complications, such as cirrhosis or cancer.[14]

## Antiviral Therapy

There are seven drugs approved for treatment of chronic hepatitis.[12] Interferon (IFN) is a signal protein produced by infected or cancerous cells to bolster the immune response of neighboring cells.[38] Interferon alpha (IFN-α) therapy is an approved antiviral for HBV and HCV infection. Both standard IFN-α and pegylated IFN-α (an IFN derivative with a longer half-life in the body)[39] are administered via subcutaneous injection.[5] INF-α, either alone or in combination with the nucleoside analog lamivudine, lowers viral load and normalizes ALT levels.[9] IFN alone may reduce the incidence of cirrhosis, hepatocellular carcinoma, and liver-related deaths.[9] Side effects of IFN include fatigue, flu-like symptoms, mood changes, bone marrow suppression, and development or exacerbation of autoimmune illnesses.[9] IFN-α may be better for achieving a sustained virologic response than nucleotide analogs.[5]

## Nucleotide and Nucleoside Analogs

Nucleotide and nucleoside analogs (NUCs; lamivudine, telbivudine, entecavir, adefovir dipivoxil, and tenofovir disoproxil fumarate) interfere with HBV viral replication. Trials of NUCs in HBV patients demonstrate a decrease in viral load, ALT levels, and hepatocellular carcinoma incidence, as well as the possible reversal of HBV-mediated cirrhosis. As oral medications, NUCs are more convenient to take than IFN, but the eventual development of resistance to these drugs limits their long-term utility. Side effects, which vary by drug, include myopathy and peripheral neuropathy (telbivudine), kidney toxicity and dysfunction (tenofovir and adefovir), decreased bone mineral density (tenofovir), and lactic acidosis in patients with liver disease (entecavir).[9]

# NOVEL AND EMERGING THERAPIES

## Heteroaryldihydropyrimidines

Heteroaryldihydropyrimidines (HAPs) are antiviral compounds that have been shown to inhibit HBV replication in isolated cells and animal models. In contrast to nucleotide and nucleoside analogs, which interfere with the replication of the viral genome, HAPs prevent the proper assembly of the protein capsule that surrounds the mature virus and serves as the site of DNA replication.[40,41] They are effective against HBV mutant strains resistant to nucleotide/nucleoside analog drugs.[13] Bay 41-4109, the best studied HAP, reduced HBV viral load by about two- to three-fold in a humanized mouse model (mice with livers that contain human liver cells).[13,42] These compounds await human trials.

## RNA Interference

RNA interference (RNAi) is a cellular mechanism for controlling gene expression; it is used by cells to regulate cell development and metabolism, but can also be used to turn off the expression of foreign genes, such as those of an invading virus. Since the life cycle of HBV relies on RNA intermediates for its replication, it is sensitive to inhibition by RNAi.[39] Therapeutic RNA inhibitors have been designed to interrupt HBV DNA replication, and turn off the genes that produce the structural and regulatory proteins required for assembly of infectious HBV particles. They have shown success in decreasing virus replication in cell cultures.[16] Early results of a safety trial of the small interfering RNA NUC B1000 appear promising.[43]

## Thymosin α1

Thymosin α1 (Tα1) is an immunomodulatory peptide derived from the thymus that stimulates T cells (one of the principle immune cells) to mature and produce cytokines, as well as increases the ability of the immune system to recognize invading pathogens.[44,45] In several studies of Tα1 therapy in chronic, HBeAg-negative (low-infectivity) HBV patients, thymosin lowered the liver enzyme ALT and increased the rate of HBV DNA clearance.[45] It is better tolerated than IFN-α. While treatment with Tα1 alone does not appear to be superior to current HBV therapies,[39] it may enhance the effectiveness of antivirals and IFN when used as a combination therapy,[46,47] especially in difficult-to-treat, HBeAg-positive patients. Tα1 is approved for use as a hepatitis B treatment in 30 countries, but is not yet available in the United States.[48]

# PREVENTION

## Vaccination

The availability of HBV vaccine and anti-HBV antibodies has significantly lowered HBV infection rates throughout the world. The first HBV vaccine was introduced in 1982, along with official recommendations for its use in high-risk groups.[49] Recommendations for childhood[50] and adolescent[51] vaccination programs were published within the decade. A synthetic version of the vaccine was introduced in 1986, replacing blood-derived versions of the vaccine,[6] and a thimerosal-free version has been available since 1999.[52]

Immunization may be one way to prevent mother-to-child transmission of HBV. In an analysis of several trials of children born to infected mothers, immunization reduced likelihood of mother-to-child transfer by 72%.[22] This protective effect decreased significantly when the initial dose of vaccine was delayed more than 7 days following birth.[6,53]

As mentioned above, rates of vaccination are relatively low among high-risk populations in the United States.[11] Health care workers at risk of HBV infection are recommended to receive the vaccine. However, in a study of matriculating health care students at a U.S. university, only about 60% had been vaccinated.[54]

# NUTRITIONAL STRATEGIES FOR HEPATITIS B

Although research on specific nutritional strategies for HBV infection is not as broad as for HCV infection, evidence suggests that natural compounds can be of benefit for both conditions (see the Hepatitis C protocol for more information).

## Selenium

Selenium is an essential trace element with protective roles in the defense against free radicals, liver detoxification reactions, and immunity.[55] Chronic hepatitis patients (as well as those infected with hepatitis C virus) tend to be selenium deficient compared to uninfected counterparts. The degree of deficiency relates to the severity of HBV infection (in one study, selenium levels dropped by 50% in HBV-infected men).[56] Adequate selenium may also be associated with less liver damage in HBV-infected patients.[57] It is suggested that HBV and HCV patients be tested for selenium adequacy and supplemented if deficient.[56] Long-term selenium treatment reduced HBV infection by 77% and liver lesions by over 75% in an animal model. In an 8-year trial, treatment reduced the incidence of liver cancer in HBV patients by 35%.[58]

## Coffee and Related Compounds

Evidence from several European and Japanese studies suggests coffee consumption is associated with reduced risk of liver cancer in. Heavy coffee consumption (defined in the studies as over 3 cups daily by Europeans, or over 1 cup daily by Japanese) reduced hepatocellular carcinoma (HCC) risk by an average of 55% over 10 observational studies.[59,60] Moderate coffee consumption (≥4 cups weekly) in HBV carriers reduced hepatocellular cancer incidence by almost 60% in a separate study.[61] *Chlorogenic acid*, a compound isolated from coffee, was shown to inhibit HBV viral replication in isolated liver cells, and reduce blood levels of HBV in an animal model. Its efficacy was comparable to the nucleoside analog lamivudine.[62] Special coffee roasting procedures can retain chlorogenic acid, which is normally depleted by Dian roasting procedures. Chlorogenic acid is also supplied by *green coffee extract* supplements.

## Green Tea

Green tea and its major antioxidant component *epigallocatechin gallate (EGCG)* reduce the levels of HBV DNA and hepatitis B antigens in isolated liver cells by inhibiting the replication of HBV DNA.[63,64] A study of 204 HCC cases in Chinese individuals with HBV infection revealed that green tea consumption reduced the risk of cancer progression by nearly half.[65] But a Japanese study of 110 cases of HCC could not determine any effect of green tea consumption on cancer risk.[66]

## Zinc

Zinc, which is found in various enzymes, has a role in immunoregulation.[67] Clearance of viral infection requires the activity of T cells, which are highly dependent on zinc.[68] Levels of zinc (as well as molybdenum, manganese, and selenium) are reduced in HBV-infected children compared to healthy subjects.[67] Low serum zinc is associated with elevated blood levels of liver enzymes (aspartate aminotransferase and alanine aminotransferase; markers of liver damage) in adults.[57] In one study, children with higher serum zinc levels had a better response to interferon (IFN) therapy.[69] In another study, the response to combination therapy of zinc and IFN-α in HBV infection was not significantly different than IFN-α alone. However, researchers speculate that the lack of response may have been due to the low dose of zinc administered (7.5–10 mg).[68]

## Lactoferrin

Lactoferrin is an antimicrobial protein with inhibitory activity against several viruses, possibly through interactions with host cells or direct binding to the invading virus. The antiviral activity of lactoferrin (a major protein in milk) may partially explain the low incidence of mother-to-child transfer of HBV through breastfeeding in humans.[70] Isolated human liver cells pre-treated with bovine or human lactoferrin were resistant to HBV infection.[71] Bovine lactoferrin, as well as zinc- and iron-saturated lactoferrin, inhibited HBV replication in infected human liver cells in culture.[72]

## Iron-Sequestering Compounds

High serum and hepatic iron have been associated with a reduced response to IFN treatment and increased risk of disease progression in chronic hepatitis B patients.[73] While their efficacy in HBV treatment has not been examined, several compounds have been shown to reduce iron absorption from the gut or chelate iron from cells or body fluids; these include several *flavonoids*,[74] *pectin*,[75] *silybin from milk thistle*,[76] and *curcumin*.[77] *Lactoferrin*[78] and *green tea*[79] may also have iron-sequestering activity in addition to their antiviral activity. More information is available in the Hemochromatosis protocol.

## B Vitamins

Patients with chronic hepatitis B exhibit marked increases in oxidative stress and lipid peroxidation along with decreased antioxidant status.[80] Vitamin B1 (thiamine) is required for the formation of dihydrolipoate, an important antioxidant and cofactor in iron metabolism, two functions with relevance to HBV disease mitigation. A small study on Chinese children with chronic HBV demonstrated similar reductions in HBV DNA and hepatitis B e-antigen (HBeAg) between thiamine and standard IFN therapies. But a second study in the same population showed no effect of thiamine on HBV.[73] Chronic HBV infection reduces levels of vitamins B2 (riboflavin) and B6 (pyridoxine) in red blood cells.[81] Supplementation with these vitamins may be helpful in HBV patients, although their effects on mitigating HBV disease are unknown.[81]

## Vitamins C and E

Vitamin C and E stores are also reduced in chronic HBV patients.[82] Three small studies of vitamin E therapy in HBV-infected children and adults suggest a possible role for the antioxidant in the clearance of HBV DNA, adaptation of immune response to the viral antigen, and normalization of liver enzymes levels.[73]

## Resveratrol

In an animal model of HBV-associated liver disease, resveratrol reduced fatty changes in the liver and structural alterations of liver cells (such as degradation of mitochondria), raised cellular glutathione levels, and decreased reactive oxygen species. Additionally, resveratrol reduced incidence of HCC by 5-fold, and enhanced liver cell proliferation and liver regeneration.[83]

## Curcumin

Curcumin reduces viral replication and expression of HBV genes in isolated human hepatocytes by inhibiting the activity of the metabolic regulator PGC-1$\alpha$.[84,85] PGC-1$\alpha$, which is activated during starvation and turns on genes involved in glucose production, also increases the replication of HBV.[85]

## N-Acetyl-Cysteine

N-acetyl-cysteine (NAC) is derived from L-cysteine, a conditionally essential amino acid. This powerful antioxidant diminishes free radicals and raises glutathione levels.[86] It reduces viral load in experimental models by disrupting the assembly of HBV virus particles.[87] The few studies of NAC in HBV patients have had mixed results. Dosages of 1200–8000 mg per day were able to raise glutathione levels in chronic HBV patients or lower levels of bilirubin (high bilirubin can indicate liver dysfunction), but did not significantly affect most other markers of liver function.[88–90] Neither oral nor intravenous NAC significantly affected HBV viral load or time to patient recovery, although differences in dosages and small study populations may preclude any conclusions about NAC therapy for HBV.[91,92]

## Phyllanthus

*Phyllanthus*, a genus of plant used to treat chronic liver disease in traditional Chinese and Indian medical systems, has demonstrated inhibition of HBV viral replication and antigen synthesis in isolated cells as well as in animal models.[93] A review of several small clinical trials suggests some positive effects of *Phyllanthus* on parameters of HBV infection and significant reductions in serum HBV antigen. Several species of *Phyllanthus* were used in these trials; one of the most commonly used is *Phyllanthus amarus* at a dose of 600–1200 mg daily.[94] Fifteen trials have investigated combinations of *Phyllanthus* and antiviral drugs (INF-α, lamivudine, adefovir dipivoxil, thymosin, vidarabine), and demonstrated significant improvements associated with combination therapy over antiviral drugs alone, such as reducing blood levels of HBV DNA and HBV antigen, and increasing immune response to HBV.[95]

## Whey Protein

In addition to its anabolic benefits, long-term supplementation with whey protein may increase antioxidant status and reduce markers of liver damage.[96] An open-label study of eight chronic hepatitis B patients revealed that 12 g twice daily of undenatured whey protein reduced ALT activity in six of the patients and raised glutathione in five after 12 weeks of supplementation. Additionally, markers of lipid oxidation significantly decreased, while interleukin-2 levels and natural killer (NK) activity (both involved in immune response) significantly increased.[97]

## Astragalus

Astragalus root has a history of traditional usage in Chinese medicine for immune and liver health. It inhibited secretion of HBV antigens from isolated human liver cells infected with the virus, and reduced levels of HBV DNA in a hepatitis-B animal model.[98] A mixture of astragalus polysaccharide and another plant extract called emodin demonstrated significant reductions in HBV DNA and HBV antigens (HBsAg, HBeAg and HBcAg) in a hepatitis-B mouse model.[99] A Chinese study examined the effectiveness of astragalus and adjuvant compounds (*Bupleurum chinense*, *Salviae miltiorrhizae*, curcumin, peony, and paeoniae) (116 g daily as a tea) in 116 chronic HBV patients. Two months of treatment with the tea was clinically effective (defined as improvement in clinical symptoms—fatigue, anorexia, abdominal distension, and jaundice—and partial or full recovery of liver function) in 91% of patients, compared to 70% of controls (who took a low-dose mixture of silibinin, oleanic acid, and the herb yi-gan-ling).[100]

## Schizandra

Members of the genus *Schizandra* inhibited the secretion of virus antigens from isolated human liver cells by up to 76.5% in one experiment.[101-103] A *Schizandra*-containing herbal formulation reduced the production and secretion of HBsAg and HBeAg surface antigens (a measurement of virus particle secretion) from isolated liver cells, and reduced the growth of isolated hepatocellular carcinoma cells.[104] In a phase I trial, 23 volunteers with HBV infection took the herbal formulation daily for 10 weeks. The

average number of monocytes (a type of circulating immune cell) in the blood decreased over the course of the study, which the authors suggested may lower self-inflicted host immune response and liver cell destruction.[105]

## Milk Thistle

Milk thistle is a traditional liver tonic; the active compound in milk thistle (silymarin) has antioxidant and antifibrotic activity.[106] Although it does not affect HBV viral replication, and has yet to demonstrate a significant effect on virus-related mortality in clinical trials,[107] milk thistle may be beneficial in reducing the inflammation inherent to hepatitis that may precipitate complications such as cirrhosis or cancer.[106] Silibinin, a component of silymarin, slows the growth of isolated human hepatocellular carcinoma cells, and exhibits the strongest inhibition toward cancer cells positive for the hepatitis B virus.[108] In an animal model of hepatitis B infection, silymarin prevented the progression of precancerous lesions into hepatocellular carcinoma, but had no effect on existing cancer. Cancer developed in 80% of control animals.[109] A small trial in mixed hepatitis patients demonstrated that 480 mg silibinin daily for 7 days could significantly reduce aspartate aminotransferase (AST), alanine aminotransferase (ALT), gamma-glutamyltranspeptidase (GGT), and bilirubin, all markers of liver dysfunction.[110]

## Life Extension Suggestions

- **Green tea extract,** standardized to 98% polyphenols: 725–1450 mg daily
- **Schisandra:** 150–250 mg daily
- **N-acetyl-cysteine (NAC):** 600–1800 mg daily
- **Lactoferrin,** providing 95% of apolactoferrin (285 mg): 300 mg daily
- **Pectin:** 875–1500 mg daily
- **Milk Thistle,** standardized extract: 750 mg daily
- **Curcumin,** as highly absorbed BCM-95®: 400–800 mg daily
- **Multivitamin/multimineral complex** containing:
  - Zinc: 30 mg daily
  - Molybdenum: 100 mcg daily
  - Manganese: 1–2 mg daily
  - Selenium: 200 mcg daily
- **Vitamin B complex** containing:
  - Thiamine (vitamin B1): 100 mg daily
  - Riboflavin (vitamin B2): 50 mg daily
  - Pyridoxine (vitamin B6): 75 mg daily
- **Vitamin C:** 1000–2000 mg daily taken away from iron-containing foods because vitamin C

enhances iron absorption into the bloodstream from the digestive tract.

- **Vitamin E:** 400 IU daily with at least 200 mg gamma tocopherol
- **Trans-resveratrol:** 250 mg daily
- **Phyllanthus amarus:** 600–1200 mg daily
- **Coffee** (containing 132–172 mg of chlorogenic acid per cup); and/or **green coffee extract** (standardized to 50% chlorogenic acid): 400–1200 mg daily
- **Whey protein isolate:** 20–40 g daily
- *Astragalus membranaceus*: 450 mg daily

In addition, the following *blood tests* may be helpful:

- Hepatitis B surface antibody
- Hepatitis Be antigen

- Hepatitis B DNA
- Hepatitis panel
  - Hepatitis B surface antigen (HBsAg)
  - Hepatitis B core antibody (HBcAb)
  - Hepatitis A antibody (HAAb)
  - Hepatitis C antibody (HCAb)
- Chemistry panel and complete blood count (includes liver function tests)

## REFERENCES

References available at: www.lef.org/dpt5/ch70

# 71

# *Hepatitis C*

Hepatitis C is an infectious disease caused by the hepatitis C virus (HCV), which infiltrates the liver and other organs. It causes inflammation and damage to DNA regulatory genes.

According to a 2007 report, hepatitis C causes more deaths each year in the United States than human immunodeficiency virus (HIV). HCV is a primary reason why people need liver transplants. More than 4 million Americans are infected with HCV.[1-4]

Approximately 75–85% of people infected with HCV develop a *chronic infection* and face the risk of advanced liver fibrosis, cirrhosis, cancer, and other complications.[5]

Many people have the disease for decades before it is diagnosed. This is because HCV infection usually causes only minor symptoms until liver damage is advanced.[6]

In some cases, liver abnormalities detected during routine blood work can suggest to a physician that a patient might have an HCV infection. This may allow treatment to begin before the disease reaches a critical stage. Therefore, proactive *blood testing* could be helpful in discovering an undetected HCV infection.[7]

Though current standard of care has met with somewhat limited success and is burdened by considerable side effects, exciting findings reveal potential for underutilized drug strategies, such as *metformin* and *thymosin alpha-1*, to complement conventional treatment and improve outcomes in hepatitis C.[8-13]

In this protocol, you will learn about how the HCV is transmitted and the consequences of an infection. You will also discover that *many people may not realize they are infected*, and *early detection* can save lives. Lastly, you will find out about breakthroughs on the horizon that promise to vastly improve medical treatment outcomes as well as several natural compounds that target multiple aspects of hepatitis C.

## HOW THE HEPATITIS C VIRUS IS TRANSMITTED

HCV is transmitted primarily via exposure to infected blood or blood products. Any HCV carrier can potentially transmit the infection.[14] The most common mode of transmission is sharing contaminated needles during intravenous (IV) drug use.[15] Having had a blood transfusion before 1992 is a known risk factor as well. Other possible risk factors include body piercing, tattooing, and exposure to contaminated items such as toothbrushes, razor blades, or nail clippers.[16,17] While sexual transmission of HCV is possible, rates are low.[17-20]

Approximately 4% of infants born to HCV-infected mothers acquire the infection during childbirth. Transmission risk increases 2- to 3-fold if the HCV infected mother also has HIV. Breastfeeding does *not* increase the risk of transmission.[21]

## DISEASE COURSE AND OUTCOMES

### Acute Phase

The first 6 months of HCV infection encompass the acute phase.[22] Because it passes with few, if any signs or symptoms in most cases, this stage of the illness is usually dismissed by the patient. About 20–30% of adults with acute HCV infection may develop clinical symptoms. The symptomatic onset ranges from 3–12 weeks after exposure.[5,23] Patients may experience fever, fatigue, tenderness in the liver area, nausea or decreased appetite, and jaundice.[5,22]

### Chronic Phase

Approximately 75–85% of HCV-infected persons will progress to chronic HCV infection.[5]

The chronic phase is generally established when HCV genetic material (RNA) persists in the patient's serum for 6 months or more.[5,23]

Numerous factors appear to affect the likelihood of developing chronic HCV infection. Females are more likely to clear the virus, for example, as are people who develop jaundice during the acute phase. In contrast, the virus appears to be more likely to persist in patients co-infected with HIV.[5,23]

Although the disease is transmittable during the chronic phase through blood, HCV carriers may not recognize they have an infection for up to 20 years because symptoms during this time are often mild.[24]

While elevations of *alanine transaminase (ALT)*—a liver enzyme that increases in response to liver cell death[5]—may be observed, at least one-third of patients may exhibit normal levels.[7] Eventually, nonspecific symptoms such as fatigue usually prompt the patient to visit a physician.

### Outcomes

Within the first 20 years of infection, advanced liver disease may develop. During this timeframe, roughly 10–15% of patients develop *cirrhosis of the liver*—the replacement of healthy liver tissue by dysfunctional fibrous tissue and nodules.[5,23]

Up to 4% of patients with HCV-related liver cirrhosis develop *liver cancer* each year.[25] Liver cancer may be suspected in someone with advanced HCV-related liver cirrhosis that experiences sudden weight loss, elevation in liver function tests, or pain or fullness in the right upper abdomen.[26]

More than a third of *liver transplants* are a consequence of hepatitis C.[27,28] Although 5-year survival following transplant is good (up to 85%), most hepatitis C patients who receive liver transplants have a recurrence of the virus.[28,29]

## IRON OVERLOAD AND HCV

HCV-induced oxidative stress appears to disrupt iron balance by suppressing levels of a hormone called hepcidin, which is a regulator that helps control iron absorption.[30–32] Low hepcidin levels lead to increased iron accumulation in the liver[32,33]; this is common in HCV.[34–36] Excess iron in the liver may, in turn, create more oxidative stress, causing liver injury and fibrosis.[37,38]

In a study of the impact of iron overloading on oxidant/antioxidant systems, scientists found evidence that HCV core protein inhibits iron-induced activation of antioxidants in the liver, exacerbating oxidative stress, which could facilitate the development of liver cancer.[39] Hepatic iron depletion has been postulated to decrease the risk of hepatocellular carcinoma in patients with cirrhosis due to chronic hepatitis C.[31]

*Phlebotomy* (ie, therapeutic bloodletting) to reduce iron levels significantly improves liver enzyme levels in HCV patients,[40] and yields histologic improvements[41] as well as increased interferon efficacy in interferon nonresponders.[42,43] A comprehensive review concluded that phlebotomy enhanced patient response to interferon treatment.[44] Additional findings suggest that iron depletion may lower the risk of developing hepatocellular carcinoma.[45]

At a minimum, most hepatitis C patients should avoid supplements containing iron and seek to reduce dietary sources of iron such as red meat. *Vitamin* C facilitates iron absorption while *calcium* and *green tea* impede it. Hepatitis C patients should take their vitamin C at a different time than when eating foods with high iron levels.

## DIAGNOSIS

HCV infection is usually detected during routine blood testing. Elevated levels of the liver enzyme ALT would alert a physician to a possible infection with HCV. If a doctor suspects HCV, hepatitis C testing typically begins with a blood test to detect the presence of antibodies to the HCV.[16,46]

The disease can be diagnosed by the presence of HCV antibodies or the direct presence of the virus or viral products in the blood. If the screen is positive, a liver biopsy may also be recommended to assess the severity of the disease and guide treatment decisions.[46]

Baby boomers (people born between 1946 and 1964) in particular are urged to get tested because rates of HCV infection are particularly high in this population.[47]

## NONINVASIVE TOOLS ARE NOW AVAILABLE TO MONITOR HEPATITIS C PROGRESSION

In HCV patients, determining the degree of fibrosis progression in the liver is crucial—and new methods may make this possible without the need for an invasive liver biopsy.

One new approach synchronously combines blood tests (*FibroMeters*) and ultrasound-based transient elastography (*Fibroscan*), which are then algorithmically analyzed to yield a thorough liver fibrosis assessment.[48–51] In a large study of 1785 patients with chronic hepatitis C, the diagnostic accuracy of this new method did not differ significantly from that of current algorithms, but it provided a more precise diagnosis.[52] Also, this new combination method is much more accurate at classifying the fibrosis stage than FibroMeters or Fibroscan alone.[48]

Another noninvasive strategy is also now available for assessing liver fibrosis. *FibroTest* is a patented test that uses the results of 5 blood tests to generate a score that correlates with the degree of liver damage.[53]

In a recent study involving 1457 patients with chronic HCV, noninvasive liver fibrosis tests helped predict the 5-year survival of people with chronic HCV. Patient outcomes declined with increased liver stiffness and FibroTest values. FibroTest may facilitate an earlier prognosis so certain treatments, such as liver transplant, can be evaluated.[54] FibroTest and ActiTest (an assessment of necroinflammatory activity) are marketed in the United States as FibroSure.[50,55]

## CONVENTIONAL TREATMENT

The goal of HCV infection therapy is to slow or halt progression of fibrosis and prevent the development of advanced cirrhosis.[46]

Standard treatment for hepatitis C centers on *pegylated interferon* plus *ribavirin* (PEG-IFN/RBV).

- *Interferons* occur naturally and help the immune system recognize and attack viruses. Pegylated interferon is a chemically altered interferon that remains active in the body for a long time and helps mount robust immunity against HCV.

- *Ribavirin* is an antiviral drug that interferes with viral replication.

- The combination of the two drugs is more effective than either alone.

During PEG-IFN/RBV treatment, physicians routinely test levels of liver enzymes, HCV antibodies, and the virus itself in the bloodstream. Monitoring these levels can help measure the effectiveness of treatment and determine prognosis.[46,56,57]

This combination treatment is ineffective in over 40% of HCV patients, leaving these individuals to seek additional approaches to eradicate the virus and/or protect against its damaging effects. Moreover, the contraindications and severe side-effects associated with interferon (eg, depression, anemia, leukopenia, and sepsis) can make treatment challenging.[46,58]

Sustained virologic response is the surrogate marker to evaluate the effectiveness of treatment. If HCV treatment is successful, the patient will achieve a sustained virologic response; this occurs when HCV RNA cannot be detected in serum 24 weeks after treatment ends.[58]

## PROTECTING AGAINST RIBAVIRIN-INDUCED ANEMIA WITH ANTIOXIDANTS

Ribavirin (RBV) can damage red blood cell membranes and cause anemia.[59,60] This can negatively impact treatment response by necessitating a dose reduction, or force the patient to stop treatment altogether.[61,62]

*Oxidative stress* contributes to ribavirin-induced breakdown of red blood cell membranes,[59] so therapies that aim to quench reactive free radicals have piqued the interest of researchers.

Antioxidants tested on patients with ribavirin-induced anemia have yielded promising results.[63] In chronic HCV patients, 100 g daily of tomato-based functional food (containing high levels of natural antioxidants) in addition to standard combination treatment decreased the severity of ribavirin-related anemia and increased patient tolerance to the full dose of ribavirin. Specifically, 8.7% of the functional food group had to decrease their daily dose of ribavirin versus 30.4% in the control group.[64]

In another study of chronic HCV patients, adding a high daily dose of *vitamins C* (2000 mg/day) and *E* (2000 mg/day) to combination interferon alpha-2b/ribavirin treatment prevented ribavirin-induced anemia.[65] In yet another study, while vitamins C (750 mg/day) and E (500 mg/day) in addition to standard treatment for 26 weeks did not suppress ribavirin-induced anemia, the prevalence of dose reduction was much lower in the vitamin group (14.3%) versus the control group (47.1%). Additionally, only 7.1% of the vitamin group discontinued treatment compared to 35.3% of the control group.[66]

## EMERGING THERAPIES

Only about 40% of patients with HCV genotype 1 infection (the most common genotype in North America)

achieve sustained virologic response with PEG-IFN/RBV therapy.[58,67] Therefore, rigorous research efforts are aimed at developing more effective treatment strategies.

### Direct-Acting Antivirals (DAAs)

Telaprevir and boceprevir, direct-acting antivirals (DAAs) that inhibit HCV replication, received Food and Drug Administration approval in 2011. They are used in combination with PEG-IFN/RBV to treat chronic genotype 1 HCV infection.[68,69]

**Telaprevir.** In chronic HCV-infected patients who had either not been treated or for who conventional treatment was unsuccessful, adding telaprevir to PEG-IFN/RBV therapy resulted in significantly higher sustained virologic response rates.[67,70]

The rate of chronic HCV infection is notably high in the African American population.[71] Research showed when telaprevir was used in combination with PEG-IFN/RBV in African Americans, the sustained virologic response rate was 61% versus 25% without telaprevir.[72]

Additional evidence indicates that using telaprevir may shorten treatment time.[73] Being able to shorten treatment duration is extremely important, as some patients stop complying with treatment over time or may need to stop treatment due to adverse events.[68,74] If prolonged exposure to these therapies can be minimized, this might encourage patient compliance.

**Boceprevir.** Adding boceprevir to PEG-IFN/RBV treatment has also yielded major improvements in sustained virologic response rates.[75] In previously untreated patients, treatment with boceprevir plus PEG-IFN/RBV therapy yielded high sustained virologic response rates in most patients at 28 weeks; boceprevir was also found to be safe and effective for up to 48 weeks (when necessary). Having a 4-week lead-in period of PEG-IFN/RBV treatment before adding boceprevir yielded a better sustained virologic response as well as decreased viral breakthrough and relapse over a 48-week duration.[76]

Limitations of DAAs include a greater frequency of adverse events than PEG-IFN/RBV,[77] complex dosing regimen,[74] potential for drug–drug interactions,[77] and the emergence of treatment-resistant HCV strains.[68,78–80] Also, neither drug is equally effective against all HCV genotypes. New therapies are being developed to address a broader range of genotypes.[81]

### Metformin: More Than a Diabetes Drug

Life Extension has been reporting on the benefits of metformin for years. New research indicates metformin, normally used to treat diabetes, may be a useful therapy for HCV patients. In vitro data suggest that metformin may have a suppressive effect on HCV replication.[82] In women with HCV genotype 1 infection who were found to exhibit insulin resistance, taking metformin in addition to standard HCV therapy resulted in a doubled sustained virologic response and greater decrease in viral load compared to placebo in the first 12 weeks of treatment.[83] A number of other clinical studies have also shown improved sustained virologic response rates among insulin-resistant HCV patients receiving metformin in addition to standard therapy.[11,12] Metformin use was also correlated with a significantly better prognosis among 99 diabetic HCV patients with cirrhosis. Compared to nonuse, metformin treatment was associated with an 81% reduction in risk of hepatocellular carcinoma and a 78% reduction of liver-related death or need for liver transplant.[13]

### Ezetimibe: A Cholesterol-Lowering Drug That Inhibits HCV Viral Entry

New findings reveal certain cholesterol medications may be useful in HCV treatment. Niemann-Pick C1-like 1 (NPC1L1) receptors are important mediators of cholesterol absorption in the human body. Interestingly, scientists recently found NPC1L1 receptors also help the HCV virus enter cells.

The cholesterol drug *ezetimibe* specifically targets NPC1L1 receptors. Researchers tested its effects on HCV and found it *inhibits infection by all major HCV genotypes*. Moreover, in mice with human liver grafts, ezetimibe slowed the establishment of HCV genotype 1b infection. These findings represent a breakthrough discovery by identifying an entry factor for HCV and revealing a new treatment target.[84]

### Interferon-Free Treatment

In a 2012 Phase II study, patients were treated with an investigational interferon-free therapy (combination of protease inhibitor BI 201335 and polymerase inhibitor BI 207127) with and without ribavirin and for varying treatment durations. Treatment for 28 weeks resulted in a viral cure in nearly 82% of patients with HCV genotypes 1a CC and 1b infection, the most common genotypes in Asia and Europe. Moreover, 68% of all patients in the study achieved a viral cure, including individuals with genotype 1a non-CC, which is normally very difficult to treat. If proven to be a viable treatment option, interferon-free therapy would eliminate interferon's side effects. This, in turn, would potentially encourage patient compliance.[85]

### HCV Vaccination on the Horizon

A February 2012 report states that Michael Houghton, one of the scientists who discovered HCV in 1989, developed a *vaccine* from a strain of HCV. The results have been overwhelmingly positive—patients who received this vaccine produced antibodies that neutralized all known strains of HCV, a feat previously thought impossible given the virulence of HCV. Although further testing will be needed, and it would likely take 5–7 years before the vaccine could receive approval, preliminary findings are encouraging.[86]

### Thymosin Alpha-1

Life Extension has been reporting on the benefits of thymosin alpha-1 since the early 1980s. This immune-boosting agent has been studied for its potential role in treating cancer and viral hepatitis. Study results suggest thymosin alpha-1 in addition to PEG-IFN/RBV treatment may improve the efficacy of treatment in patients who were previously not responsive to therapy.[8,9] Other study findings have indicated taking thymosin in addition to standard HCV treatment might lower the rate of relapse.[10] Moreover, thymosin alpha-1 shows promise as a potential adjuvant therapy in difficult-to-treat patients with HCV, but more studies are needed.[87] In another trial among 552 hepatitis C patients who were nonresponders to standard care, addition of two 1.6-mg subcutaneous injections of thymosin alpha-1 per week to PEG-IFN/RBV for 48 weeks resulted in a 41% sustained virologic response compared to 26% in placebo recipients.[88]

## TARGETED NATURAL THERAPEUTICS

### Boosting Liver Glutathione and Easing Oxidative Stress

*Glutathione* acts as a cellular detoxifier and helps prevent damage from free radicals.[89] However, glutathione depletion is a common finding among HCV-infected patients.[90] The following compounds may help to increase glutathione levels.

**N-acetyl-cysteine.** N-acetyl-cysteine (NAC) is derived from L-cysteine, a conditionally essential amino acid. This powerful antioxidant diminishes free radicals and raises glutathione levels.[91] In conventional medicine, NAC has been used to treat acetaminophen poisoning. In children with acute liver failure from causes other than acetaminophen poisoning, receiving NAC was associated with a shorter hospital stay, greater incidence of liver recovery, and better survival after transplantation.[92] In an early trial, addition of NAC to interferon boosted glutathione levels in white blood cells of patients with chronic hepatitis C and normalized ALT levels in 41% of interferon nonresponders.[93] While more recent trials have been unable to confirm the therapeutic role of NAC in chronic hepatitis C, they have established that it is very well tolerated.[94,95]

**S-adenosyl-L-methionine.** S-adenosyl-L-methionine (SAMe), a methyl donor for numerous methylation reactions, has been studied for its antidepressant properties.[96] SAMe also regulates glutathione synthesis.[97] In HCV-infected patients who were nonresponders to previous antiviral therapy, adding SAMe to a PEG-IFN/RBV regimen improved early viral response.[98] In a separate trial, SAMe and trimethyglycine (another methyl donor) were given along with PEG-IFN/RBV to chronic hepatitis C patients. The treatment resulted in an early virologic response (EVR) in 59% of subjects, whereas PEG-IFN/RBV alone had previously achieved only a 14% EVR.[99]

**Lipoic acid.** This free-radical scavenger helps to repair damage caused by oxidative stress, assisting in the regeneration of important antioxidants such as glutathione and vitamin E.[100] In animals, lipoic acid has been found to prevent fatty liver disease.[101] In human trials, administration of antioxidant blends containing lipoic acid was shown to favorably modulate liver enzymes, HCV RNA levels, and liver biopsy score in HCV patients.[102,103]

**Whey protein.** Whey protein boosts glutathione levels and improves the functioning of the immune system.[104] In an animal model of hepatitis, whey protein supplementation attenuated chemical-induced liver enzyme elevations.[105] Moreover, a clinical study found oral whey protein reduced viral load, decreased inflammation, lowered ALT levels, and exerted other beneficial effects in compensated chronic HCV-infected patients.[104]

**Selenium.** Selenium is an essential component of glutathione peroxidase, an enzyme that protects cells from free radical damage.[106] Patients with hepatitis C or B have been found to have lower serum selenium concentrations than healthy individuals.[106] Moreover, selenium deficiency is thought to contribute to insulin resistance in people with HCV-related chronic liver disease; and reduced

selenium levels have been observed in patients with hepatocellular carcinoma.[107,108]

**Glutathione.** A 1989 study found consumption of oral glutathione increased plasma glutathione levels.[109] Preclinical trials found oral glutathione increases glutathione levels in tissues such as the lungs, liver, and kidneys.[110–114]

## Targeting Excess Iron Levels

**Lactoferrin.** Lactoferrin, an iron-binding glycoprotein, may be beneficial as an adjunctive treatment for serum iron overload in hepatitis patients. Lactoferrin is a potent antioxidant, antiviral agent, and scavenger of free iron.[115] In addition, it is directly involved in the upregulation of natural killer cell activity, making it a natural mediator of immune function.[115] As an immune mediator, lactoferrin may work synergistically with interferon to reduce viral load.[116] In another study among patients with chronic HCV, lactoferrin alone significantly lowered the HCV RNA titer and improved efficacy of subsequent treatment with interferon and ribavirin.[117]

**Green tea.** Epigallocatechin-3-gallate (EGCG) from green tea has been found to interrupt the first step of HCV infection by blocking the virus from entering target cells. In addition, EGCG inhibited cell-to-cell transmission of HCV. Both of these effects were observed regardless of the genotype tested. These findings carry important implications for the prevention of HCV reinfection in liver transplant patients.[118] In addition, green tea has been shown to inhibit iron absorption in intestinal cells[119] and accumulation in liver tissue,[120] which can contribute to excessive oxidative stress.

**Elemental calcium.** Calcium inhibits iron absorption.[121] Taking 600 mg of elemental calcium can reduce iron absorption by as much as 60%.[122]

## Additional Natural Liver Protection

**Milk thistle.** Silymarin and its chief active ingredient, silibinin, are derived from milk thistle, a member of the daisy family. Both substances help the liver avoid toxic damage and regenerate after injury.

- **Silymarin.** Findings from several studies suggest that silymarin has potential antiviral,[123] antioxidant,[124] anti-inflammatory,[123,125] and antifibrotic[126] effects within the liver. It may also improve liver enzyme levels in HCV patients.[127]

  In a cell culture study, silymarin inhibited entry of HCV into cells, inhibited viral RNA and protein expression, and decreased cell-to-cell transmission of HCV.[128]

A clinical study involving 1145 HCV-infected participants showed patients using silymarin had fewer liver-related symptoms and somewhat higher quality-of-life scores.[129] Doses greater than 700 mg may improve bioavailability of silymarin; and oral doses of up to 2.1 g per day have been found to be safe and well tolerated.[130]

- **Silibinin.** The antioxidant, antifibrotic, and metabolic effects of silibinin have been demonstrated in numerous studies.[131,132] Silibinin also has antiviral capabilities.[133,134]

The clinical efficacy of oral silibinin in active chronic hepatitis C has not yet been clearly established.[131,135] However, intravenous silibinin effectively treated HCV reinfection following liver transplantation in a small number of patients in one trial,[136] and helped 85% of nonresponders to standard of care achieve undetectable HCV RNA levels in another.[137] Likewise, administering high doses of silibinin intravenously in addition to PEG-IFN/RBV therapy lowered viral loads in HCV-infected patients who were previous nonresponders to treatment[134]; and 1400 mg of intravenous silibinin daily for 14 days successfully induced sustained virologic response (SVR) in a 57-year-old liver transplant patient.[138]

A medical literature review found no significant side effects with silybin phytosome at doses up to 10 g per day, and no significant interactions with other medications.[131]

**Polyenylphosphatidylcholine.** Polyenylphosphatidylcholine (PPC) is a major component of essential phospholipids.[139] In addition to improving liver enzymes in HCV,[140] PPC replenishes levels of SAMe, a precursor to the potent antioxidant glutathione.[141] PPC protects against liver damage[139] and improves liver function.[140,142] In animal studies, it has demonstrated antioxidant, cytoprotective, anti-inflammatory, and antifibrotic effects, inhibiting oxidative stress and the development of alcoholic liver disease.[139,140] Numerous double-blind, placebo-controlled clinical trials have shown essential phospholipids improve chronic hepatitis among human subjects.[143]

***Schisandra chinensis.*** Berries from the *Schisandra chinensis* (*S. chinensis*) plant contain active ingredients that protect the liver.[144] Crude *Schisandra* and its extracts have traditionally held a role in Chinese and Japanese medicine,[144] and *S. chinensis* has been used

to treat chemical and viral hepatitis.[145] A study examining the effects of a Japanese herbal combination containing *S. chinensis* indicated that *Schisandra* fruit could inhibit HCV infection.[146] The seed extract from *S. chinensis* appears to have liver-detoxifying capabilities; components of the seed extract are thought to have anticancer, anti-inflammatory, liver-protective, anti-HIV, and immunomodulating effects.[147]

**Licorice root extract.** Licorice root extract (glycyrrhizin) is known to exert an antiviral effect against HCV.[148] In Japanese HCV patients, the long-term use of glycyrrhizin has shown to be helpful in preventing inflammation, liver cirrhosis, and hepatocellular carcinoma.[149,150] The broad anti-inflammatory activity[151] and antioxidant capabilities[152] of glycyrrhizin have also been observed. Adding a nutritional supplement containing vitamin C, glycyrrhizic acid, and other antioxidants to standard PEG-IFN/RBV treatment has been linked to a notably higher rate of biochemical and histologic improvements in patients with chronic HCV.[153,154] In chronic HCV patients, oxidative stress and immunologic parameters showed marked improvement following treatment with this blend.[153]

A preparation known as Stronger Neo-Minophagen C (SNMC) contains glycyrrhizin as an active component and has been used in Japan for more than 30 years to treat chronic hepatitis.[150] In animals with HCV, SNMC has been found to prevent fatty liver disease[155] and protect liver cells against carbon tetrachloride-induced oxidative stress by restoring depleted glutathione levels.[156] A possible side effect associated with ingestion of large amounts of licorice is hypertension[157]; therefore, blood pressure should be monitored regularly.

**Vitamin D.** Diminished vitamin D levels have been observed in HCV patients.[158,159] Low serum vitamin D levels are associated with severe fibrosis, as well as a low sustained virologic response to PEG-IFN/RBV treatment in patients with chronic HCV infection[159]; and vitamin D supplementation has been found to enhance HCV response to PEG-IFN/RBV therapy.[160] In a recent study involving patients with HCV genotypes 2–3 receiving PEG-IFN/RBV treatment, supplementing with oral vitamin D significantly improved viral response. Twenty-four weeks after treatment, 95% of the treatment (vitamin D) group was HCV RNA negative versus 77% of the control group.[161]

**Coffee.** A recent study showed patients with advanced HCV-related chronic liver disease who drank 3 or more cups of coffee each day were about 3 times more likely to respond to PEG-IFN/RBV treatment than nondrinkers. These patients were previous nonresponders to interferon treatment.[162] Published study reports have documented an association between coffee consumption and lowered risks of liver cirrhosis,[163,164] hepatocellular carcinoma,[165,166] liver disease progression in HCV infection,[167] and lower serum ALT activity.[168] Population studies have shown coffee drinking reduces the risk of clinically significant chronic liver disease.[169] These effects may be due in part to the antiviral activity of *chlorogenic acid*, a coffee polyphenol found in especially high concentrations in *green coffee extracts*.[170]

**Zinc and zinc-carnosine.** Zinc has HCV-inhibiting capabilities.[171] Zinc supplementation has resulted in a higher reported rate of HCV eradication among patients receiving interferon treatment,[172] decreased gastrointestinal disturbances and hair loss, and improved fingernail health in patients with chronic HCV. It may also improve patient tolerance to IFN-alpha-2a and ribavirin.[173]

A chelate compound consisting of *zinc* and *L-carnosine* may induce antioxidative functions in the liver, thereby decreasing liver cell injury.[174] Supplementation with chelated zinc-carnosine has been found to lessen the degree of liver damage and improve long-term outcome of patients with chronic HCV infection or liver cirrhosis.[175] In patients with HCV-related chronic liver disease, it appears to have a beneficial anti-inflammatory effect on the liver by decreasing iron overload.[176] In addition, fewer gastrointestinal side effects were observed when zinc-carnosine supplementation was added to combination PEG-IFN/RBV therapy.[177]

**Curcumin.** Curcumin is a yellow pigment present in the curry spice turmeric. It possesses antioxidant, anti-inflammatory, antifungal, antibacterial, and antiproliferative capabilities.[178–180] In addition, curcumin has been found to exert antiviral activity against a variety of viruses including HIV,[181] influenza virus,[182] and coxsackievirus.[183] One team of researchers found curcumin reduces HCV gene expression, and combining curcumin with IFN-alpha treatment had "profound inhibitory effects" on HCV replication. The authors concluded curcumin may be valuable as a novel anti-HCV agent.[184] Curcumin has also been shown to protect against liver cancer.[185]

**Quercetin.** Quercetin is a flavonoid present in fruit, vegetables, wine, and tea that has antioxidant and anti-inflammatory properties. Studies indicate that it also possesses antihypertensive, antibacterial, antifibrotic, antiatherogenic, and antiproliferative properties.[186] Quercetin has also been found to attenuate HCV virus production.[187,188]

**L-carnitine.** Chronic HCV patients received PEG-IFN/RBV plus the amino acid L-carnitine or PEG-IFN/RBV alone for 12 months. A significant improvement in sustained virologic response was observed in 50% of the L-carnitine group versus 25% of the non–L-carnitine group.[189] Supplementing PEG-IFN/RBV treatment with L-carnitine has also been associated with decreased mental and physical fatigue, as well as improved health-related quality of life in patients with chronic HCV. These latter outcomes could potentially improve patient compliance with PEG-IFN/RBV treatment.[190]

## Life Extension Suggestions

### Boosting Liver Glutathione and Easing Oxidative Stress
- **N-acetyl-cysteine (NAC):** 600–1800 mg daily
- **S-adenosylmethionine (SAMe):** 200–1200 mg daily in divided doses
- **R-lipoic acid:** 300–600 mg daily
- **Whey protein isolate:** 20–40 g daily
- **Natural vitamin E:** 400 IU daily with at least 200 mg gamma tocopherol
- **Vitamin C:** 1000–2000 mg daily (on an empty stomach)
- **Selenium:** 200–400 mcg daily
- **Glutathione:** 50–150 mg daily

### Targeting Excess Iron Levels
- **Lactoferrin (apolactoferrin):** 300 mg daily
- **Green tea extract** (standardized to 98% polyphenols): 725–1450 mg daily
- **Calcium:** 700–1200 mg daily with iron-containing foods to block iron absorption

### Additional Natural Liver Protection
- **Milk thistle,** standardized extract: 750 mg daily
- **Polyenylphosphatidylcholine (PPC):** 1800–2700 mg daily
- **Schisandra chinensis standardized extract:** 250 mg daily
- **Licorice root extract:** 25–50 mg daily
- **Vitamin D:** 5000–8000 IU daily, depending on blood levels of 25-OH-vitamin D
- **Green coffee extract** (standardized to 50% chlorogenic acid): 200–1200 mg daily
- **Zinc** (as zinc chelate and zinc-L-carnosine): 30–50 mg daily

- **Curcumin** (as highly absorbed BCM-95®): 400–800 mg daily
- **Quercetin** (as quercetin glycoside derivatives and free quercetin): 250–500 mg daily
- **L-carnitine:** 500–2000 mg daily

In addition, the following *blood tests* may be helpful:

- 25-hydroxyvitamin D serum iron ferritin chemistry panel

- Complete blood count (CBC) hepatitis C virus
- Quantitative, real-time PCR hepatitis C virus antibodies

## REFERENCES

References available at: www.lef.org/dpt5/ch71

# 72

# Herpes and Shingles

In their lifetimes, most human beings will be exposed to a herpesvirus. This family of viruses (*Herpesviridae*) has been implicated in a wide range of diseases and conditions, including chickenpox, oral or facial herpes, genital herpes, mononucleosis, and corneal blindness. It is also likely that we have not yet discovered all herpesviruses. One variety was discovered as recently as 1990, and researchers still are not sure which diseases, if any, it causes in humans.

Herpesviruses are distinguished by their ability to lay dormant, or "hide" in the human body after primary infection. They then reappear during periods of reactivation. The mechanism of reactivation is not really understood. Although there is no effective cure for herpes, many studies have shown that herpes reactivation is more common among patients with compromised immune systems, suggesting that a strong immune system is a good defense against herpes reactivation. To manage herpes, physicians try to reduce the number and severity of outbreaks.

Among the most well-known herpesviruses are the following.

## THE HERPES FAMILY OF VIRUSES

### Herpes Simplex Virus 1 (HSV1)

HSV1 is extremely common, with the vast majority of adults showing evidence of exposure to the virus (eg, antibodies in their blood), even if they are not positive for HSV1.[1] This form of the virus is most often associated with oral or facial lesions that appear during childhood, although it can also cause genital infection.

### Herpes Simplex Virus 2 (HSV2)

Researchers estimate that about 20% of the U.S. population has antibodies to HSV2.[1] This form of the virus is closely associated with genital herpes. Genital herpes caused by HSV2 is twice as likely to reactivate and recurs 8–10 times more frequently than genital infection with HSV1.[1]

### Varicella-Zoster Virus

This extremely common virus is responsible for chickenpox infections (varicella) and shingles (herpes zoster).

Up to 90% of people are attacked by this virus, about half of them between ages 5–9 years. Almost all clinical cases of chickenpox are diagnosed in children and adolescents younger than 14 years. For more information on varicella-zoster virus, see the Chickenpox and Shingles section in this chapter.

Although herpes infection is primarily associated with oral, facial, or genital herpes, the herpesvirus can also cause infections in the following ways:

- **Herpetic whitlow.**  Infection of the finger.
- **Herpes gladiatorum.**  Also known as traumatic herpes, herpes gladiatorum can cause infection anywhere on the chest, ears, face, and hands. This form of herpes is sometimes associated with wrestling because the rough contact between wrestlers helps spread the virus.
- **Herpes of the eye.**  The most common cause of corneal blindness in the United States.
- **Infection of the central or peripheral nervous systems.**  The herpesvirus accounts for up to 20% of sporadic viral encephalitis (swelling of the brain due to a virus) cases in the United States. Herpes can also cause herpetic meningitis.
- **Infection of the internal organs.**  This includes herpes infection of the esophagus (HSV esophagitis), lungs (HSV pneumonitis), and liver.
- **Neonatal herpes.**  Neonates (infants <6 weeks) can contract herpes during birth (if their mothers are infected with the virus) or if they are handled by someone with oral or facial herpes. Neonates are the most likely to have herpes infections that affect the central nervous system or internal organs. Mortality among neonates with untreated herpes is 65%.[1]

Genital herpes, which may be the most highly publicized form of the disease, is a widely misunderstood condition. Many people believe that genital herpes is only transmissible during active outbreaks of herpes (when herpes lesions are visible). They may also believe that herpes is relatively rare. In fact, herpes is much more common than many assume. Many people with herpes antibodies (those exposed to the virus) are not aware they have the disease; they suspect the condition only when they have seen pictures of herpetic lesions. Also contrary to popular belief, herpes is not transmitted exclusively by direct contact with active lesions. It can be transmitted by people without manifestations of the disease, but who are shedding the virus or have either subclinical symptoms or tiny lesions not visible to the naked eye. Studies have shown that HSV2 can be located on the genital tract regardless of the presence of symptoms.[1] Condoms have been shown to reduce the transmission of herpes during periods of nonsymptomatic shedding.

Herpes symptoms depend on the form of the disease. Oral or facial herpes is often accompanied by inflammation of the gums and throat during the initial outbreak. Children with this condition may have fever, malaise, inability to eat, irritability, and lesions in and around the mouth. Genital herpes is accompanied by similar symptoms, as well as lesions on the genitals. Among newly infected women, the cervix and urethra are usually involved. If the central or peripheral nervous systems are infected, a fever and neurologic symptoms are often present during periods of virus activation.

Because herpes sometimes resembles other diseases (especially herpes affecting the skin, mouth, or central nervous system), it can be challenging to diagnose. The most common diagnostic method is to isolate the virus in a tissue culture or demonstrate HSV antibodies or DNA in scrapings from active lesions.

The herpes family also includes the following viruses:

## Cytomegalovirus

Initial infection with cytomegalovirus (CMV) usually occurs during childhood and adolescence, but typically goes undetected. In healthy adults, the primary infection is usually mild and may present as fever, muscle pain, fatigue, and elevated liver enzymes. CMV may be dangerous in people with weakened immune systems, such as organ transplant recipients and people with HIV/AIDS. The virus is spread from person to person through direct contact, sexual intercourse, or blood transfusion(s). CMV is excreted in saliva, urine, semen, cervical secretions, and feces.[2]

## Human Herpesvirus 6

Human herpesvirus 6 (HHV6) is the primary cause of roseola infantum, a common childhood disease characterized by high fever and a red, raised rash on the neck and trunk.[3] Among older adults, it can also cause a mononucleosis-like syndrome. HHV6 can be found in secretions of healthy individuals.[3]

## Human Herpesvirus 7

Human herpesvirus 7 (HHV7) was discovered in 1990. Although no diseases have been conclusively linked to HHV7, it might be associated with pityriasis rosea, a benign skin condition characterized by scaly, pink, or dry raised capsules. Like HHV6, HHV7 can also be found in secretions of healthy individuals.[4]

## Human Herpesvirus 8

Human herpesvirus 8 (HHV8) is associated with Kaposi's sarcoma.[5,6] Latent HHV8 may target tumor suppressor pathways, leading to cell proliferation and tumor formation in people with weakened immune systems (eg, HIV patients).[7–9]

## Epstein-Barr Virus

Epstein-Barr virus (EBV) is the most common cause of infectious mononucleosis, which is characterized by fever, sore throat, and swollen lymph nodes. Complete recovery may take months.[10] Infection is common, with about 95% of the population having antibodies against the virus by age 30 years. EBV is transmitted via exchange of saliva containing the virus.

# CHICKENPOX AND SHINGLES

Chickenpox and shingles are both caused by the varicella-zoster virus, and infection is strongly reminiscent of infection with either HSV1 or HSV2. However, unlike HSV1 or HSV2, the virus is often transmitted via the respiratory tract.

Chickenpox is an extremely common and highly contagious childhood disease. It is usually benign, with an incubation period of up to 21 days (after initial infection) and a disease course of 14–17 days. During the time the varicella-zoster virus is most active, the patient has characteristic skin lesions. The lesions cause intense itching, with a risk of infected lesions due to scratching. Disease severity and number of lesions varies from person to person. Adults with the disease and a weakened immune system might run a fever. In fact, adult chickenpox is considerably more dangerous than the benign childhood variety. Adults are more likely to have symptoms (eg, headache and pain) as a result of chickenpox. A form of pneumonia (varicella pneumonia) is seen in about 20% of adults who contract chickenpox.[1] The virus can also cause brain inflammation.

Chickenpox will likely become less of a health issue. Since 1995, children in large numbers across the United States have been vaccinated against the varicella-zoster virus. The results of this vaccination program have been dramatic: hospitalizations have declined by 88% and direct medical expenditures by 74%.[11] These benefits were seen across all age groups.

However, researchers still do not know the impact of the chickenpox vaccine on shingles. Shingles, which occurs when the varicella-zoster virus reactivates (usually in adulthood), is characterized by a painful skin rash. Reactivation occurs in about 15% of people who have had chickenpox, and most often in people aged 60–69 years, although it can occur in any age group.

Some researchers have hypothesized that vaccination in childhood would actually make an adult more susceptible to shingles later in life. However, this has yet to be proven in clinical studies.[12] In the meantime, vaccination against herpes zoster in adults has been shown to reduce the incidence of shingles.[13]

Shingles is 9 times more likely to develop in those infected with HIV. In the early stages of HIV infection, shingles symptoms are fairly typical.[14] In more advanced infection, herpes zoster may take the form of repeated episodes of severe, prolonged, and sometimes atypical disease (such as varicella-zoster virus retinitis). Shingles is also more common in immunocompromised children and adults (including organ transplant recipients and chemotherapy patients). It is important to treat these patients early and aggressively with antiviral drugs.

Like chickenpox, shingles is characterized by skin lesions. The lesions may be accompanied by severe, sometimes debilitating pain. An outbreak of shingles usually lasts 7–10 days. It can take up to 2 weeks for the skin to appear and feel normal. Herpes zoster can also infect the nerves in the eye. This serious condition can result in blindness if not treated with antiviral therapy.[15–20]

Pain associated with shingles that persists more than 3 months after other symptoms subside is known as postherpetic neuralgia. The characteristics of postherpetic neuralgia are spontaneous aching and burning, intermittent shooting pains, and extreme sensitivity.[21] Postherpetic neuralgia is more common in older people. However, at least 50% of patients older than age 50 years who had shingles report some degree of pain months after the resolution of the skin rashes.[1] Several drug classes are used to treat postherpetic neuralgia, including tricyclic antidepressants[22] and painkillers (eg, acetaminophen, glucocorticoids, and lidocaine).

## CONVENTIONAL TREATMENT OF HERPES

### Antiviral Drugs

Conventional treatment of herpes relies on antiviral drugs shown to reduce the severity of outbreaks and, in some cases, reduce the likelihood of transmission. These drugs include the following.

**Acyclovir.** Acyclovir interferes with the virus' ability to replicate.[1] Common side effects include nausea, vomiting, headache, diarrhea, dizziness, fatigue, anorexia, edema, and sore throat.[23]

**Valacyclovir.** Valacyclovir (ie, the salt version of acyclovir) becomes acyclovir after being metabolized by the liver. Valacyclovir has a bioavailability 3–5 times greater than oral acyclovir. Common side effects are similar to acyclovir and include nausea, vomiting, headache, dizziness, and abdominal pain.[23]

**Famciclovir.** Famciclovir is a precursor to the antiviral drug penciclovir. Penciclovir works in a similar manner to acyclovir. Side effects are the same as those for acyclovir and valacyclovir.

These antiviral drugs may be given intravenously or orally, depending on the severity and location of the outbreak. They are effective in treating both herpes and shingles. In addition to these antiviral drugs, a number of topical medications are used in the treatment of herpes infections of the eye. These include trifluridine, vidarabine, idoxuridine, acyclovir, penciclovir, and interferon.

In recent years, clinicians have discovered strains of acyclovir-resistant herpes. Because the drugs are closely related, acyclovir-resistant strains of herpes are also cross-resistant to valacyclovir and famciclovir. These strains are most often detected in patients with weakened immune systems, such as those with HIV or AIDS.[1] In these cases, treatment with a very powerful antiviral called foscarnet, which must be administered with an intravenous (IV) pump, is sometimes effective. Foscarnet can cause severe adverse effects, including kidney disorders.

## NOVEL APPROACHES TO HERPES TREATMENT

### Cimetidine: A Novel Approach

Cimetidine (Tagamet®), an over-the-counter drug, helps reduce the severity of herpes outbreaks (especially in patients with shingles), as well as reduces the time of active infection. It works by temporarily inhibiting T-suppressor cells. T-suppressor cells downregulate the immune system after the pathogen has been destroyed. Because of the inhibitory effect on T-suppressor function, cimetidine therapy is contraindicated in patients with organ transplants or autoimmune disorders.[24]

The following studies appear to demonstrate the effectiveness of cimetidine against herpes:

- A combined in vitro/in vivo study evaluated the effect of cimetidine on herpes zoster. Treatment with cimetidine shortened the median time to initial pain reduction and complete resolution of pain. It also promoted more rapid healing of skin lesions than symptomatic treatment.[25]

- In 221 shingles patients given 200 mg of cimetidine 3 times during the day and 400 mg at night, disease duration was reduced. It was suggested that use of cimetidine should begin during the prodromal period (ie, the time when appearance of early symptoms may mark the onset of the condition).[26]

- Patients with herpes labialis (oral lesions) and herpes keratitis (herpes infection of the eye) showed a shortened duration and frequency of infection after treatment with cimetidine.[27]

- A case report in Canada appeared to show that cimetidine therapy reduced the expected length of the active phase of herpes zoster from 35 days to 10 days.[28]

- A paper presented at Michigan State University concluded that patients with herpes zoster given cimetidine exhibited enhanced immunity.[24]

Cimetidine is sold over the counter. Refer to the package insert for possible drug interactions.

## Herpes Vaccines on the Horizon

Although condoms and antiviral drugs can lower the risk of contracting herpes, the ultimate goal is a herpes vaccine that would inoculate the population against the virus.

Researchers have made significant progress in developing a herpes vaccine. An investigational vaccine resulted in a significant reduction of genital herpes in women never exposed to the virus.[29] For unknown reasons, this particular vaccine did not protect men.[30]

While it appears that effective herpes vaccines are on the horizon, there are still significant research questions to answer, such as who should be vaccinated, when, and whether a vaccine that suppresses symptoms prevents human transmission of the virus.[31]

## Herpes and the Immune System

Herpes-specific T-cell immunity may be related to reactivation. Animal studies have shown that ultraviolet light, a weakened immune system, and trauma all contribute to reactivation of the virus.[1] At this time, there are no drugs or agents that can cause a latent virus to stay hidden forever. The number and frequency of reactivation events depends on the site, nutrition, and immune status of the host.[32,33]

Life Extension's approaches herpes management based on the premise that a strong immune system can help reduce viral reactivation. People with herpes can benefit from a nutritional regimen of supplements that studies suggest may fight the virus directly, as well as support a healthy immune system.

### WHAT YOU HAVE LEARNED SO FAR

- The herpes family includes several related viruses, including HSV1, HSV2, and varicella-zoster virus. These viruses are extremely common, with the majority of the U.S. population showing antibodies to viruses in the herpes family.

- Herpesviruses are distinguished by their ability to go into clinical dormancy, or period that they hide in the body before becoming reactivated. Herpes outbreaks are often characterized by skin lesions, fever, and other symptoms.

- The varicella-zoster virus is responsible for chickenpox in children. After the initial outbreak, the virus can enter a long period of latency and reappear in the sixth decade of life as shingles.

- Both HSV1 and HSV2 can cause oral lesions, facial lesions, or genital disease. Herpesvirus can also infect the central nervous system, internal organs, and eyes. Neonatal herpes is usually passed from infected mother to child during birth.

- Contrary to popular belief, genital herpes can be transmitted even when active lesions are not visible and symptoms not present. People with the disease can shed the virus or may have lesions that are not readily visible.

- Conventional herpes treatment relies on antiviral drugs that have powerful side effects. These drugs can help lessen the severity of outbreaks.

- Reactivation is associated with a weakened immune system, so patients with herpes might consider an immune-boosting nutritional program to strengthen their immune systems. Many supplements have been proven to fight herpes by boosting the immune system or interfering with the virus's ability to penetrate cell walls.

# TARGETED NATURAL INTERVENTIONS

Although there is no cure for herpesvirus infection, various supplements have shown the ability to reduce severity and frequency of outbreaks. This might be due to their ability to support a healthy immune system (a weakened immune system has been associated with herpes reactivation).

Antioxidants are particularly important immune-boosting supplements. Multiple clinical studies support the theory that antioxidants are of benefit in the management of herpesviruses.[34–37]

## Vitamin A and Beta-Carotene

Vitamin A plays a role in protecting the skin and mucous membranes from invasion of microorganisms. In 178 HIV-positive women with genital herpes, who were neither pregnant nor taking oral contraceptives, decreased vitamin A levels were closely associated with increased cervical HSV shedding.[38]

Experimental studies have documented vitamin A's effectiveness against other herpesviruses. The strong antiproliferative activity exerted by retinoids (vitamin A derivatives) indicates these compounds may be useful tools in the management of EBV–related disorders in immunosuppressed patients.[39]

Beta-carotene is the major precursor of vitamin A.[40] Studies show that long-term beta-carotene supplementation may be beneficial for immune, viral, and tumoral surveillance in aging individuals. In a controlled, double-blind study, the effects of 10–12 years of beta-carotene supplementation on natural killer (NK) cell activity were evaluated. Although no significant difference was seen in NK cell activity in middle-aged groups, elderly men who took supplemental beta-carotene had significantly greater NK cell activity than the control group receiving placebo.[41]

## Vitamins C and E

Vitamin C (ascorbic acid) is important in maintaining immune status. Vitamin C can strengthen white blood cell function and boost interferon levels. It is a free radical scavenger,[42] protects tissues from oxidative stress, and enhances the actions of vitamin E.[43]

In one clinical trial, a water-soluble bioflavonoid/ascorbic acid complex (600–1000 mg of bioflavonoids and 600–1000 mg of ascorbic acid taken 3–5 times daily) was shown to be effective in reducing recurrent HSV1, reducing blisters and preventing disruption of vesicular membranes. Remission of symptoms was observed in 4 days.[44]

In another randomized, double-blind, placebo-controlled study on the topical treatment of recurrent mucocutaneous herpes, a pharmaceutical ascorbic acid formulation with antimicrobial properties (Ascoxal®) demonstrated the antiviral effects of vitamin C. A cotton pad soaked in the Ascoxal® solution was firmly pressed on the lesion for 2 minutes, 3 times (with 30-minute intervals in between), for 1 day only. The treatment resulted in markedly reduced symptoms and fewer days of scab formation.[45]

High levels of vitamin C can protect levels of vitamin E in tissue and may contribute to the immune system enhancement of vitamin E.[46]

Vitamin E is a powerful antioxidant and free radical scavenger. A double-blind, placebo-controlled study looked at the effect of Vitamin E to boost immune function in healthy individuals >65 years. Supplementation with vitamin E for 4 months improved clinically relevant indices of cell-mediated immunity.[47]

## Zinc and Selenium

Zinc plays many roles in basic cellular function, including DNA replication, RNA transcription, cell division, and cell activation. Zinc is a specific activator of T cells, T-cell division, and other immune cells. Zinc also functions as an antioxidant and stabilizes membranes against the oxidative effect of other minerals (eg, iron and copper) by increasing the levels of catalase, superoxide dismutase, and glutathione-S-transferase. Zinc-deficient patients display reduced resistance to infection.[48]

In a double-blind, placebo-controlled, randomized clinical trial that evaluated the effect of a zinc oxide/glycine cream on facial herpes in 46 patients, treatment reduced or shortened the duration of cold sore lesions (5 days) compared to placebo (6.5 days) when applied within 24 hours of symptom onset. The cream also reduced the severity of symptoms, particularly blistering, soreness, itching, and tingling.[49]

Selenium, an antioxidant with immune system–boosting properties, may help suppress the reactivation of herpesviruses by increasing immunity. A number of studies have shown that the combination of zinc and selenium enhances immunity in the elderly. A pioneering study found that seniors taking modest doses of a multivitamin/multimineral supplement containing zinc and selenium showed a general reduction in infection and required antibiotics for significantly fewer days annually.[50]

A well-designed, randomized, placebo-controlled, double-blind study found that seniors taking zinc and selenium had significantly fewer infections over a 2-year period, but vitamin supplementation alone did not have a major effect.[51] The zinc and selenium supplement cut the number of infections by nearly two-thirds compared to placebo.

## L-Lysine

L-lysine, an essential amino acid, has been studied for its ability to reduce the reactivation rate of herpes.[52,53] It works by inhibiting the action of L-arginine during viral replication. Proteins within herpes are rich in L-arginine. An altered ratio of L-lysine to L-arginine, in favor of L-lysine, has been studied for its ability to inhibit the virus. While the results of some studies have been mixed, the following studies have shown L-lysine's ability to inhibit herpes:

- In a double-blind, multicentered, placebo-controlled study evaluating L-lysine for the prevention and treatment of recurrent herpes infection, one group received 1000 mg of L-lysine 3 times daily for 6 months. This group had significantly fewer outbreaks, less severe symptoms, and more rapid healing. The researchers said that L-lysine was an effective agent for reducing the occurrence, severity, and symptoms of herpes.[54]

- In a second prospective, randomized, double-blind, placebo-controlled, cross-over study, oral intake of L-lysine (1248 mg daily) decreased the recurrence of herpes simplex in people with healthy immunity. A daily dose of 624 mg was not effective. L-lysine may also decrease the severity of symptoms associated with recurrences. Neither dosage shortened healing time.[55]

- In a double-blind clinical study examining the long-term prophylactic efficacy of L-lysine supplementation for herpes labialis, volunteers with a history of frequent outbreaks were recruited. The treatment group received daily oral supplements of 1000 mg of L-lysine. The L-lysine treatment group had significantly fewer outbreaks than the control group. Volunteers taken off L-lysine generally showed a significant increase in the recurrence of lesions. Data revealed fewer lesions when a person's serum L-lysine concentration exceeded 165 nanomoles per milliliter (nmol/mL) and increased significantly as concentration levels fell below 165 nmol/mL. These results suggest that prophylactic L-lysine may be useful in managing selected cases of recurrent herpes labialis.[56]

Foods rich in L-lysine include legumes, eggs, yogurt, fish, and chicken.[57,58] Taking L-lysine with vitamin C and bioflavonoids together has been shown to reduce the risk of herpetic outbreaks.[57]

## Propolis

Propolis, a natural product from bees, is comprised of a complex of antiviral chemicals (especially flavonoids).

In one study, propolis extract was tested against the herpesvirus both in vitro and in experimental animals. In the in vitro study, propolis caused a 50% reduction in herpes infection. Administration of propolis before or at time of infection yielded the most significant results. However, even when added 2 hours after infection, propolis still yielded 80–85% protection. In the animal portion of the study, a weak propolis solution prevented the appearance of herpes symptoms in rats and corneal herpes in rabbits.[59]

In a multicentered and randomized study, 90 men and women with recurrent genital HSV2 were divided into two groups to compare the healing ability of propolis ointment (with natural flavonoids) to that of acyclovir ointment and placebo. Ointments were applied 4 times daily for 10 days. At day 10, 80% of patients in the propolis group healed. Forty-seven percent in the acyclovir group healed, and 40% in the placebo group healed. Investigators concluded that an ointment containing flavonoids was more effective in healing genital herpetic lesions and in reducing local symptoms than ointments containing either acyclovir or placebo.[60]

## Thymus Extract

Thymus extracts have immune system–enhancing and restorative properties.[61] In a randomized, placebo-controlled study, immunodeficient patients with recurrent HSV1 cold sores were given bovine thymus extract (Thymostimulin) for 6 months; the thymus extract group had only 17 recurrences versus 62 in the control group. A significant increase in total white blood cells, lymphocyte count, and T-cell numbers was detected. Thymus extract may be useful in reducing the risk of viral reactivation in people with weakened immune systems.[62]

## Lactoferrin

Numerous studies have shown that lactoferrin, a whey protein found in human milk as well as an antimicrobial, has powerful antiherpetic properties. Lactoferrin works by reducing the ability of HSV1 and HSV2 to penetrate cell walls.[63] Studies show that lactoferrin:

- Reduces the appearance of skin lesions in herpes-infected mice.[64]
- Works synergistically with acyclovir.[65]
- Lowers the risk of herpes keratitis (herpes infection of the eye) among herpes-infected mice.[66]

## Curcumin

Curcumin, a component of the curry spice turmeric, significantly inhibits the growth of HSV1 in cell culture. In a laboratory experiment, cells were cultured, either pretreated with curcumin or left untreated, then administered HSV1. Curcumin significantly reduced the growth of HSV1 in the treated cells, as determined by the number of plaques, size of plaques, and viral counts, compared with untreated cells. Results indicate that curcumin aids cells in resisting HSV1 infection and slows HSV1 replication (growth). The antiviral effect is due to suppression of HSV1 gene expression.[67]

## Fucoidan Extract

*Undaria fucoidan* extract has been shown to inhibit replication of herpes by stimulating ingestion of the virus by macrophage cells and boosting the number of antibody-producing B cells.[68,69] In an early phase, open-label trial, oral *Undaria fucoidan* was administered to 15 individuals of various ages (from less than 10 years up to 72 years) suffering from herpetic infections including herpes type 1 (cold sores), herpes type 2 (genital herpes), herpes zoster (chicken pox; shingles), and Epstein-Barr virus (mononucleosis). The *Undaria* dosage approximated typical daily seaweed intake in Japan. *Undaria* increased the healing rates of active herpes virus infections in all 15 subjects. Individuals with chicken pox and shingles noted reduced pain and more rapid resolution of skin lesions. In the laboratory, scientists found that *Undaria* extract increased the growth of infection-fighting T cells in culture. Scientists postulated that *Undaria*'s ability to increase T-cell growth in the laboratory may be related to its ability to enhance immunity in human subjects.[70]

Laboratory studies of the same fucoidan preparation revealed potent antiviral activities against human herpes virus types 1 and 2, and against cytomegalovirus, a common infection in individuals with compromised immune systems.[71,72] Animal studies reveal that *Undaria fucoidans* prevent virus binding with host cells and inhibit viral replication, while simultaneously stimulating host-defensive immune responses.[73,74]

## Dehydroepiandrosterone

Reactivation of herpes and shingles has been associated with a weakened immune system. Among older people more likely to get shingles, a reduced immune response might be caused by age-related changes in steroid hormones.[75,76]

Dehydroepiandrosterone (DHEA), a steroid hormone, is known to decline as people age. In a 1997 study,[77] scientists proposed that oral administration of DHEA among elderly men would result in activation of their immune systems. Nine healthy men with an average age of 63 years were treated with a placebo for 2 weeks, followed by 20 weeks of DHEA (50 mg daily). After 2 weeks on oral DHEA, serum DHEA levels increased 3- to 4-fold. These levels were sustained throughout the study. Compared to placebo, DHEA administration resulted in the following:

- 20% increase in insulin-like growth factor (IGF)-I, which is thought to be responsible for some of the antiaging, anabolic effects that DHEA has produced in previous human studies.

- 35% increase in the number of monocyte immune cells.

- 29% increase in the number of B cells and 62% increase in B-cell activity.

- 40% increase in T-cell activity, even though the total numbers of T cells was not affected.

- 50% increase in interleukin-2 (IL-2).

- 22–37% increase in the number of NK cells and a 45% increase in NK cell activity.

- No adverse effects; however, this was a short study with few subjects.

DHEA has been shown in numerous human and animal studies to boost immune function via several different mechanisms.[78–80] A study demonstrated that when older female mice were treated with DHEA, several markers of immune function improved.[81]

## Garlic

Garlic (*Allium sativum*) has substantial antiviral activity. Fresh garlic extract, in which thiosulfinates are the active components, was virucidal against every virus tested, including HSV1 and HSV2. The predominant thiosulfinate in fresh garlic extract is allicin.[82]

## Life Extension Suggestions

- **Comprehensive multivitamin:** per label instructions
- **Cimetidine (Tagamet®):** 600 mg daily and 400 mg at bedtime (800 mg at bedtime if you cannot take cimetidine throughout the day)
- **Vitamin A:** 20 000 IU daily during outbreaks; 2500–5000 IU for maintenance
- **Beta-carotene:** 25 000 IU daily for 7–10 days during outbreaks
- **Vitamin C:** 5–10 g of esterified or buffered vitamin C during outbreaks
- **Vitamin E:** 400 IU daily (with 200 mg gamma tocopherol)
- **Zinc:** 30 mg daily
- **Lactoferrin:** 300–900 mg daily during an outbreak; 300 mg daily for maintenance
- **Selenium:** 200 mcg daily
- **L-lysine:** 700–1400 mg daily to suppress outbreaks
- **Propolis:** 500–2000 mg daily during outbreaks
- **Thymus extract:** 580 mg daily
- **Garlic extract:** 1200–4800 mg daily
- **DHEA:** 100–200 mg daily if an outbreak appears imminent and during outbreaks until lesions disappear (blood testing is recommended after DHEA therapy to ensure adequate levels)

In addition, the following blood testing resources may be helpful:

- **Cytomegalovirus (CMV) antibodies, IgM:** detects recent (acute) infection
- **Cytomegalovirus (CMV) antibodies, IgG:** detects previous exposure

## REFERENCES

References available at: www.lef.org/dpt5/ch72

# 73

## High Blood Pressure

High blood pressure is a silent epidemic that threatens the lives of 1 in every 3 American adults. Of those taking blood pressure medications, control rates vary between *less than half* to only *two thirds*.[1,2] This means that the majority of those diagnosed with hypertension spend most of their day with blood pressure levels that are dangerously elevated. Since increased blood pressure is a major risk factor for *heart disease, stroke, congestive heart failure*, and *kidney disease*, it acts as an accomplice in *millions* of additional deaths each year.[3]

Mainstream medicine has *fallen fatally short* of relieving high blood pressure. A major problem is that mainstream medicine's definition of what constitutes acceptable blood pressure levels is far too high. The medical establishment defines high blood pressure (*hypertension*) as *over 139/89 mmHg*. However, in 2006, researchers found that blood pressure levels ranging from *120–129 mmHg systolic/80–84 mmHg diastolic* were associated with an *81% higher* risk of cardiovascular disease compared to levels of *less than 120/80 mmHg*. Moreover, blood pressure levels of *130–139/85–89 mmHg* were associated with a *frightening 133% greater* risk of cardiovascular disease compared to levels *below 120/80 mmHg*.[4] Worse yet, studies suggest that conventional physicians are unlikely to treat hypertension until levels exceed *160/90 mmHg*, a level that *dramatically* increases the risk of disease and death.[5]

Controlling blood pressure means radically reducing disease risk. Studies have estimated that reducing blood pressure by 10/5 mmHg, to no lower than 115/75, can reduce the risk of death due to stroke by 40% and the risk of death due to heart disease or other vascular causes by 30%.[6] In individuals 40 to 70 years old, each 20/10 mmHg increment over 115/75 *doubles* the risk of heart attack, heart failure, stroke, or kidney disease.[6,7] Based on these and other data, Life Extension recognizes that for many individuals, a target blood pressure of 115/75 mmHg yields the best benefits.[7]

The development and progression of high blood pressure is complex and *multifactorial*. Thus, effective management is rarely achieved through a single intervention. Instead, optimal management often requires a *broad-based approach* including lifestyle modification, nutritional components, pharmaceutical medication(s), and regular self-monitoring. These approaches will be discussed in detail throughout this protocol.

## UNDERSTANDING BLOOD PRESSURE

Blood pressure is a measurement of the force exerted upon blood vessel walls by blood as it flows through the arteries. High blood pressure occurs when there is an increase of force against the arterial wall, with potentially damaging consequences.

Since the heart has distinct "beats," the pressure of oxygenated blood in the arteries is not continuous, but varies between two values, one when the heart is contracting, and one when the heart is relaxing. As

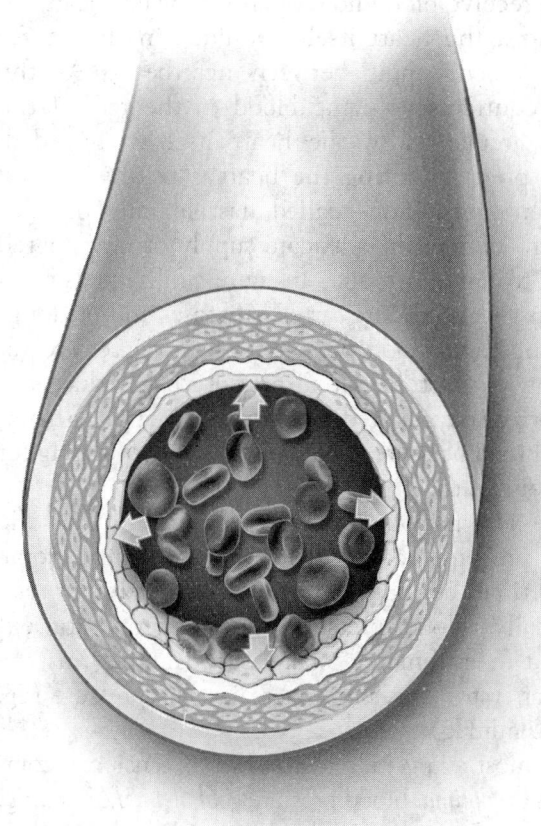

Blood pressure is the measurement of force applied to the artery walls

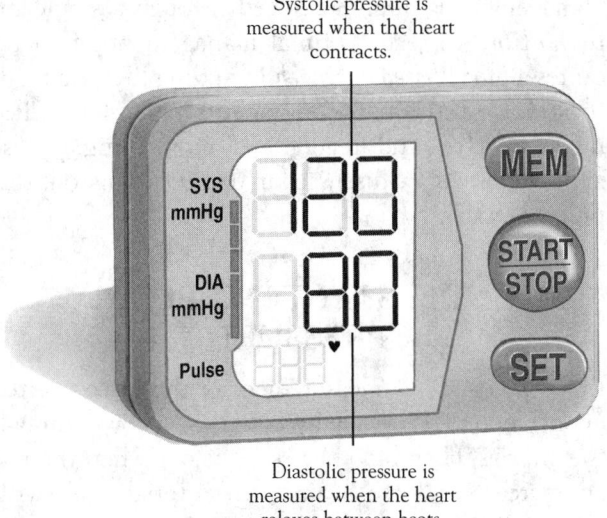

Systolic pressure is measured when the heart contracts.

Diastolic pressure is measured when the heart relaxes between beats.

the heart contracts, blood is expelled from the left ventricle under the greatest force; this upper pressure limit is the *systolic* blood pressure.

Following contraction of the heart, the aortic valve closes, which prevents blood from flowing backward into the heart, and helps maintain pressure in the arteries. This allows the heart muscle to relax and fill with blood. Unlike all other organs, which receive blood flow when the heart "beats" or contracts, the heart itself is unique in that it receives blood supply between heartbeats. As the heart contracts to pump blood to the rest of the body, circulation to the heart itself is impeded. Blood pressure during the heart's "resting" period between contractions, called diastole, must be sufficient to deliver an adequate supply of oxygenated blood to cardiac tissue. In aging individuals with pre-existing coronary artery disease and/or long-standing high blood pressure, overly aggressive reduction of diastolic blood pressure can reduce the delivery of oxygenated blood to the heart. The diastolic blood pressure should be close to 75 mmHg for optimal health.

The alternation between systolic and diastolic blood pressure occurs with every heartbeat, some 60–80 times per minute in the average adult at rest. Clinically, blood pressure measurements are expressed in millimeters of mercury (mmHg), as the ratio of systolic pressure over diastolic pressure (eg, 120/80 mmHg).

For most aging individuals, Life Extension recommends an *optimal* blood pressure *goal of 115/75 mmHg*. However, those aging individuals with long-standing hypertension and/or coronary artery disease should be aware that a rapid, overly aggressive reduction of

blood pressure, in particular diastolic blood pressure, should be avoided.

## HOW IS BLOOD PRESSURE REGULATED?

Blood pressure in the circulatory system is controlled three ways: (1) the force and rate at which blood leaves the heart (cardiac output), (2) the diameter and flexibility of the blood vessels though which blood flows (peripheral resistance); and (3) the total volume of blood in the circulatory system. All three work in concert to maintain a steady long-term pressure, while allowing for short-term increases to address cardiovascular needs.

Increasing the rate at which the heart beats, and the force at which blood leaves the heart results in a greater flow of blood and an increase in pressure, thus allowing the short-term increase in circulation that may be necessary during exercise, or in adapting to stress. Increases in cardiac output can be triggered by signals from the brain, or in response to stress hormones, such as epinephrine (adrenaline).

*Peripheral resistance* describes the increase in blood pressure caused by blood vessels themselves. The more resistance to blood flow, the greater the amount of blood pressure needed to overcome this resistance. Arteries actively modulate their resistance by constriction, which decreases the diameter of the vessel (vasoconstriction) and increases blood pressure, or dilation (vasodilation), which lowers resistance and blood pressure. Vasoconstriction and vasodilation are also short-term mechanisms to regulate blood pressure, and are under the control of several hormones. Aging causes arteries to lose their elasticity, which explains why the majority of aging people have above optimal blood pressure readings. Since it is "normal" for people's blood pressure to rise with age, interventions are usually required to keep it in safe ranges. People should not be surprised to learn that they need to take steps to bring their blood pressure under control—it is a part of normal aging for most of us.

The last mechanism for blood pressure regulation is through blood volume. Blood is a suspension of cells in an aqueous medium; its volume can therefore be modified by altering water content. Increasing the amount of water in the blood increases volume and the pressure it exerts. Reducing water content lowers blood pressure. Changes in blood volume are long-term mechanisms for blood pressure control.

Aside from the influence of neural triggers on heart rate, much of blood pressure control is performed by the *kidneys.* By controlling the balance of water and salt, the kidneys influence blood volume, lending long-term blood pressure control. The kidneys also produce hormones that act remotely to increase blood pressure through vasoconstriction of arteries. Kidney function can become impaired as people age, which is another reason why blood pressure may increase as we grow older. A major reason for kidney impairment is hypertension, so those starting with mild kidney problems have elevated blood pressure that then inflicts more kidney damage resulting in still higher blood pressure readings. Excess blood glucose (above 99 mg/dL) is another major cause of kidney damage. Fasting glucose levels should be kept *below* 86 mg/dL for overall disease prevention (optimal range: 70–85 mg/dL).

Central to the kidney's control of blood pressure is the renin-angiotensin-aldosterone system, a hormone system that works together to control blood pressure. Renin is an enzyme produced in the kidneys in response to low blood volume, depletion of sodium chloride, and stress. The production of renin leads, in turn, to the production of angiotensin II, a hormone that increases blood pressure. Angiotensin II increases blood pressure in the following ways:

- Causing the kidneys to retain sodium and water, which increases blood volume

- Causing the vasoconstriction of small blood vessels, which increases arterial blood pressure

- Inhibiting bradykinin (ie, a hormone that relaxes blood vessels)

- Stimulating the production of additional hypertensive (blood pressure raising) hormones in the adrenal and pituitary glands

- Indirectly acting on the central nervous system to increase thirst and the craving for salt, both of which are necessary for increasing blood volume

## HYPERTENSION AND ENDOTHELIAL DYSFUNCTION: A DEADLY DUAL THREAT TO VASCULAR HEALTH

In recent years, researchers have made tremendous strides in understanding the connection between high blood pressure and various cardiovascular diseases. It turns out that elevated blood pressure damages arteries at a basic level—the endothelium. Endothelial dysfunction is linked with the development of cardiovascular events.

Arteries are made up of three layers. The outer layer is mostly connective tissue that provides support to the inner two layers. The middle layer is smooth muscle that contracts and expands to facilitate circulation and maintain optimal blood pressure. The inner layer, or endothelium, is composed of a thin layer of cells that protects the integrity of the artery, promotes blood clotting in case of injury, and helps prevent damaging molecules such as low-density lipoproteins (LDLs) and triglycerides from penetrating the wall of the artery. When the endothelial layer is damaged, the result can be a thickened arterial wall and the abnormal aggregation of white blood cells. Sensing an injury, the endothelium stimulates a healing response that ultimately leads to an atherosclerotic plaque.[8,9]

Elevated blood pressure has been shown to contribute significantly to endothelial dysfunction. High blood pressure causes functional alterations in the endothelium that, in turn, are associated with decreased arterial mobility and increased stiffness in the arterial wall.[10] When the arteries become "stiff" or hardened, and can no longer contract and dilate sufficiently, additional stress is placed on the heart's main pumping chamber, the left ventricle. As a result, the left ventricle may be enlarged (left ventricular hypertrophy).[11] Left ventricular hypertrophy is often the first sign that damage from uncontrolled high blood pressure has started to occur.[12] If left untreated, ventricular hypertrophy may evolve into congestive heart failure.

The degree of endothelial dysfunction correlates with target organ damage.[13] As a result, physicians measure the effects of high blood pressure by looking at target organ damage. In other words, treatment decisions are based on how much damage high blood pressure is causing to organs such as the kidneys, eyes, or heart.

The intimate relationship that exists between high blood pressure and endothelial dysfunction highlights the need to address both of these phenomena as separate, yet unified contributors to cardiovascular disease. In fact, the network of interrelated cardiovascular risk factors includes a myriad of additional components that must be addressed to truly reduce cardiovascular risk. More information on the multifactorial nature of cardiovascular disease can be found in the *Life Extension Magazine* article titled "How to Circumvent 17 Independent Heart Attack Risk Factors."

## HYPERTENSION AND RELATED DISEASE RISK

While increases in blood pressure from the resting rate are expected under certain conditions such as excitement, stress, or physical exertion, a prolonged elevation in blood pressure can be detrimental. Sustained high pressure within the cardiovascular system compromises the integrity of vessels, leading to vascular damage and failure of the organs that the vessels supply.[14] Short of this, even modest, sustained increases in blood pressure elevate the risk of several diseases, including arteriosclerosis, stroke, chronic kidney disease/ failure, peripheral arterial disease (PAD), aneurysm, and vision loss. Hypertension is a more important risk factor for coronary artery disease than high non-HDL cholesterol, elevated C-reactive protein, high serum triglycerides, or obesity.[15–17] Even so, one cannot completely reduce cardiovascular risk without controlling *all* of their risk factors.

The current definition of hypertension is based on the risk of serious complications and the methods of their management.[7] While the threshold used to define hypertension has been >139/89 mmHg for decades, several published studies reveal that blood pressure should be kept around *115/75 mmHg* in order to truly protect against cardiovascular disease.[18–20]

Hypertension is classified as *primary* and *secondary* based on underlying cause. Primary hypertension, the most frequent and preventable type, arises from a number of underlying contributing factors.[21, 22] Inadequate intake of nutrients including potassium, magnesium, vitamin D, and vitamin K may also play a role. Secondary hypertension represents only about 5–10% of hypertension cases, and results from an underlying condition, usually associated with diseases of the kidneys, endocrine, vascular, or central nervous system. Although antihypertensive drugs are sometimes used to manage secondary hypertension, correcting the underlying cause can often lead to a cure.[21]

*Prehypertension* is a *"predisease"* state, which carries an increased risk of progression to hypertension. Those in the 130/80 to 139/89 mmHg blood pressure range (which is already dangerously high) are twice as likely to develop clinical hypertension (which means much higher blood pressure readings) as those with lower values.[23,24] Despite the availability of studies indicating that individuals within this blood pressure range are at increased risk of developing clinical hypertension as well as heart disease, mainstream medicine usually opts *not* to treat blood pressure with pharmaceutical drugs at this level.

*Stage 1 and Stage 2 hypertension*, defined as 140–159/90–99 and >160/100 mmHg, respectively, carry the greatest risk of cardiovascular disease. The two stages of hypertension differ in their conventional medical treatments, with stage 2 hypertensive patients usually requiring the most aggressive intervention using combinations of antihypertensive drugs.

## SOME CAUSES OF SECONDARY HYPERTENSION[7,21]

### Renal

- Chronic kidney disease
- Renal vascular disease
- Renin-producing tumors

### Endocrine

- Primary aldosteronism (secretion of excess aldosterone, a hormone that increases salt retention)

- Hypo- or hyper-thyroidism
- Adrenocortical hyperfunction (oversecretion of adrenal hormones)
- Acromegaly (secretion of excessive growth hormone)

### Neurogenic

- Acute stress-related hypertension
- Spinal cord damage/quadriplegia

### Vascular

- Rigidity or narrowing of the aorta

### Hypertension induced by drugs

- Oral contraceptives
- Steroid therapy
- Sympathomimetic drugs (decongestants, appetite suppressants)
- Nonsteroidal anti-inflammatory drugs (NSAIDs) and COX-2 inhibitors
- Immunosuppressants
- Erythropoietin
- Amphetamines

### Miscellaneous

- Obstructive sleep apnea
- Nutrient deficiency
- Pregnancy-induced hypertension

## RISK FACTORS FOR HIGH BLOOD PRESSURE

Advancing age, gender, family history, and genetic predisposition all contribute to the development of high blood pressure. However, they are considered nonmodifiable risk factors, meaning that it is not possible to reduce the risk that these factors pose by taking preventive action. Modifiable risk factors, on the other hand, also contribute significantly to the development of high blood pressure, but *can* be addressed through preventive action. Modifiable risk factors for hypertension include:

- **High sodium intake.** According to emerging hypotheses, excess sodium appears to alter the balance between excitatory and inhibitory adrenergic receptors in such a way that favors vasoconstriction, leading to increased blood pressure.[25] A 2011 study found that individuals with hypertension consume significantly more sodium each day than those without high blood pressure.[26] Overindulging with salt also increases the risk for stroke, kidney disease, and cardiovascular disease.[27,28] In order to avoid the hypertensive effects of sodium, intake should be limited to 2.4 g of sodium, or 6 g of sodium chloride (table salt) daily.[7]

- **Low potassium intake.** Adequate potassium intake helps balance the hypertensive effects of sodium. Diets containing excess sodium require ample amounts of potassium-rich foods to help mitigate the hypertensive consequences of modern sodium overindulgence. The suggested potassium intake for adults is 4.7 g daily, but most Americans consume far less.

- **Obesity and insulin resistance.** Body weight gain accounts for as much as 75% of the risk for high blood pressure.[29] Nearly 70% of Americans are overweight. As body fat mass increases, blood volume increases as well, which contributes to increased blood pressure. Insulin resistance, which often occurs in tandem with obesity, contributes to vascular resistance and increased blood pressure.[30]

- **Stress.** Stressful situations cause the release of hypertensive (blood pressure-raising) hormones, such as *epinephrine*. As chronic stress causes the continual release of hypertensive hormones, sustained elevations in blood pressure become dangerous. A study following government employees who participated in disaster relief efforts in the Niigata Prefecture of Japan after the 2004 earthquake found that those with the most stressful workloads were much more likely to develop high blood pressure. Individuals under the greatest stress were also more likely to gain weight and have high cholesterol levels.[31]

- **Sedentary lifestyle, smoking, and too much alcohol.** All of these behaviors increase the risk of high blood pressure. Light alcohol consumption does confer benefits for cardiovascular health, while heavy alcohol ingestion increases the risk of hypertension. Therefore, intake should be limited to 2 drinks daily for men and 1 drink daily for women.[7]

Although conventional physicians usually consider the aforementioned risk factors, mainstream medicine has overlooked two important contributors that may play a significant role in blood pressure regulation—vitamin K and vitamin D.

- **Low vitamin D intake.** Insufficient intake of this hormone-like vitamin is implicated in the pathology of high blood pressure along with numerous other diseases. Studies suggest that vitamin D might target many of the factors that contribute to hypertension including suppressing renin (a hypertensive enzyme) and protecting kidney function.[32] In a review of 10 randomized controlled trials, vitamin D supplementation was shown to mildly reduce blood pressure. Moreover, individuals with higher blood levels of vitamin D were at less risk of developing cardiovascular disease.[32] Life Extension suggests that all individuals maintain a blood 25-hydroxyvitamin D level of 50–80 ng/mL.

- **Low vitamin K intake.** Vitamin K is required to maintain soft and pliable arterial walls. Inadequate vitamin K intake can result in an accumulation of calcium in the arterial wall, leading to hardening of the arteries and increased peripheral resistance.[33] Ensuring adequate vitamin K intake allows for proper allocation of calcium *into* the bones to maintain skeletal integrity and *away* from the arterial wall, helping prevent the arterial "stiffness" that robs so many aging individuals of proper circulation.

## PHARMACEUTICAL THERAPIES FOR HYPERTENSION

Conventional management of hypertension begins with lifestyle modification, followed by the possible addition of one or more antihypertensive drug therapies to achieve a target blood pressure goal of less than *140/90* mmHg (<130/80 mmHg for persons with diabetes or renal disease). As described earlier, studies show that blood pressure >115/75 mmHg can increase risk of vascular disease. However, it is also important to consider that overly aggressive blood-pressure lowering in aging individuals with pre-existing, longstanding hypertension or other cardiovascular disease may be dangerous.

Thus, a blood pressure reduction regimen must be accompanied by close supervision and careful monitoring of blood pressure throughout the day. A diligent plan encompassing regular at-home blood pressure monitoring and regular health care practitioner–patient interaction will ensure optimal risk reduction and patient safety.

Antihypertensive drugs lower blood pressure by attenuating one or more of the blood pressure–regulating mechanisms. Major "classes" of antihypertensive drugs are variably defined, but the most widely prescribed can be grouped into three categories based on their activities.

### Diuretics

Reduction of blood volume is the first target of conventional antihypertensive therapies. Diuretics (thiazide diuretics, loop diuretics, potassium-sparing diuretics) are the most commonly prescribed drugs in this category. Diuretics exert effects on the kidneys to increase the excretion of water. This drop in blood volume results in a drop in pressure.

Adverse effects of thiazide diuretics include sexual dysfunction, glucose intolerance, gout, low potassium level (hypokalemia), and low sodium level (hyponatremia). Conventional doctors often overlook the depletion of vital magnesium that can be caused by diuretics. Many patients do better by starting with the angiotensin II receptor blockers described later in this chapter. Those who require diuretic drugs should supplement with plenty of magnesium and potassium if dietary intake is low (dietary intake of magnesium is usually too low even for those who do not take diuretic drugs).

## Cardioinhibitory Drugs

Cardioinhibitory drugs decrease the rate and force with which the heart pumps, reducing cardiac output and lowering blood pressure.

*Beta blockers* lower heart rate and blood pressure by blocking the beta adrenoceptors. Normally, these adrenoceptors sense the hormones epinephrine (adrenaline) and norepinephrine in the blood, and then respond by increasing heart rate and constricting blood vessels outside the heart. Beta blockers disrupt this interaction.

Beta blockers are contraindicated in individuals with COPD (chronic obstructive pulmonary disease) and asthma. Side effects include a worsening of blood glucose control (in diabetics), elevated triglycerides, and lower high-density lipoprotein (HDL—sometimes called the "good" cholesterol) levels. These drugs may exacerbate depressive symptoms, cause erectile dysfunction, and are associated with sleep disturbances, fatigue, and lethargy.

A second group of drugs, calcium channel blockers, specifically bind to and block the channels (cellular pores) that allow calcium to flow into cardiac muscle cells. Since muscle fibers require calcium for contraction, reducing the availability of calcium in cardiac muscle lowers the force at which the heart contracts, lowering blood pressure. Additionally, certain calcium channel blockers, which are less specific toward calcium channels in the heart, also have vasodilating properties.

Side effects commonly associated with calcium channel blockers include flushing of the face and neck, headache, edema (swelling; usually in the ankles and feet), dizziness, fatigue, and skin rash.

## Vasodilators

Vasodilators increase the diameter of vessels, lowering their resistance and the pressure required to move blood through them. There are several types with differing mechanisms. Angiotensin-converting enzyme (ACE) inhibitors stop the activity of ACE, the enzyme that catalyzes the final step in the synthesis of the hypertensive hormone *angiotensin II*. By lowering levels of angiotensin II, ACE inhibitors promote the dilation of blood vessels, increasing the excretion of water and sodium from the kidneys, thereby lowering blood volume. Frequent side effects of ACE inhibitor use include dizziness, fatigue, weakness, headache, and persistent dry cough.

Renin inhibitors, another group of vasodilators, also reduce angiotensin II levels at the first step of its synthesis. This class of drugs is associated with several side effects, which include diarrhea, dizziness, flu-like symptoms, fatigue, and cough.

The effects of angiotensin receptor blockers (ARBs) are similar to ACE inhibitors. Instead of reducing the levels of angiotensin II, however, they reduce its bioactivity, preventing it from interacting with receptors on the surface of cells and signaling hypertensive effects.

In addition to efficiently lowering blood pressure,[34] a comprehensive review of published studies, which examined data for nearly 150 000 subjects, revealed that use of an angiotensin receptor blocker was associated with a 10% reduction in the likelihood of suffering a stroke, heart failure, or developing diabetes.[35]

Angiotensin receptor blockers also convey some surprising additional benefits. Studies show that suppressing the signaling of angiotensin receptors may blunt oxidative stress and encourage the activation of genes associated with enhanced longevity. Amazingly, animals genetically engineered not to express the primary angiotensin receptor were shown to *live 28% longer* than normal animals.[36] Moreover, these animals have a greater number of mitochondria, the cellular components that provide the energy needed to function with youthful vigor.[37] Other data indicate that angiotensin receptor blockers may help modulate the immune system in ways that discourage autoimmunity, suppress inflammation, and slow the progression of cardiovascular disease independent of their effects on blood pressure.[38]

Angiotensin receptor blockers may cause dizziness, headache, or elevated blood levels of potassium (hyperkalemia). Emerging evidence also suggests that some drugs in this class may cause severe gastrointestinal problems resembling celiac disease.[39] However, most individuals do not experience these effects.

For many people with hypertension, taking an individualized daily dose of an *angiotensin receptor blocker* can keep blood pressure readings in optimal ranges over a 24-hour period.

Alpha blockers prevent the binding of norepinephrine to *alpha adrenoceptors*, which are located on vascular smooth muscle cells within blood vessel walls. They function much like beta blockers do in the heart, preventing the contraction of blood vessels in response to stress hormones. This class of medication can sometimes cause dizziness, lightheadedness, or fainting upon arising from a sitting or lying position.

## LETHAL MISCONCEPTION ABOUT ANTIHYPERTENSIVE DRUGS

A properly functioning heart is of little consequence without the means to maintain a predictable pressure throughout the circulatory system. A dangerous assumption made by doctors is that once a day dosing with an antihypertensive drug will keep a patient's blood pressure under control over an entire *24-hour period*. The reality is that these drugs will wear off in many patients within 12 to 18 hours, leaving the body vulnerable to dangerous daily blood pressure spikes. Few physicians understand that it is during periods of the day when blood pressure spikes above *115/75* mmHg that damage is inflicted. Therefore, keeping blood pressure suppressed for even 18 hours leaves patients exposed to the damaging effects of hypertension for 6 hours every day.

The best way to effectively monitor blood pressure is with an at-home blood pressure monitor. If one takes a 50-mg dose of *losartan* in the morning, and blood pressure exceeds 115/75 at any time of the day thereafter, they should consult their physician about taking a second dose of losartan in the evening to ensure all-day blood pressure control. Those who take Benicar® usually only need a once-daily dose of 10–20 mg.

It does not matter what drug or natural therapy one employs to lower blood pressure. The objective is to use at-home blood pressure devices to achieve blood pressure readings no higher than *115/75* mmHg throughout a 24-hour period.

## BLOOD PRESSURE MEDICATIONS MAY CONFER GREATER PROTECTION IF TAKEN AT BEDTIME IN SOME POPULATIONS

A 2011 study revealed that dosing schedules for antihypertensive medications may influence their efficacy.[40]

In 661 patients with chronic kidney disease, ambulatory blood pressure was measured at baseline and then tracked for over 5 years after adjusting medication scheduling according to one of two regimens. In the first group, all antihypertensive drugs were taken upon awakening, while a second group took at least one medication at bedtime. Not only did the second group have lower blood pressure during sleep, but a significantly greater percentage of them gained control over their daytime blood pressure compared to the morning dosing group.

After analyzing the study data, researchers uncovered a *dramatic* reduction in the risk of cardiovascular events and associated mortality—those taking blood pressure meds at bedtime had only about *one third the risk* versus those taking all their blood pressure meds in the morning. Moreover, each 5-mmHg reduction in blood pressure during sleep was tied to a *14% reduction* in cardiovascular events during the follow-up period.

While this study clearly shows that those with chronic kidney disease and hypertension benefited from a bedtime dosing regimen, it does not necessarily mean that a similar effect will be observed in other populations. However, Life Extension suggests that everyone taking a blood pressure-lowering drug consult with their health care provider as to whether adjusting their dosing regimen to include at least one of their meds at bedtime may be wise.

## DIETARY AND LIFESTYLE APPROACHES TO MANAGING BLOOD PRESSURE

Dietary modifications aim to balance macro- and micronutrient intake to favorably influence the body's inherent blood pressure-regulating systems.

Weight management, increased physical activity, limitation of alcohol consumption, and dietary modification (particularly the reduction of dietary sodium) are among the best studied, and most effective lifestyle changes for blood pressure management. A body mass index (BMI) between 18.5 and 24.9 carries the lowest risk of hypertension. Reductions of systolic blood pressure by 5–20 mmHg per 10 kg (22 pounds) of weight loss have been observed in several studies.[41,42] Regular exercise has been associated with average reductions in blood pressure of 3.2 mmHg (systolic) and 3.5 mmHg (diastolic) in thousands of subjects across many studies.[43-45] Limitation of alcohol consumption ($\leq$ 2 drinks per day for men, less than this for women) can further reduce systolic blood pressure by 2–4 mmHg.[45]

A sodium-restricted diet (<1.5 g/day) can significantly reduce blood pressure. The DASH (Dietary Approaches to Stop Hypertension) eating plan has been shown to lower systolic blood pressure by 8–14 mmHg, and is included among suggested dietary guidelines.[46,47] The first DASH eating plan focused on fruits, vegetables, and whole grains, was especially high in fiber (31 g/day) and potassium (4.7 g/day), and low in animal products. Ironically, the original DASH was not a low-sodium diet (allowing up to 3 g/day), but nonetheless had blood pressure-lowering effects.[48]

**Fiber.** How dietary fiber (both soluble and insoluble) reduces blood pressure is poorly understood. Possible mechanisms include a reduction of the glycemic index of foods and the attenuation of insulin response (insulin plays a role in blood pressure regulation). Soluble fibers may also increase mineral absorption (such as calcium, magnesium, and potassium) by several mechanisms.[49] A comprehensive review of 24 randomized, controlled clinical trials examined the effects of fiber in people with both normal and high blood pressure. They demonstrated modest reductions in systolic (1.13 mmHg) and diastolic (1.26 mmHg) blood pressure at an average dose of 11.5 g fiber/day.[50] Another review found an average reduction in both systolic and diastolic blood pressure in trials conducted among patients with hypertension (systolic 5.95 mmHg and diastolic 4.20 mmHg) and in trials with a duration of intervention ≥8 weeks (systolic 3.12 mmHg and diastolic 2.57 mmHg).[51]

**Protein.** Results from a comprehensive review of hypertension studies indicate an association between low dietary protein intake and elevated blood pressure.[52] A recent review of 46 studies demonstrated the effects of plant protein on reductions in blood pressure (up to a 1.4-mmHg reduction in systolic blood pressure and a 1-mmHg reduction in diastolic blood pressure for every 11 g of plant protein consumed daily). The blood pressure-lowering effect was stronger in both middle-aged and hypertensive individuals, as well as those with a high initial BMI.[53] The mechanism for the blood pressure-lowering effect of protein is unclear. It may increase sodium (and water) excretion from the kidneys, increase blood concentration(s) of arginine (the precursor to nitric oxide), or improve insulin sensitivity (especially if it replaces carbohydrates in the diet).[52]

**Caloric restriction (CR).** CR is the chronic reduction of dietary calories (typically 30%, but sometimes up to 50% in some protocols), without malnutrition.[54] Restriction in energy intake slows down the body's growth processes, causing a focus on protective repair mechanisms. The overall effect is an improvement in several measures of health.

Observational studies have tracked the effects of calorie restriction on lean, healthy individuals, and have demonstrated that a moderate calorie restriction (22–30% decrease in caloric intake from normal levels) improves cardiac function as well as reduces markers of inflammation and risk factors for cardiovascular disease

(LDL-C, triglycerides, blood pressure).[55–58] Reductions of systolic blood pressure (5–10 mmHg) and diastolic blood pressure (4–6 mmHg) have been observed in studies of individuals with normal and high blood pressure that adopted a caloric-restricted regimen.[59–62]

# RESTORING YOUTHFUL HORMONE BALANCE TO CONTROL BLOOD PRESSURE

The risk of developing primary hypertension is significantly higher in postmenopausal women and men older than 55 years of age. As hormone levels decline with age, the risk of high blood pressure and heart disease rise.

Vascular endothelium and smooth muscle cells have sex steroid receptors.[63] Research has supported bioidentical hormone restoration of estrogen, progesterone, and testosterone for use in the management of blood pressure and overall cardiac health.

Sex hormones stimulate endothelial cell growth, inhibit smooth muscle proliferation contraction, and relax the vascular endothelium via nitric oxide and prostacyclin.[64] When hormones are present in youthful concentrations, vascular function in patients with high blood pressure may be modulated.[65]

Japanese scientists found that a group of menopausal women treated with estriol for 12 months had a significant decrease in both systolic and diastolic blood pressure.[66] Another placebo-controlled study demonstrated that estriol replacement for 30 weeks improved flow-mediated dilation, a measure of arterial relaxation.[67] Estriol accomplishes these effects by strongly activating nitric oxide signaling systems and stabilizing atherosclerotic plaques.[68]

In a 2-year-long study involving postmenopausal women, hormone replacement therapy (HRT) (upon initiation of treatment) was able to quickly and significantly lower blood pressure.

Moreover, the effects were maintained over the 2-year period as women receiving HRT displayed significantly lower blood pressure at 12- and 24-month checkups.[69]

Likewise, in males, low testosterone levels are predictive of hypertension and cardiovascular disease risk.[69] Life Extension suggests that aging men maintain free testosterone levels of 20–25 pg/mL for optimal health.

If you are interested in learning more about the numerous benefits of restoring hormone concentrations to youthful levels, see Life Extension's Female Hormone Restoration and Male Hormone Restoration protocols.

# NUTRIENTS TO SUPPORT HEALTHY BLOOD PRESSURE LEVELS

Nutritional approaches to hypertension management mirror many of the strategies of pharmaceutical therapies. The inclusion of specific dietary compounds with blood pressure-lowering (hypotensive) or cardioprotective properties can significantly support cardiovascular health.

Several dietary compounds can also lower blood pressure through the mechanism of *antioxidation*. Hypertension is associated with an increase in oxidative stress and the activity of pro-oxidant enzymes. Oxidative stress can inactivate the vasodilation signal nitric oxide by converting it into the peroxynitrite free radical. Several hypotensive antioxidants appear to function by reducing this oxidative damage, and preserving the bioavailability of nitric oxide.

## Cardioinhibitory and Cardiotonic Nutraceuticals

**Magnesium.** As early as the 1950s, the hypotensive effects of magnesium were a focus of speculation based on findings showing that drinking hard water (which is high in magnesium and other minerals) is associated with lower cardiovascular mortality.[70] Dozens of observational studies have demonstrated that magnesium intake is associated with lower blood pressure, and hypertensive individuals have lower intakes of magnesium than those with normal blood pressure.[70] Magnesium may lower blood pressure both by acting like a natural calcium channel blocker and serving as a cofactor for the production of the vasodilator *prostaglandin E1*.[71]

Interventions using magnesium have shown modest effects on blood pressure. An analysis of 12 controlled trials containing over 500 patients demonstrated that supplemental magnesium for 8 to 26 weeks led to an average decrease in diastolic blood pressure of 2.2 mmHg.[72] A comprehensive analytical review of 44 human studies of supplemental magnesium showed that it may enhance the blood pressure lowering effect of anti-hypertensive medications in early-stage hypertensive subjects. Patients treated with medications continuously over 6 months saw significant further decreases in systolic and diastolic blood pressure with magnesium supplementation as low as 230 mg daily.[73]

Daily supplementation with 300 to 500 mg of elemental magnesium is vital for those taking diuretic drugs. Absorption of magnesium into the bloodstream is not particularly effective. Higher blood magnesium levels may be achieved by taking 2000 mg of *magnesium threonate* daily, even though its elemental magnesium is relatively low.[74]

**Hawthorn (Crataegus laevigata, Crataegus monogyna, Crataegus oxyacantha).** Hawthorn is a traditional cardiovascular tonic that has been in use since the Middle Ages. Hawthorn extracts are believed to exhibit mild blood pressure lowering activity by multiple mechanisms, including the dilation of coronary and peripheral blood vessels, inhibition of ACE, antioxidative and anti-inflammatory effects, and mild diuretic activity.[75,76] It also improves cardiac oxygen consumption.[77]

Three trials have supported the potential blood pressure-lowering activity of Hawthorn extracts. A small randomized controlled study of 36 untreated, mildly hypertensive, middle-aged subjects compared standardized hawthorn extract (500 mg) and magnesium (600 mg), both separately and in combination for 10 weeks. There was a small decrease in diastolic blood pressure in the hawthorn group.[78] In a second larger study, 92 middle-aged hypertensive participants were randomized to take standardized hawthorn extract or placebo 3 times daily for 4 months. Hawthorn demonstrated a significant decrease in both systolic and diastolic blood pressure.[79] In the third study, a group of 39 patients with type 2 diabetes took hawthorn extract in conjunction with existing blood pressure or blood sugar-lowering drugs. Test participants receiving 1200 mg hawthorn extract daily for 16 weeks saw a 2.6-mmHg drop in diastolic blood pressure from baseline values, while the control group saw no change.[78]

## Regulation of Blood Volume

**Potassium.** Potassium is one of the most abundant electrolytes in the body. Due to their antagonistic roles in metabolism, the balance of sodium and potassium plays a critical role in blood pressure regulation. Potassium increases excretion of sodium from the kidneys (reducing blood volume) and reduces the sensitivity of blood vessels to vasoconstriction by angiotensin II.[80]

Evidence from observational studies and clinical trials consistently indicate that high levels of potassium are associated with lower blood pressure.[71] Four comprehensive reviews of potassium trials report average reductions in systolic blood pressure of 2.4–5.9 mmHg and diastolic blood pressure of 1.6–3.4 mmHg when supplementing with potassium for 2–8 weeks.[72,81-83] The degree of blood pressure lowering appears to be dose dependent, with the largest decreases in blood pressure occurring at the high end of the dosage range (daily doses of 1.9–4.7 g were used in the trials).

The adequate intake (AI) of potassium is 4.7 g daily for adults. Most adults have a median dietary intake substantially lower than this (2.8–3.3 g daily in men and 2.2–2.4 g daily in women).[84] Less than 3% of the population consumes the AI.[85] It should be noted that the amount of potassium in over-the-counter supplements is typically <100 mg, so individuals with high blood pressure should consume potassium rich foods to ensure AI.

**Calcium.** In addition to magnesium and potassium, population-based studies suggest a role for calcium in the prevention of hypertension, possibly through its ability to promote sodium excretion, balance the concentrations of other minerals (particularly magnesium and potassium), and its role in the activity of smooth muscle cells in blood vessels.[86,87] In a review of 40 randomized controlled trials, an average daily calcium dose of 1200 mg was associated with a reduction in systolic (1.9 mmHg) and diastolic (1.0 mmHg) blood pressure. In persons with habitually low calcium intake (<800 mg/day), the hypotensive effect was even greater (2.6/1.3 mmHg).[88]

## Antioxidants

**Coenzyme Q10 (CoQ10).** As a critical component of mitochondrial function and energy production, CoQ10 has a central role in proper cardiac function.[89] Within blood vessels, CoQ10 may directly contribute to the functionality of vascular smooth muscle cells,

allowing them to properly dilate.[90] As a lipid-soluble antioxidant, CoQ10 may quench free radicals and spare levels of vasodilatory nitric oxide.[91]

In two separate reviews of human CoQ10 studies (a total of 12 studies comprising 328 hypertensive patients), *all* showed improvements in blood pressure.[91,92] Three randomized, controlled trials of CoQ10 (100–120 mg daily for up to 8 weeks) demonstrated mean decreases in systolic and diastolic blood pressure of 11 mmHg and 7 mmHg, respectively, while open-label trials revealed slightly larger average decreases (–13.5/–10.3 mmHg).[91]

CoQ10 (at 200 mg daily) has also been shown to improve blood pressure and blood sugar control in type 2 diabetics when combined with the cholesterol-lowering drug fenofibrate.[93] CoQ10 may lead to modest reductions in diastolic blood pressure in chronic kidney disease patients when combined with fish oil.[94]

**Carotenoids.** Epidemiologic evidence suggests that the risk of hypertension decreases as the concentration of four serum carotenoids (α- and β-carotene, lutein/zeaxanthin, and β-cryptoxanthin) increases.[95] In addition, *lycopene* (a carotenoid) has demonstrated hypotensive activity in a human intervention study. A small crossover study of 31 patients with stage 1 hypertension taking 250 mg of a lycopene-enriched tomato extract for 8 weeks demonstrated significant reductions in blood pressure (–10/–4 mmHg), while no changes in blood pressure were observed during the placebo period. Thiobarbituric acid-reactive substance (TBARS), a marker for oxidative stress, also decreased during the test period.[96]

**Chlorogenic acid.** Chlorogenic acid from *green coffee* (unroasted coffee beans) is a hypotensive antioxidant, likely increasing the availability of nitric oxide (for vasodilation) by inhibiting enzymes that form reactive oxygen-free radicals.[97] The roasting of coffee reduces the effects of *chlorogenic acid* on blood pressure. Still, the activity of chlorogenic acid remaining in roasted coffee is enough to counteract some of the hypertensive effects of caffeine, explaining why coffee consumption raises blood pressure less than an equivalent amount of caffeine alone.[98] Green coffee bean extract supplements are available to provide standardized doses of chlorogenic acid with minimal amounts of caffeine.

Two multicenter, randomized controlled trials investigated the effects of various doses of chlorogenic acid on volunteers with mild hypertension. In the first, 117 male volunteers were randomized into 3 dosage groups (46 mg, 93 mg, or 185 mg) of green coffee extract versus placebo once daily for 28 days. At study end, average reductions in systolic blood pressure

**Table 1. Top 10 Foods Highest in Potassium**

| Food | Serving Size | Potassium Content (mg) |
|---|---|---|
| Tomato paste, without salt added | 1 cup | 2657 |
| Orange juice, frozen concentrate, unsweetened, undiluted | 6 fl-oz. | 1436 |
| Beet greens, cooked, boiled, drained, without salt | 1 cup | 1309 |
| Beans, white, mature seeds, canned | 1 cup | 1189 |
| Dates, deglet noor | 1 cup | 1168 |
| Milk, canned, condensed, sweetened | 1 cup | 1135 |
| Tomato puree, without salt added | 1 cup | 1098 |
| Raisins, seedless | 1 cup | 1086 |
| Potato, baked, flesh and skin, without salt | 1 potato | 1081 |
| Grapefruit juice, white, frozen concentrate, unsweetened, undiluted | 6 fl-oz. | 1002 |

U.S. Department of Agriculture 2007.[84a]

from baseline (4.7 mmHg and 5.6 mmHg for the medium- and high-dose groups, respectively) varied significantly from placebo. Differences in diastolic blood pressure from the placebo group were also observed in the medium- and high-dose groups (–3.2 mmHg and –3.9 mmHg, respectively).[99] The second trial, with a similar design and duration, tested 4 doses of green coffee bean extract standardized to chlorogenic acid (0 mg, 82 mg, 172 mg, or 299 mg) in 203 pre- and stage-1 hypertensive volunteers (male and female). Green coffee bean extract had an anti-hypertensive effect on systolic blood pressure in a dose-dependent manner (ranging from –2.7 mmHg to –3.3 mmHg for the low and high doses, respectively). Diastolic blood pressure reduction was consistent across all dosages (approximately 3 mmHg).[100]

**Vitamin C.** Vitamin C is an essential water-soluble antioxidant vitamin in humans. It is thought to exert hypotensive effects through an improvement in endothelial function, reduction in arterial stiffness, and its ability to bind the angiotensin receptor (thereby lowering its ability to bind angiotensin II).[101] Higher plasma levels of vitamin C are associated with lower blood pressure.[102] In observational studies, individuals with the highest plasma ascorbic acid (vitamin C) concentrations had 4.66 mmHg lower systolic blood pressure and 6.04 mmHg lower diastolic blood pressure than those with the lowest concentrations.[103]

Intervention studies with vitamin C in hypertensive adults have shown mixed results. Several small studies have shown modest reductions in systolic (1.8 to 4.5 mmHg) and diastolic (2.8 mmHg) blood pressure at doses of 500–2000 mg daily,[104–109] while others failed to reveal significant effects.[110–112]

## Vasodilators

**Grape seed extract.** Grape seed extract contains *oligomeric procyanidins (OPCs)* that support vasodilation through an increase in nitric oxide production and ACE inhibition.[113] Two 4-week studies of standardized grape seed extract (150 mg or 300 mg) in prehypertensive patients with metabolic syndrome demonstrated a marked reduction in systolic and diastolic blood pressure. The reduction averaged –12/–7 mmHg between the two studies and did not significantly differ between the two dosages.[114,115] Another trial is underway as of August 2011.[116]

**Pomegranate.** Pomegranate contains several bioactive antioxidant polyphenols, including *punicalagins*. Pomegranate juice consumption (50 mL [1.7 oz.] daily) has been associated with decreases in systolic blood pressure of 8 *mmHg* in a 2-week study,[117] and *21 mmHg* in a 1-year study.[117]

In addition to its potent antioxidant activity (it has been shown to reduce LDL oxidation and increase levels of the cellular antioxidant glutathione),[118] pomegranate polyphenols also function as ACE inhibitors. Reductions in ACE activity by 36% have been demonstrated after 2 weeks of pomegranate juice consumption.[117]

**L-arginine.** An amino acid, L-arginine serves as the main raw material for the production of the vasodilator nitric oxide. Low cellular levels of L-arginine and nitric oxide are evident in individuals genetically predisposed to hypertension, likely due to inefficient transport of L-arginine across the cellular membrane.[119] Test diets rich in arginine-containing foods, or supplemented with arginine, demonstrated decreases in blood pressure (6.2 mmHg systolic, 5.0–6.8 mmHg diastolic) when compared to control diets in a short-term human study.[120] Reductions in systolic and diastolic blood pressure were also observed in a pilot trial where kidney transplant patients were supplemented with 18 g daily of arginine,[121] as well as in a small controlled trial with diabetic patients.[122]

**Soy isoflavones.** Soy isoflavones have been suggested to increase arterial vasodilation, improve endothelial function, and decrease blood pressure, possibly by reducing oxidative stress and increasing the availability of nitric oxide.[123] Two analyses of 25 randomized controlled trials confirm the effect of isoflavone intake on reductions in blood pressure. In the first analysis, 14 clinical trials with 789 participants (both with normal blood pressure and pre-hypertension) revealed that a daily ingestion of 25–375 mg of purified soy isoflavones for 2–24 weeks decreased systolic blood pressure by an average of 1.92 mmHg compared with placebo.[124] Decreases in systolic blood pressure were greater in studies of longer duration (3.45 mmHg in studies longer than 3 months).

A second analysis of 11 trials (with a total of 549 participants) looked at isoflavone intake from soy protein, revealing a similar average reduction of systolic (2.5 mmHg) and diastolic (1.5 mmHg) blood pressure when compared to placebo.[125] These trials used a narrower range of isoflavone dosage (65–153mg daily). Within the trials utilized in this analysis, the blood pressure-lowering effects of soy isoflavones were greatest in hypertensive patients and in trials lasting longer than 3 months.

**Olive leaf** (*Olea europaea*). Olive leaf has traditionally been used to treat high blood pressure, atherosclerosis, and diabetes.[126] The leaves contain the active compounds *oleuropein* and *oleacein*, which may function as a vasodilator and ACE inhibitor, respectively.[127]

They also contain ursolic and oleanic acids, two compounds shown to promote normal heart rhythm and lower cardiac output (acting as beta blockers) in rats.[128] Olive leaf extract has also shown calcium channel-blocking activity.[129]

Despite traditional usage, controlled human clinical trials on olive leaf extract have, until recently, been equivocal.[130,131] Two studies using a standardized commercial extract, however, have produced promising results. The first was an open-label, controlled study using 20 pairs of identical twins with borderline hypertension. Supplementation with 1000 mg of olive leaf extract over 8 weeks resulted in a decrease of up to *19/10 mmHg* within pairs. Within pairs of subjects, differences in blood pressure could be observed at a lower dosage of 500 mg.[132] In the second, more recent study, 148 stage-1 hypertensive patients were randomized to captopril (a prescription ACE Inhibitor) or olive leaf, 500 mg twice daily. After 8 weeks, mean reductions from baseline were –11.5 and –13.7 mmHg (systolic) and –4.8 and –6.4 mmHg (diastolic) in the olive leaf and captopril groups, respectively, indicating that olive leaf extract was nearly as effective as the prescription drug for lowering blood pressure. The olive leaf extract group also demonstrated reductions in serum total cholesterol (2.8%) and triglycerides (7.8%), as well as a borderline statistically significant reduction in LDL-cholesterol (2.9%).[133]

## Other Hypotensive Dietary Factors

**Vitamin D.** Vitamin D has several direct and indirect effects on cardiovascular health. It contributes to the maintenance of blood pressure by suppressing the production of renin in the kidneys (lowering angiotensin II production).[134] It can also suppress parathyroid hormone and proinflammatory cytokines, which are both associated with cardiovascular disease. The endothelial cells, which line the insides of blood vessels, have receptors for vitamin D, which suggests a direct effect of vitamin D on vascular metabolism. Several observational studies have revealed an increased risk for hypertension when comparing persons with the lowest and highest vitamin D intake. An analysis of 18 studies revealed a 16% reduction in the risk of hypertension for every 16 ng/mL increase in serum vitamin D.[135] According to data from the National Health and Nutrition Examination Survey (NHANES), nearly 75% of light-skinned, and up to 90% of dark-skinned Americans are vitamin D insufficient.[138]

Interventions using vitamin D have demonstrated modest results for lowering blood pressure. A review of 11 randomized, controlled vitamin D intervention trials (including over 700 subjects) demonstrated a small reduction in systolic (3.6 mmHg) and diastolic (3.1 mmHg) blood pressure at daily doses of 800–2500 IU.[137] Supplemental D2 and D3 exhibited an average systolic blood pressure reduction of 6.2 mmHg, while alfacalcidol (a synthetic, activated analogue of vitamin D3) had no effect. A second review of vitamin D trials, including 2 newer studies, revealed a mean systolic blood pressure reduction of 2.44 mmHg.[138]

Life Extension suggests that all individuals maintain a blood 25-hydroxyvitamin D level of 50–80 ng/mL. Doing so often requires daily supplementation with 5000–8000 IU of vitamin D. Supplemental doses should always be based on an individual's blood test results.

**Vitamin K.** *Atherosclerosis* is a leading cause of disability and death in advanced capitalist societies. Many factors are involved in the initiation and progression of atherosclerosis. Vascular assaults including homocysteine or oxidized LDL can initially damage the inner arterial lining (the endothelium).[139] To repair this damage, the endothelium accumulates *collagen* that forms a cap over the injury site.[140]

These endothelial collagen caps attract calcium that accumulates (calcifies) and forms a hard material resembling bone; this is why atherosclerosis is sometimes referred to as "*hardening of the arteries.*" Ultimately, this process suppresses vascular flexibility and causes narrowing of the passage through which blood must flow, leading to increased blood pressure. Calcification of the coronary arteries markedly increases heart attack risk as well.[141]

Studies reveal that vitamin K plays an indispensable role in the balance of calcium deposition as it relates to both skeletal *and* vascular health. Vitamin K ensures that adequate calcium remains in the bones for strength while keeping calcium out of the arteries to maintain flexibility.[142-144] A substantial volume of research shows that *insufficient* vitamin K2 *accelerates* arterial calcification.[144] Animal models indicate that supplemental vitamin K is able to *reverse* arterial calcification.[145]

**Garlic.** Garlic's promotion of cardiovascular health has been substantiated by several human trials, particularly its hypotensive activity and ability to induce favorable blood lipid profiles. Garlic also reduces systolic and diastolic blood pressure in hypertensive individuals, as well as systolic blood pressure in persons with normal blood pressure. A recent review and analysis of 11 controlled human trials showed a mean systolic decrease of 4.6 mmHg in the garlic group compared to placebo, while the mean decrease in hypertensive subjects was 8.4 mmHg for systolic and 7.3 mmHg for diastolic.[146]

**Fish Oil.** Fish oil is a source of the omega-3 fatty acids eicosapentaenoic acid (EPA) and docosahexaenoic acid (DHA). EPA and DHA are made to a very limited degree in the human body from alpha linolenic acid, but are nonetheless *essential* for several metabolic processes. Aside from reductions in the risk of cardiovascular mortality and nonfatal cardiovascular events,[147] fish oil fatty acids show reductions in blood pressure. In an analysis of 36 clinical trials on the effects of omega-3 supplementation in over 2000 individuals with normal and high blood pressure, a median intake of 3.7 g daily of fish oil demonstrated an average blood pressure reduction of 2.1 mmHg (systolic) and 1.6 mmHg (diastolic).[148] The effects were greater in hypertensive individuals, with average reductions of 4 mmHg (systolic) and 2.73 mmHg (diastolic). Omega-3 fatty acids from fish oil have also demonstrated modest hypotensive activities in diabetic patients. A review and analysis of 5 small randomized controlled trials revealed a mean blood pressure reduction of 1.69/1.79 mmHg.[149]

Sesame lignans (including sesamin and sesamolin) are found in sesame seeds and sesame oil. Several animal studies have reported that sesame lignans suppress the development of hypertension.[150–152] When used as a substitute for other types of cooking oil, sesame oil (about 35 g daily as part of meal preparation) exhibited significant reductions in systolic (20 mmHg) and diastolic (18 mmHg) blood pressure in 40 middle-aged, diabetic, hypertensive patients after a period of 45 days. These changes disappeared after switching back to groundnut or palm oil.[153] A larger study of similar design (356 hypertensive patients on the calcium channel blocker nifedipine) produced similar reductions in systolic and diastolic blood pressure from baseline values. Sesame oil further increased the hypotensive efficacy of nifedipine (reducing blood pressures by an average of almost 15/10 mmHg over the drug alone).[154] A small randomized controlled trial of purified sesamin supplementation (30 mg, 2 times daily for 4 weeks) in 25 middle-aged, prehypertensive subjects decreased systolic blood pressure by 3.5 mmHg and diastolic by 1.9 mmHg.[154]

Sesame lignans may lower blood pressure due to their suppression of the vasoconstrictor 20-hydroxyeicosatetraenoic acid (20-HETE). A 30% reduction in 20-HETE levels has been observed in humans after 5 weeks of sesamin supplementation (39 mg daily).[155] Sesame lignans may also lower blood pressure through antioxidant activity (sparing nitric oxide from oxidation).[156]

**Whey protein peptides.** Whey protein peptides have antioxidant potential and display blood pressure lowering properties.[157–159] They also contribute to blood vessel relaxation and reduced "stiffness."[160] The discovery that antioxidant status directly affects angiotensin availability further explains how whey proteins may fight elevated blood pressure.[161] Human studies of whey-rich or whey-enriched milk products demonstrate convincing reductions in blood pressure compared with placebo- or casein-supplemented patients.[160,162,163]

In recent years, scientists have found that whey proteins exert substantial direct angiotensin-converting enzyme (ACE)-inhibiting effects.[164–166] In the human stomach and intestine, some whey protein breaks down into very specific, short amino acid chains (peptides) that function as efficient ACE inhibitors.[167–169] Laboratory studies consistently show that blood pressure is reduced in hypertensive animals given whey protein derivatives.[170,171] This effect is attributed, in part, to ACE inhibition. The ACE-inhibitory effect is substantially less powerful than those of prescription drugs. However, some people encounter side effects with those drugs.[172] Whey protein derivatives, by contrast, can be used for long periods of time without adverse side effects. Other studies suggest that these active milk components also inhibit the release of other vessel-constricting molecules such as endothelin-1, offering a second pathway for blood pressure control.[173]

## Life Extension Suggestions

High blood pressure is very dangerous, often going unnoticed by its victims until it strikes a devastating blow such as a heart attack or stroke. Therefore, the first step in the management of hypertension is regular self-monitoring with an at-home blood pressure cuff. A multimodal approach, combining dietary changes, increased exercise, nutritional supplements, and pharmaceutical drugs should be utilized to maintain blood pressure as close to *115/75 mmHg* as possible for optimal protection.

Many nutritional ingredients that modulate blood pressure do so in much the same way as some pharmaceutical agents. Therefore, it is important to consult with your physician before embarking on a nutritionally based blood pressure management regimen, especially if you are already taking blood pressure medication(s).

While a number of nutrients have shown varying degrees of blood pressure lowering effects, many aging people will require at least one class of antihypertension prescription medication(s). Lifestyle modification and nutritional supplementation may enable a lower dose of antihypertensive drug(s) or elimination of medication if 24-hour blood pressure readings of 115/75 mmHg are achieved.

## Cardioinhibitory and Cardiotonic Nutrients (Controlling the force at which the heart pumps)
- **Magnesium:** 350–1500 mg daily
- **Hawthorn berries:** 2–3 g daily

## Regulation of Blood Volume (Blood is mostly water, so its volume is dynamic; therefore, interventions that help control water storage can modulate blood pressure as well)
- **Potassium:** 99 mg daily (or more) when instructed to do so by a health-care professional, based on blood test results
- **Calcium:** 1000–1200 mg daily

## Antioxidants (Reducing oxidative stress helps maintain the ability of blood vessels to dilate, a critical step in blood pressure regulation)
- **CoQ10:** 100–300 mg daily (ubiquinol form of coenzyme Q10)
- **Lycopene:** 15–30 mg daily
- **Green coffee**, standardized extract: 400–1200 mg daily
- **Vitamin C:** 1000–2000 mg daily

## Vasodilators (Compounds that enhance the production or activity of nitric oxide and help the blood vessels dilate, allowing for reduction in blood pressure)
- **Grape extract** (containing seed and skin extracts): 150 mg daily

- **Pomegranate extract**, standardized to 30% punicalagins: 400 mg daily
- **L-arginine:** 1600 mg, 3 times daily between meals
- **Soy isoflavones:** 135–270 mg daily
- **Olive leaf extract:** 500–1500 mg daily

## Other Hypotensive Dietary Factors
- **Vitamin D:** 5000–8000 IU daily (depending on blood test results)
- **Vitamin K:** 2100 mcg daily (as 1000 mcg K1, 1000 mcg MK-4, and 100 mcg MK-7)
- **Garlic**, standardized extract: 1500–6000 mg daily
- **Fish oil** (with sesame lignans and olive polyphenols): 2000–4000 mg daily
- **Whey protein peptides:** 1700–3400 mg daily

In addition, the following *blood testing* resources may be helpful:

- Female panel or Male Panel
- Cortisol AM/PM
- Vitamin D, 25-Hydroxy
- RBC Magnesium
- CoQ10 (coenzyme Q10)
- Omega Score®

## REFERENCES

References available at: www.lef.org/dpt5/ch73

# 74

# HIV/AIDS

Quality of life for human immunodeficiency virus/acquired immunodeficiency syndrome (HIV/AIDS) patients has *dramatically* improved in recent years with the advent of sophisticated new therapies, and scientific innovation is unraveling the mysteries of HIV at an expeditious rate. Cutting-edge treatments under investigation at the frontiers of science are redefining the discussion of HIV/AIDS, and "cure" is no longer a four-letter word in the minds of some leading HIV researchers.[1]

Having identified multiple aspects pivotal in controlling HIV infection and developing antiretroviral drugs to target many of them, the scientific community has made tremendous strides in the management of latent HIV. The mortality rate for HIV-positive individuals has declined considerably and continues to do so.[2-4]

Alas, the indispensable antiretroviral drugs themselves cause a number of troubling side effects. Patients treated with long-term antiretroviral therapy usually develop, among other concerns, *lipodystrophy*, *insulin resistance*, and increased *cardiovascular risk*. Unfortunately, these drug-induced conditions diminish patients' quality of life and contribute to an increased rate of cardiovascular events and *diabetes*.[5-8]

Life Extension believes that a major gap in conventional HIV treatment regimens is the failure to aggressively manage patients' cardiometabolic risk by using evidence-based drugs like *metformin*, and scientifically studied natural compounds like *green coffee extract* and omega-3 fatty acids from *fish oil*. Moreover, *hormone restoration therapy* appears to promote healthy fat redistribution and improve body composition in male HIV patients, and is associated with lower risk of death in HIV-positive women.

In this Life Extension protocol, you will learn some basics of the biology of the human immunodeficiency virus and how it destroys the immune system of its host. You will also discover a number of natural compounds that may improve your quality of life by targeting several antiretroviral drug-related side effects, and read about avant-garde medical therapies that aim to improve the outlook for HIV patients even further in the not-so-distant future.

## UNDERSTANDING HIV/AIDS

HIV *causes* AIDS by destroying CD4+ "helper T cells." In healthy individuals, helper T cells organize immune responses that protect the body from infection. When HIV invades the human system, it binds to co-receptors (typically CXCR4 or CCR5) on the surfaces of CD4+ cells and macrophages, and introduces viral genetic material into these cells.

Once HIV has gained entry into the host cell, viral RNA is *reverse transcribed* into viral DNA and combines with the DNA of the host cell—so as the infected cell replicates, so, too, does the virus.[9] Reverse transcription from viral RNA to viral DNA is a target for some antiretroviral drugs. As CD4+ cell levels become depleted with advancing HIV infection, viral replication within macrophages, dendritic cells, and other cell types sustains viral load.

HIV can be categorized based on its interaction with surface co-receptors during attachment and entry into host cells. Three primary entry methods comprise a large percentage of HIV cases—R5, which utilizes the receptor CCR5 to gain entry; X4, which uses the CXCR4 co-receptor; and X4R5, which uses both.[10]

Given the dependency on these cell-surface co-receptors for entry, some strains of HIV are unable to infect individuals who harbor mutations in the gene encoding the co-receptor. These people are resistant to the subtype(s) of HIV that would normally utilize a wild-type receptor to gain entry into host cells.

In addition to attacking the immune system, HIV has the ability to escape immune attack. During cell replication, some HIV viruses mutate at such a rapid rate that they become unrecognizable to the immune system. This enables the virus to keep multiplying and also allows for further mutations. Furthermore, viral DNA that enters the chromosome of the infected cell (where it combines with the cell's own DNA by the action of the HIV-integrase enzyme) may remain in a latent state. As a result, it can remain undetected by the immune system.[9,11] This has presented a tremendous obstacle for achieving complete elimination of the disease.

As HIV continues to survive and replicate within its human host, it eventually weakens the immune system; this leaves the infected individual susceptible to opportunistic infections, including *Pneumocystis pneumonia* (PCP), tuberculosis, herpes simplex virus, and Kaposi's sarcoma.[9,12]

## DISTINGUISHING BETWEEN HIV-1 AND HIV-2

The widely used term "HIV" generally refers to HIV-1, the most prevalent form worldwide. However, two types have been identified: HIV-1 and HIV-2. Both are transmitted via the same routes,[13] both are associated with similar opportunistic infections, and both cause AIDS.[14] However, HIV-2 has a lower viral load,[14-16] is less pathogenic,[15,16] generally progresses more slowly than HIV-1,[16,17] and is mostly confined to West Africa.

The breakdown of the immune system from HIV-2 infection is less dramatic and occurs at a slower rate than it does with HIV-1.[18] Also, neutralization escape—that is, the ability to mutate and dodge an attack from neutralizing antibodies—is less common in HIV-2 infections.[19] Thus, characteristics of HIV-1 including a higher viral load, greater pathogenicity, and the ability to escape neutralization more often, contribute to its widespread prevalence.

Both types of HIV appear to have originated from simian immunodeficiency viruses (SIVs) in chimpanzees (*Pan troglodytes*) and sooty mangabeys (*Cercocebus atys*; SM).[20,21] SIVs are retroviruses that infect primates; certain strains of SIV are thought to have mutated into HIV and subsequently infected humans.[20,22]

## TRANSMISSION

HIV can be transmitted via exposure to contaminated body fluids, such as blood,[23,24] semen,[23,25] or breast milk.[26-29] Potential routes of transmission include blood transfusions,[30] intravenous drug use,[24,31] and unprotected sexual intercourse[32]; HIV-infected females can transmit the virus to their children in utero,[33,34] during delivery,[34] or via breastfeeding.[35]

Anal sex is associated with a much higher risk of HIV transmission than vaginal sex. One factor that may contribute to this is that the rectum contains a thin membrane (the lamina propria) that harbors an abundance of HIV target cells—and only one layer of tissue separates these target cells from the rectal lumen.[36,37]

Although oral sex generally presents a relatively low risk of HIV transmission,[38] the risk of transmitting HIV increases if the mouth or genitals contain cuts or open sores (eg, recent dental work) that could provide an entryway for the virus.[39] Similarly, the risk of transmission during anal or vaginal sex increases in the presence of sexually transmitted diseases, such as herpes or syphilis, that produce ulcers or sores that compromise mucosal integrity, leaving the individual more susceptible to infection.[40,41] Additional risk factors include sexually transmitted infections such as gonorrhea or chlamydia, which produce genital inflammation that can weaken mucosal barriers that would normally help shield the body from infection. Gonorrhea also interferes with CD4 cell activation and proliferation, potentially increasing the opportunity for infection.[42]

Uncircumcised men are at higher risk of contracting HIV than those who are circumcised. This may be because the foreskin possesses numerous Langerhans cells, which contain a protein called *langerin*. Langerin helps protect the body from HIV infection by quickly degrading the virus. However, if a viral onslaught occurs and the cells run out of available langerin, these cells become viral transporters for infection and deliver the virus to lymph nodes. Thus, removing the foreskin diminishes the opportunity for the Langerhans cells to promote viral infection as transporters.[43,44]

## SYMPTOMS/COURSE OF DISEASE

HIV progression comprises the acute, latent, and late/advanced stages. The acute stage comprises the first few weeks after infection, during which time the patient may experience "flu-like" symptoms including headache, nausea, sore throat, or fever[45]; other possible symptoms include swollen lymph nodes, muscle pain, and oral and esophageal sores. As HIV enters and replicates within CD4+ cells in the immune system, the viral load increases sharply, and there is a corresponding dip in the number of CD4+ cells, and an increase in CD8+ cells in the blood. During this stage, the patient is extremely infectious.

This phase usually ends a few weeks later, when the immune system is able to mount an effective response—the viral load decreases, and the number of CD4+ rises again, marking the beginning of the latent stage. At this point, the disease enters a period of clinical dormancy that could last for many years, although it can be much shorter in some patients. During this time, there may be no symptoms, and the carrier may be entirely unaware that he or she is carrying HIV. The virus, however, still continues to progress.

As CD4+ cell count decreases below 350 cells per microliter, patients often develop constitutional symptoms, such as fatigue and night sweats, and become more prone to various infections. When the immune system is no longer able to fight off the infection, the advanced stage begins and is characterized by CD4+ cell counts below 200 cells per microliter, the development of opportunistic infections, and a severely impaired immune system, all of which culminate into AIDS.[45]

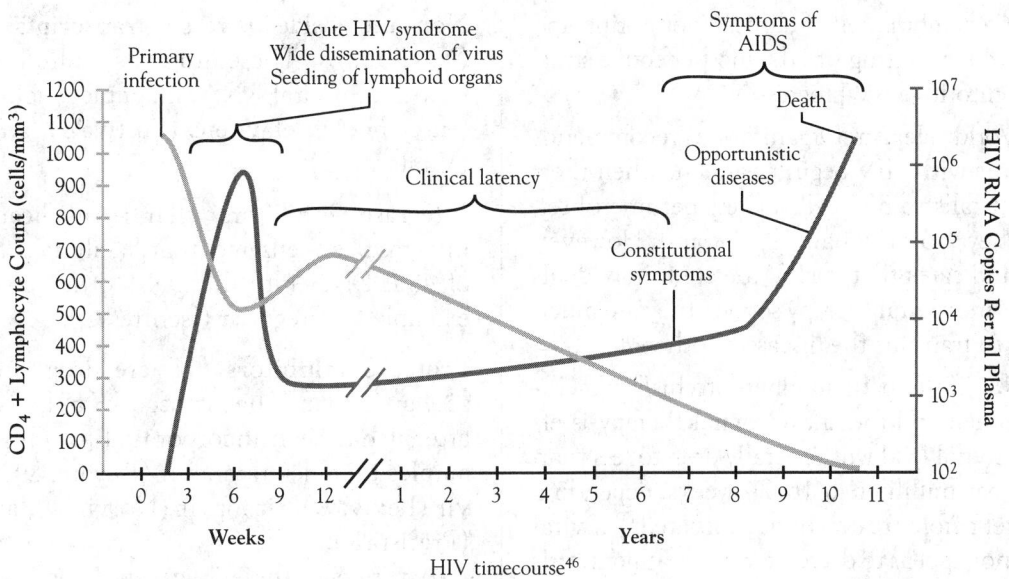

HIV timecourse[46]

## DIAGNOSIS

The diagnosis of HIV typically begins with a test that detects natural antibodies produced against the virus. If the antibody test result is positive, a more sensitive test is performed, such as a Western blot analysis or indirect immunofluorescence assay (a test that uses fluorescent compounds so that HIV antibodies present in the blood glow fluorescent green when placed under ultraviolet light).

The human body generally does not produce HIV antibodies until several weeks after infection, so if antibody tests are administered prior to that point, they may return false-negative results. This is particularly worrisome given that people with HIV appear to be most infectious during the acute stage.[47–49] Consequently, patients with a negative test result are encouraged to be tested again 3 months later, as well as 6 months later. Virologic tests, which detect the actual virus or components thereof, are useful for identifying acute infection in patients who test negative for HIV antibodies.[50]

Current diagnostic options for detecting HIV include the following:

- **Viral load tests.** These tests measure the quantity of HIV in the blood. Examples include the polymerase chain reaction (PCR) test, which can identify HIV by detecting its genetic material.

- **P24 antigen test.** This test detects the p24 antigen, a protein produced by HIV. Detectable levels of p24 are produced during the early stages of HIV infection, making this a useful test in cases where an asymptomatic patient is suspected to have HIV (eg, because of high-risk behaviors) and tests negative for antibodies.[51]

- **Fourth-generation assay.** In 2010, the Food and Drug Administration approved a new "fourth-generation" test called the ARCHITECT HIV Ag/Ab Combo Assay. This test detects both the p24 antigen and HIV antibodies, with the goal of facilitating early diagnosis of the infection. It has demonstrated high diagnostic sensitivity and specificity in detecting HIV.[52–54]

- **Nucleic acid tests.** Nucleic acid tests (NATs) can identify HIV infection approximately 12 days before antibodies become detectable.[55] This allows for earlier detection of the virus, which could prevent the spread of the infection due to early awareness. In a study of more than 3000 people who were tested for HIV, using NAT improved the detection yield by 23% compared with a rapid HIV test.[56]

- **Rapid tests.** Rapid HIV tests present an affordable option that allows for easy sample collection (eg, via oral swab or finger prick) and produces results in just 15 minutes. However, they are associated with a high rate of false-positive results. Consequently, patients who test positive with a rapid test should then be checked via a conventional HIV test to confirm the diagnosis.

Once an HIV infection has been diagnosed, key measures used for evaluation and monitoring are as follows:

- **CD4+ cell count.** This is considered the hallmark of disease progression. In healthy individuals, CD4 count usually range from 500 to more than 1000 cells per microliter; when these levels drop below 200, it is a criterion for AIDS.[57] In addition to being an indicator of disease progression, CD4 count can help assess when to start antiretroviral therapy. A trial found that a combination of clinical monitoring and CD4+ cell count testing was the most effective strategy for monitoring HIV progression.[58]

The World Health Organization recommends that patients with HIV begin treatment when their CD4 count falls to 350 cells or less per microliter, even if they do not have symptoms. However, evidence indicates that if HIV-infected individuals initiate antiretroviral therapy sooner, they are much less likely to transmit the disease to others.[59]

- **Viral load.** If the patient adheres to his/her medication regimen and the antiretroviral therapy is effective, the viral load will generally drop to less than 50 copies per milliliter in 16–24 weeks, depending on the level before treatment was initiated.[60] If viral load does not appear to decrease with treatment, this could be a sign of drug resistance.

- **Drug resistance.** These tests determine whether a strain of HIV is resistant to any anti-HIV medications. During genotypic testing, for example, the genetic structure of the HIV sample is studied for mutations that are recognized as creating HIV resistance to certain drugs. During phenotypic testing, the HIV is exposed to different concentrations of various antiretrovirals to determine resistance.

Patients who test positive for HIV should also undergo screening for other conditions that are associated with HIV, including other sexually transmitted diseases, tuberculosis, and hepatitis B.[61]

## TREATMENT

### Antiretroviral Drugs

Patients today have access to an arsenal of powerful antiretroviral drugs to decrease the viral load.

**Entry inhibitors.** These drugs bind to CCR5 receptors on immune cells, preventing HIV from attaching to them and initiating infection. An example is maraviroc (Selzentry®).

**Fusion inhibitors.** Fusion inhibitors block the gp41 protein on the surface of HIV, which prevents it from fusing with the host cell.[62] An example is enfuvirtide (Fuzeon®).

**Nucleoside/nucleotide reverse transcriptase inhibitors (NRTIs/NtRTIs).** These medications interfere with HIV's ability to be imported into the DNA of healthy immune cells by limiting reverse transcription of viral RNA into viral DNA. Examples include abacavir (Ziagen®), emtricitabine (Emtriva®), lamivudine (Zeffix®), tenofovir (Viread®), and zidovudine (Retrovir®).

**Non-nucleoside reverse transcriptase inhibitors (NNRTIs).** These drugs also inhibit reverse transcription of viral RNA. Examples include etravirine (Intelence®), efavirenz (Sustiva®), and nevirapine (Viramune®).

**Integrase inhibitors.** These medications inhibit integrase, an enzyme that facilitates the insertion of viral DNA into the DNA of infected cells.[63] An example is raltegravir (Isentress®).

**Protease inhibitors.** These drugs inhibit protease, an enzyme that is used to help assemble HIV after it has been incorporated into host DNA. Examples include atazanavir (Reyataz®), fosamprenavir (Lexiva®), ritonavir (Norvir ®), and darunavir (Prezista®).

A variety of these drugs, and others, are often used in combination to manage HIV; this strategy is referred to as highly active antiretroviral therapy, or HAART. Drug regimens are typically chosen based on a number of factors, including patient tolerability, patient genetic background, and physician experience.

## A LANDMARK DISCOVERY

Antiretroviral drugs do not completely eliminate the virus—a patient receiving HAART can still infect others, for example, through needle sharing or sexual intercourse. However, breakthrough findings emerged in 2011 with the HIV Prevention Trials Network (HPTN) 052 clinical trial, which found that if a heterosexual with HIV initiates antiretroviral treatment early (prior to the advanced stages of the disease), this can reduce the likelihood of sexual transmission to uninfected partners by a staggering 96%. These monumental findings suggest that, in addition to treating HIV infection, antiretroviral drugs may also *dramatically* decrease the likelihood of transmission of HIV between heterosexual partners if taken early enough. The study compared "early" participants who began antiretroviral treatment immediately at the beginning of the study, versus those who initiated treatment when their CD4+ counts fell to 250 cells/mm$^3$ or less, or when they experienced an AIDS-associated illness.[59] As the authors carry out further research, these findings represent a groundbreaking discovery in HIV management.

Challenges of antiretroviral treatment include the following:

- **Drug resistance.** Combining protease inhibitors and reverse transcriptase inhibitors into drug "cocktails" has been extremely effective at decreasing viral load in patients with HIV.[64] As noted earlier, however, HIV can mutate at a rapid rate during cell replication; this can give rise to resistant strains of the virus that do not respond to treatment. Patients can mitigate this risk by adhering to their medication schedules, as nonadherence encourages the development of resistant strains of HIV. Inadequate drug treatment (ie, consisting of just one or two drugs, versus a broader combination) can also promote resistance.[65-67] Drug resistance tests, which establish whether an HIV strain is resistant to certain medications, can provide guidance for selecting optimal drug combinations for each patient and could be useful for revising combination therapies in cases where treatments begin to fail.

- **Toxicity/side effects.** A significant concern with antiretroviral drugs is their high toxicity and negative side effects, which range from nausea and diarrhea to more serious complications, including liver abnormalities and insulin resistance.[68] In many cases, a patient may not be able to tolerate one or more drugs. Moreover, these medications have been found to increase oxidative stress, overwhelming the body's antioxidant supplies. Until less toxic therapies are developed, patients can support their health by optimizing other, more controllable areas of the overall treatment package, such as engaging in moderate physical activity and maintaining optimal nutrition.

**Note:** *Some preliminary human data indicates that milk thistle extract may support liver health in HIV/ HCV co-infected patients.[69] Additionally, a write-up of a single case involving a man with HIV/HCV co-infection reports eradication of both infections after 2 weeks of intravenous infusions of silymarin, a group of active constituents from milk thistle.[70] More study is needed before firm conclusions can be drawn.*

- **Insulin resistance and other cardiometabolic abnormalities.** Long-term antiretroviral drug therapy has been associated with a number of metabolic side effects, including insulin resistance and diabetes.[5-7] Impaired glucose metabolism in antiretroviral-treated HIV patients, in turn, contributes to an increased risk of cardiovascular disease and other major comorbidities. In order to maintain the best quality of life, HIV patients must strive to keep these metabolic risks in check by controlling their glucose levels.

Life Extension recommends the antidiabetic drug *metformin* to maintain optimal glucose metabolism during healthy aging, as well as in various disease states.[71] Several studies suggest that metformin effectively combats HAART-associated cardiometabolic risk as well.

In a year-long trial involving 50 HIV-infected patients who had been treated with antiretroviral drugs

for an average of 6 years and had developed metabolic syndrome, metformin treatment significantly slowed the rate of coronary artery calcification compared to lifestyle modification.[72] Moreover, metformin alone significantly improved insulin sensitivity, and when combined with lifestyle modification, boosted levels of HDL ("good") cholesterol.

In addition to improving insulin sensitivity, metformin also appears to promote healthy fat distribution, which is typically deregulated in HAART-treated HIV patients. A small, 6-month trial in nondiabetic HIV-positive patients revealed that metformin therapy reduced abdominal fat accumulation, lowered blood pressure, and raised HDL cholesterol, supporting the cardioprotective role of the drug in this population.[73]

Studies show that though some other diabetic drugs may control insulin sensitivity in HIV patients, they do not reduce overall cardiovascular risk as effectively as metformin. In one investigation involving 37 patients, rosiglitazone tempered insulin resistance similarly to metformin, but only metformin suppressed postprandial lipemia, an independent cardiovascular risk factor.[74]

A small study published in *the Journal of the American Medical Association* found that metformin was safe and well-tolerated in HIV patients at a dose of 500 mg twice daily.[75] This trial further showed that metformin reduced visceral abdominal fat, which poses greater cardiometabolic risk than subcutaneous abdominal fat, without affecting liver function and causing only mild gastrointestinal discomfort in some patients.

*Green coffee* extract has emerged as a powerful glucose control agent as well. Unroasted coffee beans, once purified and standardized, produce high levels of *chlorogenic acid* and other beneficial polyphenols that can suppress excess blood glucose levels. Human clinical trials support the role of *chlorogenic acid*–rich green coffee bean extract promoting healthy blood sugar control and reducing disease risk.

Scientists have discovered that *chlorogenic acid* found abundantly in *green coffee bean extract* inhibits the enzyme *glucose-6-phosphatase* that triggers new glucose formation and glucose release by the liver.[76,77] Glucose-6-phosphatase is involved in dangerous postprandial (after-meal) spikes in blood sugar.

In another significant mechanism, *chlorogenic acid* increases the signal protein for insulin receptors in liver cells.[78] That has the effect of increasing *insulin sensitivity*, which in turn drives down blood sugar levels.

In a clinical trial, 56 healthy volunteers were given an oral glucose tolerance test before and after a supplemental dose of green coffee extract. The oral glucose tolerance test is a standardized way of measuring a person's after-meal blood sugar response. In subjects not taking green coffee bean extract, the oral glucose tolerance test showed the expected rise of blood sugar to an average of 144 mg/dL after a 30-minute period. But in subjects who had taken 200 mg of the green coffee bean extract, that sugar spike was significantly reduced to *124 mg/dL—a 14% decrease*.[79] When a higher dose (400 mg) of green coffee bean extract was supplemented, there was an even *greater* average reduction in blood sugar—up to nearly 28% at 1 hour.

> **Note:** *Metformin and green coffee extract may not be appropriate for patients who are experiencing malabsorption. Patients with malabsorption should consult a qualified health care provider before using metformin or green coffee extract.*

## Cytokine Therapy

Cytokines are cell-signaling proteins used by the immune system to orchestrate immunologic activity. By secreting cytokines, cells of the immune system are able to modify the number and/or activity of other immune cells throughout the body. Cytokines are needed to mediate responses to infection and injury, and to ensure hemostatic immune balance during healthy conditions. During HIV infection, however, cytokine signaling becomes irregular.[80,81]

CD8+ cytotoxic T cells are necessary to destroy HIV-infected cells, while CD4+ T-helper cells are necessary to organize defense against pathogens. In late-stage HIV, CD8+ cells become dysfunctional and CD4+ cell numbers decline dramatically, allowing HIV to replicate rampantly and impairing the body's ability to respond to infections. Thus, upon progression to AIDS, most patients succumb to opportunistic infections. Research suggests that suboptimal production and signaling of γ-chain cytokines (IL-2, -4, -7, -9, -15, and -21) contributes significantly to immunological failure in HIV-infected patients.[81]

Armed with this knowledge, scientists have begun developing cutting-edge therapies that capitalize on the ability of exogenous recombinant cytokines to reinvigorate immune function lost to HIV infection. Currently, clinical trials with IL-2 and -7 have shown promising results,[82–84] and preliminary data with IL-15 and -21 is encouraging.[85–87] A growing body of evidence indicates that cytokines, especially in combination, may become an important tool in augmenting CD4+ cell populations and CD+8 function in HAART-treated HIV patients.

Moving forward, researchers hope to begin assessing efficacy of various combinations of recombinant γ-chain cytokines in HIV patients. Clinical trials are underway; any HIV patient interested in participating in a trial should speak with their health care provider(s) and visit www.clinicaltrials.gov to identify trials that they may be eligible for.

## Hormones: Striking the Right Balance

Hormones appear to have a profound impact on conditions associated with HIV.

**Growth hormones.** Body fat distribution disorders, including lipoatrophy (fat loss in select areas) and lipohypertrophy (fat accumulation in select areas), are common among people with HIV/AIDS.[88,89] Lipoatrophy usually occurs in the patient's buttocks, limbs, and face, whereas lipohypertrophy is characterized by visceral fat accumulations, or fat accumulations in the abdomen, mid-upper neck, mammary area, and/or above the pubic region.[88] These physical changes can have a negative impact on self-perception and quality of life. Moreover, antiretroviral drug therapy is associated with the development of these conditions, a factor that could dissuade patients from taking their medications.[88–90] Prolonged exposure to thymidine analogs, for example, particularly stavudine (d4T), is considered a risk factor for developing lipohypertrophy and lipoatrophy.[88]

This disturbance in fat metabolism, commonly referred to as "lipodystrophy syndrome," is associated with various metabolic changes, including insulin resistance and dyslipidemia (excessive amounts of fat in the blood).[88] Mounting evidence suggests that growth hormone plays a role in the pathogeneses of these phenomena,[89–92] and numerous study findings have indicated that using hormone replacement therapy may help to combat these metabolic challenges.

In HIV-infected individuals with accumulations of abdominal fat, an independent association was found between lowered secretions of growth hormone and higher levels of fasting glucose and triglycerides. This suggests that enhancing the amount of growth hormone may be beneficial for such patients.[93] Additional support for this hypothesis came from a study by Benedini and colleagues, who found that people with HIV who had syndromes of fat accumulation benefited from significant reductions in body fat, as well as increased lean tissue, following growth hormone treatment.[94] A review of several randomized controlled trials revealed that the use of growth hormone–axis drugs successfully decreases visceral fat tissue mass and increases lean body mass in people who have HIV-associated lipodystrophy.[95] A review by Leung and Glesby found that analogs of the growth hormone/growth hormone–releasing hormone axis seemed particularly effective at decreasing visceral fat tissue in patients with HIV.[96]

**Testosterone.**   Testosterone has many important functions in the body, including its roles in fat distribution and muscle mass.[97–99] However, low testosterone levels are common in patients with HIV.[100–102]

Low testosterone levels are associated with the loss of lean body mass, lost muscle mass, and an increased incidence of wasting.[101,103] In many studies, patients with HIV who received testosterone treatment found that it helped stop the loss of lean body and muscle mass.[101] A study of HIV-infected male patients using HAART indicated that sex hormones participate in fat distribution changes, as well as insulin sensitivity, among male patients with HIV-lipodystrophy.[104]

The beneficial effects of testosterone treatment in HIV-infected patients have been reported in a number of studies. A systematic review and meta-analysis by Kong and Edmonds found that testosterone therapy increased lean body mass more than placebo, and that a greater increase occurred when the testosterone was administered intramuscularly.[105] In a review of anabolic steroids for the treatment of weight loss in people with HIV, Johns and associates found a potential relationship between the use of anabolic steroids and small increases in lean body mass and body weight. However, the authors did not formally recommend testosterone treatment due to study limitations, as well as the lack of knowledge regarding potential benefits and adverse effects of long-term anabolic steroid use, target populations for the therapy, and the best regimen.[106] In HIV-infected men with abdominal obesity and low testosterone, taking 10 g of testosterone each day for 24 weeks corresponded with a greater reduction in total, whole body, and abdominal fat mass, as well as a more substantial increase in lean mass, compared with participants who took a placebo.[107]

**DHEA.**   Dehydroepiandrosterone (DHEA) is an adrenal steroid hormone that exerts influence within a variety of biological systems either directly, or via its metabolites, which include androgens and estrogens. With respect to the immune system, studies have shown that the number of CD4+ cells correlates positively with serum DHEA levels, and negatively with cortisol levels in HIV patients.[108] Other data indicate that antiretroviral drug therapy may cause a drop in serum DHEA levels.[109] In a study that followed 34 HIV-positive men for nearly 3 years, lower DHEA and higher cortisol levels were associated with increasing lipodystrophy severity.[110]

In clinical trials, DHEA treatment has enhanced overall quality of life,[111] improved the steroid hormone profile,[111] and eased depressive symptoms[113] in HIV patients. The effects of DHEA administration on CD4+ and CD8+ levels in humans remain unclear, but DHEA treatment does not appear to result in negative outcomes in HIV trials.

Men and women who would like more information about maintaining healthy hormone levels should review Life Extension's Male Hormone Restoration and Female Hormone Restoration protocols.

**Female hormone restoration.**   In a review of patient data from 84 cases of HIV in women older than 40, use of hormone replacement therapy was associated with a strong reduction in risk of death.[114] In fact, the risk reduction for hormone replacement therapy was as strong as that associated with antiretroviral drug use in this trial.

## DEVELOPING A CURE

The medical community has not yet found a cure for HIV/AIDS, but a striking case from Berlin may provide valuable insights into potential treatment strategies. Due to a genetic mutation (known as CCR5-delta32), some people do not express chemokine receptor 5 (CCR5), a co-receptor for HIV, on their CD4+ cells. These individuals are naturally resistant to R5 HIV infection. In the Berlin case, a patient with leukemia and HIV received a stem cell transplant from an individual with this mutation.[115] Since the stem cell treatment, which occurred several years ago, doctors have not found any evidence of HIV. This finding has prompted further study in an attempt to replicate these results and ultimately develop a cure.

In 2011, Sangamo BioSciences announced a cell-based method for reducing HIV viral load, harnessing the potential therapeutic power of the CCR5 mutation. The process involves the temporary cessation of antiretroviral treatment, the removal of T cells containing the CD4 receptor, and the exposure of these cells to an enzyme to knockout the gene for the CCR5 co-receptor. Following this treatment, the cells are reintroduced into the patient, where they appear to function normally. In preliminary experiments, this method has been found to boost CD4 cell counts in people with HIV and may also be useful for controlling viral load. One HIV-infected patient in these experiments was able to maintain a controlled viral load even without HAART.[116]

Numerous other investigations have been carried out to devise a cure, including attempts to produce an HIV vaccine. Kang and colleagues developed the

SAV001 vaccine, which is now undergoing clinical trials. The SAV001 vaccine is made by genetically modifying the virus so that it is no longer pathogenic. From there, the virus undergoes further deactivation via radiation and chemical treatments. Testing this vaccine in clinical trials will take a few years, but if it proves successful, it will represent one of the greatest developments in the history of HIV/AIDS research.

## DIETARY AND LIFESTYLE CONSIDERATIONS

Optimal nutrition is important for maintaining a healthy immune system and preserving overall general health. However, several factors make this a challenge for people with HIV. Weight loss and malnutrition are common due to complications such as anorexia, changes in metabolism, malabsorption, and chronic diarrhea.[117] HIV-related factors such as depression, loss of appetite, impaired taste or smell, or stomach upset (from treatment or from co-infections) may prevent affected individuals from eating enough.[117,118] Even people with HIV who consume adequate diets may experience chronic diarrhea and/or vomiting from drug treatments or opportunistic infections, leading to nutrient loss.[117] Combined, these factors can lead to nutrient deficiency, which can impair immune function and lower the body's resistance to infection.[118,119] New infections, in turn, can further impair nutritional status, creating a vicious cycle that promotes the progression of the disease.[118] Moreover, some individuals with HIV may have increased nutrient requirements for other reasons, including pregnancy, or because they are infants or growing children. These issues underscore the importance of ensuring adequate intake of vitamins and other nutrients to maintain health.

Other steps toward optimal health include maintaining a healthy lifestyle—avoiding the use of illicit drugs, alcohol, and tobacco, as well as engaging in moderate physical activity. In moderation, being active has been found to support immune function, reduce the potential for metabolic abnormalities, and decrease the risk of acute infection. It can also boost muscle mass, which may be useful for countering HIV-related lipodystrophy.[118] Regular physical activity is associated with decreased levels of skeletal muscle inflammatory proteins, as well as reductions in several other important markers of inflammation. These markers bear strong correlations with adverse conditions such as cardiovascular and metabolic diseases (eg, insulin resistance), underscoring the value of moderate physical activity. Moderate activity can

also eliminate obesity. This presents additional health-related benefits, particularly since obesity is associated with impaired immune function, along with a host of other health problems.[120] Prolonged (>1.5 hours), high-intensity exercise is not recommended for people with HIV, as it may have an immune-suppressing effect.[121]

## TARGETED NATURAL INTERVENTIONS

Given the deteriorating effects of HIV/AIDS progression on the immune system and nutrient status, it is not surprising that nutritional supplements have been shown to be extremely beneficial in patients with HIV. Taking vitamin supplements lowered the risk of HIV disease progression in several studies.[122–126] The use of vitamin supplements has also been associated with improved pregnancy outcomes in HIV-infected pregnant women,[122,127] increased appetite in HIV-infected children,[128] and better health and survival of children with HIV.[129–131]

In addition, nutritional supplements have been found to improve comorbidities associated with HIV. In HIV-infected patients being treated for tuberculosis (TB), for example, the consumption of micronutrients (vitamins A, B complex, C, and E, plus selenium) corresponded with a lower risk of TB recurrence and a significantly lower incidence of peripheral neuropathy (a side effect of TB treatment); this treatment also raised CD4+ and CD3+ counts.[132] In a study of children with HIV, a daily supplement of vitamins A, B complex, C, D, E, and folic acid, plus zinc, iron, and copper (at levels based on recommended daily allowances) corresponded with faster recovery from diarrheal episodes and pneumonia.[133]

### Antioxidants

Antioxidants are widely known for their health benefits and may be particularly important for people with HIV. In 1985, the Life Extension Foundation® was among the first organizations to propose that patients with HIV/AIDS would benefit from taking high doses of antioxidants. Since then, many scientific studies have examined a wide range of nutrients and supplements for use in HIV/AIDS.

Under normal circumstances, metabolic processes in the body generate free radicals. At low/moderate concentrations, these reactive oxygen species are not harmful, but instead have a variety of beneficial functions. At high concentrations, however, they become extremely destructive. Normally, the human body keeps these levels in check by neutralizing free radicals with its own natural antioxidant defense system. However, some conditions can boost the production of free radicals and create oxidative stress—a condition in which the body's antioxidant defenses are unable to neutralize the overwhelming quantity of free radicals being produced. This can lead to cellular damage and the development of disease.[134]

HIV is associated with substantial oxidative stress,[135–142] and reactive oxygen species participate in the progression of HIV to AIDS.[139] As HIV progresses, antioxidant levels decline.[143,144] Compounding this problem further is the fact that various HIV treatments have been shown to increase oxidative stress.[141,145–147] Combined, these factors create an unhealthy environment that could be further exacerbated by the inadequate intake or poor absorption of nutrients commonly associated with HIV.[148,149] Antioxidant micronutrient deficiencies are common among people with HIV.[150] Reduced serum levels of vitamins E (a powerful antioxidant) have been associated with a higher risk of developing AIDS.[151]

Antioxidant supplements have been found to counteract some of the damaging effects associated with HIV. Taking supplemental vitamin E (800 IU per day) and vitamin C (1000 mg daily) for 3 months lowered oxidative stress among patients with HIV and produced a trend toward a decrease in viral load.[150] High serum levels of vitamin E have been linked with a slower progression of HIV.[151] In a large study in Tanzania involving 1075 pregnant women with HIV, taking a daily multivitamin combination consisting of vitamins C (500 mg), E (30 mg), and various B vitamins and folic acid improved CD4, CD3, and CD8 cell counts and lowered the risk of fetal death, low birth weight, preterm birth, and small size for gestational age.[127]

Other antioxidants have also shown beneficial effects in people with HIV. A study involving 331 AIDS patients found that when patients received supplements including various carotenoids (natural pigments with antioxidant properties) as well as multivitamins and minerals, mortality rates were lower and CD4 T-cell counts were higher compared with patients who received the same supplementation without the carotenoids.[152] In HIV-infected patients following a stable HAART regimen, the use of broad-spectrum, high-dose micronutrient supplementation with antioxidants corresponded with a 24% increase in CD4 cell count.[153] Other important antioxidants that have been highlighted in the HIV literature include:

**Glutathione.** Glutathione, because it appears to interfere with HIV's entry into its target cells, is thought to be an extremely important antioxidant.[154] Glutathione deficiency—a common finding in HIV[155]—is associated with compromised T-cell function and decreased

survival.[156] Some nutrients that offer a host of health benefits also assist in the production of glutathione. One of these is N-acetylcysteine.

**N-acetylcysteine.** N-acetylcysteine (NAC) is of particular interest for people with HIV/AIDS because it reinstates glutathione levels and has been found to maintain glutathione concentrations,[123,157] improve T-cell counts, and reduce viral load in patients with advanced AIDS.[157–159] In many studies, the use of NAC oral supplements has correlated with better quality of life and patient well-being.[160] A study involving 81 HIV-infected patients showed that 8 weeks of oral NAC supplementation correlated with significant improvements in whole blood glutathione concentrations as well as increased T-cell glutathione levels.[161] NAC is known for exerting antioxidant effects against the activity of glycoprotein 120 (gp120), an HIV protein that induces oxidative stress during the infection of macrophages (a type of white blood cell).[162]

**Green tea.** Green tea leaves contain compounds called catechins, which have powerful antioxidant properties. The most abundant catechin in green tea, epigallocatechin gallate (EGCG), has also been found to suppress HIV.[163] Kawai and colleagues found that EGCG can bind to T cells and block the virus from attaching to them.[164] When HIV comes into contact with a helper T cell in the human body, glycoprotein 120 (gp120) on its surface binds to a CD4 receptor on the surface of the T cell, ultimately leading to infection.[165] In several studies, EGCG blocked the attachment of gp120 to CD4 cells with varying degrees of inhibition.[164,166] EGCG also appears to lower the risk of HIV transmission—normally, fibrils in human sperm collect HIV viruses and deliver them to target cells. EGCG inhibits this activity and degrades the fibrils, thereby lowering transmission risk.[167] EGCG has also been found to inhibit a variety of HIV subtypes at physiologic concentrations without damaging human cells.[165] When coupled with other nutrients (vitamin C or lysine), green tea extract inhibited the production of HIV in chronically infected T cells; in latently infected cells, combining the green tea extract with vitamin C and amino acids resulted in significantly greater suppressive action than when any of the three were applied individually.[168]

**Lipoic acid.** This powerful antioxidant plays a central role in the defense against free radicals.[169] It also recycles other important antioxidants, including glutathione,[169] and decreases intracellular signaling that promotes inflammation.[170] Taking a 300-mg supplement of alpha lipoic acid 3 times per day for 6 months significantly elevated blood glutathione levels in a group of HIV-infected men and women aged 44–47 years.[171] In the lab, alpha lipoic acid has been shown to inhibit HIV replication.[172] Its ability to scavenge reactive oxygen species has been found to block nuclear factor-kappa B, a transcriptional activator that is instrumental in the regulation of HIV gene expression.[173] In a study by Merin and associates, applying alpha-lipoic acid to cells infected with HIV completely stopped "initiation of HIV-1 induction by [tumor necrosis factor-alpha]."[174]

**Carnitine (acetyl-L-carnitine).** The antioxidant acetyl-L-carnitine (ALC) boosts immune function and helps the body convert fat into energy. A number of studies have reported positive effects of ALC supplementation in people with HIV, especially its positive impact on the side effects of certain antiretroviral drugs. People with HIV who use the NRTIs zalcitabine, didanosine, or stavudine often experience peripheral neuropathy (peripheral nerve damage) and myopathy (muscle tissue disease).[175] These outcomes have been observed in other NRTIs as well and can discourage patients from adhering to their medication regimens.[175] However, ALC may help to mitigate these effects.

ALC is known to be involved with peripheral nerve regeneration.[176] In a small study by Osio and associates (n = 20), taking 2000 mg of oral ALC each day for a month led to significant reductions in pain intensity scores among HIV-infected patients taking antiretroviral therapy.[177] A larger study involving 90 HIV-positive patients with antiretroviral toxic neuropathy found that taking 500 mg of ALC intramuscularly twice per day for 14 days resulted in statistically significant improvements in weekly mean pain ratings versus placebo. When these patients subsequently took 1000 mg of oral ALC twice per day for 6 weeks, symptomatic improvements were observed.[178] In a cohort study involving 21 HIV patients with NRTI-related neuropathy who were reviewed after receiving acetyl-L-carnitine for a mean of 4.3 years, 13 of the 16 patients who completed the study reported "very much or moderate" symptomatic improvement, and 9 were pain-free.[179] Hart and associates observed that when HIV-infected patients with antiretroviral toxic neuropathy took ALC treatment, 76% of patients experienced reductions in neuropathic pain.[176] In a small study involving 21 participants, receiving 3000 mg of ALC daily for 24 weeks corresponded with improvements in subjective pain ratings.[180] A very small review and meta-analysis of 14 studies that described various analgesics did not find a significant benefit of taking

1 g of ALC daily in treating HIV-associated sensory neuropathy; the authors pointed out that this review was limited by the small number of eligible studies as well as the differences in study designs and size, which made comparisons across studies difficult.[181]

## Vitamins

Certain vitamins have amassed a notable amount of clinical evidence to highlight their potential supplemental value in people with HIV.

**Vitamin D.** Vitamin D has a multitude of important functions within the human body, including its roles in supporting proper immune function, regulating bone metabolism, and maintaining calcium and phosphorus homeostasis.[182,183] In people with HIV, vitamin D deficiency is common, as is lower-than-normal bone mineral density.[4,184–191] Additionally, people with HIV appear to be at an increased risk of osteopenia and osteoporosis.[184,190,192] In a review of the medical literature, McComsey and colleagues concluded that HIV infection should be regarded as a risk factor for bone disease.[193]

Deficient levels of vitamin D in HIV-infected individuals may be due to the virus itself[185,190] as well as the effects of antiretroviral treatment.[184,185,189,190,194–197] Tenofovir, for example, is a widely used NRTI that is associated with low bone mineral density[198–201] as well as increased levels of parathyroid hormone (PTH).[202] (Increased PTH levels are associated with decreased bone mineral density.[202]) Non-nucleoside reverse transcriptase inhibitors (NNRTI) have also been implicated in vitamin D deficiency; one in particular—efavirenz—has been linked to low concentrations of 25-hydroxyvitamin D (the form of vitamin D measured to determine vitamin D status in the human body).[187,189,203]

As people with HIV continue to live longer, bone loss prevention becomes an even more prominent consideration in this aging population.[192] Some studies have shown a correlation between vitamin D status and CD4 counts,[186,203–206] while others did not find this relationship.[187,207] Interestingly, some studies that detected vitamin D deficiencies in HIV patients found that *uninfected* individuals also had low levels of vitamin D.[186,187] In the United States, vitamin D deficiency is highly prevalent in the general population, regardless of HIV status.[187]

**Beta-carotene/vitamin A.** Beta-carotene, a plant pigment found in colorful fruits and vegetables, is converted into vitamin A in the body. It plays important roles in human growth, vision, and its support of the immune system. In people with

HIV who were given 100 000 IU of vitamin A from beta-carotene daily for 4 weeks, white blood cell counts rose 66% and T-helper cells rose slightly. Six weeks after cessation of the beta-carotene treatment, the immune-cell measurements returned to pretreatment levels.[208] In a Uganda study involving 181 children with HIV, vitamin A supplementation was associated with significantly lower mortality rates as well as improvements in chronic diarrhea and persistent cough.[129] In another study, 687 children in Tanzania with pneumonia received 400 000 IU of vitamin A at baseline, as well as 4 months after discharge, and then 8 months after discharge. None of the children showed any signs of vitamin A deficiency when they started treatment. Vitamin A supplementation was associated with a 49% drop in mortality and a 92% decrease in diarrhea-related deaths. Plus, AIDS-related deaths plummeted 68%.[130] In a population in South Africa that is not generally vitamin A deficient, children with HIV-infected mothers received 50 000 IU of vitamin A at ages 1 month and 3 months, 100 000 IU at 6 months and 9 months, and then 200 000 IU at 12 months and 15 months; this resulted in a significant reduction in morbidity from diarrheal disease.[131] In a U.S. study involving HIV-infected children, the use of vitamin A supplementation prior to influenza vaccination muted the increase of HIV viral load postimmunization.[209]

Kennedy-Oji and associates observed improved weight retention among South African HIV-infected women with vitamin A supplementation.[210] Conversely, vitamin A deficiency in HIV-positive women has been associated with increased mother-to-child transmission of the infection.[211] However, the potential value of vitamin A supplements in pregnant women with HIV remains questionable, particularly as some studies have indicated that vitamin A supplementation may increase the HIV load in breast milk,[212] and may potentially elevate the risk of HIV transmission from mother to child.[213] A review of studies encompassing 6517 women with HIV in South Africa, Zimbabwe, Malawi, and Tanzania found that vitamin A supplement use among HIV-infected pregnant women correlated with improved birth weights; although the review found no evidence that vitamin A supplements increase the risk of mother-to-child transmission of HIV, the authors pointed out the moderate quality of scientific evidence in these studies.

**B vitamins.** B vitamins are responsible for an array of important functions within the body, including proper functioning of the brain and immune system.[214,215] A number of reports have documented the beneficial effects of B vitamin supplementation in people with HIV. In a study involving 281 HIV-infected patients, taking vitamin B6 (>2 times the RDA), vitamin B1 (>5 times the RDA), or vitamin B2 (>5 times the RDA) was independently associated with improved survival.[216] In 108 HIV-infected men tracked over an 18-month period, low B12 levels at the beginning of the study were significant predictors of faster disease progression (as determined by CD4 cell count); although the development of B12 deficiency corresponded with a drop in CD4 cell count, the normalization of vitamin B12 levels corresponded with higher CD4 cell counts.[217]

### Additional Support

Compelling evidence has also been accumulating for the following:

**Omega-3 fatty acids.** Omega-3 fatty acids are essential oils—they are not made in the body and must be consumed from external sources. Their anti-inflammatory and immune-modulating capabilities make them a valuable component of general health[218]; additionally, they appear to have therapeutic value for people with HIV who suffer from high triglyceride levels. A number of published medical reports have described changes in lipid metabolism, increased levels of serum triglycerides, and low levels of HDL cholesterol in people with HIV; moreover, combination antiretroviral treatment is reported to be a risk factor.[219–222] A combination of dieting and omega-3 supplements (6 g/day) was found to cause a major drop in serum triglycerides and levels of arachidonic acid.[223] A small systematic review found that varying doses of omega-3 fatty acids caused significant reductions in triglyceride concentrations in people with HIV who were taking antiretroviral therapy.[224] A study involving 48 HIV-infected patients (47 males, 1 female) with HAART-associated hypertriglyceridemia found that a 12-week course of omega-3 fatty acids (4 g/day) led to significant reductions in triglyceride levels compared with placebo.[224] Wohl and associates found that omega-3 fatty acids (in the form of fish oil supplements) plus dietary and exercise counseling lowered fasting triglyceride levels in HIV-infected patients with hypertriglyceridemia taking antiretroviral medication; however, the difference was not significant compared with participants who received counseling without the fish oil supplements.[226] In other studies of HIV-infected patients with elevated triglyceride levels who were using antiretroviral therapy, omega-3 supplementation was associated with significant decreases in triglycerides.[227–229]

**Whey protein.** Whey protein contains all essential and nonessential amino acids, which are important for maintaining an adequate immune system response. Whey is also an important supplement to help boost the body's synthesis of glutathione, and various therapeutic benefits, including its immune-enhancing properties, make it of great interest to people with HIV.[230] In a study involving 41 HIV-infected patients, those who received 40 g of whey protein each day benefitted from a CD4 count increase of 31 cells per microliter, versus the control group, which showed a decline of 5 cells per microliter over the same 12-week period.[231] Whey protein has been found to improve immune function, elevate cellular glutathione levels, and maintain muscle mass.[230,232] Although large randomized controlled trials will impart greater insights into the potential benefits of whey protein in patients with HIV, the results so far are encouraging.[232]

**Lactoferrin.** Lactoferrin is derived from whey protein. It has been found to inhibit viruses by binding to viral receptor sites, thus preventing the virus from infecting healthy cells.[234] In vitro studies show that lactoferrin is an effective inhibitor of HIV entry.[235–237] It may also effectively inhibit initial HIV infection by blocking uptake into epithelial cells and transfer from dendritic cells to CD4+ cells.[238]

One study that compared 22 asymptomatic and 45 symptomatic patients with HIV to 30 healthy control subjects found that plasma lactoferrin levels were decreased in patients infected with HIV.[239] In a 6-month trial involving 22 HIV-1-infected children, oral lactoferrin caused a small decrease in viral load and an increase in CD4+ cell numbers; lactoferrin plus antiretroviral therapy was more effective than lactoferrin alone.[240]

**Coenzyme Q10 (CoQ10).** CoQ10 is present in all cells of the human body and is essential for proper cell function. Low levels of CoQ10 have been detected in people with HIV, and one study found that the level of CoQ10 deficiency corresponds with the stage of HIV infection.[241] CoQ10 supplementation increases a number of immune parameters, including T-cell counts,[242,243] an important consideration in HIV. A known antioxidant, it has also been found to contribute to the improvement of antioxidant defenses in HIV-infected men when administered as part of a regimen consisting of various antioxidants.[244] In a case study involving a 52-year-old man with HIV, the patient suffered from drug-related skeletal myopathy caused by zidovudine. Daily supplementation of CoQ10 led to recovery, allowing the patient to continue his HIV drug treatment.[245] Cherry and associates

tested a water-soluble formulation of CoQ10 on cultured rat cells and found that it was effective in preventing neurotoxicity caused by d4T (stavudine; the HIV medication most commonly associated with neuropathy).[246] Although studies on the effects of CoQ10 in HIV are limited, findings so far highlight this as a promising area for further study.

**Selenium.** Selenium is required for proper immune system function[247] and facilitates a multitude of antioxidant activities in the body.[248,249] It also decreases the effect of inflammatory cytokines, which may reduce the risk of developing neurological damage, Kaposi's sarcoma (a common HIV-associated cancer), and wasting syndrome.[250] In people with HIV, selenium deficiency has corresponded with disease progression to AIDS or death.[247,250,251] Shor-Posner and colleagues found that among HIV-infected drug users, low selenium was a significant risk factor for developing mycobacterial disease.[252] The HIV-inhibiting effects of selenium have also been observed in human cell cultures.[253,254] In human studies, selenium supplementation has been found to reduce the incidence of diarrhea and decrease the number of patient hospitalizations.[255,256]

**Zinc and magnesium.** On average, patients with HIV/AIDS who have low zinc levels have a higher viral load and lower T-cell counts.[257,258] A U.S. study of 231 HIV-infected adults found that taking zinc supplements every day for 18 months reduced the rate of diarrhea by more than 50% compared with placebo and lowered the risk of immunological failure by 400% (CD4 T-cell counts of <200 cells per microliter). However, it did not affect viral load, nor did it have an impact on mortality.[259,260] In a literature review of six human studies involving 1009 participants, the use of zinc supplements appeared to decrease opportunistic infection among adults and children with HIV. Only the adults were found to have higher CD4 counts; no adverse events were reported for adults or children from using zinc supplementation.[261]

Some antiretroviral drugs appear to chelate magnesium post-interaction with integrase. Therefore, supplemental magnesium may ensure that magnesium levels are not depleted.[262]

**Probiotics.** The human gut contains naturally growing bacteria that possess an array of beneficial functions. These include their ability to provide essential nutrients to the body; break down foods that are otherwise indigestible, via fermentation reactions, for example; and prevent the growth of harmful pathogens.[263,264] However, the gut is largely compromised in patients with HIV. Acute HIV infection is marked by the dramatic depletion of CD4+ cells from the gastrointestinal (GI) tract. The GI tract is believed to be a particularly attractive target for HIV replication because the CD4 cells it contains are primarily CD4+ memory cells, which are preferential targets for HIV replication. (CD4+ "memory" cells are named as such because they "remember" antigens they previously encountered; this allows them to mount a more rapid response in subsequent encounters.) Moreover, CD4+ cells in the GI tract express substantial amounts of CCR5—a receptor commonly used by HIV to enter and infect cells.[265,266] As HIV depletes the gut of immune cells, intestinal epithelial permeability generally increases, and the human host becomes increasingly vulnerable to microbial invasion and disease progression.[267]

Probiotics are living microorganisms that when provided in sufficient quantities, impart health benefits. Certain strains of probiotics are associated with reduced inflammation[268–270] and permeability,[271–273] both of which are of notable interest for patients with HIV. In several studies involving people with HIV/AIDS, consuming probiotics was associated with improvements in CD4 cell counts.[274–276] More recently, Hummelen and colleagues found that adding probiotics to micronutrient-fortified yogurt did not boost CD4 cell count after 1 month, versus the same preparation without the added probiotics; the added probiotics were well tolerated, however, and no adverse events were reported.[277] Larger clinical studies with longer follow-up periods are needed to fully assess the impact of probiotic supplementation on people with HIV, but results so far are promising.

## Life Extension Suggestions

### Glutathione Boosters
- **N-acetylcysteine:** 600 mg twice daily
- **Vitamin C:** 1000 mg, 3 times daily
- **Selenium:** 200–400 mcg daily
- **R-lipoic acid:** 210 mg twice daily

### Antioxidants
- **Beta-carotene:** 5000 IU daily
- **Natural vitamin E:** 100–400 IU alpha-tocopherol and 200 mg gamma-tocopherol daily
- **Green tea,** standardized extract: 725–1450 mg daily
- **CoQ10,** as ubiquinol: 200 mg daily

### Micronutrients
- **Zinc:** 30 mg daily
- **Magnesium:** 140–500 elemental mg of highly absorbable magnesium

- **B-complex vitamin:**
  - **Thiamine (B1):** 75–125 mg daily
  - **Riboflavin (B2):** 50 mg daily
  - **Niacin (B3):** 50–190 mg daily
  - **Folate** (preferably as L-methylfolate): 400–1000 mcg daily
  - **Vitamin B12:** 300–600 mcg daily
  - **Biotin:** 300–3000 mcg daily
  - **Pantothenic acid:** 100–600 mg daily

### Supporting Immune Function and Targeting the HIV Viral Lifecycle
- **Vitamin D:** 5000–8000 IU daily, based on blood test results
- **Lactoferrin** (as apolactoferrin): 300–600 mg daily

### Combating Antiretroviral Side Effects
- **Acetyl-L-carnitine:** 1000–2000 mg daily
- **Green coffee extract:** 200–400 mg before meals, up to 3 times daily
- **Fish oil** (with olive polyphenols): providing 1400 mg EPA and 1000 mg DHA daily
- **Whey protein isolate:** 30–60 g of whey protein daily in two or three divided doses
- **Milk thistle extract,** standardized to 80% silymarin: 750 mg daily
- **Probiotics:** per label instructions

### Hormonal Therapies
- Bioidentical hormone replacement therapy: based on blood test results; review Life Extension Male and Female Hormone Restoration Therapy protocols
- Growth hormone replacement: under physician supervision
- DHEA: based on blood test results; doses typically range from 15–25 mg daily for women, and 25–75 mg daily for men

In addition, the following *blood testing* resources may be helpful:

- Female Panel or Male Panel
- Vitamin D, 25-Hydroxy
- Glutathione

## REFERENCES

References available at: www.lef.org/dpt5/ch74

# 75

# Homocysteine Reduction

Homocysteine is an amino acid that inflicts damage to the inner arterial lining (endothelium) and other cells of the body.

In 1968, a Harvard researcher observed that children with a genetic defect that caused them to have sharply elevated homocysteine levels suffered severe atherosclerotic occlusion and vascular disorders similar to what is seen in middle-aged patients with arterial disease. This was the first indication that excess homocysteine might be an independent risk factor for heart disease.

Life Extension has identified elevated homocysteine as one of 17 independent risk factors for cardiovascular disease. Any one of these risk factors can initiate and propagate vascular disease. Among such risk factors, homocysteine's role in cardiovascular and cerebrovascular disease continues to be misunderstood by mainstream medicine.

Much of this confusion stems from highly publicized results of clinical trials that used B vitamins to reduce blood levels of homocysteine yet failed to prevent cardiovascular events in people with advanced atherosclerosis.[1,2] The Life Extension Foundation® believes these studies were seriously flawed, most notably because they used doses of B vitamins that were too low to reduce homocysteine to Life Extension's recommended optimal range of <7–8 µmol/L. At present, medical testing laboratories consider a homocysteine number between 11–15 µmol/L as the upper limit of "normal" despite robust clinical data to the contrary.[3,4] Consequently, many doctors remain misinformed as to the optimal target range for homocysteine and the doses of homocysteine-lowering nutrients required to achieve this optimal range.

## HOMOCYSTEINE BASICS

All homocysteine in the body is biosynthesized from methionine, an essential amino acid found abundantly in meats, seafood, dairy products, and eggs. Vegetables, with few exceptions (eg, sesame seeds and Brazil nuts), are low in methionine; even such protein-rich legumes as beans, peas, and lentils contain relatively small amounts of methionine compared to animal-derived foods.

Homocysteine exists in several forms[5]; the sum of all homocysteine forms is termed "total homocysteine." Protein-rich diets contain ample amounts of methionine and consequently produce significant levels of homocysteine in the body.[6]

Homocysteine is metabolized through two pathways: remethylation and transsulfuration. Remethylation requires folate and B12 coenzymes; transsulfuration requires pyridoxal-5'-phosphate, the B6 coenzyme.[7]

## HOMOCYSTEINE METABOLIC PATHWAYS

The remethylation pathway requires vitamin B12, folate, and the enzyme 5,10-methylenetetrahydrofolate reductase (MTHFR). In the kidney and liver, homocysteine is also remethylated by the enzyme betaine homocysteine methyltrans]teine via the demethylation of betaine to dimethylglycine (DMG). The transsulfuration pathway requires the enzyme cystathionine-synthase (CBS) and vitamin B6 (pyridoxal-5'-phosphate). Once formed from cystathionine, cysteine can be utilized in protein synthesis and glutathione (GSH) production.

Active folate, known as 5-MTHF or 5-methyltetrahydrofolate, works in concert with vitamin B12 as a methyl-group donor in the conversion of homocysteine back to methionine.

Normally, about 50% of homocysteine is remethylated; the remaining homocysteine is transsulfurated to cysteine, which requires vitamin B6 as a co-factor. This pathway yields cysteine, which is then used by the body to make glutathione, a powerful antioxidant that protects cellular components against oxidative damage.

Vitamin B2 (riboflavin) and magnesium are also involved in homocysteine metabolism. Thus a person needs several different B-vitamins to help keep homocysteine levels low and allow for it to be properly transformed into helpful antioxidants like glutathione. Without B6, B12, B2, folate, and magnesium, dangerous levels of homocysteine may build up in the body.

Blood levels of total homocysteine increase throughout life in men and women.[8] Prior to puberty, both sexes enjoy optimally healthy levels (about 6 µmol/L). During puberty, levels rise, more in males than females,[9,10] reaching on average almost 10 µmol/L in men and more than 8 µmol/L in women.[11] As we age, mean values of homocysteine continue to rise and the concentrations usually remain lower in women than in men.[11]

The higher total homocysteine concentrations seen in the elderly may be caused by many factors including malabsorption of B12 or a suboptimal intake of B vitamins (especially vitamin B12), reduced kidney function, and medications that reduce the absorption of vitamins (as in the case of H2 receptor antagonists or proton-pump inhibitors reducing B12 absorption)[12] or increase the catabolism of the vitamins (as in the case of metformin reducing blood levels of B12 and folic acid).[13] Certain diseases are associated with higher homocysteine levels, as can such lifestyle factors as smoking,[14] coffee consumption,[15] and excessive alcohol intake.[16] Lack of exercise, obesity, and stress are also associated with hyperhomocysteinemia.

## WHAT IS A HEALTHY HOMOCYSTEINE NUMBER?

Clinical testing laboratories consider a homocysteine value of 5–15 μmol/L as healthy. The Life Extension Foundation® believes that an upper limit of 15 μmol/L is too high for optimal health. Studies indicate that adults with homocysteine values ≥6.3 μmol/L are at increased risk of atherosclerosis (Homocysteine Studies Collaboration), heart attack and stroke.[17] Homocysteine levels in the blood can increase due to age,[18] prescription drug use (see the "Drugs that Raise Homocysteine Levels" section), declining ability to absorb vitamin B12,[19] deteriorating kidney function,[20] smoking,[14] alcohol,[16] coffee consumption,[21] obesity,[22] declining levels of physical activity,[4] and inheriting a genetic polymorphism known as the MTHFR C677T variant in methylenetetrahydrofolate reductase (MTHFR).[23] After age 50, a more practical target value for homocysteine is <7–8 μmol/L. Depending upon other factors, you may require larger-than-usual intakes of B vitamins to achieve a healthy blood level of homocysteine. Data from published studies reveal that there is no safe "normal range" for homocysteine. Epidemiological studies have shown that higher homocysteine levels are associated with higher risk, even at levels that are considered "normal."[24] Life Extension recommends a target of <7–8 μmol/L because published data, as well as the Foundation's experience with homocysteine in tens of thousands of members over more than 30 years, indicate that this threshold target is a realistic goal when taking optimal amounts of vitamins B6, B12, folate, TMG, and other homocysteine-lowering nutrients.[25]

The MTHFR C677T gene polymorphism is the single most important genetic determinant of blood homocysteine values in the general population. More than 40% of Hispanics and 30–38% of whites living in the United States inherit at least one copy of this gene,[26] which impairs their ability to fully activate (methylate) folic acid to 5-methyltetrahydrofolate, the bioactive form of the B vitamin. Individuals who inherit this gene variant from both parents have a significantly higher (14–21%) risk of vascular disease than those who do not.

For this affected group, taking the bioactive folate supplement, 5-MTHF, may be a better strategy. 5-MTHF is clinically tested, is highly bioavailable,[27] can cross the blood–brain barrier,[28] and is unlikely to mask a vitamin-B12 deficiency as folic acid can do.[29] Those who carry this gene variant can safely reduce their risk of homocysteine-related health problems using an inexpensive, nonprescription natural folate supplement.

## HOMOCYSTEINE AND HEALTH

### Homocysteine and Alzheimer's Disease

In a 2002 study published in the *New England Journal of Medicine*, dementia developed in 111 study participants of which 83 were diagnosed with Alzheimer's disease over an 8-year follow-up. In those with a plasma homocysteine level >14 μmol/L, the risk of Alzheimer's disease nearly doubled. Investigators concluded, "An increased plasma homocysteine level is a strong, independent risk factor for the development of dementia and Alzheimer's disease."[30]

### How Elevated Homocysteine Leads to Vascular Damage

If unhealthy levels of homocysteine accumulate in the blood, the delicate lining of an artery (endothelium) can be damaged.

Homocysteine can both initiate and potentiate atherosclerosis. For example, homocysteine-induced injury to the arterial wall is one of the factors that can initiate the process of atherosclerosis, leading to endothelial dysfunction and eventually to heart attacks and strokes.[31,32] Several studies have shown that homocysteine can inflict damage to the arterial wall via multiple destructive molecular mechanisms.[19,33,34]

### Homocysteine Is Linked to Congestive Heart Failure

Small clinical studies have shown that patients with congestive heart failure (CHF) suffer from elevated plasma homocysteine levels.[35] Based on preclinical evidence that the myocardium may be especially susceptible to homocysteine-induced injury,[36] and based on observations linking homocysteine to oxidative stress[37] and to left ventricular remodeling,[38,39] it has been hypothesized that elevated plasma homocysteine levels would increase the risk of CHF. Accordingly, researchers investigated the relationship of plasma homocysteine concentration to the risk of CHF in a community-based sample of adults (2491 adults, mean age 72 years, 1547 women) who participated in the well-known Framingham Heart Study during the 1979–1982 and 1986–1990 examination periods and who were free of CHF or prior myocardial infarction at baseline. In one study that examined patients without any manifestation of coronary heart disease at baseline, investigators found that the association of plasma homocysteine levels with risk of CHF was maintained in men and women and concluded "an increased plasma homocysteine level independently predicts risk of the development of CHF in adults without prior myocardial infarction."[40]

### Reducing Homocysteine for Migraine Relief

Migraine is a debilitating disease that can be associated with elevated blood levels of homocysteine.[41-43]

A recent study showed that treatment with B-complex vitamins, including 5-MTHF, could provide relief for migraine sufferers including those with the MTHFR C677T genotype,[44] which typically limits the clinical effectiveness of supplemental folic acid since individuals with this genotype do not effectively convert folic acid to its active form. People with the C677T genotype consistently have higher levels of homocysteine than those with the normal C677C genotype. Headache frequency and pain severity were also reduced. The treatment proved successful in reducing homocysteine levels and migraine disability in study participants with the MTHFR C677T genotype. Researchers have long suspected that migraine headaches have a genetic component because migraine sufferers often have family members who also have the condition. Studies suggest that up to 12% of those living in the United States and Western Europe have this genetic link to migraine.[45]

### Homocysteine's Role in Macular Degeneration

Studies of homocysteine's role in age-related macular degeneration (AMD: both wet and dry types) reveal a strong link between the compound and the disease.

In a group of 2335 study participants who had evidence of AMD as detected from retinal photographs, researchers found that homocysteine blood levels >15 μmol/L were associated with an increased likelihood of AMD in participants aged <75 years. They also found a similar association for blood levels

of vitamin B12 <125 pmol/L among all study participants. In participants with homocysteine levels 15 μmol/L, *low serum B12 was associated with nearly fourfold higher odds of AMD.*[46]

In a larger and more recent study, Harvard researchers enrolled 5442 women who were at high risk for cardiovascular disease. The women were given a placebo or 2.5 mg folic acid, 50 mg vitamin B6, and 1 mg vitamin B12 daily. After an average of >7 years of treatment and follow-up, researchers recorded 55 cases of AMD in the B-vitamin treatment group and 82 in the placebo group. Investigators concluded that in women at high risk of cardiovascular disease, daily long-term supplementation with folic acid, B6, and B12 may reduce the risk of AMD.[47]

### Homocysteine Linked to Hearing Loss

A number of published studies suggest that hearing loss may be linked to plasma homocysteine levels, which could be reduced by folic acid supplementation.

One study conducted from September 2000 to December 2004 in 728 older men and women in the Netherlands (which does not have mandatory folic acid fortification) found that at initiation, the median threshold for hearing in the low frequency range (0.5–kHz) was 11.7 decibels (dB), and 34.2 dB in the high frequency range (4–8 kHz). By the end of the study, the thresholds had increased for both folic acid and placebo groups. In other words, a louder noise was required to get study participants to hear it. However, the increase was lower in the supplemented group in the low frequency range (1.0- versus 1.7-dB increase for folic acid and placebo groups, respectively). There was no significant difference in threshold decline in the higher frequency region. Thus, folic acid supplementation slowed the decline in hearing of the speech frequencies typically associated with aging.[48]

Researchers studied the levels of homocysteine in 28 male patients (mean age 37) with noise-induced hearing loss. Homocysteine levels of subjects with noise-induced hearing loss were significantly higher compared to healthy controls, suggesting a causal link between increased homocysteine levels and noise-induced hearing loss.[49]

### Flawed Studies Lead to Confusion over B Vitamins and Heart Disease

A 2010 review of several large randomized, double-blind, placebo-controlled trials that used various B-vitamin therapies for reducing cerebrovascular risk (VISP study[50]) and secondary cardiovascular disease risk (HOPE 2,[51] NORVIT,[52] WAFACS,[53] and WENBIT[54] studies) concluded that B-vitamin treatments effectively decrease plasma homocysteine levels and stroke risk, although such treatments failed to reduce cardiovascular risk.[2] A meta-analysis of randomized clinical trials comprising 16 958 participants with preexisting vascular disease found that folic acid supplementation had no effect on the risk of cardiovascular disease or all-cause mortality.[55]

Critical examinations of such studies that failed to show a reduction of cardiovascular events in patients treated with B vitamins have revealed numerous design and methodological flaws including limited statistical power, relatively short duration of follow-up, and insufficient number of cardiovascular events.[56-58] In addition, 3 of the studies were secondary prevention trials and therefore were not designed to test the ability of B vitamins to prevent heart attacks in healthy people. The most egregious flaw in these trials, however, is that *they all failed to use high enough doses of B vitamins to reduce study participants' homocysteine levels to the optimal target range of <7–8 μmol/L.*

Additional B-vitamin studies in patients undergoing balloon angioplasty and vascular stenting reveal the critical importance of lowering homocysteine levels to Life Extension's recommended optimal target range. Two studies that failed to use high enough doses of folic acid, B6, and/or B12 to achieve optimal homocysteine reduction saw restenosis rates rise in some patients who received vitamin therapy.[59,60] In contrast, a prospective, double-blind, randomized trial (the "Swiss Heart Study") examined the effects of folic acid, vitamin B6, and vitamin B12 treatment in 553 patients who underwent angioplasty.[61] Investigators observed a significant reduction in the need for revascularization of the target lesion at 1 year (9.9% in the treatment group versus 16.0% in the control group). Significantly, the Swiss Study is the *only* randomized controlled trial to date in which treatment reduced study participants' average plasma homocysteine levels (7.5 μmol/L) to within the range recommended by the Life Extension Foundation® (<7–8 μmol/L).

## Stroke Protection from B-Vitamin Therapy

The 2009 HOPE-2 trial for homocysteine therapy and stroke risk, which randomized 5522 adults with known cardiovascular disease to a daily treatment regimen of B-vitamin therapy (2.5 mg of folic acid, 50 mg of vitamin B6, and 1 mg of vitamin B12) for 5 years, *achieved reduction in stroke risk of 25%.*[51] HOPE-2 was the first large randomized, double blind, placebo-controlled trial to use clinically adequate doses of vitamin B12. It included high-risk

participants with and without history of cerebrovascular disease drawn from countries with and without folic acid food fortification. *Significantly, homocysteine concentration decreased by 2.2 μmol/L in the B-vitamin therapy group and increased by 0.80 μmol/L in the placebo group.*

Another meta-analysis that focused on a subset of 7 of 12 randomized studies added a randomized trial from China to assess the efficacy of folic acid supplementation in stroke prevention. Study investigators found that folic acid supplementation significantly reduced the risk of stroke by 18%.[62]

## Additional Studies on Homocysteine Reduction and Vascular Disease

A number of controlled studies that found positive effects of B-vitamin therapy on vascular disease yielded the following results:

- Folate supplementation improved arterial function in patients with peripheral arterial disease.[63] Two measures of arterial health, brachial pressure index (ABPI) and pulse wave velocity (PWV), were measured; ABPI improved significantly in all patients receiving folate compared with controls, while PWV improved significantly in individuals receiving an active form of folic acid (5-MTHF), and tended to be improved in those taking folic acid compared with controls.

- Twenty hypercholesterolemic adults taking Lovastatin® were given a daily folate supplement (5 mg) for 8 weeks while 20 patients received a placebo[64]; only the folate-supplemented group experienced decreased blood levels of homocysteine.

- Reducing blood levels of homocysteine through B-vitamin therapy was shown to improve endothelial function in renal transplant recipients with hyperhomocysteinemia.[65] Investigators assigned 36 stable renal transplant recipients with hyperhomocysteinemia to either a B-vitamin treatment group (5 mg folic acid, 50 mg vitamin B6, and 1000 mg vitamin B12 daily) or to a control group (placebo only) for 6 months. Investigators found that homocysteine significantly decreased in the B-vitamin treatment group compared with baseline (12.6 versus 20.1 μmol/L); no significant changes in homocysteine levels were observed in the control group. Vasodilatation responses were significantly improved in the treatment group compared to controls.

- Folic acid treatment in patients undergoing hemodialysis (10 mg 3 times weekly after dialysis treatment for 6 months) lowered plasma homocysteine levels while it significantly increased total plasma antioxidant capacity levels.[66] Twenty patients receiving placebo treatment showed no statistically significant effect on any of the parameters studied.

- A study treated liver transplant recipients with 5-methyltetrahydrofolate (5-MTHF; 1 mg) versus folic acid (1 mg) versus placebo in an 8-week, double-blind, placebo-controlled trial. Investigators observed a significant decrease of total serum homocysteine in the 5-MTHF group by week 8; they found no significant decrease of total serum homocysteine in either the folic acid group or the placebo group. The effects of 5-MTHF (active folate) were found to be significantly more potent than folic acid at lowering elevated homocysteine levels in liver transplant recipients.[67]

- A randomized study in 103 patients at increased risk of heart attack or stroke investigated the effect of daily supplementation of folic acid (5 mg) on carotid artery intima-media thickness (IMT). Study participants were randomized to receive either a daily dose of 5 mg folic acid or placebo. After 18 months of folic acid supplementation, participants in the active treatment group saw their homocysteine levels significantly reduced, compared to a significant increase in the placebo group. *Investigators noted significant regression of carotid IMT in the treatment group* compared to significant IMT progression in the placebo group.[68]

- A controlled study was carried out to assess whether folic acid supplementation could produce a reduction in homocysteine levels and improvement in endothelial function in patients with unstable angina (UA) and hyperhomocysteinemia.[3] Investigators treated patients with 5 mg of folic acid for 8 weeks, rechecking homocysteine, folic acid, and vitamin B12 levels at the end of 4 and 8 weeks. Plasma homocysteine levels were significantly higher in patients with UA than in patients without UA at baseline (19.2 versus 10.7 μmol/L), whereas plasma levels of folic acid and vitamin B12 were significantly lower. After 8 weeks of folic acid supplementation, homocysteine levels were reduced by 55.3% in the 22 UA patients with hyperhomocysteinemia. Flow-mediated dilation, an indirect measure of endothelial function, also improved significantly after 8 weeks of treatment with folic acid.

- A 2008 study examined carotid artery atherosclerosis as determined by measurements of carotid intima-media thickness (IMT) and plaque calcification in 923 patients with vascular disease or diabetes.[69] Study investigators found an inverse association between plasma folate and plaque calcification score; there was a trend toward an inverse association with IMT as well.

# TARGETED NUTRITIONAL STRATEGIES

## N-Acetyl-Cysteine

Research studies have documented the homocysteine-lowering effect of the nutraceutical, N-acetyl-cysteine (NAC), which can lead to a highly significant reduction in cardiovascular events, owing to the ability of NAC to lower plasma homocysteine levels and improve endothelial function. Researchers believe that NAC displaces homocysteine from its protein carrier in the blood. This promotes the formation of cysteine and NAC disulfide molecules with high renal clearance, thereby removing homocysteine from plasma.[70,71]

A 2007 study randomized 60 patients with hyperhomocysteinemia and confirmed coronary artery disease to folic acid 5 mg, NAC 600 mg, or placebo daily for 8 weeks. Folic acid and NAC supplementation both lowered homocysteine levels and improved endothelial function. Folic acid decreased homocysteine from 21.7 μmol/L to 12.5 μmol/L and NAC decreased homocysteine from 20.9 μmol/L to 15.6 μmol/L. Both treatments improved endothelium-dependent dilation compared to placebo.[72]

In a double-blind crossover design study, Swedish investigators gave NAC supplements to 11 patients with high plasma lipoprotein(a), which is an independent risk factor for cardiovascular disease.[73] While investigators observed no significant effect on plasma lipoprotein(a) levels, they did find that plasma levels of homocysteine were significantly reduced during treatment with NAC by *an astounding 45%.*

One study examined the effect of oral NAC supplementation in 9 young healthy females and found that the supplement induced a rapid and significant decrease in plasma homocysteine levels and an increase in whole blood concentration of the antioxidant glutathione. Study investigators concluded that NAC might therefore be a highly efficient nutraceutical for reducing blood levels of homocysteine.[74]

## Omega-3 Polyunsaturated Fatty Acids (PUFAs)

A growing body of research on marine lipids, rich in omega-3 polyunsaturated fatty acids (PUFAs), reveals that omega-3 rich fish oil supplementation can reduce elevated homocysteine levels.

A 2010 animal model study examined the effect of fish oil rich in omega-3 PUFAs on homocysteine metabolism. Three groups of randomly divided rats were fed olive oil, tuna oil, or salmon oil for 8 weeks. The level of plasma homocysteine was significantly decreased only in the group fed tuna oil, rich in omega-3 PUFAs. It is not clear why the salmon oil did not reduce homocysteine as it too is rich in omega-3 PUFAs.[75]

A 2009 randomized double-blind placebo-controlled clinical trial conducted on 81 patients with type 2 diabetes assigned each patient either 3 capsules of omega-3 fatty acids (3 g) or a placebo every day for a period of 2 months. Homocysteine levels in the treatment group declined as much as 3.10 µmol/L; glycosylated hemoglobin (HbA1C, a measure of long-term sugar levels in the blood) decreased in the treatment group and increased in the control group.[76]

## Taurine

Supplementing with the amino acid taurine can protect against coronary artery disease by favorably modulating blood levels of homocysteine. Research suggests that taurine can block methionine absorption from the diet, thereby reducing available substrate for homocysteine synthesis.[77] One animal study found that taurine normalized hyperhomocysteinemia and reduced atherosclerosis by 64% over control animals and reduced endothelial cell apoptosis by 30%.[78] Study investigators also observed that taurine supplementation reduced left main coronary artery wall pathology due to a favorable effect on plasma total homocysteine and apoptosis.

A study of 22 healthy middle-aged women (33–54 years) found that after taurine supplementation (3 g daily for 4 weeks), plasma homocysteine levels exhibited a significant decline, *from 8.5 µmol/L to 7.6 µmol/L*. The investigators concluded that sufficient taurine supplementation might effectively prevent cardiovascular disease.[79]

## Trimethylglycine and Choline

Trimethylglycine (TMG) was originally called betaine after its discovery in sugar beets in the 19th century. TMG serves as a methyl donor in a reaction converting homocysteine to methionine. It is commonly used for reducing high homocysteine levels though it has yet to be effectively studied to determine its full cardiovascular benefits through its ability to lower homocysteine.[80]

A 2009 study examined the effect of betaine (TMG) supplementation on atherosclerotic lesion progression in apolipoprotein E-deficient mice.[80] After a 14-week treatment with TMG, analyses revealed that the higher dose of TMG was related to smaller atherosclerotic lesion area. Compared with mice not treated with TMG after 14 weeks, mice receiving 1%, 2%, or 4% TMG had 10.8%, 41%, and 37% smaller lesion areas, respectively. TMG supplementation also reduced aortic expression of the inflammatory cytokine, tumor necrosis factor-alpha (TNF-α) , in a dose-dependent way. These data suggest that in addition to its homocysteine-lowering action, TMG may also exert its antiplaque effect by inhibiting aortic inflammatory responses mediated by TNF-α.

Data from the Framingham Offspring Study found that intakes of TMG and choline (choline is metabolized to TMG in the body) were inversely related to circulating homocysteine concentrations, particularly among participants with low folate intake or among those who consumed alcoholic beverages.[81] Other studies have shown that choline deficiency in mice and humans is associated with increased plasma homocysteine levels after consuming methionine.[82] A Finnish study of TMG supplementation showed that a daily supplement of 6 g TMG for 12 weeks reduced blood homocysteine values in healthy subjects by approximately 9%.[83]

## S-Adenosyl-L-Methionine

S-adenosyl-L-methionine (SAMe), biosynthesized from methionine and ATP, functions as a primary methyl group donor in a variety of reactions in the body and is directly involved in homocysteine synthesis and metabolism. Taking supplemental SAMe promotes the conversion of homocysteine to cysteine and glutathione, thus lowering homocysteine levels.[84] One study found that taking SAMe supplements increased the activity of 5-MTHF, a major co-factor involved in the metabolism of homocysteine.[85]

In effect, SAMe acts as a "switch" to control enzymes involved in the remethylation and transsulfuration pathways of homocysteine metabolism.[86] Since some of the SAMe's methyl groups are used in the body's production of creatine (an energy substrate used primarily by skeletal muscle), it has been suggested that supplementing one's diet with creatine would free up SAMe's methyl groups to favorably modulate homocysteine levels.[87] One study found that lab animals maintained on creatine-supplemented diets exhibited significantly lower (~25%) plasma homocysteine levels than controls.[88] Those who use SAMe should make sure they are taking supplemental folate, B6 and B12 to ensure that SAMe promotes the conversion of homocysteine to beneficial compounds in the body.

## Riboflavin

Vitamin B2 (riboflavin) has long been known to be a determinant of plasma homocysteine levels in healthy individuals with the 5-MTHFR C677T gene variant that causes hyperhomocysteinemia.[89] Homocysteine is highly responsive to riboflavin (riboflavin is required as a co-factor by MTHFR), specifically in individuals with the MTHFR 677 TT genotype.[90]

A 4-week randomized placebo-controlled double-blind trial found that 10 mg/day oral riboflavin supplementation for 28 days lowered plasma homocysteine concentrations in 42 subjects (60–94 years) with low riboflavin status.[91]

## B Vitamins

A 2-year randomized clinical trial (known as VITACOG) completed in 2010 found that the accelerated rate of brain atrophy in elderly patients suffering from mild cognitive impairment could be significantly slowed by treatment with homocysteine-lowering B vitamins.[92]

Researchers at Oxford University randomized study participants to receive either placebo or a combination of folic acid (0.8 mg/day), vitamin B12 (0.5 mg/day) and vitamin B6 (20 mg/day) for 24 months. A subset of participants agreed to have cranial MRI scans at the start and finish of the study for the purpose of measuring the change in rate of atrophy of the entire brain.

A total of 168 participants (85 in active treatment group; 83 receiving placebo) completed the MRI section of the trial. Results showed that the B-vitamin treatment response was related to baseline homocysteine levels; participants in the B-vitamin treatment group with the highest levels of homocysteine ($\geq$13.0 $\mu$mol/L) at the start of the trial experienced half the brain shrinkage over 2 years compared to those participants with the highest homocysteine blood levels at the start of the trial and who received the placebo.

This important study demonstrated that the accelerated rate of brain atrophy seen in approximately 16% of elderly patients suffering from mild cognitive impairment[93] could be significantly slowed by simple treatment with folic acid and vitamins B6 and B12.

### WHAT YOU NEED TO KNOW

- Elevated blood levels of homocysteine have been linked with a wide range of health disorders including heart disease, stroke, macular degeneration, hearing loss, migraine, brain atrophy, dementia and cancer.
- A high-protein diet, especially one that includes red meats and dairy products, is also high in methionine, the parent compound of homocysteine. Following such a diet can increase blood levels of homocysteine.
- Numerous factors, including prescription drug use, smoking, coffee and alcohol consumption, advancing age, genetics, and obesity contribute to elevated homocysteine levels.
- Many people carry a genetic variation that is linked with elevated homocysteine levels. People carrying this gene variant suffer from an impaired ability to metabolize folic acid to its active form, but may achieve a significant reduction in plasma homocysteine by taking an active folate (5-MTHF) supplement.
- Vitamin B2, B6, and B12 supplements as well as those containing choline and TMG work together with active folate to maintain homocysteine levels within a healthy range.
- As humans grow older, homocysteine levels increase substantially. However, although these increased levels are "normal," they are still associated with higher risk of various health problems.
- Although some clinical testing laboratories consider homocysteine levels of up to 15.0 $\mu$mol/L as normal, Life Extension believes this is too high for optimal health and therefore recommends keeping homocysteine levels <7–8 $\mu$mol/L.
- People taking active folate can achieve plasma folate levels 700% higher than by taking an ordinary folic acid[27] supplement and may therefore more effectively lower elevated homocysteine levels.

A program of regular exercise may help people recovering from a heart attack, bypass surgery, or angioplasty to modestly reduce homocysteine levels.

**Ordinary B-vitamin supplements and folate-rich foods may not be enough to lower homocysteine.** Even though folic acid–fortified foods are ubiquitous, and despite peoples' best efforts to insure adequate intake of the vitamin through supplementation, many individuals run the risk of not obtaining sufficient amounts of folate necessary to achieve healthy blood levels of homocysteine unless they supplement with bioactive folate. Cooking and food processing destroy natural folates.[94] Although red blood cells can retain folate for 40–50 days following discontinuation of supplementation, synthetic folic acid is poorly transported to the brain and is rapidly cleared from the central nervous system.[95]

Many people who take ordinary B-vitamin supplements are unable to sufficiently lower their homocysteine levels enough to prevent disease.[96] Fortunately, there is hope for those with seemingly intractable homocysteine levels. One study found that giving L-methylfolate (5-MTHF; also called *active folate*) to patients with coronary artery disease resulted in a *700% higher plasma concentration of folate-related compounds compared to folic acid.*

This difference was irrespective of the patient's genotype.[27]

5-MTHF is the predominant biologically active form of folate in cells,[97] blood,[98] and cerebrospinal fluid.[95] Until recently, 5-MTHF was available only in prescription medicines and medicinal food products. Now, this active form of folate, which provides increased protection against homocysteine-related health problems, is available as a dietary supplement. This form of the vitamin is unlikely to mask a vitamin B12 deficiency, a well-known shortcoming of folic acid. Since 5-MTHF is *the only form of folate used directly by the body*, it does not have to be converted and metabolized to be clinically useful, as does synthetic folic acid.

Synthetic folic acid, as used in ordinary dietary supplements and vitamin-fortified foods, must first be converted in cells to active L-methylfolate in order to be effective. These steps require several enzymes, adequate liver and gastrointestinal function, and sufficient supplies of niacin (vitamin B3), pyridoxine (B6), riboflavin (B2), vitamin C, and zinc.[99]

The low dose requirements for 5-MTHF make it a relatively inexpensive supplement with superior clinical benefits over folic acid. People who would benefit from taking active folate include:

- Those who desire to take advantage of 5-MTHF as a part of their antiaging strategy due to its potency, low cost, and bioavailability
- Those with elevated risk factors for cardiovascular disease
- Those taking drugs known to interfere with the absorption or metabolism of folate
- People with the gene variant 5-MTHFR C677T

Individuals with the 5-MTHFR C677T polymorphism are at higher risk of cardiovascular disease, stroke, preeclampsia (high blood pressure in pregnancy), and birth defects that occur during the development of the brain and spinal cord (neural tube defects). The mutation replaces the DNA nucleotide cytosine with thymine at position 677 in the MTHFR gene (nucleotides are the building blocks of DNA). This change in the MTHFR gene produces a form of the enzyme, methylenetetrahydrofolate reductase, which is thermolabile, meaning its activity is reduced at higher temperatures.

A daily dose of 0.8 mg 5-MTHF is typically used in research studies to achieve a clinically beneficial reduction in elevated plasma homocysteine concentrations. In some cases, doses as low as 0.2–0.4 mg have been shown to achieve this effect.[100]

## DRUGS THAT RAISE HOMOCYSTEINE LEVELS

A number of prescription drugs and natural compounds can elevate blood levels of homocysteine by interfering with folate absorption or metabolism of homocysteine. These include:

- **Caffeine**[101]: Cafcit®, Cafergot®, Esgic®, Excedrin Migraine®, Fioricet®, Fiorinal®, Norgesic®, Synalgos-DC®
- **Cholestyramine**[102]: Questran®, Questran Light®, Cholybar®
- **Colestipol**: Cholestid®[103]
- **Fenofibrate**[104]: Antara®, Fenoglide®, Lipofen®, Lofibra®, Tricor®, Trilipix®
- **Levadopa**[105]: Parcopa®, Sinemet®, Stalevo®
- **Metformin**[106]: ActoPlus Met®, Avandamet®, Fortamet®, Glucophage® Glucovance®, Glumetza®, Janumet®, Metaglip®, Prandimet®, Riomet®
- **Methotrexate**[106]: Rheumatrex®
- **Niacin**[106]: Advicor®, Ocuvite®, Cardio Basics®, CitraNatal®, Niaspan®, Simcor®
- **Nitrous oxide**[107]
- **Pemetrexed**[108]: Alimta®
- **Phenytoin**[109]: Dilantin®, Phenytek®
- **Pyrimethamine**[110]: Daraprim®, Fansidar®
- **Sulfasalazine**[111]: Azulfidine®

## FOR MORE INFORMATION

To learn more about the conditions associated with hyperhomocysteinemia, refer to the following chapters:

- Congestive Heart Failure
- Atherosclerosis and Cardiovascular Disease
- High Blood Pressure
- Diabetes
- Thyroid Regulation

### Life Extension Suggestions

#### General Suggestions

- **Avoid methionine-rich foods:** Avoid red meats and dairy products in particular. Although methionine is an essential amino acid, it is also suspected to indirectly promote atherosclerotic plaque growth by increasing homocysteine levels.
- **Exercise:** In a cardiac rehabilitation program following bypass surgery, angioplasty, or heart attack, 76 participants experienced a modest 12% reduction in homocysteine just by engaging in a program of regular exercise.[112]
- **Decrease or eliminate:** Alcohol, coffee (filtered and unfiltered), and smoking.
- **Weight loss:** Obesity is associated with higher homocysteine.

The following nutrients can provide an effective means of reducing homocysteine:

- **Folate/folic acid,** with several options:
  - **5-MTHF/L-methylfolate (active folate):** 800–1000 mcg daily; certain individuals may require up to 5 mg daily (under medical supervision). This is the best choice for those with higher homocysteine levels, those with the MTHFR 677TT genotype, and those who are not getting their homocysteine levels low enough with regular folic acid.
  - **Natural folate:** 800–1600 mcg. This form is becoming more popular in high-end multivitamins and is the form found naturally in food.
  - **Folic acid:** 1–2 mg is another option that has been used for years to reduce homocysteine levels. However, if a 2-mg dose does not help to reduce homocysteine levels, then consider using the active folate (5-MTHF) form instead.
- **N-acetylcysteine (NAC):** 600–1800 mg daily
- **SAMe (S-adenosylmethionine):** 400 mg, 2–4 times daily
- **Taurine:** 1000–3000 mg daily
- **TMG (trimethylglycine):** 2000–6000 mg daily
- **Vitamin B12 (cobalamin):** 1–2 mg daily
- **Vitamin B2 (riboflavin):** 10–100 mg daily
- **Vitamin B6 (as pyridoxal-5'-phosphate):** 100–200 mg daily
- **Zinc:** 30–60 mg daily
- **Micronized creatine:** 500 mg (in capsule form), 4–8 times daily
- **CDP choline:** 250–500 mg daily. Alternatively, you can use 1–3 teaspoons of liquid choline chloride daily mixed with 2 oz of juice, 1 tablespoon of pure lecithin granules daily, or 250 mg of a-GPC daily.

If this protocol is not successful at lowering your homocysteine level, a weekly 1-mg vitamin B12 injection may be necessary (this requires a prescription).

In addition, the following blood testing resources may be helpful:

- Chemistry Panel and Complete Blood Count (CBC)
- Vitamin B12 and Folate
- Omega Score®

# PRECAUTIONS

The precautions listed below are primarily related to taking very high doses of B vitamins and nutrients that modulate homocysteine levels in the blood. Individuals who take a number of dietary supplements as part of their life extension strategy should account for all products that contain B vitamins when calculating how much of the vitamin they are ingesting each day.

## Folic Acid

Folic acid, when administered as a single agent at chronic doses above 1000 mg daily, may obscure the detection of vitamin B12 deficiency (specifically, the administration of folic acid may reverse the hematological manifestations of B12 deficiency, including pernicious anemia, while not addressing the neurological manifestations). Research has shown that 5-MTHF is less likely than folic acid to mask vitamin B12 deficiency.[29]

## Fibrate Therapy

Prescription fibrates may induce urinary TMG loss (common in patients with metabolic syndrome or diabetes mellitus).[113] Loss of TMG can increase blood levels of homocysteine because TMG supplies methyl groups during methionine/homocysteine metabolism and therefore can modulate plasma homocysteine levels. TMG supplementation could be considered in conjunction with fibrate therapy.

## Creatine Supplementation

A 2009 study found that high-dose creatine supplementation (21 g daily) in patients with coronary artery disease was associated with an 11–20% increase in homocysteine concentration.[114] Individuals supplementing with creatine at typical doses (5–10 g daily) are unlikely to experience elevations in homocysteine. However, high-dose creatine supplementation (>20 g daily) should be associated with regular monitoring of homocysteine levels.

## Balloon Angioplasty and Vascular Stenting

People undergoing balloon angioplasty and vascular stenting should lower their homocysteine levels to <7–8 μmol/L in order to reduce the risk of restenosis (see the section titled "Flawed Studies Lead to Confusion over B Vitamins and Heart Disease").

## Medical Foods Containing 5-MTHF

A number of drugs and medical food products on the market contain very high amounts (5 mg or 5000 mcg) of 5-MTHF and should be used under the supervision of a health care practitioner.

---

## REFERENCES

References available at: www.lef.org/dpt5/ch75

# 76

# *Hypoglycemia*

Hypoglycemia is diagnosed when blood glucose levels fall to abnormally low levels. Under normal conditions, and despite wide variations in food intake and energy expenditure, the body maintains a very narrow range of blood glucose levels.[1]

This careful balance is partly regulated by two hormones, insulin and glucagon, which have opposite effects. Both are produced in the pancreas in small clusters of cells called the islets of Langerhans. High blood levels of glucose stimulate the secretion of insulin, which results in cellular uptake of glucose, and subsequent lowering of blood glucose.

Low blood levels of glucose stimulate the secretion of glucagon from the liver. Glucagon stimulates a rise in blood glucose through two processes. First, glycogen (the animal version of starch) in the liver is metabolized into glucose. A normal liver stores relatively small amounts of glucose as glycogen, so glycogen stores can be depleted fairly quickly. Most people's glycogen stores are virtually gone within 24 hours of no caloric intake. When glycogen levels are low, or when energy needs are high, fatty acids and amino acids are converted into glucose in the liver and kidneys through the process of gluconeogenesis. Adrenal glands also play a role in increasing blood glucose. The hormone epinephrine stimulates glycogen breakdown, and cortisol promotes gluconeogenesis.

## TYPES AND CAUSES OF HYPOGLYCEMIA

Hypoglycemia is a result of any disorder that causes abnormal restrictions in the production of glucose by the liver or kidneys, or that causes an abnormal increase in glucose uptake by the cells.[2] Hypoglycemia can be divided broadly into 3 categories: reactive, drug induced, and fasting.

Reactive hypoglycemia occurs within 4 hours after eating if glucose levels rise too rapidly because of underlying conditions (eg, increased absorption of glucose from the small intestine). In response, the body overexcretes insulin, which drives the glucose from the blood, resulting in hypoglycemia. It may be caused by the following factors[3]:

- Increased sensitivity to counterregulatory hormones (eg, epinephrine)
- Deficiency in glucagon release
- Polycystic ovary syndrome
- Rare enzyme deficiencies (eg, hereditary fructose intolerance and galactosemia)

Drugs used in the treatment of diabetes (eg, insulin and sulfonylurea) are the most common cause of drug-induced hypoglycemia. These drugs are used to lower blood glucose levels. When used in excess, blood glucose levels drop rapidly and markedly, leading to hypoglycemia.[3] Alcohol-induced hypoglycemia can result from alcohol ingestion after fasting long enough to exhaust glycogen stores, making liver glucose output dependent on gluconeogenesis. Hypoglycemia can be induced by blood alcohol levels well below legal driving limits.[2]

Fasting hypoglycemia occurs after strenuous exercise or during an extended period between meals. It is relatively uncommon among healthy people. Fasting hypoglycemia can occur in people who drink heavily, have liver disease, and in children with genetic enzyme abnormalities that disrupt sugar metabolism.[3]

Hypoglycemia may also be caused by other factors[3]:

- Certain types of tumors secrete insulin-like growth factor, which acts in a manner similar to insulin.
- Autoimmune disorders may cause abnormal insulin secretion.
- Addison's disease, which affects the pituitary and adrenal glands, and chronic illnesses (eg, hepatic, renal, or cardiac failure or sepsis), which cause inadequate glucose to be delivered to the body's cells, may also cause hypoglycemia.

## SYMPTOMS OF HYPOGLYCEMIA

The symptoms of hypoglycemia can be divided into two categories.[3]

### Neurogenic Symptoms

Neurogenic symptoms, which include sweating, shakiness, tachycardia, and anxiety due to secretion of adrenal hormones (mainly epinephrine), are the earliest signs of hypoglycemia.

### Neuroglycopenic Symptoms

Neuroglycopenic symptoms include weakness, tiredness, or dizziness; difficulty with concentration; confusion;

blurred vision; fatigue; seizure; loss of consciousness; and in extreme cases, coma and death.

# DIAGNOSING HYPOGLYCEMIA

If hypoglycemia is suspected, diagnosis will be made by measuring glucose levels in the blood. If glucose levels are too low (usually below 60 mg/dL), the person is diagnosed hypoglycemic. To test for reactive hypoglycemia, blood glucose should be measured while symptoms are present. A blood glucose level below 70 mg/dL at the time of symptoms, followed by relief after eating, will confirm the diagnosis.

In standard tests for measuring blood glucose in the context of hypoglycemia, the person undergoes a supervised fast lasting 48–72 hours. This test is usually performed in a hospital to ensure safety. During that time, measurements of blood glucose, insulin, glucagon, cortisol, and other components of the glucose control system are measured. The pattern of results can help physicians diagnose the underlying cause of hypoglycemia. For example, persistently high insulin levels might suggest an insulin-secreting pancreatic tumor, while low glucose with low insulin levels and normal levels of ketones (markers of fatty acid breakdown) might suggest a disorder in lipid metabolism. Many other patterns may occur during such a fast, and each provides another clue to help the physician determine the cause of an individual's hypoglycemia.

# CONVENTIONAL TREATMENT

Treatment of hypoglycemia depends on the underlying cause; no single drug is used. The goal is to uncover the underlying cause and treat it, if possible.

In the case of reactive hypoglycemia, treatment usually focuses on dietary changes. For instance, people who suffer from hypoglycemic episodes after eating should eat small meals and snacks about every 3 hours, exercise regularly, eat a wide variety of foods, limit sugar, and eat plenty of high-fiber foods. These changes will help keep blood glucose levels stable throughout the day.

The following medications may be used to treat hypoglycemia.

## Diazoxide

The usual treatment of hypoglycemia caused by overdose of insulin or sulfonylurea drugs is the oral consumption of glucose or sucrose. However, several studies[4,5] have shown that diazoxide together with glucose is more effective in correcting hypoglycemia than glucose alone, and also reduces the amount of glucose needed. Diazoxide acts by inhibiting release of insulin, making this medication useful in the treatment of

conditions such as insulin-secreting tumors, in which too much insulin from internal sources is present.

## Glucagon

Since glucagon acts in a contrary fashion to insulin, it is used to treat severe hypoglycemic reactions due to insulin, particularly when oral consumption of glucose or sucrose is not possible. Glucagon treatment is not effective in people who have been fasting or have been hypoglycemic for a prolonged period; glucagon can act only by releasing glucose from glycogen stores, and if these are depleted by prolonged fasting, there is nothing to release.[6]

# DIETARY AND SUPPLEMENTAL THERAPY

A well-balanced diet will help normalize blood sugar levels. Usually a regimen moderate in protein, unrefined carbohydrates (eg, whole-grain products and vegetables, which are slow to be absorbed), and fats is recommended. Foods high in rapidly absorbed sugars should be avoided. This diet can help prevent reactive hypoglycemia due to a sudden influx of glucose into the blood.

Acute hypoglycemia therapy focuses on immediately raising the blood sugar level. Any substance containing carbohydrates (eg, saltine crackers, fruit juice, or hard candy), if taken at the beginning of a hypoglycemic episode, will help raise blood sugar quickly and ease the severity of an attack. A severe hypoglycemic attack is therefore a good time to consume rapidly absorbed simple sugars. Fruit juice, glucose syrup, or sugary soft drinks can be lifesaving. Milder attacks can be managed with foods that contain complex carbohydrates, which are less rapidly absorbed. However, these should not be used by a person having a severe attack (ie, a diabetic with an insulin reaction).

The use of a fiber supplement before meals also helps control the rate of absorption of dietary carbohydrates. Alcohol, caffeine, tobacco, and other stimulants should be avoided because they are capable of precipitating a hypoglycemic attack. Frequent small meals are recommended to control the amount of carbohydrates entering the system and prevent rapid declines in blood glucose levels.

The following nutrients have been shown to help normalize blood glucose levels.

## Chromium

Chromium is widely recognized as an essential trace element. It has multiple effects on insulin levels. Chromium has been widely studied (in the context of type 2 diabetes) for its ability to lower blood sugar levels at higher doses by increasing insulin sensitivity.[7] However, studies have also shown that chromium can help enhance glucagon secretion.[8]

## Amino Acids

Glutamine, the most abundant amino acid in the human body, is involved in more metabolic processes than any other amino acid.[9] Few clinical trials have been conducted to determine whether glutamine supplementation can increase glucose levels. Amino acid infusions, however, are known to raise glucagon levels, which produces an increase in glucose in otherwise healthy individuals.[10] Hypoglycemia was induced by insulin infusions in diabetic and nondiabetic subjects in two studies. The participants then received amino acid mixtures. The results indicated a sharp rise in glucagon secretion in normal participants and a modest rise in diabetic participants.[11]

A study in an animal model demonstrated that the liver's ability to produce glucose from certain amino acids was increased during insulin-induced hypoglycemia. Glucose levels increased in animals given the amino acid infusion, but not in control animals given only a saline infusion.[12]

## N-Acetylcysteine

N-acetylcysteine (NAC) is an amino acid with antioxidant properties. It has been shown to alleviate hypoglycemia in rodents exposed to toxic chemicals by preventing the rapid loss of glucose. For example, in one study of rats exposed to a toxin that causes hypoglycemia, administration of 200 mg/kg NAC prevented depletion of glucose.[13] In another study of rats exposed to arsenic, which is known to cause hypoglycemia, administration of 163.2 mg/kg of NAC daily prevented hypoglycemia.[14]

## Life Extension Suggestions

If you are diabetic and using medications, talk to your physician immediately if you experience hypoglycemic symptoms. You may need your medication adjusted.

The following supplements are suggested for assistance in maintaining normal blood glucose levels:

- **Chromium:** 200–500 mcg daily
- **L-glutamine powder:** 3–5 g daily between meals
- **N-acetylcysteine (NAC):** 500 mg daily

## REFERENCES

References available at: www.lef.org/dpt5/ch76

# 77

# *Immune System Strengthening*

Age, stress, and poor nutrition can sap our immune system of its effectiveness. Influenza provides one example; during young adulthood, when the body can mount a robust immune response to this common virus, influenza is rarely fatal. Among the elderly, however, the virus is associated with significant rates of death and hospitalization.[1]

The impact of aging on the immune system is profound. As people age, a number of critical immune system components including cellular response, antibody production, and response to vaccines are reduced or slowed. At the same time, susceptibility to infection and cancer is increased. Some of this increased susceptibility to disease is linked to chronic inflammation, which is associated with many disorders of aging.[2–4]

Age, however, is not the sole culprit in reduced immune function. There is no question that exercise, stress, and nutritional status play an important role in maintaining a healthy immune system. Consider the following research findings.

- Dietary deficiencies and malabsorption alter metabolism and exacerbate chronic disorders. An imbalance in the intake of dietary fat, carbohydrate, and protein can contribute to the development of disease(s).[5] On the other hand, there is overwhelming evidence of the benefits of a good diet on reducing the risk of many chronic diseases.[5,6]

- Malnutrition causes a decline in immune function and increases susceptibility to infection.[7–9] Likewise, a vitamin or mineral deficiency can suppress immune system function.[9] Correct choices of supplements, vitamins, minerals, fatty acids, probiotics, and botanicals have been shown to boost immunity and may also reduce the risk of disease(s) in healthy individuals.[10]

- Psychological health influences the immune system and the course of many diseases.[11] Depression, stress, and anxiety increase the production of proinflammatory chemicals in the blood, which in turn can compromise, depress, or suppress the immune system.[12–20]

- High levels of anxiety are associated with decreased immune function.[11,17,21,22]

- Chronic stress can provoke long-term increases in proinflammatory chemicals. For example, caregiving for a relative with a serious medical condition results in long-term immune suppression among women.[18]

- Chronic stress from persistent marital problems, burnout at work,[23] and lengthy unemployment[24] can lead to immune alterations that persist for years.[17, 25–28.]

Life Extension believes that all aging people should take action to bolster their immune systems. This includes reducing negative psychological stress; following a physician-approved, moderate, long-term exercise program; and following a diet as well as consuming nutrients that have been shown to enhance immune response and promote health.

## THE IMMUNE SYSTEM: HOW IT WORKS

The immune system is an elegant and complex set of components that combine to fight disease, infection(s), and various pathogens. A healthy immune system distinguishes organisms in the body as "self" or "nonself." An intact immune response identifies pathogens as "nonself" and rapidly destroys them. A depressed immune system, by contrast, will allow invading organisms to flourish.

When the immune system mistakenly recognizes a "self" cell as "nonself" and mounts an immune response, it can result in an autoimmune disorder (eg, rheumatoid arthritis).

In general, the body has two primary defense mechanisms: natural immunity and acquired immunity. Natural immunity is the "first responder" to attack. Natural immune response relies on various white blood cells and physical barriers to block or immediately attack any foreign invader and attempt to destroy it.

Acquired immunity, on the other hand, involves antibodies created in response to specific foreign antigens. This sort of response requires a few days for the body to recognize the invader and manufacture antibodies against it. Once the body has manufactured a particular antibody for a specific invader, the immune system response is faster and more effective the next time that invader appears.[29,30]

The natural immune system relies on a host of weapons to protect the body, including various kinds of white blood cells (see Table 1). These natural defenses include the following organs, chemicals, and processes.

## Table 1:    Major Cells of the Immune System[29,124]

| Cell | Activity |
|---|---|
| **Lymphocytes** | |
| Natural killer cells | Destroy a variety of tumor cells and antibody-coated target cells; not antigen specific. |
| Cytotoxic T (CD8+) cells | Secrete cytokines that attract macrophages and increase their phagocytic activity; destroy target cells that display the same antigen that activated their progenitor cell; lyse infected cells by releasing toxins. Cytotoxic T cells fight foreign invaders by destroying cells that display the antigen which activated its progenitor cells (immunologic surveillance). |
| Helper T (T4+) cells | Stimulate cellular immunity and inflammation; secrete cytokines that stimulate proliferation of B cells and other T cells; amplify antibody production by plasma cells. |
| Suppressor T cells | Suppress activity of naïve (unstimulated) and effector T cells. |
| Memory T cells | Recognize antigens that have invaded in the past, which allows for a larger and more rapid response when there is a second encounter with that antigen. |
| B lymphocytes (B cells) | Differentiate into antibody-producing plasma cells; process and present antigen to helper T cells; display immunoglobulin and class II MHC antigens. |
| Plasma cells | Main antibody-secreting cells. |
| Memory B cells | Descendants of B cells that remain after an immune response. |
| **Phagocytes** | |
| Macrophages | Phagocytize antigens, then process and present them to T cells for destruction; attack dead and defective blood cells; secrete cytokines that induce proliferation of B and T cells. |
| Neutrophils | Major defense against bacteria; first on scene to fight infection. |
| Eosinophils | Active against parasites and commonly elevated in allergies. |
| Dendritic cells (interdigitating reticular cells) | Process and present antigens to T and B cells; most potent stimulators of T cell responses. |
| Antigen-presenting cells | Engulf antigens, process them internally, and then display fragments of them on their surface; surface markers alert other immune cells that there is an invader. Identified antigen-presenting cells: dendritic cells, macrophages, and B lymphocytes. |

## Physical and Chemical Barriers

The body's first lines of defense are the skin and mucous membranes, which prevent the entrance of many pathogens. There are also many secondary barriers. For example, tears, sweat, and saliva combat some bacteria; also, the hydrochloric acid as well as protein-digesting enzymes secreted by the stomach are lethal to many, but not all pathogens.[29,30]

## Inflammation and Fever

Inflammation is a nonspecific response to infection or tissue injury. The 4 signs of inflammatory response are redness, swelling, heat, and pain. Inflammation begins when cells release certain cytokines, including interleukin (IL)-1, IL-6, and tumor necrosis factor-alpha (TNF-α).[29,30]

## Phagocytic Cells

Phagocytic cells engulf and destroy foreign cells. Phagocytic cells are white blood cells and include neutrophils, eosinophils, and macrophages; they have short lives and must be continually replenished by the body. Neutrophils and macrophages are very important aspects of the innate defenses of the body.[29,30]

## Natural Killer Cells

Natural killer cells destroy certain cancer cells and a variety of pathogens. Killer cells are active secretors of interferon, an important and potent protein. Natural killer cells attach directly to the surfaces of infected cells and cause them to burst. They can also kill a pathogen by making its outer membrane leak.[29,30]

## Antimicrobial Proteins

Infected immune cells produce interferon, which causes healthy cells to produce antiviral proteins. There are more than 30 distinct antiviral proteins. When an individual complement (immune system) protein is activated by infecting organisms, it triggers a cascade that activates other complement proteins. Activated proteins can destroy bacteria while sparing host cells or cause the infected cells to become engulfed by phagocytic cells.[29,30]

## Cytokines

Cells use chemical messengers (ie, cytokines) to communicate and share information; each chemical sends a different message to other cells. Cytokines regulate immunity, inflammation, and the production of white blood cells. There are dozens of cytokines; each performs a specific set of activities against specific target cells. They can act in concert or in opposition. Cytokines are often produced in a cascade; in other words, a cytokine stimulates its target cells to make additional cytokines. TNF-α, IL-1, IL-6, and type I interferon are important cytokines in the regulation of natural immunity.

## Acute-Phase Proteins

Acute-phase response is activated during critical illness. When phagocytic cells bind pathogens, they release proinflammatory cytokines. This response enables the body to recognize invaders before immune responses have been fully activated. Acute-phase proteins promote inflammation and stimulate phagocytes to move where they are needed.

## Inflammation, Free Radicals, and Cytokines

Although acute inflammation is an important immune system response, chronic inflammation has also been linked to many diseases, including heart disease. Besides being associated with proinflammatory cytokines, inflammation may be related to the overproduction of free radicals.[29]

A free radical is an atom or group of atoms (ie, a molecule) with unpaired electrons. Free radicals are extremely unstable and react easily with other molecules, thereby changing their chemical composition. Oxygen is especially susceptible to free radical formation. Free radicals derived from oxygen are known as reactive oxygen species (ROS), or oxidants.

When the body has increased levels of ROS (ie, when it is experiencing oxidative stress), widespread damage may result. At high concentrations, free radicals can damage fats, proteins, and nucleic acids. They can also cause cell death, gene mutations, and cancer. Several diseases may be the result of cellular and genetic damage caused by free radicals, including several immune disorders.[31]

In order to reduce the damage caused by elevated free radicals and cytokines (both part of the natural immune system), the body fights back by producing antioxidants and hormones (eg, cortisol) to suppress the immune system.[32] Antioxidants are valuable because they pair with unstable free radicals, thereby limiting the damage free radicals can inflict on other cells.

## WHAT YOU HAVE LEARNED SO FAR

- The immune system declines as we age, making us more susceptible to various diseases and pathogens.
- Immune system health is closely related to stress, frequency of exercise, and nutritional status. Poor intake of vital nutrients is closely associated with depressed immune response and increased rate of disease.
- The immune system has two primary defense mechanisms: natural, which uses white blood cells and physical barriers to protect against disease, and acquired, in which specialized cells generate antibodies to defend against specific pathogens.
- Inflammation is caused by multiple factors, including microorganisms, physical stress, tissue death, and inappropriate immune response. Chronic inflammation is linked to diseases such as heart disease. Inflammation is mediated by cytokines and free radicals. It is an important immune system response, but can also be dangerous because a chronic inflammatory state is linked to various diseases of aging.
- Free radicals are unstable molecules that readily react with other molecules, especially oxygen, to change their chemical composition. Antioxidants are used by the body to scavenge for free radicals and limit the amount of damage they can cause.

# NUTRITION, IMMUNITY, AND GENETICS

Researchers are just now beginning to understand how genes affect nutrition and overall immunity. It turns out that the overall risk of contracting many diseases is influenced by genetics.[33] A new field of nutritional genomics explores the interaction of nutrition, genes, and environmental factors (including diet).[5]

This emerging field of science evolved from the Human Genome Project, which mapped the human genome and identified many genes that cause disease.

The association between diet and chronic diseases such as atherosclerosis, diabetes, obesity, and cancer is well known.[5,34-36] Nutrients supplied by food are an important variable in gene expression. Deficiency of some essential nutrients can alter metabolism and the structure of DNA.[5] A well-studied example of the relationship between genetics and diet is type 2 diabetes. This condition is associated with a sedentary lifestyle, being overweight, and ethnicity. Although some individuals are genetically predisposed to this condition, many can control symptoms through exercise and a change in diet.[5]

In the future, genetic testing might be able to help in the creation of nutritional programs tailored to each individual's genetic makeup; thus, may help people fight disease and stay healthy.

# SUPPORTING A HEALTHY IMMUNE SYSTEM

A healthy immune system grows ever more important as we age, and immune status is closely associated with nutrition, exercise, and stress reduction. Older people and people with compromised immune systems should talk to their physician about exercising, reducing stress, and designing an active, immune-boosting nutritional program.

## Vitamin D

Adults (and children) with higher vitamin D levels contract substantially fewer cold, flu, and other viral infections.[37-39] Vitamin D down-regulates the expression of proinflammatory cytokines while up-regulating the expression of antimicrobial peptides in immune cells.[40] This biological mechanism explains why vitamin D confers such dramatic protection against common illnesses.

## Glutathione Boosters

Glutathione is probably the body's most important cellular defense against free radical damage. It is a free radical scavenger and major antioxidant.

Low levels of glutathione are linked to many diseases. Malnutrition and aging[41] deplete glutathione. Glutathione is also involved in one of the major liver detoxification pathways.

Glutathione is produced in the body, but not easily absorbed when taken orally. Instead, glutathione precursors may be used by the body to increase glutathione[42] Glutathione precursors include glutamine, N-acetylcysteine (NAC), and S-adenosyl-L-methionine (SAMe).[43] It can also be up-regulated by lipoic acid as well as vitamins C and E.

## Glutamine

Glutamine is the most abundant amino acid in the body. Glutamine depletion causes down-regulation of glutathione levels in the body, and dietary supplementation increases these levels.[44] Glutamine has immunoregulatory activities.[44,45] Lymphocytes and macrophages use glutamine at a very high rate.[46] Glutamine stimulates lymphocyte production and killer immune cell activity.[47-50]

Glutamine depletion slows wound healing and increases the risk of organ failure under certain conditions.[51] Endurance athletes whose muscles do not fully recover between workouts have decreased glutamine levels.[52,53] Some scientists believe that intense physical exercise or stress due to trauma, burns, or sepsis (blood infection) forces the body into glutamine debt, which temporarily compromises immune function.[46]

## S-Adenosyl-L-Methionine

S-adenosyl-L-methionine (SAMe) is a natural amino acid present throughout the body. It is crucially important

because it is involved in dozens of chemical reactions, including the synthesis of DNA and RNA, proteins, melatonin, creatine, and many others. Being an important energy source,[54] SAMe is intrinsically related to the synthesis of glutathione.

## N-Acetylcysteine

N-acetylcysteine (NAC) acts as an antioxidant and is recommended for conditions that increase oxidative stress or decrease glutathione levels.[55] NAC has a protective effect on DNA and is a powerful free radical scavenger. It increases the synthesis of glutathione only when there is a demand, and is thought to concentrate only in tissues where it is required.[55] NAC can modulate the concentrations of certain cytokines. In laboratory studies, it has increased IL-1 and IL-2 levels when they are at low concentrations and decreased these cytokines at higher concentrations.[56] It also demonstrated an ability to inhibit cell growth and proliferation in cancer cell lines,[57] and prevent the transformation of carcinogens into more toxic compounds.[58,59]

## Antioxidants

Because of their ability to scavenge free radicals, antioxidants are important immune-system boosters. Supplementation with antioxidants like vitamins C, E, and B vitamins may improve immune function,[60] and supplementation with vitamin A stimulates antibody-mediated immune responses.[61]

**Vitamin E.** Vitamin E is a powerful fat-soluble antioxidant. It protects cellular membranes of the immune system and other cells by trapping free radicals, and enhances the effectiveness of lymphocytes.[10]

**Vitamin C.** Vitamin C (ascorbic acid) is a key component of the immune system and antioxidant defense.[62-64] It prevents the production of free radicals and reduces DNA damage in immune cells. Moreover, vitamin C down-regulates the production of proinflammatory cytokines and participates in recycling vitamin E.[65]

**B vitamins.** B vitamins indirectly contribute to antioxidant defenses and have considerable influence on immune function. Vitamins B12 and B6 are cofactors in the creation of cysteine, a key component in glutathione synthesis. Deficiencies in B vitamins and vitamin E create abnormalities in immune response.[66]

**Lipoic acid.** Lipoic acid is a potent antioxidant with antiviral, free-radical-quenching, and immune-boosting qualities. It is unusual because it is soluble in both fat and water,[63] and is active in both its oxidized and reduced forms.[67] Lipoic acid is able to regenerate other antioxidants (eg, vitamins C and E) and raise glutathione levels significantly.[68-71]

**Coenzyme Q10.** Coenzyme Q10 (CoQ10), synthesized from the amino acid tyrosine, is present in high quantities in the heart muscle. CoQ10 has shown a wide range of benefits. It is an essential cofactor in the production of adenosine triphosphate (ATP), which is the primary source of energy for all the body's cells. Levels of CoQ10 decline naturally as humans age, which may be related to increased lipid peroxidation. CoQ10 is a powerful antioxidant and scavenger of free radicals. It inhibits lipid peroxidation and works synergistically with vitamin E.[72] CoQ10 has an important role in the stimulation of the immune system and improves several parameters of immune function.[73]

**Whey protein.** Whey protein is isolated from milk. Proteins in whey are highly available to the body, and whey protein contains potent antioxidants. Its antioxidant activity is due to its high concentrations of glutamate and cysteine, which are precursors to glutathione.[74] Whey also contains several substances that enhance the immune system, including the following:

- Beta-lactoglobulin, which modulates lymphatic responses[75]
- Alpha-lactalbumin, which has a direct effect on B and T lymphocytes and has the ability to reduce oxidative stress
- Lactoperoxidase, which reduces toxic hydrogen peroxide[76,77]

Lactoferrin, a major component of whey protein, also acts as an antioxidant.[78] It can inhibit the absorption of bacteria through the intestinal wall. Whey protein can activate natural killer cells.[79] In the laboratory, lactoferrin inhibited metastasis of cancer cells in mice,[80] and increased IL-2 and natural killer activity.[81]

## Minerals

**Copper, zinc, and selenium.** Metallic micronutrients such as copper, zinc,[82] and selenium influence the activity of antioxidant enzymes and can reduce oxidative stress. Among children, deficiencies of zinc, copper, and selenium have been linked to immune deficiency and infection.[83]

Selenium is involved in several key metabolic pathways.[84-86] Glutathione peroxidase, the enzyme that recycles glutathione, depends on the presence of selenium for its antioxidant activity.[87] Although plant food is a major dietary source of selenium (eg, garlic is rich in selenium), the highest concentration of dietary selenium occurs in meat.

Zinc deficiency is linked to impaired immune function, partly because of decreased T-lymphocyte and B-lymphocyte function. Zinc has shown the ability to decrease inflammation and the production of IL-2.[88] Copper and zinc together have been shown to stimulate internally produced antioxidants such as glutathione and superoxide dismutase (SOD).[89]

## Dehydroepiandrosterone

Dehydroepiandrosterone (DHEA) is produced by the adrenal glands. DHEA has over 100 metabolites and is used by the body for estrogen and testosterone production.

Blood levels of DHEA rise until they peak in the third decade of life, then rapidly decline. Endocrinologists and antiaging researchers have been focusing on this decrease in DHEA, which in turn produces a decline in other steroidal hormones.

Animal experiments suggest that DHEA has many biological effects, including anticancer, immune-enhancing, neurotrophic, and general antiaging effects.[90] A published review article of DHEA supplementation in men found convincing research showing positive effects of DHEA on the cardiovascular system, body composition, skin, central nervous system, sexual function, and immune system.[91]

On the cellular level, DHEA exerts its actions on peripheral target tissues either indirectly (following its conversion to androgens, estrogens, or both) or directly, as a steroid hormone.[92] Lower DHEA levels are associated with decreased production of IL-2 and an increase in the presence of IL-6, which is a proinflammatory cytokine.[93] A study was performed on younger and older men to compare DHEA blood levels and peripheral blood mononuclear cells (PBMCs) in populations of varying ages. The results showed significant changes in sex steroid metabolism by human PBMCs with aging, which may represent a link to age-associated changes in the immune system.[93]

Immunomodulatory effects of DHEA in various autoimmune diseases have been studied. Relative reductions in DHEA have been noted in patients with rheumatoid arthritis, systemic lupus erythematosus, HIV and AIDS, sepsis, and trauma.[94] Overall, DHEA blood levels have been used as diagnostic factors in evaluating the impact of aging on the immune system. Supplemental DHEA has been clinically valuable when used to restore youthful hormonal blood levels in aging, stressed, and immune-compromised individuals.[95]

One of DHEA's metabolites, 7-Keto® DHEA, has also been studied for its ability to support the immune system. A study found that 4 weeks of 7-Keto® DHEA supplementation improved immune function in elderly men and women.[96] In this randomized, double-blind, placebo-controlled study, 22 women and 20 men over the age of 65 took either 100 mg of 7-Keto® twice daily or a placebo. The 7-Keto® group had a significant decrease in immune suppressor cells and a significant increase in immune helper cells. The 7-Keto® group also saw reductions in diastolic blood pressure and an increase in neutrophils, the first white blood cells to respond to infection.

## Polyunsaturated Fatty Acids

Polyunsaturated fatty acids, such as the omega-3 fatty acids found in fish oil and flaxseed oil, have been studied for their anti-inflammatory action.[10] Polyunsaturated fatty acids reduce the inflammatory response caused by TNF-α.[97,98]

Most people in the United States have an imbalance in the ratio of omega-3 to omega-6 fatty acids because of diets high in animal fat and vegetable oils high in omega-6 (eg, corn oil). This imbalance has been associated with inflammation.[99] The ratio can be improved by taking supplemental omega-3 fatty acids. Omega-3 fatty acids have also been shown to:

- Counteract suppression of the cellular immune system[98]
- Suppress TNF-α production and have an anti-inflammatory effect[100]

## Probiotics

The gastrointestinal tract relies on live bacteria (microflora) to help support a robust immune response. These probiotic bacteria help prevent foreign bacteria and allergens from passing through the intestinal wall and are important to the overall health of the intestinal immune system.[101-103] Probiotics are found in foods such as yogurt and kefir, which enhance the microflora in the gut by providing additional probiotic bacteria.[104,105] The most commonly used probiotic bacteria are lactobacillus and bifidobacterium in yogurts.

Probiotics also strengthen the intestinal immunological barrier. Lactobacillus stimulates natural immunity by improving phagocytic and natural killer immune cell activity.[10]

## Grape Seed Extract

Chemicals in grape seeds known as proanthocyanidins have potent antioxidant and immune-boosting properties.[106-108] They increase the activity of internal antioxidants such as glutathione and SOD.[109]

The antioxidants in grape seed extract are twice as potent as vitamin E and 4 times as potent as vitamin C.[107,108] In laboratory studies, proanthocyanidins increased the power of natural killer cells, enhanced the production of IL-2, and decreased production of IL-6.[110]

## Green Tea Extract

Green tea extract, which contains a class of compounds known as catechins, has become increasingly popular as scientists learn more about its antioxidant and free radical–scavenging abilities. One of the most potent catechins in green tea is epigallocatechin-3-gallate.[111] Green tea extract is also rich in vitamins C and B.[112,113]

Green tea has a positive influence on lipid metabolism and exerts anticancer effects. Green tea modulates the inflammatory processes and protects against DNA damage.[114] The catechins from green tea demonstrate considerable antioxidant activity[111] and are potent free radical scavengers.[115,116]

## Hyperimmune Egg Extract

Hyperimmune egg extracts provide unique immune protection. Long ago, agricultural scientists discovered that they could immunize hens against germs that threaten humans. This immunity was then passed on by the hen to her egg.[117-119] Concentrated protein extracts from those so-called "hyperimmune eggs" confer some immunity to humans who consume them.[120,121]

## Andrographis

Healers in Asia and India have long prescribed the bitter herb *Andrographis paniculata* for the treatment of ailments ranging from infections and inflammation to colds and fevers.[122] Researchers have isolated a number of the herb's active ingredients. Chief among these are andrographolides, which are phytochemicals believed to exert their effects, in part, on tissues of the blood cell-producing bone marrow and/or spleen. One such compound, andrographanin, enhances the ability of certain white blood cells to recognize and neutralize foreign cells (eg, tumor cells and viruses).[122]

## Beta Glucan

Beta glucans can naturally boost the immune system by optimizing its response to diseases and infections. Because the body does not produce beta glucans naturally, the only way to get them is through outside sources. Studies have shown that beta glucans act as immunomodulator agents, meaning they trigger a cascade of events that help regulate the immune system, making it more efficient. Specifically, beta glucans stimulate the activity of macrophages, which are versatile immune cells that ingest and demolish invading pathogens and stimulate other immune cells to attack.[123] Macrophages also release cytokines, chemicals that when secreted enable immune cells to communicate with one another. In addition, beta glucans stimulate lethal white blood cells (lymphocytes) that bind to tumors or viruses, and release chemicals to destroy it.

## Life Extension Suggestions

- **Comprehensive multivitamin:** per label instructions
- **Selenium:** 200–400 mcg daily
- **Zinc:** 30–90 mg daily
- **Vitamin D:** 5000–8000 IU daily (depending on blood levels of 25-OH-vitamin D)
- **Vitamin C:** 1000–5000 mg daily
- **Garlic extract:** 1200 mg daily
- **Andrographis extract:** 25–150 mg daily 30 minutes before a meal
- **Beta glucan** (highly purified beta 1,3/1,6 glucan): 100–600 mg daily 30 minutes before a meal
- **Whey protein isolate:** 20–40 g daily

- **DHEA:** 15–25 mg daily for women; 25–75 mg daily for men (depending on blood test results)
- **L-carnitine:** 1–2 g daily
- **CoQ10** (as ubiquinol): 100–200 mg daily
- **Lactoferrin (apolactoferrin):** 300 mg daily
- **Probiotics:** per label instructions
- **Fish oil** (with olive polyphenols): providing 1400 mg EPA and 1000 mg DHA daily
- **Thymus extract:** per label instructions
- **Grape extract** (containing seed and skin extracts): 150 mg daily
- **Green tea extract** (standardized to 98% polyphenols): 725 mg daily
- **NAC:** 600–1800 mg daily
- **R-lipoic acid:** 300–600 mg daily
- **Hyperimmune egg extract:** per label instructions

In addition, the following *blood tests* may provide helpful in formation:

- Vitamin D, 25-Hydroxy
- Chemistry panel and complete blood count (CBC)

## REFERENCES

References available at: www.lef.org/dpt5/ch77

# 78

# Inflammation (Chronic)

Of the 10 leading causes of *mortality* in the United States, *chronic low-level inflammation* contributes to the pathogenesis of at least seven. These include heart disease, cancer, chronic lower respiratory disease, stroke, Alzheimer's disease, diabetes, and nephritis.[1–9]

Inflammation has classically been viewed as an *acute* (short-term) response to tissue injury that produces characteristic symptoms and usually resolves spontaneously. More contemporary revelations show *chronic* inflammation to be a major factor in the development of degenerative disease and loss of youthful functions.

*Chronic inflammation* can be triggered by cellular stress and dysfunction, such as that caused by excessive calorie consumption, elevated blood sugar levels, and oxidative stress. It is now clear that the destructive capacity of *chronic* inflammation is unprecedented among physiologic processes.[10]

The danger of chronic, low-level inflammation is that its *silent* nature belies its *destructive* power.

In fact, stress-induced inflammation, once triggered, can persist undetected for years, or even decades, propagating cell death throughout the body. Due to the fact that it contributes so greatly to deterioration associated with the aging process, this silent state of chronic inflammation has been coined "inflammaging."

Chronic low-level inflammation may be *threatening your health* at this very moment, without you realizing it. In this protocol you will learn about low-cost blood tests that can assess the inflammatory state within your body. You will also discover novel approaches that combat chronic inflammation to help avoid age-related health decline.

## THE INFLAMMATORY PROCESS

### The Acute Inflammatory Response

Inflammation, the adaptive immune response to tissue injury or infection, plays a central role in metabolism in a variety of organisms.[11]

At its most basic level, an acute inflammatory response is triggered by (1) tissue injury (trauma, exposure to heat or chemicals) or (2) infection by viruses, bacteria, parasites, or fungi. The classic manifestation of acute inflammation is characterized by four cardinal signs. Redness and heat result from the increased blood flow to the site of injury. Swelling results from the accumulation of fluid at the injury site, a consequence of the increased blood flow. Finally, swelling can compress nerve endings near the injury, causing the characteristic pain associated with inflammation. Pain is also important to make the organism aware of the tissue damage. Additionally, inflammation in a joint usually results in a fifth sign (impairment of function), which has the effect of limiting movement and forcing rest of the injured joint to aid in healing.

A well-controlled acute inflammatory response has several protective roles:

- Prevents the spread of infectious agents and damage to nearby tissues
- Helps remove damaged tissue and pathogens
- Assists the body's repair processes

However, a third type of stimuli, *cellular stress and malfunction*, triggers *chronic inflammation*, which, rather than benefiting health, contributes to disease and age-related deterioration via numerous mechanisms.

## Cellular Stress and Chronic, Low-Level Inflammation

*Mitochondria*—cellular organelles responsible for generating biochemical energy in the form of *adenosine triphosphate* (ATP)—are a fundamentally necessary component of life in higher organisms. In fact, in the case of sophisticated multicellular life forms, organismal viability depends on optimal mitochondrial function. Paradoxically, mitochondrial processes can also bring about a tissue-destroying inflammatory mediator known as *the inflammasome*; this phenomenon is provoked by damaged and dysfunctional mitochondria.[12]

*Mitochondrial dysfunction* arises consequent of exposure to exogenous (eg, environmental toxins, tobacco smoke) and endogenous (eg, reactive oxygen species) stressors, and as a result of the aging process itself. For example, a byproduct of mitochondrial energy generation is the creation of *free radical molecules*. Free radicals can damage cellular structures and initiate a cascade of proinflammatory genetic signals that ultimately results in cell death (apoptosis), or worse, uncontrolled cell growth—the hallmark of cancer.

Aging is associated with declining mitochondrial efficiency and increased production of free radical molecules. Recent research identifies this age-associated aberration of mitochondrial function as a principle actuator of chronic inflammation.[13] Specifically, mitochondrial dysfunction brings about inflammation as follows:

1. Accumulation of free radicals induces mitochondrial membrane permeability.

2. Molecular components normally contained within the mitochondria leak into the *cytoplasm* (intracellular fluid in which cellular organelles are suspended).

3. Cytoplasmic *pattern recognition receptors* (PRRs), which detect and initiate an immune response against intracellular pathogens, recognize the leaked mitochondrial molecules as potential threats.

4. Upon detection of the potential threat, PRRs form a complex called the inflammasome that activates the inflammatory cytokine *interleukin-1β*, which then recruits components of the immune system to destroy the "infected" cell.[14]

These four steps represent a simplified scheme of mitochondrial dysfunction leading to cellular destruction; however, intracellular free radicals are not the only inducers of inflammatory cell death.

Circulating sugars, primarily *glucose* and *fructose*, are culprits as well. When these "blood sugars" come in contact with proteins and lipids, a damaging reaction occurs that forms compounds called *advanced glycation end products* (AGEs). AGEs bind to the cell-surface receptor called *receptor for advanced glycation end products*, or RAGE. Upon activation, RAGE triggers the movement of the inflammatory mediator *nuclear factor kappa-B* (NF-κB) to the nucleus, where it activates numerous inflammatory genes.[15] Advanced glycation end products are primarily formed *in vivo*, and glycation is exacerbated by elevated blood sugar levels. However, dietary AGEs also contribute to inflammation; they are abundant in foods cooked at high temperatures, especially red meat.[16,17]

Additional biochemical inducers of a chronic inflammatory response include:

• *Uric acid (urate)* crystals, which can be deposited in joints during gouty arthritis; elevated levels are a risk factor for kidney disease, hypertension, and metabolic syndrome[18,19]

• *Oxidized lipoproteins* (such as LDL), a significant contributor to atherosclerotic plaques[20]

• *Homocysteine*, a non-protein-forming amino acid that is a marker and risk factor for cardiovascular disease, and may increase bone fracture risk[21]

Together, these proinflammatory instigators promote a perpetual low-level chronic inflammatory state called *parainflammation*.[11]

Although it progresses silently, parainflammation presents a major threat to the health and longevity of all aging humans. Chronic, low-level inflammation is associated with common diseases including cancer, type 2 diabetes, osteoporosis, cardiovascular diseases, and others. Thus, by targeting the myriad physiological variables that can inaugurate an inflammatory response, one can effectively temper chronic inflammation and reduce their risk for inflammatory diseases.

## MARKERS AND MEDIATORS OF INFLAMMATION

Following is a list of some of the most prominent markers of inflammation used in research and diagnosis. Some can be detected by blood tests.

### Tumor necrosis factor alpha

Tumor necrosis factor alpha (TNF-α) is an intercellular signaling protein called a cytokine, which can be released by multiple types of immune cells in response to cellular damage, stress, or infection. Originally identified as an anti-tumor compound produced by macrophages (immune cells),[22] TNF-α is required for proper immune surveillance and function. Acting alone or with other inflammatory mediators, TNF-α slows the growth of many pathogens. It activates the bactericidal effects of neutrophils, and is required for the replication of several other immune cell types.[23] Excessive TNF-α, however, can lead to a chronic inflammatory state, can increase thrombosis (blood clotting) and decrease cardiac contractility, and may be implicated in tumor initiation and promotion.[7]

### Nuclear factor kappa-B

Nuclear factor kappa-B (NF-κB) is important in the initiation of the inflammatory response. When cells are exposed to damage signals (such as TNF-α or oxidative stress), they activate NF-κB, which turns on the expression of over 400 genes involved in the inflammatory response.[23] These include other inflammatory cytokines, and proinflammatory enzymes including *cyclooxygenase-2* (COX-2) and *lipoxygenase*. COX-2 is the enzyme responsible for synthesizing proinflammatory prostaglandins, and is the target of nonsteroidal anti-inflammatory drugs (NSAIDs) (ibuprofen, aspirin) and COX-2 inhibitors (Celebrex®).

### Interleukins

Interleukins (IL) are cytokines that have many functions in the promotion and resolution of inflammation. Pro-inflammatory interleukins that have been the subject of most research include IL-1β, IL-6, and IL-8. IL-1β helps immune cells to move out of blood vessels and into damaged or dysfunctional tissues. IL-6 has both proinflammatory and anti-inflammatory roles, and coordinates the production of compounds required during the progression and resolution of acute inflammation. IL-8 is expressed by both immune and nonimmune cells, and helps attract neutrophils (immune cells that can destroy pathogens) to sites of injury.

## C-reactive protein

C-reactive protein (CRP) is an acute-phase protein, one of several proteins rapidly produced by the liver during an inflammatory response. Its primary goal in acute inflammation is to coat damaged cells to make them easier to recognize by other immune cells.[24] CRP elevation above basal levels is not diagnostic on its own, as it can raise in several cancers, rheumatologic, gastrointestinal, and cardiovascular conditions, and infections.[25] Elevation of CRP (as determined by a high-sensitivity CRP assay or hs-CRP) has a strong association with elevated risk of cardiovascular disease and stroke.[26]

## Eicosanoids

Eicosanoids are "local" messages produced by cells that are proximal to the site of inflammation, and are meant to travel short distances (locally within the same organ, to neighboring cells, or sometimes only to different parts of the same cell) in order to elicit immune defenses.[27] These are in contrast to the cytokine factors mentioned above (interleukins, TNF-α), which are "long-distance messages." Eicosanoids are produced by cells at the site of inflammation and released into the blood, carrying information about the inflammatory response throughout the body. There are several families of eicosanoids (including prostaglandins, prostacyclins, leukotrienes, and thromboxanes) that are created by most cell types in all major organ systems. Aside from their roles in inflammation (and anti-inflammation), prostaglandins have a variety of functions in cell growth, kidney function, digestion, and the constriction and dilation of blood vessels. Thromboxanes are important mediators of the blood-clotting process. Proinflammatory leukotrienes are important for recruiting and activating white blood cells during inflammation, and are best studied for their role in airway constriction and anaphylaxis.

Cells produce eicosanoids using unsaturated fatty acids that are part of their cell membranes. The fatty acid starting materials for eicosanoid synthesis are the essential fatty acids linoleic acid (omega-6) and its derivative arachidonic acid (AA); and alpha-linolenic acid (an omega-3) and its derivatives *eicosapentaenoic* acid (EPA) and *docosahexaenoic* acid (DHA). While generalizations about roles of these fatty acids in eicosanoid synthesis should be approached cautiously, the most potent inflammatory eicosanoids are produced from omega-6 fatty acids (linoleic and arachidonic acids). Diets high in omega-3 fatty acids are associated with lower biomarkers of inflammation and cardiovascular disease risk; proposed mechanisms include the production of less inflammatory or anti-inflammatory eicosanoids and through the cyclooxygenase and lipoxygenase enzymes.[28]

## Cyclooxygenases and lipoxygenases

Cyclooxygenases (COX) and lipoxygenases (LOX) are enzymes that catalyze the first steps required by eicosanoids to be synthesized from unsaturated fatty acids. Cyclooxygenases initiate the conversion of omega-3 and omega-6 derivatives into one of the many prostaglandins or thromboxanes. The interest in COX enzyme metabolism comes from the fact that its inhibition leads to decreased prostaglandin synthesis, and therefore a reduction in inflammation, fever, and pain. The analgesic and anti-inflammatory activity of aspirin and the NSAIDs (like ibuprofen and naproxen) is due to their inhibition of COX enzymes. There are two COX enzymes with well-defined roles in humans (COX-1 and COX-2). COX-2 has the most relevance to the inflammatory process; it is normally inactive, but is turned on during inflammation and stimulates this process of inflammation by creating proinflammatory prostaglandins and thromboxanes.

Lipoxygenases convert fatty acids into proinflammatory *leukotrienes*, important local mediators of inflammation. Several potent inflammatory leukotrienes are produced by 5-LOX in mammals. Lipoxygenase enzymes, and the proinflammatory factors they produce, have a fundamental role in the inflammatory process by aiding in the recruitment of white blood cells to the site of inflammation. They also stimulate local cells to produce cytokines, which amplifies the inflammatory response.[27] Thus, LOX enzymes may be involved in a wide variety of inflammatory conditions, and represent an additional target for anti-inflammatory therapy.

While COX and LOX enzymes are most often associated with proinflammatory processes, it is important to remember that both enzymes also produce factors that inhibit or resolve inflammation and promote tissue repair (including the prostacyclins and lipoxins). The proper transition from the pro- to anti-inflammatory activities of the COX and LOX enzymes is important for the progression of a healthy inflammatory response.

## RISK FACTORS FOR CHRONIC INFLAMMATION

Several risk factors increase the likelihood of establishing and maintaining a low-level inflammatory response.

## Age

In contrast to younger individuals (whose levels of inflammatory cytokines typically increase only in response to infection or injury), older adults can have consistently elevated levels of several inflammatory molecules, especially IL-6 and TNF-α.[9] These elevations are observed even in healthy older individuals. While the reasoning for this age-associated increase in inflammatory markers is not thoroughly understood, it may reflect cumulative mitochondrial dysfunction and oxidative damage, or may be the result of other risk factors associated with age (such as increases in visceral body fat or reductions in sex hormones).

## Obesity

Fat tissue is an endocrine organ, storing and secreting multiple hormones and cytokines into circulation and affecting metabolism throughout the body. For example, fat cells produce and secrete both TNF-α and IL-6, and visceral (abdominal) fat can produce these inflammatory molecules at levels sufficient to induce a strong inflammatory response.[29,30] Visceral fat cells can produce three times the amount of IL-6 as fats cells elsewhere,[31] and in overweight individuals, may be producing up to 35% of the total IL-6 in the body.[32] Fat tissue can also be infiltrated by macrophages, which secrete proinflammatory cytokines. This accumulation of macrophages appears to be proportional to BMI, and appear to be a major cause of low-grade, systemic inflammation and insulin resistance in obese individuals.[33,34]

## Diet

A diet high in saturated fat is associated with higher proinflammatory markers, particularly in diabetic or overweight individuals.[35,36] This effect was absent in healthy individuals.[37–39] Diets high in synthetic trans-fats (such as those produced by hydrogenation) have been associated with increases in inflammatory markers (IL-6, TNF-α, IL-8, CRP) in some studies,[40,41] but had no effect in others.[42,43] The increases in markers of inflammation due to synthetic trans-fats may be more pronounced in individuals that are also overweight.[42]

General dietary overconsumption is a major contributor to inflammation and other detrimental age-related processes in the modern world. Therefore, eating a calorie-restricted diet is an effective means of relieving physiologic stressors. Several studies show that calorie restriction provides powerful protection against inflammation.[44,45] For more information about the metabolic benefits of eating fewer calories, readers should refer to the Caloric Restriction protocol.

## Low Sex Hormones

Among their many roles in biology, sex hormones also modulate the immune/inflammatory response. The cells that mediate inflammation (such as neutrophils and macrophages) have receptors for estrogens and androgens that enable them to selectively respond to sex hormone levels in many tissues.[46] A notable example is that of *osteoclasts*, the macrophages that reside in skeletal tissue and are responsible for breaking down and recycling old bone. Estrogens turn down osteoclast activity. Following menopause, lowered estrogen levels cause these bone depleting cells to maintain their activity, breaking down bone faster than it is rebuilt. This is one of the factors in the progression of osteoporosis.

Experiments in cell culture have demonstrated that testosterone and estrogen can repress the production and secretion of several proinflammatory markers, including IL-1β, IL-6, TNF-α, and the activity of NF-κB.[47–49] These observations have been corroborated by observational studies that have linked lower testosterone levels in elderly men to increases in inflammatory markers (IL-6 and IL-6 receptor).[50,51] Several studies have shown an increase in inflammatory IL-1β, IL-6, and TNF-α following surgical or natural menopause.[52,53] Conversely, the preservation of sex hormone levels is associated with reductions in the risk of several inflammatory diseases, including atherosclerosis, asthma in women, and rheumatoid arthritis in men.[46] Hormone replacement therapy (HRT) may partially exert its protective effects through an attenuation of the inflammatory response. Reductions in the risks of coronary heart disease and inflammatory bowel disease in some individuals, as well as levels of some circulating inflammatory cytokines (including IL-1B, IL-8, and TNF-α) has been observed in some studies of women on HRT.[53–55]

## Smoking

Cigarette smoke contains several inducers of inflammation, particularly reactive oxygen species. Chronic smoking increases production of several proinflammatory cytokines (TNF-α, IL-1β, IL-6, IL-8), while simultaneously reducing production of anti-inflammatory molecules.[56] Smoking also increases the risk of periodontal disease, an independent risk factor for increasing systemic inflammation.[57]

## Sleep Disorders

Production of inflammatory cytokines (TNF-α and IL-1β) appears to follow a circadian rhythm and may be involved in the regulation of sleep in animals and humans.[58] Disruption of normal sleep can lead to daytime elevations of these proinflammatory molecules. Plasma levels of TNF-α and/or IL-6 were elevated in patients with excessive daytime sleepiness, including those with sleep apnea and narcolepsy.[58] These elevations in cytokines were independent of body mass index or age,[59,60] although persons with higher visceral body fat were more likely to have sleep disorders.[61]

## Other Inciting Factors

Periodontal disease can produce a systemic inflammatory response that may affect several other systems, such as the heart and kidneys.[62,63] It is by this mechanism that periodontal disease is thought to be a risk factor for cardiovascular diseases.[64]

Stress (both physical and emotional) can lead to inflammatory cytokine release (IL-6); stress is also associated with decreased sleep and increased body mass (stimulated by release of the stress hormone cortisol), both of which are independent causes of inflammation.[65]

The maintenance of a proper inflammatory response may also involve the central nervous system. The recently identified vagal immune reflex senses inflammatory molecules through a network of nerves (branches of the vagus nerve) and sends this information to the brain. If the brain determines that the inflammatory response is too great, it sends signals to the site(s) of inflammation to attenuate the response.[66] Preliminary data suggest that depressed nerve activity may be associated with exaggerated inflammatory responses seen in sepsis.[67] Smoking, itself a risk factor for inflammation, also decreases activity of the vagus nerve.[68]

## EXCESS BLOOD GLUCOSE FUELS INFLAMMATORY FIRES

When glucose is properly utilized, our cells produce energy efficiently. As cellular sensitivity to *insulin* diminishes, excess glucose accumulates in the bloodstream. Like spilled gasoline, excess blood glucose creates a highly combustible environment from which oxidative and inflammatory fires chronically erupt.

Excess glucose not used for energy production converts to *triglycerides* that are either stored as unwanted *body fat* or accumulate in the blood where they contribute to the formation of *atherosclerotic plaque*.

As an aging human, you face a daily onslaught of excess *glucose* that poses a grave risk to your health and longevity. Surplus glucose relentlessly reacts with your body's proteins, causing damaging *glycation* reactions while fueling the fires of *chronic inflammation* and inciting the production of destructive *free radicals*.[69–71]

### Avert Glycation and Inflammation by Controlling Glucose Levels with Green Coffee Extract

Unroasted coffee beans, once purified and standardized, produce high levels of *chlorogenic acid* and other beneficial polyphenols that can suppress excess blood glucose levels. Human clinical trials support the role of *chlorogenic acid*-rich green coffee bean extract in promoting healthy blood sugar control and reducing disease risk.

Scientists have discovered that *chlorogenic acid* found abundantly in green coffee bean extract inhibits the enzyme *glucose-6-phosphatase* that triggers new glucose formation and glucose release by the liver.[72,73] Glucose-6-phosphatase is involved in dangerous postprandial (after-meal) spikes in blood sugar.

In another significant mechanism, *chlorogenic acid* increases the signal protein for insulin receptors in liver cells.[74] That has the effect of increasing *insulin sensitivity*, which in turn drives down blood sugar levels.

In a clinical trial, 56 healthy volunteers were challenged with an oral glucose tolerance test before and after a supplemental dose of green coffee extract. The oral glucose tolerance test is a standardized way of measuring a person's after-meal blood sugar response. In subjects not taking green coffee bean extract, the oral glucose tolerance test showed the expected rise of blood sugar to an average of 144 mg/dL after a 30 minute period. But in subjects who had taken 200 mg of the green coffee bean extract, that sugar spike was significantly reduced, to just *124 mg/dL—a 14% decrease*.[75] When a higher dose (400 mg) of green coffee bean extract was supplemented, there was an even *greater* average reduction in blood sugar—up to nearly 28% at 1 hour.

Ensuring that fasting glucose levels stay *between 70 and 85 mg/dL* and 2 hour post-meal glucose levels remain *under 125 mg/dL* can help combat chronic inflammation.

## DISEASES ASSOCIATED WITH CHRONIC INFLAMMATION

### Cardiovascular Disease (CVD)

Inflammation is an integral part of atherosclerosis (recall that oxidized low-density lipoprotein cholesterol stimulates the inflammatory response). Circulating inflammatory cytokines are predictive of peripheral arterial disease, heart failure, atrial fibrillation, stroke, and coronary heart disease.[9,26]

### Cancer

Several studies have established links between chronic low-level inflammation and many types of cancer, including lymphoma, prostate, ovarian, pancreatic, colorectal, and lung.[7,76] There are several mechanisms by which inflammation may contribute to carcinogenesis, including alterations in gene expression, DNA mutation, epigenetic alterations, promotion of tumor vascularization, and the expression of proinflammatory cytokines that have roles in cancer cell proliferation.[7,77]

### Diabetes

The infiltration of macrophages into fat tissue and their subsequent release of proinflammatory cytokines into circulation occur at a greater rate in type 2 diabetics than in nondiabetics.[33,35,78] Proinflammatory cytokines clearly decrease insulin sensitivity.[2]

## Age-Related Macular Degeneration (AMD)

An evaluation of 11 population-based studies encompassing over 41 000 patients demonstrated a clear association between elevated serum CRP levels (>3 mg/L) and the incidence of late onset AMD.[79] The risk of AMD in these high-CRP patients was increased over two-fold compared to patients with CRP levels <1 mg/L.

## Chronic Kidney Disease (CKD)

The chronic, low-grade inflammation in CKD can lead to the retention of several proinflammatory molecules in the blood (including cytokines, AGEs, and homocysteine).[6] The reduced excretion of proinflammatory factors by the diseased kidney can accelerate the progression of chronic inflammatory disturbances elsewhere in the body, such as the cardiovascular system.

## Osteoporosis

Inflammatory cytokines (TNF-α, IL-1β, IL-6) are involved in normal bone metabolism. Osteoclasts, the cells that break down (resorb) bone tissue, are a type of macrophage and can be stimulated by proinflammatory factors. Systemic elevations in proinflammatory cytokines push bone metabolism towards resorption, and have been observed to induce bone loss in persons with periodontal disease, pancreatitis, inflammatory bowel disease, and rheumatoid arthritis.[3] An increase in the levels of inflammatory cytokines is also a mechanism by which menopause stimulates bone loss.

## Depression

There is a small, yet significant association between elevated IL-6 and CRP in depressed patients, which has been observed in many population studies.[80] It is unclear whether inflammation leads to stress or vice versa, and there are data supporting both hypotheses.[81,82]

## Cognitive Decline

Several observational studies have linked chronic low-level inflammation in older adults to cognitive decline and dementia, including vascular dementia and Alzheimer's disease.[9] One study found that people with the highest CRP and IL-6 levels (>2.4 pg/mL) had a ~30–40% increased risk of cognitive decline compared to those with the lowest levels (<1.4 pg/mL).[83] Inflammatory markers can be elevated before the onset of cognitive dysfunction, indicating their potential relevance as a prognostic tool in high-risk individuals.[9]

## Others

Elevations in circulating inflammatory cytokines are associated with several other conditions, both inflammatory (rheumatoid arthritis, IBD/Crohn's disease, pancreatitis) and noninflammatory (anemia, fibromyalgia, frailty, sarcopenia/cachexia/muscle wasting).[4,35,84–86] Again, whether inflammation incites these conditions or results from them is unclear, and requires further investigation.

# CONVENTIONAL MEDICINE TYPICALLY OVERLOOKS CHRONIC INFLAMMATION

Chronic inflammation or parainflammation is generally not treated on its own by mainstream physicians. Interventions in conventional medicine are usually only undertaken when the inflammation occurs in association with another medical condition (such as arthritis). Currently, conventional preventive medical approaches to inflammation are limited to the use of CRP to predict cardiovascular disease in high-risk subjects, and the prophylactic use of drugs like aspirin to inhibit the inflammatory cascade linked to thrombosis (uncontrolled blood clotting). Indeed, the potentially asymptomatic nature of low grade inflammation is such that elevations of proinflammatory cytokines may progress undetected for some time, only being discovered after they have had time to cause enough cellular damage to produce disease symptoms. As future studies solidify the association between inflammatory mediators and different diseases, early detection of cytokine aberrations and anti-inflammatory therapy to reduce disease risk may gain more mainstream acceptance.

## TESTING BLOOD FOR INFLAMMATORY FACTORS

The following two blood tests are inexpensive and good markers of systemic inflammation. They can be used to detect the presence of chronic inflammation and monitor the success or failure of various anti-inflammatory regimens:

| Pro-Inflammatory Marker | Optimal Ranges |
| --- | --- |
| High-sensitivity C-reactive protein (CRP) | <0.55 mg/L in men <br> <1.50 mg/L in women |
| Fibrinogen | 200–300 mg/dL |

The following blood tests are expensive and help identify specific factors causing systemic inflammation:

| Cytokine Testing | Normal Ranges (LabCorp) |
| --- | --- |
| Tumor necrosis factor alpha (TNF-α) | <8.1 pg/mL |
| Interleukin-1 beta (IL-1β) | <15.0 pg/mL |
| Interleukin-6 (IL-6) | 2–29 pg/mL |
| Interleukin-8 (IL-8) | <32.0 pg/mL |

# DRUG STRATEGIES TO COMBAT CHRONIC INFLAMMATION

## Pentoxifylline

Pentoxifylline is a drug used to treat conditions involving poor circulation to the brain, limbs, and other areas perfused by small blood vessels. The drug effectively modulates properties of both blood vessels *and* red blood cells thanks to its action as a nonselective *phosphodiesterase* inhibitor. Phosphodiesterase inhibition is a clinically important mechanism in many additional aspects of human physiology as well, so pentoxifylline has been studied in a wide range of applications ranging from diabetic complications and nonalcoholic liver disease, to endometriosis and cardiac surgery.[87–90]

The potent anti-inflammatory properties of pentoxifylline were a secondary discovery, and still are not fully understood. Studies have revealed, however, that pentoxifylline modulates TNF-α signaling, which probably contributes to the considerable suppression of inflammation it has evoked in several human trials.[91] In a recent trial, 400 mg of pentoxifylline taken twice daily significantly suppressed hs-CRP, fibrinogen, and TNF-α levels in patients with chronic kidney disease; subjects' renal function improved with treatment as well.[92] In patients with HIV-related vascular dysfunction, pentoxifylline lessened leukocyte adhesion—a process that contributes to cardiovascular disease by allowing inflammatory cells to infiltrate the endothelial lining of blood vessels.[93] Given by IV-infusion, pentoxifylline lowered TNF-α levels and pain intensity following surgical removal of kidney stones.[94]

Pentoxifylline dosage varies depending on individual circumstances and clinical application; however, 400 mg taken twice daily has consistently tempered inflammation in diverse human trials. For example, administered at this dose for 1 month to 30 diabetic individuals with high blood pressure, not only did pentoxifylline quell inflammation (20% reduction in CRP levels and an 11% improvement in erythrocyte sedimentation rate [measure of inflammatory tendency of a blood sample]), but it also bolstered plasma antioxidant status, as evidenced by a 20% reduction in malondialdehyde levels (measure of oxidative stress) and a nearly 5% increase in glutathione levels, a powerful antioxidant.[95]

## Metformin

The regulation of energy metabolism and inflammation are closely associated; this is evidenced by the coincidence of metabolic disorders (obesity, diabetes) and low-grade inflammation.[96] Metformin may reduce the activity of inflammatory cytokines by increasing the production of IL-1β receptor *antagonist (IL1Rn)*, a protein factor which interferes with proinflammatory signaling of IL-1β.[97] It may also promote favorable CRP levels, although not to the same extent as weight loss.[96,98] A randomized controlled trial of hypertensive and dyslipidemic patients taking 1700 mg/day of metformin for 12 weeks demonstrated a 26.7% reduction in IL-6 and 8.3% reduction in TNF-α from baseline levels, a degree of reduction similar to that of the potent statin drug rosuvastatin (Crestor®).[99] The anti-inflammatory effects of metformin appear to be rapid; reductions in circulating TNF-α, IL-1β, CRP, and fibrinogen were observed after only 30 days in a larger study of 128 type 2 diabetic patients with dyslipidemia.[100]

## Aspirin

Aspirin has been used as an anti-inflammatory therapy long before the molecular mechanics of inflammation had been discovered; it is now well characterized as an inhibitor of cyclooxygenase enzymes. The modification of COX molecules by aspirin has important implications for cardiovascular health. Blood platelets use cyclooxygenase to produce thromboxane A2, a proinflammatory molecule that is an important signal during the initial stages of the clotting process. The inhibitory effect of aspirin on COX enzymes in platelets can partially explain its protective effects against the complications of several disorders, including hypertension, heart attack, and stroke.[101] Aspirin's inhibition of cyclooxygenase also helps explain its potential effect on cancer risk reduction as observed in several studies,[102–105] as COX-2 also appears to have roles in increasing the proliferation of mutated cells, tumor formation, tumor invasion, and metastasis, and may contribute to drug resistance in some cancers.[106] Aspirin has also been shown to reduce the activity of NF-κB in vitro[107] and lower levels of multiple inflammatory markers (TNF-α, CRP, IL-6) in patients with cardiovascular disease.[108–111]

Unlike many other NSAIDs, the effects of aspirin on COX enzymes are permanent for the life of the COX enzyme. Interestingly, it appears that rather than rendering the enzyme inactive, aspirin modifies the function of COX. Aspirin stops the enzyme from producing proinflammatory prostaglandins, and enables it to begin producing anti-inflammatory molecules called resolvins.[112]

## Low-Dose Statin Drugs

Statins are thought to reduce inflammation by a mechanism distinct from their effects on cholesterol metabolism—they interfere with the function of cytokine receptors on the surface of white blood cells. Therefore, proinflammatory signals in the blood are unable to provoke a response from white blood cells, and they are prevented from further stimulating inflammation.[113,114] Results of the JUPITER trial presented the strongest evidence for statins as anti-inflammatory therapy; in this study of over 17000 healthy middle-aged men and women with elevated levels of the inflammatory marker CRP but normal levels of blood lipids, 20 mg/day of rosuvastatin reduced CRP levels by over half, in addition to reducing heart attack and stroke incidence.[115] Smaller studies have looked at the effect of statins on other inflammatory markers as well. A randomized controlled trial of hypertensive and dyslipidemic patients taking a lower dose (10 mg/day) of rosuvastatin for 12 weeks demonstrated a ~22% reduction in IL-6 and 13% reduction in TNF-α from baseline levels.[99] A second uncontrolled study of simvastatin demonstrated more modest reductions in IL-6, but no changes in TNF-α from the statin treatment.[116] To generate a substantial anti-inflammatory effect using statin drugs alone requires a high dose that is more likely to induce side effects than lower-dose statin therapy.

## DIETARY AND LIFESTYLE APPROACHES TO REDUCE CHRONIC INFLAMMATION

Inflammation itself is not a disease, but is featured, to varying degrees, in adverse health conditions. Information on strategies and research regarding the reduction of inflammation characteristic to specific health conditions are featured in corresponding Life Extension protocols: Allergies, Age-Related Macular Degeneration, Cancer Adjuvant Therapy, Atherosclerosis and Cardiovascular Disease, Gout and Hyperuricemia, Inflammatory Bowel Disease (Crohn's and Ulcerative Colitis), Arthritis-Osteoarthritis, Arthritis-Rheumatoid, and Osteoporosis. What follows is a summary of dietary and supplemental approaches to addressing general chronic inflammation and parainflammation. As many types of general inflammation often occur without additional symptoms, most of the strategies listed below are based on their ability to reduce circulating inflammatory cytokines, the hallmark of the parainflammatory state.

### Macronutrients and Energy Balance

Macronutrient content (particularly the types and levels of carbohydrates and fats) can have a significant effect on the progression of inflammation (as measured by increases in proinflammatory markers). Diets with relatively high glycemic index (GI) and glycemic load (GL) have been associated with elevated risk of coronary heart disease, stroke, and type 2 diabetes mellitus, particularly among overweight individuals, and have been associated with modest increases in proinflammatory markers in multiple studies.[117] In a study of over 18 000 healthy women ≥45 years old without diagnosed diabetes, high GI and GL diets resulted in a

small but significant increase in hs-CRP (+12% for high GI) over low GI diets.[118] In the Danish Hoorne study,[119] for every 10-unit increase in dietary GI, circulating CRP was increased by 29%. As discussed previously, some dietary fats (particularly saturated and synthetic trans-fats) increase inflammation occurrence, while omega-3 polyunsaturated fats appear to be anti-inflammatory.[40]

Since fat tissue (especially abdominal fat) expresses inflammatory cytokines, obesity can be a major cause of low-grade, systemic inflammation.[33,34] Thus, it is important that total energy intake be proportional to energy expenditure to avoid the deposition of abdominal fat. Obesity-induced increases in inflammatory cytokines appear to be reversible with fat loss.[120] In a dramatic example, weight loss (by adjustable gastric banding) in a group of 20 severely obese individuals reduced IL-6 by 22% and CRP by almost half.[121]

An inflammatory index, developed by a group from the Arnold School of Public Health at the University of South Carolina, scored 42 common dietary constituents based on their ability to raise serum CRP.[122] Constituents (such as saturated fat, tea polyphenols, or vitamin D) were given either a positive (anti-inflammatory) or negative (proinflammatory) score, the magnitude of which was weighted based on the volume of inflammation research on the isolated ingredient. Human clinical data were weighted more than animal data, and clinical trials more than observational studies. The scores were then verified by comparing them to nutrient intakes and CRP levels from a group of 494 volunteers over the course of 1 year. Among the most anti-inflammatory nutrients (based on the model and study data) were magnesium, beta-carotene, turmeric (curcumin), genistein, and tea; the most proinflammatory included carbohydrates, total and saturated fat, and cholesterol. The index may provide a useful metric for accessing the overall inflammatory potential of an individual diet.

### Exercise

Energy expenditure through exercise lowers multiple cytokines and proinflammatory molecules independently of weight loss. While muscle contraction initially results in a proinflammatory state, it paradoxically lowers systemic inflammation. This effect has been observed in dozens of human trials of exercise training in both healthy and unhealthy individuals across many age groups.[123]

### Fiber

In an analysis of seven studies on the relationship between weight loss and hs-CRP, increased fiber consumption correlated with significantly greater reductions in hs-CRP concentrations.[120] In these studies, daily fiber intakes ranging from 3.3 to 7.8 g/MJ (equivalent to about 27–64 g/day for a standard 2000-kilocalorie [kcal] diet) reduced CRP from 25% to 54% in a dose-dependent fashion. These results should be interpreted carefully, as only two of the seven studies were specifically designed to examine the effects of fiber independently.[120] The Women's Health Initiative failed to detect an effect of fiber consumption on hs-CRP, but found that greater intake of dietary soluble and insoluble fiber (>24 g/day) was associated with lower levels of IL-6 and TNF-α.[124]

## Micronutrients

**Magnesium.** In two large observation studies (the Women's Health Initiative and Harvard Nurses Study), greater magnesium intake was associated with lower hs-CRP, IL-6, and TNF-α receptor, a measure of TNF-α activity.[117,125] Data from the Multi-Ethnic Study of Atherosclerosis failed to find significant differences in IL-6 or CRP levels between individuals with the highest and lowest magnesium intakes, but did find a significant association between greater dietary magnesium and the lower levels of the inflammation-associated proteins homocysteine and fibrinogen.[126] Magnesium was rated as the most anti-inflammatory dietary factor in the Dietary Inflammatory index, which rated 42 common dietary constituents on their ability to reduce CRP levels based on human and animal experimental and observation data.[122]

**Vitamin D.** Vitamin D appears to exert anti-inflammatory activity by the suppression of proinflammatory prostaglandins and inhibition of the inflammatory mediator NF-κB.[127] Although intervention studies of its anti-inflammatory activity in humans are lacking, several observational studies suggest vitamin D deficiency may promote inflammation. Vitamin D deficiencies are more common among patients with inflammatory diseases (including rheumatoid arthritis, inflammatory bowel disease, systemic lupus erythematosus, and diabetes) than in healthy individuals.[128] They also occur more frequently in populations that are prone to low-level inflammation, such as obese individuals and the elderly.[129] Vitamin D levels can drop following surgery (a condition associated with acute inflammation) with a concomitant rise in CRP.[130] Low vitamin D status was associated with elevated CRP in a study of 548 heart failure patients[131] and with increases in IL-6 and NF-κB in a group of 46 middle-aged men with endothelial dysfunction.[132]

**Vitamin E.** Vitamin E functions as an antioxidant in the body. Specifically, vitamin E is incorporated into low-density lipoprotein (LDL) particles and protects them against oxidative damage; it seems to guard against atherosclerosis via other mechanisms as well.[133] The *gamma-tocopherol* form of vitamin E appears to complement the anti-inflammatory action of *alpha-tocopherol*. Gamma-tocopherol has been shown to inhibit COX-2 and attenuate IL-1β signaling.[134,135] In a small clinical trial on subjects with metabolic syndrome, the combination of gamma-tocopherol and alpha-tocopherol effectively suppressed C-reactive protein and TNF-α levels compared to placebo.[136] In this study, the combination of both tocopherols performed better than either alone, prompting the investigators to remark "*the combination of [alpha-tocopherol] and [gamma-tocopherol] supplementation appears to be superior to either supplementation alone on biomarkers of oxidative stress and inflammation and needs to be tested in prospective clinical trials…*"

**Zinc and selenium.** Zinc- and selenium-containing antioxidant proteins (such as superoxide dismutase and glutathione peroxidase) reduce reactive oxygen species (free radicals), which indirectly inhibits NF-κB activity and prevents the production of several inflammatory enzymes and cytokines. Zinc can also inhibit NF-κB in a more direct manner.[137,138] Zinc supplementation is associated with decreases in inflammation in populations that are prone to zinc deficiency, such as children and the elderly.[139,140] Low-level inflammation and circulating proinflammatory factors (CRP, TNF-α, IL-6, and IL-8) were reduced in elderly subjects by moderate zinc supplementation in several studies.[141–143] Like zinc, selenium deficiencies are common in chronic inflammatory states associated with disease (such as sepsis),[144] where selenium supplementation has been associated with reductions in inflammation and better patient outcomes.[138]

## Other Dietary Factors

**Resveratrol and pterostilbene.** The exact mechanism by which resveratrol exerts anti-inflammatory activity has not been established, although it inhibits a variety of proinflammatory compounds (cyclooxygenase, TNF-α, IL-1β, IL-6, NF-κB) in animal models and human cell culture.[145,146] The related compound pterostilbene has demonstrated similar inhibition of inflammatory markers in cell culture.[147] Modulation of the inflammatory immune response likely contributes to resveratrol's protective role in animal models of heart disease, cancer, acute pancreatitis, and inflammatory bowel disease.[148] Resveratrol may be protective against general, low-level parainflammation as well. When taken with a single high-fat, high-carbohydrate meal (930 kcal), resveratrol (100 mg) prevented the sharp post-meal increases in markers of oxidation and inflammation in a small crossover study of 10 healthy volunteers. For example, synthesis of IL-1β increased by 91% over 5 hours following the test meal; with resveratrol, this increase was significantly less (29%).[149]

**Curcumin.** Extensive in vitro and animal studies have examined the effects of curcumin on experimentally-induced inflammatory diseases (atherosclerosis, arthritis, diabetes, liver disease, gastrointestinal disorders, and cancers) and disease markers (lipoxygenase, cyclooxygenase, TNF-α, IL-1β, NF-κB, and others).[150,151] Fewer human studies have examined curcumin's effects on patient-oriented outcomes in inflammatory diseases, but most of the small randomized controlled trials of curcumin have consistently shown patient improvements in several inflammatory diseases, including psoriasis, irritable bowel syndrome, rheumatoid arthritis, and inflammatory eye disease.[152,153]

**Tea polyphenols.** The anti-inflammatory effects of green and black tea polyphenols have been substantiated by dozens of in vitro and animal studies.[154] The polyphenols EGCG and theaflavin exert their anti-inflammatory effects through the inhibition of the NF-κB signaling pathway, which decreases expression of several inflammatory proteins (lipoxygenase, cyclooxygenase, TNF-α, IL-1β, IL-6, and IL-8) in cell culture experiments.[155] EGCG also inhibits the production and release of histamine, a key mediator of allergic and inflammatory response in vitro.[156] In observational studies of tea consumption, >2 cups of tea/day (black or green) was associated with a nearly 20% reduction in CRP compared to non-tea drinkers, and significantly lower levels of two other inflammatory markers (serum amyloid A and haptogen, which are elevated in coronary heart disease).[157] In clinical interventions, black tea appears to be more successful in reducing inflammatory markers than green.[117] A 25% reduction in CRP was also observed in a small trial of healthy, nonsmoking men consuming a black tea extract (equivalent to 4 cups of tea/day) for 6 weeks.[158] A similar average reduction was observed in a larger study of healthy individuals at high risk for coronary heart disease, but revealed a more dramatic 40-50% reduction in CRP among individuals with the highest starting CRP values (>3 mg/L).[159]

**Carotenoids.** In the Women's Health and Aging Study, participants with the highest blood levels of α-carotene and total carotenoids were significantly more likely to have lower IL-6 levels than participants with low carotenoid levels at the onset of the study.[160] Participants with the lowest blood levels of α- and β-carotene, lutein/zeaxanthin, or total carotenoids were more likely to experience increases in IL-6 over a period of 2 years.

**DHEA.** Low levels of sex hormones are associated with systemic increases in inflammatory markers[9]; DHEA (dehydroepiandrosterone), an adrenal steroid hormone, is the precursor to the sex steroids testosterone and estrogen. DHEA is abundant in youth, but steady declines with advancing age and may be partially responsible for age-related decreases in sex steroids.[161] In cell culture and animal models, DHEA can suppress inflammatory cytokine activity, in some cases more effectively than either testosterone or estrogen.[162] Chronic inflammation may itself reduce DHEA levels.[163] DHEA supplementation in elderly volunteers (50 mg/day for 2 years) significantly decreased TNF-α and IL-6 levels as well as lowered visceral fat mass and improved glucose tolerance (both associated with inflammation) in a small study.[164]

**Fish oil.** Fish oil is the best source of the omega-3 fatty acids eicosapentaenoic acid (EPA) and docosahexaenoic acid (DHA), which can only be synthesized to a limited extent in humans. Omega-3 fatty acids have been well studied for their prevention of cardiovascular disease and mortality in tens of thousands of patients; the anti-inflammatory effects of omega-3s contribute to this activity.[165] They have also proven successful at improving patient outcomes in scores of studies of other inflammatory diseases, particularly asthma, inflammatory bowel disease, and rheumatoid arthritis.[166,167]

The association between greater fish oil/omega-3 consumption and reduced systemic inflammation is substantiated by data from several large observational trials. In 855 healthy participants from the Health Professionals Follow-Up Study, intake of omega-3 fatty acids was associated with lower plasma levels of markers of TNF-α activity; interestingly, high intake of both omega-3 and omega-6 fatty acids (which are usually assumed to be proinflammatory) was associated with the lowest level of inflammation.[168] The Nurses' Health Study 1 cohort of 727 women revealed lower concentrations of inflammatory markers (including CRP and IL-6) among those in the top 20% of omega-3 consumption compared to those who consumed the least amount.[169] In the ATTICA study of over 3000 Greek men and women without any evidence of cardiovascular disease, participants who consumed over 300 g of fish/week had, on average, 33% lower CRP, 33% lower IL-6, and 21% lower TNF-α than participants who did not consume fish.[170] In a sample of 5677 men and women without cardiovascular disease from the Multi-Ethnic Study of Atherosclerosis (MESA) cohort, long-chain omega-3 intake (from fish or supplements) was associated with reduced plasma concentrations of multiple inflammatory markers (including CRP, IL-6, and TNF-α receptor, a measure of TNF-α activity).[171]

**N-acetyl cysteine.** Activation of the NF-κB pathway plays a central role in the activation of inflammatory cytokine genes; N-acetyl cysteine (NAC) inhibits NF-κB in cell culture, lowering expression of cytokines such as

## Figure 1. Arachidonic Acid's Destructive Cascade

To better understand the pathways by which arachidonic acid can cause
arthritic, carcinogenic, and cardiovascular conditions, the flow chart below
shows how arachidonic acid cascades down into damaging compounds in the body.

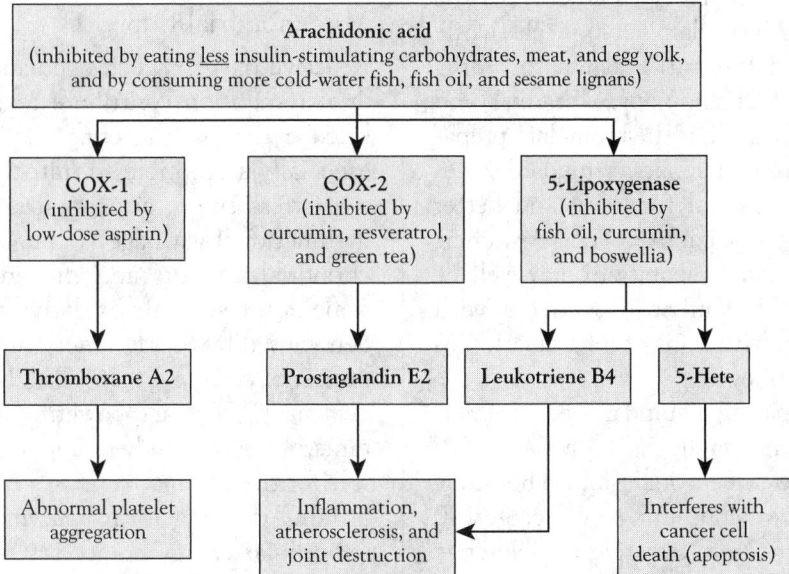

IL-6 and IL-8.[172,173] Data establishing the effects of NAC on lowering chronic inflammation in humans are limited, but show promise. NAC supplementation for 8 weeks demonstrated modest, but statistically significant decreases in circulating IL-6 levels in patients with chronic kidney disease.[174] The effects were more pronounced in persons with significant inflammation at the start of the study (as measured by hs-CRP). NAC also reduced markers of systemic inflammation in a small study of patients with burn injuries.[175]

**Boswellia.** *Boswellia serrata* (frankincense) is a traditional antiarthritic in Ayurvedic medicine; its anti-inflammatory properties have been attributed to the specific inhibition of 5-LOX and reduction in the production of proinflammatory leukotrienes by boswellic acids, a constituent of the *Boswellia* gum resin.[176] In cell culture, both crude and highly purified *Boswellia* extracts inhibited the production of proinflammatory TNF-α and IL-1β.[177] One of the boswellic acids, *acetyl-11-keto-beta-boswellic acid* (AKBA), was an inhibitor of NF-κB activity in mice,[178] while a topical mixture of the four most abundant boswellic acids decreased inflammation in a rodent inflammation model.[179] A recent systematic review of human trials of *Boswellia* for inflammatory conditions revealed that the small number of randomized controlled trials on the extract have produced encouraging results for its use for asthma and osteoarthritis,[180] warranting larger studies to confirm the extract as an effective therapy. Standardized *Boswellia* extracts (30% AKBA) have been effective in mitigating pain in osteoarthritis patients[181]; when combined with nonvolatile *Boswellia* oil, the standardized

extract (called AsprèsFlex™, or Aflapin®) demonstrated improved activity at a lower concentration.[182] The use of *Boswellia* extracts for inflammatory bowel diseases has been investigated in multiple clinical trials, although results have been mixed.[183–185]

**Sesame lignans.** The observation that sesame oil could decrease the production of arachidonic acid in fungi and rat liver cells led to the identification of the sesame lignans (sesamin, sesamolin, sesaminol) as specific inhibitors of Δ5 desaturase (delta-5-desaturase), one of the enzymes used in the synthesis of arachidonic acid.[186] By inhibiting Δ5 desaturase, sesame lignans may reduce the synthesis of proinflammatory prostaglandin, leukotrienes, and thromboxanes, each of which require arachidonic acid as a starting material.[187] In animal models, diets high in sesame seed oil reduced production of the proinflammatory prostaglandins PGE-1 and -2, as well as thromboxane B2.[188] In humans, 5 weeks of sesamin supplementation (39 mg/day) reduced the production of the proinflammatory vasoconstrictor 20-hydroxyeicosatetraenoic acid (20-HETE, a product of the enzyme 5-LOX) by 30%.[189] This potential anti-inflammatory property of sesame lignans may partially explain its observed hypotensive (blood pressure-lowering) activity.[190]

**Bromelain.** The anti-inflammatory activity of the proteolytic enzyme preparation bromelain has been attributed to its ability to reduce COX-2 activity, decrease prostaglandin and thromboxane synthesis, lower circulating fibrinogen levels, and reduce cellular adhesion of proinflammatory white blood cells to the sites of inflammation.[191] Human trials of bromelain for inflammatory conditions have yielded promising results.[192] In a blinded study from Germany, researchers divided 90 patients with painful osteoarthritis of the hip into two groups: one half received an oral enzyme preparation containing bromelain for 6 weeks while the other half received the anti-inflammatory drug diclofenac (sold under the brand name Voltaren® and generic names). They found that the bromelain preparation was as effective as diclofenac in standard scales of pain, stiffness, and physical function, and better tolerated than the drug comparator. The researchers concluded, "[the bromelain preparation] may well be recommended for the treatment of patients with osteoarthritis of the hip with signs of inflammation as indicated by a high pain level."[193]

Another study comparing a standardized commercial enzyme preparation containing bromelain with diclofenac reached the same conclusion. The study reported the supplement containing bromelain (90 mg, three times daily) to be as effective as diclofenac (50 mg, twice daily) in improving the symptoms of osteoarthritis of the knee. Patients reported comparable reductions in joint tenderness, pain and swelling, and improvement in range of motion at the end of the study. The investigators found bromelain to be as good as diclofenac on a standard pain assessment scale and better than the drug in reducing pain at rest (41% for bromelain versus 23% for the drug), improving restricted function (10% for bromelain versus 0% for the drug), being rated by more patients in improving symptoms (24% for bromelain versus 19% for the drug), and being evaluated by more physicians as having good efficacy (51% for bromelain versus 37% for the drug). In summary, the investigators determined bromelain to be an effective and safe alternative to NSAIDs such as diclofenac for painful osteoarthritis.[194]

In further research from the United Kingdom, a 3-month study looked at the dose-dependent effects of bromelain, either 200 mg or 400 mg/day in volunteers with mild acute knee pain. Pain evaluation was based on patient symptom scores, which were reduced by 41% in the 200-mg bromelain group and 59% in those receiving 400 mg of bromelain, indicating a dose–response relationship. This was also observed for scores of stiffness and physical function, which decreased significantly in the higher-dose bromelain group compared with those receiving 200 mg. The researchers also noted that overall psychological well-being was significantly improved in both bromelain groups, leading to their conclusion that this natural therapy may be effective in improving general well-being as well as symptoms in otherwise healthy adults suffering from mild knee pain.[195]

In animal models and cell culture experiments, bromelain has consistently demonstrated a variety of anti-inflammatory properties.[196–199]

## Mitochondrial Support

Reactive oxygen species generated during mitochondrial respiration contribute to inflammation, as outlined earlier in the chapter. Aging individuals are especially susceptible to mitochondria-related oxidative stress since mitochondria become increasingly dysfunctional with age. Taking steps to support mitochondrial integrity and efficiency can help alleviate some of the systemic oxidative and inflammatory burden caused by poorly functioning mitochondria. Two nutrients, *coenzyme Q10* (CoQ10) and *pyrroloquinoline quinone* (PQQ) are powerful mitochondrial protectants,[200,201] and studies support an anti-inflammatory role for these compounds.

PQQ is a cofactor for enzymes critically important for cellular energy homeostasis and redox balance.[202] Several studies have shown that PQQ exerts a protective effective during circumstantial mitochondrial stress and increased oxidative load.[201,203] In one study, rats given a diet supplemented with PQQ displayed greater energy expenditure and, remarkably, increased mitochondrial density in liver tissue. PQQ supplemented rats also had lower triglycerides and their hearts were more protected against lack of oxygen than rats that had not been given PQQ.[204] During periods of limited oxygen supply to cardiac tissue, a dramatic spike in oxidative stress and subsequent inflammation damages cells; the findings from this animal model indicate that PQQ can stave off this inflammatory cell destruction by preserving mitochondrial efficiency in adverse conditions.

Coenzyme Q10 is an indispensable intermediary in mitochondrial ATP production. Studies have shown that CoQ10 levels are low during inflammatory conditions. In one investigation, patients with septic shock were found to have CoQ10 levels substantially lower than healthy individuals, and, among patients, lower CoQ10 levels correlated with higher levels of an inflammatory mediator called VCAM.[205] In an animal model in which rats were given drinking water with added fructose, an experiment that led to obesity, diabetes, and other inflammatory complications, CoQ10 supplementation attenuated the inflammatory response by decreasing hepatic expression of CRP and other inflammatory mediators.[206] Laboratory experiments indicate that CoQ10 modulates the expression of several hundred genes, many involved in inflammatory signaling.[207] Of particular significance, one experiment showed that CoQ10, at physiologically relevant concentrations, was able to blunt induced TNF-α by more than 25% via modulation of the NF-κB signaling pathway.

## Guarding Against Inflammatory Glycation Reactions

The role of elevated blood sugar and glycation end products in initiating an inflammatory storm was discussed earlier in the chapter. Fortunately, in addition to reducing caloric intake to suppress both fasting and post-meal glucose concentrations, some natural compounds ameliorate the glycation process and may help rein in the sugar-induced inflammatory cascade. Chief among these antiglycation nutrients are *benfotiamine*, a member of the B-vitamin family, and *carnosine*, an amino acid.

*Benfotiamine* has been used to target diabetic complications since the mid 1990s.[208] More recent evidence continues to support its use as a powerful protector against blood sugar-induced tissue damage. In a clinical trial, 165 subjects with diabetes were randomized to receive benfotiamine at either 300 or 600 mg/day, or a placebo for 6 weeks. After the intervention period, those taking benfotiamine exhibited improvements in neuropathic pain in a dose-dependent fashion.[209] An animal model found that benfotiamine relieved neuropathic pain by powerfully suppressing inflammation.[210] Moreover, laboratory experiments have shown that in addition to blocking glycation reactions, benfotiamine may regulate inflammation more directly by modulating COX and LOX enzyme activity.[211]

*Carnosine* exerts a range of favorable biochemical effects within the body; it powerfully blunts glycation reactions and eases oxidative stress.[212] In addition, several experiments have revealed a marked ability of carnosine to suppress inflammation in various cell types.[213-215] Unfortunately, carnosine levels decline as much as 63% between ages 10 and 70.[216] Furthermore, in patients with type 2 diabetes, skeletal muscle carnosine content is markedly lower than in healthy control subjects.[217] When carnosine is administered as a supplement to animals with chemically induced diabetes, it is able to protect delicate retinal cells from inflammatory complications related to high blood sugar.[218]

## Life Extension Suggestions

### General Support
- **Magnesium**: 100–800 elemental mg of highly absorbable magnesium
- **Vitamin D**: 5000–8000 IU daily (depending on blood test results; optimal blood levels are between 50 and 80 ng/mL)
- **Vitamin A**: 500 IU acetate and 4500 IU beta-carotene daily

- **Natural Vitamin E**: 100–400 IU alpha-tocopherol and 200 mg gamma-tocopherol daily
- **Fish oil** (with olive polyphenols and sesame lignans): providing 1400 mg EPA and 1000 mg DHA daily
- **Zinc**: 30 mg daily
- **Selenium**: 200 mcg daily
- **DHEA**: 15–25 mg daily for women, and 25–75 mg daily for men (depending on blood test results)

### Antioxidants
- *Trans*-resveratrol: 100–500 mg daily
- *Trans*-pterostilbene: 0.5–50 mg daily
- **Green tea extract**, standardized to 98% polyphenols: 725–1450 mg daily
- **Black tea extract**, standardized to 25% theaflavins: 350 mg daily
- **N-acetylcysteine**: 600–1200 mg daily

### Mechanism-Specific Support
- **Curcumin** (as highly absorbed BCM-95®): 400–800 mg daily
- **Boswellia serrata extract** (as highly absorbed AsprèsFlex™), standardized to 20% AKBA: 100 mg daily
- **Bromelain** (enteric coated): 500–1000 mg daily

### Optimizing Glucose Levels and Targeting Advanced Glycation End Products
- **Green coffee extract**, standardized to 50% chlorogenic acid: 200–400 mg before each meal, up to 3 times daily
- **Benfotiamine**: 150–1000 mg daily
- **L-carnosine**: 500–1500 mg daily

### Supporting Mitochondrial Function
- **Pyrroloquinoline quinone**: 10–20 mg daily
- **CoQ10** (as ubiquinol): 100–200 mg daily

In addition, the following *blood tests* should be considered:

- Male or Female Panel (includes glucose, C-reactive protein, LDL, homocysteine, sex hormones, and many other important tests)
- Fibrinogen
- Vitamin D, 25-Hydroxy
- Cytokine Panel
- Omega Score®

## REFERENCES

References available at: www.lef.org/dpt5/ch78

# 79

# Inflammatory Bowel Disease (Crohn's and Ulcerative Colitis)

"Inflammatory bowel disease" describes a collection of conditions affecting the digestive tract. *Crohn's disease* and *ulcerative colitis* are by far the most prevalent and thus are the focus of this protocol.

Inflammatory bowel disease is a result of *immunologic imbalances* at the interface of the *intestinal lumen* (the "hollow" part of the digestive tract through which food passes) and the *intestinal epithelium* (the inward-facing surface of the intestinal wall). Suppressing inflammation is the chief goal of both conventional *and* integrative treatment. However, potent immunosuppressive medications employed in inflammatory bowel disease,

such as *glucocorticoids*, are laden with side effects; which greatly limits their long-term efficacy.[1-3]

On the other hand, several natural interventions such as *omega-3 fatty acids*, *vitamin D*, and *probiotics* *modulate* immune cell function without impairing infection-fighting ability, which is one of the many side effects of *TNF-inhibitors*, another class of drugs used in inflammatory bowel disease.[2]

Patients with inflammatory bowel disease are predisposed to *colon cancer*. Even between disease flares, low-level inflammation irritates and damages intestinal tissue, which can lead to malignancy. This subclinical inflammation also propagates systemically, which can increase cardiovascular risk.[4,5] Therefore, not only is it imperative that patients with inflammatory bowel disease have regular colon cancer screenings, but also that they monitor inflammatory markers in their blood such as *C-reactive protein* (CRP) and *interleukin-6* (IL-6). In this protocol, you will learn how several natural ingredients powerfully regulate gut immunity and complement the action of conventional treatments to quench the fires of inflammatory bowel disease. You will also discover several convenient *blood tests* that can help identify nutritional deficiencies due to *malabsorption*—a

## Inflammatory Bowel Disease (IBD)

Crohn's Disease

Ulcerative Colitis

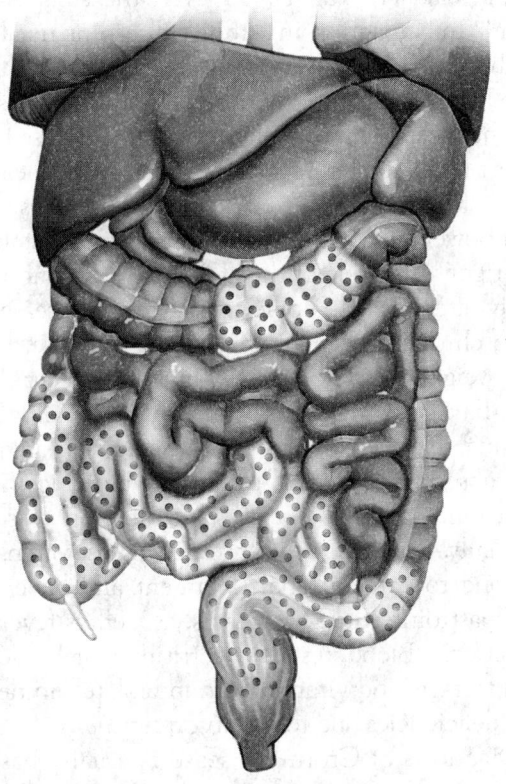
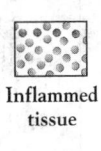
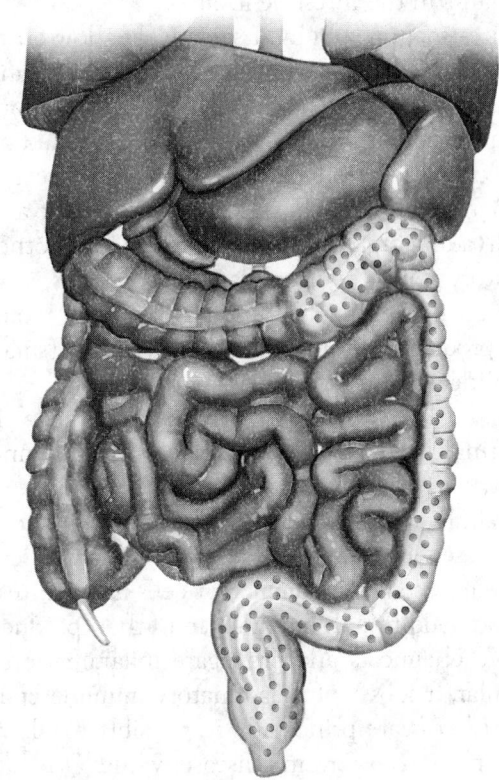

Inflammed tissue

common problem in inflammatory bowel disease. By integrating dietary strategies, evidence-based nutritional support, and pharmaceutical therapeutics one can develop a comprehensive program to help manage inflammatory bowel disease during both disease flares *and* periods of remission.

## ANATOMY OF THE DIGESTIVE TRACT AND IMMUNOLOGY OF INFLAMMATORY BOWEL DISEASE

The digestive tract consists of a single long tube that has many folds and convolutions and extends from the mouth to the anus. The tube is divided into distinct parts (such as the esophagus, stomach, small intestine, and large intestine), each with a specific structure and function. Solid organs such as the liver and pancreas are also considered portions of the digestive system.

The hollow parts are responsible for breaking down large portions of food into small molecules that can be readily absorbed into the circulation. The sterile bloodstream is separated from the mass of nutrients, toxins, and organisms in various parts of the hollow digestive tract by only a very thin layer of cells, collectively called the *intestinal mucosa*. This delicate and complex lining is responsible for secreting substances that aid in digestion and absorption of nutrients, and for defending the body against the toxins and other contaminants in the intestine itself.

The intestinal mucosa must selectively allow entry of beneficial molecules while excluding toxins and organisms that could be harmful. To do this, the mucosa is equipped with several kinds of cells including secretory cells that produce a layer of mucus to trap contaminants, immune cells that directly attack and destroy invading organisms (macrophages), and other inflammatory cells (neutrophils, killer T cells, and others) that respond to the presence of foreign molecules by producing proinflammatory *cytokines* (small cell-signaling protein molecules).[6]

During healthy conditions, the immune cells in the intestinal lining cope with invaders quickly and efficiently, without producing excessive amounts of localized inflammation. However, in inflammatory bowel disease, inflammation becomes uncontrolled. Cytokines released by inflammatory cells in the intestine attract additional immune cells that produce destructive chemicals and propagate inflammation.[7] In particular, a subset of inflammatory immune cells called *Th17 cells* are principally responsible for driving inflammation in Crohn's disease, while *Th2 cells* drive inflammation in ulcerative colitis. A number of factors cause Th17 and Th2 cells to produce excessive

inflammation including penetration of the intestinal epithelium by gut microbes, composition of the intestinal microbiota, injury to the intestinal wall, insufficient mucus layer production, and allergies or sensitivities to foods. Genetics contribute to inflammatory bowel disease susceptibility, but the immune response as well as the intestinal microenvironment and diet can be modified to mitigate inflammatory propensity, even in genetically predisposed individuals.

Since the inflammatory reactions taking place in the gut can promote systemic inflammation people with IBD should monitor levels of inflammatory cytokines in their blood. Cytokine testing can be used as a measure of the effectiveness of anti-inflammatory therapies, and can also help determine risk for other conditions associated with inflammation, such as atherosclerosis. Cytokine blood profiles measure tumor necrosis factor-alpha (TNF-$\alpha$), interleukin-1 (beta) (IL-1b), and interleukin-6 (IL-6).

## CROHN'S DISEASE: BACKGROUND AND DIAGNOSIS

Crohn's disease can attack any portion of the digestive tract, although inflammation most commonly occurs in the lower portion of the small intestine, known as the *ileum*. The disease can cause ulcerations within the intestine that can erode into surrounding tissues such as the bladder,[8] vagina,[9] or even the surface of the skin.[10] Inflammation in Crohn's disease is not limited to the intestine—some people who have Crohn's disease have inflammation of the eyes and joints as well.

The most common symptoms of the disease include severe abdominal pain with or without diarrhea. Diarrheal stool may be mixed with blood, mucus, and/or pus. Bowel movements are often painful. Cramping in the right lower side of the abdomen is common, especially after meals. People with Crohn's disease often have chronic low-grade fever, poor appetite, fatigue, and weight loss. Skin rashes may also occur. People who have Crohn's disease often have some degree of anemia, related to poor iron, folic acid, and/or vitamin B12 absorption and due to chronic blood loss. Those with mild Crohn's can eat and function reasonably normally, while those with severe disease often fail to respond to conventional treatment and have persistent gastrointestinal symptoms, as well as fevers, and infections. Blood tests for ferritin, which measures iron storage, and vitamin B12 and folate can help detect deficiencies due to malabsorption.

Diagnosis of Crohn's disease is usually based on a patient's medical history and symptoms. Diagnostic tests may be used to confirm the disease and to distinguish it from ulcerative colitis. Such tests include x-rays (with contrast material such as barium), colonoscopy, and endoscopy.

No blood test can diagnose Crohn's disease, but routine testing is usually done to detect anemia, infection, degree of inflammation, and determine liver function. Certain markers of inflammation, such as erythrocyte sedimentation rate (ESR) and C-reactive protein (CRP) may be used to follow a patient's course over time. The anti-*Saccharomyces cerevisiae* antibody (ASCA) blood test is sometimes used to help differentiate Crohn's disease from ulcerative colitis.[11]

There is a high prevalence of celiac disease in people with Crohn's disease.[12] Celiac disease blood testing such as tissue transglutaminase and antigliadin antibodies should be considered in Crohn's.

## ULCERATIVE COLITIS: BACKGROUND AND DIAGNOSIS

Ulcerative colitis is characterized by inflammation of the large intestine (colon) that leads to episodes of bloody diarrhea, abdominal cramping, and even fever. Unlike Crohn's disease, ulcerative colitis usually does not affect the full thickness of the intestine and rarely affects the small intestine. The disease usually begins in the rectum or sigmoid colon and spreads partially or completely through the large intestine.

Ulcerative colitis typically begins gradually, with abdominal pain and diarrhea that is sometimes bloody. In more serious cases, diarrhea is severe and frequent. Fever, loss of appetite, and weight loss occur. The severity of the disease depends on how much of the colon is involved. For many patients, there may be long periods with no symptoms at all, followed by flare-ups.

A definitive diagnosis can be made by direct examination of the colon by sigmoidoscopy (examination of the lower portion only) or colonoscopy (examination of the entire colon, the preferred approach). Both procedures can be used to take a biopsy of intestinal tissue, which can reveal important information about the degree and extent of inflammation and help rule out other causes of symptoms. A barium enema x-ray of the colon may also be required at some point in the course of colitis to determine the extent of involvement. Once diagnosed, ulcerative colitis can be categorized based on disease severity as follows:

- **Severe.** Severe ulcerative colitis, which involves the entire colon, is the least common form of the disease. Symptoms consist of profuse bloody diarrhea (occurring 6 or more times per day), often with a sustained fever and tachycardia (rapid heart rate). Severe anemia, increased white blood cell count, and decreased serum albumin levels are also characteristic symptoms.

- **Moderate.** Symptoms consist of recurrent diarrhea, small amounts of blood in the stool, possible low-grade fever, mild anemia, and minimal signs of inflammation. Moderate ulcerative colitis responds quickly to appropriate therapies. However, repeated attacks of equal or increased severity can occur, which can significantly increase the risk of developing colon cancer later.

- **Mild.** Mild ulcerative colitis is the most common form of the disorder, occurring in about 50% of patients. In most cases, ulcerative colitis will be limited to the lower portion of the colon and the rectum. Systemic complications are uncommon and the primary symptom is rectal bleeding.

## CONVENTIONAL TREATMENT OPTIONS

Conventional treatments for IBD depend on disease location and severity, complications, and response to prior treatments. The goals of therapy are to control inflammation, correct nutritional deficiencies, and relieve symptoms such as abdominal pain, diarrhea, and rectal bleeding. It is important to note that an early diagnosis is associated with greater efficacy of less-aggressive drug regimens and thus a less oppressive burden of side effects. Therefore, seeing a physician as soon as symptoms emerge is suggested. Therapy may include drugs, surgery, or a combination of approaches.

### Drug Treatments
The following drugs can be used to treat IBD:

#### Anti-Inflammatory Drugs

- Aminosalicylates are drugs that contain 5-aminosalicyclic acid (5-ASA) and help control local inflammation of the gut. These drugs are primarily used to treat mild to moderate IBD and help with remission maintenance.[13] Adverse effects include nausea, vomiting, heartburn, diarrhea, and headache. 5-ASA agents such as olsalazine, mesalamine, and balsalazide have fewer adverse effects and may be used by people who cannot take sulfasalazine. Balsalazide is converted in the colon to mesalamine, and has been shown to reduce bowel inflammation, diarrhea, rectal bleeding, and stomach pain.[14] 5-ASA agents are given orally or rectally (through an enema or in a suppository), depending on the location of the inflammation. Sulfasalazine interferes with folate absorption, so those taking this drug should also supplement with folate.[15] Use of aminosalicylate drugs or antibiotics may deplete vitamin K in IBD patients, and oral supplementation of this vitamin relieves this problem.[16]

- *Glucocorticoids or corticosteroids* (such as prednisone and hydrocortisone) reduce inflammation. They are used to treat more severe cases of IBD and to end acute attacks. Glucocorticoids can be given orally, intravenously, or rectally (through an enema or in a suppository), depending on the location of the inflammation. These drugs can cause serious adverse effects, including increased risk of infection, diabetes, high blood pressure, bone loss, kidney suppression, and ulcers. Less serious adverse effects include weight gain, acne, facial hair, and mood swings. They are not recommended for long-term use and are typically replaced with 5-ASA drugs once remission has been induced. Calcium and vitamin D may help combat glucocorticoid-induced bone loss.[17]

### Immune System Suppressors

- **Azathioprine and Mercaptopurine.** These antimetabolites prevent replication of inflammatory T-cell lines. They are used to treat people with IBD who have not responded to 5-ASAs or glucocorticoids, or who are dependent on glucocorticoids. However, antimetabolites are slower acting than other types of drugs. Anyone taking these drugs should be monitored for complications such as pancreatitis, hepatotoxicity, reduced white blood cell count, and an increased risk of infection. A genetic test known as thiopurine methyltransferase (TMPT) genotyping can help predict who will have severe adverse effects from these drugs.[18]

- **Cyclosporine.** This drug inhibits T-cell–mediated immune responses, thus reducing the immune reaction that underlies inflammation. It blocks a number of inflammatory cytokines, including TNF-α and various interleukins. Because cyclosporine is associated with significant risk of toxicity, its use is limited to severe ulcerative colitis or Crohn's disease.

- **Methotrexate.** The cancer chemotherapy drug methotrexate is used in Crohn's patients that are steroid dependent or have not responded to glucocorticoids.[19] It can be given orally or by weekly injections under the skin or into the muscles.[20] Methotrexate is most effective for maintenance of remission when given as an injection.[21] This drug also interferes with folate metabolism. Folate should be supplemented with it, particularly to help prevent colorectal cancer, which this drug otherwise promotes.[21,22]

- **Biologics/TNF-α Inhibitors.** During flare-ups, levels of the inflammatory cytokine TNF-α become elevated. This has led to interest in antibodies such as infliximab, adalimumab, certolizumab pegol, and golimumab that block TNF-α. These have all been shown to induce and maintain remission including mucosal healing and restoration of gut barrier function.[23–25] However, these drugs are very expensive, have not been shown to prevent colectomy in severe ulcerative colitis,[26] and may cause autoimmune diseases, cancer, infections, and viral reactivation syndromes including shingles.[27]

- The following immunosuppressive agents may be considered as well: tacrolimus, mycophenolate mofetil, and thalidomide.

### Others

- **Cromolyn Sodium.** This drug is modified from the natural compound known as khellin and works as a mast cell–stabilizing anti-inflammatory. One clinical trial found that daily administration of 200 mg cromolyn sodium rectally for 15 days induced remission in almost all patients with ulcerative colitis, and this was maintained in 93% of them when they took 240 mg daily for 2–3 years.[28] In another trial, oral cromolyn sodium at a dose of 1500 mg daily relieved diarrhea more effectively than an elimination diet (in which problematic foods are avoided) in patients with irritable bowel syndrome.[29] This indicates that cromolyn may ameliorate reactivity to some foods, a factor that possibly drives some inflammation in inflammatory bowel disease. As is so often the case with drugs that are off-patent and thus not very profitable, no company or government has seen fit to fund further research on this safe and cheap drug for inflammatory bowel disease.

- **Naltrexone.** Originally developed to help treat heroin addiction, lower doses of naltrexone have shown a range of remarkable immunological activities. A placebo-controlled study on the use of low-dose naltrexone (4.5 mg/day at bedtime) suggested that the drug could resolve mucosal inflammation and induce clinical remission in patients with moderate-to-severe Crohn's disease.[30] This confirms one earlier uncontrolled study of low-dose naltrexone's efficacy for Crohn's disease.[31] Naltrexone appears to relieve inflammatory bowel disease in part by decreasing expression of proinflammatory cytokines and promoting tissue repair.[32] At low dosages, the drug may cause drowsiness, but other side effects are uncommon.

## Surgery

In severe cases of Crohn's disease, abscesses can develop in chronically inflamed tissues. These abscesses can grow and tunnel through tissue barriers to produce *fistulas*, or channels between organs. Almost half of patients who have Crohn's disease develop perianal disease involving anal fissures, perianal abscesses, and fistulas. These symptoms seldom respond well to conventional therapies.[33,34] Surgery may be required in a high percentage of these patients.[35] Complications are frequent.

Surgery may also be recommended to remove severely inflamed portions of the intestinal tract. The goal of surgery is to preserve as much of the intestine as possible. Surgery commonly involves the colon or small intestine. Occasionally, the end of the intestine that has been left in place will need to be brought to the skin's surface to allow waste excretion. When this procedure involves the small intestine, it is called an ileostomy. If the procedure involves the colon, it is called a colostomy. Although Crohn's disease may recur after surgery, the symptoms are likely to be less severe and less debilitating than they were previously.[36] Elemental diets (in which simple molecules like glucose and individual amino acids replace whole foods) have been shown to reduce recurrence of Crohn's disease when employed after surgery.[37,38]

Newer surgeries, however, have been developed that can preserve fecal continence by using part of the ileum to create a pouch that is connected to the intact rectal sphincter.[36] In a thorough review, the use of probiotic supplements was able to significantly reduce the occurrence of pouchitis, or inflammation of the reservoir formed upon surgical creation of an ileoanal pouch, by 96% compared to placebo after surgery among ulcerative colitis patients.[39]

# DIETARY AND LIFESTYLE CONSIDERATIONS

Lifestyle changes and nutritional supplementation synergize to promote healthy digestion and absorption while simultaneously reducing the inflammation and damage associated with inflammatory bowel disease (IBD).

## Crohn's Disease

Since aspirin increases the risk of Crohn's disease (but not ulcerative colitis), people with Crohn's disease should consider avoiding the medication.[40]

The GI tract of individuals with Crohn's disease may also be exceptionally sensitive to the negative effects of smoking. Smoking among those diagnosed with Crohn's disease may increase the risk of flare ups, impede remission, and increase the overall severity of the condition necessitating more invasive treatments.[41] The following steps may help patients with Crohn's disease first reduce their symptoms and then begin long-term repair of the damage caused by their disease:

**Avoid Troublesome Foods.** Remove all foods that precipitate symptoms. In one study of Crohn's disease patients, an elemental diet was followed by food reintroduction with one new food daily. If any food reintroductions led to symptoms such as diarrhea or pain, they were excluded. This approach was more effective than glucocorticoids in preventing relapse of Crohn's disease in this trial.[42] A trial diet of just organic meat, spelt, butter, and organic tea was found to be superior to a low-fat, high-carbohydrate, low-fiber diet for people with Crohn's disease.[43] Long-term remission was achieved in 31% of Crohn's patients in one study solely using an elimination diet.[44] Other evidence suggests Crohn's disease patients are more reactive to certain foods.[45,46] Some research suggests a reduced carbohydrate diet (84 g/day) may be associated with better outcomes in Crohn's disease.[47] Also, elevated levels of trans-fats have been found in the adipose (fat) tissue of people with Crohn's disease.[47,48] Baker's yeast should be avoided in those with elevated yeast antibodies, and has been shown to aggravate Crohn's disease in some research.[49]

Following a diet based on blood *IgG antibody testing* for food sensitivities has been shown to reduce stool frequency in Crohn's patients.[50] In one trial, Crohn's disease symptoms were shown to be aggravated by diverse foods differing among study participants. Elimination of the problematic foods was helpful on an individual basis, but the bothersome foods were not the same for all subjects, underscoring the need to identify specific foods that cause symptoms.[51] More information about testing for food allergies and sensitivities is available in the Allergies protocol.

**Supplement to Correct Potential Nutritional Insufficiencies.** The diets of most patients who have

IBD are deficient in one or more vitamins or minerals.[52] Vitamin D and vitamin K deficiencies are frequently found in those with Crohn's disease, as well as deficiencies in iron, vitamin B6, carotene, vitamin B12, and albumin (protein).[53–55] Patients with Crohn's disease are usually under increased oxidative stress and have lower levels of antioxidant vitamins. Supplementation with vitamins C and E reduces oxidative stress.[56]

**Balance Intestinal Microbiota.** A normal healthy intestine contains about 100 trillion microorganisms.[57] In a diseased intestine, these bacteria are often not present in adequate amounts and/or have been replaced by pathogenic organisms. Balancing microbiota consists of taking mixtures of friendly bacteria (probiotics), which may include *Bifidobacteria* and *Lactobacilli* to promote continued repopulation with these beneficial bacteria.[58] The probiotic yeast *Saccharomyces boulardii* may be considered as well. The role of probiotics in inflammatory bowel diseases is expounded upon below.

In children and adolescents who have Crohn's disease, a semielemental diet has been shown to be as effective as glucocorticoids in maintaining remissions.[59] In one study of IBD, 44% of the study population went into remission by consuming an elemental diet.[60,61] An elemental diet has also been shown to decrease inflammatory parameters in IBD intestinal tissue. The elemental diet also reduces intestinal permeability in those with Crohn's disease.[62,63] When coupled with individualized elimination of food triggers, elemental diets reduce the relapse rate of Crohn's disease.[64] In another trial involving 268 Crohn's disease patients, an elemental diet was associated with a reduced hospitalization rate.[65]

Those who use conventional elemental diets are sometimes noted to develop micronutrient deficiencies, such as of selenium.[66] Therefore, supplementation with a high-quality multivitamin/mineral, among other nutrients discussed below, may be pertinent.

## Ulcerative Colitis

Sulphate-reducing bacteria (SRB) have been implicated in the development of ulcerative colitis through the harmful effects of hydrogen sulfide, a waste product of their respiration.[67,68] Hydrogen sulfide is toxic to the colon-lining cells, and is associated with ulcerative colitis. Hydrogen sulfide may, in particular, interfere with butyrate metabolism, a critical nutrient for colon cells produced by beneficial bacteria.[69] Also, higher exposure to sulfur dioxide air pollution was associated with higher rates of ulcerative colitis in one study.[70] Ulcerative colitis has also been associated with a higher dietary intake of sulfur-containing foods. Removing foods rich in sulfur-containing amino acids (such as milk, eggs, and cheese) is associated with benefits in ulcerative colitis.[71–73]

# NUTRITIONAL AND ALTERNATIVE THERAPY

Inflamed intestines may not absorb nutrients properly. Therefore, people with IBD are prone to malnutrition and vitamin deficiencies.[74–77]

**Probiotics.** Variation in the population of microorganisms within the digestive tract is capable of altering immune cell function locally and systemically. One study describes a novel probiotic organism that can directly produce *interleukin-10* (IL-10), an anti-inflammatory cytokine that promotes immune tolerance.[78–80] Furthermore, ingestion of probiotic bacteria can blunt the effects of pathogenic bacteria via various mechanisms including, competing for epithelial receptor binding, and enhancing the barrier function of the gut.[78,81,82] Some probiotics also produce butyrate—a short-chain fatty acid important for health of cells within the colon wall.[83]

Clinical trials of probiotic use in IBD populations have indicated beneficial effects. Duration of trials and organisms employed has varied, but there have been several instances of positive results.[84] A 2011 trial using a probiotic (*Bifidobacterium breve*) as well as a prebiotic (galacto-oligosaccharide) demonstrated a marked improvement in clinical status of people with ulcerative colitis.[85] Clinical trials in Crohn's disease showed that supplements supplying 50 billion organisms per day or higher improved gut health.[86,87] In one trial, relief was so great for two subjects they were able to discontinue glucocorticoid medication.[86] Other research suggests that probiotics may suppress the likelihood of colorectal cancer development, a major concern for patients with IBD.[88]

Another organism that has shown promise in IBD is *Saccharomyces boulardii*, a probiotic yeast. Several trials have proven the efficacy of *S. boulardii* for ameliorating infectious diarrhea and other gastrointestinal problems.[89] Moreover, specifically relevant to IBD, *S. boulardii* appears to modulate the inflammatory response in the intestinal epithelium, reducing TNF-α and IL-6.[90] This same study showed that *S. boulardii* promotes intestinal tissue repair and immune tolerance in cell samples from patients with IBD. In a randomized, placebo-controlled clinical trial, *S. boulardii* lessened intestinal permeability in Crohn's disease patients when it was added to conventional therapy.[91] Supplementation with *S. boulardii* appears to generally be safe and effective in a variety of pathologic states.[92]

**Omega-3 Fatty Acids.** The two most prominent omega-3s, *eicosapentaenoic acid* (EPA) and *docosahexaenoic acid* (DHA), are found in cold-water fish.[93] Omega-3 fatty acids are powerful immunoregulatory agents that reduce circulating inflammatory cytokines and decrease the cytotoxicity of natural killer cells.[94-98] Additionally, in one animal study, α-linolenic acid (a plant-derived omega-3 fatty acid) suppressed expression of *adhesion molecules*, which are important in inflammation, immune responses and in intracellular signaling events.[99,100]

In clinical trials, fish oil supplementation improves the fatty acid profile in Crohn's disease and ulcerative colitis patients, and is associated with lower levels of inflammatory mediators.[101-103] These changes have some correlation with remission from disease flares.[104,105] Fish oil may also reduce the dosage of glucocorticoid drugs needed to cause a remission.[105] *Enteric-coated* fish oil was found to be helpful in one study of Crohn's disease patients by reducing the rate of relapse.[106]

The majority of Americans have unhealthy high ratios of omega-6s to omega-3s in their blood—an imbalance strongly associated with inflammatory diseases.[107] Life Extension recommends that the omega-6 to omega-3 ratio be kept *below 4:1* for optimal health[108]; this may be especially important for IBD patients. You can assess your omega-6 to omega-3 ratio using a convenient blood test called the *Omega Score® test*.

**Vitamin D.** Vitamin D is another powerful immunomodulator. Experimental models have shown that T-cells express a vitamin D receptor, and that lack of vitamin D signaling causes T-cells to produce higher levels of inflammatory cytokines. Moreover, vitamin D is required for development of subsets of T-cells that are important in suppressing inflammation specifically in the gut.[109,110] Patients with IBD often have low vitamin D levels, as revealed by low levels of serum 25-hydroxyvitamin D.[111] Many other lines of evidence connect low vitamin D levels with IBD as well.[112,113] Administration of 25-hydroxyvitamin D3 or calcitriol (fully activated vitamin D3, a very potent substance available only by prescription) lowered measures of inflammation and improved bone health in 37 patients with Crohn's disease in remission.[114] Taking 1200 IU of vitamin D3 per day showed a trend toward a lower relapse rate (from 29% to 13% [$P = 0.06$]) compared to placebo in one double-blind trial involving 94 Crohn's disease patients in remission.[115] Moreover,

bone loss is a major concern for IBD patients—both the disease and glucocorticoids used to treat it contribute to poor bone health. Supplementation with vitamin D has been shown to maintain bone density in Crohn's disease.[116]

Life Extension suggests maintenance of 25-hydroxyvitamin D levels within the range of *50–80 ng/mL*. Testing your vitamin D blood level is inexpensive and convenient. A 25-hydroxyvitamin D blood test should be performed regularly by those supplementing with vitamin D to ensure that they stay in the optimal range.

**Antioxidants.** Normal digestion produces a host of reactive oxygen and nitrogen species (also known as free radicals), against which the intestinal mucosa maintains an extensive defense system of antioxidants. When presented with excessive oxidant stress, however, the mucosal barrier can sustain damage and become leaky, setting the stage for inflammation.[117,118]

In addition, inflammation itself produces large quantities of reactive species, and a destructive cycle can be perpetuated. In patients who have IBD, there are high levels of reactive oxygen species in the intestines, which contributes to the damage caused by the disease.[117] In one study, the antioxidant capacity of individuals with IBD was found to be significantly lower than those without the disease.[119] Some research has shown that an antioxidant combination of vitamin A, vitamin C, vitamin E, and selenium in combination with fish oil can reduce certain inflammatory markers in Crohn's disease.[120,121] Moreover, IBD patients had significantly lower levels of carotenoids and vitamin C, in their blood.[122]

**Curcumin.** The efficacy of the turmeric extract curcumin as an anti-inflammatory agent in a variety of settings is well-documented. Prominent among its multiple effects is the inhibition of *nuclear factor kappa-B* (NF-κB) signaling. NF-κB is a signaling protein that drives production of myriad inflammatory cytokines including interleukin-1b (IL-1b) and interleukin-6 (IL-6). Since NF-κB and related cytokines are central in IBD pathology, curcumin has been investigated as an intervention.[123] In one study, curcumin helped reduce symptoms of Crohn's disease and ulcerative colitis in a small group of patients, many of whom were able to discontinue aminosalicylates and/or glucocorticoids.[123,124] Curcumin coupled with aminosalicylates reduced recurrence of acute flares and symptom severity compared to placebo plus aminosalicylates in a group of 82 ulcerative colitis patients. In the curcumin group, the relapse rate during 6 months of therapy was 4.6%, while in the control group it was over 20%.[125]

**Boswellia.** Resin from the Boswellia genus of tree contains a powerful anti-inflammatory compound called *acetyl-11-keto-β-boswellic acid* (AKBA). One double-blind clinical trial found that boswellia was as effective as mesalamine at improving symptoms of Crohn's disease with far fewer side effects.[126] One trial has also found boswellia as effective as sulfasalazine for inducing remission from ulcerative colitis in 30 patients.[127] This confirmed an earlier report of efficacy of boswellia for ulcerative colitis patients.[128] However, another double-blind trial involving 108 Crohn's disease patients did not find boswellia superior to placebo for maintaining remission.[129] An improved extract called AprèsFlex™, or Aflapin®, which combines AKBA with other nonvolatile boswellia oils, demonstrated improved anti-inflammatory activity at a lower concentration when compared to other preparations standardized to the same percentage of AKBA.[130]

**Wormwood.** A standardized extract of wormwood (*Artemisia absinthium*), a bitter herb native to the Mediterranean region, has been studied in patients with Crohn's disease. Compared to placebo it was much more effective at maintaining remission in patients who tapered off their medications.[131] The reason for this may be because wormwood blocks TNF-α,[132] a potent proinflammatory cytokine.

**Aloe Gel.** The mucilaginous gel found in the interior of aloe leaves has been used traditionally for ulcerative colitis for many years. One double-blind, randomized trial found that aloe gel at a dose of 3 oz twice a day ended acute flares in ulcerative colitis patients better than placebo without adverse effects.[132] Aloe gel's immunomodulating, gut healing, and inflammation-quelling properties may all play a role in its efficacy.[133]

**Selenium.** Selenium is a trace element that is essential for the function of a number of selenium-dependent enzymes. Selenium deficiency is common in people who have IBD.[134–136] Supplementation helps alleviate this problem, based both on increases in serum selenium and improved glutathione peroxidase function.[137]

**Butyrate.** Butyrate (also known as butyric acid) is a short-chain fatty acid produced when intestinal fiber is metabolized by certain bacteria. Experimental models have shown that oral butyrate ameliorates inflammation in ulcerative colitis.[138] One mechanism by which butyrate may function is to inhibit the activation of the proinflammatory cell–signaling component *nuclear factor kappa B* (NF-κB).[139] In clinical trials, oral butyrate has provided relief in both Crohn's *and* ulcerative colitis.[140–141] In one trial, nearly 70% of

subjects with Crohn's disease responded to a dose of 4 grams (g) of enteric-coated butyrate tablets daily for 8 weeks. Of those responders, 53% achieved remission and their levels of NF-κB and another inflammatory factor—IL-1b—decreased significantly.[141]

**L-Carnitine.** The amino acid carnitine is necessary for proper cellular metabolism, and insufficient carnitine levels particularly affect cells that require a great deal of energy, such as those of the immune system. Several experiments have shown that carnitine modulates production of inflammatory mediators and that insufficient carnitine levels are associated with greater production of inflammatory cytokines.[142,143] Indeed, in a clinical trial involving 36 dialysis patients, 1 g/day L-carnitine supplementation led to a 29% reduction in CRP levels and a 61% reduction in IL-6 levels.[144] With respect to the gut, L-carnitine significantly blunted the inflammatory response to oxygen deprivation and restoration in intestinal tissue in an animal model.[145] In a randomized, placebo-controlled trial involving 121 subjects with ulcerative colitis, *propionyl-L-carnitine*, at 1–2 g daily, led to greater remission rates than placebo when added to conventional therapy.[146] In the group receiving 1 g of carnitine daily, the rate of remission was 55%, while in the placebo group it was only 35%.

**Glutamine.** A conditionally essential amino acid, glutamine is the major fuel for the enterocytes (intestinal absorptive cells). Oral glutamine supplementation can stabilize intestinal permeability and mucosal integrity.[147] A study demonstrated that glutamine can help improve capillary blood flow in inflamed segments of the colon in animals with colitis.[148] Moreover, glutamine levels are low in people with moderate-to-severe Crohn's disease.[149] In a randomized clinical trial, a 0.5 g/kg body weight daily dose of glutamine for 2 months decreased intestinal permeability and improved morphology in patients with Crohn's disease.[150] However, the clinical benefit of glutamine supplementation may be limited to periods of remission, as another trial found that glutamine supplementation during a disease flare did not improve intestinal permeability.[151]

**Melatonin.** Although melatonin is known as a hormone that helps synchronize sleep–wake cycles, it has also been shown to be produced in the digestive tract in quantities far larger than in the brain.[152] Melatonin reduces TNF-α levels.[153] Numerous *in vitro* and animal studies have suggested that melatonin can reduce inflammation in IBD.[154] Melatonin synthesis increases in IBD patients and higher levels are associated with lower symptoms, suggesting it is part of the body's attempt to reduce excessive inflammation.[155] In a double-blind trial of 60 patients with ulcerative colitis being treated with mesalazine, half were randomized to take melatonin and half to take placebo for 1 year.[156] Inflammation and clinical symptoms rose in the placebo group while the melatonin group remained in remission. This confirms an earlier, uncontrolled study showing that melatonin was helpful for patients with Crohn's disease and ulcerative colitis.[157] Caution is warranted, though—at least one case study has been published in which melatonin caused a flare of ulcerative colitis that did not respond to glucocorticoids.[158]

**Dehydroepiandrosterone (DHEA).** This hormone plays an important role in preventing chronic inflammation and to maintain healthy immune function. Published studies link low levels of DHEA to chronic inflammation, and DHEA has been shown to suppress levels of proinflammatory cytokines and protect against their toxic effects.[159,160] DHEA has been shown to suppress damaging IL-6 levels.[161]

The deficiency of DHEA in inflammatory diseases also implies a deficiency in peripheral tissue of various sex hormones for which DHEA serves as a precursor. These hormones, both estrogenic and androgenic, are known to have beneficial effects on muscle, bone, and blood vessels. However, mainstream therapy with glucocorticoids lowers androgen levels. Consequently, researchers argue that hormone replacement for patients who have chronic inflammatory diseases should include not only glucocorticoids but also DHEA.[161,162]

**Vitamin K.** This vitamin is used by the body to regulate blood clotting. A deficiency in vitamin K can result in bruising or bleeding. Patients with IBD are frequently deficient in vitamin K. One study showed that 31% of patients who had ulcerative colitis or Crohn's disease had a vitamin K deficiency.[16] Low vitamin K activity was linked with higher Crohn's disease activity in one study.[53] Vitamin K deficiency in IBD patients is associated with lower bone density as well.[53,163]

**Fiber.** Greater intake of dietary fiber is linked with lower incidence of Crohn's disease,[164] while higher sugar consumption is associated with increased risk.[165] A diet low in refined sugar and high in dietary fiber has been shown to have a favorable effect on the course of Crohn's disease and does not lead to intestinal obstruction compared to a normal diet.[166]

Fermentation of dietary fiber by intestinal bacteria is the major source of short-chain fatty acids, such as butyrate, and various studies have shown that vegetable fibers are helpful at preventing flares of ulcerative colitis.[167]

## Folate and Colon Cancer Risk in Ulcerative Colitis

People with ulcerative colitis are at increased risk of colon cancer.[168] It is assumed that chronic inflammation is what causes cancer in ulcerative colitis. This is supported by the fact that colon cancer risk increases with longer duration of colitis, greater anatomic extent of colitis, and the concomitant presence of other inflammatory manifestations.[169] Folate deficiency and an increased level of homocysteine have been linked to greater colon cancer risk in IBD.[170]

In a comprehensive review involving data from 13 studies and over 725 000 subjects, each 100-mcg/day increase in folate intake was associated with a 2% decrease in colon cancer risk.[171] Other evidence highlights multiple ways that folate might protect against colon cancer in ulcerative colitis.[172] However, data are conflicting as other studies have come to differing conclusions. For example, another review found that long-term folic acid supplementation was associated with increased colon cancer risk.[173]

Deficiencies in folate and B12 are often observed in IBD.[174] Supplementing the diet with vitamin B12 enables the body to metabolize folate better and avoids masking a vitamin B12 deficiency. Vitamin B12 supplementation is important, particularly for older people (when it is less effectively absorbed) and for vegetarians, especially vegans, who obtain little B12 from their diet. More information is available in the Colorectal Cancer protocol.

## INFLAMMATORY BOWEL DISEASE AND ELEVATED HOMOCYSTEINE LEVELS

A number of studies have shown that patients with IBD are more likely to have elevated homocysteine levels. A comprehensive review of published studies found that the risk of having high homocysteine levels was over *4 times greater* in IBD patients compared to controls.[175] In one study, more than 55% of patients with IBD had elevated homocysteine levels.[176] The greatest risk factor for elevated homocysteine in patients with IBD is reduced folate levels.[177] Vitamin B12 deficiencies are also frequently encountered.[178]

The elevated homocysteine level that is typical in patients with IBD contributes to a 3-fold higher risk of blood clots and vascular disease.[179,180] It also helps explain why patients with IBD are more likely to have early atherosclerosis.[181]

Certain drugs used to treat IBD, such as methotrexate, are antimetabolites for folic acid, which may help explain why so many patients are deficient in folic acid. Supplementation of folic acid reduces adverse effects caused by methotrexate as well.[21]

Genetic studies have found that alterations in folate metabolism are associated with IBD.[182] Therefore, IBD patients may benefit from supplementation with *5-methyltetrahydrofolate*, the active form of the nutrient.

More information about managing homocysteine levels is available in the Homocysteine Reduction protocol.

## Inflammatory Bowel Disease and Bone Loss

Osteoporosis is a serious complication of IBD that has not received adequate recognition despite its high prevalence and potentially devastating effects.[183,184] Osteoporosis can be caused by IBD itself, or it can be an adverse effect of glucocorticoid treatment. Data derived from a retrospective survey of 245 patients with IBD suggest that the prevalence of bone fractures in people with ulcerative colitis and Crohn's disease is unexpectedly high, particularly in patients who have a long duration of disease, frequent active phases, and high cumulative doses of glucocorticoid intake.[185,186] Low vitamin D and K levels have also been correlated to higher rates of osteoporosis in IBD patients.[187] Bone-density measurements to predict fracture risk and define thresholds for prevention and treatment should be performed routinely in patients with IBD.[188] Glucocorticoids can also contribute to the risk of osteoporosis because of their effects on calcium and bone metabolism. Glucocorticoids suppress calcium absorption in the small intestine, increase calcium excretion by the kidneys, and alter protein metabolism. Patients with Crohn's disease who take glucocorticoids have a higher risk of fractures compared to those who do not.[189] Nutrients that can help protect against bone loss include calcium, magnesium, vitamin D, and vitamin K. For more information, see the Osteoporosis protocol.

## Inflammatory Bowel Disease and Blood Clot Risk

Inflammatory bowel disease patients are at increased risk of forming blood clots—primarily venous thromboembolism.[190-192] These clots can break off and lodge in the blood vessels in the lungs, potentially causing death. Moreover, use of glucocorticoids by IBD patients potentiates clotting propensity.[190] Conventional medicine often relies on warfarin or heparin to mitigate thrombotic risk in IBD patients, but these drugs are prone to cause negative side effects and require clinical monitoring.[193] Vitamin E, vitamin D, and resveratrol may all help offset the risk of clotting in IBD patients, though specific clinical trials are lacking.[194] IBD patients should review the Blood Clot

Prevention protocol for further discussion of strategies to mitigate risk for blood clots.

## Life Extension Suggestions

- **Probiotics**: per label instructions
- *Saccharomyces boulardii*: 250 mg twice daily
- **Fish oil** (with olive polyphenols): At least 1400 mg/day of EPA and 1000 mg/day of DHA
- **Vitamin D**: 5000–8000 IU daily, depending on blood test results
- **Comprehensive multivitamin**: per label instructions
- **Zinc**: 30 mg daily
- **Vitamin C**: 500–2000 mg day
- **Natural vitamin E**: 100–400 IU alpha-tocopherol and 200 mg gamma-tocopherol daily
- **Vitamin A**: 500 IU acetate and 4500 IU beta-carotene daily
- **Vitamin K**: 2100 mcg daily; providing K1, MK-4, and MK-7
- **B-complex vitamins** (many of these should be included in high potency multi-vitamin supplements):
  - Thiamine (B1): 75–125 mg daily
  - Riboflavin (B2): 50 mg daily
  - Niacin (B3): 50–190 mg daily
  - Folate (preferably as L-methylfolate): 400–1000 mcg daily
  - Vitamin B6 (preferably as pyridoxal-5-phosphate): 75–105 mg daily
  - Vitamin B12: 300–600 mcg daily
  - Biotin: 300–3000 mcg daily
  - Pantothenic acid: 100–600 mg daily
- **Selenium**: 100–200 mcg daily
- **Iron**: 15–60 elemental mg daily (depending on ferritin blood test results)
- **Curcumin** (as highly absorbed BCM95®): 400–800 mg daily
- **Boswellia serrata** (as highly absorbed Apres-Flex™): 100 mg daily
- **Propionyl-L-carnitine**: 1000–2000 mg daily
- *Trans*-resveratrol: 100–500 mg daily
- **Wormwood**; standardized extract: per label instructions
- **Aloe gel**: 3 oz twice daily (not the same as aloe juice, which is much more dilute)
- **Soluble fiber**: 5–15 g daily
- **Melatonin**: 0.3–5 mg before bed (sometimes up to 10 mg)
- **DHEA**: 15–25 mg daily for women, and 25–75 mg daily for men (depending on blood test results)

In addition, the following *blood tests* can provide helpful information:

- **C-reactive protein (CRP)** (Available in the Male or Female Panel): Assesses systemic inflammation quantitatively
  - Optimal range: under *1.5* mg/L for women; under 0.55 mg/L for men
- **Erythrocyte sedimentation rate (ESR)**: A functional assessment of the inflammatory tendency of a blood sample
- **Omega Score®:** Assesses the blood fatty acid profile
  - Optimal range: omega-6 to omega-3 ratio <4:1
- **Vitamin D, 25-Hydroxy**: Assesses vitamin D status
  - Optimal range: 50–80 ng/mL
- **DHEA** (Available in the Male or Female Panel)
  - Optimal range: 350–490 µg/dL for men and 275–400 ug/dL for women
- **IgG antibodies**: Quantitatively assesses systemic immunoreactivity to foods

- **Cytokine Panel**: Assesses levels of the inflammatory mediators interleukin 1B (IL-1b), IL-6, IL-8, and TNF-α
- **Ferritin**: Assesses stored iron status to help detect anemia due to iron malabsorption
- **B12 and Folate**: Determines B12 and folate status; useful for detecting anemia
- **Celiac Disease Antibody Screen**: Assesses for possible celiac disease

## REFERENCES

References available at: www.lef.org/dpt5/ch79

# 80

# *Influenza*

## PREAMBLE

If you are reading this because you have developed influenza symptoms, it is critical that you act quickly to halt the rapid replication of viruses occurring in your body at this very moment. Go to the nearest health food store or pharmacy and purchase:

1. **Zinc lozenges.** Take 2 zinc lozenges (13–24 mg of zinc in each lozenge) immediately and again every 2–3 hours for 1–2 days. Then slowly reduce the dose until symptoms dissipate.
2. **Garlic.** Take 9000–18000 mg of a high-allicin garlic supplement each day until symptoms subside. Take with food to minimize stomach irritation.
3. **Vitamin D.** If you do not already maintain a blood level of *25-hydroxyvitamin D* over 50 ng/mL, then take 50000 IU of vitamin D the first day and continue for 3 more days. Slowly reduce the dose to around 5000 IU vitamin D daily. If you already take around 5000 IU of vitamin D daily, then you probably do not need to increase your intake.
4. **Cimetidine.** Take 800–1200 mg daily in divided doses. Cimetidine is a heartburn drug that has potent immune-enhancing properties. (It is sold in pharmacies over the counter.)
5. **Melatonin.** 3–50 mg at bedtime.

*Do not delay implementing the above regimen.* Once a flu virus infects too many cells, it replicates out of control and strategies like zinc lozenges will not be effective. Treatment must be initiated as soon as symptoms manifest.

The flu is a highly contagious, potentially *deadly* viral infection of the nose, throat, and lungs. It is caused by a number of *influenza* virus strains.[1-3] The flu is responsible for over 200000 hospitalizations and thousands of deaths annually in the United States.[3-6]

In the majority of flu cases the illness is self-limiting with recovery typically within 2 weeks.[1,7,8] However, some groups are at high risk for developing flu-related complications (eg, bacterial pneumonia), including people 65 or older, people with certain medical conditions (eg, asthma, COPD, diabetes), and those with weakened immune systems.[1,9,10]

Although *vaccination* is the most effective and inexpensive flu *prevention* measure, conventional *treatment* strategies for severe cases of influenza are mainly limited to certain classes of antiviral drugs (eg, neuraminidase inhibitors such as oseltamivir [Tamiflu®]).[11-13] However, among otherwise healthy individuals, these antiviral drugs are only associated with a modest 1-day decrease in flu duration.[14] This might be because antiviral therapy is often initiated *too late* after symptom onset to avert severe illness. Tamiflu® may be especially effective when initiated within 24–48 hours of contracting influenza virus.

Life Extension recommends *early and aggressive action* at the first sign of flu symptoms. Unfortunately, people often wait until they are very sick before seeking influenza treatment. This delay can preclude rapid eradication of the infectious agent. In some cases, treatment delay can be lethal.

This protocol will discuss the nature of the influenza virus, how it is spread, and how its transmission can be prevented. Conventional flu prevention and treatment strategies will be examined, as will novel drug strategies that may reduce severity of symptoms during influenza infection. Several scientifically studied natural therapies that may prevent or ease symptoms of the flu will also be reviewed.

## SIGNS AND SYMPTOMS OF THE FLU

Influenza, commonly called the "flu," is a respiratory infection that is different from the "common cold" or the "stomach flu".[15] Influenza is primarily characterized by inflammation of tissues that line the nasal cavity, throat, the inner surface of the eyelids (ie, conjunctiva), and the lungs.[16-19] Common clinical symptoms of influenza include a sudden onset of fever, fatigue, headache, and muscle aches.[20] Although both the flu and the common cold are caused by a viral infection of the respiratory system, symptoms of the common cold rarely include severe fever, headaches, or extreme exhaustion.[15] More information is available in the Common Cold protocol.

## UNDERSTANDING INFLUENZA

Influenza viruses are classified based on their protein composition. They are divided into types A, B, and C, with type A having numerous subtypes.[15,21] Among the three types of influenza, type A viruses are the most dangerous to humans and are associated with the most severe disease.[15] Influenza type C is less problematic because most people acquire antibodies to influenza C early in life.[22]

In nature, the flu virus continuously mutates.[15] Every year or so, these mutations can create completely new viruses that are often not harmful.[21]

## Common Cold versus the Flu: Comparison of Characteristics[70,119,190–192]

| Feature | Colds | Flu |
| --- | --- | --- |
| Etiologic agent | >200 viral strains; rhinovirus most common | 3 strains of influenza virus: influenza A, B, and C |
| Site of infection | Upper respiratory tract | Entire respiratory system |
| Symptom onset | Gradual: 1–3 days | Sudden: within a few hours |
| Fever, chills | Occasional, low grade (<101° F) | Characteristic, higher (>101° F), lasting 2–4 days |
| Headache | Infrequent, usually mild | Characteristic, more severe |
| General aches, pains | Mild, if any | Characteristic, often severe and affecting the entire body |
| Sore throat | Common, usually mild | Sometimes present |
| Cough, chest congestion | Common; mild to moderate, with hacking, productive cough | Common; potentially severe dry, nonproductive cough |
| Runny, stuffy nose | Very common, accompanied by bouts of sneezing | Sometimes present |
| Fatigue, weakness | Mild, if any | Usual, may be severe and last 2–3 weeks |
| Extreme exhaustion | Rarely | Frequent, usually in early stages of illness |
| Season | Year-round, peaks in winter months | Most cases between November and February |
| Antibiotics helpful? | No, unless secondary bacterial infection develops | No, unless secondary bacterial infection develops |

However, sometimes mutations can alter viral structure in such a way that the virus can suddenly jump the barrier between species and infect humans. In fact, it is the precise assortment of surface proteins that will dictate the severity of each influenza strain.[15] This can occasionally result in the formation of a novel flu virus that is better able to evade the host's immune system, becoming more dangerous to humans.[15] These mutations can also allow influenza to evolve resistance to conventional antiviral drugs.[23]

### Transmission of the Influenza Virus

The flu virus is mostly spread by tiny droplets (ie, aerosols) that are expelled when a person sneezes, coughs, or even speaks. These droplets contain virus-laden respiratory secretions and can transmit influenza if they land in the mouths or noses of bystanders. Also, an individual might become infected by touching their mouth, eyes, and/or nose after previously touching a surface where the virus has landed.[24]

Once the virus has found its way to the host respiratory tract, it will attempt to invade the epithelium (ie, cells that line the tissue surface).[23] Within 4–6 hours of invading a cell, the influenza virus will begin to replicate and the host cell will begin to release large numbers of replicated virus progeny in a process known as "virus shedding." These released viruses are then free to invade any nearby susceptible cells, thus starting a new replication cycle in each newly infected cell. The time from initial infection to symptomatic illness (ie, incubation period) ranges from 1–4 days, with an average of 2 days.[21] The contagious period generally begins 24 hours prior to symptom onset and can continue for up to a week after becoming sick. Young children

and those with a weakened immune system may be contagious for longer periods.[1]

### Influenza among Populations (Epidemics and Pandemics)

When disease outbreaks are confined to one geographical area, they are referred to as *epidemics*.[21] An epidemic is upgraded to a *pandemic* once it has spread to a large number of people in other countries or continents through person-to-person contact.[15,21,25] Out of the three influenza pandemics that occurred during the 20th century, the most deadly was the Spanish flu (influenza type A/H1N1) of 1918–1919, which caused approximately 50 million deaths worldwide.[26–28] In 1997, the novel avian influenza virus (H5N1) first began infecting humans in China and has since been sporadically transmitting from birds to humans across a wide geographical area including Asia, Europe, and Africa.[26] The H5N1 is currently considered to be the most deadly influenza virus that has crossed the species barrier.[29]

The first pandemic of the 21st century was attributed to the swine-origin influenza A (H1N1) virus, which was originally identified in April 2009 in Mexico.[30,31] The H1N1 epidemic spread quickly and was confirmed worldwide in just a few weeks, forcing the World Health Organization (WHO) to officially declare it a pandemic on June 11, 2009.[30] Although most cases of H1N1 resulted in a self-limited respiratory illness, this infection also caused severe progressive pneumonia and death, even among young healthy individuals.[30–32] Moreover, most of the deaths that resulted from H1N1 occurred among individuals younger than 65 years.[21] As of August 2010, the WHO reported that H1N1 had crossed into at least 214 countries and was responsible for approximately 18 500 deaths worldwide.[33] Research suggests the true mortality rate may be 15 times higher than originally reported.[34]

## Seasonal Influenza

Seasonal influenza is also a major public health threat in the United States, as it is associated with significant suffering and death each year.[35] The seasonal flu is a term used to describe the annual outbreaks of influenza that largely occur in late fall and winter in temperate climate regions.[15,36]

Annual flu outbreaks are known for having a significant impact on not only the infected individual, but also society as a whole.[37] For example, 5–20% of the U.S. population is infected by the seasonal flu each year.[15] Globally, seasonal influenza epidemics account for 3–5 million severe cases of illness.[38] and up to 1 million deaths each year.[39] In the United States, seasonal influenza is associated with more than 200 000 hospitalizations and thousands of deaths each year[3,6,40]; thus, it represents a significant economic burden with up to about $5 billion annually in medical costs.[23,41,42]

Although a majority of the suffering and death attributable to seasonal influenza is due to infections among the elderly,[23] seasonal influenza has been known to cause clinical illness and hospitalization in all age groups.[43] Outbreaks of seasonal influenza generally begin abruptly, with a surge in clinical cases of pediatric fever and respiratory illnesses, which is followed by a similar surge in symptoms among adults. These seasonal outbreaks usually last for about 3 months, and spread within a community during a 2–3 week peak period.[23]

Among otherwise healthy adults, seasonal influenza is typically associated with about 6–8 days of clinical symptoms such as sudden fever, general fatigue, headache, or muscle aches.[1,20,37] Additional common symptoms can include dry/unproductive cough, sore throat, and a runny/stuffy nose.[1,21] The seasonal flu can also cause more serious complications, such as secondary bacterial pneumonia, ear infections, sinus infections, dehydration, and worsening of chronic medical conditions including asthma, diabetes, and congestive heart failure.[1] Among those in the workforce, seasonal influenza infection is associated with an average of 4–5 days of sick leave each year.[37] In fact, taking sick leave for influenza is recommended in order to decrease the risk of transmission.[37]

## The Role of Cytokines

Cytokines are a multifunctional group of signaling proteins that regulate immune and inflammatory responses and are released by cells in response to infection. With most infections, the release of cytokines is controlled in order to maintain a balance between killing the virus and minimizing damage to healthy cells.[44,45] However, when certain severe types of influenza A virus (such as H5N1) invade endothelial cells and begin to proliferate, the cells will occasionally flare out of control and mount an excessive host immune response.[46] Also called a *cytokine storm*, this clinical phenomenon involves the massive overproduction of inflammatory cytokines, such as tumor necrosis factor (TNF), interferons (IFN), colony-stimulating factors (CSFs), and interleukins (ILs).[44,47–49]

---

### CYTOKINE STORM

Cytokine storm—a massive inflammatory response mounted by a robust immune system in response to a pathogen—is a predictor of suffering and death, especially among young, otherwise healthy individuals with highly competent immune systems.[50] Although cytokine storms are associated with tissue destruction in the lungs,[51] autopsy studies of H5N1 patients have shown that this dysregulation of cytokines might also be the cause of multiple-organ tissue damage.[52] The initiation of a cytokine storm is not only limited to H5N1, but is also associated with a wide assortment of viral, bacterial, and immunologic diseases.[53]

One potential method for controlling cytokine storms is to restrict the host's immune response, in order to reduce the self-inflicted inflammatory damage.[45,47] However, this has been met with little success. Other therapeutic strategies are aimed at reducing inflammation.[44] Agents shown to suppress excessive cytokine production include fish oil, green tea,[54] black cumin seed oil,[55–58] and Vitamin D.[59]

---

## FLU PREVENTION

### Vaccination

In an effort to reduce the burden of influenza, the World Health Organization Global Influenza Surveillance Network (WHO GISN) tracks and analyzes the epidemiology and antigenic specificity (or surface protein characteristics) of circulating influenza viruses in order to figure out which strains are appropriate vaccine candidates.[60,61]

According to conventional experts, vaccination is the most effective and least expensive intervention for preventing influenza.[13] The Centers for Disease Control and Prevention (CDC) recommends that all individuals over the age of 6 months be vaccinated yearly.[1] However, vaccination does not guarantee flu prevention.[62–64] Public health agencies must correctly determine which influenza strains are likely to be most prevalent during upcoming flu seasons. Strains thought unlikely to cause an outbreak in the coming season are not included in vaccines. Sometimes one of the strains not included in the vaccine can unexpectedly cause an outbreak and the population will not be protected.[65,66]

## Other Considerations

Other important nonpharmaceutical interventions for preventing influenza can be recalled by using the acronym "WHACK," as in "WHACK the Flu"[67–69]:

---

Wash or sanitize your hands frequently.
Home is where you should be when you are sick.
Avoid touching your eyes, nose, and mouth.
Cover your coughs and sneezes with a tissue or the inner crook of your elbow.
Keep your distance from sick people when possible or wear a mask.

---

In addition to avoiding those infected with influenza, the CDC also recommends all linens, eating utensils, and dishes used by sick individuals be thoroughly washed in a dishwasher or by hand with soap and water prior to being used by anyone else.[24]

## CONVENTIONAL FLU TREATMENT

Treatment of the flu typically aims to ease symptoms and prevent complications. In many cases, over-the-counter medicines can relieve symptoms such as aches and fever. However, this approach may not be sufficient for those at high risk for flu-related complications. In high-risk cases, such as hospitalized people with severe illnesses, antiviral therapy is employed.[70]

The decision to initiate antiviral drug therapy for the treatment of influenza depends on a number of factors, such as individual patient characteristics, the time elapsed since symptoms began, as well as the prevalence and virulence of influenza circulating in the surrounding community.[23,71,72] The goal of treatment with antiviral drugs is to reduce signs and symptoms of influenza and prevent hospitalizations or death in patients with severe disease.[73]

The antiviral drugs most commonly used to treat influenza include *neuraminidase inhibitors* (eg, oseltamivir [Tamiflu®] and zanamivir [Relenza®]) and *adamantanes* (eg, amantadine [Symmetrel®] and rimantadine [Flumadine®]).

**Neuraminidase inhibitors.** Neuraminidase inhibitors interfere with viral neuraminidases, which promote viral infection of healthy cells, drive inflammation, and mitigate viral inactivation by respiratory mucus.[74] They produce gastrointestinal side effects such as nausea and

vomiting in about 10% of those who take them and have rarely been reported to cause bronchospasm in asthmatics.[75] They should be administered within 24–48 hours of symptom onset.

**Adamantanes.** Adamantanes are thought to exert antiviral action by inhibiting the release of viral genetic material into the host cell via interfering with uncoating of the virus particle.[76] These drugs can cause potentially serious side effects, such as heart rhythm irregularities, hallucinations, and respiratory distress, especially in the elderly or those with impaired kidney function.[75] Over recent years, the CDC has made recommendations for or against use of adamantanes for treatment or prevention of the flu, depending on which strain is actively circulating in the population. For example, during the 2005–2006 flu season and 2009 H1N1 outbreak, the CDC recommended against the use of adamantanes.[77,78]

Patients infected with a highly pathogenic (such as, H5N1) or resistant form of influenza may be prescribed the antiviral drug *ribavirin* (eg, Copegus®, Rebetol®, Virazole®).[79] Ribavirin, although not directly indicated for influenza, has multiple potential clinical applications (due to its broad spectrum antiviral activity) and has been used to treat influenza on a limited basis.[80–82] Adverse effects of ribavirin may include nausea, joint and muscle pain, bone marrow depression, heart rhythm irregularities, and pancreatitis.[75]

One of the most important things to know before taking antiviral drugs is how long it has been since the onset of influenza-like symptoms. In general, antiviral drug treatment should be started within 48 hours of symptom onset[83]; clinical studies have demonstrated little benefit when these agents are given outside this time window.[71] However, results of a survey of patients at an internal medicine clinic showed only 13% reported calling their physician within 48 hours after initial symptom onset.[84]

The CDC recommends that antiviral drug treatment only be used in select patient populations.[85] This may be because most cases of seasonal influenza are self-limiting,[8] because antiviral drugs can cause side effects, and because the drugs are only capable of decreasing symptoms by 1 day among healthy individuals.[86] However, individuals who are hospitalized, severely ill, or at high risk of infection should be treated with an antiviral drug within 48 hours of symptom onset. High-risk groups may include children <2 years and adults ≥65 years, the immunocompromised, the morbidly obese (ie, body mass index [BMI] ≥40), and long-term care residents. High-risk groups may also be prescribed antiviral drugs on a preventive basis. Although antiviral medications are between 70–90% effective for preventing influenza infections, they should not be used capriciously because they can promote the emergence of resistant viral strains.[85] Since influenza is caused by a virus and not a bacterium, taking antibiotics is not recommended and could lead to unwanted side effects and/or a future antibiotic-resistant infection.[87]

# NOVEL FLU TREATMENT STRATEGIES

## Cimetidine

The over-the-counter drug cimetidine is a histamine receptor type 2 (H-2) blocker approved by the Food and Drug Administration (FDA) for inhibition of gastric acid secretion or gastric and duodenal ulcer disease.[88,89] Cimetidine has also been shown to augment the immune system. It appears to accomplish this by mitigating the effects of specialized immune cells called T-regulatory cells, which normally suppress immunity.[90–93] Since cimetidine enhances the immune system, it may be beneficial for combating various infections and has been utilized as an immune modulator for the treatment of several diseases such as herpes simplex infections and mucocutaneous candidiasis.[94,95] However, since cimetidine stimulates proinflammatory cytokines and inhibits regulatory T cells,[93] it may exacerbate the development of a cytokine storm and should be avoided by individuals at risk for cytokine storm.

## Statin-Class Drugs

Statins (eg, simvastatin, atorvastatin, and lovastatin) reduce serum lipids (ie, cholesterol) and are used to prevent and treat vascular diseases.[96] Further research into the actions of statin drugs has revealed that these drugs can down-regulate inflammatory immune responses to certain influenza viruses.[97,98] A 2007 study found that moderate-dose statin users had a dramatically reduced risk of mortality from influenza and chronic obstructive pulmonary disease (COPD) compared to non-statin users.[99] Furthermore, a 2012 study revealed that statin use may be linked with reduced mortality in patients hospitalized with influenza.[97]

# TARGETED NATURAL INTERVENTIONS

In addition to consuming a healthy, balanced diet and exercising regularly, the following natural interventions may help avoid influenza infection or ease flu symptoms.[100–102]

## Vitamin D

Vitamin D has a significant role in the regulation of the human immune system and may reduce the risk of certain viral and bacterial infections by modulating immune response to such pathogens.[103,104] Vitamin D blood levels appear to be related to respiratory infections, in that a 4-ng/mL increase in vitamin D levels correspond to about a 7–10% decrease in infection risk.[105,106] Furthermore, vitamin D deficiency may be linked to an increased risk of influenza and respiratory tract infection.[103,107] In one clinical trial, 1200 IU daily of vitamin D3 reduced incidence of seasonal influenza by about 67% in school children compared to children not taking any vitamin D–containing supplements.[108] Similarly, in a 3-year trial, postmenopausal African American women taking 2000 IU of vitamin D daily reported significantly fewer incidence of influenza compared to those taking a placebo.[109]

Vitamin D is derived in the skin from its precursor 7-dehydrocholesterol following stimulation by ultraviolet B (UVB) light (eg, sunlight). It is then eventually converted to 1,25-dihydroxyvitamin D3, which combines with vitamin D receptors to trigger an immune response that may be effective against influenza infection.[110] Studies suggest that vitamin D also helps prevent excessive expression of inflammatory cytokines.[59,106] Because of this, it may help to prevent the occurrence of cytokine storm.[111]

Life Extension suggests an optimal 25-hydroxyvitamin D blood level of 50–80 ng/mL. If you do not already maintain a blood level of *25-hydroxyvitamin D* over *50 ng/mL*, then take *50 000 IU* of vitamin D the first day and continue for 3 more days. Slowly reduce the dose to around 5000 IU vitamin D daily. If you already take around 5000 IU of vitamin D daily, then you probably do not need to increase your intake.

## Vitamin C

In order to protect against infections (particularly viral), the human immune system requires a sufficient daily intake of vitamin C. Vitamin C enhances the production and action of white blood cells; for example, it increases the ability of neutrophils (a type of white blood cell) to attack and engulf viruses.[112–114] Daily 1-g doses of vitamin C have been shown to reduce the incidence and severity of a cold.[115] Additionally, very high doses of vitamin C administered before or after symptom onset have been shown to reduce reported cold and flu symptoms. Among asymptomatic young adults 18–30 years of age, three 1000-mg doses of vitamin C daily, or hourly doses of

1000 mg vitamin C for the first 6 hours after symptom onset followed by 1000-mg doses of vitamin C 3 times daily in symptomatic individuals, reduced reported flu and cold symptoms by 85% compared to placebo.[116]

## Zinc

Zinc is required for numerous metabolic processes and serves as a cofactor for a large number of enzymes.[117,118] Zinc plays an important role in maintaining healthy immune function.[119] Zinc deficiency, which is common among the elderly, can impair cell-mediated immunity. This, in turn, can increase the risk of infection. Rectifying zinc deficiency through supplementation has been shown to be efficacious for a variety of infections. This is because zinc affects the expression of interleukin-2, which helps the immune system ward off viruses.[119] In a comprehensive analysis of the effects of zinc lozenges on viral upper respiratory tract infections, doses greater than 75 mg daily were shown to reduce symptom duration by 20–42%. The authors of this study emphasized that doses lower than 75 mg daily did not shorten sickness duration.[120]

## Selenium

Selenium serves as a powerful antioxidant in nearly all human tissues.[121] In addition, selenium boosts the immune system and can provide protection against some pathogens.[121,122] Data show that selenium deficiency promotes the spread of influenza by increasing its virulence, and increases susceptibility to viral infection by interfering with human influenza-induced host defense responses.[123–125] An animal model showed a selenium-deficient diet was associated with significantly higher mortality from influenza than a selenium-supplemented diet.[126]

## Vitamin E

Vitamin E is not only a potent antioxidant, but it is also involved in a variety of physiologic processes, ranging from cognitive performance to immune function.[127] For example, vitamin E supplementation has been shown to enhance certain functions of the human immune system and decrease influenza virus titers in preclinical models of influenza.[128] Animal studies have shown that vitamin E deficiency may precipitate viral genome changes that increase virulence and may contribute to greater severity of influenza.[102]

## Lactoferrin

Lactoferrin is an iron-binding component of whey protein.[119,129] It is known to possess some immune-modulating effects as well as an ability to exert a broad spectrum of activity against bacteria, fungi, protozoa,

and viruses.[119,129] Laboratory studies reveal that lactoferrin inhibits viral infection by interfering with the ability of certain viruses to bind to cell receptor sites and prevents entry of viruses into host cells.[130,131] Lactoferrin may be beneficial for alleviating symptoms or complications of viral infections, like the flu, because it suppresses free radical–mediated damage and decreases availability of essential metals to microbial cells pathogens.[119]

## Elderberry

The purplish-black fruits of the elderberry plant are a rich source of antioxidants and have long been considered a folk remedy for the treatment of influenza.[132] Clinical studies have revealed that the extract of elderberry appears to be a safe, effective, and cost-efficient treatment option for those infected with influenza. Laboratory research indicates this clinical effect is achieved through elderberry's ability to interfere with the replication process of the influenza virus.[133] A 2009 study demonstrated that elderberry extract was capable of inhibiting influenza H1N1 infection by binding to the outside of the virus and keeping it from invading host cells.[134]

## Green Tea

Green tea, which contains a powerful antioxidant called epigallocatechin gallate (EGCG), has been utilized as a medicinal product for the last 4700 years.[54,135] EGCG has a variety of beneficial properties with regard to influenza. For example, it has been shown to directly kill the influenza virus and decrease the number of viruses found in blood during chronic viral infection. In addition, EGCG can decrease flu-like symptoms by reducing inflammation.[54] The antiviral effects of green tea have been demonstrated for nearly all age groups.[54,136,137]

## Beta-Glucans

Beta-glucans are naturally-occurring glucose polymers that constitute the cell walls of certain plants and fungi.[138–140] These polysaccharides have been shown to increase host immune defense and are associated with enhanced macrophage and natural killer cell function.[138,141]

Korean researchers demonstrated anti-viral properties of beta-glucans against influenza in a swine model. In this experiment, one group of piglets received beta-glucans for 3 days before being infected with swine flu, while another group received only placebo. The lungs of piglets not given beta-glucans showed significantly more damage than those that received beta-glucans. Furthermore, piglets pretreated with beta-glucan had significantly higher concentrations of natural immune-enhancing substances, including interferon-gamma, in fluid obtained from the lungs within a week of infection. Researchers concluded that beta-glucans reduced signs of lung disease and the viral replication rate in the piglets.[142]

In another experiment, young piglets were exposed to porcine reproductive and respiratory syndrome virus. White blood cells were then removed and exposed to varying concentrations of beta-glucans. Beta-glucans increased the production of interferon-gamma in a dose-dependent manner, leading scientists to conclude that soluble beta-glucans may enhance innate viral immunity.[143]

## Andrographis

*Andrographis paniculata*, an annual plant used as a medicinal herb among Asian cultures for centuries, has been reported to have anti-inflammatory, anti-hypertensive, antiviral, and immune-modulating properties.[144,145] Chief among andrographis's active constituents are *andrographolides*. Chinese researchers showed that an andrographolide called *andrographanin* enhances mobility of white blood cells in response to cytokine stimulation,[146] which may allow for more efficient immune response against pathogens. A 2009 study found that an extract of andrographis enhanced immune function, as well as reversed drug-induced immunosuppression.[147] In a clinical trial conducted on 540 people diagnosed with influenza, andrographis was shown to speed flu recovery and reduce the risk of complications.[148]

## Probiotics

Probiotics are "friendly" microorganisms that confer health benefits to the host.[149–151] Clinical studies suggest that certain probiotics may help prevent viral respiratory tract infections by modulating the immune system. Probiotics may also be useful for treating influenza, given their association with a reduction in severity and duration of symptoms caused by common upper respiratory tract infections.[150,152–155]

Probiotics may be useful for managing infectious diseases because of their potential for stabilizing the microflora of the gut, enhancing resistance against pathogenic colonization, and modulating immune function.[153] For example, a probiotic strain of *Bacillus coagulans* has been shown to significantly increase T-cell production upon experimental exposure of blood samples from healthy people to an influenza A virus.[155,156] Probiotics, such as *Lactobacillus plantarum*, have also demonstrated immune-stimulating effects

that may help improve influenza vaccination responses among the elderly.[157]

## Reishi

Reishi mushrooms attack and reverse *immunosenescence*—age-related decline in immune system function—through the combined effects of 3 compounds: a group of long-chain carbohydrates called polysaccharides, a unique protein named LZ-8, and a small group of steroid-like molecules called triterpenes.[158–160] Reishi mushrooms' immune-stimulating effects play directly into their ability to fight off both bacterial and viral infections.[161] Both polysaccharide and triterpene components of the mushrooms contribute to this activity.[162,163] Reishi extracts have been shown to inhibit growth of a number of bacterial germs, especially infections of the urinary and digestive tracts. They also enhance the activity of standard antibiotics in treating bacterial infections. Scientists evaluated combinations of Reishi with four different antibiotics, and found an additive effect in most cases. And true synergy (the effect of both exceeds the combined effects of either alone) was demonstrated with the combination of Reishi and cefazolin, a common antibiotic for surgical infections.[164]

But it is in the realm of viral disease that Reishi mushrooms truly flex their muscles.[165,166] In laboratory cell cultures, Reishi mushrooms stop or slow growth of influenza, HIV, hepatitis B, and many other viruses.[165–168] Additional laboratory studies have shown that extracts from Reishi are especially effective against viruses in the *herpes virus* family, which include not only the well-known oral and genital herpes infections, but also the viruses that cause chickenpox and shingles, and the Epstein-Barr virus, a viral cause of certain lymphomas.[162,165,166,169,170] In human studies, supplementation with Reishi dramatically shortens the time until symptomatic relief by more than 50% in people with oral or genital *herpes*, and in people with *shingles*, the excruciating adult sequel to childhood chickenpox infection.[171,172]

## Immune-Modulation Hormones

**Dehydroepiandrosterone.** Dehydroepiandrosterone (DHEA), a multifunctional steroid hormone derived from cholesterol, has antiviral activity and enhances host resistance to infections.[173–178] The enhanced immune response conferred by DHEA allows it to have activity against a wide range of viral, bacterial, and parasitic infections.[179,180] Low levels of DHEA have been shown to suppress the host's antibody response by altering cytokine production (eg, TNF-alpha and

IL-10).[180] Higher baseline DHEA levels appear to result in better immunization against influenza.[181,182] In a 20-week clinical trial, 50 mg of DHEA daily bolstered white blood cell populations among aging men. Immune cell activity was enhanced as well.[183]

**Melatonin.** Melatonin is a hormone produced in the brain by the pineal gland. In addition to regulating the sleep–wake cycle and acting as an antioxidant, melatonin is also capable of influencing the state of the immune system both directly and indirectly. Melatonin has been shown to combat many types of viral infections.[184–186] While the mechanism behind melatonin's involvement with immune function is still being studied, research has shown that its binding to immune-governing cells called T-helper cells can trigger a cascade of events leading to an enhanced immune responsiveness. In addition, melatonin administration can increase the production of antibodies.[187] In some instances, melatonin also acts as an anti-inflammatory mediator[188]; thus, may be preventive or supportive for cytokine storm. Because age-related impairment of the immune system usually begins to occur around age 60 and coincides with decreased melatonin concentrations, melatonin supplementation may be beneficial among seniors.[189]

## Life Extension Suggestions

- **Vitamin C:** 5000–20 000 mg daily in divided doses to bowel tolerance
- **Andrographis paniculata extract:** 25 mg daily (increase up to 150 mg as needed)
- **Beta-glucan:** 100 mg daily (increase up to 600 mg as needed)
- **Zinc lozenges:** 2 zinc lozenges (13–24 mg of zinc in each lozenge) immediately and again every 2–3 hours for 1–2 days. Then slowly reduce the dose until symptoms dissipate.
- **Vitamin D:** If you do not already maintain a blood level of 25-hydroxyvitamin D over 50 ng/mL,

then take 50 000 IU of vitamin D the first day and continue for 3 more days. Slowly reduce the dose to around 5000 IU of vitamin D daily. If you already take around 5000 IU of vitamin D daily, then you probably do not need to increase your intake.

- **Vitamin E:** 400 IU daily with at least 200 mg gamma tocopherol
- **Dehydroepiandrosterone (DHEA):** 200–400 mg early in the day. This is much higher than normal, but DHEA has shown some unique benefits in boosting one's ability to mount a stronger immune response and also protect against dangerous inflammatory cytokine responses that sometimes occur in response to viral infections.
- **Melatonin:** 3–50 mg at bedtime
- **Elderberry:** 2400–4800 mg daily or 1–4 tablespoons daily
- **Lactoferrin:** 1200 mg daily
- **High-allicin garlic:** 9000–18 000 mg daily
- **Reishi mushroom,** standardized extract from fruiting body and spore: 1130 mg daily
- **Black cumin seed oil:** 1000 mg daily
- **Probiotics:** per label instructions
- **Green tea extract,** standardized to 98% polyphenols: 725–1450 mg daily
- **Selenium:** 200–400 mcg daily

### Over-the-Counter Drug Support

- **Cimetidine:** 800–1200 mg daily in divided doses. Cimetidine is a heartburn drug that has potent immune-enhancing properties.

In addition, the following *blood tests* may be helpful:

- Vitamin D, 25-Hydroxy
- Cytokine panel

## REFERENCES

References available at: www.lef.org/dpt5/ch80

# 81

# Insomnia

Insomnia is the most common sleep disorder, affecting one in four people.[1–3]

It is well-known that sleep problems can significantly *diminish quality of life*. However, many people may not realize that insomnia and short sleep duration correlate with various health problems including *cardiovascular disease*, *anxiety*, and potentially *cancer*.[4–8] Insomnia also increases *mortality* in adults.[9,10]

Despite the dramatic toll insomnia takes on individuals and populations, conventional treatment options remain far from ideal. In fact, in 2012, a well-controlled study revealed an association between popular *hypnotic sleep aids*, such as zolpidem (Ambien®), eszopiclone (Lunesta®), and temazepam (Restoril®), and *a more than three-fold increased risk of death*.[11]

These alarming findings highlight the need for safe and effective strategies to improve sleep quality, especially since up to 10% of adults in the United States use hypnotic sleep aids.[11] We should note, however, that those using hypnotic sleep aid drugs often have poor overall sleep quality, which could be the factor causing the sharply increased risk of death. Hypnotic sleep aids are by no means a cure for chronic insomnia.

In this protocol, you will learn about the causes of sleep problems and simple lifestyle changes that can improve your sleep quality.[12,13] You will also discover that some emerging therapies have achieved prolonged sleep quality improvements in studies, with potentially fewer side effects than some popular sleep drugs.[14] In addition, you will read about several *natural compounds* that can modulate the biology of sleep and may be safer than some pharmaceutical options.

## TYPES OF INSOMNIA

### Transient Insomnia

Transient insomnia, lasting a few days to a week, can be triggered by many things (eg, excess environmental noise, medications, and extreme temperatures). One type of transient insomnia is jet lag, in which traveling through time zones causes a temporary disruption of the body's circadian rhythm.[15]

### Acute Insomnia

Acute insomnia may last for several weeks. Common triggers include emotional stress or conflict, environmental changes, or anxiety associated with going to bed. Acute insomnia can also be triggered by the same things that trigger transient insomnia.[3,16]

### Chronic Insomnia

Chronic insomnia, which may last for months or years, can have profound effects on health, quality of life, productivity, and safety.[17]

## INSOMNIA INCREASES DISEASE RISK AND EXACERBATES EXISTING CONDITIONS

Insomnia can lead to elevated levels of cortisol, epinephrine, and other "stress" hormones.[18,19] Elevated levels of cortisol can cause weight gain, weaken the immune system, and increase risk of developing diabetes and osteoporosis.[20–22]

In addition, insomnia triggers the release of chemicals (eg, interleukin-6 [IL-6] and tumor necrosis factor-alpha [TNF–α]) that promote *inflammation*, which is associated with arthritis, inflammatory bowel disease, heart disease, and other conditions.[23]

Insomnia can exacerbate *chronic pain* conditions by causing heightened sensitivity to pain and interfering with the body's ability to modulate central pain signals.[24] As a result, poor sleep can increase the amount of pain perceived by people with chronic pain disorders (eg, osteoarthritis and fibromyalgia). Therefore, treating insomnia may help reduce pain in individuals with chronic pain disorders.

A study reported that among healthy individuals, average sleep duration of 6 hours or less per night was associated with a four-fold increased risk of *stroke* compared to sleep duration of 7–8 hours.[25]

## WHAT CAUSES INSOMNIA?

In many cases, insomnia may be a consequence of another *underlying medical problem*.

### Mental Health Issues

Insomnia is a symptom of many mental health problems, including *anxiety*, *depression*, and bipolar disorder.[26–28]

Not only can mental health disorders trigger insomnia, but insomnia can be a major risk factor for mental health issues. Data indicate that insomnia complaints are a major predictor for onset of depressive disorder within 1–35 years.[27]

Insomnia is also linked to certain psychological personality traits, such as social introversion and repression of feelings.[29]

**Psychophysiologic insomnia (PPI).** PPI, a type of chronic insomnia, is associated with excessive worrying specifically focused on not being able to sleep. It appears to be linked to hyperarousal when going to bed.[18,30,31] The hypothesis behind it is that afflicted individuals have a hard time relaxing and settling down when they go to sleep, resulting in "racing thoughts." They then focus on their difficulty falling asleep, which results in anxiety that further disturbs sleep. Over time, poor sleep and worrying about sleeping can become associated with going to bed, resulting in a pattern of chronically poor sleep that affects daytime activities. Some believe that in addition to heightened arousal, individuals with PPI may have some dysfunctional neurologic inhibitory mechanisms that would normally help the mind "dis-engage" from daytime thought patterns,[32] preventing them from falling asleep.

## Physical Health Issues

Many conditions are associated with insomnia, including musculoskeletal problems, cardiovascular disease, gastrointestinal and urinary problems, neurologic problems, respiratory problems, immunologic problems, and cancer.[27,33–37]

## Hormonal Imbalances

Levels of sex hormones (ie, estrogen, progesterone, and testosterone) may have a significant impact on sleep. This is especially true for women; the incidence of sleep disturbances rises to 40% at 3 years after menopause.[38] Studies have found that hormone replacement therapy in menopausal women can significantly improve sleep.[39,40]

The relationship between sleep and hormone levels occurs in men as well; lower levels of testosterone correlate with increased severity of obstructive sleep apnea (a particularly serious sleep disorder).[41] People with trouble sleeping should have their hormone levels tested. It used to be thought that higher testosterone levels in men worsened sleep apnea, but more recent studies show it is low testosterone that is associated with sleep disturbances in aging men.[42,43]

## Medications

Medication-induced insomnia can be caused by a wide variety of drugs, including decongestants, monoamine oxidase inhibitors (MAOIs), selective-serotonin reuptake inhibitors (SSRIs), corticosteroids, chemotherapeutic agents, calcium channel blockers, beta-agonists, and theophylline.[44–47]

## Stimulants

Stimulants (eg, *caffeine* and *nicotine*) contribute to insomnia by making it harder for the brain to achieve the state of relaxation needed for sleep. The half-life (amount of time it takes the body to break down 50% of a dose) of caffeine is between 3 and 7 hours; larger amounts and/or repeated doses of caffeine lead to slowed caffeine clearance, causing caffeine's effects to last even longer.[48] As a result, caffeine consumption can impair sleep for many hours. Although, some studies have found that mild caffeine consumption in the morning does not impair sleep.[49]

Nicotine use and nicotine withdrawal can contribute to insomnia.[50] Even those undergoing nicotine replacement therapy (to quit smoking) experience the adverse effects of nicotine on sleep.[51]

While most people think of *alcohol* as a sedative, it increases dopamine release within the brain, which has a stimulating effect.[52] Chronic alcohol use is associated with insomnia, as is alcohol withdrawal.[53]

## Lifestyle

*Shift work sleep disorder* is a type of insomnia in which nonstandard work schedules (such as rotating shifts, on-call work, or permanent night shifts) trigger a disconnect between the body's *circadian rhythm* and time.[54]

---

### OBSTRUCTIVE SLEEP APNEA—A HIDDEN EPIDEMIC WITH DEADLY CONSEQUENCES

Obstructive sleep apnea is a common and potentially lethal sleep disorder. It results from the upper airway collapsing during sleep, reducing oxygen flow. The resulting low oxygen in the bloodstream arouses the individual, resulting in disrupted sleep (even if they do not fully remember awakening). Between 2% and 7% of adults have obstructive sleep apnea, causing poor sleep quality, snoring, and intractable fatigue.[55–56]

This underdiagnosed and often overlooked sleep disorder represents a major risk factor for cardiovascular disease, the leading cause of death in American adults. Data indicate obstructive sleep apnea is associated with a 68% increase in coronary heart disease in men.[57] Obstructive sleep apnea may also be associated with increased cholesterol, hypertension,[56,58] type 2 diabetes,[59] cancer mortality,[60] stroke and death.[61]

---

## NONPHARMACOLOGIC THERAPIES

### Improving Sleep Hygiene

One of the most widely used behavioral therapies is improving *sleep hygiene*. There is a correlation between good sleep hygiene and reduced daytime sleepiness.[12,62] Sleep hygiene encompasses a number of behaviors and environmental factors that contribute to good quality sleep.[12–13] Consider the following sleep hygiene measures:

- Minimize the amount of light, noise, and changes in temperature in the bedroom.

- Avoid eating large meals before bed. Indigestion can make falling asleep difficult.

- Limit the amount of stimulants (eg, caffeine, nicotine, and alcohol) consumed during the day, especially close to bedtime.

- Avoid vigorous exercise during the two hours prior to sleep.

- Avoid bedtime activities not related to sleep (eg, watching TV, reading, or listening to the radio).

- If worrying about falling asleep and the time, cover the alarm clock to avoid anxiety.

## Sleep Restriction to Reset Circadian Rhythms

Sleep restriction therapy limits the amount of time spent in bed (including naps) to increase the biological need for sleep at night. A study comparing sleep hygiene therapy plus sleep restriction to sleep hygiene therapy alone found that sleep restriction improved *sleep efficiency*, a measure of the proportion of time spent in bed that resulted in sleep.[63,64] This process usually begins by restricting the time spent in bed to the amount of time estimated that one should spend sleeping. For example, a person who stays in bed for 9 hours but only sleeps 6 will initially restrict time in bed to 6 hours. This causes mild sleep deprivation in the beginning. However, the sleepiness it creates trains the body to fall asleep more quickly. As the body adjusts, people can extend the amount of time spent in bed by 15–20 minutes until they are able to get a full night's sleep without spending extra time in bed.[64]

## General Lifestyle Considerations

General lifestyle considerations that may benefit people with insomnia include[13]:

- Getting regular exercise

- Developing a sleep ritual aimed at improving relaxation and resolving emotional dilemmas before going to bed. Resolving stress may help improve sleep quality. People with insomnia should also review the Stress Management protocol.

# CONVENTIONAL PHARMACOLOGIC TREATMENT

## Over-the-Counter Medication

One of the most common types of over-the-counter (OTC) sleep medications is antihistamines, such as doxylamine (Unisom®) and diphenhydramine (Benadryl®). Antihistamines block the receptors that respond to histamine; this reduces congestion, sneezing, coughing, and allergy symptoms. Centrally, blockade of histamine receptors causes sedation; thus antihistamines can be used as sleep aids.

Despite the widespread use of these OTC drugs, there are significant concerns regarding their efficacy and safety. Although some studies have found that these OTC drugs can improve sleep, there are few well-designed trials to definitively determine their efficacy.[65] Diphenhydramine can remain in the body for long periods of time, resulting in sedation the following day. In addition, the human body can build up a tolerance to the effects of antihistamines. Evidence appears to suggest that antihistamines may be useful for insomnia for short periods of time, but not efficacious in treating chronic insomnia.[65]

## Benzodiazepines

Benzodiazepines (eg, alprazolam [Xanax®], clonazepam [Klonipin®], and diazepam [Valium®]) composed the cornerstone for the treatment of insomnia until the 1990s. These medications enhance the effect of the neurotransmitter gamma-aminobutyric acid (GABA), which is one of the main inhibitory neurotransmitters in the brain.[66] Studies have found that benzodiazepines are able to reduce the amount of time users need to fall asleep.[67,68]

Benzodiazepines can be classified based on their duration of action. Short-acting benzodiazepines are more likely to cause withdrawal symptoms, whereas long-acting ones are more likely to leave users feeling groggy and produce a "hangover" feeling,[66] as well as paradoxical rebound anxiety.

## Nonbenzodiazepines

Nonbenzodiazepines, also called benzodiazepine-like drugs, such as zalelplon (Sonata®), zolpidem (Ambien®), and eszopiclone (Lunesta®), are the next generation of sleep aids.[66] Zaleplon, one of the first nonbenzodiazepines developed for the treatment of insomnia, has been proven to be effective in reducing the amount of time it takes to fall asleep.[69,70] Its short half-life (1 hour) also reduces the risk of lasting effects the following morning. However, this may make it less useful for people who wake up during the night.[69] Zolpidem's half-life (about 2.5 hours) may make it more effective at reducing the amount of time it takes to fall asleep and stay asleep. In order to improve zolpidem's effectiveness for maintaining sleep, "modified release" and "extended release" formulations have been designed. Studies have found that modified release forms are very effective at improving sleep, with over 92% of individuals reporting that zolpidem helped them sleep when taken 3–7 nights per week; also, that it may not affect performance the next day.[71,72] Eszopiclone has also been shown to be effective at improving sleep.[73,74]

There are some significant risks associated with taking these drugs. For example, zolpidem can cause sleep-walking, sleep-driving, and eating while sleeping.[75] In addition, sedative hypnotics increase the risk of depression, and long-term effects on the brain are not known.[76] Moreover, in 2012, a well-controlled study revealed an association between *popular hypnotic sleep aids*, such as zolpidem (Ambien®), eszopiclone (Lunesta®), and temazepam (Restoril®), and *a more than three-fold increased risk of death*.[11] We should note, however, that those using hypnotic sleep aid drugs often have poor overall sleep quality, which could be the factor causing the sharply increased risk of death. Hypnotic sleep aids are by no means a cure for chronic insomnia, despite ads run on national TV claiming miraculous sleep improvement.

## Antidepressants

Many antidepressants such as doxepin (Silenor®), a histamine receptor antagonist with tricyclic antidepressant properties; trazodone (Desyrel®), a serotonin antagonist and reuptake inhibitor; and amitriptyline (Elavil®), a tricyclic antidepressant, are used to treat insomnia because they have sedative properties.[77–79] Doxepin has been found to increase sleep time without causing significant adverse effects.[80,81] Some data have shown that trazodone, functioning as a mild hypnotic, may temporarily help people fall asleep.[82] However, there are few well-designed studies that demonstrate its effectiveness. Trazodone can cause significant side effects such as dizziness as well as slowed thinking and movement the next day. Therefore, its risks may outweigh its benefits, particularly in those more susceptible to these side effects (eg, the elderly).[83] Although amitriptyline is commonly prescribed by physicians as a sleep aid, data regarding its effectiveness for the treatment of primary insomnia is limited.[84]

---

## CYCLING SLEEP MEDICATIONS TO PREVENT TOLERANCE

Developing drug tolerance is a significant concern for many people who need long-term pharmacologic sleep support. Some experts suggest avoiding drug tolerance by alternating the type of sleeping medication used. Here is a potential prescription drug schedule to treat chronic insomnia for a person who has never taken prescription sleeping pills:

- Valium, 2.5 mg, taken only at bedtime for 30 days
- During the next 30-day cycle, 5–10 mg Ambien® taken only at bedtime
- During the next 30-day cycle, 1–3 mg Klonopin® taken only at bedtime

At some point, patients may find that they do better by taking Valium® one night, Ambien® the next night, and Klonopin® or Lunesta® the third night. The drug Sonata® in a 5- to 10-mg dose provides about 5 hours of sleep and can be helpful on occasions when only a limited amount of sleep time is available. If heavy alcohol is consumed, these types of drugs should be avoided on the same night.

A person with chronic insomnia must develop a close relationship with a physician who understands that some people need sleep medications on a routine basis or their lives will be miserable and they will be at a higher risk of contracting a serious degenerative disease.

---

# NOVEL AND EMERGING TREATMENTS

## Targeting Melatonin Receptors

*Ramelteon* (Rozerem®) is an insomnia medication that binds to and activates receptors (MT1 and MT2) for melatonin.[85] It has a higher affinity for the receptors than melatonin itself and a half-life of just over 1 hour.[86–88] Studies have found that ramelteon is effective at reducing the amount of time it takes to fall asleep and increasing the amount of time people stay asleep.[88–91] Few side effects have been demonstrated in humans. Studies also indicate a low potential for abuse.[88]

## Selective MT2 Drugs

The particular melatonin receptor *MT2* has been shown in animal studies to be important for promoting deep sleep.[92,93] Drugs that specifically target the MT2 receptor are beginning to emerge. Two of these novel medications, IIK7 and UCM765, have increased the amount of deep sleep in mice.[92–93] However, human research needs to be done to confirm safety, efficacy, and potency.

## 5-HT2 Receptor Antagonists

Serotonin (5-hydroxytryptamine or 5-HT) is a neurotransmitter with diverse roles during sleep and wakefulness. It exerts activities by binding to and activating various 5-HT receptors whose biological roles depend on tissue distribution (eg, central vs. peripheral), structural variations, interaction with other compounds (eg, melatonin), and the environment (eg, light/dark cycle).[94,95]

With regard to sleep, two 5-HT receptors are of particular interest: 5-HT2A and 5-HT2C. Activation of these receptors interferes with deep sleep.[95] Therefore, some emerging therapeutics attempt to reduce signaling through these receptors to facilitate high-quality sleep.[96,97]

While both animal and human data suggest that blocking 5-HT2A/C signaling appears to be a promising mechanism for improving sleep quality, more research is needed.[96,97]

---

## NOVEL USE OF AN ANESTHETIC TO RESET SLEEP RHYTHMS

*Propofol* is a rapid, short-acting anesthetic that is often administered intravenously for the induction and maintenance of anesthesia.

Electroencephalography (or EEG, a technique that measures the brain's electrical activity) confirms that there are distinct differences between sleep and sedation. Anesthetic agents (eg, propofol) can induce activity in areas of the brain important for regulating sleep, particularly in people with insomnia.[14]

Clinical trial subjects receiving a 2-hour infusion of propofol for 5 consecutive nights showed improvement in sleep onset latency (ie, amount of time needed to fall asleep), quality of sleep, ease of waking up, and behavior after awakening. These improvements persisted for 6 months, suggesting that the benefits of propofol could continue long after the initial treatment. In addition, the subjects showing no response to traditional agents such as zopiclone or zolpidem before study treatment were able to effectively use them on occasion after treatment, suggesting that propofol restored the brain's response to conventional sleep aids.[14] The study showed that using propofol for a short period of time (at the same time each night) could help reset the body's natural circadian rhythm, providing long-term benefits for people with chronic refractory insomnia.

Life Extension is funding a propofol sleep study, but there are no sleep centers currently offering propofol, which requires strict medical vigilance and adherence to safety protocols to avoid dying of a propofol overdose as Michael Jackson did. The therapeutic use of propofol, administered under carefully controlled clinical conditions, is separate and distinct from the irresponsible use of propofol by incompetent healthcare personnel in the absence of adequate cardiopulmonary monitoring.

## TARGETED NATURAL INTERVENTIONS

### Amino Acids and Hormones

**Melatonin.** Melatonin, a hormone made in the pineal gland, is highly correlated with the body's sleep–wake cycle. In humans, elevated melatonin levels coincide with the body's normal time for sleeping. Low melatonin levels have been linked to insomnia, particularly in the elderly. In a clinical review, serum melatonin levels were reported to be significantly lower (and the time of peak melatonin values delayed) in elderly subjects with insomnia compared to age-matched normal controls.[98]

Several studies have found that melatonin supplementation is able to improve sleep. One study found that melatonin helped reduce the amount of time needed to fall asleep.[99] Other studies have found that it improves sleep quality and alertness after sleep,[100] as well as reduces the number of times subjects wake up during the night.[101] Despite these successful studies, melatonin is not always an effective solution for those with severe chronic insomnia.

**L-tryptophan.** L-tryptophan is an amino acid that serves as a precursor for serotonin and melatonin.[102,103] L-tryptophan supplements may increase the amount of melatonin made by the pineal gland, thus facilitating sleep.[104] Early studies found that 1 g of L-tryptophan could reduce the amount of time needed to fall asleep.[105] Like melatonin, L-tryptophan levels decrease with age.[104] Therefore, L-tryptophan supplementation may aid in the treatment of elderly insomnia.

Animal studies have found that tryptophan supplementation reduced activity at night and led to other biological changes that are conducive to sleep, such as a lower core body temperature and reduced levels of interleukin-6 (an inflammatory cytokine).[106] In one small human clinical trial, intravenous infusion of L-tryptophan caused dramatic increases in plasma melatonin levels and had a sleep-inducing effect, regardless of whether it was administered during the day or night.[107] In addition, L-tryptophan may help alleviate some forms of depression, which can exacerbate insomnia.[108]

### Minerals

**Magnesium.** Magnesium is a mineral that plays a role in cellular communication and regulation of circadian rhythms.[109] As sleep restriction increases, intracellular magnesium concentrations decline.[110] Magnesium supplementation combined with melatonin and zinc has been shown to improve sleep in the elderly.[111] Another trial found that magnesium supplementation helped relieve insomnia related to restless legs in subjects with a mean age of 57 years.[112] A form of magnesium known as *magnesium threonate* may be beneficial for sleep since it has been shown to penetrate the blood–brain barrier more efficiently than other forms of magnesium.[113,114]

**Zinc.** Zinc may also play a role in facilitating sleep.[111] Research found that women with the highest levels of zinc in their bodies slept for longer periods of time than women with the lowest levels.[115] As mentioned above, when combined with melatonin and magnesium, zinc also supported quality of sleep in the elderly.[111] Among children with attention-deficit/hyperactivity disorder, zinc (in combination with magnesium and omega-3 and omega-6 fatty acids) helped relieve problems falling asleep.[116]

## Herbal Support

**Valerian.** Valerian is a sedative herb that has been used since the 18th century for the treatment of insomnia.[117] The putative mechanism of valerian root is interaction with the GABA system in the brain, thus helping reduce brain activity and allowing users to fall asleep more easily. Valerian affects the transport and liberation of GABA, modulating GABAergic signaling. Valerian also improves quality of sleep; one study demonstrated that valerian increases the percentage of time participants spend in slow-wave sleep. This is significant because slow-wave sleep is considered the most refreshing.[118] One study compared the effects of 600 mg of valerian to the commonly prescribed tranquilizer oxazepam. During 6 weeks of treatment, valerian showed comparable efficacy to 10 mg of oxazepam.[119] Evidence also suggests that the side effect profile of valerian is superior to commonly prescribed sleep aids. In one small study, subjects taking valerian reported none of the mood-altering or negative cognitive effects demonstrated by diazepam.[120] The typical dose of valerian is about 300–600 mg, 30–120 minutes before going to bed to sleep.[117] It may take up to 2 weeks of daily usage for the full sedative effect of valerian to manifest.[121]

**Chamomile.** Chamomile is a popular herb often used as a tea to promote sleep and relaxation.[122,123] It was noted in a study on rats that chamomile had a mild hypnotic effect (much like benzodiazepines) and improved sleep onset latency,[124] although it is not clear how it has this effect. One clinical trial found that chamomile improved daytime functioning of humans with sleep problems.[123] More research needs to be done to determine the benefits and drawbacks of using chamomile for sleep.

**Passionflower.** *Passiflora incarnate (P. incarnata)*, a member of the passiflower genus *Passiflora*, is best known for its sedative and anxiety-reducing effects.[125] The active compounds in *P. incarnata* appear to interact with the GABA and opioid systems.[126–128] In an animal model, *P. incarnata* was shown to reduce anxious behavior.[127] Additionally, another animal model found that passionflower-derived compounds were able to prevent diazepam dependence in mice when given along with the drug over a 3-week period.[129] More human studies are needed to evaluate the effectiveness and safety of passiflora products.

**Ashwagandha.** *Withania somnifera*, also known as ashwagandha, is an Indian herb that may be beneficial for treating insomnia. This herb has been best characterized for its effects on stress, as several animal studies have found that it is able to improve the ability to handle stress and can significantly reduce anxiety.[130–132] Because emotional stress can be a significant contributor to insomnia, using ashwagandha to reduce stress may help improve sleep. This herb has also been found to directly improve sleep in animal models; it appears to do so by increasing GABAergic activity.[133]

**Lemon Balm.** Lemon balm is an herb traditionally used for its calming and anxiety-reducing effects.[134,135] One double-blind, placebo-controlled, randomized study showed that 600 mg of lemon balm improved mood and significantly increased self-ratings of calmness.[136] Lemon balm has also been investigated in the treatment of sleep problems. A study found that a combination of valerian and lemon balm was able to treat sleeping disorders in children. About 81% of them experienced improvement of their symptoms after taking the study preparation.[137]

**Lavender (as essential oil aromatherapy).** Aromatherapy is an alternative medicine practice that utilizes plant oils to treat health problems. Lavender oils have been extensively studied for the treatment of insomnia. Studies have found that lavender oil improves sleep quality[138,139] and reduces feelings of drowsiness after awakening.[140]

## Additional Natural Therapy

**Bioactive milk peptides.** Select peptides, made by breaking down milk proteins with enzymes, may relieve stress related sleep disorders.[141] These bioactive peptides were able to increase the amount of time spent sleeping and reduce the amount of sleep needed after just two weeks of treatment.[142] Lactium, one of the trade names for this uniquely formulated product, is sometimes combined with melatonin to improve sleep by taking advantage of the sleep promoting effects of both bioactive milk peptides and melatonin.

## Life Extension Suggestions

### Amino Acids and Hormones
- **Melatonin:** 0.3–5 mg before bed (sometimes up to 10 mg)
- **L-Tryptophan:** 500–1500 mg daily or as recommended by a healthcare practitioner

### Vitamins and Minerals
- **Magnesium:** 140 mg daily as magnesium-L-threonate; 320 mg daily as magnesium citrate
- **Zinc:** 30–90 mg daily

### Herbal Support
- **Valerian:** 300–600 mg, 30–120 minutes before bed
- **Ashwagandha extract:** 200 mg daily

- **Lemon balm:** 300–600 mg daily
- **Chamomile tea:** Per label instructions
- **Passiflora** (passion flower): Per label instructions
- **Lavender oil** (as aromatherapy): Per label instructions

### Additional Natural Therapy
- **Bioactive milk peptides:** 150 mg daily

## REFERENCES

References available at: www.lef.org/dpt5/ch81

# 82

# *Irritable Bowel Syndrome (IBS)*

Irritable bowel syndrome (IBS) is a very common gastrointestinal disorder, estimated to be present in about 11–15% of the global population.[1–5] Typical IBS symptoms include chronic abdominal pain, bloating, and varying bouts of diarrhea and constipation. The condition is generally associated with a reduced quality of life.[3] IBS is a functional disorder, and as such has not been consistently linked to tissue damage or other biological markers that can be tested clinically.[3,6] It is thought to be largely underdiagnosed.[2,3,7,8]

IBS should not be confused with inflammatory bowel disease (IBD). IBD includes Crohn's disease and ulcerative colitis, which are characterized by inflammatory lesions in the intestines.[9] For more information on IBD, see Life Extension's Inflammatory Bowel Disease (Crohn's and Ulcerative Colitis) protocol.

Many are unaware that multiple factors may cause or exacerbate IBS symptoms. For example, stress, anxiety, depression, food sensitivities, small intestinal bacterial overgrowth, and hormonal fluctuations are all associated with IBS.[10–14]

Treatment of psychological conditions in IBS patients is especially important because irritable bowel symptoms often persist despite drug therapy if these issues are not addressed.[15–22]

This protocol will discuss the causes of and risk factors for IBS along with its diagnosis and conventional treatment; emerging drug strategies will be examined as well. The important role of dietary and lifestyle modification will be reviewed, and data on scientifically studied natural compounds that may alleviate IBS symptoms will also be presented.

## CAUSES AND RISK FACTORS

The cause(s) of IBS are not clear.[6] Stress, altered gut bacteria, genetics, and food sensitivities may all be involved.[23] One theory proposes that altered serotonin metabolism within the gastrointestinal (GI) tract and/or abnormalities in pain perception pathways causes hypersensitivity to abdominal pain,[3,24,25] while other hypotheses have pointed to stress-induced inflammation,

gastroenteritis, and a history of traumatic events as factors that contribute to the development of IBS.[8,23]

### Disrupted Brain–Gut Communication

Some evidence suggests that altered communication between the brain and gut may contribute to pain hypersensitivity and/or motility disturbances in IBS.[26–29] The mechanisms behind these phenomena are unclear, but some studies have identified altered autonomic and central nervous function in individuals with IBS.[29–31] Another study employed magnetic resonance imaging to examine the brains of people with IBS and identified some structural changes that may contribute to enteric hypersensitivity.[32] Stress and anxiety appear to contribute, at least in part, to gut hypersensitivity via modulation of neural pain-processing pathways by glucocorticoid hormones, which are also called "stress hormones."[10] Another aspect of this impaired brain-gut communication may stem from altered levels of chemical messengers called neurotransmitters. Levels and activity of the neurotransmitter *serotonin* in particular appear to be somewhat abnormal in people with IBS.[33,34]

### Small Intestinal Bacterial Overgrowth

Small intestinal bacterial overgrowth (SIBO) is a condition characterized by overgrowth of microbes in the small intestine. As a result, fermentation of food begins before it has been thoroughly digested and absorbed, which can lead to gas formation.[35,36] SIBO is more common in people with motility disturbances, low stomach acid production, and bowel obstruction.[35] The prevalence of SIBO in IBS varies across studies, but estimates range from about 20–84%.[11–13]

### Medications That May Contribute to IBS Development

Certain medications may contribute to the development of IBS.[37] Proton pump inhibitors (eg, omeprazole [Prilosec®]), which are used to treat heartburn, can alter intestinal barrier function, affect intestinal microflora, and are known to have a positive association with IBS.[37] Similarly, many common analgesics, such as nonsteroidal anti-inflammatory drugs (NSAIDs), are known to damage the intestinal epithelium, an important barrier against harmful substances. This tissue damage may compromise intestinal permeability.[38] Although broad-spectrum antibiotics are designed to target systemic infections, antibiotics are known to alter the colonic flora.[39] Indeed, a study showed that the use of broad-spectrum antibiotics, particularly macrolides (eg, erythromycin) or tetracyclines (eg, tetracycline, doxycycline), was associated with IBS development.[39]

## Food Sensitivities

Food sensitivities may have a role in IBS. See the *Dietary Considerations* section of this protocol for an exploration of this topic.

**Gluten sensitivity.**   Gluten is a protein component of some grains, especially wheat. Sensitivity to gluten is common and is associated with a spectrum of symptoms ranging in severity from minor skin conditions to severe gastrointestinal compromise in the case of celiac disease.[40-43] Some evidence suggests gluten sensitivity potentially contributes to IBS symptoms.[40,44] Although evidence is not yet strong enough to support a recommendation that all IBS patients avoid gluten, findings from at least one study indicate that using a blood test to detect *immunoglobulin G (IgG) antibodies* against components of wheat may help identify patients with diarrhea-predominant IBS (IBS-D) who are likely to respond positively to a gluten-free diet.[45]

## Postinfectious IBS

Some cases of IBS arise following a gastrointestinal infection, usually with a bacterial or parasitic pathogen.[46] This is called postinfectious IBS, or PI-IBS, and occurs in up to about 30% of individuals who contract an acute gastrointestinal infection.[47,48] Symptoms of PI-IBS typically resemble IBS-D.[47] Irritable bowel symptoms are thought to arise following enteric infection due to inflammatory damage to the gut epithelium, which increases intestinal permeability; alterations in intestinal flora may also contribute.[48-50] Some estimates suggest as many as one-third of all IBS cases may arise postinfection.[51]

## Hormone Fluctuations

Some evidence suggests a potential role for sex hormone imbalance(s) in IBS. For example, women often experience worsening of IBS symptoms near menstruation, which coincides with natural changes in sex hormone levels.[52,53] One study found that women with IBS have generally lower estradiol levels than their healthy counterparts.[54] However, postmenopausal women have fewer symptoms compared to women who are still menstruating.[4]

## SYMPTOMS AND DIAGNOSIS

The cardinal symptom of IBS is abdominal pain that is relieved with defecation and associated with a change in stool frequency or appearance.[55] Pain or discomfort associated with IBS typically "flares" for 2–4 days intermittently. Other symptoms not directly associated with the GI tract have been reported in some IBS patients, including headache, backache, and lethargy. People with IBS frequently experience symptoms for years after diagnosis; however, IBS does not increase risk for more serious conditions like colon cancer.[25]

Subcategories of IBS include *constipation-predominant* (IBS-C) and *diarrhea-predominant* (IBS-D), with the former associated with fewer than three bowel movements per week and the latter associated with more than three bowel movements per day.[2]

Diagnosing IBS is complex and often involves multiple tests to rule out several other diseases that may be associated with IBS-like symptoms such as hyperthyroidism, celiac disease, lactose or fructose malabsorption, IBD, microscopic colitis, colon cancer, and/or pancreatic cancer.[2,6,56] A complete blood count and blood chemistry panel may be ordered as well to asses for anemia or other abnormalities.[6]

The Rome III criteria have been developed in order to help facilitate accurate diagnosis of IBS.[57-59]

According to the Rome III criteria, a diagnosis of IBS requires recurrent abdominal pain or discomfort at least 3 days per month during the past 3 months associated with two or more of the following[8,59,60]:

- Improvement with defecation
- Onset associated with a change in stool frequency
- Onset associated with a change in stool appearance

## CONVENTIONAL TREATMENT

IBS treatment aims to alleviate predominant symptoms, such as diarrhea, constipation, or abdominal cramping.[8]

### Bulking Agents

Bulking agents (ie, dietary fiber) are frequently used to treat both subtypes of IBS. Insoluble fiber facilitates defecation by reducing transit time, or the time it takes for the remains of ingested food to be excreted. While defecation generally alleviates IBS symptoms, a comprehensive review found conflicting effects of bulking agents on IBS severity.[7,61] A potential side effect of fiber supplements is bloating,[3] which can exacerbate certain IBS types who have difficulty evacuating their bowels.

### Laxatives

Laxatives and stool softeners are commonly used to treat IBS-C.[3,7] These treatments typically provide rapid relief, but are not recommended for long-term use as they can cause electrolyte imbalances by enhancing the excretion of fluids.[62] The most common laxatives work by osmosis, that is, they draw fluid into the intestine producing softer stools that are easier to pass. Polyethylene glycol (MiraLAX®) is one of the most studied laxatives; it has been shown to be superior to lactulose (another osmotic laxative).[63] Lubiprostone (Amitiza®) is a prostaglandin E1 analog that draws fluid into the intestine by directly acting on the ClC2 chloride receptor. Lubiprostone is indicated for IBS-C in the United States.[7,64] Lubiprostone acts quickly to facilitate defecation, relieve discomfort, and resolve abdominal pain.[65,66]

## Antispasmodic Medications

Antispasmodics relax the smooth muscle of the lower GI tract and may be helpful in IBS, especially for abdominal pain, although more data from high quality randomized controlled trials are needed to thoroughly assess their effectiveness.[3,7,61] In studies conducted in Europe, alverine (Spasmonyl®), which blocks signaling through a specific serotonin receptor called 5-HT1a, was effective at relieving abdominal pain and discomfort in IBS patients when combined with the oral antifoaming agent simethicone (Gas-X®).[67] However, alverine was shown to be ineffective when used alone.[68] Antagonists of either muscarinic acetylcholine or 5-HT1a receptors exert direct antispasmodic effects, whereas simethicone reduces gas/flatulence and is not an antispasmodic.[67] Propantheline (Probanthine™) is an anticholinergic antispasmodic medication used to treat IBS.[69]

## Serotonergics

**Centrally acting.** Antidepressants are another class of therapeutic agents that can be used in IBS treatment.[7] They do not address the underlying condition, but instead reduce feelings of discomfort. These drugs have demonstrated a modest degree of success.[61] The selective serotonin reuptake inhibitor (SSRI) paroxetine (Paxil®) has shown some benefits,[70] although results with another SSRI, citalopram (Celexa®), suggest that efficacy might be limited to IBS sufferers who are also clinically depressed.[71] The dual serotonin norepinephrine reuptake inhibitor (SNRI) duloxetine (Cymbalta®), on the other hand, is efficacious in nondepressed IBS patients, but is typically limited to IBS-D since constipation is a potential side effect.[72] Tricyclic antidepressant drugs like amitriptyline inhibit peristalsis and can markedly worsen constipation-predominant IBS.

**Locally acting.** Alosetron (Lotronex®), which blocks an intestinal serotonin receptor called the 5-HT3 receptor, is used to treat IBS-D.[25,73] One randomized clinical trial in women with severe IBS-D showed significant beneficial effects of alosetron versus placebo, whereby every measured aspect of quality of life improved (eg, emotional, mental health, sleep, energy, etc.) and workplace productivity increased.[73] However, alosetron may cause significant side effects including severe constipation and loss of blood flow to the colon.[74,75] Alosetron is indicated for use in women with severe IBS-D who have not responded to other therapies,[3] and not women with IBS-C.

## Other Treatment Considerations

**Small intestinal bacterial overgrowth.** Evidence suggests that SIBO may contribute to IBS symptoms in some patients.[35,76] The gold standard for diagnosing SIBO is microbial investigation of fluids collected from the small intestine. Other noninvasive testing such as hydrogen and methane breath tests are more commonly used. Antibiotics are a mainstay in SIBO therapy; however, probiotics are becoming an increasingly appreciated option.[77,78]

**Balancing hormones.** Premenopausal women often experience IBS symptom exacerbation around menstruation, which may be related to fluctuations in sex hormone levels.[52,53] Using blood testing to assess hormone levels and, if necessary, working with an experienced, integrative physician to appropriately balance hormone levels may represent a potential solution, though studies have yet to test this hypothesis.

# NEW AND EMERGING THERAPIES

## Linaclotide

Linaclotide (Linzess®) activates a receptor in cells on the intestinal surface called the guanylate cyclase 2C receptor, which stimulates intestinal fluid secretion and softens the stool making it easier to pass. Linaclotide is effective in attenuating IBS-C, chronic constipation, and abdominal discomfort.[79] Linaclotide was approved by the Food and Drug Administration (FDA) for the treatment of IBS-C in August 2012; an indication shared by only one other drug (Lubiprostone [Amitiza®]). Linaclotide and lubiprostone treat both constipation and pain, whereas traditional laxatives do little to relieve abdominal pain.[80] In 2 large randomized clinical trials, linaclotide safely and effectively treated bowel and abdominal symptoms associated with chronic constipation.[79]

## Mesalazine

Some evidence implicates low-level inflammation and immune system activation in IBS.[81,82] Although the specific contributions of inflammation to IBS symptoms are not fully understood, the aspirin-like anti-inflammatory drug mesalazine (also known as mesalamine and 5-aminosalycylic acid, 5-ASA), which is used in the treatment of IBD,[83] has successfully relieved IBS symptoms in clinical trials.[84] In one trial, 360 subjects with varying types of IBS were treated with 500 mg of mesalazine 4 times daily or standard therapy for 28 days. Mesalazine treatment led to significant reductions in pain and symptom duration in most IBS subtypes. In addition, the treatment normalized stool patterns among subjects with IBS-D and lessened infiltration of immune cells into bowel mucosa.[85] In an earlier proof-of-concept study conducted on 20 IBS patients, treatment with 800 mg mesalazine 3 times daily for 8 weeks led to marked reductions in the number of immune cells present upon examination of colonic biopsy specimens and improved subjects' general well-being.[86]

# DIETARY CONSIDERATIONS

Dietary considerations such as reducing daily intake of caffeine and fatty foods may benefit individuals with IBS.[8] Individuals with IBS are often aware of some foods that exacerbate symptoms; thus, they may be able to improve symptoms by avoiding those foods.[6] The following specific diets may help manage IBS symptoms. Each involves the selective exclusion of one or more types of food.

## FODMAPs (Fermentable Oligosaccharides, Disaccharides, Monosaccharides, and Polyols)

A low-FODMAP diet is based on the hypothesis that impaired carbohydrate absorption allows excess undigested carbohydrates to reach the lower GI tract (large intestine). There, undigested carbohydrates stimulate the growth of pathogenic microbes, leading to excess gas, diarrhea, and constipation.[87] Theoretically, the restriction of fermentable foodstuffs deprives the dysbiotic gut flora of their energy source and results in decreased symptoms.

Foods typically avoided on a low-FODMAP diet include fructo-oligosaccharides (eg, wheat, rye, onions, garlic, artichokes), galacto-oligosaccharides (eg, legumes), lactose (eg, milk), fructose (eg, honey, apples, pears, watermelon, mango), sorbitol (eg, apples, pears, stone fruits, sugar-free mints/gums), and mannitol (eg, mushrooms, cauliflower, sugar-free mints/gums). In one study, IBS sufferers assigned to a low-FODMAP diet experienced significant improvement in their symptom response (ie, bloating, abdominal pain, and flatulence) relative to a standard diet group.[88,89]

These results are supported by a later study showing that IBS patients who were guided to eat a low-FODMAP diet experienced a significant decrease in abdominal pain.[87]

## Gluten-Free

While a gluten-free diet is required for patients with celiac disease, there is a wide spectrum of nonceliac gluten sensitivities that present like IBS.[90] Gluten is found in grains (eg, wheat, barley, rye), breads, pasta, and so on. Similar to the gluten-free diet, the low-FODMAP diet also restricts gluten. Both diets are used to manage food sensitivities, suggesting that gluten sensitivity might be a more common contributor to IBS symptoms than previously thought.[91] In one double-blind, randomized, placebo-controlled study of IBS sufferers who specifically did *not* have celiac disease, the addition of gluten worsened abdominal pain, bloating, fatigue, stool consistency, and overall symptoms of IBS.[92]

---

## FOOD SENSITIVITIES AND IBS

Many features of IBS are similar to food sensitivities. A food allergy or food sensitivity is an inappropriate immune response to one or more components of the diet. Following ingestion, the immune system "attacks" particles of the problematic food(s). This "attack" is mediated by *antibodies*, which are components of the immune system that normally identify pathogens and trigger an immune response. In the case of food sensitivities or food allergies, antibodies mark certain food particles as pathogens and initiate a wider immune response that can lead to tissue inflammation and/or dysfunction.

Conventionally recognized "food allergies" are primarily mediated by 2 specific types of antibodies: *immunoglobulin E (IgE)* and *immunoglobulin A (IgA)*. However, evidence suggests that "food sensitivities," which are triggered primarily by the *immunoglobulin G (IgG)* antibody, may contribute to intestinal disorders as well, although mainstream medicine typically refutes this hypothesis. The reduction in IBS symptoms seen following the elimination of IgG-positive foods attests to the viability of this theory.[93]

In one study, IBS patients were tested for IgG antibodies against a variety of foods, including chicken, wheat, soybeans, and rice.[14] They were then assigned to diets that excluded the foods to which they were IgG positive. In almost every case, this resulted in a significant improvement, which was reversed when the troublesome foods were reintroduced.[14] Similar findings were discovered in a 2012 study that demonstrated the existence of an IgG-mediated food sensitivity.[91] In this study, IgE testing was important to exclude food *allergy*, whereas IgG testing was important to diagnose food *sensitivity*. Taken together, these findings suggest that specific elimination diets may be successful and that *IgG food sensitivity testing* may help identify foods that contribute to IBS.[94]

## LIFESTYLE CONSIDERATIONS

### Stress Reduction

Stress associated with early life adverse events is implicated in the etiology of IBS[95]; about 50% of individuals who seek IBS treatment have depression or anxiety.[25] This relationship appears to be bidirectional, meaning that IBS may cause stress, and stress may contribute to IBS symptoms. This cycle may be partially attributed to enhanced sympathetic nervous system ("fight or flight") signaling in IBS patients relative to healthy controls.[96]

IBS symptoms appear to respond positively to stress reduction. In one study, a meditation-based intervention known as mindfulness-based stress reduction (MBSR) reduced the severity of IBS and stress symptoms in IBS patients, although improvements in mood and quality of life were similar to those of a control group of IBS patients who were placed on a waiting list for MBSR.[97] Furthermore, psychological therapies—including cognitive therapy, dynamic psychotherapy, and hypnotherapy—have been deemed highly effective in relieving global symptoms of IBS by the American College of Gastroenterology Task Force on IBS.[98]

### Exercise

Exercise also appears to be beneficial for IBS patients. In one study, subjects who engaged in 20–60 minutes of moderate to vigorous physical activity 3–5 days per week experienced a marked improvement in quality of life that was associated with reduced IBS severity.[99]

### Acupuncture

Some clinical trials suggest that acupuncture may alleviate IBS symptoms,[100–102] but a 2012 comprehensive review found that evidence remains inconclusive.[103] Although more trials are needed, acupuncture may be a useful adjunct to conventional IBS treatment and is not likely to cause significant side effects.

## TARGETED NATURAL INTERVENTIONS

### IMMEDIATE RELIEF FROM CONSTIPATION-PREDOMINANT IBS

Some cases of *IBS-C* are caused by *insufficient peristalsis*, which means there is not enough colon contractile activity to completely evacuate the bowels.[104] Instead of reverting to laxatives, there are specific nutrients that, if taken at the right time, can induce healthy colon peristaltic action without producing adverse effects.

On an empty stomach, certain nutrients will induce powerful colon peristalsis. One combination is taking several teaspoons of a *buffered vitamin C* powdered mix that contains in each teaspoon, 4000 mg of vitamin C, 365 mg of potassium, and 55 mg of magnesium. The powder should be mixed in 8 oz. glasses of water or the juice of a freshly squeezed grapefruit; wait for the fizzing to stop before drinking. This convenient product sold by several vitamin companies contains magnesium and potassium salts mixed with ascorbic acid which induces an evacuation of bowel contents within 30–90 minutes. Depending on the person, a few teaspoons (or, in some cases, 1–2 tablespoons) of this *buffered vitamin C powder* can produce a powerful but safe laxative effect.

Another popular approach is to use several teaspoons (or 1–2 tablespoons) of *effervescent magnesium ascorbate crystals* that will evacuate the bowel within 30–90 minutes if taken on an empty stomach with several glasses of water. This powdered formula provides 3000 mg of vitamin C and 170 mg of magnesium in each teaspoon, which is healthier than commercial laxatives that are abused by so many. The dose of *buffered vitamin C powder* or *effervescent magnesium ascorbate crystals* needs to be individually adjusted so it will not cause day-long diarrhea.

Nutritional laxatives such as ascorbic acid mixed with magnesium and potassium salts are becoming more popular with people who have constipation that is resistant to fiber therapies.

## Peppermint Oil/Caraway Oil

Peppermint oil is a natural antispasmodic. In one study, an enterically coated preparation of 225 mg peppermint oil taken twice daily was shown to reduce all IBS symptoms by over 50% in three-fourths of the patients, whereas only 38% of the placebo group improved.[105] In another well-designed study, 187 mg of a similar peppermint oil product taken 3 times daily for 8 weeks led to a significant improvement over placebo with regard to abdominal discomfort, abdominal pain, and quality of life, but not in terms of diarrhea, constipation, or bloating.[106] IBS patients treated with peppermint oil in yet another study reported benefits including decreased abdominal pain, less bloating and flatulence, decreased stomach growling, reduced stool frequency, and improved stool consistency.[107]

In a clinical study using a fixed combination of peppermint and caraway oil, 45 patients with nonulcer dyspepsia, the majority of whom had IBS, were studied in a double-blind, placebo-controlled trial. The test group took one enteric-coated capsule 3 times daily for 4 weeks. While all patients complained of moderate to severe pain before treatment, 42% of the patients in the test group were pain-free 2 weeks after taking the combination therapy. Only one patient in the placebo group reported freedom from pain. After 4 weeks of treatment, 63% of those that received the combination formula were pain-free compared to 25% in the placebo group, and 89% showed improvement in the combination formula group versus 45% in the placebo group.[108]

## Probiotics

Probiotics are microorganisms that may provide health benefits to their host when administered at sufficient levels.[109]

A pathogenic alteration in the gut microflora—*dysbiosis*—is one consistent finding associated with both IBS-D and IBS-C, which can cause or exacerbate IBS symptoms in a variety of ways.[110,111] Dysbiosis is associated with increased intestinal permeability whereby pathogens, toxins, or undigested foods that are not usually absorbed are able to pass into the bloodstream. This can trigger abdominal pain and altered bowel habits.[112] Dysbiosis can also lead to aberrant immune system activation, resulting in the release of cytokines that increase abdominal pain perception and alter bowel habits.[112]

Dysbiosis associated with IBS produces an abnormally high amount of gas in response to certain foods, particularly those high in fermentable carbohydrates.[113] This results in an increase in abdominal bloating, abdominal pain, and flatulence that is reversed by avoiding those foods.[89] Probiotic supplementation may help rebalance intestinal flora and alleviate IBS symptoms.

A particularly important type of probiotic—*bifidobacteria*—is found in reduced quantities in the GI tracts of both IBS-C[111] and IBS-D[114] sufferers relative to healthy individuals.[115] In one study, probiotic *Bifidobacterium infantis* 35624, in a dose of 10 billion colony-forming units (CFUs), significantly improved abdominal pain/discomfort, abdominal bloating/distension, and difficulty with bowel movements in women with IBS after only 4 weeks.[116] In a randomized clinical trial, IBS patients treated with 1 billion CFUs of *bifidobacteria* (a relatively low dose) experienced significant improvements in abdominal discomfort, bloating, and urgency relative to those who received placebo.[117] This treatment resulted in a significant improvement in quality of life and mental health.[117]

Another more robust finding supporting probiotic use in IBS comes from a study of the probiotic *Lactobacillus plantarum* DSM 9843. In this study, 20 billion CFUs were administered daily for 4 weeks to IBS sufferers. Flatulence resolved rapidly, and improvements in overall GI function remained long after supplementation was discontinued.[118]

Collectively, these data suggest probiotics are effective in treating IBS, with strains of bifidobacteria being more favorable than lactobacilli, as lactobacilli are actually increased in certain populations with SIBO[119] and IBS,[120,121] correlating with worse symptoms.[122]

## Artichoke

Artichoke leaf has been used since Roman times as a traditional medicine that supports digestive function. It has been shown to promote the production of bile that helps digest dietary fats and reduce spasms and flatulence. In one study, two capsules of 320 mg artichoke leaf extract taken 3 times daily almost completely eliminated abdominal pain, cramps, bloating, flatulence, and constipation in a population of IBS sufferers who also exhibited nonspecific GI discomfort or dyspeptic syndrome.[123] This was later confirmed and accompanied by a significantly improved quality of life in artichoke leaf extract-supplemented patients with functional dyspepsia.[124] In another study, consumption of 320 or 640 mg of artichoke leaf extract daily for 2 months significantly attenuated IBS symptoms and improved quality of life.[125]

## Melatonin

Melatonin is a multifunctional hormone that exhibits a variety of beneficial effects in gastrointestinal disorders independent of its more widely known effects on sleep.[126] In one study of IBS patients with sleep disturbances, 3 mg of melatonin taken prior to bedtime for 2 weeks significantly decreased abdominal pain and rectal sensitivity.[127] These findings were confirmed in a larger double-blind, placebo-controlled crossover study in which 3 mg of melatonin reduced abdominal pain and bloating in women with IBS.[128] In a study that examined a wider array of symptoms, besides improving bowel function, melatonin was also associated with a marked reduction in lethargy in a group of IBS sufferers.[129]

## Additional Support

**Curcumin.** In one large nonplacebo-controlled trial, consumption of 72 or 144 mg *Curcuma longa* extract daily for 8 weeks significantly reduced IBS prevalence and improved quality of life.[130]

***Saccharomyces boulardii.*** The probiotic yeast *Saccharomyces boulardii* was shown in one study to improve quality of life measures among subjects with IBS after 4 weeks of treatment.[131]

**Stress-modifying natural therapies.** Several natural compounds, including *adaptogenic herbs* (eg, Rhodiola, Bacopa, *Holy Basil*, Ashwagandha and *Cordyceps*) and stress-response–modifying nutrients such as phosphatidylserine, may benefit IBS sufferers by mitigating stress.

For example, *Rhodiola rosea* is effective in alleviating a variety of psychological conditions, including irritability, anxiety, and loss of zest for life.[132] As such, it might offer relief to IBS sufferers, although this has yet to be empirically tested. Similarly, some IBS patients exhibited altered dynamics of the stress hormone cortisol,[133] which may be corrected by an omega-3 fatty acid-enriched phosphatidylserine supplement.[134-136]

Research on *Bacopa monnieri* indicates that it has adaptogenic effects and can significantly decrease stress-related anxiety.[137,138] *Bacopa* (in combination with another herb) was found to be particularly beneficial in IBS-D in a 6-week randomized, controlled trial.[139]

More stress-reduction strategies are discussed in Life Extension's Stress Management protocol.

## Life Extension Suggestions

- **Buffered vitamin C powder or effervescent magnesium ascorbate crystals:** Take on a completely empty stomach and allow at least 30–90 minutes for these peristalsis-inducing nutrients to evacuate the bowel. This is for IBS of the *constipation* type only.
- **Probiotics:** per label instructions
- **Fiber:** 7 g daily

- **Peppermint oil/caraway oil:** per label instructions
- **Artichoke leaf extract:** 500–1500 mg daily
- **Melatonin:** 0.3–5 mg before bed (sometimes up to 10 mg)

### Additional Therapies

- **Curcumin,** as highly absorbed BCM-95®: 400–800 mg daily
- **Holy basil:** 1200 mg daily
- **Ashwagandha:** per label instructions
- **Cordyceps:** per label instructions
- **Bacopa monnieri:** per label instructions
- **Rhodiola extract,** root, standardized to 3% rosavins (7.5 mg): 250 mg daily
- **Phosphatidylserine:** 100 mg daily
- ***Saccharomyces boulardii:*** 500 mg daily

In addition, the following *blood tests* may be helpful:

- Food safe allergy test
- Celiac disease antibody screen
- Female Basic Hormone Panel or Female Comprehensive Hormone Panel
- Chemistry panel and complete blood count (CBC)

## REFERENCES

References available at: www.lef.org/dpt5/ch82

# 83

# Jet Lag

Almost everyone who has traveled across more than a few times zones in one trip has experienced the debilitating effects of jet lag. While travel across vast distances is now rapid, convenient, and commonplace, we are still saddled with biological limitations arising from millions of years of evolution. The distress associated with jet lag results when the body's internal clock, or circadian rhythm, becomes desynchronized with the external time zone.

Jet lag is characterized by unpleasant symptoms, including insomnia, sleepiness, impaired performance, diminished alertness, irritability, depressed mood, and gastrointestinal distress.[1] Symptoms of jet lag are slightly more dramatic for travelers heading east. In addition, older individuals are likely to suffer more from its effects.[2]

The human circadian rhythm (characterized by rising and falling hormone levels, undulating body temperature, and the familiar sleep–wake cycle) is linked to the rising and setting of the sun. Through its production of melatonin (ie, the circadian hormone), the pineal gland plays a crucial role in circadian rhythm.

Research suggests that the jet aircraft environment itself may also contribute to jet lag. In a recent experiment, researchers simulated the mild oxygen deprivation (hypoxia) that occurs in pressurized aircraft cabins during long-duration flights at altitudes between 8000 and 12 000 feet. Participants were assessed for changes in melatonin levels. Scientists found a significant decrease in the nightly peak of melatonin, prompting speculation that hypoxia induced by cabin air contributes to postflight fatigue after long flights and to the clinical disorder of jet lag.[3]

## JET LAG'S EFFECTS ON THE MIND AND BODY

Symptoms of jet lag may include malaise, decreased strength and efficiency, decreased ability to remember or concentrate, gastrointestinal disturbance, headache, irritability, loss of appetite, tiredness during the day, and sleeplessness at night.[4-9] Scientists have documented that even elite athletes' performance suffers from jet lag, and some world travelers may experience depression after long flights.[7,10-12]

Researchers have documented that jet lag affects normal daily changes in blood pressure and heart rate, alters otherwise normal changes in body temperature, and disrupts the normal ebb and flow of the stress hormone cortisol. These alterations in normal functions may last for a week or more.[7,13,14] For instance, long-distance flight crews experiencing chronic jet lag may have significantly elevated cortisol levels compared to those of controls. This elevation in cortisol correlates with deficits in cognitive performance.[13]

In addition, jet lag may trigger more serious conditions.[15] Researchers in Israel have investigated the relationship between jet lag and major psychiatric disorders. Conducted at a mental health center in Jerusalem, the study involved 152 patients who had been hospitalized for psychiatric disorders within a 6-year period. Researchers assigned patients to one of two groups, based on the number of time zones they crossed while traveling to Israel. Only those patients who were mentally healthy at the time of travel or who had been free of any psychiatric symptoms for at least 1 year before travel were included in the study. The team documented a significant correlation between crossing 7 or more time zones and a relapse of psychiatric disorders.[6,15]

Researchers in France have investigated whether chronic disruptions of the circadian rhythm could hasten cancer growth. Working with mice, they entrained one group to a normal rhythm of 12 hours of daylight followed by 12 hours of darkness. A second group of rodents repeatedly underwent 8-hour advances of the light–dark cycle every 2 days. Both groups were injected with cancerous cells known to cause tumors in mice. Compared with mice kept on a normal sleep–wake cycle, the jet-lagged mice experienced faster tumor growth.[16]

Among humans, scientists have observed that frequently jet-lagged individuals and night-shift workers whose circadian cycles are routinely disrupted are more prone to disease than people who adhere to a normal sleep–wake cycle. Shift workers, for instance, are at increased risk of experiencing cardiovascular, gastrointestinal, and reproductive dysfunction, and are more prone to developing clinical depression.[17-23] There is also a correlation between sleep and proper immune function, so insomnia related to jet lag may increase susceptibility to infection.[24]

## COMBATING JET LAG WITH MELATONIN

Most scientifically sound methods for reducing the effects of jet lag are based on 2 facts:

1. In healthy individuals, circadian rhythm is synchronized with daylight.

2. Effects of the daylight–dark cycle on circadian cycle are mediated by melatonin.

Specifically, melatonin is secreted by the pineal gland in response to the absence of light. Melatonin triggers a cascade of chemical and physiologic responses that ultimately result in sleep, usually within about 30 minutes. As dawn breaks and light begins to impinge on the brain's "circadian pacemaker," melatonin production drops off dramatically, and the waking portion of the daily sleep–wake cycle begins.

Strategies to manipulate the sleep–wake cycle, such as those used to alleviate symptoms of jet lag, therefore depend on strategic manipulation of exposure to bright light and intake of supplemental melatonin at key times. Some studies have also examined the usefulness of stimulants (eg, caffeine).

### Jet Lag: A Dangerous Deficiency in Melatonin

Melatonin's role in human health is far more profound than once suspected. We now know that melatonin has remarkable properties as an antioxidant and a modulator of immune system functioning. As an antioxidant, it works on several levels. Production of the body's natural antioxidant enzymes (eg, superoxide dismutases, peroxidases, catalase, and glutathione peroxidase) is promoted by melatonin. Also, melatonin triggers other cell-signaling pathways that result in decreased production of harmful, inflammation-producing chemicals (eg, nitric oxide synthases and lipoxygenases).

Melatonin receptors are found throughout the body, including the gastrointestinal and reproductive tracts. It is now known that melatonin is produced by a number of tissues, including skin, gut, liver, kidney, and white blood cells.[25-27]

Another study examined the effects of pineal gland removal on the skin of laboratory rodents. Changes in skin thickness and texture, among others, were seen in animals whose pineal glands had been removed, but not in control animals that underwent a sham operation. When supplemental melatonin was given to the affected rodents, their skin dramatically improved. These results suggest that melatonin is a highly efficient antiaging factor; as its levels decrease with age, melatonin use may minimize age-related skin changes.[28]

Other studies have suggested that melatonin plays an important role in preserving neurological function in rats with spinal cord injuries.[29,30] Melatonin has been studied as a support for age-associated neurologic disorders.[31] Some of its metabolites are believed to improve mitochondrial functioning and quell inflammation.[32]

Thus, melatonin plays an indispensable role in synchronizing the body's internal clock with the external environment and is also a vital component of overall health and well-being.[33] Jet lag, which involves a disruption not only of the sleep–wake cycle but of melatonin secretion as well, is not to be underestimated as a potential threat to health.

## THE "CHRONOSENSE": AN INTERNAL TIMEKEEPER

Melatonin, which stimulates sleep, is only part of the equation when it comes to jet lag. Light is also a major factor in regulating the natural circadian clock. German researchers have proposed a previously unsuspected role for the eye in the function of the circadian clock. While structure and function of the eye as the sensory organ of vision are well known, it apparently also serves as an organ of time sense.[34]

This role relies on a sensory pigment that allows non-image-forming photoreception in mammals. Researchers refer to the nexus of this photopigment and retinal nerve as the "chronoreceptor," which mediates the sense of time, or "chronosense." Although the exact photopigment responsible for chronoreception has not yet been identified with certainty, a chemical called melanopsin is emerging as a likely candidate.[34-36]

These newly discovered chronoreceptors provide the brain with readings that correspond to changes in the intensity of both natural and artificial light. Light signals travel from the eye through a small subset of retinal ganglion cells to a region of the hypothalamus (specifically, to the suprachiasmatic nucleus), and from there to the pineal gland. The suprachiasmatic nucleus is also the site of the circadian pacemaker.

Scientists in Brazil demonstrated that the chronosense, or light–dark entrainment, occurs even in blind primates otherwise unresponsive to visible light. This finding suggests the biological importance of adjusting circadian rhythm to the daily light–dark cycle.[35] The importance of chronosense was further supported when researchers discovered that newborns are functionally blind at birth, yet the newborn retina is nevertheless sensitive to light, and there is a

functioning connection between the chronoreceptors and the circadian pacemaker in the brain.[37]

# MINIMIZING JET LAG: A PLAN OF ATTACK FOR RAPID REENTRAINMENT

In 2003, leading British jet lag researchers published a review of clinical trials that used bright light with and without melatonin in an effort to hasten circadian rhythm reentrainment after simulated or actual flights crossing more than 5 time zones. They cited 10 randomized, controlled trials that compared the effects of melatonin versus placebo in participants undergoing simulated or actual long-distance travel.[38]

Eight of 10 trials found a clear reduction in jet lag when melatonin was taken. Five of the studies recorded global jet lag scores between zero (none) and 100 (extreme). The mean score after placebo was 48. Mean score after melatonin was 25, indicating that jet lag severity was reduced by about half among melatonin users.

Scientists concluded that 2–5 mg of melatonin taken at bedtime after arrival is an effective means of minimizing jet lag.[38] Melatonin administration at bedtime should probably continue for the following 2–4 days for maximum effectiveness. In addition, careful attention to meal times and light exposure may hasten reentrainment. Conversely, inappropriate meal times, injudicious use of alcohol or caffeine, and exposure to bright light at the wrong times may hinder the process.

Light was identified as the most important external cue. Specifically, after a westward flight, it is important to stay awake during daylight hours at the new destination and sleep only after it gets dark. After an eastward flight, it is important to remain awake in the morning but avoid bright morning light. It is also recommended to be outdoors as much as possible in the afternoon at the new destination.

Getting some moderate exercise[39] and perhaps indulging in sightseeing at times when bright light exposure is advised may also reinforce the reentrainment process. Doses of melatonin ranging between 0.5 mg and 5 mg are similarly effective in facilitating reentrainment, but one research team found that participants fall asleep more rapidly and sleep somewhat more soundly after 5 mg melatonin than after 0.5 mg. The team also reported that fast-acting rather than timed-release forms of melatonin are more effective for reentrainment purposes.[40]

It is unclear whether alcohol or caffeine affects adaptation, and the answer may at least partially depend on what an individual is accustomed to. But, these beverages appear more likely to hinder than help adaptation. It is recommended, therefore, that alcohol and caffeine be used sparingly, at best, until full reentrainment is achieved.[38]

# AN ALTERNATE STRATEGY: PREENTRAINMENT

Preentrainment is another strategy to help avoid jet lag. Preentrainment is the technique of adjusting to a new time zone before departure. Researchers in Chicago conducted a study in 2003 using 28 healthy young participants who received one of three protocols, all designed to advance each subject's habitual sleep schedule by 1 hour per day, for 3 days, with or without the use of morning bright light. The goal was to arrive at the new destination with circadian rhythms already partially reentrained to local time, thus minimizing jet lag symptoms and facilitating full reentrainment after arrival.[41]

On each of the 3 study days, participants were exposed to differing amounts of morning light for the first 3.5 hours after waking. Normal wake time was incrementally advanced 1 hour each day, simulating the wake time of eastward time zones. Phase shifting (reentrainment of the circadian cycle toward the destination goal) was measured by monitoring changes in melatonin content of saliva before and after each light session.

As expected, participants who received the greatest amount of bright light upon waking experienced the most dramatic phase shift, which equaled about 2 hours. Even intermittent bright light, which allows a subject enough time to conveniently perform morning chores (eg, showering), resulted in a phase shift of nearly 2 hours with minimal side effects and only a slight reduction in sleep duration.[41]

The scientific team proposed that its 3-day treatment may be especially helpful to eastward travelers, particularly those who travel across multiple time zones and arrive in the morning. They cited previous studies confirming the benefit of early morning bright light exposure, showing that appropriately timed bright light can increase the phase advance more than dim light.[39,41-44]

In early 2005, the same research team conducted a follow-up study.[45] The goal was again to phase shift participants before an anticipated long-haul eastward flight. As in the previous study, participants were subjected to bright light therapy upon waking for 3 days. In this study, however, participants were divided into 2 groups. One group was awakened

2 hours earlier than their usual wake time each day; the second group was awakened 1 hour earlier than usual each day. Both groups were exposed to intermittent bright light therapy for 3.5 hours each morning upon waking.

Participants' phase advances were measured by monitoring changes in saliva melatonin content. Participants who altered their wake time by 2 hours experienced a mean phase shift of 1.9 hours versus 1.4 hours for the group waking up 1 hour earlier. The advantage of advancing the wake schedule by 2 hours was not statistically significant compared with the 1-hour approach. In fact, participants in the 2-hour group eventually experienced misalignment between circadian rhythms and sleep schedules and had difficulty falling asleep. This did not occur among participants in the 1-hour group.[45]

Researchers speculated that a schedule alternating 15 minutes of bright light followed by 15 minutes of dim light might work as well, or better than the study's 30 minutes bright/30 minutes dim protocol because it is the initial pulse of bright light that has the greatest effect on entrainment.[45] Finally, the study's authors noted that the recent discovery that the human circadian system is most sensitive to short wavelength (blue) light of about 460 nanometers (nm) might mean that lamps of lesser intensity and with a greater concentration of this blue light may work as well, or better than a standard, commercially available bright light.

## Preentrainment with Light and Melatonin

In late 2005, the same research team published the results of a study in which varying doses of supplemental melatonin, administered in the afternoon, were added to participants' bright light exposure upon waking.[46] Participants received four 30-minute sessions of exposure to bright light from a light box, alternated with 30 minutes of dim room light. This schedule was intended to allow participants the flexibility of completing morning chores conveniently. In the afternoon, participants received either 0.5 mg or 3.0 mg melatonin. Wake time was advanced by 1 hour each day for 3 days.

Results were similar to those reported in the 2003 study. Participants phase advanced by about 2.5 hours, with no appreciable jet lag symptoms. No statistically significant difference was found between participants receiving the smaller or larger doses of melatonin.[46] Thus, morning bright light exposure and an afternoon dose of melatonin of at least 0.5 mg, combined with an incremental advance in wake time of 1 hour per day for 3 days prior

to travel, may be the most effective approach to preventing, or at least ameliorating jet lag before flying across more than 5 time zones.

## Life Extension Suggestions

Jet lag is the bane of modern travelers, but its debilitating effects can be minimized with proper planning. Eastward flight generates far more severe jet lag than westward flight, but the reentrainment procedures outlined here should work for travel in either direction. The following procedures are suggested:

- Attempt to schedule your arrival for morning or early afternoon, if possible.
- Attempt to depart fully rested.
- Expose yourself to (carefully timed) bright daylight.
  - Such light exposure should not commence until 2 hours before normal wake time. For example, if you normally rise at 7 a.m., do not expose yourself to light at the destination until the time that corresponds to 5 a.m. at your departure point. Thus, on a 7-hour eastward flight, do not expose yourself to light until noon at your destination.
- Take 0.5–5.0 mg supplemental *melatonin* within 3 hours of desired bedtime at the destination.
- Sleep in absolute darkness, to the extent possible.
- Avoid caffeine after noon.

To beat jet lag on a long-distance eastward trip, consider the following preentrainment procedure. This strategy requires taking action at least 3 days before departure. While flights across more than 5 time zones are of greatest concern, preentrainment may be useful for flights that cross as few as 2 or 3 time zones. For two time zone flights, begin 2 days before departure.

- For each of the 3 days before departure, set the alarm for 1 hour earlier than usual wake time.
- Immediately upon waking each day, expose yourself to bright light.
- For 3.5 hours after waking each morning, including the morning of departure, alternate 30 minutes of exposure to bright light with 30 minutes of exposure to ordinary room light.
  - Perform morning chores requiring mobility (eg, showering, shaving, etc.) during bright-light phases.
  - Tasks such as working on a computer, applying makeup, or gardening outdoors without a hat

or sunglasses may be completed during bright-light phases, as long as full bright-light exposure is not compromised.

- Take 0.5–3.0 mg supplemental *melatonin* in late afternoon (3–5 hours before desired bedtime).
- Attempt to retire to bed 1 hour earlier than usual.
- Attempt to sleep in absolute darkness.
- Repeat procedure, again setting wake time another hour earlier than usual, for 2 more days.

By day 3 you should be waking 3 hours earlier than usual.

- Avoid caffeine after noon.

## REFERENCES

References available at: www.lef.org/dpt5/ch83

# 84

# *Kidney Health*

For many years, the Centers for Disease Control and Prevention (CDC) has listed kidney disease as one of the top 10 causes of death by disease in the United States. Kidney disease also plays a significant role in hypertension and diabetes, 2 other diseases also included on the CDC's list of top 10 causes of death each year. End-stage renal (kidney) disease (ESRD) is growing at a rate of 4–8% each year in the United States. Someone with advanced ESRD may require either therapeutic or regular dialysis, or both, and may eventually require a kidney transplant. When kidney function is reduced to 10–15% or less, dialysis is started in ESRD patients. Sometimes ESRD patients are placed on a waiting list for a kidney transplant.

According to statistics compiled by the National Institute of Diabetes and Digestive and Kidney Diseases (NIDDK),[1] kidney conditions such as inflammation, kidney stones, and cancer affected over 2.5 million persons; ESRD affected 424179 people; polycystic kidney diseases affected 600000 people; and other urinary conditions such as kidney infections, bladder infections, and cystitis affected millions more, costing billions of dollars in medical care funded by public and private individuals.[2–4]

Due to the limited scope of this protocol, we will briefly describe some of the more common kidney disorders and treatments. However, 2 conditions will be described in greater detail: *autosomal dominant polycystic kidney disease* (ADPKD) and *kidney stones*. ADKPD is a common human genetic disease, resulting in many cases of ESRD, and eventually the need for kidney transplantation. Kidney stones affect approximately 10% of the U.S. population at some point in their lives.[5] Unfortunately, about 60% of persons with a kidney stone will develop another stone. It has been reported by the NIDDK that urinary stones account for more than 1.3 million physician visits in a single year.[6]

Attention to overall kidney health is essential. If you have healthy kidneys, take care of them. Educate yourself about how to do this. We will provide information in the paragraphs that follow to assist you in being proactive in maintaining healthy kidneys. If you have a condition (eg, diabetes or hypertension) that poses a threat to your kidneys, seek a qualified medical professional to treat and control these conditions. Carefully follow monitoring and treatment advice. Information will also be provided to assist in supporting kidneys that have already sustained damage.

## KIDNEY FUNCTION

Kidneys are bean-shaped organs that act as sophisticated filters to remove organic waste products from the blood and then excrete these products, along with excess salt and water, from the body through the urine. We are normally born with 2 kidneys located on either side of the lower back, just below the rib

**Anatomy of the Kidney**

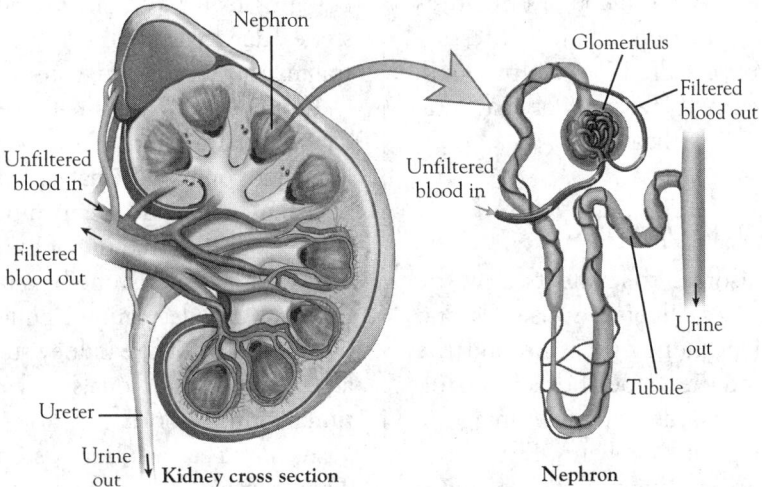

Unfiltered blood in

Filtered blood out

Nephron

Ureter

Urine out

**Kidney cross section**

Glomerulus

Filtered blood out

Unfiltered blood in

Urine out

Tubule

**Nephron**

cage. Kidneys are such incredibly well-functioning organs that only one normal, healthy kidney is required for good health. Each kidney is 4–5 inches long, weighs about 6 oz, and contains about 1 million nephrons (ie, the working units of the kidney responsible for waste removal).[7] As part of our normal aging process, kidney function diminishes as the number of functional nephrons is reduced.

Kidneys play a role in controlling the acid-base balance in the body and helping to control blood pressure. Another function of the kidneys is to produce hormones such as erythropoietin, which regulates the production and release of red blood cells from bone marrow.

Each day, kidneys filter approximately 200 quarts of blood, producing about 2 quarts of waste products and water.[7] The waste products and excess water pass from the kidneys, through the ureters (tubes that connect the kidneys to the bladder), and into the bladder where they are briefly stored before being eliminated as liquid waste via the urine. Filtered waste products include normal organic material from the breakdown of cells, proteins, excess food by-products, and various minerals, as well as individual waste excretions from cells of the body. Alcohol, drugs, excess protein, minerals, and ingested toxins are also filtered by the kidneys. These toxic agents can have a dramatic, destructive effect on the health and function of the kidneys.

The rate of blood flow through the kidneys is about 20% of the total blood pumped by the heart each minute.[8]

Kidney function is often measured by using routine blood and urine tests to indicate gross problems. These tests measure creatinine levels, possible blood in the urine, blood urea nitrogen (BUN), proteinuria (protein in the urine), and mineral content, including calcium, magnesium, phosphorus, sodium, potassium, oxalic acid, and other elements. If blood or urine tests indicate improper kidney function, additional testing using conventional x-rays, needle biopsy, ultrasound, computed tomography scan (CT scan), or magnetic resonance imaging (MRI) is indicated.[9]

# KIDNEY DISORDERS

Kidney disease is any disorder that affects how the kidneys function. A list of all of the diseases and conditions that can affect kidney function and the possible causes are beyond the scope of this protocol. However, some of these disorders include analgesic nephropathy, chronic nephritis, diabetes, ESRD, hypertension, infection, injury, kidney stones, lupus erythematosus, and ADPKD.[9]

Symptoms of renal disease can include frequent headaches and urination, itching, poor appetite, fatigue, burning bladder, anemia, baggy eyes, nausea and vomiting, swollen or numb hands or feet, poor concentration, darkened skin, and muscle cramps.[9]

## Kidney Stones (Calculi)

Kidney stones (or calculi) are a common and incredibly painful condition. It is estimated that 10% of the U.S. population will pass a kidney stone at some time in their lives. Men have more kidney stones than women, and white people are more prone to kidney stone formation than black people. The incidence of kidney stones is higher in the summer. This may be because people perspire more in the summer; as a result, urine becomes more concentrated.

A kidney stone is a solid, rock-like type of material that has formed or is present in the kidneys, ureters, or bladder. A kidney stone is formed from mineral substances that precipitate from urine. Kidney stones can stay in the kidney or travel down the urinary tract. Small stones are sometimes passed from the body with either a small or large degree of pain. Larger stones may lodge in the ureter, bladder, or urethra, blocking urine flow and causing extreme pain.[7]

Most kidney stones contain calcium combined with either oxalate or phosphate. Calcium stones are formed when extra calcium is not eliminated in the urine. Another type of kidney stone is a *struvite stone*, which can form following a urinary infection. *Uric acid stones* form when there is too much acid in the urine. A rare type of kidney stone is made up of cystine. Evidence shows that cystine-based stones tend to be inherited (the result of a genetic disease).[7]

Kidney stones vary widely in size, from a grain of sand to the size of a golf ball. Although most kidney stones are quite small, they can grow to a size that is life threatening or requires surgical removal. Some large kidney stones, due to age of the patient or danger of associated trauma to a vital organ, cannot be surgically removed.

Kidney stones are usually yellow or brown in color. Their structure and texture can be smooth or jagged. Another common visual characteristic is a crystalline appearance with different mineral striations appearing throughout the structure of the stone. Examination and testing of a kidney stone by a urologist (ie, specialist in urology) can determine significant information about possible cause of the kidney stone, and perhaps suggest a remedy for individuals with potential to form additional kidney stones.[7]

As noted earlier, kidney stones tend to be inherited. They can also be associated with geographic factors. Therefore, people living in tropical climates may be at greater risk for kidney stone formation due to the way bodies manage water in a tropical setting. Perspiration often becomes the prevalent method of how the body excretes water in tropical or very hot conditions, and urination may decline slightly due to urine being stored longer in the urinary tract. Most people do not drink enough water; in tropical areas, this is even more significant. Excessive perspiration becomes more significant while engaging in physical labor or strenuous sports in hot conditions. The body loses large amounts of water during excessive perspiration. For example, a NFL lineman can lose up to a gallon of water (or up to 10 lb of water weight) during a 4-hour game. Therefore, sufficient water intake is both a preventive and a therapeutic measure.

Symptoms of a kidney stone attack include sudden extreme pain in the lower back, side, or groin; blood in the urine; fever and chills; vomiting; a bad odor or cloudy appearance to the urine; and a burning sensation during urination. Any of these symptoms require evaluation by a physician. Pain in the lower back, side, or groin can also indicate that a kidney stone is moving or there is a serious urinary tract blockage that requires immediate medical intervention. Kidney stone episodes frequently include urinary tract infections (UTIs). Recurrent, untreated UTIs can eventually cause permanent kidney damage and reduced kidney function.

Passing a kidney stone can be as simple as drinking large amounts of liquid and running up and down stairs or jumping up and down vigorously to dislodge the stone. This practice uses the basic physics of gravity to get the stone moving so that it can be passed normally. If possible, catch the stone in a strainer or retrieve it to be examined by a nephrologist or urologist.[7]

**Medical intervention for kidney stones.** Many kidney stones pass from the body naturally. However, more complex procedures are required to assist stones that cannot be passed or remove stones that are growing larger.[7] Either lithotripsy or surgical removal of the stone is used when a kidney stone is firmly lodged in the ureters, bladder, or urethra. In the past, these stones represented a significant health concern because the only way to remove them was invasive surgery with a high risk of postoperative infection. It is now possible for urologists to avoid surgery, except when there is no alternative. Newer methods to remove kidney stones include ureteroscopy, tunnel surgery, extracorporeal shock wave lithotripsy (ESWL), and percutaneous lithotripsy. These methods break the stone into smaller pieces so it can be removed or passed through the urinary tract.[7]

**Preventing kidney stones.** Research into the prevention of recurrent kidney stones has produced many helpful dietary guidelines, nutritional protocols, and lifestyle changes that can reduce or eliminate the potential for recurring kidney stones. They may also help pass a recurrent stone faster and with less difficulty.

In 1997, a double-blind study was conducted to determine if potassium/magnesium citrate would prevent recurrent formation of calcium oxalate kidney stones.[10] Sixty-four patients with a history of renal calculi were given 42 mEq potassium, 21 mEq magnesium, and 63 mEq citrate or a placebo daily for 3 years. New renal calculi formed in 63.6% of patients receiving placebo. Patients receiving potassium/magnesium citrate presented with 12.9% recurrent renal calculi. The study concluded that "potassium/magnesium citrate effectively prevents recurrent calcium oxalate stones, and this treatment given for up to 3 years reduces risk of recurrence by 85%."[10]

Two major studies have shown that calcium should not be reduced for patients with a history of kidney stones.[11,12] It was originally postulated that patients with a history of renal calculi should limit their calcium intake. Newer findings contradict this restriction and offer scientific evidence that uncombined intestinal oxalic acid is the real culprit for calcium oxalate kidney stones.[13]

Harvard researchers studied nearly 92000 nurses over a 12-year period to determine the relationship between calcium intake and occurrence of renal calculi (the well-known Harvard Nurses' Health Study). The study concluded that those nurses who consumed diets higher in calcium were at lower risk for kidney stones.

The reason this type of dietary modification reduced the chance of kidney stones was relatively simple. A high percentage of kidney stones are comprised of calcium and oxalic acid, which form calcium oxalate *inside the kidneys*. Oxalic acid is able to pass through the intestinal wall, into the blood, and enter the kidneys where it has a chance to combine with calcium. Calcium oxalate, when normally combined *inside the digestive tract*, does not pass through the intestinal wall and into the blood, but is eliminated with other waste products. Therefore, when combined with dietary or supplemental calcium inside the intestinal tract, oxalic acid will never reach the kidneys; thus, calcium oxalate kidney stones cannot be formed.

The *Harvard Nurses' Health Study* presented the following important findings: dietary calcium intake from food or supplements reduced the risk of renal calculi; calcium supplementation must be taken with food and in small dosages (<400 mg); plant foods high in calcium, fiber, vitamins, minerals, antioxidants, and some protein were an excellent source of dietary phytochemicals.

Another study conducted in South Africa found that "mineral water containing calcium and magnesium deserves to be considered as a possible therapeutic or prophylactic agent in calcium oxalate kidney stone disease."[14] A French mineral water containing 202 ppm calcium and 36 ppm magnesium was selected as the delivery method. Twenty males and females with previously formed calcium oxalate renal calculi and 20 healthy males and females participated in the study. Each subject provided daily 24-hour urine collection samples during the study. Mineral water was ingested over a 3-day period; then, participants switched to tap water. The cycle was repeated at least twice by each subject. Males with a history of calcium oxalate renal calculi received the most benefit, showing 9 risk factors favorably affected by the mineral water containing calcium and magnesium.[15]

Recommendations to avoid kidney stones include[16]:

- Drink more water. Try to drink at least 12 full glasses of water each day. Drinking extra water helps flush substances that form stones from the kidneys.

- It is not necessary to eliminate coffee, tea, and colas from your diet, but limit caffeine because it can increase fluid loss. Consider drinking ginger ale, lemon-lime soda, and fruit juices.

- Follow your physician's recommendations about dietary limitations. If you form uric acid stones, your physician will probably ask you to eat less meat because meat breaks down to form uric acid.

- Follow your physician's recommendations about taking medicines to prevent kidney stone formation.

## Autosomal Dominant Polycystic Kidney Disease (ADPKD)

ADPKD is one of the most common genetic diseases in humans. It is a systemic disease caused by at least 3 different genes: PKD1, PKD2, and PKD3. However, most mutations are found in the PKD1 gene.[17,18] ADPKD is a very serious disease. Worldwide, it is responsible for 8–10% of all cases of ESRD. Patients with ADPKD develop cysts in both kidneys. These cysts continue to grow over the lifetime of the patient and ultimately lead to hypertension, reduced kidney function, and eventually renal failure. Poor kidney function in ADPKD patients accounts for many kidney transplants each year.

According to the Polycystic Kidney Disease (PKD) Foundation (Kansas City, www.pkdcure.org), 60% of individuals with ADPKD develop kidney failure or ESRD. The only treatment is dialysis or transplant. Interestingly, because ADPKD is genetic in origin, persons who receive kidney transplants do not reacquire their genetic mutation with transplanted kidneys. Common symptoms are frequent infections, blood in the urine, and back pain.

Polycystic kidney disease (PKD) may occur at birth, during childhood or adulthood. Congenital polycystic disease can be detected at birth and may affect all or only small parts of one or both kidneys. Childhood PKD can cause death after a few years due to liver and kidney failure. In some adults, the disease may be present at birth, but not manifest any symptoms until young adulthood or middle age. In adults, it can affect either one or both kidneys.[19] PKD is characterized by autonomous cellular proliferation, pockets of fluid accumulation within the cysts, and intraparenchymal fibrosis of the kidney. Other clinical observations include renal failure, liver cysts, and cardiac valve abnormalities.[20]

The traditional method of diagnosing ADPKD has been detecting renal cysts via ultrasound, CT, or MRI of the kidneys. The challenge in diagnosing ADPKD is to detect it in people with the defective gene, but who may not have symptoms or show any developed cysts. Newer methods of DNA testing can now identify individuals who carry the defective gene, but are not symptomatic. For example, every member of 4 Chinese families with a known history of ADPKD showed unique DNA patterns.[21] DNA diagnostic testing methods have value for patients with existing ADPKD, as well as for presymptomatic patients.

ADPKD progresses to end-stage renal insufficiency before the age of 73 years in about 50% of affected patients.[22] It remains a mystery as to why some patients are affected by numerous cysts that form inside the proximal and distal tubules, while others are spared. The formation of cysts begins in early childhood, affecting less than 1% of tubules as a consequence of mutated DNA. The risk factors associated with PKD include gender (males progress more quickly than females), race (black patients progress more rapidly than whites), and other contributing factors such as hypertension and proteinuria. These factors can aggravate and accelerate PKD through to end term.[22]

Because hypertension (a common and serious factor of ADPKD) usually occurs early in the disease (ie, before renal function begins to decrease), Doppler ultrasonography has been used to assess renal vascular resistance (RVR) by measuring resistive and pulsatility indices. In a study of 42 patients with ADPKD and 65 control subjects, it was found that Doppler indices reflect increased RVR in those patients with ADPKD and that renal function disturbance did manifest systemic arterial hypertension.[23] The abnormality of the kidneys in these patients was easily observed using ultrasound. However, this method did not show ADPKD potential for patients if renal cysts were not present. DNA testing is required to determine whether a patient carries the PDK1 and PDK2 chromosomes.

Cardiovascular complication is a very common cause of death for persons with ADPKD. After examining the relationship of known cardiovascular risk factors, hypertension, and ADPKD, researchers noted that left ventricular hypertrophy (LVH) is an important risk factor for premature cardiovascular death in persons with essential hypertension.[24] Hypertension occurs frequently and early in ADPKD patients. In 116 adult ADPKD patients and 77 healthy controls, a higher frequency of LVH was found in ADPKD men (46% versus 20%) and women (37% versus 12%) compared to control subjects.[24] LVH in ADKPD patients was associated with higher systolic and diastolic blood pressure. According to the researchers, the role of blood pressure as a contributing factor to LVH in ADPKD patients may be partly due to early onset and inadequate treatment.

The possibility is being explored that ADPKD may have an emerging infectious disease component as well. Research has shown fungal DNA in kidney tissue and cyst fluids of ADPKD patients, but not in healthy kidneys of persons without ADPKD.[25] In a differential activation protocol assay, researchers showed bacterial endotoxin and fungal beta-D-glucans in cyst fluids from human kidneys with PKD. Tissue and cyst fluids were examined for fungal components and the serologic tests showed *Fusarium*, *Aspergillus, and Candida* antigens. Researchers concluded that "endotoxin and fungal components, sphingolipid biology in PKD, the structure of PKD gene products, infection, and integrity of gut function [will establish a mechanism] for microbial provocation of human cystic disease."[26]

# FACTORS AFFECTING KIDNEY FUNCTION

Adults lose kidney function and capacity with normal aging. A number of factors, including drug reactions and degenerative disease not endemic to the kidneys, may bring added stress.

## Analgesics

An analgesic is any medicine intended to kill pain. Analgesics that contain narcotics are for more severe pain and require a prescription from a physician. However, many analgesics can be purchased over-the-counter (OTC) (aspirin, ibuprofen, acetaminophen, and naproxen). OTC analgesics rarely present a problem for most people if the recommended dosage is taken. However, some conditions (eg, chronic kidney disease [CKD]), long-term use, or taking them in combination with other analgesics make OTC analgesics dangerous. Analgesics such as aspirin, ibuprofen, acetaminophen, and naproxen have been attributed to incidence of acute kidney failure in persons with lupus erythematosus or chronic renal conditions, persons of advanced age, or persons who have had a recent binge of alcohol consumption.[7]

Painkillers that combine 2 or more analgesics (eg, aspirin and acetaminophen together) with caffeine or codeine are more likely to cause kidney damage. These mixtures are often sold in powder form. Single analgesics (eg, aspirin) are less likely to cause kidney damage.[7] More research is required to determine whether aspirin or acetaminophen contributes to kidney failure, or whether people with ailments that predispose them to kidney failure are more likely to use painkillers. It is recommended that each patient be considered individually with respect to their risk of kidney failure, length of time painkiller will be taken, and other existing illnesses, particularly in the elderly and persons with chronic conditions.[27] If possible, avoid acetaminophen-based analgesics, as these may be most toxic to the kidneys.

## Autoimmune

Glomeruli, tiny blood vessels in nephrons where blood is filtered in the kidneys, can become inflamed by autoimmune disorders (eg, Goodpasture syndrome and lupus erythematosus). When an autoimmune disorder occurs, the body attacks itself with its own immune system. In the kidneys, this type of inflammation is called glomerulonephritis.[19,28] While glomerulonephritis is usually caused by an autoimmune disorder, it can also be caused by infection (eg, streptococcal bacterial).

## Congenital and Genetic

Congenital abnormalities of the kidneys are not uncommon. Sometimes the 2 kidneys are joined together at their base. Some people are born with only one kidney, both kidneys on the same side of the body, or underdeveloped kidneys that barely function. Polycystic kidney disease is a genetic condition that may manifest at birth, but often appears in young adult-hood or middle age.

## Drug Reactions

Acute kidney damage can result from an allergic reaction to a drug, taking large quantities of a drug (eg, painkillers) for a long period of time, taking outdated tetracyclines, taking potent antibiotics, accidental ingestion of poisons, toluene inhalation (eg, industrial exposure and glue sniffing), or combining prescription drugs, OTC drugs (aspirin, acetaminophen, ibuprofen, naproxen sodium), and alcohol.[7] Regular blood tests to assess kidney function are recommended for anyone taking medicine known to damage the kidneys or with a condition that puts them at risk for developing kidney disease.

## Homocysteine

Discovered in 1932, homocysteine is a sulfur-containing amino acid normally found in small amounts in the blood of healthy persons. Homocysteine is derived from dietary protein (meat, milk, eggs) and is metabolized in the liver using vitamins B6 and B12. High levels of homocysteine can result from genetic disease (homocystinuria), kidney disease, hyperthyroidism, psoriasis, systemic lupus erythematosus, drug treatment for chronic diseases, and dietary vitamin deficiencies (folic acid, B6, B12).[29]

Homocysteine levels, which tend to increase with age, are higher in men than women. High homocysteine levels can be very damaging to kidneys and the vascular system.[30-32] Accumulation of toxic homocysteine has been associated with the development of cardiovascular disease (atherosclerosis, stroke, heart attack), pulmonary embolism and deep venous thrombosis, dementia (Alzheimer's disease, multi-infarct dementia), and ESRD.[29,30,32-35] Cardiovascular disease (CVD), common in patients with CKD, is responsible for the majority of morbidity and mortality in patients.[32]

As early as 1969, researchers began to make clinical observations linking elevated homocysteine to vascular diseases.[36] Subsequent investigations confirmed these observations.[29,37-41] In CVD, there is evidence that elevated homocysteine levels are related to arterial wall damage, but the mechanism is unclear.[29] It may be that homocysteine has a toxic effect on the endothelial (cellular) lining of blood vessels. Data from a study of 14916 healthy U.S. physicians with no prior history of heart disease demonstrated that highly elevated homocysteine levels are associated with a more than three-fold increase in the risk of heart attack over a 5-year period.[39] The Framingham Heart

Study (1041 elderly subjects) and other studies have also confirmed that elevated homocysteine is an independent risk factor for heart disease.[41-45]

Kidneys do not filter homocysteine properly; therefore, blood homocysteine levels increase in kidney disease patients (sometimes 3–4 times higher than normal).[43,45-47] Homocysteine is consistently elevated to very high levels in patients who require dialysis.[32] Plasma homocysteine concentrations often decrease after dialysis.[29] To further help lower homocysteine levels, dialysis patients often require high levels of nutrients, including folic acid, vitamin B12, TMG (also known as betaine or trimethylglycine), and vitamin B6.[29,32,43,47-52]

Folic acid was used in a study conducted in 82 patients undergoing dialysis 3 times weekly for 4 weeks (hemodialysis, 70 patients; peritoneal dialysis, 12 patients).[30] Results demonstrated that in both groups, homocysteine concentration was reduced by 35% after taking 2.5–5 mg of folic acid after each dialysis treatment.

As noted earlier, although dialysis has the effect of lowering homocysteine levels, folic acid further reduced homocysteine levels and, more importantly, had long-term effects even after supplementation was withdrawn.[30]

Although the relationship between CVD and CKD is convincing, therapeutic strategies appear to be underused in the care of patients with kidney disease. CVD and CKD have similar traditional (diabetes, hypertension, dyslipidemia, obesity) and nontraditional (hyperhomocysteinemia, anemia, disturbed mineral metabolism, parathyroid excess) risk factors. Because these risk factors are also specific to kidney disease and are modifiable, they should be identified and treated in persons with CKD.[32] Patients with mild hyperhomocysteinemia have no clinical signs and are typically asymptomatic until the third or fourth decade of life.[29]

For some time, physicians have recognized the danger(s) of homocysteine, and have recommended use of vitamin supplements to lower homocysteine levels.[29,52] The "normal range" used by commercial laboratories is 5–15 μmol/L of blood. However, epidemiological data reveal that homocysteine levels above 6.3 μmol/L result in a steep, progressive risk of heart attack, with each 3-unit increase equaling a 35% increase in risk for heart attack.[50,53] There may be no safe "normal range" for homocysteine. A survey in Cardiologia reported that the average American's homocysteine level is 10 μmol/L.[54]

For many persons, daily intake of TMG (500 mg), folic acid (800 mcg), vitamin B12 (1000 mcg), vitamin

B6 (100 mg), choline (250 mg), inositol (250 mg), and zinc (30 mg) will keep homocysteine levels in a safe range. Unfortunately, without a homocysteine blood test, it is impossible to know if the proper amounts of nutrients are being taken. Therefore, the only way to ascertain that your homocysteine level is below 7 is to have a blood test. Sometimes treatment must be individualized for complicated conditions. High levels of homocysteine can require up to 6 g of TMG or vitamin B6 (in cystathione-B synthase deficiencies).

## Hypertension

High blood pressure (or hypertension) creates a significant risk factor for kidney failure. This risk factor is amplified for persons with ADPKD. After investigating the 24-hour blood pressure profile of ambulatory patients, particularly to measure nocturnal fall of blood pressure, researchers found that in ADPKD patients, the reduction in nocturnal blood pressure was attenuated (lessened), indicating increased risk for kidney damage.[55] Further studies are needed to evaluate the contribution of nocturnal hypertension on the overall progression of renal failure. However, in another related study of untreated children, it was found that nocturnal hypertension was a major risk factor for renal deterioration.[56]

## Impaired Blood Supply

Any condition that impairs blood flow to the kidneys (eg, diabetes mellitus, hemolytic uremic syndrome, physiologic shock, lupus erythematosus) can damage or cause obstruction of small blood vessels in the kidneys.

## Infection

A kidney may become infected when the flow of urine is restricted in the urinary tract.[7] An obstruction may lead to stagnation of urine in the kidney that allows infection to spread into the bladder. Possible causes of an obstruction are a congenital defect, kidney stone, bladder tumor, or enlargement of the prostate gland. Tuberculosis of the kidney occurs when infection is carried by the blood to the kidney from somewhere else in the body (usually the lungs).

## Inflammatory Cytokines

Destructive cell-signaling chemicals called inflammatory cytokines contribute to degenerative, inflammatory, and autoimmune diseases.[57,58] Degenerative diseases (congestive heart failure, anemia, rheumatoid arthritis, fibrinogen formation, fibrosis, diabetes, asthma, lupus, psoriasis) appear to be factors in or possible underlying causes of kidney failure and disease.

People with multiple degenerative disorders often exhibit excess levels of pro-inflammatory markers in their blood. Therefore, seemingly unrelated inflammatory or autoimmune diseases can have a common link to kidney disease (ie, inflammatory cytokines). In kidney failure, inflammatory cytokines restrict circulation and damage nephrons (the filtering units of the kidneys).

For those with degenerative diseases, particularly multiple ones, cytokine profile and C-reactive protein blood tests are highly recommended (available through your own physician or Life Extension National Diagnostics, Inc.). If the cytokine test reveals excess levels of cytokines—tumor necrosis factor-alpha (TNF-α), interleukin-1b (IL-1b)—nutritional supplementation, dietary modifications, and low-cost prescription medications (pentoxifylline or PTX) are advised. See Life Extension's Inflammation (Chronic) protocol for a discussion of systemic inflammation and recommendations for reducing inflammatory conditions.

## Metabolic

Kidney stones are more common in middle age and usually caused by excessive concentrations of substances such as calcium, uric acid, or cystine in the urine.[7] Hyperparathyroidism, cystinuria, and hyperoxaluria are rare, inherited metabolic disorders that can cause kidney stones. In cystinuria, too much of the amino acid cystine can lead to the formation of stones made of cystine. In patients with hyperoxaluria, the body produces too much of the salt oxalate. Excessive oxalate in the urine cannot be dissolved, crystals settle out, and stones form. Absorptive hypercalciuria occurs when the body absorbs too much calcium from food. Extra calcium ends up in the urine, and the high levels cause calcium oxalate or calcium phosphate crystals to form in the kidneys or urinary tract. Other causes are hyperuricosuria (a disorder of uric acid metabolism), gout, excess vitamin D intake, and blockage of the urinary tract. Certain diuretics ("water" pills) or calcium-based antacids, by increasing the amount of calcium in the urine, can increase the risk of kidney stone formation.[7]

## Tumors

Tumors in the kidneys, either benign or malignant, are rare. When malignant, the most common type is renal cell carcinoma, particularly in adults over 40 years.

## Other

Urinary tract infections (UTIs) are frequently occurring health conditions caused by various urinary systemic infections, sexual contact, bacteria entering the kidneys via the bloodstream or urethra, kidney stone blockages, and kidney damage.[19] Infection can lead to impaired kidney function. Therefore, a kidney infection should be treated immediately to prevent more serious disease. A direct blow to the kidneys can also cause extensive damage (eg, a car accident, industrial accident, sports injury, or accidental fall).[9]

# CONVENTIONAL MEDICAL TREATMENTS

Treatment of kidney disease is a complex issue and depends on the type, underlying cause, and duration of the disease. Treatment usually starts with addressing the original cause (eg, inflammation). Inflammation from infection is treated with antibiotics. Inflammation caused by an immune reaction is more difficult to treat. In this case, immunosuppressant drugs (corticosteroids) are used in an attempt to control the immune reaction.

In the case of acute kidney failure, treating the underlying cause may return the kidneys to normal function. Sometimes dietary restrictions (less salt and protein) are required until the kidneys are better able to handle these substances. Diuretic medicines help the body excrete more water and salt. However, with chronic kidney failure, medicines are used to stop the disease from progressing to ESRD.

When kidney disease does not respond to treatment with dietary restrictions and medications, dialysis or kidney transplantation are the next treatments to consider.[19] Dialysis is a technique used to remove waste products from the blood and excess fluid from the body (in the case of renal failure). Kidney transplantation is a surgical procedure in which the diseased kidney (sometimes both kidneys) is removed and replaced with a healthy kidney from a donor.[28]

Four percent of the U.S. population is at risk for kidney disease. An annual physical checkup should include blood levels of creatinine, BUN, and urine protein levels. Small elevations of creatinine can be an early sign of kidney disease. According to the National Kidney Foundation,[59] 11 million Americans have elevated blood levels of creatinine. Healthy kidneys remove creatinine, but when kidney function diminishes, creatinine levels in the blood rise. Early detection leads to early treatment, which can help prevent kidney disease from advancing to a more serious stage. Diabetes is the leading cause of CKD, followed by hypertension. See your physician regularly and follow prescribed dietary and drug treatment to control blood sugar levels and blood pressure.[59] Treatment options for conditions that can lead to kidney disease include numerous prescription drugs and treatment protocols. See the following Life Extension protocols: Diabetes, Immune System Strengthening, Atherosclerosis and Cardiovascular Disease (sections on Homocysteine and Hypertension), Thyroid Regulation, and Urinary Tract Infection (UTI) for additional information on specific conditions and treatment.

## Protecting Kidneys Against Inflammatory Attack

Pentoxifylline (PTX) is a prescription drug approved by the Food and Drug Administration (FDA) to treat peripheral vascular disease. The standard dose is 1200 mg daily to improve circulation. To suppress proinflammatory cytokines often involved in age-related renal impairment, a lower dose of 400 mg twice daily can be used.

**Note:** *Refer to pentoxifylline precautions in the summary section before using this drug.*

A controlled study on human diabetics with advanced renal failure showed that 400 mg daily of PTX reduced TNF-α levels by approximately 35%. In the PTX group, a measurement of kidney impairment was reduced 59%. There were no changes in those given placebo. Researchers noted that inflammatory cytokines such as TNF-α have long been implicated in the development and progression of diabetic kidney failure.[60] Organ failure induced by TNF-α has been confirmed by other studies.[61]

In advanced kidney failure, anemia can be induced by an inflammatory cytokine attack on erythropoietin, the major natural hormone responsible for red blood cell (RBC) production. In a group of 7 anemic patients with advanced renal failure, PTX suppressed TNF-α and reversed the anemic state.[62]

## Kidney Dialysis

Kidney dialysis is a medical treatment used to filter out waste products from the blood. Dialysis has been proven to be an effective technique for removing waste and extra fluid from the body. According to the annual report of the U.S. Renal Data System, 400 000 persons in the United States were using dialysis treatment in 2009.[63] Dialysis treatment permits these people to live relatively normal lives within the limitations of their disease.

The 2 types of dialysis methods are hemodialysis and peritoneal dialysis. The most common technique is hemodialysis, accounting for slightly over 85% of dialysis treatment. The remaining 15% of patients use peritoneal dialysis.[6] Neither is uncomfortable and both are equally effective in removing wastes and extra fluids from the body. The choice is usually based on preference or level of convenience desired by the patient in consultation with appropriate medical professionals.

Even for dialysis patients, kidney failure can cause other health-related problems over time, including high blood pressure (including a latent nocturnal factor), bone disease, anemia, and nerve damage. As kidney function declines past the minimum threshold, kidney transplant becomes the only hope for patients with advanced ESRD.

Studies on human dialysis patients indicate that a high number of free radicals are formed in response to dialysis and antioxidant supplements can protect against this damage.[64–66]

## Transplantation

Statistical surveys of medical facilities, which occur yearly, indicate that kidney transplantation accounted for 13483 transplant operations in 1999.[6] In the United States, many people live with a functioning kidney as a result of transplantation. However, it is very difficult to obtain accurate statistics on the number of people living with a functioning kidney transplant at any given time. Unfortunately, each year patients die while awaiting a matching donor kidney. According to the NIDDK,[6] as of November 2, 2001, there were 50305 people awaiting a kidney transplant. To be a potential candidate for kidney transplantation, a person must have kidney function estimated to be below 15% and must not be positive for certain diseases, such as unstable coronary artery disease, infection, or glomerulonephritis (ie, inflammation of the tiny blood vessels in the nephrons where blood is filtered in the kidneys). It is usually caused by an autoimmune disease, but can also be caused by infection.

A study was conducted to determine if a very-low-protein diet could defer renal replacement therapy (RRT) in patients with chronic renal failure. High protein intake is known to be stressful for the kidneys and over time, can be a contributing factor to a slow, pervasive decline in kidney function. Two groups of patients were put on a very-low-protein diet (0.3 g/kg) combined with supplemental amino acids. The patients were well-motivated RRT candidates who were closely monitored for nearly 1 year. During the course of the study, indications of malnutrition did not occur, and the patients were able to maintain acceptable kidney function (glomerular filtration rate or GFR <10 mL/min or <15/mL/min for diabetic patients).[67]

**Note:** *Since 1973, Medicare has picked up 80% of ESRD treatment costs, including the costs of dialysis and transplantation and of some medications. To qualify for benefits, a patient must be insured or eligible for benefits under Social Security or be a spouse or child of an eligible American. Private insurance and state Medicaid programs often cover the remaining 20% of treatment costs.*

# NATURAL AND ADJUVANT TREATMENTS

## Dietary Management

In the early stages, careful dietary management may slow down the process of kidney disease. A diet low in sodium, potassium, and phosphorus, 3 substances regulated by the kidneys, is essential in managing kidney disease. Other dietary restrictions (eg, reducing protein) may also be required. Your physician might suggest you consult a renal dietitian with special training in diets for persons with kidney disease. Vegetarians have diets that are naturally high in potassium and phosphorus; therefore, need good nutritional advice. If required to limit phosphorus, sodium, or protein, remember the following:

- Phosphorus is especially high in dairy products (eg, milk, cheese, ice cream), dried beans and peas, nuts and peanut butter, some salt substitutes, cocoa, beer, and cola soft drinks.

- Sodium is especially high in table salt, canned soup, processed cheese, snack foods, prepared and "fast foods," pickles, olives, sauerkraut, and smoked and cured food (eg, ham, bacon, luncheon meat).

- Protein is especially high in food from animal sources (eg, poultry, meat, seafood, eggs, and dairy products). Protein is found in smaller amounts in food from plant sources (eg, bread, cereal, grain, vegetables, and fruit).

However, a certain amount of phosphorus, sodium, and protein is necessary for good health. To keep yourself healthy, it is important to learn to read labels and make better choices. For example, non-dairy creamers and milk substitutes are a good way to lower dietary phosphorus.

Avoid losing too much weight. It is important to maintain a good caloric intake because calories give you energy. If limiting protein, get more calories from other food sources including[68]:

- Unsaturated fats from oils (eg, canola or olive oil)
- Simple carbohydrates (eg, honey, jam, and jelly)

*Note: The recommendations for using sugar may not be appropriate for diabetics or overweight individuals. If you are diabetic, consult your physician or renal dietitian for alternative recommendations.*

## Dietary Supplements

Dietary supplements are often recommended by physicians and renal dietitians.[69] Their recommendations are guided by regular blood testing utilized to monitor kidney function. Always speak with a physician or renal dietitian before using or adding any supplements or herbal products.

**Multivitamins.** In addition to a diet containing appropriate nutrients and protein, a comprehensive multivitamin is often required to replace vitamins lost during dialysis treatments.[69]

**B vitamins.** Vitamins B6, B12, and folate (folic acid) are members of the B-vitamin group. B vitamins are known for having many beneficial qualities, including promoting growth, improving heart function, lowering homocysteine, protecting against atherosclerosis caused by excess homocysteine, helping with the formation and regeneration of red blood cells (thus preventing anemia), and increasing energy as well as endurance.[70]

The formation of *advanced glycation end products* (AGEs) is a well-established factor in the onset and progression of kidney disease.

A *formidable* AGE antagonist is the vitamin B6 compound *pyridoxamine*. A plethora of research confirms its power to halt formation of AGEs.[71–73] Evidence has also emerged that pyridoxamine drastically limits formation of equally deadly *advanced lipoxidation end products* (ALEs)—another catalyst for kidney disease.[74–76]

A convincing body of research on pyridoxamine therapy in *humans* with CKD has also emerged in recent years. In 2007, researchers set out to determine optimal interventions to halt the progression of kidney disease in diabetics.[77] They conducted two 24-week multicenter placebo-controlled trials in patients with known *diabetic nephropathy*—treatment of which is known to delay the onset of ESRD in diabetics. Doses of pyridoxamine ranged from 50–250 mg twice daily.

Pyridoxamine significantly inhibited the waste product creatinine, one of the key biomarkers of kidney dysfunction and a predictor of kidney failure. Urinary levels of inflammatory cytokines were also significantly lower in the treated group compared to controls.

In 2009, the FDA classified pyridoxamine as a drug, putting it out of reach for many Americans suffering from this deadly condition. No one should be forced to bear the *outrageous* burden of costly pharmaceuticals and their toxic side effects when a perfectly safe alternative exists.

Fortunately, an equally safe option exists; that is, another form of vitamin B6 known as *pyridoxal-5-phosphate* (P5P) that also exerts potent anti-AGE effects. P5P has been shown to prevent the progression of diabetic kidney disease in pre-clinical models.[78] In fact, as far back as 1988, it was used by a German research group to reduce blood lipids in humans with CKD.[79]

**Vitamin C.** Vitamin C is an antioxidant that helps keep many different types of tissues healthy. Vitamin C, which helps wounds and bruises heal faster, may aid in preventing infection.[69]

**Vitamin D.** Additional vitamin D, which promotes the absorption of calcium along with calcium supplements, may also be recommended. Some physicians prescribe vitamin D in a pill form called vitamin D3.[69]

**Vitamin E.** Supplementation with vitamin E may protect the kidneys from free-radical damage, a major factor in renal health. In experiments using rats, it was found that a dietary deficiency of vitamin E caused progressive and pronounced renal damage.[51] Vitamin E has been shown to restore tubular flow to rats with severe kidney disease by suppressing the free radicals that cause tubulointerstitial damage.[80]

**Calcium.** Calcium (along with vitamin D) helps keep bones healthy. Calcium is also used to bind to dietary phosphorus. Speak to a physician about taking calcium.[69]

**Phosphorus.** The proper amount of phosphorus is needed for healthy bones. As noted earlier, when kidneys do not work properly, blood levels of phosphorus can get too high, causing calcium to be taken from the bones. This results in the bones becoming weak. It is important to keep phosphorus and calcium balanced to maintain strong bones.[81]

**Potassium.** Another kidney function is to maintain the right amount of potassium. Potassium plays an essential role in keeping the heartbeat regular and other muscles working properly; however, high blood levels of potassium are to be avoided. In order to help control potassium levels, avoid foods high in potassium.[82]

**Iron.** Because red blood cells carry oxygen to all tissues and organs throughout the body, low levels of oxygen may result in reduced performance of vital organs (including the kidneys). Anemia (ie, a low level of red blood cells) is common in people who have kidney disease. Healthy kidneys produce a hormone called erythropoietin (EPO). EPO stimulates the bone marrow to produce red blood cells. However, diseased kidneys often do not make enough EPO; therefore, bone marrow makes fewer red blood cells. Other common causes of anemia include loss of blood during hemodialysis and low levels of iron and folic acid. Anemia often starts in the early stages of kidney disease and tends to worsen as the disease progresses. It has been shown that nearly everyone with end-stage kidney failure has anemia.[83]

A CBC (complete blood count) measures the hematocrit (Hct) (ie, percentage of blood consisting of red blood cells) and amount of hemoglobin (Hgb) in the blood. If at least half of normal kidney function (ie, serum creatinine >2 mg/dL) has been lost and Hct is low, the most likely cause of anemia is decreased EPO production. The National Kidney Foundation's Dialysis Outcomes Quality Initiative (DOQI) recommends that a detailed evaluation of anemia in men and postmenopausal women on dialysis should begin when Hct falls below 37%. For women of childbearing potential, evaluation should begin when Hct falls below 33%.

If no other cause for EPO deficiency is found, it can be treated with a genetically engineered form of the hormone (usually injected under the skin 2–3 times per week). Hemodialysis patients who cannot tolerate EPO injections in their skin can receive EPO intravenously during dialysis treatment. However, intravenous dosing requires a larger, more expensive dose that may not be as effective.

Because EPO alone will not relieve the effects of anemia if iron levels are too low, many people who require EPO treatment also need iron supplementation. Iron can be taken in a pill form; however, according to the NIDDK, iron pills often do not work as well in people with kidney failure as intravenous iron. Iron supplements should only be taken if prescribed by a physician based on blood results.[69]

In addition to EPO and iron, some people also need vitamin B12 and folic acid supplements. Supplementation with EPO, iron, and appropriate B vitamins help raise hemoglobin levels resulting in most kidney disease patients feeling better, having more energy, and living longer.[83]

**L-carnitine.** L-carnitine is an amino acid that has proven effective in providing cellular energy to both healthy individuals and those with chronic diseases. For patients in a predialysis stage, undergoing dialysis, or post-transplant, nutritional supplementation with L-carnitine lost during dialysis may reduce the side effects of common renal problems (eg, cardiomyopathy

and blood platelet aggregation) and may also help improve the patient's perception of overall quality of life.

General muscle weakness is a common complaint among patients undergoing hemodialysis. One study that measured serum L-carnitine found that hemodialysis lowered L-carnitine levels and posed new problems for patients.[84] This study measured muscle atrophy (via nerve conduction and velocity testing) and found indications of "neurogenic atrophy of the muscles." This well-known type of muscle weakness was further studied by doctors in Japan who reported that low dosages of L-carnitine (500 mg daily) showed improvement in 20 of 30 patients studied for 12 weeks. The patients reported less muscle weakness, general fatigue, cramps, and aches. This study concluded that low doses of L-carnitine could improve muscle weakness and should be considered as a prolonged adjuvant therapy for dialysis patients.[85]

ESRD affects every aspect of a patient's life. Therefore, improved quality of life is very important for dialysis patients, potentially affecting compliance with medical, nursing, and nutritional prescriptions. In one study, patients were given the Medical Outcomes Study Short Form to assess quality of life before taking L-carnitine and at 1.5-month intervals for the duration of the study.[86] This double-blind study was conducted on 101 patients who received L-carnitine or placebo just before and immediately after dialysis. After 3 months of supplementation (1 g of L-carnitine before and after every hemodialysis treatment), patients reported an "improved vitality and general health." It was noted that serum albumin concentration was directly correlated with the patients' feelings of well-being.

A study of L-carnitine therapy on erythropoiesis and blood platelet aggregation was conducted in patients with chronic renal failure. The 22-month study divided the patients into 3 groups (group 1 received erythropoietin alone, group 2 received erythropoietin and L-carnitine, and group 3 received L-carnitine alone). Iron concentration and platelet count measured in urea concentration were relatively unchanged. However, it was noted that L-carnitine therapy caused a "significant rise in collagen-induced platelet aggregation" after 2 months.[87]

**Coenzyme Q10.** Because of tremendous blood flow and high concentration of metabolic toxins continuously circulating through the kidneys, they are the site of extraordinary oxidative stress, which is known to contribute to progressive kidney damage and its complications (eg, high LDL and increased cardiovascular disease risk).[88]

CoQ10 *fortifies* the body's natural antioxidant capacity and reduces levels of oxygen free radicals, indicating its important defense against CKD. CoQ10 has been used experimentally to control hypertension and kidney disease in laboratory animals *since the early 1970s*.[89,90]

Human studies have shown that CoQ10 levels substantially decline, while markers of oxidation (eg, malondialdehyde) are dramatically *elevated* in kidney disease patients with even mild renal dysfunction.[91] Decreased CoQ10 levels also make circulating *lipoproteins* (eg, LDL) more vulnerable to oxidative damage, which in turn increases risk for further cardiovascular damage, adding to renal burden and substantially increasing risk of kidney disease.[92]

Kidney disease patients that undergo transplantation typically have marked disturbances in lipid profiles as a result of tremendous oxidative stress. The European group supplemented their patients with 30 mg of CoQ10 3 times daily for 4 weeks; then, they monitored levels of oxidation factors (such as *malondialdehyde*), natural antioxidant enzymes in the body, and lipid profiles.[93]

Significant improvements were seen after 4 weeks, with a reduction in LDL, increase in beneficial HDL, and decrease in the presence of inflammatory cells. These results suggest a potentially dramatic improvement in both quality of life and survival rates for patients whose disease has progressed to the point of kidney failure (ie, requiring transplantation or dialysis). They also bode well for those with early-stage kidney disease.

Animal studies have also shown that CoQ10 can protect kidney tissue from numerous nephrotoxic drugs, including *gentamicin*, a powerful antibiotic with a notorious propensity for causing kidney damage.[94,95]

**Silymarin.** Silymarin is extracted from milk thistle (*Silybum marianum*), a plant rich in the flavonolignans silychristin, silydianin, silybin A, silybin B, isosilybin A, and isosilybin B, which are collectively known as the *silymarin complex*.

This safe, natural compound has a long history as a traditional therapy for liver and kidney conditions.[96,97] It has been used in Western medicine for more than a quarter of a century as the treatment of choice for serious kidney injury resulting from severe mushroom poisoning, owing to its potent antioxidant and nephron-protective effects.[98] In fact, it was noted in 1979 that kidney injury by mushroom poisoning in animals pretreated with silymarin can be almost entirely prevented.[99] These effects make it a natural choice for protection against drug-induced kidney damage, since so many drugs can act like poisons, exerting extreme oxidant stress on kidney tissue.

Mushroom poisons (mycotoxins) are among the most deadly natural toxins known. Their kidney toxicity is surpassed only by some of the most aggressive chemotherapy agents. Physicians have therefore looked to silymarin as a potential "renoprotective" agent for patients undergoing chemotherapy.

Silymarin is also protective against several classes of nephrotoxic drugs, in particular *cisplatin and Adriamycin®*, two of the most potent chemotherapeutic drugs—but also two of the most damaging to the kidney owing to oxidative damage and severe inflammation.[91,100,101] Researchers around the world have found that silymarin and its components reduce and often entirely prevent kidney damage caused by these drugs.[102–105]

**Curcumin.** Curcumin is a potent antioxidant extract from the spice turmeric (*Curcuma longa*). It has a wide range of health benefits: antiviral, anti-inflammatory, anticancer, and cholesterol-lowering. A study in rats investigated the effect of curcumin on nephrosis caused by Adriamycin® (ie, a drug commonly used in chemotherapy).[106] Results indicated that curcumin "remarkably" prevented kidney injury caused by Adriamycin®. The researchers in this study stated that their data demonstrated that curcumin offered protection "by suppressing oxidative stress and increasing kidney glutathione content and glutathione peroxidase activity." They suggest that administration of curcumin offers promise in the treatment of nephrosis caused by Adriamycin®.

Another group studied the effect of curcumin on streptozotocin-induced diabetes. Streptozotocin is also a commonly used chemotherapy drug. Their data "suggested that dietary curcumin brought about significant beneficial modulation of the progression of renal lesion in diabetes." This benefit of dietary curcumin on diabetic nephropathy may be mediated by its ability to lower blood cholesterol levels.[107]

**Ginkgo biloba.** Already known for its antioxidant effects, ginkgo biloba may also protect small blood vessels against loss of tone, prevent capillary fragility, inhibit atherosclerosis, and treat diabetic vascular disease. Gentamicin-induced nephrotoxicity in rats was studied.[108] Gentamicin is an antibiotic used to treat serious infections. Unfortunately, it can cause kidney damage and irreversible hearing loss. This study found that gentamicin treatment increased levels of blood urea and serum creatinine. However, they also found that ginkgo biloba extract (GBE) protected the rats from gentamicin-induced nephrotoxicity by preventing changes in blood urea, serum creatinine, and creatinine clearance.

In another study, the effects of GBE on the development of hypertension, platelet activation, and renal dysfunction in deoxycorticosterone acetate-salt hypertensive rats were examined. After 20 days, the rats fed a 2% GBE diet had attenuated development of hypertension.[109]

In yet another study in rats, encouraging results of co-administration of cisplatin (ie, an effective anti-neoplastic [cancer killing] agent used for treating solid tumors) and GBE were reported.[110] However, cisplatin can also cause hearing loss and nephrotoxicity. This study concluded that co-administration of cisplatin with GBE was beneficial to ameliorate cisplatin-induced toxicity without attenuating the antitumor activity of cisplatin.

**Resveratrol.** The considerable advance in our understanding of the cyclical relationships between oxidative stress, endothelial dysfunction, inflammation, atherosclerosis, and CKD points to resveratrol as an intervention in the chain of events that ultimately lead to renal failure.[111]

Italian researchers are among the leaders in resveratrol research. One group published remarkable research demonstrating the impact of resveratrol on preserving kidney structure and function in rats exposed to *ischemia/reperfusion* injury.[112,113]

Japanese and Indian urologists followed that up in 2005 and 2006 with reports detailing the mechanisms by which resveratrol combats oxidative damage following reperfusion, markedly reducing kidney dysfunction.[114–118] Overwhelming bacterial infections (sepsis) are a common cause of kidney failure in the intensive care unit and following surgery or trauma. Turkish physiologists demonstrated that resveratrol can reduce or prevent both kidney and lung injury in septic rats.[119]

Resveratrol's unmatched antioxidant and anti-inflammatory potential has been tapped in studies of its ability to prevent drug-induced kidney damage as well. Nephrotoxicity in rats exposed to the antibiotic gentamicin was significantly reduced and more rapid healing of injured kidney tissue was attained using resveratrol, with dramatic reduction in markers of oxidant injury.[120] A team of toxicologists in Brazil demonstrated its kidney protective power against cisplatin, the powerful chemotherapy agent responsible for drug-induced kidney damage.[121] Finally, by pretreating the animals with resveratrol, Indian pharmacologists were successful in protecting animal kidneys from damage caused by cyclosporine A, another common chemotherapy and immune suppressant drug.[116]

Since diabetes is the leading cause of kidney disease—and because the damage it inflicts is largely mediated by free radical production resulting from destructive alteration of proteins by glucose (glycation)—researchers have explored resveratrol as a preventive in diabetic kidney damage. Indian pharmacologists have shown that they could significantly attenuate kidney damage in rats with experimentally induced diabetes, even 4 weeks after the diabetes was induced.[122]

**Lipoic acid.** Lipoic acid is a powerful antioxidant with few known side effects.[123] Lipoic acid has been successfully employed in the laboratory to block oxidative damage caused by ischemia/reperfusion injury, thereby opening the door to another effective treatment for this common cause of acute kidney failure.[124] In 2008, researchers showed that they could reverse all adverse effects on renal function and lab abnormalities following experimental ischemia/reperfusion injury in animals.[125]

Lipoic acid has been comprehensively studied worldwide for its power to prevent or mitigate drug-induced kidney damage. Lipoic acid is an effective kidney-protective agent against damage inflicted by Adriamycin®,[126,127] the immunosuppressive drug cyclosporine A,[123,128,129] and even acute toxic doses of the pain reliever acetaminophen. In studies of protection against cyclosporine toxicity, lipoic acid also helped normalize blood lipid abnormalities.[130]

Nephrologists at Georgetown University examined lipoic acid in the context of diabetic kidney disease. Their results showed it can improve renal function in diabetes by lowering sugar levels.[131]

They have also demonstrated that lipoic acid lowers proteinuria (ie, protein loss in urine) and improves kidney structure and function in diabetic laboratory animals by reducing oxidative stress.[131]

**Green tea.** The effects of green tea tannin to ameliorate cisplatin-induced renal injury in rats were studied.[132] They found that green tea tannin suppressed the cytotoxicity of cisplatin, "the suppressive effect increasing with the dose of green tea tannin." Additional testing showed rats given green tea tannin had decreased blood levels of urea nitrogen and creatinine and decreased urinary levels of protein and glucose, indicating less kidney damage. This study concluded that "based on the evidence available, it appeared that green tea tannin eliminated oxidative stress and was beneficial to renal function." Earlier, researchers reported that green tea tannin was found to be beneficial for the kidney under oxidative stress.[133,134] In 1991, it was found that green tea had antiviral activity, inhibiting rotaviruses and enteroviruses in rhesus monkeys.[135]

**Soy.** There is evidence that dietary phytoestrogens have a beneficial role in CKD.[136,137] Nutrition intervention studies demonstrated that consuming soy-based protein and flaxseed reduced proteinuria and attenuated renal functional or structural damage in both animals and humans. Study results are encouraging and further investigations are needed. Three groups of researchers investigated the effects of a soy protein diet on polycystic kidney disease.[138–140] Although the studies were conducted in rats and mice, research teams suggested that soy protein-based diets had beneficial effects in polycystic kidney disease: soy diet prevented significant elevation in serum creatinine in diseased versus normal animals[140]; soy protein was effective in retarding cyst development, and this beneficial effect may be unrelated to genistein (an isoflavonoid present in soy protein) content[138]; dietary protein level and source significantly affected polycystic kidney disease, with the effects being most pronounced in female animals fed low protein diets and soy protein-based diets.[139]

**Taurine.** Taurine, abundant in the brain, heart, gallbladder, and kidneys, plays an important role in health and disease in these organs. Taurine, an amino acid that has been shown to protect against experimentally induced lipid peroxidation of the renal glomerular and tubular cells, may alleviate tubular disorders such as glomerular impairment.[141] It is also thought to lower blood pressure by balancing the ratio of sodium to potassium in the blood. Taurine may also regulate increased nervous system activity that can contribute to high blood pressure. It has been noted that some people with type 1 diabetes appear to be deficient in taurine.[142]

**Trimethylglycine (betaine).** Trimethylglycine (TMG) plays a role in the manufacture of carnitine and serves to protect the kidneys from damage.[143] TMG has been reported to play a role in reducing blood levels of homocysteine, a toxic breakdown product of amino acid metabolism believed to promote atherosclerosis. The main nutrients involved in controlling homocysteine levels are folic acid, vitamins B6 and B12; TMG, however, has been reported to be helpful in some individuals whose elevated homocysteine levels did not improve with these other nutrients. TMG has also shown to be helpful in certain rare genetic disorders involving cysteine metabolism.[144–149] Its primary use as a nutritional supplement is in supporting proper liver function and possibly reducing the risk of urinary tract infections.

## SUMMARY

Kidneys are remarkably resilient organs that with prompt medical attention can sometimes recover normal function from acute trauma as a result of injury, drug overdose, or poisoning. However, there are forms of kidney disease that include conditions that can either *rapidly or slowly* reduce kidney function over several years, producing few or no symptoms. Damage from these conditions is not reversible. When kidney function is reduced to less than 10–15%, dialysis is required. When dialysis can no longer support kidney function, kidney transplantation is required.

If you have healthy kidneys, protect them. Eat a healthy diet, drink a lot of water, pay careful attention to use of OTC medication(s) (particularly when combined with prescription medication or other OTC products), consume alcohol responsibly (OTC or prescription drugs can be very damaging to the kidneys when combined with alcohol), protect kidneys from sports-related injury, and consider taking protective supplements and nutrients to support overall kidney health.

As part of an annual physical, request creatinine and BUN be checked, along with urine protein levels. Small elevations of creatinine can be an early sign of kidney disease. Early detection leads to early treatment, which can occur at a stage when treatment may help prevent kidney disease from advancing to a more serious stage.

Because diabetes is the leading cause of CKD, followed by hypertension, see your physician regularly and follow prescribed dietary and drug treatment to control blood sugar and blood pressure levels.[59] Refer to Life Extension's Diabetes and High Blood Pressure protocols for additional information.

Prevent kidney stones by increasing water intake to 12 full glasses daily, limiting caffeine (eg, coffee, tea, and colas) because it increases fluid loss, increasing dietary calcium, and including appropriate calcium/magnesium supplementation (taken only with food).

Research into gene therapy holds great hope for genetic kidney diseases. Of particular interest is research on the PKD1 gene, which is responsible for 85% or more of all ADPKD cases. ADKPD, often progressing to kidney failure in young adulthood or middle age, results in kidney transplantation for many individuals.

If you have early stage or CKD, follow the dietary recommendations of your physician or renal dietitian. For example, a diet low in sodium, potassium, and phosphorus, 3 substances regulated by the kidneys, is essential in managing kidney disease. Other dietary restrictions (eg, reducing protein) may be required depending on the cause of kidney failure and type of treatment being used (eg, dialysis). Patients with chronic kidney failure may also need to limit their fluid intake.

## Life Extension Suggestions

Follow your physician's recommendations concerning the addition of daily dietary supplements. Multivitamins, minerals, and other supplements may be prescribed or recommended to help replace essential nutrients lost during dialysis treatments. Consult medical professionals experienced in treating kidney disorders and follow their treatment recommendations carefully. Establish appropriate dietary habits. The following supplements are supportive of overall kidney health. The recommendations are for healthy individuals. If you have any form of kidney disease, consult your physician before adding or changing any supplements you may currently be taking.

- **Complete multivitamin:** per label instructions
- **B-complex vitamin:** per label instructions
- **Pyridoxal 5'-phosphate (P5P):** 100 mg daily
- **Vitamin C:** 1000–2000 mg daily
- **Vitamin D:** 5000–8000 IU daily (depending on blood test results; optimal levels are between 50 and 80 ng/mL)
- **Vitamin E:** 400 IU alpha-tocopherol and 200 mg gamma-tocopherol daily
- **Calcium:** 200–1200 mg daily
- **Iron:** 300 mg of iron protein succinate, equivalent to 15 mg of elemental iron per capsule daily
- **L-carnitine:** 500–2000 mg daily
- **CoQ10,** as ubiquinol: 100–200 mg daily
- **Silymarin:** 100–600 mg daily
- **Curcumin,** as highly absorbed BCM-95®: 400–800 mg daily
- **Ginkgo biloba,** standardized extract: 120 mg daily
- **Resveratrol:** 100–250 mg daily
- **R-lipoic acid:** 300–600 mg daily
- **Green tea,** standardized extract: 725 mg daily
- **Soy extract,** containing up to 60 mg of isoflavones: twice daily
- **Taurine:** 2–3 g daily
- **TMG (trimethylglycine):** 500–2500 mg daily
- **Omega-3 fish oil:** 1400 mg EPA and 1000 mg DHA daily
- **Dehydroepiandrosterone (DHEA):** 25–50 mg daily (based on blood test results)
- **Nettle:** 120–240 mg daily

- **N-acetyl cysteine (NAC):** 600–1800 mg daily
- **Vitamin K:** 2100 mcg of vitamin K as 1000 mcg K1 and 1100 mcg K2 (as MK-4 and MK-7)
- **Magnesium:** 200 mg–1000 mg daily

In addition, the following *blood tests* may provide helpful information.

- C-peptide
- Chemistry panel and complete blood count (CBC)
- Cystatin-C
- Homocysteine
- Cytokine panel
- C-reactive protein

### Overlooked Prescription Drug

Kidneys are especially vulnerable to attack by proinflammatory cytokines. *Pentoxifylline* (PTX) is a drug that has been shown to protect against this type of kidney damage. The suggested dose of PTX is 400 mg twice daily.

PTX should not be used in patients with bleeding disorders such as those with recent cerebral or retinal hemorrhage. Patients taking Coumadin® should have more frequently monitored prothrombin time. Those suffering from other types of bleeding should receive frequent physician examinations. Furthermore, consider having a physician evaluate coagulation status to see what effect PTX has on template bleeding time. This is an inexpensive test that relates to the biological effect of PTX or other agents like aspirin (nonsteroidal anti-inflammatory agents) on platelet function. All of these agents affect platelet aggregation and this effect can be manifested in a prolonged template bleeding time. According to 2 studies, PTX should be avoided by Parkinson's patients. It is important to note that the body uses TNF-α to acutely fight infection(s). If patients are showing any sign of infectious disease, drugs like Enbrel® that inhibit the effects of TNF-α are temporarily discontinued. A FDA advisory states that patients should be tested and treated for inactive, or latent tuberculosis prior to therapy with another TNF-α inhibiting therapy (eg, infliximab). Since PTX, fish oil, and nettle directly suppress TNF-α, perhaps these agents should be temporarily discontinued during the time when one has an active infection.

For more information, contact the National Kidney Foundation, (800) 622-9010 or http://www.

kidney.org; the American Foundation for Urologic Disease, (800) 828-7866 or www.access.digex. net/~afud; and the National Kidney and Urologic Diseases Information Clearinghouse, (301) 654-4415 or e-mail nkudic@info.niddk.nih.gov; (website) www.niddk.nih.gov.

## REFERENCES

References available at: www.lef.org/dpt5/ch84

# 85

# *Leukemia*

Leukemia refers to cancers that begin in the blood-forming cells of the body. These abnormal cells grow and multiply in an uncontrolled way. As the disease progresses, leukemic cells move through the bloodstream and invade other organs, such as the spleen, lymph nodes, liver, and central nervous system. In the United States, more than 30 000 new cases of leukemia are diagnosed every year, and adult onset accounts for 90% of the new cases.[1]

Risk factors for leukemia include advanced age, poor nutrition, previous chemotherapy and radiation treatment for other cancers, and smoking. Medical treatment for leukemia primarily revolves around chemotherapy and radiation therapy. Nutritional supplements help support the healthy function of the immune system, and in particular, the white blood cells in leukemia patients. In addition, some nutritional supplements are able to kill leukemia cells. Key examples include vitamin A, genistein from soy extract, and curcumin from turmeric.

## TYPES OF LEUKEMIA

Leukemia can be classified into 4 major types based on whether the disease is acute or chronic and according to the type of white blood cell affected:

- Acute myelogenous leukemia (AML)
- Chronic myelogenous leukemia (CML)
- Acute lymphocytic leukemia (ALL)
- Chronic lymphocytic leukemia (CLL)

Myelogenous leukemia involves myeloid cells, granulocytes (neutrophils, basophils, and eosinophils), and monocytes (macrophages). Lymphocytic leukemia involves T and B cells (lymphocytes).

## LEUKEMIA CASES IN THE UNITED STATES

In the United States, leukemia occurs more frequently in males than females.[2–4] In addition, Caucasians are more likely to develop leukemia than African Americans and Hispanics.[1,5]

Table 1

| Type of Leukemia | Number of New Cases/Year | Average Age at Diagnosis (years) |
|---|---|---|
| AML | 10 000 | 65 |
| CLL | 7800 | >50 |
| CML | 4500 | 67 |
| ALL | 4000 | <10 |

With the exception of ALL, leukemia is generally associated with aging. Furthermore, the behavior of leukemia in older individuals differs from that seen in younger people. For example, AML occurring in older individuals is more resistant to chemotherapy than AML in younger patients.[6]

## HOW DOES LEUKEMIA DEVELOP?

All cancers begin with damage to the cells' deoxyribonucleic acid (DNA). Within a cell, DNA is found in structures called chromosomes, which are themselves made up of segments called genes. Leukemia begins with DNA damage in the white blood cells, which protect the body from infections. In leukemia, DNA damage can occur through chromosome translocations (shifting and rearrangement of chromosome segments) or mutations. Any one type of leukemia can have several genetic abnormalities at its core—this further complicates the interaction with other healthy genes, as well as the individual's nutritional status in the development of leukemia.[7,8]

## RISK FACTORS

Inherited, abnormal genes account for a small proportion of leukemia cases.[9–11] However, in most cases, the DNA damage that eventually results in the onset of leukemia is brought about by interactions between genes, age, and a variety of environmental or lifestyle factors such as nutrition and exposure to chemicals.[7,8]

### Age

Since up to 70% of leukemia cases are in those over 50, age can be considered the biggest risk factor for developing leukemia.[12,13] The chromosomes of white blood cells in older people are more fragile than those in young adults and are more vulnerable to the types of DNA damage (eg, free radical damage) known to cause leukemia.[14,15]

A diet rich in fruits and vegetables and other antioxidants can help guard against DNA damage caused by free radicals.[16] However, the ability of the elderly to repair DNA damage is poor and is associated with suboptimal micronutrient status.[12,17] The metabolism of elderly people is altered in such a way that while they continue to efficiently absorb macronutrients such as fats and proteins, absorption of micronutrients such as vitamins B12 and D are compromised, leading to malnutrition.[13] Suboptimal levels of micronutrients can cause DNA damage associated with leukemia and limit the ability to repair this damage.[17,18]

## Nutrition

Diets lacking in essential micronutrients are as detrimental as cigarette smoking in the cause of cancer and can cause the same kind of DNA damage as exposure to radiation.[17] Deficiencies is several micronutrients, including folic acid and vitamins B12 and B6 may contribute to leukemia.[18]

Folic acid deficiency causes chromosome breaks,[12] and is a risk factor in the development of ALL. In folic acid deficiency, efforts to repair damaged DNA are compromised and lead to breakages in genes (chromosome breaks).[18–20] Deficiencies in vitamins B12 and B6 are thought to act in the same way as folic acid deficiency in increasing the risk for both adult and childhood ALL.[18]

There is a possible relationship between the restricted nutrient intake of slimming diets and the development of acute leukemia.[21] Another theory is that phenol and hydroquinone (chemicals mainly ingested from meat and protein-rich diets, known to produce DNA damage) and antibiotics may cause leukemia.[22]

## Chemotherapy

Chemotherapy, used for the treatment of other cancers, can cause DNA damage and increase the risk of developing some form of leukemia. For example, chemotherapy for the treatment of other cancers is the major recognized cause of AML in the young, referred to by clinicians as secondary or treatment-related AML.[23] Treatment-related AML is associated with therapy for breast cancer, ovarian cancer, Hodgkin's disease and non-Hodgkin's lymphoma, and accounts for up to 20% of AML cases.[24,25] Treatment with epipodophyllotoxins (etoposide and teniposide) is associated with the development of secondary AML.[26,27] Cyclosporine A, used to treat suppressed red blood cell production, is associated with the development of secondary leukemia.[28]

## Radiation

Exposure to high doses of radiation causes leukemia by inducing DNA damage through translocations.[29] Population studies show a link between radiation exposure from nuclear testing between 1951 and 1962 in the

United States and the onset of leukemia.[30,31] The incidence of leukemia was high in the United States in the years during and immediately after the nuclear testing. Utah showed high increases (up to 5 times the norm) in leukemia rates, which persisted as late as the 1980s.[30,31] Exposure to radiation is linked to acute and myeloid leukemia in children.[30] The association between radiation exposure and leukemia was noted in survivors of the atomic bomb in Japan[32] and in people who lived near nuclear reactors in the Chernobyl disaster of 1986.[33] Leukemia caused by radiation typically appears 10 years after exposure.[34]

## Chemicals

Long-term or occupational exposure to benzene is a cause of acute leukemia.[35,36] Long-term exposure to herbicides, pesticides, and other agricultural chemicals is linked to an increased risk of developing leukemia.[37] Hair dyes contain chemicals that cause cancer and are associated with leukemia,[38] particularly the long-term use of permanent dyes.[39]

## Smoking

Cigarette smoke contains leukemia-causing chemicals like benzene.[40] Although smoking in the young is associated with modest increases in the risk of developing leukemia, in those over 60, smoking is associated with a 2-fold increase in risk for AML and a 3-fold increase in risk for ALL.[41]

## Genetics

Children with Down's syndrome have a 10–20 times higher risk of developing leukemia than the general population.[11] This risk is not confined to childhood years and extends through adulthood. There are also inherited disorders (eg, Fanconi's anemia and Bloom's syndrome) characterized by genetic instability and inability to repair DNA damage that are associated with an increased risk of leukemia.[9,10]

## Viruses

Acute T-cell leukemia is associated with infection by the human T-cell leukemia virus (HTLV); human lymphotrophic virus-1 causes leukemia in humans. In infected individuals, HTLV proteins attach themselves to proteins in the lymphocytes responsible for regulating cell growth and corrupt their functions, resulting in the uncontrolled cell growth of leukemia.[42] This type of leukemia is rare in the United States; it is generally found in Asia and parts of the Caribbean.

# DIAGNOSIS

Symptoms associated with leukemia include weakness, fatigue, unexplained weight loss, pain, (abdominal, bone, and joint), abnormal bleeding, infection, fever, excessive bruising, and enlarged spleen, lymph nodes, and liver.

The first step in diagnosing leukemia is a complete blood count (CBC). With a diagnosis of leukemia, further testing of cell samples obtained by bone marrow aspiration or lumbar puncture determines the specific type of leukemia. Specific treatment is then targeted for leukemia based on a number of factors, including results of genetic tests and leukemic cell sub-type.

## WHAT YOU HAVE LEARNED SO FAR

- Leukemia is a collective name for cancers of the white blood cells that grow, multiply, and change uncontrollably.
- Leukemia occurs through damage to the genes, such as chromosome translocations or mutations.
- Leukemia can be chronic or acute and occur in myeloid or lymphocytic white blood cells.
- Risk factors for leukemia include environmental or lifestyle factors such as nutrition, smoking, exposure to chemicals, viruses, radiation, and previous chemotherapy or radiotherapy treatment for other cancers.
- Diagnosis is made from results of blood and bone marrow tests.
- Leukemia is more prevalent in the aged who have altered metabolism causing micronutrient deficiencies and reduced bone marrow function.[43]
- Vitamin D3, curcumin, green tea, and soy extracts help support healthy cell growth, function, and maturation in patients with leukemia.

# CONVENTIONAL MEDICAL THERAPY

## Chemotherapy and Radiotherapy

Chemotherapy agents attack rapidly dividing cells; however, they do not distinguish leukemia cells from other rapidly dividing but noncancerous cells. As a result, chemotherapy harms healthy red and white blood cells, blood-clotting platelets, hair follicles, and cells lining the gastrointestinal tract, thus creating unpleasant side effects.

The damage to white blood cells increases the risk of infection. Medications known as colony-stimulating factors (CSFs) increase white blood cell counts and are often given in combination with chemotherapy.[44,45] The use of CSFs in leukemia is discussed in the Immunomodulators and Immune Enhancers section.

Successful treatment with chemotherapy and severity of associated side effects in leukemia may be positively influenced by nutritional status. Antioxidant levels are reduced in leukemia patients undergoing chemotherapy.[46] Low levels of antioxidant intake are associated with increases in adverse effects of chemotherapy in children with ALL.[46] Vitamins C, E, and beta-carotene are associated with reduced toxicity from chemotherapy and lower frequencies of infections.[46,47] A discussion on chemotherapy, nutritional support, and natural strategies to counteract the associated side effects can be found in the Chemotherapy protocol.

Radiotherapy kills leukemia cells by exposing them to ionizing radiation that damages cell DNA. In clinical practice, radiotherapy is typically used in 4% of leukemia cases.[48] This is partly due to chemotherapy alternatives.[49] Irradiation of the spleen is sometimes used in the treatment of leukemia patients with enlarged spleens.[49,50]

## Interferon Therapy

Interferons (IFNs) are a group of naturally occurring substances sometimes used in the treatment of chronic leukemia.[51,52] IFN reduces the growth and reproduction of leukemia cells and enhances the immune system's response to cancer (see Immunomodulators and Immune Enhancers section). IFN is particularly useful when used as a maintenance therapy in patients after partial or complete remission. Use of IFN in combination with all-trans retinoic acid (a synthetic vitamin A analog) may prolong the lives of patients with promyelocytic and other forms of leukemia.[53,54]

## Stem Cell Therapy

As the chemotherapy required to kill leukemia cells also damages the rapidly dividing blood-forming cells, stem-cell therapy replenishes bone marrow. Stem cell therapy is the transplantation of stem cells into the patient's bone marrow following chemotherapy and/or radiation therapy to kill the leukemia cells.[55-57] Stem cells may be obtained from the patient (autologous) or from a donor (allogeneic) who is a close tissue match to the patient.[55-57] Autologous stem-cell therapy is rare due to the challenge of ensuring that the removed stem cells are not contaminated with leukemia cells. Stem cells can be obtained either by bone marrow aspiration or by a procedure called apheresis (also called peripheral blood stem-cell [PBSC] transplant), through which the cells are removed from the peripheral blood system. This type of therapy is still in the experimental stages.

## Inhibiting Cell-Signaling Pathways

Early in disease progression, many types of leukemia produce certain inflammatory and immunosuppressive cytokines (chemical messengers) and use cell-signaling pathways.

For example:

- Vascular endothelial growth factor (VEGF) is considered essential for leukemia cell growth, survival, and spread.[58] Expression of high VEGF levels is associated with shortened survival in CLL patients.[59]

- Basic fibroblast growth factor (bFGF) is a potent mitogen (growth signal) and is essential for blood vessel growth and spread of cancer cells.[60]

- Hepatocyte growth factor (HGF) stimulates the growth and spread of leukemia cells.[61] HGF is particularly overexpressed in AML, CML, CLL, and chronic myelomonocytic leukemia.[61]

- Tumor necrosis factor-alpha (TNF-α) is a proinflammatory cytokine significantly elevated in all leukemias except for AML and myelodysplastic syndromes.[61]

- Interleukin-6 (IL-6) is a proinflammatory and immunosuppressive cytokine. Elevated serum IL-6 is associated with a poor prognosis and shortened survival in CLL.[62]

Types of leukemia that overexpress these cytokines are in the following table.[58,60–62]

| Disease | Cytokines Overexpressed |
| --- | --- |
| Chronic myeloid leukemia | VEGF, bFGF, HGF, TNF-α, IL-6 |
| Acute myeloid leukemia | VEGF, bFGF, HGF |
| Chronic myelomonocytic leukemia | VEGF, bFGF, HGF, TNF-α |
| Acute lymphoblastic leukemia | bFGF, HGF, TNF-α |
| Chronic lymphocytic leukemia | VEGF, bFGF, HGF, TNF-α, IL-6 |
| Myelodysplastic syndromes | VEGF, bFGF, HGF |

## Regulating Normal Cell Growth

The drug Gleevec® (formerly STI571) slows proliferation and causes apoptosis in Bcr-Abl cell lines and fresh leukemic cells from "Philadelphia chromosome positive" (Ph+) CML. Gleevec® (imatinib mesylate) is indicated for the treatment of patients with Ph+ CML in blast crisis, accelerated phase, or chronic phase after failure of IFN-alpha therapy. Although Gleevec® is approved by the Food and Drug Administration (FDA), its effectiveness is continuously evaluated. The latest findings can be found on the website

www.gleevec.com. It is interesting that a drug that functions through a mechanism similar to certain dietary supplements (eg, curcumin and genistein) was put on the FDA's "fast track" for approval.

## Immunomodulators and Immune Enhancers

Substances that enhance the function of the immune system are used to support the conventional treatment of leukemia with chemotherapy and radiotherapy. These substances fall into 3 main categories:

- Hematopoietic growth factors
- Cytokines (glycoprotein messengers)
- Immunotoxins

The use of growth factors such as granulocyte-colony stimulating factor (G-CSF) during chemotherapy elevates the number of normal white blood cells, thus enabling patients to tolerate high chemotherapeutic doses and reducing infections.[44,45] G-CSF (filgrastim, Neupogen®) treats low neutrophil counts (neutropenia) during CML therapy.[63] Another growth factor, granulocyte macrophage-colony stimulating factor or GM-CSF (sargramostim, Leukine®), blocks the migration of myeloid cells and leukemia spread.[64]

Cytokines are glycoprotein messengers that enhance the function of immune cells. The use of IFN in the treatment of chronic leukemia is common.[51,52] The use of the cytokine IL-2 in AML and CML patients reportedly improves immune responses.[65]

Antibodies specifically targeted to molecules present on the surface of AML cells exhibit antileukemic responses in clinical studies.[66–68] The binding of an antibody to a leukemia cell marks the cell as a target for destruction. Antibodies can be attached to cytotoxic agents that can be selectively delivered to leukemia cells.[67,68] Antibody therapy is beneficial in treating CLL[69] and hairy cell leukemia.[70]

Cancer vaccines present an opportunity to manipulate the immune system into attacking leukemia cells.[71] Research on this therapeutic option is still in the experimental stage and has focused on solid tumors.

### DRUGS TO REDUCE THE SIDE EFFECTS OF CHEMOTHERAPY

**Neulasta® and GM-CSF.** The frequency and duration of low white blood cell counts (low neutrophil counts) that is caused by chemotherapy can be reduced by the use of medications such as Neulasta® (G-CSF, also known as pegfilgrastim) and GM-CSF.[63,72–74] In clinical trials, Neulasta® reduced the frequency of infections, hospitalizations, and enabled continuing use of chemotherapy doses that normally would be reduced as a result of chemotherapy-associated neutropenia.[75]

**Procrit® and Epogen®.** Anemia (low red blood cells) associated with both leukemia and chemotherapy can be treated using Procrit® and Epogen® (epoetin alfa, also known as recombinant human erythropoietin).[76,77] In clinical assessments, epoetin alpha improved anemia in 77% of CLL patients.[76]

# HORMONES AND METABOLISM

The development of acute leukemia is accompanied by abnormalities in levels of cholesterol and some lipids.[78–80] In particular, AML and ALL patients have low levels of high-density-lipoprotein (HDL) cholesterol.[78–80] Upon treatment, cholesterol levels return to normal in patients that respond to treatment, suggesting that cholesterol could be used as a marker to monitor chemotherapy.[78–80] Research using specific types of leukemia cells (HL-60 cells) and showing that cholesterol is required for cells to progress through cell division[81] may explain the link between low cholesterol levels and acute leukemia that is characterized by the failure of cells to reach maturity.

Levels of the anti-inflammatory hormone cortisol are elevated in AML, CML,[82,83] and CLL[84] patients. These high levels of cortisol, a powerful immunosuppressive agent, are associated with impaired immune cell responses[82,84] and may be partially responsible for the immune dysfunction seen in these patients.

## DHEA

The hormone dehydroepiandrosterone (DHEA) has been shown to favorably alter inflammatory cytokines such as interleukin-2 (IL-2) in leukemic mice.[85] DHEA favorably modulated the immune dysfunction that occurred during leukemia retrovirus infection in old mice[86] and prevented leukemia growth.[87]

DHEA might be effective in supporting healthy immune function in leukemia patients with a DHEA deficiency, which can be determined by a blood test.[88] DHEA is contraindicated in both men and women with certain hormone-related cancers.

# NUTRITIONAL THERAPY

## Apigenin

A flavone (ie, a class of flavonoids) that is present in fruits and vegetables (eg, onions, oranges, tea, celery, artichoke, and parsley), has been shown to possess anti-inflammatory, antioxidant, and anticancer properties. Many studies have confirmed the cancer chemopreventive effects of apigenin.[89]

Apigenin has shown to induce apoptosis in leukemia cells.[90,91] In addition, apigenin inhibited the growth of human leukemia cells and induced these cells to differentiate (they became healthy mature cells).[92,93] Topoisomerases are enzymes involved in many aspects of leukemic cell DNA metabolism (eg, replication). In one study, apigenin was shown to inhibit topoisomerase-catalyzed DNA irregularities.[94]

## Astragalus

Astragalus, an herb used for centuries in Asia, has exhibited immune-stimulatory effects. Astragalus potentiates lymphokine-activated killer cells.[95] One study found that astragalus could partially restore depressed immune function in tumor-bearing mice,[96] while another concluded that "astragalus could exhibit anti-tumor effects, which might be achieved through activating the … anti-tumor immune mechanism of the host."[97]

Astragalus has also shown to be beneficial against leukemia. It was observed in a clinical trial that astragalus induced apoptosis in a chronic myeloid leukemia cell line.[98]

## Coffee

Coffee, especially brews enriched with chlorogenic acid, protect cells against the DNA damage that leads to aging and cancer development.[99–101] Growing tumors develop the ability to invade local and regional tissue by increasing their production of "protein-melting" enzymes called matrix metalloproteinases. Chlorogenic acid—present in coffee—strongly inhibited matrix metalloproteinase activity.[102,103] In addition, chlorogenic acid induced apoptosis in CML cells.[104]

## Vitamins D3, E, K2, and B12

Vitamin D3 and its analogs may help certain leukemia cells (AML) to become, or differentiate into, normal cells.[105] However, a monthly complete blood count (CBC) to monitor serum calcium, and kidney and liver function, is necessary to prevent vitamin D3 toxicity.

Vitamin E levels are lower in CML patients compared to healthy individuals.[106] Vitamin E (as the succinate salt), in combination with vitamin D3, promotes cell maturation in HL-60 leukemia cells.[107]

Vitamin K2 analogs help normalize leukemia cells.[108] Vitamin K2 supplementation taken alone or with all-trans retinoic acid (ATRA) therapy may benefit myelogenous leukemia.[109]

Deficiency of vitamin B12 causes chromosome breaks and is a risk factor for ALL.[18,19] Vitamin B12 supplementation is thought to reduce chromosome damage that leads to ALL.[18]

## Soy Extract

Soy extracts contain high levels of genistein, an inhibitor of protein tyrosine kinase, an enzyme that becomes dysfunctional in cancer cells. Protein tyrosine kinase activity is reduced by genistein, subsequently impeding the growth of cancer cells.[110,111]

Studies have shown that genistein increased the potency of the chemotherapeutic agent bleomycin against the leukemia cell line HL-60 and reduced the damage this agent normally causes to normal lymphocytes, thus it may reduce normal tissue toxicity associated with chemotherapy.[112]

The benefits of soy extract may be more significant in leukemia cases with a mutant p53 gene, making the leukemia cells more sensitive to chemotherapy. For example, genistein derived from soy extracts has been shown to increase expression of the gene that helps suppress cancer cell growth (ie, normal p53 tumor suppressor gene) in solid tumors that acts to protect the body from cancer development.[113]

The presence of mutant p53 genes is determined by a pathologist's examination of leukemia cells. Consult your physician to determine if the pathologist performing an immunohistochemistry test for mutant or functional p53 discovered mutant p53; alternatively ask your physician to perform this test via Genzyme Genetics (formerly IMPATH Laboratories; www.genzymegenetics.com).

## Curcumin

An extract of the spice turmeric, curcumin acts in combination with the soy isoflavone genistein to reduce the number of leukemia-promoting properties, such as growth signals and pro-inflammatory cytokines that are over-produced in leukemia.[114]

Curcumin has been shown to:

- Inhibit production of bFGF, a potent growth signal for cancer cells that is known to be overproduced in AML, CML, and ALL.[114]

- Increase expression of the cancer-protective p53 gene in leukemia cell lines, thus making them more susceptible to cell death.[115]

- Reduce the production of the inflammatory cytokine TNF-α, which is overproduced in CML and ALL.[116]

## Green and Black Tea

Epigallocatechin gallate (EGCG) in green tea blocks the production of VEGF, considered essential for leukemia growth and spread.[117] EGCG may be particularly useful in CLL, a leukemia type that relies heavily on VEGF for its survival. EGCG significantly increased the rate of cell death in 8 out of 10 CLL samples.[117] Green tea blocks the proliferation of lymphocytes from adult T-cell leukemia patients.[118] Theaflavins found in black tea have also been shown to be as potent as EGCG from green tea in blocking proliferation of leukemia cell lines.[119]

## Essential Fatty Acids (EPA, DHA, and GLA)

Several leukemias are associated with abnormally high levels of the inflammatory cytokines TNF-α and IL-6.[61,62] Docosahexaenoic acid (DHA) and gamma-linolenic acid (GLA) are essential fatty acids that suppress these dangerous inflammatory cytokines.[120,121] The use of GLA and DHA have been shown to improve the response of leukemia to chemotherapy.[122] GLA and eicosapentaenoic acid (EPA) have been shown to cause death in HL-60 leukemia cells.[123] Furthermore, a phase 1/2 clinical study in humans with solid cancer also showed that DHA may improve responses to paclitaxel and carboplatin chemotherapy.[124]

Essential fatty acids DHA and EPA are derived from fish, primrose, and borage oils.

## Antioxidants (Lipoic Acid and L-Ascorbic Acid)

Lipoic acid is a powerful antioxidant with antiaging effects.[125,126] Exposure of the Jurkat leukemia cell line to lipoic acid increased cell death (apoptosis) of the cancer cells but did not affect lymphocytes from normal healthy individuals.[127] Lipoic acid activates the enzyme caspase that drives a particular type of apoptotic cell death.[127] Lipoic acid helps crippled, damaged immune cells (such as those of cancer patients) to function more normally.[128]

Research shows that lipoic acid, used in combination with vitamin D3, helps support normal (versus cancerous) growth and maturation of leukemia cells.[107]

Laboratory tests show L-ascorbic acid inhibits proliferation of HL-60 leukemia cells and supports their normal (versus cancerous) growth and maturation.[129] In fact, L-ascorbic acid is being assessed for the treatment of AML because laboratory tests showed that it blocked growth of 3 AML cell lines and fresh leukemic cells from 3 AML patients.[46,130]

Whether use of antioxidants antagonizes or supports chemotherapy agents may depend on the type of leukemia, drug used, and dose of antioxidant. People undergoing chemotherapy should discuss the use of antioxidants with an oncologist and refer to the Chemotherapy protocol.

## NUTRITIONAL SUPPLEMENTATION FOR SPECIFIC FORMS OF LEUKEMIA

**Promyelocytic leukemia.** The use of retinoic acid (derived from vitamin A) and its synthetic derivatives, often in combination with vitamin D3, is well established in promyelocytic leukemia. This strategy takes into account the underlying genetic problems in this type of leukemia.[131,132]

**Chronic myeloid leukemia.** Several dietary supplements share similarities with Gleevec®,[133,134] the FDA-approved drug for CML. These include curcumin,[135] genistein from soy extracts,[110] catechin from green tea, and alkylglycerols from shark liver oil,[117,136] all of which inhibit the activity of protein tyrosine kinase, an enzyme that is abnormal in CML cells. In addition, curcumin inhibits the production of growth factors and chemical messengers that are abnormal in CML, therefore reducing the leukemic cell's ability to multiply and grow.[114,116] Ajoene, a garlic extract, has been shown in some studies to have activity against CML cells.[137]

**Acute myeloid leukemia.** Some studies have suggested that curcumin and genistein can block growth of AML cells by interfering with growth factors that are overproduced in AML cells.[114,138,139] L-ascorbic acid is being clinically tested for AML after encouraging laboratory tests.[130] Studies have shown that resveratrol and ajoene are capable of killing AML cells.[137,140–142] Moreover, ajoene has been shown to kill chemotherapy resistant AML cells that present particular difficulties in the older patients.[143]

**Acute lymphocytic leukemia.** Curcumin and genistein have been shown to possess the ability to block inflammatory substances, such as TNF-α, that are observed in high levels in ALL.[114,116,138,139]

**Chronic lymphocytic leukemia.** EGCG from green tea, curcumin from turmeric, and genistein from soy extracts have all been shown to block the production of growth factors, such as VEGF,[110,114,117] typically seen in high levels in CLL.[59] Essential fatty acids have been shown to suppress other inflammatory factors, such as IL-6 and TNF-α, seen in high levels in CLL.[120,121]

## Panax Ginseng

Panax ginseng, also known as Korean ginseng, has been used in China for thousands of years as a popular remedy for various diseases including cancer.[144] Researchers observed that panax ginseng extract suppressed growth in human promyelocytic leukemia cells by inducing apoptosis.[145,146] Also, the ability of vitamin D to induce differentiation (ie, the process by which cancer cells transform into cells that appear to be normal to a greater degree, and therefore less aggressive) of leukemic cells was enhanced by panax ginseng.[147]

## Polysaccharide-K

Polysaccharide-K (PSK), which is a specially prepared polysaccharide extract from the mushroom *Coriolus versicolor*, has been studied extensively in Japan where it is used as a nonspecific biological response modifier to enhance the immune system in cancer patients.[148–150] PSK suppresses tumor cell invasiveness by downregulating several invasion-related factors.[151] PSK has been shown to enhance natural killer (NK) cell activity in multiple studies.[152–155]

The Coriolus mushroom has demonstrated antileukemic effects. In one study, Coriolus suppressed the proliferation of leukemic cells by greater than 90%.[156] Other studies have confirmed these findings with the mechanism of action mediated via apoptosis.[157,158]

## Reishi

The active constituents of reishi mushroom include polysaccharides, a unique protein named LZ-8, and triterpenes.[159–161] Among its broad-spectrum immune-boosting effects are the following:

- Reishi promotes specialization of dendritic cells and macrophages, which are essential in allowing the body to react to new threats, vaccines, and cancer cells.[162–166]

- Reishi's effects on dendritic cells have been proven to boost the response to tetanus vaccine; the mushroom's proteins are also under investigation as "adjuvants" to emerging cancer DNA vaccines and other immune-based cancer treatments.[163,167–169]

- Reishi polysaccharide triggers growth and development of bone marrow, where most immune cells are born; following bone marrow eradication by chemotherapy, reishi increased production of both red and white blood cells.[170] Reishi polysaccharides provide immune-boosting function to various types of circulating cancer-killing white blood cells.[160]

- Reishi increases numbers and functions of virtually all cell lines in the immune system, such as NK cells, antibody-producing B cells, and the T cells responsible for rapid response to a new or "remembered" antigen.[164,171,172]

Laboratory and animal studies confirm that reishi stimulates an appropriate anticancer immune response while quashing a cancer-promoting inflammatory one. A few small human studies have demonstrated reishi's ability to enhance immune function in patients with advanced cancers.[173–175]

Reishi extracts have also proven useful in inducing cell death in various "white blood cell cancers" such as lymphoma, leukemia, and multiple myeloma.[176] In each of these cancer types, reishi mushroom extracts have been shown to prevent new tumors from arising, and in many cases to shrink existing tumors or precancerous masses.[177–180] These effects, because they may stop a tumor in its tracks before it ever reaches a detectable or dangerous size, can be considered successful cancer prevention by immunosurveillance.[177,178]

## Shark Liver Oil

Alkylglycerols are naturally occurring ester-lipids that were first isolated from shark liver oil and used in the treatment of children with leukemia.[181] Treatment of cancer cells with alkylglycerols lowered the cancer cell's ability to reproduce and invade healthy cells.[182] Animal studies show that alkylglycerols curtail tumor growth by blocking cancer-cell blood vessel growth.[183] Alkylgylcerols also inhibit protein kinase C, a protein critical in cell proliferation that is often deregulated in malignancy.[136] Shark liver oil is the main source of alkylglycerols and could be taken in a dosage of up to 100 mg, 3 times daily for 3 months without side effects.[136] Shark liver oil should not be consumed without first consulting your physician.

## Sulforaphane

Sulforaphane, which is an isothiocyanate, is most highly concentrated in broccoli as well as in other cruciferous vegetables (eg, Brussels sprouts, cabbage, and cauliflower).

Sulforaphane detoxifies potential carcinogens, promotes apoptosis, blocks the cell cycle required for cancer cell replication, prevents tumor invasion into healthy tissue, enhances NK cell activity, and combats metastasis.[184–187] Research has also demonstrated that sulforaphane is among the plant chemicals most potently capable of blocking the cancer-producing effects of ultraviolet radiation.[188]

In a clinical trial, sulforaphane enhanced the efficacy of imatinib (a drug used in the treatment of CML) against leukemia cells.[189] It has also triggered apoptosis in leukemia cells.[190]

## Garlic Extract (Ajoene)

Ajoene, a natural sulfur-containing compound extracted from garlic, has antileukemia properties.[137,142,143] Ajoene has antithrombotic and cholesterol-lowering properties but has not been tested clinically. Laboratory tests show ajoene blocks division and growth of leukemia cell lines, lowers cholesterol biosynthesis through HMG-CoA-reductase inhibition, and causes death of CML cells.[137]

Ajoene enhances the ability of 2 chemotherapeutic agents (cytarabine and fludarabine) to kill human AML cells that were previously resistant to chemotherapy.[137,143] Ajoene is a promising new therapy for relapsed AML and AML in the elderly, which are more resistant to chemotherapy. Pure garlic supplements contain ajoene.

## Vitamin A

Oral administration of vitamin A analogs as well as synthetic vitamin A derivatives help support normal growth and maturation of cells and are associated with remission rates as high as 90% when used to treat certain types of leukemia.[131,132,191] Fat-soluble vitamin A (retinyl palmitate) has been used to maintain long-term survival of children with AML.[192] Vesanoid (Tretinoin®), a vitamin A analog that inhibits cell division and allows myeloid cells to reach maturity and attain normal function, is approved for treatment of certain leukemias.[193]

Studies have shown that chemotherapy drug resistance may be overcome using vitamin A derivatives in combination with vitamin D3 and its analogs.[194–197]

Vitamin A is available as the prescription drug retinol (which is a vitamin A alcohol). Oral administration of water-soluble vitamin A may inhibit deficiency in those with malabsorption, a low protein intake, active infection, or undergoing antibiotic therapy. A monthly blood test to measure serum concentration of vitamin A is necessary to monitor for vitamin A-induced liver toxicity. Animal studies show that vitamin E protects against vitamin A toxicity and increases assimilation and storage of vitamin A.[198,199]

Supplementation with vitamin A in patients being treated with synthetic retinoids or vitamin A analogs (mimics) for cancer should be avoided because of the potential toxicity with the combination. Supplementing with vitamin A to support healthy cell growth and maturation may be considered *only* after consultation with your physician if you are also being treated for leukemia with synthetic vitamin A derivatives.

## Resveratrol

Resveratrol, a plant polyphenol found in grapes and red wine, has been shown in scientific studies to inhibit the growth of leukemia cell lines. Resveratrol reduces the growth of AML cell lines and causes death in HL-60 leukemia cells.[200] Resveratrol has been shown to block the proliferation of fresh AML cells taken from the bone marrow of 5 newly diagnosed patients.[140,141] Exposure of the leukemia cell line U937 to concentrations of resveratrol similar to those found in red wine blocked cell proliferation, but in this case, did not increase cell death of these abnormal cells.[201]

Studies of resveratrol in humans suggest that it is safe,[202] but appropriate human doses for leukemia therapy have not been determined. However, a study in mice showed resveratrol, taken orally, only showed potential antileukemic activity at high doses of 80 mg/kg body weight.[203] Supplementation with resveratrol to support healthy cell growth and maturation should be done *only* after consulting with your physician if you are also being treated for leukemia.

## Folic Acid

Studies have suggested that supplementing a woman's diet with folate during pregnancy protects the child from childhood ALL,[204] and that abnormalities in the genes responsible for folate metabolism are a known risk factor for adult and childhood ALL.[19] However, folic acid supplementation during leukemia treatment should be approached with caution because it may interfere with the chemotherapy drugs being used to treat the leukemia.

The best example of this is the drug methotrexate. Methotrexate, a chemotherapy drug used to treat many different types of cancers (including certain types of leukemias), works by competing with folic acid for a key enzyme used in cell growth. Since cancer cells grow much faster than normal cells, methotrexate works by interfering with the cancer cells' ability to grow quickly. For example, methotrexate is used to treat childhood ALL.[205,206] However, supplementing with folic acid may interfere with methotrexate's ability to limit cancer cell growth.

If a patient with leukemia or other cancer is being treated with methotrexate, or another antifolic acid drug that is actually a folate analog, then folic acid supplementation should be avoided because it may interfere with methotrexate's anticancer effect.

## Melatonin

Melatonin, a hormone produced by the pineal gland during nighttime hours, regulates sleep and waking cycles in humans.[207] Additionally, it helps support the immune system by stimulating lymphocyte activity.[208]

The use of melatonin supplements in leukemia treatment was initially approached with caution.[209] However, studies show that melatonin may augment the efficiency of leukemia treatment.[210,211] A study in animals showed that melatonin sensitized a chemotherapy-resistant leukemia cell line (P388) to treatment.[210] Furthermore, a clinical study showed that melatonin supplementation supported the treatment of leukemia with the cytokine IL-2.[211] Melatonin supplementation and co-treatment with autologous or allogeneic cells has been proposed as a model for control of malignant beta-cell leukemia.[212] The use of melatonin to support a healthy neuroendocrine system should be used with caution and *only* after consultation with your physician if you are being treated for leukemia.

## TRACKING YOUR PROGRESS

### Monthly Blood Tests

Because all leukemia therapies produce individual responses based on factors such as the type of leukemia, patient's age, nutritional status, and the presence of other diseases, monthly blood testing to monitor progress is recommended. Patients treated for leukemia should work closely with their physician to follow the results of blood and other tests to determine the best treatment course.

The following tests are valuable:

**Cholesterol levels.** Low cholesterol returned to normal physiologic levels with response to treatment in AML and CML.[78–80]

**Total lipid profiles.** Monitoring of lipids can play a role in assessing response to treatment as these lipids have been observed to be abnormal at leukemia diagnosis.[80,213]

**Cortisol levels.** Increased levels in AML, CML, and CLL are associated with immune dysfunction.[82–84] Monitoring cortisol levels in cancer patients may be useful in observing the psychological impact of the disease and associated treatment on the individual.[214]

**DHEA levels.** Abnormal levels may be associated with immune cell dysfunction.[88] Baseline levels can be determined by radioimmunoassay before DHEA supplementation, shown to correct impaired immune function in animal models.[86,87]

**Coagulation profile.** Blood-clotting parameters are usually abnormal in leukemia. Tests may show low levels of platelets, increased prothrombin time (PT), partial thromboplastin time (PTT), and/or decreased fibrinogen.[215] Response to therapy is often accompanied by normalization of these blood tests with increased fibrinogen and decreased PTT.[216,217]

**Hemoglobin levels.** Anemia is common in patients with leukemia, and this can be monitored by periodically measuring hemoglobin status. Hemoglobin levels less than 11g/dL are typically seen with leukemia.[218]

**Cytokine panel.** Tests in patients with leukemia typically reveal that blood levels of proinflammatory cytokines, such as interkeukin-6 (IL-6), interleukin-8 (IL-8), interleukin-1 beta (IL-1ß), and tumor necrosis factor-alpha (TNF-α) are elevated.

**Genetic profile.** p53[113,219,220] and Bcr-Abl tyrosine kinase.[221]

**Blood smears.** Assessments of blood cell shape and size show the presence of leukemia cells by highlighting irregularities in cell shape and structure.

**Bone marrow tests.** Samples taken by aspiration can detect leukemic cells in bone marrow and monitor treatment effectiveness.

**X-rays.** Leukemia progression can be monitored by x-rays to detect disease spread to the lymph nodes, lungs, bone, and joints. Magnetic resonance imaging (MRI) can detect brain metastases.[222]

**Abdominal sonography.** This is a diagnostic imaging method used to monitor the effect of treatment through detection of enlarged spleen (splenomegaly) and abdominal lymph nodes.[223]

**Physical examinations.** Physical examinations play a very important role in monitoring the response to treatment and checking for relapse following leukemia remission, including the presence of enlarged lymph nodes or an enlarged spleen.[224]

---

## FOR MORE INFORMATION

Leukemia patients may wish to read these protocols and design a program that will address the full range of their cancer problems:

- Chemotherapy
- Cancer Radiation Therapy
- Cancer Adjuvant Therapy
- Complementary Alternative Cancer Therapies
- Blood Disorders (Anemia, Leukopenia, and Thrombocytopenia)

For general information on all aspects of leukemia:

- The American Cancer Society, (800) ACS-2345
- The Leukemia & Lymphoma Society, (800) 955-4572, http://www.leukemia-lymphoma.org/hm_lls

## Life Extension Suggestions

Leukemia patients should consult their physicians before using any nutritional supplements while receiving conventional medical treatment. In addition, leukemia patients using nutritional supplements should enlist the assistance of their physicians to ensure the implementation of blood tests and diagnostic procedures that are essential for monitoring the effectiveness of any adjuvant therapy for leukemia. Life Extension suggests:

- **Apigenin:** 20–50 mg daily
- **Astragalus:** 2000–4000 mg daily
- **Green coffee bean extract:** 200–400 mg (standardized to contain chlorogenic acid) 3 times daily
- **Vitamin A:** 40 000–50 000 IU daily[225,226]
- **Vitamin D3:** 16 000 IU, 3 times per week[227]
- **Curcumin:** three 800-mg capsules up to 3 times daily, 2 hours apart from all medications[228]
- **Green tea:** 725 mg of green tea extract (containing 93% polyphenols, 34% epigallocatechin gallate) 3 times daily; or 10 cups of Japanese green tea[229,230]
- **Soy extract:** containing 50 mg of isoflavones twice daily[231]
- **Lipoic acid:** 600 mg orally 3 times daily[232]
- **Vitamin E:** 400 IU daily[225]
- **Vitamin B12:** 1 mg daily[233]
- **L-Ascorbic acid:** 2000 mg daily[225]
- **Shark liver oil:** 1500–3000 mg (containing 20% alkylglycerols [300–600mg]) daily in divided doses[136]
- **Essential fatty acids:** 700 mg GLA, 4.8 g EPA, and 4.9 g DHA daily[234,235]
- **DHEA:** 50 mg daily for men; 25 mg daily for women[236]
- **Resveratrol:** 25 mg daily[237]
- **Folic acid:** up to 1 mg daily[238]
- **Melatonin:** 20 mg before bedtime[211]
- **Panax ginseng:** 200–600 mg daily standardized to contain 4–7% ginsenosides
- **PSK (from the mushroom *Coriolus versicolor*):** 3 g daily
- **Reishi:** 980–3000 mg daily standardized to contain 13.5% polysaccharides and 6% triterpenes
- **Sulforaphane:** 400–1600 mg daily of a broccoli extract
- **Garlic:** 600 mg of aged garlic extract twice daily[137]

---

## REFERENCES

References available at: www.lef.org/dpt5/ch85

# 86

# Liver Degenerative Disease

Compared to other health conditions, it is striking how little attention is given to diseases of the liver, particularly considering the rising level of concern about health and health-related environmental issues. *Hepatoprotection* (or protection of the liver) should be of intense interest because the liver plays a critical role in all aspects of metabolism and overall health.

This protocol will present intriguing information about the role of the liver and why a well-functioning liver is essential for overall health and quality of life. Additionally, you will learn about ways to support healthy liver function, identify environmental hazards that constantly challenge the detoxification capacity of the liver, and the effects of alcohol on the liver.

Some beneficial herbs will also be described. In Europe and Asia, herbal liver remedies have been in common use for decades—perhaps even centuries. The effectiveness of the herbs used in these remedies has been validated through research and clinical studies. These herbs generally contain antioxidants, membrane-stabilizing and bile-enhancing compounds, or substances that prevent depletion of sulfhydryl compounds, such as glutathione.

## WHAT DOES THE LIVER DO?

The liver is located on the right side of the body, in the upper abdomen. In humans, it is the second largest organ of the body, weighing about 4 lbs (skin is the largest organ). Even while exposed to tremendous potential for damage, the liver performs a multitude of essential functions: metabolizing, detoxifying, and regenerating. It does an extraordinary job of keeping us alive and healthy by metabolizing the food we eat (ie, breaking it down into useful parts) and protecting us from the damaging effects of numerous toxic compounds we are exposed to on a daily basis. Several times each day, our entire blood supply passes through the liver. At any given time, about a pint of blood is in the liver (or 10% of the total blood volume of an adult).[1] In addition, the liver has impressive restorative capabilities and is the only organ in the body capable of regenerating itself when part of it has been damaged.

The metabolizing functions of the liver are numerous. The liver is intricately involved in carbohydrate, fat, and protein metabolism; the storage of vitamins and minerals; and in many essential physiologic processes. The liver is also involved in several regulatory mechanisms that control blood sugar and hormone levels. It synthesizes proteins (eg, plasma albumin, fibrinogen, and most globulins), lipids and lipoproteins (phospholipids, cholesterol), as well as bile acids that are excreted in the detoxification process.[1]

Other important functions of the liver include production of prothrombin and fibrinogen (two blood-clotting factors) and heparin (a mucopolysaccharide sulfuric acid ester that helps prevent blood from clotting within the circulatory system). The liver also processes glucose into glycogen and stores it until muscles need energy; when released, glycogen becomes glucose in the bloodstream. Some glucose is also converted and stored as fat.

Additionally, the liver produces and secretes bile (stored in the gallbladder) that is needed to break down and digest fatty acids, and produces blood protein and hundreds of enzymes needed for digestion and other bodily functions. As the liver breaks down proteins, it produces urea, which it synthesizes from carbon dioxide and ammonia. Urea is the primary solid component of urine, and it is eventually excreted by the kidneys. Essential trace elements such as iron and copper as well as vitamins A, D, and B12 are also stored in the liver.

The detoxifying function is an essential part of human body metabolism, with the liver playing a key role in the process. Toxic chemicals, of internal and external origin, constantly bombard the liver. Even normal everyday metabolic processes produce a wide range of toxins neutralized in the liver.

The regenerating capacity of the liver is one of the most intriguing survival mechanisms of the body. The liver is an incredibly resilient organ. Up to 75% of its cells can be surgically removed or destroyed by disease before it ceases to function.[2] As with some other organs, the liver has been designed with an excess of tissue to protect it from damage or loss of function. The healthy parts of the liver have an amazing capacity to regenerate new, healthy liver tissue to replace damaged liver tissue.

## CONDITIONS LEADING TO LIVER DAMAGE

Symptoms that are indicative of reduced liver function or possible liver damage include general malaise, fatigue,

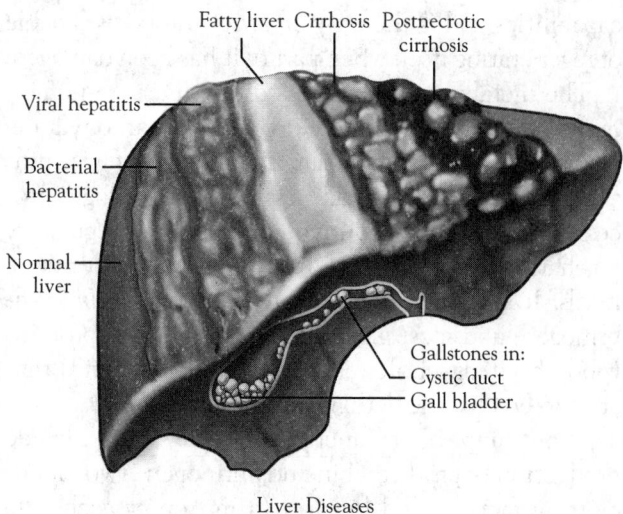

Liver Diseases

digestive disturbances (eg, constipation), allergies and chemical sensitivities, weight loss, jaundice, edema, and mental confusion. Generalized pruritus (itching), nausea, and vomiting can also result from impaired liver function. Causes of liver damage are numerous and may include congenital defects (malformed or absent bile ducts), obstructed bile ducts (cholestasis), autoimmune disorders, metabolic disorders (hemochromatosis, Wilson's disease), tumors, toxins (drugs, overdoses, poisons), alcohol-related conditions (cirrhosis), bacterial and parasitic infections, and viral infections (hepatitis B and C). This section discusses several chronic disorders and diseases that can lead to degenerative liver damage without proper diagnosis and treatment.

## Cholestasis

Cholestasis is interruption or stagnation of bile flow in any part of the biliary system, beginning with the liver. Cholestasis has several causes, including obstruction of the bile ducts by the presence of gallstones or a tumor, drug and alcohol use, hepatitis, and existing liver disease.[3] In the United States, an important cause of cholestasis and impaired liver function is the consumption of alcohol. Other common causes of cholestasis are viral hepatitis and drugs, particularly steroidal hormones (including estrogen and oral contraceptives).

Cholestasis can cause alterations of liver function tests, indicating cellular damage. In the initial stages of liver dysfunction, standard tests (serum bilirubin, alkaline phosphatase, SGOT, LDH, GGTP, etc.) may not be sensitive enough to be of value for complete, early diagnosis. However, measurement of serum bile acids is a safe, sensitive test to determine the functional capacity of the liver. Treatment for cholestasis includes surgery resulting in unobstructed bile flow

from the liver. Drug-induced cholestasis will generally disappear if the causative drug is discontinued. There is no specific treatment for cholestasis caused by hepatitis. However, bile flow will improve slowly if inflammation of the liver can be resolved.

## Wilson's Disease

Wilson's disease is an inherited disorder characterized by the liver's inability to metabolize copper, resulting in the accumulation of excessive amounts of copper in the brain, liver, kidney, cornea, and other tissues. The resulting copper accumulation and toxicity result in liver disease and brain damage in some patients. Although deposits of copper begin at birth, it may be some time until symptoms of liver disease become evident. Patients, generally between the ages of 10–40 years, present symptoms of liver disease, a movement disorder associated with neurologic disease, behavioral abnormalities, or often a combination of these. Blood testing will reveal elevated liver enzymes. Symptoms of hepatitis and cirrhosis may be evident. Secondary injury from an accumulation of copper in the body may include kidney damage, neurologic disorders, hemolytic anemia, and osteoporosis.

Copper also accumulates in other organs (particularly the brain) and may result in difficulty with speech, trembling, writing problems, unsteady gait, depression, suicidal impulses, and loss of mental functions. Other organs may also be damaged by copper overload. Copper can accumulate in the cornea of the eye and cause a characteristic brown pigmentation called Kayser-Fleischer rings. Hemolytic anemia, a low blood count related to damaged red blood cells, may occur in patients with Wilson's disease. There may also be injury to the kidneys from copper overload. Finally, severe bone disease from osteoporosis can occur in patients with Wilson's disease.

If left untreated, Wilson's disease will cause increasing damage to organs, especially in the liver and brain. D-penicillamine is a copper chelating agent administered to remove excess copper and prevent further accumulations. Trientine may also be used as a copper chelating agent. Both drugs are administered with vitamin B6 (see Life Extension's *Heavy Metal Detoxification* protocol for additional information on chelation). Foods high in copper content such as shellfish, nuts, chocolate, liver, and mushrooms must be avoided.

Because Wilson's disease can be effectively treated, it is extremely important for physicians to learn to recognize and diagnose the disease. Treatment options have evolved rapidly in the last few years, with zinc now being an important choice in most situations.

Researchers consider zinc to be so important in the treatment of Wilson's disease that they refer to it as being "the drug of choice."[4]

Wilson's disease requires management by a physician. Self-treating this condition with zinc is not recommended.

## Autoimmune Hepatitis

Autoimmune hepatitis is associated with an increase in circulating autoantibodies and gammaglobulin resulting in progressive inflammation of the liver. The symptoms of type 1 autoimmune hepatitis (the most common) are characterized by the presence of antinuclear antibodies and a resemblance to symptoms of systemic lupus erythematosus. The disease occurs most commonly in females during adolescence or early adulthood. Other autoimmune disorders may be present with autoimmune hepatitis including thyroiditis, ulcerative colitis, vitiligo (loss of skin pigmentation), and Sjögren's syndrome (characterized by dry mouth and eyes).

Fatigue, abdominal discomfort, aching joints, itching, jaundice, enlarged liver, and spider angiomas (blood vessels) on the skin are the most common symptoms. More severe complications of liver disease may occur as the disease progresses.

Up to 80% of patients have long-term survival with appropriate treatment. Prednisone and azathioprine are usually administered to treat immunosuppression. The treatment goal is to control rather than cure the disease.

## Hepatitis B

In the United States and Europe, approximately 1.25 million people are chronically infected with the hepatitis B virus (HBV).[5] About 5–10% of those with acute hepatitis B will develop chronic infection. The remainder will recover and develop antibodies to the virus that make them immune from further viral activity.[6,7] At least 1 million chronically infected individuals die each year of complications due to HBV-related diseases, especially liver cancer and cirrhosis. In the entire world, about 5% of the population (or 350 million people) have chronic hepatitis B.[8]

Hepatitis B causes inflammation of the liver resulting from infection with a DNA-type virus. The infection is passed via blood products, as in transfusions or the sharing of contaminated needles. It may also be acquired by exposure to bodily fluids in addition to blood, during sexual intercourse, and in transmission from mother to fetus. About 5–10% of volunteer blood donors show evidence of having prior hepatitis B—meaning that they once had hepatitis B, and may or may not still be infected with the viral agent.

The incidence of hepatitis B is increased in dialysis patients, IV drug users, persons with AIDS, transplant recipients, and patients frequently receiving blood transfusions (eg, those with leukemia or lymphoma). When acute hepatitis occurs, symptoms include weakness, nausea, vomiting, body aches (myalgias), diarrhea, fever, joint pain (arthralgia), jaundice (yellow discoloration of the skin and whites of the eyes), loss of appetite, weight loss, loss of interest in tobacco products, and sometimes an itchy skin rash. The average duration of symptoms of acute hepatitis B is 1–3 months. During the final phase of symptoms, the body begins to build immunity against the hepatitis B infection and does become immune 90% of the time.[6] In the other 10%, however, a state of persistent infection occurs for more than 6 months. These persons are designated as having chronic hepatitis B. A liver biopsy is done in those patients with chronic hepatitis B; about one-third have chronic active hepatitis and two-thirds have chronic persistent hepatitis. Of these 2 types, chronic active hepatitis is more aggressive with a more rapidly progressing course.

Two forms of therapy are now licensed for use in chronic hepatitis B infection: interferon-alpha and lamivudine (Epivir). A vaccine for hepatitis B now exists and is frequently given to newborns, oversea travelers, and other people at risk of exposure (*refer to Life Extension's Hepatitis B protocol for more information and specific therapies*).

## Hepatitis C

Hepatitis C can be transmitted by blood and blood product transfusion. Up to 170 million persons are infected worldwide. In the United States, more than 4 million people are infected with the hepatitis C virus (HCV). Most liver transplants in the United States are a result of hepatitis C. Hepatitis C has a frightening tendency to result in chronic hepatitis, resulting in cirrhosis (15–20% of those infected) or hepatocellular carcinoma (primary liver cancer).[9]

HCV is an RNA virus, spherical and enveloped in a lipid (fatty) outer envelope, which can be transmitted by narcotics use, transfusion of blood products, and exposure of medical personnel to infected patients. In some cases, the reason one contracts hepatitis C cannot be determined. The HCV inflicts most of its damage by latching onto molecules of iron and generating free-radical damage to liver cells. These free radicals can induce liver inflammation, cirrhosis, and primary liver cancer via oxidative attacks on liver cells.

Successful eradication of the HCV from the body often requires that iron levels in the liver and blood be at very low levels. In many cases, high stores of iron in the liver preclude successful therapy against the HCV. It is desirable to reduce iron levels in the body before initiating treatment with conventional (interferon and ribavirin) therapy. Despite substantial scientific evidence, few physicians implement iron-depletion therapy when treating hepatitis C. This partially accounts for the high failure rate to eradicate the virus.

In patients with hepatitis C, particularly those who are HIV-positive, a systemic depletion of glutathione is present, especially in the liver. This depletion may be a factor underlying resistance to interferon therapy. This finding represents a biological basis for taking supplements that boost cellular glutathione levels. Glutathione is a critical factor in protecting liver cells against free-radical damage.

Standard therapy for hepatitis C has consisted of ribavirin combined with interferon. However, a combination therapy of peginterferon alpha-2b and ribavirin is currently the standard of care (refer to Life Extension's Hepatitis C protocol for more information and specific therapies).

## Hemochromatosis

Hemochromatosis is a hereditary disorder in which too much iron is absorbed from the diet resulting in free-radical damage to the liver, heart, and pancreas. It is estimated that over 1 million Americans suffer from the disease. If diagnosed early, hemochromatosis can be controlled by phlebotomy (giving blood) until stored iron levels are reduced. High levels of antioxidants and herbal detoxifiers are usually recommended to neutralize free radicals generated by excess iron. Chelation therapy is an alternative treatment in which a synthetic amino acid is administered intravenously to bind and extract unwanted metals from the body. People with hemochromatosis must avoid iron-fortified foods, cast-iron cookware, and red meat. Symptoms may not appear until middle age, after multiple organ damage has occurred. Due to blood loss from menstruation and pregnancy, the disease is less prevalent in women than men (refer to Life Extension's Hemochromatosis protocol for more information and specific therapies).

## Steatosis, Steatohepatitis, and Cirrhosis

Steatosis (fatty liver) is a common finding in biopsy of the human liver. Fatty liver is a condition in which fat accumulates within the liver cells (hepatocytes) without causing any specific symptoms. Fatty liver is defined as either more than 5% of cells containing fat droplets or total lipid exceeding 5% of liver weight.

Fatty liver is usually a long-standing chronic condition, occurring in association with a wide range of causes—exposure to poisonous and toxic substances, taking certain drugs, and drug abuse (injecting recreational drugs)[10]—although in clinical practice, the majority of cases are the result of excessive alcohol, diabetes, and obesity. Less common are occurrences of acute fatty liver during pregnancy or in response to the administration of tetracyclines, acetaminophen, prescription drugs, and toxins.

Our understanding of fatty liver has advanced considerably. At one time, fatty liver was believed to be a benign, reversible condition. However, clinical studies now demonstrate that fatty liver, whether from alcoholic or nonalcoholic origin, can lead to inflammation, cell death, fibrosis (steatohepatitis), and perhaps progress to cirrhosis. Cirrhosis is the irreversible end result of fibrous scarring, a response by the liver to a variety of long-standing inflammatory, toxic, metabolic, and congestive damage processes (refer to Life Extension's Cirrhosis and Liver Disease protocol for more information and specific therapies).

As stated earlier, in the Western world, alcohol is a common cause of fatty liver and the second most common cause of cirrhosis. However, there are considerable differences among individuals in the degree of liver damage produced by excessive alcohol intake. There seems to be no correlation between the incidence and severity of fatty liver and the amount, type, or duration of alcohol abuse. In some individuals, it is unclear why fatty liver, whatever its etiology, never progresses to steatohepatitis and cirrhosis.

Obesity is considered to be the most common cause of nonalcoholic steatohepatitis (NASH). There is evidence to suggest that liver disease can actually be considered to be a complication of obesity. However, no major prospective longitudinal studies of NASH have been carried out. Generally, it seems that the risk of progression to cirrhosis is low for nonobese individuals, but significant among obese individuals. Unfortunately, there is also no predictable correlation between symptoms, abnormality of liver function tests, and severity of liver tissue damage.

As early as 1985, a study of 50 unselected, obese subjects admitted to a hospital for weight reduction found that 10% had normal livers, 48% had fatty livers, 26% had steatohepatitis, 8% had fibrosis, and 8% had cirrhosis.[11] Obesity was defined as being 21–130% above ideal body weight.

Among patients with fatty liver related to obesity, it has been observed that rapid weight loss caused by dieting and intestinal bypass surgery actually increased the risk for developing steatohepatitis. The resulting increase in the concentration of fatty acids and/or ketones within the liver severely augmented the generation of free radicals.[12]

A study indicated that obesity also increases susceptibility to endotoxin-mediated liver injury.[13] Endotoxins are cell wall components produced by intestinal Gram-negative bacteria thought to play a role in liver injury induced by alcohol and other hepatotoxins. Under normal conditions, endotoxins are absorbed into portal venous circulation and detoxified by the liver. Hepatic dysfunction interferes with this clearing mechanism and amplifies the negative activities of endotoxin, such as lipid peroxidation, reduced P-450 function, and impairment of the immune system.

Researchers summarized the following insights on the mechanisms of steatohepatitis[14]:

- Its development requires a double hit, the first producing steatosis, the second a source of oxidative stress capable of initiating significant lipid peroxidation. This concept provides a rationale for both the treatment and prevention of disease progression in steatosis of alcoholic and nonalcoholic causes. Management strategies should ideally be directed at reducing the severity of steatosis and at avoiding and removing the triggers of inflammation and fibrosis. Specific treatment modalities for at-risk individuals might include sensible weight reduction, cessation of exposure to toxins and treatment with antioxidants and inhibitors of peroxisomal β-oxidation.

## Toxic Damage to the Liver

The *external* environment contributes most to the load of toxins that the liver has to detoxify. Today, the burden on the liver is heavier than ever before. Additionally, nutritional deficiencies and imbalances from unhealthy eating habits add to the production of toxins, as do alcohol and many prescription drugs, further increasing stress on the liver and requiring a strong detoxification capacity. Surprisingly, even unprocessed organic foods can have naturally occurring toxic components that require an effective detoxification system.

Toxic chemicals are found in the food we eat, water we drink, and air we breathe, both outdoors and indoors. In a study by the Environmental Protection Agency (EPA), chemicals such as p-xylene, tetrachloroethylene, ethylbenzene, and benzene were documented as "everywhere present" in the air.[15] Listed as "often present" were chloroform, carbon tetrachloride, styrene, and p-dichlorobenzene. A customary trip to a gas station or dry cleaner (as well as smoking) results in elevated levels of inhaled toxins.

The Food and Drug Administration (FDA) has found an alarming level of chlorinated pesticides in food. Dichlorodiphenyldichloroethylene (DDE) was found in 63% or more of 42 food samples, even though dichlorodiphenyltrichloroethane (DDT) and DDE have been banned in the United States since 1972; DDE is a breakdown product of DDT. Unfortunately, toxic chemicals used anywhere in the world can move easily around the globe (ie, they are carried by the wind). There is enough evidence of a connection between chemical exposure and chronic health problems for us to be aware that herbicides, pesticides, household chemicals, food additives, etc. pose serious health concerns.

When the liver's detoxification system is overloaded, the liver does not function properly; thus, toxins we are exposed to accumulate in the body. These toxins affect us in numerous ways, and have damaging effects on many bodily functions, particularly the immune system, causing chronic health problems. It is not surprising that an overburdened and undernourished liver can be a root cause of many chronic diseases.

Cancers are also thought to be a result of the effects of environmental carcinogens (eg, cigarette smoke, chemical fumes, toxic exhaust, and airborne particulates), particularly if combined with deficiencies of nutrients required for optimal functioning of the detoxification and immune systems. A study of chemical plant workers in Turin, Italy analyzed the association of bladder cancer according to occupation (ie, textiles, leather, printing, dyestuffs, tire and rubber goods production). Highest risks were for the leather, dyestuffs, and tire production industries. An association was found for cancer and the aromatic amines, with the risk being estimated at 10% for those occupations consistently associated with bladder cancer. Researchers also found that there was a multiplicative effect of relative risks for persons in high-risk occupations who also smoked cigarettes.[16]

## HOW THE LIVER DETOXIFIES

The liver has 3 main *detoxification* pathways:

- *Filtering* the blood to remove large toxins.
- *Enzymatically* breaking down unwanted chemicals. This usually occurs in 2 steps, with Phase I modifying the chemicals to make them an easier target for the Phase II enzyme systems.
- *Synthesizing* and *secreting* bile for excretion of fat-soluble toxins and cholesterol.

*Filtering* the blood is an essential detoxifying function of the liver. As noted earlier, total blood supply passes through the liver several times a day and at any given time, about a pint of blood is in the liver being detoxified. Blood detoxification is critical because blood is loaded with bacteria, endotoxins, antigen-antibody complexes, and other toxic substances from the intestines. A healthy liver clears almost 100% of bacteria and toxins from blood before the blood enters general circulation.

The second essential detoxifying role of the liver involves a two-step *enzymatic process* for the neutralization of unwanted chemical compounds, such as drugs, pesticides, and enterotoxins from the intestines. Even normal body compounds such as hormones are eliminated in this way. Phase I enzymes directly neutralize some of these chemicals, but many others are converted to intermediate forms then processed by Phase II enzymes. These intermediate forms are often much more chemically active and thus, more toxic than the original substances. Therefore, if the Phase II detoxification system is not working properly, the intermediates linger and cause damage.

Phase I detoxification involves a group of 50-100 enzymes named the cytochrome P450 system. These enzymes play a central role in the detoxification of both exogenous (beginning outside the body, such as drugs and pesticides) and endogenous (coming from inside the body, such as hormones) compounds, as well as in the synthesis of steroid hormones and bile acids.

A side effect of this metabolic activity is the production of free radicals (ie, highly reactive molecules that will bind to cellular components and cause damage). The most important antioxidant for neutralizing these free radicals is glutathione, which is needed for Phase I and Phase II detoxification. When exposure to high levels of toxin produces so many free radicals from Phase I detoxification that glutathione is depleted, Phase II processes dependent on glutathione cease. This causes an imbalance between Phase I and Phase II activity, causing severe toxic reactions as a result of the build-up of toxic intermediate forms.

Phase II detoxification involves conjugation (ie, a protective compound becomes bound to a toxin). Besides glutathione conjugation, the other pathways are amino acid conjugation, methylation, sulfation, sulfoxidation, acetylation, and glucuronidation. These enzyme systems need nutrients and metabolic energy to function. As noted earlier, if liver cells do not function properly, Phase II detoxification slows down and increases the load of toxic intermediates.

The third essential detoxifying role of the liver is *synthesis and secretion of bile*. The liver manufactures approximately a quart of bile daily. Bile serves as a carrier to effectively eliminate toxic substances from the body. In addition, bile emulsifies fats and fat-soluble vitamins in the intestine, improving their absorption. When excretion of bile is inhibited (cholestasis), toxins stay in the liver longer, subjecting the liver to damage.

## FREE-RADICAL DAMAGE AND LIPID PEROXIDATION

Oxidative damage from the production of free radicals has far-reaching consequences. Lipid peroxidation describes fats that have been chemically damaged by oxygen free radicals. Cell membranes consist mainly of layers of phospholipids. As free radicals attack the cell membrane, injury and eventual death to the cell occur due to DNA strand breakage. DNA is the cellular blueprint required for replication. Oxidative stress also affects circulating lipids in the body including cholesterol, 80% of which is produced in the liver. Peroxidized cholesterol has been shown to damage arteries, leading to atherosclerosis; a growing body of evidence supports a role for lipid peroxidation in the continued development of liver damage.

While cell damage in the human liver is likely multifactorial, free radicals have been implicated in a variety of liver diseases, particularly in the presence of iron overload, ethanol consumption, and ischemia/reperfusion injury, either initiating or perpetuating liver damage. Additionally, free radical-initiated lipid peroxidation appears to play a role in hepatic fibrogenesis.[17] The role of free radicals is significant in toxic liver injury often induced by drugs and chemicals. Damage is first caused by the toxin itself and then is continued when the toxin is metabolized by the liver.[18]

## CONVENTIONAL MEDICAL THERAPY

Liver damage caused by degenerative conditions is *irreversible*. There are no commonly accepted, effective, conventional drug therapy regimes to *prevent* or *reverse* liver damage. Treatment primarily consists of identifying the underlying cause(s), determining possible steps to slow or stop progression of degeneration, and manage symptoms. One causal factor is alcohol: stopping alcohol intake will help stop progression. Ending the use of hepatotoxic drugs and removing sources of environmental toxins will also stop progression. The possible presence of metabolic diseases (eg, hemochromatosis, Wilson's disease) should be investigated. Identifying the presence of hepatitis viruses is essential. Because obesity plays an important role in fatty liver, attention to weight control is essential.

Conventional drug therapies can include:

## Colchicine

Colchicine, a generic drug used to treat gout, also inhibits collagen (a protein in the body the makes up scar tissue) and has produced some improvement in liver function and patient survival.[19]

## Corticosteroids

Corticosteroids reduce inflammation and have been helpful in improving liver function and symptoms; however, they have potentially serious side effects.[3] If taking a corticosteroid, measures must be taken to monitor adverse side effects such as edema, hypertension, diabetes mellitus, osteoporosis, and ulcers.

## Malotilate

Malotilate (a drug developed in Japan) prevents damage to liver cells (and cirrhosis) induced in laboratory animals. It has been shown by several researchers to prevent induced liver damage, accumulation of collagen, and morphologic changes (such as accumulation of inflammatory cells and fibrosis and to reduce ethanol induced lesions).[20-22]

## Alpha Interferon (Intron A) and Ribavirin (Rebetol and Virazole)

Alpha interferon and ribavirin are antiviral drugs used in treating hepatitis viruses. These drugs are a mainstay for some persons.[23] However, some patients are not responsive, experience relapse after the antiviral drugs are discontinued, or have great difficulty handling the side effects.[24] Newer alpha interferon drugs are pegylated, meaning they contain polyethylene glycol combined with interferon. *PEG-Intron®* was approved by the FDA in January 2001 for once-weekly therapy for the hepatitis C virus. Another drug, PEGASYS® was approved by the FDA in October 2002 as therapy for treating the hepatitis C virus.

## Gene Therapy

Gene therapy as a treatment option is the subject of research, but even if research indicates that gene therapy appears feasible, human trials are years away.

## Therapies to Help Relieve Itching

Itching is a very troublesome symptom for patients with liver disease. It is also a very difficult symptom to manage for physicians. The reason why patients with liver disease itch is not understood. One thought is that certain substances accumulate in the blood as a result of liver disease and cause itching. The nature of these substances is under investigation, but some evidence suggests that normal substances found in blood plasma (eg, endogenous opioids known as enkephalins) for some unknown reason cause itching in liver disease patients. Itching/scratching studies have also shown that some patients manifest scratching in a 24-hour rhythm (circadian), suggesting that neurotransmitters in the brain may cause itching.[25] At this time, the following treatments are available for itching secondary to liver disease.

**Cholestyramine.**   Cholestyramine (taken with food) and Naltrexone can help relieve itching.[19] High doses of Naltrexone are toxic for the liver, but low doses appear to be safe.

**Phototherapy.**   Phototherapy (light therapy) has been helpful in reducing itching.[19]

# NATURAL THERAPIES

Scientific literature reports the results of research using natural or alternative treatments for liver conditions. Note that the vast majority of natural or alternative treatments act by having an antioxidant effect. As with almost all disease processes, research has demonstrated that good *antioxidant* levels are necessary for optimum health and to protect from physical assaults of trauma and disease. Some therapies listed in the following section also act by having an effect on the immune system (an *immune-modulating* effect). Other therapies have *anti-inflammatory* benefits. Additionally, some agents act by having both antioxidant mechanisms and immune modulating mechanisms.

For the liver to continue to perform essential functions, even when damaged, a healthy intake of vitamins, minerals, and essential trace elements from dietary sources such as fruits and vegetables is important. However, few people can consistently include enough fruits and vegetables in their daily diets to protect from degenerative conditions, especially those related to age-related diseases, toxic agents, carcinogens, inflammatory agents, free-radical damage, and immune suppression. As an adjunct to maintaining a healthy diet, supplements can:

1. Maintain healthy metabolic functioning

2. Neutralize free-radical damage

3. Increase levels of glutathione, the liver's natural antioxidant

4. Detoxify the liver

## Supplements that Maintain Metabolic Health

**Vitamin B complex.**   Vitamin B complex is a group of vitamins (B1, thiamine; B2, riboflavin; B3, niacin; B5, pantothenic acid; B6, pyridoxine; and B12, cyanocobalamin) that differ from each other in structure and the effect they have on the human body. The B vitamins play a vital role in numerous essential processes including enzyme activities (thiamine, riboflavin, niacin, pantothenic acid, pyridoxine). These enzyme activities have many roles and are involved in the metabolism of carbohydrates and fats, functioning of the nervous and digestive systems, and production of red blood cells. The B vitamins have a synergistic effect with each other.[2] They are found in large quantities in the human liver as well as in many foods and yeast.

**Folic acid.**   Folic acid, an important member of the B-complex family, reduces harmful levels of homocysteine (ie, a sulfur-containing amino acid known to be a major culprit in heart disease). The liver uses folic acid to facilitate healthy methylation patterns that are essential components of enzymatic detoxification. Decreased folate (folic acid) is also associated with increased levels of lipoperoxidases (ie, an indicator of increased oxidative stress). Therefore, folic acid is potentially beneficial if there is ongoing oxidative damage.[26]

**Choline.**   Another B-complex vitamin is choline, essential for the use of fats in the body. It comprises a large part of acetylcholine (a nerve signal carrier). Choline also stops fats from being deposited in the liver and helps move fats into the cells. Choline deficiency can lead to degenerative diseases such as cirrhosis with associated conditions such as bleeding, kidney damage, hypertension (high blood pressure), hypercholesterolemia (high blood levels of cholesterol), atherosclerosis (cholesterol deposits in blood vessels), and arteriosclerosis (hardening of the arteries).[3]

**Acetyl-L-carnitine.**   Acetyl-L-carnitine has been shown to convert some hepatic parameters to more youthful levels. Acetyl-L-carnitine is the biologically active form of the amino acid L-carnitine that has been shown to protect cells throughout the body from age-related degeneration. By facilitating the youthful transport of fatty acids into the cell mitochondria, acetyl-L-carnitine facilitates conversion of dietary fats to energy and muscle. Acetyl-L-carnitine has also been shown to regenerate nerves,[27] provide protection against glutamate and ammonia induced toxicity to the brain,[28] and reverse the effects of heart aging in animals.[29]

## Antioxidants That Reduce Free-Radical Damage

**Vitamin C.**   Vitamin C is a potent antioxidant found naturally in many fruits and vegetables. Vitamin C has protective effects against liver oxidative damage, particularly when used in combination with vitamin E. Researchers have found inadequate levels of vitamin C in patients with degenerative diseases. They noted that supplementation in rats lowered plasma and liver lipid peroxidation, normalized plasma vitamin C levels, and raised vitamin E above normal levels.[30]

**Vitamin E.**   Vitamin E protects the lipid membrane from oxidative damage. Adequate vitamin E levels also protect cholesterol from oxidative damage. Oxidized cholesterol damages arteries and contributes to atherosclerosis.[31] Hepatocytes incorporate vitamin E into lipoproteins, which then transport it to various tissues in the body.

**Coenzyme Q10.**   Coenzyme Q10 (CoQ10) is an antioxidant that is protective for a liver that has been damaged by ischemia (reduced blood flow).[32] CoQ10 is also an important component of healthy metabolism. It protects the mitochondria and cell membrane from oxidative damage and helps generate ATP, the energy source for cells. CoQ10 is absorbed by the lymphatic system and distributed throughout the body. Japanese researchers studied the effects of the toxic drug hydrazine on liver cells. Hydrazine caused remarkable increases in intracellular levels of reactive oxygen species in hepatocytes, which were suppressed by CoQ10.[33]

**N-acetyl-cysteine.**   N-acetyl-cysteine (NAC) is an amino acid that acts as an antioxidant or free-radical scavenger. Most scientific articles related to liver protection with NAC emphasize this effect. NAC is frequently used in medical settings to treat liver toxicity associated with ingesting Tylenol® (also poisonous mushrooms).[34,35]

**Lipoic acid.**   Alpha-lipoic acid is an antioxidant shown to decrease the amount of hepatic fibrosis associated with liver injury. Both of these mechanisms suggest it has promise for cirrhosis. Because alpha-lipoic acid is fat soluble, it can penetrate the cell membrane to exert therapeutic action. It has been shown to effectively scavenge harmful free radicals, chelate toxic heavy metals, and help prevent mutated gene expression.[36] Another of its most beneficial functions is enhancing the effects of other essential antioxidants including glutathione, which is vital to a healthy liver.[37,38] Alpha lipoic acid consists of 2 different forms (isomers) that have vastly different properties.

The "R" form is the biologically active component (native to the body) that is responsible for lipoic acid's phenomenal antioxidant effect. The "S" form is produced from chemical manufacture and is not very biologically active. Alpha lipoic acid supplements consist of the "R" and "S" form in a 50/50 ratio. That means a 100 mg alpha lipoic acid supplement is providing 50 mg of the biologically active "R" form. The human body normally produces and uses R-lipoic acid, the active form.

**Selenium.**   Selenium is a trace element that acts by several mechanisms, including detoxifying liver enzymes, exerting anti-inflammatory effects, and providing antioxidant defense. The presence of selenium helps induce and maintain the glutathione antioxidant system.[39]

**Zinc.**   Zinc is an essential dietary nutrient used in numerous protective drugs and preparations. Zinc helps remove copper from the body and is used as an adjuvant treatment in Wilson's disease.[4]

**Schisandra and melon pulp concentrate.**   As the body loses its natural primary antioxidant mechanisms, it accumulates lipid peroxidation products, and liver mitochondria begin to fail. Purified extract from a non-GMO *Cucumis melo* melon has been found to be rich in superoxide dismutase (SOD), the first enzyme in the body's mitochondrial oxidant protection system.[40,41] Melon-derived SOD quickly converts primary free oxygen radicals into hydrogen peroxide. That hydrogen peroxide must be rapidly converted into water to complete the mitochondrial oxidant detoxification process. That task is handled by a second liver-protective agent, an extract of the Chinese vine *Schisandra chinensis*.

## Protecting and Improving Liver Function

**S-adenosylmethionine.**   S-adenosylmethionine (SAMe), a methylation agent (a methyl group donor), is necessary for the synthesis of glutathione. Medical studies have shown that SAMe has beneficial antioxidant effects on the liver and other tissues, particularly in protecting and restoring liver cell function destroyed by the hepatitis C virus. SAMe decreases the production of liver collagen, which leads to the formation of fibrous tissue.[42] SAMe is found naturally in every cell of the body. It is synthesized from a combination of the amino acid L-methionine, folic acid, vitamin B12, and trimethylglycine, provided all these ingredients are present and performing.[43]

**Phosphatidylcholine.**   Phosphatidylcholine is a type of fat that is part of cell membranes. Phosphatidylcholine, one of the most important substances for liver protection and health, is a primary constituent of cell membranes. Phosphatidylcholine acts by several mechanisms: exerting potent antioxidant effects; inhibiting the tendency of stellate cells to progress to cirrhosis; decreasing apoptotic death of liver cells and thereby prolonging the life of liver cells; stabilizing the cell membrane, thus improving the integrity and function of the liver cell; and exerting an antifibrotic effect related to the breakdown of collagen (not only slowing the progression of fibrosis, but also encouraging regression of existing fibrosis).[44–47] A special form of phosphatidylcholine called polyenylphosphatidylcholine (PPC) has been shown to prevent the early changes in the damaged liver from occurring before the actual development of cirrhosis.[48]

**Silymarin.**   Silymarin (also known as milk thistle or *Silybum marinum*) is a member of the aster family (*Asteraceae*). The active extract of milk thistle is silymarin,[49] a mixture of flavolignans, including silydianin, silychristine, and silybin, with silybin being the most biologically active. Silymarin has proven to be one of the most potent liver-protecting substances. Its main routes of protection appear to be the prevention of free-radical damage, stabilization of plasma membranes, and stimulation of new liver cell production. It has also been shown to inhibit lipid peroxidation and prevent glutathione depletion induced by alcohol and other liver toxins, even increasing total glutathione levels in the liver by 35% over controls.[50] Early studies show that silymarin has the ability to stimulate protein synthesis, resulting in production of new liver cells to replace older, damaged ones.[51,52] Studies also demonstrate the benefits of silymarin for protection from numerous toxic chemicals.

**Branched-chain amino acids.**   Branched-chain amino acids (BCAAs) (leucine, isoleucine, and valine) are considered to be *essential* amino acids because humans cannot survive unless these amino acids are present in their diet. BCAAs are needed for the maintenance of muscle tissue and appear to preserve muscle stores of glycogen (stored form of carbohydrates that can be converted into energy). Dietary sources of BCAAs are dairy products and red meat. Whey protein and egg protein supplements are other sources. Most diets provide the daily requirement of BCAAs for healthy people. However, in cases of physical stress, energy requirements increase (in persons with cirrhosis, in particular). Studies on alcoholic cirrhosis patients have shown benefits from supplementing valine, leucine, and isoleucine. These branched-chain amino acids can enhance protein synthesis in liver and muscle cells, help restore liver function, and prevent chronic encephalopathy.[53,54] In studies, BCAAs have also been shown to have therapeutic value in adults with cirrhosis of the liver. According to the researchers, BCAAs seem to be the preferred substrate to meet this requirement.[55]

## Life Extension Suggestions

- **Thiamine (B1):** 40–100 mg daily
- **Riboflavin (B2):** 50 mg daily
- **Niacin (B3):** 200–500 mg daily
- **Pantothenic acid (B5):** 500–1000 mg daily
- **Vitamin B6:** 75–250 mg daily
- **Vitamin B12:** 1000–5000 mcg daily
- **Folate:** 800–1000 mcg daily
- **Vitamin C:** 1000–6000 mg daily
- **Acetyl-L-carnitine:** 1000–2000 mg daily
- **N-acetyl-cysteine (NAC):** 600–1800 mg daily
- **R-lipoic acid:** 240–480 mg daily
- **Milk thistle** (standardized extract): 750 mg daily
- **L-glutathione:** 250–500 mg daily
- **Vitamin E:** 400 IU daily with at least 200 mg gamma tocopherol
- **Coenzyme Q10** (as ubiquinol): 100–300 mg daily
- **S-adenosylmethionine (SAMe):** 800–1200 mg daily
- **Zinc:** 30 mg daily
- **Selenium:** 200–400 mcg daily
- **Polyenylphosphatidylcholine (PPC):** 1800–2700 mg daily
- **Branched-chain amino acids (BCAAs):** 2400 mg daily
- **Schisandra extract** (standardized to 9% total schisandrins [22.5 mg]): 250 mg daily
- **Melon pulp concentrate:** 10 mg daily

## REFERENCES

References available at: www.lef.org/dpt5/ch86

# 87

# Lung Cancer

Each year, an estimated 93 000 men and 82 000 women in the United States will be diagnosed with lung cancer, with a median age of 70 years.[1,2] To date, the prognosis is grim for most forms of lung cancer as the 5-year overall survival rate of only 14% has hardly changed in the past 50 years.[3] Cigarette smoking is the main cause of lung cancer; however, nonsmokers also develop the disease due to genetics, secondhand smoke, and exposure to toxins and radon gas.[4,5]

Novel approaches are urgently needed that reverse, suppress, or prevent lung cancer development.[6] Early detection offers the best chance for long-term survival.[7] The conventional choices of treatment include surgery, chemotherapy, and radiotherapy, and depend on the type and stage of the cancer.[8] Irrespective of the treatment method used, complementary therapy, such as nutritional supplementation and the use of bioresponse modifiers, is an important addition to traditional treatment that could help control symptoms, enhance quality of life, and improve overall survival.[9]

## WHAT IS LUNG CANCER?

Lung cancer is a disease in which cells in the lungs begin to grow out of control and interfere with normal lung functions such as breathing. The vast majority of lung cancer cases fall into one of 2 categories: non-small-cell lung cancer (NSCLC) and small-cell lung cancer (SCLC).

### Non-Small-Cell Lung Cancer

NSCLC is the most common type of lung cancer, making up nearly 80% of all cases. This type of lung cancer grows and spreads more slowly than the other major type and is therefore more treatable. NSCLC is divided into 3 subtypes: squamous cell carcinoma, adenocarcinoma, and large cell carcinoma. The 5-year survival rate for patients with NSCLC is less than 25%.[1]

### Small-Cell Lung Cancer

Small-cell lung cancer (SCLC) accounts for 20% of all lung cancer cases. Its small cells can rapidly reproduce to form large tumors that quickly spread to the lymph nodes and other parts of the body. This type of lung cancer is almost always caused by smoking or secondhand smoke. Initially, SCLC responds well to chemotherapy and radiotherapy treatment. However, less than 5% of SCLC patients survive 5 years past diagnosis; a patient with untreated SCLC has an average survival time of 2–3 months.[10]

### Mesothelioma

Mesothelioma is diagnosed when cancer cells are found in pleural fluid or tissue. It is associated with asbestos exposure (70% of cases), and asbestos workers have a lifetime risk of 8%; tumors arise 20–40 years after asbestos exposure. Mesothelioma has a poor prognosis; 75% of patients die within 1 year and a 5-year survival of about 5%. Long-term survival has been reported in 50% of patients who receive a combination of surgical removal of cancer followed by chemotherapy during surgery and intraperitoneal chemotherapy soon after surgery.

## CAUSES OF LUNG CANCER

Lung cancer is a multistep process that involves cancer-causing agents (environmental carcinogens), inherited genes, and tumor promoters (eg, inflammatory mediators).[11-13] Cigarette smoking may cause as many as 90% of male and 79% of female lung cancers.[14]

### Smoking

Cigarette smoke contains potent cancer-causing derivatives of nicotine, and nicotine itself is directly involved in lung cancer development.[15] Smoking cessation is difficult because nicotine is highly addictive; however, nicotine replacement therapy combined with Zyban® (bupropion) enables a higher smoking-cessation rate.[16] Medicinal herbal tea made from cloves and milk vetch reduces smoking withdrawal symptoms and increases the rate of smoking cessation.[17] In 2006, the Food and Drug Administration approved a new smoking-cessation drug called Chantix® (varenicline). This new drug is the first prescription medication approved for smoking cessation in almost a decade. It works by partially activating the nicotine receptors in the brain, thus reducing the craving for nicotine and reducing withdrawal symptoms. It also reduces the satisfaction gained by smoking, which may lessen addiction.

**Nonsmokers get lung cancer too.** Nonsmokers make up 10–15% of all lung cancer cases.[18] Many nonsmokers who develop lung cancer appear to carry a genetic tendency.[19]

## Genetics

A two- to three-fold increase in lung cancer risk is associated with having a relative with lung cancer.[20] Adults with retinoblastomas (inherited mutations in the retinoblastoma-1 [RB1] gene) and those with Li-Fraumeni syndrome (inherited mutations in the tumor suppressor p53 gene) may develop lung cancer (typically bronchial cancers) at a higher rate than the general population, suggesting a family association.[21,22] The p53 and RB1 genes are both mutated in more than 90% of SCLCs, while p53 is mutated in more than 50% and RB1 in 20% of NSCLCs.[23,24]

## Exposure to Toxins and Viruses

Indoor exposure to secondhand smoke, radon gas, asbestos, and heavy metals (eg, arsenic, nickel, chromium, iron oxide) and exposure to petrochemicals, polycyclic aromatic hydrocarbons, and human papillomavirus all cause lung cancer.[5,11,25–27]

# UNDERSTANDING AND REDUCING YOUR RISK

## Smoking and Secondhand Smoke

More than 90% of lung cancers are unquestionably caused by tobacco and the 4000 cancer-causing substances in cigarette smoke.[28] The risk of developing lung cancer increases 20- to 40-fold for lifelong smokers and 1.5-fold for people with long-term passive exposure to cigarette smoke. Population studies show that approximately 15% of heavy smokers will ultimately develop lung cancer but that, interestingly, 85% of heavy smokers will not develop lung cancer because of innate differences in cancer susceptibility, or in other words, genetics. If a family member has lung cancer, chances are your genes render you susceptible to cancer, and you should stop smoking.

The lung cancer death rate is related to the total number of cigarettes smoked, and the risk for a man smoking 2 packs daily for 20 years is 60- to 70-fold the risk run by a nonsmoker. Among individuals who smoke 15 or more cigarettes per day, reducing smoking by 50% significantly reduces the danger of lung cancer.[29] In addition, stopping smoking may prolong survival of cancer patients.[14]

To reduce risk:

- Stop smoking. Use nicotine replacement therapy, Zyban®, counseling, and herbal tea made of cloves and milk vetch.[17] A smoking-cessation drug, Chantix® (varenicline), is available by prescription.

- Increase intake of citrus fruits and tomatoes, which are high in beta-cryptoxanthin, lycopene, alpha-carotene, and lutein.[30–33]

- With the approval of your physician, take aspirin regularly.[34]

- Take folate and vitamin B12, which improve abnormal bronchial cell growth in smokers.[35]

- Consume green tea, whose polyphenols prevent DNA damage in lung cells exposed to oxidants from cigarette smoke.

- Test your home for radon gas.

## Dietary Factors

A low intake of fruits and vegetables and consumption of red meat and preserved and fatty foods increase risk.[36,37] Therefore, your diet should consist mostly of vegetables, fruits, raw foods, and fresh fish.[38,39] However, the genes one inherits play an important role in individual susceptibility to lung cancer.[40]

- The overall risk of lung cancer decreases by one-half among those with a high intake of lettuce and cabbage, even among current smokers.[39]

- Chinese leek (*Allium tuberosum Rottler*), also known as Chinese chives, reduced lung cancer metastasis (spread) in mice by 40% and prevented cancer cell growth in experimental conditions.[41]

See the section titled "Preventing Lung Cancer" for more recommendations.

**Genetics.** Especially among nonsmokers, a genetic predisposition increases an individual's susceptibility to cancer-causing agents (carcinogens) in the environment. Nonsmokers with a close family member stricken by cancer might reduce their lung cancer risk by about 25–50% by taking the following steps:

- Increasing intake of darkly colored vegetables and fruits.

- Consuming carotene-containing fruits and vegetables—spinach, kale, carrots, cantaloupes, and sweet potatoes.[42,43]

## Lung Disease

Lung diseases such as chronic obstructive pulmonary disease and infections such as tuberculosis, human papilloma virus, and *Microsporum canis* (skin fungus) are linked with a proinflammatory state and a high risk of lung cancer.[40,44] Although most of these conditions are easily diagnosed and fairly well managed, smoking cessation is a must.

## Environmental Carcinogens

Certain elements in the environment further increase one's risk of developing lung cancer. See the discussion under the section titled "Exposure to toxins and viruses."

# DIAGNOSING LUNG CANCER

Approximately 5–15% of lung cancers are discovered in the course of a routine chest x-ray of people with no symptoms. However, more than 50% of new lung cancer cases will be diagnosed by the presence of symptoms that indicate cancer spread (metastasis).

### Symptoms

Lung cancer symptoms are caused by tumor growth in the lungs, invasion or obstruction of nearby structures, and tumor growth in lymph nodes and in distant sites after cancer spreads through the blood. Symptoms include worsening or chronic cough, shortness of breath, wheezing, coughing up blood, back pain, and weight loss.

### Screening

Screening methods include examination of a sputum (spit) sample, chest x-ray, and low-dose spiral computed tomography (CT) lung scanning. A biopsy of the tumor tissue is necessary to confirm a diagnosis of lung cancer. Physical examination, bone scans, brain CT, and bone marrow examination are performed when SCLC is suspected. Positron emission tomography scans are also useful in detecting cancer spread.

## WHAT IF LUNG CANCER IS DETECTED?

### Blood Tests

Blood tests should measure levels of electrolytes (sodium, potassium, calcium, magnesium, phosphorus, chloride, and bicarbonate), indicators of liver function (aspartate aminotransferase, alanine aminotransferase, prothrombin time, bilirubin, and alkaline phosphatase), and level of lactate dehydrogenase.

A complete blood count will determine most of these values. However, the prothrombin time is a separate test that measures how quickly the blood clots. A prolonged prothrombin time, in the absence of vitamin K deficiency, and an elevated D-dimer level are associated with a poor outcome after surgery for lung cancer.[45,46] An elevated alkaline phosphatase level suggests cancer spread to the bone. Blood tests

can be performed via Life Extension National Diagnostics, Inc.: http://www.lef.org/bloodtest/.

## WHAT YOU HAVE LEARNED SO FAR

- Smoking is the major cause of lung cancer; thus, most lung cancers are preventable.
- Genetics, secondhand smoke, human papillomavirus infection, an unhealthy diet, and exposure to chemicals, heavy metals, and radon gas cause lung cancer in nonsmokers.
- All these risk factors are modifiable.
- Symptoms include worsening or chronic cough, shortness of breath, wheezing, coughing up blood, back pain, and weight loss.
- Tests for lung cancer include sputum sample, chest x-ray, and computed tomography lung scanning, but a biopsy is needed for diagnosis.
- In the past 50 years, the 5-year survival rate for lung cancer has not improved significantly.
- A healthy lifestyle and diet (citrus fruits, tomatoes, spinach, carrots, cantaloupes, and sweet potatoes), in addition to supplementation with folate and vitamin B12, may help prevent lung cancer.

# STAGING OF LUNG CANCER

How extensive or advanced a cancer is can be determined by "staging," which is important in determining the proper treatment approach. NSCLC is staged according to tumor size, whether lymph nodes are affected, and whether the cancer has spread (metastasized). NSCLC has 5 stages, numbered 0 through 4 with 0 being the earliest stage and having the best chance of cure and 4 being the most advanced.

SCLC is divided into 2 stages: limited disease (25–30% of cases), in which the cancer is limited to the chest and nearby lymph nodes, and extensive disease (70–75% of cases), in which the cancer extends beyond the chest.

# PROGNOSIS FOR LUNG CANCER

Lung cancer generally has a grim prognosis, which can be defined by means of the blood tests mentioned above as well as the following tests.

### Tumor Markers

Tumor markers are substances produced by cancer cells. They reflect the presence or absence of cancer, and indicate whether a cancer returns (recurs) after treatment. Measuring the following 6 tumor markers is essential to daily lung cancer management. They are measured either by blood testing or testing the tumor biopsy sample.

**Carcinoembryonic antigen.** High carcinoembryonic antigen (CEA) levels in the blood (>10 ng/mL before and after surgery) are linked with poor survival.[47]

**Neuron-specific enolase.** Neuron-specific enolase (NSE) in the tumor biopsy sample is a significant predictor of survival.[48,49]

**Sialyl Lewis X-i antigen.** Sialyl Lewis X-i antigen (SLX) identifies the presence of lung metastasis.[50]

**Serum cytokeratin fragment 21.1.** Serum cytokeratin fragment 21.1 (CYFRA) diagnoses NSCLC, especially squamous cell and adenocarcinoma.[51]

**Squamous cell carcinoma antigen.** Some 85% of patients with squamous cell carcinoma antigen (SCC) levels higher than 2 ng/mL have squamous tumors.[52]

**Pro-gastrin-releasing peptide.** High levels of pro-gastrin-releasing peptide (ProGRP) are found in SCLC patients, and this test is more specific than NSE for SCLC.[53]

### Cyclooxygenase-2

Cyclooxygenase-2 (COX-2) is associated with a worsening prognosis in lung cancer. Therefore, COX-2 inhibitors, taken as either prescription medication or nutritional supplements, may be beneficial in addition to standard treatments and in the prevention of lung cancer.[54] COX-2 inhibitors enhance the cancer-killing effects of chemotherapy and radiation therapy in lung cancer cell lines with high levels of COX-2.[55]

Advanced lung cancer patients who took Celebrex® (celecoxib, 200 mg twice daily), medroxyprogesterone (500 mg twice daily), and oral food supplementation for 6 weeks had stable weight (±1%) or gained weight and had significant appetite improvement and relief from nausea and fatigue.[56] Consequently, clinical trials are currently assessing Celebrex® alone for preventing lung cancer in heavy smokers and Celebrex® in combination with chemotherapy or after radiation therapy in lung cancer treatment. More information on ongoing clinical trials may be found at www.clinicaltrials.gov.

The following may also inhibit the effects of COX-2:

- Eicosapentaenoic acid (EPA) from fish oil,[57] alpha-tocopheryl succinate,[58] and a tea made from clove[59] hinder COX-2 in lung cancer cells.
- Aspirin also slows down COX-2 activity in lung cancer cells and may prevent tobacco carcinogenesis.[60]

### Gene Abnormalities

Mutations in K-ras genes are associated with a poor prognosis in NSCLC,[61,62] while tumor amplification of c-myc is associated with a poor prognosis in SCLC[63] and shorter survival in NSCLC.[64] The p16/CDKN2 gene is abnormal in 10% of SCLCs and in more than 50% of NSCLCs, and its detection may improve early diagnosis.[65]

Detection of K-ras mutations may help predict treatment outcome. For example, tumors in patients with a mutant ras gene are more difficult to kill with radiation than are tumors in people without the mutation. K-ras mutations can be detected in blood, sputum, lavage fluids, stool sample,[66] and the tumor itself. Testing may be available through the Harvard Medical School-Partners Healthcare Center for Genetics and Genomics Laboratory for Molecular Medicine (www.hpcgg.org) or LabCorp (www.labcorp.com). Several gene therapies are under investigation.

- Perillyl alcohol, found in lavender, cherries, and mint, slowed down ras activity and prevented lung cancer in experimental studies. Because it stimulated lung cancer cell death, it is being tested in clinical trials as an anticancer agent.[67,68]
- Theaflavins and epigallocatechin gallate (EGCG), black tea components, alter c-myc levels, resulting in a decreased occurrence and delayed onset of pre-invasive lung cancers.[55,69]
- Grape seed proanthocyanidins alter c-myc activity and protect against tobacco-induced death of healthy cells.[70]

## TREATING LUNG CANCER

Treatment methods depend on the type of lung cancer. SCLC is treated with chemotherapy with or without radiotherapy, as surgery is unlikely to control the cancer in most cases. NSCLC, if contained within the lung area, may be cured with either surgery or radiotherapy. Alternatively, certain chemotherapy agents are beneficial in specific cases.

### Surgery

The goal of surgery is to remove as much of the cancer as possible in order to prevent recurrence, increase the effectiveness of chemotherapy and radiotherapy if needed, and use the cancer cells to make a vaccine if required.

**SCLC.** Approximately 25% of SCLC patients with a single lung nodule (ie, limited disease) can be cured with surgery.[71,72] The 5-year survival rate of stage 1 patients with a peripherally located tumor who undergo cancer surgery is 44.9%, compared with 11.3%

for conventionally treated patients (ie, those treated with chemotherapy or chemoradiotherapy).[73] However, studies show surgery will not benefit most SCLC patients.[74]

Complete lung (pulmonary) function tests should be performed before surgery because part of a lung lobe or an entire lung may be removed. The Cancer Surgery protocol provides information on nutritional supplementation in preparation for surgery and recuperation afterwards.

**NSCLC.** Fewer than 25% of patients with NSCLC are diagnosed with early-stage disease and are best treated by surgery.[54] The 5-year survival rate of NSCLC patients who undergo complete removal of cancer via surgery is 33%.[75]

The combined effects of the season in which surgery is performed and recent vitamin D intake are associated with the survival of early-stage NSCLC patients. Some 56% of NSCLC patients who have surgery during summer and have the highest vitamin D intake (from sunlight) have remissions lasting more than 5 years, compared with 23% of patients who have surgery during winter and have the lowest vitamin D intake.[76] Therefore, if regular exposure of the skin to sunlight (which makes vitamin D in the body) is not possible before cancer surgery, then increased vitamin D intake or supplementation is suggested as an alternative.

Surgical removal of lung cancer causes a significant reduction of total plasma antioxidant capacity in lung cancer patients during the first postoperative day.[77] An antioxidant-rich diet is therefore recommended after surgery.

If cancer returns after surgery, it usually occurs within 2 years and involves cancer spread to the brain, bones, and liver. Treatments after surgery, such as chemotherapy or radiotherapy (or both), have been tested; unfortunately, they generally do not improve survival rates for most advanced lung cancer patients.[54]

## Radiation Therapy (Radiotherapy)

The goal of radiotherapy is to kill any cancer cells remaining after surgery and cure patients with early-stage lung cancer if they are not suitable for surgery or refuse it. It is also used to relieve symptoms in advanced cancer patients.[78]

In the past, radiotherapy after surgery had an unfavorable effect on survival. A meta-analysis found that the risk of death increased by 21% and the 2-year survival rate fell 7 points (from 55 to 48%) with radiation therapy after surgery.[79] However, in those studies, most patients were treated with older

technology (cobalt-60).[80] The newer radiotherapy technologies, such as intensity modulated radiotherapy, four-dimensional proton beam therapy, image guided radiotherapy, three-dimensional conformal radiotherapy, and radiation seeds (brachytherapy), reduce lung and heart damage (eg, pneumonitis and fibrosis) significantly and when combined with nutritional supplements, improve overall survival.[78,81–86]

**SCLC.** Radiation therapy to the chest area is used to treat SCLC that has spread to bone and the central nervous system, and it improves survival in patients with limited-stage disease but not those with widespread disease. Whole-brain radiation therapy decreases the occurrence of cancer spread to the central nervous system but does not affect survival.[87]

**NSCLC.** Radiation therapy combined with alpha-tocopherol (a type of vitamin E) and pentoxifylline (Trental®) improves survival in stage 3B NSCLC.[78,82,88] Sixty-six patients were treated with alpha-tocopherol (300 mg twice daily) and Trental® (400 mg 3 times daily) during radiotherapy, followed by 300 mg alpha-tocopherol and 400 mg Trental® daily for 3 months after radiotherapy. In patients who received Trental® and alpha-tocopherol, 1- and 2-year overall survival rates were 55% and 30%, respectively, and most patients survived at least 18 months. In patients treated with radiotherapy alone, 1- and 2-year overall survival rates were significantly lower, 40% and 14%, respectively, with a median survival of 10 months.[88] Trental® is safe and effective in preventing lung damage caused by radiotherapy.[86]

Several nutritional supplements may also mitigate the effects of radiotherapy:

- Coenzyme Q10 and vitamin E have protective effects against heart damage (cardiotoxicity) caused by radiation.[89]

- Proteolytic enzymes were given systemically to 44 patients with lung cancer undergoing radiation treatment (and polychemotherapy). It prevented lung damage, specifically fibrosis.[90]

See the Cancer Radiation Therapy protocol for information on other nutritional supplements (taurine, L-arginine, and vitamin A) that help radiotherapy kill cancer cells without damaging normal, healthy cells or causing heart or lung damage or other side effects, thus improving the success of radiotherapy for lung cancer. The protocol also provides a list of proton beam therapy centers in North America.

## Chemotherapy

The goal of chemotherapy is to treat lung cancer with drugs that have a specific toxic effect on cancer cells and result in direct cancer death. It is sometimes used before surgery to shrink inoperable tumors to make them operable. In these cases the response rates vary from 50 to 60%.

Unfortunately, chemotherapy cannot selectively destroy cancer cells; it damages healthy cells too, resulting in many serious and often life-threatening side effects (such as low blood cell counts, immunosuppression, and heart damage). The Chemotherapy protocol outlines nutritional supplements and prescription drugs that mitigate the well-known adverse effects of specific chemotherapy drugs.

**SCLC.** A customized chemotherapy approach including chemosensitivity testing (see the Chemotherapy protocol) is critical to determine which chemotherapy combinations will be effective in killing these cancers, particularly in early-stage SCLC. Tailoring chemotherapy to the unique characteristics of patients and their tumor should improve treatment outcome, provided that patients are in fairly good health.[91] The chemotherapy drugs cisplatin and etoposide, or oral topotecan (Hycamtin®) with intravenous cisplatin, are used to treat SCLC, resulting in 1- and 2-year survival rates of 31% and 5–20%, respectively, depending on the stage of the cancer.[92]

**NSCLC.** In patients with early-stage NSCLC completely removed by surgery, cisplatin plus Navelbine therapy after surgery (without radiotherapy) significantly prolonged survival (94 versus 73 months) compared with surgery alone, but not without severe toxicities (low white blood cell counts, nausea, vomiting, and fatigue) and 2 deaths among 242 patients. The 5-year survival rates were 69% and 54%, respectively.[93] By contrast, chemotherapy with alkylating agents (mainly cyclophosphamide or nitrosourea in combination with methotrexate) after surgery is detrimental to survival (producing a 15% increased risk of death) and should not be used to treat NSCLC after surgery. Furthermore, the use of radiotherapy in combination with chemotherapy after surgery is not recommended as a treatment for patients with completely removed NSCLC.[94]

The following supplements may optimize the effects of chemotherapy:

- Polysaccharopeptide (PSP), from the mushroom *Coriolus versicolor*, helps lessen symptoms and prevents decline in immune status of lung cancer patients undergoing chemotherapy or radiotherapy.[95]

- Low molecular weight heparin, an anticoagulant, improves survival in patients with SCLC undergoing chemotherapy with Cytoxan®, Ellence® (epirubicin), and Oncovin® (vincristine). Median overall survival was 8 months with chemotherapy alone and 13 months when low-molecular-weight heparin was added to chemotherapy.[96]

- *Scutellaria baicalensis* is used in traditional Chinese medicine and increases blood cell production during chemotherapy (when it is typically reduced, resulting in side effects). It also intensifies bone-marrow activity (erythro- and granulo-cytopoiesis) and the numbers of circulating red and white blood cell precursors.[97,98] Lung cancer patients who took *Scutellaria baicalensis* extract during chemotherapy had a beneficial increase in the number of immunoglobulins and maintained their relative number of T cells.[98]

- Coenzyme Q10 protects the heart from damage typically caused by doxorubicin, cytoxan, and 5-fluorouracil.[89]

- A clinical study tested the efficacy of high-dose multiple antioxidants (ascorbic acid 6100 mg daily; dl-alpha-tocopherol [vitamin E], 1050 mg daily; and beta-carotene, 60 mg daily) in addition to chemotherapy (Taxol® and carboplatin) in 136 advanced NSCLC patients. The overall survival rates at 1 year were 32.9% in the chemotherapy-alone group and 39.1% in the antioxidants-plus-chemotherapy group. At 2 years, the two groups' survival rates were 11.1% and 15.6%, respectively.[99]

**Hormones and chemotherapy.** Advanced-stage NSCLC patients who have had no previous surgery or chemoradiotherapy may benefit from a combination of hormones and oral chemotherapy. Treatment with melatonin, vitamin D, retinoids, somatostatin, bromocriptine, and the chemotherapy drug Cytoxan® improved survival and quality of life (relieved cough, shortness of breath, pain, fatigue, and insomnia) in NSCLC patients. Median survival time was 12.9 months (range, 1.5–33.5 months), and the overall survival rates at 1 and 2 years were 51.2% and 21.1%, respectively.[100]

**Customizing chemotherapy to the patient.** The concept of customized chemotherapy involves predicting how well proposed chemotherapy drugs will kill a patient's cancer or lower the patient's risk of adverse effects[101] before they are given to the patient. It is critical to extending survival time.[102] Molecular markers in patients' tumors can help predict response to specific chemotherapy drugs.

- Iressa® treatment is linked with favorable survival in NSCLC patients whose tumors have low levels of ribonucleotide reductase.[91,103]

- The ability of 5-fluorouracil to kill lung cancer cells depends on the activity of dihydropyrimidine dehydrogenase and thymidylate synthase in patients' tumors.[104,105]

- The responsiveness of NSCLC to Iressa® and Tarceva® depends on the presence of epidermal growth factor receptor (EGFR) mutations in the tumor.[106]

- The response to Taxol® and Navelbine® depends on tubulin III and stathmin mRNA levels in tumor cells. High levels of tubulin III are associated with a poor response to chemotherapy and a shorter progression-free survival.[107]

- If the tumor shows BRCA1 and ERCC1 (genes involved in DNA repair pathways), then cisplatin, carboplatin, and taxanes will not be effective in killing the tumor, resulting in poor survival.[108,109]

For more details, see the Chemotherapy protocol.

# INTEGRATIVE CANCER THERAPY

## Hormones

Estrogens and peptide hormones play important roles in the development and progression of lung cancer, whereas melatonin and thyroid hormones are pivotal in the stabilization and inhibition of lung cancer in men.[110,111]

**Estrogens.** Whether produced in the body or obtained through hormone replacement therapy, estrogens may be involved in lung cancer development and progression.[112,113] Lung cancer tissue contains an abundance of estrogen receptors, which are not found in normal lung tissue, thus opening up a possibility of antiestrogen therapy for patients with advanced lung cancer displaying estrogen receptors in their tumors.[114]

If a patient's lung cancer displays estrogen receptors, then reducing estrogen levels in the body (because estrogen stimulates cancer growth), in addition to standard treatments, is potentially beneficial. Because body fat is a source of estrogen, it is important to establish and maintain a healthy weight.[115] In addition, the following nutritional supplements with natural antiestrogen properties show promise:

- Melatonin has multiple antiestrogen actions and decreases estradiol levels in the body.[116,117]

- Vitamin K2 (menaquinone), known for its blood coagulation effects, decreases the ratio of estradiol to estrone, slowing down estrogen activity.[118]

Furthermore, estrogen levels in the body can be lowered by counteracting obesity (see Obesity and Weight Loss protocol) and keeping a low-fat diet.[119–121]

**Peptide hormones.** Peptide hormones act as growth factors and increase lung cancer growth.[122] For example, SCLC and NSCLC both produce gastrin-releasing peptide (GRP), neurotensin and adrenomedullin, which are growth factors that increase lung cancer growth.[122] However, growth factor antagonists prevent SCLC growth in vitro and have been studied in phase 3 clinical trials.[123] These growth factor antagonists may provide new treatments for SCLC patients in the future.

**Melatonin.** The most widely investigated anticancer hormone is melatonin.[124] It has been used both alone and in combination with most standard cancer treatments because it improves both survival and quality of life.[125] Advanced lung cancer patients show a progressive reduction in melatonin levels,[126] and their daily sleep-wake patterns are disrupted.[127,128] However, even in patients for whom no other standard treatment is offered, melatonin with aloe vera extract stabilizes the cancer growth and improves survival.[128]

In a study of 100 lung cancer patients randomized to receive either chemotherapy alone or chemotherapy with melatonin (20 mg/day orally), the 5-year survival rates were significantly higher for the group of patients who received melatonin. In addition, no patient treated with chemotherapy alone was alive after 2 years, whereas 5-year survival was achieved in 3 of 49 patients (6%) treated with chemotherapy and melatonin. Furthermore, lung cancer patients treated with melatonin tolerate chemotherapy better and have less-serious side effects.[129–131]

**Thyroid hormones.** Thyroid stimulating hormone (TSH) controls 25% of the body's metabolism, thereby affecting how quickly cells (including cancer cells) grow and die. Therefore, making the thyroid underactive (a condition known as hypothyroidism) by reducing TSH levels in the body may slow down cancer growth. Hypothyroidism can be achieved artificially with the prescription drugs propylthiouracil (PTU) or Tapazole®.

A patient originally diagnosed with metastatic lung cancer (ie, lung cancer that had spread throughout the body) was admitted to the hospital because of a rare complication of underactive thyroid disease (ie, hypothyroidism) called myxedema coma. This rare clinical condition can be caused by insufficient thyroid hormone (T4) replacement, infection, cold exposure, trauma, or the drug amiodarone (which causes thyroid hormone abnormalities).[132] The myxedema coma occurred just 2 months after the patient was diagnosed with metastatic lung cancer. On examination for myxedema coma, the patient was found to have no evidence of remaining cancer, and 5 years later the lung cancer had still not returned (ie, he remained in remission). It was concluded that spontaneous remission (complete permanent disappearance) of the lung cancer had occurred due to a severe deficiency of thyroid hormone; in other words, thyroid hormone deprivation had induced total tumor cell death.[133,134]

If a lung cancer patient also has hypothyroidism or subclinical hypothyroidism, it may be wise to avoid taking too much thyroid hormone to correct this condition. By contrast, if a lung cancer patient has an overactive thyroid (hyperthyroidism), it is essential to reduce the levels of the thyroid hormones triiodothyronine (T3) and T4 to normal (or lower) as quickly as possible (typically with PTU or Tapazole®) because hypothyroidism or inadequate thyroid hormone replacement prolongs survival of lung cancer patients, and in some cases, causes spontaneous remission of the lung cancer.[135] TSH, T3, and T4 can be measured by a simple blood test.

## COMPLEMENTARY ALTERNATIVE THERAPIES

Vitamin and mineral supplementation is associated with longer survival and quality of life in NSCLC patients. Median survival is 4.3 years for NSCLC patients who supplement with vitamins and minerals versus 2 years for those who do not use such supplements.[136] As the statistics on conventional treatment outcomes for lung cancer remain disappointing, vitamin and mineral supplementation combined with complementary alternative therapies should be considered to help control lung cancer, maintain quality of life, and prolong survival.[28] It is particularly important for advanced lung cancer patients to incorporate novel and integrative nutritional supplementation into their treatment regimens.

### Apigenin

Apigenin, a flavone (ie, a class of flavonoids) that is present in fruits and vegetables (eg, onions, oranges, tea, celery, artichoke, and parsley) has been shown to possess anti-inflammatory, antioxidant, and anticancer properties. Many studies have confirmed the cancer chemopreventive effects of apigenin.[137]

Apigenin inhibits expression of vascular endothelial growth factor (VEGF) and angiogenesis in lung cancer cells.[138] It was observed in a study that apigenin suppressed the proliferation of lung cancer cells and increased their susceptibility to antitumor drugs.[139]

### Astragalus

Astragalus, an herb used for centuries in Asia, has exhibited immune-stimulatory effects. Astragalus potentiates lymphokine-activated killer cells.[140] One study found that astragalus could partially restore depressed immune function in tumor-bearing mice,[141] while another concluded that "astragalus could exhibit antitumor effects, which might be achieved through activating the ... anti-tumor immune mechanism of the host."[142]

In a 2003 study, individuals with advanced lung cancer received injectable astragalus. The 1-year survival rate was 46.8% in the astragalus group compared to 30% in the control group.[143] In 2006, researchers conducted a review to evaluate evidence from trials using Astragalus-based herbal medicine combined with platinum-based chemotherapy in patients with advanced non-small cell lung cancer. The researchers identified 12 studies with a total of 940 subjects that reported a 33% decreased risk of death at 1 year in those receiving astragalus-based Chinese herbal combinations compared to chemotherapy alone. Additionally, 9 studies were identified with a total of 768 subjects that reported a 27% decreased risk of death at 2 years in favor of those receiving astragalus-based Chinese herbal combinations compared to chemotherapy alone.[144]

### Vitamin D

As previously outlined in the "Surgery" section, vitamin D improves survival in early-stage NSCLC patients.[76] Therefore, vitamin D supplementation is recommended for lung cancer patients planning to undergo surgery, particularly during the winter season, and especially for those with darker skin, and for vegans who have limited sun exposure. Experimental studies show that vitamin D protects against lung cancer progression by preventing cancer spread (metastases).[145] Sources of vitamin D include sunlight, milk, and dark-colored fish.

### Adenosine Triphosphate (ATP)

Adenosine triphosphate (ATP) is produced in the body and provides energy to cells. In nonrandomized studies involving advanced NSCLC patients, ATP infusions slowed weight loss and deterioration of quality of life.[146] A randomized trial showed that

ATP infusions (20–75 mg/kg/min for 30 hours at 2- to 4-week intervals) have beneficial effects on weight, muscle strength, energy levels, and quality of life in patients with advanced NSCLC.[147]

Intravenous ATP infusions work by restoring liver energy levels in patients with advanced lung cancer[148] and counteracting tissue loss.[149] ATP is taken up by red blood cells and reaches levels 50–70% above baseline concentrations at approximately 24 hours.[150] In addition, preclinical studies showed that ATP administration may improve the anticancer effects of chemotherapy,[151] radiotherapy,[152] and may also have protective effects against tissue damage caused by radiation.[153]

## Green Tea

A phase 1 clinical trial in advanced NSCLC patients determined that high doses of green tea extract (3 g/m² daily) are well tolerated and stabilize cancer in some patients.[154] Based on their results, the researchers proposed that green tea extract might be useful in preventing cancer progression in those at high risk for lung cancer relapse (following completion of treatment for early-stage lung cancer) or in those at high risk of developing a second cancer. In addition, green tea extract could be considered in combination with standard chemotherapy agents in advanced lung cancer.[154]

Green tea extract can be taken safely for at least 6 months at an oral dose of 7–8 Japanese cups (120 mL), 3 times daily.[155] The side effects of green tea extract are caffeine related. However, preclinical studies found that caffeine contributes to the prevention of tumor growth.[156,157] Therefore, decaffeinated green tea extract may be less effective.

## Alpha-Tocopherol

High levels of alpha-tocopherol (50 mg), if taken during the early critical stages of lung cancer initiation, may prevent lung cancer development.[158] Alpha-tocopheryl succinate hinders the initiation and progression of lung cancer by preventing COX activity and blocking inflammatory responses mediated by prostaglandin E2.[58]

## Pomegranate

Pomegranate, which is rich in antioxidants, has gained widespread popularity as a functional food (ie, has health benefits). The health benefits of the fruit, juice(s), and extract(s) have been studied in relation to a variety of chronic diseases, including cancer.[159,160] Pomegranate extract provides significant protection against experimentally induced lung cancer. Researchers observed that 8 months of pomegranate supplementation reduced lung tumor formation by 66% in mice exposed to lung carcinogens.[161] Another study found that pomegranate fruit extract inhibited the formation of tumor growth in mice implanted with lung cancer cells, leading the authors to conclude that "pomegranate fruit extract can be a useful chemopreventive/chemotherapeutic agent against human lung cancer."[162]

## Polysaccharide K (PSK)

PSK, which is a specially prepared polysaccharide extract from the mushroom *Coriolus versicolor*, has been studied extensively in Japan where it is used as a nonspecific biological response modifier to enhance the immune system in cancer patients.[163–165] PSK suppresses tumor cell invasiveness by downregulating several invasion-related factors.[166] PSK has been shown to enhance NK cell activity in multiple studies.[167–170]

In a clinical trial, individuals with stages 1–3 lung cancer received radiation therapy with or without PSK. Researchers observed that the 5-year survival was 39% in the PSK group compared to 17% in the control (stages 1 and 2) and 26% in the PSK group compared to 8% in the control (stage 3).[171] Similar results were obtained by these same researchers in a previous study.[172]

## Quercetin

Quercetin is a flavonoid found in a broad range of foods, from grape skins and red onions to green tea and tomatoes. Quercetin's antioxidant and anti-inflammatory properties protect cellular DNA from cancer-inducing mutations.[173] Quercetin traps developing cancer cells in the early phases of their replicative cycle, effectively preventing further malignant development and promoting cancer cell death.[174] Furthermore, quercetin favorably modulates chemical signaling pathways that are abnormal in cancer cells.[175,176]

Quercetin inhibits the growth of lung cancer cells.[174,177] In one experiment, laboratory rats were treated with quercetin (25 mg/kg body weight) before exposure to benzo(a)pyrene, a powerful environmental carcinogen found in cigarette smoke, charbroiled foods, and automobile (particularly diesel) exhaust, making it among the most common pollutants in the environment. While untreated rats developed lung cancers, those supplemented first with quercetin showed no such findings.[178]

## Selenium

Selenium protects against lung cancer, especially in populations in which average selenium intakes are low.[179–181] Family members of lung cancer patients were found to have selenium levels significantly lower than those of healthy controls.[182] At pharmacologic doses, selenium may act as an adjuvant treatment for lung cancer.[183] A phase 3 multicenter clinical trial is investigating whether daily selenium supplementation is effective in preventing the growth of new tumors in NSCLC patients whose tumors were surgically removed; details are available at www.clinicaltrials.gov.

## Novel Nutritional Supplements

The following nutritional supplements have been investigated in lung cancer patients and found to be without adverse effects; however, optimum doses have not yet been established:

- N-acetylcysteine[184,185]
- R-lipoic acid[186]
- Zinc[187]
- Magnesium[188]
- *Scutellaria baicalensis*[97,98]

The following nutritional supplements have shown promising affects against lung cancer in experimental studies, although clinical studies have not yet been carried out:

- Curcumin[189]
- Ginseng[190]
- Garlic[191]
- Lycopene[192]
- GLA[193]
- Silibinin[194]
- Grape seed proanthocyanidins[70]
- Black tea polyphenols[69]
- Genistein from soy[195,196]

Lung cancer patients are invited to call Life Extension at 1-800-544-4440 for updated information on optimal dosages of the above nutrients.

# PREVENTING LUNG CANCER

To lower the risk of lung cancer, the following interventions are recommended.

## Stop Smoking

Smokers should stop smoking (by using nicotine replacement therapy, Zyban®, and counseling) because at present there are no known dietary changes that can guarantee prevention or lower the occurrence of lung cancer in smokers. Medicinal herbal tea made from cloves and milk vetch reduces smoking withdrawal symptoms and increases the rate of smoking cessation.[17]

## Test Your Home for Radon

Read the section titled "Causes of Lung Cancer" to learn why this is important and to find important sources for more information.

## Take Aspirin

Take aspirin regularly if your physician approves.[34]

## Monitor Your Diet

Smokers, ex-smokers, and people who have never smoked should all consume 5 or more servings of colorful vegetables (including raw, darkly colored, and root vegetables) and fruits daily to achieve serum levels of micronutrients associated with the lowest risk of lung cancer. A diet rich in tomatoes, tomato-based products (containing lycopene), citrus fruits, and carotenoids (lutein, zeaxanthin, beta-cryptoxanthin, and retinol) reduces the risk of lung cancer.[197] Egg yolk is a bioavailable source of lutein and zeaxanthin.[198] Good food sources of carotenoids are spinach, kale, carrots, cantaloupes, cherries, and sweet potatoes.

Phytoestrogens (plant estrogens) from food sources are associated with a decrease in the risk of lung cancer in both current smokers and people who never smoked, but less so in former smokers. Food phytoestrogens include isoflavones, phytosterols, and lignans. High intake of the lignans enterolactone and enterodiol and use of hormone therapy are associated with a 50% reduction in the risk of lung cancer.[199] The soy isoflavone genistein significantly prevented lung tumor formation and cancer metastasis in mice.[200] Phytoestrogens are also available as nutritional supplements.

## Consider Antioxidants

Studies examining the role of antioxidants in lung cancer have gained significant attention. In the 1990s, a study was launched to determine if alpha-tocopherol and beta-carotene could reduce the risk of cancer, particularly lung cancer. The study, however, indicated that lung cancer incidence increased among people who took beta-carotene. These results were later replicated in a study that tested a combination of beta-carotene and vitamin A. Additional studies found that beta-carotene raised the risk of lung cancer among smokers.[201]

However, newer studies have examined the role that dosage plays and found that low-dose antioxidants, including beta-carotene, in combination with additional antioxidants may reduce the incidence of lung cancer. One study tested the effectiveness of daily, low-dose antioxidant supplementation with vitamins (vitamin C, 120 mg; vitamin E, 30 mg; and beta-carotene, 6 mg) and minerals (selenium, 100 mcg; and zinc, 20 mg) in reducing the frequency of cancers. After 7.5 years of supplementation, this low-dose antioxidant regimen lowered total cancer occurrences and deaths in men but not in women.[202] Based on these study results, Life Extension recommends that people at high risk for lung cancer avoid high doses of beta-carotene but supplement with low-dose antioxidants to reduce their risk of lung cancer.

## Add Folate and Vitamin B12

Folate and vitamin B12 reduce abnormal bronchial cell growth in smokers.[35]

## Take Alpha-Tocopherol

In the Alpha-Tocopherol, Beta-Carotene Cancer Prevention Study, higher serum alpha-tocopherol status was associated with lower lung cancer risk. Alpha-tocopherol supplementation may reduce the risk of lung cancer associated with increased smoking exposure for some people more than for others, depending on hereditary factors.[203]

## Drink Green Tea

Consumption of green tea by nonsmoking women is associated with a reduced risk of lung cancer, and the risks decrease with increased consumption.[204] Experimental studies consistently show that green tea and its polyphenols (eg, EGCG) can slow the growth of, and kill, lung cancer cells.[205]

# FOR MORE INFORMATION

The complications related to lung cancer treatment can be acute (such as low blood cell counts) and chronic (heart and lung damage). For more information, please refer to the following protocols:

- Cancer Surgery
- Chemotherapy
- Cancer Vaccines and Immunotherapy
- Blood Disorders (Anemia, Leukopenia, and Thrombocytopenia)
- Heavy Metal Detoxification

## Life Extension Suggestions

For optimal results, nutritional supplements or dietary changes should be introduced before starting lung cancer treatment.

Life Extension suggests:

- **Apigenin:** 20–50 mg daily
- **Astragalus:** 2000–4000 mg daily
- **Coenzyme Q10:** 100–400 mg daily
- **Folate:** 800–1600 mcg daily
- **Green tea extract:** up to 5.7 g daily
- **Melatonin:** 20 mg nightly
- **Multivitamin-multimineral supplement** (without copper): per label instructions
- **N-acetylcysteine:** 1200 mg daily
- **Perillyl alcohol:** 2050 mg, 4 times daily
- **Pomegranate:** 280–375 mg daily of punicalagins
- **PSK** (from the mushroom *Coriolus versicolor*): 3 g daily
- **PSP** (from the mushroom *Coriolus versicolor*): 2 g daily
- **Quercetin:** 1000–3000 mg daily
- **R-lipoic acid:** 300 mg daily
- **Selenium:** 200–400 mcg daily
- **Vitamin B12:** 500–1000 mcg daily
- **Vitamin C:** 2500 mg daily
- **Vitamin D:** 800 IU daily
- **Vitamin E:** 400 IU daily with at least 200 mg gamma tocopherol
- **Vitamin K2:** 10 mg daily
- **Proteolytic enzymes:** 3 tablets, 2 times daily, at least 45 minutes before meals
- **Zinc:** 20 mg daily

### Innovative Drug Strategies

- **ATP intravenous infusion:** 20–75 mg/kg per minute for 30 hours at 2–4 week intervals (must be performed by a qualified physician)
- **Celebrex®:** 200 mg twice daily
- **Medroxyprogesterone:** 500 mg twice daily
- **Trental®** (pentoxifylline): 400 mg, 3 times daily
- **PTU or Tapazole®, low-molecular-weight heparin, nicotine replacement therapy (eg, Zyban®), and aspirin:** Appropriate dosages of these pharmaceutical drugs should be discussed with your treating physician.

### REFERENCES

References available at: www.lef.org/dpt5/ch87

# 88

# Lupus: Systemic Lupus Erythematosus (SLE)

Lupus is a systemic *autoimmune* disease driven by *inflammation* in which the immune system indiscriminately attacks "self-tissues" throughout the body. It is estimated that more than 16000 people are diagnosed with lupus each year in the United States. Approximately 1.5 million Americans, and 5 million people worldwide, currently live with lupus.[1]

Lupus autoimmunity can cause variable symptoms from person to person. Parts of the body frequently affected by lupus include the skin, kidneys, heart and vascular system, nervous system, connective tissues, musculoskeletal system, and other organ systems.

The immune system is the primary facilitator of lupus; therefore, its treatment requires a strategy that successfully targets immune cells. Unfortunately, conventional medicine typically relies on global *immune suppression* to accomplish this goal, inadvertently predisposing patients to potentially *deadly* infections and a host of troubling side effects.

However, advancements in medical technology in recent years have led to the development of promising new medical therapies for lupus. These include the use of *monoclonal antibodies* targeted against cells of the immune system responsible for lupus autoimmunity, and *stem cell therapy*, which aims to replace aberrant immune cells with healthy immune cells in order to suppress autoreactivity.

Moreover, mounting evidence suggests that *vitamin D* may be a critical *missing link* in virtually all autoimmune diseases, including lupus. Vitamin D is capable of *modulating* the activity of immune cells, and studies have identified widespread vitamin D *deficiency* in lupus patients.[2,3] For example, one study found that a mere *1.2%* of lupus patients had adequate vitamin D levels, compared to 45% of healthy controls[4]; another found that *lower* vitamin D levels were linked with more *aggressive* lupus autoimmunity.[5]

Life Extension's strategy is centered on *easing inflammation* and combines several scientifically studied nutrients to complement the *immunomodulatory* role of vitamin D. Additionally, avoiding inflammatory foods high in omega-6 fatty acids in favor of healthy omega-3s provides a nutritional foundation ideal for balancing an inappropriately reactive immune system.

## EPIDEMIOLOGY

The population most affected by lupus is women of childbearing age—that is, women between the ages of 15 and 44 years.[1] Lupus is also more likely to develop in African-American, Asian-American, Native-American, and Latina women compared to Caucasian women.[6] However, it is possible for lupus to develop in people of any age group, race, or either gender.

Women with lupus are more likely to have high-risk pregnancies than those without this chronic disease. One study found that these women have a 3- to 7-fold greater risk of developing low platelet levels (thrombocytopenia), infection, and blood clots (thrombosis).[7] Women who experience a "flare" within 6 months of conception are much more likely to experience complications during the pregnancy affecting their own health. Additionally, the fetuses and neonates of individuals who experience a flare during pregnancy are more likely to have complications.[8] Consequently, doctors generally advise women with lupus to plan pregnancies after 12–18 months of remission, and definitely not before 6 months of remission.[9]

## TYPES OF LUPUS

The term "lupus" commonly refers to systemic lupus erythematosus (SLE), but there are other types of lupus as well, each with distinct signs and symptoms.[10]

### Systemic Lupus Erythematosus

This is the disease often simply referred to as "lupus." The word "systemic" refers to the fact that connective tissues throughout the body are affected; "erythematosus" is a clinical state in which red, raised patches develop on the skin. When referring to lupus elsewhere in this chapter, we are referring to this form of the disease.

### Discoid Lupus Erythematosus

This form of lupus is distinct from SLE in that the symptoms are only skin related; discoid lupus erythematosus causes a red rash, often developing on the face and/or scalp. People with discoid lupus often also have SLE, or develop SLE in the future.

### Drug-Induced Lupus

Certain medications can potentially cause lupus, but the condition generally goes away after stopping the triggering drug. The medications that can possibly cause drug-induced lupus include some oral contraceptive drugs, certain blood pressure–lowering drugs, and antibiotics and antifungal medications.

Specific drugs most frequently associated with drug-induced lupus include:

- Procainamide (antiarrhythmic)
- Hydralazine (antihypertensive)
- Quinidine (antiarrhythmic)

### Neonatal Lupus

As the name indicates, this form of lupus develops in newborn infants. This form of lupus is quite rare, and is caused by autoantibodies being transmitted from a mother with lupus to the baby.[11] Although most of the babies born of women with lupus are healthy,[6] more than half of infants with neonatal lupus have problems with their skin, heart, and/or gallbladder.[12,13] Neonatal lupus may spontaneously resolve over the first few months of life, but can sometimes cause serious complications. Death occurs in approximately 10% of neonatal lupus cases, the major causes of which are typically pneumonia or heart complications.[13]

## LUPUS SIGNS, SYMPTOMS, AND DIAGNOSIS

Lupus is a complex disease with varying manifestations. Some people have many symptoms; others have only a few. The symptoms in some individuals are severe, while those in others remain mild. Both genetic (inherited) and environmental factors influence the development and severity of lupus symptoms.

Because of these characteristics, doctors sometimes have difficulty in correctly diagnosing lupus.

People with lupus have periods in which they are feeling well, called *remission*, and periods of worsening symptoms, called *flares*. Lupus patients can often predict the onset of flares due to specific warning signs, such as worsening fatigue and/or onset of headache, fever, dizziness, rash, and/or pain.[14] Being able to recognize warning signs is important because catching and treating flares early can prevent them from becoming severe.

The most commonly occurring symptoms of lupus include[10,15]:

- Intense fatigue
- Painful and/or swollen joints
- Muscle pain
- Red rash on the face and/or in response to sitting in the sun
- Pain in the chest after taking a deep breath
- Unexplained fever
- Edema (swelling), often in the legs or around the eyes
- Mouth sores
- Unexplained hair loss
- Raynaud's phenomenon, which is characterized by cold fingers and/or toes that are pale or purple in color.

In 1982, the American College of Rheumatology published a method for doctors to use for diagnosing lupus (Table 1). They then updated these criteria in 1997, and they have remained the same ever since. Lupus is generally diagnosed when an individual exhibits 4 or more of the criteria.

**Table 1:   Eleven Criteria Used in Diagnosis of Lupus, by American College of Rheumatology***

| Criterion | Signs/Symptoms | Test |
|---|---|---|
| Malar rash | Red rash on the cheeks and the bridge of the nose; often called a "butterfly rash" | Physical exam, medical history |
| Discoid rash | Raised, hard patches of scaly skin | Physical exam, medical history |
| Photosensitivity | Red skin rash caused by exposure to sunlight | Physical exam, medical history |
| Oral ulcers | Sores in the mouth, usually painless | Physical exam, medical history |
| Nonerosive arthritis | Inflammation in 1 or more joints, making them feel tender and swollen. Cartilage, which is protective tissue surrounding the bone, remains intact | Physical exam, medical history, x-ray |
| Pleuritis and/or pericarditis | Inflammation of lung or heart lining, respectively; may cause pain when breathing deeply; growing tired easily | Lung function test; chest x-ray to look for fluid in the lungs; cardiac stress test; echocardiogram, which uses sound waves to visualize the heart |
| Neurologic disorder | Reduced or abnormal brain function, headaches, seizures, memory loss, difficulty concentrating | Physical exam, medical history, brain MRI (magnetic resonance imaging); produces high-resolution image of the brain |

**Table 1:   Eleven Criteria Used in Diagnosis of Lupus, by American College of Rheumatology\*—cont'd**

| Criterion | Signs/Symptoms | Test |
|---|---|---|
| Kidney disorder | Usually no symptoms; signs are blood or high levels of protein in the urine | Urinalysis |
| Blood disorder | Anemia (low red blood cell levels) with associated fatigue, dizziness, shortness of breath; increased susceptibility to infection; slow clotting, excessive bleeding | CBC (complete blood count); test for abnormal cell counts of platelets, red blood cells, lymphocytes, and/or leukocytes |
| Immunologic disorder | Possible increased susceptibility to infection, inflammation in various organ systems | Assorted tests to detect antibodies from a blood sample |
| Positive antinuclear antibodies | Possible increased susceptibility to infection, inflammation in various organ systems | ANA (antinuclear antibody) test; test for the presence of antibodies that bind the cell nucleus, which is where the DNA that makes up genetic material is stored |

\*These criteria are based on the common lupus signs and symptoms. Lupus is diagnosed when any 4 or more criteria are present.[15,16]

Doctors assess lupus severity by calculating a *systemic lupus erythematosus disease activity index* (SLEDAI) score. Based on the presence or absence of various lupus signs and symptoms over the preceding 10 days, a total score is calculated. For example, protein present in the urine would result in 1 point, and another point would be added if a new rash had appeared. One point is assigned for each symptom or sign present and the greater the score, the more severe the disease at that time. A mild or moderate flare is defined as a change in the SLEDAI score of ≥3 points; a severe flare is diagnosed when the SLEDAI score has increased by ≥12 points.[15,16]

## LUPUS PATHOPHYSIOLOGY

### Inflammation and Tissue Injury

The principal cause of lupus-mediated tissue injury is inflammation triggered by *autoantibody complexes*.

B cells, so-called because these immune cells originate in the bone marrow, produce and secrete the antibodies, which are specialized proteins that bind to other molecules. The immune system generates millions of different antibodies that target an extremely large variety of molecules on the surface of microbes, such as bacteria and viruses. The antibody binds its specific molecule on a microbe in similar fashion to a key in a certain lock. When the "key" (antibody) and "lock" (microbe) fit together, the antibody sticks tightly to the microbe and marks it to be removed from the body. In people with lupus, many of the B cells secrete *autoantibodies*, which means that these antibodies bind to molecules on otherwise healthy tissues instead of molecules on microbes.

T cells, which are generated in the thymus, produce various proteins called cytokines that help B cells grow, become activated, and stimulate B cells to produce antibodies. Other immune cells, including macrophages and neutrophils, migrate to the site of inflammation and produce tissue damaging *reactive oxygen species* (ROS), as well as engulf microbes and cells through a process called *phagocytosis*. One of the ways that macrophages know when to engulf a microbe is by sensing that antibodies are stuck to their surface. All of these cells collectively are called leukocytes or white blood cells because of their lack of color. B and T cells are a subset of leukocytes called lymphocytes.

The types of self-molecules ("the lock") that stick to autoantibodies ("the key") vary in each case of lupus. Self-molecules common in lupus often are associated with the cell nucleus, which is the compartment within a cell that contains DNA and other proteins that make up genes.

Lupus-mediated tissue damage can be summarized as follows:

1. B cells become activated and produce autoantibodies that bind various self-molecules.

2. Activated T cells produce proteins called cytokines that help activate more B cells.

3. Large complexes of antibodies stuck to self-molecules are formed.

4. These complexes become lodged in various tissues throughout the body, such as the kidney and joints.

5. The complexes cause an influx of neutrophils, macrophages, and other B cells and T cells into the tissue.

6. Proinflammatory cells secrete damaging reactive oxygen species and more proteins that cause tissue damage.

7. If the inflammation is not treated and persists over time, the tissue may become permanently damaged.

## VITAMIN D BALANCES IMMUNE REACTIVITY IN AUTOIMMUNE DISEASES

Vitamin D intervenes in the process of autoimmunity by tilting the properties of T and B cells toward "tolerance" of self tissues. Tolerance is a phenomenon orchestrated by a variety of highly specialized cytokines and other cell-signaling molecules.

Early in the developmental process of immune cells, they are directed to become either "effector" or "regulatory" immune cells. In other words, they become immune cells that *promote* tissue destruction, or those that *suppress* tissue destruction.

Patients with lupus have elevated numbers of effector cells and lower numbers of regulatory cells.[17] Moreover, the regulatory cells of lupus patients are malfunctional.[17] Vitamin D exerts multiple actions at the cellular level to balance the population of effector cells and regulatory cells.[18] In a 2012 study, 20 lupus patients with initially low vitamin D blood levels received 100000 International Units (IU) of vitamin D weekly for 4 weeks, followed by 100000 IU monthly for 6 months. The treatment resulted in significantly increased vitamin D blood levels (from 18 ng/mL at baseline to 51 ng/mL at 2- and 6-month follow-ups), decreased effector T cell counts and anti-DNA antibodies, and increased regulatory T-cells. Over the 6-month follow-up period, no disease flares were noted (Terrier 2012).[18] These lines of evidence establish a very strong case for the importance of maintaining sufficient vitamin D blood levels to combat lupus disease activity. Life Extension suggests an optimal vitamin D blood level of 50–80 ng/mL (measured as 25-hydroxyvitamin D).

## Kidneys

Kidney disease is a common complication in people with lupus; in fact, almost 50% of those with lupus have some degree of kidney disease.[6] Like other affected tissues in lupus, damaging inflammation from autoimmune attack causes a kidney disease called *lupus nephritis*.

The circulatory system delivers blood to the glomeruli, which are the small filtering units of the kidneys, through small capillaries. Glomeruli help to regulate blood pressure and electrolytes by removing or reabsorbing fluids and salt according to the body's needs. In people with lupus, the large autoantibodies/antigen complexes that circulate in the blood can become lodged in the glomeruli and cause damaging inflammation. The onset of kidney complications generally occurs at least 5 years after the onset of lupus symptoms.

A healthy kidney only allows small molecules like salts to be removed from the body, and allows large protein molecules to remain in the blood. However, kidney disease—including that caused by lupus nephritis—causes proteins to leak out of the kidney into urine. High levels of protein in the urine, clinically called *proteinuria*, are indicative of kidney damage. A normal level of protein in a 24-hour urine sample is below 300 mg.[19]

### Heart and Cardiovascular

People with lupus are at a significantly increased risk of developing coronary artery disease (CAD). One study found that women between the ages of 35 and 44 who had lupus were 50 *times* more likely to have a heart attack than counterparts without lupus.[20] Additionally, heart disease is one of the most common causes of death for people with lupus.[21] This increased heart disease risk in people with lupus is caused by a several different factors,[22] including:

• Lupus-mediated inflammation can directly damage the endothelium, the lining of blood vessels, ultimately leading to atherosclerosis.

• Type 2 diabetes, high blood pressure, and high cholesterol, are more likely to be present in people with lupus, all of which make the risk of heart disease greater.

• People with lupus are often less active because of various symptoms such as fatigue, joint pain, and muscle pain. A low degree of activity is associated with unhealthy weight gain and high blood pressure, both of which are risk factors of heart disease.

People with lupus should be sure to do everything they can to take care of their heart and vascular system. The *Life Extension Magazine* article titled "How to Circumvent 17 Independent Heart Attack Risk Factors" is an excellent resource to help ensure that every risk factor for cardiovascular disease is addressed.

### Nervous System

Lupus may also damage the nervous system. The possible signs and symptoms include confusion, excessive tiredness, seizures, difficulty concentrating, and/or headaches.[23] The exact mechanisms causing nervous system damage in lupus are still being investigated, but are likely due to 2 principal factors[10,24]:

• Specific autoantibodies may inappropriately target molecules on nerve cells, causing inflammation and subsequent nerve damage.

• Inflammation in and around blood vessels prevents the delivery of the nutrients and oxygen nerves need to stay healthy.

Additional signs and symptoms of nervous system involvement in lupus include a very stiff neck reminiscent of meningitis, a high fever, psychosis, and/or seizures.[25] Severe neurologic disease in lupus can lead to coma and even death, and therefore immediate emergency medical attention should be sought at the first sign of these symptoms.

## Muscles

Lupus also causes muscle pain, but fortunately, the strength of the muscle is not affected. Up to 16% of people with lupus experience this painful symptom, which commonly affects the arms and upper thighs.[26]

## Bones

Loss of bone density is more common in people with lupus, which can lead to osteoporosis and a greater risk of fracture. The disease itself, and/or disease-related inactivity, can contribute to osteoporosis risk. However, exercise is often difficult or painful for individuals with lupus because of joint and muscle pain and stiffness. Additionally, certain conventional medications used to treat lupus, such as corticosteroids, can also accelerate bone loss.[6]

## Blood Disorders

These disorders are, unfortunately, very common in people with lupus. Four potentially severe lupus-associated complications are blood count abnormalities. Blood cell counts are typically measured as number of cells in 1 mm$^3$ (cubic millimeter) of blood.

*Anemia:* Too few red blood cells. A complete blood count (CBC) is a common blood test in which all of the blood cell types are counted in a fixed volume. Normal results for men are 4.7–6.1 million red blood cells per microliter of blood, and normal results for women are 4.2–5.4 million red blood cells per microliter.[27]

*Thrombocytopenia:* Too few platelets in the blood. Platelets are small cell fragments that, when activated, stick together to form blood clots. Too few platelets may cause a delay in clot formation and excessive bleeding. Normal levels are between 150 000 and 450 000 platelets per cubic millimeter[28]; thrombocytopenia in context of lupus is defined as platelet levels below 100 000 per cubic millimeter.[29]

*Leukopenia:* A reduced level of leukocytes, also called white blood cells due to their lack of color. Defined as a count below 4000 per cubic millimeter.[29] Leukopenia increases the risk of potentially severe infections.

*Lymphopenia:* A reduced level of a subset of white blood cells called lymphocytes, defined as a count below 1500/mm$^3$.[29] B and T cells fall broadly into the leukocyte group and can be more specifically defined lymphocytes. Lymphopenia also increases the risk of severe infections.

## The Hormone Connection

The link between sex hormones and lupus disease activity has been the subject of debate for decades. The fact that women are considerably more likely to develop autoimmune diseases than men suggests that steroid hormones, especially estrogen and progesterone, influence the immune system.

Estrogen actions tend to be proinflammatory, while the actions of progesterone, androgens, and glucocorticoids are anti-inflammatory.[30] Studies have documented low progesterone levels in women with lupus, suggesting that a relative imbalance in favor of estrogen may contribute to immune reactivity in some female patients.[31]

Accordingly, studies in women with lupus revealed an increased rate of mild- to moderate-intensity disease flares associated with estrogen-containing hormone replacement therapy.[32] Experimental studies have suggested that testosterone may suppress immune reactivity in lupus animal models and in cells from patients with lupus.[33,34]

Based on the available data, Life Extension suggests that women with lupus evaluate their sex hormone levels and ensure that progesterone and testosterone levels are sufficient. If progesterone or testosterone levels are found to be low, women should consider using bioidentical progesterone and/or testosterone creams to restore levels to a normal range.[35]

# CONVENTIONAL MEDICINE'S APPROACH TO LUPUS TREATMENT

Since lupus potentially targets multiple organ systems, the type of treatment should be tailored for each individual person. Doctors may prescribe 1, 2, or more medicines at a time to maximize treatment response. An effective overall treatment strategy includes maintaining a healthy lifestyle—which may include conventional medicine, complementary medicine, exercise, good nutrition, and avoiding smoking and excessive sunlight—in order to reduce the frequency and severity of lupus flares. It is important to consider both the positive and detrimental effects of any treatment type before commencing a treatment plan.

## Anti-Inflammatory Drugs

Several categories of conventional medications are available that reduce inflammation, which is the chief cause of symptoms in lupus. Many of these medicines are often quite effective at reducing symptoms and preventing severe flare-ups. Unfortunately, these medicines are commonly associated with significant adverse long-term side effects.

### Corticosteroids

Corticosteroids (glucocorticoids) are one type of steroid with powerful, anti-inflammatory effects. Synthetic corticosteroids mimic the effects of natural corticosteroids produced in the body and effectively reduce inflammation in people with lupus.

The most common corticosteroid medicine prescribed to treat lupus is *prednisone*. It may be taken orally in pill form, or injected into the skin to treat rashes, or intramuscularly (IM) to treat muscle inflammation. Other corticosteroids include hydrocortisone, dexamethasone, and methylprednisolone.

The possible side effects of corticosteroids include easy bruising, fat redistribution leading to an increase in fat around the abdomen, weight gain and insulin resistance, and psychological changes ranging from irritability and depression to euphoria. They may also lead to increased risk of complications from diabetes, high blood pressure, and glaucoma, and may cause elevated triglyceride and cholesterol levels. If taken over the long term, corticosteroids cause bone loss and therefore lead to an elevated risk of bone fracture. Due to effects on triglyceride and cholesterol, long-term corticosteroid use could also contribute to an increased risk for atherosclerosis.[36]

Due to these potentially severe side effects, the lowest dose of corticosteroids that provides symptom relief is prescribed. Injected corticosteroids are typically used only to treat very severe disease flares; once symptoms come under control, oral administration is resumed.[36-37]

### NSAIDs

Like corticosteroids, nonsteroidal anti-inflammatory drugs (NSAIDs) also suppress inflammation. However, NSAIDs are less effective for individuals with severe lupus than corticosteroids. NSAIDs, of which there are more than 20 types available, are both anti-inflammatory and analgesic, meaning they provide pain relief as well as reduce inflammation. Examples of NSAIDs include ibuprofen and naproxen. Although adverse effects are possible, and these risks are elevated in people with lupus, administration of NSAIDS with close monitoring by physicians can be helpful.[38]

NSAIDs operate by inhibiting the secretion of leukotrienes and prostaglandins that cause inflammation and pain. Possible side effects include stomach upset, nausea, and even gastrointestinal bleeding, fluid retention, kidney damage, and increases in blood pressure and heart attack risk.[39]

---

*Aspirin* may be particularly helpful in individuals who have antiphospholipid antibodies, which can make blood particularly "sticky" and prone to clotting. In the case of patients who are discovered to have antiphospholipid antibodies without any known thrombotic problems, the question of preventive (prophylactic) treatment is unresolved. Currently, aspirin is the general recommendation.[40]

Due to aspirin's blood-thinning, anti-inflammatory, and analgesic effects, doctors may recommend taking low-dose aspirin to reduce the risk of heart disease in people with lupus and relieve the pain of aching joints.[41]

---

## Antimalarial Drugs

Although the original purpose was to treat the parasitic disease malaria, it was discovered more than 50 years ago that antimalarial drugs were also effective in treating the symptoms of lupus through minor immune suppression. In people with lupus, these drugs have been shown to reduce inflammation in the lining of the lung (pleurisy) and heart (pericarditis), improve joint and muscle pain, and reduce fever and fatigue. Examples of antimalarials include chloroquine, hydroxychloroquine, and quinacrine.[42-44]

Possible side effects include gastrointestinal symptoms like nausea, vomiting, diarrhea, and stomach cramps; headache, dizziness, and irritability; and the skin may darken in color and become very dry.[44]

## Immune System Modulators

Immune system modulators treat lupus by altering the number or function of immune cells. As lupus is an immune-mediated disease, this approach is often effective.

Some immune system modulating drugs globally suppress the immune system, and are thus called immunosuppressives. While the self-reactive immune cells are suppressed, the cells that fight against infections are also inhibited, which can lead to increased susceptibility to infections. Potentially severe side effects may occur with all immunosuppressive drugs. Examples of commonly prescribed immunosuppressive drugs are discussed in following sections.

### Cyclophosphamide

Cyclophosphamide has been used for several decades and is quite effective in treating lupus-related kidney disease. However, the side effects of cyclophosphamide can be severe and include nausea, vomiting, infertility, and hair loss. One study indicates that low-dose cyclophosphamide is still effective in treating individuals with lupus nephritis.[45]

## Mycophenolate Mofetil

This medicine is newer, more effective, and causes fewer side effects than cyclophosphamide. Due to these positive characteristics, mycophenolate mofetil has replaced cyclophosphamide as the first-line drug for the treatment of lupus.[46–48]

## Azathioprine

Azathioprine is an immunosuppressive drug that also has fewer severe side effects than cyclophosphamide, and overall, data suggest that it is similar in effectiveness.[49]

## Monoclonal Antibodies

When an antibody "sticks" to the surface of a cell, it either blocks its function and/or tags the cell for removal from the body. Scientists have taken advantage of this quality of antibodies to design ones that stick to and induce the clearance of many different cell types, including B and T cells.

Monoclonal antibodies are created through a complex process involving culturing specialized immune cells with disease-specific stimuli (antigens) and purifying the antibodies that are produced as a result.

Monoclonal antibodies represent one of the greatest advancements in lupus treatment in recent history. The advent of monoclonal antibodies targeted towards receptors on the surface of B-cells allows physicians to turn the immune system against itself, in a sense, and eradicate self-reactive B-cells that underlie lupus pathology.

The Food and Drug Administration (FDA) has approved a few of these drugs to treat some diseases, especially certain types of cancer. Monoclonal antibodies also show promise as drugs to treat lupus.

One monoclonal antibody drug recently approved by the FDA to treat lupus is *belimumab*, which targets *B-cell activating factor* (BAFF), a protein involved in activation, differentiation, and proliferation of B cells.[50–52] The FDA's approval of belimumab for the treatment of lupus is a groundbreaking achievement, as this is the first new drug developed specifically for lupus that has been approved for the last 50 years.[50] Belimumab is co-marketed by Human Genome Sciences and GlaxoSmithKline under the name Benlysta®, with cost estimates exceeding $30 000 annually. However, insurance should cover this therapy in most cases, as few new therapeutic options for lupus exist.[53]

*Rituximab* is also a monoclonal antibody drug that targets a receptor on B-cell surfaces called *CD20*, thereby causing the immune system to destroy B cells. It was originally approved to treat lymphoma, and may be effective in other diseases characterized by too many or malfunctional B cells, including lupus.

Currently, studies are mixed as to whether this drug is effective in treating lupus.[54] Rituximab is not approved to treat lupus, but is often used off-label for this purpose by many physicians.

Other monoclonal antibody drugs that may be effective in treating lupus and are still being studied include epratuzumab, abetimus, ocrelizumab, and atacicept, all of which target B cells.[54] Additional drugs are being developed and tested with targets such as T cells and proinflammatory proteins.

Currently, monoclonal antibody drugs face several challenges and may cause adverse reactions in some patients. However, scientists are quickly elucidating the role of particular proteins and receptors in the molecular physiology of lupus, and it is very likely that monoclonal antibody therapy will become much more efficacious in the near future.

## A Novel Approach: Stem Cells

A stem cell is unique in that it is a nonspecific cell type and has the potential to develop into many different types of specialized cells. These cells can divide and produce another stem cell to replenish themselves or grow into specialized cells, such as nerve cells, brain cells, or B cells.

Stem cell transplantation has the potential to revolutionize the treatment of several types of diseases. In this procedure, stem cells are taken from a person, grown in the laboratory into specialized cells, and then transplanted back into the individual to replace diseased cells. To treat lupus, one approach is to take blood stem cells from a person with lupus and grow them in the laboratory into healthy new B and T cells that do not attack self-tissues. The next step is to replace the autoimmune B and T cells in an individual with the individual's own new, healthy B and T cells.

This general approach is called *autologous hematopoietic stem cell transplantation*. The word "autologous" refers to the fact that the transplanted blood cells are derived from the person's own stem cells; "hematopoietic" refers to the fact that the type of stem cell used is the precursor of blood cells like B and T cells. As of 2011, approximately 200 stem cell transplantations for the treatment of lupus have taken place.[55]

Data regarding the safety and efficacy of autologous stem cell transplantation is not yet plentiful, but some studies suggest that this treatment approach may be promising.

For example, in one small clinical study conducted in China, the disease status of almost 65% of patients did not get any worse over 7 years.[56] A comprehensive review of several studies that investigated autologous hematopoietic stem cell transplantation revealed that, in total, 81% of those that survived at least 3 years beyond the procedure showed some positive response to treatment.[57] However, it is important to note that this analysis also found that an average of 11% of people who participated in these types of studies ultimately died because of transplant-related causes.

Stem cell transplantation is currently reserved for individuals with very severe disease who have not responded to conventional lupus treatments. In this population specifically, a remarkable 50% probability of 5-year, disease-free survival was achieved in the 2 largest studies to date exploring stem cell transplantation as a therapeutic option for lupus.[55]

## THE INFLUENCE OF LIFESTYLE ON DISEASE ACTIVITY

Lifestyle, including diet, physical activity, and stress levels, can have a potent effect on many chronic diseases, including lupus. A healthy lifestyle is an important factor in preventing flares, reducing disease severity, and improving overall quality of life.

The level of stress an individual with lupus experiences can significantly affect disease. Whether this stress comes from work, finances, relationships, or from managing this chronic disease, it can trigger flares or worsen lupus severity. A recent study found that the people with lupus who had a greater ability to cope with stress reported better quality of life.[58] Additional data suggest that people who participate in a short stress-management program may have less pain.[59]

Ultraviolet (UV) light from the sun can cause or exacerbate the skin lesions often associated with lupus, and therefore avoiding or reducing exposure to the sun may be necessary for some people to avoid triggering these symptoms. One study found that photosensitivity was tightly linked with lupus disease, irrespective of the type of lupus, the level of serum autoantibodies, and use of anti-inflammatory medications.[60] Fortunately, avoiding sun exposure or applying sunscreen is quite effective in preventing the damaging effects of UV light.[61] Ironically, the need to avoid exposure to sunlight may exacerbate the widespread vitamin D deficiency in lupus patients.

Exercising regularly is important for everyone's health, but is especially important for individuals with lupus. Exercise helps prevent inflamed joints from becoming excessively stiff and keeps muscles, bones, and cartilage strong.[62] Physical activity has also been shown to improve physical fitness in individuals with lupus, but can also help improve feelings of depression and overall quality of life.[63] Exercise can be daunting to those who are already feeling ill because of lupus, but remaining active is an important part of remaining as healthy as possible, even during flares. Those feeling too ill for more vigorous exercise can participate in gentle range-of-motion exercises so that muscles and joints can remain as flexible as possible.

One small pilot study with individuals with lupus confirmed that both aerobic exercise and the more gentle range-of-motion exercises are safe for people with lupus and did not worsen signs or symptoms.[64]

## NUTRITION AND LUPUS DISEASE ACTIVITY

### Vitamin D

Vitamin D is an essential nutrient, and the precursor to the active form is produced in the skin after absorbing ultraviolet light. Other sources of vitamin D include fatty fish like salmon and mackerel; fortified foods like margarine, milk, and breakfast cereals; and vitamin D supplements.[65]

Studies have shown that vitamin D may be important in reducing the risk of lupus.[66] It has been shown that higher blood levels of vitamin D are associated with less severe lupus disease activity.[67]

Two observational studies found that women with systemic lupus erythematosus have significantly lower levels of 25-hydroxy vitamin D.[2,68] Another study found that while 22% of healthy control women had a deficiency in vitamin D, 69% of women with lupus exhibited a deficiency in this vitamin.[5]

Reduced levels of vitamin D in people with lupus may be due to 1 or both of 2 possible scenarios: (1) the deficiency is related to the disease itself, or (2) the deficiency is caused/exacerbated by avoiding sun exposure due to increased photosensitivity of individuals with lupus.

As discussed above, lupus and some of its treatments can cause bone loss and lead to osteoporosis. Healthy levels of vitamin D are necessary to help the body absorb calcium and keep bones as strong as possible and this is especially important in individuals with lupus.

Life Extension suggests that 25-hydroxyvitamin D levels be kept between 50 and 80 ng/ml for optimal health. This usually necessitates supplementation with 5000–8000 IU of vitamin D daily for most individuals. However, supplemental doses should always be determined based on blood test results.

### Fish Oil

The oil from fatty fish, such as mackerel, tuna, salmon, and halibut, is especially rich in omega-3 fatty acids.[69]

Fish oil is rich in 2 types of omega-3 fatty acids: docosahexaenoic acid (DHA) and eicosapentaenoic acid (EPA).

Omega-3 fatty acids, also sometimes referred to as polyunsaturated fatty acids (PUFAs), promote health in a number of ways. EPA and DHA are of particular interest in autoimmune diseases, including lupus.

Similar to vitamins, the body needs EPA and DHA, but can only produce them in very limited quantities. Therefore, these fatty acids must be included in the diet in adequate amounts.[70]

Recent evidence has revealed a critical role for EPA and DHA in establishing balanced immunity in autoimmune disease. Experimental studies found that EPA was able to induce immune cells into a regulatory phenotype, thus countering the action of aggressive effector immune cells.[71]

Two clinical studies found that taking fish oil reduced lupus severity.[72,73] Another study found that taking fish oil reduced the level of serum lipids in people with lupus,[74] which may be useful as they are at a greater risk of developing heart disease.

The ratio between inflammatory omega-6 fatty acids and anti-inflammatory, omega-3 fatty acids in the blood is of critical importance in autoimmune diseases. If the ratio is too high, disease activity may increase.[75] Life Extension recommends that everyone strive to maintain an *omega-6 to omega-3 ratio of 4:1 or lower*. Readers can learn more about the importance of the omega-6 to omega-3 ratio and how to test it in the *Life Extension Magazine* article titled "Optimize Your Omega-3 Status."

## Minerals and Vitamins
### Vitamin E

There are several forms of vitamin E, 4 tocopherols and 4 tocotrienols, each of which has different levels of activity in the human body. Vitamin E has been shown to reduce several different markers of inflammation in the body, including inflammatory cytokines.[76] Since inflammation is responsible for the widespread tissue damage in lupus, antioxidant vitamins may aid in prevention or delay of the disease.

Vitamin E helps stabilize membranes of lysosomes, or immune cells that contain destructive enzymes used to fight intruders. When membranes are unstable, these enzymes cause damage to surrounding healthy tissue. Vitamin E can help prevent the onset of auto-immune attacks by stabilizing membranes of lysosomes.[77] The symptoms of mice with lupus that were treated with vitamin E greatly improved. The mice lived longer, immune cell activity was normalized,

anti-DNA antibodies were reduced, and kidney function improved.[78]

One study indicates that vitamin E can reduce the level of autoantibodies in lupus patients,[79] but further studies are needed to confirm these effects. A case report of 2 patients indicates that a topical formula containing vitamin E improves the health of skin in people with discoid lupus erythematosus.[44]

### Vitamin A

The active form of vitamin A, called retinol, is important for healthy skin, bones, and soft tissues,[80] and supports healthy immune function.[81] Since people with lupus have an abnormally functioning immune system and a higher risk of osteoporosis, healthy vitamin A levels are especially important for this population. Interestingly, one study showed that people with lupus consumed less vitamin A in their diets than age-matched healthy controls, which may contribute to a vitamin A deficiency.[82]

Consumption of beta-carotene, a vitamin A precursor, is an ideal way to ensure that vitamin A levels are sufficient while simultaneously avoiding vitamin A toxicity. The body will convert beta-carotene into active vitamin A as necessary and excrete any excess.

## Plants and Herbs
### Curcumin

Curcumin, a bioactive derivative of the spice turmeric, has been tested over the last several years for its antioxidant, anticancer, and anti-inflammatory clinical properties. Curcumin decreases the ability of lupus autoantibodies to bind their specific antigens an average of 52%.[83] The damaging inflammation of lupus-mediated injury is facilitated by the binding of autoantibodies to protein and nucleic acid antigens. Therefore, successful blocking of antigen/autoantibody binding suppresses inflammation before it even begins.

Experimental studies have revealed a considerable role for curcumin in modulating inflammatory crosstalk between cells of the immune system by suppressing cytokines such as IL-1β, IL-6, IL-12, and TNFα.[84] Moreover, a recent animal model of an autoimmune disease identified NF-κB suppression as a key mechanism behind curcumin's anti-inflammatory action.

A clinical trial tested the effects of curcumin in 24 patients with the lupus-associated kidney disease lupus nephritis. One group of patients took 500 mg of turmeric daily over a 3-month period, which is equivalent to a daily curcumin dose of 22.1 mg. Compared to the placebo control group, the turmeric group exhibited significant improvement in proteinuria.[85]

Although some clinical studies have been conducted showing some signs and symptoms are reduced in some autoimmune diseases such as multiple sclerosis and rheumatoid arthritis, clinical studies have not yet been conducted to determine if curcumin has a similar effect with lupus.[84] However, these results are promising and suggest potential beneficial effects of curcumin in people with lupus.

### Ginkgo

*Ginkgo biloba*, or more simply "ginkgo," is an herb that has been used for thousands of years in traditional Chinese medicine. This nutrient is often prepared by making an extract from the dried leaves. Such extracts contain high concentrations of molecules called flavonoids and terpenoids, which are antioxidants and improve blood flow, respectively.[86]

A clinical study revealed that taking 120 mg of *Ginkgo biloba* extract 3 times per day for 10 weeks significantly reduced the number of Raynaud's phenomenon attacks, a set of symptoms that often affect people with lupus.[87]

### Pine Bark Extract

There is evidence that extract from the bark of the pine tree (*Pinus pinaster*) helps improve lupus inflammation, although more information is likely needed to make definite conclusions about this ingredient.

One study found that administration of pine bark extract reduced oxidative stress and improved lupus signs and symptoms in 6 patients that received the supplement in addition to prescription medications compared to a placebo group.[88] Specifically, the patients who took pine bark extract exhibited a reduction in the SLEDAI score, meaning that disease as a whole was reduced.

## Other Natural Therapies

### Dehydroepiandrosterone (DHEA)

DHEA is a hormone naturally produced by the adrenal gland and is converted into sex hormones. In addition to being produced in the body, DHEA is also present in the Mexican yam, from which it is extracted for use as a nutritional supplement.[80]

Low levels of DHEA-s, a plentiful metabolite of DHEA in humans, have been observed in patients with lupus and other inflammatory diseases.[89] DHEA and its various metabolites exert considerable influence over immune system activity by regulating production of multiple cytokines including IL-2, IL-1, IL-6, and TNFα.[89]

In a clinical trial, when individuals with lupus took 200 mg of DHEA daily for 24 weeks, the number of patients who experienced lupus flares was significantly reduced.[90] In another study, the same investigators showed that taking 200 mg of DHEA daily for 24 weeks reduced blood levels of the cytokine IL-10, which enhances antibody production.[91] This reduction in IL-10 may have contributed to the reduced incidence of lupus flares seen in the first study.

Another double-blind, randomized, controlled trial involving 41 women found that 6 months treatment with 20–30 mg DHEA daily improved mental and emotional well-being in lupus patients.[92] Also, at a dose of 200 mg daily, DHEA improved bone mineral density in postmenopausal women with lupus.[93]

Life Extension suggests that DHEA-s blood levels be kept between 350 and 490 µg/dL for men and 275–400 µg/dL for women in order to achieve optimal immunomodulatory action.

## PLANTS TO AVOID

### Alfalfa

The seeds of the alfalfa plant have the potential to cause transient lupus-like symptoms, including autoimmune-related anemia, in certain people and primates.[94-95] Alfalfa seeds are rich in the amino acid L-canavanine, which was shown to be the responsible triggering agent in humans, and in certain types of mice.[94,96] Due to these potential effects, people with lupus should avoid alfalfa seeds.

### Echinacea

*Echinacea* is an herb that has long been used to promote a strong immune system to prevent infections like the flu and colds.[97] Considering that lupus is a disease characterized by an overactive immune system, people with lupus would likely benefit from staying away from *Echinacea*, which has been shown to be an immune system stimulant. While studies have not yet been conducted to determine the effect of *Echinacea* specifically on lupus, case studies have shown that taking this herb can exacerbate the severity of other autoimmune diseases.[98] Additionally, a number of studies have shown that *Echinacea* can induce human immune cells to secrete proinflammatory cytokines that are known to play a role in lupus disease.[99] People with lupus should avoid *Echinacea*.

### Tripterygium wilfordii (*Thunder God Vine*)

Some reports exist in the scientific literature suggesting that using thunder god vine, a Chinese herbal, may ameliorate symptoms associated with autoimmune diseases.[100] Due to these reports, thunder god vine is sometimes suggested by alternative health sources to those with lupus. However, Life Extension has reviewed the available scientific literature and concluded that in most cases, the risk outweighs the potential benefit with this plant.

Several reports of severe toxicity and even death associated with the use of thunder god vine are available, and it appears that the dose required for clinical effectiveness is very close to that required to cause toxicity.[101,102] Another report linked thunder god vine use with low bone mineral density in women.[103]

Life Extension does not suggest that use of *Tripterygium wilfordii* outside a clinical setting. If a healthcare practitioner decides to use this therapy with patients, only a standardized extract of the skinned root should be used, as other parts of the plant are highly toxic.[104]

## Life Extension Suggestions

Life Extension's strategy is centered upon *easing inflammation* and combines several scientifically studied nutrients to complement the *immunomodulatory* role of vitamin D. Additionally, avoiding inflammatory foods high in omega-6 fatty acids in favor of healthy omega-3s provides a nutritional foundation ideal for restraining an overactive immune system.

- **Vitamin D:** 5000–8000 IU daily, depending on blood test results
- **Fish oil** (with olive polyphenols): 1400 mg EPA and 1000 mg DHA daily
- **Vitamin E,** as high gamma tocopherol mix with sesame lignans: 359 mg daily
- **Vitamin A,** as beta-carotene: 3000–5000 IU daily

- **Curcumin,** as BCM-95®-enhanced absorption curcumin: 400–800 mg daily
- **Ginkgo biloba,** standardized extract: 120–360 mg daily
- **Pine bark extract:** 75–200 mg daily
- **Dehydroepiandrosterone (DHEA):** 25–200 mg daily (depending on blood levels of DHEA-s)

In addition, the following blood testing resources may be helpful:

- Antinuclear Antibody (ANA)
- Urinalysis
- Chemistry Panel and Complete Blood Count (CBC)
- Vitamin D, 25-Hydroxy
- Omega Score®
- Rheumatoid Factor (RF)
- Female Panel / Male Panel

## REFERENCES

References available at: www.lef.org/dpt5/ch88

# 89

# Lymphoma

More than 60 000 Americans were diagnosed with some form of lymphoma in 2004, and more than 20 000 died from their disease. Lymphomas are linked to a variety of risk factors, including diet, medical history, environmental exposure to chemicals, and infections. To date, conventional medical treatment for lymphoma has been based on combinations of chemotherapy, radiotherapy, and stem cell therapy. However, new treatments for lymphoma now add to these traditional therapies the use of substances that can specifically target the delivery of radiotherapy to lymphoma cells (radioimmunotherapy) or activate the immune system to kill lymphoma cells (chemoimmunotherapy).

Nutritional supplements with demonstrated activity against lymphoma cells include curcumin, genistein from soy extract, vitamins A, C, D, and E, green tea, resveratrol, ginger, fish oil, and garlic. These supplements can be used to complement conventional drugs, and they can be closely monitored for effectiveness with a range of blood tests and diagnostic procedures described in this protocol.

## WHAT IS LYMPHOMA?

The lymphatic system consists of organs such as the lymph nodes, thymus gland, spleen, and bone marrow, which participate in the production and storage of infection-fighting white blood cells (lymphocytes), as well as in the network of vessels that carry these white blood cells around the body. Lymphomas are cancers of the white blood cells (lymphocytes) within the lymphatic system.

There are 2 types of lymphoma[1]:

• Hodgkin's lymphoma, also known as Hodgkin's disease (HD)
• Non-Hodgkin's lymphoma (NHL)

The diagnosis, staging,[2] and general symptoms[3] of lymphoma are summarized in Table 1.

Hodgkin's lymphoma begins in the lymph nodes and is characterized by the presence of Reed-Sternberg cells, which are large, cancerous cells that increase in number with disease progression.[4,5] Evidence suggests that B lymphocytes (B cells), the infection- and tumor-fighting cells that produce antibodies, produce Reed-Sternberg cells.[4-6] However, T lymphocytes (T cells) have also been implicated in rare cases.[5]

Although it can affect any lymph tissue, HD most commonly affects the supraclavicular, high-cervical, or mediastinal lymph nodes.[3] There are 5 different types of Hodgkin's lymphoma.

NHL describes all lymphoma types without Reed-Sternberg cells.[7,8] NHL develops as a result of malignant B and T lymphocytes (white blood cells). B-cell lymphomas are more common and account for over 85% of NHL cases.[7] There are at least 29 different types of NHL; the main types, which can be further classified into subtypes, are summarized in Table 2.

**Table 1: Lymphoma: Symptoms, Diagnosis, and Staging**

|  | Hodgkin's Lymphoma | Non-Hodgkin's Lymphoma |
|---|---|---|
| Symptoms | Swollen lymph nodes<br>Fever<br>Night sweats<br>Weight loss | Swollen lymph nodes<br>Excessive sweating<br>Severe itching<br>Weight loss |
| Diagnosis | Magnetic resonance imaging (MRI)<br>Computed tomography (CT)<br>Tissue biopsy | Similar to that of HD |
| Staging | Ann Arbor Staging Classification system:<br>4 stages (1, 2, 3, and 4)<br>Stage 1: Least serious<br>Stage 4: Most serious<br>or<br>HD is also classified as type A (no symptoms)<br>and B (with fever, sweats, and weight loss) | The Working Formulation:<br>Low grade (slow growing)<br>Intermediate grade<br>High grade (fast growing)<br>or<br>The Revised European American Lymphoma (REAL) system:<br>Indolent (slow growing)<br>Aggressive (fast growing)<br>Highly aggressive |

## Table 2: Different Types of Non-Hodgkin's Lymphoma and Malt (Mucosa-Associated Lymphoid Tissue) Lymphoma

| NHL types | Characteristics |
| --- | --- |
| B-cell lymphoma | Lymphoma cells have characteristics similar to B cells |
| Burkitt's lymphoma | Associated with a viral infection; common in Africa |
| Cutaneous T-cell lymphoma | Initially involves the skin and lymph nodes |
| Diffuse lymphoma | Lymphoma cells are evenly spread throughout the lymph nodes |
| Follicular lymphoma | Lymphoma cells are concentrated in clusters/follicles in the lymph node |
| High-grade lymphoma | Progresses rapidly if left untreated |
| Low-grade lymphoma | Progresses slowly if left untreated |
| MALT lymphoma | Originates in the intestinal lining |
| Mantle cell lymphoma | Originates in the mantle zone of the lymph node |
| T-cell lymphoma | Lymphoma cells have characteristics similar to T cells |

## LYMPHOMA OCCURRENCE

New cases of Hodgkin's lymphoma represent less than 1% of all cancer cases in the United States. By contrast, NHL is the fifth most common cancer after lung, breast, colorectal, and prostate cancers.[9] Moreover, NHL is among the top 5 causes of cancer-related death,[10,11] and is the leading cause of cancer death in males aged 15–54.[12] U.S. cases of lymphoma for 2004 are summarized in Table 3.[13]

Lymphoma is generally more common in men than in women.[9,14] The incidence of lymphoma also varies by race. Statistics indicate that African Americans are less likely to develop lymphoma than Caucasians.[9,15]

## GENETIC ABNORMALITIES IN LYMPHOMA

Like all cancers, lymphoma begins with damage to the cell's deoxyribonucleic acid (DNA), the molecules

## Table 3: Lymphoma Cases in the United States in 2004 (U.S. National Cancer Institute Seer Data)

| Lymphoma Type | New Cases in 2004 | Deaths in 2004 |
| --- | --- | --- |
| Hodgkin's lymphoma | 7880 (4330 males; 3550 females) | 1320 |
| Non-Hodgkin's lymphoma | 53 370 (28 850 males; 25 520 females) | 19 410 |

containing all the information that determine the structure and function of cells. Within each cell, DNA is housed in structures known as chromosomes, which are made up of sections called genes.

The development of lymphoma begins with damage to the DNA of T cells and B cells (lymphocytes), immune cells that protect the body from infections.[5,7] DNA damage that can start cancer development occurs in genes called oncogenes or tumor-suppressor genes, which play important roles in maintaining a balance between cell death and cell growth.

Excessive cell growth occurs in lymphoma as a result of malfunction of the proteins that control cell growth (leading to permanent cell division) and cell death (making the cell insensitive to normal signals to die). Numerous genetic abnormalities have been implicated in the malfunction of cell controls. Two critical proteins involved in lymphoma development are bcl-2 and bcl-6.

The identification of these genetic irregularities has important implications for treating lymphoma, as it indicates potential targets for manipulation with pharmaceutical drugs or nutritional supplements. For example, pharmacologic agents capable of inactivating bcl-6 can cause increased cell death (apoptosis) in lymphoma cells.[16] Furthermore, in clinical studies, an agent that targets bcl-2 has also been shown to have efficacy in NHL patients.[17]

## CAUSES OF LYMPHOMA

The cause of lymphoma is still a subject of much debate, and many lymphoma patients do not have obvious risk factors.

### Hodgkin's Lymphoma

**Epstein-Barr and herpes viruses.** The Epstein-Barr virus is thought to cause one third of all HD cases.[18] In addition, HD patients often show high numbers of herpes-infected cells.[19] These viruses are thought to contribute to the development of lymphoma[19] and are also linked to the development of NHL.[20,21]

**Weakened immune system.** Individuals with suppressed immune systems associated with HIV (human immune deficiency virus) infection appear to be at higher risk of developing HD.[22,23]

### Non-Hodgkin's Lymphoma

Factors that play a role in susceptibility to NHL include nutrition, medical history, environment, and use of medications.

**Diet/nutrition.** NHL is more common in individuals with weakened immune systems.[24,25] Clinical studies have now shown that diets rich in animal protein and fats, which are thought to diminish immune function,[26-28] are associated with an increased risk of developing NHL.[24,29-31] Clinical studies have also shown that diets rich in fruits and vegetables, which are thought to enhance immune cell function,[32-34] are associated with a reduced risk of developing NHL.[25,35]

**Medical history.** Evidence suggests that some medical conditions or procedures, especially those that reduce immune system activity, increase the risk of developing NHL. These include:

- Blood transfusions and organ transplantation
- Diabetes
- Celiac disease
- Hepatitis C
- Epstein-Barr virus
- Gastric ulcers (*Helicobacter pylori*)
- HIV
- HTLV (human T-lymphotropic virus)
- Herpes

Numerous studies have examined the link between blood transfusions and the development of NHL. However, the data are conflicting, with some studies showing that allogeneic blood transfusions (ie, from other people/donors) are associated with a 2-fold increase in the risk of developing NHL.[36,37] Similarly, the risk of NHL is thought to increase in organ transplant patients,[37] most likely as a result of post-transplant immunosuppression.

In older women, adult-onset (type 2) diabetes of long duration has also been shown to increase the risk of developing NHL.[38] Other clinical studies have also shown that diabetes sufferers are at greater risk of developing NHL,[39] presumably because diabetes impairs the efficiency of the immune system.[40,41]

Celiac disease, a condition characterized by inflammation of the intestinal lining due to sensitivity to a protein called gluten (found in wheat and rye), is also associated with increased risk of developing NHL, particularly localized in the gut.[42-44]

Hepatitis C virus, a common infection in the United States, is linked to the development of B-cell NHL,[45,46] MALT lymphoma,[47] and a rare type of NHL known as primary hepatic lymphoma.[48] Interestingly, this association appears to have some geographical variations, although some studies do not support it.[49,50]

*Helicobacter pylori* infection, normally associated with peptic ulcers, is also linked to the development of gastric MALT lymphomas.[51,52]

The immunosuppression caused by infection with HIV is associated with a greater risk of developing NHL.[53-55] The incidence of NHL in HIV-positive individuals is 60 times greater than that observed in the general population.[55]

The human T-lymphotropic virus, a close relative of HIV, is also known to cause T-cell lymphomas.[56]

**Environment.** Exposure to pesticides and herbicides is associated with an increased risk of developing NHL, particularly in rural farming communities where these substances are used routinely.[57-59] Asthmatics exposed to pesticides have a higher risk of developing NHL compared to nonasthmatics.[60] Chemicals known as dioxins, which are emitted from solid waste incinerators, are thought to increase the risk of NHL.[61] Contamination of drinking water with nitrates is also thought to increase the risk of developing NHL,[62] although other studies show that contamination levels would have to be very high to pose this risk.[63]

**Medications.** Long-term use of medications such as conventional hormone replacement therapy (primarily unopposed estrogens with synthetic, equine-derived estrogens), certain antibiotics, and pain relievers is associated with an increased risk of certain types of NHL.[64-66] In particular, individuals with rheumatoid arthritis who are long-term users of aspirin and other nonsteroidal anti-inflammatory drugs (NSAIDs) have a greater risk of developing NHL.[67]

---

## WHAT YOU HAVE LEARNED SO FAR

- Lymphomas are cancers of the lymphatic tissues that are involved in storage and distribution of infection- and tumor-fighting white blood cells.
- Because lymph tissue is found throughout the body, lymphoma can begin in almost any part of the body and spread to almost any tissue or organ.
- Risk factors linked to the development of lymphoma include diet, medical history, certain viruses, chemical exposure, and conditions that weaken the immune system.
- Swollen lymph nodes and weight loss are possible signs of lymphoma.
- Tests that examine the lymph nodes are used to detect and diagnose lymphoma.
- Medical treatment for lymphoma traditionally has been based on combinations of chemotherapy, radiotherapy, and stem cell therapy.
- Innovative treatments include radioimmunotherapy and chemoimmunotherapy.
- Nutritional supplements that can be used to complement conventional treatments include curcumin, genistein in soy extract, vitamins A, C, D, and E, green tea, resveratrol, ginger, fish oil, and garlic.

## CONVENTIONAL THERAPY

Currently, medical treatment for lymphoma revolves around the following therapies:

- Chemotherapy
- Radiotherapy
- Stem cell therapy

A discussion of how chemotherapy and radiotherapy agents kill blood cancers, and the use of stem cell therapy, is available in the Leukemia protocol.

The standard chemotherapy regimen for NHL, known as CHOP, combines 4 agents: cyclophosphamide, doxorubicin, vincristine, and prednisone.[68–70] Although CHOP has been the accepted "gold standard" for NHL chemotherapy treatment for the past 30 years, its delivery was optimized with a change to a 14-day dose-dense schedule, which increased clinical responses compared to the traditional 21-day schedule.[70] A study showed the effectiveness of another chemotherapy combination (carmustine, doxorubicin, etoposide, vincristine, and cyclophosphamide, plus mitoxantrone, cytarabine, and methotrexate with a factor known as BAVEC-MiMA) for NHL treatment.[71]

The standard chemotherapy combination for HD is known as ABVD (doxorubicin, bleomycin, vinblastine, and dacarbazine).[68]

The use of these chemotherapy agents is often combined with radiotherapy[72] and stem cell therapy.[73]

### Side Effects of Conventional Therapy

Chemotherapy often has a side effect of reducing white blood cell count to very low levels, thereby leaving the patient vulnerable to infections.[74] As with other cancers, the risk of developing lymphoma increases sharply with increasing age.[75] Changes in the aging body reduce the patient's ability to tolerate standard chemotherapy and radiotherapy regimens that are often better suited to the relatively more robust immune systems of young adults.

In particular, the aging body experiences a decline in its ability to make new white blood cells.[76] The use of chemotherapy in elderly patients therefore aggravates this problem because it destroys patients' normal white blood cells, leaving them prone to infections. Readers should refer to the Chemotherapy protocol for a range of prescription drugs that can be taken to reduce this negative side effect of chemotherapy. Readers should also refer to the protocol titled Blood Disorders (Anemia, Leukopenia, and Thrombocytopenia) for other practical guidelines on dealing with reduced white and red blood cells.

Heart disease (cardiomyopathy) is the most important long-term toxicity of Adriamycin® (doxorubicin) administration, which is used to treat both NHL and HD. Several clinical studies suggest that some changes in the heart's electrical activity caused by Adriamycin® may be prevented by coenzyme Q10 (CoQ10) supplementation.[77,78] CoQ10 supplementation has a protective effect on cardiac function during therapy with Adriamycin® in lymphoma patients.[79,80] Some investigators believe that simultaneous CoQ10 and vitamin E supplementation is indicated during Adriamycin® therapy in order to reduce its toxicity and prevent fatal congestive heart failure.[80]

## NEW AND UPCOMING THERAPIES FOR LYMPHOMA

New treatments for lymphomas largely involve the use of established chemotherapy and radiotherapy agents in combination with methods that capitalize on innate features of the immune system. Successful treatment of lymphoma must take into account the patient's age and the role of nutrition in helping the body tolerate and recover from cytotoxic treatments.

### Immunotherapy

B cells, and therefore all lymphomas of B-cell origin, have a molecule on their surface known as CD20.[81] Rituxan® (rituximab) is an antibody designed to bind to CD20 on lymphoma cells.[82] Upon the binding of Rituxan®, a process known as antibody-dependent cell cytotoxicity (ADCC) is initiated; this causes the immune system to destroy the lymphoma cell. Because normal B cells also have CD20 on their cell surface, use of Rituxan® leads to their destruction as well, and patients suffer from low B-cell numbers for approximately 6 months; however, these numbers return to normal 9–12 months after treatment.[82]

In the United States, Rituxan® is already available for the treatment of low-grade or follicular, relapsed NHL.[82] Studies suggest that Rituxan® is also effective against diffuse, large B-cell lymphoma.[83]

### Chemoimmunotherapy

Studies have shown the use of Rituxan® in combination with CHOP chemotherapy to be more effective than CHOP chemotherapy alone in elderly patients with diffuse large B-cell lymphoma.[84] This therapy is also effective in previously untreated mantle cell lymphoma and aggressive recurrent pediatric B-cell large-cell NHL.[85,86]

## Radioimmunotherapy

Radioimmunotherapy is the use of antibodies that target the CD20 molecule on lymphoma cells to specifically deliver the radiation required to destroy the cancer cell.[87] Two such radio-labeled antibodies to CD20 (iodine-131 tositumomab and yttrium-90 [$^{90}$Y] ibritumomab tiuxetan) have been tested against NHL.[88] In 2002, $^{90}$Y ibritumomab tiuxetan was approved in the United States for the treatment of relapsed or refractory low-grade, follicular, or transformed lymphoma; it is commercially available as Zevalin®.[88–92] The second radioimmunotherapy agent, I-131 tositumomab, has also been approved in the United States and is commercially available as Bexxar®.[91]

According to a recent *New York Times* report, 2 potentially life-saving drugs, Zevalin® and Bexxar, are languishing in obscurity, largely due to market forces. These drugs have been approved by the Food and Drug Administration (FDA) for the treatment of lymphoma, including NHL, the fifth most common cancer in the United States. However, only about 10% of eligible patients are receiving the drugs, despite some remarkable results among those few who have been treated with them. Although patients are more likely to respond to Zevalin® or Bexxar than to older, more commonly-used lymphoma treatments—and the newer drugs are better tolerated, with fewer side effects[93]—oncologists have been slow to embrace them.

Part of the problem stems from the fact that the drugs are the first members of a promising new class of treatments, known as radioimmunotherapies. These drugs utilize cutting-edge monoclonal antibody technology to deliver radioactive particles directly to tumor cells. However, while radioactivity is the key to their effectiveness, it is also a stumbling block that has rendered many oncologists reluctant to prescribe them. Due to their radioactivity, they must be administered in a hospital setting. As a result, oncologists must abandon financial incentives they might otherwise reap for prescribing older chemotherapy drugs and coordinate their efforts with additional clinicians. Patients taking the new drugs must also be monitored for changes in blood cell counts.

A single treatment may cost about $25 000, but one treatment is often all that is required to effect remission. The more common alternative—treatment with months of chemotherapy followed by a commonly prescribed drug, Rituxan®—costs about the same.

But Bexxar or Zevalin® are often more effective at stopping the deadly disease. A study found the drugs offer "impressive clinical outcomes (approximately 20%–40% complete response rates and 60%–80% overall response rates for patients with [non-Hodgkin's lymphoma]."[94] Another study reported similar results.[95] An older study compared the newer drugs to Rituxan® and found an overall response rate of "80% for the [Zevalin®] group versus 56% for the [Rituxan®] group." The same study found that 30% of Zevalin® patients experienced complete remission, as opposed to 16% of patients receiving Rituxan®.[96]

Advocates worry the drugs' makers may abandon production if physicians do not overcome their reluctance to use them soon. They hope the as-yet-unreleased results of ongoing clinical trials, designed to assess the efficacy of the drugs among large groups of patients, may finally convince oncologists to embrace their use. According to the *New York Times*, some lymphoma patients have been forced to take matters into their own hands, demanding access to the drugs, often with remarkable results.

## Vaccine Therapy

The use of vaccination as a treatment for lymphoma is also being investigated. Further details on vaccine therapy for lymphoma can be found in the Cancer Vaccines and Immunotherapy protocol.

# NUTRITIONAL THERAPY

Nutritional supplements with demonstrated activity against lymphoma cells include:

## Curcumin

Curcumin, an extract from the spice turmeric, blocks the growth of various types of lymphoma cells, including Burkitt's lymphoma and EBV B-cell lymphomas.[97–99] In addition to arresting the growth of lymphoma cells, curcumin also causes lymphoma cell death by reducing the levels of some genes (c-myc, bcl-2) and mutant p53 proteins.[97,98,100] Curcumin has an additional benefit in that it blocks the production of growth factors that cancer cells require to invade other organs.[101] Clinical studies have shown curcumin supplements to be safe in doses of up to 3.6 g per day.[102]

## Soy Extract

Genistein, found in soy extracts, induces cell death in lymphoma cells.[103,104] It increases the effectiveness of chemotherapy for lymphoma by making cells more susceptible to agents that cause lymphoma cell death.[12] Genistein also reduces the ability of cancer cell spread (angiogenesis) by blocking the production of proteins (angiogenesis growth factors) that cancer cells need to form new blood vessels.[101]

## Vitamins A and D

Natural and synthetic vitamin A (also known as retinoids) promote normal cell differentiation and have been used to treat T-cell lymphomas.[105–107] Vitamin D blocks the growth of lymphoma cells.[108]

## Green Tea

Green tea, which contains epigallocatechin gallate (EGCG), triggers lymphoma cell death.[109,110] In addition, EGCG from green tea reduces the ability of lymphoma cells to invade other organs by blocking the production of growth factors, such as vascular endothelial growth factor (VEGF) and the glycoprotein messenger interleukin-8 (IL-8), which lymphoma cells need to spread.[101]

## Vitamins C and E

In experimental studies, vitamin C has improved the effectiveness of chemotherapy in inducing lymphoma cell death.[111–113] Vitamin E supplements boost the function of immune cells capable of killing lymphoma cells.[114–116] Alpha-tocopheryl succinate, a semisynthetic analogue of vitamin E, is a potential adjuvant in cancer treatment.[117]

## Reishi

The active constituents of Reishi mushrooms include polysaccharides, a unique protein named LZ-8, and triterpenes.[118–120] Among its broad-spectrum immune-boosting effects are the following:

- Reishi promotes specialization of dendritic cells and macrophages, which are essential in allowing the body to react to new threats, vaccines, and cancer cells.[121–125]

- Reishi's effects on dendritic cells have been proven to boost the response to tetanus vaccine; the mushroom's proteins are also under investigation as "adjuvants" to emerging cancer DNA vaccines and other immune-based cancer treatments.[122,126–128]

- Reishi polysaccharide triggers growth and development of bone marrow, where most immune cells are born. Following bone marrow eradication by chemotherapy, reishi increased production of both red and white blood cells.[129] Reishi polysaccharides provide immune-boosting function

to circulating cancer-killing white blood cells of various types.[119]

- Reishi increases numbers and functions of virtually all cell lines in the immune system, such as natural killer cells, antibody-producing B cells, and the T cells responsible for rapid response to a new or "remembered" antigen.[123,130,131]

Laboratory and animal studies confirm that reishi stimulates an appropriate anticancer immune response while quashing a cancer-promoting inflammatory one. A few small human studies have demonstrated reishi's ability to enhance immune function in patients with advanced cancers.[132–134]

Reishi extracts have also proven useful in inducing cell death in various "white blood cell cancers" such as lymphoma, leukemia, and multiple myeloma.[135] In each of these cancer types, reishi mushroom extracts have been shown to prevent new tumors from arising, and in many cases to shrink existing tumors or precancerous masses.[136–139] These effects, because they may stop a tumor in its tracks before it ever reaches a detectable or dangerous size, can be considered successful cancer prevention by immunosurveillance.[136,137]

## Resveratrol

Resveratrol, a naturally occurring substance found in grapes, blocks the growth of lymphoma cells and also increases their rate of cell death.[140,141] Resveratrol sensitizes chemotherapy-resistant lymphoma cells to treatment with paclitaxel-based chemotherapy.[142] Resveratrol also reduces the production of growth factors such as VEGF and IL-8, and theoretically should be beneficial in reducing the ability of lymphoma cells to spread to other organs.[101]

## Ginger

Extracts from ginger, known as galanals A and B, induce cell death in human lymphoma cells.[143]

## Fish Oil

Eicosapentaenoic acid (EPA) found in fish oil induces cell death in lymphoma cells.[144–146] Omega-3 fatty acids in fish oil normalized elevated blood lactic acid in a dose-dependent manner, increasing disease-free survival and survival time for dogs with stage 3 lymphoma.[147]

## Garlic

Garlic extracts can induce death in lymphoma cells.[148,149] In a study, conjugation of a garlic extract to the antibody rituximab (which targets lymphoma cells) led to the death of these cells.[148]

# BLOOD TESTS

Patients are advised to consult their physicians about the following blood tests that can be used to monitor the effectiveness of conventional medical treatment and nutritional supplements for lymphoma.

## Cancer Cell Markers

Several nutritional supplements, including curcumin and ginger extracts, work by reducing the production of proteins such as p53 and bcl-2. Production of these proteins could be monitored to assess the continued effectiveness of therapy.[97,98,143,150,151]

## Angiogenesis Markers

Supplements of green tea, curcumin, resveratrol, and genistein work in part by blocking the production of growth factors, such as VEGF and IL-8, that cancer cells need to spread to other organs.[101] Patients using these nutritional supplements could routinely monitor these growth factors in their blood samples to assess the effectiveness of their therapy and check for disease progression. Reductions in VEGF levels have been linked to treatment response in lymphoma patients.[152]

## Interleukin-6 (IL-6)

Patients could also monitor levels of the cytokine (messenger) IL-6, as reductions in its levels have been linked with treatment response and can be used to forecast survival.[152]

## Beta-2-Microglobulin

Levels of this protein are elevated in lymphoma patients, and monitoring it can be used to assess treatment response and disease progression; levels less than 3.0 mg/L are associated with remission.[69,153]

## Lactate Dehydrogenase

Levels of the enzyme lactate dehydrogenase (LDH) are elevated in lymphoma patients before treatment, and monitoring it can be used to assess response to treatment and forecast survival.[69,154]

## Molecular Monitoring

Lymphoma cells can be detected in samples of blood and bone marrow. However, when these cells are present in very low numbers, molecular monitoring using a technique known as polymerase chain reaction (PCR) is recommended to determine response to treatment and check for remission.[155]

## Calcium Levels

Patients using vitamin D supplements should be monitored for vitamin D toxicity, which can result in abnormally high calcium levels in the blood.[156]

*Physical examination and diagnostic imaging should also be utilized to detect and/or monitor disease progression.*

# FOR MORE INFORMATION

Lymphoma patients may wish to consult the following protocols for additional information.

- Leukemia
- Cancer Radiation Therapy
- Chemotherapy
- Blood Disorders (Anemia, Leukopenia, and Thrombocytopenia)

## Life Extension Suggestions

Lymphoma patients should consult their physicians before using any nutritional supplements while receiving conventional medical treatment. In addition, lymphoma patients using nutritional supplements should enlist their physicians in ensuring the use of blood tests and diagnostic procedures that are essential in monitoring the effectiveness of any adjuvant therapy for lymphoma.

- **Curcumin:** up to 3.2 g daily[102]
- **Soy extract** (containing up to 60 mg of isoflavones): twice daily[157]
- **Vitamin A:** 40000–50000 IU daily[158,159]
- **Vitamin D3:** 16000 IU, 3 times weekly[160]
- **Green tea:** 725 mg, 3 times daily; or 10 cups of Japanese green tea[161,162]
- **Vitamin C:** 2000 mg daily[158]
- **Vitamin E:** 400 IU daily[158]
- **Resveratrol:** 20–40 mg daily[163]
- **Ginger:** up to 6 g daily[164]
- **Fish oil:** 4.8 g of EPA/DHA daily[165]
- **Garlic:** 600 mg of aged garlic extract twice daily
- **Reishi:** 980–3000 mg daily standardized to contain 13.5% polysaccharides and 6% triterpenes

## Blood Test Availability

Cancer cell markers (tumor antigen profile) can be determined via Genzyme Genetics (www.

genzymegenetics.com) and may be ordered by a physician calling (800) 966-4440.

Tests for angiogenesis markers (eg, VEGF) and chemical messengers (IL-6 and IL-8) are available at UCLA's Jonsson Comprehensive Cancer Center (http://www.cancer.mednet.ucla.edu/).

Lactate dehydrogenase (LDH), calcium levels (part of a Chemistry Panel/Complete Blood Count), and IL-6 blood tests are available via Life Extension/National Diagnostics, Inc., and may be ordered by

calling (800) 544-4440 or online at http://www.lef.org/bloodtest/.

X-rays, scans, and physical examinations can be arranged through your physician.

## REFERENCES

References available at: www.lef.org/dpt5/ch89

# 90

# *Male Hormone Restoration*

The significance of testosterone for male sexual function is apparent to most Life Extension members. New insights, however, underscore the critical role that testosterone plays in maintaining youthful neurologic structure and alleviating depression, as well as inducing fat loss in those who are unable to reduce body weight regardless of diet and exercise.

Recent studies have demonstrated that low testosterone in men is strongly associated with metabolic syndrome, type 2 diabetes, cardiovascular disease,[1] and an almost 50% increase in mortality over a 7-year period.[2]

Restoring testosterone to youthful ranges in middle-aged, obese men resulted in an increase in insulin sensitivity as well as a reduction in total cholesterol, fat mass, waist circumference and proinflammatory cytokines associated with atherosclerosis, diabetes, and the metabolic syndrome.[3–5] Testosterone therapy also significantly improved erectile function[6] and improved functional capacity, or the ability to perform physical activity without severe duress, in men with heart failure.[7]

## FACTORS THAT AFFECT TESTOSTERONE LEVELS IN MEN

**DHEA.** Dehydroepiandrosterone (DHEA) is a hormone produced from cholesterol that then follows one of two pathways, both involving two-step enzymatic conversions, to yield either estrogens or testosterone. Thus, levels of DHEA can have a role in determining levels of estrogen and testosterone, although DHEA alone is seldom enough to sufficiently restore testosterone levels in aging men.

**Aromatase.** One of the most important factors that affect testosterone levels and the ratio between testosterone and estrogen is the *aromatase* enzyme. Aromatase converts testosterone to estrogen, further depleting free testosterone levels and increasing estrogen levels.

**Obesity.** Obesity and associated hyperinsulinemia suppress the action of luteinizing hormone (LH) in the testis, which can significantly reduce circulating testosterone levels,[8] even in men under the age of 40.[9] In addition, increased belly fat mass has been correlated with increased aromatase levels.[10]

The vicious circle of low testosterone and obesity has been described as the *hypogonadal/obesity cycle*. In this cycle a low testosterone level results in increased abdominal fat, which in turn leads to increased aromatase activity. This enhances the conversion of testosterone to estrogens, which further reduces testosterone and increases the tendency toward abdominal fat.[11,12]

**Sex Hormone–Binding globulin (SHBG).** Most testosterone circulating in the bloodstream is bound to either *sex hormone–binding globulin* (SHBG) (60%) or albumin (38%). Only a small fraction (2%) is unbound, or "free."[13]

Testosterone binds more tightly to SHBG than to albumin.[14] Consequently, only albumin-bound testosterone and free testosterone constitute the bioavailable forms of testosterone, which are accessible to target tissues and carry out the actions of the essential hormone.[13] Thus the bioavailability of testosterone is influenced by the level of SHBG.

Aging men experience both an increase in aromatase activity and an elevation in SHBG production. The net result is an increase in the ratio of estrogen to testosterone and a decrease in total and free testosterone levels.[15] As will be discussed below, it is crucial that this skewed ratio be balanced.

**Liver Function.** The liver is responsible for removing excess estrogen and SHBG, and any decrease in liver function could exacerbate hormonal imbalances and compromise healthy testosterone levels. Thus it is important that aging men also strive for optimal liver function.

## EFFECTS OF AGE-RELATED DECLINE IN TESTOSTERONE LEVELS AND TESTOSTERONE THERAPY

The exact cause of the age-related reduction in testosterone levels is not known, but is likely the result of a combination of factors, including:

- Increasing body fat (especially belly fat, and therefore increasing aromatase activity)
- Oxidative damage to tissues responsible for the production of testosterone
- Reduction in testicular testosterone synthesis
- Declining levels of precursor molecules, such as DHEA
- Nutritional status and liver function

The consequences of declining testosterone levels are striking.

**Body Composition and Inflammation.** Testosterone affects fat cell metabolism and fat loss in several ways: inhibiting fat storage by blocking a key enzyme called lipoprotein lipase that is necessary for the uptake of fat into the body's fat cells; stimulating fat burning by increasing the number of specific receptors on the fat-cell membrane that release stored fat; increasing insulin sensitivity; enhancing growth of muscle fibers; and decreasing fat deposits. All of these effects promote lean body mass and reduce fat mass.[16,17] Placebo-controlled trials have demonstrated both significant increases in lean body mass and decreases in fat mass after varying courses of testosterone treatment in older men. In these studies, the greatest favorable changes in body composition were seen in participants with low baseline testosterone levels who received testosterone therapy for ≥12 months.[18]

Emergent evidence suggests that maintaining youthful testosterone levels may help aging men avert a variety of inflammation-mediated disease, such as atherosclerosis and arthritis. By powerfully suppressing the activity an enzyme called *5-lipoxygenase*, testosterone calms a fundamental proinflammatory pathway involved in the synthesis of signaling molecules known as *leukotrienes*.[19] Leukotrienes are derivatives of the proinflammatory omega-6 fatty acid *arachidonic acid*; these molecules underlie much of the inflammatory development of asthma and bronchitis, and play a role in the pathology of cardiovascular disease and diabetes as well.[20,21]

In a study involving 184 men with low testosterone levels, 18 weeks of testosterone replacement therapy suppressed markers of inflammation including IL-1β, TNF-α, and C-reactive protein. Moreover, when compared to men who received a placebo control, men receiving testosterone replacement exhibited significant decreases in body weight, and BMI, and waist circumference.[22] The reduction in waist circumference indicates that testosterone reduces fat accumulation around the trunk of the body; this is particularly important since central fat mass and is strongly associated with increased susceptibility to inflammatory diseases and mortality.[23]

**Musculoskeletal System.** Bone integrity rests upon a balance between bone formation and bone resorption, which is controlled by multiple factors, including levels of estrogen and testosterone.[24,25] In a clinical trial, testosterone increased bone mineral density in elderly men.[26] Testosterone supplementation also has a positive effect on muscle metabolism and strength.[27] This positive effect is undiminished with age.

**Central Nervous System (CNS).** Key to aging well is an optimistic outlook on life and the ability to engage in social and physical activity. However, low levels of testosterone have been associated with depression and other psychological disorders.[28] To make matters worse for aging men, many conventional antidepressant medications suppress libido. Some experts suggest that testosterone therapy might reduce the need for the antidepressant medications entirely.[29,30] Furthermore, testosterone treatment often increases feelings of well-being.[31]

Cognition and alertness are also governed, in part, by testosterone's effects on the CNS.[32] Low testosterone levels have been shown to correlate with lower scores on various psychometric tests,[33] and similar effects have been reported in men undergoing androgen (male hormone) deprivation therapy for prostate cancer.[34]

Testosterone also acts as an endogenous neuroprotective agent, able to support neuron integrity against a variety of toxic insults, including oxidative stress.[35,36] In addition, testosterone has been shown to reduce β-amyloid accumulation, an important pathophysiologic factor in Alzheimer's disease.[37,38]

Testosterone improves neuron survival in brain regions vulnerable to neurodegenerative disease. This may explain the association of low testosterone levels in men with neurodegenerative diseases.[39,40] Studies demonstrate testosterone loss occurred 5 to 10 years prior to Alzheimer's disease diagnosis. This suggests low testosterone is an important risk factor for Alzheimer's disease.[41,42] In a clinical study of 36 men recently diagnosed with Alzheimer's disease, intramuscular testosterone treatment with 200 mg every 2 weeks for up to 1 year was associated with improvement in both overall cognitive ability as well as critical visual-spatial function.[43].

**Glucose and Lipid Metabolism.** Testosterone also has been linked to metabolic function in the body. Specifically, studies have found inverse associations between the severity of metabolic syndrome, a condition characterized by excess abdominal fat, high cholesterol and high blood pressure that predisposes one for cardiovascular disease, and low plasma testosterone.[18,44] A clinical study demonstrated that men with low testosterone levels are twice as insulin resistant as their counterparts with normal testosterone levels, and 90% met the criteria for the metabolic syndrome.[45]

There also appears to be an inverse relationship between low testosterone levels and diabetes in men.[46] Men with diabetes have lower testosterone levels compared to men without a history of diabetes.[47] The

Third National Health and Nutrition survey of 1413 men showed that men initially ranked in the lowest one-third with respect to either free or bioavailable testosterone were approximately 4 times more likely to have prevalent diabetes compared to those ranked in the top one-third, after researchers adjusted the results for age, race/ethnicity, and adiposity.[48]

**Cardiovascular Health.** While conventional thought has been that because more men die from heart attacks than women, the disparity must have something to do with testosterone. However, research is pointing out that, in fact, the opposite may be true. Low levels of testosterone appear to be correlated with several cardiovascular risk factors, including atherogenic lipid profiles, insulin resistance, obesity, and a propensity to clot.[49] In addition, recent research is showing a clear relationship between low testosterone levels and increased incidence of cardiovascular disease and mortality in men.[2]

**Prostate Health.** Compared to younger men, older males have much more estradiol (a potent form of estrogen) than free testosterone circulating in the body. These rising estrogen and declining androgen levels are even more sharply defined in the prostate gland.

Estrogen levels increase significantly in the prostate with age, and estrogen levels in prostate gland tissues rise even higher in men who have benign prostatic hyperplasia (BPH).[50–52]

An important study indicates that testosterone is beneficial for the prostate gland in the vast majority of cases. In this study researchers looked at multiple parameters, including prostate volume, prostate-specific antigen (PSA) levels, and lower urinary tract symptoms in a group of men with low or low-normal testosterone levels.[53] Of the 207 men studied, 187 responded favorably to testosterone treatment.

# THE IMPORTANCE OF HORMONE TESTING

Millions of aging men have the dual conditions of low testosterone and high cholesterol. Conventional physicians prescribe cholesterol-lowering drugs to reduce cholesterol, when, in fact, the age-related rise in cholesterol might simply be the body's way of increasing hormone levels by supplying the raw materials necessary to make hormones.[54] Researchers at the Life Extension Foundation have successfully treated high cholesterol levels through a program of bioidentical hormone replacement therapy.

Life Extension believes that comprehensive tests, along with a careful physical examination,

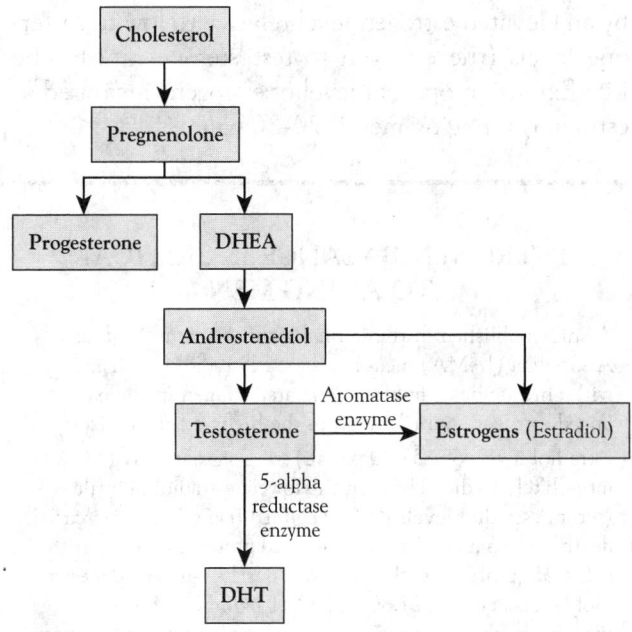

Simplified Hormone Cascade

are essential in detecting hormonal imbalances in aging men.

The so-called "normal" levels of testosterone in older men reflect population averages. The Life Extension Foundation believes that most aging men would prefer not to accept the loss of youthful vigor as normal. Instead, we suggest that a more valid optimal level for all men would be in the upper one-third of the reference range used for men aged 21–49 years, and that any supplementation should aim to restore hormone levels to that range. The current Life Extension optimal level of free testosterone is 20–25 pg/mL.

When measuring testosterone levels, it is critical to determine the levels of both *free* and *total* testosterone to understand the cause of any observed symptoms of deficiency.[55]

Because of difficulties with equipment standardization and interlaboratory variability, it is recommended that physicians consistently use the same local laboratories and gain familiarity with the accuracy, precision and definition of normal values for the assays offered in their communities.[13]

It is also important to remember that blood levels of both free and total testosterone vary widely among individuals, making it difficult to establish a general baseline on which to prescribe a standardized treatment protocol. However, levels are quite consistent within individuals, and thus it is important that men have multiple tests over time to determine trends and individual thresholds for treatment.

Finally, during the initial testing, it is also imperative to test estrogen levels. Many of the unwanted effects of male hormone imbalance are actually caused by an elevated estrogen level relative to low testosterone levels (the estrogen to testosterone ratio). The Life Extension optimal level of estrogen (measured as estradiol) for aging men is 20–30 pg/mL.

## ESTROGEN BALANCE IS CRITICAL TO AGING MEN

A study published in the *Journal of the American Medical Association* (JAMA) measured blood estradiol in 501 men with chronic heart failure. Compared to men in the balanced estrogen quintile, men in the highest quintile (serum estradiol levels of ≥37.40 pg/mL) were significantly (133%) more likely to die. Those in the lowest estradiol quintile (serum estradiol levels <12.90 pg/mL) had a 317% increased death rate compared to the balanced group. The men in the *balanced* quintile—with the fewest deaths—had serum estradiol levels between 21.80 and 30.11 pg/mL.[56] This is the ideal range that Life Extension has long recommended that men strive for.

An epidemic problem that we at Life Extension observe in aging men is insufficient free testosterone, ie, <20–25 pg/mL of serum. When accompanied by excess estradiol (>30 pg/mL of serum), this can signal excess aromatase enzyme activity.

## TESTOSTERONE REPLACEMENT THERAPIES

Optimal testosterone treatment usually requires a physician's prescription. Integrative physicians typically prescribe bioidentical testosterone creams (available from compounding pharmacies). Conventional physicians are more likely to prescribe prepackaged, testosterone patches and/or gels from pharmaceutical companies that have sought Food and Drug Administration approval for the mass commercialization of their products.

All forms of bioidentical testosterone have the same molecular structure and will increase free and total testosterone in the blood. The major difference is that prepackaged versions could cost up to 10 times more per dose than compounded versions. Furthermore, prepackaged testosterone gels are sold only in a limited number of doses, whereas compounded testosterone can be formulated at virtually any dose the physician feels is clinically necessary and useful.

## USING HORMONE REPLACEMENT WISELY

If a man opts for testosterone therapy (available orally or as an injection, subcutaneous implant, topical cream, gel, or skin patch), he should keep several facts and precautions in mind[57,58]:

- Hormone replacement should not be initiated without comprehensive testing.
- The patterns and trends over time of multiple hormone levels, (for instance free testosterone, total testosterone, and estrogen), determine the specific hormone replacements required.
- It may not be safe to use large amounts of testosterone in any form without also using aromatase-inhibiting supplements or medications.
- Because of the risk of worsening prostate cancer, careful screening, including a digital rectal examination and prostate specific antigen (PSA) screening, must be done before starting any hormone replacement program. However, recent research indicates that low endogenous testosterone levels may present a greater risk for prostate cancer than higher levels.[59,60] If a man already has prostate cancer, however, testosterone replacement should be delayed until the underlying cancer is eradicated.
- A man contemplating hormone replacement, whether through a prescription or supplements, should work closely with a qualified physician to plan a rational treatment approach that includes continued monitoring and screening.
- There is no "one size fits all" treatment. Individuals vary, and hormone replacement can be a simple or complex process and often requires careful attention to signs and symptoms, as well as laboratory testing.

## BOOST TESTOSTERONE AND SUPPRESS ESTROGEN LEVELS NATURALLY

For men who choose not to (or are advised not to) use hormone replacement therapy, nutrients can play a vital role in a comprehensive program designed to reduce the impact of aging on sex hormone production and metabolism. The following is a list of nutrients that are part of the Life Extension Foundation's comprehensive male hormone restoration program:

### Essential Nutrients for Optimal Testosterone Production

**Zinc.** This mineral is involved in almost every aspect of male reproduction, including testosterone metabolism, sperm formation, and sperm motility.[61] A prime example of the usefulness of zinc was illustrated in a study of 37 infertile men with decreased testosterone levels and associated low sperm counts.[62] The men were given 60 mg of zinc daily for 45–50 days. In the majority of patients, testosterone levels significantly increased and mean sperm count rose from 8 million to 20 million. Some men require higher levels of zinc to adequately suppress aromatase.

**L-Carnitine.** L-carnitine is an amino acid derivative that may be more active than testosterone in aging men who have sexual dysfunction and depression caused by an androgen deficiency.[63] Both testosterone and carnitine improve sexual desire, sexual satisfaction, and nocturnal penile tumescence, but carnitine is more effective than testosterone in improving erectile function, nocturnal penile tumescence, orgasm, and general sexual well-being. L-carnitine was also more efficacious than testosterone for treating depression.[63]

**DHEA.** DHEA is an important hormone that tends to be depleted steadily with age.[64] A 2006 study assessing DHEA supplementation in men of average 65 years of age found that the men experienced significant increases in testosterone and significant decreases in low-density lipoprotein.[65]

**Tribulus.** *Tribulus terrestris,* also known as puncture vine, contains the active ingredient protodioscin, which is reportedly converted to DHEA in the body.[66] This DHEA-boosting activity may account for puncture vine's reputation as an aphrodisiac in its native Europe and Asia. While some animal studies appear to confirm the ability of tribulus to improve sexual function, no reliable human trials have taken place.[67,68]

**Antioxidants.** One reason testosterone production may decline with advancing age is oxidative damage in the tissues that produce testosterone. A study examining the role of antioxidants in male hormone imbalance in aging men noted that antioxidant supplements (including vitamins A and E, zinc, and selenium) all supported testosterone production.[69]

## Natural Products Keep Aromatase and/or Sex Hormone–Binding Globulin (SHBG) in Check

**Chrysin.** The bioflavonoid chrysin is a natural aromatase inhibitor.[70] Bodybuilders have used chrysin as a testosterone-boosting supplement, because it minimizes the conversion of testosterone to estrogen. Although chrysin has low oral bioavailability,[71] its bioavailability may be significantly enhanced by co-administration with the black pepper extract, piperine, thus enhancing its actions as an aromatase inhibitor.[72]

**Quercetin.** One study showed that red wine inhibits aromatase, thus inhibiting the conversion of testosterone to estrogen. The study attributed this effect to the quercetin and other ingredients.[73]

**Nettle Root.** Lignans contained in nettle root extract may help prevent the binding of *sex hormone–binding globulin* to testosterone. This may help ensure that free testosterone is available for promoting male vitality and youthful sexual function.[74,75] Nettle root extract is used extensively, either in combination with saw palmetto[76] or by itself[77] for relief of BPH symptoms.

**Fish Oil.** A study examined how the essential fatty acids EPA and DHA affected SHBG levels in men 43 to 88 years of age.[78] After controlling for other variables, the researchers concluded that both EPA and DHA decreased levels of SHBG in middle-aged and elderly men.

**Protein.** While adequate protein consumption is vital to maintaining muscle mass, it is also important in maintaining testosterone levels. A study examined the relationship between diet and SHBG, and found that diets low in protein in men 40–70 years old may lead to elevated SHBG levels and consequently decreased testosterone bioactivity.[79]

## Natural Products to Support Sexual Function

**Muira Puama.** Muira puama, *Ptychopetalum olacoides,* grows in the Amazon region of Brazil. It is considered an aphrodisiac and an effective treatment for impotence. It has been studied by Jacques Waynberg,[80] a prominent medical sexologist at the Institute of Sexology in Paris. In one of his studies, men with loss of libido received 1.5 g/day of muira puama for 2 weeks. Sixty-two percent rated the treatment as having a dynamic effect, and 52% with erectile dysfunction rated the treatment as beneficial. In another study, muira puama treatment was given to 100 men, aged 18 years or older, with impotence and/or loss of libido. A significantly increased frequency of intercourse was reported in 66% of the men. Of the 46 men who complained of loss of desire, 70% reported libido intensification. The stability of erection during intercourse was restored in 55% of men, and 66% of men reported a reduction in fatigue. Other reported beneficial effects included improved sleep and morning erections.

**Maca.** Maca has been used among indigenous people in the Andes region for centuries. It is a reputed aphrodisiac and fertility enhancer. Peruvian researchers conducted a randomized, placebo-controlled double-blind study on a small group of men aged 21–56. Results showed that, versus placebo, maca improved subjective reports of male sexual desire. Subjects consumed either 1500 mg or 3000 mg of maca, or placebo, for 3 months. After 8 weeks, improvements were noted in sexual desire among the subjects who consumed maca.[81]

## Natural Products to Support Prostate Health

**Indole-3-Carbinol (I3C).** I3C protects against dangerous estrogen metabolites and subsequent prostate cancer. An adequate intake of I3C, through vegetables such as broccoli, Brussels sprouts, and cabbage, or via supplements, may be very helpful for aging men in both keeping undesirable estrogen metabolites such as 16-alphahydroxyestrone in check and decreasing their risk of prostate cancer. Studies have demonstrated that I3C increases the ratio of 2-hydroxyestrone to 16-alpha-hydroxyestrone. For men, this very well might mean a decrease in prostate cancer risk.[82,83] In a study that examined the association of prostate cancer risk with estrogen metabolism, the authors said, "results of this case-control study suggest that the estrogen metabolic pathway favoring 2-hydroxylation over 16-alpha-hydroxylation may reduce risk of clinically evident prostate cancer,"[84]

**Pygeum.** A bark extract from the native African cherry tree *Pygeum africanum*, has been used in Europe to treat BPH since 1960, and is currently the most commonly used therapeutic agent for this condition in France.[85] One theory for the anti-BPH action of pygeum involves the conversion of testosterone to *dihydrotestosterone* (DHT), a potent testosterone metabolite that may exacerbate BPH, via the enzyme 5-a-reductase.[86] A recent study identified that N-butylbenzene-sulfonamide (NBBS) was isolated from P. africanum as a specific androgen receptor (AR) antagonist. NBBS inhibits AR- and progesterone receptor (PR)-mediated transactivation, as well as endogenous PSA expression and growth of human prostate cancer cells.[87]

**Saw Palmetto.** In Europe, saw palmetto (*Serenoa repens*) has been used extensively as a drug for reducing symptoms of BPH. Saw palmetto has multiple mechanisms of action: inhibition of *5-alpha-reductase*; inhibition of DHT binding to the androgen receptor; reduction of the inflammatory component of prostate growth (by inhibiting COX-2 and an enzyme called 5-lipoxygenase); and induction of apoptosis and inhibition of prostate cell proliferation.[88–91] Its clinical benefits for prostate enlargement include reduced nocturnal urinary urgency,[92] decreased residual urine volume in the bladder,[93] and less discomfort from urination symptoms.[94]

# TESTOSTERONE AND PROSTATE CANCER: THE MYTH

For more than 60 years, the medical establishment erroneously conjectured that testosterone replacement therapy increased risk of developing prostate cancer. This fear has made it standard practice for physicians to deprive hypogonadal male patients of testosterone replacement that could otherwise provide them with a world of cardiovascular, musculoskeletal, cognitive, metabolic, and other health benefits, as discussed above.

Remarkably, though, it appears that, in most cases, the opposite is true—lower levels of endogenous testosterone present a greater risk of prostate cancer than higher levels.[95] A review of data from the National Institutes of Health revealed that, in men of advancing age, "*high testosterone levels are not associated with an increased risk of prostate cancer, nor are low testosterone levels protective against prostate cancer.*"[59]

A collaborative review of 18 prospective studies compared serum concentrations of androgen and estrogen in 3886 men with prostate cancer with those in 6438 healthy controls. The results showed *no significant associations between the risk of prostate cancer and sex hormone levels.*[60]

In more than 500 men diagnosed with prostate cancer (followed over a mean of 8.7 years), high androgen levels were actually associated with a *decreased* risk of aggressive prostate disease, compared with no change in the risk of nonaggressive disease. Overall, levels of any steroid hormones (except estradiol) were not correlated with the risk of aggressive prostate cancer.[96]

Abraham Morgentaler, an associate clinical professor at the Harvard Medical School, in his book *Testosterone for Life*, convincingly makes the case for the benefits and safety of high testosterone versus the dangers of low testosterone. He also goes back to the original 1941 Nobel Prize–winning research[97] about testosterone and shows how these data have been misinterpreted and unquestioned for over 70 years.

## Life Extension Suggestions

*Step One:* Testing

It is critical that men undergo comprehensive medical testing before embarking on a hormone modulation program. First, a baseline blood PSA must be taken to rule out existing prostate cancer (for more information, see the Prostate Cancer protocol). Then, free and total testosterone and estradiol tests are needed to make sure that testosterone is not being excessively converted into estrogen. If estrogen levels are too high, the use of aromatase inhibitors can reduce the rate at which testosterone converts to estrogen in the body. Follow-up testing for estrogen, testosterone, and PSA levels are needed to rule out prostate cancer and fine-tune your program. Additional tests that should be considered include:

- Complete blood cell count and chemistry profile, including liver and kidney function, glucose, minerals, lipids and thyroid-stimulating hormone (TSH)

- DHEA
- Luteinizing hormone (LH) (optional)
- SHBG (optional)
- Dihydrotestosterone (optional)

Blood for these tests may be drawn at your physician's office or directly at a laboratory in your area. Information about ordering these tests on your own may be obtained by calling 1-800-208-3444. These tests will yield crucial information that can help you design a program tailored to your unique situation.

**Step Two:** Interpreting the Results

**Free testosterone:** The Life Extension Foundation believes that direct testing for free testosterone is the best way to test for testosterone activity, as free testosterone is the active form of the hormone and comprises only about 2% of total testosterone.

The Life Extension Foundation recommends that men strive for a free testosterone level that is in the upper one-third range for men aged 21 to 49 years. The range of free testosterone serum level is 20–25 picograms per milliliter (pg/mL), using our current testing methodology.

There are five reasons that free testosterone levels may be low:

1. Too much testosterone is being converted to estrogen through the activity of aromatase.
2. Too much free testosterone is being bound by SHBG. This would be especially apparent if a man's total testosterone level is in the high normal range but his free testosterone level is low.
3. The pituitary gland, which controls testosterone production through the production of luteinizing hormone (LH), is not secreting enough LH to stimulate gonadal production of testosterone. In this case, total testosterone would be low.
4. The testicles (gonads) have lost their ability to produce testosterone, despite adequate amounts of LH. In this case, the level of LH would be high despite a low testosterone level.
5. The DHEA level is abnormally low.

**Estrogen:** Measured as estradiol, should be kept in a range of 20–30 pg/ml. If a man's estrogen level is elevated, it could be associated with:

- Increased aromatase activity, often caused by increased abdominal fat.
- The liver is failing to remove excess estrogen, possibly because of heavy alcohol intake. In men, heavy alcohol intake has been shown to boost estrogen levels within the liver.[98]

If a man's estradiol level is >30 pg/mL, it should be reduced by using aromatase-inhibiting drugs or nutrients. (Optimal estradiol levels are 20–30 pg/mL.)

| Hormone | Optimal Range |
|---|---|
| DHEA | 350–490 µg/dL |
| Estradiol | 20–30 pg/mL |
| Total testosterone | 700–900 ng/dL |
| Free testosterone | 20–25 pg/mL |

**Step Three:** Correcting Abnormal Levels

Ultimately, the ideal program will depend on the results of various tests. Below are some common scenarios and solutions to correct hormone imbalances.

**Low free testosterone, high estradiol, mid total testosterone:** This situation suggests excessive aromatase activity, which converts free testosterone to estrogen. Inhibition of aromatase and reduction in aromatase-containing tissue (fat) is indicated. Suggestions include:

- **Chrysin**: 1500 mg daily
- **Piperine**: 10 mg daily to enhance absorption of chrysin
- **Zinc**: 50–90 mg daily
- **Acetyl-L-carnitine**: 1000–2000 mg daily
- **Muira puama**: 850 mg daily
- **Quercetin**: 500–1000 mg daily
- Lose weight to reduce aromatase activity.
- Reduce or eliminate alcohol intake to enable excess estrogen removal by the liver.
- Review all current medications to see if they might be interfering with healthy liver function. Common medications that affect liver function are nonsteroidal anti-inflammatory drugs (NSAIDs) (eg, naproxen, ibuprofen, acetaminophen, and aspirin); the statin class of cholesterol-lowering drugs (eg, simvastatin, atorvastatin); some heart medications; some blood pressure-lowering medications; and some antidepressants. Drugs being prescribed to treat the symptoms of testosterone deficiency (such as statins and certain antidepressants) may actually aggravate the testosterone deficit, thus making the cholesterol problem or depression worse. However, do not discontinue any prescription medicine without consulting your physician.
- If all of the above fail to increase free testosterone and lower excess estradiol, consider discussing with your physician the use of the aromatase inhibitor anastrozole (Arimidex) at the very low dose of 0.5 mg twice per week.

**Low free testosterone, low estrogen, high total testosterone:** This situation suggests excessive SHBG levels, making sufficient testosterone unavailable to target tissues. The elevation of SHBG explains why some older men who are on testosterone replacement therapy do not report a long-term beneficial effect; that is, the administered testosterone becomes bound by SHBG and is not bioavailable to cellular receptor sites where it would normally produce an effect. Suggestions include:

- Inhibit aromatase by following some of the recommendations in the previous section, since low testosterone and high estrogen are involved in excess SHBG activity.
- Take the following supplements:
  - **Chrysin**: 1500 mg daily
  - **Nettle root extract**: 240 mg daily
  - **Pygeum extract**: 100 mg daily
  - **Cruciferous vegetable extract (I3C)**: 400 mg daily
  - **Fish oil**: 2000 mg daily (at least 700 mg EPA, 500 mg DHA)
  - **DHEA**: 15–75 mg daily, followed by blood tests in 3–6 weeks

**Low free testosterone, low estrogen, low testosterone:** This situation suggests low production of testosterone, with resultant low conversion to estrogen. Suggestions include:

- Use testosterone patches or creams. Do not use testosterone injections or tablets. If tests reveal low levels of LH, ask your physician about the possibility of using human chorionic gonadotropin (HCG). HCG functions in a manner similar to that of LH, thus helping to stimulate the Leydig cells of the testes to produce more testosterone.
- Take **DHEA**: 15–75 mg daily
- **Tribulus fruit extract** (40% saponins): 450 mg daily

*General Nutrients to Boost Sexual Function*

A number of nutrients have been studied for their ability to boost testosterone and/or treat conditions such as erectile dysfunction and loss of libido. This nutrient group includes antioxidants, which may function by reducing oxidative damage to testosterone-producing tissues.

- **Selenium**: 200 mcg daily
- **Vitamin E**: 400 IU daily with at least 200 mg of gamma-tocopherol
- **Vitamin D**:[99] 5000–10000 IU daily
- **Protein Powder**: 10–20 g daily
- **Maca Powdered Extract**: 1500–3000 mg daily

In addition, the following blood testing resources may be helpful:

- Male Comprehensive Hormone Panel or Male Basic Hormone Panel

## REFERENCES

References available at: www.lef.org/dpt5/ch90

# 91

---

# *Meningitis*

---

Meningitis is inflammation of the tissue covering the brain and spinal cord (the meninges). Reports of the illness date back to the 16th century; the disease was first accurately described in 1805.[1] Meningitis is characterized by swelling of the meninges; increased pressure inside the skull blocks the flow of blood to the brain, starving the brain of nutrients and oxygen. Encephalitis, which is actual inflammation of the brain, can occur along with meningitis.

People with meningitis usually have fever, severe headache, and stiff neck accompanied by neck pain. Almost any type of movement can cause the neck pain, and it may be impossible to lower the chin to the chest. Seizures are associated with acute forms of the disease. In severe cases, meningitis can be fatal.

Other symptoms include nausea and vomiting, dizziness, sensitivity to light, rashes, and weakness. Babies and older adults may not experience stiff neck. However, babies may lose their appetite, have a shrill cry, and be difficult to soothe, or conversely may be extremely sleepy or lethargic.

Symptoms such as tiredness and lightheadedness can last for several months after recovery from the acute form of the disease. Resulting problems range from headache, nausea, loss of balance, and stiff neck to brain damage and hearing loss. Long-term complications include brain damage, hearing loss, vision problems, and persistent seizures.

---

### WARNING!

If meningitis is even remotely suspected, seek immediate medical assistance.

Bacterial meningitis is not a disease to be taken lightly. It is a degenerative, rapidly progressing disease that can result in death or permanent disability. If bacterial meningitis is suspected, patients are urged to see a doctor (go to a hospital emergency department if necessary) for appropriate testing and prompt intravenous antibiotic treatment. Patients with suspected meningitis should get medical care as quickly as possible.

## DIAGNOSING MENINGITIS: THE SPINAL TAP

If a person has symptoms of meningitis, his or her physician may order a lumbar puncture, commonly called a spinal tap.

During a spinal tap, a needle is placed in the lumbar (lower) portion of the spinal canal and a small sample of cerebrospinal fluid (CSF) is removed. After the CSF is removed, it is cultured (the sample of CSF is incubated for a few days under conditions that promote the growth of microorganisms). If bacteria grow in the fluid, the type of bacteria causing the meningitis can be determined, and the most effective antibiotic can be prescribed.

Because viral meningitis is caused by a virus and not a bacterium, there will be no growth in the culture medium. This is why viral meningitis is also sometimes called aseptic meningitis.

## CAUSES OF MENINGITIS

Meningitis is usually caused by infection from a bacterium or virus that has penetrated the nervous system. Most cases of meningitis are caused by bacterial or viral infection, although meningitis can also be caused by other conditions, such as allergic reactions to drugs, fungi, or parasites.

Viral meningitis is responsible for most cases of meningitis and is also usually (although not always) less severe than bacterial meningitis.

Bacterial meningitis is a serious disease that can cause death or permanent brain damage if not treated by a physician immediately. Acute bacterial meningitis is most common in children aged 1 month–2 years. However, localized outbreaks can occur in self-contained groups living in close quarters, such as college students living in dorms or people living in military barracks. Elderly people and those with compromised immune systems (eg, patients with HIV/AIDS) are also at risk.

Although the mortality rate from bacterial meningitis has dropped in recent years, the Centers for Disease Control and Prevention (CDC) report that 10–14% of people with bacterial meningitis die, and 11–15% of people who recover are disabled.[2]

## TYPES OF MENINGITIS

### Bacterial Meningitis

Many people who carry bacteria associated with meningitis will never develop the disease. In some people, however, for reasons not fully understood, the bacteria will migrate through the body's outer immune defenses (eg, through nasal passages) and into the bloodstream.[3]

Acute bacterial meningitis is dangerous and needs to be diagnosed and treated with antibiotics as quickly as possible. In the past, it was fatal in more than 50% of cases. However, with better and earlier treatment, fatality has dropped to 10–14%. Nevertheless, about 15% of survivors have long-term disabilities, including hearing loss and brain damage.[2] If acute bacterial meningitis is suspected, the person should see a physician and receive treatment immediately.

The most common strains of bacteria that cause meningitis are *Streptococcus pneumoniae* (*S. pneumonia*) (about 50% of bacterial cases), *Neisseria meningitidis* (*N. meningitidis*) (about 25% of bacterial cases—and up to 60% in cases that involve children), and *Listeria monocytogenes* (about 10% of bacterial cases—almost exclusively in newborns and elderly).[4]

In recent years, common causes of bacterial meningitis have changed because of vaccines that targeted *Haemophilus influenzae* (*H. influenza*) and, to a lesser extent, *N. meningitidis*.[5] Previously, these two bacteria were responsible for most bacterial meningitis infections. *H. influenzae* type b used to be the most common cause of meningitis in infants; however, since the *H. influenzae* serotype b (Hib) vaccine was introduced in 1985; the number of children in the United States who get meningitis from this organism has decreased by 95%.[6,7] Today, *S. pneumoniae* accounts for about half of all bacterial cases.

Symptoms classically associated with bacterial meningitis include fever, headache, and stiff neck. In more than 75% of cases, changes in mental status occur, ranging from lethargy to coma, although some patients may become agitated and even combative. Nausea, vomiting, and sensitivity to light are also common symptoms. Seizures occur in up to 40% of patients.

There are several classes of drugs used to treat bacterial meningitis, including antibiotics, inflammation suppressors, and pain relievers. Antibiotics are used to kill the organism causing the infection. The other treatments are used to manage symptoms associated with the disease. If seizures occur, anti-seizure drugs (eg, phenobarbital and phenytoin) may be administered. When patients have trouble breathing, they may be administered oxygen, or may require assisted ventilation.

In the future, anti-inflammatory medications are expected to play a larger role in meningitis therapy.[8] The inflammatory reaction associated with meningitis is at least partly modulated by proteins in the brain called tyrosine kinases.[9,10] They are involved in inflammatory reactions in the brain and in the movement of bacteria across the blood–brain barrier. Inhibitors of tyrosine kinases, including supplements such as genistein, may decrease the severity of inflammation and the ability of bacteria to cross the blood–brain barrier, which could possibly prevent infection and limit damage.[10]

## Viral Meningitis

Viral meningitis is the most common form of the disease.[11] About 90% of cases (in which the virus has been identified) are caused by enteroviruses, mostly coxsackieviruses and echoviruses.[12]

It used to be difficult to identify which virus was causing viral meningitis; also, once bacteria were ruled out, further tests were not commonly done. However, because of the West Nile virus (which can also cause meningitis), more tests using the polymerase chain reaction technique have been performed to identify the viruses. Epstein-Barr virus has also been found in the CSF of patients with meningitis.[13] The viruses that cause measles, mumps, and chickenpox can also cause meningitis. Vaccines against these diseases may be partly responsible for the decrease in viral meningitis in children.[14]

Mollaret's meningitis is a rare, recurrent viral meningitis that is painful but not generally life-threatening. The herpes simplex viruses, HSV1 and HSV2, have been associated with Mollaret's meningitis.[15]

Viral meningitis is generally treated with analgesics, bed rest, and fluids. Acyclovir or valacyclovir, drugs used to treat herpes, may be useful for treating Mollaret's meningitis.[15]

As with bacterial meningitis, the inflammatory cascade is an important contributor to damage caused by viral meningitis, and anti-inflammatory therapy will probably develop into an important part of therapy in the near future.[3]

## Other Types of Meningitis

Meningitis can also occur after certain medical procedures, such as catheter-based intervention for cerebral aneurysm.[16] Chemical meningitis can occur as a result of drug use. In these nonbacterial or viral conditions, the disease is characterized chiefly by inflammation, making anti-inflammatory therapy potentially more important.

Chronic meningitis can occur after infections with tuberculosis, Lyme disease, AIDS, or syphilis, as well as in noninfectious disorders such as some cancers of the brain or blood (eg, leukemias and lymphomas).[6]

Fungal infections are usually only a problem in people with weakened immune systems, such as people with AIDS or who have had their spleens removed. Usually the fungus responsible is a species of Cryptococcus, an encapsulated yeast.[6] These infections start when a person breathes in fungal spores from contaminated soil; the infection in the lungs is usually cleared by the immune system. Only when the immune system is weak do these infections progress to meningitis.

## FOR MORE INFORMATION

For more information on strengthening the immune system or on HIV/AIDS, please see the following protocols:

- Immune System Strengthening
- HIV/AIDS

# TREATMENT AND PREVENTION OF MENINGITIS

If bacteria are the cause, meningitis will be treated with intravenous antibiotics. If the patient is very sick and bacterial meningitis is suspected (but not yet proven with a culture), antibiotics are generally started before the specific bacteria are identified. In most cases, 2 or more antibiotics will be prescribed to kill the bacteria. Treatment may also include analgesics to relieve fever and pain, corticosteroids to decrease inflammation, and fluids to maintain electrolytes and prevent dehydration.

In recent years, anti-inflammatories for the treatment of bacterial meningitis have attracted significant attention. Although this form of the disease is caused by bacteria, the majority of damage resulting from meningitis is associated with an inflammation cascade touched off by an immune system response.

Antibiotics are used to treat only bacterial infections, therefore they are ineffective in treating viral meningitis (also, overuse of antibiotics leads to drug resistance). People usually recover from viral meningitis in a couple of weeks. Treatment includes analgesics for pain and fever, rest, and fluids to prevent dehydration. There are 25 000–50 000 hospitalizations in the United States from viral meningitis each year.[12]

In recent years, researchers have made a number of advances against meningitis, ranging from the introduction of vaccines (that target the pathogens that cause meningitis) to a deeper understanding of how inflammation is crucial to the disease process. During meningitis, the immune system is activated to produce a host of proinflammatory chemicals, including tumor necrosis factor-alpha (TNF-$\alpha$) and various interleukins.[3] This immune-modulated inflammation causes

much of the damage associated with meningitis. In the future, anti-inflammatories are expected to play a major role in conventional meningitis therapy.[3]

Because meningitis is contagious, people should practice good hygiene. Although organisms are spread by breathing them in and are rarely contracted by touching contaminated surfaces, washing hands frequently and thoroughly is still suggested.

See a doctor if you have been exposed to someone with meningitis. Close contact with a person who has bacterial meningitis is enough to warrant prophylactic (preventive) antibiotic therapy.

## WHAT YOU HAVE LEARNED SO FAR

- Meningitis is an inflammation of the tissue lining of the brain and spinal cord, and is usually caused by bacteria or viruses. Viral meningitis is more common, and generally less severe, than bacterial meningitis.
- The major symptoms of meningitis are severe headache, neck pain, and fever.
- Bacterial meningitis is a severe problem that requires immediate medical assistance and intravenous antibiotic treatment. If untreated or not treated promptly, bacterial meningitis can lead to death or brain damage.
- Viral meningitis has no specific treatment, but people usually recover at home with analgesics, rest, and fluids.
- Anyone who suspects that they or someone they know (especially a child) has meningitis should see a doctor or go to a hospital emergency department immediately.
- Inflammation associated with meningitis is caused by a widespread immune response to the invading bacteria or virus. The majority of damage resulting from meningitis is associated with inflammation Thus, it is likely that anti-inflammatories may play a significant role in future therapy.

# NUTRITION'S ROLE IN MENINGITIS

Although much of the research is still preliminary, exciting discoveries are being made on the role of nutrients in meningitis, especially anti-inflammatories and antioxidants. Evidence suggests that much of the damage caused by bacterial meningitis is due to overactivation of the immune system.[3] This immune response is thought to be caused primarily by bacterial endotoxin, a poison (present in the bacteria) released when the bacterial cell disintegrates. Studies have clearly shown that the degree of severity of bacterial meningitis is linked to the level of endotoxin.[17]

Once in the bloodstream, an endotoxin binds to a protein, appropriately called endotoxin-binding protein. This alters the endotoxin, enabling it to activate macrophages and other inflammatory cells. Once activated, these cells secrete proinflammatory chemicals including TNF-$\alpha$, interleukin 1(b), and interferon. At the same time, immune system cells called neutrophils are activated, releasing yet more inflammatory chemicals and enzymes, which damage blood vessels and the inner lining of body cavities.[18] The result is widespread inflammation and damage.

By looking at the disease as an inappropriate immune response that touches off an inflammatory cascade, researchers are studying exciting new therapies to reduce the damaging consequences of meningitis. While these studies are ongoing, Life Extension believes that nutrients that fight inflammation can safely be considered in helping reduce the inflammation associated with meningitis.

## Nutrients That Fight Inflammation

**Genistein.** Genistein is an isoflavone and phytoestrogen. It inhibits the activity of tyrosine kinases, which are directly involved in both the inflammation associated with meningitis and the ability of bacteria to cross the blood–brain barrier. This suggests that genistein may help reduce the severity of the disease and have a preventive effect.[10]

**Essential fatty acids.** Essential fatty acids, including omega-3 and omega-6 fatty acids, have powerful anti-inflammatory effects. A proper ratio of omega-3 fatty acids, including eicosapentaenoic acid (EPA) and docosahexaenoic acid (DHA), to omega-6 fatty acids (linoleic acid) is vital to good health. Omega-3 fatty acids have been shown in hundreds of published studies to reduce inflammation through the reduction of prostaglandin E2, a hormone-like chemical that promotes inflammation. Although there have been no studies that examined the use of essential fatty acids in meningitis, if recent research implicating widespread inflammatory damage in meningitis withstands scientific scrutiny, supplementing with EPA and DHA may have some benefit.

**Perilla leaf extract.** Perilla leaf extract contains luteolin and rosmarinic acid, both of which have demonstrated anti-inflammatory effects in animal studies.[19] Again, although no studies have been performed testing Perilla leaf extract's effect on meningitis, the extract's anti-inflammatory effects may have some benefit.

**Rosmarinic acid.** Rosmarinic acid is contained in large amounts in Perilla leaf extract. Studies have shown it to have anti-inflammatory action through the inhibition of cytokines and other inflammatory mediators in human asthma subjects.[20]

## Antioxidants

Antioxidants have also attracted attention among meningitis researchers. Studies have found that meningitis patients have oxidative stress caused by reactive nitrogen species in bacterial meningitis.[21]

**Superoxide dismutase.** In a mouse model of bacterial meningitis, the internal antioxidant superoxide dismutase (SOD) was studied for its ability to limit oxidative stress that caused damage to the ears. SOD, given by injection, was found to significantly reduce damage to the cochlea.[22]

**Vitamin C.** Two studies have explored the relationship between the antioxidant vitamin C and bacterial meningitis. In some cases, CSF of children with meningitis showed elevated levels of vitamin C, while other studies showed a marked deficiency in vitamin C, suggesting that vitamin C is involved in the body's defense against free-radical–associated damage.[23,24] Vitamin C's decrease in CSF of patients with bacterial meningitis seems to be correlated with the increase in reactive molecules in the brain.[21,25] Together, these results suggest that vitamin C supplementation may be helpful in treating patients with bacterial meningitis.

**Melatonin.** Melatonin is another nutrient studied in association with meningitis. The CSF of patients with viral meningitis tends to have higher concentrations of melatonin. This suggests that melatonin may play an immunomodulatory role in viral meningitis.[26] In an exciting new animal study, rabbits received melatonin at 20 mg/kg of body weight. Researchers found that rabbits, given melatonin simultaneously with infection, had higher levels of SOD and lower levels of dangerous reactive nitrogen species. This suggests that melatonin had protective effects against infection.[27]

## A Word from Life Extension

Life Extension and its founders have devoted themselves to pushing the knowledge of health beyond rigid, conventional boundaries. Although individual components of the information given here have been published in studies, there have been no clinical trials to support these recommendations in their entirety. In some cases, we are basing our recommendations on observations gleaned from decades of experience.

However, these supplements may help ward off an infection in the first place, which would naturally reduce the chances of developing meningitis.

The following have been used at the first sign of a viral or bacterial infection.

**Cimetidine (Tagamet®).** An over-the-counter heartburn drug that also boosts immune function by reducing T-suppressor cells[28]; 800 mg each day is the recommended dose.

**Zinc.** A number of studies have shown that if zinc lozenges are taken within 24 hours of the onset of cold symptoms, the severity and duration of the cold are reduced.[29] Take 2 lozenges (24 mg each) every 2 hours when awake. This is a very high dose of zinc and should be continued for only a few days to avoid toxic side effects.

**Lactoferrin.** A daily dose of 1200 mg may boost natural killer cell activity and can kill certain viruses.[30,31]

**High-allicin garlic.** In the dose of 9000 mg once or twice a day. This potent form of garlic will cause painful stomach-esophageal burning if you do not eat food right afterward. An intake of 9000 mg of this kind of garlic will cause you to reek of a strong sulfur odor, but saturating the body with this pungent garlic is the objective. Garlic has shown direct virus-killing effects in a number of published studies.[32,33]

**Aged garlic extract.** This type of garlic, at a dose of 3600 mg daily, has unique immune-boosting properties (independent of high allicin garlic).[34]

**Dehydroepiandrosterone (DHEA).** A dose of 200–400 mg early in the day may boost the immune system. DHEA has shown powerful immune-enhancing and antiviral properties.[35,36]

**Melatonin.** At a high dose, 10–50 mg at bedtime, melatonin may help boost the immune system[37] and facilitate deep, restorative sleep, which is needed to fend off infection.

## Life Extension Suggestions

- **Complete multivitamin:** per label instructions
- **Vitamin C:** 2.5–6.0 g daily
- **Genistein:** 135 mg soy isoflavone concentrate, standardized to supply 55.5 mg isoflavones and 28 mg genistein
- **Fish oil,** with olive polyphenols and sesame lignans: providing 1400 mg EPA and 1000 mg DHA daily
- **Rosmarinic acid:** 100–200 mg daily, containing 50–100 mg of Perilla leaf extract
- Natural plant complex providing **superoxide dismutase (SOD)** activity: 2100 mg daily
- **Melatonin:** 10–50 mg at night

## REFERENCES

References available at: www.lef.org/dpt5/ch91

# 92

# Metabolic Detoxification

Detoxification ("detox") has broad connotations ranging from the spiritual to the scientific, and has been used to describe practices and protocols that embrace both complementary (fasting, colonic cleaning) and conventional (chelation or antitoxin therapy) schools of medical thought—as well as some that push the boundaries of scientific plausibility (such as ionic foot detoxification).

In the context of human biochemistry (and this protocol), detoxification can be described with much more precision; here it refers to a specific metabolic pathway, active throughout the human body, that processes unwanted chemicals for elimination. This pathway (which will be referred to as metabolic detoxification) involves a series of enzymatic reactions that neutralize and solubilize toxins, and transport them to secretory organs (like the liver or kidneys), so that they can be excreted from the body. This type of detoxification is sometimes called xenobiotic metabolism, because it is the primary mechanism for ridding the body of xenobiotics (foreign chemicals); however, detoxification reactions are frequently used to prepare unneeded endobiotics (endogenously produced chemicals) for excretion from the body.

Excess hormones, vitamins, inflammatory molecules, and signaling compounds, among others, are typically eliminated from the body by the same enzymatic detoxification systems that protect the body from environmental toxins or clear prescription drugs from circulation. Metabolic detoxification reactions, therefore, are not only important for protection from the environment, but central to homeostatic balance in the body.

This protocol describes nutritional approaches for general optimization of metabolic detoxification; it is designed to provide a foundation for proper function of this critical system. Specific health concerns may require supplementary detoxification "intervention" protocols (such as heavy metal detoxification, or alcohol-induced hangover prevention).

## TOXIN AND TOXICANT EXPOSURE

Toxins are poisonous compounds produced by living organisms; sometimes the term "biotoxin" is used to emphasize the biological origin of these compounds. Human-made chemical compounds with toxic potential are more properly called toxicants. Toxins and toxicants can exert their detrimental effects on health in a number of ways. Some broadly act as mutagens or carcinogens (causing DNA damage or mutations, which can lead to cancer), others can disrupt specific metabolic pathways (which can lead to dysfunction of particular biological systems such as the nervous system, liver, or kidneys).

The diet is a major source of toxin exposure. Toxins can find their way into the diet by several routes, notably contamination by microorganisms, human-made toxicants (including pesticides, residues from food processing, prescription drugs, and industrial wastes), or less frequently, contamination by toxins from other "nonfood" plant sources.[1,2] Some of the toxic heavy metals (lead, mercury, cadmium, chromium), while not "man-made," have been released/redistributed into the environment at potentially dangerous levels by human activity, and can find their way into the diet as well. Microbial toxins, secreted by bacteria and fungi, can be ingested along with contaminated or improperly prepared food.

Even the method of food preparation has the potential for converting naturally occurring food constituents into toxins.[3] For instance, high temperatures can convert nitrogen-containing compounds in meats and cereal products into the potent mutagens benzopyrene and acrylamide, respectively. Smoked fish and cheeses contain precursors to toxins called N-nitroso compounds (NOCs), which become mutagenic when metabolized by colonic bacteria.

Outside of the diet, respiratory exposure to volatile organic compounds (VOCs) is a common risk that has been associated with several adverse health effects, including kidney damage, immunologic problems, hormonal imbalances, blood disorders, and increased rates of asthma and bronchitis.[4]

One of the greatest sources of nondietary toxicant exposure is the air in the home.[5] Building materials (such as floor and wall coverings, particle board, adhesives, and paints) can "off-gas" releasing several toxicants that can be detected in humans.[6] For example, a toxic benzene derivative commonly used in disinfectants and deodorizers was detected in 98% of adults in the Environmental Protection Agency's (EPA) "TEAM" study.[7] In another EPA study, three additional toxic solvents were present in 100% of human tissue samples tested across the country.[8]

Newly built or remodeled buildings can have substantial amounts of chemical "off-gassing," giving rise to what has been called "sick building syndrome."[9]

Carpeting is an especially big offender, potentially releasing several neurotoxins; in testing of over 400 carpet samples, neurotoxins were present in >90% of the samples, quantitatively sufficient in some samples to cause death in mice.[10] Ironically, shortly after the TEAM report, 71 ill employees evacuated the new EPA headquarters in Washington, DC, claiming health problems, which were eventually attributed to the 27,000 square feet of new carpet.[11]

Carpets also trap environmental toxins; the "Non-Occupational Pesticide Exposure Study" (NOPES) found an average of 12 pesticide residues per carpet sampled, and determined that this route of exposure likely provides infants and toddlers with nearly all of their nondietary exposure to the notorious pesticides DDT, aldrin, atrazine, and carbaryl.[12]

## AVOIDING TOXIN/TOXICANT EXPOSURE

While it is not possible to completely eliminate toxin/toxicant exposure from all sources, there are ways to minimize it:

- Limit the introduction of VOCs in the home by using VOC-free cleaning products, low-VOC paints, and choosing throw rugs instead of new carpeting.[13]
- Store food in bisphenol A (BPA)–free or phthalate-free containers, and avoid reheating foods in plastic containers.
- Look for organic produce, which is grown without pesticides, and will contain less residue than conventionally produced fruits and vegetables (although be aware that organic produce isn't necessarily "pesticide free").[14]
- Washing fruits or vegetables can decrease some pesticide residue, although it is not effective against all pesticide types,[15] and commercial fruit and vegetable wash solutions may not be any more effective than water alone.[16] Peeling skins off of produce may help to further lower pesticide levels.
- Limit intake of processed foods. Even ones that are free of synthetic preservatives may contain detectable amounts of toxic compounds that were introduced (by chemical transformation) during processing. For example, numerous toxins are produced by the high temperatures used to manufacture some processed food ingredients.[17]
- Although the risk of acute toxicity from undercooking meat (food poisoning) is likely a greater risk than toxin exposure from overcooking it, there are ways to reduce toxin production during meat preparation: avoid direct exposure of meat to open flame or hot metal surfaces; cook meat at or below 250 °F via stewing, braising, crock-pot cooking (slow food preparation methods that utilize liquid); and turn meat often during cooking, avoid prolonged cooking time at high temperatures, and refrain from consuming charred portions.[18]

## OVERVIEW OF XENOBIOTIC METABOLISM

The driving force in the evolution of sophisticated metabolic detoxification systems was actually fairly straightforward and dependent on the ability of water to act as a "solvent" to dissolve substances.

Since cellular membranes are primarily lipid based and impermeable to most water soluble (scientifically: "polar") substances, the transport of water-soluble compounds into a cell requires specialized transport proteins. By placing the appropriate transport proteins on the cell membrane, a cell will only allow desirable water-soluble molecules to enter, and will prevent entry of water-soluble toxins. This same paradigm also applies when the cell needs to excrete unwanted water soluble compounds (like cellular wastes); they exit the cell by a similar mechanism.

In contrast to water-soluble compounds, the lipid cell membrane presents little barrier to lipid-soluble compounds, which can freely pass through it. Potentially damaging lipid-soluble toxins can therefore gain free access to cellular interiors, and are much more difficult to remove.

The metabolic detoxification systems address this problem by converting lipid-soluble toxins into inactive water-soluble metabolites. The "solubilization" of a toxin is accomplished by enzymes that attach (conjugate) additional water-soluble molecules to the lipid-soluble toxin at specific attachment points. If the toxin does not contain any of these attachment points, they are first added by a separate set of enzymes which chemically transform the toxin to include these molecular "handles." Following the solubilization reactions, the chemically-modified toxin is transported out of the cell and excreted.

These three steps or phases of removing undesirable or harmful lipid-soluble compounds are performed by three sets of cellular proteins or enzymes, called the phase I (transformation) and phase II (conjugation) enzymes, and the phase III (transport) proteins.

Phase I, II, and III metabolisms have different biochemical requirements and respond to different metabolic signals, but must work in unison for proper removal of unwanted xenobiotics (such as toxins or drugs) or endobiotics (such as excess hormones). Enzymes of the phase I, II, and III pathways have several characteristics that make them well suited for their important roles.[19] Unlike most other enzymes, detoxification enzymes (1) can react with many different compounds, broadening the number of toxins that a single enzyme can metabolize; (2) are more concentrated in areas of the body that are most directly exposed to the environment (like the liver, intestines, or lungs); and (3) are inducible, meaning that their synthesis can be increased in response to toxin exposure.

The liver is the primary detoxification organ, as it filters blood coming directly from the intestines and prepares toxins for excretion from the body. Significant amounts of detoxification also occur in the intestine, kidney, lungs, and brain, with phase I, II, and III reactions occurring throughout the rest of the body to a lesser degree.

# THE THREE PHASES OF DETOXIFICATION

**Phase I detoxification—enzymatic transformation.** Under most circumstances, phase I enzymes begin the detoxification process by chemically transforming lipid-soluble compounds into water-soluble compounds in preparation for phase II detoxification. The bulk of the phase I transformation reactions are performed by a family of enzymes called the cytochrome P450s (CYPs).

CYP enzymes are relatively nonspecific, and each has the potential to recognize and modify countless different toxins. After all, a mere 57 human CYPs must be able to detoxify any potential toxin that enters the body.[20] However, the cost of this versatility is speed: CYPs metabolize toxins very slowly compared to other enzymes. For instance, compare the predominant CYP3A4, which metabolizes 1–20 molecules per second,[21] to superoxide dismutase (SOD), which metabolizes over a million molecules per second. Major sites of detoxification overcome the slower speed by producing large amounts of CYPs; CYPs may represent up to 5% of total liver proteins, and similar large concentrations can be found in the intestines. CYPs are among the most well-studied and best-characterized detoxification proteins due to their role in the metabolism of prescription drugs, and to their role in metabolizing endogenous biochemicals (eg, aromatase, which transforms testosterone to estradiol, is a CYP).[22]

Several other enzymes contribute to the phase I process as well, notably the flavin monooxygenases (FMOs, responsible for the detoxification of nicotine from cigarette smoke), alcohol and aldehyde dehydrogenases (which metabolize drinking alcohol), and monoamine oxidases (MAOs, which break down serotonin, dopamine, and epinephrine in neurons and are targets of several older antidepressant drugs).[23]

**Phase II detoxification—enzymatic conjugation.** Following phase I transformation, the original lipid-soluble toxin has been converted into a more water-soluble form; however, this reactive intermediate is still unsuitable for immediate elimination from the cell for a couple of reasons: (1) phase I reactions are not sufficient to make the toxin water-soluble enough to complete the entire excretion pathway, and (2) in many cases, products from the phase I reactions have been rendered more reactive then the original toxins, which makes them potentially more destructive than they once were. Both of these shortcomings are addressed by the activities of the phase II enzymes, which modify phase I products to both increase their solubility and reduce their toxicity. The activation of the phase II enzymes is responsible for the antimutagenic and anticarcinogenic properties of the metabolic detoxification systems. It is widely accepted that phase II enzymes protect against chemical carcinogenesis, especially during the initiation phase of cancers.[24]

At the genetic level, the production of most phase II enzymes is controlled by a protein called nuclear factor erythroid-derived 2 (Nrf2), a master regulator of antioxidant response.[25] Under normal cellular conditions, Nrf2 resides in the cytoplasm (the liquid inside cells within which the cells components are contained) of the cell in an inactive state.[26] However, the presence of oxidative stress (triggered by metabolism of toxins by CYPs) activates Nrf2, allowing it to travel to the cell nucleus.[27] In the cell nucleus, Nrf2 turns on the genes of many antioxidant proteins, including the phase II enzymes.[28] In this way, Nrf2 "senses" oxidative stress or the presence of toxins in the cell, and allows the cell to mount an appropriate response. Nrf2 regulates the activity of genes involved in the synthesis and activation of important detoxification molecules including glutathione and superoxide dismutase (SOD). It also plays an important role in initiating heavy metal detoxification, and the recycling of CoQ10, a potent antioxidant.[29–31]

Certain dietary constituents (including *sulforaphane* from *broccoli* and *xanthohumol* from *hops*) may also directly activate Nrf2 and stimulate antioxidant enzyme activity; this may partially explain their beneficial effects on detoxification.[32]

There are several families of phase II enzymes that differ significantly in their activities and biochemistry. In several cases, phase II enzymes exhibit redundancy—a particular xenobiotic or endobiotic can be detoxified by more than one phase II enzyme.

**UDP-glucuronlytransferases** (UGTs) catalyze glucuronidation reactions, the attachment of glucuronic acid to toxins to render them less reactive and more water soluble. There are several different UGTs that are distributed throughout the body, with the liver being the major location. In humans, many xenobiotics, environmental toxicants, and 40–70% of clinical drugs are metabolized by UGTs.[33] The plasticizer bisphenol A[34] and benzopyrene (from cooked meats)[35] are two notable examples of UGT substrates (a substrate is a molecule upon which an enzyme acts). Intestinal UGTs may affect oral bioavailability of several drugs and dietary supplements, and may be responsible for chemoprevention in this tissue.[36]

**Glutathione S-transferases** (GSTs) catalyze the transfer of glutathione (a significant cellular antioxidant) to phase I products. GSTs play a major role in the metabolism of several endobiotics, including steroids, thyroid hormone, fat-soluble vitamins, bile acids, bilirubin, and prostaglandins.[37] GSTs can also function as antioxidant enzymes, detoxifying free radicals[38] and oxidized lipids or DNA.[39] GSTs are soluble enzymes that are ubiquitous in nature and in humans, forming about 4% of the soluble protein in the human liver and present in several other tissues (including brain, heart, lung, intestines, kidney, pancreas, lens, skeletal muscle, prostate, spleen and testes).[40,41] Products of GST conjugation can be excreted via bile, or can travel to the kidneys where they are further processed and eliminated in urine.

**Sulfotransferases** (SULTs) attach sulfates from a sulfur donor to endo- or xenobiotic acceptor molecules. This reaction is important both in detoxification reactions, as well as normal biosynthesis (eg, the addition of sulfate to chondroitin and heparin is catalyzed by specific SULTs).[42] SULTs play a major role in drug and xenobiotic detoxification, and the metabolism of several endogenous molecules (including steroids, thyroid and adrenal hormones, serotonin, retinol, ascorbate, and vitamin D).[43] SULTs in the placenta, uterus, and prostate are thought to play a role in the regulation of androgen levels.[44] In contrast to other phase II enzymes, SULTs can convert a number of procarcinogens (such as heterocyclic amines from cooked meats) into highly reactive intermediates that may act as chemical carcinogens and mutagens.[45]

While the UGTs, GSTs, and SULTs catalyze the bulk of human detoxification reactions, several other phase II enzymes contribute to the process to a lesser, but still important extent:

- Methyltransferase enzymes: Methyltransferase enzymes catalyze methylation reactions using S-adenosyl-L-methionine (SAMe) as a substrate. COMT (catechol O-methyltransferase) is a major pathway for eliminating excess catecholamine neurotransmitters (such as adrenaline or dopamine). Methylation reactions are one of the few phase II reactions that decrease water solubility.[46]

- Arylamine N-acetyltransferases (NATs): NATs detoxify carcinogenic aromatic amines and heterocyclic amines.[47]

- Amino acid–conjugating enzymes: Acyl-CoA synthetase and acyl-CoA amino acid N-acyltransferases attach amino acids (most commonly glycine or glutamine) to xenobiotics. The food preservative benzoic acid is one example of a toxin metabolized by amino acid conjugation.[48]

**Phase III detoxification—Transport.** Phase III transporters are present in many tissues, including the liver, intestines, kidneys, and brain, where they can provide a barrier against xenobiotic entry, or a mechanism for actively moving xenobiotics and endobiotics in and out of cells.[49] Since water-soluble compounds require specific transporters to move in and out of cells, phase III transporters are necessary to excrete the newly formed phase II products out of the cell. Phase III transporters belong to a family of proteins called the ABC transporters (for ATP-Binding Cassette[50]), because they require chemical energy, in the form of ATP, to actively pump toxins through the cell membrane and out of the cell.[51] They are sometimes called the multidrug resistance proteins (MRPs), because drug-resistant cancer cells use them as protection against chemotherapy drugs.[52]

In the liver, phase III transporters move glutathione, sulfate, and glucuronide conjugates out of cells into the bile for elimination. In the kidney and intestine, phase III transporters can remove xenobiotics from the blood for excretion from the body.[53]

## BALANCE OF PHASE I AND PHASE II REACTIONS

The products of phase I metabolism are potentially more toxic than the original molecules, which does not present a problem if the phase II enzymes are functioning at a rate to rapidly neutralize the phase I products as they are formed. This, however, is not always the case. Factors that increase the ratio of phase I to phase II activity can upset this delicate balance, producing harmful metabolites faster than they can be detoxified, and increasing the risk of cellular damage. Some of the factors include diet (some foods and supplements increase phase I enzyme activity), smoking and alcohol consumption (both induce phase I), age (which can decrease phase II UGT, GST, and SULT activity), sex (premenopausal women show 30–40% more phase I CYP3A4 activity than men or post-menopausal women), disease, and genetics.[54]

An illustrative (and unfortunately common) example of the consequences of phase I/phase II imbalance is toxicity caused by overdose of the analgesic acetaminophen (paracetamol)—the active ingredient in Tylenol®. Acetaminophen toxicity is the most common cause of liver failure in the United States.[55] With a normal therapeutic dose of acetaminophen, the drug is predominantly detoxified by the phase II UGT and SULT enzymes. A small amount of the drug is detoxified by a third mechanism: it is first transformed into the toxic metabolite NAPQI (N-acetyl-p-benzoquinoneimine) by phase I CYP enzymes, and this intermediate is detoxified by conjugation with glutathione using the phase II enzyme GST.

During acetaminophen overdose, the UGT and SULT enzymes become quickly overwhelmed. Proportionately more of the drug undergoes the third detoxification mechanism (transformation to NAPQI and conjugation by GST). Eventually, activity of the phase II GST enzyme slows as glutathione stores become depleted,[56] and NAPQI is produced faster than it can be detoxified. Rising levels of NAPQI in the liver cause widespread damage, including lipid peroxidation, inactivation of cellular proteins, and disruption of DNA metabolism.[57] Treatment for acetaminophen overdose involves the timely replenishment of glutathione stores through administration of the precursor amino acids for glutathione synthesis (most commonly N-acetyl cysteine).[58]

# ADDITIONAL ASPECTS OF THE DETOXIFICATION PROCESS

Several other mechanisms work in concert with the phase I, II, and III enzyme systems to improve their efficiency or extend their functionality. While not officially characterized as part of xenobiotic metabolism, they are nonetheless important for reducing or mitigating toxin exposure.

*Bile secretion* is a critical digestive process for the absorption of dietary fats and fat-soluble nutrients, but also functions as the major mechanism for moving conjugated toxins out of the liver and into the intestines, where they can be eliminated.

*Antioxidation* is a necessary protective measure against the harsh phase I oxidation reactions, which frequently produce free-radical byproducts. The production of antioxidant enzymes, many of which are under the same genetic regulation (by Nrf2) as the phase II enzymes, is important for minimizing this free-radical damage.

*Heavy metal toxicity* can lead to oxidative damage by direct generation of free radical species and depletion of antioxidant reserves.[59] Mercury, arsenic, and lead, for example, effectively inactivate the glutathione molecule so that it is unavailable as an antioxidant or as a substrate for xenobiotic detoxification[60]; lead can also reduce the activity of the enzymes that recycle glutathione.[61] One method for heavy metal removal is their chelation by the cellular proteins metallothioneins (MTs), which have a high capacity to bind various reactive metal ions, such as zinc, cadmium, mercury, copper, lead, nickel, cobalt, iron, gold, and silver.[62] One molecule of MT can bind 7–9 zinc or cadmium ions (or any combination of these two), up to 12 copper ions, and up to 18 mercury ions.[63] Cellular stress (particularly oxidative stress), turns up MT production, which, like the phase II enzymes, is stimulated by the activity of Nrf2.[64]

*Prevention of absorption* through trapping of potential toxins (such as surface adhesion to another molecule in the gut, like activated charcoal or kaolin clay[65]) is an effective means of mitigating exposure; this mechanism has the requirement of some dietary adsorbent to be taken while the toxin is in transit in the GI tract. Uptake of potential toxins and their detoxification by beneficial colonic microflora could have a similar effect.

## WHAT YOU NEED TO KNOW ABOUT METABOLIC DETOXIFICATION

- Detoxification is the metabolic process of removing unwanted lipid-soluble compounds from the body.
- These "unwanted" compounds can be foreign (such as an environmental toxicants) or endogenous (toxins, such as excess hormones) in nature.
- Detoxification reactions occur throughout the body, with the liver being the predominant detoxifying organ.

Detoxification reactions follow three steps or "phases" that have the ultimate goal of converting the toxin into an inert, water-soluble form for excretion.

**Phase I** reactions transform the toxin into a chemical form that can be metabolized by the phase II enzymes. Phase I reactions are performed primarily by cytochrome P450 enzymes.

**Phase II** reactions conjugate (attach) the toxin to other water-soluble substances to increase its solubility. Each of the different types of phase II enzymes catalyzes a different type of conjugation reaction.

- UDP-glucuronlytransferases (UGTs) catalyze the glucuronidation of most clinical drugs, and several environmental toxins

- Glutathione-S-transferases (GSTs) conjugate toxins with the antioxidant glutathione; they can also directly detoxify free radicals
- Sulfotransferases (SULTs) catalyze sulfonation reactions; they may also be important for controlling sex hormone levels

Other types of phase II reactions that are used less frequently include methylation and amino acid conjugation reactions.

**Phase III** detoxification involves the transport of the transformed, conjugated toxin into or out of cells. Various phase III transport proteins work in concert to shuttle toxins from different parts of the body into bile or urine for excretion.

Following detoxification reactions, the toxins are removed from the body by excretion as follows:

- Products of liver detoxification often leave the body by being secreted into the intestines in bile, but can sometimes be transported into the bloodstream for processing by the kidneys.
- The cells that line the intestines can detoxify toxins as they are absorbed, and release them back into the intestinal lumen.
- The kidneys can filter and further process toxins from circulation, excreting them from the body as urine.

## DIETARY MODIFICATION OF METABOLIC DETOXIFICATION

Given the sheer number of diverse enzymes and transport proteins involved in metabolic detoxification and its related pathways, it is no surprise that detoxification depends on, and is sensitive to, a large number of dietary factors.

Macronutrient and micronutrient intake influences phase I and II systems. Protein deficiency decreases CYP metabolism, while high-protein diets increase it.[66] The opposite effects are observed for carbohydrates; the effects of lipids on CYP metabolism are unclear. Efficient phase I reactions require sufficiency in several micronutrients. Deficiencies in vitamins A, B2, and B3, C, and E; folate; iron; calcium; copper; zinc; magnesium; and selenium have all been shown to decrease the activities of one or more phase I enzymes, or slow the transformation of specific drugs.[67]

The diverse set of phase II enzymes requires an equally diverse set of essential nutrients, especially B vitamins, as cofactors.

The reduced glutathione for GST conjugation depends on adequate dietary sulfur-containing amino acids (methionine or cysteine), vitamin B6 for the conversion of methionine to cysteine, as well vitamins B2 and B3 for the activity of glutathione reductase, which recycles oxidized glutathione.

The methylation reactions use *SAMe* as a substrate; which, in turn, is synthesized through folate- and vitamin B12–dependent enzymatic reactions.

The conjugation reactions of the NATs and amino acid acyltransferases use the cofactor acetyl-coenzyme A (acetyl-CoA), which is synthesized from vitamin B5 using enzymes that themselves depend on multiple B vitamins.

Several phase II reactions require the energy molecule ATP in some fashion. For example, the chemical cofactors for the phase II methylation, sulfonation, glucuronidation, and glutathione conjugation reactions are all made using ATP; these ATP-mediated reactions are magnesium dependent.

*Flavonoids* have been extensively studied in vitro and in animal models for their ability to lower the activity of CYPs, and increase phase II enzyme activities (except for SULTs, which they tend to inhibit).[68] The inhibition of CYP activity by naringenin (the principal flavonoid in grapefruit) has been well documented in humans[69]; hence, the recommendation to avoid grapefruit when taking prescription drugs. Other flavonoids that have demonstrated mild inhibition of multiple CYPs in animal models include genistein, daidzein, and equol from soy,[70,71] and theaflavins from black tea.[72]

*Green tea extracts* and the *quercetin* derivatives isoquercetin and rutin are an exception to most other flavonoids, green tea tannins can increase CYP activity in vivo,[73] but also increase phase II activity (GST and UGT). Similarly, the quercetin derivatives were demonstrated to increase intestinal and liver CYPs in rats; quercetin had no effect on CYPs in this experiment.[74]

*Nrf2 activators:* A wide variety of dietary components have been shown in vitro or cell culture to activate Nrf2 and directly increase activity of phase II enzymes. These include epigallocatechin gallate (EGCG),[75] resveratrol,[76] curcumin[77] and its metabolite tetrahydrocurcumin, which has greater phase II activity,[78] cinnamaldehyde,[79] caffeic acid phenylethyl ester, alpha lipoic acid,[80] alpha tocopherol,[81] lycopene,[82] apple polyphenols (chlorogenic acid and phloridzin),[83] gingko biloba,[84] chalcone,[85] capsaicin,[86] hydroxytyrosol from olives,[87] allyl sulfides from garlic,[88] chlorophyllin,[89] and xanthohumols from hops.[90] The beneficial effects of these phytochemicals have been demonstrated in numerous animal and human studies, particularly chemopreventative and antioxidant abilities. These effects may be explained by their indirect stimulation of antioxidant enzyme production and phase II detoxification through Nrf2 signaling.[91]

*Isothiocyanates derived from glucosinolates* are reactive sulfur compounds with potent chemopreventive properties. The prototypical member is sulforaphane, a constituent of broccoli that is the subject of several human cancer trials.

Isothiocyanates such as sulforaphane and indoles such as indole-3-carbinol (I3C) are among the most potent natural inducers of phase II detoxification enzymes.[92] Sulforaphane and a derivative of I3C both directly activate Nrf2,[93] which increases the production of several protective enzymes, including GSTs, UGTs, glutamate-cysteine ligase (which synthesizes glutathione), and NQO1.[94] I3C derivatives are also strong inducers of many phase I and II enzymes, and thus are among the most well-studied phytochemicals for detoxification, as well as cancer prevention.[95–99]

Compounds from the Japanese horseradish **Wasabi japonica**,[100,101] and benzyl isothiocyanate (BITC)[102] from **cruciferous vegetables** similarly stimulate phase II enzyme activity via Nrf2 activation. Both sulforaphane and BITC also lower CYP activity.[103]

**Sulfur constituents from garlic** are inhibitors of various CYPs,[104] and induce GST and NQO1 activity in gastrointestinal tissues in rats.[105] By activating Nrf2, components in garlic were able to reverse the depletion of antioxidant enzymes caused by a toxic metal compound in the livers of laboratory rats.[106]

**D-limonene** (from citrus oil) has been investigated for anticancer activity in uncontrolled human trials and animal studies with some success[107]; part of this chemopreventive activity is due to the induction of phase I and phase II enzymes. In rats, D-limonene has been shown to increase total CYP activity,[108] intestinal UGT activity,[109] and liver GST and UGT activity.[110,111]

**Calcium D-glucarate** is present in many fruits and vegetables, and can be produced in small amounts in humans.[112] When activated in the gut, it functions as an inhibitor of beta-glucuronidase, an enzyme produced by colonic bacteria and intestinal cells. In the intestines, beta-glucuronidase removes (deconjugates) glucuronic acid from neutralized toxins—essentially reversing the reaction catalyzed by UGTs. Deconjugation reverts the toxin to its previous dangerous form, and allows it to be reabsorbed. Elevated beta-glucuronidase activity has been associated with increased cancer risk.[113]

**Chlorophyllin** is a chlorophyll derivative[114] that inhibits CYP activity[115] and stimulates GST activity in cell culture and rodent models.[116] The unique chemical structures of chlorophyllin and chlorophyll enable them to bind and "trap" toxins in the gut preventing their absorption. In animal models, chlorophyllin and chlorophyll lower the bioavailability and accelerate the excretion of several environmental carcinogens.[117–119] Toxin trapping may partly explain the results of a human trial of residents in Qidong, China, an area with a high incidence of liver cancer due to exposure to aflatoxin (a toxin produced by species of the fungus Aspergillus). Among the 180 people who took 100 mg of chlorophyllin 3 times daily, urinary levels of DNA-aflatoxin conjugates (a marker for DNA mutation) went down 55% compared to untreated people.[120]

Certain strains of **probiotic bacteria** may minimize toxin exposure by trapping and metabolizing xenobiotics or heavy metals.[121] Examples include the detoxification of aflatoxin and patulin (two toxins produced by Aspergillus, a type of mold species),[122] the metabolism of heterocyclic amines and dimethylhydrazine,[123] and the binding of lead and cadmium.[124] Additionally, the production of the short-chain fatty acid butyrate by lactic acid bacteria (from the fermentation of dietary fiber) has been shown to stimulate GST production in intestinal cell culture; this may also contribute to some of the anticarcinogenic properties of dietary fiber.[125]

**N-acetyl cysteine** (NAC) can provide an alternative source of sulfur for glutathione production. It is a free radical scavenger on its own, effective at reducing oxidative stress, particularly due to heavy metal toxicity.[126] Because it can directly replenish glutathione stores, NAC is more effective than methionine at preventing liver damage,[127] and is the current treatment for acetaminophen toxicity. It is an effective treatment for acute liver failure due to nonacetaminophen drug toxicity as well.[128]

**Milk thistle** (Silybum marianum), the most well-researched plant in the treatment of liver disease,[129] contains a mixture of several related polyphenolic compounds called silymarin. Silymarin promotes detoxification by several complementary mechanisms. The antioxidant capacity of silymarin can lower the liver oxidative stress associated with toxin metabolism, particularly lipid peroxidation[130], which has the effect of conserving cellular glutathione levels.[131] Like NAC, silymarin can protect against acetaminophen toxicity (possibly by the similar mechanism of preserving glutathione levels). Silymarin, however, may be a more effective antidote than NAC for acetaminophen toxicity if the treatment is delayed (in an animal model, it was effective when administered up to 24 hours after overdose).[132]

Phase III transporters, while important for removing toxins from healthy cells, can also decrease the effectiveness of pharmaceutical therapies by increasing their clearance. This can be especially problematic with chemotherapy drugs, to which phase III transporters enable cancer cells to become resistant. Therefore, stimulation of phase III activity may not always be desirable.

Dietary factors can have differing effects on phase III transporters. For example, apple polyphenols[133] and sulforaphane (at levels equivalent to about two servings of broccoli)[134] both stimulate the activity of the phase III proteins. In contrast, the curcumin metabolite tetrahydrocurcumin decreases the activity of the phase III transporters in human cervical carcinoma and breast cancer cell lines.[135] Resveratrol decreases phase III protein synthesis, which prevents acute myeloid leukemia cells from becoming resistant to the chemotherapy drug doxorubicin in cell culture.[136] *Silibinin*, the chief constituent of milk thistle,[137] is also a phase III inhibitor, both in vitro and in vivo.[138]

**Bile flow:** As a major carrier of toxins from the body, proper bile flow is a critical final step in the metabolic detoxification process. Impairment of bile flow (cholestasis), resulting from dysfunction within the liver or blockage of the bile duct, can result in the buildup of liver toxins and liver injury. Cholestasis can also be the result of the detoxification process itself; there is increasing evidence that the detoxification and excretion of clinical drugs into the bile can produce cholestatic liver disease.[139] Artichoke has been used for centuries in folk medicine as a liver protectant and to stimulate bile flow (choleresis), and is the best-studied herbal choleretic agent.

*Artichoke* contains several antioxidants that can protect against oxidative liver damage, as well as caffeoylquinic acids, which have been shown to stimulate bile flow in animal models.[140] Caffeoylquinic acids may also be responsible for the choleretic properties of yarrow,[141–143] fennel,[143] and dandelion.[144] Andrographis, garlic, cumin, ginger, ajowan (carom seed), and curry and mustard leaf have also been shown to stimulate bile flow or bile acid production in rodent models.[145–148]

## Life Extension Suggestions

- **N-acetyl cysteine:** 600 mg 1–3 times daily
- **Green Tea extract**, standardized to EGCG: 725 mg daily
- **Quercetin:** 250–500 mg daily
- **B-vitamin complex:** Per label instructions
- **Magnesium:** 300–600 mg daily
- **Broccoli extract,** standardized to glucosinolates: 400 mg once or twice daily, with meals
- **I3C** (indole-3-carbinol): 80–160 mg daily
- **SAMe:** 400 mg 2–3 times daily; take with cofactors B12, B6, and folic acid
- **Milk thistle extract,** standardized to silymarin and silibinins: 750 mg daily
- **R-lipoic acid:** 240–480 mg daily
- **Calcium-D-glucarate:** 140–300 mg daily
- ***Trans*-resveratrol:** 250 mg daily
- **Curcumin:** 400 mg daily, with meals
- **Chlorophyllin:** 100 mg 3 times daily with food
- **Artichoke extract:** 500 mg daily
- **Probiotics:** Per label instructions

## REFERENCES

References available at: www.lef.org/dpt5/ch92

# 93

---

# *Migraine Headache*

---

Migraine headaches are recurrent, painful headaches often accompanied by nausea, photophobia (ie, light sensitivity) and/or phonophobia (ie, sound sensitivity). A migraine is often unilateral and pulsating, and may occur with or without an aura.[1–8]

About 23 million adults in the United States are reported to experience migraine headaches, and they are one of the most common complaints encountered by neurologists in day-to-day practice.[9,10] Nonetheless, migraine disorder remains a commonly *underdiagnosed* and *undertreated* condition.[11–14]

Conventional pharmacologic migraine treatments often meet with limited success and may have intolerable side effects or be contraindicated with other common coexisting conditions.[15–18]

On the other hand, avoiding migraine triggers such as *intense emotional stress*, *poor sleep habits*, and *unbalanced hormone levels* may reduce the occurrence of attacks.[6,19,20] In addition, there are a variety of safe and effective natural treatment approaches available for migraine management.[21]

Upon reading this protocol, you will learn what causes migraine and how conventional medicine treats migraine headaches. You will also discover how to avoid common migraine triggers and read about natural options that can help you manage migraine headaches.

## WHAT IS A MIGRAINE HEADACHE?

Migraine headache is often described as intense throbbing or pulsating head pain that interferes with a person's ability to go about normal daily functioning.[3,22] Migraine headache pain is often made worse by physical activity.[23]

Migraine sufferers frequently describe the pain as being limited to one side of the head.[24] However, some people do experience migraines on both sides of the head.[25] Migraine is commonly associated with nausea, as well as light and/or sound sensitivity.[26] Although migraine duration varies from patient to patient, a typical attack lasts for several hours, and sometimes persists for up to several (eg, 2–3) days.[23]

Various physical and/or psychological changes sometimes precede the onset of a migraine headache by a few hours to a few days. This phase of a migraine is called *prodrome*. The experience of prodrome varies from person to person but can include such things as appetite changes, loss of balance, mood changes, tiredness, neck stiffness, and changes in alertness. The prevalence of a distinct prodrome phase is not entirely clear because studies have reported differing rates, but a significant portion of migraineurs indicate that they experience symptoms that predict the onset of migraine. Individuals who have experienced migraine preceded by prodrome in the past may be able to recognize an impending headache based on their prodrome symptoms and plan accordingly for the next hours or few days by taking steps such as avoiding rigorous or stressful activity and ensuring they have an adequate stock of migraine relief medication.[27]

Approximately 25% of migraineurs will experience a premigraine phenomena called *aura*, which is a neurologic abnormality causing mostly visual, but also other sensory and/or movement disturbances that manifests within a few hours of a migraine headache.[28,29] Most experts believe that migraine aura is caused by a phenomenon in the brain called cortical spreading depression (CSD), a slowly progressing wave of excitability followed by long-lasting neuronal inhibition.[30]

## WHAT CAUSES MIGRAINE?

In the early years of migraine research, scientists believed that the headache portion of a migraine resulted from the dilation of blood vessels, while the aura portion of migraine was caused by vasoconstriction.[31] However, more recent evidence suggests that these vascular changes are not the cause of migraine, but rather an epiphenomenon that accompanies the pain.[22] Today, migraine is viewed as a result of complex dysfunction within the central nervous system.[32] Various factors that contribute to this dysfunction are reviewed below.

### Serotonin

The neurotransmitter serotonin (5-hydroxytryptamine [5-HT]) plays a role in the development of migraine attacks. This conclusion is supported by evidence indicating that migraine patients tend to have low levels of serotonin in their brains.[33] Additional support for this theory is found in data indicating that tricyclic antidepressants, which increase serotonin signaling, reduce the frequency of migraine attacks.[31]

Furthermore, melatonin, an active metabolite of serotonin,[34] has also been found to be deficient among migraine patients,[35,36] and melatonin supplementation has resulted in symptom improvement among some migraine patients.[37]

Although the exact mechanism linking low serotonin levels to migraine pathology has not yet been fully described,[38] researchers have hypothesized that serotonin may interfere with pain processing in the brain. Serotonin also affects the dilation and contraction of blood vessels in the brain.[31]

Although low serotonin levels may give rise to an attack, some evidence suggests that elevated serotonin levels may contribute to migraine pathology *during* an attack.[39,40] Due to the complexity of serotonin's role in migraine, further study is needed to fully characterize the effects of modulating serotonin levels and/or signaling in migraine patients.

## The Role of Hormones

Migraine disproportionately affects women—females make up about 70% of all migraine patients—suggesting a potential hormonal link.[41]

Although many hormonal events in a female's life may influence the occurrence of migraine (eg, menarche, menstruation, pregnancy, and menopause),[42] menstruation appears to be the most important. For example, 70% of female patients who experience migraine report some type of menstrual link.[43] A phenomenon called *estrogen withdrawal*, which occurs in the late luteal phase of the menstrual cycle and is characterized by an abrupt decline in estrogen levels, is likely an important migraine trigger in some women.[44,45]

Fluctuations in estrogen levels associated with migraine produce biochemical changes in prostaglandin production, prolactin release, and endogenous opioid regulation.[20,46]

Prostaglandin E2 (PGE-2) is a well-defined mediator of fever and inflammation. PGE-2 increases vasodilatation and thereby induces pain. Estrogens increase the production of PGE-2. An excess of estrogens, deficit of progesterone, or dominance of estrogens can cause increased production of PGE-2, resulting in migraine.

Elevation of the prolactin level or increased sensitivity to prolactin leads to a decreased level of prostaglandin E1 (PGE-1). Patients with migraine may have prostaglandin-induced hypersensitivity to prolactin. PGE-1 is a substance that in fact improves the microcirculation and leads to the development of collateral circuits with a consequent improvement in local hemodynamics.

If a patient has a dominance of PGE-2, vasodilatation of major arteries with spasm of collateral circuits would be expected, which in turn can cause pain. Restoration of hormonal levels and balance between them can stabilize levels of prostaglandins.

Steroid hormones also influence the metabolism of calcium and magnesium. Estrogens regulate calcium metabolism, intestinal calcium absorption, and parathyroid gene expression and secretion, triggering fluctuations across the menstrual cycle. Alterations in calcium homeostasis have long been associated with many affective disturbances.

Clinical trials in women with premenstrual syndrome have found that calcium supplementation may help alleviate most mood and somatic symptoms. Evidence to date indicates that women with symptoms of premenstrual syndrome have an underlying calcium abnormality.[47] A low brain magnesium level can be an expression of neuronal hyperexcitability of the visual pathways and thus would be associated with a lowered threshold for migraine attacks.[48] Clinically, it is known that magnesium supplementation relieves premenstrual problems (eg, migraine, bloating, and edema) that occur late in the menstrual cycle, and that migraine, particularly in women, is associated with deficiencies in brain and serum magnesium levels. Testosterone was not shown to produce any significant alteration in magnesium levels, but estrogens and progesterone do.[49]

Among women with menstrual-related migraines, using hormone therapy to minimize monthly declines in estrogen concentration may be effective in preventing migraine attacks.[50] Studies suggest that nonoral routes of estrogen therapy, such as a topical cream to be applied to the skin, are more likely to improve migraine than oral estrogens.[44]

More information about hormone testing and restoration is available in the Female Hormone Restoration protocol.

---

## THE NEUROHORMONAL AND METABOLIC DYSBALANCE HYPOTHESIS OF MIGRAINE

Some researchers suspect that an important cause of migraine is an *imbalance* between estrogens and *progesterone* levels, rather than the absolute levels of these hormones. Indeed, therapies aimed at improving the ratio of estrogens to progesterone have successfully relieved severe menstrual migraine in preliminary reports.[51]

Some innovative physicians believe that consideration should be given to the balance of other sex hormones as well, including *testosterone, dehydroepiandrosterone (DHEA)*, and *pregnenolone.*[20]

According to the neurohormonal and metabolic dysbalance hypothesis of migraine, migraine is not a single disorder, but a collection of disorders involving faulty hormonal feedback in the *hypothalamic-pituitary-adrenal-gonadal axis*.

Contributing to this hormonal abnormality is an imbalance between two of the three arms of the autonomic nervous system (the sympathetic and parasympathetic nervous systems), which causes a decline in the brain's pain threshold. Because of disequilibrium between intra- and extracellular calcium and magnesium, the polarity of the cell membrane is changed, which affects the electrical stability of the cell membrane and sensitivity to neurohormonal impulses (steroid hormones, melatonin, and serotonin).

Although well-controlled clinical trials designed to test the hypothesis that comprehensive hormone testing and balancing may relieve migraine headaches are lacking, several case reports present positive outcomes using this novel approach.[20]

One link between hormonal imbalance and migraine may stem from the opposing roles of *estrogen* and *progesterone* within the brain. While estrogen stimulates neural excitability, progesterone exhibits inhibitory actions in central neurons.[52] Therefore, imbalance between these neuromodulatory hormones may give rise to physiological conditions that alter susceptibility to migraine.[52]

Tailored *hormonal replacement therapy (HRT)* aimed at minimizing estrogen/progesterone imbalance and stabilizing estrogen levels may be effective for preventing migraines among pre- and post-menopausal women.[43,53–55] In the words of some forward-thinking migraine researchers, "[C]linical experience strongly supports the notion that migraine can be managed only when levels of all the basic hormones—pregnenolone, DHEA, testosterone, estrogen, and progesterone—are optimal with the physiological cycle."[56]

Women suffering migraines without relief through conventional medical treatments should consider comprehensive hormone testing and restoration of hormonal balance using *bioidentical hormone replacement therapy*.

# DIAGNOSIS

History and physical examination are used to diagnose migraine headaches.[4,8,31,57–59]

Migraine headache is often misdiagnosed as sinus headache or tension-type headache.[58] This is especially true when the headache complaints are not accompanied by the typical features of migraine such as nausea, light/sound sensitivity, and exacerbation upon physical activity.[31]

Some less common but potentially more serious disorders, including subarachnoid hemorrhage, intracranial mass lesions, and cerebral vasculitis, among others, can cause migraine-like symptoms. Therefore, it is important that your doctor rule out other possible causes of headache, especially in the absence of history of migraine.[2,59–61]

When physicians are not sure that migraine is the proper diagnosis, tests such as computerized tomography (CT), magnetic resonance imaging (MRI), and a spinal tap (lumbar puncture) may be used to help rule out other possible conditions.[61,62]

# CONVENTIONAL TREATMENT

Most migraine treatment plans involve both *acute* and *preventive* strategies.[63]

## Acute Treatment

The goal of acute or abortive treatment is to relieve the intensity and/or duration of an imminent or ongoing migraine as quickly as possible.[64]

First-tier options for acute migraine management may include *nonsteroidal anti-inflammatory drugs (NSAIDs)* and/or mild analgesics (eg, acetaminophen or aspirin).[64,65] *Caffeine*, due to its vasoconstrictive properties, is sometimes combined with aspirin and/or acetaminophen as well.[66] However, these options may not be sufficient for treating severe migraines, in which case a variety of drugs in the triptan class may be considered.[64]

The *triptan drugs* (eg, sumatriptan, rizatriptan, eletriptan, and almotriptan) act on several specific mechanisms of a migraine headache, such as promoting vasoconstriction and blocking pain pathways in the brainstem. Triptans mediate these effects by activating certain serotonin receptors in cranial blood vessels.[67]

Although the triptans are arguably the most effective treatment for acute relief of a migraine headache (ie, the "gold standard"), they have a number of side effects.[68] For example, triptans should be avoided (when possible) in patients who are at risk for cardiovascular events and stroke (ie, patients with heart disease). Furthermore, triptans require careful monitoring because they are known to interact with a large number of other commonly used medications.[69]

Other drugs that may be used to treat migraine include *ergot alkaloids*, which cause blood vessel constriction, *opioids*, and, less commonly, *corticosteroids*.[70]

Medicating as early as possible during migraine increases the chances of successfully aborting an attack or reducing its intensity.[71]

## Preventive Treatment

The main goals of preventive therapy are to reduce migraine frequency, severity, and duration, as well as improve responsiveness to acute treatment(s). Preventive treatment options include headache trigger avoidance, daily medication, physical therapy, and/or behavioral therapy.[72]

Drugs used to prevent migraines include blood pressure medications (eg, beta blockers, calcium channel blockers, ACE inhibitors, and angiotensin receptor blockers), tricyclic antidepressants (eg, amitriptyline [Elavil®]), and anticonvulsants (eg, valproate [Depakote®], gabapentin [Neurontin®], and topiramate [Topamax®]). These drugs should be started at low doses, and given adequate time to reach peak effectiveness. Therefore, depending on the chosen medication, a proper drug trial could take anywhere from 4 weeks to 3 months to take effect.[73]

Ironically, taking too much migraine prevention medication for too long can lead to "medication overuse headache." Medication overuse headache can become a chronic, self-perpetuating condition called *chronic daily headache*, in which patients experience daily headaches caused by medication overuse, but continue to use medication to relive the headaches. To prevent medication overuse headache, migraine patients should (on average) limit use of NSAIDs to ≤15 days a month and limit triptan or over-the-counter combination analgesic use to ≤9 days a month.[74,75]

## LIFESTYLE CONSIDERATIONS

Although there is a wide variety of acute and preventive drugs available for treating migraines, many patients will not experience significant symptom relief unless healthy lifestyle modifications are made.[76] The following lifestyle interventions may prevent migraines[77–81]:

- avoidance of caffeine, nicotine, red wine, and other migraine triggers
- stress reduction (see the Stress Management protocol)
- improving sleep hygiene (see the Insomnia protocol)
- massage therapy
- chiropractic manipulation
- acupuncture
- getting sufficient exercise
- frequent stretching

## DIETARY INTERVENTIONS

A significant association between dietary intake and migraine incidence exists; one out of every four migraine patients reports that certain foods can trigger an attack.[82] Furthermore, the avoidance of food allergies and/or sensitivities may reduce or eliminate migraine symptoms for some patients.[83]

Common nutritional migraine triggers include[84]:

- *Monosodium glutamate (MSG)* is a commonly used flavor enhancer found in some soups and Chinese food.

- *Nitrites* are preservatives found in processed meats such as hot dogs.
- *Tyramines* are natural compounds found in wines and aged foods (eg, cheeses).
- *Phenylethylamine* is a stimulant compound found in chocolate, garlic, nuts, raw onions, and seeds.

Many of these nutritional migraine triggers have vasoactive properties (causes constriction or dilation of blood vessels),[85] which is why they may contribute to migraine attacks.

Other potential dietary triggers include cow's milk, wheat, eggs, alcohol, artificial sweeteners, citrus fruits, pickled products, and vinegar.[86,87]

It is important to note that not all migraine patients are susceptible to the aforementioned nutritional triggers; thus the complete elimination of these items is not always necessary.[86] In order to identify nutritional triggers, experts suggest the use of food diaries because they are simple and inexpensive. Removal of trigger foods is associated with a reduction in migraine headaches.[88]

In addition, food allergy and sensitivity testing to measure immunologic reactivity to foods may allow for identification of potential migraine triggers.[87,89,90]

In addition to the above triggers, dietary fasting for longer than 4 hours should also be avoided (when possible) since it has been linked to an increased risk of migraine.[91,92]

## TARGETED NUTRITIONAL INTERVENTION

Natural therapies (eg, dietary supplements) are well tolerated, and many have been shown to reduce migraine symptoms.[21,93]

**Butterbur root.** Butterbur (*Petasites hybridus*) is a plant that flourishes in moist conditions, and has been used for a wide range of medicinal purposes in Europe since ancient times.[94] Butterbur extracts possess analgesic, anti-inflammatory, antispasmodic, and vasodilatory properties, which may explain their efficacy for migraine prevention.[94,95] Butterbur root extract (standardized to 15% petasins) has been shown to be both safe and effective for the prevention of migraines.[94,96,97] In one study, researchers split 245 patients into three groups to receive: 75 mg of butterbur extract twice a day, 50 mg of butterbur extract twice a day, or placebo. At the end of a 4-month treatment period, those taking the 75 mg dosage experienced a whopping 48% reduction, on average, in the frequency of migraine attacks.[97]

Butterbur is so effective for reducing the frequency and severity of migraine attacks that the *American Academy of Neurology (AAN)* and the *American Headache Society (AHS)* have recommend it as an effective treatment for migraine.[98]

**Coenzyme Q10.** Coenzyme Q10 (CoQ10) is a potent antioxidant[99] and an important component of cellular energy production. Researchers have found that organs with a high metabolic rate, such as the brain, appear to quickly deplete CoQ10 stores, potentially leading to a deficiency.[100]

CoQ10 (at doses of 100–300 mg daily) has been shown to be beneficial for preventing and reducing the frequency of migraine attacks among adults.[21,101] These actions are attributed to CoQ10's potential to interfere with inflammatory mechanisms and mitochondrial dysfunction, both of which have been implicated in the migraine process.[101]

**Riboflavin.** Riboflavin (ie, vitamin B2) contributes to cell growth, enzyme function, and energy production.[102] High-quality data indicate that riboflavin is effective for the prevention of migraine among both children and adults,[103,104] and may decrease the need for traditional rescue medications.[104] It is believed that riboflavin's beneficial effects are due to its ability to enhance mitochondrial energy production,[105] which is based on data indicating that riboflavin is especially effective among migraine patients with mitochondrial genetic abnormalities.[106]

One study involving 23 participants showed that supplementation with 400 mg riboflavin daily reduced headache frequency by an impressive 50% at 3 months, with improvement persisting through 6 months.[104] Riboflavin is also cost-effective and has a minimal side effect profile.[103]

**Feverfew.** Feverfew (*Tanacetum parthenium*) is a small, daisy-like flower with a distinctively strong, bitter odor.[107] Recent evidence has revealed that feverfew inhibits the production of several inflammatory mediators that may be involved in migraine, including arachidonic acid, cyclooxygenase-2, TNF-α, IL-1, and MCP-1. Due to these anti-inflammatory properties, feverfew's use in the management of migraine attacks is promising.[107–109] However, a review of randomized controlled trials revealed mixed results for the effectiveness of feverfew.[110] For example, a study that used dried leaf revealed a decrease in the frequency of migraines while another using a $CO_2$ extract did not show significant benefit.[110] A combination of ginger and feverfew has also been shown to be effective for migraine prevention with minimal side effects.[111,112] A dosage of 100–300 mg up to 4 times daily is recommended.[113]

**Magnesium.** Magnesium modulates many important neural and vascular processes involved in the development of a typical migraine attack. Migraine patients commonly exhibit low magnesium levels (in the serum, tissue, and lymphocytes), especially during an attack.[114–116] Furthermore, magnesium deficiency can trigger cortical spreading depression (CSD), platelet aggregation, vasoconstriction, and substance P release, all of which have been implicated in migraine pathology.[116] A dosage of 600 mg of magnesium daily has been shown to be effective for the prevention of migraine attacks,[117] and is inexpensive and well-tolerated.[116] In combination with CoQ10, vitamin B2, and ginkgo, magnesium has been shown to significantly decrease the number of migraine headaches.[118] Although not yet proven in clinical trials, a form of magnesium called *magnesium-L-threonate* may be ideal for people with migraine because experimental data indicate that it enters the central nervous system more efficiently than other forms of magnesium.[119]

**Melatonin.** Melatonin is a natural compound produced by the pineal gland that helps regulate the sleep–wake cycle (ie, circadian rhythms), and has been clinically shown to possess potent antioxidant and analgesic properties.[120] Since melatonin is often found in lower-than-normal levels among migraine patients (especially during an attack), it is thought that it may play an important role in migraine pathology.[35,121]

Some researchers hypothesize that migraines are triggered by an irregularity in pineal gland function.[122] When this imbalance is corrected through melatonin supplementation, some migraine patients experience an improvement in symptoms.[37] In one clinical study, melatonin supplementation trended toward a two-thirds reduction in number of migraine attacks.[123] This response rate may have been more statistically significant if the researchers used a larger dose of melatonin (3 mg instead of 2 mg), and if treatment was extended for a longer period of time (12–16 weeks, instead of 8 weeks).[124] Melatonin has been found to be safe and associated with few or no side effects.[122]

**S-adenosylmethionine (SAMe).** SAMe is a nutritional supplement derived from the amino acid methionine and adenosine triphosphate, a nucleic acid.[125] It is a naturally occurring substance produced by the body to perform a variety of important biochemical processes, especially involving the central nervous system (CNS).[126] Some data suggest that long-term supplementation with SAMe may relieve pain among migraine sufferers, possibly due to its ability to increase serotonin.[127,128]

**L-tryptophan.** The amino acid L-tryptophan is a precursor to serotonin. Several lines of evidence indicate that low serotonergic signaling within the brain may precipitate migraine.[38] Therefore, supporting serotonin synthesis by providing precursors like L-tryptophan may help avoid physiologic conditions that promote migraine headache. Indeed, in an older clinical trial, supplementation with 2–4 grams of L-tryptophan daily was as effective at preventing migraine attacks as the medication methysergide.[129] Also, a more recent trial found that dietary tryptophan depletion caused exacerbation of migraine symptoms.[130]

**Miscellaneous Beneficial Ingredients.** The following list of natural ingredients may also be useful for managing migraine symptoms, although definitive clinical data are lacking:

- Ginkgo biloba[21]
- Lipoic acid[131]
- Vitamin B6[132]
- Ginger[133]

## Life Extension Suggestions

- **Butterbur root**, standardized extract: 150 mg daily
- **Riboflavin:** 400 mg daily
- **Ginger root**, standardized extract: 250 mg daily

- **Coenzyme Q10** (as ubiquinol): 100–300 mg daily
- **Feverfew** (dried leaf): up to 1200 mg daily in divided doses
- **Magnesium:** 140 mg daily as magnesium-L-threonate; 320 mg daily as magnesium citrate
- **Melatonin:** 0.3–5 mg before bed (sometimes up to 10 mg)
- **S-adenosylmethionine (SAMe):** 200–1200 mg daily
- **Ginkgo biloba**, standardized extract: 120 mg daily
- **R-lipoic acid:** 300–600 mg daily
- **Vitamin B6** (as pyridoxal-5-phosphate): 100 mg daily
- **L-tryptophan:** 500–2000 mg daily

In addition, the following *blood tests* may provide helpful information:

- Food Safe Allergy Test
- Magnesium (RBC)
- Female Comprehensive Hormone Panel/Male Comprehensive Hormone Panel or Female Basic Hormone Panel/Male Basic Hormone Panel

## REFERENCES

References available at: www.lef.org/dpt5/ch93

# 94

# Multiple Sclerosis

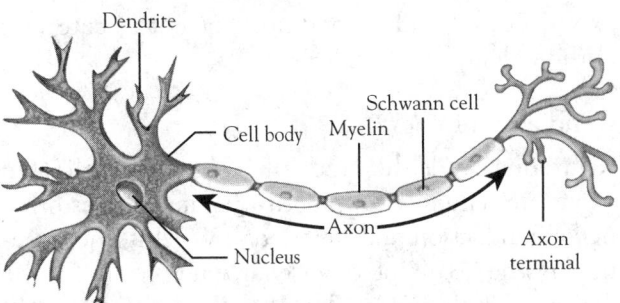

Anatomy of a Neuron

**M**ultiple sclerosis (MS) is a disease of autoimmunity and inflammation characterized by destruction of the *myelin sheath* that insulates and protects neurons. When a patient experiences an "attack," or episode of increased disease activity, the resulting impairment of neuronal communication can manifest as a broad spectrum of symptoms, affecting sensory processing, locomotion, and cognition.

Scientific research suggests that both genetic and environmental factors contribute to the development of the disease. Current medical treatments for MS include potent immunosuppressive drugs, which reduce immune function, and anti-inflammatory medications as well as invasive procedures such as plasma exchange, which attempts to reduce inflammatory mediators in a patient's blood.

Largely ignored and discounted by mainstream medicine, nutrients offer immune-modifying benefits that can help complement pharmacologic and clinical interventions and improve quality of life for MS patients.

Furthermore, mounting evidence suggests that vitamin D may be a *missing link* in virtually all autoimmune diseases, including MS. This single vitamin has the ability to *modulate* the immune system in ways that even pharmaceutical drugs cannot. A multitude of epidemiologic studies have revealed that individuals with low levels of vitamin D in their blood are at considerably increased risk for developing MS; in fact, up to 90% of MS patients are *deficient* in vitamin D.[1]

## UNDERSTANDING MULTIPLE SCLEROSIS

Within the central nervous system (CNS) (brain and spinal cord) a vast network of neurons are constantly communicating amongst themselves, and with the peripheral nervous system (outside of the brain and spinal cord), to control every aspect of human function, from sight and hearing, to cognition and mobility. The efficiency and accuracy of communication between individual neurons forms the basis for our ability to do things as diverse as complete simple daily tasks and comprehend complex philosophical or mathematical ideas.

Neuronal communication is similar to the transmission of an electrical current through a series of wires. Droves of neurons work together to deliver messages to every corner of the body by transmitting signals along their long, cylindrical midsections called *axons* and passing it on to the next neuron. This is repeated until the message reaches its destination. Like electrical wires, neuronal axons require insulation to ensure that they are able to transmit a signal accurately, and at high speeds. Specialized cells called *oligodendrocytes* provide this insulation to neurons by wrapping the axons in an insulating material called *myelin*. Without this *myelin sheath*, neuronal communication becomes nearly impossible, and neurons become susceptible to damage.

Multiple sclerosis is a disease which ultimately leads to the inability of neurons to communicate among themselves. Because MS is not selective for specific neurons, and can progress through the brain and spinal cord randomly, each patient's symptoms may vary considerably.

During the initial stages of the disease, symptoms often emerge for a finite time before regressing for an extended period.

## PATHOLOGY OF DISEASE PROGRESSION

### Demyelination

Multiple sclerosis (MS) is an immuno-inflammatory disease in which immune cells enter the CNS and destroy the myelin sheath. Immune cells, which become activated through complex mechanisms, migrate into the CNS and attack the myelin sheath. The resultant demyelination is thought to be carried out by T lymphocytes, B lymphocytes, and macrophages, 3 primary classes of immune cells routinely found in MS lesions.[2]

Loss of myelin followed by subsequent lack of neural communication and neuronal death is accepted as the primary cause of disability in MS patients.[3] Axonal transection, or the severing of axons, occurs under conditions of both acute and chronic demyelination.[4-6]

## Remyelination

Remyelination is the process by which demyelinated axons are naturally rewrapped with myelin, restoring nerve conduction and functionality.[7] This phenomenon is the result of oligodendrocytes repairing the damage to the myelin sheath that occurs during an episode of increased disease activity. However, as the disease progresses over years (usually decades), the oligodendrocytes begin to lose their ability to repair the damage, and symptoms become progressively worse and episodes more frequent due to remyelination failure. In addition to developing therapies that slow MS disease progression, many laboratories are developing novel therapeutics that aim to promote remyelination and reverse existing CNS damage.

## Inflammation

In addition to immune-mediated loss of myelin, another characteristic feature of MS is inflammation caused by a class of white blood cells called T cells.[8,9] Some of the damage in the CNS is directly carried out by 2 subpopulations of T lymphocytes called *T helper 1* and *T helper 17*, which produce proinflammatory factors.[10] Recent studies have identified that chemical mediators, interleukin-23 (IL-23) and granulocyte macrophage colony-stimulating factor (GM-CSF), contribute to the autoimmune characteristics of these T cells. Data suggest that absence of these pro-inflammatory signals was sufficient to prevent inflammation in the brain.[11] This suggests that therapeutic strategies directed at blocking the production of inflammatory mediators could be effective for treating MS.

## Vitamin D and Multiple Sclerosis: A Panacea?

Mainstream medicine has *failed* to recognize the pivotal role of vitamin D in *regulating* the overactive immune system in MS patients.

More than 30 years have passed since vitamin D was originally hypothesized to be an important environmental determinant of the prevalence of MS.[12,13] During the 3 decades following the initial linking of vitamin D and MS, evidence has continued to mount. It is now known that MS occurs more frequently in individuals with lower blood levels of vitamin D. A study published in the prestigious *Journal of the American Medical Association* found that, compared to those with the highest vitamin D blood levels, those with the lowest blood levels were 62% more likely to develop MS.

MS attacks occur less frequently during seasons corresponding with the highest exposure to sunlight; since vitamin D synthesis depends on exposure of the skin to sunlight, the summer months also bring the highest blood levels of vitamin D.[14] A recent study has quantified the impact of vitamin D blood levels on risk for MS relapse: *For each 4 ng/ml increase in 25-hydroxy vitamin D in the blood, the risk for MS relapse is reduced by 12%.* The investigators who conducted this study concluded: "Clinically, raising 25-hydroxy vitamin D levels by 20 ng/ml could halve the hazard of a relapse."[15]

Vitamin D mediates these disease-modifying effects through complex and powerful interactions with the immune system. Hostile immune cells, which attack the myelin sheath, are calmed upon exposure to vitamin D. In fact, when aggressive immune cells taken directly from MS patients are exposed to the active form of vitamin D, the cells divide and reproduce much more *slowly*, indicating that vitamin D has the ability to *impede* the aberrant autoimmunity that is a driving force in MS.

However, vitamin D does more than just arrest damaging immune cells; it also *supercharges protective* immune cells.

*T-reg* cells are specialized components of the immune system that help keep immunity *balanced*. If too few T-reg cells are present, the immune system becomes *overactive*, as in autoimmune diseases like MS. Vitamin D *increases* the number of *protective* T-reg cells, restoring equilibrium to an overactive immune system.[16]

In a randomized controlled trial, supplementation with doses of vitamin D ranging from 10000 IU to 40000 IU daily over the course of 52 weeks resulted in a reduction in relapses and a reduction in the number of aggressive immune cells in patients with MS.[17]

Despite robust findings across a range of studies on the link between vitamin D and MS, mainstream medicine and the federal government have only just recently begun to realize the need to initiate federally funded trials. A large scale, randomized, controlled clinical trial to assess the effects of vitamin D in MS is now recruiting; the study is expected to be complete in 2014.[1]

Life Extension® members should not be surprised if vitamin D emerges as a frontline treatment for MS in the coming years. However, instead of waiting for mainstream physicians to begin recommending vitamin D to MS patients, Life Extension® suggests that *all* individuals monitor their blood levels of 25-hydroxyvitamin D and maintain a blood level of *50–80 ng/mL*. This is because low vitamin D levels are also an emerging risk factor for numerous other diseases, such as type 1 diabetes, heart disease, and rheumatoid arthritis.[18-22] The amount of supplementation required to achieve this blood level varies, but it appears that many individuals require supplementation of *5000–8000 IU* of vitamin D each day to reach these levels.

More information about the role of vitamin D in health is available in the compelling Life Extension Magazine article entitled "Startling Findings About Vitamin D Levels in Life Extension® Members."

## RISK FACTORS FOR MS

### Genetics and Family History

Studies have established a definitive role for genetics as contributing factor for developing MS. The most compelling data reveal that while unrelated adopted siblings have a 0–2% disease risk, identical twins demonstrate a 25% disease risk.[23] Several studies have identified susceptibility genes related to many aspects of immune function.[24-28] While these genetic links are helpful in understanding MS population clusters, findings such as the 25% disease risk among identical twins and the geographic distribution of MS, suggest that up to 75% of MS must be attributable to nongenetic or environmental factors.

### Infection

Infection is one of the more widely suspected nongenetic risk factors for MS. Data suggests that, in genetically predisposed individuals, exposure to an infectious agent may lead to MS.[29] One common theory, molecular mimicry, proposes that presentation of foreign antigens that are molecularly similar to self-antigens leads to an autoimmune response.[30,31] In other words, viruses involved in the development of autoimmune diseases could possibly display very similar proteins to the proteins found on nerves making these nerves also a target for antibodies. Investigators have probed the involvement of several viruses, including herpes simplex virus (HSV), rubella, measles, mumps, and Epstein Barr virus (EBV).[32] Currently, the strongest evidence for the involvement of an infectious agent implicates EBV. Virtually all patients who have MS are infected with the EBV.[32] Further, levels of antibodies to EBV are strongly correlated with the risk of developing the disease.[33]

### Vitamin D

Considering the regulatory role that vitamin D plays in immune system reactivity, it is not surprising that population-based studies have consistently found lower levels of vitamin D in the blood of patients with MS compared to healthy control subjects.

Data from the Nurses Health Study (>92000 women followed 1980–2000) and the Nurses Health Study II (>95000 women followed 1991–2001), support the notion of a protective effect for vitamin D against the risk of developing MS. The incidence of MS was 33% lower in women who consumed the most vitamin D as compared to those who consumed the least. In addition, those that consumed at least 400 international units (IU) daily of vitamin D from supplements had an astounding 41% lower incidence of MS.[18]

In a recent study, researchers at the University of California, San Francisco discovered low 25-hydroxyvitamin D blood levels in African Americans with MS as compared to controls.[34] The senior author, who is also the associate director of UCSF Multiple Sclerosis Center concluded, "It seems relatively clear low vitamin D levels are a risk factor for developing multiple sclerosis."

### Hormones

Studies have shown that MS is more common in women than men, and that the disease course is affected by the fluctuation of steroid hormones during the female menstrual cycle.[35] It is also widely reported that MS patients who become pregnant experience a significant decrease in relapses, enabling women who have MS to bear children safely.[36] Animal models of MS have shown that the pregnancy hormone, estriol, can ameliorate disease and can cause an immune shift.[36,37] Other studies note that pregnant women who have MS tend to experience a rebound of their disease within 3 months postdelivery.[38]

These findings suggest that hormones can regulate the course of MS, and this theory is further supported by research demonstrating that steroid hormones, such as estrogens, testosterone, progesterone, and dehydroepiandrosterone (DHEA) can modulate the immune system.[39-41]

The specific relationship of hormones to the disease process of MS is complex, with ratios between the individual hormones also playing a role. For example, during a human study that examined the presence of MS lesions by magnetic resonance imaging (MRI), patients with high estradiol and low progesterone levels had more lesions that those who had low levels of both hormones. Further, patients with a high estrogen to progesterone ratio had a significantly greater number of "active" inflamed lesions than patients who had a low ratio.[42] These studies suggest that maintaining youthful *hormone balance* may ease the symptoms of MS.

A study from Italy provided further evidence that abnormal hormone levels may play a role in the development of MS. The investigators measured hormone levels in 35 women and 25 men with MS and in 36 people without the disease. Women with low testosterone levels were found to have more brain tissue damage, as determined using magnetic resonance imaging (MRI). The women with MS had lower levels of testosterone throughout their monthly cycle compared to women who did not have the condition. Testosterone levels did not vary between men with MS and unaffected men. However, men with MS who had the highest levels of the female hormone estradiol were found to have the greatest degree of brain tissue damage.[43]

More information about optimizing and balancing hormone levels can be found in Life Extension's Male Hormone Restoration protocol and the Female Hormone Restoration protocol.

## Organic Solvents

In the mid-1990s, researchers in Sweden evaluated 13 studies investigating the connection between solvent exposure and autoimmune disease. Organic solvents include chemicals such as toluene, paint thinner, and acetone, the latter of which is commonly found in nail polish remover. Ten of those studies indicated a significant relationship between organic solvent exposure and MS. All of the analyses suggested that exposure to solvents increases a person's relative risk of developing MS.[44] In another study, scientists analyzed the occupational health records of more than 57000 workers in Norway, covering a 16-year period. They concluded that workers, such as painters, who are routinely exposed to organic solvents, had twice the risk of developing MS than those who were not occupationally exposed. These results were compatible with the hypothesis that organic solvents are a possible risk factor for MS.[45]

Individuals interested in protecting themselves from organic solvents and other environmental toxins should read Life Extension's Metabolic Detoxification protocol.

## Food Sensitivities

Sensitivities to certain foods may also play a role in the development or exacerbation of MS. Antibodies to gluten, which is a protein found in wheat, are more common in patients with MS.[46,47] MS is also most prevalent in areas where consumption of wheat gluten and milk are also high.[48] This relationship led scientists to explore a possible link between antibodies produced to bovine milk proteins and the ability of those antibodies to cross-react to the protective sheaths around nerves triggering an MS episode. Indeed, this immunologic cross-reactivity has been demonstrated in the laboratory in rodents that have MS.[49,50] Further investigations have revealed that in MS patients, higher levels of these antibodies are produced within the CNS.[51] Additional studies are still needed to understand how this cross-reactivity plays into the development and progression of MS.

To help rule out food sensitivities, Life Extension® suggests blood testing such as the food safe allergy test and the celiac disease antibody screen. Call 800-226-2370 for more information on how to obtain this type of testing. Additional information about food allergies is available in the Life Extension Magazine article entitled "What's Really Making You Sick?"

## Smoking

A recently published literature review, evaluating more than 3000 MS cases and 450000 controls, supports the emerging consensus that smoking increases the risk of developing MS by approximately 50%.[52] It is unlikely that smoking alone accounts for the worldwide variation in MS prevalence, and thus, the interplay between genetic markers and smoking has also been investigated. One such study reported that smokers with 2 known genetic markers for MS had 2 times the risk for developing MS than their nonsmoking counterparts.[53] Another study has also verified that smokers diagnosed with MS but in remission have 3.5 times the risk of reactivating and progression of their disease than their nonsmoking counterparts.[54,55]

# SYMPTOMS AND DIAGNOSIS

MS can affect people of all ages; however, the average age of disease onset is between 20 and 40 years.[48] Fatigue, numbness in the limbs, impaired vision, muscle weakness, loss of balance, and bladder dysfunction are frequent symptoms.

Symptoms of MS vary widely, depending on the location of affected nerve fibers.[48]

Symptoms affecting mobility tend to appear early in the course of MS and they may include weakness, clumsiness, leg dragging, stiffness, and a tendency to drop objects.

- Common sensory symptoms include numbness, sensations of heaviness, tingling, and electrical sensations.

- Visual symptoms are also common, affecting more than one third of all people who have MS. The classic visual disturbances, such as blurred or foggy vision and eyeball pain, usually appear early in the course of the disease.

- MS can also interfere with the nerves that supply the vestibular apparatus in the inner ear, which is where balance is perceived. This can result in dizziness, nausea, and vomiting.

- In the later stages of the disease, involvement of the genitourinary tract may result in loss of bladder, sexual, and bowel function.[56]

- Over 40% of MS patients suffer from changes in memory, reasoning, spatial perception, and verbal fluency.[57]

- Symptoms of MS are often triggered or worsened by an increase in body temperature.

- MS is a tremendously variable and unpredictable disease. Different patients will experience different symptoms, rates of disease progression, and responses to treatment.

## Four Disease Courses Identified in MS

- **Progressive relapsing** (PR) MS, which is the least common disease course, shows progression of disability from onset but with clear acute relapses, with or without full recovery. Approximately 5% of people with MS appear to have PRMS at diagnosis.

- **Secondary progressive** (SP) MS begins with an initial relapsing-remitting disease course, followed by progression of disability. Typically, secondary-progressive disease is characterized by: less recovery following attacks, persistently worsening functioning during *and between* attacks, and accompanied by progressive disability. Many patients with relapsing-remitting MS do develop SPMS ultimately.

- **Primary progressive** (PP) MS is characterized by progression of disability from onset, without plateaus or remissions or with occasional plateaus and temporary minor improvements. A person with PPMS, by definition, does not experience acute attacks. 10% of diagnosed MS are PPMS.

- **Relapsing-remitting** (RR) MS represents 85 percent of clinical diagnoses of the disease. It is characterized by clearly defined acute attacks with full recovery or with residual deficit upon recovery. Periods between disease relapses are characterized by a lack of disease progression.

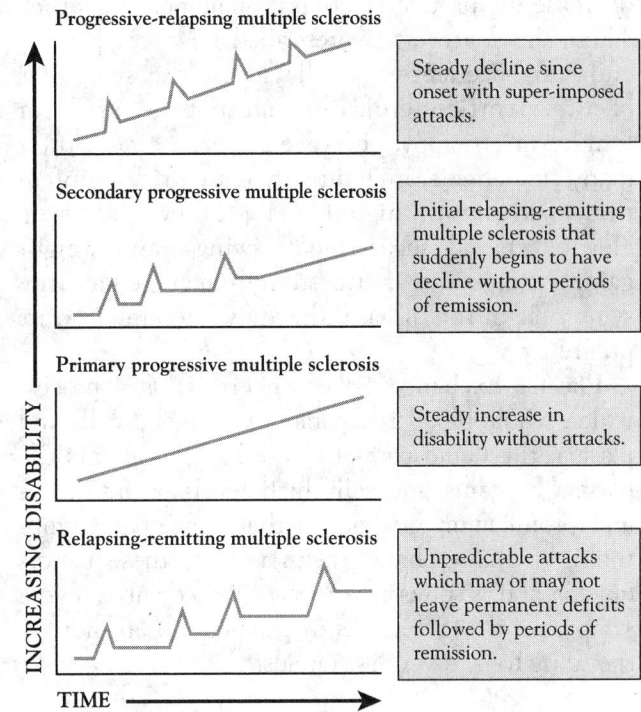

Progression of the 4 courses of MS over time

Progressive-relapsing multiple sclerosis — Steady decline since onset with super-imposed attacks.

Secondary progressive multiple sclerosis — Initial relapsing-remitting multiple sclerosis that suddenly begins to have decline without periods of remission.

Primary progressive multiple sclerosis — Steady increase in disability without attacks.

Relapsing-remitting multiple sclerosis — Unpredictable attacks which may or may not leave permanent deficits followed by periods of remission.

INCREASING DISABILITY

TIME

## Diagnosis

No single test gives a definitive diagnosis for MS, and variable symptoms and disease course make early diagnosis a challenge. Most presumptive diagnoses of MS are based on the clinical symptoms seen in an acute attack. These presumptions are then supported by a combination of diagnostic imaging with magnetic resonance imaging (MRI), antibody testing of the fluid found in the CNS, measurements to evaluate how efficiently nerves conduct impulses (since demyelination slows nerve conduction), and evaluation of how the symptoms progress through time.[58]

## CONVENTIONAL THERAPIES

A cure for MS has yet to be discovered, and although recent efforts have brought advances in available treatments, substantial room for improvement remains. Presently, conventional medical treatment typically focuses on strategies to treat acute attacks, to slow the progression of the disease, and to treat symptoms.

### Conventional Medical Treatment to Modify Course of Disease

**Corticosteroids.** For acute MS flares, corticosteroids such as methylprednisolone are commonly administered in high doses to suppress the immune system and decrease the production of proinflammatory factors. These drugs are often prescribed for short periods and can be effective at alleviating the symptoms of MS. Corticosteroids should not be used for long-term therapy, however, because of their many side effects, including increased risk of infection, *osteoporosis*, high blood pressure, cataracts, elevated blood sugar, mood swings, and weight gain. Also, while corticosteroids may reduce the symptoms of the disease, they have no effect on its progression.[59]

**Plasma Exchange (Plasmapheresis)** is a process which whole blood is separated into blood cells and plasma, the liquid part of blood. In MS patients the plasma contains unusually high levels of antibodies and proinflammatory factors that exacerbate symptoms. Plasma exchange helps remove these factors quickly and is sometimes used to help combat severe symptoms of MS relapses in people who are not responding to intravenous steroids.

## Conventional Medical Treatment to Modify Course of Disease

**Beta interferons** (Avonex®, Betaseron®) reduce inflammation and slow progression of the disease, but like many medications used in conventional medical treatment of MS, the mechanism of action is poorly understood.[60,61] This specific treatment may be accompanied by adverse effects such as suicidal depression, liver damage, flu-like symptoms, and injection site reactions[62]

**Glatiramer acetate** (Copaxone®) is an MS treatment that yields fewer adverse side effects than beta interferon while still remaining clinically effective. Glatiramer has a chemical structure similar to the protective myelin sheath around nerves and serves as a decoy for antibodies that would otherwise attack this sheath.[63] Side effects may include flushing, rapid heartbeat, nausea, shortness of breath after injection, and injection-site reactions.[64]

**Mitoxantrone** (Novantrone®) and **Fingolimod** (Gilenya®) are immunosuppressants. Clinical data show that these drugs can slow the rates at which disability progresses and the rate at which new lesions form in the brain and spinal cord. These therapies, however, are not used as a first-line treatment as they can cause severe side effects including heart disease, leukemia, decreased white blood cell counts, and increased rates of infection.[65]

**Natalizumab** (Tysabri®) is thought to block a protein that allows white blood cells to enter the brain and spinal cord and cause disease progression in MS.

Due to an association with 3 cases of a potentially fatal infection of the CNS,[66] this is a controversial drug that is only available for patients enrolled in the Tysabri Outreach Unified Commitment to Health (TOUCH) program.[67] This medication is reserved for people who do not see results from other types of treatments.

**Dalfampridine** (Ampyra®) is a medication approved in 2010 that increases the ability of nerve cells to conduct impulses.[68] This drug represents a new class of therapies that is aimed at addressing neurologic deficits directly.

## Medications to Treat Symptoms

**Muscle relaxants.** Multiple sclerosis patients may experience painful or uncontrollable muscle stiffness or spasms, particularly in the legs. Muscle relaxants such as baclofen (Lioresal) and tizanidine (Zanaflex) may improve muscle spasticity. However, baclofen may increase weakness in the legs, and tizanidine may cause drowsiness or a dry mouth.

**Medications to reduce fatigue.** Drugs such as amantadine (Symmetrel) may help reduce fatigue.

**Other medications.** Medications may also be prescribed for depression, pain, and bladder or bowel control problems that may be associated with MS.

## Medications on the Horizon

There are approximately 20 experimental therapies that are on the pathway to approval by the Food and Drug Administration (FDA). Investigators are making progress toward developing treatments that may be capable of protecting the CNS as well as encouraging repair of brain and spinal cord lesions. Many of these drugs are potentially valuable as treatments for MS, but are months or years from traversing all phases of the FDA process.

*Laquinimod* has been shown to decrease proinflammatory factors and increase factors that promote nerve protection without increasing risk of infection. Laquinimod was well tolerated by most patients, with only a few reports of adverse effects.[69]

*Alemtuzumab* (*Campath®*) is an antibody specific for mature white blood cells that targets them for destruction by the immune system. This drug is approved for the treatment of certain types of lymphoma and leukemia. In one study, it was shown to be more effective than beta interferon in reducing disability progression and relapse rate, however, the trial was discontinued early due to serious side effects.[70]

*Fumaric acid* is a substance that has been used in the treatment of psoriasis and shows promise in MS to decrease white blood cell infiltration into the spinal cord.[71]

## THERAPY AND REHABILITATION TO IMPROVE QUALITY OF LIFE

In addition to one or more drug-based therapies, MS patients will often participate in rehabilitation programs intended to maintain or improve their ability to perform at home and at work. More specifically, these programs focus on general fitness and aim to address problems related to mobility, speech and swallowing, and cognitive deficits.

Common rehabilitation strategies include:

- Physical therapy: Practices that aid mobility and functionality through structured physical activity on a scheduled basis.

- Occupational therapy: Skills aimed at using work, self-care, and leisure activities to foster development and limit disability.

- Speech therapy: Work with speech therapists can help MS patients overcome speech and language difficulties and help with troublesome swallowing.

- Cognitive rehabilitation: Assistance in managing difficulties with memory, high-order thinking, and perception. A variety of cognitive rehabilitation options are available. For example, playing chess regularly is a great way to promote neuronal function and communication; computer-based "brain training" programs are also helpful.

- Vocational rehabilitation: Support in making career plans, gaining job skills, and approaches to remaining gainfully employed.

## MULTIPLE SCLEROSIS NUTRITIONAL PROTOCOL

### Overview

Most patients that employ complementary treatments for MS do so as an accompaniment with conventional drug treatments and find both classes of therapy to provide clinical benefits.[72] The following section outlines key details and evidence-based findings concerning the latest complementary approaches to treating MS.

### Vitamin D

As previously mentioned, mainstream medicine has overlooked a critical missing link in MS management—vitamin D. This hormone-like vitamin is capable of safely interacting directly with the genome to modulate a variety of physiologic functions, including aspects of immune function involved in autoimmune diseases like MS.

Two human clinical trials demonstrated that individuals with MS using vitamin D tended to have fewer relapses and less inflammation.[17,73,74] In a 1-year vitamin D study, the recurrence rate of MS "attacks" was 27% lower compared to baseline.[74] In another large-dose, vitamin D trial, MS patients given 28000–280000 IU weekly were found to have fewer active lesions during the 28-week study.[75] In light of the accumulating epidemiologic and clinical evidence of the importance of vitamin D in this disease, supplementing the diet with vitamin D appears to be a low-cost means to address this risk.

### Omega-3 Fatty Acids

Omega-3 fatty acids (FAs) are polyunsaturated FAs that cannot be synthesized in humans and therefore must be provided via dietary sources. Both plant and animal foods are potential sources of omega-3 FAs. For example, linolenic acid, found in flaxseed, flaxseed oil, and preferably, fish and fish oils, have very high levels of EPA and DHA.

A small study that was focused on the effects of omega-3 FAs on MS found that immune cells from treated patients and healthy controls produced significantly fewer proinflammatory cytokines after 3 months of treatment with 6 g of fish oil per day.[76] One double-blind, placebo-controlled study exists to date looking at the effect of omega-3 FAs on MS disease progression. In this study 312 patients were given either fish oil or olive oil placebo for 2 years. The results of this trial exhibited a trend toward decreased disease severity in the omega-3 FA group when compared with controls.[77] More recent studies have shown that MS patients given 10 g of fish oil per day for 3 months exhibited significantly reduced levels of matrix metalloproteinase-9 (MMP-9), a factor correlated with disease progression, and also had greater concentrations of omega-3 FAs in their red blood cell membranes.[78] Other work has shown that MS patients, while on a low-fat diet with omega-3 FA supplementation, experienced significantly reduced fatigue and lower relapse rates.[79] Based on clinical data and patient accounts, omega-3 FAs appear to be well tolerated and safe with no reports of adverse events.

### Linoleic Acid and Omega-6 Fatty Acids

Linoleic acid is converted to gamma-linolenic acid (GLA), a beneficial omega-6 FA, after it is taken orally. However, this conversion is occasionally impaired, especially during inflammatory disease states.[48,80] GLA has been shown to quell inflammation, and research involving an animal model of MS has demonstrated that GLA administration significantly improved clinical outcomes when compared with control treatment.[81]

Some studies have shown significantly reduced relapse rates and disease progression scores, while others have found no differences between treatment and control groups.[81–83] A closer look at the data from these trials revealed that patients with lower levels of disability at the beginning of the trial exhibited a smaller increase in disability over the study period than did controls. In addition, linoleic acid was found to reduce the severity and duration of MS episodes in patients at all levels of disease severity.[84]

### Selenium and Vitamin E

Patients who have MS tend to have abnormally low levels of glutathione peroxidase, a powerful endogenous antioxidant.[85,86]

Researchers in Denmark conducted a small study in which patients with MS were given an antioxidant mixture containing approximately 2000 mcg of selenium, 2 g of vitamin C, and 480 mg of vitamin E, once a day for 5 weeks. Although glutathione peroxidase levels were initially lower in patients with MS than in normal control subjects, after 5 weeks of antioxidant therapy, levels of this antioxidant enzyme increased five-fold and reported side effects were minimal.[85] "[O]xidative stress plays an important role in pathogenesis of multiple sclerosis. This finding also suggests the importance of antioxidants in diet and therapy of MS patients."[87]

### N-acetylcysteine (NAC)

An effective strategy for increasing the body's supply of the powerful antioxidant glutathione is taking the oral supplement N-acetylcysteine (NAC), a potent antioxidant that serves as a precursor to glutathione[48,88] NAC's potential benefit in the context of MS has been noted by some researchers.[48,89]

In a rodent MS model, NAC was able to diminish clinical symptoms and pathologic evidence of CNS injury and attenuate inflammation.[90]

### Lipoic Acid

Lipoic acid (LA) is a dietary supplement with antioxidant properties and has been studied specifically in MS. Reactive oxygen species (ROS), generated primarily by immune cells, are implicated as mediators of demyelination and nerve damage.[91,92] Known to cross the blood–brain barrier, LA decreases the activity of intercellular adhesion molecule-1 (ICAM-1), which is thought to play a role in the pathogenesis of MS. It is believed that ICAM-1 and other adhesion molecules are responsible for allowing certain proinflammatory immune cells such as T lymphocytes to enter the CNS, paving the way for induction or exacerbation of inflammation and tissue damage.[93–95]

In an animal MS model, LA produced a significant reduction of demyelination and infiltration of the CNS by T lymphocytes.[96–98] Other researchers have followed up on these studies. In a pilot clinical trial, 37 patients with MS were randomly assigned to receive various doses of LA (up to 2400 mg/day) or placebo. After 2 weeks, patients were assessed for levels of ICAM-1 and tolerability of high-dose LA. In addition to being well tolerated by patients, LA treatment was associated with reduced ICAM-1 levels and reduced T-cell migration into the CNS.[99]

### Coenzyme Q10

The antioxidant coenzyme Q10 (CoQ10) is an essential part of healthy mitochondrial function and energy production with potential usefulness in treating MS. Decreased levels of CoQ10 are associated with many disease states, including heart disease, cancer, and neurodegenerative diseases.[100,101] CoQ10 was low in patients with MS.[102] Several clinical trials of CoQ10 have been performed in neurodegenerative disease, such as Parkinson's disease, Huntington's disease, Alzheimer disease, Friedreich's ataxia, and amyotrophic lateral sclerosis.[103] CoQ10 is a powerful lipid-soluble antioxidant that is also capable of regenerating the antioxidant capacity of vitamin E in the body. Based on clinical evidence, CoQ10 appears to be well tolerated and safe, with potential usefulness in the management of MS.

### Vitamin B12

Some data suggest that patients with MS have abnormally low levels of vitamin B12 in their cerebrospinal fluid, blood serum, or both.[104] In fact, clinical vitamin B12 deficiency and MS share remarkably similar characteristics, occasionally rendering correct diagnosis difficult.[105] Notably, vitamin B12 plays a key role in the generation of myelin. Thus, for decades, integrative physicians have prescribed B12 injections for patients who have MS.

Data suggest that patients given vitamin B12 supplements have experienced clinical improvements in their symptoms.[48] For example, in the

United Kingdom, researchers investigated the effects of 6 months of vitamin B12 (1 mg/week injection) on 138 patients with MS. The researchers concluded that the clinical course of patients with MS improved after beginning vitamin B12 treatment.[106]

## Gingko Biloba

Gingko biloba extracts are primarily composed of flavonoids and terpenoids and have been reported to have properties that can influence neural activity and improve cognitive performance. While controlled trials of the effects of Gingko biloba on cognitive function have generated inconsistent findings, more recent studies found encouraging results for patients with MS.[107–109] In one study, patients received 120 mg of Gingko biloba extract or placebo twice per day for 12 weeks. Patients taking gingko biloba exhibited improved measures of attention and reported fewer difficulties with memory.

## Green Tea—Epigallocatechin-3-Gallate (EGCG)

Epigallocatechin-3-gallate (EGCG) is one of many active ingredients of green tea reported to have beneficial effects on the nervous and immune systems. In an animal study of MS, ECGC was found to prevent severity of clinical signs by decreasing inflammation and protecting nerve cells.[110] According to animal research, green tea has the ability to significantly increase regulatory T cells, which are critical to providing balance to the immune system and suppressing autoimmunity.[111]

## Curcumin

*Curcumin* is an active component of turmeric, a popular Indian spice. Laboratory studies have demonstrated that curcumin has potent anti-inflammatory effects.[112] A research group carrying out animal studies has demonstrated exciting findings that curcumin treatment results in a significant reduction in disease severity and a reduction in duration of acute attacks.[113] In a followup study, laboratory researchers found that curcumin not only suppressed disease severity, but also was associated with reduction of levels of interleukin-17 (IL-17), a cytokine that has been directly implicated in the progression of MS.[114]

## SWANK DIET

Dr. Roy Swank first proposed a connection between increased consumption of saturated animal fat and the incidence of MS in 1950.[115] He conducted a study that enrolled 208 patients

with MS in the early 1950s, all of whom had experienced at least 2 acute relapses, and followed their progress over 34 years.[116] In this study, patients maintained the diet now called the Swank diet, which consists of <15 g/day of saturated animal fat, 10–15 g/day of vegetable oil, 5 g/day of cod liver oil, and 1 multivitamin (full details below). Long-term follow-up results from this study indicate that the patients adhering to the Swank diet experienced reduced MS disease activity and progression of disability when compared to patients who did not follow the regimen. While these results are encouraging, this trial is criticized for its lack of a proper control group and non-blinded design. Nevertheless, the Swank diet remains one of the most popular complementary approaches to treating MS.

### Swank Low-Fat Diet: Detailed Guidelines

- Saturated fat should remain <15 g per day
- Unsaturated fat should be approximately 20–50 g per day
- No red meat should be consumed during the first year
- After the first year, a maximum of 3 oz of red meat per week
- Dairy products must have 1% butterfat or less
- Processed foods containing saturated fat should not be eaten
- A source of omega-3, a multivitamin, and a mineral supplement are recommended daily
- Wheat, gluten, or dairy product quantities are not restricted, unless they are foods that cause allergies or reactions.

## Hormone Therapy

Because women often experience improvement of MS symptoms while pregnant, hormone therapy using estrogen has been studied as a treatment for the disease. In human studies, estriol treatment (8 mg/day) in nonpregnant women with MS was associated with reduced lesion numbers and lesion volumes and when treatment ceased, these values returned to levels observed before treatment.[37] Patients given estriol also had enhanced cognitive function. With respect to immune studies, estriol was associated with reduced proinflammatory and increased anti-inflammatory cytokine production and these changes correlated well with the reduced formation of lesions.[39]

Other studies have shown that male MS patients treated with 10 mg of testosterone exhibited improved cognitive performance and reduced brain atrophy, although MRI data showed no change in lesion formation.[117] In another similar study, testosterone treatment in males was associated with reduced production of inflammatory cytokines and increased production of neuroprotective factors.[118]

There is currently debate among researchers about the role of hormones with MS and how that relationship may be exploited as a means of therapy. Some studies argue for hormone replacement as a new therapeutic approach.[119] More information can be found in Life

Extension's protocols on Male Hormone Restoration Therapy and Female Hormone Restoration Therapy.

## Life Extension Suggestions

Recent advancements in the understanding and treatment of MS have improved the prognosis and quality of life of MS patients. People with MS have a substantial ability to affect the course of their illness.

### Neuronal support and immune regulation

- **Vitamin D3**: 5000–8000 International Units (IU) daily, depending on blood levels of 25-OH-vitamin D
- **EPA/DHA:** 700–1400 mg of EPA and 500–1000 mg of DHA daily
- **GLA:** 900 mg daily of borage oil
- **Turmeric extract** (curcumin): 400–1200 mg daily
- **Vitamin B12:** 1000–5000 micrograms (mcg) daily in the form of sublingual methylcobalamin

### Antioxdiants

- **NAC:** 600–1200 mg daily with 1800 mg of vitamin C
- **Vitamin E:** 400 IU daily
- **Selenium:** 400 mcg daily
- **Lipoic acid** (preferably R-lipoic acid): 240–600 mg daily
- **CoQ10** (as ubiquinol): 100–200 mg daily

### Additional Support

- **Green tea,** standardized to EGCG: 700–2100 mg daily
- **Ginkgo biloba extract:** 120–240 mg per day

Hormonal therapy with *bioidentical hormones* may also be considered. Before bioidentical hormonal therapy is initiated, *hormone blood testing* is important. For more information on hormone testing, call 1-800-226-2370.

In addition, the following blood testing resources may be helpful:

- Vitamin D, 25-Hydroxy
- Omega Score®
- Food Safe™ Allergy
- Female Panel / Male Panel
- Female Comprehensive Hormone Panel/Male Comprehensive Panel

## REFERENCES

References available at: www.lef.org/dpt5/ch94

# 95

# *Muscular Dystrophy*

Muscular dystrophy (MD) is a family of genetic disorders characterized by progressive muscle weakness, loss of muscle function, and wasting. Despite many years of intense research and heavy publicity aimed at conquering this tragic disease, patients rarely survive past 30 years of age.

The many forms of MD are distinguished on the basis of their chief characteristics. They may be categorized according to the ways that symptoms manifest (eg, where muscle weakness occurs primarily), at what age symptoms commence, or in what manner the disorder is inherited. For instance, Duchenne muscular dystrophy (DMD), the most common form, is passed only from a female to her son(s). In addition to being the most common form of MD, DMD (also known as Meryon's disease) is the second most common childhood genetic disease, afflicting one of every 3330–3500 boys born worldwide.[1]

DMD is also defined by the specific genes it affects. There are many other varieties of MD, characterized by the muscular groups involved, age of onset, and other criteria. Most forms of MD result from mutations in genes that ordinarily code for a variety of proteins and enzymes associated with the structure and function of muscle cells. DMD and Becker MD, for example, are associated with a deficiency of the protein dystrophin. Other MDs are associated with deficiencies in additional proteins.[2] Half of congenital MD cases, for instance, involve a deficiency of merosin.[3]

Unless otherwise noted, DMD will be considered representative of the general MD family of diseases and referred to in particular. Although specifics may not apply to all forms of MD, the general principles involved are similar. It should be noted, however, that there is wide variability among specific subtypes of MDs in terms of the age of onset, patterns of skeletal muscle involvement, rate of complications (eg, heart damage), rate of progression, and mode of inheritance.[2]

## UNDERSTANDING MUSCULAR DYSTROPHY

To understand MD, it is necessary to delve into the molecular realm of genes and cells, where an inheritable mutation of a specific gene results in failure to produce a viable protein. Dystrophin, the protein affected in DMD, is a minor, yet crucial component of every muscle cell. It forms part of the flexible framework of filaments, tubules, and other structures within the cell. This network, called the cytoskeleton, provides every cell with structure, shape, and function. Communications within the cell depend on the compounds of the cytoskeleton to work properly; so when dystrophin or any other component fails to function, there is serious disruption of the cell's ability to operate.

Among patients suffering from any of the MDs, serum levels of creatine kinase (an enzyme involved in energy storage and expenditure) rise. It has been proposed that the absence of dystrophin in MD patients' muscle may lead to damage of muscle cell membranes. Cell membranes are responsible for the selective passage of various nutrients, gases, and waste. Damage to muscle membranes is believed to allow creatine kinase to escape from cells into the bloodstream.[4] There is some indication that supplementation with creatine may delay or alleviate some of the muscle deterioration associated with MD.[5,6]

DMD is associated with a notable loss of muscle mass. As muscle cell membranes degrade, fibers are replaced first by connective tissue and then by fat. In time, only residual areas of muscle fibers remain, adrift in a pool of fat. Usually beginning with the upper thigh and buttocks muscles, and eventually including muscles associated with breathing and specialized muscle cells of the heart, the progressive loss of muscle function ultimately forces patients to rely on wheelchairs and ventilators until death comes at approximately 20 years of age. Death is usually due to respiratory failure, although heart problems may also contribute.[4]

Dystrophin has also been identified in the brain, although its function in that organ remains unclear. In any event, its absence appears to also affect neurological function in patients with DMD, as they are known to experience cognitive and intellectual deficits, as well as occasional emotional problems and a reading disability similar to a common type of dyslexia.[4,7-9]

## TREATMENT OPTIONS

Numerous treatments for MD have been proposed and investigated, but results have been largely disappointing. Few approaches offer even marginal improvements in prognosis, but there is some cause for hope. Recent research suggests that certain approaches may delay degeneration, prolonging life and providing a more comfortable existence. In the long run, it is likely that gene therapy offers the best hope for an actual cure. However, this line of inquiry is in its infancy, and many obstacles remain to be overcome before a true cure for this deadly genetic disease is achieved. Other future treatments may include transplantation of stem cells or muscle precursor cells that will proliferate and replace defective, dystrophin-deficient muscle cells.[1]

The lack of a true cure renders the development of palliative treatments (ie, intended to improve quality of life and reduce symptoms) all the more important. Scientists are still learning about dystrophin deficiency and how to minimize its effects. Currently, several approaches promise some modest benefits.

## Steroid Therapies

Normal growth and maintenance of muscle mass is accompanied by some degradation and regeneration of muscle tissue, but this process is grossly imbalanced in MD. Regeneration fails to keep pace with inflammation and disintegration. By definition, anabolic steroids enhance muscle building, so steroids have been investigated for their potential in MD. However, anabolic steroids (eg, the male hormone testosterone) also tend to be androgenizing; they trigger masculinization effects, which in addition to beefing up muscle, include promotion of beard and body hair growth, maturation of genitalia, and development of acne, among others.

Early attempts to harness the potential of testosterone were only partially successful. While initially improving muscle mass, testosterone failed to increase strength, and the numerous side effects became problematic.[10] Later attempts with synthetic anabolic steroids, such as those abused by body builders and some unscrupulous professional athletes, have yielded mixed results. Synthetics (eg, norethandrolone and methandrostenolone) provided some initial benefits, but young boys experienced premature development of secondary sex characteristics; far worse, when treatment was halted, rapid and severe deterioration in muscle mass and function ensued.[1]

Newer synthetic steroids (eg, oxandrolone) offer fewer side effects and the promise of decreased muscle degeneration.[11,12] Oxandrolone provides benefits on two fronts: while enhancing muscle building (like other anabolic steroids), it also interferes with the binding of the hormone cortisol to glucocorticoid receptors on muscle, thus preventing muscle breakdown. Among burn victims who received this treatment, increases in lean body mass (largely muscle) continued for up to 6 months after treatment ceased. This bodes well for MD patients, for whom withdrawal

of anabolic steroids is often accompanied by rapid decline in muscle mass.

Glucocorticoid drugs, including corticosteroids (eg, prednisone and deflazacort), have become fairly standard treatment for MD.[13,14] Among other things, they have been shown to delay degeneration of heart function. At best, they improve motor function and delay breakdown of existing muscle.[15] Studies show these drugs may prolong the time a patient can walk as well as delay the onset of spinal curvature (scoliosis), which is a common development in the progression of MD.[16] However, improvements tend to be short-lived (lasting an average of 6 months to 2 years) and side effects range from growth suppression and excessive weight gain to osteoporosis. Like all existing treatments for the various forms of MD, glucocorticoids are ultimately powerless to halt the eventual progression of the disease.

## Nutritional Support

Nutritional support, although often overlooked, is especially important in order to improve quality of life. Antioxidants and anti-inflammatories offer some benefit. So does exercise, especially early in life. However, studies have shown that the ability of affected muscle to regenerate and repair itself may quickly become overwhelmed, at which point further exercise becomes counterproductive.

**Creatine.** Long used as a supplement by bodybuilders to enhance strength and endurance, creatine may also benefit MD patients. Creatine is an "energy precursor" naturally produced by the body.[17] Transformed by the body into phosphocreatine, it enters muscle cells and promotes protein synthesis while reducing protein breakdown. In healthy individuals, creatine has been shown to enhance endurance and increase energy levels by preventing depletion of the body's primary energy-storage compound, adenosine triphosphate (ATP).[18] Among MD patients, studies have suggested that supplemental creatine can improve muscle performance and strength, decrease fatigue, and slightly improve bone mineral density.

A small, randomized, double-blind, placebo-controlled crossover study in Belgium assessed the effects of creatine supplementation in 12 boys afflicted with DMD and 3 with Becker MD.[5] Participants received either 3 g creatine or placebo daily for 3 months, followed by a 2-month washout period. They then received the opposite substance for another 3 months. After each phase of the study, doctors assessed strength, bone and joint health, and fatigue levels.

The boys receiving placebo exhibited no change in maximum voluntary muscle contraction (a quantitative measure of strength). Likewise, resistance to fatigue remained unchanged, while joint stiffness worsened by 25%. After taking creatine for 3 months, the boys' strength increased by 15%, resistance to fatigue doubled, and joint stiffness remained unchanged. Furthermore, a biochemical marker of bone tissue degradation decreased by two-thirds.

Among the 5 boys able to walk at the beginning of the study, bone mineral density increased by 3% after the creatine supplementation phase of the study. MD patients frequently suffer from osteoporosis, in which bone mineral density declines, rendering bones fragile.

A somewhat larger study conducted in Ontario, Canada assessed the effects of daily creatine supplementation (100 mcg/kg of body weight) on 30 participants for 4 months. Again, researchers found that bone degradation decreased when participants were taking creatine, and strength (measured by dominant hand–grip strength) increased. The same was not true during the placebo phase. Researchers noted that creatine was well tolerated, and fat-free mass increased.[19]

Other studies on patients with myotonic dystrophy have been somewhat less encouraging, although creatine may still be of some benefit for them. In one German study, scientists randomly assigned 34 myotonic patients to receive either 10.6 g creatine daily or placebo. After 8 weeks, researchers concluded that "creatine supplementation was well tolerated, without relevant side effects." However, there was no statistically significant improvement in muscle strength or daily-life activities.[20]

Another double-blind crossover study considered creatine's effects on a variety of MD types, including 12 facioscapulohumeral, 10 Becker, 8 DMD, and 6 limb-girdle MD patients. After 8 weeks, patients who received creatine exhibited "mild but significant improvement in muscle strength and daily-life activities." Creatine was well tolerated throughout the study.[21]

In another study, Austrian researchers administered creatine to one 9-year-old boy with DMD for more than 5 months. The patient subsequently demonstrated "improved muscle performance." Magnetic resonance imaging of calf muscle function supported this finding.[6]

Another study examined the effects of creatine supplementation alone and in combination with the corticosteroid prednisolone on mouse models of MD. The study also investigated the effects of conjugated linoleic acid, alpha-lipoic acid, and hydroxyl-beta-methylbutyrate, alone and in combination with creatine and prednisolone. Each of the supplements showed some benefit when given alone, but the combination of all 4 with the corticosteroid "provided the most consistent evidence of efficacy." Efficacy, or effectiveness of therapy, was assessed in terms of increased strength and decreased fatigue, among other parameters.[22]

**Green tea.** Green tea has been credited with diverse benefits (eg, protection of the skin from damaging rays of the sun,[23–25] protection against numerous cancers, improvements in cardiovascular health, and protection against neurologic decline).[26,27]

Recently, scientists in Switzerland published the results of a study conducted on mouse models of MD. These "mdx" mice were fed ordinary food, food containing green tea extract, or green tea's major bioactive polyphenol compound, epigallocatechin gallate (EGCG). After feeding the animals for either 1 or 5 weeks, researchers examined the rodents' muscle tissue microscopically for signs of damage associated with the progression of their MD-like disease. Researchers concluded that "diet supplementation . . . with green tea extract or [EGCG] protected muscle against the first massive wave of necrosis and stimulated muscle adaptation toward a stronger and more resistant phenotype."[28]

Green tea polyphenols, such as EGCG, are known to be powerful antioxidants. Because inflammation is involved in the degradation of muscle tissue in MD, oxidative stress is believed to play a role in this process. Green tea and its active constituents may improve MD prognosis by reducing this oxidative stress.[29] In an earlier experiment with mdx mice, the same Swiss team gave them varying concentrations of green tea extract for 4 weeks, beginning at birth. Upon examining various muscles, they determined that the extract significantly reduced degradation of certain muscles and noted that higher doses correlated with greater inhibition of decline. There was also biochemical evidence that green tea extract reduced oxidative stress in muscle cells. The effective dose of extract used in this study corresponds to about 7 cups of brewed green tea per day in humans, rendering its use in DMD patients feasible.[29]

**Coenzyme Q10.** Coenzyme Q10 (CoQ10; also called *ubiquinone*) is a powerful antioxidant and mitochondrial respiratory chain cofactor. It possesses membrane-stabilizing properties and is capable of penetrating cell membranes and mitochondria. Mitochondria serve as cellular powerhouses, generating energy to power life's many processes. Muscle cells expend a great deal of energy and are rich in mitochondria. As an essential cofactor, CoQ10 acts to facilitate a complex series of reactions that occur within the mitochondria. Known as the respiratory chain, these chemical reactions ultimately supply energy, which may be stored for later use or readily expended.

Given its importance in this process, scientists wondered if supplemental CoQ10 might improve the prognosis of MD patients, who suffer from declining muscle strength and deficient energy metabolism within muscle cells. Scientists at the University of Texas conducted double-blind investigative trials of daily CoQ10 supplementation in a dozen patients with a variety of MDs, including DMD and Becker, limb-girdle, and myotonic dystrophy. Participants received either 100 mg CoQ10 daily for 3 months or placebo. A second trial, with a comparable treatment protocol, enrolled 15 patients with a similar mix of MD. The scientists concluded that participants' physical performance was "definitely improved" and added, "patients suffering from these muscle dystrophies and the like, should be treated with [Coenzyme] Q10 indefinitely." Although patients received 100 mg CoQ10 daily and the treatment was considered effective and safe, researchers noted that the most effective dose is probably larger.[30]

Further evidence of the link between MD and CoQ10 deficiency was reported by Italian researchers who investigated CoQ10 levels in myotonic dystrophy patients. "Serum CoQ10 appeared significantly reduced with respect to normal controls," they reported. In subsequent experiments on patients with Steinert's myotonic dystrophy, they discovered that patients with the greatest degree of genetic mutation tended to have the lowest CoQ10 levels; suggesting CoQ10 deficiency is indeed related to deficient energy metabolism of muscle cells in MD patients.[31,32]

**Calcium and vitamin D.** By the time they reach 10 years of age, many boys with MD will have lost the ability to walk. Confined to a wheelchair, they inevitably develop bone-weakening osteoporosis, although the process often begins before becoming wheelchair bound.[33,34] In fact, although bone density in MD has received relatively little attention, one study investigated bone health in 32 DMD patients and found that bone mineral density in all patients was lower than normal for children of comparable ages. This indicator of declining bone health was especially advanced in patients on corticosteroid therapy. The scientists also found that patients had lower-than-normal levels of a form of bioactive vitamin D.[35] Although no formal clinical trials have been conducted on providing supplemental vitamin D and calcium to MD patients, the practice has been recommended by at least one MD researcher.[4]

In normal individuals, vitamin D and calcium are known to play a crucial role in the maintenance of healthy bone mineralization and density. Although vitamin D is generated within the body in response to adequate sunlight, exposure to sufficient sunlight to guarantee an adequate supply of vitamin D may be problematic. This is especially true in northern latitudes during winter months; research shows that winter sunlight is northern latitudes is too weak for the body to generate adequate vitamin D.[36] Even in southern latitudes, vitamin D levels may drop sufficiently during winter to contribute to osteoporosis among otherwise healthy aging men and women.[37]

**Glutamine.** Glutamine is involved in many metabolic processes. It is an important energy source for many cells.

Some researchers have suggested that glutamine may be "conditionally essential" in DMD because the ability to synthesize glutamine is impaired in MD patients.[38] Scientists in Florida administered oral glutamine to 6 boys with DMD and monitored indicators of protein synthesis as well as degradation. They concluded that "acute oral glutamine administration might have a protein-sparing effect" in the boys.[39]

More recently, a larger, double-blind, placebo-controlled clinical trial looked at the effects of 6 months of supplementation with oral glutamine and creatine on 50 boys with MD. Results were tantalizing but ultimately inconclusive. Researchers noted that "although there was no statistically significant effect of either therapy based on manual and quantitative measurements of muscle strength, a disease-modifying effect of creatine in older Duchenne muscular dystrophy, and creatine and glutamine in younger Duchenne muscular dystrophy cannot be excluded." Both treatments were well tolerated.[40]

**Arginine and utrophin.** The most prevalent forms of MD are caused by lack or inadequacy of the cytoskeletal protein dystrophin. A related protein, utrophin, is not affected by the MD mutations responsible for dystrophin deficiency. Because utrophin is 80% similar to dystrophin, and evidence suggests that it may fulfill many of the same functions as dystrophin, scientists proposed that utrophin may serve as an effective substitute for dystrophin in the muscle cells of MD patients. Therefore, any substance that promotes an increase in production of utrophin may be of benefit in treating MD.

In the late 1990s, French scientists showed that feeding supplemental arginine to mdx mice enhanced production of utrophin.[41] They also showed that this increase was likely mediated by arginine-fueled production of nitric oxide (NO), which plays an important role in blood vessel function and is generally lower in people with MD.[42] In subsequent experiments, the same team demonstrated that both healthy and MD-model muscle cells can be prompted to produce greater amounts of utrophin by supplying the NO substrate, arginine, or an NO donor compound.[43]

A team of scientists in the Unites States investigated this effect and came to similar conclusions. They administered L-arginine (the bioactive form of the amino acid) to both normal and mdx mice. Muscle cells from treated mdx mice were less susceptible to exercise-induced damage, and the animals exhibited decreased muscle cell death. An increase in utrophin was also noted in muscle cells of treated mice, which contributed to a decrease in muscle degradation.[44]

Aside from stimulating production of utrophin, arginine and other chemicals that increase NO may also benefit MD patients by stimulating muscle regeneration. Brazilian scientists administered mdx mice a drug that served as an NO donor, while other mice received placebo or other drug treatment for 20 days. Muscle fiber regeneration was increased by 20% only in the mice given the NO-donor drug, isosorbide dinitrate (ISD). Researchers concluded that "NO derived from ISD stimulated and/or recruited satellite cells. Pharmacological treatment with ISD could be clinically useful for improving muscle regeneration in Duchenne muscular dystrophy."[45]

Canadian scientists published the results of a study suggesting the combination of arginine and deflazacort (a standard corticosteroid drug used in the treatment of MD) is more beneficial than deflazacort alone. Mdx mice were treated for 3 weeks with deflazacort, placebo, or deflazacort plus arginine. They were subsequently assessed for evidence of muscle degeneration and regeneration initiated by 24 hours of voluntary exercise. Although deflazacort alone prevented the progressive loss of function that ordinarily occurs in such mice, the deflazacort plus arginine combination yielded still more impressive protection from exercise-induced muscle damage and "induced a persistent functional improvement in distance run." According to the scientists, these results offer a new treatment option that might improve quality of life.[46]

**Taurine.** There is some evidence that the amino acid taurine may be of benefit in the symptomatic treatment of MD. Taurine is abundant in normal skeletal muscle and believed to exert both long- and short-term control over the functionality of ion channels.[47] These channels serve as passageways between the interior and exterior environment of a cell. An excessive influx of calcium ions into MD muscle cells is believed to play a significant role in the inflammation and pathology associated with the disease.[48] Accordingly, regulation of ion channel function would appear to play an important role in the management of MD.

In ordinary laboratory rodents, it has been shown that aging is associated with biochemical changes that decrease muscles' ability to contract. These changes are accompanied by a decrease in muscle cell taurine content. When taurine becomes depleted in adult rat muscle cells, biochemical changes similar to those seen in aged rats occur. When aged rats are fed supplemental taurine, these changes may be reversed.[49]

Building on this preliminary research, Italian scientists investigated taurine's potential to influence muscle status in mdx mice. To test taurine's effect(s) in MD, researchers treated mdx mice with taurine or other substances for 4–8 weeks. The animals were subjected to chronic exercise on a treadmill, an activity known to worsen symptoms of MD. Afterward, animals were evaluated for various indicators of declining or improving muscle functionality. "Exercise produced a significant weakness," researchers reported. But taurine "counteracted the exercise-induced weakness." Among the substances tested, this counteraction effect was strongest for taurine. "The results predict a potential benefit of taurine . . . for treating human dystrophy," the researchers concluded.[50,51]

## Anti-Inflammatory Therapy

Inflammation is playing an increasingly large role in the research regarding MD. Physicians are steadily gaining knowledge and insight into inflammatory changes responsible for much of the actual damage associated with many diseases, including MD. This progress opens up the possibility for new, targeted treatment(s) that would interfere with the inflammatory cascade, thus limiting muscle damage and slowing the disease. Although most of this research remains speculative, there appears to be great promise in anti-inflammatory therapies for MD.[52]

Scientists have shown that chronic inflammation in DMD results from the coordinated activity of numerous components, including cytokine and chemokine signaling, white blood cell adhesion, and complement system activation, among others.[53]

**Omega-3 fatty acids.** The omega-3 fatty acids eicosapentaenoic acid (EPA) and docosahexaenoic acid (DHA), primarily obtained from fish oil, have repeatedly been shown to exert anti-inflammatory effects when consumed in sufficient quantities.[54,55] Omega-3s are crucial components of cell membranes, where they contribute to stabilization and healthy function.[56] Accordingly, at least one scientist has proposed that supplemental omega-3 fatty acids may be of some benefit in the nutritional support of MD patients.[4]

## Life Extension Suggestions

The following supplements may be beneficial to MD patients:

- **Creatine:** 1000–3000 mg daily on an empty stomach
- **Green tea extract** (standardized to 98% polyphenols): 725–1450 mg daily
- **CoQ10** (as ubiquinol): 100–300 mg daily
- **Vitamin D:** 5000 IU–8000 IU daily; individualize dosing based on results of vitamin D testing
- **Calcium:** 700–1200 mg daily
- **Glutamine:** 1000 mg daily
- **Arginine:** 900–2700 mg daily
- **Taurine:** 1000–3000 mg daily
- **Omega 3 fatty acids from fish oil:** 1400 mg EPA and 1000 mg of DHA daily

In addition, the following *blood tests* may provide helpful information:

- Female Panel or Male Panel
- Creatine Kinase
- CoQ10 (Coenzyme Q10)

## REFERENCES

References available at: www.lef.org/dpt5/ch95

# 96

# Myasthenia Gravis

Myasthenia gravis is an autoimmune disorder characterized by muscle weakness. The disease tends to strike women more often than men (ratio of about 3 to 2, respectively), usually affecting women between the ages of 20 and 40.[1] After about age 50, both sexes tend to be equally affected.[2]

Myasthenia gravis is progressive and can affect any muscle group; however, people afflicted with the disease often have weakness of face, tongue, and neck. This muscle weakness might result in double vision or drooping eyelids, which along with difficulty chewing, swallowing, and talking, are characteristic symptoms of myasthenia gravis.

## CAUSES OF MYASTHENIA GRAVIS

The underlying cause of myasthenia gravis is unknown. However, there is likely a genetic component, and clear evidence exists that the disease is somehow related to abnormalities in the thymus gland. Even though an exact cause has not been determined, the disease course is fairly well understood.

Myasthenia gravis affects the neuromuscular junction, or the area where nerve endings communicate with skeletal muscles. At the neuromuscular junction, nerve endings transmit impulses across a tiny space (synapse) to the muscle, causing it to contract. When a nerve impulse travels down the nerve, a neurotransmitter (ie, acetylcholine) is released from vesicles in the nerve ending into the synapse and bathes acetylcholine receptors located on the muscle side of the synapse, causing the muscle to be stimulated and contract.

The reaction is short-lived; in a very brief time, acetylcholine in the receptor is metabolized into its components (acetate and choline) by the enzyme acetylcholinesterase. Any remaining acetylcholine diffuses away from the receptors.

With myasthenia gravis, this normal impulse transmission is disrupted by T-cell–mediated autoantibodies that target and block the body's own acetylcholine receptors. If enough receptors are blocked by autoantibodies, then the muscle contraction will be weak, causing the principal symptoms of myasthenia gravis.

The disease also affects the synapse in other ways besides blocking the acetylcholine receptors. On the muscle side of the synapse, acetylcholine receptors are normally grouped closely in tight synaptic folds. In myasthenia gravis, however, the autoantibodies work in concert with complement proteins (also part of the immune system) to damage and spread out the receptors and widen the synaptic folds. The result is fewer receptors.

In recent years, several interesting theories have been advanced to explain myasthenia gravis. Up to 90% of people with myasthenia gravis suffer from some form of abnormality in the thymus gland. The thymus gland is where T cells—the chief immune cells involved in myasthenia gravis—are produced and "schooled." About 70% of people with myasthenia gravis have an enlarged thymus gland (hyperplasia), and 20% have usually benign thymic tumors (ie, thymomas).[3] By studying cells from thymomas and tissue from the thymus gland, scientists have begun to develop a unified theory that might one day explain the cause of myasthenia gravis.

According to this theory, myoid cells in the thymus might be responsible for the autoimmune reaction seen in myasthenia gravis. Myoid cells are muscle-like cells within the thymus gland. Recent studies have shown that T cells are first sensitized against myoid cells within the thymus. This has 2 effects. First, it causes the microscopic thymus changes seen in early-onset myasthenia gravis, which occurs before the age of 40 years. These changes resemble those eventually seen in skeletal muscles. Second, the sensitization of T cell antibodies to myoid cells causes the formation of germinal centers, which are key facilitators in the autoimmune reaction against acetylcholine receptors.[4,5]

Building on this work, researchers have looked more recently at the role of inflammatory cytokines in myasthenia gravis. In several studies, scientists have discovered that the expression of acetylcholine receptors is modified by inflammatory cytokines such as tumor necrosis factor-alpha (TNF-$\alpha$). These proinflammatory chemicals have been implicated in other autoimmune diseases (eg, multiple sclerosis and Lou Gehrig's disease). In one study, researchers found that cytokine activity was enhanced in the myasthenia gravis thymus, possibly influencing acetylcholine-receptor expression and contributing to initiation of the autoimmune response.[6] While this research is still preliminary, it offers novel therapeutic targets for the treatment of myasthenia gravis.

## SYMPTOMS OF MYASTHENIA GRAVIS

People with myasthenia gravis generally experience specific muscle weakness (such as in the eye), especially with repeated use of the muscles. This weakness often has a characteristic pattern, that is, face and head muscles are involved early in the disease. Drooping eyelids and double vision are the most common early complaints.[7] People afflicted may also have difficulty chewing, facial weakness that affects their smile, and a nasal quality to their voice due to weakness in the palate.

Progression of the disease is variable, with periods of remission followed by exacerbation(s). In about 85% of cases, the weakness will progress to a generalized weakness affecting large muscle groups.

At some point in the illness (usually within 2–3 years after diagnosis), 12–16% of myasthenia gravis patients will experience a crisis episode, in which the weakness becomes so severe that breathing is compromised and respiratory assistance is required.[8,9] This eventuality is most likely in people with tongue and mouth weakness or a thymoma.[8-10]

Myasthenia gravis is distinguishable from congenital myasthenic syndromes. These syndromes are caused by genetic defects in the acetylcholine receptor and other components of the neuromuscular junction. Although they share symptoms, the illnesses respond differently to treatment(s).

## AGGRAVATING FACTORS FOR MYASTHENIA GRAVIS

Myasthenia gravis is frequently associated with chronic infections of any kind. These infections may cause a myasthenia gravis crisis or exacerbate existing conditions by provoking a T-cell–mediated immune response. Other aggravating factors for myasthenia gravis are discussed in following sections.

### Hormone Fluctuation

One study documented a relationship between the female menstrual cycle and myasthenia gravis. Of the women studied, 67% reported exacerbation of their symptoms 2–3 days prior to the menstrual period. These exacerbations frequently required therapeutic changes.[11] Both progesterone and estrogen levels are lowest at that time of the cycle.

### Pesticides

Many pesticides contain organophosphorus chemicals that inhibit the acetylcholinesterase enzyme.

Although these agents may produce a cholinergic crisis in anyone excessively exposed, myasthenia gravis patients on antiacetylcholinesterase medication are especially susceptible. Halides (like chlorine and fluorine) may pose additional risk for myasthenia gravis patients. In one case report, an individual exposed to chlorine gas subsequently developed generalized myasthenia gravis.[12] Fluoride is also implicated, and fluoridated water may trigger a myasthenia gravis crisis or contribute to long-term deterioration, with extreme exhaustion and muscle weakness.[13]

## DIAGNOSIS

Physicians may suspect myasthenia gravis in anyone with characteristic weakness. Once suspected, various tests may be ordered to confirm the diagnosis.

### Ice Test

This is a quick test that does not require special equipment and can be performed in the physician's office. After covering the patient's eye with an icepack for a couple of minutes, the physician will look for improvement in eyelid drooping. Any improvement may point toward a myasthenia gravis diagnosis.

### Acetylcholinesterase Inhibition

Because acetylcholine receptors are blocked in myasthenia gravis, drugs that increase the amount of acetylcholine can be used to test for the disease. Edrophonium is a fast-acting acetylcholinesterase inhibitor that, when administered intravenously, will produce immediate and temporary relief of muscle weakness in myasthenia gravis patients by sparing existing acetylcholine. Edrophonium acts quickly (within 30 seconds) and lasts for about 5 minutes.

### Immunohistochemistry of Blood

Antiacetylcholine receptor antibodies are detectable in the serum of about 85% of people with myasthenia gravis. However, they are present in only about 50% of people with symptoms confined to eye muscles.[7] More recently, antibodies to muscle-specific kinase (MuSK) have been discovered in about 70% of patients who test negative for antiacetylcholine receptor antibodies, yet suffer from classic symptoms of myasthenia gravis.[14] MuSK is a protein that helps organize acetylcholine receptors on the muscle cell surface, and this test is emerging as a helpful diagnostic tool if no autoantibodies are detected when symptoms of the disease are present.

### Electrophysiologic Studies

Nerve conduction studies may be used to detect muscle responses to mild stimuli. Patients with myasthenia gravis will demonstrate progressively smaller or weaker responses. Although this is the most specific nerve test for myasthenia gravis, it is not indicative in all cases and can be performed only on certain muscles.

### Thyroid Tests and Thymic Imaging

A number of tests might be conducted to assess the health of the thyroid and thymus glands. These include a computed tomography chest scan to reveal a thymoma or enlarged thymus gland and thyroid function tests to detect hyperthyroidism.

## CONVENTIONAL TREATMENT

Conventional treatments for myasthenia gravis are discussed in following sections.[15]

### Acetylcholinesterase Inhibitors

These drugs work by blocking the enzyme that normally destroys acetylcholine in the synapse, which allows existing acetylcholine more time to interact with available receptors. The result is stronger and more complete muscle contractions. Excessive use of antiacetylcholinesterase drugs can have fatal side effects. The most commonly used acetylcholinesterase inhibitors in myasthenia gravis are pyridostigmine and neostigmine.

### Thymectomy

Dozens of studies support the use of thymectomy (surgical removal of the thymus gland) to treat myasthenia gravis patients.[16] There is some debate, however, over how effective the procedure is among patients without a thymoma: one review suggested no benefit from thymectomy in myasthenia gravis patients who lacked a thymoma.[17] Other reports suggest that the procedure is especially valuable in early-onset myasthenia gravis.[3] Following a thymectomy, patients often report that symptoms lessen and, in some cases, disappear completely.

### Immunosuppressants

Immunosuppressants are often used in myasthenia gravis to blunt the overactive immune response. These drugs might include glucocorticoids such as prednisone, azathioprine, cyclosporine, and others. Although they are effective in many patients, careful management of patients on long-term glucocorticoid therapy is crucial because of the significant side effects associated with these drugs. Glucocorticoid use over the long term is associated with significant metabolic side effects, including central obesity, impairment of insulin sensitivity, and bone loss.

### Plasmapheresis

Plasmapheresis separates plasma, which contains the autoantibodies, from red blood cells, which then return to the body. This treatment temporarily improves symptoms and is especially valuable in preparation for surgical removal of the thymus. Several studies have reported that plasmapheresis is tolerated well in patients. The most common side effects are reversible hypotension (low blood pressure) and mild tremor. Several studies indicated that infection and mortality rates due to plasmapheresis were negligible, and all patients had immediate benefit from the procedure.[18,19]

### Intravenous Immunoglobulin

High-dose intravenous human immunoglobulin (IVIg) has emerged as a therapy for various neurologic diseases, including myasthenia gravis. Rather than expunging abnormal antibodies from the blood, the procedure floods the body with gamma globulin antibodies from several donors. In controlled clinical trials, IVIg was effective in treating chronic inflammatory demyelinating polyneuropathy.[20] IVIg has also produced improvement in some patients with myasthenia gravis.[21,22] IVIg therapy generates temporary relief lasting weeks to months. Studies comparing plasmapheresis and IVIg found that although both treatments demonstrated a clinically significant effect in patients with chronic myasthenia gravis, the improvement had a more rapid onset after plasmapheresis than after IVIg.[21]

## NUTRITIONAL SUPPORT

Many traditional therapies are somewhat successful in managing myasthenia gravis, but often at a price. Side effects of prescription drugs, especially glucocorticoids, can be serious and even life threatening. Complementary nutrients may offer ways to address myasthenia gravis and attack it from several angles while limiting adverse effects. The following nutrients have been shown to suppress the overactive immune response or enhance the action of acetylcholine.

### Vitamin K

Vitamin K may have a regulatory effect on myasthenia gravis. This fat-soluble vitamin has been shown to decrease levels of the proinflammatory cytokine interleukin-6,[23] which is involved in myasthenia gravis pathogenesis and correlates with acetylcholine receptor antibody production.[24]

## Dehydroepiandrosterone

Dehydroepiandrosterone (DHEA) is a hormone produced by the adrenal glands that can be converted into estrogen and testosterone. One study sought to detect a possible effect of DHEA in the pathogenesis of experimental myasthenia gravis. DHEA administered to rats resulted in a decrease in antibodies against acetylcholine receptors and an inhibition of the antibody-secreting cells. The authors concluded that these results encourage future study of DHEA treatment in human myasthenia gravis.[25]

## Huperzine A

Huperzine A is an active component of Chinese club moss (*Huperzia serrata*). Huperzine A is a reversible, highly effective, and highly selective inhibitor of the acetylcholinesterase enzyme.[26] Several experiments have demonstrated that huperzine A can intensify muscular contractions.[27] Research on 128 cases of myasthenia gravis indicated that 99% of the clinical symptoms were controlled or improved after treatment with huperzine A.[28]

## Creatine

Many studies have investigated creatine supplementation to enhance muscle power and strength, both in normal participants and patients with various neuromuscular diseases. A case study was performed to determine the effects of creatine supplementation in a myasthenia gravis patient taking glucocorticoids. After creatine supplementation (5 g daily) and training, the patient demonstrated increases in body weight, lean muscle mass, and muscle strength. The authors concluded that resistance exercise plus creatine supplementation may promote gains in strength and lean muscle mass in myasthenia gravis patients.[29]

## Choline and Lecithin

Choline is critical to normal membrane structure and function. Lecithin (phosphatidylcholine), abundant in nerve cell membranes, is required for nerve growth and function. Lecithin is a safer means of dietary choline supplementation than is choline itself. Additionally, it is fully compatible with pharmaceuticals and other nutrients. Bioavailability of lecithin is high; about 90% is absorbed over 24 hours. Also, lecithin is

an excellent emulsifier that enhances the bioavailability of coadministered nutrients.

Choline is a precursor of acetylcholine biosynthesis. Consumption of supplemental choline has been shown to increase acetylcholine release and enhance cholinergic function.[30] A subsequent trial of oral choline ameliorated symptoms in patients with tardive dyskinesia, a disease associated cholinergic dysfunction. The authors suggested a role for dietary precursors in treating diseases associated with neurotransmitter abnormality.[30] Another study of choline supplementation in 5 patients with tardive dyskinesia produced similar results. Both choline and lecithin increased blood choline levels and improved abnormal movements in all patients. Lecithin had fewer adverse effects than choline.[31] Choline and lecithin supplementation may be an effective means of increasing the levels of acetylcholine in myasthenia gravis patients; thus relieving symptoms or preventing myasthenic episodes.

## Additional Support

Besides the supplements mentioned above, there are many nutrients with a profound impact on muscle function or that can moderate the production of inflammatory cytokines, which have been implicated in myasthenia gravis. Although these supplements have not yet been studied in the context of myasthenia gravis, there may nevertheless be justification to experiment with them and see if beneficial results are obtained, provided there is no contraindication. As always, a supplement regimen should be monitored by a qualified physician familiar with your particular condition. Supplements that might help with muscle function or reduce inflammation include *branch chain amino acids, coenzyme Q10, fish oil, NADH, vitamin E,* and minerals such as *calcium* and *potassium*. The *B vitamin complex* is also highly involved in cellular function as well as acetylcholine production and may help boost acetylcholine levels.

Many people report that dietary modification helped their myasthenia gravis. While these claims are not supported in peer-reviewed studies, some patients with myasthenia gravis advocate a raw food or gluten-free diet. As long as adequate nutrition is maintained (a multivitamin is probably a good idea), these diets can be attempted under the supervision of a qualified physician.

## Life Extension Suggestions

- **Multivitamin/multinutrient:** per label instructions of a broad-spectrum, multinutrient formula containing the B-complex vitamins; vitamins A, C, D, and E; grape seed extract; citrus bioflavonoids; and more

- **Huperzine A:** 50 mcg daily
- **Vitamin K:** 2.1 mg daily
- **DHEA:** 15–75 mg daily to start, followed by blood testing in 3–6 weeks to make sure that optimal levels of this hormone are maintained
- **Creatine:** taken in 2 phases (in conjunction with weight training): the loading phase (higher dosage) and the maintenance phase (dose of 2–5 g daily)
- **Lecithin granules:** 1 heaping tablespoon daily, with meals
- **Thymus capsules:** per label instructions (only for people whose thymus gland has been removed)
- **Coenzyme Q10 (as ubiquinol):** 100–200 mg daily
- **Fish oil:** 1400 mg EPA and 1000 mg DHA daily

- **Calcium:** 200–1200 mg daily
- **Potassium:** 99 mg daily (or more) when instructed to do so by a health-care professional, based on blood test results.
- **NADH:** 5 mg daily
- **Branched chain amino acids (BCAA):** per label instructions

In addition, the following *blood tests* may provide helpful information:

- Chemistry panel and complete blood count (CBC)
- Thyroid panel (TSH, T4, Free T4, Free T3)

## REFERENCES

References available at: www.lef.org/dpt5/ch96

# 97

# Myofascial Syndrome

*Myofascial: from the Greek myelos, meaning marrow (muscle) and from the Latin fascia meaning bandage or band*

Myofascial syndrome (MFS) is a musculoskeletal condition characterized by painful foci of muscle called trigger points (TrPs). MFS became better known based on the work of Janet Travell, a White House physician for many years.

MFS has often been confused with fibromyalgia because they both involve muscle pain. Trigger points of MFS differ from tender points of fibromyalgia in that they may be just about anywhere, whereas the tender points of fibromyalgia are in a specified pattern. When a physician presses on a tender point in fibromyalgia patients, they describe exactly that—tenderness. When a physician pushes a trigger point in MFS, the trigger point elicits an involuntary "twitch" response. Additionally, the patient may experience referred pain (ie, pain that radiates to an area away from the trigger point itself). The painful trigger point area is in the muscle or junction of the muscle and fascia. Hence, myofascial pain is usually associated with a taut band, indicating a "ropey" thickening of muscle tissue.

The fascia is a tough connective tissue that spreads throughout the body in a 3-dimensional web from head to foot without interruption. The fascia surrounds every muscle, bone, nerve, blood vessel, and organ of the body, all the way down to the cellular level. Therefore, malfunction of the fascial system due to trauma, posture, or inflammation can create a "binding down" of the fascia, resulting in abnormal pressure on nerves, muscles, bones, or organs.

Much of the pain that accompanies MFS is due to inadequate blood flow to the trigger point area (ischemia) that inhibits the ability of the muscle to eliminate metabolic wastes (eg, lactic acid and potassium). These accumulated metabolic byproducts combined with inadequate oxygen flow to the affected area then build up, stimulating nearby nerve endings that lead to trigger point pain.

## DISTINGUISHING MFS FROM FIBROMYALGIA

What distinguishes MFS from fibromyalgia is that MFS is not usually associated with poor sleep or chronic fatigue, although some patients may have a little bit of both. Trigger points of MFS do not go away by getting the patient to sleep better. Since a patient can have both fibromyalgia and MFS, treating the fibromyalgia may improve things. However, persistent painful areas may be the result of MFS. For example, a patient may experience headaches and have classic fibromyalgia. Following the fibromyalgia protocol makes the patient feel much better, but the headache persists. Upon reexamination, the patient's physician finds the same mid-trapezoidal trigger points described above, greater on the right than the left. It turns out that the patient carries a heavy laptop every day on the right shoulder. When the trigger point is pressed on very firmly, the patient develops neck pain that evolves into a migraine. Treating the trigger point and having the patient stop carrying the laptop for a while will result in resolution of the headaches. What has been described is, of course, the ideal diagnostic situation. Some patients may not develop the migraine right there in the office. However, anyone with unexplained headaches should have an evaluation for the presence of trigger points. The same is true for any persistent muscular pain that appears to be nondermatomal in origin.

## CAUSES OF MFS

Causative factors of MFS include the following:

- Repetitive motions; excessive exercise; muscle strain due to overactivity
- Lack of activity (eg, leg or arm in a sling)
- Nutritional deficiencies
- Nervous tension or stress
- Generalized fatigue
- Sudden trauma to muscles, ligaments, or tendons
- Hormonal changes (eg, premenstrual syndrome or menopause)

## A LINK TO DEPRESSION AND ANXIETY

Many painful conditions, including headaches, migraines, temporomandibular joint (TMJ) pain, and muscle pain improve when trigger points associated with MFS are identified and treated. However, chronic pain may affect people emotionally, and many people with MFS experience depression or anxiety disorders. It may be beneficial to consult a mental health professional in addition to a regular physician.[1] (See Life Extension's Depression, Anxiety, and Stress Management protocols for additional information.)

Antidepressants are often prescribed for the treatment of MFS. At low doses, medications, such as tricyclic antidepressants relax muscles, improve sleep, and help regulate neurotransmitter activity that contributes to associated pain. At higher doses, they will help relieve depression, but have side effects that often preclude long-term use.

## TREATMENT

Janet Travell developed a technique to map out myofascial pain regions and their associated trigger points; the technique is used to either inject a local anesthetic with a mild anti-inflammatory steroid solution into the trigger point or to break up the trigger point with a needle. The exact pathology of the trigger point is not entirely understood. It is clear, however, that treating the trigger point is responsible for resolving many types of pain patterns.

Janet Travell's work coincides with acupuncture points. The trigger points and associated pain radiation areas have been co-related by an acupuncture researcher. Eighty-seven percent of Travell's trigger points and their associated pain areas lie on acupuncture meridians and correlate with known acupuncture points. Additionally, acupuncturists describe a certain grabbing of the needle (taking Chi), which correlates with the twitch response described by Travell. When a trigger point is properly needled, there is a visible "grab" observed by the practitioner and a feeling of a grabbing or slight contraction around the needle experienced by the patient. These techniques had been utilized by the Chinese for thousands of years before finally being introduced by Travell into Western medicine.[2]

The acupuncture points He Gu (near the wrist where the thumb and forefinger join) and Yin Men (back of the thigh) were found to increase blood flow and reduce MFS-related pain.[3] Most studies, however, seem to indicate that although acupuncture is an effective short-term treatment for chronic pain due to MFS, there is limited evidence that acupuncture will be effective in the long-term, and further human studies need to be conducted.[4,5] One study on the use of amitriptyline in people with temporomandibular joint (TMJ) pain and MFS seemed to show that while the beneficial effects of these pain treatments were reduced over time, muscular pain was still manageable more than 1 year after treatment.[6] Amitriptyline is a tricyclic antidepressant drug with many side effects that preclude long-term use in most people.

For refractive cases of MFS, a homeopathic solution of Traumeel® and/or a mild narcotic called buprenorphine injected into the trigger point(s) may be employed.

Travell's technique of injecting corticosteroids and/or local anesthetics into trigger points appears to be effective in reducing muscle pain. Japanese researchers conducted studies on 40 women with chronic lumbar, shoulder, or neck myofascial pain. Using Travell's technique, each woman was given an injection of diluted anesthetic or saline placebo, and their pain levels were measured. In another portion of the study, 21 outpatient volunteers were given different dilutions of different anesthetics in each shoulder. The researchers concluded that the most suitable type of local anesthetic is lidocaine or mepivacaine, and the most effective water-diluted concentration is 0.2–0.25%.[7]

Trigger points may require multiple treatments that necessitate excessive amounts of steroids over time. Some physicians feel that local anesthetics may irritate the muscle tissue, and multiple injections into the same trigger point may aggravate the problem.

Buprenorphine, a mild narcotic with agonist and antagonist properties, has a very low addiction liability (if any), indicating it can be used for a long period of time without developing serious withdrawal symptoms. Buprenorphine acts rapidly on depression, reducing pain, and inducing sleep; thus, it is effective for conditions with multiple symptoms (eg, MFS).[8]

Buprenorphine is available as an injectable, 0.3-mg ampule dose. The dosage is variable. Because buprenorphine is poorly absorbed orally, larger dosages must be used. Oral buprenorphine liquid is withdrawn or shaken from the ampule and held under the tongue as long as possible. Compounding pharmacies can make up buprenorphine for sublingual use as a troche (ie, lozenge). Both forms, the ampules and troches, are expensive. For pain that prevents sleep, start with 2–6 ampules sublingually or 0.5–2 mg as a sublingual troche. For treating depression-related pain throughout the day, begin with 2–6 ampules (or 0.5–2 mg as a sublingual troche) every 4–6 hours. As with most medications, begin with a low dose and increase slowly until the smallest dose that proves effective is reached. Do not be concerned about addiction.

Buprenorphine, when diluted and injected into trigger points, may have a local pain-reducing action or in some way help to directly break up the trigger point. Additionally, buprenorphine is a mild narcotic analgesic that makes repetitive injections more tolerable for the patient. The dosage of Traumeel®, since it is homeopathic, is not critical. One to two ampules a session may be adequate, depending upon the number of trigger points and volume of the solution. The proportion works out to 1 ampule per 10 cc of saline. Since buprenorphine has a systemic action and may produce drowsiness, no more than 2 ampules per session are usually used, again depending upon the volume. Some patients, especially those who are obese, may tolerate more than 2 ampules per session. The dilution is one-half to two ampules (0.15–0.6 mg) per 20 cc of saline depending upon patient response and the number of trigger points treated per session. It is advised to begin with the lower concentrations.

Injections are usually 2–4 cc per trigger point. The patient must be driven home after treatment due to the potential for sedation. For really difficult-to-treat trigger points, the Edegawa technique involves taking a 60-cc syringe filled with saline (salt water) and injecting it rapidly through an 18-gauge (large) needle. Anywhere from 10 cc to the full 60 cc may be used for a particularly recalcitrant trigger point. It is believed that rapid influx of saline pulls muscle fibers apart where they cross the trigger point, resulting in a breakup of the trigger point itself.

If saline injections fail, Traumeel® and buprenorphine may be added to the saline. This combination is recommended at the outset due to the safety of the two preparations, the possible direct actions of both agents on the trigger point, and the systemic pain-killing properties of buprenorphine. After all, multiple injections of large volumes of fluids into the muscle tissue are painful. The dilution is 6 ampules of Traumeel® and 1–2 ampules of buprenorphine per 60 cc of saline. Each trigger point may require anywhere from 10–60 cc of fluid as previously described. The amount must be found empirically. No matter how many trigger points are treated, it is suggested that no more than 3 ampules per session of buprenorphine be used because of the potential for sedation. However, some patients, especially those who are obese, may require and tolerate more. There is no need to worry about addiction. See Life Extension's Pain (Chronic) protocol for more information.

# TARGETED NUTRITIONAL AND LIFESTYLE INTERVENTIONS TO REDUCE SYMPTOMS OF MFS

## S-Adenosylmethionine

The supplement S-adenosylmethionine (SAMe) has been shown to be specifically effective as a therapy to reduce chronic pain and depression associated with fibromyalgia.[9] SAMe is synthesized in the body from the amino acid methionine. The enzyme methionine S-adeno-syltransferase (MAT) catalyzes a reaction between methionine and adenosine triphosphate (ATP) to form SAMe. SAMe has been tested for depression caused by a variety of diseases, including Parkinson's

disease, fibromyalgia, cancer, cardiovascular disease, and rheumatoid arthritis. Researchers have used SAMe successfully in conjunction with drug and alcohol withdrawal.

In a study, 44 fibromyalgia patients took 800 mg of SAMe for 6 weeks. Results showed that SAMe reduced pain at the tender points, as well as fatigue, morning stiffness, and resting pain.[10]

## Dietary Changes to Improve Symptoms

Patients with MFS are encouraged to employ proper basic nutrition and supplementation. Women with MFS have been found to have higher cholesterol levels than women without MFS, but no conclusive link has been made between blood lipid levels and MFS.[11] The following dietary recommendations will improve overall health:

- Limit intake of stimulants (caffeine) and depressants (alcohol) due to their potential to disrupt neurologic and metabolic function.

- Limit intake of refined sugars to avoid fluctuation of blood sugar levels, mood swings, lowered energy, and lowered immunity.

- Consume whole foods such as fruits and vegetables that contain phytochemicals and fiber. Fiber is helpful for maintaining digestive regularity. Eat slowly, chewing food well.

- Increase intake of cold-water fish that supply essential fatty acid building blocks (gamma linolenic acid [GLA] and eicosapentaenoic acid [EPA]) needed for cell membrane maintenance and function.

- Increase intake of probiotic cultures from food or supplements. Probiotics are "healthy" bacteria that normally reside in the gastrointestinal tract. "Healthy" bacteria aid proper digestion of food and prevent absorption of ingested toxins.

- Drink plenty of water (preferably purified) to ensure adequate fluid levels.[12]

## Amino Acid Supplementation

Phenylalanine is one of the 20 essential amino acids that must be obtained from the diet. It is a necessary precursor for neurotransmitter biosynthesis and may be helpful in relieving chronic pain. The amino acid tyrosine is synthesized in the body from phenylalanine. It is a precursor to the biosynthesis of the neurotransmitters epinephrine, norepinephrine, and dopamine. Tyrosine has been used as an antidepressant because it positively affects the neurotransmitters required to prevent depression. Supplementing with these 2 amino acids may be beneficial to people with

MFS. Vitamins B6 and C are cofactors in the bioconversion of these amino acids to their neurotransmitter receptors.

## Exercise

With the help of a physical therapist or other health care professional, exercises can be designed that will avoid causing undue stress and pain to sensitive trigger points while improving physical fitness. In addition to promoting overall fitness, physical activity assists in maintaining flexibility, building muscle strength, and helping protect joints. Walking, bicycling, swimming, and some types of weight-bearing exercises are good examples of physical activity that may be appropriate. It is important to note that lack of exercise can lead to brittle bones as well as causing muscles to become smaller and weaker. In particular, people with MFS should avoid repetitive weight-bearing exercises involving affected area(s). Gentle stretching of muscle groups should be done daily to their full range of motion within the limits of pain.

## SUMMARY OF TREATMENT MODALITIES

- Trigger point therapy: myofascial release therapy, myotherapy, massotherapy spray, and stretch technique (stretching of the muscles with a vapocoolant spray, where a coolant is sprayed on the trigger point to lessen the pain, then the muscle is stretched). This is often done by a physical therapist.

- Trigger point injections: local anesthetics (eg, lidocaine) are injected directly into trigger points. Trigger point injection has been shown to be one of the most effective treatment modalities to inactivate trigger points and provide prompt relief of symptoms.[13]

- Dry needling: the use of a needle without injecting anything. TrP injections and dry needling mechanically disrupt the trigger point. The use of lidocaine is no more effective, but reduces soreness after injection.

- For MFS, there is no role for injected steroids.

- Acupuncture is recommended as a treatment option for patients with associated musculoskeletal conditions.[14]

- The application of ice packs will numb the affected area, providing temporary relief.

- Chiropractic or osteopathic manipulation treatment.

- Physical therapy (hands-on).

- Elimination of stress; biofeedback; counseling for depression that may result from chronic pain.

- Follow good basic nutrition.

- Buprenorphine is a mild narcotic that can safely relieve multiple symptoms of MFS. Contact a compounding pharmacy to make a sublingual preparation. Buprenorphine must be prescribed by a physician.

- Consider regular exercise under the guidance of a healthcare professional to maintain cardiovascular and musculoskeletal fitness.

## Life Extension Suggestions

Patients with unexplained persistent headaches or muscle pain should be examined for the presence of trigger points. Consult with a healthcare professional familiar with the various techniques used to relieve pain associated with trigger points. Make sure that both you and your physician find the source of the trigger points and seek ways to prevent recurrence. Look for repetitive injury as the cause before deciding that stress is the etiology. If stress is the etiology, it is most important to find ways of relieving it, or MFS pain will reoccur.

- **Vitamin C:** 1000–2000 mg daily
- **Vitamin B6:** 75–250 mg daily
- **D,L-phenylalanine:** 1000 mg daily
- **Tyrosine:** 1000 mg daily
- **S-adenosylmethionine (SAMe):** 800–1200 mg daily
- **Omega 3 fatty acids from fish oil:** 1400 mg EPA and 1000 mg of DHA daily
- **Gamma-linolenic acid (GLA):** 1300 mg daily
- **Probiotics** containing *Lactobacillus* and *Bifidobacterium* strains: per label instructions

## REFERENCES

References available at: www.lef.org/dpt5/ch97

# 98

# *Nail Health*

Nails are important for many reasons, including aesthetic appeal. They can also serve as important barometers offering clues to a person's overall health. Indeed, conditions as seemingly benign as increased nail thickness, horizontal white lines in the nails, or nail concavity (spooning) may be an indication of a variety of problems (eg, anemia, endocarditis, connective tissue disorders).[1] Common nail complaints include brittle, dry nails, and infection with a variety of pathogens.

Aging can cause slowed nail growth as well as brittle, dull, or yellowish nails. Other significant causes of nail abnormalities include environmental factors (eg, exposure to chemicals, polishes, or harsh detergents; prolonged water exposure; reaction to adhesives used in artificial nails; use of certain medications), and injury or trauma (eg, striking fingers with a hammer, closing fingers in doors, stubbing a toe, wearing ill-fitted footwear, biting nails habitually).

In many cases, treating nail disorders is frustrating for physicians and patients alike. Nail disorders such as fungal infections are difficult to treat, and healing is slow. Worse yet, a few of the common prescription medications used to treat nail disorders have potentially significant side effects, especially liver damage. Natural agents, such as vitamin E, shown to support strong nails may offer the same benefits as prescription drugs, without the risk of serious side effects. If a nail condition is caused by underlying disease (eg, diabetes), seek treatment for that condition immediately.

## ANATOMY OF NAILS

Nails are composed of a hard, strong protein called keratin, as well as small amounts of sulfur, calcium, fats, and water. The nail plate (ie, visible part of the nail) protects the sensitive nail bed underneath it. The folds of skin surrounding the nail on 3 sides are nail folds. Within the nail plate is the cuticle, which is connected to the nail folds and nail plate, and the lunula (ie, whitish, half-moon-shaped area at the base of the nail). Nails grow from the matrix, an area under the cuticle, at a rate averaging one tenth of an inch per month. Healthy nails grow continuously; serious illnesses can leave behind tell-tale signs called growth arrest lines, also known as Beau's lines.

Some of the most commonly reported nail problems are also among the most bothersome (aesthetically and emotionally), even though many of them are not medically serious. Others, such as yellow nail syndrome, may be caused by a serious underlying disease. Below are some of the more common complaints.

### Paronychia

Paronychia infection of the nail folds can be caused by bacteria, fungi, or viruses. This condition can cause pain, redness, and swelling of the nail folds. It may be seen in people who keep their hands in water for extended periods.

### Brittle Nails

Brittle nails are one of the most common complaints. They are generally characterized by vertical splitting or separation of the nail plate at the end of the nail. This is often a consequence of aging as the flow of moisture and natural oils to the nail bed declines.

### Ingrown Toenail

Ingrown toenails typically affect the great ("big") toe and occur when a corner of the nail curves downward into the skin. This condition can be very painful and lead to infection. Ingrown toenails are usually caused by improper nail trimming, poor posture, or tight shoes. Nails should always be cut longer than the tips of the toe to prevent the advancing edge of the nail plate from "digging in" to the soft tissue of the nail folds.

### Nail Psoriasis

This nail abnormality occurs primarily in people with psoriasis of the skin; it is seen in about 80% of people with inflammatory arthritis associated with psoriasis, especially when the arthritis affects the toes and fingers. Characteristics include yellow-red discoloration of the nail, pitting, separation of the nail plate from the nail bed, crumbling or splitting of the nail plate, and subungual hyperkeratosis.[2]

### Onychomycosis

Approximately 7% of adults in North America contract this fungal infection. Onychomycosis invades the nail plate, causing the nail to separate from the nail plate (onycholysis) and chalky debris to form under the nail plate.[3,4] More than 90% of cases are caused by one of 2 pathogens: *Trichophyton rubrum* or *Trichophyton mentagrophytes*. Factors that have an important effect on the development of onychomycosis include increasing age; genetics; and the presence of diabetes, acquired immunodeficiency syndrome, or peripheral arterial disease.[5] One multicenter study reported that diabetics are nearly 3 times more likely to develop onychomycosis than nondiabetics; also, up to one-third of diabetics may develop nail fungus.[6]

## Pitting

The formation of tiny depressions in the nail plate is known as pitting; it can be caused by any localized skin condition that interrupts natural growth of the nail. Pitting occurs in up to 50% of people with psoriasis; it is also a common problem in people with connective tissue disorders (eg, *Alopecia areata*, *Incontinentia pigmenti*, pemphigus, Reiter's syndrome, and sarcoidosis).

## White Nails (Terry's Nails)

This nail abnormality is characterized by a white nail bed with a pink band that is 1–2 mm wide at the tip. In most cases, all the fingernails are affected, although it can affect a single finger. White nails affects about 80% of people with severe liver disease.[1] It is also seen in people with type 2 diabetes, chronic renal failure, or congestive heart failure and is associated with advancing age.[7]

# CONVENTIONAL TREATMENT

Most nail abnormalities are associated with underlying medical conditions and resolve as those conditions are treated. Infections of the nails, such as with fungus or bacteria, are a significant exception in that they may respond to specific treatment. Although both topical and oral medications are available, topical agents typically are not very effective because infections are usually under the nail, and topical medications cannot penetrate the nail plate.[8] For paronychia, or nail infection, antibiotics and surgical drainage of the infected nail fold may be recommended.[9]

For nail fungus, one of 2 oral medications is usually prescribed: Lamisil® (terbinafine) or Sporanox® (itraconazole). The use of these drugs is associated with liver toxicity, however. In rare cases, liver failure and death have occurred, especially among people with severe underlying systemic conditions.[10] Use of these drugs should be closely monitored by a physician.

## Lamisil®

In an open-label, randomized, multicenter trial, 75 patients aged 65 or older who had moderate to severe onychomycosis were treated with 250 mg Lamisil® daily for

12 weeks. Half also underwent 4 sessions of aggressive debridement (surgical removal of fungus). At the 48-week follow-up, 64% of the patients had mycologic cure and reported that the drug had been well tolerated. Those who also underwent debridement appeared to fare better than those who did not.[11]

In a comparative, randomized study of 30 patients with onychomycosis, either Lamisil® or Sporanox® was administered for 16 weeks, and patients were followed up for 36 weeks. At the end of follow-up, little or no nail deformity was seen in 86.7% of the Sporanox® group and 100% of the Lamisil® group. Reported side effects included nausea, abdominal cramps, back pain, flu-like syndrome, and headache.[12]

While Lamisil® alone has proven to be effective in onychomycosis, researchers have found that Lamisil® combined with topical ciclopirox nail lacquer is more effective than Lamisil® alone. Eighty patients with onychomycosis received either oral Lamisil®, 250 mg daily for 16 weeks, or the same Lamisil® protocol plus ciclopirox nail lacquer applied once daily for 9 months. After 9 months of follow-up, the infection cleared in 64.7% of the Lamisil®-only patients and 88.2% of those who got the combination therapy.[13]

## Sporanox®

Use of Sporanox®, both alone and in combination with another medication, has proven effective in the treatment of onychomycosis. One study reported significant results when patients used 100 mg daily for 6 months,[14] and another study found that pulse therapy (200 mg daily for 1 week per month over 5.6 ± 4.3 months) resulted in a 62% cure rate overall.[15]

Use of Sporanox® pulse therapy and amorolfine 5% solution nail lacquer was examined in a randomized study. Forty-five patients received 2 pulse treatments plus amorolfine for 6 months, and another 45 patients received 3 pulse treatments of Sporanox® without amorolfine. The investigators found that the combination treatment was as safe and effective as Sporanox® alone, with less cost per patient.[16]

For patients prone to onychomycosis, treatment may never completely eliminate the disease.[17,18] In fact, treatment fails in 25–40% of onychomycosis cases.[19] Combining drug therapies (an oral and topical medication) or combining drug therapy with mechanical debridement can be successful.

## Treating Nail Psoriasis

Oral drug treatment of nail psoriasis remains problematic due to the high cost of the drugs (eg, methotrexate, acitretin, and cyclosporine) as well as their potential for systemic complications. Several topical medications may be helpful. Calcipotriol, for example, has proved effective for psoriatic nails and can be used in chronic cases.[20] In one study, a combination of 1% 5-fluorouracil cream and 20% urea resulted in improvement of more than 50% of the clinical signs of nail psoriasis in 59 patients.[21] Side effects of topical agents may include burning, tingling, and swelling at or near application sites.

For serious ingrown toenails that have not responded to topical or oral medications, surgery is an option. Several types of operations that use a modification of the Zadik method and artificial skin have proven effective.[22]

# NUTRITIONAL THERAPY FOR HEALTHY NAILS

Natural remedies for nail treatment are up against the same obstacles as prescription agents: it is difficult to deliver healing agents to the site of infection. However, a few nutrients stand out for their ability to support strong, healthy nails.

## Silicon

Silicon is an essential trace mineral that is vital to healthy bones and skin. It helps facilitate the formation of collagen, which is necessary for strength and healthy development of epithelial and skeletal connective tissue. In a study, silicon was examined for its ability to improve skin and nail health in women with sun-damaged skin. Chronic exposure to sunlight has been shown to damage connective tissue, which causes loss of elasticity in skin. In this randomized, double-blind, placebo-controlled study, women were given 10 mg daily of either a bioavailable silicon or placebo. Measurements of skin and nail health were taken throughout the study. At the end of 20 weeks, women taking silicon had decreased skin roughness and less-brittle nails and hair, showing that silicon had a significantly positive effect on nails, skin, and hair.[23] This study used a stabilized orthosilicic acid, which is the form of silicon with the greatest bioavailability.

## Vitamin E

The results of several small studies show that vitamin E can be effective in the treatment of nail changes in yellow nail syndrome, which also has profound effects on heart and lung function that must be treated separately.[24] A few studies found that high doses (800–1200 IU daily for several months) were effective in some patients[25–27]; another study focused on topical vitamin E used twice daily for 12 months, which also provided noticeable results.[24]

## Biotin

In one study, supplementation with the B-complex vitamin biotin increased nail thickness by 25% in 63% of participants with brittle nails. Nearly all patients had improved hardness and firmness after taking 2.5 mg biotin daily for an average of 5.5 months.[28] In another study, researchers reported that patients taking biotin daily for 3–6 months experienced a significant decrease in brittleness and splitting.[29] Increased nail thickness was evident after biotin supplementation in yet another study, in which progress was identified using scanning electron microscopy.[30]

## Protein

Protein, consisting of amino acids chains, is a building material for new nails. Researchers have found an association between protein deficiency and nail abnormalities such as Muehrcke's lines (ie, paired, white, transverse lines that appear on the nail plate). Muehrcke's lines appeared in individuals with low blood protein levels (ie, albumin level less than 2 g/dL, or 20 g/L), but when protein levels were normalized, the white bands disappeared.[1] Protein from sources that provide a variety of amino acids have also been shown in studies to increase the health and strength of the nail plate.[31]

## Iron

Iron-deficiency anemia, which affects 20% of women and 50% of pregnant women, can cause brittle nails if it becomes severe. A blood test should be used to diagnose iron-deficiency anemia in people with brittle nails. Supplemental iron should be taken under the supervision of a physician.

## Zinc

Zinc deficiency has been associated with poor nail health, manifesting as deformed nails, hangnails, inflamed cuticles, and white spots in the nail plate. A few small studies have shown that supplementation with oral zinc can help resolve nail abnormalities in yellow nail syndrome.[32,33]

## L-Cysteine

L-cysteine is a conditionally essential amino acid, one of only 3 sulfur-containing amino acids. The others are taurine (which can be produced from L-cysteine) and L-methionine, from which L-cysteine can be produced in the body by a multistep process.

L-cysteine is an important component of keratin, hair, and nails.

## PREVENTION: PROPER NAIL CARE

To help achieve and maintain healthy looking nails, consider the following guidelines:

- Use cotton-lined rubber gloves when doing dishes or using harsh chemicals, then wash hands with a gentle soap and dry them thoroughly (perspiration buildup inside gloves can set the stage for fungal infections). Renew and replace gloves frequently to reduce possible fungus accumulations.
- Avoid biting your nails or picking at your cuticles.
- Keep nails clipped slightly longer than the tip of finger or toe to prevent hangnails or ingrown nails.
- To avoid ingrown toenails, wear shoes with a toe box that does not squeeze your toes together.
- Try to keep your nails short, square-shaped, and slightly round on the top. It is best to trim brittle nails after a bath (they will be more supple then) and apply moisturizer.
- If your nails are very brittle, avoid nail polish.
- If your nails or cuticles are dry, consider moisturizing them at bedtime and wearing cotton gloves while you sleep.
- Use nail polish remover no more than twice a month. If necessary, touch up nails with polish.
- Mend split or torn nails with nail glue or clear polish.

To avoid fungal infections, follow these tips:

- Wear shower shoes or flip-flops in communal showers.
- Make sure your feet and body are thoroughly dried.
- Avoid sharing towels or clothing.
- Use nonirritating soaps and detergents.

### Life Extension Suggestions

- **Orthosilicic acid** (a source of bioavailable silicon): 10 mg daily
- **Vitamin E:** 400 IU alpha-tocopherol and 200 mg gamma-tocopherol daily
- **Biotin:** 600–5950 mcg daily
- **Iron:** If testing reveals iron-deficiency anemia, consult your physician for dosage.
- **Zinc:** 30 mg daily
- **L-cysteine:** 500 mg daily
- **Whey protein:** 17–34 g daily

In addition, the following *blood test* may provide helpful information:

- Iron and total iron binding capacity (TIBC)

## REFERENCES

References available at: www.lef.org/dpt5/ch98

# 99

---

# *Neuropathy (Diabetic)*

---

Millions of people are living with some form of neuropathy. The term neuropathy means a condition in a nerve or group of nerves that causes pain and dysfunction. There are many different causes of neuropathy and a broad range of symptoms.

Unfortunately, there is no single good treatment for most neuropathies, and many have no known cause. A number of prescription drugs are used, but all have side effects, and none can correct the underlying nerve defect causing the pain. Nutrient therapy offers a promising alternative for people who want to avoid the side effects of prescription drugs.

Neuropathies can originate either within the central nervous system (ie, central neuropathies, such as Guillain-Barre syndrome) or in peripheral nerves, which lie outside the central nervous system. These are called peripheral neuropathies and account for the majority of cases. They can have many causes (eg, toxins, alcohol, and metabolic disease). Diabetes is the most common cause of peripheral neuropathies.

## WHY NEUROPATHY HURTS

In all forms of neuropathy, there is abnormal stimulation of nerves or damage that results in pain. Peripheral nerves are sensitive conduits that carry impulses from extremities back to the central nervous system (ie, the spinal cord and brain). Impulses are transmitted along nerves by changes in the electrical charge of the cell membrane caused by movement of ions such as sodium, potassium, and calcium. Impulses are transmitted between nerves by neurotransmitters such as acetylcholine and substance P, which is responsible for transmitting pain impulses. For protection, most nerves are covered with a thin sheath called myelin, which is made from choline and lipids. Myelin functions like the rubber wrapping around an electrical cord: it insulates the nerve fibers and prevents abnormal transmissions.

Depending on the nature of the specific neuropathy, some part of this system breaks down. In diabetic neuropathy, for example, there is a change in the microvascular network supplying the nerve with nutrients. This lack of blood supply and nutrients causes the nerve to function abnormally. Diabetic neuropathy tends to occur in more than one nerve area (polyneuropathy) and may cause loss of sensation and pain that typically worsens at night. In severe cases, diabetics can suffer from autonomic neuropathy. In this case, the autonomic nervous system, which controls automatic body functions, is affected with possibly serious consequences, including gastrointestinal problems, bladder-emptying problems, abnormal heart rhythms, and even sudden death.[1]

Neuropathies can also be caused by specific nutritional deficiencies (eg, vitamin B12) and infectious diseases (eg, syphilis).

Pain associated with neuropathy can be very intense and may be described as cutting, stabbing, crushing, burning, shooting, gnawing, or grinding. In some cases, a minimal stimulus such as a light touch can trigger severe pain, or pain may be felt even in the absence of any stimulus. If a problem with the motor nerve has continued over a length of time, muscle shrinkage (atrophy) or lack of muscle tone may be noticeable.

## OPTIONS FOR TREATING NEUROPATHIES

Unfortunately, treatment options for most neuropathies are less than ideal. The following are some of the common strategies:

- For diabetic neuropathy, blood glucose control is essential because glucose causes high levels of oxidative stress throughout the body. In animals, antioxidant therapy, with glutathione and other antioxidants, has been shown to help prevent neuropathy.[2]

- Vitamin B12 deficiency can cause peripheral neuropathies, optic neuropathies, and pernicious anemia. This condition is typically treated with vitamin B12 shots. Additionally, folic acid deficiency has been linked to various neuropathies and is usually treated with supplementation.[3]

- For neuropathies caused by an autoimmune disorder (eg, rheumatoid arthritis, lupus, or Guillain-Barre), treatment is generally aimed at the underlying inflammatory condition.

- For neuropathies caused by nerve pressure, treatment focuses on relieving the source of the pressure. This strategy may include ergonomic changes to alter any repetitive motions or positions (such as at a keyboard) that caused the neuropathy, or even surgery to relieve internal pressure. Carpal tunnel syndrome is a common cause of neuropathies in the wrist and hand.

- For neuropathy caused by exposure to toxic metals (eg, lead and mercury) or medications, treatment focuses on reducing exposure to the offending substance and reducing blood levels of any toxins. Antioxidants are also frequently used to reduce oxidative stress.

## Medications

A number of medications may also be prescribed or recommended to help deal with the pain. The most common ones are pain relievers (eg, over-the-counter medications such as ibuprofen) and other nonsteroidal anti-inflammatory drugs. Because of the risk of serious liver and kidney toxicity, Life Extension does not recommend long-term use of acetaminophen for treatment of neuropathies. Aspirin is also frequently suggested for mild neuropathy.

For more serious neuropathies, drugs such as gabapentin (Neurontin®), carbamazepine (Tegretol®), and phenytoin (Dilantin®) may be prescribed. These drugs were originally developed to treat epilepsy, but also work to reduce the pain associated with neuropathy. Their main side effect is dizziness. In one study, the combination of gabapentin and B vitamins was shown to effectively and significantly reduce pain and improve quality of life.[4]

Pentoxifylline (PTX) is a prescription drug approved by the Food and Drug Administration (FDA) to treat peripheral vascular disease. PTX is prescribed to improve the flow properties of blood by decreasing its viscosity. Aging causes a progressive decline of blood delivery to the tissues. Those with diabetes experience accelerated circulatory deficit. In a study on diabetic rats, 2 weeks of PTX administration resulted in a correction of nerve conduction deficit, amounting to 56.5% in the sciatic motor nerve and 69.8% in the saphenous sensory nerve. PTX restored the microvascular deficit by 50.4%.[5] This study indicates that PTX may be of particular benefit to diabetics, especially those suffering from neuropathy, kidney disease, and other vascular disorders.

Research also suggests that triiodothyronine (Cytomel), a drug used to treat hypothyroidism, is also effective at regenerating damaged peripheral nerves. In animal studies, administration of Cytomel regenerated nerve axons after surgical transection of the sciatic nerve, although the mechanism of action remains unclear.[6] Researchers believe that Cytomel administration may have therapeutic potential in cases of peripheral neuropathy by enhancing nerve regeneration.[7]

Antidepressants are sometimes used. These drugs may have side effects (eg, dry mouth, nausea, tiredness, constipation, and weight gain) that discourage people from continuing their medication, although the side effects tend to be less severe than those of anticonvulsants.

In the most severe cases, opiates such as oxycodone (OxyContin®) may be prescribed. Because of their reputation for dependency, many physicians hesitate to prescribe opiates for pain, even when they are an appropriate therapy. If prescribed opiates, carefully follow the dosing instructions.

Unfortunately, none of these medications can actually fix the underlying nerve damage; they can only reduce the pain associated with neuropathies.

## Alternative Therapies for Neuropathy

The following nondrug therapies have been shown to reduce pain associated with neuropathy:

**Transcutaneous electrical nerve stimulation.** In this therapy, small electrodes placed on the skin deliver tiny electrical impulses to specific nerve pathways. This treatment is effective for some types of pain.

**Biofeedback.** During biofeedback, people learn how to control body responses to reduce pain. Biofeedback is taught with a special machine in a hospital or medical center. Afterward, people learn how to control these responses by themselves.

**Acupuncture.** Acupuncture is a traditional Chinese method of pain relief in which tiny needles are placed in specific spots to relieve tension and stress. Acupuncture has shown specific benefit in treating peripheral diabetic neuropathy.[8]

**Hypnosis.** Hypnosis for pain relief works best on adults who are willing and motivated participants in their own therapy. It must be performed by a qualified professional.

**Relaxation and visualization techniques.** These exercises range from deep breathing to imaginary "escapes" from pain. Classes are available through local hospitals and yoga centers to help people learn how to control their pain in this way.

# NUTRITIONAL OPTIONS FOR NEUROPATHY

If the cause of neuropathy is known and treatable, then managing the underlying condition is the best option. In many neuropathies, however, no specific cause will ever be identified. In addition, many of the causes of neuropathies are themselves not readily treatable. A number of supplements have been shown to interfere with the underlying mechanisms of a variety of forms of neuropathy.

## Acetyl-L-Carnitine

Acetyl-L-carnitine is known to have neuroprotective properties. Two studies found that acetyl-L-carnitine can limit neuropathy associated with some chemotherapy drugs.[9,10]

It has also been shown to limit neuropathy associated with diabetes. In 2 randomized, placebo-controlled clinical trials, acetyl-L-carnitine, in daily doses of 500 mg and 1000 mg, was shown to yield significant reductions in pain.[11]

In 2 related studies of diabetic nerve degeneration and neuropathy, acetyl-L-carnitine accelerated nerve regeneration after experimental injury. In the first study, diabetic animals treated with acetyl-L-carnitine maintained near normal nerve conduction velocity without any adverse effects to glucose, insulin, or free fatty acid levels, suggesting that acetyl-L-carnitine can hasten nerve regeneration in the context of diabetes.[12] In another study, carnitine was shown to correct a number of nerve dysfunctions in animals with chemically induced diabetes.[13]

In a human trial, acetyl-L-carnitine appeared to help prevent or slow cardiac autonomic neuropathy in people with diabetes.[14] In a large, multicenter human trial, L-carnitine improved nerve conduction velocity and reduced pain associated with diabetic neuropathy over a 1-year period.[15]

## Lipoic Acid

As a powerful antioxidant, lipoic acid positively affects important aspects of diabetes, including prevention, blood sugar control, and the development of long-term complications such as disease of the heart, kidneys, and small blood vessels.[16–23] It has also been shown to reduce pain associated with diabetic neuropathy.[24] Studies include the following:

- Clinical trials of diabetics with symptoms caused by nerve damage affecting the heart showed significant improvement taking 800 mg oral alpha-lipoic acid daily without significant side effects.[25,26]

- In another study, 23 diabetic patients were treated with 600 mg alpha-lipoic acid, delivered intravenously daily for 10 days, followed by 600 mg oral alpha-lipoic acid for 60 days. At the end of the study, all participants showed significant improvements in cranial neuropathy, as well as improvements in both peripheral and autonomic neuropathy, which affects internal organs.[27]

- In another study, 26 patients with type 2 diabetes were given 600 mg alpha-lipoic acid daily for 3 months. At the end of the study, 20 patients experienced a significant regression of neuropathic symptoms, while 5 patients experienced a complete cessation of all symptoms. Alpha-lipoic acid was especially beneficial in women as well as thinner and younger patients.[28]

## N-Acetylcysteine

N-acetylcysteine (NAC) is a powerful antioxidant and a precursor to glutathione, an intrinsic antioxidant. Animal studies have shown that NAC can inhibit diabetic neuropathy and protect against neuropathies caused by chemotherapy drugs.[29,30]

## Curcumin

Researchers are continuing to discover the benefits of curcumin, which is the yellow pigment that gives turmeric its distinctive golden hue. In a study of inherited peripheral neuropathies, curcumin was shown to relieve neuropathy by causing the release of disease-associated proteins that are produced by a mutated gene.[31] Curcumin has also shown promise in animal studies of diabetic neuropathy and as a neuroprotective agent in central nervous system diseases.[2]

## Omega-6 Fatty Acids

The body ordinarily makes the gamma linolenic acid (GLA) it needs from linoleic acid, an omega-6 fatty acid found in foods. Among diabetics, however, the body is not able to make sufficient GLA, and it must be supplemented.[32–34]

GLA improves diabetic neuropathy if given long enough to work. In one double-blind, placebo-controlled study, 111 people with mild diabetic neuropathy received either 480 mg GLA daily or placebo.[35] After 12 months, the group taking GLA was doing significantly better than the placebo group. Good results were seen in 2 smaller studies as well.[36,37]

## Omega-3 Fatty Acids

Omega-3 fatty acids are found in high quantities in cold water fish (eg, salmon) and are widely consumed for their anti-inflammatory properties. Omega-3s are essential fatty acids and are important components of cell membranes, including the delicate myelin sheath that protects nerves. Studies have shown that omega-3 fatty acids, including eicosapentaenoic acid (EPA) and docosahexaenoic acid (DHA), are able to reduce demyelination in the nerves of diabetic animals, which reduces neuropathic pain.[38]

## Vitamin B1 and Benfotiamine

Some animal studies have shown a decrease in pain with the combination of vitamins B1 (thiamin), B6, and B12.[39-41] The fat-soluble form of vitamin B1, called benfotiamine, has been used effectively to treat alcoholic and diabetic neuropathies. The most marked pain relief from benfotiamine occurred in patients with diabetic neuropathy after only a 3-week trial period.[42-44]

### Vitamin B6

Vitamin B6 (pyridoxine) inhibits glycosylation of proteins,[45] one of the major risk factors for developing diabetic neuropathy. Diabetes patients with neuropathy have been shown to be deficient in vitamin B6 and benefit from supplementation.[46] Interestingly, neuropathy caused by vitamin B6 deficiency is indistinguishable from diabetic neuropathy.

### Vitamin B12

Neuropathy caused by vitamin B12 (cobalamin) deficiency is characterized by numbness of the feet, pins-and-needles sensations, or a burning feeling.[47,48] Supplementation that restores normal B12 levels is part of a successful treatment for diabetic neuropathy.[49] In a review of clinical trials conducted between 1954 and 2004, vitamin B12, as well as combination therapy of vitamin B12 and methylcobalamin, was shown to reduce pain.[50]

The most common forms of supplemental B12 are cyanocobalamin or hydroxycobalamin. The natural form of B12 found in food is methylcobalamin (or a similar form, adenosylcobalamin). The structure of B12 is very complex, with numerous methyl groups attached. Methyl groups ($CH_3$) are used in beneficial methylation reactions, such as those that reduce homocysteine. Methylcobalamin appears to be the most effective form to protect the nerves.

### Vitamin C

Insulin facilitates the transport of vitamin C into cells, decreasing capillary permeability and improving wound healing. Diabetes depletes intracellular vitamin C, which deprives a diabetic of vitamin C's cellular protection.[51] Vitamin C levels have been shown to be reduced in diabetic patients.[52]

### Capsaicin

Derived from hot peppers, capsaicin has been shown to reduce chronic pain by reducing the stimulation of pain receptors. It is often applied as a cream. Initially, capsaicin may cause a prickly, hot sensation that results in many people discontinuing use. However, once this first phase passes, capsaicin is effective. It has been documented to reduce the pain associated with

diabetic neuropathy without adversely affecting glucose control.[24]

### Vitamin E

Vitamin E is a powerful antioxidant that reduces levels of free radicals and oxidative stress. In a placebo-controlled, double-blind, randomized study of 21 patients with type 2 diabetes, large doses of vitamin E were studied for their ability to reduce neuropathy. During the 6-month study, patients were given either 900 mg vitamin E or placebo, and then measured for nerve conduction and function. Researchers found that mild to moderate defective nerve conduction was improved with high-dose vitamin E, which suggested patients with neuropathy might experience a reduction in symptoms.[53]

These results appear to not be limited to diabetic neuropathy. In a case study of a 24-year-old man with a progressive disease and peripheral neuropathy, daily supplementation with high-dose vitamin E for 2 years slowed disease progression and produced significant improvement in his neuropathy.[54]

---

### FOR MORE INFORMATION

Additional protocols that might be of interest include:

- Diabetes
- Pain (Chronic)

---

### SUMMARY

Whether or not the cause of neuropathy is known, it can be a debilitating condition that seriously impacts quality of life. If the cause is known, the first strategy should be to address the underlying condition. If neuropathy is caused by alcohol, cocaine, medication, or environmental toxins, exposure to those agents should be limited if possible. Do not discontinue prescription medications without permission from your physician, but inquire whether it may be possible to find a substitute therapy for a neuropathy-causing drug. In the event that neuropathy is caused by heavy metals (eg, mercury or lead), chelation therapy may be useful. In addition, administration of Cytomel, a synthetic thyroid hormone, may boost peripheral nerve regeneration. Before taking Cytomel, have your thyroid hormone levels tested.

Because diabetes is a common cause of peripheral neuropathy, diabetics are strongly encouraged to read the Diabetes protocol. Strict glucose control is very important, and diabetics must be aware that any substance ingested may affect their blood sugar levels. An aggressive program of dietary supplementation should not be launched without the supervision of a qualified physician.

## Life Extension Suggestions

- **Fat-soluble vitamin B1 (benfotiamine):** 250–1000 mg daily
- **Acetyl-L-carnitine:** 1000–2000 mg daily
- **R-lipoic acid:** 240–480 mg daily
  OR
  **Alpha-lipoic acid:** 500–1000 mg daily
- **NAC:** 600–1800 mg daily
- **Curcumin** (as highly absorbed BCM-95®): 400–800 mg daily

- **Gamma linolenic acid (GLA):** 299–1495 mg daily
- **Fish oil** (with olive polyphenols): 4000 mg daily, providing at least 1400 mg EPA and 1000 mg DHA
- **Vitamin B6** (as pyridoxal-5'-phosphate): 100–200 mg daily
- **Vitamin B12 (methylcobalamin):** 1–2 mg daily
- **Vitamin C:** about 2000–4000 mg daily
- **Vitamin E:** 400 IU daily (with around 200 mg gamma tocopherol)

## REFERENCES

References available at: www.lef.org/dpt5/ch99

# 100

# Non-Alcoholic Fatty Liver Disease (NAFLD)

Roughly one-third of the American population suffers from *nonalcoholic fatty liver disease* or NAFLD.[1-3] Many of its victims do not know they have it. NAFLD can go undetected for years and may eventually progress to inflammation and scarring of the liver (cirrhosis) and, in some cases, full-blown liver failure.

A formerly rare condition, its rapid emergence has been linked to skyrocketing rates of metabolic syndrome and "diabesity," the term that many experts use for co-occurring diabetes and obesity.[3-5]

While poor dietary choices are often to blame, cutting-edge research suggests that hidden genetic factors may also play a role, as some people do not metabolize polyunsaturated fats properly, resulting in fatty deposits in the liver.[6]

As mainstream medicine continues to struggle in the search for drugs to manage this widespread condition, emerging scientific evidence has shed light on effective natural interventions that may halt or even *reverse* its progress.

## FAT OVERLOAD, LIVER DAMAGE, AND THE INFLAMMATORY STORM

NAFLD is defined as deposition of fat in the liver cells of patients with minimal or no alcohol intake and with no other known cause.[7] The term "NAFLD" refers to a group of related and progressive conditions closely associated with overweight and obesity.[2]

NAFLD starts off as a low-level disturbance characterized by dull right upper-quadrant abdominal discomfort and fatigue in most patients, but it is hardly benign.[8] Early NAFLD can ultimately progress to a more serious condition, *nonalcoholic steatohepatitis* or NASH.[9] About a third of people with NAFLD will develop NASH,[8] and about 20% of people with NASH will go on to liver fibrosis and cirrhosis, with its accompanying risk of liver failure and even liver cancer.[2,8,10] Overall, people with NAFLD stand a 12% increased risk of liver-related death over 10 years.[8]

NAFLD has multiple interrelated causes. Primary mechanisms include obesity leading to steadily increasing insulin resistance coupled with an overabundance of circulating fatty acids. These factors fuel one another in a destructive cycle.[4] Together with advanced glycation end-products (AGEs), these events lead to increased oxidant stress and ultimately inflammation, cell death, and fibrous destruction of liver tissue.[3,4,8]

An overload of fatty acids and abnormal lipid profiles factor so heavily in the onset of NAFLD that they're now referred to as "lipotoxicity" because of the ways they directly poison liver tissue.[9,11,12] And as fat builds inside liver cells, they begin churning out a storm of fat-related cytokines known as *adipokines*, which fan the inflammatory flames of the metabolic syndrome and NAFLD.[1]

Of course, what we eat is as important as the calories it contains. One of the major bad actors in today's world is fructose, found in high quantities in high-fructose corn syrup.[13] Fructose promotes formation of new fat molecules in the liver, blocks breakdown of existing fats, stimulates free radical production, and promotes insulin resistance.[14] An increasing number of studies are linking increased fructose consumption with NAFLD, and even with its deadlier consequence, nonalcoholic steatohepatitis (NASH).[15] Patients with NAFLD consume 2–3 times as much fructose as do control patients, even corrected for body weight.[16]

## DIAGNOSIS OF NAFLD

In order to make a diagnosis of NAFLD, a physician considers both clinical data about the patient, and, when appropriate, data from a liver biopsy (for definitive diagnosis). The first indication that NAFLD might be present is rarely a symptom, but rather a finding of elevated levels of liver enzymes in the blood, indicating early liver cell damage. Other treatable causes of liver disease must be ruled out by appropriate testing (eg, hepatitis B or C), and other liver functional parameters (eg, blood clotting factors) should also be measured. Some physicians will do an imaging study such as a liver ultrasound, but normal appearance of the liver does not rule out NAFLD. Alcoholic fatty liver, which can closely resemble NAFLD, must be ruled out. This can be done by reliably establishing the absence of substantial alcohol intake (less than 20–40 g of alcohol per day, equivalent to 2–3 drinks). If and when there is concern that the more dangerous condition, NASH, is present, then liver biopsy must be performed to establish a definitive diagnosis.[17]

## TREATMENT OF NAFLD

Despite a growing understanding of the pathology of NAFLD, scientists have been persistently baffled in their attempts to prevent and treat it with drug therapies. Lifestyle interventions such as steady, gentle weight loss and regular exercise have been the only interventions that offered any hope at all.[2,9] Insulin-sensitizing drugs, while theoretically of value, have proved disappointing in clinical trials.[18,19]

The only successful *pharmaceutical* intervention for dealing with NAFLD has been metformin, which will be examined below.

Cholesterol-lowering drugs like statins have no proven benefit to date.[4] Further studies are needed to determine whether bariatric surgery to induce weight loss benefits patients with NAFLD.[9,20]

---

### WHAT YOU HAVE LEARNED SO FAR

- One in three Americans now suffers from the stealth condition known as nonalcoholic fatty liver disease or NAFLD.
- NAFLD may go undetected for years, and may progress to liver inflammation and scarring (cirrhosis) or full-blown liver failure.
- While chiefly driven by poor dietary choices linked to metabolic syndrome and "diabesity," genetic factors can also play a role in NAFLD's progress.
- Medical science has proved relatively helpless at preventing or treating NAFLD and NASH, leaving millions of Americans vulnerable to their effects.

---

## NUTRITIONAL AND SUPPLEMENTAL SUPPORT

In contrast to the failure of most pharmacologic therapies, numerous nutritional approaches show real promise in slowing the development and progression of NAFLD. In particular, Life Extension has identified 8 interventions with scientifically validated effectiveness.

**Vitamin E.** Scientists began a series of studies on NASH (the advanced middle stage of NAFLD) and vitamin E in 2004. Based on their knowledge that NASH arises from persistent insulin resistance and oxidative stress, they examined the effects of pioglitazone (Actos®), an insulin-sensitizing drug, and vitamin E. Patients receiving both vitamin E (400 IU per day) and pioglitazone (30 mg per day) had improvements in more parameters than did patients on vitamin E alone.[21]

In a follow-up study, subjects received either vitamin E (800 IU per day) or pioglitazone (30 mg per day), or placebo, for 96 weeks.

Both treatments improved levels of liver cell-injury markers in blood, and both reduced liver fat levels and inflammation. But only vitamin E produced significant improvements in the appearance of liver tissue on biopsies.[22] Here are some clues that explain these otherwise startling results.

Vitamin E is a powerful antioxidant, and an obvious choice once the role of oxidant stress was made clear in NAFLD.[23] People with fatty liver disease and NASH have depressed levels of vitamin E in their blood, the result of increased oxidation.[24,25] Even relatively low-dose vitamin E (450 IU/day) can reduce circulating liver enzymes, a chemical marker of liver cell injury.[26,27]

Important animal studies refine our understanding of how vitamin E works. One study provided the first evidence that vitamin E can prevent NAFLD before it develops, largely by reducing oxidative stress, inflammation, and liver cell death by apoptosis.[28] Another study demonstrated a vitamin E-related reduction in oxidative damage and tissue levels of the inflammatory mediator TNF-α, while beneficially reducing PPAR-gamma activity.[29] This wealth of animal and now human data clearly supports daily use of 800–1200 IU of vitamin E for prevention and treatment of NAFLD and NASH.

**Omega-3 Fatty Acids.** Just as vitamin E fights the oxidant and inflammatory components of NAFLD, the omega-3 fatty acids attack the problem of lipotoxicity, while contributing considerable anti-inflammatory activity of their own.[12] People and experimental animals with insufficient omega-3 in their diets are prone to NAFLD and type 2 diabetes, suggesting that supplementation might reverse (or prevent) the process.[12,30–32]

Increasing the amount of unsaturated fats like omega-3s in cell membranes is associated with improved insulin sensitivity.[33] And supplementation with omega-3–rich fish oil results in activation of the important metabolic sensor, called PPAR-alpha, in liver cells, suppressing production of new fat molecules.[34] Omega-3s also contribute to improved insulin sensitivity, a reduction in serum triglycerides, and stimulation of fat utilization in liver tissue and skeletal muscle.[35]

A long-term human trial, using 1000 mg per day of omega-3, revealed significant decreases in serum markers of liver cell damage, triglyceride levels, and fasting glucose. Most impressively, supplemented patients display improvement of their liver's appearance and blood flow on ultrasound exams, providing graphic evidence of supplement benefits.[36] Another study found that supplementation with 751 mg eicosapentaenoic acid (EPA) and 527 mg docosahexaenoic acid (DHA)

3 times daily for 24 weeks decreased triglyceride levels in individuals with NAFLD.[37] Olive oil also decreases accumulation of triglycerides in the liver during NAFLD, but fish oil provided better antioxidant activity.[38] Olive oil also independently improves postprandial triglyceride levels in blood and upregulates glucose transport in the liver. At the same time, it improves insulin resistance by decreasing liver inflammation.[39] And long-term consumption of olive oil enriched with omega-3 fats in patients with NAFLD is able to improve liver texture on ultrasound exams, while improving serum markers of liver injury and increasing protective adiponectin levels.[40]

Clearly the omega-3 fatty acids have earned their designation as an innovative therapy for nonalcoholic fatty liver disease.[41]

**Metformin.** Because of the central role of insulin resistance in the development of NAFLD and NASH, it makes sense to evaluate insulin-sensitizing drugs for their prevention.[42,43] No oral antidiabetic drug has as broad a spectrum of action, and as hefty a safety record, as the drug metformin, which is finding a host of new applications outside of diabetes itself.[44,45]

Studies of metformin for NAFLD and NASH have multiplied in the past few years. Metformin, 500 mg 3 times daily for 6 months, produced dramatic improvements in liver blood flow and velocity as detected by Doppler ultrasound exams.[46] A similar dose of metformin (20 mg/kg body weight for 1 year, or approximately 1450 mg/day for a 160-pound person) produced reductions in blood markers of liver cell death.[47] On the other hand, improved insulin sensitivity has repeatedly been shown in patients with NASH and NAFLD who take metformin, and many studies have now shown sustainable improvements in liver chemistry measurements.[42,48] And a recent study showed significant reduction in the prevalence and severity of fatty liver after 6 months' treatment with 850 mg metformin twice daily in obese adolescents.[49]

Metformin is an ideal drug for combination studies because of its safety and compatibility with other therapies. The combination of metformin with the potent antioxidant N-acetyl cysteine (NAC) for 12 months improved liver chemistry results, measurements of insulin resistance, and liver appearance on biopsy.[50]

Recent evidence shows that metformin blocks the induction of cellular stress proteins in cultured liver cells, protecting them from death induced by fatty acids.[51] This novel mechanism adds to metformin's already impressive array of multitargeted effects on metabolism and fatty liver disease.

**S-Adenosylmethionine (SAMe).** Their constant exposure to oxidant and toxic stresses makes liver cells especially vulnerable to depletion of *glutathione* (GSH), a natural antioxidant that participates in many liver detoxification reactions.[52,53] The nutrient SAMe can replenish GSH levels and restore liver cell protection to normal.[54] In individuals with alcoholic or nonalcoholic liver disease, supplementation with 1200 mg SAMe daily increased liver glutathione levels.[55] Studies using agents that increase SAMe levels are known to reduce severity of NAFLD.[52,56]

SAMe and other liver antioxidants improve levels of liver enzymes, an early marker of cell damage.[57] SAMe supplements improve microscopic features of NAFLD associated with fatty degeneration, inflammation, and tissue death. And SAMe also downregulated damaging proinflammatory genes in an animal model of NAFLD.[54]

A major discovery about SAMe is that it directly stops progression of relatively mild NAFLD to dangerous NASH. NASH develops as the result of "second hits," that is, additional events that damage liver cells after NAFLD has already developed; one of those "hits" is steady depletion of SAMe.[58] This has led to interest in using SAMe to prevent NASH from developing in people who already have NAFLD.[59]

**N-Acetyl Cysteine (NAC).** Another molecule that supports and replenishes the natural antioxidant glutathione is N-acetyl cysteine (NAC), a versatile sulfur-rich compound that prevents liver damage following acetaminophen poisoning.[60] It rapidly restores depleted glutathione levels, sparing liver cells from the effects of oxidant damage.[61-63]

An NAC derivative, called SNAC, was recently shown to prevent onset of NAFLD in rats fed a liver disease-inducing diet.[64] In humans, the combination of NAC (1200 mg/day) with metformin (850–1000 mg/day) improved liver appearance and reduced fibrosis in patients with NAFLD.[50] And, given to rats with NAFLD, NAC stimulates regeneration of healthy liver cells in animals that have part of the liver removed.[65]

**Silymarin (Milk Thistle).** Extracts of milk thistle have long been used for liver protection. Silymarin is composed of 6 major active molecules such as silybin, which are known as flavolignans, having exceptional antioxidant and anti-inflammatory activity.[66,67]

One very effective combination is silymarin plus vitamin E and phospholipids (such as phosphatidylcholine); this approach improves the overall antioxidant activity of the compound.[68] In animal studies the combination limited liver depletion of the natural antioxidant glutathione, and reduced mitochondrial stress damage.[69] Human trials have shown that a preparation providing 376 mg silybin, 776 mg phosphatidylcholine, and 360 mg vitamin E produces therapeutic effects in patients with a variety of different forms of liver damage, improving insulin resistance, reducing liver fat accumulation, and reducing blood levels of markers of liver scarring.[70–72]

**Phosphatidylcholine and PPC**. Phospholipids—fat molecules with phosphate groups attached—are major constituents of cell membranes in mammals. One of the most important phospholipids in humans is *phosphatidylcholine* (PC). Higher amounts of PC in cell membranes help to assure membrane integrity in the face of oxidative and other stresses; they also help limit the progression of NAFLD into NASH.[73]

A particularly rich source of PC molecules is a mixture called *polyenylphosphatidylcholine* (PPC), derived from soybeans.[74] PPC supplements in animals attenuate nonalcoholic liver fibrosis and even accelerate its regression.[75] PPC appears to exert this effect in part by blocking oxidant damage to cell membranes.[76–78] A separate mechanism is reduction in the high cholesterol levels that precede NAFLD formation.[79] PPC also prevents proliferation of scar tissue in NAFLD and other forms of liver toxicity.[80] And PPC restores liver cell levels of SAMe, providing additional liver protection.[81]

**Resveratrol**. Resveratrol protects liver tissue against the ravages of alcoholic fatty liver disease through its antioxidant effects, buffering the impact of alcohol.[82] It also activates 2 critical signaling molecules, SIRT1 and AMPK, which are inhibited by alcohol, and are also dysfunctional in metabolic syndrome.[83–86] Those effects make it highly promising for prevention of NAFLD, the liver manifestation of metabolic syndrome. In animal studies, resveratrol activates AMPK, which in turn reduces liver fat accumulation, suppresses new liver fat formation, and reduces insulin resistance.[87–89]

## Life Extension Suggestions

NAFLD and NASH are progressive conditions that require patient collaboration with a qualified physician. Because the liver metabolizes many nutrients and drugs, it is important that liver patients not add any substances to their regimen without cooperation and close monitoring by a qualified physician. The goals of therapy are:

- Reduce the accumulation of fat in liver tissue by decreasing new fat synthesis and increasing utilization of existing fat stores in the liver.
- Minimize free radical production, and enhance free radical scavenging in liver tissue.
- Reduce or eliminate the inflammatory responses of fat-infiltrated liver tissue to prevent progression of NAFLD to the more deadly NASH, which is a precursor of liver failure.

The following have been shown to boost liver health and help manage NAFLD:

- **Vitamin E:** 800 IU daily includes at least 200 mg gamma tocopherol
- **Omega-3 fatty acids:** 700 mg EPA and 500 mg DHA daily
- **Metformin:** 500 mg 3 times daily
- **S-adenosylmethionine (SAMe):** 1200 mg daily
- **N-acetyl cysteine (NAC):** 1200 mg daily
- **Silymarin** (milk thistle extract): 900 mg daily
- **Polyenylphosphatidylcholine (PPC):** 900 mg daily
- *Trans*-**resveratrol:** 500 mg daily

In addition, the following blood testing resources may be helpful:

- Chemistry Panel and Complete Blood Count (CBC)
- Hemoglobin A1C (HbA1C)
- Insulin (Fasting)
- Omega Score®

## REFERENCES

References available at: www.lef.org/dpt5/ch100

# 101

---

# *Obesity and Weight Loss*

---

A startling 60–75% of the adult population in the United States is overweight or obese.[1] Around the world, the prevalence of obesity has nearly *doubled* from 1980 to 2008.[2]

Being overweight or obese significantly increases the risk of multiple *debilitating diseases* including cardiovascular disease, arthritis, high blood pressure, and malignancies such as breast, prostate, pancreatic and colon cancer.[3-6] Excess body weight also affects mobility, interferes with restful sleep, contributes to digestive disorders, and can contribute to an overall lower quality of life than that enjoyed by lean individuals.[7-10] Obesity results in shortening of the life span by an average of *8–10 years* compared with people at normal weight. For every *33 extra lb*, risk of early death increases by around 30%.[11]

For many aging obese individuals, the struggle to achieve a healthy body weight becomes a veritable battle against biology as a number of metabolic processes promote weight gain despite genuine efforts to decrease food consumption and increase energy expenditure.[12-14]

Scientific investigations have shed light on the biology of weight loss in recent times. It turns out the battle against the bulge is much more complex than the overly simplistic "eat less food to lose weight" message often promoted by government health agencies.

In 2009, Life Extension described the *Nine Pillars of Successful Weight Loss*. Each of the nine pillars represents a fundamental insight into sustainable weight. If any weight loss strategy is to be successful, it must evolve beyond the conventional cliché that weight loss only requires a reduction in food consumption. Instead, successful weight management requires a paradigm that acknowledges the multifactorial nature of obesity.

The *Nine Pillars of Successful Weight Loss* that should not be overlooked if healthy weight management is to be achieved are:

1. *Restore insulin sensitivity*
2. *Restore youthful hormone balance*
3. *Control rate of carbohydrate absorption*
4. *Increase physical activity*
5. *Restore brain serotonin/suppress hunger signals*
6. *Restore resting energy expenditure rate*
7. *Restore healthy adipocyte (fat cell) signaling*
8. *Inhibit the lipase enzyme*
9. *Eat to live a long and healthy life*

This protocol will detail the biological underpinnings of obesity and weight gain. Consideration will be given to each *pillar of successful weight loss* in the context of obesity risk factors in order to highlight the inadequacies of typical weight loss strategies. Methods of utilizing novel natural compounds and strategically incorporating some pharmaceutical options to support critical metabolic factors for long-term weight management will be discussed.

## REGULATION OF BODY WEIGHT

Our system of energy balance evolved to ensure that a healthy person maintained adequate reserves of body fat to sustain life through repeated times of food scarcity, including famine. Food energy abundance is a relatively recent phenomenon, quite dissimilar to the vast majority of time over the past 100000 years. In fact, body weight maintenance is achieved by the very complex and interrelated interaction of neurologic and hormonal factors, with the goal of increasing appetite and preserving body fat when energy stores are low. Within the brain, a region called the *hypothalamus* monitors and integrates neurologic signals and modulates appetite accordingly. Sensory cells located within the stomach walls that detect stretching of stomach tissue can directly signal satiety to the brain through nerve impulses. Indirectly, blood levels of glucose, fatty acids, and amino acids (components of proteins) stimulate the perception of satiety in brain centers and depress eating behavior. Additionally, a variety of hormones released at various levels of the gastrointestinal tract perform numerous functions in the balance of energy intake and utilization. *Insulin* (released from the pancreas and critical for the uptake of glucose into cells) and *cholecystokinin (CCK)* (secreted by the upper part of the small intestine and important for triggering release of digestive enzymes and bile) are also potent satiety signals.[15]

In addition, *fat stores* in the body are able to relay the overall state of energy storage to the brain through the secretion of the hormone *leptin*.[15] Leptin is secreted into the blood by adipose (fat) cells in proportion to their levels of stored fats. It travels to the brain and acts on the hypothalamus, stimulating the release of neurotransmitters that signal satiety, and suppressing those that signal hunger. Thus, leptin released by adipose tissue provides the brain with information on long-term energy economy, and allows it to adjust food intake accordingly.[16] However, this intricate system of appetite control can become perturbed in obesity, as excess fat stores contribute to chronically elevated leptin levels. This leads to down regulation of cellular sensitivity to the effects of leptin, a physiologic state known as *leptin resistance*. Weight loss efforts put forth by obese individuals may be undermined by failure of the leptin system to suppress their appetite, resulting in excessive hunger.[17]

Another hormone derived from fat cells, called *adiponectin*, is an *antiobesity* signaling molecule; adiponectin signaling is disrupted in obesity-related diseases and states of insulin resistance.[18] Evidence suggests that leptin and adiponectin can work together to combat insulin resistance.[19–21] *Optimizing fat cell signaling* thus represents an important aspect of any comprehensive weight-loss strategy.

*Resting energy expenditure* (REE) also influences weight gain and progression to obesity. REE is the rate at which metabolic activity burns calories during periods of rest or inactivity. Having a low REE may contribute to weight gain or make it difficult to lose weight. Studies show that REE is directly related to serum adiponectin levels, and higher leptin levels (as occurs in leptin resistance) are associated with decreased REE.[22] Aging is also associated with decreased REE.[23,24] These findings suggest that boosting REE could be a valuable strategy to mitigate age-related weight gain.

# CAUSES AND RISK FACTORS FOR OBESITY

Weight gain and progression to obesity can be caused by energy imbalances.[25]

Aging can negatively affect the balance of energy input and expenditure in several ways. The natural aging process is associated with hormonal changes, particularly *decreases in sex and thyroid hormones*, which contribute to a decrease in metabolism and energy expenditure. Advancing age is also associated with reduced insulin sensitivity, which may interfere with appetite control.[16,26] With age also comes a decrease in physical activity, which further reduces energy expenditure. Only about a quarter of Americans aged 65 to 74 exercise daily; this drops to less than 1 in 10 at age 85.[27] Obesity and decreased mobility in the aging individual may have reciprocal effects on one another; age-related increases in weight and reductions in muscle mass lead to decreased mobility and energy expenditure. In a review of 28 population studies of older obese individuals, all but one showed significant associations between obesity and reduced mobility.[28]

## Sex Hormone and Thyroid Hormone Insufficiencies/Imbalances

Levels of sex hormones (such as testosterone and dehydroepiandrosterone [DHEA]) decline with age in both genders. This may lead to an increase in fat mass, reduction in lean body mass, or central fat redistribution.[29,30] Similarly, declining *thyroid hormone levels* are associated with reduced metabolic rate, and thus obesity.[14]

In men, free testosterone levels sharply decline between the ages of 40 and 80. Both free and total testosterone levels are significantly lower in overweight and obese men compared to those with weights in a normal range across all ages.[31] Men with low testosterone levels (hypogonadism) develop increased fat mass, and testosterone replacement therapy in hypogonadal men reduced fat mass by 6% in one study.[32,33]

Obesity and low testosterone have a complex relationship; low testosterone can be considered both a cause *and* consequence of obesity.[31] In men, increases in fat mass may also increase the *conversion* of testosterone to *estrogen* by the enzyme *aromatase*.[34] While this conversion is a normal phenomenon, aromatization occurs more readily in fat tissue, and is increased by obesity, age, inflammation, insulin, leptin, and stress.[35] Thus, in older men with excessive abdominal fat, the ratios of testosterone to estrogen are lower than in younger men. Elevated estrogens, similar to low testosterone levels, are associated with increased abdominal fat.[34] If a blood test reveals elevated estrogen (estradiol) levels in a man, a physician may prescribe an *aromatase-inhibiting drug* such as anastrozole (Arimidex®).

In women, estrogen levels decline suddenly with menopause. Hormone replacement has shown modest increases in lean body mass and reductions in waist circumference and abdominal fat in some, but not all studies of postmenopausal women.[36–38]

The thyroid is a central regulator of metabolism; it integrates signals from the brain and secretes thyroid hormone (thyroxine or T4) to influence metabolism in a variety of tissues.[14] Thyroid dysfunction can affect body weight and composition, body temperature, and energy expenditure independent of physical activity. Depressed thyroid function (hypothyroidism) has been associated with decreased thermogenesis (conversion of stored energy into heat) and metabolic rate, as well as weight gain.[14]

Clinical studies have shown that treatment of hypothyroidism with thyroxine may lead to weight loss, and population studies suggest that low T4 levels and high TSH levels are both associated with higher body mass index (BMI).[39] Depressed thyroid activity is also more common as people age; hypothyroidism in the general population is 3.7%, but is 5 times more common in individuals aged 80 or older when compared to 12 to 49 year-olds.[40]

A significant number of patients with morbid obesity display elevated *thyroid-stimulating hormone* (TSH) levels. TSH is produced in the brain by the pituitary gland, then travels to the thyroid and stimulates the production of thyroid hormone. Increased blood levels of TSH may indicate thyroid dysfunction and are associated with the progression of obesity.[41] For example, in one Norwegian study of over 27 000 individuals older than 40, TSH correlated with BMI: for every unit that TSH increased, BMI increased by 0.41 in women and 0.48 in men.[39]

## Insulin Resistance and/or Leptin Resistance

In addition to being a result of obesity, elevated levels of the hormones leptin and insulin in obese individuals may be indicative of a *resistance* to their activities. Insulin is a hormone that helps facilitate cellular uptake of glucose, primarily in the muscles, liver, and adipose tissue. When insulin resistance develops, glucose levels are no longer efficiently controlled by the action of insulin and blood levels become elevated, predisposing the insulin-resistant individual to several chronic diseases associated with aging.[42] Moreover, while higher levels of both leptin and insulin normally suppress the desire to eat and stimulate energy expenditure, they are unable to perform this function in resistant individuals.[43]

- *Insulin resistance* is a consequence of sustained hyperinsulinemia (high insulin levels) and is complicated by chronic inflammation and obesity.[8,44,45] Strategies aimed at *improving insulin sensitivity* are an integral part of the *nine pillars of successful weight loss*. These strategies can include use of a low-cost prescription drug called *metformin*, which is approved for the treatment of type 2 diabetes and can also help reduce body fat, and natural compounds that help promote healthy insulin signaling.[46,47]

- Similarly, *leptin resistance* results from sustained periods of high leptin secretion associated with high fat stores. In obese individuals, leptin may lose its ability to be transported into the brain.[48] An interaction between leptin and the inflammatory biomarker *C-reactive protein* (CRP) in cell culture suggests a role of chronic inflammation in leptin resistance and the loss of appetite control. In an animal model of

obesity, infusions of CRP countered the appetite-suppressing effects of leptin. The scientists who conducted these experiments postulated that CRP may bind to leptin and inhibit its physiologic functions.[49] Based on these findings, interventions that ease inflammation, such as the plant compound *curcumin* and *omega-3 fatty acids* from fish oil, may help combat the detrimental effects of leptin resistance.[50–53] In addition, the mango-like fruit of *Irvingia gabonensis*, a tree found in Africa, has also been shown to combat leptin resistance and lower CRP levels.[54,55]

## Overeating and Dining Out

Increases in daily average food consumption significantly contribute to weight gain in the United States.[56] Data from the National Health and Nutrition Examination Survey (NHANES) show a significant increase in average daily energy intake between 1971 and 2000, amounting to 168 calories per day for men and 335 calories per day for women. Without increased expenditure, this represents potential theoretical weight gains of 18 lb per year for men and 35 lb per year for women.[25] A separate study estimates a 350-calorie-per-day increase for children (about one can of soda and a small order of French fries) and a 500-calorie-per-day increase for adults (about one large hamburger) over our daily calorie intake in the 1970s.[56]

Eating outside the home can encourage overconsumption, especially of calorie-dense, nutrient-poor foods. Spending on food away from home has almost doubled in the last half century, rising to almost one-third of a person's calories in the United States.[12] Half of Americans eat out 2 or more times per week, and 20% of males and 10% of females eat commercially prepared foods 6 or more times per week.[57]

People have a decreased ability to make healthy food choices away from home for several reasons. They tend to increase their consumption proportional to the amount of food they are served, and average portion sizes have been steadily increasing over the last 30 years.[58,59] Choices for foods consumed away from home are also influenced by marketing and the relative abundance of high-calorie, low-nutrient choices compared to healthier ones. Fast food restaurants may also play into inherent weaknesses in human cognitive capacity. Reasoned decisions are time-consuming; therefore, people often depend on automatic choices when they are hungry. When glucose levels are low, or a person is distracted or preoccupied, they tend to make less healthy food choices and are often unaware of the quality of food they have consumed. Although attempts have been made to provide point-of-sale nutritional labeling in many restaurants, there has been limited evidence of effect.[12]

In an effort to avoid the caloric excess to which so many restaurant-goers succumb, suppression of *hunger signals* is likely to be of great benefit. To this end, several natural compounds, including *saffron extract*, *L-tryptophan*, and *pine nut oil*, as well as the pharmaceutical drug *lorcaserin (Belviq®)* may be of benefit; each of these compounds is discussed in detail later in this protocol.

Another strategy to counter the excessive amount of calories encountered when dining out involves "*preparing your body to eat*" by taking measures to reduce the rate at which fats and carbohydrates are *absorbed*. Supplementing with *green coffee extract* before meals can slow carbohydrate absorption, helping to *reduce after-meal spikes in glucose levels*.[60] These after-meal glucose spikes inflict damage to cells via multiple mechanisms and have been linked to cardiovascular disease, cancer, Alzheimer's disease, and kidney failure. Also, a pharmaceutical drug called *orlistat* (Alli®, Xenical®) can help *reduce the absorption of fats* by inhibiting an enzyme called *lipase*.[61,62] Targeting after-meal spikes in blood levels of glucose (postprandial glycemia) and fatty acids (postprandial lipemia) is a critical step toward averting cardiovascular disease, for which obesity is a leading risk factor.[63-66]

### Altered Serotonin Signaling, Chronic Stress, and Appetite

Low levels of the neurotransmitter serotonin, typically associated with depression, may be associated with weight gain. Serotonin interacts with receptors in the brain that regulate feeding behavior.[67] When brain levels of serotonin are increased, the desire to eat is decreased; as serotonin levels drop, appetite is stimulated.[68] Mimicking the serotonin-receptor interaction has been the target of several antiobesity drugs developed over the last 4 decades.[69] Moreover, studies have shown that obese individuals have low levels of *tryptophan*, a precursor to serotonin, in their blood.[70] These findings suggest that *restoring serotonin signaling* may be a way to combat hunger cravings that can preclude weight loss.

While stress is an important adaptation essential for survival, long-term stress can be damaging. *Chronic stress* can compromise the function of hormonal, gastrointestinal, and immune systems.[71] Exposure to chronic stress has been associated with obesity and metabolic syndrome in human and animal studies.[13] Stress increases production of the hormone *cortisol*, which when combined with access to abundant food, promotes the development of visceral obesity.[72]

Cortisol promotes weight gain in several ways. Visceral fat tissue contains a high number of cortisol receptors and responds to circulating cortisol by increasing fat cell growth and lipid storage.[73] Cortisol may also stimulate the neurotransmitters that signal hunger and decrease the activity of leptin, which signals satiety.[74] Activation of the stress response appears to stimulate the human appetite for highly palatable, energy-dense foods,[75] which may explain the association between emotional stress and increased food intake.[13] A comprehensive overview of strategies to mitigate the negative effects of stress is available in the Stress Management protocol.

---

## IMPORTANT OBESITY-RELATED TESTS

Knowledge of one's overall risk enables the selection of an appropriate weight loss strategy. For example, sufficient levels of thyroid hormone are necessary to minimize obesity risk; thyroid insufficiency can be treated with hormone replacement. Low levels of testosterone and estrogen are associated with weight gain in men and women, respectively, and sufficient DHEA is essential for sex hormone production. High cholesterol, high blood pressure, and chronic inflammation are all risk factors for one or more of the obesity-related diseases.

Life Extension offers comprehensive blood test panels designed specifically to assess factors that may influence weight loss. Two versions are available; one for men (Male Weight Loss Panel) and one for women (Female Weight Loss Panel).

**See table on next page**

---

## CONSEQUENCES OF OBESITY

### Chronic Inflammation

Obese individuals have higher levels of inflammatory markers. Sustained, low-level inflammation has been implicated in the pathogenesis of several significant diseases, including heart disease, cancer, diabetes, and Alzheimer's disease.[76-79] Fat tissue can act much like an endocrine (hormonal) gland, storing and secreting hormones and *cytokines* (signaling proteins involved in triggering the inflammatory response) into circulation and affecting metabolism throughout the body. Abdominal visceral fat cells may produce inflammatory molecules such as *tumor necrosis factor-alpha (TNF-α)* and *interleukin-6* at levels sufficient to induce an inflammatory response.[7,80] In overweight individuals, abdominal fat cells may be producing up to 35% of the total interleukin-6 in the body.[81] Fat tissue can also be infiltrated by macrophages (cells of the immune system that mediate inflammation), which secrete proinflammatory cytokines. This accumulation of macrophages appears to be proportional to BMI, and may be a major cause of low-grade, systemic inflammation and insulin resistance in obese individuals.[44,45]

## Important Obesity-Related Tests

| Test | Standard Reference Range | Optimal Level |
|---|---|---|
| Thyroid-stimulating hormone (TSH) | 0.4–5.0 µIU/mL | 1.0–2.0 µIU/mL |
| Free thyroxine (T4) | 0.82–1.77 ng/dL | Upper third of reference range |
| Free triiodothyronine (T3) | 2.0–4.4 pg/mL | 3.4–4.2 pg/mL |
| Total cholesterol | 100–199 mg/dL | 160–180 mg/dL |
| LDL cholesterol | 0–99 mg/dL | <100 mg/dL |
| HDL cholesterol | >39 mg/dL | ≥50 mg/dL |
| Triglycerides | 0–149 mg/dL | <80 mg/dL |
| Sex hormone binding globulin (SHBG) | *Men*<br>Age 20–49: 16.5–55.9 nmol/L<br>Age >49: 19.3–76.4 nmol/L<br>*Women*<br>Age 20–49: 24.6–122 nmol/L<br>Age >49: 17.3–125 nmol/L | 30–40 nmol/L<br><br><br>60–80 nmol/L |
| Dehydroepiandrosterone sulfate (DHEA-S) | *Men*<br>Age 20–24: 211–492 µg/dL<br>*Women*<br>Age 20–24: 148–407 µg/dL | 350–490 µg/dL<br><br>275–400 µg/dL |
| Total testosterone | *Men*<br>348–1197 ng/dL<br>*Women*<br>8–48 ng/dL | 700–900 ng/dL<br><br>35–45 ng/dL |
| Free testosterone | *Men*<br>Age 20–29: 9.3–26.5 pg/mL<br>*Women*<br>0.0–2.2 pg/mL | 20–25 pg/mL<br><br>1–2.2 pg/mL |
| Estradiol | *Men*<br>7.6–42.6 pg/mL<br>*Women*<br>Premenopausal: varies<br>Postmenopausal:<br><6.0–54.7 pg/mL | 20–30 pg/mL<br><br>Premenopausal: varies<br>Menopausal/ postmenopausal:<br>30–100 pg/mL |
| Progesterone | *Women*<br>Premenopausal: varies<br>Postmenopausal:<br>0.1–0.8 ng/mL | Premenopausal: varies<br>Menopausal/ postmenopausal:<br>2–6 ng/mL |
| C-reactive protein (high sensitivity) | Low risk: 1.0 mg/L | *Men*<br><0.55 mg/L<br>*Women*<br><1.5 mg/L |
| Insulin | 2.6–24.9 µIU/mL | <5 µIU/mL |
| Glucose (fasting) | 65–99 mg/dL | 70–85 mg/dL |
| Blood pressure (optimal) | 120/80 mmHg | 115/75 mmHg |

TSH, *thyroid-stimulating hormone; LDL, low-density lipoprotein; HDL, high-density lipoprotein; DHEA-S, dehydroepiandrosterone sulfate; µIU/mL, microunits per milliliter; mg/dL, milligrams per deciliter; mg/L, milligrams per liter; µg/dL, micrograms per deciliter; ng/dL, nanograms per deciliter; ng/mL, nanograms per milliliter; pg/mL, picograms per milliliter; nmol/L, nanomole per liter; mmHg, millimeters of mercury.*

## Cancer

Obesity is a risk factor for several types of cancer. White adipose tissue (ie, "bad fat") can secrete a variety of hormones and growth factors that may stimulate cancer cell growth. Experimental cancer models in animals suggest that tumors may recruit healthy cells from elsewhere in the body (including white fat) to build the blood vessels critical for the progression of tumor growth.[82]

Postmenopausal breast cancer risk increases with obesity, possibly through effects on systemic inflammation or increases in circulating insulin and insulin-like growth factor 1 (IGF-1), both of which can promote tumor growth.[83] Obesity increases gastric and esophageal cancer risk; mechanisms for this also include increased insulin and IGF-1 signaling, as well as increased incidence of gastroesophageal reflux disease

(GERD).[84] Population studies have implicated obesity as a risk factor for liver cancer (hepatocellular carcinoma). Along with obesity, nonalcoholic fatty liver disease (NAFLD), an increase in fat stores in the liver, is a hallmark of metabolic syndrome; the inflammation and liver fibrosis associated with fatty liver can progress into hepatocellular carcinoma.[85] Central obesity has been reported as a risk factor for colorectal cancer. Comprehensive reviews have estimated that colorectal cancer risk increases by 7% as BMI increases by 2 points, or 5% for each inch of waist circumference above normal.[8] Again, circulating growth factors and inflammatory cytokines are thought to contribute to the increase in abnormal cell proliferation. Some evidence suggests that the satiety hormone leptin may also play a role in colorectal cancer progression; cell culture studies have shown that leptin can increase the growth and proliferation of colon adenocarcinoma cells.[86]

Obesity may increase thyroid cancer risk; the rise in thyroid cancer incidence parallels that of obesity, although studies that explore the relationship between these 2 diseases have conflicting results.[87] The effect of obesity on thyroid cancer may be due to increased insulin/IGF-1 expression; thyroid stimulating hormone levels are sensitive to insulin and IGF-1 levels, and all 3 hormones work together to stimulate thyroid activity. Increases in IGF-1 have been correlated with increased thyroid tumor diameter, and insulin resistance has been shown to be more frequent in thyroid cancer patients than cancer-free controls.[88]

## Insulin Resistance

Insensitivity of tissues to circulating insulin (ie, insulin resistance), which is a hallmark of type 2 diabetes and metabolic syndrome, has obesity as a major risk factor. While moderate postmeal increases in insulin are normal and signal tissues to take up glucose and store it as glycogen and fat, overconsumption can lead to accelerated increases in fat mass and excessive insulin production (ie, hyperinsulinemia). Sustained hyperinsulinemia activates inflammatory pathways, which can lead to insulin resistance; although the mechanisms of this phenomenon are not clearly understood.[8,89] The appetite suppressing activity of insulin may be abolished in insulin-resistant obese individuals,[43] which can promote further weight gain by removing this important appetite control mechanism.

## High Blood Pressure

Increased blood pressure elevates the risk of several other diseases, including atherosclerosis, heart attack, heart failure, stroke, chronic kidney disease, and vision loss.[90–92] Excessive adipose tissue can increase blood pressure by several possible mechanisms: aside from its effect on inflammation, fat cells can be a source of the hypertensive proteins *renin* and *angiotensinogen*, and *angiotensin converting enzyme*, all of which work together to increase blood pressure by promoting water retention and causing constriction of blood vessels.[93] Fat tissue also produces the satiety hormone leptin, which, in combination with the renin-angiotensin and sympathetic nervous systems, may influence blood pressure by causing the kidneys to retain sodium and water; high leptin levels are also related to insulin resistance, itself a risk factor for hypertension.[93,94] Compared to normal weight individuals, overweight individuals are 1.7 times as likely to have hypertension, while for obese individuals, the risk is 2.6-fold.[9] A BMI between 18.5 and 24.9 carries the lowest risk of hypertension. Reductions of systolic blood pressure by 5–20 mmHg per 22 lb of weight loss have been observed in several studies.[95,96]

## Arthritis

Excess weight puts additional mechanical stress on the joints. Obesity has been unequivocally associated with osteoarthritis risk, particularly in weight-bearing joints such as the knee and hip. In an analysis of 21 studies on obesity and knee osteoarthritis incidence, a 5 point increase in BMI was associated with a 35% increase in osteoarthritis risk; this effect was more significant in women than men (38% versus 22%, respectively).[97]

## Gastroesophageal Reflux Disease

Gastroesophageal reflux disease (GERD) is a condition that develops when the reflux of stomach contents into the esophagus causes troublesome symptoms (heartburn) and/or complications (esophageal cancer).[98] Increased body mass and abdominal adiposity increases pressure on the stomach and lower esophagus. This can stress the lower esophageal valve, which is responsible for retaining acid in the stomach. When this valve is compromised, it loses its ability to maintain a seal against gastric reflux. Sustained abdominal pressure due to central obesity can also increase risk of hiatal hernia (the forcing of part of the stomach above the diaphragm into the chest cavity), another risk factor for gastric reflux.[99] Among seven studies that examined the relationship between body mass and GERD complications, overweight individuals averaged a 43% increase, and obese individuals a 94% increase, in GERD symptoms over individuals with a normal body mass.[100] Exposure to stomach acid also increases the rate of neoplastic alterations (abnormal cellular proliferation) within the esophagus, leading to the higher incidence of esophageal adenocarcinoma observed in overweight individuals in most of these studies.

## Sleep Disorders

Obesity is the strongest contributor to obstructive sleep apnea, a breathing disorder that occurs during sleep and causes symptoms ranging from restless sleep to low blood oxygen (hypoxemia). About 70% of people with obstructive sleep apnea are obese, and about 40% of obese individuals have sleep apnea. Among individuals with BMIs over 60, the prevalence of sleep apnea is 90%. Obese individuals are more likely to suffer from night eating syndrome or sleep-related eating disorder, disorders characterized by symptoms ranging from excessive nighttime hunger to unconscious nocturnal eating. The prevalence of these eating disorders among obese persons is 6–16%, as compared to 1.5% in the general population. Narcolepsy (excessive daytime sleepiness) is also more common in obese individuals.[101]

Poor sleep quality is more than just a consequence of obesity. Rather, a *vicious cycle* in which obesity leads to impaired sleep leads to increased appetite leads to obesity may complicate weight loss efforts for many individuals. Studies show that sleep deprivation, as can occur when one's sleep is suboptimal due to obesity-related phenomena such as sleep apnea, is associated with increased appetite.[102] In an insightful magnetic resonance imaging experiment, researchers showed that a brain region called the *anterior cingulate cortex* appears to be more responsive to anticipation of food following sleep deprivation as compared to a full night of sleep. Increased neural activity in this brain region is associated with obesity, and its level of activation correlated with appetite in this study.[103] Thus, improving *sleep hygiene* and ensuring that restful, restorative sleep is attained is an integral aspect of successful weight loss. A number of strategies for improving sleep quality are discussed in the Insomnia protocol.

# DIAGNOSIS AND ASSESSMENT OF OBESITY

## Diagnosis

Obesity is typically diagnosed and defined by analysis of body size, weight, and composition. *BMI* is the most commonly accepted metric for defining obesity; it is a surrogate measurement of adiposity, calculated as body mass (in kilograms) divided by height squared (in meters). Alternatively, it can be calculated in Imperial units as [weight (in lb)/height$^2$ (in inches)] × 703.[104]

The World Health Organization (WHO) definitions of overweight and obese are BMIs of ≥25 and ≥30 kg/m$^2$, respectively.[105]

**WHO Classification of Weight Status by BMI**[106]

| Status | BMI, kg/m2 |
| --- | --- |
| Underweight | <18.5 |
| Normal range | 18.5–24.9 |
| Overweight | 25–29.9 |
| Obese class I | 30–34.9 |
| Obese class II | 35–39.9 |
| Obese class III/morbid obesity | ≥40 |

Although BMI is strongly correlated with total body fat, it is not without limitations. For example, there are significant racial considerations that can influence its interpretation (eg, Asians typically carry more body fat, and Africans less, than Caucasians at any particular BMI). BMI overestimates body fat content for individuals with high muscle mass (such as athletes). Additionally, BMI cannot measure some changes in body composition; for example, the concurrent loss of lean muscle and increase in body fat in aging individuals might not result in a change in their BMI.[107] Alternative measurements (eg, skin-fold thickness and waist-to-hip ratio) have been suggested as more accurate methods for body fat estimation, but in terms of predicting clinical outcomes, BMI has shown similar accuracy to these techniques and remains an acceptable measurement despite its shortcomings.[108] BMI can be combined with waist circumference measurements, which can estimate an individual's abdominal fat content (abdominal or visceral fat is a greater risk factor for obesity-related diseases than total body fat). Waist circumference measurements of >102 cm (40 in.) for men and >88 cm (35 in.) for women carry high risk of obesity-associated disease (eg, type 2 diabetes, cardiovascular disease, and hypertension).[104]

## STUDY FUNDED BY LIFE EXTENSION FOUNDATION® REVEALS INADEQUACIES OF CONVENTIONAL BMI MEASUREMENTS

The most widely used tool to assess weight-related health status is the calculated *BMI*, despite several shortcomings. Although a number of studies and analyses have established relatively consistent associations between various BMI ranges and risk of several diseases, the technique is unable to provide an accurate determination of body fat percentage.[109,110] This leads to inevitable oversights as to obesity-related risks given the variation in adipose tissue distribution among individuals.

Scientists at the frontiers of obesity research recognize the inadequacy of relying on calculated BMI measurements and are vigorously investigating methods to circumvent its short-comings.

A groundbreaking 2012 study supported by a grant from the nonprofit Life Extension Foundation® meticulously examined the discrepancy between BMI-diagnosed obesity and obesity determined as a function of body fat content assessed by *dual energy x-ray absorptiometry (DXA)*, a highly accurate, albeit expensive and cumbersome method of measuring body fat. This study evaluated 11 years of records pertaining to nearly 1400 patients for whom DXA-determined body fat and BMI measurements had been captured.

The results showed that BMI was a poor indicator of body fat content and may result in the underdiagnosis and under-treatment of individuals at risk for obesity-related diseases. Measurement of BMI alone was shown to be especially prone to underestimation of obesity in aging women: 48% of women classified nonobese by BMI calculation were found to be obese when body fat percentage was determined by DXA.

The authors of this study simultaneously examined correlates between blood levels of *leptin* and DXA-determined body fat content; they found that leptin levels emulated the DXA findings in many cases.

Therefore, the researchers suggest that blood levels of leptin can *complement* calculated BMI measurements to improve detection of obesity. For example, if a person has a "normal" BMI, but very high leptin levels, they may still be at risk for obesity-related diseases and may benefit from antiobesity intervention. Likewise, if a person with a BMI typically classified as "overweight" has low leptin levels, they may be at lower risk and not require aggressive antiobesity intervention.[111]

While direct measurement of body fat by DXA remains a premium choice for determination of obesity-related disease, its high cost and limited availability make it an unreasonable option for many people. Emerging evidence suggests, however, that augmenting a calculated BMI measurement with leptin blood testing may help physicians determine patients' risks with improved clarity.

# CONVENTIONAL OBESITY MANAGEMENT

A National Institutes of Health panel established recommendations for the treatment of obesity based on BMI, waist circumference, and overall disease risk.[104] The Panel recommends low-calorie or very-low calorie diets as the cornerstone of any weight-loss strategy, such as to create a deficit of 500–1000 calories/day and a weight loss of 1–2 lb/week. Lifestyle modification and weight loss are the recommended methods for lowering blood pressure and blood lipids (low-density lipoprotein [LDL], total cholesterol, and triglycerides) in overweight/obese individuals, and for lowering blood glucose in overweight type 2 diabetes patients. The panel further recommends 30–45 minutes of moderate physical activity, 3–5 days per week, to promote weight loss and decrease abdominal fat.

Weight loss drugs may be incorporated into the weight loss plan for obese individuals (BMI ≥30) with no other risk factors or obesity-related diseases (eg, hypertension, heart disease, diabetes), or for over-weight individuals with a BMI of ≥27 and obesity-related risk factors or diseases. Weight loss surgery is reserved for class III obese individuals (BMI ≥40), or class II individuals (BMI ≥35) at high risk of obesity-associated mortality and when noninvasive methods have failed.[104,112]

## Pharmaceutical Therapy

The drugs in this section are approved by the Food and Drug Administration (FDA) for the treatment of obesity.

**Orlistat.** While pharmaceutical approaches to obesity have traditionally addressed appetite suppression, orlistat (Alli®, Xenical®) works by *decreasing fat absorption* from the gut. It binds and inactivates pancreatic lipase, the enzyme responsible for breaking down dietary triglycerides into fatty acids so they can be absorbed through the intestinal wall.[113]

Sixteen trials have observed orlistat's effects in over 10 000 subjects, and have shown an average annual weight loss of 6.4 lb when used over 12 months. It has been shown to reduce the incidence of diabetes, lower total and LDL cholesterol and blood pressure, and improve blood sugar control in patients with diabetes, while only slightly lowering high-density lipoprotein (HDL, or "good" cholesterol) concentrations.[114] The most common side effects of orlistat include diarrhea, flatulence, bloating, abdominal pain, and indigestion.[69] Although rare, serious liver damage has been reported from orlistat usage.[115] Life Extension suggests taking fat-soluble nutrients such as vitamins D, E, and K, lutein, zeaxanthin, and fish oil at the time of the day furthest from the last orlistat dose, since it may impair their absorption.

**Lorcaserin.** Lorcaserin is a selective serotonin receptor agonist, specifically the 5-HT2C receptor, enhancing the satiating effects of serotonin in the central nervous system. Lorcaserin acts more selectively on serotonin receptors than the fenfluramine antiobesity drugs that were introduced in the 1970s and withdrawn in 1997 due to increased risk of cardiac valvular disease. Lorcaserin acts on the 5-HT2C receptor, showing roughly 100-fold greater selectivity for the 5-HT2C receptor than the 5-HT2B receptor, and demonstrated no increase in the rate of valvular disease after 2 years of treatment.[69]

In two phase 3 trials, lorcaserin treatment of 6380 nondiabetic patients aged 18–66 years with a BMI of 27–45 for 1 year resulted in a 5.8% weight loss, compared to 2.5% with placebo.[69] Lorcaserin was FDA-approved in June 2012 under the brand name Belviq®, making it the first antiobesity drug to be approved since orlistat in 1999.[116] The most frequent side effects for lorcaserin are headache, dizziness, and nausea. Also, there may be some potential for abuse due to the drug's hallucinogenic properties; the Drug Enforcement Administration (DEA) has thus proposed regulating lorcaserin as a schedule IV substance.[117]

**Phentermine/topiramate.** Topiramate is an approved antiepileptic drug with appetite-suppressant activity; phentermine is an amphetamine that has been available in the United States as a short-term, prescription weight-loss treatment. The combination has been investigated as an antiobesity therapy; in a 28-week randomized trial, phentermine plus topiramate (92 mg/15 mg and 46 mg/7.5 mg doses) demonstrated a 9.2% weight loss compared to a 6.4% weight loss with topiramate alone, 6.1% for phentermine alone, and 1.7% for placebo.[69]

Phentermine/topiramate was FDA-approved under the brand name Qsymia® in July 2012.[118] The combination is also in clinical development for sleep apnea syndrome and type 2 diabetes.[119] Potential side effects include depression and cognitive complaints, potential cardiovascular risk, and an increase in heart rate.[120]

## Bariatric Surgery

Bariatric surgical procedures modify the size or course of the gastrointestinal tract to attenuate the appetite. Five bariatric procedures have been developed, although the 2 most common (Roux-en-Y gastric bypass and laparoscopic gastric band) represented about 49% and 42% of procedures in the United States in 2008, respectively. Gastric bypass reduces the stomach to a small pouch and bypasses part of the small intestine. The laparoscopic gastric band fits around the upper part of the stomach, also creating a smaller stomach pouch that limits food consumption. A newer procedure, sleeve gastrectomy, is increasing in popularity; it only removes part of the stomach, but leaves its connection to the intestines intact.[121]

Bariatric procedures reduce hunger and caloric intake, and have resulted in average weight losses of 20–35%, depending on surgical technique. They have also been shown to affect food preferences by a yet unknown mechanism; gastric banding usually limits consumption of breads and pasta, and gastric bypass reduces intake of sweet and fatty foods and possibly increases vegetable consumption. Several studies of bariatric surgery in diabetic patients have demonstrated a reduction in high blood sugar levels and insulin resistance, and reduced the need for blood sugar-lowering medications. Most of these procedures are permanent, require lifelong follow-up, and are not without surgical risk. Because they dramatically alter gastrointestinal anatomy and physiology, they can also lead to malabsorption and deficiency of certain nutrients (particularly vitamin B12, iron, folate, calcium, vitamin D, zinc, and copper).[121]

# NOVEL AND EMERGING THERAPIES FOR OBESITY

## Temporary Surgical Procedures/Endosleeves

The duodenojejunal bypass sleeve (DJBS) is a flexible, nutrient-impermeable plastic sleeve that is surgically inserted into the upper part of the small intestine (duodenum). The sleeve serves as a barrier to nutrient absorption, simulating the effect of a Roux-en-Y gastric bypass, but is a reversible procedure.[122] By preventing absorption in the part of the small intestine closest to the stomach, the sleeve may also delay gastric emptying and stimulate satiety.[123] DJBSs are temporary devices for weight loss; in human trials they were left in place for 3 months and successfully removed, resulting in the loss of 22–24% of excess weight. Complications include esophageal tears, bloating, upper gastrointestinal bleeding, and movement of the sleeve.[123]

## Metformin

Metformin, a first-line antidiabetic drug with a long history of safety and efficacy, has shown promising results as an antiobesity therapy. While not currently approved for weight loss, studies have shown average weight losses between 4.4 and 6.6 lb, reaching up to 19.8 lb in some studies. Metformin also has the added benefit of being known to prevent progression to diabetes in prediabetic patients.[115] Metformin may also reduce the activity of inflammatory cytokines; low-grade inflammation is associated with the incidence of metabolic disorders (eg, obesity and diabetes).[124,125] Finally, metformin can produce many of the gene expression changes associated with long-term caloric restriction in animal models, possibly due to its influence on insulin or IGF-1 signaling.[126]

## Acarbose

Acarbose (Precose®) is an oral antidiabetic agent that delays glucose release from complex carbohydrates by inhibiting the activity of the enzyme alpha-glucosidase, and can lead to a reduction of postmeal blood glucose levels.[127] Two comprehensive reviews of more than 30 randomized, double-blind, placebo-controlled trials with a minimum acarbose treatment course of 12 weeks have shown its ability to significantly improve glycemic control and lower glycated hemoglobin (HbA1c) in type 2 diabetic patients.[128] The first of the two analyses (seven acarbose studies)[127] demonstrated lower triglyceride levels and systolic blood pressure in the acarbose treatment group, and a significant effect on reducing the risk of heart attack and other cardiovascular events. Across these studies, there was a slight average reduction in body weight of 2.4 lb among type 2 diabetic patients on acarbose therapy compared to 1.8 lb for the placebo group; BMI data also showed a similar modest reduction with acarbose treatment. In the second review,[128] the weight-lowering effects of acarbose were not clinically significant.

# NINE PILLARS OF SUCCESSFUL WEIGHT LOSS

Rebalancing energy intake and expenditure to lose weight, by reducing caloric intake and increasing physical activity, is requisite for any weight loss regimen. However, alterations in metabolism, including age-related hormonal changes, can complicate successful weight loss by necessitating dramatic reductions in caloric intake that are difficult to sustain.[16,29,40,74] Therefore, it is important to consider a multimodal approach to weight loss, in which low-calorie diet and exercise are augmented by steps to restore optimal levels of steroid and thyroid hormones, promote insulin sensitivity, and modulate macronutrient absorption. By this approach, one might not only increase their chance of successful weight and body fat loss, but also potentially reduce many of the other risks associated with obesity such as cardiovascular disease and cancer.

## Eat for a Long and Healthy Life

**Caloric restriction.** Caloric restriction is the dramatic reduction of dietary calories to a level short of malnutrition.[129] Restriction of energy intake slows down the body's growth processes, and causes it to instead focus on protective repair mechanisms; the overall effect is an improvement in several measures of wellbeing. Even in lean, healthy individuals, moderate caloric restriction (22–30% decreases in caloric intake from normal levels) improves heart function, reduces markers of inflammation (eg, C-reactive protein and TNF-α), reduces risk factors for cardiovascular disease (eg, LDL-C, triglycerides, and blood pressure), and reduces diabetes risk factors (eg, fasting blood glucose and insulin levels).[130–133] The multicenter CALERIE trial on the effects of calorie-restricted diets in otherwise healthy, overweight volunteers has shown that moderate caloric restriction can reduce several cardiovascular risk factors (LDL-C, triglycerides, blood

pressure, and C-reactive protein) in addition to promoting weight loss.[134]

It is important to remember that as more calories are eliminated from the diet, dietary levels of essential nutrients drop and may need to be replaced; in studies of four popular diet plans that limited calories to 1100–1700 per day (including the NIH and American Heart Association-recommended "DASH diet"), all were found to be on average only 43.5% sufficient in recommended daily intakes (RDIs) for 27 essential micronutrients values, and deficient in 15 of them.[135] Eating for a long and healthy life likely involves calorie restriction and nutrient supplementation. Refer to the Life Extension protocol on Caloric Restriction for additional information on energy-restricted diets and a comprehensive list of nutrients that may simulate caloric restriction.

## Increase Physical Activity

Increased physical activity promotes weight loss by addressing both sides of the energy balance equation. It increases energy expenditure leading to reduced body weight and fat mass, and exercise reduces appetite at least in the short term by delaying gastric emptying, or possibly increasing the body's sensitivity to hormones that control appetite such as cholecystokinin.[136] It may also protect against the insulin resistance associated with obesity.[137] Several intervention studies in both young[138] and older adults have shown small-to-moderate decreases in body weight, fat mass, and/or waist circumference with regular, moderate exercise (30–45 minutes of moderate exercise, 3–5 times per week), especially when combined with reduced calorie diets. Exercise may also offset some of the lean muscle loss associated with weight loss in older individuals; loss of lean body mass is associated with decreased independence among this group.[139]

## Restore Resting Energy Expenditure

**Black coffee consumption.** Black coffee consumption has been associated with reductions in body weight; it adds fluid to the diet without adding additional calories, and contains compounds (eg, chlorogenic acid and caffeine) that may promote weight reduction.[140,141] In a large population study of almost 60 000 healthy men and women over a 12-year period, coffee consumption was associated with less weight gain in women.[142] While some of this may have been attributable to caffeine content, the same study also revealed modest associations between greater decaffeinated coffee consumption and less weight gain, suggesting other components of coffee may also protect against weight gain. Intervention studies have reported similarly positive results. In one study, 33 healthy volunteers saw slight reductions of body weight and body fat following 4 weeks of consumption of 750 mL of brewed coffee per day that contained both green and roasted coffee constituents.[143] In a second study, 15 overweight and obese volunteers consumed 11 g per day of instant coffee enriched with 1000 mg chlorogenic acid (approximately 5 cups coffee per day) for 12 weeks and saw reductions in body weight of almost 12 lb, compared to a loss of 3.7 lb among volunteers who drank regular instant coffee.[144]

**Green tea polyphenols.** Green tea has exhibited anti-inflammatory activity in dozens of laboratory and animal studies,[145] as well as cholesterol-lowering effects in human trials (averaging about 9 mg/dL of LDL cholesterol decrease across 4 studies).[146] The effect of green tea on body composition has been the subject of at least 21 unique trials. Two analyses of these trials suggest a modest effect of green tea on body weight.[147–149] In an analysis of 11 randomized, controlled trials of green tea consumption for 12–13 weeks duration, green tea decreased body weight by about 3 lb compared to controls in Asian participants.[148] A second analysis of 15 randomized trials demonstrated that consumption of green tea catechins with caffeine produced a greater decrease in BMI and body weight compared to controls.[149]

**Fucoxanthin.** Fucoxanthin is a carotenoid from brown seaweed that has been shown to reduce white fat levels in animal models, by increasing energy expenditure through the activation of the thermogenic factor mitochondrial *uncoupling protein 1 (UCP1)*.[150,151] In a 16-week trial of 151 obese, premenopausal women with and without NAFLD, consumption of a combination of 2.4 mg fucoxanthin and 300 mg of *pomegranate seed oil*, along with a reduced calorie diet (1800 calories/day), resulted in a significant reduction of body weight compared to placebo (an average of 12.1 lb lost in NAFLD patients and 10.8 lb lost in non-NAFLD patients).[152] Serum triglycerides and C-reactive protein levels also dropped in both groups taking fucoxanthin/pomegranate seed oil compared to control.

**Fish oil.** Fish oil, a rich source of the omega-3 fatty acids eicosapentaenoic acid (EPA) and docosahexaenoic acid (DHA), can only be synthesized to a limited extent by humans but are nonetheless essential for several metabolic processes. Omega-3 fatty acids have been well studied for the prevention of cardiovascular disease and their ability to lower inflammation and reduce hypertension; these processes are all associated with the progression of obesity and metabolic syndrome.[153,154]

Some evidence suggests EPA and DHA may promote thermogenesis.[155] Omega-3 fatty acids from fish oil may have protective effects against weight gain independent of their blood-pressure-lowering and anti-inflammatory roles. When combined with regular aerobic exercise, 6 g per day of fish oil for 12 weeks demonstrated significantly lowered triglycerides, increased HDL cholesterol, improved endothelium-dependent arterial vasodilation, and improved arterial compliance in a study of 75 overweight volunteers.[156] Additionally, both fish oil and exercise independently reduced body fat, albeit modestly. Incorporating lean or oily fish, or fish oil, into energy-restricted diets (1600 calories per day) resulted in about 2.2 lb more loss of weight over 4 weeks than diets without fish in a group of 138 overweight and obese men.[157]

**Capsaicin/cayenne.** Capsaicin is a major "spicy" constituent of chili peppers (eg, cayenne). Regular intake of chili peppers delays oxidation of serum lipids, which contributes to reducing the risk of cardiovascular disease.[158] Because of the sensation of heat and increased energy expenditure when eaten, chili peppers are thought of as potential interventions for obesity management.[159] Capsaicin has been studied as a potential thermogenic compound in 10 long- and short-term studies, mostly in Asian populations where it is more commonly consumed. Results of capsaicin studies are mixed; it appears to significantly increase energy expenditure (up to 30% in some studies) and decrease appetite and energy intake, but these results are more robust in Asian participants than Caucasians.[160]

Another compound that may increase resting energy expenditure is 3-acetyl-7-oxo-dehydroepiandrosterone (*7-Keto® DHEA*). For more information, see the discussion on restoring youthful hormone balance later in this protocol.

## Restore Healthy Adipocyte (Fat Cell) Signaling

**Irvingia gabonensis.** *Irvingia gabonensis* is a mango-like West African fruit; extracts of its seeds have been shown to reduce fat stores and promote healthy blood lipid and fasting blood glucose levels.[161] *Irvingia gabonensis* extracts are thought to work by inhibiting adipogenesis (ie, the development of fat cells) by down-regulating a protein involved in activating fat cell growth and proliferation. Three randomized controlled trials have investigated Irvingia extracts in healthy volunteers; all have demonstrated its ability to significantly decrease body fat stores, weight, and waist circumference.[54,162,163] When compared to placebo, healthy overweight and/or obese volunteers taking 150 mg of *Irvingia gabonensis* seed extract before meals for 10 weeks exhibited a significantly greater decrease in body fat percentage (6.3% versus 1.9%), body weight (28.2 lb versus 1.5 lb), and waist circumference (–6.37 in versus –2.09 in), as well as significant drops in total and LDL cholesterol, C-reactive protein, and fasting blood glucose.[54] These kinds of results are seldom duplicated outside the clinical study setting, however.

***Sphaeranthus indicus* and mangosteen (*Garcinia mangostana*).** Mangosteen has long been used as a diabetic treatment in Southeast Asia; modern investigations suggest antioxidant and anti-inflammatory activities, especially in white adipose tissue.[164] *Sphaeranthus indicus* (*S. indicus*) has been widely used in Ayurvedic medicine for a variety of ailments, and has been studied for its anti-inflammatory, blood sugar-lowering, and lipid-lowering activities in animal and cell culture models.[165] In a trial of 60 obese volunteers, 30 were randomized to receive 800 mg per day of the *S. indicus* and mangosteen combination for 8 weeks, while maintaining a restricted 2000 calorie per day diet and exercising (walking) for 30 minutes, 5 times per week. After 8 weeks, the group receiving the dual plant extract exhibited significant reductions in body weight (11 lb versus 3.3 lb for placebo), BMI (2.05 versus 0.5 for placebo), waist circumference (4.05 inches versus 2.02 for placebo), as well statistically significant reductions in total cholesterol, serum triglycerides, and serum glucose.[166]

## Restore Brain Serotonin/Suppress Hunger Signals

**Tryptophan.** Tryptophan is an essential amino acid and precursor to serotonin, a neurotransmitter involved in gastrointestinal function as well as mood and feeding behavior. Increases in brain levels of serotonin signal satiety, while decreases signal the desire to eat.[68] Multiple studies have shown that calorie-restricted diets, while successful at reducing weight, also reduce circulating tryptophan levels by 14–23%. This may lead to reduced serotonin synthesis, increased hunger, and a reduction in the probability of maintaining weight loss.[167] In a study of 10 healthy, young, normal-weight men, 2- and 3-g doses of tryptophan reduced energy intake compared to placebo when taken before a buffet-style meal.[168] In 10 obese subjects, 1, 2, or 3 g of tryptophan taken 1 hour before a plated meal reduced calorie consumption in a dose-dependent manner.[169]

**Saffron.** Extracts of saffron stigma (*Crocus sativus*) have been studied for a variety of applications, including pain relief, anti-inflammation, and memory enhancement. In animal models, high doses of saffron have been shown to possess an antidepressant-like activity, which may explain its potential for reducing the desire to eat. In a study of 60 healthy, mildly overweight women on an unrestricted diet, 176.5 mg of saffron stigma extract per day for 8 weeks produced an average weight loss of about 2 lb. Much of this weight reduction is attributed to a reduction in snacking frequency; at the study's end, individuals on the saffron supplement reported having 5.5 snacks per week (compared to 8.9 snacks per week in the placebo group), a reduction in snacking frequency of 55% from pretrial levels.[170]

**Pine nut oil.** Pine nut oil, which contains a constituent called *pinolenic acid*, has been shown to reduce food intake. When doses of pine nut oil ranging from 2–6 g were given to overweight female subjects prior to a buffet-style meal, food consumption was reduced up to 9% compared to placebo. The researchers suggested that this reduction of food intake was attributable to pine nut oil's satiating effects, which may be mediated via modulation of cholecystokinin (CCK) and other appetite-suppressing compounds.[171]

## Control Rate of Carbohydrate Absorption

**Green coffee extract.** Green coffee extract, an *antioxidant-rich* mixture from unroasted coffee beans, has been shown to temper deadly *after-meal spikes in glucose* and to combat insulin resistance in animals.[60,172–174] Higher intakes have been associated with weight loss benefits.[141]

To determine conclusively whether green coffee bean extract has an *antiobesity* benefit, scientists set up a randomized, double-blind, placebo-controlled, linear dose, crossover study on humans.[60] In a crossover study, participants are cycled through different phases of treatment and placebo. In this case, subjects took a high dose of *green coffee bean extract* for 6 weeks, a lower dose of *green coffee bean extract* for 6 weeks, and a placebo for 6 weeks in a randomized, double-blind manner. Between phases, there was a 2-week "washout" period, making the entire study 22 weeks long. Crossover studies are considered sound, because each person in the test group serves as his or her own control. This improves the chances of getting an accurate result, because it eliminates the possibility of the outcome reflecting a difference between the active and control groups. To ensure the findings were more representative, the investigation enlisted both men and women.

Participants were restricted to those who were classified as obese or preobese, because people who have these conditions are subject to obesity's *metabolic effects* and find weight loss difficult to achieve. To further ensure that any effect on weight, body fat, or BMI could be solely attributed to the extract, there were *no significant changes in dietary calories* or dietary percentages of carbohydrates, fat, and proteins at any time during the study. There were also no significant changes in exercise. Daily 350-mg capsules of *green coffee bean extract* were the only intervention, although in a non-study situation, people seeking weight reduction would ideally combine *green coffee bean extract* with lower calorie consumption and greater physical activity to promote maximum weight loss.[60]

During the high-dose phase, subjects took 350 mg of extract, 3 times daily. The lower dose phase included 350 mg of extract taken twice daily.[60] The placebo phase involved a 350-mg dose taken 3 times daily of an inert capsule containing an inactive substance. The striking results were published in January 2012[60]; over the 22-week trial, investigators found that all subjects experienced a reduction in body weight, BMI, and body fat during both the high-dose and low-dose phases of the study, but not in the placebo phase. After 12 weeks of administering 350 mg of green coffee bean extract 3 times a day, the scientists found that:

- Weight decreased by over 17.6 lb on average—with some subjects losing more than 22.7 lb.
- BMI decreased by an average of 2.92.
- Body fat percentage decreased by an average of 4.44%, with some subjects dropping their body fat percentage by 6.44%.
- Heart rate decreased by a significant average of 2.56 beats per minute.

The substantial antiobesity impact was clearly reflected in the finding that a remarkable 37% of participants who were assessed as having preobesity (25–30 BMI) at the start of the study had their condition reversed to the normal weight range.

A study follow-up showed that, contrasting with food-restriction diets, a surprising 87.5% of the test subjects were able to maintain their weight loss after completing the study. No side effects were observed. This and other studies demonstrate the importance of *"preparing your body to eat"* by taking *green coffee bean extract* before each meal. The dual effects of reducing *after-meal glucose* and inducing meaningful *weight loss* make it a supplement that virtually every aging person should take before eating.

In 2011, a detailed review of three studies of green coffee extract (180–200 mg per day) for 4–12 weeks in a total of 142 overweight volunteers demonstrated an average reduction in body weight of 5.4 lb compared to placebo.[141]

A compound called *chlorogenic acid* may be largely responsible for the weight loss benefits associated with green coffee extract. Chlorogenic acid is not found in great quantities in most conventional coffee beverages, since the roasting process dramatically reduces its content (although methods of retaining or re-infusing chlorogenic acid into roasted coffee have been developed). Chlorogenic acid has been shown to reduce glucose absorption in healthy volunteers,[144] which may be one way green coffee extract combats weight gain.[175] Moreover, chlorogenic acid may control glucose via inhibition of an enzyme called *glucose-6-phosphatase*, which is involved in the generation of glucose by the liver through a process known as *gluconeogenesis*.[176,177] Inhibition of gluconeogenesis may help normalize fasting glucose levels.

One compelling study showed that people not taking green coffee extract had glucose levels of 130 mg/dL 1 hour after sugar ingestion. In study subjects taking 400 mg of green coffee extract, glucose levels dropped to 93 mg/dL after sugar ingestion.[174] The difference between having a postload glucose reading of 93 mg/dL compared to 130 mg/dL is about a 70% reduction in heart attack risk.[178]

**Seaweed extracts.** Extracts from kelp (*Ascophyllum nodosum*) and bladderwrack (*Fucus vesiculosus*) have been demonstrated to inhibit the activity of the digestive enzymes alpha-amylase (α-amylase) and alpha-glucosidase (α-glucosidase)[179]; inhibition of these enzymes interferes with the digestion of dietary starches and may reduce or slow the absorption of high glycemic carbohydrates.[180] A proprietary composition of demineralized polyphenols from brown seaweed was examined in 23 volunteers for its ability to reduce postmeal blood glucose and insulin secretion following consumption of a carbohydrate-containing meal. When taken just prior to the consumption of a meal containing 50 g of carbohydrates (from bread), 500 mg of the seaweed extract was associated with a 12.1% reduction in insulin excretion and a 7.9% increase in insulin sensitivity when compared to placebo.[179]

**White kidney bean extract (*Phaseolus vulgaris*).** White kidney bean contains an inhibitor of α-amylase (ie, a pancreatic digestive enzyme required for the conversion of starches to simpler sugars in animals).[181] By inhibiting α-amylase, absorption of starch from the diet is attenuated; individuals can still include a reasonable carbohydrate proportion in their diet but lessen or slow the absorption of high glycemic carbohydrates.[180] Ten clinical trials have investigated the carbohydrate-blocking activity of *Phaseolus vulgaris* extracts. In 3 randomized, controlled studies, overweight and obese volunteers taking Phaseolus extracts (at doses ranging from 445 mg for 4 weeks to 3000 mg for 8–12 weeks) exhibited reduced body weights compared to controls (ranging from 1.9–6.9 lb lost). A fourth study showed a loss in body weight only among participants who consumed the greatest amount of carbohydrates. Additional trials demonstrated significant weight loss over time, as well as reductions in plasma triglycerides and postmeal blood glucose.[181]

**L-arabinose.** Sucrose (common sugar) is composed of two simple sugar molecules, glucose and fructose. It is poorly absorbed in the intestine in this form. In order to be utilized, it must first be broken down by the digestive enzyme *sucrase*. Blocking the enzymatic action of sucrase therefore reduces uptake of sucrose.

Researchers have identified a potent sucrase inhibitor called *L-arabinose*. L-arabinose, an indigestible plant compound, cannot be absorbed into the blood. Instead, it remains in the digestive tract and is eventually excreted.[182,183] By blocking metabolism of sucrose, L-arabinose inhibits the spike in blood sugar and fat synthesis that would otherwise follow a sugar-rich meal.[183] In animal models, L-arabinose virtually eliminated the rise in blood sugar following administration of sucrose, with blood glucose levels rising only 2% higher than in control animals that did not receive sucrose. L-arabinose did not exert any effect on serum glucose levels in control animals that did not receive sucrose.[184]

L-arabinose has been shown to be safe in both short- and long-term studies, and may contribute to lowered levels of glycosylated hemoglobin (hemoglobin A1C [HbA1c]), a measure of chronic exposure to sugar in the blood. A study concluded that combining L-arabinose and white kidney bean extract not only smoothed out postprandial glucose spikes and reduced insulin levels, it lowered systolic blood pressure as well.[185]

**Glucomannan.** Glucomannan is a soluble fiber derived from *Amorphophallus konjac*. It is thought to prolong gastric emptying time, which has several antiobesity outcomes. It may increase satiety, reduce body weight, reduce the postmeal rise in plasma glucose, suppress liver cholesterol synthesis, and increase the elimination of cholesterol-containing bile acids.[186] An analysis of 14 randomized, controlled studies of glucomannan usage by 531 hyperlipidemic, diabetic, or obese adults and children demonstrated its ability to affect modest reductions in body weight (an average reduction of 1.8 lb across all studies), when supplied at dosages between 3 and 15 g per day.[187] Additionally, glucomannan demonstrated significant average reductions in total cholesterol

(–19.28 mg/dL), LDL cholesterol (–15.99 mg/dL), triglycerides (–11.08 mg/dL), and fasting blood glucose (–7.44 mg/dL). *Propolmannan* is the name of a well-studied glucomannan soluble fiber.

---

## PROPOLMANNAN AND THE ROLE OF BILE ACIDS IN DIETARY FAT ABSORPTION

*Bile acids* are excreted from the liver into the small intestine where they facilitate the *absorption* of dietary *fats* into the bloodstream. Dietary fat absorption is dependent on bile acids and the *lipase enzyme*. An intact soluble fiber binds to bile acids in the small intestine, thus helping impede absorption of dietary fats (while simultaneously reducing serum LDL and total cholesterol).

Specially processed, *propolmannan* is a plant-derived polysaccharide fiber. Propolmannan is patented in 33 countries as a purified fiber that does not break down in the digestive tract.

Published research reveals propolmannan's ability to not only increase the amount of bile acids in feces, but also reduce the rate of carbohydrate absorption and subsequent glucose/insulin spike in the blood. When propolmannan is taken before meals, consistent and significant reductions in blood triglyceride, LDL, and total cholesterol are observed.[188]

---

### Restore Youthful Hormone Balance

*Hormone replacement therapy*, using natural compounds like *dehydroepiandrosterone (DHEA)* and *Armour® thyroid*, may help aging individuals overcome some of the barriers that insufficient or imbalanced hormone levels pose against successful weight loss. Comprehensive blood testing to assess hormone levels should be undertaken before beginning a hormone restoration regimen under the care of an experienced physician. The Male Weight Loss Panel or Female Weight Loss Panel are designed specifically to assess blood parameters that may influence weight loss. More information is available in the protocols on Male and Female Hormone Restoration, as well as the Thyroid Regulation protocol.

**DHEA and 7-Keto® DHEA.** Low levels of sex hormones are associated with obesity,[29] as well as systemic increases in inflammatory markers.[189] Dehydroepiandrosterone (DHEA) is an adrenal steroid hormone, a precursor to the sex steroids testosterone and estrogen. DHEA is abundant in youth, but steadily declines with advancing age and may be partially responsible for age-related decreases in sex steroids.[190] DHEA supplementation (50 mg per day for 2 years) in elderly volunteers significantly lowered visceral fat mass and improved glucose tolerance, as well as decreased levels of inflammatory cytokines in a small study.[191] High-dose DHEA induced thermogenesis, decreased body fat without decreasing food intake, and decreased glucose levels in animal models; and *7-Keto® DHEA* (3-acetyl-7-oxo-dehydroepiandrosterone) was shown to be 4-fold more thermogenic than DHEA.[192] It may work by increasing the shuttling of energy substrates into the mitochondria for conversion into heat/energy, and may act on the same enzyme systems as the thyroid hormone T3.[192,193] In human studies, overweight volunteers taking 100 mg of 7-Keto® DHEA twice daily lost significantly more weight and body fat than did the placebo group (6.3 lb versus 2.2 lb, respectively, and reductions in body fat of 1.8% versus 0.57%).[194] This weight reduction may be related to 7-Keto® DHEA's effect on increasing REE. In overweight subjects maintained on a calorie-restricted diet, 7 days of treatment with 7-Keto® DHEA increased REE by 1.4% (equivalent to an extra 115 calories burned per day), whereas subjects taking placebo saw their REE decrease by 3.9%.[195] Studies in healthy volunteers demonstrated that 7-Keto® DHEA does not activate the androgen receptor and is not converted to other androgens or estrogens in the body.[196]

## Restore Insulin Sensitivity

Restoring the function of insulin at the cellular level is paramount to combatting diseases related to chronically elevated glucose levels. Several medical strategies can help accomplish this. *Metformin* is a blood-sugar-regulating drug used to treat diabetes[197]; doses ranging from 250–850 mg 3 times daily with meals may help facilitate weight loss and promote insulin sensitivity. A physician should be consulted before a metformin regimen is initiated. Restoring youthful levels of *testosterone* may help men improve their insulin sensitivity as well.[198] In addition, a number of natural strategies may help improve insulin sensitivity.

**Chromium.** Chromium is an essential trace mineral and cofactor to insulin. Chromium enhances insulin activity and has been the subject of a number of studies assessing its effects on carbohydrate, protein, and lipid metabolism.

**Magnesium.** Magnesium is an essential trace mineral with several potential protective activities against obesity-associated diseases. Population studies suggest a relationship between low magnesium and increased risk of metabolic syndrome and diabetes,[199] and a controlled trial has demonstrated its ability to decrease fasting insulin concentrations by 2.2 µIU/mL in otherwise healthy overweight volunteers.[200] Additionally, magnesium may enhance satiety.[201]

## Inhibit the Lipase Enzyme

The lipase enzyme is responsible for facilitating the absorption of dietary fats. Taking steps to reduce the activity of the lipase enzyme may reduce the total amount of dietary fat absorbed. The pharmaceutical drug *orlistat* (Alli®, Xenical®), a lipase inhibitor, is sometimes prescribed by physicians as part of a weight management plan. In addition, the following natural intervention may help control fat absorption.

**Green tea.** Green tea is rich in powerful antioxidants called catechins. Studies have shown that green tea extracts are able to inhibit the activity of the lipase enzyme and reduce absorption of fats from the intestine.[202,203] In an animal model of obesity induced by a high-fat diet, supplementation with the green tea catechin *epigallocatechin gallate* (*EGCG*) attenuated insulin resistance and reduced cholesterol levels. Moreover, 16 weeks of treatment with EGCG mitigated increases in body weight, body fat, and visceral fat compared to no treatment. The researchers postulated that these antiobesity effects may have been conferred in part by a reduction in fat absorption, which was obviated by increased fecal lipid content in animals that received the extract.[204] Another experiment showed that EGCG reduced the incorporation of lipids into fat cells, suggesting that green tea not only combats fat absorption from the gut, but also acts at the cellular level to combat fat storage.[205] A similarly designed trial in animals showed that 17 weeks of supplementation with EGCG offset some of the metabolic effects of a high-fat, Western-style diet including body weight gain and symptoms of metabolic syndrome; it also reduced markers of inflammation. Again, these results were partly attributed to reduced fat absorption.[206] In a human trial among moderately obese subjects, 3 months of supplementation with a green tea extract standardized to catechins reduced body weight by 4.6% and waist circumference by 4.4%; study investigators also cited the ability of green tea constituents to reduce the activity of the lipase enzyme as a mechanism behind the observed metabolic benefits.[207]

## Life Extension Suggestions

### Eat to Live a Long and Healthy Life

Life Extension encourages anyone striving to lose weight to consider adopting a calorie-restricted, but nutrition-dense diet. A detailed explanation of this type of dietary pattern is presented in the Caloric Restriction protocol.

## Increase Physical Activity

Increasing physical activity is one of the most effective means of attaining a negative energy balance, which facilitates weight loss. Physical exercise should be undertaken regularly in accordance with one's overall health and mobility. Anyone with a physical impairment, such as extreme obesity or severe osteoarthritis, should consult a healthcare provider prior to embarking on an exercise regimen.

## Restore Resting Energy Expenditure

- **Green tea extract:** 725–1450 mg daily with meals
- **Fucoxanthin:** 200 mg, 3 times daily
- **Fish oil** (with olive polyphenols): providing 1400 mg EPA and 1000 mg DHA daily
- **Cayenne:** 600 mg once or twice daily with meals

## Restore Healthy Adipocyte (Fat Cell) Signaling

- *Irvingia gabonensis:* 150 mg twice daily
- *Sphaeranthus indicus* and mangosteen (*Garcinia mangostana*): 800 mg daily

## Restore Brain Serotonin/Suppress Hunger Signals

- **L-tryptophan:** 500–1500 mg daily
- **Saffron extract:** 88–176 mg daily
- **Pine nut oil:** 3000–6000 mg daily

## Control Rate of Carbohydrate Absorption and Glucose Synthesis

- **Green coffee extract as GCATM** (standardized to 50% chlorogenic acid): 350 mg, 3 times daily (before meals)
- **Seaweed extracts** (from *Ascophyllum nodosum* and *Fucus vesiculosus*): 250 mg daily
- **White kidney bean extract:** 445 mg before carbohydrate containing meals
- **L-arabinose:** 550 mg before carbohydrate containing meals
- **Propolmannan:** 1000–2000 mg before meals

*Pharmaceutical support:*

- **Acarbose:** 25–100 mg before meals

## Restore Youthful Hormone Balance

- **Dehydroepiandrosterone (DHEA):** 15–25 mg daily for women; 25–75 mg daily for men (depending on blood test results)
- **7-Keto® DHEA:** 100 mg twice daily

*Pharmaceutical support:*

- **Natural (bioidentical) hormone replacement therapy** (if needed): as directed by an experienced physician
- **Thyroid hormone replacement therapy** (if needed): as directed
- **Aromatase inhibitor** (if needed; men only): 0.5 mg twice weekly until estradiol levels are between 20–30 pg/mL of blood

## Restore Insulin Sensitivity

- **Chromium:** 500–1000 mcg daily
- **Magnesium:** 160–800 mg daily

*Pharmaceutical support:*

- **Metformin:** 250–850 mg before meals (no more than 3 times daily)

## Inhibit the Lipase Enzyme

- **Green tea extract** (standardized to 98% polyphenols): 725–1450 mg daily

*Pharmaceutical support:*

- **Orlistat (Alli®, Xenical®):** 60–120 mg before meals (no more than 3 times daily)

In addition, the following *blood testing* resource may be helpful:

- Male Weight Loss Panel or Female Weight Loss Panel

## REFERENCES

References available at: www.lef.org/dpt5/ch101

# 102

# Obsessive-Compulsive Disorder (OCD)

Obsessive-compulsive disorder (OCD) is a type of anxiety disorder in which people suffer from recurrent, unwanted thoughts or ideas (obsessions); engage in repetitive, irrational behaviors or mental acts (compulsions); or both. Among people with OCD, carrying out compulsive behavior tends to ease feelings of anxiety while repressing compulsive behavior causes stress.

According to the National Institute of Mental Health, OCD affects about 2.3% of the U.S. population aged 18–54 years (ie, approximately 3.3 million Americans). An additional 1 million children and adolescents have the disorder. The condition typically begins during early childhood or adolescence and affects men and women equally.[1]

Up to two-thirds of people with OCD suffer from additional psychiatric conditions. These conditions, including depression, eating disorders, personality disorder, attention deficit disorder, and other anxiety disorders (eg, social phobia and separation anxiety disorder) can make it difficult for physicians to diagnose and treat OCD due to overlapping symptoms. Of these additional conditions, major depressive disorder appears to be the most common, affecting up to 55% of OCD patients. Bipolar disorder affects as many as 30% of OCD patients, while social phobia impacts 23%.[2,3]

There are many types of obsessions; the most common include repeat thoughts about contamination (by dirt or germs), repeat doubts (eg, whether a door is locked or an appliance left on), need for order or exactness, fear of harming someone, inappropriate or frightening sexual thoughts or imagery, and repeat thoughts of certain images, words, or sounds. In an attempt to relieve the anxiety caused by these thoughts, people with OCD may engage in compulsive behaviors such as excessive showering or hand washing, repeat checking to make sure doors are locked, rearranging objects for order or symmetry, and counting items over and over. Although adults recognize, at least sometimes, that their obsessions and compulsions are unreasonable, children with OCD typically are not capable of this same realization.[4]

There are no diagnostic tests for OCD. A clinical diagnosis of the disorder requires that the behaviors be extreme enough to interfere with everyday activities (take more than 1 hour per day) or significantly interfere with a person's relationships, health, social functioning, or occupational functioning. For example, up to 70% of people report problems with family relationships, and more than half report interference with social and work relationships.[5–8] As a result, most people with OCD struggle to rid themselves of obsessive thoughts and stop compulsive behaviors.

## DIAGNOSTIC CRITERIA FOR OCD

Based on the American Psychiatric Association's *Diagnostic and Statistical Manual of Mental Disorders*, fourth edition (DSM-IV):

A. Obsessions, as defined by the following:

- Recurrent and persistent thoughts, urges, or images that an individual perceives as inappropriate and intrusive and that are associated with distress or anxiety

- Such thoughts, urges, or images are not just excessive worries about actual problems

- Individuals make attempts to suppress or ignore these thoughts, urges, or images, or to neutralize them by engaging in other behaviors or thoughts

- Individuals recognize that the persistent thoughts, urges, or images are a product of their mind and are not imposed by an outside force

Compulsions, as defined by the following:

- Repetitive behaviors (eg, hand washing, showering, arranging) or mental acts (eg, counting, repeating words silently) that individuals feel driven to perform in response to an obsession or according to rules they feel compelled to follow rigidly

- Such behaviors or mental acts are done to prevent or reduce anxiety or to prevent the occurrence of a dreaded situation or event, even though the behaviors or mental acts are not realistically connected to the things they are designed to neutralize or prevent

B. At some point during the course of the disorder, the individual recognizes that the obsessions or compulsions are excessive or unreasonable. (This criterion does not apply to children.)

C. The obsessions or compulsions cause significant anxiety or distress, consume more than 1 hour per day, or significantly interfere with people's normal lifestyle, occupational or academic functioning, or typical relationships or social activities.

D. If another disorder is present, the nature of the individual's obsessions or compulsions is not limited to it (eg, preoccupation with food in eating disorders, hair pulling in trichotillomania, preoccupation with sexual fantasies or impulses in paraphilia, or obsessive guilt in major depressive disorder).

E. The obsessions and/or compulsions are not the direct physiologic result of a substance (eg, medication, a drug of abuse) or a general medical condition.

## ORIGINS OF OCD

Although the exact cause of OCD is unknown, a combination of environmental, cognitive, and biological factors appear to be involved. A deficiency of serotonin (a neurotransmitter in the brain that assists with the transmission of electrical messages among nerve cells) has been proposed as at least a partial explanation. Serotonin deficiency has also been implicated in anxiety, depression, and other psychiatric disorders. Various neuroimaging studies also suggest that an electrical dysfunction in certain brain regions may contribute to OCD.[9] This observation is supported by comparisons of brain activity taken by single photon emission computed tomography and positron emission tomography from healthy controls and people with OCD. Investigators have also suggested that OCD, tic disorders, or both may be caused by an autoimmune response to streptococcal bacteria in some susceptible children.[10]

Genetic factors may also play a role in the development of OCD. People with a first-degree relative (ie, parent, sibling) with OCD, for example, have a five-fold greater risk than others of developing the condition.[11] A comprehensive review of studies of twins shows that in children, genetic factors account for 45–65% of the risk of developing OCD.[12] In another study, researchers identified a gene variant that doubles a person's risk of developing OCD.[13]

## TREATMENT OF OCD

Because OCD is one of several anxiety disorders believed to be mediated by serotonin transmission, treatment often focuses on boosting levels of serotonin. A high density of serotonin receptors is located in areas of the brain involved in the mediation of fear and anxiety (eg, the hippocampus and amygdala), and stimulation of these receptors is believed to reduce activity in these neurons, thus reducing the fear response. Therefore, OCD treatment typically involves substances that support availability of serotonin, including pharmaceuticals and nutritional supplements.

Drugs currently used to treat OCD and other anxiety disorders usually fall into one of 3 categories: selective serotonin reuptake inhibitors (SSRIs), tricyclic antidepressants, and benzodiazepines. The Food and Drug Administration (FDA) has ordered that a black box warning appear on the label of all antidepressants, advising consumers that use of these drugs carries an increased risk of suicidal thoughts and behaviors in children and adolescents.

### Drugs Used to Treat OCD

**SSRIs.** SSRIs inhibit the reuptake of serotonin (5-hydroxytryptamine, or 5-HT) into nerve terminals, which allows serotonin to remain available to stimulate a large number of 5-HT receptors. This results in an elevation in mood and a reduction in anxiety symptoms. Clomipramine was the first FDA-approved SSRI for OCD. Other SSRIs, including fluoxetine, fluvoxamine, paroxetine, and sertraline, have shown similar efficacy.

Although SSRIs tend to cause fewer side effects than older antidepressants (tricyclics, for example), they are not without side effects. Some people experience nausea, diarrhea, agitation, or stomach upset when they begin taking SSRIs, but these symptoms usually disappear after a few weeks. Approximately 15–20% of patients who take SSRIs have significant insomnia, and sexual dysfunction (decreased libido, delayed or absent orgasm) is a problem for many individuals as well. Weight gain may occur in some patients.

**Tricyclic antidepressants.** Tricyclic antidepressants work by inhibiting the reuptake of norepinephrine (a neurotransmitter in the brain) and inhibiting some serotonin reuptake. Tricyclics used in the treatment of OCD include amitriptyline and clomipramine. Milder side effects may include dizziness, drowsiness, dry mouth, and weight gain, while dangerous adverse effects include cardiac arrhythmias and seizures. Tricyclic use is associated with weight gain to a much greater degree than SSRIs.

**Benzodiazepines.** Benzodiazepines are used to induce sedative, muscle-relaxant, anticonvulsant, and antianxiety effects. Benzodiazepines have largely been replaced by SSRIs in the treatment of OCD and other anxiety disorders, although are still used in some cases.

### Hormones and OCD

A number of studies have shown that people with OCD are likely to have abnormal hormone levels and that hormones may play a role in triggering or worsening OCD.[14] For instance, several research groups have noticed that women with OCD tend to experience worse symptoms during premenstrual periods, when estrogen levels are highest.[15] Estrogen is known to promote anxiety and other feelings that may exacerbate OCD. Among men, at least one case report exists of successful treatment with antiandrogenic therapy that greatly reduced the levels of sex hormones.[16]

Based on these studies, comprehensive hormone testing and correction may be warranted on an individual basis. Women who are estrogenic, or have elevated levels of estrogen, may consider progesterone therapy to balance high estrogen levels. Progesterone is known to inhibit anxiety and seizure activities in other diseases and, although it has not been tested specifically in OCD, may help reduce symptoms.[17]

Additionally, the pineal hormone melatonin is well known to induce sleep in humans. At least one study has shown that people with OCD tend to have depressed melatonin levels, along with elevated levels of the stress hormone cortisol.[18]

## Nonpharmaceutical Approaches

Other treatment approaches, including psychotherapy, exercise, and relaxation methods, can be used in addition to pharmaceutical and nutritional therapies or as treatment options if conventional medications have failed.

**Psychotherapy.** Some people with OCD have had success with specific types of behavioral therapy. One approach, called exposure and response prevention (ERP), appears to have long-lasting effects and work best in patients who are highly motivated and have a positive attitude about treatment. ERP involves having patients deliberately confront their feared object or idea, then refrain from either acting out or ritualizing to obtain relief. Compulsive hand washers, for example, may be asked to touch an object they believe is contaminated and then may be urged to avoid washing for several hours until the anxiety has decreased.

In a study, 113 patients with OCD took part in group exposure and response prevention therapy for either 7 or 12 weeks. The investigators found that improvements in obsessions, compulsions, and depression were evident in both treatment groups at the end of treatment and long-term follow-up; also, that the outcomes did not differ significantly between the two groups.[19]

To see how ERP compares to medication (clomipramine) or placebo or when combined with clomipramine, a multisite, randomized, controlled trial was conducted for 12 weeks in 122 adults with OCD. The investigators were interested in response (defined as a decrease in symptoms) or remission (minimal symptoms after treatment). At the end of treatment, there were significantly more responders and remitters in both ERP groups than in the clomipramine-alone or placebo groups. In terms of remission alone, 58% achieved it in the ERP-plus-clomipramine group, 52% in the ERP-alone group, 25% in the clomipramine-only group, and none achieved remission in the placebo group.[20]

Not all patients with OCD benefit from or tolerate the ERP approach. For them, cognitive interventions may be an option. Cognitive behavioral therapy for OCD, in which patients attempt to change their beliefs and thinking patterns, has been investigated. A study compared the efficacy of ERP therapy and cognitive-behavioral therapy in 59 patients with OCD. The patients were randomly assigned to receive ERP therapy or cognitive-behavioral therapy for 12 weeks. At post-treatment and 3-month follow-up, recovery status in both groups ranged from 58–76%, but there was no significant difference between the two groups.[21]

**Exercise.** The healing power of exercise is often touted by health care professionals, and various studies support this recommendation. In a review of 3 separate meta-analyses, investigators found that patients who participated in at least 21 minutes of daily aerobic exercise experienced a reduction in anxiety.[22] A second study noted that regular exercise may help people who suffer from OCD, phobias, and other psychiatric disorders. When the investigators examined studies of anxiety disorder and exercise dating back to 1981, they found that strength training, running, walking, and other forms of aerobic exercise help relieve mild to moderate depression and may also help treat anxiety and substance abuse.[23]

**Relaxation techniques.** Beginning in the 1970s, evidence has accumulated that relaxation techniques (eg, meditation and self-hypnosis) can reduce stress and anxiety.[24] One problem with relaxation studies is compliance and the accompanying high drop-out rates. This problem, however, does not negate the fact that meditation and other relaxation techniques, when practiced regularly, can be effective in relieving stress and producing feelings of calm.

Clinical studies and observations of experts show that yogic breathing, meditation, and good posture enhances mood, stress tolerance, well-being, and mental focus.[25] A study found a specific kundalini yoga protocol to be effective in treating OCD as well as a broad range of anxiety disorders.[26]

**Hormones.** Both men and women may consider comprehensive hormone testing to see whether they are suffering from abnormal hormone levels. If so, bioidentical hormone therapy may be recommended. For more information on bioidentical hormone testing, please see the Female Hormone Restoration or Male Hormone Restoration protocols.

# NUTRITIONAL THERAPY

While a balanced, nutrient-rich diet and adequate sleep are standard recommendations for general good health, sleep and diet are especially important for people with OCD. Certain herbs and nutritional supplements act directly on the nervous system, promoting relaxation and feelings of tranquility. Others may relax tense muscles, ease stress-related headaches, soothe gastrointestinal upset, and encourage restful sleep.

## Tryptophan

The amino acid tryptophan is a precursor to serotonin. It has been shown that serotonin-promoting tricyclic antidepressants and SSRIs are successful in treating OCD and that tryptophan is effective in the treatment of other anxiety disorders. Thus, researchers have hypothesized that tryptophan supplementation might reduce OCD symptoms while tryptophan depletion might exacerbate them.

In one study, depletion of tryptophan in patients with OCD resulted in more significant sleep disturbances (altered rapid eye movement parameters, decreased total sleep time) than experienced by healthy controls.[27] However, several other studies have shown that depletion of tryptophan has no effect on OCD or Tourette's syndrome symptoms, although some mood-lowering changes were reported.[28,29] The fact that researchers observed a different response in OCD than depression and panic disorder trials suggests that OCD treatment may depend less on the availability of serotonin and more on changes that occur further along in the synthesis of serotonin. Another possible explanation is that the tryptophan-depletion study in OCD did not introduce a challenge, as was done in the panic disorder studies and which may have triggered a relapse in symptoms.[30]

In a double-blind, placebo-controlled study, researchers found that acute tryptophan depletion caused patients to experience significantly greater subjective distress when provoked with triggering situations.[31]

## Inositol

Inositol, a nutrient related to the vitamin B complex, is necessary for the proper formation of cell membranes. Among inositol's many functions is its ability to affect nerve transmission, aid in the transportation of fats within the body, facilitate the action of various methylating agents, and play an important role in reproduction, embryogenesis, and prevention of neural tube defects (eg, spina bifida).

In a crossover trial comparing inositol supplementation to placebo, 13 patients with OCD took inositol and placebo for 12 weeks (6 weeks each). Patients experienced a significant reduction in OCD symptoms taking inositol compared with the weeks taking placebo.[32]

## St. John's Wort

St. John's wort is an herb with a history of successful treatment for depression and other psychological disorders. Its value in the treatment of OCD may lie in its ability to selectively inhibit reuptake of serotonin, thus, act as an SSRI.[33] Researchers have also hypothesized that St. John's wort reduces production of cytokines induced by substance P, a neuropeptide known to cause depression and anxiety.[34]

## N-Acetylcysteine

N-acetylcysteine (NAC) is a nutritional supplement used in the treatment of many compulsive disorders (including OCD). Researchers have found that NAC works for such hard-to-treat problems as pathologic gambling and compulsive hair-pulling (trichotillomania).[35]

## L-Theanine

L-theanine (delta-glutamylethylamide) (in green tea), despite containing caffeine, is known to have a calming effect. A study demonstrated that L-theanine may be capable of antagonizing the stimulant effects of caffeine on brain activity in a laboratory rat model.[36]

One advantage of theanine is that it readily crosses the blood-brain barrier. Research shows that this ability allows theanine to directly stimulate production of alpha brain waves, which promotes deep relaxation. In one study, for example, researchers found that 50–200 mg theanine given to volunteers resulted in the production of alpha waves within 40 minutes of ingesting the amino acid.[37]

## Life Extension Suggestions

- **L-theanine:** 100–400 mg daily
- **Inositol:** 4 g in 3 divided doses daily
- **L-tryptophan:** 500–1500 mg taken in the evening on an empty stomach
- **St. John's wort:** 300–600 mg daily
- **Melatonin:** 0.3–5 mg before bed (sometimes up to 10 mg)
- **N-acetylcysteine (NAC):** 1200–1800 mg daily

In addition, the following *blood tests* may provide helpful information:

- Female Panel
- Male Panel

## REFERENCES

References available at: www.lef.org/dpt5/ch102

# 103

# Organ Transplantation

The increased frequency of organ transplant operations over the decades has given rise to some startling statistics: 5-year survival of transplanted tissue is only 50% for lung transplants, 67% for liver transplants, and not much better for other organs.[1] These bleak statistics are attributable to the destruction of transplanted tissue by the host's (tissue recipient's) immune system, which ultimately leads to the rejection of the transplanted organ.

Despite the widespread use of immunosuppressive drugs and advancements in medical technology, the immune system remains a formidable factor in successful organ transplantation.[2]

Certain aspects of the immune system are responsible for suppressing inflammation and inhibiting transplant rejection. Important inhibitory components of the immune system are $T_{reg}$, (or T-regulatory cells). The inflammatory cytokines IL-1β, IL-2, IL-6, IL-15, IL-21, and TNF-α, by inhibiting the function of $T_{reg}$ cells and promoting the activation of cytotoxic T cells, are responsible for the intensity of the attack against the transplanted tissue by the host's immune system.[3]

New findings demonstrate that calcineurin inhibitors (CNIs), immunosuppressive drugs widely prescribed to transplant patients, fail to address an important underlying cause of transplant rejection—insufficient levels of protective $T_{reg}$ cells.

Several nutrients have been shown in peer-reviewed studies to target the specific inflammatory cytokines that are dually responsible for the stimulation of aggressive T cells and the suppression of protective $T_{reg}$ cells.

## IMMUNOLOGICAL RESPONSE TO FOREIGN TISSUE

Transplanted tissue contains molecular components of the donor's immune system, known as the major histocompatibility complex (MHC), coupled with antigen-presenting cells (APCs), which interact with the host's immune system. Donor APCs, with the help of MHCs, present peptides (sections of proteins) derived from the transplanted tissue to specialized receptors, called CB8 receptors, on certain T cells (white blood cells involved in cellular immunity) of the host. The host's T cells recognize that the peptide is foreign and begin traveling through the body in search of cells that contain this peptide.

The host's T cells are now "activated" and programmed to destroy the cells of the transplanted tissue. As the activated T cells travel, they secrete inflammatory cytokines that serve to recruit and activate additional T cells to help destroy the foreign cells. Importantly, these cytokines stimulate a particularly aggressive class of T cells, called Th17 cells, as well. This process culminates in the initiation of an inflammatory storm that triggers the host's immune system to mount a full-fledged assault against the transplanted tissue.

## INFLAMMATORY CYTOKINES AND $T_{REG}$ CELLS: PIVOTAL ROLES IN TISSUE TOLERANCE

The immune system is more than a "seek-and-destroy" mechanism. Certain aspects of the immune system are responsible for suppressing inflammation and inhibiting the tissue destruction caused by activated T cells. These inhibitory components of the immune system are known as T-regulatory, or $T_{reg}$ cells. $T_{reg}$ cells are the counterbalance to aggressive, activated T cells. Without $T_{reg}$ cells, our immune system would constantly attack our own tissue. In fact, the role of $T_{reg}$ cells in suppressing autoimmune diseases (eg, diseases in which the immune system attacks the body's own tissue, such as rheumatoid arthritis, lupus, Crohn's disease, psoriasis, etc.) has been well documented.[4]

$T_{reg}$ cells are critical to the tolerance of an *allograft* (genetically nonidentical transplant—all human transplants are allografts, unless the organ is taken from an identical twin). The more $T_{reg}$ cells present in circulation, the weaker the attack against the transplanted tissue.[5] Ironically, the same inflammatory cytokines that stimulate aggressive T cells also suppress $T_{reg}$ cells, promoting the attack against the transplanted tissue from two angles.

$T_{reg}$ cells and T cells originate in the thymus, a specialized organ located just behind the sternum, between the lungs. Here, nonfunctional *progenitor* cells develop (differentiate) into either the immunomodulatory $T_{reg}$ cells or the aggressive *cytotoxic* T cells, depending on cytokine exposure.

Exposure to high levels of the inflammatory cytokines Il-1β, IL-6, or IL-21 causes progenitor cells to develop into aggressive T cells, while exposure to sufficient levels of a highly specialized *anti-inflammatory* cytokine, called *transforming growth factor-β*

(TGFβ), induces differentiation into $T_{reg}$ cells. Significantly, it has been shown that high levels of IL-6 inhibit the ability of TGFβ to effectively induce differentiation of progenitor cells to $T_{reg}$ cells, leading to an increase in the number of allograft-destroying cytotoxic T cells..[3,6]

The roles of the inflammatory cytokines IL-1β, IL-2, IL-6, IL-15, IL-21, and TNF-α in transplant rejection have been well-studied. By inhibiting the function of $T_{reg}$ cells and promoting the activation of T cells, these cytokines are responsible for the intensity of the attack against the transplanted tissue by the host's immune system.[3]

One of the most effective strategies for modulating an overaggressive immune response against transplanted tissue is to target the specific inflammatory cytokines that are dually responsible for the stimulation of aggressive T cells and the suppression of protective $T_{reg}$ cells.

---

### WHAT YOU HAVE LEARNED SO FAR

- Organ transplantation involves surgically replacing a failing organ with a healthy organ from a donor.
- The donated organ does not contain the same DNA as the recipient of the transplant. Therefore, the recipient's immune system recognizes that the donated organ is foreign and tries to eliminate it, leading to transplant rejection.
- Multiple inflammatory cytokines, like IL-1 β, IL-2, IL-6, IL-15, IL-21, and TNF-α, stimulate cytotoxic T cells to attack the transplanted organ.
- T regulatory cells, or $T_{reg}$ cells, help to calm the attack against the transplanted tissue by suppressing the activity of cytotoxic T cells.
- The same inflammatory cytokines that stimulate the aggressive cytotoxic T cells also inhibit the action of the protective $T_{reg}$ cells, contributing to transplant rejection from two angles.
- Targeting specific inflammatory cytokines responsible for stimulating cytotoxic T cells and suppressing $T_{reg}$ cells is a rational approach to reducing the overaggressive immune response to transplanted tissue.

---

## NATURAL COMPOUNDS THAT TARGET PROINFLAMMATORY CYTOKINES INVOLVED IN TRANSPLANT IMMUNOLOGY

### Curcumin

Studies of curcumin, a principle component of the Indian spice turmeric, have identified it as a potent anti-inflammatory agent.[7] In particular, numerous studies have revealed the ability of curcumin to target several cytokines involved in transplant rejection, including IL-1, IL-2, IL-6, IL-21, and TNF-α.[8–11]

An experimental study found that curcumin, in combination with cyclosporine, significantly improved survival time in animals that received a cardiac transplant from donors with incompatible genotypes. Animals treated with curcumin and cyclosporine survived for an average of 28.5–35.6 days after receiving a transplant, compared to untreated animals, which survived an average of only 9.1 days. The effect of the combination of curcumin and cyclosporine was greater than the effect of either one alone. The authors concluded that curcumin is efficacious as a novel adjuvant for immune system modulation both in vivo and in vitro.[12]

To more closely examine the immunomodulatory effects of the spice, researchers analyzed the effects of curcumin on lymphocytes of renal transplant patients who were experiencing transplant rejection. They found that the use of curcumin dose dependently decreased interferon-alpha (an inflammatory cytokine) induction in cultures from patients experiencing acute rejection (38.3–18.3%) and those experiencing chronic rejection (40.6–12.9%), when compared with corresponding untreated cultures. Furthermore, the team also noted that curcumin was able to inhibit activation of nuclear factor kappa B (NF-κB), an inflammatory transcription factor, and inhibit proliferation of T cells, having a synergistic effect when combined with cyclosporine. The researchers concluded that curcumin was a pharmacologically safe adjuvant to be used with cyclosporine, and can effectively suppress inflammatory cytokine induction after renal transplant.[13]

Curcumin has also been shown to combat acute renal failure and related oxidative stress caused by chronic administration of cyclosporine in an animal model. Researchers administered a dose of curcumin, equivalent to roughly 145 mg for a 60-kg human, to animals, along with cyclosporine for 21 days. It was shown that curcumin markedly reduced elevated levels of thiobarbituric acid–reactive substances (markers of oxidative stress), significantly attenuated renal dysfunction, increased the levels of the antioxidant enzymes superoxide dismutase and catalase, and normalized altered renal morphology in cyclosporine-treated animals.[14]

### Fish Oil

Omega-3 fatty acids, also known for their potent anti-inflammatory properties, are capable of suppressing the inflammatory cytokines IL-1, IL-2, IL-6, IL-15, and TNF-α.[15–18]

Researchers examined the endothelial function, as measured by endothelium-dependent vasodilation, of seven cardiac transplant patients who consumed 5000 mg of EPA plus DHA daily for 3 weeks and compared the results to those of seven cardiac transplant control patients who did not receive fish oil. The researchers found that endothelium-dependent vasodilation was significantly improved in the fish oil group (+14% to +15%), while it worsened in the control group over the study period (−1 to −9%).[19]

In another study, researchers examined the effect of 6 g of fish oil taken daily for 1 month in 40 cyclosporine-treated patients who had received a transplanted kidney. It was found that fish oil–treated patients showed a significantly better recovery of renal function after a histologically confirmed rejection episode compared to control. The researchers went on to conclude that "dietary supplements with fish oil favorably influence renal function in the recovery phase following a rejection episode in cyclosporine-treated renal transplant recipients."[20]

To evaluate the perioperative safety of fish oil in a transplant population, researchers evaluated hemodynamic, biochemistry, and hematologic parameters in kidney recipients who received intravenous fish oil for 5 days postoperatively. The researchers concluded that "administration of [omega-3 fatty acids] is safe in organ donors and in kidney recipients."[21]

In 2008, researchers found that dietary fish oil significantly reduce the severity of rejection to transplanted small bowel tissue in an animal model. They also found that fish oil favorably altered the expression of several genes involved in allograft rejection, and reduced the rate of apoptosis of graft cells. They went on to conclude that "omega-3 polyunsaturated fatty acids can suppress the rejection to mucosal cells of allograft at the time of chronic rejection in small intestinal transplantation, which may be significant in increasing the surviving rate of allograft, delaying the chronic dysfunction, and prolonging the lifetime of both allograft and acceptor."[22]

Additionally, fish oil was shown to stimulate production of the very important *anti*-inflammatory cytokine transforming growth factor-β (TGFβ) and decrease the level of circulating cytotoxic T cells in pregnant women receiving 500 mg DHA and 150 mg EPA daily. Fish oil supplementation was associated with reduced production of multiple inflammatory cytokines.[23]

## Resveratrol

Studies conducted on resveratrol provide strong evidence that suggests it can help quell the cytokine storm and prolong the survival of transplanted tissue. Resveratrol has been shown to attenuate the action of the cytokines IL-1β, IL-2, IL-6, and TNF-α.[24–27]

Resveratrol, at a dose equivalent to 967 mg for a 60-kg human, was shown to significantly increase survival time of animals that received a genetically incompatible liver transplant. Furthermore, resveratrol also reduced levels of cytotoxic T cells.[28]

In a skin graft model, used to study transplant rejection, rats supplemented with relatively small doses of resveratrol, equivalent to approximately 5 mg for a 60-kg human, had notable prolongation of the time period before their skin grafts were rejected. Only approximately 20% of the allografts in the control group survived >9 days postoperation, compared to 100% of the grafts in the group receiving resveratrol. The researchers noted that resveratrol significantly reduced infiltration of T cells and necrosis in graft tissue.[29]

## Green and Black Tea Polyphenols

Compounds in green and black tea have been identified as particularly powerful anti-inflammatory agents.[30] Studies have shown that components of tea are potent inhibitors of IL-1β, Il-2, IL-6, and TNF-α.[31–34]

Cardiovascular health is a major concern for transplant recipients, especially because cyclosporine, an immunosuppressive drug widely used after organ transplantation, is known to impair endothelial function.[35]

Black tea consumption was shown to dramatically improve endothelial function, as measured by flow-mediated vasodilation and brachial artery diameter, in a study of renal transplant patients aged 25–50 years. The researchers went on to conclude that "based on our study, short-term consumption of black tea may improve endothelial function and endothelium-dependent arterial vasodilation in renal transplant recipients."[36]

## Quercetin

The flavonoid quercetin is found in significant quantities in apples, onions, grapes, and citrus fruits. Quercetin is known to modulate the action of several inflammatory cytokines that are of particular concern to transplant recipients, including IL-1β, IL-2, IL-6, IL-15, and TNF-α.[37–41]

Quercetin, in combination with vitamin E, has also been shown in vitro to combat the hepatotoxic effects of cyclosporine. Researchers found that the combination attenuated cyclosporine induced oxidative stress by restoring the activity of the antioxidative enzymes glutathione peroxidase and catalase.

They concluded that "our data demonstrates that vitamin E and quercetin play a protective role against the imbalance elicited by cyclosporine between the production of free radicals and antioxidant defence systems, and suggests that a combination of these two antioxidants may find clinical application where cellular damage is a consequence of reactive oxygen species."[42]

Considering the cytokine suppressive effects of quercetin, a team of researchers evaluated the impact of quercetin on the proliferation of T cells. The team found that quercetin significantly inhibited T-cell proliferation, suggesting that it may be effective in reducing transplant rejection. They concluded that the "results suggest the potential use of these select phytochemicals for treating autoimmune and transplant patients..."[43]

## Vitamin D

Published studies in recent years have revealed an astonishing number of benefits attributable to vitamin D. Among these benefits, modulating the activity of multiple inflammatory cytokines is especially important in the context of organ transplantation.

Researchers recently discovered that vitamin D was able to prevent a cyclosporine mediated increase in the inflammatory cytokines IL-1β, IL-6, and TNF-α in an animal model.[44] Vitamin D, in combination with cyclosporine, significantly reduced production of IL-2 and the proliferation of T cells, and vastly prolonged allograft survival in an animal model of liver transplantation. The authors of this study went on to conclude that vitamin D is effective as an adjunct to immunosuppressive therapy for the prevention and treatment of liver graft rejection.[45]

A very important 2009 study shed light on just how critical vitamin D supplementation is for transplant recipients. Researchers examined the relationship between blood levels of the active form of vitamin D (1,25-dihydroxy vitamin D) and 1-year mortality rates of heart transplant patients.

They found that "one-year mortality was 3.7 per 100 person-years in the tertile with the highest 1,25-dihydroxy vitamin D concentrations, 13.2 per 100 person-years in the intermediate tertile and 32.1 per 100 person-years in the tertile with the lowest 1,25-dihydroxy vitamin D concentrations." This means that the mortality rate was over 8 times *higher* at 1 year post-transplant in the group with the *lowest* one-third blood levels of active vitamin D compared to the group with the *highest* one-third levels of active vitamin D. The researchers also found that higher blood levels of vitamin D were associated with lower levels of the inflammatory marker C-reactive protein, as well as the cytokine TNF-α.[46]

# THE TH17:T_REG RATIO: A LIMITATION OF IMMUNOSUPPRESSIVE PHARMACEUTICAL DRUGS

The ratio of a particularly aggressive subclass of T cells, called Th17 cells, to $T_{reg}$ cells is highly reflective of the tendency of the immune system to react aggressively toward transplanted tissue.

It is known that $T_{reg}$ cells have *anti-inflammatory* properties and cause quiescence of an overaggressive immune response and prolongation of transplant function. Furthermore, Th17 cells are *proinflammatory* and can exacerbate the immune response in transplant rejection.[6,47,48]

In October 2010, researchers confirmed that decreasing the Th17:$T_{reg}$ resulted in increased allograft survival in an animal model. The team administered TGFβ directly to mice that had received transplants of pancreatic islet cells. Administering TGFβ resulted in a decrease in IL-6 activity and number of Th17 cells in circulation, and an increase in circulating $T_{reg}$ cells, prolonging allograft survival time. The researchers concluded that targeting IL-6 activity and lowering the Th17:$T_{reg}$ ratio "provides a promising approach for inducing transplant tolerance..."[49]

Incorporating this recent understanding of immune tolerance and inflammatory pathology, researchers examined the impact of calcineurin inhibitors (CNIs) on the level of allograft protecting $T_{reg}$ cells circulating in 32 liver transplant recipients. Their study revealed that CNIs significantly *reduced* the level of $T_{reg}$ cells in circulation, compared to healthy control patients not receiving a CNI. The data led the team to conclude that CNIs hampered progression toward a tolerance-inducing Th17:$T_{reg}$ profile.[50]

These new findings demonstrate that the most commonly prescribed immunosuppressive drugs in transplant patients fail to address an important underlying cause of transplant rejection—insufficient levels of protective $T_{reg}$ cells.

# GRAPE SEED EXTRACT FAVORABLY ALTERS THE TH17:T_REG RATIO

An October 2010 study revealed that a proanthocyanidin-rich grape seed extract is highly effective in reducing the ratio of Th17:$T_{reg}$ and modulating an overaggressive immune response. Researchers observed that grape seed extract favorably altered the

Th17:T$_{reg}$ ratio in both animal (murine) and human cell lines.[51]

In taking their research a step further, the scientists examined the effect of grape seed extract on the clinical symptoms of mice with collagen-induced arthritis, a model highly sensitive to the Th17:T$_{reg}$ ratio. They found that grape seed extract effectively attenuated clinical symptoms, confirming that the extract was a potent immunomodulator. The authors concluded that "by potently regulating inflammatory T-cell differentiation, grape seed extract may serve as a possible novel therapeutic agent for inflammatory and autoimmune diseases."

Another study showed that dietary supplementation with blueberry extract (also high in proanthocyanidins) was highly effective in prolonging the survival of transplanted dopamine neurons, which are exceptionally delicate, in an animal model of Parkinson's disease. The researchers also noted that the mice receiving blueberry extract exhibited better mobility and coordination than did the control group, which was not receiving blueberry extract.[52]

# TARGETING RESIDUAL EFFECTS OF ORGAN TRANSPLANTATION AND SIDE EFFECTS OF IMMUNOSUPPRESSIVE PHARMACEUTICAL DRUGS

Avoiding tissue rejection is not the only challenge facing transplant recipients. Many other complications frequently arise as a result of receiving a transplant and taking immunosuppressive drugs.

In nearly all transplant cases, the vasculature of the transplanted organ functions less optimally than that of the host's native tissue. This often leads to cardiovascular complications, such as blood clots and hypertension.[53,54] It is vitally important that the health and function of the endothelial cells (cells that line the inside of blood vessels) in recipients of an organ transplant be maintained.

## Controlling Homocysteine

Maintaining a low level of homocysteine is very important for transplant patients. Homocysteine is an amino acid derivative that damages endothelial cells and contributes to the pathogenesis of atherosclerosis.

A study published in October 2010 found that higher homocysteine was a predictor of death from any cause in 378 renal transplant recipients, even after the researchers adjusted for multiple confounding factors. Subjects with the lowest one-third homocysteine

level (<13.1 µmol/L) were much more likely to be alive 3000 days post-transplant than those with the highest one-third homocysteine levels (>18.5 µmol/L). The researchers also noted that subjects taking a CNI had higher levels of homocysteine than subjects not taking a CNI (mean 16.3 µmol/L vs. 14.3 µmol/L), suggesting that CNIs, like cyclosporine, might raise homocysteine.[55]

Fortunately, there are several nutraceutical ingredients that have been shown to effectively control homocysteine in transplant patients.

## B6, B12, and 5-Methyltetrahydrofolate

In evaluating 98 renal transplant patients, researchers found that, not only were high levels of homocysteine correlated with chronic allograft dysfunction, but intake of vitamin B6, as well as higher blood levels of the active form of folate, 5-methyltetrahydrofolate, were associated with lower levels of homocysteine and improved vascular health. The researchers noted that "increased folate and vitamin B6 intakes seem to reduce homocysteine concentrations among transplant patients...and could contribute to reducing the risk of chronic allograft dysfunction."[56]

In 56 renal transplant recipients, the combination of 50 mg B6, 400 mcg B12, and 5 mg folic acid daily, for 6 months, was found to significantly *reduce* levels of homocysteine (from 21.8 µmol/L to 9.3 µmol/L vs. no change in the placebo group) and carotid intima-media thickness, a marker of atherosclerosis (from 0.95 mm to 0.64 mm, average 32% reduction) while the placebo group showed a marked *increase* in carotid intima-media thickness (from 0.71 mm to 0.87 mm) over the trial period.[57]

A study of 730 renal transplant patients provided unique insight into the importance of vitamin B12 and active folate in this population. Researchers in this study noted that higher levels of plasma B12 and active folate are likely associated with a survival advantage seen in kidney transplant patients who have a genetic predisposition to having higher levels of these vitamins in circulation.[58]

## N-Acetyl Cysteine

The antioxidant N-acetyl cysteine, especially in combination with B vitamins, has been shown to lower homocysteine levels and improve endothelial function.[59]

In 12 children who received liver transplants, intravenous infusions of N-acetyl cysteine (70 mg/kg), in combination with prostaglandin-E1, were administered daily for 6 days starting immediately postoperation. The combination reduced the severity of rejection episodes within the first 3 months after the transplant, compared to a control group who did not receive infusions.[60]

Intravenous N-acetyl cysteine (5 g over 4 hours) was shown to dramatically reduce levels of homocysteine (from 15.5 μmol/L to 3.36 μmol/L) in 11 renal transplant patients with healthy levels of B12 and folate. The team reported no adverse effects attributable to N-acetyl cysteine. This study highlights both the safety and efficacy of N-acetyl cysteine in renal transplant patients.[61]

An animal model of cyclosporine-induced kidney toxicity found that N-acetyl cysteine was protective against the nephrotoxic effects of cyclosporine. Animals receiving cyclosporine alone showed significant increases in oxidative stress, as measured by levels of the reactive species nitric oxide and malondialdehyde, significant decreases in superoxide dismutase and glutathione peroxidase activity and notable kidney morphologic changes, while animals receiving N-acetyl cysteine with cyclosporine did not manifest these changes.[62]

In an in vitro study conducted on cells taken from lung transplant recipients, N-acetyl cysteine was able to reduce the genetic expression of the inflammatory cytokine TNF-α, which contributes to transplant rejection. The authors concluded that "the therapeutic use of antioxidant compounds could, therefore, be of interest in conditions such as lung transplantation, in which oxidative stress and inflammation can contribute significantly to the loss of allograft function."[63]

## Cocoa and Pomegranate Polyphenols

Researchers, in double-blind, placebo controlled fashion, examined the impact of polyphenols derived from cocoa on the vascular health of 22 heart transplant recipients. Researchers evaluated endothelial function, as measured by endothelium-dependent coronary vasomotion and coronary artery diameter, 2 hours after subjects consumed 40 g of dark chocolate, providing 15.6 mg of polyphenols. Cocoa polyphenols were found to significantly increase coronary artery diameter (from 2.36–2.51 mm) and improve coronary vasomotion (+4.5% vs. –4.3% in placebo group). Furthermore, the researchers also saw a significant reduction in platelet adhesion in the polyphenol group (from 4.9% to 3.8%), compared to no change in the placebo group, indicating a decreased risk of blood clot formation and hypertension.[64]

Polyphenols from pomegranate, also known to support endothelial function,[65] were administered to animals at a dose equivalent to approximately 500 mg for a 60-kg human for 21 days. Researchers found that pomegranate polyphenols significantly reduced cyclosporine-induced hepatic oxidative stress, as measured by levels of thiobarbituric acid–reactive substances and activity of the antioxidative enzymes glutathione-S-transferase, superoxide dismutase, and catalase. The team concluded that "the results of this study indicate that [pomegranate polyphenols] might play an important role in protecting [against] cyclosporine-induced oxidative damage in the liver."[66]

## CoQ10

Daily supplementation with 90 mg of CoQ10 for 4 weeks resulted in significant improvements in cardiovascular health, as measured by HDL, LDL, and total cholesterol levels, in 11 renal transplant patients. Furthermore, the researchers found that CoQ10 did not adversely affect blood levels of cyclosporine, highlighting the safety of CoQ10 in transplant patients taking cyclosporine.[67] These data suggest that CoQ10 could safely combat the side effects of cyclosporine, which is known to cause oxidative damage and unfavorably alter cholesterol levels.[68]

## Vitamins C and E

A double-blind trial examining the effect of supplementation with a combination of 500 mg vitamin C and 400 IU vitamin E, twice daily, showed that the vitamins slowed the progression of coronary arteriosclerosis in heart transplant patients. Over a period of 1 year, patients receiving vitamins C and E (n = 19) experienced no increase in average intima-media index, while patients receiving a placebo (n = 21) saw an 8% increase.[69]

In a randomized, placebo-controlled fashion, researchers studied the effects of 2000 mg of vitamin C on the vascular function of 13 renal transplant patients. They found that vitamin C significantly improved endothelium-dependent dilation (1.6–4.5%), and also enhanced the antioxidant capacity of the subject's blood, as measured by the time required to oxidize lipids in vitro.[70]

The widely prescribed immunosuppressive drug, cyclosporine, is known to cause oxidative damage, and is associated with an unhealthy lipid profile.[68] Vitamin E was effective in reducing cyclosporine-induced mitochondrial damage to porcine renal endothelial cells,[71] and, in combination with quercetin, was shown to be protective against hepatotoxicity caused by cyclosporine, as measured by the level of thiobarbituric acid-reacting substances, and activity of glutathione peroxidase and catalase, in an animal model.[42]

It is important to note that, in at least one study, the combination of vitamins C and E was shown to reduce blood levels of cyclosporine by roughly 30% in heart transplant recipients who were taking 500 mg vitamin C twice daily and 400 IU vitamin E twice daily. These researchers went on to state that "although more detailed pharmacokinetic analysis is necessary to clarify the exact mechanism of this interaction, physicians who take care of transplant recipients should be aware that more frequent cyclosporine concentration monitoring is warranted after initiating these anti-oxidant agents."[72]

## L-Arginine

The amino acid L-arginine has been shown in multiple studies to improve the function of endothelial cells.[73,74]

A 2010 study of 22 heart transplant patients found that supplemental L-arginine, 6 g twice daily, improved endothelial function, as measured by the nitric oxide to endothelin ratio, and increased submaximal exercise capacity, as measured by a 6-minute walk test (distance walked increased from 525 m to 580 m). Significantly, the researchers also noted that supplemental L-arginine improved subjects' overall quality of life score, as measured by standardized questionnaire.[75]

## Probiotics

A study of 777 liver transplant recipients found that surgical site infection occurred in 37.8% of patients. These infections resulted in, on average, roughly 24 additional days of hospital stay, $159 967 in extra expenses, and a 10% increase in mortality.[76] Furthermore, postoperative infections have been associated with a significantly higher incidence of graft loss due to rejection.[77]

A randomized, placebo-controlled trial of 95 liver transplant recipients examined the effects of probiotics (10 billion colony-forming units), in combination with fiber, on postoperative infection rates. The researchers found that infection occurred in only 13% of the patients receiving probiotics and fiber, while in the control group 48% of patients developed infections.[78]

In order to duplicate these impressive results, the same lead researcher conducted another similar study shortly thereafter. This time the team studied the effect of probiotics, in combination with fiber, against fiber alone, on postoperative infection rates in 66 liver transplant recipients. The group receiving the combination of probiotics and fiber had an infection rate of only 3%, while in the group receiving solely fiber, postoperative infection occurred in 48% of the patients.[79]

## Magnesium

Magnesium wasting is common in transplant patients, especially those who receive a transplanted kidney.[80]

Low levels of magnesium have been shown to potentiate the toxic effects of cyclosporine and reduce allograft survival.[81]

In a study of 14 hypomagnesemic renal transplant patients, magnesium supplementation at a dose of 400–1200 mg daily for 3 months, was shown to significantly improve total and LDL cholesterol levels, glucose metabolism, and restore levels of magnesium. The researchers concluded that magnesium replenishment was effective for combating magnesium wasting and important for maintaining the health of renal transplant patients.[82]

---

### WHAT YOU NEED TO KNOW

- The overaggressive immune response against transplanted tissue results in very poor 5-year survival rates for transplanted organs.
- Targeting specific inflammatory cytokines, like IL-1 β, IL-2, IL-6, IL-15, IL-21, and TNF-α, which impair the activity of protective $T_{reg}$ cells and stimulate cytotoxic T cells, is a rational approach to calming the overaggressive immune response and supporting healthy function of transplanted tissue.
- Several nutrients target these inflammatory cytokines and favorably alter the ratio of highly aggressive Th17 cells to transplant-protecting $T_{reg}$ cells.
- The most widely prescribed immunosuppressive drugs to transplant patients, calcineurin inhibitors, fail to promote the activity of protective $T_{reg}$ cells and have been shown to be highly toxic.
- Many nutrients safely address the residual effects of organ transplantation such as infection, poor endothelial function and aggressive atherosclerosis, and combat side effects of immunosuppressive drugs.

---

### SUMMARY

Organ transplantation offers individuals with critically injured or failing organs a means to improve the quality of their lives and extend their life span. However, receiving a transplanted organ comes with many challenges.

Because a donated organ does not contain the DNA of the tissue recipient, the immune system of the host recognizes the transplanted organ as pathologic and attempts to eliminate it. This ongoing battle between the donated tissue and the host's immune system ultimately results in the destruction of the transplanted tissue. Thus, recipients of a transplant must take side-effect–laden immunosuppressive drugs in order to preserve the transplanted organ for as long as possible.

Life Extension has identified multiple nutraceuticals, which, based on peer-reviewed scientific evidence, target specific aspects of the immune response involved in tissue rejection, as well as help combat side effects of immunosuppressive drugs.

## Life Extension Suggestions

- **Curcumin:** 400 mg daily
- **Fish oil:** 4000–6000 mg daily
- *Trans*-**resveratrol:** 250–500 mg daily
- **Tea polyphenols:** 725 mg daily
- **Quercetin:** 250–500 mg daily
- **Vitamin D3:** 5000 IU daily
- **High proanthocyanidin grape seed extract:** 100 mg daily
- **Standardized pomegranate extract:** 500 mg daily
- **Vitamin B6** (as pyridoxal 5'-phosphate): 100 mg daily
- **Vitamin B12** (as methylcobalamin): 1000–5000 mcg daily
- **Folate** (as 5-methyltetrahydrofolate): 1000 mcg daily
- **N-acetyl cysteine:** 600–1200 mg daily
- **CoQ10** (as ubiquinol): 100 mg daily
- **Vitamin C:** 1000–2000 mg daily
- **Gamma tocopherol vitamin E:** 350 mg daily
- **L-arginine:** 2000–6000 mg daily
- **Probiotics:** Per label instructions
- **Magnesium:** 500 mg daily

In addition, the following blood testing resources may be helpful:

- Vitamin D, 25-Hydroxy
- Cytokine Panel
- Vitamin B12 and Folate
- Homocysteine
- RBC Magnesium
- Coenzyme Q10 (CoQ10)

---

## SAFETY CONSIDERATIONS

- Consult with your physician before you begin taking any dietary supplements.
- Avoid grapefruit juice and St. John's wort; both alter the rate at which your body metabolizes immunosuppressive drugs, and can significantly alter levels of these drugs in your system due to their ability to interact with drug metabolizing CYP450 enzymes. A study found that 250 mL of grapefruit juice increased blood concentrations of cyclosporine roughly 25%. In another study, St. John's wort decreased concentrations of cyclosporine by 46%.[83,84]
- A combination of 500 mg of vitamin C and 400 IU of vitamin E was shown, in one study, to decrease blood levels of cyclosporine.[72] Based on these data, patients contemplating supplemental vitamin C and E, at these dosages, should have blood concentrations of cyclosporine checked on a regular basis.
- A study reported that supplemental colostrum caused a 71-year-old man, who was 7 years post–liver transplant, to develop severe allograft rejection, requiring hospitalization.[85] Based on this evidence, avoiding supplemental colostrum is suggested if you have had an organ transplant.

---

## REFERENCES

References available at: www.lef.org/dpt5/ch103

# 104

# *Osteoporosis*

Osteoporosis, defined as a reduction of bone mass or bone density, was long viewed as a disease unique to aging women, and has been treated primarily with conjugated equine estrogens (CEEs) in hopes of mitigating the decline in endogenous female hormone levels that occurs during menopause.[1,2] Sadly, much of what conventional wisdom held true about osteoporosis turns out to be flawed; it is now clear that osteoporosis (like many age-related conditions) is not a disease with a singular cause affecting a specific population. Rather, it is a multifaceted disease driven by a barrage of interrelated factors, and must be addressed as such for optimal prevention and treatment.[3]

Today we realize that osteoporosis not only impacts the lives of women, but of men as well; fully one third of those affected by the condition are males (about 2.8 million of them as of 2011), and that number is likely to grow as the population ages.[4–6] Indeed, one out of every four men will sustain an osteoporotic fracture during their lifetime.[7] Conventional physicians have been slow to recognize the prevalence of osteoporosis in men; as a result the diagnosis is often delayed even more than it is in women, allowing the disease to progress to an advanced stage before it is detected.[8]

Scientific advancements have revealed that the etiology of osteoporosis stems not only from hormonal imbalances, but oxidative stress, elevated blood sugar, inflammation, and components of the metabolic syndrome as well.[3,8–10]

Overlooked by mainstream medicine is the critical role that micronutrients play in bone health. For instance, emergent research on vitamin K has attracted great scientific interest through the revelation of its involvement, along with vitamin D, in both bone health and atherosclerosis, a condition to which osteoporosis is intimately related.[11,12] In fact, these two conditions can be thought of as mirror images of one another.[13,14] Osteoporosis is characterized by loss of calcium from bones, shifting them from their healthy hard state to a diseased state of softness. Atherosclerosis, on the other hand, is characterized by excessive influx of calcium into arterial walls, shifting them from their healthy flexible state to a diseased state of hardness. Insufficiency of vitamin K contributes to this unhealthy balance.

Similarly underappreciated contributors to bone loss in both men and women are advanced glycation end products (AGEs); byproducts of high blood sugar. AGEs interact with proteins in bone causing impaired mineralization and increases in the number of osteoclasts—bone resorbing cells. Moreover, AGEs encourage vascular calcification by activating a specialized receptor called RAGE, which recruits calcium into vascular smooth muscle cells, leading to hardening of the arteries. This relationship between elevated blood sugar, osteoporosis, and atherosclerosis comprises a vicious cycle linking the conditions in a manner unknown to the majority of mainstream physicians.[10,15–17]

Pharmaceuticals, such as Actonel® or Fosamax®, have shown limited success and are associated with some potentially serious side effects including atrial fibrillation and osteonecrosis of the jaw.[18,19] These drugs work chiefly by inhibiting the cells responsible for breaking down bone tissue, but neglect multiple other factors responsible for osteoporosis.[20,21] Although these drugs do increase bone density, the fact that they disrupt the natural cycle of regeneration and resorption—which is important for bone strength—is poorly appreciated.[22]

An integrative approach, based on the human body's finely tuned relationship with its environment and the nutrients that support bone health, makes much more sense.[8,23] This realization has led to an awakening to the tremendous potential of nutrient and mineral supplements along with hormonal optimization in the prevention and management of osteoporosis. The myriad complexities of osteoporosis necessitate the need to integrate pharmaceutical, nutritional, and lifestyle interventions in order to maintain bone health into advancing age.

## THE TRUTH ABOUT OSTEOPOROSIS: MULTIPLE CAUSES, MULTIPLE TARGETS

Most of us assume that bones are like pieces of rocks or hard shells. However, bone is a living tissue, constantly undergoing demolition and renewal as it responds to changing forces in the environment.[24,25] Bone is also the body's primary reservoir of the calcium needed for a wide variety of biological processes.[26] Bone is now recognized as an endocrine organ, secreting compounds that function like hormones throughout the body.[27]

Bones are made of crystals of calcium salts in a protein matrix. Specific cells, called osteoblasts, produce the matrix and attract calcium compounds to form new bone, while a different set of cells, called osteoclasts,

Normal Bone Architecture

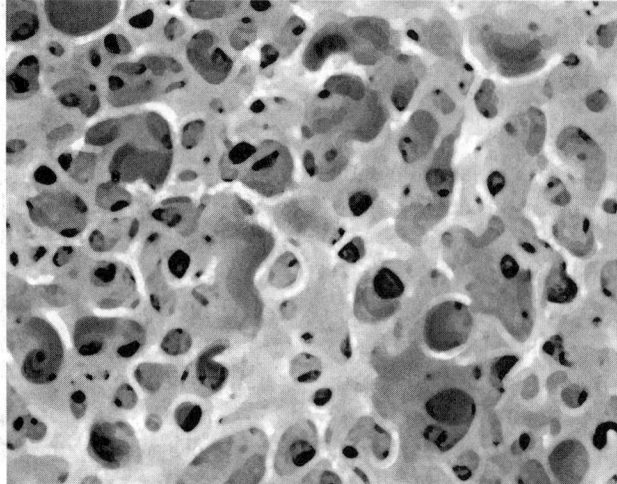

Osteoporotic Bone Architecture

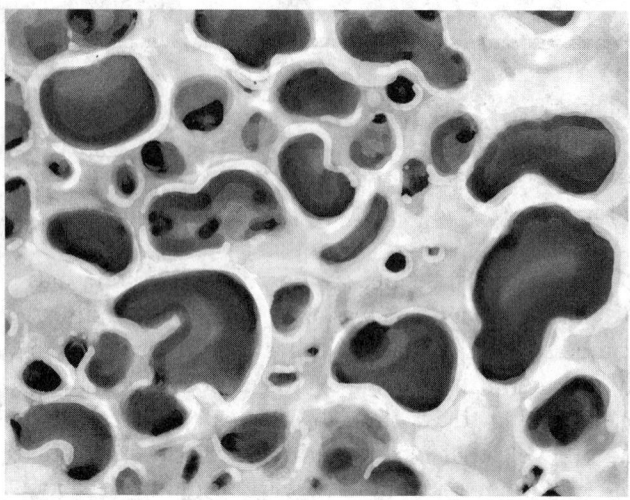

resorbs the bone tissue to allow new shapes and structures to form in response to gravity and the pull of muscles. This process of remodeling helps repair microdamage that occurs as a result of daily activity and prevents the accumulation of old fragile bone.[24,25,28]

At the simplest level, osteoporosis occurs when more bone is resorbed than formed.[29,30] There are multiple causes for osteoporosis including suboptimal nutrition, age-related hormonal imbalance, and lack of weight-bearing exercise, to name a few.[25]

**Sedentary Lifestyle.** Perhaps the earliest contributing lifestyle factor is lack of weight-bearing exercise, as many as 20% of young and middle aged women already have an abnormal spinal curvature related to bone loss in their vertebrae, a situation that only gets worse as one ages.[31,32] A sedentary lifestyle reduces the constant forces that bone needs to experience in order to continue its normal process of remodeling.[33] Studies show that both women and men who engage in regular exercise have much lower risk of osteoporosis and fracture.[34,35]

**Vital Hormones.** Estrogen and testosterone, among others, are hormones that promote bone formation and regulate bone resorption. When these hormone levels drop, osteoporosis can occur. At puberty, bone production increases dramatically, producing the growth spurt of the early teen years. This effect seems to be driven mostly by estrogens, the "female" hormones, in both boys and girls.[36,37] Near the end of puberty, androgens, the "male" hormones, increase in both women and men. The androgen surge fuses the bone growth plates, with the result being that the bones can no longer elongate. Young adults generally maintain a steady-state balance in which new bone formation is nearly equal to bone resorption.

Sex hormones also remain at roughly steady levels throughout young adulthood and early middle age.[37] After about the age of 35, however, the total amount of bone in the body begins to diminish. In women, the process begins fairly sharply with the onset of menopause, when estrogen levels drop dramatically. In postmenopausal women, bone is lost both from the inner and outer surfaces of bones, as bone resorption by osteoclasts exceeds the already reduced new bone formation by osteoblasts. In men, however, new bone formation on the outer surface of bone keeps pace with resorption on the inner surface for much longer.[38] This obvious connection probably accounts for the fact that osteoporosis was thought for so long to be a problem unique to women, and may account for the fact that men begin to suffer fractures from osteoporosis about a decade later than women,[39] but similar factors are involved.[40]

The discovery that primary control of bone mineralization in both men and women is mediated by estrogens not only enhances our understanding of how osteoporosis occurs in men, but also has dramatic implications for how we can prevent and treat it.[36]

**Sex Hormone-Binding Globulin.** Sex hormone-binding globulin (SHBG), a protein produced primarily in the liver, serves to bind estrogen and testosterone.[41] It has long been known that declining estrogen levels in both sexes are significant contributors to bone mineral loss with aging. Experts now recognize that the steady rise in SHBG with aging is directly correlated with bone loss and osteoporosis in both men and women.[42,43] As a general rule the higher the SHBG level, the *less* estrogen is available to contribute favorably to bone health.

Evidence indicates that the SHBG molecule itself plays another key role in the body, as it conveys essential signals to the heart, brain, bone, and adipose (fat) tissue that ensure their optimal function.[44] There is even a special SHBG receptor molecule on cell surfaces that functions much like the ubiquitous vitamin D receptor protein, helping cells communicate with one another.[45,46] In other words, SHBG itself functions much like a hormone.

New studies are finding a direct role for SHBG and its cell surface receptor in bone loss.[47] The association is so strong that some experts are now suggesting routine measurement of SHBG as a useful new marker for predicting severity of osteoporosis.[47]

**Insulin Resistance, Blood Sugar, and Glycation.** Bone functions as an endocrine organ secreting compounds that act like hormones.[27] Healthy production of bone matrix protein increases insulin sensitivity in other tissues.[27,48] Conversely, people with the metabolic syndrome who are insulin resistant have poorer bone quality and an increased risk of osteoporotic fracture.[49,50] Metabolic syndrome also raises SHBG levels, further reducing bioavailable levels of estrogen and testosterone.[51]

Research suggests that advanced glycation end products, or AGEs, are implicated in bone loss. AGEs are formed when proteins interact with glucose molecules to form damaged structures in the body. One study examined the proteins in osteoporotic bones to determine if there was damage by AGEs. More AGEs present resulted in fewer bone-building osteoblasts.[52] It is suggested that limiting AGE formation by maintaining a healthy blood sugar level may slow the osteoporotic process.[53]

**Oxidation and Inflammation.** Oxidation of fatty acids and other molecules produces reactive oxygen species that directly and indirectly impair new bone formation and promote excessive bone resorption.[54,55] In a similar fashion, chronic inflammation hastens the absorption of existing bone while impeding normal production of new bone.[30] Fat cells produce a steady efflux of inflammatory cytokines while diminishing cells' insulin sensitivity; both factors further impede normal bone production.[56,57]

**Vitamin K.** For healthy, mineral-rich bone to form, healthy bone matrix protein must be produced.[58,59] Over the past decade scientists have realized that vitamin K is an essential co-factor for production of the major bone protein, osteocalcin.[58,60] Vitamin K–dependent enzymes produce changes in osteocalcin that allow it to tightly bind to the calcium compounds that give bone its incredible strength.[58,59,61]

**Calcium and Vitamin D.** Many other environmental and nutritional factors contribute to the gradual development of osteoporosis. The role of low intake of vitamin D and calcium are well known.[62,63] Adequate calcium intake is required to allow healthy bone remodeling and prevent osteoporosis. Vitamin D promotes intestinal absorption of calcium, and also regulates how much calcium enters and leaves bone tissue in response to the body's other calcium requirements.

**Trace Minerals.** While bone is primarily composed of matrix protein and calcium compounds, small amounts of other trace minerals are essential for normal bone function. These include magnesium, which regulates calcium transport; silicon, which reverses loss of calcium in the urine; and boron, which interacts with other minerals and vitamins and also has anti-inflammatory effects.[64–69]

The conventional model of osteoporosis predicts that simple restoration of declining sex hormone levels and provision of modest amounts of calcium and vitamin D should be sufficient to prevent osteoporosis. When those steps fail (which they inevitably do), conventional medicine resorts to suggesting that osteoporosis must be an inevitable consequence of aging.

Life Extension's position, however, is much more nuanced and incorporates the truth about the complex, interrelated factors that genuinely contribute to osteoporosis. Life Extension recommends a lifelong commitment to an active lifestyle, and supplementation with targeted vitamins, minerals and nutrients that quench reactive oxygen species (ROS), reduce inflammation, control obesity and insulin resistance, promote healthy bone matrix protein synthesis, and supply sufficient trace minerals to support healthy bone.

## RISK FACTORS FOR OSTEOPOROSIS

The risk factors for osteoporosis, like those for all chronic, multifactorial conditions, are many, and they interact with one another. Here is a summary of those we understand best, and that we can take steps to incorporate in prevention strategies.

**Gender.** Women are more likely to develop osteoporosis than men. This difference is related to several reasons including: the abrupt loss of estrogen at menopause, women start with a lower bone density and lose bone more quickly than men and women live longer than men.

**Age.** Increasing age is associated with falling production of estrogen and testosterone, which increases osteoporosis risk. Levels of sex hormone–binding globulin (SHBG) rise with age, binding to the sex hormones and reducing their total bioavailable levels, which further aggravates bone loss. Advancing age also means longer total exposure to chronic oxidant stress and inflammation, both of which contribute to development of osteoporosis.[55,56,70,71]

**Ethnicity.** Caucasian and South Asian people have greater risk of osteoporosis.[72,73]

**Family History.** A family history of hip fracture carries a two-fold increased risk of fracture among descendants.[74]

**Estrogen Exposure.** Women with late puberty or early menopause are at higher risk due to a decrease in estrogen exposure over their lifetime.[75,76]

**Vertigo.** Several recent studies have shown an association between "benign positional vertigo" (BPV) and lower bone mineral density.[75,77,78] The inner ear, where balance is maintained, contains tiny bone particles (otoconia) that may be affected in osteoporosis.[75] Some experts recommend that people with BPV should undergo screening for osteoporosis.[77]

**Slim Stature (Underweight).** People with a body mass index of ≤19 or small body frames tend to have a higher risk because they may have less bone mass to draw from as they age.[79]

**Obesity.** Increased body fat was long thought to be protective against osteoporosis.[80] Accumulating evidence, however, suggests that obesity-related components such as insulin resistance, hypertension, increased triglycerides, and reduced high-density lipoprotein cholesterol are all risk factors for low bone mineral density.[80,81]

**Cardiovascular Disease.** Cardiovascular disease and mortality are associated with osteoporosis and bone fractures.[11] That's not surprising since the two conditions share many mechanisms and risk factors, such as oxidant damage and inflammation.[11,82]

**Chronic Stress and Depression.** Both condition increase cortisol production, leading to suppression of sex hormone production, increased insulin resistance, and enhanced release of inflammatory cytokines.[83–85] All of these effects increase the risk of bone mineral loss and osteoporosis.[85–88]

**Other Risk Factors.** Included here are HIV infection,[89] anorexia,[90] cancer,[91,92] smoking,[93] caffeine,[94,95] and alcoholism.[96]

**Medication Use.** A variety of medications increase one's risk for osteoporosis, including the following:

- *Corticosteroids.* These immune-suppressive drugs mimic the effect of stress-induced cortisol, with all of its suppression of sex hormones, weight gain, and insulin resistance.

- *Selective Serotonin Reuptake Inhibitors (SSRIs).* Both depression and medications used in its treatment, such as SSRIs, increase the risk of osteoporosis.[86]

- *"Blood Thinning" Medications (Anticoagulants).* The drug Coumadin, used to prevent clot formation in patients with cardiovascular disease, acts to block the beneficial effects of vitamin K and is associated with decreased bone mineralization in some patients.[97] Low molecular weight heparin, an unrelated blood thinner, can also cause reduced bone mineral content.[61]

# SYMPTOMS AND DIAGNOSTIC TESTS

Anyone who is losing height with age may have osteoporosis, unfortunately, osteoporosis typically has no symptoms at all until a serious fracture occurs, usually from a relatively minor injury.[98,99] All the while, however, the disease is actually progressing, which is why early prevention is so important.[5] Diagnosis and treatment are often substantially delayed, especially in men, because the concept of male osteoporosis is still unfamiliar to many practitioners as well as patients.[5]

In women, the "dowager's hump" that is classically associated with the disease is actually also a late finding, caused by gradual collapse of the front portion of the bones of the spinal column.[32] It is predictive of decreased mobility in subsequent years.[100] Once fractures are evident, of course, they are associated with symptoms such as pain and immobility. If the hip is fractured, patients are often bedridden for weeks or months, putting them at major risk of pneumonia and blood clots. Hip fracture continues to be a leading cause of death in older adults.[72]

The current gold standard for diagnosis of osteoporosis, the so-called DEXA scan, uses dual energy x-ray absorptiometry to determine the relative bone mineral content.[101] The DEXA test is most commonly used because there are more DEXA testing devices in doctors' offices than the more advanced quantitative computed tomography (QCT), another x-ray–based apparatus for determining bone mineral density. However, studies suggest that the QCT test is much more sensitive.[102]

In one clinical study, osteoporosis was present in 63% of men at the time of diagnosis of prostate cancer, prior to any therapy. In this landmark paper, the investigators evaluated DEXA bone mineral density testing and compared it to QCT bone mineral density testing in the same patients. A significantly greater percentage of men were found to have osteoporosis by the QCT methodology than by means of the DEXA approach. DEXA bone mineral density evaluation detected osteoporosis in only 5% of men, whereas with QCT technology, 63% of men were diagnosed with osteoporosis. Using QCT technology, bone density abnormalities (osteopenia and osteoporosis) were found in 95% of men, compared to 34% of men evaluated with DEXA.[102]

Although QCT testing exposes patients to more radiation than DEXA does, the amount of radiation associated with QCT for determining bone density is roughly equivalent to that of a dental series and is approximately 50% that of a mammogram (depending on the technique used). Most important, QCT generates far less radiation exposure—orders of magnitude less than a contrast-enhanced abdominal CT scan.

The results of bone density testing are given in T-scores. These scores are developed by comparing the person being tested to a young adult of the same gender between 25 and 45 years of age. A T-score of −2.5 or lower indicates high fracture risk, or a 60% chance of fracturing a hip. For every decrease of 1 in T-score, there is a two-fold increase in risk of fracture. Individuals with a T-score of −1.1 to −2.5 are diagnosed with osteopenia, or mild bone loss. Results are also given as Z scores, which measures individual results against people of the same age, gender, and race.

DEXA and QCT scans require specialized equipment, keeping them from more widespread use in rural areas. As a result, a variety of predictive scales and scores are being developed that have similar predictive accuracy at substantially less cost. The ultrasonometric scanner,[103] Osteoporosis Prescreening Risk Assessment tool (OPERA),[104] and Osteoporosis Self-Assessment Tool (OST)[105] are a few examples.

The problem, however, with using any of these modalities is that they are useless until substantial bone mineral loss has already occurred (because they rely on measuring that loss). In most people these findings occur only after years of progressive exposure to the chronic, underlying causes of osteoporosis, such as oxidant stress, inflammation, insulin resistance, and insufficiency or deficiency of vitamins D and K.

# CONVENTIONAL TREATMENTS AND ASSOCIATED RISKS

**HRT (Hormone Replacement Therapy).** For many years, while osteoporosis was thought of as primarily a disease of post-menopausal women, treatment included conventional hormone replacement therapy (HRT) using conjugated equine estrogen (CEE) and the synthetic progestogen medroxyprogesterone acetate (MPA). Early termination of the large Women's Health Initiative trial in 2002 revealed the dramatic faults in that approach, demonstrating increased rates of breast cancer and heart attack risk in women using conventional HRT.[106,107] As a result, conventional HRT fell out of favor, because of risks associated with stroke, heart disease, and some types of cancer.

In an effort to recoup some of the beneficial effects of conventional HRT, drug companies have brought out a new class of single-targeted drugs called selective estrogen receptor modifiers, or SERMs. These drugs mimic the beneficial effects of estrogen on bone density in postmenopausal women.[108,109] Raloxifene is an example of this drug class, approved for women with osteoporosis, not men. SERMs theoretically should reduce both osteoporosis and breast cancer. While they show some promise, these drugs remain expensive and associated with side effects such as blood clots, hot flashes, and leg cramps.[110]

Life Extension suggests that women talk to their doctor about bioidentical hormone replacement instead; for details, see the Female Hormone Restoration Protocol.

**Testosterone Treatment.** When a man has osteoporosis because of low testosterone production, testosterone treatment may be recommended. The positive effects of testosterone on lumbar bone density in men were consistent.[111,112] A common misconception is that testosterone administration necessarily increases the risk of prostate cancer, in a causal fashion similar to the risk of HRT and breast cancer in women. However, a careful review of the medical literature reveals otherwise. For example, in a landmark review article published in the *New England Journal of Medicine*, the authors report *"there appears to be no compelling evidence at present to suggest that men with higher testosterone levels are at greater risk of prostate cancer or that treating men who have hypogonadism [low testosterone] with exogenous androgens increases this risk."*[113] However, since testosterone stimulates cell growth in androgen-responsive tissues, it may accelerate the growth of existing prostate cancer. Cancer-screening tests such as a PSA test are necessary before replacement therapy. Testosterone replacement therapy is contraindicated in men with active prostate cancer.[114]

**Bisphosphonates.** Bisphosphonate drugs (Actonel® and Fosamax®) are chemical mimetics of one of the mineral components of bone structure, and they help prevent bone density loss.[115] What many people do not know is that bisphosphonate focus on limiting additional bone loss, rather than building more bone. When taken up by osteoclasts, the bisphosphonates impair those cells' ability to resorb bone minerals.[115] The result is an increase in bone mineral density, but since the remodeling process is reduced, the bone may accumulate microdamage and after prolonged use can result in atypical fractures.[22,38]

Most recently, bisphosphonate drugs have been found to increase oxidant stress in the liver, as well as expression of components of the inflammatory system involving NF-κB, a critical inflammation-regulator.[116,117] That may imply that these drugs are aggravating inflammation, one of the fundamental underlying processes that contribute to osteoporosis, while superficially treating only the end result.

Few studies in this drug class have actually followed patients for >5 years, yet bisphosphonate drugs are generally considered safe by the conventional medical community.[22,38] Oral bisphosphonates can cause upset stomach, inflammation, erosion of the esophagus, and intravenous bisphosphonates have been associated with influenza-like illness.[118] More serious, rare side effects include a condition called osteonecrosis of the jaw, and an increase in atrial fibrillation, a heart rhythm disturbance.[18,19]

Reports of osteonecrosis of the jaw (ONJ) secondary to bisphosphonate (BP) therapy indicated that patients receiving BP orally were at a negligible risk of developing ONJ compared with patients receiving BPs intravenously; a landmark study of 208 patients who had taken alendronate, 70 mg once per week for 1–10 years, 9 (4%) developed jaw bone osteonecrosis. None of more than 13,500 dental patients who had not taken alendronate developed jaw bone osteonecrosis.[119] In patients taking bisphosphonates, 3–5% developed atrial fibrillation and 1–2% developed serious atrial fibrillation, with complications including hospitalization or death.[120]

There is also some evidence that prolonged treatment (more than 5 years) with bisphosphonates is associated with increased risk for esophageal cancer.[121] Experts currently advise a critical reassessment of bone density and the risk versus benefit of bisphosphonate therapy after 3-5 years of use.[122]

**Calcitonin.** Calcitonin is a hormone made by the thyroid gland, which inhibits the cells that break down bone. An intranasal salmon calcitonin (50–200 IU/day) plus oral calcium supplements was administered for 1 to 5 years to postmenopausal women for prevention of osteoporosis. The results showed bone mineral density of the lumbar spine increased by approximately 1–3% from baseline. In contrast, postmenopausal women receiving only oral calcium supplements typically had reductions in bone mineral density about 3–6%.[122]

A newly developed oral formulation of salmon calcitonin provides increased efficacy on bone based on Phase I and II clinical trials data, as compared with the nasal formulation.[123]

**Stem Cell Therapy.** Mesenchymal stem cells are easily obtainable from bone marrow by means of minimally invasive approach and can be expanded in culture and permitted to differentiate into the desired lineage. Experimental investigations of the clinical application of the adult bone marrow derived mesenchymal stem cells with bioactive molecules, growth factors have become promising.[124] A case report of mesenchymal stem cells, when percutaneously injected into knees, resulted in significant cartilage growth, decreased pain and increased joint mobility in the patient.[125]

Another study investigated the effects of systemic transplantation of human adipose-derived stem cells (hASCs) in ovariectomized mice. hASCs induced an increased number of both osteoblasts and osteoclasts in bone tissue and thereby prevented bone loss.[126]

Scientists believe that stem cells could halt osteoporosis, and promote bone growth as well as new pathways that control bone remodeling.[127]

**Calcium and Vitamin D.** These supplements may help older patients lower their risk of hip fractures (details in prevention protocol). Most people in North America, however, lack sufficient sunlight exposure to produce adequate amounts of vitamin D, so vitamin D insufficiency is widespread.[115]

---

## WHAT YOU NEED TO KNOW

- Osteoporosis is a condition in which healthy bone is lost through decreased new bone formation and increased resorption of existing bone.
- Osteoporosis was long thought to result simply from age-related reductions in sex hormones, primarily estrogen. As a result osteoporosis was only considered a disease of postmenopausal women.
- Life Extension recognizes that osteoporosis is in fact the ultimate consequence of a host of modifiable factors that accumulate over time, including chronic oxidant stress, inflammation, insulin resistance and obesity, chronic life stress that increases cortisol secretion, and nutritional deficiencies or insufficiencies of a host of vitamins, minerals and other compounds.
- As a result, Life Extension recommends a multitargeted approach to osteoporosis prevention, one that includes regular resistance exercise, weight loss, stress reduction, hormone restoration, and strategic use of nutritional supplements to restore or maintain a more youthful body milieu.
- Life Extension's supplement regimen goes beyond the simple recommendations for calcium and vitamin D provided by conventional medicine, adding supplements that

promote healthy bone protein formation, and those that reduce inflammation, protect against oxidant stress, and supply adequate amounts of trace and ultra-trace minerals.

# OSTEOPOROSIS PREVENTION AND TREATMENT PROTOCOL

In contrast with conventional medicine's reactive, after-the-fact approach to osteoporosis, Life Extension recommends a comprehensive, integrative strategy to address all of the underlying causes and exacerbating factors involved in osteoporosis. Like most chronic conditions, prevention of osteoporosis is a much better choice than treatment.

**Bioidentical Hormone Replacement Therapy.** Considering the importance of estrogen, progesterone and testosterone on bone health, Life Extension urges its members to regularly obtain a complete hormone profile. Conventional hormone replacement therapy (Premarin® and Provera®) provides hormones that are unnatural to the human body. Bioidentical hormones, on the other hand, have the same exact molecular structure as the hormones produced naturally within the body. As a result, bio-identical hormones are properly utilized, and are then able to be naturally metabolized and excreted from the body. The use of bioidentical HRT has increased during the last several years as women have sought a more natural approach to restoring hormonal balance. Generally overlooked by mainstream medicine are research findings suggesting that women may more safely benefit from individualized doses of natural estrogens and progesterone.

Estriol (a type of bioidentical estrogen), has been documented for increasing bone mineral density. A Japanese study involving 75 postmenopausal women found that after 50 weeks of treatment with 2 mg/day of estriol cyclically and 800 mg/day of calcium lactate, women had an increase in bone mineral density with no increased risk of endometrial hyperplasia (uterine tissue overgrowth that may precede cancer).[128] In a second study emanating from Japan, researchers treated postmenopausal and elderly women with 2 mg/day of estriol and 1000 mg/day of calcium lactate versus 1000 mg/day calcium lactate alone. Bone mineral density significantly increased in women who received estriol, while the women who did not take estriol experienced a decrease in bone mineral density.[129]

Similar research has confirmed these findings. In this investigation, 25 postmenopausal women were given either 2 mg/day of estriol plus 2 g/day of calcium lactate, or 2 g/day of calcium lactate alone for one year. Bone mineral density was significantly reduced in the group that received calcium alone (without estriol). In contrast, the group that received estriol plus calcium experienced a 1.66% increase in bone mineral density after one year. Furthermore, biochemical markers of bone resorption were significantly decreased in the estriol group. "*These data indicate that the acceleration of bone turnover usually observed after menopause was prevented by treatment with E3 [estriol],*" the authors of this study noted.[129]

A 2009 study compared the effects of conventional hormone replacement (conjugated equine estrogens and medroxyprogesterone) to that of estriol in 34 postmenopausal women. After 1 year of treatment, bone mineral density and lipids were measured. In both groups bone mineral density showed improvement however, women taking conventional HRT had an increase in triglycerides that was not seen in the women taking bioidentical estriol. The authors concluded that estriol might be an efficacious alternative to conventional HRT.[130]

Given the degree of evidence, maturing women should understand that bioidentical hormone replacement, when appropriately prescribed, offers an alternative to conventional hormone replacement to help relieve menopausal symptoms and optimize bone density, and that accumulating evidence suggests that bioidentical hormone replacement appears to offer advantages over conventional hormone replacement therapy.

Hormonal *balance* is critical for maintaining optimal bone metabolism and overall health. In addition to restoring estrogen, testosterone, and progesterone levels to youthful ranges, DHEA levels should also be maintained. DHEA is a hormone that is active throughout the body; it also serves as a precursor to testosterone and estrogen. Indeed, some evidence suggests that DHEA supplementation may support bone health in aging women.[131,132]

For more information on bioidentical hormone replacement, see the Female Hormone Restoration protocol.

**Isoflavones.** Isoflavones, chiefly derived from soybeans, chemically resemble estrogen; as a result they are often referred to as phytoestrogens—literally, plant estrogens.[133] Following the worrisome safety issues associated with the Women's Health Initiative showing increased cancer risk in women on synthetic hormone replacement therapy (HRT), there has been dramatically increased interest in phytoestrogens as an alternative.

The primary soy isoflavones (in order of abundance) are genistein, daidzein, and glycitein; all three have confirmed phytoestrogenic effects.[134] Genistein and daidzein have been shown in animal and human studies to contribute to increased bone mineralization and bone strength, while reducing bone resorption.[135-139] A 2002 study showed that genistein supplementation (54 mg/day) reduced urinary markers of bone turnover in a fashion similar to conventional HRT.[133] The same study demonstrated increased serum markers of bone protein formation in genistein recipients; HRT recipients actually showed decreased levels of those proteins. And animal studies show that genistein reduces bone resorption by a mechanism different from the bisphosphonate drugs and estrogen.[140] Finally, the phytoestrogen isoflavones have substantial anti-inflammatory effect, adding to their ability to break the chain of events that contribute to osteoporosis.[141]

Concerns have been raised about the possible effects of phytoestrogens on breast cancer risk, given their biochemical similarity to estrogen.[142] Long-term studies, however, have demonstrated no increased risk of cancer or precancerous changes in women taking 54 mg/day of genistein.[142] In fact, "*consumption of genistein in the diet has been linked to decreased rates of metastatic cancer in a number of population-based studies. Extensive investigations have been performed to determine the molecular mechanisms underlying genistein's antimetastatic activity, with results indicating that this small molecule has significant inhibitory activity at nearly every step of the metastatic cascade.*"[143]

A total daily isoflavone dose of about 54–110 mg for preventing loss of bone mineral content and reducing markers of bone resorption appears reasonable based upon the literature.[135,144,145]

**Vitamin K.** Vitamin K regulates several biochemical processes that require exquisite balance to function normally, including blood coagulation, bone mineralization and vascular health. Through diverse actions vitamin K holds promise in helping to prevent and manage some of the most crippling conditions associated with advancing age, including osteoporosis, coronary artery disease, and blood clots.

Vitamin K is an essential co-factor for building the protein matrix that traps calcium crystals in bone.[146,147] Like vitamin D, vitamin K is also essential for preventing calcium accumulation in arterial walls.[148] People with lower levels of vitamin K are at increased risk for calcification of major arteries.[148] Vitamin K also reduces activity of bone-resorbing cells by decreasing levels of inflammation regulating complexes.[149] Low vitamin K status and use of warfarin-like anticoagulants (which antagonize the action of vitamin K by undermining a process called carboxylation) are associated with low bone mineral density and increased fracture risk.[61,150] Vitamin K2 supplementation

(1500 mcg/day) has been shown to accelerate proper bone protein formation.[151]

Vitamin K comes in two main forms: K1 (phylloquinone) and K2 (menatetrenone, or M4). Vitamin K2 has been shown to support bone health when used as a supplement in humans.[150,152,153]

Vitamin K2 supplementation reduces the amount of circulating bone protein, a measure of inadequate bone formation.[154,155] Supplementation also increases bone mineral content and bone strength at many different body sites, although DEXA scans may or may not show improvement in bone mineral density.[156] K2 supplementation added to bisphosphonate drug therapy brings further benefit to both bone mineral density and bone protein.[157]

Some individuals with osteoporosis who may benefit from supplementation with vitamin K are also taking warfarin, and so avoid vitamin K because they are concerned that it might interfere with their anticoagulant therapy. However, low-dose vitamin K (100 mcg daily) has been shown to help stabilize the INR (clotting time) of patients on anticoagulant therapy in a small trial.[158] In fact, emergent research suggests that some the beneficial effects of vitamin K2 for promoting bone mineral density may be entirely unrelated to vitamin K-dependent carboxylation, and resistant to the antagonistic effects of warfarin.[157,160] Individuals on anticoagulant therapy who are interested in supplementing with vitamin K should discuss low-dose vitamin K with their physicians.

**Vitamin D.** Along with calcium, vitamin D is the nutrient that most people recognize as important for bone health.[161] But, even today, few people understand the powerful and complex ways that vitamin D acts to promote not only bone health, but the way the entire body handles calcium, both in healthy and in undesirable ways.[162] Vitamin D triggers absorption of calcium from the intestine and deposition of calcium in bone—and also removal of calcium from blood vessel walls. Conversely, insufficient vitamin D intake results in depletion of calcium from bones—and increased deposition of calcium in arterial walls, contributing to atherosclerosis.[163,164]

Vitamin D deficiency (or insufficiency) also causes muscle weakness and neurologic deficits, increasing the risk of falling, which of course makes fractures still more likely.[165-167] The dose of vitamin D required to achieve the neuroprotective and other non–bone-related effects are substantially higher than those required simply to achieve good calcium absorption.[168]

A validated measure of total body vitamin D status in blood is serum 25-hydroxy vitamin D (also known as 25(OH)D, or calcidiol). This measure is reported in two different units, nanomoles per liter (nmol/L) and nanograms per milliliter (ng/mL), so it is vital to check which set of units a lab is using. Vitamin D deficiency is defined as a serum 25(OH)D level of <20 ng/mL. Experts recommend a higher level of 75 nmol/L, or 30 ng/mL.[165,168] To obtain the many health benefits of Vitamin D, current scientific evidence suggests a minimum target threshold for optimal health is over 50 ng/mL or 125 nmol/L.[169–171]

The optimal dose of vitamin D has been hotly debated in recent years. More than 13 000 Life Extension® members have had their vitamin D level checked. The results from these tests provides important information about achieved vitamin D blood levels in a large group of dedicated, health-focused individuals. Vitamin D dosage as high as 5000–8000 IU per day may be required to achieve a minimum target level for optimal health in aging individuals.[172]

A new study in the journal *Anticancer Research* echoed Life Extension's recommendation, noting that traditional intakes of the essential vitamin just are not enough.[173] In a news release, the author stated, *"We found that daily intakes of vitamin D by adults in the range of 4,000 to 8,000 IU [international units] are needed to maintain blood levels of vitamin D metabolites in the range needed to reduce by about half the risk of several diseases—breast cancer, colon cancer, multiple sclerosis and type 1 diabetes."*

**Calcium.** Calcium is the predominant mineral in bone, and crystals of calcium compounds give bone its hardness and strength. Most Americans do not meet the daily adequate intake for calcium, so supplementation is generally recommended.[174] Calcium supplementation also suppresses bone resorption, further fighting osteoporotic changes.[175] Large trials of calcium supplementation, with and without vitamin D, have shown mixed results at preventing osteoporosis, but closer examination of those studies has revealed that many of the patients who got no benefit did not take the supplements regularly.[63,176,177]

Individuals at high risk or who have been diagnosed with osteoporosis may need to consume up to 1200 mg/day. Calcium supplements are available in many forms. For optimal absorption and convenience of dosing, use a combination of dicalcium malate (DimaCal®), calcium glycinate chelate (TRAACS®), and calcium fructoborate. Calcium citrate is also a water-soluble form and can be taken at any time; it is the supplement of choice for people with suppressed gastric acid secretion, such as those taking antacids and proton pump inhibitors.[174]

**Strontium.** Strontium is chemically akin to calcium, and is taken up by bone cells in an identical fashion.[178,179] Strontium ranelate, approved in Europe for postmenopausal osteoporosis,[180] is the first antiosteoporotic medicine that has dual mode of action, simultaneously increasing bone formation and decreasing bone resorption, thus rebalancing bone turnover formation.[178,181,182] Strontium ranelate 2 g daily has been well studied in postmenopausal women with osteoporosis,[183–185] significant reductions of up to 43% in the risk of hip fractures were observed over a period of 5 years.[184]

Strontium ranelate has fewer gastrointestinal side effects than bisphosphonates.[186] A pooled Phase 3 study did note a slightly increased risk of blood clot;[187] therefore antithrombotic agents like low-dose aspirin, fish oil, and aged garlic extract should be taken daily if strontium is being used to rebuild bone mass. Those on anticoagulant or antiplatelet therapy should alert their doctor if they are using strontium. A recent report associated strontium with a form of drug reaction with severe skin breakdown.[188]

Strontium ranelate has yet to be approved by the Food and Drug Administration (FDA) in the United States, however several salts of strontium such as strontium citrate or strontium carbonate are available as dietary supplements, providing close to the recommended strontium element content of strontium ranelate. Little clinical data exist to suggest that other salts of strontium will have the same effects. Despite the lack of clinical evidence, other salts of supplemental strontium are theorized to promote bone health since the cation (strontium element) is responsible for the pharmacologic effect of strontium ranelate.[189]

Worth noting, strontium is not an essential mineral (has no known physiological function in human body), dietary strontium is estimated at 2–4 mg/day from vegetables and grains,[190] and the estimated whole-body strontium content of an average (70 kg) human is 320 mg.[191] Furthermore, the uptake of heavier strontium in place of calcium into bone matrix results in a false increase in bone density as assessed by DEXA scanning, making further follow-up of bone density by DEXA harder to interpret.[185] Therefore, the pharmacological dose strontium supplements should be reserved for those with significant loss of bone density, and those on supplemental strontium should alert their physicians prior to a bone density test.[185,192]

**Magnesium.** Magnesium is an important micronutrient that regulates active calcium transport in humans, and is therefore important in bone health.[64] Older adults tend to be magnesium deficient because of diminished dietary intake and absorption coupled with increased urinary losses.[193] Chronically elevated stress hormone levels also contribute to depressed magnesium levels.[193] Together these effects conspire to damage bone health.

Magnesium supplementation in both animal and human studies reduces bone turnover, tending to favor bone formation over bone resorption.[64] The resulting improved bone mineralization contributes to a reduction in fracture frequency.[194]

**Boron.** Boron is an ultra-trace element that has been discovered to be essential for bone health.[195] Its primary effect seems to be its interactions with more prevalent minerals such as calcium and magnesium, but it also has independent anti-inflammatory effects that may contribute to its usefulness.[96]

In human studies boron deficiency caused changes in calcium metabolism that resemble those seen in osteoporosis, and which were exacerbated by low magnesium levels.[197] Animal studies show that boron supplementation stimulates bone formation and inhibits bone resorption.[198]

A daily dose of 3–9 mg of boron from calcium fructoborate, a boron-based supplement that also has antioxidant and anti-inflammatory actions, is reasonable for bone health based on the scientific literature.[69,196]

**Silica.** Silicon is one of the most abundant elements in the Earth's crust. It has few known biological functions, but recently silica (silicon dioxide) has been discovered to play an important role in bone formation and health.[67] Silicon deficiency in animals results in bone defects.[199]

Supplementation with organic silicon compounds, on the other hand, improves bone mineral density and prevents bone loss.[199,200] A human study demonstrated that the addition of organic silicon to a calcium and vitamin D3 regimen improved production of bone proteins.[68]

**Collagen.** Researchers are now discovering the vital importance of collagen for achieving optimal bone tensile strength. Collagen, a resilient type of protein molecule, makes up most of the structure of bone.[201] The spongy matrix of collagen fibers and crystalline salts within bone is crucial to absorbing compression forces to resist stress fractures, much as the tensile supports of steel bridges provide flexibility so that the bridge can withstand gale force winds and heavy traffic.

Scientists developed a new form of calcium that molecularly binds collagen. This unique form of collagen calcium chelate is designed to enhance collagen support and turnover while increasing bone mineral density and bone strength.[202]

Scientists at Tokyo University found that supplementation with collagen calcium chelate improved bone strength to a greater extent than the same amounts of calcium and collagen either given separately or together but in a nonchelated form. Specific improvements with collagen calcium chelate were seen not only in bone mineral density but just as importantly in femur (thigh bone) weight, bone collagen production, and bone flexibility and strength.

In an experimental model of osteoporosis, the test group received a low-calcium diet for one week. In addition to their low-calcium diet, some of the test group consumed a high-dose collagen calcium chelate. The cohort receiving high-dose collagen calcium chelate had an increase in femur bone weight by an impressive 9.6%, compared with the group given the same amount of calcium in nonchelated form. The test group receiving the collagen calcium chelate had dose-dependent increases in bone mineral density, which were 3.5–11.1% higher than those seen in the group receiving the same amount of nonchelated calcium. The investigators concluded that collagen calcium chelate had an additive effect on bone mineral density, better than that of calcium alone or of a simple calcium and collagen mixture.[202]

Collagen calcium chelate was also associated with increases in femur bone strength, by about 9.9–25%, compared with the group receiving the same amount of calcium.[202] Remarkably, the benefits of collagen calcium chelate were evident after only 8 weeks of supplementation. Given these encouraging results, a large clinical study is currently underway, in collaboration with the U.S. Army, to look at the effect of collagen calcium chelate on bone fractures in hard-training recruits.

**Antioxidant Vitamins.** Oxidant stress, particularly that imposed by oxidized LDL-cholesterol, is a significant contributor to bone loss in osteoporosis.[203,204] Some bisphosphonate drugs may themselves actually increase oxidant damage as well.[203] Antioxidant vitamins and other supplements, therefore, have an important role in prevention.[205,206]

The antioxidant vitamins C and E play important roles in production of proteins, development of bone-forming cells, and bone mineralization.[203,207] Vitamin C also suppresses activity of bone-resorbing cells while promoting maturation of bone-forming cells.[208] Vitamin E improves bone structure, contributing to stronger bone.[209]

Women with higher vitamin C intake have significantly better bone mineral density, so long as their calcium intake is also above 500 mg/day.[207] Postmenopausal women who took 600 mg vitamin E and 1000 mg vitamin C daily achieved stable bone mineral density compared with placebo recipients, whose density dropped over a 6-month period.[205] Similar doses of both vitamins were useful in preventing bone loss in elderly men and women.[71]

Daily doses of 1000 mg vitamin C and 600 mg of vitamin E (as mixed tocopherols) are reasonable for osteoporosis prevention; alpha-tocopherol alone is likely to be ineffective.[71,204,205,210] A recent study investigated the bone anabolic effects of Vitamin E in rats and for the first time reported that gamma isomer improves all the parameters of bone biomechanical strength, while alpha tocopherols only improved some of the parameters.[209]

**Omega-3 Fatty Acids (Fish and Flax Oils).** The omega-3 fatty acids found in fish oil (EPA and DHA) and flax oil (ALA) have powerful anti-inflammatory and antioxidant effects.[211–213] That makes them ideal candidates for inclusion in an antiosteoporosis regimen, given the role of inflammation in osteoporosis.[211] EPA and DHA also reduce activity of bone-resorbing cells, increase that of bone-forming cells, and improve calcium balance.[213]

Men and women who consume higher amounts of oily fish (tuna, mackerel, salmon, etc) have greater bone mineral density than do those with lower fish consumption.[214] Animal studies have shown increased bone mineral content and strength in animals supplemented with fish oils or the omega-3 fatty acids EPA and DHA, as well as the flax seed oil–derived ALA.[215–219] Intriguingly, fish oil plus soy isoflavone supplementation resulted in a higher weight-bearing capacity of lumbar vertebra.[216]

EPA and DHA have specific antiresorption effects on bone cells in culture, and also stimulate differentiation and activity of bone-forming cells.[220,221] Increased dietary intake of omega-3s in animals protects against bone loss by downregulating the important NF-κB inflammation-controlling complex.[212] In human studies, supplementation with EPA (omega-3) and GLA (gamma-linolenic acid, a beneficial omega-6), along with 600 mg/day of calcium, maintained spine and hip bone mineral density over 18 months, while in placebo recipients bone density fell significantly.[222] Fish oil supplements containing a total of 2.7 g/day of EPA and DHA reduced inflammatory cytokine production in humans.[211] And daily 900 mg/day of mixed omega-3 fatty acids decreased bone resorption in postmenopausal women with osteoporosis.[223]

**Curcumin.** Curcumin is a bioactive component of the Indian spice turmeric.[224] It has powerful antioxidant and anti-inflammatory actions, particularly by reducing the gene expression of the master inflammation-regulatory complex NF-κB.[224,225]

Lab studies show that curcumin decreases activity of bone-resorbing cells by reducing NF-κB expression.[225] Animal studies reveal multiple beneficial effects of curcumin on bone mineral content and structure.[226] Curcumin improves bone mineral density in rat models of postmenopausal osteoporosis, and increases bone strength.[227]

**Resveratrol.** Resveratrol is a powerful phytoalexin molecule produced by plants, especially grape vines and Japanese knotweed, for protection against oxidant stress and pathogens.[228] As the chief health-promoting component of red wine, it has achieved prominence for its ability to mimic the beneficial effects of calorie restriction on many genes that contribute to longevity and health.[229] Among the genes that resveratrol modulates are several that are crucial for bone health.

Certain stem cells can differentiate into either fat or bone tissue, depending on how their genes are regulated. Resveratrol activates genes that tip the cells to develop into bone forming cells, and suppresses those that would create fat cells.[228,230–232] Resveratrol also prevents inflammation-induced maturation of bone resorbing cells.[233] In animal studies, resveratrol supplementation results in increased bone mineral density and reduced bone resorption.[234]

**Quercetin.** Quercetin is a plant polyphenol found in a wide variety of fruits. It is a powerful antioxidant and a mild phytoestrogen as well.[235,236] Quercetin directly stimulates the differentiation and activity of bone-forming cells in laboratory studies.[237,238] It also reduces activity of bone-resorbing cells through its down-regulation of inflammation.[236]

Quercetin recently was shown to enhance activity of the vitamin D receptor in intestinal cells, which in turn helps in proper regulation of calcium metabolism.[239] Together these effects provide support for the observation that quercetin supplementation in experimental models inhibits bone loss following induced menopause.[240]

**Berberine.** Berberine is a plant alkaloid used extensively in ancient Chinese and Japanese medicine for use in promoting bone health.[241,242] Animal and laboratory studies reveal that berberine prevents decrease in bone mineral density by inhibiting the activities of bone-resorbing cells.[241] Used as a dietary supplement in experimental models, berberine resulted in an increase in bone mineral density.[243] Berberine also increases differentiation of bone-forming cells through activation of cellular signaling pathways.[244,245]

**Hops.** Hops is an herb best known for producing the typical bitter flavor of beer, and has long been known to have health benefits.[246] The active ingredients in hops have multiple biological effects, particularly in their ability to act as selective estrogen receptor modulators (SERMs). In this capacity, hops extracts may boost beneficial estrogen effects without triggering estrogen-related outcomes such as breast cancer.[247] Among their benefits are positive effects on bone mineral density and prevention of osteoporosis.[248] Hops extracts increase gene expression and differentiation of bone-forming cells in laboratory studies.[247]

## Life Extension Suggestions

- **Calcium:** 1000–1200 mg daily
- **Vitamin D:** 2000–8000 IU daily; individualize dosing based on results of Vitamin D testing
- **Magnesium:** 200–1000 mg daily
- **Vitamin K:** 2100 mcg of vitamin K as 1000 mcg K1 and 1100 mcg K2 (as MK-4 and MK-7)
- **Silica:** 5–10 mg daily
- **Boron:** 3–9 mg daily
- **Zinc:** 15–30 mg daily
- **Calcium collagen chelate:** 3000 mg daily
- **Omega-3 fatty acids:** 1400 mg EPA and 1000 mg DHA daily
- **Curcumin:** 400 mg daily
- **Resveratrol:** 250 mg daily
- **Quercetin:** 250 mg daily
- **Berberine:** 25 mg daily from 250 mg goldenseal

The following hormone-related supplements may be considered.

- **DHEA:** 15–50 mg daily, depending on blood test results
- **Isoflavones:** 52–104 mg daily
- **Hops:** 120 mg daily

**Bioidentical hormone replacement therapy** may also be considered.

Hormone blood testing is important when considering bioidentical hormone replacement therapy. For more information on hormone testing, call 1-800-226-2370.

In addition, the following blood testing resources may be helpful:

- Female Comprehensive Hormone Panel/Male Comprehensive Hormone Panel or Female Panel/Male Panel
- Vitamin D, 25-Hydroxy
- Insulin (fasting)
- Deoxypyridinoline (DPD) Cross Link Urine Test or Osteocalcin

## REFERENCES

References available at: www.lef.org/dpt5/ch104

# 105

# Pain (Chronic)

**Table 1:** *Classification of Pain and Examples*

| Classification of Pain | Examples |
|---|---|
| Severity | Mild, Moderate, or Severe |
| Duration | Acute or Chronic |
| Location | Lower back, Abdomen, or Head |
| Origin | Nociceptive or Neuropathic |
| Body system | Muscular, Neurologic, or Skeletal |
| Mechanism | Central or Peripheral |
| Diagnosis | Cancer or Non-cancer |
| Response to treatment | Opioid-responsive or Opioid-resistant |

The sensation of pain arises in the nervous system. It has a variety of causes, but the experience of pain is variable and subjective.

Pain is both *acute* as well as *chronic*. *Acute pain* is a protective mechanism that makes you aware of an injury.[1,2] In contrast to acute pain, *chronic pain* is persistent and can last for months or years. *Chronic* pain can drastically reduce quality of life. We now know that 79% of chronic pain patients report disruptions in daily activities and 67% indicate that chronic pain negatively impacts their personal relationships.[1,3,4]

Chronic pain is often resistant to conventional medical treatments.[5–7] Moreover, pharmacologic pain management of chronic pain is hindered by *grave long-term side effects*.

Opioids are wrought with adverse effects and have significant addiction potential, but poorly appreciated is that even over-the-counter pain medicines like acetaminophen and ibuprofen are linked with *liver damage, kidney damage,* and *heart attack*.[8,9]

In this protocol, you will learn about the risks of long-term pharmaceutical pain management strategies. You will also discover that several *natural compounds* have been shown to target some of the fundamental mechanisms of pain to provide relief without debilitating side effects.

## UNDERSTANDING PAIN

Acute pain follows a predictable, finite pattern and is generally short-lived and self-limiting, as well as easy to diagnose and treat. Pain that persists for longer than 3 months, and is not progressively better, is referred to as "chronic." It can be difficult to pinpoint the exact factors that cause chronic pain to persist over time.[6]

Although there are many ways to organize different types of pain, one of the most popular and accepted schemes utilizes the following eight classifications to differentiate pain complaints (see Table 1).[10]

There are 2 major categories of pain: *nociceptive* and *neuropathic*.[11]

*Nociceptive* pain guards the body against potential injury. It occurs as a result of the activation of peripheral pain receptors called *nociceptors*, which are activated by injurious stimuli. The stimuli is converted into an electrical signal, which is conveyed along nerve cells into the spinal cord or brain, where it is perceived as an unpleasant sensation.[12]

*Neuropathic* pain occurs as a consequence of either injury or dysfunction in the nervous system. It produces a variety of unusual pain sensations that have been described as burning, crushing, and "pins and needles." Unlike nociceptive pain, neuropathic pain often persists for prolonged periods of time, even after the original trauma and/or dysfunction is addressed.[13] Since neuropathic pain is more complex than nociceptive pain, it is consequently more difficult to treat.[14]

## NOCICEPTIVE PAIN AND INFLAMMATION

Inflammation and nociceptive pain go hand in hand. Inflammation is initiated upon tissue injury and sets off a cascade of biochemical reactions that prime the nervous system for pain sensing. Moreover, long-term inflammation reinforces adaptive changes in the nervous system that can cause the sensation of pain to become exaggerated or inappropriate.[15] For example, inflamed tissue (eg, an arthritic knee) may be excessively tender and even a light touch might cause pain, a phenomenon known as *allodynia*.

Nociceptive pain does not occur spontaneously, it must be *triggered* within the nervous system. This task is accomplished by specialized receptors called *nociceptors*.

When you experience an injury, several inflammatory mediators including *prostaglandins, tumor necrosis factor-alpha (TNF-α), interleukin 1β (IL-1β),* and *interleukin-6 (IL-6)* are released at the site of the injury and interact with nociceptors, facilitating the transmission of pain signals through the nervous system. If you have a chronic inflammatory condition (eg, osteoarthritis), then increased levels of inflammatory mediators at the affected site (eg, a joint), as well as systemically, predispose you to increased pain sensations.

Therefore, taking steps to ease inflammation is an effective means of interfering with the process of pain sensitization. This is why drugs like acetaminophen (the active ingredient in Tylenol®) and ibuprofen, which are anti-inflammatory in nature, relieve pain. Unfortunately, though these drugs and others like them are very effective for reducing inflammation and pain, they often cause alarming side effects, which compromises their long-term risk versus benefit profile (see section titled "The Potentially Lethal Side Effects of Over-the-Counter Pain Medications").

A variety of *natural anti-inflammatory compounds* are able to target inflammation by reducing the synthesis of inflammatory mediators or modulating inflammatory pathways. As will be discussed later, many natural compounds exert powerful anti-inflammatory activity without causing unwanted side effects. See the "Targeted Nutritional Interventions" section.

# PAIN MANAGEMENT

The scientific approach to pain management demands a stepwise approach, which utilizes lower-risk interventions first. In many cases, these lower-risk interventions are helpful for relieving chronic pain. For example, a recent review found that exercise and behavioral therapy were effective at decreasing pain and increasing functioning among patients with chronic pain.[16] Other nonpharmacologic interventions that may be useful for chronic pain include meditation, biofeedback, acupuncture, electrical stimulation, and surgery.[1] However, in those cases that do not respond to initial pain management treatment options with lower-risk interventions, patients with chronic pain may have no other choice but to initiate pharmacologic therapy.

*Pharmacologic therapy* is one of the most popular treatment options for managing chronic pain. While initial treatment recommendations will vary based on diagnosis (eg, nociceptive vs. neuropathic), the most commonly used agents include the following[17]:

- Nonopioid analgesics (acetaminophen and/or NSAIDs)
- Opioids
- Antidepressants (tricyclics and serotonin-norepinephrine reuptake inhibitors [SNRIs])
- Antiepileptic drugs (gabapentin, pregabalin, and other anticonvulsants)
- Muscle relaxants
- Topical analgesic agents

---

## THE POTENTIALLY LETHAL SIDE EFFECTS OF OVER-THE-COUNTER PAIN MEDICATIONS

In an effort to relieve suffering, many chronic pain patients turn to over-the-counter analgesics such as acetaminophen or nonsteroidal anti-inflammatory drugs (NSAIDs).[18] However, since these drugs do not require a prescription from a doctor, patients may incorrectly assume that they do not need to be as careful about dosing as they would with a prescription analgesic. Therefore, it is important for chronic pain patients to become educated about the most serious adverse side effects that can occur with popular nonprescription analgesics.[19]

Since it was first marketed in 1955, acetaminophen has become one of the most widely used analgesics in the United States. In 2008, approximately 25 billion doses of acetaminophen were sold in the United States alone.[20] Although acetaminophen can be safe when used appropriately, it can also be extremely dangerous. For example, unintentional acetaminophen overdose is responsible for approximately 15 000 hospitalizations each year, and is the leading cause of acute liver failure in the United States.[8] Patents taking acetaminophen should follow these recommendations[21]:

- Do not exceed a maximum dose of 4 g daily.
- Remember that many prescription pain medications also contain acetaminophen.
- Recognize that acetaminophen is also called APAP, paracetamol, and acetyl-para-aminophenol.
- Do not use with other NSAIDs (without medical consultation) because such combinations increase the risk of kidney toxicity.
- Do not take with alcohol, which increases the risk of liver toxicity.

NSAIDs such as ibuprofen and naproxen can significantly reduce pain associated with various conditions. However, NSAID use is also associated with significant adverse effects such as gastrointestinal bleeding, peptic ulcer disease, high blood pressure, edema (ie, swelling), kidney disease, and heart attack.[9] For example, long-term use of NSAIDs can lead to impaired glomerular filtration, renal tubular necrosis, and ultimately chronic renal failure by disrupting prostaglandin synthesis, which can impair renal perfusion.[22] Even in NSAID users without overt kidney dysfunction, subclinical irregularities in kidney function are sometimes observed.[23]

Aspirin (a type of NSAID) is commonly used to treat minor aches and pains, as well as being prescribed at low doses (ie, 81 mg daily) for heart protection and stroke prevention. Aspirin irreversibly inhibits an enzyme called cyclooxygenase-1 (COX-1) in platelets, which is why it poses a greater risk of bleeding (ie, hemorrhage) than other NSAIDs.[18] Therefore, patients taking aspirin should avoid the simultaneous use of anticoagulant drugs and/or alcohol (without talking to their doctor first). In addition to bleeding, aspirin can also cause side effects such as heartburn, nausea, vomiting, stomach ache, ringing in the ears, hearing loss, and rash.[24] See Figure 1 for more information about the role of cyclooxygenase in inflammatory reactions.

---

Despite the wide variety of pharmacologic therapies available for patients with chronic pain, a recent report published by an international panel of experts has pointed out that current conventional treatment schemes are lacking in efficacy and often impose unacceptable side effects.[7] For example, opioids are the most commonly prescribed class of medication in the United States for short-term relief of chronic pain, and yet their efficacy and negative side effect profile have many experts questioning their use in this way, especially since the increase in opioid availability has been accompanied by an epidemic of opioid abuse and overdose.[25,26] In addition to the potential for dependence, patients beginning opioid therapy should also be aware of other common side effects, which include the following[26]:

- Constipation
- Nausea
- Excessive sleepiness
- Itchiness (ie, pruritus)
- Headache
- Respiratory depression

According to the World Health Organization's (WHO) "analgesic ladder," opioids are not recommended for chronic pain unless the pain can be described as moderate to severe, and/or has not responded to previous (nonopioid) treatment approaches. Consensus guidelines only recommend opioid therapy for managing chronic (noncancer) pain once all other reasonable lower-risk and lower-cost pain management interventions have failed.[27,28]

In an effort to reduce the risk of serious adverse outcomes associated with narcotic pain relievers, Congress has recently mandated that the Food and Drug Administration (FDA) create risk evaluation and mitigation strategies (REMS), which require drug companies to develop special educational programs for physicians and for patients who are prescribed these potentially dangerous medications.[29] While opioid therapy *can* be used for chronic (noncancer) pain in a safe way, it must be initiated properly, and only in select patient populations

(ie, physicians should carefully screen for mental disorders and history of substance abuse).[28,30]

---

## OPIOIDS AND ENDOCRINE DYSFUNCTION

Evidence linking long-term opioid use to a decline in endocrine function and subsequent hormonal imbalance has been accumulating for some time now, but recent data have garnered renewed attention.[31]

The molecular structure of opioids makes them well equipped to interfere with the normal function of the endocrine system. Evidence suggests this influence occurs in the hypothalamus and pituitary gland (brain regions) and the gonads (reproductive organs). Opioids tend to decrease gonadotropin-releasing hormone (GnRH) secretion from the hypothalamus, in turn decreasing the release of luteinizing hormone (LH) and follicle-stimulating hormone (FSH) from the pituitary gland.[31]

This upstream disruption has significant implications, especially concerning the ability of the endocrine system to produce additional hormones that rely on steady levels of GnRH, LH, and FSH. As a result of this hypothalamic-pituitary-gonadal axis suppression, the long-term use of opioids is associated with the development of hypogonadism.[31,32] Opioids have also been known to reduce testosterone levels, which is associated with increased cholesterol levels and decreased insulin sensitivity.[33]

Fortunately, most of these abnormalities can be identified through hormone-level testing as well as patient history and physical examination. Table 2 summarizes some common endocrine-related problems associated with long-term opioid use[33-35]:

The three main therapeutic options available for patients experiencing these side effects follow[33]:

- Switch to a different type of opioid (ie, opioid rotation).
- Switch to a non-opioid analgesic, or
- Initiate hormone replacement therapy (HRT). A recent study among male chronic pain patients concluded that long-term testosterone replacement therapy was associated with an increased quality of life and decreased pain ratings.[36]

---

**Table 2:  Common Endocrine-Related Problems Associated with Long-Term Opioid Use**

| Men | Women |
| --- | --- |
| Decreased body hair | Infertility |
| Adrenal dysfunction | Decreased libido |
| Decreased growth hormone | Osteoporosis |
| Miscellaneous hormonal abnormalities | Depression |
| Erectile dysfunction | Missed menstrual periods |

## Centrally Acting Drugs for Pain Relief

Chronic activation of peripheral pain sensors (nociceptors), such as occurs in osteoarthritis, for example, can alter central neural pain processing over time. The ongoing nature of chronic pain, and the adaptive nature of the central nervous system both contribute to biochemical alterations that increase pain sensitivity and cause the brain to become accustomed to processing pain. This phenomenon is known as *central sensitization*.

When the central nervous system has become "sensitized" to pain, painful sensations can be augmented because they are no longer only a nociceptive response, but are now being reinforced by mechanisms within the brain and spinal cord.[37] Thus, chronic pain has a *peripheral and* a *central* element. For instance, evidence shows patients with osteoarthritis of the knee are more sensitive to pain at other sites on their body than are healthy controls.[38] This is because the brains of people afflicted with chronic pain have adapted to processing pain and have become hyperresponsive to painful stimuli.

The central element of chronic pain does not respond to traditional therapies such as anti-inflammatory drugs because they cannot modulate the transmission of pain within the sensitized central nervous system. Therefore, drugs such as antidepressants and antiepileptics can complement traditional anti-inflammatory drugs by modulating central biochemistry.

In the case of antidepressant drugs, it appears that the mechanism by which they provide pain relief is somewhat independent from their mood-altering affects,[39] while antiepileptics alter pain signaling by modulating calcium signaling in the brain, which is also a mechanism by which they control seizures.[37]

For many people with chronic pain, centrally acting drugs are effective adjuvants to traditional pain therapies. Moreover, because central processing is a critical element of neuropathic pain, centrally acting drugs are a mainstay of treatment in this setting.[40]

## NUTRITION AND PAIN

### Diet

Recent evidence suggests that certain types of dietary intervention may have significant effects on chronic pain, especially severe forms of chronic pain.[41] Also, chronic pain can result in a decreased protein intake and increased sugar and starch intake. These dietary changes result in wasting (ie, catabolic state).[41]

Although the exact parameters of an "anti-pain" diet have not yet been recommended by any clinical organization,[41] the scientific literature contains plenty of data indicating a strong link between food and pain. For example, periods of dietary fasting have been linked to the temporary relief of pain among many patients.[42] For longer-term pain relief, some experts suggest a high-protein, low-carbohydrate diet (ie, low glycemic index), which has been associated with decreases in pain sensitivity and inflammation.[43] Likewise, several studies have shown that a vegetarian/vegan diet is also beneficial to patients with chronically painful conditions.[44]

Consuming a diet rich in antioxidants may also be helpful in the relief of chronic pain. This is because antioxidants neutralize free radicals and oxidative stress, which play a significant role in persistent pain conditions and have been linked to an increase in pain sensitivity.[45]

Some researchers believe that many of these dietary interventions activate the endogenous opioid system, which is the body's natural defense against pain.[42] Moreover, documenting dietary history to ensure adequate protein intake can help chronic pain patients avoid muscle loss and weakness.[41]

## TARGETED NUTRITIONAL INTERVENTIONS

### Omega-3 Fatty Acids

Fatty acids are essential nutrients derived from dietary intake of fats. They are an important source of energy for the body, and serve a variety of other biologic functions.

Greater dietary intake of omega-3 polyunsaturated fatty acids (PUFAs) has been linked to a reduction in both inflammatory and neuropathic pain, and has been shown to be beneficial for decreasing pain associated with rheumatoid arthritis, dysmenorrhea (pain during menstruation), inflammatory bowl disease, and neuropathy.[46] Conversely, *excessive levels of omega-6 PUFAs*, such as *arachidonic acid*, are associated with inflammatory activities, an effect that can be offset by the simultaneous consumption of omega-3 PUFAs.[47]

In response to arachidonic acid overload, the body increases its production of enzymes like 5-lipoxygenase (5-LOX) to degrade arachidonic acid. Not only do 5-LOX products directly stimulate cancer cell propagation, but the breakdown products that 5-LOX produces from arachidonic acid (such as leukotriene B4, 5-HETE, and hydroxylated fatty acids) cause tissue

### Figure 1. Arachidonic Acid's Destructive Cascade

To better understand the pathways by which arachidonic acid can cause arthritic, carcinogenic, and cardiovascular conditions, the flow chart below shows how arachidonic acid cascades down into damaging compounds in the body.

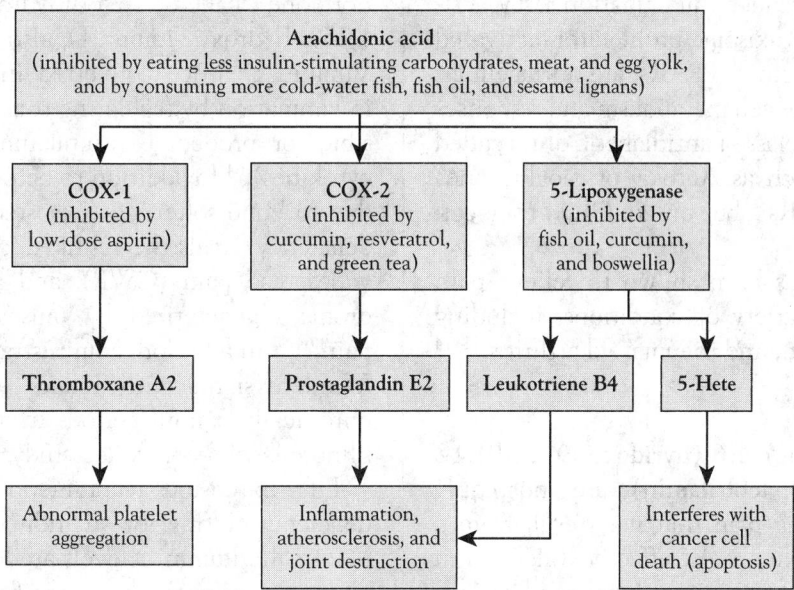

destruction, chronic inflammation, and increased resistance of tumor cells to apoptosis (programmed cell destruction).[48-57]

It is important to understand that 5-LOX is not the only dangerous enzyme the body produces to break down arachidonic acid. As seen in Figure 1, both cyclooxygenase-1 and cyclooxygenase-2 (COX-1 and COX-2) also participate in the degradation of arachidonic acid.

COX-1 causes the production of thromboxane A2, which can promote abnormal arterial blood clotting (thrombosis), resulting in heart attack and stroke.[58] COX-2 is directly involved in cancer cell propagation, while its breakdown product (prostaglandin E2) promotes chronic inflammation.[59] Most health-conscious people already inhibit the COX-1 and COX-2 enzymes by taking low-dose aspirin, curcumin, green tea, and various flavonoids such as resveratrol.

A more integrative approach to this problem, however, would be to also reduce levels of arachidonic acid, which is the precursor of 5-HETE and leukotriene.

Experts believe that *another* mechanism responsible for the anti-inflammatory effect of omega-3 PUFAs has something to do with their metabolites (ie, resolvins), which possess potent anti-inflammatory properties.[60] Resolvins bind and activate receptors on immune cells and neuronal cells leading to alterations in pain transduction in the spinal cord and a dampened inflammatory response.[15,61] The positive effect of

omega-3s on neuropathic pain has been partially explained by their ability to block voltage-gated sodium channels (VGSCs), ultimately interfering with pain signaling.[62]

Because omega-3 PUFAs are associated with positive effects on cognition, mood, and behavior,[63] they may also be beneficial to central pain processing.[64] Omega-3 supplementation can also help reduce anti-inflammatory analgesic consumption,[65] which might in turn reduce the associated risk of developing gastrointestinal side effects. Since omega-3s do not interact with most analgesic drugs, some experts recommend their concomitant use (along with conventional analgesic therapies) for the management of both inflammatory and neuropathic pain.[66]

### Gamma Linolenic Acid—The Beneficial Omega-6 Fatty Acid

Gamma linolenic acid (GLA) is a plant-derived omega-6 most abundant in seeds of an Eastern flower known as borage. Although a member of the omega-6 family, it is metabolized differently than other omega-6s.

GLA plays an important role in modulating inflammation throughout the body, especially when incorporated into the membranes of immune system cells.[67,68] Early in 2010, a team of Taiwanese researchers discovered that GLA regulates the inflammatory "master molecule" nuclear factor-kappa B or

NF-κB, preventing it from switching on genes for inflammatory cytokines in cell nuclei.[69]

A separate mechanism by which GLA and other beneficial fatty acids reduce inflammation is by activating the powerful peroxisome proliferator–activated receptor (PPAR) system.[70] PPARs are intracellular receptors that modulate cell metabolism and responses to inflammation. The class of antidiabetic drugs called thiazolidinediones (such as Actos® or pioglitazone) acts by targeting PPARs—but unlike GLA, they can be deadly.

In studies, GLA has been shown to relieve pain that results from a variety of conditions, including neuropathy, breast pain, and rheumatoid arthritis.[71-74]

## Vitamins

*Vitamins B1 (thiamine), B6 (pyridoxine), and B12 (cyanocobalamin/methylcobalamin)* are not only beneficial for managing pain that may result from a vitamin B deficiency, but are also effective (alone or in combination) with other conventional medications for various painful diseases (eg, degenerative spine disease, rheumatic diseases, low-back pain, and tonsillectomy pain).[75-77]

The administration of a mixture of vitamins B1, B6, and B12 has also been shown to reduce neuropathic pain in humans and animals,[78] and can therefore help treat peripheral neuropathies.[79] Benfotiamine (a better-absorbed derivative of vitamin B1) has also been suggested for reducing inflammatory and neuropathic pain in humans.[80] Evidence suggests that neuropathic pain plays a considerable role in many cases of chronic pain, and that B vitamins primarily provide relief by targeting pathways associated with central neural pain processing.[81]

*Vitamin C (ascorbic acid),* a versatile antioxidant, may act as another natural shield against pain. Accumulating evidence indicates that free radicals play a role in the exaggeration of pain hypersensitivity.[82] Vitamin C has been linked to a rapid and consistent antinociceptive (pain-relieving) effect in animal studies.[83] A 2011 animal study revealed that the administration of the antioxidants vitamins C and E inhibited pain related to peripheral injury. The authors concluded, "[S]upplementation or treatment with both vitamins might be an option in patients suffering from specific pain states."[82] Administration of vitamin C also reduces spontaneous pain associated with postherpetic neuralgia, which is a type of peripheral neuropathic pain.[84] Prophylactic vitamin C supplementation has also been linked to a 5-fold decrease in the incidence of complex regional pain syndrome among patients who recently underwent foot/ankle surgery (compared to no treatment).[85]

*Vitamin D* is a prohormone version of an important hormone called 1,25-dihydroxycholecalciferol or 1,25-dihydroxy vitamin D, also known as calcitriol.[86] Vitamin D, once converted into calcitriol, inhibits inflammation by regulating some of the genes responsible for producing proinflammatory mediators (ie, cytokines).[64] In addition to being associated with pain due to bone softening (ie, osteomalacia), vitamin D deficiency has also been linked to fibromyalgia, chronic widespread pain (CWP), and an unusual pain syndrome characterized by musculoskeletal and bone pain.[64,87] In addition, administration of vitamin D was found to significantly reduce pain for women with chronically painful periods in a randomized, double-blind, placebo-controlled study.[88]

Life Extension recommends routine vitamin D deficiency testing for all individuals with pain complaints. If vitamin D levels are low, vitamin D supplementation may result in significant improvements in pain.[89] Life Extension suggests that blood levels of 25-hydroxyvitamin D should be kept between 50 and 80 ng/mL for optimal health.

*Vitamin E* has been associated with a reduction in the severity of cyclic breast pain, a condition affecting as many as 69% of women.[90] It is also effective at relieving the pain associated with menstrual cramps.[91] In experimental models, supplementation with tocotrienols (a certain type of vitamin E) has been shown to improve neuropathic pain intensity associated with both diabetic and alcoholic neuropathy in animal models.[92,93] The analgesic effects of vitamin E may be partially explained through its antioxidant properties, which involve blocking the production of reactive oxygen species (ROS) that are involved in neuropathic pain. Vitamin E's analgesic effect may also be related to its ability to make the brain less sensitive to pain.[94]

## Miscellaneous Natural Compounds

*Curcumin* is the major component of turmeric, a spice that gives Indian curry its distinct color and taste. In addition to its use as a food additive, curcumin has been widely used as an herbal medicine, due to its antioxidant and anti-inflammatory properties.[95] Specifically, curcumin has been shown to reduce levels of the inflammatory mediators TNF-α, IL-1β, and IL-6, which contribute to nociceptor hypersensitivity.[96,97] Since curcumin has been shown to have analgesic effects, it may be useful for a variety of pathologic pain conditions.[98] For example, curcumin is used in India for managing traumatic and postoperative pain,[99] and has been linked to a reduction in neuropathic pain in experimental models.[100]

**Ginger (Zingiber officinale)** has analgesic and anti-inflammatory properties that soothe progressive muscle pain.[101] Certain wild ginger species have antinociceptive characteristics, and have been used traditionally to treat toothaches, muscle sprains, and swollen cuts/sores.[102] Researchers have also found that regular consumption of ginger is an effective pain reliever for arthritis patients, as well as muscle injury due to exercise.[101] For the treatment of menstrual pain, ginger has been found to be as effective as conventional analgesics such as ibuprofen.[103] Long-term administration of ginger reduced TNF-$\alpha$ expression and augmented levels of the anti-inflammatory hormone corticosterone in rats, suggesting it relieves pain by suppressing inflammation.[104]

**Proanthocyanidins** (tannins) belong to a group of chemical compounds called "flavonoids," which provide a variety of beneficial functions for humans (eg, their well-known antioxidant and anti-inflammatory effects). Grape seed is an especially rich source of proanthocyanidins, which have been associated with symptom reduction in a variety of painful diseases (eg, diabetic neuropathy and chronic pancreatitis).[105,106] Other sources of proanthocyanidins include berries, seeds, flowers, and leaves.[106] The mechanism(s) by which proanthocyanidins alleviate pain are not well understood, but some evidence indicates that central interaction with dopamine receptors may be involved.[107]

**Melatonin** is a naturally occurring hormone that is synthesized by the pineal gland and regulated by the environmental light/dark cycle.[108] Melatonin can reduce pain through its beneficial effect on sleep, as well as its analgesic properties. It is also a potent antioxidant, and has been shown to reduce the pain associated with a variety of chronically painful conditions (eg, fibromyalgia, irritable bowel syndrome, and migraine).[109] A study in infants found that melatonin powerfully relieves pain by suppressing levels of the IL-6 and other inflammatory cytokines.[110] Melatonin is such a remarkable compound that its chemical structure may be the basis of new analgesic drugs for the treatment of pain associated with cancer, headache, or even surgical procedures.[111]

**Methylsulfonylmethane (MSM)** is an organic sulfur-containing compound[112] found in a variety of fruits, vegetables, grains, and meats. Among its many beneficial functions, MSM has been shown to display anti-inflammatory and antioxidant properties.[113] MSM has been successfully used to treat pain associated with osteoarthritis (OA) of the knee,[112] and is

not typically associated with any significant adverse side effects.[114] When combined with *Boswellia serrata*, MSM significantly reduced the need for NSAIDs compared to placebo among subjects with knee osteoarthritis, suggesting that the combination exerted considerable anti-inflammatory action.[115]

**Decursinol** is a medicinal compound found in the roots of the Korean flower called **Angelica gigas Nakai (Korean angelica).**[116] It has been widely utilized in traditional Korean medicine as a treatment regimen for pain associated with menstruation, arthritis, migraine, abdominal pain, and other miscellaneous injuries.[117] Researchers suggest that decursinol may act in the central nervous system to exert its analgesic effect, or interfere with nociception.[118] Scientists report laboratory evidence showing that an active constituent derived from Korean angelica inhibits activation of nuclear factor-kappa B (NF-$\kappa$B), a DNA transcription factor that is involved in many inflammatory and disease states.[119] More recent studies indicated that coadministration of decursinol and acetaminophen resulted in synergistic effects, which enabled acetaminophen to be therapeutic at lower-than-normal doses. This acetaminophen-sparing effect implies that decursinol may inhibit the COX (cyclooxygenase) enzymes.[120]

**Capsaicin,** the compound that gives chili peppers their spicy taste, also has medicinal value as an over-the-counter topical pain reliever. It is well tolerated, and comes in a variety of formulations such as creams, gels, lotions, patches, and sticks.[121] It has been shown to be an effective analgesic for low-back pain, as well as chronic pain originating in the muscles, tendons, and ligaments.[122] Topical capsaicin has also been associated with a significant reduction in neuropathic pain.[123] Researchers believe its analgesic effect occurs as a result of its ability to reduce the amount of nerve fibers in the application area (upon long-term administration), as well as its capacity for interfering with nociception (ie, defunctionalization). Both of these actions ultimately contribute to a local decrease in responsiveness to a wide range of sensory stimuli.[124,125]

While L-phenylalanine is a naturally occurring amino acid that is a precursor to dopamine and related neurotransmitters,[126] D-phenylalanine appears to slow metabolic breakdown of endogenous opioids.[127] **DL-phenylalanine,** which is a mixture of both stereoisomers, may therefore provide an analgesic and mood-boosting effect. Some limited studies suggest that supplementation with phenylalanine might provide pain relief,[127,128] but larger, well-designed studies have failed to corroborate these early observations.[129,130] Evidence is currently insufficient to draw firm conclusions as to the pain-relieving efficacy of DL-phenylalanine.

## Boosting Serotonin Signaling

Antidepressant medications provide analgesia via various mechanisms, including by boosting levels of serotonin, which helps the brain control pain sensations.[131] Therefore, since the amino **L-tryptophan** and bioactive compounds in *saffron* may modulate serotonergic activity within the brain, some innovative scientists have proposed them as potential central pain relievers.[132,133]

## Hepatoprotective Nutrients

For those taking high doses of acetaminophen for pain relief, supplementation with hepatoprotective nutrients such as **N-acetyl-cysteine** and *milk thistle extract* may provide a means of reducing drug-induced liver damage.[134,135]

## Life Extension Suggestions

- **Curcumin** (as highly absorbed BCM-95®): 400–800 mg daily
- **B-complex vitamins** (many of these should be included in high-potency multivitamin supplements):
  - **Thiamine** (B1): 75–125 mg daily
  - **Riboflavin** (B2): 50 mg daily
  - **Niacin** (B3): 50–190 mg daily
  - **Folate** (preferably as L-methylfolate): 400–1000 mcg daily
  - **Vitamin B6** (preferably as pyridoxal-5-phosphate): 75–105 mg daily
  - **Vitamin B12**: 300–600 mcg daily
  - **Biotin**: 300–3000 mcg daily
  - **Pantothenic acid**: 100–600 mg daily
- **Fish oil** (with olive polyphenols): providing 1400 mg EPA and 1000 mg DHA daily
- **Capsaicin** (topical): Per label instructions
- **Vitamin D**: 5000–8000 IU daily, depending on blood levels of 25-OH-vitamin D
- **Ginger,** standardized extract: 150–300 mg daily
- **Korean angelica** extract: (as Decursinol-50™): 200 mg daily
- **Milk thistle,** standardized extract: 750 mg daily
- **N-acetyl-cysteine** (NAC): 600–1800 mg daily
- **Melatonin**: 0.3–5 mg before bed (sometimes up to 10 mg)
- **Methylsulfonylmethane** (MSM): 3000–6000 mg daily
- **Boswellia serrata** (as highly absorbable Après-Flex™): 100 mg daily
- **Gamma linolenic acid** (GLA): 300–600 mg daily
- **Vitamin C**: 1000–2000 mg daily
- **Proanthocyanidins** (as Pycnogenol®): 50–100 mg daily
- **Natural vitamin E**: 100–400 IU alpha-tocopherol and 200 mg gamma-tocopherol daily
- **DL-phenylalanine**: 500 mg daily
- **Saffron,** standardized extract: 180 mg daily, in two divided doses with food
- **L-tryptophan**: 500–1500 mg daily

In addition, the following blood tests may provide helpful information:

- 25-Hydroxyvitamin D
- Male or Female Panel (to assess hormone levels)
- High-sensitivity C-Reactive Protein (hs-CRP)

## REFERENCES

References available at: www.lef.org/dpt5/ch105

# 106

# *Pancreatic Cancer*

Pancreatic cancer is the fourth leading cause of cancer death in the United States and is responsible for an estimated 270 000 deaths worldwide each year.[1]

Multiple factors, including a complex and poorly understood pathophysiology and difficulty in early detection and diagnosis make successful treatment of pancreatic cancer extremely challenging. Pancreatic cancer is typically not detected until it has already reached a locally advanced or metastatic stage due to the relative lack of symptoms in early disease. Current standard of care comprises surgery if the tumor is contained within the pancreas, followed by adjuvant chemotherapy and possibly radiation. However, if the cancer has spread, conventional treatment is limited, and long-term survival rates remain very low.

The rapidly accelerating use of specialized *immunotherapies* and innovative *genetic analysis technology* represent the next generation of novel medical treatments for pancreatic cancer. The ability to *tailor* treatment based upon the unique molecular biology of a patient's cancer promises to considerably improve a currently bleak outlook.

Life Extension advocates a comprehensive pancreatic cancer management strategy including intensive cancer cell biology testing to determine which specific conventional therapies are most likely to be effective. Off-label use of pharmaceutical agents such as *metformin* and *chloroquine*, an antimalaria drug, hold promise in the treatment of pancreatic cancer as well. In addition, select nutritional ingredients can combat genetic abnormalities common in pancreatic cancer cells and offer an affordable means to *pharmacogenomically* target pancreatic cancer progression for all patients.

Life Extension Foundation® will be funding an aggressive, multidisciplinary pancreatic cancer clinical trial at the City of Hope Cancer Center. This groundbreaking trial will assess the effects of conventional chemotherapy in combination with various natural ingredients discussed in this protocol in patients with locally advanced unresectable or metastatic pancreatic cancer.

## ABOUT THE PANCREAS

The pancreas is located behind the stomach. It comprises the exocrine pancreas, which produces pancreatic enzymes that break down carbohydrates, fats, and proteins, and the endocrine pancreas, which produces the hormones insulin and glucagon that regulate how the body stores and uses food.

About 95% of pancreatic cancers begin in the exocrine pancreas, while the remaining 5% are of the endocrine pancreas. Typically, pancreatic cancer spreads first to nearby lymph nodes, then to the liver and, less commonly, the lungs.

### Alterations of Function in Pancreatic Cancer

Pancreatic cancer can alter the normal function of the pancreas by:

- Creating a deficiency of pancreatic enzymes and bile salts, thus disrupting pH.
- Causing poor absorption of nutrients from food.
- Impairing the use of pancreatic enzymes.

The pancreas secretes about 2 liters of bicarbonate (a buffer) to neutralize stomach acid in the small intestine. Reduced bicarbonate levels create an acidic microenvironment that weakens the activity of pancreatic enzymes. Some evidence suggests that antacids and an alkaline diet may be beneficial for managing symptoms associated with pancreatic cancer and its treatment.[2-4]

## CAUSES OF AND RISK FACTORS FOR PANCREATIC CANCER

While the exact cause of pancreatic cancer is not known with certainty, several factors—including smoking, nutrition, glucose levels, hormones, and genetics—are thought to be involved in its initiation and development.

Genetic susceptibility is thought to account for 10–20% of cases, but ongoing research may reveal that the role of genetics exceeds these estimates.[5] About 40% of cases are associated with inflammatory conditions caused by poor nutrition, excessive alcohol consumption, chronic pancreatitis, obesity, and chemical exposure.[6]

### Modifiable/Acquired Risk Factors

**Smoking.** Thirty percent of all pancreatic cancers are associated with smoking and tobacco use.[7] Both active cigarette or cigar smoking, as well as exposure to tobacco smoke, increase pancreatic cancer risk.

That risk, however, is reduced to levels of nonsmokers within 5–10 years of quitting. Heavy cigarette smokers and cigar smokers have roughly a 50–60% increased risk compared to nonsmokers.[8] People who smoke and drink are diagnosed with pancreatic cancer at a younger age compared to never-smokers.[9]

**Diabetes mellitus.** Long-standing diabetes (diabetes diagnosed at least 5 years prior to the diagnosis of pancreatic cancer) increases the risk of pancreatic cancer by 40–100%. Recent-onset diabetes (within 3 years) is associated with a 4- to 7-fold increase in risk, such that 1–2% of patients with recent-onset diabetes will develop pancreatic cancer within 3 years.[10,11]

**Glucose levels.** Overconsumption of sugar, sugar-sweetened soft drinks or foods, and foods that elevate after-meal blood sugar levels increase the risk of pancreatic cancer, particularly in individuals with insulin resistance.[12,13] A high glycemic load (glucose load in the blood) and fructose were associated with a greater risk of pancreatic cancer,[14] and hyperglycemia (high blood sugar/glucose levels) promotes pancreatic cancer progression in cell-based studies.[15,16]

**Dietary factors.** Dietary factors play a major role in the development of pancreatic cancer. High intake of dietary fat of animal origin, saturated fats and oils,[17] cholesterol,[18] including omega-6 fatty acids,[19] fried foods, meat, and dairy products clearly increase the risk.[20] Likewise, intake of excess calories, carbohydrates and processed meat (which are sources of dietary nitrates, nitrites and nitrosamines) increase the risk.[21,22]

**Vitamin and micronutrient deficiency.** Deficiency in folate, vitamins B6 and B12 and methionine, as well as reduced intake of vitamins C, D, and E, calcium, potassium, and selenium increase the risk of pancreatic cancer development.[23] Conversely, a high dietary intake of vitamins C, D and E, selenium, fruits, vegetables, and fiber lower the risk.[24,25] Higher vitamin D intake ( ≥600 IU/day) is associated with a 41% lower risk of pancreatic cancer compared to those with the lowest intake (<150 IU/day).[26,27]

**Folate.** Folate deficiency increases risk of pancreatic cancer due to hypomethylation of DNA.[28] Conversely, higher folate intake from food sources (or fortified foods with folic acid) and methionine decrease the risk of pancreatic cancer by 53%.[23,29]

**Periodontal disease.** Those with a history of periodontal disease have a 54–100% greater risk of pancreatic cancer. Tooth loss was positively associated with pancreatic cancer development.[30,31] In addition,

*Helicobacter pylori* (*H. pylori*) are found in dental plaque and are associated with periodontal disease and pancreatic cancer.[32]

**High body mass index (BMI) and/or obesity.** Individuals who are overweight and have a high BMI have an increased risk of developing pancreatic cancer.[33] A high BMI and hyperinsulinemia often occur together, and it is well-established that insulin promotes pancreatic cancer growth and development.[34,35] Those who are overweight or obese from the ages of 20–49 years have an earlier onset of pancreatic cancer.[36] Obesity at an older age is associated with a lower overall survival in pancreatic cancer patients.[33]

**Alcohol.** Heavy drinking (>9 alcoholic drinks per day) and binge drinking increase pancreatic cancer risk.[37,38] A significant increase in risk was seen among men consuming ≥45 g of alcohol from liquor per day.[39] Consuming more than three drinks (but not beer or wine) was associated with death from pancreatic cancer.[40]

**Chronic pancreatitis.** Chronic pancreatitis is associated with a 13- to 18-fold increase in the subsequent development of pancreatic cancer.[41,42] Chronic pancreatitis is associated with heavy alcohol consumption; approximately 10% of heavy drinkers develop chronic pancreatitis.[43]

**Chemical exposure.** Chemical exposure has been implicated in the cause of pancreatic cancer. Chemicals such as DDT (dichlorodiphenyltrichloroethane), formaldehyde, petroleum products, synthetic rubber, resins, polyesters, plastics, and styrene are involved in causing pancreatic cancer.[44,45]

**Helicobacter pylori (H. Pylori) infection.** A recent population-based case–control study and meta-analysis evaluating 2335 patients demonstrated an association between the development of pancreatic cancer and *H. pylori* infection, particularly for individuals with non–O blood types.[46,47]

## Intrinsic/Unmodifiable Risk Factors

**Age, sex, race, and ethnicity.** The disease is more common in the elderly, men, and among African Americans.[48]

**Inherited pancreatic disease.** Individuals with hereditary pancreatitis have a higher lifetime risk for developing pancreatic cancer.[49] Individuals with immediate family members affected by the disease are at increased risk (up to 57-fold with three or more family members affected) and should consider pancreatic cancer screening if it becomes available.[50,51]

## Are Hormones Involved?

Clinical studies indicate that pancreatic cancer patients have sex steroid hormone imbalances and respond to various hormonal therapies. However, the treatment outcome may be dependent on individual patient and tumor characteristics, such as hormone receptor expression.[52,53]

**Testosterone.** A recent study indicates that hormone imbalances in pancreatic cancer patients are associated with shortened survival.[54]

Male pancreatic cancer patients often have lower levels of free testosterone and progesterone and higher levels of follicle-stimulating hormone (FSH), luteinizing hormone (LH), and estradiol. Female pancreatic cancer patients often have higher levels of estradiol and lower levels of LH, FSH and progesterone.[55] In addition, pancreatic cancer patients have significantly lower testosterone/dihydrotestosterone (DHT) ratios.[56,57]

Low serum testosterone in men and excess estrogen in women are associated with shortened survival in advanced pancreatic cancer, indicating a critical need for hormone manipulation and dietary intervention. Hypogonadal males have a 3 times greater risk of death compared with those with balanced hormones.[54]

Systemic inflammation (determined by C-reactive protein [CRP] and interleukin-6 [IL-6] levels) and opioid use are associated with decreased total testosterone and free testosterone and worsened survival (opioid use almost doubles the risk of death). Furthermore, women with high estrogen showed worsened survival (2.43 times greater risk of death) compared with those with balanced hormones.[54]

Hormone levels (total testosterone, free testosterone, FSH and LH) and proinflammatory mediators (CRP, IL-6) can be measured by a simple blood test to determine hormone and inflammation status, both of which can be improved with nutritional supplementation. Studies indicate that poor nutritional status correlates with lower total testosterone levels in pancreatic cancer patients.[58]

# GENETICS AND PANCREATIC CANCER

Several key genes are overproduced and/or activated in pancreatic cancer, and these can be specifically targeted to stop tumor growth.[59] Therefore, genetic analyses may be valuable in helping to determine an optimal individualized treatment plan, involving gene targeting, to prevent cancer progression.[60] These tests can be performed by Genzyme Genetics (www.genzymegenetics.com).

## Activation of Cancer-Associated Genes (Oncogenes)

Four cancer-associated genes (oncogenes) are mutated in most cases of pancreatic cancer (K-ras, p16, p53, and MADH4 genes). Activation of the K-ras oncogene plus inactivation of tumor suppressor genes (p53, p16, DPC4, and BRCA2) are associated with the development of pancreatic cancer.[61] The transcription factors STAT3 and NF-κB (nuclear factor kappa B) are aberrantly activated in pancreatic cancer. These mutated genes, transcription factors, and inactivated tumor suppressor genes can be specifically targeted by nutritional supplements and dietary-derived targeted therapies.

Nearly 95% of all cases of pancreatic cancer have K-ras mutations, 90% have p16 mutations,[62] 75% have p53 mutations, and 55% have DPC4 mutations.[63]

**Ras genes.** Ras proteins play a central role in regulating cell growth and multiplication. Mutations in the ras genes can transform normal cells into cancerous cells that grow rapidly and form tumors. Mutations in the ras oncogene is a molecular fingerprint of this disease.[64] Smoking, alcohol, milk, and dairy consumption have been linked with the occurrence of ras mutations in pancreatic tumors.[65]

**Detection of K-ras mutations.** The detection of K-ras mutations may help to predict treatment outcome.[66] K-ras mutations are relatively easy to detect,[67] in various human tissues, including blood, intestinal fluid,[68] pancreatic fluid,[69] stool,[70,71] regional lymph nodes, and other bodily fluids, and the tumor itself.[64]

The cellular response to Ras gene activity can be inhibited in vitro by genistein, curcumin, green tea extract containing epigallocatechin gallate (EGCG),[21,72,73] and fish oil containing the omega-3 fatty acids eicosapentaenoic acid (EPA) and docosahexaenoic acid (DHA).[74]

Ras gene activity can be slowed by:

- *D-Limonene* and *perillyl alcohol*, natural monoterpenes from citrus fruits[21,75]
- *Black tea extract* containing black tea polyphenols[73]
- *Garlic's* bioactive constituent, diallyl disulfide[76,77]

**HER2 (human epidermal growth factor receptor-2).** HER2 is found in many pancreatic cancers and is associated with poor patient survival rates. Patients with HER2 overexpression tumors had significantly shorter survival times than those with HER2 normal expression tumors (median survival time, 14.7 versus 20.7 months, respectively).[78] Therefore, targeting

HER2 is crucial to improve survival of many pancreatic cancer patients.

- The tocotrienol form of *vitamin E* can cause pancreatic cancer cell death by downregulating HER2 and suppression of vital tumor cell survival pathways.[79]

- HER2 can be targeted specifically by the anti-HER2 monoclonal antibody drug trastuzumab (Herceptin®).[80]

**EGFR (epidermal growth factor receptor).** In pancreatic cancer cells, EGFR is activated and levels are up to 4-fold higher than in normal healthy pancreatic cells.[81]

- Genistein is powerful in reducing levels of EGFR[82] and disables the EGFR signaling pathway.[21]

- Curcumin and EGCG from green tea also block EGFR activity in pancreatic cancer cells.[83,84]

- The pharmaceutical agent *erlotinib* inhibits signaling of EGFR, and is approved by the Food and Drug Administration (FDA) for use in combination with gemcitibine for patients with locally advanced unresectable or metastatic pancreatic cancer.[85,86] In clinical trials, erlotinib has performed well in combination with gemcitabine and other chemotherapeutic agents,[87] but survival is not significantly prolonged. Some preliminary evidence suggests that erlotinib may improve chemosensitivity in pancreatic cancer.[88]

## Important Genes Turned Off in Pancreatic Cancer

Compared to other major types of cancer, pancreatic cancer displays a loss of activity of genes known to suppress tumor development, such as p16, DPC4, BRCA2, and most importantly p53.

**P16.** Ninety percent of pancreatic carcinomas suffer a loss of p16 function. Moreover, carriers of p16 germline mutations have a 12- to 20-fold increased risk of developing pancreatic cancer.[89]

**DPC4.** The absence of this gene is associated with more invasive cancer growth.[63] However, pancreatic cancer cells with a DPC4 homozygous (complete) deletion are sensitive to nontoxic doses of alpha-tocopherol succinate.[90]

**BRCA2.** This is the most common mutation in patients with hereditary pancreatic cancer. Carriers of BRCA2 mutations have a 3.5- to 10-fold increased risk of developing pancreatic cancer. A clinical case study suggests that patients with metastatic pancreatic carcinoma and BRCA2 mutations may have disease

that is more sensitive to camptothecin-11 chemotherapy and consequently have prolonged survival.[91]

**p53.** Because the p53 gene is a tumor suppressor gene involved in repairing damaged DNA, when the gene is inactive (turned off) or malfunctions, damaged DNA is able to proliferate and form cancerous cells.[92]

Nutritional supplements known to restore function of the p53 tumor suppressor gene include:

- *Curcumin* and *resveratrol* both upregulate p53 in pancreatic cancer cells[93,94]

- *Omega-3 fatty acids* activate p53[95]

- *Gamma-tocotrienol* reduces cell survival proteins through the p53 pathway[96]

- Red grape seed *proanthocyanidins*[97,98]

- Phytochemicals such as *genistein* from soy,[99] *indole-3-carbinol (I3C)* from cruciferous vegetables, the green tea polyphenol *EGCG*,[100,101] and *resveratrol*[94]

## Regulation of Transcription Factors

A transcription factor controls whether a particular gene is turned on (active) or off (inactive). Transcription factors can be activated or deactivated selectively by other proteins, often as a final step in the process of transmitting their signals. The presence and activity of these factors can differ in normal and cancerous tissues.

**STAT3.** STAT3 is a dormant transcription factor activated in pancreatic cancer but not in normal pancreatic tissue; it plays an important role in the progression of pancreatic cancer. Silencing of the STAT3 gene using nutritional agents such as I3C and genistein[102] may be a novel therapeutic option for treatment of pancreatic cancer.[103] Omega-3 fatty acids inhibited the proliferation of pancreatic cancer cells by decreasing STAT3 phosphorylation.[104]

**NF-kappa B (NF-κB).** NF-κB is another transcription factor activated in human pancreatic cancer, but not in normal pancreatic tissue. Blocking NF-κB activity prevents cancer invasion and spread (metastasis) in animals with tumors. Furthermore, preventing NF-κB activity reduces levels of molecules involved in tumor blood-vessel development, thereby retarding tumor growth and slowing cancer spread.[105]

- *Gamma-tocotrienols* inhibit human pancreatic tumor growth and sensitize them to gemcitabine by suppressing NF-κB-mediated inflammatory pathways linked to the formation of tumors.[106]

- *Genistein* and *curcumin* both reduce NF-κB activation.[107–109]
- The *omega-3 fatty acid* EPA inhibits NF-κB.[110]

# POSSIBLE SIGNS AND SYMPTOMS OF PANCREATIC CANCER

- Jaundice (yellowing of the skin and whites of the eyes) due to blockage of the bile duct or liver malfunction
- A gnawing pain from the stomach to the back
- Unexplained weight loss
- Fatigue, weakness, dark urine, light stools, and anorexia

# SCREENING AND EARLY DETECTION

One of the main reasons that pancreatic cancer has a poor survival rate is the inability to screen for and prevent this disease. Pancreatic cancer needs to be detected early (precancerous lesions or small pancreatic cancers) in order to improve the chance of survival. Unfortunately, premalignant lesions and early pancreatic cancers are asymptomatic and current screening strategies are ineffective and inefficient.[111]

Currently, there are no approved screening tests for pancreatic cancer. CA 19-9 is elevated in 70–90% of patients but it is not accurate enough for early detection (poor sensitivity), nor is carcinoembryonic antigen (CEA).[112] Efforts are underway to identify biomarkers with a high level of accuracy that detect pancreatic cancer at an early stage, such as early mutations in K-ras, p53, and p16, but none are yet in routine clinical use.[66]

Future screening tests might incorporate biomarkers in addition to endoscopic ultrasound (EUS), possibly contrast-enhanced,[51] or noncontrast MRI with ultrasound, which is now used in Japan.[113] In the future, proteomic analysis of pancreatic fluid aspirate will be a novel method of pancreatic cancer detection.[114]

# DIAGNOSIS

## Blood Tests

Serum tumor markers can be detected by a simple blood test and can be used in conjunction with diagnostic imaging tests for the diagnosis of pancreatic cancer and for monitoring progress after surgery. Tumor markers used include CA19-9, CEA, CA-50, CA72-4, and CA242.[115]

CA 19-9 (carbohydrate antigen 19-9) is the mainstay tumor marker and is ordered when pancreatic cancer is suspected, particularly if the patient shows signs of jaundice. CA 19-9 levels match the course of the disease following treatment.[116] A high preoperative CA19-9 level (>500–1000 IU/mL) implies more advanced disease that is not amenable to resection.[117] Additional diagnostic methods are required because this test is only 70% sensitive and 87% specific for pancreatic cancer.

The EUROPAC study is currently evaluating fasting blood glucose as a marker for early pancreatic cancer in sporadic cases[118] and molecular analysis of pancreatic juice (K-ras and p53 mutations, and p16 promoter methylation). Screening for recent onset diabetes could possibly lead to early diagnosis or reduce pancreatic cancer deaths.[119]

An alkaline phosphatase blood level that is 4–5 times the upper limits of normal (and disproportionate to the bilirubin level) may occur from tumor obstruction of the bile duct.

**Assessment of pancreatic function.** In pancreatic cancer, abnormal digestion associated with inadequate pancreatic enzymes and function (insufficiency) can occur.[120] When pancreatic enzyme levels fall below 1–2% of normal, poor nutrient digestion and incorporation occur. Poor digestion can cause significant weight loss, nutritional deficiencies, and foul-smelling or greasy bowel movements. It is also associated with changes in gastrointestinal function, such as changes in acid-base balance, bile acid metabolism, stomach emptying, and motility of the intestines.[121]

Tests for pancreatic enzyme function include:

- Lipase, amylase, chymotrypsin levels, and bicarbonate secretion[122,123]

With enzyme supplementation, weight loss and biochemical indices of malnutrition can be greatly improved.[124]

Tests for pancreatic hormone function include:

- Insulin: Fasting blood sugar levels and an oral glucose tolerance test (OGTT)[125]
- Measurement of hormone levels (insulin, glucagon, somatostatin, and pancreatic polypeptide) after a meal[126]

## Diagnostic Imaging

Poor survival in pancreatic cancer is due not to early spread but rather late diagnosis. Early diagnosis of this cancer is rare because symptoms develop gradually, and cancer is often present for many months or even years before diagnosis. Physicians use a range of imaging techniques to confirm the diagnosis. Tumor markers do not yet enable early diagnosis of pancreatic cancer.[119]

The use of endoscopic ultrasound-guided, fine-needle aspiration (EUS-FNA) for fluid collection enables physicians to detect tumor markers and abnormal cells which supplement EUS imaging in pancreatic cancer diagnosis,[127] and with a minimal risk of tumor seeding.[128] EUS-FNA can also reveal, in approximately 10% of patients, metastatic spread.[129]

## Future Methods of Diagnosis

Optical coherence tomography (OCT) imaging can reliably distinguish between low risk (benign) and high risk (potentially malignant) pancreatic cystic lesions with over 95% accuracy (specificity and sensitivity *ex vivo*). However, at the time of writing, this technique is not yet available to patients with pancreatic disease, as a minimally invasive probe for intracystic OCT imaging still needs to be developed.[130]

# PROGNOSIS

Prognostic biomarkers are indicators of the tumor's aggressiveness (or growth potential) and the patients' final outcome, regardless of the treatment used. A recent study showed that *circulating tumor cells (CTCs)* are an independent prognostic biomarker.[131] CTCs are cancer cells that detach from the primary tumor and travel in the blood, leading to cancer spread.[132] CTCs were detected in 49.3% of blood samples from patients with advanced pancreatic adenocarcinoma and their detection correlated with poor prognosis. The median progression free survival was 60.7 days in patients with positive CTC detection versus 163.6 days in those with negative CTC detection.[59] As of the time of writing, CTC analysis is currently not commercially available for pancreatic cancer.

High platelet counts are associated with poor survival.[133,134] Patients with a neutrophil to lymphocyte ratio (NLR) value of <5 have a significantly higher median survival duration compared to those with a NLR value of ≥5.[135]

# CONVENTIONAL MEDICAL TREATMENTS FOR PANCREATIC CANCER

Pancreatic cancer is one of the most challenging cancers for oncologists. Typical conventional treatments for pancreatic cancer include chemotherapy, radiation therapy, immunotherapy, biologically targeted therapies, and surgery. Chemotherapy and radiation therapy are typically not curative and provide only minor

increases in survival rates in most cases. The median survival is only 10–12 months.[108] The 5-year survival of patients who undergo conventional treatment with surgery, chemotherapy, and radiation therapy is about 20%. However, the overall 5-year survival rate is 5%, as only 15% of patients are eligible for surgery.[136] In those cases diagnosed with locally advanced unresectable or metastatic pancreatic cancer, palliative management is typically the goal.[137]

## Surgery

Only 15% of pancreatic cancer patients may be eligible for complete surgical removal of their tumors, a procedure known as a Whipple resection. This is a high-risk procedure with a mortality rate of 15% and a 5-year survival rate of only 10%.[138] The median survival time for the inoperable 85–90% of cases is often only a few months. Management of these cases is based on relieving symptoms (*palliative care*).

Various chemotherapy drugs may be used before or after surgery to remove most of the tumor. Chemotherapy combined with radiotherapy is often used in the standard treatment of pancreatic cancer.[138]

## Radiation

Radiation therapy, such as intensity modulated radiation therapy (IMRT) is used to provide symptom relief, improve pain and rarely prolongs survival.[137] Refer to the Cancer Radiation protocol for information on supporting healthy tissues during radiation therapy.

Pancreatic tumor cells with mutant ras genes are more difficult to kill with radiation than are cells with normal ras genes.[139] However, experiments showed that the FTI (farnesyl transferase inhibitor) tipifarnib (Zamestra™) made pancreatic cancer cells with a K-ras mutation more sensitive to the killing effects of radiation.[140,141] Therefore, the combination of dietary-derived ras inhibitors and radiation may offer therapeutic advantages for those undergoing radiotherapy.[142]

## Chemotherapy

Gemcitabine (Gemzar™) has been the standard chemotherapeutic agent for the past decade but it has not significantly improved the average survival rate. Furthermore, chemotherapy often causes intolerable levels of toxicity. Six months of chemotherapy with Gemzar™ after surgery improves 5-year survival from 9 to 21%.[143] Even when Gemzar™ is combined with other chemotherapy drugs (Xeloda™ or cisplatin), or targeted-therapies such as EGFR inhibitors (Tarceva™

or Cetuximab™), there is minimal improvement in survival.[136] Clinical trials with the favored, but aggressive FOLFIRINOX (chemotherapy cocktail) produced a median overall survival of 11.1 versus 6.8 months (with Gemzar™), but with significantly worse side effects.[144]

Pancreatic cancer–gemcitabine chemoresistance is associated with enhanced NF-κB activation. The well-known capacity of omega-3 fatty acids to inhibit NF-κB[110] and promote tumor cell death has the potential to restore or facilitate gemcitabine chemosensitivity.[104] Curcumin may also help circumvent chemoresistance via downregulation of NF-κB signaling.[145]

## ANTICOAGULANTS IN THE MANAGEMENT OF PANCREATIC CANCER

Increased coagulation (blood clot formation or thrombosis) is common in pancreatic cancer patients and presents a life-threatening complication.[146] Moreover, advanced pancreatic cancer is associated with a high risk of patients developing venous thromboembolism (VTE); incidence ranges from 17–57% and is associated with a poor prognosis.[147,148] Emerging clinical data strongly suggest that anticoagulant treatment may improve pancreatic cancer patient survival by decreasing thromboembolic complications as well as by separate anticancer activity.[149,150]

Pancreatic cancer is usually associated with obstruction of the bile duct, which can elevate the level of fibrinogen. Elevated fibrinogen increases the risk of thrombosis and is also associated with increased invasiveness, metastasis, and poor clinical outcome. Increased fibrinogen levels result in increased platelet aggregation and therefore increased risk of blood clotting.[151]

Aspirin inhibits platelet aggregation (ie, has antithrombotic effects) primarily by irreversibly inhibiting cyclooxygenase-1 (COX-1). Moreover, daily aspirin use (75 mg and up) for at least 5 years reduces deaths due to pancreatic cancers. The benefit increases with duration of use.[152]

Furthermore, recent data suggest that aspirin use greater than or equal to 1 day/month is associated with significantly decreased risk of developing pancreatic cancer. This association was also found for those who took low-dose aspirin for heart disease prevention.[153]

Preclinical studies confirm that aspirin significantly suppresses pancreatic cancer development by inhibiting the proliferation of pancreatic cancer cells, in vitro, through cell cycle arrest. In vivo studies show that aspirin delays the progression, and partially represses the invasion, of pancreatic cancer formation through inhibition of NF-κB activation.[154,155]

Aspirin augments the anticancer effects of gemcitabine as well as its proapoptotic effect in pancreatic cancer cells. It also inhibits proliferation of gemcitabine-resistant human pancreatic cancer cells.[156]

Data indicate that the anticoagulants low molecular weight heparin (LMW heparin) and warfarin have a beneficial effect on the treatment of patients with pancreatic carcinoma.[157,158] LMW heparin (added to gemcitabine plus cisplatinum) resulted in a significant improvement in survival over the use of chemotherapeutic agents alone (13.0 versus 5.5 months).[159] However, another recent study did not show a survival benefit of LMW heparin (nadroparin) in patients with advanced pancreatic cancer.[160] The addition of warfarin to chemotherapy increased mean survival from 2.3 to 5.0 months.[161]

Many dietary and botanical supplements have anticoagulant, antiplatelet and/or antithrombotic effects. These include omega 3-fatty acids from fish oil, vitamin E, ginger, and gingko (antiplatelet properties); dong quai and anise (anticoagulant effects); fucus (bladder wrack) (heparin-like activity); and high doses of vitamin E. However, caution should be exerted as the aforementioned can interact with standard anticoagulants and antiplatelet drugs such as aspirin, warfarin, and LMW heparin.[162]

Determining thrombotic risk with biomarker tests (via blood tests) is crucial to identify those pancreatic cancer patients at highest risk of VTE in order to improve prognosis.[163] Biomarkers associated with increased VTE risk in cancer include platelet and leukocyte counts, C-reactive protein, D-dimer, and PT time.[158]

### Biologically Targeted Therapies

It is well-known that specific gene mutations (eg, K-ras, p53) are involved in pancreatic cancer development and progression, which is why drugs have been developed to specifically target these genes. However, even patients that have a known gene mutation (eg, K-ras) respond differently to targeted treatments because the gene mutation itself can vary between patients (eg, K-ras often mutates at codons 12, 13, or 64). Therefore, when the targeted treatment is tested in genetically dissimilar patients, it often fails.[136] Clinical trials investigating therapies targeting K-ras, EGFR, vascular endothelial growth factor (VEGF), immunotherapy using tumor-associated antigens, and biologic therapy such as TNFerade™ (GenVec, Inc., Gaithersburg, MD) have all failed to substantially improve survival.[136]

In pancreatic cancer, constitutively active K-ras is found in over 95% of tumors, making it a molecular fingerprint of this cancer.[164] K-ras initiates pancreatic cancer development and is also involved in its progression. As K-ras plays such a critical role in pancreatic cancer, there has been extensive research to discover compounds that inhibit it and the pathways it affects. Researchers have tried using farnesyltransferase inhibitor (FTI) drugs to suppress the K-ras gene, but with no success; a phase 3 clinical trial with tipifarnib (Zamestra™), which targets Ras farnesylation, plus gemcitabine, did not improve survival.[136]

*For targeted therapy to work, the target must be present in the tumor cells,* even if the percentage of tumor cells harboring that mutation is small. Therefore, tumor cell gene mutation analyses would need to be performed for each patient prior to any proposed targeted treatment strategy. These molecular analyses (which are not FDA approved or widely available to pancreatic cancer patients) for the expression of drug targets (eg, K-ras, p53, etc.) and chemoresistance markers in tumor cells can be performed by independent laboratories, such as Genzyme Genetics.

## Immunotherapy/Vaccine Therapy for Pancreatic Cancer

Vaccines for pancreatic cancer are employed to prevent recurrence and/or metastasis after surgery and boost immune responses and improve clinical outcome when used in combination with chemotherapy. Several early phase 1/2 clinical trials have shown that the vaccines studied in pancreatic cancer treatment appear to be safe and well-tolerated. However, their immunogenicity (ability to produce an immune response) has been variable. The survival data indicate that induction of an immune response is correlated with prolonged survival and most clinical trials show increased survival associated with immune responses (see Table 1). Whole tumor cells were initially used to produce vaccines because the proteins expressed by tumor cells that are recognized by the immune system were unknown. However, the identification of proteins expressed by pancreatic tumors enabled the production of specific peptide vaccines such as mutant K-ras, MUC-1, vascular endothelial growth factor receptor 2 (VEGFR2), and telomerase.[165,166]

In phase 1/2 trials, vaccination of advanced pancreatic cancer patients using peptide vaccines of mutant K-ras,[167,168] MUC1,[169–171] VEGFR2,[172] or telomerase[173] was significantly associated with immune responses and in most cases, prolonged survival.

In clinical trials, patients with advanced or nonresectable pancreatic cancer have been treated by combination therapy of chemotherapy (gemcitabine) with personalized peptide vaccines[174,175] or VEGFR2.[172] Combination therapy was shown to be safe and possibly effective in patients with advanced pancreatic cancer refractory to standard treatment.[176]

**Mutant K-ras peptide vaccines.** In a recent phase 1 study using long synthetic mutant ras peptides, 23 patients were vaccinated after surgery for pancreatic cancer. Significantly, 10-year survival was 20% (four patients of 20 evaluable) versus zero (0/87) in a group of nonvaccinated patients.[168]

In another recent study of 24 patients with resected pancreatic cancer that were vaccinated with K-ras peptide in combination with *granulocyte-macrophage colony-stimulating factor* (GM-CSF), the median overall

survival was 20.3 months. However, although the vaccine was safe and well-tolerated, it did not stimulate an immunogenic response.[167]

In a phase 1/2 study of 48 patients with pancreatic cancer (38 with advanced disease and 10 postsurgery), vaccination with mutant K-ras peptides in combination with GM-CSF resulted in immune responses and prolonged survival.[177]

A phase 2 clinical trial of mutant ras peptide-based vaccine as adjuvant therapy in pancreatic and colorectal cancers was performed with 12 patients (with no evidence of disease). Five pancreatic and seven colorectal cancer patients were vaccinated with mutant ras peptide, corresponding to their tumor's ras mutation. Five of 11 patients showed a positive immune response. Furthermore, the five patients that responded had a mean disease-free survival of 35.2+ months and a mean overall survival of 44.4+ months. Researchers noted that the vaccine is safe, can induce specific immune responses, and has a positive outcome in overall survival.[178]

**MUC1 peptide vaccines.** MUC1 is a glycoprotein highly overexpressed and mutated in pancreatic tumors, providing a tumor specific antigen and target.

A phase 1/2 clinical trial evaluated a vaccine consisting of liposomal MUC1 peptide-loaded dendritic cells (DC). Twelve pancreatic and biliary cancer patients were vaccinated following surgical removal of their primary tumors. MUC1-specific immune responses were observed even in patients with pretreated and advanced disease. Vaccinated patients were followed for over 4 years, and 4 of the 12 patients were alive at that point, all without evidence of recurrence.[169]

Vaccination of 16 patients with resected or locally advanced pancreatic cancer with MUC1 peptide and SB-AS2 adjuvant (which induces a more portent immune response) resulted in low MUC1-specific immune responses in some patients. Moreover, 2 of 15 vaccinated patients were alive and disease free during follow-up at 32 and 61 months.[171]

**hTERT mRDA dendritic cell (DC) vaccine.** hTERT (human telomerase reverse transcriptase) is an ideal tumor-associated antigen with which to develop a dendritic cell (DC) vaccine.[179] Immunotherapy targeting the hTERT subunit of telomerase induces powerful immune responses in cancer patients after vaccination with single hTERT peptides. A complete remission was reported in a pancreatic cancer patient associated with the induction of hTERT-specific immune responses against several hTERT epitopes (pieces of the antigen that are recognized by the immune system).[180]

A 62-year-old female patient underwent radical surgery for a pancreatic adenocarcinoma. After relapse, she attained stable disease with gemcitabine treatment. Due to severe neutropenia, the chemotherapy was discontinued. The patient was subsequently treated with autologous DCs loaded with hTERT mRNA for 3 years. Immune parameters were monitored regularly after vaccination and clinical outcome was assessed by CT and PET/CT scans. The patient developed an immune response against several hTERT-derived antigens. At the time of writing, she showed no evidence of active disease based on PET/CT scans and continues to receive regular booster injections.[180]

**Telomerase peptide vaccines and GM-CSF.** A phase 1/2 study demonstrated the safety, tolerability, and immunogenicity of telomerase peptide (GV1001) vaccination in 48 patients with nonresectable pancreatic cancer. Immune responses were observed in 24 of 38 evaluable patients. One-year survival was 25% for the evaluable patients in the intermediate dose group. Median survival for this group was 8.6 months.[173]

GV-1001, an injectable telomerase (hTERT) MHC class II–peptide vaccine (by GemVax AS), was reported to be undergoing phase 3 clinical trials for pancreatic cancer.[181]

**HSPPC-96 (gp96, Oncophage).** A phase 1 pilot study of autologous heat shock protein vaccine HSPPC-96 (gp96, Oncophage) in patients with resected pancreatic adenocarcinoma was performed. Ten patients who received neither adjuvant chemotherapy nor radiation were vaccinated with HSPPC-96 weekly with 4 doses. Median overall survival was 2.2 years. Three of 10 treated patients were alive and without disease at 2.6, 2.7, and 5.0 years follow-up.[182] However, there have been no follow-up studies reported.

**Poxvirus vaccines targeting CEA and MUC-1.** A phase 1 clinical study of poxviruses targeting carcinoembryonic antigen (CEA) and MUC-1 in 10 patients with advanced pancreatic cancer was conducted. Results showed the poxvirus vaccine to be safe, well tolerated, and capable of generating antigen-specific immune responses in patients with advanced pancreatic cancer. Median overall survival was 6.3 months and a significant increase in overall survival was noted in patients who generated anti CEA- and/or MUC-1-specific immune responses compared with those who did not (15.1 versus 3.9 months, respectively).[183]

**Personalized peptide vaccines.** A case of complete remission of liver metastasis of pancreatic cancer, refractory to gemcitabine chemotherapy, under vaccination with a HLA-A2 restricted peptide derived from survivin peptide was reported.[184]

**Immunotherapy combined with chemotherapy.** Emerging evidence suggests that immunotherapy used in combination with conventional chemotherapy may improve clinical outcome. It is noteworthy that gemcitabine has direct antitumor (chemotherapeutic) activity but also mediates immunologic effects that are beneficial for cancer immunotherapy. Gemcitabine treatment is not immunosuppressive and may enhance responses to specific vaccines or immunotherapy; therefore, it could be combined with vaccines or other immunotherapy.[185]

**Vascular endothelial growth factor receptor 2 (VEGFR2).** VEGFR2 is an essential factor in tumor angiogenesis and in the growth of pancreatic cancer. A phase 1 clinical trial using a peptide vaccine for VEGFR2 in combination with gemcitabine for patients with advanced pancreatic cancer (metastatic and/or unresectable) was conducted. The median overall survival time of all 18 patients who completed at least one course of treatment was 8.7 months and the disease control rate was 67%.[172]

A phase 2 study of personalized peptide vaccination with gemcitabine as the first-line therapy in patients with nonresectable pancreatic cancer was performed. The reactive personalized peptides (maximum of 4 types of peptides) were administered with gemcitabine to 21 patients with untreated and nonresectable pancreatic cancer. Median survival time of all 21 patients was 9.0 months with a 1-year survival rate of 38%. Immune responses correlated well with overall survival.[175]

**Granulocyte-macrophage colony-stimulating factor (GM-CSF).** GM-CSF is a myeloid growth factor and immune-activating protein used clinically. The GM-CSF gene inserted into tumor cells has been used to immunize patients. These genetically modified tumor cells produce GM-CSF in the local environment of the tumor, specifically activating the patient's T cells.

A phase 2 trial tested the safety and effectiveness of GM-CSF–based immunotherapy given to 60 patients with resected pancreatic adenocarcinoma. The immunotherapy treatment was given 8–10 weeks after surgery followed by 5-fluorouracil (5-FU) based chemoradiation and further immunotherapy. The median survival was 24.8 months and the immunotherapy was well tolerated.[186]

**Dendritic cell (DC)-based vaccines.** Dendritic cells (DCs) are potent antigen-presenting cells and play a pivotal role in T-cell–mediated immunity and thus immunotherapy of cancer. DC-based vaccines are safe and efficient in inducing strong tumor-specific immune responses (ie, cytotoxic T-cell [CTL] responses) against tumor antigens (in vitro and in vivo).[187] The long-term outcome of DC vaccination and immunotherapy for patients with refractory pancreatic cancer has been demonstrated.[188]

Seventeen pancreatic cancer patients underwent immunotherapy in the Kyushu University and the Yakuin CA Clinic. Six patients had postoperative recurrence, 11 were inoperable due to metastasis, 16 developed chemotherapy-resistant cancers, while 1 patient had no prior chemotherapy for recurrent cancer after surgical resection because of leukopenia. Immunotherapy was combined with chemotherapy in 11 patients and without chemotherapy in 6 patients. Immunotherapy was classified into two groups: combined DC vaccination and injection of activated lymphocytes (DC vaccine therapy), or injection of lymphokine-activated killer lymphocytes (LAK) alone (LAK therapy). This immunotherapy of refractory pancreatic cancer resulted in a median survival of 9 months. DC vaccine therapy gave a significantly better survival period than LAK therapy alone. Results suggest that immunotherapy utilizing DC vaccination may prolong the survival of patients with refractory pancreatic cancer.[188]

A recent study indicates that DC vaccine-based immunotherapies combined with gemcitabine/S-1 are effective in patients with advanced pancreatic cancer refractory to standard chemotherapy.[176] In this report, 38 of 49 patients had received vaccination with WT1 peptide-pulsed DCs with or without combination of other peptides such as MUC1, CEA, and CA125. Prior to this combination therapy, 46 of 49 patients had been treated with chemotherapy, radiotherapy, or hyperthermia but without clinical effects. Of 49 patients, 2 patients had complete remission (CR), 5 had partial remission (PR), and 10 had stable disease (SD) and median survival time was 360 days. Survival of patients receiving DC vaccine and chemotherapy plus LAK cell therapy was longer than those receiving DC vaccine in combination with chemotherapy but no LAK cells. "Dendritic cell vaccine-based immunotherapy combined with chemotherapy was shown to be safe and possibly effective in patients with advanced pancreatic cancer refractory to standard treatment."[176]

Another recent pilot study showed that DC-based vaccination can stimulate an antitumor T-cell response in patients with advanced or recurrent pancreatic carcinoma receiving concomitant gemcitabine treatment.[189] In this study, patients were eligible for DC vaccination after recurrence of pancreatic cancer or as palliative care. Twelve patients received DC vaccinations and simultaneous chemotherapy. One patient developed a partial remission, and two patients exhibited stable disease. Median survival was 10.5 months and no severe side effects occurred. DC vaccination increased the frequency of tumor-reactive cells in all patients tested; however, the degree of this increase varied. The patient with the longest overall survival of 56 months had a high frequency of tumor-reactive cells, indicating that the presence of a prevaccination, antitumor T-cell

## Table 1: Vaccines for Pancreatic Cancer

| Vaccine | Patients | Response | Reference |
|---|---|---|---|
| Dendritic cell-based *with concomitant chemotherapy* (gemcitabine) | 12 advanced or recurrent pancreatic cancer | 1 PR, 2 SD, median survival 10.5 months | 189 |
| GM-CSF postsurgery *with 5-FU chemoradiation* | 60 resected pancreatic adenocarcinoma | Median survival 24.8 months | 186 |
| Dendritic cell-based loaded with WT1, MUC1, CEA, and CA125 *Gemcitabine/S-1* | 49 advanced pancreatic cancer patients refractory to standard chemotherapy | 2 CR, 5 PR, and 10 with SD; median survival 360 days | 176 |
| hTERT mRNA dendritic cell vaccination | 1 patient post chemotherapy | Complete response (ie, no evidence of active disease based on PET/CT scans) | 180 |
| Mutant K-ras long peptide | 23 resected pancreatic cancer | 10-year survival was 20% (4 patients of 20 evaluable) | 168 |
| MUC1 peptide-loaded dendritic cell | 12 pancreatic and biliary cancer patients with resected tumors | 4 of 12 patients followed for over 4 years were alive | 169 |
| 13-mer mutant ras peptide | 12 patients with no evidence of disease; 5 pancreatic and 7 colorectal | Mean DFS of 35.2+ months and mean overall survival of 44.4+ months | 178 |
| Allogeneic GM-CSF-secreting pancreatic cancer cell, alone or in sequence with cyclophosphamide | 30 advanced pancreatic cancer | Median survival in gemcitabine-resistant patients similar to chemotherapy alone | 190 |
| Telomerase peptide with adjuvant GM-CSF | 48 advanced pancreatic cancer | 1-year survival for evaluable patients in intermediate dose group was 25% | 173 |

**Table 1: Vaccines for Pancreatic Cancer—cont'd**

| Vaccine | Patients | Response | Reference |
|---|---|---|---|
| HLA-A2 restricted peptide derived from survivin antigen | 1 metastatic (liver) pancreatic cancer patient refractory to gemcitabine | Complete remission of liver metastasis with duration of 8 months | 184 |
| Personalized peptide vaccine | 11 advanced pancreatic cancer | 6- and 12-month survival rates for 10 patients who received >3 vaccinations were 80% and 20%, respectively | 191 |
| MUC1 peptide with SB-AS2 adjuvant | 16 resected or locally advanced pancreatic cancer | 2 of 15 resected pancreatic cancer patients alive and disease-free at follow-up of 32 and 61 months | 171 |
| Dendritic cell transfected with MUC1 cDNA | 10 patients with advanced pancreatic, breast, or papillary cancer | Vaccine-specific, delayed-type hypersensitivity reaction in 3 of 10 patients | 192 |
| Allogeneic GM-CSF-secreting pancreatic cancer cell | 14 resected pancreatic cancer | 3 patients had DTH responses; 3 patients remained disease-free at least 25 months after diagnosis | 193 |
| Mutant K-ras peptide with adjuvant GM-CSF | 10 resected and 38 advanced pancreatic cancer | Prolonged survival of immune responders compared to nonresponders | 177 |

DFS, disease-free survival; DTH, delayed-type hypersensitivity; PR, partial remission; SD, stable disease.

response might be associated with prolonged survival. Five patients survived 1 year or more.[189]

## THE PHARMACOGENOMICS APPROACH

In the personalized genomic approach, a patient's tumor(s) would be biopsied and undergo rapid sequencing analysis or biotyping; then, it is compared to the patient's genetic mutations so that a personalized treatment strategy could be developed. This method would quickly decipher all targets and differences among patients and their tumors, thus identifying which patients should respond to particular combinations of targeted therapies. Instead of taking a one-size-fits-all approach to pancreatic cancer, shared mutations would be matched to a particular drug. For example, HER2 amplification, which occurs in 2–3% of pancreatic cancers, might allow some pancreatic cancer patients to be candidates for anti-HER2 drugs, such as trastuzumab or lapatinib.

With a personalized genomic approach, a combination of multiple targeted therapies is most likely to be effective for patients whose tumors have been analyzed and shown to have specific markers (eg, K-ras, p53, HER2, etc.) that can actually be targeted. Repeat sequencing analysis could be performed at frequent intervals during treatment, or if new metastases or recurrent disease occurred, and treatment could be changed accordingly to take into consideration any genetic differences between the original tumor and metastatic cancer cells.

Certain genetic tests are already commercially available by direct consumer marketing to patients, even though their efficacy has not been proven in large-scale clinical trials. For example, European laboratories perform molecular analyses of tumor cells for the expression of drug targets and chemoresistance markers, from a blood sample, tumor tissues, ascites, or bone marrow. In the future, the genome of individual patients and their tumors will be available at an affordable cost.

To learn more about advanced molecular testing, refer to the *Life Extension Magazine* article titled "Designing an Individually Tailored Cancer Treatment Utilizing Advanced CTC Molecular Analysis."

## INNOVATIVE DRUG STRATEGIES

Several innovative drug strategies are being explored for the treatment of pancreatic cancer, including FDA-approved drugs that were not originally developed for pancreatic cancer treatment but have incidentally been shown to hinder its growth and progression; these include the "off-label use" of the antidiabetic drug *metformin* and the antimalarial drug *chloroquine*. It has been proposed that chloroquine and metformin could eliminate pancreatic cancer cell traits in preinvasive premalignant lesions by inhibiting the genesis and self-renewal of cancer cells.[194]

**Chloroquine.** Chloroquine (Aralen®), which is used to prevent and treat malaria worldwide, selectively stops the growth of pancreatic tumors by inhibiting "autophagy."[195] Autophagy is the process whereby cancer cells "self-eat," or cannibalize part of themselves to survive. Pancreatic cancers have a unique dependence on autophagy; that is, they require autophagy for tumor growth.[196] In pancreatic cancers, K-ras drives autophagy. Chloroquine inactivates this process of autophagy, which causes tumor regression and prolonged survival in pancreatic cancer mouse experiments.[197]

These results are immediately translatable to the clinical treatment of pancreatic cancer patients, and provide an urgently needed novel therapeutic strategy. Currently, Hopkins researchers are pushing chloroquine into clinical trials of pancreatic cancer treatment.

Furthermore, chloroquine specifically sensitizes cancer cells to radiation therapy and chemotherapy and could possibly increase the efficacy of conventional cancer therapies.[198]

Caution should be exerted by pancreatic cancer patients with hepatic impairment and/or alcoholics.

**Metformin.** Metformin has emerged as a novel treatment strategy for pancreatic cancer patients. Metformin is a drug of the biguanide class, approved for the treatment of type 2 diabetes mellitus (ie, non–insulin dependent diabetes mellitus) worldwide because of its primary antihyperglycemic effects.[199]

Many studies suggest that diabetes mellitus can cause pancreatic cancer with possible mechanisms involving insulin resistance and high levels of insulin in the blood. Moreover, successful treatment of type 2 diabetes and/or obesity reduces the risk of pancreatic cancer by reducing high insulin levels; insulin is known to stimulate cancer growth and pancreatic cancers overexpress insulin/IGF-1 receptors.[200]

Metformin reduces the risk of pancreatic cancer through antidiabetic and antitumor actions.[10] Several studies found that metformin users (including diabetics) had a significantly lower relative risk for developing pancreatic cancer.[201] It is noteworthy that a 62% reduction in the risk of pancreatic cancer in diabetic patients having taken metformin for more than 5 years was reported. By contrast, long-term insulin use in patients with longstanding diabetes mellitus was associated with an increased risk of pancreatic cancer.[202]

Clinical studies show that metformin reduces insulin resistance and increases complete tumor response rates following neoadjuvant chemotherapy for breast cancer.[203] An Italian retrospective cohort study of 3685 type 2 diabetic patients without cancer found that each 5-year metformin exposure was associated with a significant reduction in cancer death compared to insulin and sulfonylureas.[204]

A study presented at the 2011 American Society of Clinical Oncology (ASCO) meeting shows that metformin prolongs survival and decreases risk of death in patients with pancreatic malignancy and diabetes.[205] The median survival was 16.6 versus 11.5 months for metformin ever-users versus never-users, respectively.

Metformin users are cautioned to monitor their vitamin B12 and homocysteine levels, as its use causes both folate and vitamin B12 deficiency (ie, serum total B12 level ≤ 150 pmol/L) in up to 30% of diabetic patients.[201,206]

# PANCREATIC ENZYME THERAPY

Pancreatic cancer creates a deficiency of pancreatic enzymes (termed pancreatic insufficiency), bicarbonate, and bile salt, resulting in poor absorption of nutrients from food, profound weight loss, and severe malnutrition. Fortunately pancreatic enzyme supplementation can prevent this occurrence and greatly improve quality of life in these patients.[203] To avoid malnutrition-related morbidity and mortality and to improve patients' weight and nutritional status, pancreatic enzyme replacement therapy with oral pancreatic enzymes (enteric-coated minimicrospheres) at mealtimes (aimed at providing the duodenal lumen with a sufficient amount of active lipase at the time of gastric emptying of nutrients) can greatly improve quality of life.[203,204]

*Clinical studies with pancreatic enzymes.* In a randomized, double-blind trial of 21 patients with unresectable cancer of the pancreatic head region (with suspected pancreatic duct obstruction), 8 weeks of high-dose enteric coated pancreatic enzyme supplementation and dietary counseling prevented weight loss. Patients on pancreatic enzymes gained 1.2% (0.7 kg) body weight whereas patients on placebo lost 3.7% (2.2 kg). Fat absorption and daily total energy intake in patients on pancreatic enzymes improved whereas in placebo patients it worsened.[120] Aggressive pancreatic enzyme replacement is important to optimize bowel function and prevent malnutrition in pancreatic cancer patients.[205]

## COX-2 (Cyclooxygenase-2) Inhibitors

The COX-2 enzyme, a major angiogenic mediator found to be elevated in pancreatic cancer,[210] indirectly prevents cancer cells from dying.[211] Therefore, suppressing the COX-2 enzyme may inhibit pancreatic cancer cell propagation. The COX-2 inhibitor apricoxib is now being investigated for enhancing the efficacy of gemcitabine and erlotinib in pancreatic cancer treatment.[208]

Selective reduction of COX-2 levels improves response to both chemotherapy and radiotherapy without being toxic to normal healthy tissues.[213]

A well-known COX-2 inhibitor, Celebrex® has already been combined with gemcitabine and curcumin in an ongoing study in Tel Aviv.[214] Its preclinical activity in pancreatic cell lines and other cancer cell lines have been well-documented, it is commercially available, and actively investigated in many cancer studies. In the CALGB 30203 study, celecoxib was shown to confer survival advantage to lung cancer patients who overexpressed COX-2.[215,216]

In addition, the following nutritional supplements which have been shown to reduce COX-2 expression in vitro and in vivo could be employed.[217]

- *Gamma-tocotrienol* prevents the growth of human pancreatic tumors by reducing COX-2 expression.[106]

- *Omega-3 fatty acids*, in particular EPA and DHA, found principally in oily fish, inhibit production of COX-2 significantly. EPA treatment decreases intracellular levels of COX-2 protein in pancreatic tumors.[218]

- *Curcumin* downregulates COX-2 expression in pancreatic cancer cells resulting in increased tumor cell death.[219]

For a detailed discussion of COX-2 inhibition in cancer treatment, please review the protocol Cancer Treatment: The Critical Factors.

## 5-LOX (5-Lipoxygenase) Inhibitors

The 5-LOX enzyme is produced in pancreatic cancer (but not in normal pancreatic ducts) and is critical for its growth.[220] Reducing levels of 5-LOX prevents human pancreatic cancer cell lines from multiplying and induces apoptosis (cell death).[221]

**Zileuton.** Zileuton, a powerful 5-LOX inhibitor, preclinical models suggest synergy with various agents in cancer cell lines. Its use in CALGB 30203, an eicosanoid modulation clinical trial in lung cancer, was not promising in a factorial designed experiment; however, its role in pancreatic cancer has not been evaluated, and several preclinical hamster models suggest it may be active in pancreatic cancer, alone or in combination with Celebrex®.[222–224]

For a detailed discussion of 5-LOX inhibition in cancer treatment, review the protocol Cancer Treatment: The Critical Factors.

## NUTRITIONAL THERAPY AND SUPPLEMENTS

### Dietary-Derived Targeted Therapy

Biologically active extracts (from fruits, vegetables, and herbs) that specifically target cancer cell growth

provide complementary therapy options to pancreatic cancer patients who do not have time to wait for large-scale clinical trials to validate the usefulness of these dietary agents, either alone or in combination with conventional treatments.

Dietary-derived extracts with proven specific bioactivity that have been used clinically to treat pancreatic cancer patients include curcumin, genistein, EPA and DHA, alpha-lipoic acid, perillyl alcohol,[225] and antioxidants. These dietary agents contain several biologically active constituents, in addition to vitamins, minerals, and micronutrients that exert multiple anticancer effects on pancreatic cancer cells and tumors, and specifically target pathways at the molecular, cellular, and physiologic level, resulting in suppression of cancer growth, invasion, and metastasis.[21]

Other dietary-derived extracts that suppress pancreatic cancer cell/tumor growth, progression, and spread (in vivo and in vitro) include green tea (EGCG), resveratrol, pomegranate, pterostilbene, and limonene. These nutritional supplements prevent pancreatic progression and cause tumor cell death by affecting multiple intracellular signaling molecules in pancreatic cancer development such as p53, K-ras, NF-κB, EGFR, STATs, COX-2, and tumor necrosis factor-alpha (TNF-α).[226]

Studies suggest that a diet containing multiple dietary-derived bioactive agents is preferable and much more effective over single agents for the prevention and/or treatment of pancreatic cancer. For example, curcumin combined with omega-3 fatty acids, and isoflavones together with curcumin, provided synergistic inhibitory activities against pancreatic cancer.[227] Combinatorial treatment with multiple dietary-derived bioactive agents exerts superior antitumor effects than either agent alone, partly due to the specific inhibition of multiple signaling pathways (in this case Notch-1 and NF-κB).[228]

**Curcumin.** Curcumin is extracted from the Indian spice turmeric (*Curcuma longa L.*). It is one of the most important bioactive anticancer compounds and has been extensively researched for preventing and treating pancreatic cancer.

Curcumin inhibits several signaling pathways in pancreatic cancer cells at multiple levels, such as transcription factors (NF-κB, Notch-1, STAT3, and AP-1),[228,229] enzymes (COX-2, MMPs, and 5-LOX), cell cycle growth factors (cyclin D1), proliferation (Ras, EGFR, HER2, and Akt), survival pathways (β-catenin and adhesion molecules), and TNF, prostaglandin E2, and interleukin-8,[84,230] ultimately leading to increased pancreatic cancer cell death.[231] In pancreatic cancer studies, curcumin has been used as a bioactive agent in lab, animal, and phase 1, 2, and 3 human trials.

*Clinical trials with curcumin.* Phase 2 clinical trials of curcumin determined that curcumin can be safely taken by cancer patients at oral doses up to 8 g per day.[21] However, results of the most recent clinical trial using curcumin to treat advanced pancreatic cancer patients revealed that the curcumin dose of 8 g per day was difficult to tolerate (due to abdominal fullness/discomfort) and the researchers recommended that other formulations of curcumin (with improved systemic bioavailability and therapeutic efficacy) be evaluated for future trials.[232]

A phase 1/2 study of 21 gemcitabine-resistant patients with pancreatic cancer receiving 8 g daily of oral curcumin in combination with gemcitabine-based chemotherapy found the combination therapy to be safe, well-tolerated, and feasible. Median survival time after initiation of curcumin was 161 days (109–223 days) and the 1-year survival rate was 19% (4.4–41.4%).[233]

Curcumin continues to exhibit promise as an anticancer agent, as it is remarkably bioactive but also nontoxic even at high doses. Pilot phase 1 clinical trials have shown curcumin to be safe even when consumed at a daily dose of 12 g for 3 months.[93] At the 2011 ASCO Gastrointestinal Cancers Symposium, preclinical evidence was presented regarding the efficacy of curcumin.[212] Note that the forms of curcumin used in these clinical studies were not the superior absorbing forms of curcumin that are now available over-the-counter. These newer curcumin formulas absorb about 7 times better into the bloodstream, thus providing a way for patients to obtain levels of curcumin that might offer therapeutic efficacy.

**Genistein.** Genistein, an isoflavone extracted from soybeans, has been widely studied in pancreatic cancer. Genistein inhibits pancreatic cancer progression at the genetic, cellular, and physiologic level.

At the genetic level, genistein prevents pancreatic cancer growth via targeted inhibition of Ras,[234] NF-κB,[107] EGFR,[82] HER2,[235] STAT3,[103] and activation of p53.[99] At the cellular level, genistein regulates glucose metabolism.[236] At the physiologic level, genistein exerts potent antiangiogenic and antimetastatic activities by impairing the activation of hypoxia inducible factor-1 (HIF-1) and suppressing VEGF (in vivo).[237] Intratumoral hypoxia is known to lead to increased tumor aggressiveness and distant metastasis; genistein prevents this occurrence.

*Clinical trials with genistein.* A phase 2 clinical trial on the use of genistein in combination with gemcitabine

and erlotinib to treat patients with advanced or metastatic pancreatic cancer was performed. Genistein in the form of soy isoflavones at a dose of 531 mg twice daily was taken by pancreatic cancer patients. The trial showed that the addition of soy isoflavones to gemcitabine and erlotinib did not increase the survival of advanced pancreatic cancer patients.[238] The researchers speculate that the benefit of adding soy isoflavones may be limited to patients whose tumors overexpress NF-κB, thus emphasizing the urgent need for individualized treatment plans.

As of September 2011, there was a phase 1/2 clinical trial investigating the effect of a crystalline form of genistein (AXP107-11), alone and in combination with gemcitabine, in patients with advanced or metastatic cancer of the pancreas (www.clinicaltrials.gov).

The suggested dose of genistein is approximately 500 mg daily, which requires the swallowing of about five soy isoflavone concentrated capsules (3500 mg soy extract daily flavones). This should be taken in two daily doses, each consisting of about 1750 mg of soy isoflavone extract (to provide a total daily intake of 3500 mg).[239,240]

**Fish oil.** Weight loss in advanced pancreatic cancer patients (catabolic wasting or cachexia) is refractory to conventional nutritional support. However, it is well established that supplementation with fish oil, rich in omega-3 fatty acids (EPA and DHA), reverses tumor-related weight loss (cachexia). EPA modulates the inflammatory response that contributes to weight loss in cancer and thus reverses cancer cachexia.[241]

Omega-3 fatty acids, EPA and DHA, prevent pancreatic cancer progression and cause pancreatic tumor cell death by activating p53[95] and blocking the activity of Ras,[242] EGFR,[243] COX-2 and 5-LOX,[227] STAT3,[104] and NF-κB.[110]

In a phase 1 study of five pancreatic cancer cachexia patients, a mean dose of approximately 18 g per day (doses ranged from 9 to 27 g/day) of a high-purity preparation of EPA was tolerated.[244]

Fish oil supplements providing at least 2400 mg of EPA and 1800 mg of DHA daily have been recommended.[245] To reduce cachexia, an estimated 2–12 g per day of EPA is needed.[246]

*Clinical studies with fish oil.* Many clinical studies in pancreatic cancer patients show that fish oil, omega-3 fatty acids, and/or EPA supplementation reverses weight loss caused by cancer (cachexia).

In an international, multicenter, randomized trial, a nutrition prescription of a protein and energy dense, oral nutritional supplement with and without omega-3 fatty acids taken by 200 untreated patients with unresectable pancreatic cancer over an 8-week period significantly improved weight (1.7 kg), protein (25.4 g), and energy (501 kcal) intake.[247]

Consumption of a protein- and energy-dense nutritional supplement containing omega-3 fatty acids (EPA) improved body weight, lean body mass, and quality of life in patients undergoing chemotherapy.[248]

In a prospective, randomized, double-blinded clinical trial on 44 cancer patients undergoing major abdominal tumor surgery, daily fish oil and soybean oil supplementation (0.2 and 0.8 g/kg body weight, respectively) prevented weight loss and enabled a faster recovery.[249]

In a study of 24 home-living cachectic patients with advanced pancreatic cancer, the administration of an energy and protein dense oral supplement enriched with EPA, over an 8-week period, was associated with an increase in physical activity and improved quality of life.[250]

EPA enriched protein supplements improved physical activity levels and increased total energy expenditure in advanced pancreatic cancer patients, thereby increasing their quality of life.[251]

**Perillyl alcohol.** Perillyl alcohol is a naturally derived monoterpene with activity against pancreatic cancers that have a K-ras mutation. It prevents the mutated ras proteins from stimulating pancreatic cancer growth.[75] Perillyl alcohol treatment causes complete pancreatic tumor regression in animal experiments.[252] Clinically achievable concentrations of perillyl alcohol combined with a virally delivered therapeutic cytokine (adenovirus-mediated mda-7/IL-24 gene therapy [Ad.mda-7]) effectively eliminated human pancreatic cancer cells grown in mice and increased their survival.[253]

*Clinical studies with perillyl alcohol.* A pilot study of perillyl alcohol in eight pancreatic cancer patients showed that perillyl alcohol was well tolerated. Survival time was longer in patients who received full perillyl alcohol treatment (288 ± 32 days) compared to those who did not (204 ± 96 days), but this result did not achieve statistical significance. There was a trend toward greater apoptosis in tumors versus normal pancreatic tissue of patients receiving perillyl alcohol.[254]

Twelve clinical trials have investigated the use of perillyl alcohol in various types of cancer treatments. A 2050-mg dose given 4 times daily was found to be easily tolerated.[255] The minimum required antitumor dose is 1.3 g per day.[256]

**Antioxidants.** Individual variations in the capacity to defend against oxidative stress and repair oxidative DNA damage influence pancreatic cancer risk, and some of these genetic effects are modified by dietary antioxidants.[257] Moreover, antioxidant levels are reduced in pancreatic tumors compared to healthy pancreatic tissue, resulting in increases in reactive oxygen species (ROS) that are capable of stimulating cancer growth.[258,259]

**Vitamins A, C, and E.** An overview of 14 randomized trials (with a total of 170 525 patients) showed significant effects of supplementation with beta-carotene, vitamins A, C, E, and selenium (alone or in combination) versus placebo on pancreatic cancer incidence.[260]

Retinoic acid slows pancreatic tumor progression and reduces motility of pancreatic stellate cells (PSCs).[261] A study of 23 pancreatic cancer patients tested retinol palmitate (vitamin A) and beta-interferon with chemotherapy. Eight patients responded and eight patients had stable disease. For all patients, median time to disease progression and survival time were 6.1 months and 11 months, respectively. Toxicity was high, but patients who had responses and disease stabilization had prolonged symptom relief.[262]

Vitamins A, C, and E, as well as *selenium*, increase antioxidants needed to reduce free-radical damage in the body.[263] A double-blind, placebo-controlled, randomized clinical trial involving 36 cancer patients undergoing surgery for pancreatic cancer evaluated the impact of an oral nutritional supplement (enriched with antioxidants, glutamine and green tea extract) on postoperative oxidative stress. Patients received the antioxidant-enriched supplement twice the day before surgery and once 3 hours before surgery. The nutritional supplement improved total antioxidant capacity (plasma levels of vitamin C, vitamin E, selenium, and zinc) shortly after surgery and increased plasma vitamin C levels.[264]

Recent data support the use of pharmacologic doses of ascorbate in adjunctive treatment (eg, with gemcitabine) for pancreatic cancer.[265] Ascorbate induces autophagy in pancreatic cancer cells.[266]

**Vitamin D.** Pancreatic cancer patients have a high prevalence of vitamin D deficiency indicating the need for appropriate supplementation.[267] Low serum vitamin D levels, as defined by serum vitamin D levels of <32 ng/mL using Labcorp testing method for 25-hydroxyvitamin D, in pancreatic cancer patients take longer to respond to oral vitamin D supplementation compared to healthy individuals,[268] suggesting that more aggressive supplementation may be required to obtain Life Extension's optimal level of *50–80 ng/mL.*

Vitamin D3 has multiple protective effects against pancreatic cancer including antiangiogenic, antimetastatic, anti-inflammatory, and immuno-modulatory effects.[269,270]

**Melatonin.**  Recently, it was discovered that melatonin reduces pancreatic tumor cell viability by altering mitochondrial physiology.[271] Furthermore, advanced pancreatic cancer patients have abnormal circadian fluctuations in melatonin levels,[272] which should be corrected by melatonin supplementation because even low (physiologically normal) concentrations of melatonin have a proapoptotic effect on pancreatic cancer cells resulting in tumor cell death.[273]

*Clinical studies with melatonin.* A clinical study of melatonin plus immunotherapy in the treatment of 50 advanced pancreatic adenocarcinoma patients resulted in a significantly higher 1-year survival rate in the melatonin treated group than other groups tested (3/12 versus 1/38), suggesting that melatonin immunotherapy is a promising treatment of advanced pancreatic cancer.[274]

A phase 2 study of melatonin plus tamoxifen in metastatic solid tumor patients was performed. Included in the study were five pancreatic cancer patients, for whom no other standard therapy was available. Melatonin (20 mg at night) and tamoxifen (20 mg at noon) were given orally every day. Results indicated that the combination of melatonin plus tamoxifen may have some benefit in untreatable metastatic solid tumor patients.[275]

In another clinical study in which melatonin plus low-dose interleukin-2 (IL-2) was used to treat pancreatic cancer patients with a life expectancy of less than 6 months, a complete response was achieved in one pancreatic cancer patient, and a partial response in three others. Immunotherapy with melatonin and IL-2 was a well-tolerated and effective therapy for almost all advanced cancer patients with solid tumors, including those who did not respond to IL-2 alone or to chemotherapy.[276,277]

## Investigational Nutritional Supplements

Pancreatic cancer treatment advances, whether conventional or alternative, have to be proven first in the laboratory before applying them to patients. However, epidemiologic or population-based studies also provide evidence of the benefits of specific dietary interventions.

Epidemiologic studies as well as laboratory and animal experiments suggest the following nutritional components may have a role in pancreatic cancer treatment.

**Limonene.**  Limonene is extracted from citrus fruits. It has been shown to reduce growth of pancreatic cancer cells by 50%.[278,279] Limonene is well tolerated in cancer patients at doses that may have clinical activity.[280] One partial response in a breast cancer patient at a dose of $8g/m^2$/day (8 g taken twice daily) was maintained for 11 months. Three patients with colorectal cancer showed disease stabilization for longer than 6 months on d-limonene at 0.5 or 1 g twice daily.[281] The tentative dose recommendation for limonene is 7.3–14.4 g per day.[256,291] Daily consumption of d-limonene from food sources is estimated to be 16.2 mg/person/day (0.27 mg/kg body weight/day).[282]

**Selenium.**  Selenium levels were found to be reduced in 57% of pancreatic cancer patients who underwent surgery to remove the upper portion of their intestines. Many long-term survivors (>6 months) of pancreatic surgery have frank selenium deficiencies. Thus, it is recommended that micronutrient status should be regularly checked in these patients and treated where necessary.[205]

High-selenium yeast was shown to reduce cancer risk in an intervention trial.[283] Patients with previous skin cancer were supplemented with 200 mcg of selenium or placebo daily for an average of 4.5 years. At a 6-year follow-up, it was found that those in the selenium group had a significant reduction in total cancer mortality, total cancer incidence, and incidences of lung, colorectal, and prostate cancers. Additional studies utilizing selenium supplementation have shown benefit in prostate and lung cancer.[284,285]

Selenium and beta-carotene were found to restrain the growth of pancreatic tumors caused by carcinogen exposure in mice.[286] In another preclinical study, a diet high in selenium reduced the number of carcinogen-induced pancreatic cancers significantly.[287]

**Vitamin K.**  Population studies as well as animal and laboratory data suggest a role for vitamin K in cancer prevention and treatment.[288,289] In one laboratory study, vitamin K combined with the drug sorafenib strongly inhibited growth and induced apoptosis in pancreatic cancer cells.[290]

**Vitamin B6.**  Animal and epidemiologic studies have linked antitumorigenic and anti-inflammatory effects to dietary vitamin B6.[291] In a pooled analysis of data from four cohorts including 208 pancreatic cancer cases and 623 controls, subjects in the highest quartile (one-fourth) for plasma vitamin B6 concentrations were 20% less likely to have pancreatic cancer than those in the lowest quartile.[23] Among male smokers in another study, those in the lowest one-third distribution of concentrations of the active form of vitamin B6–*pyridoxal-5'-phosphate*–were about twice as likely to develop pancreatic cancer compared to those in the highest one-third.[292]

**Green tea.** In a large population-based case–control study conducted in China, it was found that drinking green tea lowers the risk of pancreatic cancer.[293]

Epigallocatechin gallate (EGCG) is the main bioactive polyphenolic constituent in green tea. Animal studies show that EGCG inhibits pancreatic tumor growth, angiogenesis, invasion, and metastasis.[100] Furthermore, EGCG suppressed the development of pancreatic tumors in Syrian hamsters.[294,295]

Increasing evidence suggests an association of chronic inflammation in cancer development in which IL-1 plays a crucial role. Recent experimental studies show that EGCG downregulates IL-1RI expression and suppresses IL-1–induced tumorigenic factors in human pancreatic cancer cells resulting in tumor cell death.[296]

EGCG's anticancer activities in human pancreatic carcinoma cells are partly via the inhibition of insulin-like growth factor-I receptor (IGF-1R).[297] EGCG (and the buckwheat flavonoid rutin) decrease induced glucotoxicity in pancreatic beta cells, preserving insulin signaling.[298] Furthermore, EGCG improves pancreatic injury in animal models of acute pancreatitis.[299] Green tea polyphenols (GTPs) prevent pancreatic fibrosis by inhibiting activated pancreatic stellate cells (PSCs). PSCs play a central role in the pathogenesis of pancreatic fibrogenesis and inflammation. EGCG inhibits PSC activation through antioxidant mechanisms[300] and prevents migration of PSCs.[301] EGCG also decreases the expression of the K-ras gene.[73]

Clinical evidence shows that green tea supplementation is safe and protective against some types of cancer.[302]

**Zinc.** Zinc is a trace element essential for normal cell growth. Zinc deficiency may have role in cancer promotion.[303]

**L-carnitine.** L-carnitine has been shown to augment the cytotoxicity of cisplatin and is involved in the mitochondrial transport of acetyl groups.[304,305]

Acetyl-L-carnitine may indirectly influence the stability of the p53 tumor suppressor gene. The activity of this gene enhances the cytotoxicity of cisplatin chemotherapy drugs. Based on this information, researchers investigated the effects of acetyl-L-carnitine in combination with cisplatin on cancer cell lines. The results revealed a significant antimetastatic activity of acetyl-L-carnitine and enhancement of the antitumor potential of platinum chemotherapy.[305]

L-carnitine deficiency is proposed to be a cause of cancer-related weight loss (cachexia). In a randomized controlled trial, advanced pancreatic cancer patients receiving 4 g of L-carnitine daily for 12 weeks gained weight (BMI increased 3.4%), while the control group continued to lose weight (BMI decreased 1.5%). Patients supplemented with L-carnitine also experienced improved nutritional status, increased overall survival, and reported better quality of life.[306]

## Complementary Alternative Therapies

**PSK (Polysaccharide K).** PSK is a protein-bound polysaccharide derived from the mycelium of the mushroom *Coriolus versicolor*.[307] In Japan, PSK is used as a nonspecific biological response modifier to enhance the immune system in cancer patients.[308]

Two patients who had unresectable pancreatic cancer were treated with combined chemotherapy using cisplatin, PSK, and UFT (uracil-tegafur). During therapy, a partial response was observed, with a remarkable decrease in tumor size and no significant side effects. From the results of these two cases, this combination chemotherapy was considered to be one of the most effective therapies available for pancreatic cancer.[309] PSK has been used as adjuvant immunotherapy for cancer at a dose of 3 g daily.[310]

Recent studies showed that PSK has strong antitumor effects via stimulation of both innate and adaptive immune pathways.[311] Furthermore, PSK activates human natural killer (NK) cells and significantly potentiates the antitumor effect of anti-HER2 monoclonal antibody therapy (in mice). Therefore, concurrent treatment of PSK and trastuzumab may be a novel way to augment the antitumor effect of trastuzumab.[312]

PSK suppresses tumor cell invasiveness by downregulating several invasion-related factors.[313] PSK enhances pancreatic cancer cell death induced by Taxotere® (docetaxel) by inhibiting docetaxel-induced NF-κB activation.[314]

**Ukrain (NSC-631570).** Ukrain is a semisynthetic derivative of the *Chelidonium majus L.* alkaloid chelidonine shown to prolong survival of pancreatic cancer patients.

In a phase 2 trial of advanced pancreatic cancer patients, Ukrain either alone or together with Gemzar® (gemcitabine) doubled median survival times.[315]

In another clinical study, Ukrain with vitamin C treatment prolonged the survival and improved the quality of life of patients with advanced pancreatic cancer. In this study, patients were administered IV therapy consisting of either vitamin C (5.4 g every second day, repeated 10 times) and Ukrain (10 mg every second day, repeated 10 times) (21 patients), or vitamin C (5.4 g every second day × 10) and normal saline (10 mL) (control group, 21 patients). The 1-year survival was 81% versus 14%, 2-year survival

43% versus 5%, and median survival 17.17 versus 6.97 months in the Ukrain versus control group, respectively. The longest survival in the Ukrain group was 54 months.[316]

Ukrain's proapoptotic activity is based on *Chelidonium majus L.* alkaloids and is mediated via a mitochondrial death pathway.[317] Ukrain is able to control the expression of some of the key mediators of tumor progression in pancreatic carcinoma cells. It downregulates matrix metalloproteinases, suggesting that it may decrease pancreatic cancer cell invasion. It also reduces tumor cell proliferation by cell cycle inhibition, via G2/M phase arrest.[318]

Seven randomized clinical trials suggest that Ukrain has curative effects on a range of cancers, including pancreatic cancer. However, the methodologic quality of most studies was poor; therefore, independent rigorous studies are urgently needed.[319]

## Alpha-Lipoic Acid/Low-Dose Naltrexone (ALA/N)

The Integrative Medical Center of New Mexico (located in Las Cruces) previously reported the long-term survival of a male patient with pancreatic cancer metastasized to the liver who was treated with intravenous alpha-lipoid acid and oral low-dose naltrexone (ALA/N) (and a healthy lifestyle program) without any toxic adverse effects. The man was alive and well 78 months after initial treatment,[320] even though he was told by a reputable oncology center in October 2002 that there was little hope for his survival.

*Clinical studies with ALA/N.* Recently three new patients with metastatic pancreatic cancer were treated with the ALA/N protocol at the same center. In 2010, it was reported that the first patient is alive and well 39 months after presenting with pancreatic adenocarcinoma with metastases to the liver. The second patient, also with pancreatic adenocarcinoma with metastases to the liver, was treated with the ALA/N protocol and after 5 months of therapy, PET scan showed no evidence of disease. The third patient, in addition to his pancreatic cancer with liver and retroperitoneal metastases, has a history of B-cell lymphoma and prostate adenocarcinoma. After 4 months of the ALA/N protocol his PET scan showed no evidence of cancer. ALA/N exerts multiple anticancer effects including reducing oxidative stress, stabilizing NF-κB, stimulating apoptosis, inhibiting tumor cell proliferation, and modulating an immune response.[321]

Berkson and colleagues[321] believe that the results from their ALA/N integrative protocol warrant clinical trials, stating that "given its lack of toxicity at

levels reported it may have the possibility of extending the life of a patient who would be customarily considered to be terminal."

The ALA-N protocol comprises alpha-lipoic acid (ALA) (300–600 mg intravenously twice weekly), low-dose naltrexone (Vivitrol™) (3–4.5 mg at bedtime), and orally, ALA (300 mg twice daily), selenium (200 mcg twice daily), silymarin (300 mg, 4 times daily), and vitamin B complex (3 high-dose capsules daily). In addition, a strict dietary regimen, stress-reduction and exercise program, and a healthy lifestyle are essential.

## Life Extension Suggestions

The goal of therapy is to strengthen pancreatic function, impede cancer growth and spread, and reduce the severity of symptoms. Various nutritional supplements outlined in this protocol have been shown to help pancreatic cancer patients by slowing disease progression or increasing quality of life.

### Guidelines for Reducing Pancreatic Cancer Risk
- Stop smoking and stop drinking alcohol.
- Avoid or reduce exposure to toxic chemicals and petroleum products.
- Maintain a healthy body weight.
- Reduce dietary intake of fried foods, red meat, meat products, and dairy.
- Increase intake of fresh fruit and vegetables, fiber, minerals, and vitamins.
- Reduce sugar consumption (glycemic load).
- Increase physical activity.
- Maintain a diet suitable for diabetics that restricts simple carbohydrates such as sugar and emphasizes complex carbohydrates (fibers) and proteins (refer to the Diabetes protocol). Protein supplements such as soy and essential fatty acids (eg, fish oils) will help by altering the dietary intake ratio of carbohydrates, proteins, and fats.

If pancreatic cancer patients are to improve their odds of achieving a remission or long-term survival, they should attempt to integrate into their conventional therapy as many of the following dietary changes and supplements as possible, but only under a physician's supervision.

### Primary Supplements:
- **Fish oil:** 700–4200 mg of EPA, 500–2000 mg of DHA daily with food
- **Curcumin:** 2400 mg daily (as highly absorbed BCM-95®)

- **Soy extract** (14% genistein): 1750 mg twice daily with food
- **Perillyl alcohol:** 2000 mg, 4 times daily
- **Vitamin A** (preformed): 3000 IU daily, with food
- **Vitamin C:** 1000–5000 mg daily in 4 divided doses
- **Vitamin E:** 400 IU daily of natural alpha tocopherol vitamin E along with 200 mg of gamma tocopherol and about 380 mg of mixed tocotrienols
- **Vitamin D3:** 5000–8000 IU daily with food. Blood levels of vitamin D3 should be regularly monitored to achieve a blood level of 50–80 ng/mL.
- **R-lipoic acid:** 300 mg twice daily
- **Melatonin:** 10–40 mg at bedtime
- **PSK:** 3 g daily
- **Multivitamin/multimineral formula without copper:** per label instructions

Life Extension also suggests a **low-dose aspirin** (81 mg) daily.

**Secondary Supplements:**
- **Selenium:** 200–400 mcg daily with food
- **Grape seed extract:** 100 mg daily
- **Silymarin:** 100–420 mg daily
- **Dietary fiber:** 30–40 g daily (from dietary and supplemental sources)
- **Green tea extract (EGCG):** 700–2100 mg daily
- **Vitamin K, providing:**
  - Vitamin K1 (phytonadione): 1000 mcg daily
  - Vitamin K2 (as menaquinone-4): 1000 mcg daily
  - Vitamin K2 (as menaquinone-7): 100 mcg daily
- **Vitamin B6** (as pyridoxal 5'-phosphate): 100 mg daily

- **Garlic** (standardized to 10 000 ppm allicin potential [12 mg]): 1200–4800 mg daily
- **D-limonene:** 7–15 g daily
- **L-carnitine:** 500–2000 mg daily
- **Acetyl-L-carnitine:** 1000–2000 mg daily
- **Zinc:** 30–60 mg daily

**Innovative Drug Strategies**

The following should be used only under a physician's supervision:
- **Metformin:** 500 mg, 3 times daily before meals
- **Chloroquine**
- **Celecoxib**
- **Zileuton**
- **Pancreatic enzymes (by prescription):** 1000–10 000 U lipase per kg of body weight per meal.[322] Delayed-release preparations (capsules containing enteric-coated microspheres, such as Creon®) are reportedly less susceptible to acid inactivation.

  **Antacids or a histamine H2-receptor antagonist (cimetidine, Tagamet®):** used to decrease the inactivation of pancreatic enzyme activity.

  **Ukrain (NSC-631570):** Ukrain is supplied as a solution ready for injection. A ukrain therapy cycle consists of 10 mg taken intravenously every other day for 20 days. A vitamin C cycle is added to the ukrain cycle, 3 g taken intravenously every other day, and 2.4 g taken orally in 3 divided doses on the same days, for 20 days.[323]

## REFERENCES

References available at: www.lef.org/dpt5/ch106

# 107

---

# *Parkinson's Disease*

---

Parkinson's disease is a degenerative disease of the central nervous system resulting from depletion of dopamine-producing cells in a region of the brain called the *substantia nigra*. A variety of genetic and environmental factors underlie this loss of brain cells. However, emergent research implicates *oxidative stress*, *inflammation*, and *dysfunctional mitochondria* as major contributors to *neurodegeneration* in Parkinson's disease.

Up to 1 million Americans live with Parkinson's disease, with 60 000 new cases being diagnosed each year. Men are more likely to be affected than women, and the risk increases substantially after age 50–60; however, 1 in 20 patients is diagnosed under the age of 40.[1,2]

Progression of the disease usually leads to characteristic symptoms such as tremors, muscle rigidity, bradykinesia (slowness and difficulty with movements), poor balance, sleep disturbances, and loss of coordination. Eventually, cognitive decline occurs, and, in advanced disease, dementia arises.

Conventional medical approaches to treating Parkinson's disease aim to replace the lost dopamine, but *fall short* of addressing the ongoing destruction of dopaminergic *neurons*. Over time, the ability of medications to replenish dopamine levels becomes overwhelmed by further loss of dopaminergic cells. Moreover, the pharmaceutical drugs typically used to alleviate symptoms of Parkinson's disease are laden with *debilitating side effects* and often worsen effects over time. Thus, the prognosis for Parkinson's disease patients relying on conventional treatment remains limited.

The mainstream medical establishment has *failed* to recognize the *urgent* need to address the multiple, interrelated pathologic features of Parkinson's disease in order to prevent further neuronal loss and slow disease progression.

Scientific innovation has led to the realization that natural compounds and some *underappreciated* pharmaceutical agents can synergize to *support mitochondrial function*, *suppress inflammation*, *ease oxidative stress*, and may improve outlook for Parkinson's disease patients.

Life Extension's approach encompasses a regimen combining conventional therapeutics to ease symptoms and *innovative* natural ingredients along with state-of-the-art pharmaceuticals to reduce the destruction of dopaminergic neurons. This approach offers Parkinson's disease patients a chance for symptomatic improvement and enhanced quality of life.

## BRIEF HISTORY, CLASSIFICATIONS, AND RISK FACTORS

James Parkinson first described the motor system disorder known today as Parkinson's disease in an 1817 paper entitled "An Essay on the Shaking Palsy."[3] In his report, Parkinson described several characteristic traits, including an abnormal posture and gait, and partial paralysis with muscle weakness; he also described the progression of the disease. The contribution of more clearly defining the condition, theretofore known as *paralysis agitans*, led to the adoption of Parkinson's last name as the moniker that remains with us today.

Since 1817, medical advancements have helped us establish a much greater understanding of Parkinson's disease. Today, clustered symptoms like tremor at rest, stiffness, slowed movement, and postural instability are classified into 1 of 2 general categories based on their cause.

### Parkinson's Disease (Primary Parkinson's)

This is the most common form of the disease; what most of us think of when we hear the term "Parkinson's." Primary Parkinson's disease has no clear external cause, and is therefore classified as *idiopathic* (without cause, arising spontaneously). Recently, however, several genes directly tied with the development of Parkinson's disease have been identified. This has led to the classification of heritable Parkinson's disease of genetic origin as *familial Parkinson's disease*, while Parkinson's disease that arises independently of genetic predisposition is referred to as *sporadic Parkinson's disease*.

Despite the fact that conventional medical dogma holds tightly to the notion that primary Parkinson's disease *truly* lacks an identifiable cause (other than genetics in familial Parkinson's disease), metabolic phenomena, such as oxidative stress, mitochondrial fatigue, and other age-related abnormalities are linked with the death of dopamine-producing *neurons*.[4]

Exposure to *pesticides* may substantially increase risk for Parkinson's disease.[5–10] In one study, higher pesticide exposure increased Parkinson's disease risk 3-fold.[10] Numerous epidemiologic studies have confirmed the association.[11,12] Toxin-induced Parkinson's symptoms may be classified as secondary rather than primary Parkinson's.[4,13]

Interestingly, pesticides seem to accumulate in the dopaminergic tract, where they inhibit mitochondrial function and lead to neuronal death.[7,14] Dopaminergic neurons are particularly susceptible to the pesticide dieldrin, which is no longer in use in the United States, but remains ubiquitous due to environmental contamination.[15] In addition to acting as neuronal and mitochondrial toxins, some pesticides also impair the breakdown of protein aggregates, like Lewy bodies.[16]

Several lines of evidence suggest that a genetic inability to properly detoxify environmental toxicants may predispose some individuals to Parkinson's disease.[17,18]

In addition, those who experience constipation throughout their lives appear to be at increased risk.[19] In one study, constipation documented in medical records as much as 20 years before disease onset was associated with a significantly increased risk.[20] Some researchers believe that this may be related to intake of drinking water—lower water intake appears to be a risk factor as well.[21] This may be linked to reduced elimination of water-soluble toxins.

Due to the strong association between pesticides and other environmental toxins with Parkinson's disease, readers are strongly encouraged to review Life Extension's Metabolic Detoxification protocol.

## Parkinsonian Syndrome (Secondary Parkinson's)

Other forms of Parkinsonism can occur as a *secondary* effect of brain tumor, drugs, toxins (eg, carbon monoxide poisoning), postencephalitis (the viral infectious disease, "sleeping sickness"). For example, another cause of Parkinsonism is brain damage sustained by repeated blows to the head such as suffered by professional prize fighters and athletes in high-impact sports like football. Traumatic events, infections, the use of certain medications, and other factors can damage the dopaminergic cells within the midbrain, leading to the same symptoms as primary Parkinson's disease.

For example, the defining basis for Parkinsonism due to *encephalitis* (brain inflammation) was a worldwide influenza pandemic in 1917. After recovering from this illness, many patients developed Parkinson's disease years later.[22] Acquired immunodeficiency syndrome (AIDS) may also lead to Parkinsonism.[23] Resuscitation from cardiac arrest (due to temporary lack of oxygen supply to the brain) and stroke can lead to Parkinsonism as well.[24]

Several centrally acting drugs, especially those that exert an effect on the dopamine system within the brain, such as antipsychotics, frequently induce secondary Parkinsonism after sustained chronic use. In fact, *drug-induced Parkinsonism* is a well-documented phenomenon.[25–27] Some antidepressants, calcium channel blockers, and the antiarrhythmic drug amiodarone can lead to Parkinsonian tremors as well.[27] Several illicit drugs can cause Parkinsonism.

Some diseases or disorders considered to cause Parkinsonian syndromes include multiple system atrophy (MSA), progressive supranuclear palsy (PSP), corticobasal degeneration (CBGD), and Pick's disease.

## SIGNS, SYMPTOMS, AND DIAGNOSIS

Dopamine is a neurotransmitter that, among other functions, allows messages to be sent to regions of the brain responsible for coordinating movement. When dopamine levels decline due to the death of dopaminergic cells, these messages no longer reach their destination, and so the regions of the brain that control movement no longer function properly. This results in loss of conscious control of movement, and, in advanced Parkinson's disease, loss of control over several other bodily functions.

The onset and course of Parkinson's disease may be different for each patient. For example, while tremor is evident is most patients, some may not experience movement complications until the disease has advanced considerably.

Initial symptoms of primary Parkinson's disease typically develop slowly and randomly as the supply of dopamine dwindles over time. In some cases, symptoms do not appear until approximately 70% of the dopaminergic cells in the substantia nigra are already destroyed.[2]

### Motor Symptoms

The onset of a slight tremor, usually in the hand, which increases in intensity over time, is often the initial sign of Parkinson's. However, roughly 30% of patients do not develop a tremor. Parkinson's patients often experience muscle rigidity or cramping that can be painful—movements as simple as turning over in bed or buttoning a shirt can become arduous, and as the disease advances, nearly impossible. Progression of Parkinson's disease leads to slowness of movement, which can cause a great deal of frustration for patients who cannot move as quickly as they would like.

"Freezing" is a frequently reported motor symptom in advancing Parkinson's. This involves the sudden onset of the inability to move at all; patients sometimes describe freezing as feeling as if their feet are stuck to the floor. Freezing is temporary and usually lasts from a few seconds to a few minutes.

## Nonmotor Symptoms

Dopamine is involved in a number of functions beyond control of movement, so loss of dopaminergic neurons (and other neurons in late-stage Parkinson's) can cause several nonmotor symptoms as well. Nonmotor symptoms usually develop at later stages of disease progression but can be equally as debilitating as motor symptoms for many patients.

Patients with advanced Parkinson's disease may experience a variety of non-motor symptoms, including incontinence, constipation, difficulty swallowing, inability to control saliva, dizziness leading to falls, excessive daytime sleepiness, intense frightening dreams, depression and/or anxiety, and hallucinations.[2] In addition, Parkinson's disease can cause perceptible pain throughout the body, which is sometimes severe.

## Dementia

Dementia and related cognitive decline is a major concern among those with advanced Parkinson's disease. Up to 75–80% of those with Parkinson's develop dementia near the end of their life.[28,29] In addition to loss of dopaminergic neurons, *cholinergic* neurons are also at risk. Cholinergic neurons produce a neurotransmitter called *acetylcholine*, which is important for cognitive function. The accumulation of protein aggregates (clumps of dysfunctional proteins) known as *Lewy bodies* within cholinergic neurons is a common characteristic of Parkinson's disease.

As Lewy bodies accumulate inside neurons, the cells can no longer function, and eventually die. Loss of acetylcholine leads to diminished attention span, blunted sensory perceptions, loss of arousal and structural changes in the synaptic junctions (the connections between neurons through which they communicate using chemical and electrical signals). Loss of *acetylcholinergic* signaling is thought to be associated with memory deficits in Alzheimer's disease as well, though the exact mechanisms are complex.[30]

Two subsets of dementia exist in the context of Parkinson's disease, *Parkinson's disease dementia* (PDD) and *dementia with Lewy bodies* (DLB). The distinction between the 2 is quite subjective and largely based on the time of dementia diagnosis in relation to onset of motor symptoms. Whether the 2 dementias are truly separate entities or simply manifestations of different points along the "Lewy body spectrum," is a hotly debated topic.[31]

## Diagnosis

Clinicians must rely on clinical experience, interpretation of symptoms, and evaluation of medical history in order to tentatively diagnose a patient as having Parkinson's disease. This is because there are no lab tests available that definitively diagnose Parkinson's disease. Parkinson's disease is a diagnosis of exclusion; in other words, the physician will first rule out other possible diagnoses before assuming Parkinson's.

If Parkinson's is suspected because the patient is exhibiting signs such as a tremor on one side of their body or rigidity with loss of postural reflexes, oftentimes *L-DOPA*, a drug used to treat Parkinson's symptoms, is administered. If L-DOPA causes the symptoms to subside, the diagnosis of Parkinson's disease can be made more confidently, yet still not definitively.

Due to the elusive nature of a definitive Parkinson's disease diagnosis, patients should be reevaluated regularly to ensure that their symptoms are not due to another neurologic disorder that causes similar symptoms.

# CAUSES, PATHOLOGIC MECHANISMS, AND LESSONS FROM BIOLOGY

## Genetics—Familial Parkinson's

Roughly 15% of Parkinson's disease patients have a first-degree relative who also has/had Parkinson's disease; this suggests that genetics play a consequential role in the development of familial Parkinson's disease.[32] Roughly 9 genetic mutations have been associated with Parkinson's disease; of these, 6 have been particularly well characterized.[32,33] Mutations in these genes are generally associated with *early onset Parkinson's disease*, which is diagnosed before age 40. Parkinson's disease of genetic origin is sometimes diagnosed in childhood.

Mutations in the following genes are associated with an increased risk of Parkinson's disease:

- SNCA[34–37]
- LRRK2[38]
- PARK2[39]
- PINK1[40–43]
- PARK7[44–48]
- ATP13A2[49–52]

Additional research is required to fully elucidate the role of genetics in Parkinson's etiology; it is likely that several additional genes involved in the pathology will be identified in the coming years. Treatments

# Anatomy of the brain and a synapse

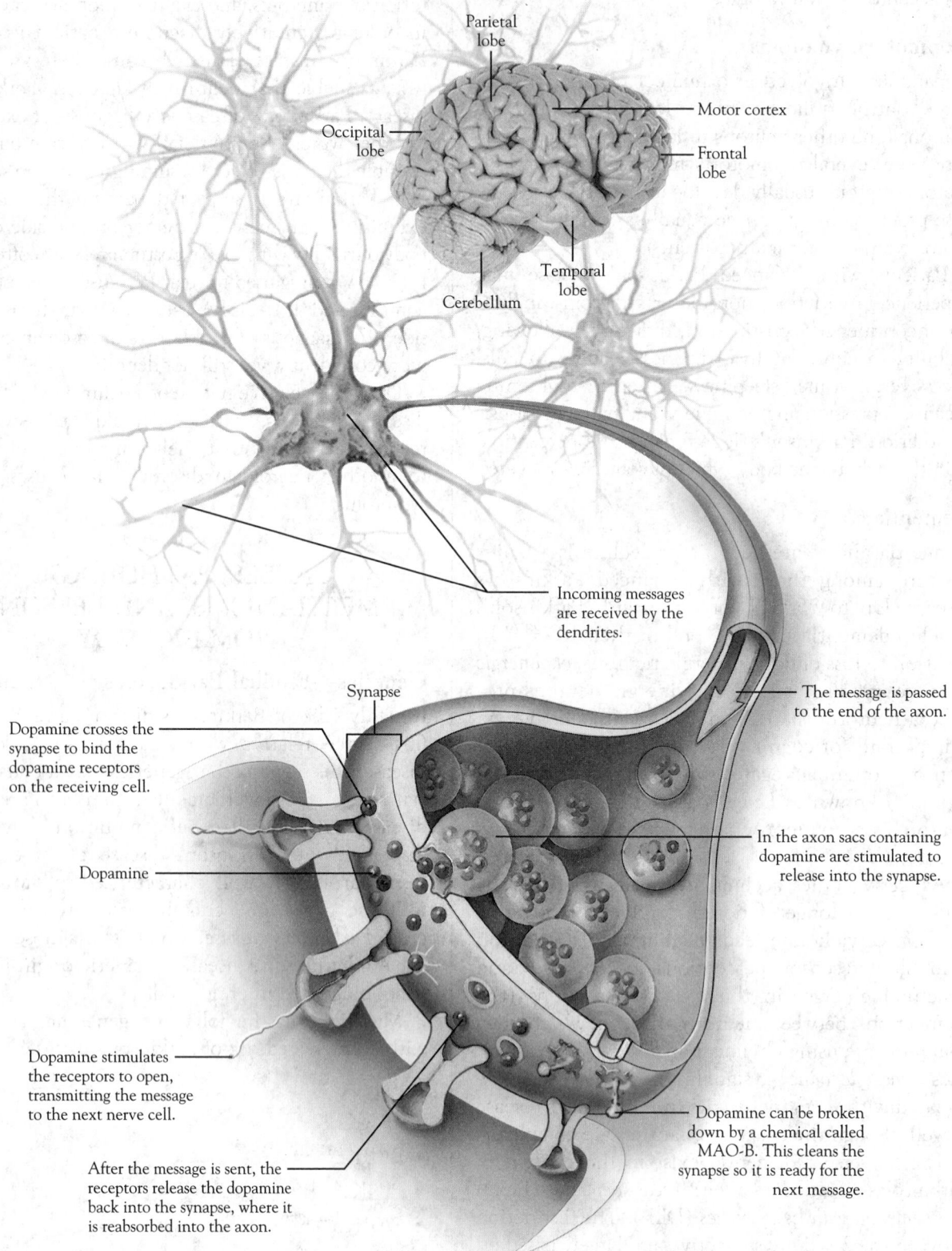

Parietal lobe

Occipital lobe

Motor cortex

Frontal lobe

Cerebellum

Temporal lobe

Incoming messages are received by the dendrites.

Synapse

The message is passed to the end of the axon.

Dopamine crosses the synapse to bind the dopamine receptors on the receiving cell.

Dopamine

In the axon sacs containing dopamine are stimulated to release into the synapse.

Dopamine stimulates the receptors to open, transmitting the message to the next nerve cell.

After the message is sent, the receptors release the dopamine back into the synapse, where it is reabsorbed into the axon.

Dopamine can be broken down by a chemical called MAO-B. This cleans the synapse so it is ready for the next message.

based on genetic therapy are likely to become more widespread and therapeutic as scientific knowledge progresses.

## GENETIC TESTING

Genetic testing for mutations known to be associated with Parkinson's disease is available through genetic health care professionals. Specifically, tests are available that check for mutations in PINK1, PARK7, SNCA, and LRRK2. Although the testing is expensive, and accuracy is a potential concern, those individuals with a family history of Parkinson's disease are encouraged to discuss genetic testing with their health care provider.

The National Human Genome Research Institute, a division of the National Institutes of Health, has compiled further information about the role of genetics and genetic testing in Parkinson's disease. This resource can also assist with the location of a *genetic counselor* near you. Their Web site is: http://www.genome.gov/10001217#4.

Individuals found to have a mutation in one or more of the genes linked to Parkinson's, as well as those with a family history of Parkinson's, should consult a Parkinson's disease specialist, and initiate nutritional and lifestyle strategies to combat neurodegeneration.

## Mitochondrial Dysfunction

A flurry of emergent research has linked *mitochondrial dysfunction* to the pathogenesis of Parkinson's disease. Mitochondrial dysfunction results in impaired ATP generation, loss of cellular repair mechanisms, and cellular inefficiency.

As mitochondria become dysfunctional they generate large quantities of *free radicals*, which contribute to *oxidative stress* that, in turn, causes further mitochondrial dysfunction. Concurrently, loss of mitochondria to oxidative damage means fewer mitochondria are available to meet the energy demands of the cell to repair damaged components. The cascade of mitochondrial dysfunction, oxidative stress, and loss of mitochondria form a continuity that ultimately leads to cell death.[53,54]

Numerous studies have clearly identified mitochondrial dysfunction as a central pathologic feature of both genetic *and* sporadic Parkinson's disease.[55,56] Moreover, many of the genes that confer predisposition to familial Parkinson's are intimately related to mitochondrial function; much of the neuronal death in Parkinson's of genetic origin is due to mitochondrial dysfunction and impaired mitophagy.[57–59] While several factors, including exposure to environmental toxins,[57,60,61] also contribute to mitochondrial dysfunction in the *substantia nigra*, age-related mutations in mitochondrial DNA are thought to be a primary culprit.[61,62] Alarmingly, dopamine itself and L-DOPA may contribute to mitochondrial toxicity in dopaminergic neurons.[63–65]

## Mitophagy, Lewy Bodies, and Alpha-Synuclein

Damaged mitochondria are continually being cleared from within the cell through a process called *mitophagy*. Mitophagy, a type of *autophagy*, is a kind of cellular recycling system that clears damaged mitochondria before they can accumulate and cause cellular dysfunction. However, *age-related* mutations in mitochondrial DNA, which cause mitophagy to become less efficient, coupled with an ever-intensifying propensity for endogenous and environmentally mediated mitochondrial damage cause the neuronal mitophagic system to become overwhelmed.[58,66] Over time, damaged mitochondria build up inside the neuron, leading to cell death. Not surprisingly, several of the genetic mutations linked to familial Parkinson's disease cause disturbances in mitophagy.[58,59]

Another toxic byproduct of mitochondrial dysfunction and impaired mitophagy is the formation of *Lewy bodies*. Lewy bodies form as reactive oxygen species derived from dysfunctional mitochondria damage structural components of the cell called *microtubules*. As microtubules are damaged, they release a protein called *alpha-synuclein*. The loose alpha-synuclein proteins then group together, or aggregate, and form a toxic mass (a Lewy body) that further damages the cell. Moreover, alpha-synuclein has been shown to directly interfere with mitochondrial function and inhibit ATP synthesis, furthering the spread of mitochondrial dysfunction in the brains of Parkinson's disease patients.[67–69] Over time, Lewy bodies spread to neighboring cells, damaging neurons within the vicinity of a dead or dying neuron.[70]

Lewy bodies share some characteristics with toxic proteins that develop in the brains of patients with Alzheimer's disease and other neurodegenerative diseases, primarily in that they cannot be broken down and cleared from the cell by normal autophagic (cellular house-cleaning) actions.

## The Role of Inflammation in Parkinson's Disease

Inflammatory responses contribute to the perpetuation of neurodegeneration in Parkinson's disease. The brain contains immune cells called microglia, which are known to be activated in Parkinson's disease.[71,72] Upon activation, microglia release inflammatory cytokines that can spread to nearby healthy neurons and cause degeneration. Dopaminergic neurons in the *substantia nigra*, the brain region most affected by Parkinson's disease, express receptors for an inflammatory cytokine called tumor necrosis factor-alpha (TNF-$\alpha$), which suggests that excess TNF-$\alpha$ released by nearby activated microglia may damage nigral dopaminergic cells.

Elevated cytokines in the brain of those with Parkinson's disease is a consequence of neurodegeneration.[73] In experimental models, exposure to the neurotoxin MPTP (a chemical used to induce Parkinson's disease in experiments) leads to death of dopaminergic neurons. Interestingly, in monkeys, inflammation is increased even years after initial exposure to MPTP.[72] This suggests that inflammation, once initiated, has long-term consequences in Parkinson's disease.

As dopaminergic cells succumb to either environmentally or genetically induced mitochondrial dysfunction, they release free radicals. These free radicals then activate nearby microglial cells, which in turn excrete inflammatory cytokines that bind to and damage nearby dopaminergic neurons. This positive feedback loop may continue over years or even decades and slowly contribute to the loss of dopaminergic neurons that leads to Parkinson symptoms.[73,74]

Epidemiological studies on the use of anti-inflammatory drugs and the risk of Parkinson's onset are conflicting. Some studies suggest a protective role of ibuprofen, but not other anti-inflammatory drugs.[75] However, a large study published in the *British Medical Journal* involving over 22 000 subjects found no association between use of any NSAID reduced risk.[76] These findings reinforce the notion that, rather than initiating dopaminergic cell death, inflammation may perpetuate it, thus contributing to Parkinson's disease progression. Life Extension believes that suppressing inflammation may slow disease progression in Parkinson's disease patients.

## SIMVASTATIN AS AN ANTI-INFLAMMATORY AND NEUROPROTECTIVE AGENT IN PARKINSON'S DISEASE

Groundbreaking research suggests that the cholesterol-lowering drug *simvastatin* may provide powerful neuroprotection in Parkinson's disease. A little-known fact is that statin drugs do more than simply lower cholesterol—they are also anti-inflammatory agents. In fact, many researchers believe that some of the cardiovascular benefits are due to their anti-inflammatory properties.[77]

Simvastatin is efficient at crossing the blood–brain barrier, and it has been shown to exert potent anti-inflammatory and neuroprotective action in the dopaminergic tract.[78,79]

In animal models, simvastatin was shown to attenuate the neurotoxicity of MPTP. In fact, simvastatin accumulated in the nigra and suppressed microglial activation, leading to reduced expression of inflammatory cytokines and increased dopaminergic neuroprotection.[80] Another animal experiment found that simvastatin was able to completely reverse the decline in dopamine receptors associate with exposure to the neurotoxin 6-hydroxydopamine.[81]

In a large human clinical study involving over 700 000 subjects, use of simvastatin was associated with a 49% reduction in the likelihood of onset of Parkinson's symptoms, as well as a 54% reduction in the risk of dementia, suggesting a substantial neuroprotective effect.[82]

Due to the emergence of strong evidence that simvastatin may have anti-inflammatory and neuroprotective actions, Life Extension encourages Parkinson's disease patients taking a cholesterol-lowering medication to talk with their doctor about switching to *simvastatin*. Even those whose cholesterol is not significantly elevated may benefit from low-dose simvastatin. People who do not take cholesterol-lowering medication should discuss this with their doctor.

Importantly, those taking any statin drug should be aware that statins deplete coenzyme Q10 (CoQ10) levels. If taking statins, supplement with CoQ10 and ensure maintenance of healthy CoQ10 blood levels by periodically having a CoQ10 blood test.

## CONVENTIONAL MEDICAL TREATMENT

For decades, the conventional standard of care for Parkinson's disease has focused on symptomatic relief. Pharmaceutical treatments for Parkinson's accomplish this by either increasing the levels of dopamine or mimicking its action. While conventional therapeutics are indispensable for improving quality of life in Parkinson's patients, they *do not provide fundamental neuroprotection or support for neuronal mitochondria*. Thus, mainstream pharmaceutical treatments cannot be expected to address the underlying cause of disease progression—neurodegeneration.

Treatment with L-DOPA causes patients to be less responsive to the medication over time, and can evoke a number of adverse side effects. However, careful dosing strategies and utilization of ancillary medications may help limit side effects and maintain the effectiveness of conventional pharmaceutical therapies.

Pharmaceutical treatment of Parkinson's disease symptoms is usually initiated when the patient has already developed some disability for which he/she needs to be treated. This is typically referred to as the *initial stage* of therapy. The primary goal of treatment during the initial stage is to limit symptoms arising from progression of the disease. However, with time, adverse side effects of the medications arise, which leads into the *secondary* treatment stage. The aim of the secondary treatment stage is to reduce Parkinson's symptoms as well as counterbalance the adverse side effects of levodopa.

## Levodopa (L-DOPA)/Carbidopa

Since approval by the Food and Drug Administration (FDA) in 1970, Levodopa (L-DOPA) has been a staple for managing Parkinson's disease symptoms. L-DOPA (the *precursor* to dopamine) is metabolized into dopamine in the body by an enzyme called *aromatic L-amino acid decarboxylase* (AADC). Dopamine itself cannot pass through the protective *blood–brain barrier*, but L-DOPA can. When L-DOPA is administered orally, a small percentage passes into the brain and is converted into dopamine. This temporary increase in dopamine levels within the brain offers relief of Parkinson's disease symptoms for a short period.

However, the body presents many obstacles that limit the efficiency of oral L-DOPA therapy. First, AADC exists outside the brain as well, which means that the majority of orally administered L-DOPA will be converted into dopamine peripherally, that is, not in the central nervous system. Therefore, L-DOPA is typically administered with an inhibitor of peripheral AADC, called *carbidopa*. Carbidopa (or another AADC inhibitor) helps to preserve orally administered L-DOPA for conversion to dopamine in the brain.

Regrettably, the use of orally administered L-DOPA over time results in diminished production of endogenous (naturally occurring within the body) L-DOPA. L-DOPA therapy is further complicated by the development of movement disorders called *dyskinesias* after 5–10 years of use in most cases.

Dyskinesias are movement disorders in which neurologic discoordination results in uncontrollable, involuntary movements. This discoordination can also affect the autonomic nervous system, resulting in, for example, respiratory irregularities.[83] Dyskinesia is the result of L-DOPA–induced synaptic dysfunction and inappropriate signaling between areas of the brain that normally coordinate movement, namely the motor cortex and the striatum.[84]

With long-term L-DOPA use (usually after about 5 years), responsiveness declines and dose adjustment is often necessary. This phenomenon leads to fluctuations in the effectiveness of L-DOPA therapy that cause the patient to experience dyskinesia as the post-dose concentration of L-DOPA peaks, and rapid reversion to severe Parkinsonism toward the end of the dosing period.

Several strategies exist for enhancing L-DOPA effectiveness. Some of these include varying combinations of L-DOPA and other medications discussed in this section as well as altering dose timing and amount. Other strategies can involve "rest periods" or "drug holidays" during which the patient abstains from L-DOPA for a short time; for instance, skipping a single dose each day may help reduce the damage caused by oxidation products of L-DOPA metabolism and maintain dopamine receptor sensitivity. Patients should never adjust their L-DOPA dose, however, without close supervision by their physician.

Other strategies for stabilizing dopamine levels include combining L-DOPA with inhibitors of enzymes that breakdown dopamine. Medications of this type include *monoamine oxidase-B (MAO-B) inhibitors*, and *catechol-O-methyltransferase (COMT) inhibitors*. By combining L-DOPA with COMT and/or MAO-B inhibitors, a physician may be able to reduce the dose of L-DOPA required to relieve symptoms, and widen dose intervals, which is more convenient for the patient.

There are a variety of ways that pharmaceuticals can be combined to deliver optimal effects in each Parkinson's case, but patient needs may vary widely. Therefore, patients should always consult an experienced physician to discuss medication combinations that may be ideal for their unique situation.

L-DOPA can produce several adverse side effects, including the following:

- Arrhythmia
- Gastrointestinal discomfort (taking L-DOPA with low protein snacks may help avoid stomach upset)
- Breathing disturbances
- Hair loss
- Confusion
- Extreme emotional variability with prevalent anxiety
- Vivid dreams
- Hallucinations
- Impaired social behavior
- Sleepiness
- Excessive libido
- Compulsive behavior (eg, reckless gambling)

L-DOPA–induced elevations in *homocysteine*, a potentially harmful amino-acid derivative, are another major concern for Parkinson's patients. High levels of homocysteine have been implicated in various cardiovascular diseases, including cerebral small vessel disease, as well as brain atrophy.[85,86]

A comprehensive review of 16 studies found that elevated homocysteine was associated with dementia and markers of neurodegeneration in patients with Parkinson's.[87]

Parkinson's disease patients taking L-DOPA should read Life Extension's Homocysteine Reduction protocol and strive to maintain homocysteine levels of *less than 7–8 µmol/L*.

## L-DOPA DRUG HOLIDAYS

Regular, chronic use of L-DOPA causes dopamine receptors within the brain to become less sensitive, leading to the eventual need for increased dosages of L-DOPA. Research suggests that taking a "drug holiday" from L-DOPA may resensitize dopaminergic receptors and lower the patient's L-DOPA requirements, or at least prevent the need for increasing L-DOPA in the near future. In a 3-year study, 15 Parkinson's patients were submitted to a 7-day L-DOPA drug holiday. Within the first 6 months following the drug holiday, symptoms improved dramatically and all of the study subjects were able to maintain a L-DOPA dose regimen of 50–70% of their preholiday dose for the entire 3-year period.[88]

Despite these promising results, there are serious risks associated with stopping L-DOPA therapy, one of which is *neuroleptic malignant syndrome*, a potentially life-threatening situation. Therefore, a drug holiday should only be initiated under the close supervision of a physician. However, at least one study suggests that use of amantadine, another drug used to alleviate Parkinson's symptoms, during an L-DOPA drug holiday may limit the severity of side effects associated with stopping L-DOPA therapy. In this study, 12 Parkinson's patients were submitted to a 3-day L-DOPA drug holiday, and during that time they were given intravenous infusions of amantadine. The subjects were then started back on the preholiday L-DOPA dose and symptomatic improvements lasting up to 4 months were noted.[89]

## Dopamine Agonists

Another method used to restore dopaminergic signaling in Parkinson's disease is medicating with a dopamine agonist. A dopamine agonist is a drug containing a molecule that binds to and activates dopamine receptors, similar to dopamine itself, thus compensating for low dopamine levels. Dopamine agonists are often used in younger patients, or in very early Parkinson's disease.

Research comparing the results of initial therapy with a dopamine agonist or L-DOPA is conflicting. Some studies suggest that initiating therapy with a dopamine agonist may delay the onset of dyskinesias as the disease progresses, while some seem to indicate that this may not be the case. Other studies suggest that initial dopamine agonist therapy delivers results

similar to those seen in L-DOPA + COMT inhibitor therapy.[90] Results from a 14-year follow-up study found that initial therapy with a dopamine agonist offered no greater benefit over standard L-DOPA therapy in the long term.[91]

Dopamine agonists pose a greater risk of serious side effects than L-DOPA and are therefore not as tolerable for some patients. Some side effects of dopamine agonists include the following:

- Euphoria
- Hallucinations
- Psychosis
- Orthostatic hypotension (low blood pressure upon standing)
- Increased orgasmic intensity
- Weight loss
- Nausea
- Insomnia
- Unusual tiredness or weakness
- Dizziness or fainting
- Twitching, twisting, or other unusual body movements
- Pathologic addiction and compulsive behavior (eg, hypersexuality, gambling)

### Selegiline and Rasagiline

**Selegiline.** Selegiline is an MAO-B inhibitor that, due to its unique chemical structure, also exerts other neuropharmacologic actions via its metabolites. By blocking the breakdown of dopamine, selegiline helps compensate for the diminished production of dopamine in Parkinson's disease. This can lead to symptomatic improvement, especially in early-stage Parkinson's.

Numerous clinical trials have confirmed the efficacy of selegiline alone and in combination with L-DOPA in early Parkinson's disease.[92–94] One study showed that selegiline was highly effective if initiated within 5 years of Parkinson's disease diagnosis, but less effective if initiated ≥10 years after diagnosis.[92]

Selegiline exerts a number of other benefits as well, including maintenance of whole-brain blood flow in depressed Parkinson's disease patients.[95] Moreover, selegiline may reduce the formation and toxicity of alpha-synuclein aggregates.[96]

**Rasagiline.** Rasagiline is a newer-generation medication based on selegiline. Laboratory studies suggest that, in addition to functioning very similarly to selegiline, rasagiline may exert a greater neuroprotective effect.[97]

Rasagiline was superior to placebo in slowing progression of Parkinson's disease in a cohort of 1176 early-stage patients. In this study, subjects receiving rasagiline were less likely than those taking placebo to need additional anti-Parkinson drugs to manage symptoms.[98] More trials need to be conducted to determine whether rasagiline is significantly more effective than selegiline for treating Parkinson's disease.

Selegiline is available via prescription in a clinically studied transdermal patch called Emsam®. Selegiline and rasagiline may cause dizziness, dry mouth, sleeplessness, and an overall stimulating effect.

# ALTERNATIVE AND EMERGING THERAPIES

In addition to the conventional standard of care, which relies heavily on L-DOPA therapy, physicians may sometimes implement other pharmaceutical agents that complement the effects of L-DOPA therapy or limit its side effects.

## Amantadine

Amantadine is an antiviral drug that exerts a number of actions in the brain. Amantadine has been shown in some studies to benefit Parkinson's patients, primarily by reducing the side effects of L-DOPA, or as an adjuvant during L-DOPA drug holidays as mentioned above, although the mechanisms are largely unclear.

In clinical studies, amantadine has been shown to temporarily reduce L-DOPA–induced dyskinesia, an effect that dissipates after about 8 months.[99,100] However, in some patients, discontinuation of amantadine appears to cause a rebound worsening of dyskinesias to an even higher intensity than before its introduction.[100]

As mentioned earlier in this protocol, at least one study suggests that amantadine may suppress side effects of L-DOPA abstinence during a drug holiday.[89] Amantadine may ease Parkinson's symptoms in some patients, but should only be initiated under physician supervision.

## Nicotine

Within the brain, there exists a grand diversity of neurotransmitter interaction and overlap. One such relationship is between the dopaminergic and cholinergic systems. For example, acetylcholine modulates dopaminergic signaling in the striatum, an area considerably impacted in Parkinson's disease.

Nicotine interacts with the cholinergic system by binding sites known as nicotinic acetylcholinergic receptors (nAChRs), which influence several functions relevant in Parkinson's disease, including dopamine signaling.[101] Moreover, loss of nAChRs accompanies many neurodegenerative disease, including Parkinson's disease, suggesting that declining cholinergic signaling is a key etiologic feature.[102]

Several studies indicate that nicotine exerts powerful neuroprotective effects via activation of nAChRs.[103] Recent data indicate that among the neuroprotective effects of nicotine is the ability to reduce alpha-synuclein aggregation, which may suppress the formation of Lewy bodies.[104]

Many epidemiologic studies have confirmed that smoking tobacco confers a substantial reduction in risk for developing Parkinson's disease.[105,106] Moreover, transdermal nicotine patches have been shown to improve cognitive functioning in patients with Parkinson's disease.[107] Other evidence suggests a therapeutic effect of nicotine in reducing L-DOPA–induced dyskinesias.[108] As of November 2012, results from at least one larger study assessing the efficacy of transdermal nicotine on motor symptoms in advanced Parkinson's disease are pending publication.[109]

Nicotine appears to have potential to deliver significant and clinically meaningful benefits in Parkinson's disease. If you have Parkinson's disease, you are encouraged to speak with your physician about potentially complementing your anti-Parkinsonian therapy with transdermal nicotine. Your doctor should help you determine an appropriate dose; the Holms study cited above used 7 milligrams (mg)/24 hrs delivered via a transdermal nicotine patch. Newer studies aim to evaluate higher doses (eg, 90 mg/week) via transdermal patch.

## Granulocyte Colony-Stimulating Factor (G-CSF)

G-CSF is a signaling glycoprotein (produced in several tissues) that stimulates the production and differentiation of white blood cells, thereby playing a significant role in immune system function. Recombinant G-CSF is frequently given to chemotherapy patients to restore levels of white blood cells that have been suppressed by treatment.

The interaction of G-CSF with the immune system is very complex. However, current evidence suggests that besides stimulating white blood cell generation, it pushes the immune system toward a less autoreactive, anti-inflammatory *TH2* phenotype rich in T-regulatory cells.[110] Due to this unique action, G-CSF may be of benefit in diseases in which inflammation contributes to the pathology.

Interestingly, receptors for G-CSF are expressed in neurons throughout the central nervous system and activation of those receptors (by G-CSF) stimulates neurogenesis and protects neurons from damage.[110,111]

In animal models of both Alzheimer's disease and Parkinson's disease, subcutaneous injections of recombinant human G-CSF suppressed inflammation in brain regions centrally involved in the pathology of each disease and stimulated the formation of new synapses.[112–114] In these studies, mice treated with G-CSF performed much better on cognitive tests than those not treated with G-CSF.

These findings are very exciting and hold promise for future research. While no human clinical trials for G-CSF in Parkinson's disease have been published as of November 2012, a phase II clinical trial is currently underway in Taiwan.[115] Results of this trial are expected sometime in 2013. If they are positive, they may lead to even larger-scale clinical trials and eventually to clinical use of G-CSF in Parkinson's disease patients.

## Stem Cells and Cell Replacement Therapy

The hallmark of Parkinson's disease is loss of dopaminergic neurons in the substantia nigra. Therefore, many therapeutic approaches have aimed at replacing lost neurons in this region using cell replacement therapy, or stem cell therapy. These therapies are largely experimental as of the current time and no large-scale clinical trials have been conducted as of yet. In fact, small-scale clinical trials have shown that benefit of replacing dopamine neurons may be questionable, and that the therapy caused severe dyskinesias in some subjects.[116]

Another major challenge associated with cell replacement therapy is ensuring survival of transplanted neurons. Thus far, this has proven extremely difficult.[117] However, further studies are underway, and advancements in research may allow for widespread use of these therapies in the not-too-distant future.

## Ablative Surgery and Deep-Brain Stimulation

A conventional therapy of last resort involves ablative surgery, or deep-brain stimulation, in which areas of the brain that are normally under control of dopamine are destroyed. This helps alleviate symptoms in some cases because when the regulatory actions of dopamine are absent, as in advanced Parkinson's disease, those regions of the brain can become dysregulated and dysfunctional.

Only a small percentage of Parkinson's patients are good candidates for ablative surgery or deep-brain stimulation, and there are many risks. Surgical options may be considered in advanced Parkinson's disease when other treatments are no longer able to control symptoms effectively.

However, researchers in the Netherlands have recently developed a method of dramatically improving the accuracy and reliability of deep-brain stimulation.[118] This may make it a more viable option in the near future.

## Cognitive Behavioral Therapy

Parkinson's disease is often accompanied by comorbid psychological disturbances such as depression and/or anxiety and psychosis (a potential side effect of anti-Parkinson medications). Treatment of psychological disturbances is limited, to some degree, due to potential interactions between pharmaceuticals used to treat Parkinson's and those used to treat other psychological conditions.

Cognitive behavioral therapy offers a highly effective, drug-free alternative for relieving psychological disturbances in Parkinson's disease patients. In one study, depressed Parkinson's patients were either clinically monitored or engaged in cognitive behavioral therapy for just over 3 years. While a mere 8% of patients undergoing clinical monitoring experienced improvements in their depressive symptoms, significant improvement was noted in 56% of those engaged in cognitive behavioral therapy.[119]

In addition to the psychological benefits, cognitive behavioral therapy may be effective for the treatment of some physical symptoms of Parkinson's disease. A 2011 study found that in patients aged ≥50 years, cognitive behavioral therapy led to a significant reduction in the incidence of urinary incontinence.[120]

Several different types of cognitive behavioral therapy are available and different styles may be appropriate in some cases while inappropriate in others. Patients with Parkinson's disease may benefit from cognitive behavioral therapy, and therefore should discuss this option with their physicians.

## Physical Therapy and Exercise

Parkinson's patients are prone to motor disturbances, such as poor balance and a greater chance of falling, which can lead to decreased mobility. As the disease progresses, engaging in structured physical therapy or exercise may be an effective way of maintaining balance and avoiding falls.[121]

Moreover, studies have shown that exercise and physical activity in general exert substantial supportive effects on brain structure and function. In fact, physical activity is associated with a decreased propensity for aging adults to develop dementia, a common problem in Parkinson's disease.[122] Experimental Parkinson's disease models demonstrate that physical activity provides neuroprotection and promotes mitochondrial integrity.[123]

Staying active is very important for Parkinson's disease patients. Those not engaged in regular physical activity are encouraged to speak with their health care provider about initiating a structured exercise or physical therapy regimen. A target goal of 75% maximum age-adjusted heart rate for a minimum of 20 minutes at least 3 times per week is ideal. However, this may not be possible for advanced Parkinson's disease patients.

## DIET

### Low-Protein Diet/Protein Meal Redistribution

L-DOPA therapy is hindered by many obstacles, one of which is excess protein (specifically, aromatic amino acids) competing with L-DOPA for transport into the brain. Therefore, some studies have evaluated the effects of engaging in protein meal redistribution, involving eating dietary protein separate from dosing with L-DOPA.

Current research indicates that protein meal redistribution may be favorable with a low-protein diet. It appears that protein meal redistribution reduces fluctuations, or "on-off periods" in response to L-DOPA therapy.[124] Taking L-DOPA at least 30 minutes before consuming protein and/or having your highest protein meal at a time when L-DOPA is not needed may be an effective strategy. However, patients should speak with their physician to determine which dieting approach is appropriate for them.

### Coffee Consumption

Coffee contains a multitude of pharmacologically active compounds, some of which have been shown to suppress oxidative stress and protect against diabetes, cancer, cognitive decline, and so on.[125] Additionally, several epidemiologic studies have found that those who consume large amounts coffee are much less likely to develop Parkinson's disease.[106,126,127]

Coffee constituents (compounds) protect brain cells, which can be extremely beneficial for Parkinson's disease patients. Coffee extracts have been shown to inhibit MAO-A and -B enzymes, a mechanism similar to that of some pharmaceutical Parkinson's therapies.[128] Experimental models suggest that coffee constituents promote neuronal development and increase antioxidant defense systems in the brain.[129,130]

*Green coffee extract* contains more of the active antioxidant compounds than brewed coffee, and may be a promising option for Parkinson's disease patients.[131] However, clinical trials have yet to confirm this potential benefit.

Intriguing research suggests that caffeine itself may be a potent anti-Parkinson agent. Upon ingestion, caffeine readily crosses the blood–brain barrier and blocks *adenosine receptors*, an effect responsible for many of its pharmacologic actions. The adenosine receptor system interacts with the dopaminergic system in several ways.[132] Experimental studies have shown that caffeine binds to presynaptic adenosine receptors causing an increase in dopamine release, thereby temporarily ameliorating some symptoms of Parkinson's disease.[133] In fact, some data from nonhuman primate studies indicate that adenosine receptor antagonists, like caffeine, may allow for a reduced dosage of L-DOPA. Data in mice also support this notion, but more studies need to be done.[134,135]

In a clinical trial, a daily caffeine dose of 100 mg was shown to reduce "freezing." However, it appeared that the subjects developed a tolerance after a few months. The researchers went on to suggest that caffeine might have therapeutic potential, but a periodic 2-week abstinence period may be required to maintain long-term effectiveness.[136]

Current evidence suggests that coffee consumption may provide some neuroprotection and pharmacologic support, with very little potential downside for Parkinson's patients.

## NATURAL INGREDIENTS TO SUPPORT NEURONAL AND MITOCHONDRIAL HEALTH

Conventional treatment of Parkinson's disease relies heavily on targeting amelioration of *symptoms*, without providing neuroprotection against continual cell death in the substantia nigra. On the other hand, various natural ingredients have been shown to *support neuronal health* and *promote mitochondrial function* in diverse ways, including suppressing *oxidative stress* and limiting *inflammation*. Many natural ingredients may have a complementary effect in combination with conventional therapies.

### CoQ10

The strong connection between defects in mitochondrial energy management and oxidative stress has led neuroscientists to explore a number of supplemental compounds with energy-enhancing, antioxidant capabilities. Excellent laboratory and clinical evidence suggests that *coenzyme Q10* (CoQ10), also known as *ubiquinone* or *ubiquinol* because of its omnipresence in living cells, is an outstanding contender in this field.[137,138] CoQ10 is used in a myriad of enzymatic reactions involving the transport of electrons from energy-supplying nutrients and their safe disposal within cells. CoQ10 deficiencies disrupt these reactions, contributing to many age-related neurodegenerative conditions. Plasma and platelet levels of CoQ10 are known to be low in patients with Parkinson's disease, suggesting a systemic deficiency state. A late 2008 study from England demonstrated for the first time that reduced CoQ10 levels are found in cortical regions of the brain of Parkinson's disease patients.[139]

In a multicenter clinical trial, 80 treatment-naïve patients with early Parkinson's disease were randomly assigned to receive either placebo or CoQ10 at daily doses of 300, 600, or 1200 mg for 16 months or until disability required drug treatment. All subjects were scored using the standard Unified Parkinson Disease Rating Scale (UPDRS), for which higher scores indicate a progressively worsening disease state. The results were compelling with a mean change of *11.99* with placebo, *8.81* with the 300-mg dose, *10.82* with the 600-mg dose, and *6.69* with the 1200-mg dose—a significant difference. All doses were well tolerated. The authors concluded that "coenzyme Q10 appears to slow the progressive deterioration of function in Parkinson's disease."[140] Two years later the same researchers showed that dosages up to 3000 mg/day of *ubiquinone* were safe and well tolerated, although plasma levels reached a plateau at 2400 mg/day.[141]

German researchers were intrigued by the aforementioned laboratory observations, which suggested that CoQ10 might not only prevent the loss of dopaminergic neurons, but could also improve functioning of the remaining cells. Their own randomized trial results were somewhat discouraging, showing no change in UPDRS scores. However, their subjects received a lower dose of CoQ10 (100 mg, 3 times daily) over just 3 months. Unlike the previous trial, they also studied patients with "mid-range" Parkinson's disease who already require L-DOPA. Therefore, they would have been by definition unable to detect significant neuroprotective effects. They did conclude, however, that the CoQ10 was safe and well tolerated.[142]

While exploring the relationship between mitochondrial dysfunction and Parkinson's disease, a group of pharmacologists in Egypt came across strong laboratory evidence supporting the need for high doses of CoQ10 either alone or *in combination with* L-DOPA therapy. They induced Parkinson's disease in rats by injecting them with a toxin known to create an accurate model of the disease. They found that the animals developed slower movements and rigidity within 20 days. Their brains also showed marked decreases in levels of dopamine and energy transfer molecules such as ATP, with increased levels of a cell death signaling protein called *Bcl-2*—identical to the brain of a human Parkinson's disease patient. Remarkably, after so much damage had already been done, treatment with CoQ10 prevented cell death, restored ATP levels, and decreased movement disorder scores. Another group of rats treated with L-DOPA alone showed symptomatic improvement but it had no effect on cell survival or energy function. The researchers concluded that "addition of coenzyme Q10 in a high dose in early Parkinson's disease could be recommended based on its proved disease-modifying role on several levels of the proposed mechanisms, including improvement of respiratory chain activity."[143]

An animal study conducted at Cornell University demonstrated CoQ10's protective qualities as it prevented dopaminergic neurons from destruction, prevented loss of enzymes that make dopamine, and prevented the development of toxic alpha-synuclein complexes that predict severe Parkinson's disease. The researchers noted that their results "provide further evidence that administration of CoQ10 is a promising therapeutic strategy for the treatment of Parkinson's disease."[144]

## Creatine

Creatine, an important amino acid-like compound that has been proposed as a neuroprotectant in supplement form, is vital to cellular energy management. Creatine deficiency is associated with neurologic damage.[145] Several animal studies have shown creatine, because of its "promitochondrial" effect, to be effective in preventing or slowing the progression of Parkinson's disease.[146–148] Influential Harvard neurologists noted that "creatine is a critical component in maintaining cellular energy homeostasis, and its administration has been reported to be neuroprotective in a wide number of both acute and chronic experimental models of neurological disease."[149]

The first human trial of creatine was performed by the Neuroprotective Exploratory Trials in Parkinson Disease (NET-PD) group at the National Institute of Neurological Disorders and Stroke (NINDS). These prestigious researchers conducted a so-called "nonfutility" trial in which they sought evidence that test substances should be submitted to larger clinical trials. They studied 200 treatment-naïve subjects who had been diagnosed within the past 5 years. Subjects were randomly assigned to receive creatine 10 g daily, the antibiotic drug minocycline (a proposed neuroprotectant) 200 mg daily, or placebo for 12 months while their scores on a standard Parkinson's disease rating scale were monitored. Based on results of the previous study, to be considered "nonfutile," a treatment had to produce at least a 30% reduction in the progression of Parkinson's symptoms. Both creatine and minocycline performed well. However, creatine showed a substantial edge in performance over minocycline. Tolerability of the treatment was 91% in the creatine group and 77% in the minocycline group. Neither group was rejected as futile indicating that there could be a benefit to more rigorous studies in the future.[150] This study was followed up by a 2008 publication that corroborated the exceptional safety and tolerability of creatine.[151]

These findings are especially encouraging when we remember that they were derived from studies of Parkinson's patients with significant damage to dopamine-producing (dopaminergic) cells.

A recent study found that creatine, in combination with CoQ10, conferred significant neuroprotection by reducing the accumulation of alpha-synuclein and suppressing lipid oxidation. In addition, animals being treated with the nutrient combination survived longer than those not being treated.[152]

Other studies have since shown that creatine, in daily doses up to 4 g, is safe and well tolerated by patients with Parkinson's disease.[153]

## Omega-3 Fatty Acids

These natural components of omega-3 fats, obtained chiefly from fish and some plant sources, exert significant anti-inflammatory action. Their concentration in nerve cell membranes decreases with age, oxidant stress, and in neurodegenerative disorders such as Parkinson's disease.[154,155] In fact, researchers in Norway have presented convincing evidence of a systematic omega-3 deficit in Parkinson's disease, Alzheimer's disease, and autism, suggesting a fundamental neurologic role for these vital fat molecules.[156,157] Supplementation with the omega-3 DHA can favorably modify brain functions and has been proposed as a nutraceutical tool in Parkinson's and Alzheimer's disease.[158]

A study from Japan found that treatment of nerve cells with omega-3 prevents *apoptosis*, the programmed cell death that occurs in part as the result of inflammatory stimuli in the brain. Interestingly,

results were a lot better when treatment was introduced *before* the chemical stresses that induced apoptosis were imposed, leading them to conclude that "dietary supplementation with [omega-3s] may be beneficial as a potential means to delay the onset of the diseases and/or their rate of progression."[159]

Canadian researchers took this study to the next level when they supplemented mice with omega-3 before injecting them with a Parkinson's inducing chemical.[160] The mice were fed either a control diet or a diet high in omega-3s for 10 months prior to injection. Control mice demonstrated a rapid loss of the dopamine-producing cells in their substantia nigra accompanied by profound declines of dopamine levels in brain tissue. These effects were prevented in the mice receiving the diet high in omega-3s.

A study of primates at the same institution demonstrated actual changes in Parkinson's symptoms, providing further compelling evidence for omega-3's protective and therapeutic effects. In this study, one group of animals was first treated for several months with L-DOPA before being given omega-3 DHA, while a second group was pretreated with omega-3 DHA before starting on L-DOPA. The study was designed this way because L-DOPA, although effective in treating Parkinson's symptoms, as stated earlier in the protocol is also known to damage dopamine-producing cells and induce dyskinesias. Omega-3 DHA reduced the occurrence of dyskinesias in both groups of monkeys, without altering the beneficial effects of L-DOPA. The researchers concluded that "DHA may represent a new approach to improve the quality of life of Parkinson's disease patients."[161]

## B Vitamins

B vitamin deficiencies have long been implicated in many neurologic disorders, including Parkinson's disease. Studies as early as the 1970s directed at demonstrating the effects of supplementation yielded discouraging results.[162-164] However, as our understanding of the close link between the toxic amino acid *homocysteine* and B vitamins grew, more targeted and mechanism-based studies became possible. Homocysteine levels are closely linked to folate and vitamin B6 and B12 status. Elevated homocysteine levels are found in cardiovascular disease as well as a variety of neurologic and psychiatric disturbances.[165-167] Also, L-DOPA treatment can itself lead to elevated homocysteine levels. As a result, more recent studies have led researchers to recommend B complex supplementation in those utilizing L-DOPA therapy.[168]

Definitive evidence supporting the benefit of this approach came from Singapore where Parkinson's disease patients, already on a stable dose of L-DOPA, were supplemented with pyridoxine (a common form of vitamin B6).[169] Mean motor and activities of daily living scores improved significantly following supplementation, and worsened again when the supplements were stopped. Low serum folate is also found in Parkinson's disease patients, especially those taking L-DOPA.[167] Canadian researchers demonstrated that a supplement containing folate and B12 could reduce plasma homocysteine levels in patients taking L-DOPA.[170]

A systematic review paper concluded that B vitamin supplementation may be of value for neurocognitive function.[171] A similar review points to recent work with the active form of vitamin B6, *pyridoxal-5'-phosphate* (P5P), noting that a number of neurologic disorders, including Parkinson's disease, offer attractive therapeutic targets for this substance.[172] The consensus among experts is that due to the deleterious effect that elevated homocysteine levels has on *both* Parkinson's itself *and* L-DOPA therapy, supplementation with folate, B6, and B12 is warranted.[173–176]

## Vitamin D

Vitamin D functions more like a hormone than a vitamin. Vitamin D receptors are expressed ubiquitously throughout the body, including on microglial cells.[177] Upon activation by vitamin D, vitamin D receptors signal for increased or decreased expression of numerous genes, many of which are immunomodulatory.[178]

Several studies have shown that higher levels of vitamin D protect against the onset of Parkinson's disease symptoms. Also, that patients diagnosed with Parkinson's have lower serum vitamin D levels than those without the disease.[179,180]

Since many of the actions of vitamin D are anti-inflammatory, Life Extension believes that maintaining optimal vitamin D blood levels (50–80 ng/mL) may quell some of the inflammatory aspects of Parkinson's disease neurodegeneration. It is likely that having optimal vitamin D levels might decrease the activation of microglial cells and reduce the release of inflammatory cytokines.

## Carnitine

Carnitine is a vital nutrient that serves as a *cofactor* in fatty acid metabolism. It helps to "ferry" large fat molecules into the mitochondrial "furnaces" where they are burned for energy, making it an important component of brain energy management and mitochondrial function.[181] There is a growing body of literature suggesting that carnitine supplementation, through its support of brain energy management, protects against Parkinson's disease.

Researchers at Mount Sinai School of Medicine were able to prevent chemically induced Parkinson's disease in monkeys by pretreating them with acetyl-L-carnitine, a readily absorbed form of the nutrient.[182] Moreover, Italian researchers have studied carnitine as a neuroprotectant in the brains of methamphetamine users. Methamphetamines cause the same basic mitochondrial destruction and free radical brain damage as that seen in Parkinson's patients.[183,184] This work has been extended in similar studies at the U.S. National Center for Toxicological Research.[185]

In an intriguing study, Chinese nutritional scientists in Shanghai explored in culture both acetyl-L-carnitine and *lipoic acid* (each alone and in combination with the other) in preventing Parkinson's disease-like changes in human neural cells. They found that both nutrients either alone or in combination, applied for 4 weeks prior to a Parkinson's disease-inducing chemical, protected the cells from mitochondrial dysfunction, oxidative damage, and an accumulation of the dangerous alpha-synuclein proteins. Notably, the combination of supplements was effective at 100- to 1000-fold lower concentrations than were required for either one acting alone. Researchers stated that "this study provides important evidence that combining mitochondrial antioxidant/nutrients at optimal doses might be an effective and safe prevention strategy for Parkinson's disease."[186]

## Green Tea

Increased tea consumption is correlated with reduced incidence of dementia and Alzheimer's and Parkinson's disease.[187] Green tea contains valuable antioxidant polyphenols known to be protective against a host of chronic age-related conditions. There is tremendous scientific interest in green tea and its active compound epigallocatechin gallate (EGCG) as a neuroprotectant in Parkinson's disease, especially since when compared to many drugs, EGCG is extremely effective at penetrating brain tissue.[188,189]

Israeli researchers showed that they could prevent the cellular changes associated with Parkinson's by pretreating mice with either green tea extracts or EGCG before inducing the disease by chemical injection.[188–190] This research has subsequently been repeated and extended in laboratories around the world.[191–195] Utilizing the brain cell cultures pretreated to develop Parkinson's-like changes, the Israeli group also showed that green tea extracts prevented activation of the inflammation-producing NF-κB system.[196] EGCG's specific anti-inflammatory properties have been demonstrated to protect cultured brain tissue from the loss of dopaminergic cells as well.[197] L-theanine, a component of green and black tea, was shown by Korean scientists to prevent dopaminergic cell death such as that seen in Parkinson's disease.[198]

Another potential benefit of green tea extract is its ability to inhibit the dopamine-degrading enzyme COMT.[199] This may help to sustain dopamine levels in ailing brain tissue, thereby reducing the severity of symptoms.

Just as we use multiple combinations of prescription drugs to capitalize on their synergistic effects, we can capitalize on green tea's neuroprotective effects in Parkinson's and other neurodegenerative diseases.[200] While more human studies are yet to be completed, green tea polyphenols have proven to exert powerful protection for dopaminergic neurons making them a key component in the prevention and treatment of Parkinson's disease.[195,201–204]

## Resveratrol

Resveratrol is a polyphenolic antioxidant compound that has shown stunning potential in preventing cardiovascular disease and prolonging life.[205–207] Not surprisingly, scientists interested in protecting brain tissue and enhancing the quality of life in aging individuals have directed their attention towards this remarkable compound.

Since dopamine itself is an oxidant compound that can contribute to the early destruction of neurons, Korean scientists studied the impact of resveratrol at preventing this paradoxical effect.[208] They found that through the loss of mitochondrial function, human neural tissue treated with dopamine underwent rapid cell death. However, exposing the cells to resveratrol for 1 hour prior to dopamine treatment prevented cell loss and preserved mitochondrial function. In addition, Canadian scientists used resveratrol to prevent neuronal cell death caused by inflammation.[209]

Resveratrol's anti-inflammatory action was further explored by Chinese researchers who at first administered a Parkinson's disease-inducing chemical to rats, then gave them oral daily doses of resveratrol for 10 weeks. They found that after only 2 weeks of supplementation, the rats demonstrated significant improvement in their movement. Also, examination of their brains showed marked reduction in mitochondrial damage and loss of dopaminergic cells. Remarkably, they also found a reduction in the levels of COX-2 and TNF-alpha (inflammatory markers). They concluded

with justifiable excitement that "resveratrol exerts a neuroprotective effect on [a chemically] induced Parkinson's disease rat model, and this protection is related to the reduced inflammatory reaction."[210]

As with green tea extracts, it appears that resveratrol's potential for preventing Parkinson's disease may reside in its multimodal mechanism of action targeting oxidant stress, inflammation, and systems such as sirtuins that are fundamental in regulating mitochondrial function and ultimately affecting longevity.[206]

Mucuna pruriens is a vine whose seeds contain a high concentration of naturally occurring L-DOPA and a variety of other psychoactive compounds.[211] Compounds in Mucuna seeds act as AADC inhibitors, mimicking the action of carbidopa and complementing the action L-DOPA in the central nervous system. In an animal experiment, Mucuna seed extract was shown to alleviate symptoms of chemically induced Parkinson's with similar efficacy to traditional L-DOPA treatment, but without inducing dyskinesia.[212] These results were repeated in another, similar trial.[211]

In a double-blind, randomized, placebo-controlled trial, Mucuna extract proved superior over standard L-DOPA/carbidopa therapy. Compared to traditional therapy, Mucuna led to a faster onset of symptom relief, longer duration of relief, and significantly fewer dyskinesias. The scientists conducting this study concluded that "[t]he rapid onset of action and longer on time without concomitant increase in dyskinesias on mucuna seed powder formulation suggest that this natural source of L-dopa might possess advantages over conventional L-dopa preparations in the long term management of [Parkinson's disease]."[213]

## Other Promising Nutrients

**Curcumin.** Curcmin, a derivative of the spices turmeric and cumin, through its potent modulation of the NF-κB system is a natural inhibitor of inflammation. It prevents chemically induced changes in lab models of Parkinson's disease and exerts significant neuroprotection.[214–221]

**Melatonin.** The antioxidant hormone melatonin (synthesized and secreted by the pineal gland) may help to reduce the accumulation of alpha-synuclein proteins while preserving the cell's ability to make dopamine. It is also an invaluable sleep aid for Parkinson's patients, who often suffer from distressing problems with sleep.[222–231]

**N-acetyl cysteine.** N-acetyl cysteine (NAC) is a precursor to the potent cellular antioxidant glutathione. In animal models, NAC prevents dopamine induced neurotoxicity and protects against some of the damaging effects of alpha-synuclein proteins.[232,233]

**Lipoic acid.** Lipoic acid, a potent reducing agent, is considered a universal antioxidant due to its amphipathic nature (both fat- and water-soluble). Lipoic acid is produced naturally within the body and contributes to xenobiotic detoxification and antioxidant protection. It also contributes to cellular energy production.[234] In addition to its ability to directly neutralize toxins and free radicals, lipoic acid bolsters levels of other cellular protectants such as glutathione and vitamin E.[235]

The low molecular weight of lipoic acid allows it to easily cross the blood–brain barrier, delivering neuroprotection within the central nervous system. Lipoic acid also combats inflammatory reactions.[235] Large-scale clinical trials have yet to be conducted in Parkinson's patients. However, given its potential for efficacy and excellent safety profile, lipoic acid should be considered as a therapeutic agent for Parkinson's disease.

**Probiotics.** Because dopaminergic signaling exerts considerable influence over intestinal function, constipation is a common problem in Parkinson's disease. In a recent clinical trial, 40 Parkinson's patients complaining of constipation were treated with *probiotics* for 5 weeks. Probiotic therapy significantly increased the number of normal stools as well as reduced the incidence of bloating and abdominal pain.[236]

## Life Extension Suggestions

Parkinson's disease is a multifactorial pathology and must be treated as such for symptomatic relief. An ideal management regimen should include the lowest possible effective dose of dopamine replacement therapy, daily use of a neuroprotective agent (such as 1 mg of rasagiline), nutrients to support mitochondrial function (such as CoQ10 and B-complex vitamins), and if possible, cardiovascular aerobic exercise with a target heart rate of 75% for a minimum of 20 minutes at least 3 times per week (to stimulate the release of neuronal growth factors in the brain). Muscle stretching and practicing either yoga or tai chi may be supportive as well.

The following nutrients target various aspects of Parkinson's disease pathology:

- **CoQ10:** 1200–2400 mg as ubiquinone, or 200–300 mg as ubiquinol
- **Creatine:** 1000–2000 mg daily
- **Omega-3 fatty acids** (from fish oil): 2000–4000 mg daily
- **Mucuna pruriens,** standardized extract: 300–1200 mg daily
- **Vitamin D:** 5000–8000 IU daily (depending on blood test results)
- **B-complex vitamins:** Per label instructions
- **Acetyl-L-carnitine:** 1000–2000 mg daily
- **Green tea,** standardized extract: 725–1450 mg daily
- **Green coffee,** standardized extract: 400–1200 mg daily
- ***Trans*-resveratrol:** 250–500 mg daily
- **Probiotics:** Per label instructions
- **Curcumin** (as highly absorbed BCM-95®): 400–1200 mg daily
- **Melatonin:** 1–5 mg daily
- **N-acetyl cysteine:** 600–1800 mg daily
- **Lipoic acid** (as R-lipoic acid): 300–900 mg daily

In addition, the following blood testing resources may be helpful:

- CoQ10 (Coenzyme Q10)
- Homocysteine
- Vitamin B12 and Folate
- Vitamin D, 25-Hydroxy
- Chemistry Panel and Complete Blood Count (CBC)
- Omega Score®

## REFERENCES

References available at: www.lef.org/dpt5/ch107

# 108

# *Periodontitis and Cavities*

There are many reasons to keep your teeth and gums healthy. Healthy teeth and gums not only look better, but also promote better eating habits and nutrition. By contrast, unhealthy, inflamed gums are associated with various diseases, including coronary heart disease and an elevated risk for heart attack, while tooth loss is linked to malnutrition.

In a healthy mouth, teeth are intact and anchored in pink with firm gums that do not bleed during brushing. A regular dental care program should include flossing and brushing twice daily, as well as regular visits to the dentist for cleaning and examination.

Gum disease and tooth loss are especially common among the elderly. Some researchers believe that malnutrition in older people may be in part due to poor dentition (the type, number, and arrangement of a set of teeth). In fact, some researchers believe that the short life span of early humans was related to tooth loss that caused starvation.[1,2]

The 3 most common problems in the oral cavity are dental caries (cavities) and the periodontal diseases gingivitis and periodontitis. These are caused by multiple factors, including plaque buildup, diet, oral hygiene, genetics, environment, and lifestyle factors. For more information on gingivitis, the most common dental disease, see Life Extension's Gingivitis protocol. Dental caries and periodontitis are discussed in this protocol.

## CAVITIES

Dental caries (cavities) occur when microorganisms build up in deposits of dental plaque and ferment dietary sugars. The byproduct of this fermentation, lactic acid, lowers the pH at the junction of the plaque layer and tooth enamel, and eventually the enamel is eroded.[3]

The layer of plaque in the mouth has recently been redefined as "biofilm."[4] Biofilm develops in a predictable pattern, whereby oral bacteria colonize areas of the gums and teeth, then spread, and eventually link with other organisms in a cohesive film. This film can occur both above and below the gum line. If left intact, it may form a hard, mineralized mass called calculus (tartar).[5] This is the hard, yellow substance that dentists scrape off with specialized equipment. Tartar contains masses of bacteria that produce lactic acid and promote tooth decay. Brushing and flossing alone cannot penetrate or remove the tartar.

One novel hypothesis for disrupting the creation of biofilm and preventing tartar involves oral vaccines that may protect the mouth against *Streptococcus mutans* (*S. mutans*), the bacteria most commonly responsible for dental caries. Human studies have shown encouraging results with antibodies designed to suppress colonization of *S. mutans* in the biofilm.[6]

The risk of developing cavities differs for each individual, based on factors such as oral hygiene, genetics, the size and shape of the teeth, resistance to infection, retention of dental plaque, and metabolism of sugar.[7,8] In addition, people with pre-existing conditions such as gum disease have a greater chance of developing cavities, and smoking can accelerate the transformation of plaque into tartar.[9] Other risk factors for dental cavities include exposure to lead,[10] polychlorinated biphenyls (PCBs),[11] and second-hand smoke.[12]

Clinically, cavities appear as blemishes on the tooth surface. If not clinically visible, they can still be detected using dental x-rays. Most dentists recommend one set of dental x-rays annually.

Waiting for tooth pain as a reason to visit the dentist is a not a good strategy for preventing cavities. In many cases, cavities are not painful because they affect only the surface layers of the tooth and do not extend into the dental pulp, which is the soft tissue inside the tooth. In more advanced cases, a cavity may extend into the pulp, causing intense pain and pulp disease known as pulpitis. Early pulpitis is generally treatable. If not treated, however, it can advance to pulp death. At this point, the tooth may stop hurting because the nerve has died. By the time a cavity has reached this stage, the tooth will most likely require extraction. Modern preventive dentistry is designed to prevent tooth decay from reaching such advanced stages.

### Fluoride: Effective against Cavities

Fluoride's role in preventing cavities has been extensively documented.[13] Teeth with adequate fluoride are resistant to acid, and studies have shown a 30–50% reduction in decay following the fluoridation of drinking water.[14]

The use of fluoride, however, is not without its side effects. The most common side effect is fluorosis. This permanent alteration causes small, barely visible white flecks on adult teeth.[15] It occurs early during tooth development, when adult teeth are just coming in.[16] To help prevent it, experts recommend:

1. Use of low-fluoride water in infant formulas
2. Adult supervision of children during brushing
3. Rigid application standards when administering fluoride supplements to children[17]

There is, however, little question that fluoride works to prevent cavities. When children between the ages of 5 and 6 years were treated with a 1.2% fluoride gel versus a placebo gel twice daily, the fluoride group showed a 40% decrease in cavities compared to the placebo group after a 2-year follow-up.[13]

# PERIODONTITIS

Periodontal diseases, including gingivitis and periodontitis, are inflammatory diseases affecting the supporting structures that anchor teeth in place (periodontium). Gingivitis and periodontitis are related conditions; if left untreated, gingivitis (inflammation of the gingival tissue [gums]) can progress to periodontitis, a more serious condition. Gingivitis is treatable and reversible, while periodontitis is irreversible and can lead to tooth loss.

Risk factors for periodontitis include smoking, stress, depression,[18] and alcohol consumption.[19] Tobacco use is an important risk factor for periodontitis.[20–23] For more specific information on risk factors for gingivitis, the most common form of gum disease, see Life Extension's Gingivitis protocol.

During periodontitis, healthy gum tissue is transformed from pink and firm, with knife-edge margins between the soft tissue and the tooth, to inflamed and red. Eventually, tissue pulls away from the tooth, allowing pockets to form. These pockets can be measured with a special probe during a standard dental check-up. Any pocket over 3 mm in depth signifies gingivitis; a pocket over 5 mm usually signifies periodontitis.

Periodontal infections frequently involve bacteria that discharge hydrogen sulfide, ammonia, amines, toxins, and inflammatory-causing enzymes that can cause tissue and tooth loss.[24] Bleeding gums, bad breath, and pain also occur.[24] Clinically, periodontitis is characterized by inflamed, red gums and deepening pockets between the tooth root and gum tissue, as well as loss of bone in the jaw. Advanced periodontal disease can be diagnosed by changes in appearance of the teeth and gums, including:

1. Noticeable loosening of teeth
2. Gum recession with tooth root exposed

3. New spaces forming between teeth
4. Food being trapped between teeth and where gums have receded
5. Constant bad taste in the mouth

Periodontal disease is usually painless until late in the disease process, when teeth are so loose that pain occurs while chewing. Retention of food in a pocket site may provoke a sudden burst of bacterial growth, resulting in a painful abscess.[25] At other times, front teeth may become so loose that they separate.

Conventional therapy for periodontal disease consists of mechanical scaling and root planing, surgical treatment, and use of various antimicrobial regimens.[25] The goal is to reduce the number of bacteria on the surface of teeth by reducing the amount of plaque. If pocket depths in the gums are ≥5 mm, large numbers of bacteria can accumulate that cannot be reached by normal oral hygiene. Periodontal surgery may then be recommended to reduce the pocket depths to 1–2 mm.[25]

Antibiotic therapy is sometimes needed when bacterial count continues to climb. In open clinical trials, tetracycline has been used successfully to treat aggressive periodontitis, either as an oral tetracycline/surgery combination,[26–28] or alone for 3–8 weeks.[29,30] Tetracycline can deplete calcium, magnesium, and iron; therefore, people on tetracycline should take a multivitamin.[31]

There are several ways to release medications directly into the periodontal pocket, including the use of long-lasting gels. These methods reduce the dose of medicine needed and deliver the antibiotic in a highly targeted fashion.[25] Devices that deliver localized antibiotics are about as effective as systemic agents in their ability to target harmful bacteria; also, people do not have to remember to take medicine, thus improving patient adherence.[32,33] These devices include Atridox®, PerioChip®, and Arestin®.[34]

# GUM DISEASE, INFLAMMATION, AND CHRONIC DISEASE

Gum disease is clearly associated with heart disease and other health-related problems. This is not necessarily due to bacterial spread from the mouth into the bloodstream, as many people think. In fact, "bacteria showers" in the bloodstream are relatively common and occur in response to brushing teeth, bowel movements, and other normal activities. These are rarely dangerous for people with healthy immune systems. Rather, the link between gum disease and other systemic diseases appears to be due to an increased inflammatory response occurring throughout the body and is triggered by inflammation in the gums. The following diseases have been associated with gum disease.

## Infective Endocarditis

Infective endocarditis is a serious, potentially fatal bacterial infection of the heart, its valves, or inner lining. It occurs when bacteria in the bloodstream are embedded on abnormal heart valves or damaged heart tissue. Dental procedures and diseases are associated with endocarditis in people with underlying congenital heart disease and in those with prosthetic heart valves or who have had other forms of heart surgery.[35-37] About 8% of cases in the United States have been associated with periodontitis or other dental diseases without an associated dental procedure. Chances of infective endocarditis following dental procedures in people with pre-existing heart conditions ranged from 1 per 3000 to 1 per 5000 procedures.[35] To prevent this condition, some heart patients are advised to take antibiotics during dental procedures.

## Cardiovascular Disease

Studies have shown an association between periodontitis and cardiovascular disease,[38-40] and suggest that periodontitis is a risk factor for cardiovascular disease.[41-43] Periodontitis is linked to heart disease by inflammation. According to the latest research, large amounts of bacteria in the gums trigger a systemic inflammatory response, with elevated levels of proinflammatory chemicals such as COX (cyclooxygenase) products, arachidonic acid, and others. These proinflammatory chemicals may contribute to atherosclerosis, which is now understood to be an inflammatory disease that affects the inner linings of arterial walls (the endothelium). Numerous studies have thus linked inflammatory gum disease to cardiovascular events such as stroke, atherosclerosis, and thickening of calcifications in the carotid artery.[44-48]

## Obesity

Obesity, a significant risk factor for numerous diseases, has been associated with periodontitis, gingivitis, and dental cavities.[49] Other conditions associated with obesity such as metabolic syndrome or syndrome X (a clustering of dyslipidemia, insulin resistance, hypertension, and type 2 diabetes) can worsen periodontitis.[50]

## Diabetes

Periodontitis is twice as prevalent in diabetics as nondiabetics.[51] Experimentally produced periodontitis

increased blood glucose levels in uncontrolled diabetic animals. Studies have linked glycation and inflammation in diabetics to worsening periodontitis. Alternatively, studies have linked the inflammatory response triggered by worsening periodontitis to amplified glycation, a damaging process that links proteins to glucose molecules and has been implicated in hardening of the arteries and other diseases.[50]

## Osteoporosis

Significant relationships exist between periodontitis and osteoporosis,[52-58] as well as tooth loss and osteoporosis.[59-62]

## Pregnancy-Related Issues

Oral infections can increase the risk of low birth weight in newborns.[63] Pregnant women with periodontitis were found to be 7.5 times more likely to have a preterm, low-birth-weight infant than pregnant women without periodontitis.[64] Pregnancy can increase the frequency, severity, and degree of gingivitis.[65,66]

## Lung Disease

Poor oral hygiene provides an ideal growth environment for anaerobic bacteria, which can cause severe pneumonia, especially in people with impaired swallowing.[67-77]

# ARE TEETH WHITENERS SAFE?

Over the past decade, sales of at-home teeth-whitening products have exploded in the United States. These products generally contain either hydrogen peroxide or carbamide peroxide, and are usually painted or brushed on, or applied in strips directly to the teeth. They are milder versions of whiteners that are used in the dentist's office, which may contain up to 35% active ingredients.

While studies have shown that these products do whiten teeth, there is some lingering concern about their safety. For example, studies have shown that peroxide from at-home whitening products penetrates the tooth enamel into the pulpy interior of the teeth.[78] In studies of human molars, these products have also been shown to adversely affect the hardness of enamel.[79,80]

So far, however, no systemic adverse effects have been demonstrated with the use of teeth whiteners containing 10% carbamide peroxide. The most common side effects are moderate tooth sensitivity and mild gum irritation that usually discontinues when the product is no longer being used.[81]

Because stronger at-home solutions containing up to 18% carbamide peroxide have not yet been extensively tested in humans, it may be advisable to use a milder at-home tooth-whitening product under a dentist's supervision.

# TOOTH LOSS, NUTRITION, AND DIET

Approximately 60% of U.S. adults are missing at least one tooth, and 10% have no teeth at all.[82] Besides the aesthetic value of a nice smile, there are harmful health repercussions of lacking functional teeth, including a greater risk of malnutrition.[83] People missing their teeth have about 20% of the chewing capacity of people with teeth, and tend to avoid eating fruits, vegetables, and whole grains.[84] This can quickly lead to malnutrition as well as serious vitamin and mineral deficiencies.

Good oral hygiene, regular tooth brushing and flossing, tongue cleaning, regular dental check-ups, and use of high-quality oral care products can prevent or reduce the risk of cavities. At the same time, because of the risk of a dangerous inflammatory response, it is important that people with gum disease protect themselves with powerful anti-inflammatories. The following nutrients support healthy gums and reduce inflammation.

## Coenzyme Q10

In one study, topical application of coenzyme Q10 (CoQ10) to periodontal pockets significantly reduced gingivitis, bleeding gums, and pocket depths after 5–7 days of treatment.[85] In another study, symptoms of gingivitis and periodontitis improved 3 weeks after beginning CoQ10 treatment.[86] Topical application of CoQ10 improved adult periodontitis alone and in combination with nonsurgical periodontal therapy.[85]

## Hydrogen Peroxide

Hydrogen peroxide, which is included in many brands of toothpaste, is valuable for its ability to reach bacteria hiding among gingival folds and gaps. Hydrogen peroxide is also added to some mouthwashes to reduce gingivitis and whiten teeth.[87] Hydrogen peroxide has been used effectively for years in dentistry.

## Essential Oils

Mouth rinses containing essential oils such as eucalyptus oil and menthol significantly reduced both gingival inflammation and bleeding when used in conjunction with fluoride toothpaste.[88] Tea tree oil

(*Melaleuca alternifolia*) is an antiseptic, fungicide, and bactericide that is effective against oral bacteria.[89,90]

Tea tree oil, used as an oral rinse, has been proven to kill bacteria.[91] In fact, research has shown that a tea tree oil concentration of 0.6% inhibited 14 of 15 oral types of bacteria. In one study, 49 subjects aged 18–60 years with severe, chronic gingivitis were divided into groups, one of which was given a gel containing tea tree oil to apply with a toothbrush twice daily. The tea tree oil group had improved gingival index and papillary bleeding index scores attributed to the herb's anti-inflammatory properties.[92]

## Folic Acid

Mouthwash containing folic acid is effective in treating gingivitis and its accompanying inflammation. Among pregnant women, who are prone to gingivitis, folate mouthwash has proven superior to oral folate supplementation in preventing gingivitis.[93-95]

## Green Tea

Green tea extract is rich in a class of antioxidants called catechins. Two in particular, epigallocatechin gallate (EGCG) and epicatechin gallate (ECG), combat oral plaque and bacteria.[96-98] These green tea polyphenols work as antiplaque agents by suppressing glucosyl transferase, which oral bacteria use to feed on sugar. Other research has demonstrated that green tea extract can kill oral bacteria and inhibit collagenase activity. Collagenase, a natural enzyme that becomes overactive in the presence of bacterial overgrowth, can destroy healthy collagen in gum tissue.

Green tea extract applied topically inhibits S. mutans bacteria in the laboratory. These bacteria have been implicated in the development of dental cavities. The scientists suggested that certain green tea extracts might be especially helpful in preventing tooth decay by inhibiting the development of bacterial plaque.[99] In a Chinese study, green tea extract was used to rinse and brush teeth. The study demonstrated that S. mutans could be inhibited completely after contact with green tea extract for 5 minutes. There was no drug resistance after repeat cultures, and researchers concluded that green tea extract is effective in reducing the risk of developing cavities.[100] Other studies have found that the catechins in green tea remain at active levels in saliva for up to 1 hour following application.[101]

Additional studies confirm the benefits of green tea in fighting gum disease, especially when combined with conventional treatments. In a pilot study, hydroxypropyl cellulose strips containing green tea catechins as a slow-release local delivery system were applied to the pockets in periodontal patients once a week for 8 weeks. The green tea catechins inhibited the bacteria *P. gingivalis* and *Prevotella* spp., and a reduction in pocket depth was observed.[102]

## Hyperimmune Egg Extract

Agricultural scientists discovered long ago that they could immunize hens against germs that threaten humans. This immunity was then passed on by the hen to the egg.[103–105] Scientists have now been able to customize eggs to provide different types of immunity. At least 24 different organisms have been used to immunize a single hen, which then lays eggs that offer passive immunity to all of the organisms.[104]

Hyperimmune egg extract has been shown to reduce the volume of dental plaque, which in turn cuts down on the total load of inflammation in the mouth.[106] Animals supplemented with hyperimmune egg against the leading bacterial cause of dental caries developed significantly lower dental caries scores than control animals.[97,107] Oral hyperimmune egg rinses have also been used successfully in humans to reduce disease-causing bacteria; the extracts remain active and present in the mouth at least overnight, offering long-standing protection.[108–110]

## Pomegranate

Researchers are finding important applications for pomegranate in the field of dental health. Clinical studies have shown that this popular antioxidant vigorously attacks the causes of tooth decay at the biochemical level.[111–115] Pomegranate attacks bacteria where they live. Research shows that by interfering with production of chemicals the bacteria use as "glue," pomegranate extract suppresses bacteria's ability to adhere to the surface of the tooth.[116,117]

A study conducted in 2007 examined the effects of a mouthwash containing pomegranate extract on the risk of gingivitis.[118] Investigators noted that pomegranate's active components, including polyphenolic flavonoids (eg, punicalagins and ellagic acid), are believed to prevent gingivitis through a number of mechanisms including reduction of oxidative stress in the oral cavity, direct antioxidant activity,[119–121] anti-inflammatory effects, antibacterial activity,[122,123] and direct removal of plaque from teeth.[113] Saliva samples were evaluated for a variety of indicators related to gingivitis and periodontitis. Subjects rinsing with pomegranate solution experienced a reduction in saliva total protein content,[118] which is normally higher among people with gingivitis,[124] and may correlate with plaque-forming bacterial content.[125]

## Cranberry

Cranberries may offer important benefits for healthy teeth and gums. The berries contain a special chemical that may inhibit and even reverse the formation of dental plaque deposits that often lead to tooth decay.[126] Cranberry constituents may also help reduce inflammation in gingival or gum tissues, which could offer protection against periodontitis.[127] These promising findings suggest that cranberry may soon find a place in dental health care regimens.

## Xylitol

Pure xylitol, a white crystalline substance that resembles and tastes like sugar, is found naturally in fruits such as plums, strawberries, and raspberries. Xylitol is used commercially to sweeten sugarless gum and candies. Xylitol has also been shown to inhibit the formation of plaque. In a double-blind and controlled study, Swedish researchers had 128 children chew gum containing either xylitol or the sweeteners sorbitol and maltitol, 3 times daily for 4 weeks. While both were effective against the buildup of dental plaque, only the xylitol-sweetened gum eliminated microbes found in saliva, particularly a strain of bacteria implicated in tooth decay.[128] Xylitol could thus be an essential ingredient in a targeted strategy to avert dental disease.

A double-blind, placebo-controlled study of 2630 children compared a standard fluoride toothpaste with one containing 10% xylitol. Over a 3-year period, children given the xylitol-enriched toothpaste developed notably fewer cavities than those using the fluoride-only toothpaste.[129]

## Probiotics

Probiotics have been defined as "living microorganisms which upon ingestion in certain numbers exert health benefits beyond inherent general nutrition."[130] Scientists have been interested in the makeup of microbes that live in the mouth (oral flora) for decades, seeking to identify factors that promote growth of healthy organisms and reduce growth of those implicated in disease and inflammation.[131–134]

Probiotics improve oral health and can help change the stubborn composition of dental biofilm and plaque.[135,136] Reducing plaque through teeth brushing is always a desirable goal; however, complete elimination is not possible. Therefore, changing the actual composition of plaque from an inflammatory cytokine-rich environment to a more benign environment (dominated by neutral or even helpful organisms) can contribute to overall systemic health.[137–139]

In laboratory studies, the probiotic *S. salivarius* helped inhibit formation of the sticky biofilm that can contribute to oral disease.[140] Building on these results, an animal study showed that the *S. salivarius* probiotic helped displace biofilm from teeth, displacing cavity-causing bacteria and inhibiting tooth decay.[141] Another experiment demonstrated how effectively a second oral probiotic protects oral health.[142] In this experiment, a form of *Bacillus coagulans* (GanedenBC30™) was shown to competitively inhibit the cariogenic (cavity-inducing) bacterium *Streptococcus mutans*, which contributes to significant tooth decay.

## Lactoferrin

Lactoferrin, a naturally occurring antimicrobial agent, is found in saliva and gingival fluid, breast milk, tears, and other bodily fluids.

This protein is a well-known immune system booster involved in the body's responses to infection, trauma, and injury.[143] Lactoferrin may bind to and slow the growth of periodontitis-associated bacteria.[144] In an animal study, locally applied lactoferrin powder appeared to support the healing of oral lesions.[145]

## Aloe Vera

Aloe vera gel packings are sometimes used by dentists after tooth extraction to reduce the incidence of infection and dry socket.[146] They have also been shown to reduce the risk of developing ulcers in the mouth.[147]

## Propolis

A 20% ethanol propolis extract was compared to antifungal agents such as nystatin, clotrimazole, econazole, and fluconazole in a study designed to assess the susceptibility of *Candida albicans*, an oral bacteria. The researchers concluded that the propolis extract could be an alternative medicine in treating candidiasis, but further studies were needed.[148]

---

### FOR MORE INFORMATION

Additional protocols that may be of interest include:

- Atherosclerosis and Cardiovascular Disease
- Homocysteine Reduction
- Diabetes

---

## The Value of Vitamin C, Vitamin D, and Calcium

Vitamin C has long been known for its ability to prevent gum disease and tooth loss. In fact, the use of vitamin C in dental disease is one of the earliest recorded uses of nutrient therapy in Western medicine. In 1747, a British Naval physician named James Lind noticed that lime juice, which is rich in vitamin C, helped prevent scurvy, which causes tooth loss. As a result, British sailors bottled lime juice for gum disease prevention. Incidentally, this practice later gave rise to the term "Limey."

Modern studies have confirmed the value of vitamin C, in conjunction with other antioxidants, in promoting good oral health. In one controlled, double-blind study of patients with periodontitis, a multivitamin combined with regular brushing resulted in significant improvements in gum health and a reduction in pockets after 60 days.[149] Clinical studies of people with vitamin C deficiencies show that gingival inflammation is directly related to ascorbic acid status, suggesting that ascorbic acid may influence the early stages of gingivitis, particularly bleeding.[150]

Researchers have also examined the value of vitamin D and calcium, which are typically used to reduce the risk of osteoporosis. Supplementation with these two nutrients reduces the rate of bone and tooth loss in postmenopausal women and men. Calcium intake of 800 mg or more daily reduced the risk of periodontitis in females.[151]

## Reducing Gum-Related Inflammation

Because of the association between gum disease and systemic inflammation, researchers have begun looking at anti-inflammatory nutrients in the context of gum disease. In one study, 30 adults with gum disease were given a variety of polyunsaturated fatty acids, including omega-3 fatty acids from fish oil (up to 3000 mg daily) and omega-6 fatty acids from borage oil (up to 3000 mg daily). At the end of the study, clinically significant improvements were measured in both gingival inflammation and depth of gum pockets.[152] Another preliminary human study found that omega-3 fatty acids tended to reduce inflammation, but called for more thorough research.[153] However, in light of the established connection between omega-3 and omega-6 fatty acids and inflammation, along with their lack of side effects, it is reasonable for people with gum disease to consider using these supplements. Other anti-inflammatory supplements include ginger and curcumin, although neither of these has been studied in the context of inflammatory gum disease.

## SUMMARY

Good oral health begins with a disciplined program of flossing, twice-daily brushing, and tongue cleaning with a tongue scraper to remove plaque and bacteria colonies on the tongue before they become incorporated in the biofilm. It is also important to visit a dentist for professional cleanings at least twice a year, and perhaps even more often. Because of the radiation associated with x-rays, Life Extension does not recommend annual dental x-rays, although occasional dental x-rays are necessary.

Avoid behaviors that contribute to gum disease and tooth decay, especially tobacco use and consumption of refined sugar. Instead, focus on consuming a diet rich in fruits and vegetables that provide important phytochemicals and nutrients. In addition, patients with gum disease and existing heart disease should monitor their levels of inflammation. C-reactive protein and homocysteine are both indicators of inflammation, which can be determined by blood tests. For more information on comprehensive blood testing, call 1-800-226-2370.

Your choice of toothpaste is also important. Today, the market is flooded with very strong toothpastes that contain high levels of hydrogen peroxide. A toothpaste is now available that has been fortified with coenzyme Q10, folic acid, tea tree oil, and other nutrients that are directly delivered to the gums each time one brushes. This novel toothpaste also contains a mild solution of 0.2% hydrogen peroxide.

A mouthwash containing pomegranate, peppermint oil, aloe and other soothing nutrients may also be helpful. In addition, a mouth spray that contains CoQ10, hydrogen peroxide, xylitol, tea tree oil and many other herbal ingredients may be very beneficial.

Patients with mouth sores (ulcers) should consider using aloe vera gel packs.

## Life Extension Suggestions

- **Coenzyme Q10** (as ubiquinol): 100–200 mg daily
- **Folic acid:** 1000 mcg daily
- **Green tea extract** (standardized to 98% polyphenols): 725–1450 mg daily
- **Vitamin C:** 1000–4000 mg daily
- **Calcium:** 900–1200 mg daily
- **Vitamin D:** 5000–10 000 IU daily
- **Fish oil** (with olive polyphenols and sesame lignans): providing 1400 mg EPA and 1000 mg DHA daily
- **Gamma-linolenic acid (GLA):** 300–600 mg daily
- **Hyperimmunized egg extract:** 3–6 tablets chewed daily on an empty stomach
- **Probiotic lozenge (*Bacillus coagulans* and *Streptococcus salivarius K12*):** 1–2 daily
- **Mouthwash** including ingredients such as pomegranate, green tea, and xylitol
- **Toothpaste** containing hydrogen peroxide, CoQ10, green tea, xylitol, lactoferrin, and folic acid
- **Herbal mouth spray** containing tea tree oil, CoQ10, hydrogen peroxide, xylitol, green tea, and additional herbal ingredients, as directed.

In addition, the following *blood tests* may be helpful:

- **Vitamin D, 25-Hydroxy**
- **C-reactive protein (CRP)**
- **Homocysteine**

## REFERENCES

References available at: www.lef.org/dpt5/ch108

# 109

# *Polycystic Ovary Syndrome (PCOS)*

Women with irregular menstrual cycles, excess facial and body hair, adult acne, weight gain, infertility, and enlarged ovaries may have polycystic ovary syndrome (PCOS), an unfortunate condition that afflicts 5–10% of women of child-bearing age and approximately 70–90% of women with irregular menstrual cycles.[1] Among its many symptoms, PCOS causes hormonal imbalances, including elevated testosterone (male hormone) and estrogen (female hormone) levels, as well as increased insulin levels.[2,3]

Although PCOS is the most common female endocrine disorder in the United States, its cause remains unclear.[4] Perhaps this is why "syndrome" is most commonly used in conventional medicine to describe PCOS since the word itself alludes to its varied signs and symptoms but does not indicate a precise cause of the condition.

However, research largely overlooked by mainstream medicine reveals a strong association between PCOS, obesity, and insulin resistance, including characteristic features of insulin insensitivity such as dyslipidemia (abnormality of metabolism of fats) and hypertension.[5,6]

If left untreated, women with PCOS often develop severe clinical manifestations, such as hirsutism (excess facial and body hair), adult acne, infertility, and depression.[7,8] Women with PCOS are at significantly higher risk for developing cardiovascular disease[9] and endometrial cancer.[10]

Integrative medicine recognizes the seriousness of PCOS, as well as the need to approach the management of PCOS as a disease of insulin resistance in order to offer hope to the millions of women who suffer from this disease. For example, metformin, an insulin-sensitizing agent that also helps to reduce excessive androgen production, promotes weight loss, restores fertility, and enhances glucose metabolism in patients with PCOS, is drastically underutilized by conventional medicine for this disease. However, management strategies commonly used to control individual symptoms of PCOS are known to have a number of undesirable side effects.[11]

For the millions suffering with PCOS, published clinical studies support the use of natural therapeutics, such as inositol and N-acetyl-cysteine (NAC), for controlling the symptoms and adverse effects.

## SYMPTOMS OF PCOS

One of the challenging aspects of diagnosing PCOS is that the signs and symptoms vary from person to person in both type and severity. Frequently, PCOS symptoms are mistaken for other medical illnesses. However, common symptoms include menstrual abnormality, excess androgen production, and polycystic ovaries.

### Menstrual Abnormality

Menstrual abnormality is the most widespread characteristic of PCOS. These include cycles longer than 35 days (fewer than 8 menstrual cycles a year), failure to menstruate for ≥4 months, and prolonged periods that may be scant or heavy.[12]

### Excess Androgen Production

Increased androgen levels are a key feature of PCOS, and may result in excess facial and body hair (hirsutism), adult acne, and male-pattern baldness (in women). Worth noting, however, is that the physical signs of androgen excess vary with ethnicity. As an example, the prevalence of hirsutism in PCOS patients is at least 40% in European and American females and even more common in darker-skinned females, but women of Asian descent may not be affected.[13]

### Polycystic Ovaries

Enlarged ovaries containing numerous small cysts can be detected by ultrasound. However, some women with *polycystic ovaries* may not have PCOS, while some women with the condition have ovaries that appear normal.[14]

## OTHER CONDITIONS ASSOCIATED WITH PCOS

### Infertility

PCOS is the most common cause of female infertility. Many women with PCOS experience infrequent ovulation or lack of ovulation altogether and may have trouble becoming pregnant. PCOS also is associated with spontaneous abortion and preeclampsia.[15]

### Obesity

Compared with women of similar age who do not have PCOS, women with PCOS are significantly more likely to be overweight or obese.[3,16] Furthermore, about half of all women with PCOS manifest central obesity, in which there is a greater deposition of visceral fat around internal organs in the abdominal region, as opposed to the fat being located on the thighs and hips. Abdominal fat distribution is associated with increased risk of hypertension, diabetes, and lipid abnormalities.[17]

## Insulin Resistance and Type 2 Diabetes

Studies have found that women with PCOS have higher incidence of insulin resistance and type 2 diabetes than age- and weight-matched controls.[3] Moreover, a majority of obese PCOS women and more than half of those of normal weight are insulin resistant,[18] and a significant number develop type 2 diabetes mellitus by the age of 40.[19]

## Acanthosis Nigricans

Acanthosis nigricans is a dark, poorly defined, velvety hyperpigmentation found on the nape of the neck, armpits, inner thighs, vulva, or under the breasts. This condition is a sign of insulin resistance, which leads to higher circulating insulin levels. Insulin spillover into the skin results in hyperplasia, an abnormal increase in skin growth.[20]

## DIAGNOSIS OF PCOS

There is no specific test to definitively diagnose PCOS. The diagnosis is one of exclusion, which means the health care provider considers all signs and symptoms to rule out other possible disorders.[14] A standard diagnostic assessment for PCOS includes a full medical history, at which time the provider will consider irregular or absent periods, obesity, hirsutism (coarse facial and body hair), and poor breast development. During a physical exam, providers typically look for physical signs of PCOS like acne, facial hair, male pattern baldness, and acanthosis nigricans.

A pelvic or transvaginal ultrasound is used to detect "follicular arrest," or the development of small (5–7 mm) follicles that never reach the preovulatory size of ≥16 mm. Although not all women with PCOS have polycystic ovaries (PCO), nor do all women with ovarian cysts have PCOS,[21] ultrasonographic scanning has substantially broadened the phenotypic spectrum of PCOS.[14]

Diagnostic criteria published by the Androgen Excess Society in 2006 require the presence of clinical or biochemical hyperandrogenism, with either menstrual dysfunction or polycystic ovarian morphology (PCOM), which are detected via transvaginal ultrasonography.[21]

Blood work is used to measure the levels of several hormones and to exclude the many possible causes of menstrual abnormalities or androgen excess that mimic PCOS. Along with tests used to measure elevated androgen levels, doctors may look for high levels of luteinizing hormones (LH) or an elevation in the ratio of LH to follicle-stimulating hormone (FSH), prolactin, thyroid-stimulating hormone (TSH), 17-hydroxyprogesterone, testosterone, and DHEA-S. Other associated conditions such as high levels of glucose, insulin, cholesterol, and triglycerides, as well as insulin resistance may also be assessed.[22]

Some doctors now screen for high levels of anti-Mullerian hormone (AMH) since it is considered a potential diagnostic marker for PCOS.[23,24] AMH is a protein released by cells that are involved with the growth of the egg follicle. AMH levels correlate with the number of antral follicles (small follicles 2–8 mm in size and appear in the beginning of the menstrual cycle) found on the ovary: the higher the antral follicle count, the higher the AMH levels.[25] Women with PCOS typically have a high number of antral follicles and correspondingly high AMH levels.[26]

## CAUSES AND RISK FACTORS FOR PCOS

PCOS was once regarded solely as a reproductive disorder affecting women of child-bearing age. Anovulation (a menstrual cycle in which ovulation does not occur) and androgen excess have been considered the hallmark diagnostic criteria of the syndrome.[14] However, insulin resistance is now identified as a significant contributor to the pathogenesis of PCOS, the metabolic and cardiovascular consequences of which are widely acknowledged within the scientific community.[11] To date, several factors involved in the development of PCOS have been identified.

## Luteinizing Hormone Secretion and Androgen Excess

Past research has emphasized the role of neuroendocrine abnormalities in the persistent and excessive secretion of luteinizing hormones (LH), one of 2 glycoprotein hormones that stimulate the final ripening of the follicles and the secretion of progesterone. Excessive LH triggers premature ovulation, disrupting the follicle's maturation process and leading to an increase in androgen production by ovarian theca cells. Some research points to increased LH as the driving force for PCOS in slender and normal body-weight women.[27]

## Hyperinsulinemia and Androgen Excess

Hyperinsulinemia produces hyperandrogenism in women with PCOS via 2 distinct and independent mechanisms. The first is by stimulating ovarian androgen production. Studies have shown that insulin acts synergistically with LH to enhance androgen production in ovarian theca cells.[28,29] The second mechanism is by directly and independently reducing serum sex hormone-binding globulin (SHBG) levels. Insulin decreases hepatic synthesis and SHBG secretion, thus increasing the amount of free, biologically active testosterone.[30] The net result of these 2 actions increases circulating free testosterone concentrations.

## Genetics and Androgen Excess

An increase in LH, as well as hyperinsulinemia, leads to an increase in androgen production by ovarian theca cells.[29] Research indicates that morphologic changes in the ovaries, including ovarian cyst development and theca-cell (steroid-producing cells in the ovaries) dysfunction, may be an indication of a genetic basis for PCOS. Researchers suspect that there is a genetically determined ovarian defect present in women with PCOS, causing the ovary to overproduce androgen.[29,31–33] Indeed, abnormal theca cell activity seems to be a primary source for excess androgens.[34]

The following risk factors are also thought to have a strong influence over the progression of PCOS.

## Obesity

Studies have found that obesity not only contributes to the development of PCOS, but arises also as a result.[16] The adipose tissue of women with PCOS is characterized by enlarged fat cells (hypertrophic adipocytes) and impairments in the body's ability to break down fat (lipolysis) and regulate insulin. Whether these abnormalities are primary or secondary to hyperandrogenism or other PCOS-related abnormalities is not yet known.[35]

## Age at Onset

Some research suggests that girls who develop pubic hair early (often before the age of 8, and a condition known as premature pubarche) have many of the signs and symptoms of PCOS. In one study that followed prepubescent girls throughout puberty, premature pubarche resulted in excess testosterone production and irregular periods consistent with PCOS, leading researchers to conclude that premature pubarche may be an early form of PCOS.[36]

## Other Risk Factors

Other risk factors that may play a role in the pathogenesis of PCOS include chronic inflammation[37]; exposure to endocrine-disrupting chemicals[38]; autoimmune disorders, especially those involving the ovaries, pancreas, thyroid, and adrenal glands[39]; and the use of medications that increase prolactin production.[40]

Putting aside etiology, women with PCOS are prone to defects in insulin signaling, which aggravates the synthesis of androgens in the ovaries and adrenal gland.[29] Excess androgens encourage insulin resistance, leading to elevated insulin levels, which in turn stimulate further androgen synthesis. This vicious cycle results in a "snowball effect" worsening PCOS symptoms and making sufferers especially susceptible to obesity and diabetes, conditions that significantly compound the syndrome's progression.[11,41]

## WHAT YOU NEED TO KNOW

- PCOS is a common female endocrine disorder.
- Although symptoms vary from person to person, it is characterized by multiple ovarian cysts, irregular, heavy or nonexistent periods, excessive facial/body hair, male pattern baldness, decreased sex drive, skin tags, infertility, depression, and weight gain.
- Insulin resistance is one of the most common features of PCOS, and a condition in which the cells of the body literally become resistant to the effects of insulin.
- The root cause of PCOS is unknown but genetic predisposition, insulin resistance, excess androgen production, and obesity all play a role.
- Since the symptoms of PCOS vary in severity and form, many treatments are used. Conventional options include drug treatments for hirsutism and acne, drugs such as clomifenem tamoxifen and gonadotrophins to induce ovulation for infertility, surgery to induce ovulation by reducing androgen levels, and promising insulin-sensitizing drugs such as metformin.
- The most important aspect of long term care of PCOS is managing cardiovascular risks such as obesity, insulin resistance, diabetes, hypertension, and elevated blood cholesterol, early recognition and intervention are considered the cornerstones of PCOS treatment.
- Emerging evidence suggests that lifestyle choices such as weight reduction and exercise, along with specific nutraceuticals targeted to safely and effectively deal with symptoms, underlying causes, and associated risk factors, might help reduce the incidence and severity of PCOS.

# CONVENTIONAL TREATMENT OF PCOS

PCOS treatment generally focuses on management of the individual's principal concerns, such as infertility, hirsutism, acne, or obesity.

## Hirsutism

- Oral contraceptive pills—estrogen–progesterone combinations—are preferably used. Estrogens lower LH levels and androgen production. Progesterone is crucial, as it may increase liver production of SHBG, reducing free testosterone levels.[42]

- Another medication called spironolactone (Aldactone®) is used as a primary medical treatment for hirsutism and female pattern hair loss since the accidental discovery of its antiandrogenic effects. Spironolactone reduces testosterone production and inhibits its action on target tissues. It is also an effective alternative treatment for acne in women. Spironolactone should not be used in pregnancy since it can disturb the growth and development of the embryo and fetus.[43]

- Even more promising are insulin sensitizers like metformin, which also holds promise for managing hirsutism in PCOS patients.[42]

## Infertility

Ovulation induction remains a milestone in the treatment of women with anovulatory infertility.[44] Clomiphene citrate (CC), an oral antiestrogen medication, is considered the first-line treatment for inducing ovulation in women with PCOS.[44]

Since insulin resistance plays a central role in PCOS, insulin reduction strategies are a possible treatment for infertility in PCOS patients.[45] For instance, if CC alone is not effective, metformin can be added to help induce ovulation.[46]

If the CC and metformin combination fails, gonadotropins—follicle-stimulating hormone (FSH) and luteinizing hormone (LH) medications that are administered by injection—may be another option.[44,47]

Aromatase inhibitors, such as anastrozole and letrozole, are a relatively new treatment for ovulation induction.[48] Aromatase inhibitors selectively block the peripheral conversion of androgens to estrogens, causing a reaction in the pituitary gland that increases FSH and optimizes ovulation. The advantage of aromatase inhibitors is that they avoid the unfavorable side effects seen frequently with antiestrogens.[49]

If medication does not work, a surgical procedure called laparoscopic ovarian drilling (LOD) may be considered. During LOD, a surgeon makes a small incision in the abdomen and inserts a tube attached to a tiny camera (laparoscope) providing detailed images of the ovaries and neighboring pelvic organs. The surgeon then inserts surgical instruments through other small incisions and uses electrical or laser energy to destroy the extra androgen-producing follicles on the surface of the ovaries. The goal of the operation is to induce ovulation by reducing androgen levels.

## Regulation of the Menstrual Cycle

Metformin improves ovulation and leads to regular menstrual cycles.

Birth control pills containing a combination of synthetic estrogen and progesterone decrease androgen production, correct abnormal bleeding, and decrease the risk of endometrial cancer as well. Low-dose birth control pills have been proven effective for regulating the menstrual cycles of those who are not trying to become pregnant.[50]

To date, there are no known clinical studies on bioidentical hormone replacement therapy (BHRT) and PCOS.

## Long-Term PCOS Management

Managing cardiovascular risks such as obesity, elevated cholesterol, high blood pressure, and diabetes is considered the most important aspect of PCOS treatment. Because medications such as metformin and thiazolidinedione improve insulin sensitivity, in 2004 Great Britain's National Institute for Health and Clinical Excellence recommended that women with PCOS who have a Body Mass Index (BMI) >25 be given metformin when other therapies fail to produce results.[51] This recommendation proved to be well founded, as metformin is known to be an effective treatment for both hyperinsulinemia and hyperandrogenism.[52–54] Indeed, metformin may be the most promising conventional medical treatment for PCOS.

---

### METFORMIN: AN UNDERUTILIZED TREATMENT FOR PCOS

- Metformin, a medication currently used to lower blood sugar, is approved by the U.S. Food and Drug Administration (FDA) to manage type 2 diabetes mellitus. Metformin inhibits liver glucose production, although it also decreases intestinal glucose uptake and increases insulin sensitivity in peripheral tissues.[55]

- Metformin improves the likelihood of ovulation in women with PCOS through a variety of actions, including reducing insulin levels and altering the effect of insulin on ovarian androgen synthesis, theca cell proliferation, and endometrial growth.[56]

- To increase metformin tolerance, patients start with 500 mg daily with food. After 1 week, the dose increases to 1000 mg for another week and then to 1500 mg daily. Clinical response is usually seen at the 1000-mg daily dose.[57] Studies have found that PCOS patients who do not respond to metformin at the 1500-mg dose respond favorably to 2000 mg.[57]

- For many years, oral hypoglycemic agents were regarded as teratogenic, and their use was contraindicated during pregnancy. However, the latest data support the safety of metformin throughout pregnancy. Researchers reported that metformin was not teratogenic and did not affect the motor or social development of infants age 3 and 6 months.[58] A 2010 study concluded that metformin improves ovulation and pregnancy rates, findings they noted while updating the Cochrane Review of insulin-sensitizing drugs (metformin, rosiglitazone, pioglitazone, and D-chiro-inositol) for women with PCOS, oligo/amenorrhea, and subfertility.[59]

- A clinical study of 50 PCOS patients reported that metformin exerts a slight but significant deleterious effect on serum homocysteine levels. Therefore, supplementing with folate is considered useful for lowering homocysteine and increasing the beneficial effect of metformin on the vascular endothelium (the inner lining of the blood vessels).[60]

## SIDE EFFECTS WITH CONVENTIONAL TREATMENTS

A pitfall of mainstream approaches to PCOS is that they are often associated with unwanted side effects.

- For trouble conceiving, doctors typically prescribe the fertility drug Clomid®. In some women, Clomid® causes no side effects. In others, side effects may include mood swings, hot flashes, breast tenderness, abdominal cramps, and nausea. Roughly 30% of women who take Clomid® experience the more serious side effects of hostile fertile mucous (HFM, a condition in which the cervical mucus become too thick to allow sperm to penetrate the cervix) and uterine lining thinning. HFM prevents conception and a thin uterine lining decreases the likelihood of implantation and may lead to early miscarriage. Both are undesirable effects of using Clomid®.

- Birth control pills are still the treatment of choice for irregular periods. However, a 2006 study concluded that birth control pills increase insulin resistance, making the symptoms of PCOS more pronounced and increase the risk of major heath complications.[61]

- In fact, many medications used in the treatment of PCOS do not adequately address the lifestyle and hormonal imbalances that are at the root of PCOS, nor do they hold much promise for managing associated cardiovascular risks and type 2 diabetes.

## PCOS NUTRITIONAL PROTOCOL

### Inositol

"Inositol" is a term used to refer to a group of naturally occurring carbohydrate compounds that exist in 9 possible chemical orientations called stereoisomers. The most common is myoinositol, which is often sold as a dietary supplement labeled simply as inositol.

Inositol, particularly myoinositol and another less common stereoisomer called D-chiro-inositol (DCI), plays a critical, but underappreciated role in insulin signaling. Conditions such as hyperglycemia and diabetes are associated with disrupted inositol signaling, leading many researchers to suggest that this may be a key pathologic feature of insulin resistance.[62,63]

Research has shown that the 3 inositol family members help to ameliorate conditions in which insulin resistance plays an important role, especially in PCOS.

**D-chiro-inositol.** DCI is perhaps the most promising inositol compound for PCOS. Our bodies produce this compound only after extensive inositol metabolism. DCI interacts with select sugars in the body to form conjugates known as inositol phosphoglycans, which play a key role in mediating insulin actions. Low levels of DCI and inositol phosphoglycans have been observed in individuals with impaired insulin sensitivity and PCOS.[64–67]

In one study, 44 overweight women with PCOS were given a daily 1200-mg dose of DCI for 6–8 weeks. During the course of the study, those who took DCI displayed significant improvements in insulin sensitivity, blood pressure, and triglyceride levels, as well as a marked decrease in serum testosterone levels. Moreover, 19 of 22 subjects receiving DCI ovulated during the study period, compared to only 6 of 22 in the placebo group. The investigators concluding statement highlights the efficacy of DCI in PCOS: "D-chiro-inositol increases the action of insulin in patients with the polycystic ovary syndrome, thereby improving ovulatory function and decreasing serum androgen concentrations, blood pressure, and plasma triglyceride concentrations."[68]

Similarly promising results were drawn from another study involving lean women with PCOS. Here, participants received 600 mg daily of DCI or a placebo for 6–8 weeks. The DCI-treated participants improved significantly, displaying a 73% decrease in testosterone levels versus no change in the placebo group. Women taking DCI also experienced reductions in insulin and triglyceride levels and blood pressure, whereas none of these changes were evident in the placebo group.[69]

Researchers looking at the effects of metformin in PCOS women concluded that the drug's benefits could be related to its ability to improve the function of DCI phosphoglycans in the body. Thus, it appears that DCI may be highly effective when used in combination with metformin for PCOS.[70]

**Myoinositol.** Myoinositol is a stereoisomer of DCI. Like DCI, it is a key factor in insulin signaling, and serves also as a precursor to DCI in endogenous inositol metabolism. It should then come as no surprise that studies using myoinositol in women with PCOS produced results as promising as those obtained with DCI.

Double-blind, placebo-controlled investigations were carried out in 42 women with PCOS, subjects receiving myoinositol fared much better when compared to the placebo group, displaying decreases in testosterone, triglycerides, and blood pressure; a significant improvement in insulin sensitivity; and a greatly increased frequency of ovulation.[71]

In another study, 20 women with PCOS were given either 2 g of myoinositol plus 200 μg folic acid, or 200 μg folic acid daily. After 12 weeks, the women taking myoinositol showed improved insulin sensitivity and androgen levels. Strikingly, all the subjects receiving myoinositol returned to normal menstrual cycles.[72]

In an Italian study of 92 PCOS patients, almost 50% showed significant weight loss and reduced leptin levels after receiving myoinositol plus folic acid (4 g myoinositol plus 400 μg folic acid). After a 14-week treatment, the myoinositol plus folic acid group lost weight, whereas the placebo group gained weight.[73]

A 6-month study involving 50 PCOS women yielded similar results and gave researchers the time to evaluate the effects of myoinositol on hirsutism. Along with decreases in testosterone and insulin levels, the participants who supplemented with myoinositol experienced a reduction in hirsutism, and improvements in skin appearance, leading researches to conclude the following: "Myoinositol administration is a simple and safe treatment that ameliorates the metabolic profile of patients with PCOS, reducing hirsutism and acne."[74]

In other well-designed clinical trials for follicular maturity and ovulation induction, myoinositol has produced promising results, cementing its position as a novel therapy for PCOS management.[75,76]

**D-Pinitol.** D-pinitol is 3-O-methyl-D-chiro-inositol that occurs naturally in several different foods, including legumes and citrus fruits.[77] D-pinitol is converted into d-chiro-inositol in the body. Like DCI, pinitol appears to favorably influence the action of insulin.[78] In a double-blind study of patients with type 2 diabetes, administration of 600 mg of pinitol twice a day for 3 months reduced blood glucose concentration by 19.3%, decreased hemoglobin A1C (HbA1C) concentration by 12.4%, and significantly improved insulin resistance.[79] In a shorter-term double-blind study, administration of pinitol at a dose of 20 mg/kg of body weight per day for 4 weeks decreased mean fasting plasma glucose concentration by 5.3%.[80]

## N-Acetyl-Cysteine

N-acetyl-cysteine (NAC) is a stable derivative of the sulfur-containing amino acid cysteine and an antioxidant that is needed for the production of glutathione, one of the body's most important natural antioxidants and detoxifiers. While cysteine is found in high-protein foods, NAC is not. A large body of evidence supports the use of NAC in women with PCOS.

- *Improving Insulin Sensitivity.* Women with PCOS frequently have an abnormally high insulin response to sugars and refined starches. A 2002 study evaluated the effect of NAC on insulin secretion and peripheral insulin resistance in women with PCOS.[81] The study subjects who had an exaggerated insulin response to a glucose challenge and were treated with NAC showed an improvement in insulin function in their peripheral tissues. The NAC treatment also produced a significant decline in testosterone levels and in free androgen index values. The researchers concluded, "NAC may be a new treatment for the improvement of circulating insulin levels and insulin sensitivity in hyperinsulinemic patients with polycystic ovary syndrome."[82]

- *Restoring Fertility.* NAC may also be useful for improving fertility in women with PCOS. In one study, NAC appeared to improve the effects of Clomid®, the widely used fertility drug. Clomid® plus NAC significantly improved ovulation rates in a study of 573 women with PCOS. According to the researchers, 52% of the study participants who took Clomid® plus NAC ovulated, whereas only 18% ovulated in the Clomid® alone group. The authors concluded: "N-acetyl-cysteine is proved effective in inducing or augmenting ovulation in polycystic ovary patients."[83]

Similarly, a study of Clomid®-resistant women has shown that NAC appears to make Clomid® more effective. In the study, 150 Clomid®-resistant women with PCOS were divided into 2 groups: one group took Clomid® and NAC. The other group took Clomid® and a placebo. In the NAC group, 49.3% ovulated and 1.3% became pregnant. In contrast, in the placebo group, only 21% ovulated and there were no pregnancies.[84]

Worth noting, the same researchers compared the effects of a NAC–Clomid® combination with the metformin–Clomid® combination on ovulation induction in anovulatory Clomid®-resistant women with PCOS. The efficacy of the metformin–Clomid® combination therapy is significantly higher than that of NAC–Clomid® for inducing ovulation and achieving pregnancy among Clomid®-resistant PCOS patients.[82]

- *Tackling Homocysteine.* Women with PCOS are often given metformin to deal with their insulin problems. But metformin may increase homocysteine levels and many women with PCOS have high homocysteine levels to begin with.[85] Elevated homocysteine is associated with coronary artery disease, heart attack, chronic fatigue, fibromyalgia, cognitive impairment, and cervical cancer. A 2009 study showed that people taking NAC for 2 months had a significant decrease in homocysteine levels.[86]

## Magnesium

Many women with PCOS have significantly low serum and total magnesium, contributing to the progression of insulin resistance to type 2 diabetes and heart disease.[87]

Magnesium insufficiency is common in poorly controlled type 2 diabetes patients. In one study, 128 patients with poorly controlled type 2 diabetes received a placebo or a supplement with either 500 mg or 1000 mg of magnesium oxide (300 mg or 600 mg element magnesium) for 30 days. All patients were treated also with diet or diet plus oral medication to control blood glucose levels. Magnesium levels increased in the group receiving 1000 mg magnesium oxide daily but did not significantly change in the placebo group or the group receiving 500 mg of magnesium. The author suggested prolonged use of magnesium in doses that are higher than usual is needed in patients with type 2 diabetes to improve control or prevent chronic complications.[88]

In a related study, 63 diabetics with below normal serum magnesium levels received either 2.5 g of oral magnesium chloride daily (providing 300 mg elemental magnesium per day) or a placebo. At the end of the 16-week study period, those who received the supplement had higher blood levels of magnesium and improved control of diabetes, as suggested by lower hemoglobin A1C (HbA1C) levels.[89]

Another study found that oral magnesium supplements helped insulin-resistant individuals avoid developing type 2 diabetes.[90] Because magnesium improves insulin-mediated glucose uptake and insulin secretion in type 2 diabetes patients, it is considered a critical mineral for women with PCOS.

## Chromium

Research shows a clear link between chromium and glucose metabolism. Indeed, chromium is one of the most widely studied nutritional interventions in the treatment of glucose- and insulin-related irregularities. Chromium picolinate specifically is the form that has been used in a number of studies on insulin resistance. Researchers at the University of Texas Health Science Center at San Antonio found that chromium picolinate (200 mcg/day) improves glucose tolerance when compared with a placebo[91] in women with PCOS.

## Lipoic Acid

Considerable evidence suggests that lipoic acid may be critical not only for maintaining optimal blood sugar levels (by helping the body use glucose), but also for supporting insulin sensitivity and key aspects of cardiovascular health, such as endothelial function. A review of experimental studies reveals that lipoic acid helps relieve several components of metabolic syndrome—a constellation of risk factors that often precedes full-blown type 2 diabetes. It appears that lipoic acid reduces blood pressure and insulin resistance, improves lipid profile, and reduces weight. Based on results of key clinical studies, scientists are sanguine about lipoic acid's potential as a therapeutic agent for individuals with metabolic syndrome.[92] Similarly positive effects have been observed in women with PCOS. In a 16-week study, women with PCOS were given 600 mg of lipoic acid twice daily, and, over the course of the study period, exhibited a sharp improvement in insulin sensitivity and a reduction in triglycerides. Lipoic acid therapy also is associated with an improved LDL-particle pattern (or "bad" cholesterol particles), indicating a reduction in cardiovascular risk.[93]

## Vitamin D

In an insightful associative study that highlighted the link between PCOS and vitamin D status, researchers found that women with higher blood levels of vitamin D were much less likely to be insulin resistant.[94] A separate study found that vitamin D when administered with metformin was helpful for regulating the menstrual cycles in PCOS women.[95]

A study conducted by researchers at Columbia University found that Vitamin D combined with calcium supplementation helped normalize menstrual cycles for 7 of 13 women with PCOS. Of the 7, 2 became pregnant and the others maintained normal menstrual cycles. These results suggest that abnormalities in calcium balance may be responsible, in part, for the arrested follicular development in women with PCOS and contribute to its pathogenesis.[96]

## Omega-3 Fatty Acids

Evidence suggests that the anti-inflammatory activity of omega-3 fatty acids ameliorates nonalcoholic fatty liver disease, a common condition in women with PCOS. In an Australian study, omega-3 fatty acid supplementation reduced liver fat content and other cardiovascular risk factors in women with PCOS, including triglycerides and systolic and diastolic blood pressure. In particular, said the researchers, omega-3 fatty acids were helpful in reducing hepatic fat in PCOS women with hepatic steatosis, which is defined as liver fat content greater than 5%.[97]

## Flax Seeds

The powerful lignans—plant compounds that have both estrogenic and antiestrogenic properties—in flaxseed may help reduce androgen levels in PCOS women. Flaxseed consumption has been shown to stimulate SHBG synthesis.[98] Changes in SHBG concentration result in relatively large changes in the amount of free and bound hormones.

In a 2007 study, daily flaxseed supplementation reduced androgen levels and hirsutism in PCOS patients, leading researchers to conclude, "The clinically-significant decrease in androgen levels with a concomitant reduction in hirsutism reported in this case study demonstrates a need for further research of flaxseed supplementation on hormonal levels and clinical symptoms of PCOS."[99]

## Cinnamon

Scientists at the U.S. Department of Agriculture (USDA) have been studying the effect of cinnamon on blood glucose for over a decade, leading to several interesting discoveries, including that of unique compounds in cinnamon bark that in laboratory studies produce a 20-fold increase in sugar metabolism.[100,101] According to one government expert, "These polyphenolic polymers found in cinnamon may function as antioxidants, potentiate insulin action, and may be beneficial in the control of glucose intolerance and diabetes."[102]

In a 2003 study, 60 diabetics taking 1, 3, or 6 g daily of ground cinnamon for 40 days lowered their fasting serum glucose by 18–29%, triglycerides by 23–30%, LDL cholesterol by 7–27%, and total cholesterol by 12–26%.[103]

A 2007 study by researchers at Columbia University found that cinnamon reduced insulin resistance in 15 women with PCOS. In the study, the women were divided into 2 groups: one group took cinnamon extract while the other group took a placebo. After 8 weeks, the cinnamon group showed significant reductions in insulin resistance while the placebo group did not. The authors did point out that, "A larger trial is needed to confirm the findings of this pilot study and to evaluate the effect of cinnamon extract on menstrual cyclicity."[104]

## Licorice Root

A 2004 study by Italian researchers investigated the effect of licorice on androgen metabolism in 9 healthy 22- to 26-year-old women in the luteal phase of their menstrual cycle and found that licorice reduced serum testosterone. The authors suggested that licorice could be considered an "adjuvant therapy" of hirsutism and PCOS. This study was the first to follow up on earlier trials, which found that an herbal formula containing licorice reduced testosterone secretion in women with PCOS.[105–107]

Spironolactone (Aldactone), an antagonist of mineralocorticoid and androgen receptors, is used as a primary medical treatment for hirsutism and female pattern hair loss. It is also associated with several side effects related to the diuretic activity of spironolactone. Interestingly, licorice was shown in a study of women with PCOS to counteract the side-effects of spironolactone when the 2 were used in combination.[108]

## Green Tea (Epigallocatechin Gallate)

Green tea may be of benefit to women with PCOS. Green tea is known to have positive effects on glucose metabolism.[109] In both human and animal studies, green tea has been shown to improve insulin sensitivity.[110,111] Animal research suggests that green tea epigallocatechin gallate (EGCG) may help prevent the onset of type 2 diabetes and slow its progression.[112] A clinical study from Japan found that daily supplementation of green tea extract lowered the hemoglobin A1C (HbA1C) level in individuals with borderline diabetes.[113] Hemoglobin A1C is a form of hemoglobin that is used to help identify plasma glucose concentration over a period of time.

Green tea also is thought to lower TNF-alpha (TNF-$\alpha$).[114] TNF-$\alpha$ or tumor necrosis factor is involved with systemic inflammation. Green tea is a potent antioxidant, and a study published in the *American Journal of Clinical Nutrition* showed that just 90 mg of EGCG before each meal increased the body's

24-hour metabolism rate by 4% and the metabolism of fat by an impressive 40%.[115]

## Spearmint

A recent study by British researchers published in the journal *Phytotherapy Research* found a positive link between spearmint tea consumption and a reduction in hirsutism in PCOS women. In the study, 42 women were divided into 2 groups: one that took spearmint tea twice a day for a 1-month period and the other a placebo herbal tea. The spearmint tea group showed significant decreases in free and total testosterone levels and an increase in LH and FSH, leading the researchers to conclude that "spearmint (tea) has the potential for use as a helpful and natural treatment for hirsutism in PCOS."[116]

## Saw Palmetto

Saw palmetto inhibits the activity of an enzyme, 5-alpha reductase, thereby reducing the conversion of testosterone to dihydrotestosterone, the more androgenic form of male hormone. This may have implications for reducing acne and excess facial and body hair, as well as male pattern hair loss. Oral administered saw palmetto has been studied as part of a formula that slowed hair loss and improved hair density in patients with testosterone related hair loss.[117]

## LIFESTYLE AND DIETARY RECOMMENDATIONS

For women with PCOS, daily physical activity and participation in a regular exercise regimen are essential for treating or preventing insulin resistance, lowering blood sugar levels, and for helping weight-control efforts.

Since a majority of PCOS women are obese, and insulin resistance plays a critical role in the development of PCOS, a diet that is high in fiber, low in saturated fatty acids and monounsaturated fat, and high in vitamins, minerals, and disease-fighting phytonutrients may reduce certain risk factors and improve overall well-being.

Additional research may determine which specific dietary approach is best for PCOS, but it is clear that *losing weight by reducing total caloric intake* benefits the overall health of women with PCOS.

A clinical study showed that short-term treatment of obese PCOS women with an ultra-low-calorie diet (350–450 kilocalories [kcal] per day) decreased androgen signaling and reduced serum insulin.[118] A study by Italian researchers concluded that comprehensive dietary change designed to lower insulin resulted in a significant decrease in testosterone, body weight, waist/hip ratio, total cholesterol, fasting blood glucose, and insulin.[119]

Diets high in monounsaturated fats have been shown to increase insulin sensitivity and lower the overall glycemic index. High-fiber foods are slowly absorbed, causing less insulin to be released; high-fiber diets increase SHBG, which binds to and lowers free testosterone; and fibers also can lower PAI-1 (plasminogen activator inhibitor, a glycosylated protein that plays a significant role in metabolic syndrome) as well as cholesterol and blood lipids.[118]

A study reported that just a moderate reduction in dietary carbohydrates reduced fasting and postchallenge insulin concentrations among women with PCOS, improving reproductive/endocrine outcomes.[120] As stated in a 2005 report, "On the balance of evidence to date, a diet low in saturated fat and high in fiber from predominantly low-glycemic-index-carbohydrate foods is recommended [in the dietary management of PCOS]."[121]

## Life Extension Suggestions

- **Myo-inositol:** 2–4 g daily
- **D-chiro-inositol:** 600–1200 mg daily
- **N-acetyl-cysteine** (NAC): 1200 mg daily
- **Lipoic acid** (as Na-RALA): 240–480 mg daily
- **Fish oil:** 2–6 g daily
- **Vitamin D:** 2000–8000 IU daily
- **Chromium:** 200–500 mcg daily
- **Magnesium:** 600–1000 mg daily
- **Saw palmetto:** 160 mg daily
- **Folic acid:** 400 mcg daily
- **Green tea:** 750 mg daily of standardized green tea extract
- **Cinnamon:** In extract form 200–300 mg; or 1–2 teaspoons ground cinnamon daily
- **Licorice root:** 500 mg daily

In addition, the following blood testing resources may be helpful:

- **Female Comphrehensive Hormone Panel or Male Comprehensive Hormone Panel; or Female Panel or Male Panel**
- **Insulin (fasting)**
- **FSH and LH**
- **Magnesium**
- **Omega Score®**
- **Vitamin D, 25-Hydroxy**

## REFERENCES

References available at: www.lef.org/dpt5/ch109

# 110

---

# *Polymyalgia Rheumatica*

---

Polymyalgia rheumatica, an inflammatory disease that usually affects women, causes muscular pain and stiffness in the shoulders, neck, and hips.[1,2]

In people with polymyalgia rheumatica, synovial membranes and bursae, which line and lubricate the joints, become inflamed, causing pain and discomfort.[3–6] Unlike the case with some other inflammatory diseases (eg, rheumatoid arthritis), no permanent damage to either the joints or muscles is associated with polymyalgia rheumatica. The disease typically resolves in a few years.

Nevertheless, during the disease course, polymyalgia is a painful condition that significantly affects quality of life. Standard conventional treatment for polymyalgia rheumatica involves nonsteroidal anti-inflammatory drugs (NSAIDs) and corticosteroids to reduce inflammation and pain. Unfortunately, this arsenal of treatment options is far from ideal. NSAIDs are rarely effective, so corticosteroids are generally used as first-line therapy. However, corticosteroid drugs are associated with significant side effects, including osteoporosis. The longer the treatment lasts, and the higher the dose(s) used, the more likely a patient will suffer serious side effects. One major goal of conventional therapy is to use the smallest dose of corticosteroids possible and taper off as soon as symptoms resolve.

Nutritional therapy offers an important adjunct approach to polymyalgia rheumatica. Even though there is a lack of serious nutritional research into polymyalgia rheumatica, the inflammatory cascade that underlies the disease is well understood. By using proven anti-inflammatory supplements, it may be possible to reduce dosages of strong prescription drugs and reduce symptoms. In addition, inflammation associated with the disease causes impairment of the adrenal hormone system, resulting in a deficiency in vital hormones that need to be replaced.

It is important to note that a significant number of people with polymyalgia rheumatica also suffer from a condition known as giant cell arteritis.[2,7] Giant cell arteritis involves inflammation of the temporal artery (a major craniofacial artery), and other arteries can also be inflamed.[8] Aneurysms can form in these weakened vessels.[9] Because the temporal artery supplies blood to the eye, blindness is a possible consequence of giant cell arteritis.[10] Up to 75% of patients with giant cell arteritis may have aortitis (inflammation of the aorta), although the condition is not always diagnosed.[9] Noninvasive imaging techniques, especially magnetic resonance imaging, have been used to determine the true degree of aortitis in patients with giant cell arteritis.[11] Because of its significant consequences, patients with polymyalgia rheumatica should be carefully monitored for signs or symptoms of giant cell arteritis.

## INFLAMMATION AND THE HPA AXIS

The hallmark of polymyalgia rheumatica is inflammation, probably caused by an autoimmune reaction in which the body's immune system is activated against itself.[12–16] In people with polymyalgia rheumatica, inflammatory chemicals (including interleukin-6 [IL-6] and tumor necrosis factor-alpha [TNF-α]) are released into the bloodstream. Besides causing the inflammation that leads to symptoms, these chemicals have a profound effect on the hypothalamic-pituitary-adrenal (HPA) axis, which is intimately involved in maintaining levels of vital hormones (eg, dehydroepiandrosterone [DHEA] and cortisol). Among people with polymyalgia rheumatica, it appears the HPA axis is depressed due to elevated levels of IL-6.[17] As a result, DHEA levels are low.[18–21]

DHEA is a vital adrenal hormone that is converted into other hormones, including estrogen and testosterone. Low levels of DHEA have been associated with a wide variety of diseases, including inflammatory, autoimmune diseases such as rheumatoid arthritis and polymyalgia rheumatica.

DHEA replacement therapy has been shown to inhibit inflammatory cytokines and decrease IL-6 levels.[22,23] In one study, DHEA administered with glutamine and arginine allowed for lower doses of prednisone (a corticosteroid) among women with polymyalgia rheumatica.[24,25] DHEA also protects against the risk of infection caused by reduced immunity in steroid-treated animals,[26] and increases bone density.[27]

## DIAGNOSIS OF POLYMYALGIA RHEUMATICA

Diagnosis of polymyalgia rheumatica requires ruling out other conditions, such as rheumatoid arthritis (RA), polymyositis, systemic lupus erythematosus, and thyroid problems.[28,29]

Polymyalgia rheumatica is rare in people less than 50 years, and patients are usually more than 60 years old.[28] It is twice as common in women as in men.[28,30] Because polymyalgia rheumatica and giant cell arteritis frequently occur in the same patients, they may represent different aspects of a single condition. Most researchers, however, think polymyalgia rheumatica and giant cell arteritis are different conditions with similar manifestations.[7,13,31,32]

The first step in diagnosing polymyalgia rheumatica is obtaining a clinical history from the patient. The main diagnostic criteria for polymyalgia rheumatica are hip and shoulder pain, coupled with exclusion of other possible causes.[29] In addition, a number of blood tests may be used to measure inflammation. For example, patients with polymyalgia rheumatica usually have an elevated erythrocyte sedimentation rate (ESR).[28,33] C-reactive protein and IL-6 are also elevated in patients with polymyalgia rheumatica.[28,29] These proinflammatory indicators, however, are elevated in response to inflammation anywhere in the body and cannot be used to definitely diagnose polymyalgia rheumatica.

If giant cell arteritis is suspected, a temporal artery biopsy is indicated, although corticosteroid treatment may start without waiting for the biopsy results.[8] Other blood vessels (including the aorta) can be visualized with magnetic resonance imaging or ultrasound to determine the extent of inflammation.

Treatment with steroids usually begins promptly. Most patients respond very quickly to corticosteroids. In fact, if symptoms do not resolve rapidly, a physician may want to conduct additional tests to determine whether the diagnosis was correct.

# CONVENTIONAL TREATMENT

## Anticytokine Therapy

TNF-α levels are elevated in patients with polymyalgia rheumatica. This important inflammatory cytokine is at the start of the inflammatory cascade.[34] In mouse fibroblasts, TNF-α increases nuclear factor kappa B (NF-κB) in the cells, which stimulate the production of IL-6.[35] Thus, blocking TNF-α may help patients with polymyalgia rheumatica avoid or reduce corticosteroid use.

In one study, 7 patients with polymyalgia rheumatica and diabetes mellitus or osteoporosis were treated with Infliximab (Remicade®), a prescription TNF-α blocker. After 6 months they experienced clinical improvement and had significantly decreased IL-6 and ESR levels.[36] The authors suggest that Infliximab may be used as a steroid-sparing agent, and it may also be useful as a first-line treatment in patients who should avoid corticosteroids.

In another study, 4 patients with polymyalgia rheumatica who had relapsed were treated with Infliximab (3mg/kg) at weeks 0, 2, and 6.[37] Three of the 4 patients went into remission by week 2, and the fourth was able to tolerate a lower prednisone dose. Together, these small-scale studies suggest that blocking TNF-α may be useful for treating polymyalgia rheumatica.

## Steroid-Sparing Drugs

A major therapeutic goal in treating polymyalgia rheumatica and giant cell arteritis is to reduce the dosage of steroid to help reduce side effects.[2] Because of the risk of blindness and other consequences of arterial inflammation (such as thrombosis and aneurysms), high doses of corticosteroids are used when giant cell arteritis is suspected. Although these high doses bring with them the additional risk of significant side effects, most clinicians feel the risk associated with giant cell arteritis justifies this approach.[10,38]

**Methotrexate.** Methotrexate is a folate antagonist with anti-inflammatory, immunosuppressive, and antiproliferative actions.[39] Studies of methotrexate in addition to prednisone have been contradictory; some studies suggest that methotrexate decreases total steroid dose needed by patients.[40,41]

Methotrexate increases homocysteine levels,[42] so people taking methotrexate should consider supplementing with vitamins B6, B12, and folate to lower homocysteine.[43,44]

**Pentoxifylline.** Pentoxifylline (PTX), an anti-inflammatory drug used for more than 20 years,[45,46] is well tolerated.[47] PTX suppresses inflammation by decreasing synthesis and secretion of cytokines, including interleukin-1, IL-6, interleukin-8, and TNF-α.[45,48–51] While no published studies of PTX in patients with polymyalgia rheumatica or giant cell arteritis exist, it is possible that PTX will be a treatment for polymyalgia rheumatica in the future. Research shows that a combination of fish oil (omega-3 fatty acids), alpha-linolenic acid, and PTX can reduce synthesis of IL-6.[52]

## Osteoporosis Prevention

Osteoporosis prevention and bone preservation are important facets of treatment for polymyalgia rheumatica. Both the disease itself and the corticosteroids used to treat it are known to increase bone loss.[53] All patients, especially postmenopausal women, need to take calcium and vitamin D to avoid problems associated with osteoporosis.[54] In some cases, prescription medications are needed to reverse osteoporosis.[55–57]

**Bisphosphonates.** Bisphosphonates are prescription drugs that slow the rate at which calcium is removed from the bones; they have been shown to increase bone mass and strength.[58]

# TARGETED NATURAL THERAPEUTICS

Data are minimal regarding the effect of many dietary supplements in polymyalgia rheumatica; perhaps because few research dollars are being directed at natural remedies for this condition. Because of significant side effects associated with drugs prescribed for polymyalgia rheumatica, however, Life Extension suggests patients do everything possible to reduce their use of these drugs, including pursuing natural remedies proven to reduce inflammatory cytokine levels.

## Calcium and Vitamin D

Calcium is important to maintain adequate serum calcium so bone demineralization can be prevented. Vitamin D or a vitamin D analog is necessary for the body to absorb and utilize calcium. Studies have shown that vitamin D analogs (alfacalcidol or calcitriol) are readily converted to active form in the body.[56,59]

## Vitamin K

Vitamin K consists of vitamins K1 and K2; vitamin K3 is a synthetic form.[60] Maintaining adequate vitamin K levels is crucial for bone mineralization, blood clotting, cell growth, and blood vessel health.[60] Vitamin K1 (phylloquinone) has anti-inflammatory effects, while synthetic vitamin K3 does not.[61]

## N-Acetylcysteine

N-acetylcysteine (NAC) is a well-known antioxidant that also helps regulate production of inflammatory cytokines. In one study, NAC modulated IL-6 production through an NF-κB mechanism.[35]

## Plant Extracts

A number of plant extracts have also been shown to decrease NF-κB, including stinging nettle extract[62]; helenalin from arnica flowers[63]; a spiroketal compound found in chamomile and *Plagius flosculosus*[64]; oleandrin from oleander[65]; resveratrol from grapes and other fruits[66]; 1'-acetoxychavicol acetate (ACA) from *Languas galanga*[67]; curcumin[68]; ergolide from *Inula britannica*[69]; rocaglamides extracted from *Aglaia*[70]; and tetrandrine from han-fang chi, a Chinese herb used to treat rheumatic disorders.[71]

## Fish Oils

The inclusion of omega-3 fish oils in the diet has shown to help with autoimmune and inflammatory diseases[72–74] by suppressing synthesis of TNF-α.[75] Vitamin E and fish oil in mice have decreased proinflammatory cytokines, including IL-6 and TNF-α.[76] Omega-3 fish oils have been useful in patients with a variety of inflammatory diseases, including rheumatoid arthritis and atherosclerosis.[73] Studies in humans with rheumatoid arthritis suggest fish oil and vitamin E decrease inflammation.[77] Moreover, fish oil supplementation has shown anti-inflammatory effects (resulting in decreased use of anti-inflammatory drugs) for patients with a variety of other chronic inflammatory diseases.[74]

## Vitamins C and E

Vitamin E is an antioxidant with anti-inflammatory actions. The alpha-tocopherol form of vitamin E can decrease inflammation that contributes to atherosclerosis. Alpha-tocopherol supplementation has been shown to decrease C-reactive protein levels.[78] Vitamin C is an antioxidant[79] that also has anti-inflammatory properties and blocks NF-κB activation by TNF-α.[80]

## Methylsulfonylmethane

Sulfur is a mineral found in several amino acids, the building blocks of all proteins in the body. Methylsulfonylmethane (MSM), a natural metabolite of dimethyl sulfoxide,[81] is used as a dietary supplement by many people. MSM is naturally found in fruits, vegetables, grains, and animals (cow's milk is a rich source).[81,82] MSM has been studied in patients with a variety of conditions, including arthritis, allergies, and fibromyalgia, among others. MSM appears to have little or no toxicity.[83]

Studies have shown that MSM can decrease pain and increase mobility in patients with osteoarthritis.[84]

## Curcumin and Ginger

Curcumin, a well-known antioxidant and anti-inflammatory, has been shown to reduce NF-κB in a wide variety of conditions, including autoimmune diseases and cancer.[85] Ginger has also been documented to reduce multiple inflammatory chemicals, including NF-κB and many others, and to be effective against a variety of inflammatory diseases, including autoimmune diseases characterized by an elevation of NF-κB.[86]

## Life Extension Suggestions

- **Omega-3 fatty acids:** 1000 mg docosahexaenoic acid (DHA) and 1400 mg eicosapentaenoic acid (EPA) daily
- **DHEA:** 15–75 mg daily to start, followed by blood testing in 3–6 weeks to ensure adequate levels
- **Arginine:** 1800 mg daily
- **Glutamine:** 1000–2500 mg daily
- **NAC:** 500–1500 mg daily
- **Vitamin E:** 400 IU daily (with 200 mg gamma tocopherol)
- **Vitamin C:** 1–3 g daily with food
- **MSM:** 1000 mg daily
- **Curcumin:** 900–1800 mg daily
- **Ginger extract:** 500–1000 mg daily
- **Topical analgesic cream:** apply to sore muscles as needed

For individuals taking corticosteroids, Life Extension suggests the following nutrients to support bone health:

- **Calcium:** 700–1200 mg daily
- **Vitamin D:** 5000–8000 IU daily; depending upon blood levels of 25-OH-vitmin D
- **Vitamin K:** 2200 mcg as 1000 mcg K1 and 1200 mcg K2 (as MK-4 and MK-7)

In addition, the following *blood testing* resources may be helpful:

- ESR (Sedimentation Rate)
- Chemistry panel and complete blood count (CBC)
- C-reactive protein (CRP)
- Interleukin 6 (IL6)

## REFERENCES

References available at: www.lef.org/dpt5/ch110

# 111

---

# *Premenstrual Syndrome*

---

Premenstrual syndrome (PMS) and related menstrual disorders are common sources of misery among menstruating women. Symptoms range from mild to severe, interfering with family activities, social activities, and work.[1]

Identifying PMS can sometimes be difficult because it covers such a wide range of symptoms. It is estimated to affect up to 50% of menstruating women, with symptoms sometimes beginning among young women aged 16–18 years, and peaking in their 20s and 30s.[2] Symptoms of PMS tend to decrease with age[3] and cease with menopause. Women who continue to experience PMS symptoms at an older age are more likely to experience menopausal symptoms.[3]

PMS can affect a number of systems and produce a wide variety of symptoms including:

- **Psychological symptoms.** Tension, depression, irritability, fatigue, panic, phobia
- **Nervous system symptoms.** Migraine, seizures, headache, dizziness, fainting
- **Symptoms affecting the skin.** Acne, boils, hives
- **Symptoms affecting the muscles and joints.** Backache, joint pain, edema
- **Respiratory symptoms.** Asthma, allergies[4]
- **Symptoms affecting the head and neck.** Sinusitis, sore throat, hoarseness
- **Urinary symptoms.** Bladder infections
- **Gastrointestinal symptoms.** Bloating, gas, food cravings
- **Symptoms affecting the breast.** Tenderness, swelling

Premenstrual dysphoric disorder (PMDD), a more severe form of PMS, occurs in 2–9% of menstruating women. Although symptoms of PMDD and PMS are similar, they are much more severe in PMDD. In fact, PMDD is characterized by symptoms severe enough to interfere with personal relationships, especially in the marital and family area.[3]

Traditional medicine is not well equipped to treat PMS. There are no unique physical findings or lab tests to diagnose PMS, and few drugs that achieve consistent results without side effects. If symptoms are mild, most women are told to use over-the-counter (OTC) painkillers (usually containing ibuprofen) and make dietary and lifestyle changes. In more serious cases, including PMDD, antidepressants are sometimes prescribed.

Hormone-based birth control pills are also frequently recommended to produce a state of anovulation (lack of ovulation). In the past, studies concerning their effectiveness have shown mixed results. However, a new form of synthetic progesterone (progestin) has shown some benefit(s). Life Extension recommends that women take natural progesterone or phytoestrogens derived from plants rather than synthetic progestin or estrogen.

Life Extension has uncovered a number of nutrients that address underlying deficiencies associated with PMS and excess levels of prostaglandins, which have been linked to symptoms of PMS. Chief among the alternative therapies for PMS is calcium, which has been used for more than 70 years in the treatment of menstrual disorders. Other therapies include magnesium, vitamin E, vitamin B6, and extract from fruit of the chaste tree.

## THE MENSTRUAL CYCLE, HORMONES, AND PMS

A normal menstrual cycle is characterized by the regular rise and fall of sex hormones, most importantly estrogen and progesterone, culminating in menstruation. The cycle is usually divided into the following 4 phases:

- **Follicular phase.** During this phase, a rise in follicle stimulating hormone (FSH) causes several follicles (each containing an egg) to begin growing on the surface of the ovary. Under the influence of the pituitary luteinizing hormone, these follicles secrete estradiol, a form of estrogen. This estrogen discourages production of FSH by a negative feedback mechanism, causing a slowdown in growth of the follicles. The estrogen also encourages endometrial (uterine lining) tissue to build up in preparation for a fertilized egg. Eventually, one follicle emerges as the dominant one.
- **Ovulation.** In this phase, the dominant follicle bursts, releasing an egg into the fallopian tube. This phase is caused by a boost in the production of luteinizing hormone. Ovulation usually occurs around day 14 of the cycle, but the timing varies from woman to woman. Once the egg is in the fallopian tube, it is available for fertilization.
- **Luteal phase.** After the egg has been released, the remaining follicle tissue is known as the corpus

luteum. During the next 2 weeks of the menstrual cycle, the corpus luteum secretes an increasing amount of progesterone to prepare the body for early pregnancy and reception of a fertilized egg. If the egg is not fertilized, progesterone levels decline.

- **Menstruation.** Menstruation is characterized by low levels of progesterone and estrogen. It occurs when the egg has not been fertilized. In this phase, the built-up portion of the uterine wall sloughs off and passes through the vagina as blood, mucus, and tissue remnants. This sloughing off is caused by contraction of the arterioles that supply the thickened endometrium with blood, as well as the contraction of endometrium smooth muscular wall. These muscular contractions cause cramping and are under the control of cyclooxygenase (COX) enzymes. COX enzymes are nonselectively inhibited by OTC nonsteroidal anti-inflammatory drugs (NSAIDs).

Among women with PMS, some form of hormonal dysfunction occurs during the luteal phase. However, PMS is still not well understood, and many theories have been proposed to explain the underlying symptoms. Until the clinical diagnosis of PMS was established, there was significant disagreement as to whether it was a legitimate medical condition.

A number of novel theories have been put forward to help explain PMS. There is evidence that in severe cases, symptoms associated with severe menstrual disorders are caused by a derangement of serotonin, an important neurotransmitter that regulates mood and behavior.[5]

Evidence also suggests decreased sensitivity of brain gamma-aminobutyric acid (GABA)-alpha receptors, increased sensitivity of brain motor cells, and disturbances of the hypothalamic-pituitary-adrenal axis, which controls stress hormone levels.[6-8] GABA-alpha is an inhibitory neurotransmitter associated with relaxation and a decrease in anxiety.

Together, these effects might account for some of the mood and motor problems commonly seen in PMS. There is also evidence that PMS runs in families, and women with PMS also tend to have a personal or family history of alcohol abuse and mood-related psychiatric disorders.[9] Also, women with a history of sexual abuse were found to be more likely to suffer from severe PMS. Studies have shown that up to 95% of women who experienced sexual abuse, often at early ages, were likely to suffer from PMS.[10]

Finally, prostaglandins (hormone-like chemicals that control various bodily functions) may play a role in PMS. Prostaglandins are known to promote smooth muscle contraction and blood vessel dilation, both of which are essential to the normal menstrual cycle. Studies have shown that prostaglandin excretion is disordered in women with PMS compared with women without PMS.[11] Prostaglandin production appears to be significantly lower in the late luteal phase of women with PMS compared with controls, based on a study of 20 women with PMS and 12 controls, while prostaglandin production is much higher in the follicular phase and early luteal phase.[12]

## Hormone Modulation and Menstrual Syndromes

The influence of hormones on PMS and menstrual syndromes has been studied extensively, often with conflicting results. Women typically suffer from PMS during the luteal phase of their menstrual cycle, which is characterized by increasing levels of progesterone and fluctuating levels of other steroid hormones. Hoping to unravel the connection between hormones and premenstrual symptoms, researchers have studied women with PMS to see whether they have abnormal levels of various hormones compared to women without PMS. In one study, researchers found that 20 women with PMS had higher levels of dehydroepiandrosterone (DHEA) and free testosterone during the luteal phase of menstruation, along with reduced levels of allopregnanolone, than did 20 controls.[13] Allopregnanolone is a metabolite of progesterone and an active neurosteroid shown to affect mood and behavior.

Using conventional estrogen-progestin (synthetic progesterone) contraceptives, many studies have examined the role of hormone therapy to control symptoms associated with PMS. These hormone preparations are used to induce a state of anovulation (no ovulation), which allows women to bypass hormonal fluctuations that occur during ovulation and thus, the accompanying symptoms.[14] Unfortunately, evidence of their effectiveness is mixed.

Some women attempt to control their symptoms with progestins, or synthetic progesterone. These drugs have consistently failed to show good results. However, a progestin called drospirenone has been introduced for the treatment of PMS. Drospirenone is derived from a source (17-alpha spironolactone) different from the progestins typically used in oral contraception. It has antimineralocorticoid activity, and thus is not associated with weight gain and fluid retention, unlike some other hormone preparations.

When it comes to hormone modulation to control symptoms of PMS, Life Extension advocates a more natural approach than can be achieved with synthetic estrogens and progestins. Natural, safe progesterones derived from yams can be used in place of progestins. In addition, phytoestrogens, or estrogen-like compounds derived from plants, have shown some efficacy in relieving PMS symptoms. In one double-blind, placebo-controlled, randomized study, phytoestrogens derived from soy were examined for their ability to reduce symptoms of PMS. After 2 months, volunteers experienced reduced headache, breast tenderness, cramps, and swelling during periods when taking soy products compared to placebo.[15]

The hormone melatonin, which is usually associated with sleep and insomnia, may also play a role in alleviating symptoms of PMS and PMDD. Melatonin, involved in a variety of mood and anxiety disorders, is intimately related to sex hormones and other hypothalamic-pituitary-adrenal-axis hormones. Studies have shown that melatonin levels are low among women with PMDD.[16]

# CONVENTIONAL TREATMENT

Conventional treatment for mild PMS usually focuses on NSAIDs, which reduce smooth muscle contractions and cramping. In addition, some of the drugs that have shown benefit, such as benzodiazepines, have risk for addiction and abuse.

## Antidepressants

Antidepressants (eg, selective serotonin reuptake inhibitors [SSRIs]) are commonly used for depression associated with PMS and PMDD.[3,17] Serotonin reuptake inhibitors that are commonly used to treat PMS include Prozac® (fluoxetine) and Zoloft® (sertraline).[9] These drugs typically require a 2–3-week phase-in period before reaching maximum effectiveness. They should be used continuously until both patient and physician agree to stop using them, and then they should be phased out gradually. They cannot be used on an "as needed" basis. Side effects associated with SSRIs include nausea, diarrhea, tremor, weight loss, and headache.

## Benzodiazepines

This class of medications is used to induce sedative, muscle-relaxant, and anticonvulsant effects.[17] Benzodiazepines have effects similar to allopregnanolone, a metabolite of progesterone that acts at the brain receptor sites where benzodiazepines operate. Xanax® (alprazolam) is a commonly prescribed benzodiazepine. However, these drugs have a serious risk of addiction and abuse.

## Nonsteroidal Anti-Inflammatory Drugs (NSAIDs)

Over-the-counter NSAIDs such as ibuprofen (Motrin®) and naproxen sodium (Aleve®) are commonly used to ease uterine cramping and breast tenderness.[14] These drugs inhibit prostaglandin synthesis.[18]

## Bromocriptine

Bromocriptine, an ergot alkaloid that blocks the release of prolactin from the pituitary gland, is often given to treat breast tenderness associated with PMS.[19]

# LIFESTYLE CHANGES TO REDUCE PMS SYMPTOMS

## Stress Reduction

Stress reduction is important to reduce symptoms of PMS and PMDD. One study determined that women with significant PMS symptoms had more stress and a poorer quality of life than women with low-grade or no PMS symptoms.[20] Stress has an effect on the hypothalamic-pituitary-adrenal axis by causing an increase in "stress" hormones with wide-ranging effects throughout the body.[21]

Women who suffer from more severe PMS may benefit from psychotherapy, massage therapy, yoga, and other alternative methods to reduce stress.

## Smoking Cessation

In a study of behavior and lifestyle factors associated with menstrual symptoms, researchers found that cigarette smoking was the lifestyle factor most highly associated with all types of measured menstrual symptoms and cycle disorders.[22] Many strategies are available to aid in smoking cessation, including group therapy, nicotine replacement patches or gums, hypnotism, and support lines.

## Exercise

Exercise seems to help reduce PMS symptoms. Both aerobic and other forms of exercise appear to be helpful.[23] Exercise also helps with weight reduction. Although obesity is not consistently associated with menstrual symptoms, endometrial hyperplasia and other gynecologic disorders are linked to overweight and obesity. Women who suffer from PMS and other menstrual disorders and who are overweight should seriously consider a weight reduction program. Mineral supplementation with chromium picolinate, which helps stabilize blood sugar levels, has been shown to help women who suffer from PMS reduce sugar cravings. Chromium picolinate has also been found to help with weight reduction.[24] For more information, see Life Extension's Obesity and Weight Loss protocol.

# NUTRITIONAL THERAPY

## Calcium and Vitamin D

Calcium has a long history in the treatment of PMS and menstrual disorders.[25] In fact, its use in symptom relief stretches back to the 1930s, when women suffering menstrual cycle problems routinely took supplemental calcium. Since then, this "folk" remedy has been tested in clinical trials with positive results.

In a study, calcium supplementation was found to be a simple and effective treatment for PMS.[26] After supplementing with calcium for 3 consecutive menstrual cycles, healthy menstruating women reported a 48% reduction in total PMS-related symptoms compared with menstruating women receiving placebo.[26]

A review study found that women receiving calcium coupled with vitamin D experienced significant relief from psychological and physical symptoms of PMS. This review confirmed that PMS represents a clinical manifestation of calcium deficiency.[27,28]

## Magnesium

Among its many functions, magnesium plays a role in maintaining parathyroid function and hormone production.[29] Magnesium deficiency has been implicated as a cause of premenstrual symptoms.[30]

A double-blind, randomized study investigated the effects of oral magnesium on premenstrual symptoms. This study noted significant changes on the Menstrual Distress Questionnaire (a measurement of menstrual distress) in women who had taken magnesium for 2 menstrual cycles.[31]

## Zinc

Researchers found that women with PMS had lower levels of zinc and higher levels of copper during the luteal phase of menstruation than menstruating women without PMS. They concluded that zinc deficiency occurs in women with PMS during the luteal phase of menstruation, and elevated copper further reduces their availability of zinc during the luteal phase.[32]

## Vitamin B6 (Pyridoxine, Pyridoxal, Pyridoxamine)

A meta-analysis was performed to evaluate the efficacy of vitamin B6. Researchers reviewed 9 placebo-controlled, published trials representing 940 women with PMS. Their conclusions showed that up to 100 mg of vitamin B6 daily is likely to be beneficial in treating premenstrual symptoms and premenstrual depression.[33]

In 1987, researchers conducted a double-blind controlled study on the effects of vitamin B6 supplementation on premenstrual symptoms experienced by 55 women who reported moderate to severe premenstrual mood changes. Study results suggested that vitamin B6 improved premenstrual symptoms related to autonomic reactions (eg, dizziness and vomiting) and behavioral changes (eg, poor performance and decreased social activities).[34]

## Vitex

Extracts of the fruits of the chaste tree (*Vitex agnus castus*) are widely used to treat premenstrual symptoms. Double-blind, placebo-controlled studies indicate that breast tenderness (one of the most common premenstrual symptoms) is beneficially influenced by this extract, also called chasteberry. In addition, numerous studies indicate that vitex extracts have beneficial effects on other psychic and somatic symptoms of PMS.[35]

A group of German researchers studied the effects of chaste tree extract versus placebo in a group of women diagnosed with PMS. Both prior to and after the treatment period, women were asked to report their symptoms of PMS and the degree of severity. Researchers evaluated the changes in reported symptoms. More than 50% of the women experienced a reduction in PMS-related symptoms. The results of this study prompted the German government to allow Vitex agnus castus to be approved for menstrual irregularities, breast pain, and premenstrual complaints.[36]

In a study comparing the efficacy of chasteberry extract with that of fluoxetine (a SSRI) on mood disorders associated with PMDD, patients responded well to both fluoxetine and chasteberry extract. However, chasteberry proved better than fluoxetine at improving physical symptoms.[37]

Researchers investigated the efficacy of using chasteberry extract to reduce breast pain related to PMS. In a placebo-controlled, randomized study, chasteberry extract was effective and well tolerated as a treatment for cyclical breast pain.[38]

## Ginkgo Biloba

In a clinical study, Ginkgo biloba was effective at reducing symptoms of anxiety and headaches. A total of 165 women aged 18–45 years were given 160 mg ginkgo extract or placebo daily from day 16 of one menstrual cycle to day 5 of the next. Symptoms of fluid retention, particularly breast tenderness, were improved, as were psychological parameters.[39]

## Vitamin E

Vitamin E is a powerful antioxidant and free radical scavenger that protects the integrity of the cellular membranes in the body. Researchers investigated the impact of D-alpha-tocopherol, a form of vitamin E, on women suffering from PMS. A daily treatment with 400 IU of D-alpha-tocopherol was administered for 3 monthly cycles. A significant improvement in physical symptoms was noted in participants treated with D-alpha-tocopherol.[40]

## Theanine

Theanine, a unique amino acid in tea, can lessen the effects of PMS. Theanine readily crosses the blood–brain barrier and exerts subtle changes in biochemistry. An increase in alpha waves has been documented, and the effect has been compared to getting a massage or taking a hot bath. Theanine does not cause drowsiness, and unlike tranquilizers, it does not interfere with the ability to think. Studies of green tea, which contains a high quantity of theanine, have shown that when given to rats, theanine modulated the release of dopamine in the brain.[41] Theanine is now available as a dietary supplement in the United States.

## Omega-3 Fatty Acids

Fatty acids play a role in mediating prostaglandins.[42] Supplementation with the right proportions of fatty acids can maximize the production of anti-inflammatory prostaglandins (E1 and E3) while suppressing proinflammatory prostaglandin (E2 and leukotriene B4). In addition to avoiding saturated fats and high glycemic foods that contribute to chronic inflammation, eating omega-3–rich foods, which provide eicosapentaenoic acid (EPA) and docosahexaenoic acid (DHA), can help control inflammation by bringing balance to essential fatty acids. In clinical studies, supplementation with omega-3 fatty acids reduced symptoms associated with PMS, including cramps.[43,44] Flax seed oil, which is derived from flax, is rich in alpha-linolenic acid. In the body, alpha-linolenic acid is converted into EPA, providing another possible source of EPA.

## Gamma-Linoleic Acid

Gamma-linoleic acid (GLA) is a long-chain polyunsaturated fatty acid found in evening primrose oil and borage seed oil. Like omega-3 fatty acids, levels of GLA are abnormal among women with PMS. For example,

one study found that levels of linoleic acid are normal or elevated in women with PMS, but levels of gamma-linoleic acid, a metabolite of linoleic acid, are low. This implies a problem with the conversion of linoleic acid to GLA.[45]

## Natural Methods to Modulate Serotonin

Among women with severe PMS, prescription antidepressants (SSRIs) are frequently prescribed. These medications inhibit the uptake of serotonin, thus making more of it available. Serotonin is an important neurotransmitter involved in the regulation of mood.

**Tryptophan.** Tryptophan, a precursor of serotonin, is sometimes used by alternative physicians to treat depression by increasing the amount of serotonin. It has been shown to significantly reduce PMS symptoms if administered during the luteal phase.[3]

**5-hydroxytryptophan.** 5-hydroxytryptophan (5-HTP), the direct precursor to serotonin, may help relieve symptoms by increasing the serotonin production. It is the intermediate step between tryptophan and serotonin. Although 5-HTP has not been studied in PMS, it has been studied in the treatment of depression.[46]

**St. John's wort.** The herb St. John's wort is sometimes recommended for PMS. St. John's wort (*Hypericum perforatum*) has gained attention as a natural antidepressant due to its role in serotonin modulation. It appears to work by multiple mechanisms, each of which is relatively weak on its own but contributes to the herb's overall effectiveness. These mechanisms include inhibiting monoamine oxidase-A and -B activity and inhibiting the uptake of serotonin, dopamine, and noradrenaline.[47] In one case study, a patient with PMDD who was unable to tolerate standard antidepressant treatment was given 900 mg of St. John's wort daily; she experienced substantial improvement in her symptoms.[48] Another observational study examined the use of St. John's wort among women with PMS. Participants took 300 mg of St. John's wort daily (standardized to contain 900 mcg of hypericin) for one menstrual cycle. The women experienced improvements in all symptom scores.[49]

## Life Extension Suggestions

Women who suffer from PMS are encouraged to reduce stress if possible. Methods might include massage or cutting back on activities whenever PMS arises. Daily exercise and weight loss (if necessary) might also help. In addition, the following supplements are suggested for women suffering from PMS:

- **Magnesium:** 160 mg of magnesium (as magnesium citrate) 2 times daily. The last dose should be taken at bedtime.
- **Calcium:** 700–1200 mg daily
- **Vitamin D:** 2000–8000 IU daily; individualize dosing based on results of vitamin D testing
- **Zinc:** 30 mg daily
- **Vitamin E:** 400 IU daily, including at least 200 mg gamma tocopherols
- **Progesterone cream:** 20–30 mg twice daily, starting on day 12 of the menstrual cycle and continuing up to day 28
- **Melatonin:** 300 mcg nightly is suggested, increasing to 10 mg if necessary
- **Soy isoflavones:** 135 mg once to twice daily, standardized to contain 40% isoflavones, including genistein, daidzein, and glycitein
- **GLA:** 299–598 mg daily
- **EPA/DHA:** 1400 mg EPA and 1000 mg DHA daily

- **Vitex berry extract:** 500–1000 mg full-spectrum extract, each dose standardized to 625 mcg agnusides
- **Ginkgo biloba extract:** 120 mg daily standardized to 28% ginkgo flavone glycosides, 7% terpene lactones, and <1 ppm ginkgolic acid
- **Theanine:** 100–400 mg daily
- **Tryptophan:** 500–1500 mg daily on an empty stomach
- **St. John's wort:** 300–600 mg, each dose standardized to 0.3% hypericin

In addition, the following *blood testing* resources may be helpful:

- Female Comprehensive Hormone Panel or Female Basic Hormone Panel

## REFERENCES

References available at: www.lef.org/dpt5/ch111

# 112

---

# Prevention Protocols

---

It used to be thought that little could be done to postpone what nature has in store for us. Today, a growing scientific consensus indicates that individuals possess a great deal of control over how long they are going to live and what their state of health will be.

Mainstream medicine has relied on simple measures of preventing disease, such as controlling hypertension, yet many doctors are coming to the realization that additional steps can be taken to protect against premature aging and death.

In fact, the results of tens of thousands of scientific studies make it abundantly clear that following the proper lifestyle can add a significant number of healthy years to the average person's life span.

The premise of taking action to maintain youthful health and vigor is based on findings from peer-reviewed scientific studies that identify specific factors that cause us to develop degenerative disease. These studies suggest that the consumption of certain foods, food extracts, hormones, or drugs will help prevent common diseases associated with normal aging.

Therefore, the concept of disease prevention can be defined as the incorporation of findings from published scientific studies into a logical daily regimen that enables an individual to attain optimal health and longevity.

Taking aggressive steps to extend one's life span is a major commitment. This Prevention protocol provides practical information about what a person can do to take advantage of the consensus of scientific knowledge obtained from the most prestigious medical journals in the world.

## THE BASIS FOR DETERMINING WHAT WORKS

People seeking to reduce their risk of disease are often overwhelmed by the volume of technical data on the subject. For the past 33 years, Life Extension has meticulously reviewed the published medical literature dating as far back as 1917; Life Extension personnel have dedicated the past 35 years to working with physicians and scientists to develop validated methods of preventing age-related disease.

Each year, Life Extension spends millions of dollars on research projects aimed at extending the healthy human life span. Since 1983, Life Extension has reviewed thousands of blood test results of members who have been following antiaging supplement, drug, and hormone-replacement programs.

Based on this vast accumulation of data, Life Extension has designed a practical disease prevention protocol that is based solely on scientific principles.

Before embarking on a program to reduce the risk of degenerative disease, it is important to know about scientific studies conducted on humans that show these therapies really work. If unaware of these published studies, you may be unlikely to methodically follow a long-term disease prevention program.

## CONVENTIONAL MEDICINE RECOMMENDS VITAMIN SUPPLEMENTS

For the greater part of the 20th century, mainstream medicine was openly hostile to the idea of healthy people taking vitamin supplements. This antivitamin position began to change in the 1990s as irrefutable evidence emerged that supplements could reduce the risk of age-related disease without inducing toxicity.

In 1998, an editorial titled "Eat Right and Take a Multi-Vitamin" was published in the *New England Journal of Medicine*. This article was based on studies indicating that certain supplements could reduce homocysteine serum levels and therefore lower heart attack and stroke risk. This was the first time this prestigious medical journal recommended vitamin supplements.[1]

An even stronger endorsement for the use of vitamin supplements was in a 2002 issue of the *Journal of the American Medical Association* (JAMA). According to the Harvard University doctors who wrote the JAMA guidelines, it appeared that people who got enough vitamins may be able to prevent such common illnesses as cancer, heart disease, and osteoporosis. The Harvard researchers concluded that suboptimal levels of folic acid and vitamins B6 and B12 are a risk factor for heart disease, colon and breast cancers; low levels of vitamin D contribute to osteoporosis; and inadequate levels of the antioxidant vitamins A, E, and C may increase the risk of cancer and heart disease.[2]

### The FDA's Suppression of Folic Acid

The Food and Drug Administration (FDA) has spent enormous resources trying to prevent people from supplementing with folic acid. The FDA argues against folic acid supplementation because the presence of folic acid in blood could mask a serious vitamin B12 deficiency. In a *JAMA* study, the authors addressed the FDA's concerns by recommending that folic acid supplements be fortified with vitamin B12 as a prudent way of gaining the cardiovascular benefits of folic acid without risking a B12 deficiency.[3]

Even though major medical journals (eg, *New England Journal of Medicine*) long ago endorsed the use of folic acid to reduce cardiovascular disease,[4] the FDA still does not accept that folic acid has any benefit other than preventing a certain type of birth defect.

A study in the *Annals of Internal Medicine* showed how fatally flawed the position of the FDA is. Data from the famous Harvard Nurses' Health Study conducted at the Harvard Medical School showed that long-term supplementation with folic acid reduces the risk of colon cancer by an astounding 75% in women. The fact that 90 000 women participated in the Harvard Nurses' Health Study made this finding especially significant. The authors of this study explained that folic acid obtained from supplements had a stronger protective effect against colon cancer than folic acid consumed in the diet. This new study helps confirm the work of Bruce Ames, the famous molecular biologist who authored numerous articles showing that folic acid is extremely effective in preventing initial DNA mutations that can lead to cancer later in life. This Harvard report, showing a 75% reduction in colon cancer incidence, demonstrated that the degree of protection against cancer is correlated with how long a DNA-protecting substance (folic acid) is consumed. Women who took more than 400 mcg of folic acid daily for 15 years experienced the 75% reduction in colon cancer, whereas short-term supplementation with folic acid produced only marginal protection.[5]

There now exists a massive body of evidence that supplementation with folic acid can prevent both cardiovascular disease and cancer, yet the FDA has proposed rules that would prohibit the American public from even learning about these benefits. Colon cancer will kill 47 000 Americans this year. It is unfortunate that the FDA did not "allow" these colon cancer victims to learn about folic acid in time.

## The Vitamin C Controversy

Some doctors still believe that vitamin C causes kidney stones; however, a report from Harvard Medical School showed no increased risk of kidney stones when evaluating 85 557 women over a 14-year study period. This report in the April 1999 issue of the *Journal of the American Society of Nephrology* showed that women who consumed 1500 mg or more daily of vitamin C were no more likely to develop kidney stones than women who consumed less than 250 mg of vitamin C

daily. The study did reveal that women who consumed 40 mg or more of vitamin B6 were 34% less likely to develop kidney stones compared to women taking fewer than 3 mg per day of B6.[6] Now that kidney stone risk has been ruled out, let us look at some of the human studies showing positive benefits to vitamin C supplementation.

In the early 1990s, several large population studies showed a reduction in cardiovascular disease in those who consumed vitamin C. The media reported on some of these findings and this favorable publicity helped push a bill through Congress that prevented the FDA from banning high-potency vitamin C and other supplements.

The most significant report emanated in 1992 from the University of California in Los Angeles (UCLA), where it was announced that men who took 800 mg per day of vitamin C lived 6 years longer than those who consumed the FDA's recommended daily allowance (RDA) of 60 mg daily. The study, which evaluated 11 348 participants over 10 years, showed that high vitamin C intake extended average life span and reduced mortality from cardiovascular disease by 42%.[7]

A study in the *British Medical Journal* evaluated 1605 randomly selected men in Finland ages 42–60 years in 1984–1989. None of these men had evidence of preexisting heart disease. After adjusting for other confounding factors, men who were deficient in vitamin C had 3.5 times more heart attacks than men who were not deficient in vitamin C. Scientists concluded that "vitamin C deficiency, as assessed by low plasma ascorbate concentration, is a risk factor for coronary heart disease."[8]

In a study in the *Lancet*, researchers at Cambridge University in England looked at serum vitamin C and length of life in 19 000 individuals. People with the lowest levels of vitamin C were twice as likely to die when compared to those with the highest serum vitamin C levels.[9] The question for those who want to achieve maximum health is: Do you want your blood to contain the lowest levels or the highest levels of vitamin C? Because being at the lowest level may double the risk of dying, we suggest you consume fruits, vegetables, and supplements that are high in vitamin C.

In a 1999 issue of the American Heart Association's journal *Circulation*, elevated homocysteine levels were shown to cause rapid onset of endothelial (arterial lining) dysfunction.[10] This type of dysfunction reduces blood flow and can facilitate a lethal arterial spasm. Vitamin C inhibited arterial dysfunction by interfering with oxidative stress mechanisms. The doctors conducting the study stated that acute impairment of vascular endothelial function can be prevented by pretreatment with vitamin C.

In a double-blind study in the *Journal of the American College of Cardiology*, the authors compared the effects of nitrate drugs in people receiving vitamin C to a placebo group not receiving vitamin C. The doctors administered nitrate drugs to healthy people and patients with coronary artery disease and then measured vasodilation response and cellular levels of cyclic guanosine monophosphate (cGMP), an energy substrate that is depleted by nitrate drugs. At day 0, all participants were measured to establish a baseline. After 3 days of vitamin C administration (2 g, 3 times daily), there was no change in either group. After 6 days of vitamin C therapy, a 42% improvement in vasodilation response was observed, and a 60% improvement in cellular cGMP levels was measured in coronary artery disease patients receiving vitamin C compared to those receiving placebo. A similar improvement occurred in the healthy subjects taking vitamin C compared to the placebo group. Doctors concluded the study by stating that "these results indicate that combination therapy with vitamin C is potentially useful for preventing the development of nitrate tolerance."[11]

In another study in the *Journal of Clinical Investigation*, the authors looked at the effects of nitrate drug therapy on human patients. Tolerance development was monitored by changes in arterial pressure, pulse pressure, heart rate, and activity of isolated patients. All patients experienced the deleterious effects of nitrate tolerance. However, when vitamin C was co-administered with nitrate drugs, the effects of nitrate tolerance were virtually eliminated. The most significant improvement was a 310% improvement in the arterial conductivity test. The nitrate drugs induced a dangerous upregulated activity of platelets, but this too was reversed with vitamin C supplementation.[12] The researchers indicated that vitamin C may be of benefit during long-term, nonintermittent administration of nitrate drugs in humans.

Chronic heart failure is associated with reduced dilating capacity of the endothelial lining of the arterial system. Scientists tested heart failure patients by high-resolution ultrasound and Doppler to measure radial artery diameter and blood flow. Vitamin C restored arterial dilation response and blood flow velocity in patients with heart failure. Scientists determined that the mechanism of action was that vitamin C increased the availability of nitric oxide, an important precursor to cGMP.[13]

In 1998, another effect of vitamin C on coronary artery disease was discovered. A study in the *Journal of the American College of Cardiology* showed that low plasma ascorbic acid levels independently predict the presence of an unstable coronary syndrome in heart disease patients. According to the doctors, study results showed that the beneficial effects of vitamin C in treating coronary artery disease may result, in part, by an influence on arterial wall lesion activity rather than a reduction in the overall extent of fixed disease.[14]

Published research findings suggest that vitamin C may reduce mortality in coronary artery disease patients, increase life span, and possibly eliminate the effects of nitrate tolerance in those taking nitrate drugs. Although not recognized in the medical establishment as a therapy for coronary artery disease, there now exists an accumulated wealth of evidence that vitamin C has beneficial effects in the treatment of heart-related illnesses.

Historically, mainstream medicine has ridiculed vitamin C supplementation. Today, conventional medicine says that only 200 mg per day of vitamin C is needed, despite findings showing that high doses of vitamin C are required to produce optimal benefit. Meanwhile, the FDA continues to hold the position that no more than 90 mg daily for men and 75 mg daily for women of vitamin C is needed.

## Saturating the Bladder

The most frequent criticism regarding supplemental vitamin intake is that it produces "expensive urine," because water-soluble vitamins, such as vitamin C and the B vitamins, are excreted into the bladder within hours of ingestion. For years, Life Extension has contended that these vitamins are beneficial in spite of their rapid excretion; moreover, it is desirable to have a bladder full of vitamins because certain vitamins inhibit chemicals that cause bladder cancer. In the September 1996 issue of the *American Journal of Epidemiology*, a study on the risk of bladder cancer in vitamin takers showed the following[15]:

- High intake of vitamin A and beta-carotene was associated with a 48% reduction in bladder cancer incidence compared to the lowest levels of vitamin A and beta-carotene intake.

- People taking higher amounts of vitamin C had a 50% reduced rate of bladder cancer. Those who took 502 mg or more of vitamin C daily had a 60% reduction in bladder cancer compared to those who took no vitamin C.

- For those who took multivitamin supplements for at least 10 years, the reduction in bladder cancer was 61% compared to people who took no vitamin supplements.

- High intake of fried foods was associated with double the risk of bladder cancer.

It appears from this study that even low-potency "one-a-day" supplements (which do not protect against other types of cancer) can at least protect against bladder cancer.

## Protecting Vision

Studies show that antioxidant supplements reduce the risk of cataracts. One study in the *American Journal of Epidemiology* evaluated 410 men for 3 years to ascertain the association between serum vitamin E and the development of cortical lens opacities (cataracts). Men with the lowest level of serum vitamin E had a 3.7 times greater risk of this form of cataract compared to men with the highest serum level of vitamin E.[16]

Although cataracts are usually treatable, a disease called wet macular degeneration is not. Those who eat spinach and collard greens have low rates of macular degeneration, and extracts from these vegetables thought to protect against this blinding disease are now available in dietary supplements that contain lutein and zeaxanthin.

## Keeping Arteries Clean

In a study reported in the *American Journal of Clinical Nutrition*, antioxidant status was assessed and carotid artery occlusion was measured in 1187 men and women 59–71 years of age without any history of coronary artery disease or stroke. The results showed that the higher the level of vitamin E in red blood cells, the lower the risk of carotid atherosclerosis. In men with the highest levels of carotid atherosclerotic plaques, the lowest levels of vitamin E, selenium, and carotenoids were found. Scientists concluded by stating: "Our findings give some epidemiologic support to the hypothesis that lipid peroxidation and low antioxidant status are involved in the early stages of atherosclerosis."[17]

A study in the journal *Atherosclerosis* showed that people who took a 900-mg garlic supplement daily for 4 years had 5–18% less plaque build-up in their carotid arteries compared to the placebo group. The women in the treatment group showed a 4.6% decrease in carotid plaque volume over a 4-year period, whereas the placebo group showed a 5.3% increase in artery-clogging plaque.[18]

There are more studies showing that atherosclerosis can be prevented than for any other degenerative disease. Because more people die or become disabled from vascular diseases than any other cause, it would appear prudent to follow a program that would reduce one's risk of suffering a vascular-related heart attack or stroke.

## Are You Concerned about Cancer?

Fear of cancer is a major reason why people take dietary supplements. As has already been shown, there is a compelling body of evidence that cancer risk can

be reduced by taking the proper supplements over an extended period of time.

An article in *JAMA* showed that 200 mcg of supplemental selenium per day reduced overall cancer mortality by 50% in humans compared to a placebo group not receiving supplemental selenium. This 9-year study demonstrated that a low-cost mineral supplement could cut the risk of dying from cancer in half in certain individuals.[19]

In a 1999 issue of the *Journal of the National Cancer Institute*, associations between intakes of specific nutrients and subsequent breast cancer risk were investigated in 83 234 women participating in the Harvard Nurses' Health Study. Breast cancer risks were significantly lower in women who consumed alpha-carotene, beta-carotene, lutein/zeaxanthin, and vitamins A and C. Among premenopausal women who consumed moderate amounts of alcohol (a known risk factor in breast cancer), beta-carotene lowered risk. Premenopausal women who consumed 5 or more servings of fruits and vegetables daily had a modestly lower risk of breast cancer than those who had less than 2 servings daily.[20]

A study in the March 1999 issue of *Cancer Research* reported that the tomato extract lycopene was the most effective nutrient shown to protect against the development of prostate cancer. This study, started in 1982, followed 578 men for 13 years. Lycopene strongly reduced prostate cancer risk and more importantly, lowered the risk for aggressive cancer. This study confirmed many previous studies showing that lycopene can help prevent pancreatic, prostate, and a host of other cancers.[21] A surprising finding revealed at the April 1999 meeting of the American Association of Cancer Research showed that 30 mg of lycopene supplements daily slowed the growth of existing prostate cancer and lowered serum prostate-specific antigen (PSA) readings by 20%.

Men with high intake of vitamin E were 35% as likely to develop colorectal adenomas as men with low vitamin E intake.[22] Adenomas are neoplastic lesions that are considered precursors to colon cancer. In a related study in the February 1999 issue of *Diseases of the Colon and Rectum*, the use of multivitamins, vitamin E, and calcium supplements were found to be associated with a lower incidence of recurrent adenomas in 448 patients with previous neoplasia who underwent follow-up colonoscopy. This study found a protective effect against the recurrence of precancerous adenomas when any vitamin supplement was used.[23] On this same subject, a report in the American Journal of Epidemiology showed that women with high folate intake were 40% less likely to develop adenomas of the colon than women with low folate intake.[22]

For those who already have cancer, the research shows a prolongation of life span with proper supplementation.

In a study in *Cancer Letters*, animals with malignant tumors given high doses of vitamins C and E and selenium manifested a significant prolongation of the mean survival time. Complete remission of tumors developed in 16.8% of the animals. Low-dose administration of these vitamins failed to exert any beneficial effect on mean survival time of the animals. Results indicated that high doses (megadoses) of vitamins C and E in combination with other carefully selected antioxidants are likely needed in order to achieve sufficient prevention and treatment of malignant diseases. This study indicated that low-potency supplements are of little value.[24]

In a study in *Cancer Research*, vitamin E succinate was shown to inhibit growth and induce apoptotic cell death of estrogen receptor-negative human breast cancer cells.[25] These findings suggest that vitamin E succinate may be of clinical use in the treatment and possible prevention of human breast cancers.

Research clearly shows the risk of cancer is reduced in those who supplement with adequate amounts of nutrients, such as selenium, folate, carotenoids, vitamins, and other plant extracts.

## Reducing Mortality

One of the most compelling reports that high-potency supplements extend life span in humans was in the August 1996 issue of the *American Journal of Clinical Nutrition*. This study involving 11 178 elderly people attempted to establish the effects of vitamin supplements on mortality. The use of vitamin E reduced the risk of death from all causes by 34%. Effects were strongest for coronary artery disease, where vitamin E resulted in a 63% reduction in death from heart attack. In addition, use of vitamin E resulted in a 59% reduction in cancer mortality. When the effects of vitamins C and E were combined, overall mortality was reduced by 42% (compared to 34% for vitamin E alone).[3] These results provided significant evidence about the value of vitamin supplementation, yet the media failed to report on it. What made this study so credible was that:

- It compared people who took low-potency "one-a-day" multiple vitamins to those who took higher-potency vitamins C and E. Previous studies measuring the life expectancy of the "one-a-day" crowd did not show significant benefits, thereby causing most doctors to conclude there is no value in vitamin supplementation. In this new report, those taking "one-a-day" multivitamins did not do any better than people taking nothing at all, which supports Life Extension's position

that higher doses of antioxidants than those found in conventional supplements are required to reduce the risk of heart disease and cancer.

- It lasted 9 years. Most studies that attempt to evaluate the benefits of vitamin supplementation are for shorter time periods. It should be noted, however, that the famous Harvard Nurses' Health Study found that vitamin E reduced coronary artery disease mortality by more than 40% after only 2 years.

- It included 11 178 people, a larger group than most previous studies.

## Controlling Aging

The National Academy of Sciences published 3 reports showing that the effects of aging may be partially reversible with a combination of acetyl-L-carnitine and lipoic acid.[26] One of these studies showed that supplementation with these two nutrients resulted in a partial reversal of the decline of mitochondrial membrane function while consumption of oxygen significantly increased. This animal study demonstrated that the combination of acetyl-L-carnitine and lipoic acid improved ambulatory activity, with a significantly greater degree of improvement in the old rats compared to the young ones. Human aging is characterized by lethargy, infirmity, and weakness. There is now evidence that supplementation with two over-the-counter supplements can produce a measurable antiaging effect.

The second study published by the National Academy of Sciences showed that supplementation with acetyl-L-carnitine and lipoic acid resulted in improved memory in old rats. Electron microscopic studies in the hippocampus region of the brain showed that acetyl-L-carnitine and lipoic acid reversed age-associated mitochondrial structural decay. In the third National Academy of Sciences study, scientists tested acetyl-L-carnitine and lipoic acid to see if an enzyme used by the mitochondria as biologic fuel could be restored in old rats. After 7 weeks of supplementation with acetyl-L-carnitine and lipoic acid, levels of the enzyme carnitine acetyl-transferase were significantly restored in the aged rats. Supplementation also inhibited free radical-induced lipid peroxidation, which enhanced the activity of the energy-producing enzyme in the mitochondria. The scientists concluded that feeding old rats acetyl-L-carnitine and lipoic acid can ameliorate oxidative damage and mitochondrial dysfunction.

## Hormone Replacement

Proper hormone replacement can produce an immediate improvement in quality of life and prevent many diseases. Dehydroepiandrosterone (DHEA) is one of several important hormones whose production in the body diminishes rapidly as people age past 35 years. There now exists a wide body of evidence that supplementation with DHEA can prevent many degenerative diseases, while improving feelings of well-being and alleviating depression.

In the October 1996 issue of the journal *Drugs and Aging*, an overview of published studies on DHEA revealed the following[27]:

- In both humans and animals, the decline of DHEA production with aging is associated with immune depression, increased mortality, increased risk of several different cancers, loss of sleep, and decreased feelings of well-being.

- DHEA replacement in aged mice significantly normalized immune function to youthful levels.

- DHEA replacement has shown a favorable effect on osteoclasts and lymphoid cells, an effect that may delay osteoporosis.

- Low levels of DHEA inhibit energy metabolism, thus increasing the risk of heart disease and diabetes mellitus.

- Studies conducted on humans show essentially no toxicity at doses that restore DHEA to youthful levels.

- DHEA deficiency may expedite the development of some diseases that are common in the elderly.

Hundreds of additional studies have substantiated DHEA's role as an antiaging hormone-replacement supplement. In a study published in *Biological Psychiatry*, DHEA was tested on middle-aged and elderly patients with major depression. DHEA was administered for 4 weeks in doses of 30–90 mg daily. This level of dosing elevated DHEA serum levels to those observed in younger people. Depression ratings, as well as aspects of memory performance, significantly improved. These data suggested that DHEA may have antidepressant and promemory effects and corresponded with previous human studies in which DHEA supplementation (50 mg daily) significantly elevated mood in elderly people.[28]

For specific information on antiaging hormone replacement, *refer to the Male Hormone Restoration, Female Hormone Restoration, and DHEA Restoration Therapy protocols.*

## Life Extension Suggestions

Life Extension's Prevention protocols consist of the 12 most important supplements for the average person to take every day to reduce risk of contracting the degenerative diseases of aging.

**Note:** *The Prevention protocol is for healthy people. Those seeking to treat an existing disease may refer to the many specific disease prevention protocols contained in this book.*

### Life Extension's Top 12 Steps for Achieving Ultimate Health

1. Supplement your diet with a multivitamin/multinutrient formula
2. Ingest plenty of omega-3 fatty acids
3. Maintain optimal CoQ10 blood levels
4. Optimize your vitamin D blood levels
5. Optimize mitochondrial function
6. Restore youthful hormone balance
7. Preserve brain function
8. Support bone health
9A. Maintain healthy prostate function (for men only)
9B. Support breast health (for women only)
10. Inhibit inflammation with curcumin
11. Fill in the missing gaps with oil-based nutrients (eg, gamma tocopherol and vitamin K)
12. Maintain optimal blood glucose levels

**Bonus: Benefit from low-dose aspirin therapy

## REFERENCES

References available at: www.lef.org/dpt5/ch112

# 113

# Prostate Cancer: Overview

## INTRODUCTION TO DR. STRUM'S PROSTATE CANCER UPDATE

When I was diagnosed with advanced prostate cancer in September 1991, I thought my life, as I had envisioned it, was over. Instead, I have found a whole new universe of living and, in doing so, have come to terms with my own mortality.

Transformation is what is possible when we are faced with a life-threatening illness. When the unthinkable happens to us and we are faced with our mortality, we have an opportunity to transform our lives.

Acceptance of our situation is the first milestone we must pass before we can truly begin the process of healing. For me this translates into doing everything I can to understand the entire process of my illness and what I can do to become well. While I do not blame myself for my diagnosis, it has been valuable for me to take an introspective look at my life in relation to the kinds of stressors or environmental exposures that may have played a role. Sometimes it is not until we are on the reef that we realize it is there.

Fortunately for us, the cancer patient today has many more resources available than there were just a few years ago. What follows by Dr. Stephen Strum is an update of the treatment of prostate cancer. I have known Steve for over 10 years. He is one of the precious few who have brought a new and compassionate dimension to the patient/physician relationship.

*Frederick Mills*
Prostate Cancer Survivor
Founding Member of Educational Council
for Prostate Cancer Patients

## PROSTATE CANCER UPDATE

Stephen B. Strum, M.D., F.A.C.P.

## GENERAL INTRODUCTION

In this edition of Disease Prevention and Treatment, I will discuss prostate cancer (PC), using the metaphor of a military incursion—needing to have a focused, strategic approach, deployed in a systematic, problem-solving manner. The purpose of such a metaphor is to bring to the student of this disease a different perspective that will hopefully provide new insights which will lead to victories in our battles against this disease. The reason for such a departure from the conventional formal discussion of PC is that this latter academic approach is not being translated into winning strategies for the man with PC. The battle is being lost because we, the generals, are not translating what has been published in medical journals and discussed at national meetings into real-time preventive, diagnostic, evaluatory, and treatment tactics. Medical pragmatism—the art of being practical and using common sense—is not being practiced.

The battle to prevent this disease, diagnose it earlier, and treat it effectively is also not occurring at the proper pace largely because men are not taking an active role in winning this war. As we are learning in our war against terrorism, you defeat the enemy by recognizing their presence early (not late), preventing their buildup, learning their location, and eradicating them with the proper weaponry. There are too many men, already diagnosed with PC, who are not taking an active role in their own recovery. Many believe that because they are consulting a professional with a medical degree (who may also command a generous salary), all or part of this equates with getting the very best advice and treatment. Wrong. In today's rapid-pace world, where medicine is practiced with 15-minute office visits and where physicians are too busy to read and translate much of what is being published, the patient and his partner must not take a passive role and assume that all that can be done is being done.

My recommendations, therefore, either to patients with PC or to their loved ones, will be those of a counselor or guide, offering practical advice based on 20 years of working on the front lines of PC management. I do not hesitate in telling you that for the vast majority of men diagnosed with PC, a successful outcome can be realized. But the principles you are about to learn must become part and parcel of the strategic approach used by the patient/partner/physician (PPP) team. The patient and his partner have the most to gain as well as the most to lose when encountering PC. They must expend serious energy to win this particular war. In doing so, they learn the art of battle; they are brought closer together and evolve in their lives; and other intertwined health issues are brought to light and healed. This is the beauty of such an approach. Are you willing to invest in the time to help yourself? Are you worth it?

The most important take-home lesson that I can tell you within the pages that follow relates to your ability to use concepts. It is through the use of concepts—the structural framework of our thinking—that we intelligently plan a strategy of success.

**Table 1: Comparison of a Military Campaign with PC Strategy**

| Winning a Military Campaign | Defeating PC |
|---|---|
| 1 Preventing War | 1 Preventing PC |
| 2 Basic Military Training | 2 Getting Help to Understand Biological Principles |
| 3 Military Information (Intel) | 3 The Importance of the Medical Record |
| 4 Early Recognition of Enemy Activity | 4 Early Diagnosis of PC |
| 5 Assessment of the Enemy | 5 Risk Assessment of the PC Patient |
| 6 Knowing Pros and Cons of Weaponry | 6 Understanding Pros and Cons of Treatment Options |
| 7 Understanding Enemy Vulnerability | 7 Learning Principles Underlying Tumor Growth |
| 8 Stopping Supply Lines to the Enemy | 8 Antiangiogenesis Treatments, Dietary Changes |
| 9 Stabilizing Key Arenas of Conflict | 9 Focus on Bone Integrity, Biomarkers, etc. |
| 10 Supporting the Troops | 10 Supportive Care of the Patient |
| 11 Boosting Morale of Troops | 11 Fostering a Will to Live, Empowering the Patient |

As stated in the introduction, defeating PC is a military campaign. Winning a military campaign, or a war against PC, involves concepts such as prevention, basic training, military intelligence (Intel), early recognition of enemy activity, assessment of the strength of the enemy, an understanding of the pros and cons of the weapons in our arsenal, stabilization of key areas of conflict, stopping supply lines to the enemy, supporting our troops, and other issues common to a military arena (see Table 1). A strategy for success, be it in a military war or a war against PC, simply involves adding factual information to a sound conceptual framework.

The approaches used in a winning strategy, whether for a military campaign or a medical battle, are superimposable. That which occurs in the life of a cell is reflected in society as well.[1] Cellular battles are but a microcosm of what takes place on a more macromolecular level within the individual, his community, his country, the planet, and the universe. This is reflected repeatedly throughout the entire history of humankind.

# 1. PREVENTING WAR: PREVENTING PC

Most students of either campaign will maintain that prevention is the key to being truly victorious. There is

no argument there. However, the desire to understand the principles and importance of preventive tactics does not appear to be a top priority for most people until the harsh reality of war or cancer is present. For example, the appreciation of terrorism in America was not brought home until September 11, 2001. This appreciation of the enemy may take the form of seeing the reality of cancer up close and personal when a father, brother, or other family member is diagnosed with PC or another malignancy. Otherwise, the motivation to learn and utilize prevention tactics does not seem to be part of human reality for the vast majority of us. What can we do to foster an appreciation of the value of preventing PC?

## Hereditary PC: Risk Factors

Out of every 100 men diagnosed with PC, approximately 5 will have hereditary PC (HPC).[2] HPC is defined by any one of the following 3 criteria:

• Three successive generations with members having PC

• Three first-degree relatives, for example, a father and 2 brothers, 3 brothers, or a father and 2 sons with PC

• Two relatives with PC diagnosed before age 55[3]

It is not surprising that the incidence of hereditary breast cancer (BC) is also about 5% of the total population of BC patients—the same incidence as that of HPC.[4]

**Genetic transmission from father to son and father to daughter.** HPC is transmitted by a gene from father to son and from father to daughter and then to her son. When HPC is present, nearly half the male offspring will have PC, and many of these will develop PC before age 55. In fact, HPC accounts for approximately 43% of PC diagnosed before the age of 55 years.[3,5,6]

Since transmission of the gene may also occur from father to daughter and then to her son, a sound medical history includes information about the health of the maternal grandfather as well as maternal uncles and maternal cousins regarding any history of PC. Studies of PC within families show a stronger familial inheritance pattern than colon or BC.

**Value of intensified surveillance in high-risk situations.** Most importantly, procedures to routinely test the first-degree relatives of those having HPC have yielded an eight-fold higher detection of PC than that found in the general population.[7] Soon, genetic testing for chromosomal abnormalities found in HPC may become commercially available. Patients' interest in testing HPC similar to that available for BC appears great when there exists a family history of such disease.[8,9]

**Increased risk of male breast cancer and colon cancer in male offspring and breast cancer in female offspring.** It should also be emphasized that men with a history of BC in their family are also at greater risk for developing PC, just as women with a family history of PC are at greater risk for developing BC.[10] Since both PC and BC share common genes, it is not surprising that men who are carriers of the gene associated with BC (BRCA1 or BRCA2) are at a greater risk for developing male BC in addition to PC and colon cancer.[4,11–13]

Therefore, greater vigilance is suggested when a history of PC or BC is present.

**What are the tests for high-risk persons?** Currently, most physicians who focus on PC as their main specialty will recommend routine prostate-specific antigen (PSA) testing starting at age 40. This is important to establish objective findings that indicate a healthy prostate. In subsequent paragraphs, this will be shown to equate with a baseline PSA of less than 2.0 and often less than 1.0 ng/mL. In a population in which there is a family history of PC, such as has been described, PSA testing should be commenced at age 35 with yearly testing for a few years to establish a trend or profile. Then, if the PSA remains below 1.0 ng/mL, consideration for testing every 2–3 years can be considered. Vigilance on the part of the empowered patient, partner, and physician will also involve digital rectal examination (DRE) at reasonable intervals and tracking of the PSA over time. If any persistent PSA increase is noted, determinations of PSA velocity, PSA doubling times, free PSA percentage, and additional testing that will be discussed in subsequent sections must be done. Moreover, a baseline colonoscopy and stool testing for microscopic blood (hemoccult) would be a reasonable consideration in such men starting at age 40 rather than at age 50.

## General Preventive Measures

Besides laboratory testing, physical examination, and investigative procedures to rule out the presence of PC and other diseases, an action plan to prevent their development should be considered. These types of preventive measures are preemptive, or defensive measures. The most apparent of these relates to what we eat and drink.

There is no doubt that what we put into our bodies relates to the health of our cells. It is obvious that food

intake is associated with delights to our senses of sight, smell, and taste. However, on a survival level, food is the necessary fuel source for all the cells of the human body. The quality and quantity of the food, water, and air we put into our bodies clearly have serious ramifications. There are major parallels between human nutrition and a high-performance engine:

- The kind of fuel we add to high-performance engines
- The fuel-to-air ratios that occur within the combustion chambers
- The metabolic breakdown products resulting from internal combustion
- The wear and tear on the engine due to driving habits
- The preventive measures used to increase engine life

The human body is certainly no less of a high-performance engine than that of an airplane or car. Yet, although we appreciate the preventive maintenance that is part of the strategy of engine survival, we are inconsistent when we too often ignore the needs of our own bodies—that is, until we have signs of engine breakdown. As many of us love our cars and care for them, we must do the same with our bodies.

**Lycopenes and their critical role in cancer prevention.** The relationship between lycopene ingestion and the health of the prostate is well-established. Lycopene consumption has been found to decrease not only the risk of PC in multiple studies,[14–16] but also the risk of BC[17] and pancreatic and stomach cancer,[16] as well as lung cancer.[18]

**Tomato-based products are the richest sources of lycopene.** In these positive studies that correlated lycopene consumption with decreased risk of PC, the lycopene sources were tomato-based products. The richest sources of lycopene in the U.S. diet are ketchup, tomato juice, and pizza sauce; these account for over 80% of the total lycopene intake of Americans.[19] In one study from Athens, Greece, the authors concluded that the incidence of PC in Greece could be reduced by about 40% if the population increased the consumption of tomatoes, reduced the intake of dairy products, and substituted olive oil for other added lipids.[20]

**Lycopene consumption correlates with blood and tissue lycopene levels.** The correlation between increased tomato-based consumption of lycopenes and decreased risk of PC and other cancers is also found in the laboratory, where serum levels of lycopene are correlated with lycopene intake. The same holds true in studies for which tissue levels of lycopene have been studied in prostate pathology specimens.[16,17]

Lycopene concentrations in the serum of healthy men are typically 0.60–1.9 nmol/mL.[21] Biochemically, lycopene is composed of 2 main chemical structures or isomers: all-trans-lycopene and cis-isomers. Tomato sauce contains primarily all-trans-lycopene (83% of total lycopene). The ingestion of tomato sauce results in substantial increases in total lycopene levels in both the serum and prostate tissue and a substantial increase in all-trans-lycopene in prostate tissue but with relatively smaller increases in the serum.[22] Serum lycopene levels are predominantly composed of the cis-isomer of lycopene, which represents 58–73% of the total serum lycopene, while the all-trans-isomer composes 27–42% of the serum lycopene.[21]

Among 72 studies identified, 57 reported that higher tomato intake or blood lycopene levels reduced the risk of cancer at a defined anatomic site; 35 of these associations were statistically significant.[23] The evidence for a benefit was strongest for cancers of the prostate, lung, and stomach. Data were also suggestive of a benefit for cancers of the pancreas, colon and rectum, esophagus, oral cavity, breast, and cervix. The relative risk (RR) was determined, comparing high tomato intake or high lycopene levels with low tomato intake or low lycopene levels. In such comparisons, about half of the RR was close to 0.6 or lower.[23] In another study, the odds of contracting aggressive PC were significantly lower when plasma lycopene levels were high. Plasma lycopene levels were divided into 5 quintiles. The highest level, the fifth quintile, showed an odds ratio (OR) of 0.56.[14] These findings add up to about a 40% reduction in risk of being diagnosed with these cancer types for those with high tomato intake or the highest plasma lycopene levels.

**The proof of the pudding is not in the eating but in the assimilation.** The proof of the pudding, in the matter of dietary issues, relates more to how we assimilate what we have eaten rather than just a history of having eaten something. It should not be surprising then that the correlation between serum or plasma lycopene levels and a lower incidence of PC is greater than the correlation between the oral intake of lycopenes and PC incidence. In a study, significant reductions in PC incidence were observed with higher plasma concentrations of the following carotenoids: lycopene (OR 0.17) and zeaxanthin (OR 0.22) when comparing highest and lowest quartiles.[24] This translates into about an 80% reduction in PC incidence when the highest blood levels of either lycopene or zeaxanthin are achieved.

**Lycopenes and strawberries lower risk, especially for aggressive and extra-prostatic PC.** A dietary history of significant lycopene and/or strawberry consumption correlated with a lower risk of aggressive and extra-prostatic PC.[14] The lycopene source that was found to be most significant in most epidemiologic studies was the tomato, in the form of tomato sauce, stewed tomatoes, and pizza sauce. In one large-scale study involving 812 new cases of PC over the years 1986–1992 with matched controls, of the 46 fruits and vegetables or related products significantly associated with lower PC risk, 3 of the 4 identified were related to lycopene—tomato sauce, tomatoes, and pizza. In this study, the combined intake of tomatoes, tomato sauce, tomato juice, and pizza (accounting for 82% of lycopene intake) was associated with a reduced risk of PC for consumption frequency greater than 10 versus less than 1.5 servings per week. Lycopene intake was also associated with a 53% reduced risk for advanced PC (stages 3 and 4). The other non-lycopene product identified with significantly lower PC risk was strawberries.[15]

A large, prospective study on male health professionals found that consumption of 2–4 servings of tomato sauce per week was associated with about a 35% risk reduction of total PC and a 50% reduction of advanced (extra-prostatic) PC. Tomato sauce was by far the strongest predictor of plasma lycopene levels in this study.[25] These associations persisted in analyses controlling for fruit consumption, vegetable consumption, and olive oil use and were observed separately in men of Southern European or other Caucasian ancestry.[26]

**Lycopene inhibits cancer cell growth by gene upregulation of connexin 43.** Lycopene functions as a very potent antioxidant. In this regard, lycopene can trap singlet oxygen and reduce mutagenesis (gene mutations) in the Ames test. Other mechanisms of lycopene action may be operative as well. Lycopene at physiologic concentrations can inhibit human cancer cell growth by interfering with growth factor receptor signaling and cell-cycle progression—specifically in PC cells—without evidence of toxic effects or apoptosis of cells.[27] Studies of human and animal cells have identified connexin 43, a gene whose expression is upregulated by lycopene and which allows direct intercellular gap junctional communication (GJC). GJC is deficient in many human tumors and its restoration or upregulation is associated with decreased proliferation.

**Lycopene is synergistic with vitamin D, inhibiting tumor cell proliferation and enhancing differentiation.** The combination of low concentrations of lycopene with 1,25-dihydroxyvitamin D3 exhibits a synergistic effect on inhibition of cell proliferation, and differentiation, and an additive effect on cell-cycle progression in the HL-60 promyelocytic leukemia cell line, suggesting some interaction at a nuclear or subcellular level.[18]

**Lycopenes reduce cardiovascular risk factors.** Lycopene levels decrease with advancing age. However, in contrast to other carotenoids, they are not found to be reduced by smoking or alcohol consumption.[16,19] Lycopenes also have an inhibitory effect on cholesterol synthesis and may enhance LDL degradation. Available evidence suggests that intimal wall thickness and risk of myocardial infarction are reduced in persons with higher adipose tissue concentrations of lycopene.[19]

**Lycopene levels may be associated with decreased insulin-like growth factor levels.** The consumption of cooked tomatoes was substantially and significantly associated with reduced insulin-like growth factor-1 (IGF-1) levels, with a mean change of −31.5% for an increment of 1 serving daily. The authors concluded that the strongest known dietary risk factor for PC (lycopene deficit, as reflected in a reduced intake of cooked tomatoes) is somehow related to an important endocrine factor (IGF-1) in the cause of this disease.[28] However, in another study, IGF-1 was not associated with any dietary factor studied, such as total fat, carbohydrate, protein, dairy products, tomatoes, or calcium.[29]

**Suggested ways to increase lycopene consumption and plasma levels.** The easiest way I have found to combine a healthy intake of lycopenes into my diet is by using marinara sauce on various foods. For example, at breakfast, an egg white omelet containing eggplant and bell peppers (ratatouille omelet) covered with marinara sauce is a healthy source of protein, contains a substantial fiber content, and is restricted in the amount of simple carbohydrates. Stewed tomatoes can be served as a vegetable side dish with lunch or dinner.

**Dietary fat increases PC growth rates.** There are studies showing that dietary fat increases tumor growth rates in an animal model of human PC. In a mouse model of PC involving androgen-sensitive human prostatic adenocarcinoma cells (LNCaP cells), mice fed a 40.5% fat diet had mean tumor weights more than 2 times greater than mice fed a 21% fat diet. The 40.5% fat diet approximates that found in the average American male diet, which has been determined to be 36%.[30]

The slower tumor growth associated with the low-fat diet occurred even after the formation of measurable tumors when the diets were changed from 40% fat to 21% fat. Serum PSA levels also were highest in the 40.5% fat group and lowest in another group fed only 2.3% fat.[30]

**Reduction of total calorie consumption decreases tumor size by decreasing VEGF, angiogenesis, and IGF-1, and increasing apoptosis.** The emphasis on dietary fat per se has lessened our focus on the importance of caloric overconsumption. Fat excess, however, is linked to excessive calorie consumption, since fat contains twice as many calories, gram for gram, as protein or carbohydrate.

I believe that diet should be regarded as having serious biochemical relevance to the health of the individual. You are, for the most part, what you eat (or at least what you assimilate). Western societies, especially the United States, are consumers of excessive calories. Excessive caloric consumption, especially coupled with a sedentary lifestyle, is a significant factor that adversely affects longevity.

An important study demonstrated that energy intake (caloric intake) modulates the growth of prostate tumors in 2 animal models: the androgen-dependent Dunning R3327-H adenocarcinoma in rats and the androgen-sensitive LNCaP human adenocarcinoma in severe combined immunodeficiency (SCID) mice.[33] Specifically, decreasing calorie consumption (energy restriction) by 20–40% from the control animals fed ad libitum resulted in:

- Increased PC cell apoptosis (programmed cell death)
- A two- to three-fold reduction in PC angiogenesis as measured by microvessel density
- A decrease in vascular endothelial growth factor (VEGF) expression
- A decrease in circulating levels of IGF-1
- A significant decrease in tumor size

Therefore, all of these findings were benefits observed in the calorie-restricted group. This study showed that the nutritional status directly or indirectly influenced interaction between tumor cells and local blood vessels by changing the expression of angiogenic growth factors. In the Dunning model, energy (calorie) restriction resulted in a striking inhibition of VEGF expression. In the LNCaP model, there was little baseline expression of VEGF. However, there was an almost three-fold reduction from the baseline IGF-1 levels in blood samples from LNCaP-bearing mice that were subjected to energy restriction.

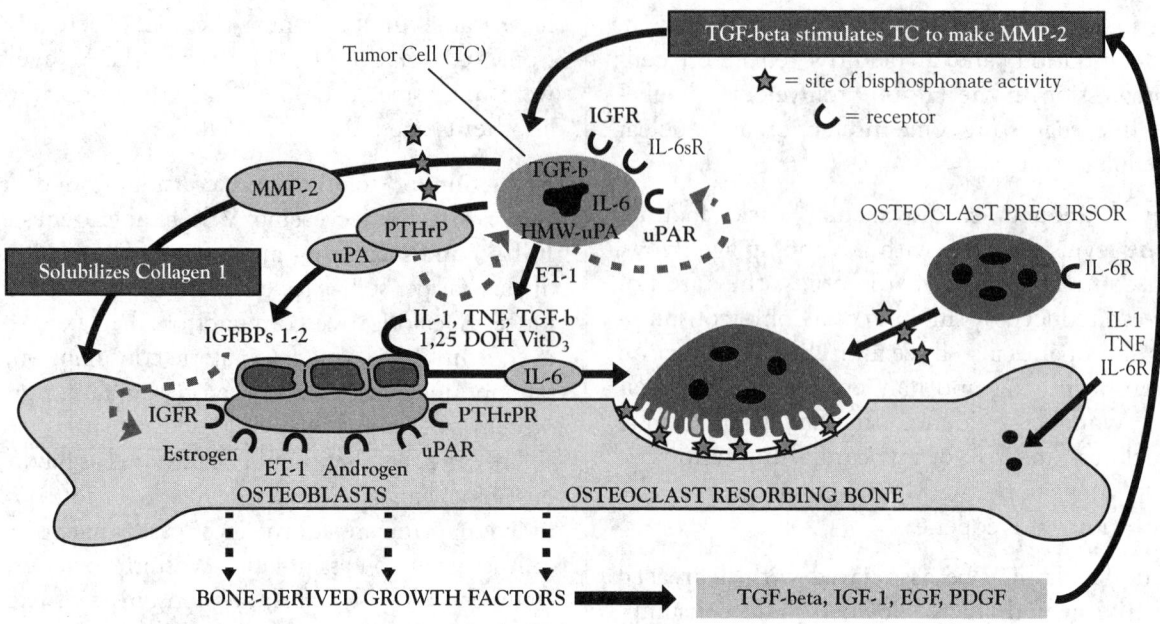

Figure 1. **The Signaling Pathways between Tumor Cell and Bone Elements.** This is a hypothetical portrayal of the tumor and bone tissue and the interactions of their cellular products. For example, PTHrP (parathyroid hormone-related protein) is one of two principal calcium-regulating hormones, but it also promotes bone breakdown. PTHrP is secreted by the neuroendocrine (NE) cells within the prostate. These NE cells are up-regulated by IL-6. PTHrP interacts with the osteoblast to stimulate IL-6 production and interacts with uPA to release IGF-1. Receptors for IL-6 on premature osteoclasts activate their maturation to fully operational osteoclasts that are able to breakdown bone.[31,32]

## IGF-1 levels stimulate PC growth, upregulate uPA, and stimulate angiogenesis.

- IGF-1 and uPA increases aggressive PC growth
- GLA and EPA inhibit uPA

Higher IGF-1 levels are associated with a four-fold greater risk of developing PC.[34] IGF-1 is a known mitogen (stimulator of cell division and tumor growth) for PC. IGF-1 receptors are found on the PC cell as well as on osteoblasts.[35] IGF-1 stimulates the PC cell to make uPA (urokinase-type plasminogen activator), a cell product implicated in the invasiveness and metastasis of PC. The uPA receptors are on the PC cell and on osteoblasts. IGF-1 adds further insult by also acting as an angiogenic growth factor.[36] A detailed illustration of these and other interactions is shown in Figure 1.

Gene expression of IGF-1 and its receptor are inhibited by 5-alpha-reductase inhibitors such as Proscar®.[37]

**IGF-1 and uPA act together to increase aggressive PC growth.** There are studies demonstrating that elevations of uPA and its receptor are associated with non-organ-confined PC at radical prostatectomy (RP), disease progression with metastases, and a poorer overall survival.[38] uPA works closely with IGF-1 and its receptors, cleaving IGF-1 from its binding proteins. uPA is also part of an autocrine pathway for the PC cell, allowing uPA to stimulate PC cell growth and make more uPA at the same time.

**Good news! GLA and EPA inhibit uPA.** Of interest is the fact that uPA production is inhibited by gamma-linolenic acid (GLA) and eicosapentaenoic acid (EPA).[39] GLA and EPA, which are essential fatty acids, are among the important players in the prevention of disease and in maintenance of health. This is discussed by Barry Sears, Ph.D., in Omega Rx Zone.[40] Sears beautifully presents the interconnection between restriction of calories, along with dietary adjustments of carbohydrate, protein, and fat intake, and the production of a class of fatty acids called eicosanoids. An understanding of these issues is fundamental to our ability to prevent disease and maintain or recapture health.

**More advantages to caloric restriction and avoidance of hyperinsulinemia.** Sears stresses the importance of caloric restriction by means of limiting the intake of high-density carbohydrates such as bread, pasta, grains in most cereals, and starches such as those found in potatoes. This reduction of caloric intake by lowering high-density carbohydrate intake decreases the stimulation of the pancreas to make insulin and limits all the adverse side effects associated with increased insulin levels (hyperinsulinemia).

Caloric restriction has been shown to be an important factor in augmenting the immune system and improving longevity. It reduces free radical production, which if otherwise unchecked, damages DNA and oxidizes polyunsaturated fats. Caloric restriction increases levels of superoxide dismutase (SOD), glutathione, melatonin, DHEA, peroxidase, and catalase. The latter substances are important defense mechanisms in our body known to decrease with age. Caloric restriction is instrumental in lowering the production of cortisol. Cortisol is associated with increased stress levels, and an imbalance in cortisol production leads to immune deficiency and bone loss through resorption, leading to osteopenia and osteoporosis, as well as muscle breakdown and aging of the skin.

Calorie restriction, as proposed by Sears and others, has been shown to also reduce advanced glycosylated end-products (AGEs). These are carbohydrate-protein complexes associated with hyperinsulinemic states and with cardiovascular disease, Alzheimer's disease, kidney disease, and other degenerative states.

We need to rethink how much food we need to eat. Our ideal body weight should be taken seriously. If we were to do this alone, we would eliminate most cases of diabetes, hypertension, hypercholesterolemia, stroke, heart disease, and a significant amount of cancer from our lives and those of our loved ones. Healthy people should consume 500 calories per meal and 100 calories per snack. Modifications of this are based on the level of disease activity, age, and body surface area. Nutritional software and nutritional counseling should be an integral part of our approach to good health.

**Insulin-stimulating carbohydrate is the damaging subcomponent of carbohydrate.** If hyperinsulinemia is crucial to the development of many of our biochemical problems—from arthritis to neurodegenerative disease to cancer—then controlling the carbohydrate loads we subject our bodies to should be a major tool in maintaining good health. Carbohydrates can be characterized by the amount of insulin-stimulating carbohydrate (ISC) that they contain. ISC is the total carbohydrate content (in grams) minus the amount of fiber (in grams) it contains. An example is 1 cup of broccoli containing a total of 7 g of carbohydrate, of which 4 g are fiber. The difference between the two equals the ISC content or 3 g. Fruits and vegetables, which are high in fiber, generally have a lower ISC content than do starches, grains, and pasta. Therefore, analogous to PSA (benign-related versus cancer-related) and to cholesterol (total cholesterol versus LDL versus HDL), any

intelligent discussion on carbohydrates must specify the components in question.

**High-density carbohydrates should be minimized.** An important variable in nutrition relates to the quantity or volume of food that we eat at each meal. Therefore, we need to specify carbohydrate intake as a function of ISC per unit volume of food. A serving of mashed potatoes (1 cup) containing a total of 40 g of carbohydrate, with 2 g being fiber, would have the difference—38 g—as ISC. The same serving of broccoli containing a total of 7 g of carbohydrate, with 4 g being fiber, would have 3 g of ISC per serving. The ISC per unit serving, comparing mashed potatoes to broccoli is therefore 38 versus 3. Carbohydrates that deliver a high insulin-stimulating effect per unit serving are termed high-density carbohydrates. Carbohydrates that are proportionally higher in fiber and lower in ISC per unit serving are called low-density carbohydrates. In our PC analogy, PSA density would relate to carbohydrate density.

**Glycemic index further modifies the concept of ISC content: the glycemic load.** Insulin release is also related to the rapidity of increase of the blood sugar after ingestion of carbohydrates. The concept of glycemic index is used to account for this variable. The glycemic index measures the rate of carbohydrate entry into the bloodstream. Factors relating to the glycemic index of a particular food include the following:

- The amount of fiber it contains
- The amount of fructose the carbohydrate contains relative to the amount of glucose
- The amount of fat eaten with the carbohydrate

High fiber and increased amounts of fructose (sugar from fruits) both function to lower the glycemic index. Fat consumed with carbohydrates will also mollify the glycemic effect and lower the glycemic index. Sears ties this nicely together by using the concept of glycemic load (GL): the amount of insulin-stimulating carbohydrate multiplied by the glycemic index of the carbohydrate (ISC × GI).

**Volume of food eaten.** An additional factor that must also be accounted for is the volume of carbohydrate ingested. You might be looking intelligently at the total carbohydrate content, noting the fiber content and determining the grams of ISC. You might even be smart enough to have memorized the glycemic indices of many of the foods you eat to determine the GL. However, if you double or triple the volume of carbohydrate you eat, you can still be over-stimulating the production of insulin. These topics relating to balancing protein, carbohydrate, and healthy fats are discussed in the Omega Rx Zone by Sears.

**Eicosanoid balance.**    Eicosanoids are hormones made within the membrane of each and every cell—all 60 trillion cells in the human body. Eicosanoids are 20-carbon structures. Eicosanoids have autocrine, paracrine, and endocrine effects. That is, they affect the very cell that produces the eicosanoid (autocrine effect) as well as nearby cells (paracrine effect) and distant cells (endocrine effect). As with every aspect of biology, balance is a critical issue relating to good health as well as the development and progression of various diseases. Likewise, eicosanoid balance plays a central role that puts this desired biological endpoint at the hub of the integrative medicine wheel. Eicosanoids, and the balance of good versus bad eicosanoids, can be seen as the heart and soul, muscle, bone, and sinew, literally and figuratively, of holistic medicine.

Clearly pertinent to a discussion of PC is the fact that the first eicosanoids isolated in 1936 by Ulf von Euler were prostaglandins—eicosanoids isolated from the prostate gland. Eicosanoids are the oldest hormones, tracing their origin back 500 million years ago to production by sponges. Hormones are messengers involved in communication between cells. A hormone is formally defined as a substance, usually a peptide or steroid, produced by one tissue and conveyed by the bloodstream to another to affect physiologic activity, such as growth or metabolism. All of medicine—in fact, all of life—represents issues of communication and balance. Such is the case at every level of existence. This is true for the cell, tissues, an organism, a human individual, family, community, society, nation, planet, and the universe. If there was ever a guiding principle that is truly holistic, it is the principle of communication and balance.

**Arachidonic acid metabolites increase PC growth, invasion, and metastasis.**    Eicosanoid synthesis involves the release of arachidonic acid (AA) from cell membrane phospholipids by an enzyme called phospholipase A2 (PLA2). AA then undergoes metabolism by cyclooxygenases (COXs) and lipoxygenases (LOXs). AA is an omega-6 fatty acid that is known to generate free radicals and is considered an unfavorable eicosanoid. Specific metabolites of AA, for example, PGE2 and 5-HETE, are created through the actions of the enzymes COX-2, 5-LOX, 12-LOX, and 15-LOX. These metabolites are examples of bad

eicosanoids and have been implicated in PC growth and metastasis.[41,42] In a study of human PC in which 5-LOX and its metabolite 5-HETE were evaluated in both malignant and benign prostate tissue within the same patient, both 5-LOX and 5-HETE were significantly overexpressed in the PC tissue.[43] In other words, specific eicosanoids are modulators of tumor cell interactions with certain host components within the context of cancer growth, invasion, and spread.

The administration of PGE2 to prostate, breast, and colon cancer cells resulted in increased cellular proliferation. Some studies have shown that stimulation of PC growth is related more to COX-2 and a resultant increase in angiogenesis than to PGE2.[44]

**Inhibition of AA and its metabolites causes PC apoptosis.**    Laboratory studies have shown a significant reduction in cancer cell invasiveness by inhibitors of PLA2, as well as general COX inhibitors such as ibuprofen (Motrin®) and specific COX-2 inhibitors.[45] In this particular study, the mechanism of action was related to a reduction in angiogenesis factors called matrix metalloproteinases (MMPs). Other studies have shown a significant role for COX-2 inhibition in PC with demonstration of reduction in microvessel density of the tumor related to a decrease in VEGF, a potent angiogenesis factor.[46] Apparently, within the center of PC tumors a state of lower oxygen tension exists (hypoxic center) which stimulates VEGF. COX-2 inhibition seems to be able to prevent this hypoxia-induced upregulation of VEGF and angiogenesis. An ibuprofen derivative called Flurbiprofen® inhibited PGE2 and reduced PC cell growth by inhibiting upregulation of COX-2.[47]

Multiple papers have shown that inhibition of 5-LOX leads to PC apoptosis.[48–51]

**EPA and DHA lower PC risk.**    EPA, an omega-3 fatty acid, has been shown to suppress AA formation by inhibiting the enzyme delta-5-desaturase.[52] Some epidemiologic studies have shown that high intakes of EPA and DHA lower PC risk substantially.[53] Other studies have shown a reduction in PC risk only with a decrease in the ratio of AA to EPA (AA:EPA).[54] A combination of GLA and EPA administered to humans was shown to strongly increase serum EPA and DGLA levels and reduce AA formation and AA metabolites such as leukotrienes.[52]

Foods rich in EPA include coldwater fish such as tuna, sardines, herring, swordfish, and salmon. Commercially available pharmaceutical-grade fish oils also contain large amounts of EPA and DHA.

## The Eicosanoid Pathways

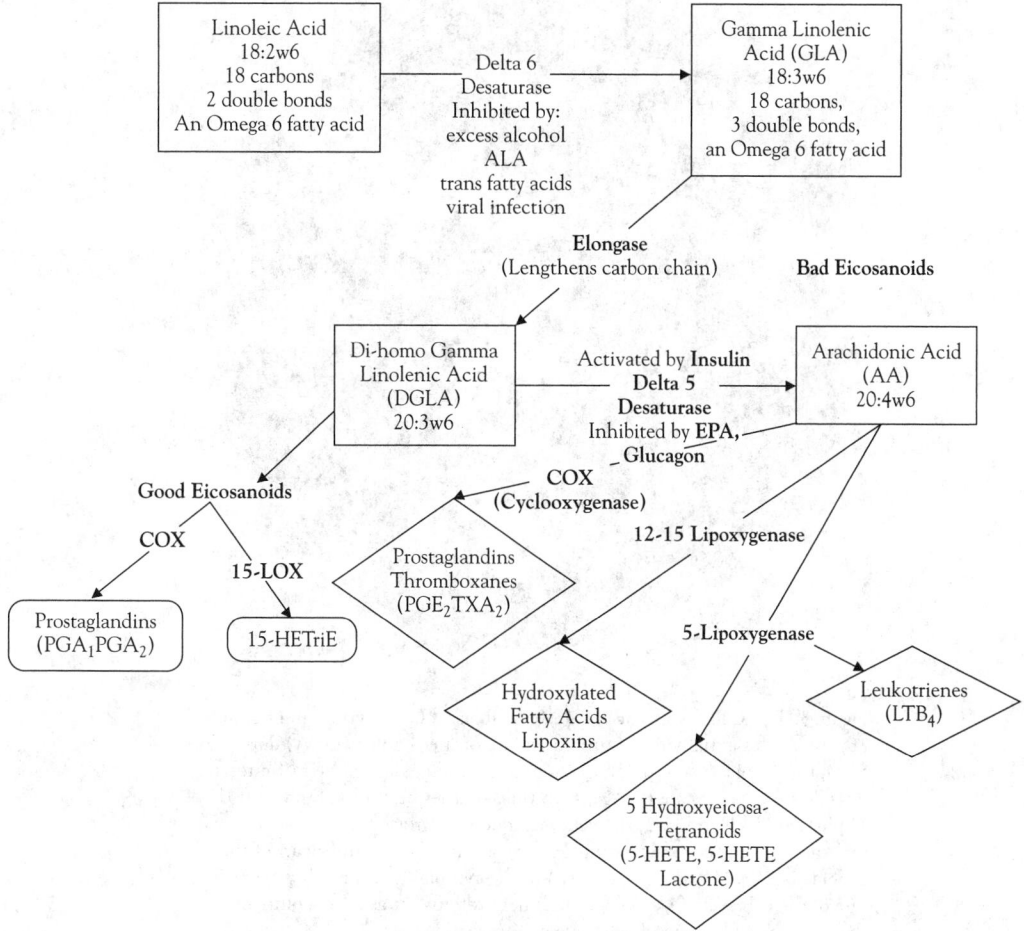

Figure 2. **The Eicosanoid Pathways—An Abridged Version.** The pathways to good versus bad eicosanoids are dictated by whether DGLA metabolism favors arachidonic acid (AA) production and the generation of bad eicosanoids or instead is shunted preferentially toward favorable eicosanoids of the PG1 series (PGA$_1$ and PGA$_2$).

**Selenium prevents PC in select patients.** Measures to prevent PC must be a routine part of the counsel that general practitioners and internists give their patients. Selenium intake of at least 200 mcg daily should be a consideration in the prevention of PC. Low plasma selenium is associated with a four- to five-fold increased risk of PC.[55] In addition, levels of plasma selenium also decrease with age, resulting in middle-aged to older men being at a higher risk for low selenium levels. Ideally, baseline levels of selenium should be obtained before beginning routine selenium supplementation. It would make sense to begin such a micronutrient and mineral assessment at age 25 and perhaps every 10 years thereafter.

The studies of selenium supplementation and its role in preventing PC need continued clarification. In one study, selenium supplements provided benefit only for those individuals who had lower baseline plasma selenium levels.[56] Other subjects with normal or higher levels did not benefit and had a slightly increased risk for PC. Studies showed that selenium reduced the incidence of PC in men 63%.[56,57] The mechanism of selenium anti-PC activity appears related to selenium's antiproliferative effect against PC. Selenium affects the cell cycle (see Figure 3) with upregulation of cell-cycle regulators such as p21 and p27, resulting in a decrease in PC growth due to G1 arrest and up to an 80% reduction in the S-phase of PC growth.[58]

**Selenium enhances cell kill with Taxol® and Adriamycin® chemotherapy.** Selenium also has been shown to have a significant antineoplastic effect on breast, lung, liver, and small intestinal tumor cells. Supplementation with selenium enhanced the chemotherapeutic effects of Taxol® (paclitaxel) and Adriamycin® (doxorubicin) in these cells beyond

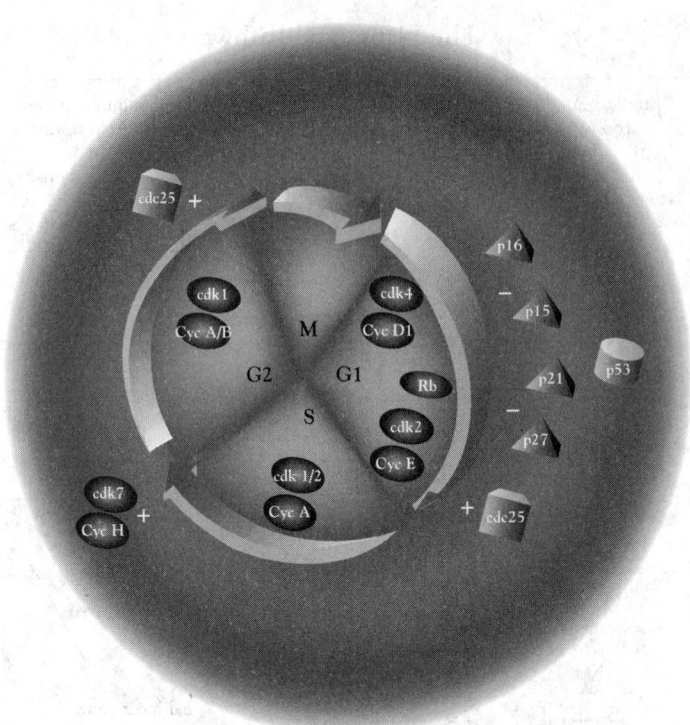

Figure 3. **The Cell Cycle and Its 4 Major Phases.** Cell division is an orderly process that essentially relates into doubling of the genome (DNA) during the S (synthesis) phase and then halving of that genome during the M (mitosis) phase. The G phases are the "gaps" in time—either before the S phase (G1) or M phase (G2). During G1, the genome undergoes growth and preparation for replication in the S phase; during G2, preparation for splitting apart of the genome occurs. Multiple proteins (p) in the cytoplasm of the cell govern the rate of the cell cycle (eg, p21, p27). Other proteins act as checkpoint controls that prevent replication of defective cells (eg, p53).

that seen when the chemotherapeutic drugs were used alone. In studies of the PC cell lines LNCaP and PC-3, the addition of Taxol® or Adriamycin®, in combination with selenium, caused small but significant inhibition of the PC cell growth. In the cited studies, the optimal inhibition of tumor growth occurred when the plasma selenium level was between 4–40 ng/mL after 72 hours of treatment.[59]

**Vitamin E isomers alpha- and gamma-tocopherol plus selenium combine to reduce PC risk.** A large-scale study of almost 11 000 men in Maryland showed that the protective effects of high selenium levels, and similarly that of the alpha-tocopherol isomer of vitamin E, were only observed when the concentrations of the gamma tocopherol isomer of vitamin E were also high.[60] In this study, the risk of PC declined with increasing concentrations of alpha-tocopherol, with the highest concentration associated with a 68% PC risk reduction. For gamma-tocopherol, men with levels in the highest fifth of the distribution had a five-fold greater reduction in the risk of developing PC than men in the lowest fifth ($p = 0.002$). The

observed interaction between alpha-tocopherol, gamma-tocopherol, and selenium suggested that combined alpha- and gamma-tocopherol supplements, used in conjunction with selenium, should be considered in future PC prevention trials.

**Vitamin E succinate inhibits PC cell growth and PSA expression.** In another study, vitamin E succinate inhibited cell growth of PC cells in the LNCaP line by suppressing androgen receptor expression and PSA expression. The combination of Eulexin® (flutamide) with vitamin E succinate resulted in a more significant inhibition of LNCaP cell growth.[61] The same investigators demonstrated that selenomethionine also showed an inhibitory effect on LNCaP cell growth but that this appeared to be independent of androgen receptor or PSA pathways.

**Vitamin E reduces incidence of PC in smokers in 2 separate studies.** A study of over 29 000 male smokers in Finland, ages 50–69, disclosed a 32% decrease in the incidence of PC (95% confidence interval [CI] = –47 to –12%). This was observed among the subjects who had received 50 mg daily of alpha-tocopherol ($n = 14564$) in contrast with those not receiving it ($n = 14569$). Mortality from PC was 41% lower among men receiving alpha-tocopherol (95% CI = –65% to –1%). Among subjects receiving beta-carotene ($n = 14560$), PC incidence was 23% higher (95% CI = –4% to 59%) and mortality was 15% higher (95% CI = –30% to 89%) compared with those not receiving it ($n = 14573$). In this study, long-term supplementation with alpha-tocopherol substantially reduced PC incidence and mortality in male smokers.[62]

An important issue is whether this benefit of alpha-tocopherol, and possibly other tocopherols, is limited to smokers or those who have recently quit smoking. A report showed significant benefit only to smokers or those recently quitting smoking in a study involving 47780 U.S. male health professionals who received at least 100 IU of supplemental alpha-tocopherol. In this population, the risk of metastatic or fatal PC was reduced 56%. In the nonsmoking population, there were no beneficial findings of statistical significance.[63] In a study on the relationship of green and yellow vegetable consumption to risk reduction in cancer development, a significant reduction was again found to occur only in smokers. The cancers studied included those of the mouth and pharynx, esophagus, stomach, liver, larynx, lung, and urinary bladder.[64]

**Vitamin E reduces VEGF levels.** A follow-up study involving the Finnish smokers compared VEGF levels in patients receiving alpha-tocopherol with those in the placebo group. There was an 11% reduction in VEGF levels in the alpha-tocopherol group as compared with a 10% increase in the placebo group ($p = 0.03$).[65]

**Vitamin E lessens adverse effects on PC growth due to dietary fat in vitro.** Research studies have shown that vitamin E reduces growth rates of PCs resulting from a high fat diet. Tumor growth rates were highest in the animals fed a 40.5%-kcal fat diet (the typical American diet). Tumors in animals fed 40.5%-kcal fat plus vitamin E were the same as those fed a 21.2%-kcal fat diet (an ideal fat level).[66]

**High consumption of dairy products and calcium increase risk of PC.** A study in Sweden examined the relationship of dairy products, dietary calcium, phosphorus, and vitamin D with risk of total, extraprostatic, and metastatic PC. The results indicated that calcium intake was an independent predictor of PC (RR = 1.91) for calcium intakes of greater than or equal to 1183 mg daily versus less than 825 mg daily. This was especially the case for metastatic tumors with a RR equal to 2.64, controlling for age, family history of PC, smoking, and total energy and phosphorus intakes. The authors concluded

that high consumption of dairy products was associated with a 50% increased risk of PC.[67]

A second study in the United States involved 1012 cases of PC among 20885 men over an 11-year follow-up period. Men consuming greater than 2.5 servings daily of dairy products had a RR of 1.34 for PC after adjustment for baseline age, body mass index, smoking, exercise, and randomized treatment assignment in the original placebo-controlled trial. Compared with men consuming less than or equal to 150 mg calcium daily from dairy products, men consuming greater than 600 mg of calcium daily had a 32% higher risk of PC. The results support the hypothesis that dairy products and calcium are associated with a greater risk of PC.

Also noted was that at baseline, men who consumed greater than 600 mg of calcium daily from skim milk had lower plasma 1,25(OH)(2)D(3) concentrations than did those consuming less than or equal to 150 mg of calcium daily (71 compared with 85 pmol/L or 30.06 pg/mL compared with 35.64 pg/mL; $p = 0.005$).[68]

The RR for the diagnosis of advanced PC was noted to be 2.97 in men with daily calcium consumption of greater than or equal to 2000 mg versus less than 500 mg.[69] The same was true for the risk of metastatic PC, but with a stronger RR of 4.57. (A RR of 4.57 means a 4.57 times greater risk of contracting PC.) Calcium from food sources and supplements independently increased risk of PC.

**High fructose consumption decreases risk of PC.** In the same study referenced above, high fructose intake was found to be related to a lower risk of advanced PC (multivariate RR, 0.51). Fruit intake was associated with a RR of advanced PC (RR = 0.63; 5 versus 1 serving daily), and this association was accounted for by fructose intake. Nonfruit sources of fructose similarly predicted lower risk of advanced PC.[69]

**Boron consumption lowers PC occurrence.** Men who ate the greatest amount of boron were 54% less likely to develop PC compared to men who consumed the least amount of boron. This information was presented in the annual Experimental Biology Conference in Florida in 2001. The study was led by Cui et al. from the UCLA Medical Center and compared dietary patterns of 95 men with PC with those of 5720 males without cancer.[70] The more boron-rich foods consumed, the greater the reduction in risk of being diagnosed with PC. Those men in the highest quartile of boron consumption had a 54% reduction in PC. Boron-rich foods include plums, grapes, prunes, avocados, and nuts such as almonds and peanuts. A serving of 100 g of prunes (6 dried prunes) has 2–3 mg of boron and 6.1 g of fiber.[71]

**Diet and supplement studies versus cancer risk: confounding findings affecting interpretation.** The lifestyle characteristics of supplement users are certainly a potential bias in studies investigating the benefits versus risks of vitamins, minerals, and dietary habits. A study evaluated supplement users and found that, among men, supplement users had the characteristics detailed in Table 2.[72]

The health-minded nature of users of vitamins, mineral supplements, and dietary plans may well confound what we think we know about the relationship of such integrative health measures and investigations dealing with RR and OR of diseases such as PC as well as other malignant and nonmalignant processes.

# 2. GETTING HELP TO UNDERSTAND BIOLOGICAL PRINCIPLES ABOUT PROSTATE CANCER

To master the tactical approaches and be victorious in your battle with PC is challenging. In such a context that involves a major crisis in your life, you need to have guidance in multiple shapes and forms.

## Support Groups

If you belong to an interactive support group, this can be a great beginning. These are some of the largest:

- Us Too International, Inc., (800) 808-7866; www. ustoo.com

- Man-to-Man, (800) 227-2345; www.cancer.org

- Patient Advocates for Advanced Cancer Treatments, (616) 453-1477; www.paactusa.org

I have attended many support group meetings, and the level at which each support group functions is highly variable. Some are informal meetings—more akin to chat groups relating personal experiences. Others are more scientific, with guest speakers involved in the diagnosis and treatment of PC. I hope that more support groups evolve into workshops that focus on each of its members—one at a time—using a scientifically objective approach with working forms. In such an idealized setting, an invited professional speaker would

be asked to orient his or her talk around selected case histories (called clinical vignettes) pertaining to individuals in the support group.

Let's face it. Everyone at the support group meeting is there because of a perceived threat involving his or her life as it relates to PC. They are present because they are seeking answers to their problems. Therefore, every PC patient-oriented meeting should have patient outcome as the prime directive. Patients should understand that they learn about their particular problem through the understanding of concepts that, more often than not, also apply to them. When such lessons are taught as a story of an actual human being, the lesson is reinforced and becomes memorable. Such an approach translates science into practical issues of value that are more understandable to the individual man with PC and to his partner.

Resolution of problems and prevention of problems unrecognized (or yet to develop) should be the prime directive of such organizations. Working together as a team (or army) to help one another is an effective way to teach all members of this platoon some valuable lessons about PC and hopefully about the spirit of human unity. Those that approach PC in such a manner will increase the likelihood that critical crossroads will now be approached in an intelligent fashion and crossed successfully. Instead of hearing about patients and physicians making the same mistakes repeatedly, we would hear more and more success stories. We do not want to fulfill the warning that the philosopher Santayana posed when he said:

*Those who cannot remember the past are condemned to repeat it.*

In my 20 years of counseling patients and physicians about PC, the same mistakes are made far too often. Using an objective format to gather data and presenting such data to your support group veterans should be the modus operandi of support groups. This will be discussed later in detail.

Also, and of great importance, working together elevates the individuals and the group. The mindset of the man with PC changes from "me against the disease" to "we against the disease." This fosters feelings of human

**Table 2: The Profile of Vitamin/Mineral Supplement Users**

| Characteristic of Supplement Users | Odds Ratio | 95% Confidence Interval |
|---|---|---|
| Twice as likely to have had a PSA test | 2.2 | 1.3–3.7 |
| Take aspirin regularly | 1.7 | 1.1–2.6 |
| Statistically significantly more likely to exercise regularly | 1.7 | 1.2–2.4 |
| Eat 4 or more servings of fruits and vegetables daily | 2.4 | 1.6–3.8 |
| Follow a low-fat diet pattern | 1.7 | 1.1–2.6 |
| Believe in a connection between diet and cancer | 1.9 | 1.4–2.9 |

unity. It is within this human unity, or humanity, that hope for humankind lies.

*Our humanity lies in our human unity.*

Without unity, we are all individuals fighting a lonely battle. With it, we can conquer anything. Support groups, then, should elevate and evolve the individuals within them. Support groups should have a task force mentality, objectify patient information, and resolve critical issues for the individual, while at the same time accomplishing this for the group. How can this be done?

## Field Guides

If we are striving to develop a group mentality and can pool our individual talents, we can now enter the phase of synergy. This can be facilitated by using the skills of those who can organize thought and details and share such organizational thinking with others. Manifestations of this are in books, medical articles written for the PC patient and partner, PC-specific newsletters, websites, and Internet-based tools. Suggestions for these elite materials, the field guides, are provided at the end of this protocol.

To summarize these points, a winning strategy for the individual soldier and his corps is to understand as much as possible about his situation in the context of the battle. His PC-fighting training, if you will, mandates his reading the manuals and doing his homework.

*The only place where success comes before work is in the dictionary.*

The concept of synergy empowers this foundational tactic. Therefore, the individual man with PC, his partner, and corps of patients in his support group must be working in the spirit of harmony. In essence, at this crossroads, the motivation for the patient and his partner is simply survival and quality of life. It comes down to the same old story: "We are only as strong as we are united, as weak as we are divided."[73]

## A Key but Often Missing Link

There is no doubt whatsoever that the outcomes of patient longevity and quality of life can be changed for the better with the relatively simple first steps described earlier. The major drawback, as I see it, is bringing the professional health care team into the equation: the third element of PPP. There are reasons for this difficulty that are worthy of some speculation.

The education of the physician is based on competition for scholastic grades in college and in medical school. The ego—the unhealthy aspects of ego—is encouraged by repetitive challenges to the student,

intern, resident, and junior staff regarding esoteric information and medical trivia. Individuals selected out of premedical candidates are often those who are accomplished at memorization of such material. The deans of medical schools are not accomplishing their mission in finding large numbers of outstanding physicians. This lies in the failure of not selecting more students who are driven by the passion to fix the individual and society. True physicians—sincere healers—all have a common denominator: a caring soul that is awed by the wonder of creation and the study of life. With such a constitution, these individuals have a passion to fix problems. This said, the fortunate patients are those able to find the real physicians.

Added to this demanding situation is another serious issue. A physician involved in the totality of cancer medicine cannot adequately cover the waterfront as it relates to all the different types of cancer. A physician must realize his limitations. In the first 10 years of my life as a general medical oncologist diagnosing and treating adult malignant conditions, I have strived to succeed in the impossible task of understanding how to best treat cancers of the breast, colon, lung, stomach, pancreas, ovary, head and neck, and brain, as well as sarcomas, lymphomas, and leukemias.

*A man has got to know his limitations.*

I should have realized from my medical school and postgraduate work on Hodgkin's disease that understanding one malignancy was in itself a formidable task. Becoming a master of 20 different malignancies is an impossible task that does not allow for an optimal outcome for the patient presenting with one particular type of cancer. How can this not be realized by the medical profession and the medical societies? It is as clear as day. Therefore, my advice to the man and his partner faced with a diagnosis of PC is to undertake the challenge of learning as much as possible about the disease, ideally in concert with a proactive and interactive support group and to do this while working with a medical doctor copartner who is hopefully specialized in the management of PC.

## What Specialist to Choose?

Patients and their partners routinely ask me, "Should I seek care under the aegis of a urologist, medical oncologist, or a radiation oncologist?" My initial response is to select an outstanding physician (no matter what his or her label or tag is) who manifests the characteristics of a real healer. With this said, I must be forthright in stating that there is a reality—in general—that the amount of time and focus spent on the patient will be such that the following ranking will most often be found to be true.

Medical Oncologist > Radiation Oncologist > Urologist

Medical oncologists and radiation oncologists are internists who have subspecialized in medical oncology and radiation oncology, respectively. Urologists are specialists in surgery. The nature of these specialties, their modus operandi, is quite different. During the junior and senior years in medical school, while we puzzled about which specialty to choose, one of the classic jokes was:

Surgeons do everything, but know nothing.
Internists know everything, but do nothing.
Psychiatrists do nothing and know nothing.
Pathologists know everything and do everything, but too late.

As silly as these stereotypes are, this joke always brings smiles to the faces of all physicians because there are inherent elements of truth present; surgeons are indeed oriented around operating—that is their modus operandi, literally and figuratively.

Therefore, in the best of all worlds, find a medical oncologist who is intensely focused on PC. Such a physician must have the patient's best interests at heart. This is the ideal teammate for the PC patient and his partner. To paraphrase Scott Peck, M.D., in *A World Waiting to Be Born*, a good act is that which appears good to an ideal observer, "a being who is more knowledgeable than you, more objective than you, yet who still cares."[74]

As with BC care or any life-threatening illness, the primary intervention of the man diagnosed with PC or suspected to have PC should be with an objective, caring, and highly informed physician—the medical oncologist trained in the area of PC. He or she is the least biased concerning which treatment the patient should be considering. He or she has a broader scope of knowledge regarding oncology and internal medicine. He or she will spend more time dealing with concepts as they relate to PC rather than with procedures.

*The good physician knows his patients through and through, and his knowledge is bought dearly. Time, sympathy, and understanding must be lavishly dispensed, but the reward is to be found in that personal bond, which forms the greatest satisfaction of the practice of medicine. One of the essential qualities of the clinician is interest in humanity, for the secret of the care of the patient is in caring for the patient.*

—Sir Francis Weld Peabody, Lecture to Harvard Medical Students, 1927

Some of the statements made above will meet with disapproval by some of my colleagues. Nevertheless, they are true. In today's world, we desperately need more integrity.

Assuming that medicine evolves to a point where physicians specializing in areas such as PC become more plentiful, the PC patient and partner must find a like-hearted and like-minded physician.

The real challenge then is for the medical profession and society to foster an increasing population of physicians meeting these qualifications, for the number of such physicians is far too small to meet the demands of 170 000–200 000 men in the United States each year who are newly diagnosed with PC. An estimate of the number of men with PC in the United States today is somewhere in the 6–9 million range.

## What Does This Mean for Patients?

- To win this battle, you must foster an understanding of the basic biological principles involved in PC. Just as a new recruit into the army becomes savvy by means of education from experienced field officers and fellow soldiers, the new patient with PC (the newbie) needs to obtain information from a supportive cast.

- The PC patient and partner must act as a team, reinforcing its growing understanding and, in time, sharing its knowledge with the community of other PC patients and partners.

- Reality is a tough concept, but an understanding of the limitations of the current medical care of the PC patient is mandatory to prevent major and minor casualties. The diagnosis and initial care plan is often made by the urologist and not a more integrative physician such as a medical oncologist focused on PC. To win a war, one needs a strategist familiar with all aspects of the battle.

- PC necessitates organizational thinking, with strategy and serious focus on biological events as they relate to tumor/host interactions. A successful military campaign requires sound military intelligence. Similarly, a successful medical campaign requires organizational thinking which is rooted in solid medical intelligence.

## 3. MILITARY INFORMATION (INTEL): THE IMPORTANCE OF THE MEDICAL RECORD

### The Medical Record—The Key to Organizational Thinking

Ask a captain of any ship or airplane about the importance of a detailed log or ask a real physician about the crucial role of the medical chart or record and you will get the same response:

*The Chart is a must to ensure the integrity of the Ship.*

The medical record is the patient's story. More important than that, it is the chronology of medical events put to music, and the music is reflected in the biological expressions of the health and disease processes. It is simply a statement of whether or not the orchestra is in harmony or in discord.

The entire clinical story of the patient informs the listening physician; it provides clues to elucidate a fuller story—a closer approximation to the truth—as well as the caring and informed physician can understand it. This really is a manifestation of medical common sense. But, as Thomas Paine once said:

*Common sense is not so common.*

When the PPP team is involved in a logical and common sense approach to analyzing and resolving the patient's problem, a medical symphony evolves. This medical symphony has different movements to it. These movements are separate, and yet they overlap at the same time. The following discussion is described and illustrated fully in Appendix F (starting on page F27) of *A Primer on Prostate Cancer, The Empowered Patient's Guide (The Primer)* by Strum and Pogliano. *The Primer* is available through Life Extension at 1-800-544-4400 or www.lefprostate.org, through amazon.com, and Barnes & Noble. A review of the important movements is described in the following.

**Basic information.** This is routine information to identify the patient. It is, in essence, name, rank, and serial number. It is very basic data that often fall into administrative details, for example, age, birth date, full address information, spouse or significant other's name, and the names of physicians with their specialty and contact information. It should also include any medical diagnoses that are likely to have some interactive role with PC.

**Prediagnostic history.** When we talk about the diagnosis of any kind of cancer, we refer to the microscopic diagnosis obtained after a biopsy or sampling of tissue. Data in the prediagnostic category relate information about biological expressions of PC that precede the diagnosis of PC. Such information might include the dates and PSA values prior to a diagnosis of PC. It might also include results of the free PSA percentage, calculations of PSA velocity (PSAV), and PSA doubling time (PSADT).

**Diagnosis and staging.** This movement relates key baseline information of prognostic significance. This includes the baseline PSA and PAP, the Gleason score, gland volume, core involvement, and clinical stage. The Gleason score must be validated by an expert in PC pathology. This section of the medical record also contains the critical biologic expressions that are used in the algorithm section. Examples of various medical inputs in this category are shown in Table 3.

Therefore, to assess the reality of the military campaign, a good intelligence officer will gather information crucial to understanding the reality of the battle being faced. This part of the winning strategy overlaps with early recognition of the enemy and assessment of enemy strength (and weakness).

For example, in the clinical data shown in Table 3, the patient's baseline PSA (bPSA) of 35 already suggests that we have a minimal chance that the PC is confined to the prostate. The high level of PSA is equivalent with a large tumor volume. These findings are unfortunately reinforced by those of the DRE where the clinical stage was T3a (indicating extracapsular extension on one side of the prostate), along with the findings showing that of the 6 biopsy cores taken, all 6 showed PC. Moreover, the percentage of individual core involvement was also very high with one core showing 100% involvement of PC and the remaining 5 cores having a total of 220% involvement, for an average core involvement of these 5 cores of 44%.[75] Again, this is indicative of a large tumor volume.

The Narayan stage assesses whether the microscopic findings of PC were limited to one side of the prostate gland (B1) versus both sides (B2). Again, the B2 Narayan stage reinforces our understanding of the enemy insofar as a larger tumor volume.[76] This is clearly not going to be a situation where watchful waiting is a rational consideration or one where the first tactic would involve surgery, radiation therapy, or cryosurgery. The PAP blood test is above 3.0, and this finding would point to a high risk of failure from RP[77] or of progression after radiation therapy, even with newer advances involving 3D conformal radiation therapy (3DCRT) or intensity modulated radiation therapy (IMRT) with or without seed implantation.[78]

The gland volume (GV) has relevance to what therapy is selected, as does the American Urologic Association (AUA) symptom index—an objective scoring system that quantifies lower urinary tract symptoms.

The gathering of this medical information allows a clearer understanding of what the patient's outcome is. In a situation that is far more favorable than this one, a patient at the time of diagnosis of PC presents with a PSA of 9 ng/mL with a Gleason score of (3,3) that has been read by an expert in PC pathology. His clinical stage based on the DRE reveals nothing to suggest PC, that is, T1c clinical stage. Moreover, he has a favorable percentage of PC core involvement with less than 50% of the biopsy cores sampled showing cancer.[79]

However, his GV is extremely large at 80 cc. Too often, at the time of the patient's diagnosis via transrectal ultrasound of the prostate, the GV is not recorded by the urologist. The patient's assessment is incomplete because the GV is a critical issue in PC diagnosis and management.[80–83] The large GV in this example would adversely affect the outcome of the patient undergoing treatment with radiation therapy (external beam and/or brachytherapy) or cryosurgery.[84–88] This would be especially true in the setting of an AUA symptom index greater than 20, a maximum urine flow of 10 mL per second or less, and even a GV greater than 40 g or cc.[89] However, controversy in this area remains.[90]

These data inputs are evolving as we understand more and more about the biological story and what is most important for a successful clinical outcome.

**Data used for algorithms and nomograms.** The gathering of this medical information is important to supply at baseline prior to any treatment. This information is critical in the treatment strategy selected by the PPP team. The calculations involved in such algorithms have been simplified by the use of software programs such as PC Tools I and II on websites such as the PCRI (Prostate Cancer Research Institute) at www.pcri.org and Kattan nomogram at www.mskcc.org.

The key baseline data necessary for many of the standard algorithms/nomograms currently in use include the data inputs mentioned in the Diagnosis and Staging section. Other data that may become available during the PC patient's course are applicable to additional algorithms involving PSA recurrence after surgery or radiation. This would involve Gleason score at RP, ploidy (DNA analysis) at RP, presence or absence of lymph node involvement at RP, PSAV and PSADT after RP, time to PSA recurrence after RP, history of use of ADT (androgen deprivation therapy), dose of RT employed, and other data. The risk assessment provided by the use of algorithms and nomograms is discussed in more detail in Section 5, Risk Assessment of the PC Patient.

**A detailed clinical chronological review (DCCR).** In my opinion, this is the most important part of the medical record for the PC patient. This is because the DCCR represents an incorporation of all prior information into a medical story that is clear to the physician, patient, and his partner (PPP). The DCCR uses a combination of a timeline and information relating to major events to present the key crossroads in the patient's history as it relates to PC. Treatments are designated as "Rx" and bolded for emphasis.

---

**Table 3: An Example of Data Important in the Diagnostic and Staging Phase of PC**

This is a hypothetical data set from a patient diagnosed with PC on 1/12/99. It objectifies key points of medical information by means of presenting this in a table with standard categories known to be of significance in the outcome of PC care.

| 1/12/1999 | 35 | 3.5 | 6/6 | (4,3) | (4,3) | Diagnostic Labs | Bostwick |
|---|---|---|---|---|---|---|---|
| PC diagnosis date | bPSA | bPAP | Cores with PC/ cores biopsied | Gleason score (GS) original | Gleason score expert review | Original GS Reviewer ID | Expert GS Reviewer ID |
| T3a | 80 cc | Diploid | 100% | 10.19 | Negative | Positive* | Negative |
| Clinical stage (CS) | Gland volume (GV) | Ploidy | % greatest core involved | Tumor volume calculation | Bone scan + vs – | ProstaScint scan + vs – | CT scan + vs – |
| B2 | 0.44 | 4 | 320% | Misc: | | | |
| Narayan stage | PSA density | AUA score | Sum % all cores involved | ErMRI/spec info: Not Done | | | |

\* Uptake of isotope in right obturator and right internal iliac lymph nodes (done at University Hospitals of Cleveland).
Staging specifics: indicate dates, findings (if abnormal); additional miscellaneous information of importance

Ideally, the PPP add information to this part of the PC medical record, encouraging its use as an important navigational tool for the entire team. Using the DCCR as a means of conveying medical information focuses energy on areas of concern. This avoids generic suggestions, for example, operate, radiate, or do nothing, and thus it engenders the need for substantial evidence to support the choice(s) of particular evaluations and/or treatments. Such an approach would help improve the outcome of the patient and ease his path to that outcome. This is the essence of good treatment strategy. You must do your homework. All of this is illustrated in *The Primer*.

**Flow sheets (a powerful graphic tool that warrants emphasis).** Flow sheets are critical in understanding the patient's response to treatment. Flow sheets, compulsively maintained, detail the treatment strategy and its response. The flow sheet, accurately kept by the physician, and ideally understood by the patient and his partner, is the nitty-gritty worksheet that conveys the success or lack of success of treatment.

Flow sheets are critical to the management of any patient, no matter what illness the PPP may encounter. Unfortunately, the concepts involved with flow sheets although simple, are often totally missed by many doctors. The flow sheet employs the concept of time in relation to treatment and correlates this with parameters (indicators) of response.

Simply put, the flow sheet gives a timetable of the patient's medications and correlates them with laboratory and radiologic studies (response parameters) to point out any changes reflecting either the presence or absence of the desired biological effect. At the same time, body system functions are monitored using laboratory tests. This monitors any developing drug toxicity or tissue damage that may be due to the treatment and/or disease. An example of this would be John Doe treated with flutamide and Lupron® for metastatic PC. An example of his flow sheet is shown in part in Tables 4A and 4B (and in full on page F37 of *The Primer*).

Note how the flow sheet acts as a treatment record and how the columns show the time-related effects of therapy on the complete blood count (CBC) (hematocrit dropping), which was due to androgen-deprivation therapy (ADT). The desired therapeutic effect on the PSA is also clearly shown. The worsening liver function test (SGPT, a liver enzyme) is forecasting problems secondary to liver toxicity, which may be due to flutamide. The flow sheet is declaring this in advance because the physician or patient can see the test result going from low normal to high normal before entering the flagged abnormal range. Alkaline phosphatase (due to bone

metastases) is showing a response to ADT and is falling from the initial 456 toward the normal range (= 125). Even after reaching the normal range, the alkaline phosphatase continues to drop lower. The concepts here relate to baseline, trends, the issue of changes within the normal range, and treatment versus response parameter.

The empowered patient and partner obtain hard copies of any laboratory data generated in the physician's office along with copies of any flow sheets. The team is encouraged to carefully review and understand these forms. A true physician welcomes such a request. The same applies to all consultation reports.

**Summary/surveillance sheets.** Lastly, as part of medical event recording, an overall assessment of the patient's total health is needed. While the patient may be having a great response to his PC treatment, his bone mineral density may be worsening.[91] If the medical campaign is to be successful, the battle needs to be won on all fronts.

Table 5 is an example of what I have used in medical practice to monitor patients. It makes little sense to put a patient through intensive treatment for PC if his cardiovascular status is deteriorating[92] or if he has a second malignancy[93] that has gone undiagnosed because of a tunnel-vision approach to the patient's care. Table 5 presents this concept of surveillance and reminds the PPP when the last such test was performed. The patient's flow sheets would show the actual results of such examinations.

## What Does This Mean for Patients?

- To win the battle against PC, you must obtain information that is highly important in deciding the outcome of this biological interaction. Medical intelligence (Intel) is as important to the survival of the patient as military intelligence is to the survival of the soldier and the success of the campaign.

- The PC patient and partner must again act as a team, reinforcing each other with their growing knowledge. In time, for the paradigm to be fulfilled, they must share this newfound knowledge with the community of other PC patients and partners.

- Being aware of the importance of medical Intel gathering and how it is organized, the patient and partner can work together with their fellows to extend influence that will affect the nature of information gathering and record keeping done by physicians.

## Table 4A:   The Flow Sheet Objectifies Medical Intel

This is a hypothetical example of a flow sheet that should be employed in the care of all patients, whether or not they have PC. This objective approach to care presents the variables of TIME and MEDICATIONS or other TREATMENTS used in the context of PARAMETERS OF OUTCOME. Such an objective correlation enables us to better decide whether the treatment is a success. The inclusion of critical laboratory data that reflect whether the medical campaign is going as planned is shown in Part A of this form. Additional parameters to tell us about outcomes that might relate to radiologic and/or pathology studies are shown in Table 4B.

| Month/Day | 2/1 | 2/28 | 3/28 | 4/25 | 5/23 |
|---|---|---|---|---|---|
| Flutamide | 250 mg TID | 3 | 3 | Hole | Resume |
| Lupron | 7.5 mg | 7.5 mg | 7.5 mg | 7.5 mg | 7.5 mg |
| Proscar® | 5 mg BID | 3 | 3 | 3 | 3 |
| Fosamax® | | | 70 mg/wk | 3 | 3 |
| Procrit® | 10 K q WK | 3 | Hold | 3 | 3 |
| Vasotec® | 5 mg QD | 3 | 3 | 3 | 3 |
| Prilosec | 20 mg QD | 3 | 3 | 3 | 3 |
| Silymarin | | | | 200 mg QD | |
| WBC | 5.5 | 5.9 | 5.7 | 6.3 | 6.0 |
| PMNs I LYMPHS | I | I | I | I | I |
| HCT % | 37 | 36 | 39 | 37 | 35 |
| PLATELETS | 180 | 212 | 188 | 234 | 177 |
| Na⁺ I K⁺ | I | I | I | I | I |
| BUN I CREAT | I | I | I | | I |
| GLUCOSE/ LDH | | | | | |
| CA⁺⁺ I PHOS⁻ | I | I | I | I | I |
| Albumin I Globulin | I | I | I | I | I |
| Bilirubin I Alk PHOS | I 456 | I 245 | I 188 | I 143 | I 92 |
| SGOT I SGPT | 18 I 18 | 20 I 24 | 26 I 33 | 55 I 78 | 35 I 40 |
| PSA I PAP | 122 I 29 | 60 I 12 | 14 I 2.5 | 0.5 I 2.2 | <0.05 I 2.0 |
| TESTO I SHBG | 345 I | <20 I | <20 I | I | I |
| PYRILINKS-D (Dpd) | 4.3 | | 6.5 | 4.0 | |
| DHEA-S I Androstenedione | 89 I 125 | I | I | I | I |
| Prolactin I DHT | 8.9 I 55 | I | I <30 | I | I |
| CEA I CGA I NSE | 2.0 I 4.8 I 7.8 | I | I | I | I |
| Weight | 160 | 162 | 163 | 168 | 170 |

## Table 4B:   The Flow Sheet (Back Side)

The reverse side of the flow sheet is shown in part. It reflects the same concept of using a parameter—a biological endpoint—as a measuring stick to gauge the results of the selected therapy. Again, this objectifies what is being done and reduces personal bias. The flow sheets, if attended to correctly and diligently, answer this question: "Is the treatment being used on me working?"
Chest X-rays

1/23/01: normal
9/17/01: normal

Endorectal MRI + Spectroscopy; Plain MRI, CT (Specify)
CT HEAD:
CT CHEST:
CT Abdomen/ Pelvis: 9/17/01 no lymph node enlargement in pelvis or abdomen; liver normal
ENDORECTAL MRI + SPECTROSCOPY: 1/15/01: gland volume 24 cc, no ECE, concordant MRI and MRS abnormalities in R and
    L base, R midgland and R apex. No regional nodes seen.
Ultrasound (Including TRUSP)
12/22/99: gland volume 30 cc; hypoechoic lesions in R and L base; capsule intact, no SV involvement
Nuclear Medicine (BS, bone scan; PS, ProstaScint scan; PET, positron emission tomography)
BS #1: 1/22/01: No abnormal uptake in bones, normal scan
Pathology Reports (Include Pathology Number)

- In an enlightened world, and certainly in a society with today's technological advances, physicians should be graded on their care of patients. This should be carried out by an on-site task force that surveys the medical records and the actual hands-on care delivered by physicians to their patients in the medical office and in the hospital.

**Table 5: Summary/Surveillance Form**

| Procedure | Date | Date | Date | Date | Date | Date | Date | Date |
|---|---|---|---|---|---|---|---|---|
| Physical Exam | | | | | | | | |
| DRE | | | | | | | | |
| Past/Fam/Soc Hx | | | | | | | | |
| Chest X-ray | | | | | | | | |
| EKG | | | | | | | | |
| Urine Analysis | | | | | | | | |
| OB X 3 | | | | | | | | |
| Colonoscopy | | | | | | | | |
| Pyrilinks-D | | | | | | | | |
| Bone density | | | | | | | | |
| ProstaScint | | | | | | | | |
| Bone Scan | | | | | | | | |
| Stress EKG | | | | | | | | |
| Eye Exam | | | | | | | | |
| Skin Exam | | | | | | | | |
| US-TSH | | | | | | | | |
| Homocysteine | | | | | | | | |
| Ferritin | | | | | | | | |
| Flu Vaccine | | | | | | | | |
| Pneumovax | | | | | | | | |

# 4. EARLY RECOGNITION OF ENEMY ACTIVITY: EARLY DIAGNOSIS OF PC

In the prior 3 sections, I have presented:

- The use of measures that have been shown to prevent PC
- Medical references for using preventive measures in PC
- The need for interactive assistance in obtaining basic medical comprehension and the associated reference tools that can provide this
- How an organized medical log ties all relevant information together in an integrative fashion

Given this groundwork, what can be said about an early diagnosis of PC?

It seems uncanny that today we are still debating the virtues of an early diagnosis of PC by means of PSA-associated tools and the DRE. I would chalk this up as a reflection of the old saying:

*Don't confuse the message with the messenger.*

or its alternate expression,

*Don't confuse the mission with the man.*

The problem is not with the early diagnosis of this disease but with what we do with the realization of such a diagnosis in the following contexts:

**The patient's overall biological setting**

1. The skills and lack of skills of the medical professionals available to the patient
2. The constraints, if any, of the patient's personal finances or medical insurance

**The patient's wishes in response to such a diagnosis**

For example, if we were to discuss an 85-year-old man with far-advanced Alzheimer's disease, it makes no sense to pursue a diagnosis of PC unless we have reasons to believe that such a diagnosis would substantially benefit the patient. In a different situation, if a patient is diagnosed with PC and his biological findings, for example, PSA velocity and doubling times, indicate a very small tumor volume and stability of the biological process, then both nutritional and lifestyle changes can be suggested to slow the biological process. This often allows the patient to outlive the PC. We can use a strategy of watchful waiting (WW). WW does not mean ignoring biological parameters. Perhaps the term WW should have been replaced long ago with the term objectified ongoing observation (OOO). Currently, more and more medical articles are pointing out the value of using a rational approach to OOO by listening to the biology of PC.[94–100]

We should not tell patients that making a diagnosis of PC is dangerous because of the morbidity and mortality of various invasive therapies when such therapies in the hands of the upper echelon of medical practitioners are not at all significantly associated with such adverse findings in the overwhelming majority of patients.[101,102]

One paradox of our modern times is the involvement of insurance carriers in the medical decision-making processes such as screening for PC, the staging of PC, and what treatment choices are available to the patient. It is not so surprising that the insurance companies wish to control this, but it is incredibly painful to observe that the physicians working for such companies would allow their professional training and judgment to be overridden by the economic needs of the insurance carrier. I believe that this reflects a conflict of interest on the part of those physicians. In my opinion, this conduct violates the Hippocratic Oath and is certainly a violation of human rights that is being tacitly accepted and therefore condoned in a supposedly sophisticated society.

Ironically, if the advisers to those insurance companies would read medical literature more carefully, they would be utilizing ways to prevent significant disease, diagnose disease early when present, and avoid the very expensive costs associated with a late diagnosis of PC and other diseases. I would attribute this to short-term vision and being "penny-wise and pound-foolish." In my experience, the frightening aspect of this control over disease management by some insurance companies is that they are deferring active treatment until the patient is so far advanced that death often precedes any chance to do the patient good. I believe that the economics of the insurance carrier has invoked the pathologic concept that "death is cost-effective." I have seen this too often to regard it as an aberration in dealing with organizations so motivated. Consumer advocacy and safeguarding are badly needed. The expression *caveat emptor* or "let the buyer beware" is operative here.

The patient's wishes—that is, the informed and educated patient and partner's wishes—must be taken into account. One unusual but true story that relates to this is that of a patient who was recently diagnosed with PC. His sex life was not at all important to him in comparison to the necessity of his feeling assured that the entire prostate gland and surrounding tissues were removed at the time of RP. Although he expressed this to his physician, and specifically his decision not to have a nerve-sparing procedure, the patient was disappointed and depressed when he realized that he had been subjected to a bilateral nerve-sparing procedure. This was not what the patient wanted. This is the only time that I have personally witnessed a man who was unhappy about having erections after a RP. The patient's wishes had been discounted and ignored by the physician.

With all of these situations discussed, what relatively simple and inexpensive tools can be used to discern that PC might be present?

## PSA Density Higher Than 0.15 ng/cc Should Raise Concern about PC

If a determination of the volume of the prostate has been made by ultrasound or some other radiologic technique, we can calculate the PSA density (PSAD) or the amount of PSA (expressed in nanograms) for each cubic centimeter of the prostate volume. The PSAD is simply the serum PSA value divided by an accurate gland volume determination.

$$PSAD = Serum\ PSA \div Gland\ Volume\ (per\ TRUSP\ or\ Endorectal\ MRI)$$

Some physicians are incredibly astute in having the ability to estimate the gland volume within 10% of more objective gland volume determinations that are obtained using radiologic studies such as transrectal ultrasound of the prostate (TRUSP) or endorectal magnetic resonance imaging (endorectal MRI). PSAD results of 0.15 ng/cc or greater are more consistent with a diagnosis of PC than if the PSAD is less than this.[103–105] There is very little in medicine that is an absolute guarantee, a definite yes or no. Therefore, it is strongly suggested that a combination of modalities be used to enhance the accuracy of any kind of assessment. This combined modality analysis was the basis for the breakthrough approaches of Oesterling[106] and Partin[107] and the many subsequent analyses that we use in a comprehensive risk assessment for the individual patient.

## PSAD of Transition Zone More Accurate Than PSAD for Diagnosis of PC

A recent improvement to the value of the PSAD is doing a PSAD of the transition zone (TZ) of the prostate; this is called PSAD-TZ. The zonal anatomy of the

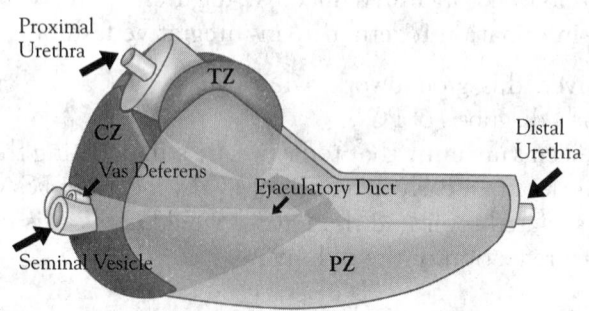

**Figure 4. The Zonal Anatomy of the Prostate.** The prostate gland shown here is a lateral or side view, as if the patient were being viewed from his right side. The Transition Zone (TZ) is on both sides of the proximal portion of the urethra and runs parallel to this portion of the urinary channel. The TZ is separated from the Central Zone (CZ) and Peripheral Zones (PZ) by fibro-muscular tissue called the "surgical capsule." The TZ increases in the aging male when benign prostatic hyperplasia (BPH) occurs. (Modified from Lee and Torp-Pedersen.[108])

prostate was proposed originally by McNeal.[109] He divided the prostate into 3 glandular zones: transition, central, and peripheral zones (see Figure 4). The PSAD-TZ has been shown to be more accurate than a simple PSAD of the entire prostate gland.

PSAD-TZ = Serum PSA ÷ Gland Volume (per TRUSP or Endorectal MRI of TZ)

In a prospective study of 559 patients, 217 men with PC and 342 with histologically confirmed benign prostatic hyperplasia (BPH) were evaluated with PSA, PSAD, PSAD-TZ, and percent free PSA. Multivariate analysis and ROC curves showed that PSA-TZ and percent free PSA (f/t PSA) were the most powerful and highly significant predictors of PC. Areas under the receiver operating characteristics (ROC) curve for PSA-TZ and percent free PSA were 0.827 and 0.778, respectively ($p = 0.01$). The combination of f/t PSA with PSA-TZ (area under curve [AUC] = 88.1%) significantly increased the AUC as compared to each of the other parameters alone as well as their combination ($p = 0.02$). The next best combinations were PSA-TZ + PSAD, PSA-TZ + PSA, and f/t PSA + PSA.

**Note:** *Accuracy is measured by the area under the ROC curve. An area of 1 represents a perfect test: an area of 0.5 represents a worthless test. A rough guide for classifying the accuracy of a diagnostic test is the traditional academic point system:*

0.90–1 = excellent

0.80–0.90 = good

0.70–0.80 = fair

0.60–0.70 = poor

0.50–0.60 = fail

See review in Tape TG: Interpreting diagnostic tests, University of Nebraska Medical Center at http://gim.unmc.edu/dxtests/ROC3.htm.

With regard to an individual test, PSA-TZ followed by f/t PSA and PSAD were the most powerful single predictors of PC in patients having a serum PSA between 4–10 ng/mL. The f/t PSA plus PSA-TZ was the most effective combination.[110] The same findings held true for PSA values of 2.5–4 ng/mL.[111]

## PSA Velocity Reflects the Biological Activity of the PC Process

The PSAV is a statement of how fast the PSA is accelerating. It is the rate of change of PSA calculated per year of time. Therefore, if the PSA on 1/1/98 was 0.5 ng/mL and on 7/1/98 it was 1.0 ng/mL and then rose to 2.0 ng/mL on 1/1/99, the PSAV would be 1.5 ng/mL per year. The PSADT would be 6 months because the PSA is consistently doubling every 6 months. The faster the PSAV, the shorter the PSADT. Such PSA kinetics are additional inputs of information for the observant physician and/or the empowered patient and partner. Results of such tests should raise or lower suspicion about the presence of a pathologic process, that is, PC.[112–114] It is important to emphasize that combining multiple sensory, or data inputs, enhances our understanding of the biology of disease. If it looks like a zebra, walks like a zebra, and has stripes, it probably is a zebra. The ability to manipulate multiple sensory inputs into an action plan for improved diagnosis and survival is a hallmark of higher-level thinking. Too often, in medicine or in life, we try to hang all of our hats on one hook. The PSAV has also been shown to be an important determinant in survival in patients with Androgen Independent PC (AIPC) or so-called hormone refractory PC.[115]

The more data points in these determinations and the longer the time period over which a trend is maintained, the greater the validity of such calculations.[116,117] The important concept underlying the above is the persistent generation of PSA by the tumor cell population reflecting itself in the bloodstream and determined by repeated testing.

## PSA Doubling Time Reflects Tumor Growth

The PSAV tells us how rapidly the PSA is increasing per year. The PSADT tells us the length in months it takes for the PSA to double in amount. All of the mathematical derivatives of serial PSA testing are expressing the biological process.[118] The average PSADT of PC is approximately 48 months, or 4 years. Men with an absolutely healthy prostate gland do not have any appreciable PSADT; their PSA levels remain essentially flat over decades of observation. Men with BPH have very slow PSA doubling times—usually over 12 years.

Men presenting with historical data showing PSADT of less than 12 years must be presumed to have PC until proven otherwise.[119] The PSADT in men with histologically established PC is a valuable tool in:

- The management of PC (watchful waiting versus active treatment)[100,120,121]

- The prediction of extent or stage of disease[122]

- The correlation of PSADT with normal versus abnormal DNA (ploidy)[123]

- The probability of local recurrence and metastatic disease after local treatment[124-127]

The same concept of the PSA doubling time paralleling the biological growth rate of the tumor may be applied to other biological markers of PC malignancy. Biomarkers such as PAP (prostatic acid phosphatase), CEA (carcino-embryonic antigen), CGA (chromogranin A), and NSE (neuron-specific enolase) may be expressed in PC variants that usually are associated with high Gleason scores; for example, 8–10.[128,129] In such patients, the expression of PSA in the blood or serum may not be great. This has been referred to as the PSA leak.[130] The PSA leak in high Gleason score PC is relatively low. For example, a Gleason score of 10 has a PSA leak of approximately 1.0 mg/cc versus 4.0 mg/cc for a Gleason score of 6.

Therefore, in patients with a Gleason score of 8–10, the PSA becomes less of a reliable marker of disease activity. Some tumors may show evidence of dedifferentiation and express relatively little PSA despite other findings of PC activity such as a progressive bone scan, bone pain, and elevations in alkaline phosphatase and lactic dehydrogenase (LDH) as well as other tests. This is uncommonly seen in newly diagnosed PC unless the disease has been diagnosed late and the chance of mutation affecting the PC population has occurred. Such patients with a late diagnosis often present with PSA levels greater than 20 and not uncommonly greater than 50. The probability of disease outside the prostate is greater in such patients, again reflecting the more aggressive nature of the PC cell population.

Therefore, we learn about a tumor based on the biological activity it manifests. The same principle involving biomarker kinetics has value in the monitoring of patients with various common malignancies

### Table 6. Biomarkers That May Reflect Tumor Activity in Major Cancers and Blood Diseases

Biomarkers are products of the tumor cell that play a functional role in the growth, spread, or sustenance of the tumor cell population. As tumor activity increases, tumor volume also increases, which often is mirrored in the level of the biomarker.

| Cancer Type | Major Marker(s) | Secondary Marker(s) |
|---|---|---|
| Prostate | PSA, PAP, testosterone, prolactin | CGA, CEA, NSE, TGF-b1, IL-6sR, CA 125 |
| Breast | CA-15-3, CA 27-29, CEA, TPA | BCA225, CA 549, MCA |
| Lung (non–small-cell lung cancer) | CEA, CA-125 | |
| Lung (small cell lung cancer) | CGA, NSE | |
| Colon | CEA, CA19-9, CA 72-4 | |
| Gastric | CEA, CA 19-9 | CA 72-4 |
| Pancreatic | CEA, CA-19-9 | CA 72-4 |
| Testicular | AFP, bHCG | |
| Ovarian | CA-125 | DM-70K |
| Lymphoma | IL2-receptors, LDH | TK |
| Myeloma | IgG, IgA, IgM, light chains | IgD, IgE |
| Hepatocellular carcinoma | AFP | |

### Table 7: Ejaculation Increases the Serum Prostate-Specific Antigen Concentration[132]

A patient undergoing PSA testing might be inadvertently channeled into a full PC work-up—with biopsies—if attention was not paid to his history of sexual activity with ejaculation prior to the drawing of the blood sample for PSA. If his apparent PSA was 2.0, this effect is substantial in all time periods up to 48 hours. If the apparent PSA was 2.5, the corrected PSA would only have significance for the ejaculation 1 hour prior to laboratory testing. The bottom line is: Do not do PSA testing within the 48-hour period following ejaculation.

| Apparent PSA (ng/mL) | Hour(s) Prior to PSA Testing When Ejaculation Occurred | Corrected PSA (ng/mL) |
|---|---|---|
| 2.0 | 1 | 1.2 |
| | 6 | 1.7 |
| | 24 | 1.8 |
| | 48 | 1.6 |
| 2.5 | 1 | 1.7 |
| | 6 | 2.2 |
| | 24 | 2.3 |
| | 48 | 2.1 |

(see Table 6). Important concepts in the use of biologic markers are to obtain blood at baseline after the diagnosis is established to see what markers the tumor is producing and to monitor the patient's course after treatment to ensure that any elevated marker(s) have returned to normal levels and that they remain there.[131] This is the same principle used in the evaluation of PC and monitoring the response to all types of therapy. This is a simple tool that should be regarded as an excellent means of assessing biological activity.

## Effect of Pressure on the Prostate Gland and PSA Elevation

In testing the PSA over periods of time, we hope that the same laboratory is being used and that confounding circumstances are not present. The latter would include physical activity that puts pressure on the prostate and falsely elevates the PSA, such as bicycle riding, motorcycle and horseback riding, and any instrumentation of the rectum, such as an endorectal ultrasound probe or endorectal MRI study.[133] The issue of the effect of strenuous exercise unrelated to pressure on the prostate gland and elevation of PSA readings remains controversial. Most studies do not show any elevation of PSA based on exercise alone,[134] and some studies report no effect of bike riding on elevating the PSA.[135]

Knowing that the PSA obtained is a valid result and that it was not influenced by an activity that puts vigorous pressure on the prostate or by instrumentation of the rectum that affects the nearby prostate has serious implications relating to the presence of PC.

## Ejaculation Can Increase the PSA

Moreover, we know that ejaculation within 48 hours preceding the PSA blood draw can elevate the PSA. The closer the time of ejaculation prior to obtaining the PSA specimen, the more falsely elevated the PSA will be.[133]

Table 7 shows a hypothetical patient with first-time PSA values of 2.0–2.5, where the effects on ejaculation may have accounted for elevations in PSA leading to further investigations (including prostate biopsies) that might have been unnecessary.

## Importance of the First-Time PSA Value

The importance of obtaining a valid PSA determination is pertinent to whether a physician suggests further studies that may involve invasive procedures such as transrectal ultrasound with biopsies of the prostate. The absolute value of the first-time PSA also has implications insofar as the presence or absence of PC. A first-time PSA value of less than 2.0 ng/mL is uncommonly associated with PC.[136,137]

In a study of 11 022 subjects with an initial PSA of less than 2 ng/mL, fewer than 2.6% (287) converted to a PSA of 4 ng/mL during the 3-year follow-up period. In contrast, in 1912 subjects with initial PSAs of 2.0–2.99 and in 1147 subjects with initial PSAs of 3.0–3.99, the conversion rate to a PSA of 4.0 or higher was 23.6% and 66.0%, respectively[136] (see Table 8).

## Free PSA Percentage

One additional biological consideration in the prediagnostic phase of PC is the understanding that the total PSA is composed of subunits that have special significance in raising or lowering our index of suspicion about the presence of PC. Consider an analogy of PSA being like a pepperoni pizza with the normal production of PSA from benign prostate cells represented by the basic pizza dough and cheese; this is the free PSA or benign-related PSA. The PSA associated with PC is reflected by the pepperoni; this is the complexed PSA or cancer-related PSA. The relationship of benign-related PSA to cancer-related PSA is commercially measured in a test called the free PSA percentage, which essentially reflects the ratio of benign-related PSA (free PSA) to total PSA (free plus complexed PSA).

Therefore, the greater the amount of complexed PSA there is, the lower the free PSA percentage and the more concerned we are that PC is present. The larger the amount of free PSA, the more likely the process is a benign-related one. The statistical cut-off

**Table 8: First-Time PSA Levels Relate to Risk of Progressive PSA Rise and PC Diagnosis**

If the first PSA level is less than 1.0 or 2.0, one has only a 1.2% or 4.5% chance of the PSA rising to 4.0 within the following 3 years, respectively. At first-time PSA levels of up to 2.99 or 3.99, the risk increases to 23.6% and 66%, respectively.

| | First-Time PSA Ranges in Nanograms per Milliliter (ng/mL) | | | |
| | 0–0.99 | 1–1.99 | 2–2.99 | 3–3.99 |
|---|---|---|---|---|
| Patient Number | 6378 | 4644 | 1912 | 1147 |
| Mean Age | 62.8 | 63.4 | 64.5 | 64.6 |
| PSA = 4.0 by Year 3* Number (%) | 77 (1.2%) | 210 (4.5%) | 451 (23.6%) | 757 (66.0%) |

*Cumulative by year.

point where we feel less concerned that PC is present is at a free PSA percentage of 25% or higher.[138]

The free PSA percentage is a valid test when the PSA is as low as 2.51 ng/mL.[139] The free PSA percentage can even be used at total PSA levels as low as 2.0 ng/mL when special statistical tools (artificial neural nets) are employed to analyze clinical and laboratory patterns associated with a high probability of PC.[140] The combination of free PSA percentage with other tools such as PSAD-TZ is a highly accurate method to diagnose PC and is independent of the potentially confounding factors of age and prostate gland volume (to be discussed later).[112]

Table 9 should be helpful to those concerned about a diagnosis of PC and whether their risk of having PC should justify undergoing a TRUSP with guided biopsies of the prostate gland.[141]

The following data are based on a study population of 428 men. This table shows only results in the PSA ranges 2.5–4.0 and 4.1–10.0. Readers may refer to the original publication[141] or to the software program at www.pcri.org (PC Tools I) if their particular data fall outside of that presented in Table 9. Note that for a specific total PSA range and free PSA percentage, the risk of PC increases with increasing age groups.

## The Dimension of Time—The Importance of Trends

The so-called prediagnostic history often provides laboratory information that when properly analyzed indicates a high probability that PC was already present but unfortunately not suspected or perhaps not pursued to establish an earlier diagnosis. We know, for example, that PSAV determinations of greater than 0.75 ng/mL a year should raise a red flag as to the presence of PC. For accuracy in analysis, such calculations should be made using one PSA assay, for example, Tosoh, DPC, Hybritech, and Bayer, among others, which is being run in the same laboratory facility.

PSAV and PSADT determinations are most valid when the PSA testing interval selected for the analysis is approximately 6 months or more. However, what is important to stress in this context is the PSA trend or slope over time. Serial PSA values showing a progressive increase in PSA should always raise concern that a biological process is occurring. It is the rapidity of such an increase that will suggest if this is a malignant or a benign process.[142]

PSA increases over time associated with a healthy prostate are tiny. They amount to average increases of less than 0.1 ng/mL a year (range 0.055–0.128) of PSA in the blood.[143–145] Therefore, the use of PSAV thresholds of greater than 0.75 ng/mL a year is quite generous in raising concern about the presence of PC. Table 10 shows my PSA values over the course of 10 years.

The PSA trend or slope (also referred to as PSA kinetics or dynamics) is a far more important biological expression than any one PSA absolute value. Such kinetic values express active changes in the status of the PC

**Table 9:** Correlation of Patient Age, Total PSA, and Free PSA Percentage with the Probability of Having PC

| Patient Age | Total PSA | Percentage of Free PSA | | | |
| | | 6.0–6.9% | 7.0–14.9% | 15.0–25% | >25% |
| | | Probability of Prostate Cancer (%) | | | |
|---|---|---|---|---|---|
| 50–59 | 2.5–4.0 | 84 | 23 | 10 | 2 |
| 60–70 | 2.5–4.0 | 94 | 47 | 25 | 6 |
| 71 and older | 2.5–4.0 | 96 | 57 | 33 | 9 |
| 50–59 | 4.1–10.0 | 87 | 28 | 12 | 3 |
| 60–70 | 4.1–10.0 | 95 | 52 | 29 | 7 |
| 71 and older | 4.1–10.0 | 97 | 62 | 38 | 11 |

**Table 10:** Stability of PSA Over 10 Years of Testing in Dr. Stephen Strum

These PSA values were obtained over a 10-year span. They show minimal changes, which are consistent with the known literature on minute increases in PSA in the healthy prostate. The PSA slope in such situations is essentially flat. Earlier PSA levels dating back to 1987 were in the 0.7–0.8 range, but unfortunately these records were lost by Dr. Strum's former primary physician. (Always keep a backup of your medical records!)

| Date | 11/2/92 | 3/5/94 | 5/1/94 | 4/2/95 | 5/17/96 | 4/13/97 | 1/26/98 | 2/19/98 | 5/14/99 |
|---|---|---|---|---|---|---|---|---|---|
| PSA | 0.75 | 0.83 | 0.83 | 1.0 | 0.82 | 0.7 | 0.75 | 0.83 | 0.6 |
| Date | 8/4/99 | 9/6/00 | 8/31/01 | 9/4/02 | | | | | |
| PSA | 0.73 | 0.571 | 0.66 | 0.75 | | | | | |

patient over the dimension of time. Realizing that aberrations in laboratory testing do occur should mandate that, when a major change is found in a laboratory test result, repeat testing for validation purposes should be required until a definite trend is clearly seen. Too often, patients with PC are ready to make major changes in their evaluation or management based on one or two PSA changes. This also applies to other biomarkers such as PAP (prostatic acid phosphatase), CGA (chromogranin A), CEA (carcinoembryonic antigen), and NSE (neuron-specific enolase), which the physician may be using to monitor the PC patient.

TRENDS ARE IMPORTANT IN BOTH THE EVALUATION AND MANAGEMENT OF ANY ILLNESS—INCLUDING PROSTATE CANCER.

## What Does This Mean for Patients?

In prior paragraphs, it was emphasized that first-time PSA levels of less than 2.0 are uncommonly associated with PC and that, in such patients, PSA testing can be done every 2–3 years. Patients with first-time values of PSA that are less than 4.0 ng/mL but at least 2.0 ng/mL should not be regarded as having a PSA within the normal range. The guidelines for a normal first-time PSA are up to 1.9 ng/mL.

It was also pointed out that the PSA and its derivatives, such as PSAV, PSADT, PSAD (total gland and for transition zone), and free PSA percentage, are instrumental in our understanding of biological reality. It is akin to the story of the three blind men feeling different parts of one elephant and describing 3 entirely different animals. What is needed in the elephant story, in the management of PC and other health issues, in a military campaign, and in the management of any world challenge, is an integrative way of thinking, which fosters unified concepts and embodies principles of synergy and harmony.

We also presented findings on the free PSA percentage; it can be done on PSA levels as low as 2.0. This finding, coupled with the information on first-time PSA readings being significant when the PSA is found to be 2.0 or higher, should lead to an earlier diagnosis of PC and greater probability of cure.

Additional reading on the subjects of free PSA, PSADT, and PSAV can be found in *The Primer* published by Life Extension Media and available at www.lef.org.

## 5. RISK ASSESSMENT OF THE PC PATIENT

Once a diagnosis of PC is established by means of tissue biopsy and microscopic findings showing PC, the foundation of the medical record should have further information added to it to allow for an even greater understanding of the patient's true status. In this context, status refers to the actual extent of disease, or stage of disease. Is the PC really confined to the prostate gland or does it penetrate the capsule of the prostate or perhaps invade local surrounding tissues such as the seminal vesicles and nearby lymph nodes? Are there any clues that the PC has spread or metastasized to more distant lymph nodes or bone?

The orientation of most specialists will be toward recommending a local therapy to eradicate PC within the gland. This is the essence of the reasoning behind the surgical removal of the prostate—RP. The other approaches toward treating PC with curative intent may be slightly more regional, but most are still designed to primarily treat the prostate gland. For example, external beam radiation therapy (EBRT) will include not only the prostate gland itself, but also a margin around the gland to kill any tumor cells that may be in this area trying to escape and spread to more distant sites. The same is true for the iceballs created by cryosurgery.[146] The critical concept here is that local measures treat local disease. The determination of the true extent or stage of the disease is one of the critical variables in the strategy of successful treatment of PC. For example, if the disease is present outside the prostate gland in tissues such as the seminal vesicle or nearby regional lymph nodes (the obturator or internal iliac lymph nodes), an RP will have a significantly diminished chance in curing the patient with PC. The same is true for RT or cryosurgery. For such therapies to have a great chance of cure, the cancer must be within the scope of the scalpel, boundaries of the radiation ports of therapy, and periphery of the iceball(s) created by cryosurgery.

An additional limiting factor for radiation therapy and cryosurgery is the amount of PC. The tumor volume has a bearing on the ability of RT or cryosurgery to destroy the entire tumor mass.[81,147,148] This second variable in the equation may relate to the penetrating ability of the radiation particle used (photon < proton < neutron)[149–151] or the understanding that the core of a large tumor has a diminished oxygen supply (a hypoxic center) that confers resistance (called radioresistance) to the treatment.[152,153] This actually may not be as critical a factor in cryosurgery as it is in RT. These aspects of RT are discussed and illustrated in detail in *The Primer*. The reader is recommended to review pages 90–127 of *The Primer* to better understand these concepts.

A third variable, one under-discussed with the patient for obvious reasons, is the variability in skill of the physician, regardless of the specialty. Some physicians are just plain outright talented artists, while others are average in skill and still others are below average.

Unfortunately, all physicians quote the outstanding literature on a particular treatment but very few present to the patient their own scorecard of performance statistics.

There are additional variables relating to diagnosis and staging. The number of these biological observations is increasing as we learn more and more about the cancer process. Some of these variables are discussed in the following sections.

### Baseline PSA and Baseline PAP Are Keystones in Our Understanding of PC

*The Primer* goes into great depth on the importance of the baseline PSA and PAP. Let me make a few salient points. The PSA is a blessing. There are no other common malignancies that forecast their development through such a simple and inexpensive blood test as the PSA. But there are limitations to the PSA, as there are with everything in life.

*Everything in life is a two-edged sword.*

One major limitation of the PSA is that it is a laboratory test, which makes it subject to error and to conditions that elevate the PSA and possibly result in false alarms. However, one can state safely that a healthy prostate is one not subject to progressive or persistent elevations of PSA. In such situations, if PC is not the underlying cause, then prostatitis or BPH is the cause. These conditions significantly affect the quality of life of many men. Many scientists involved with PC research also believe that prostatitis may be a precursor to PC.[154,155]

In regard to the laboratory errors that may occur with PSA; these may occur with all tests. The rule of thumb is that if a test shows a reading at any time that is of concern, the test should be repeated and then repeated again after a short period of time to confirm whatever trend now seems apparent. It is this persistent trend that is so important in declaring the presence of biological conditions that should concern us.

### PSA Leak Is Relatively Low in Undifferentiated PC

Another aspect of the PSA that may be misleading is in the setting of patients with a low PSA level that is associated with a high Gleason score—for example, (4,3) or higher. The problem here is that high Gleason score lesions, having a significant component of Gleason grade 4 or 5 PC, do not secrete as much PSA into the blood as lower grade lesions. This is called the PSA leak. Table 11 shows the PSA leak as a function of average (weighted) Gleason grade.

Here is where the Gleason score is very important in elaborating on the significance we give the PSA during the initial and subsequent evaluations of the patient. I have seen patients present with Gleason scores of 9 and 10 with low levels of PSA and yet they had large tumor volumes reflecting PC that was outside the prostate gland and not amenable to cure with local therapy.

### Table 11: PSA Leak Versus Weighted Gleason Grade[130]

The weighted Gleason grade is applicable when there are multiple core biopsies showing various Gleason scores. In such a setting, an average weighted Gleason score is determined. Half of that number would be the weighted Gleason grade. If all biopsy cores indicate (3,3), it makes no difference; the average weighted Gleason grade would, of course, be 3. In this table, an undifferentiated PC with a Gleason score of 10 would have an average Gleason grade of 5 (bolded) and a PSA leak of only 0.93, or approximately 1 (both bolded). In contrast, the most common Gleason score (3,3) having a weighted Gleason grade of 3 would have a PSA leak that is 4.26, or approximately 4 times higher. That means that for each cubic centimeter of PC, the Gleason score 10 lesion is leaking one-fourth the amount of PSA into the serum.

| Gleason Grade (weighted) | PSA Leak (rounded off) | PSA Leak (exact) |
|---|---|---|
| 5 | 1 | 0.93 |
| 4.5 | 1.5 | 1.36 |
| 4 | 2 | 1.99 |
| 3.5 | 3 | 2.92 |
| 3 | 4 | 4.26 |
| 2.5 | 6 | 6.23 |
| 2 | 10 | 9.12 |
| 1.5 | 15 | 13.33 |
| 1 | 20 | 19.49 |

A Microsoft Excel software program for tumor volume (which can be found on the PCRI website at www.pcri.org) shows the above relationships clearly. The program requires the b (baseline) PSA, gland volume, and Gleason score. The PSA leak is calculated from the weighted Gleason grade. The outputs of this program give you benign PSA, PC-related PSA, and calculated tumor volume. Additional integrated programs give you probability of organ-confined disease, probability of cure with RP, and likelihood of freedom from biochemical relapse at 20 months after RT.

## Gleason Score versus Gleason Grade

The Gleason score is composed of 2 grades: primary grade and secondary grade. The primary grade is the preponderant glandular pattern of PC as seen under the microscope. By definition, it composes a minimum of 51% of the picture and possibly as much as 95% of the picture. In contrast, the secondary grade must represent at least 5% and as much as 49% of the glandular architectural pattern.

The most common Gleason score seen in biopsies obtained during contemporary times is (3,3). Gleason scores of (4,4), (4,5), (5,4), and (5,5) make up about 17% of all PC cases.[153] The Gleason score of 7 is a special situation that has significant implications depending on whether the 7 is a (3,4) or a (4,3). This distinction is based solely on the amount of Gleason grade 4 PC present. As previously stated, a (3,4) could have as little as 5% Gleason grade 4 disease or as much as 49%. In contrast, a Gleason score of (4,3) must, by definition, have at least 51% Gleason grade 4 disease and possibly as much as 95% (since there must be at least 5% of Gleason grade 3 PC in a [4,3] lesion). A major difference in prognosis has been found for patients with a Gleason score of (3,4) versus (4,3) located within the RP specimen.[154-156] The Partin Tables for 2001 have different readings of risk assessment for Gleason score (3,4) versus (4,3) on the diagnostic biopsy specimen.[160] This distinction is easily seen when using the PC Tools II software program developed by Dr. Glenn Tisman (available on the PCRI website at www.pcri.org).

In the hands of expert pathologists, focused only on PC pathology, the Gleason score identification is one of the most important biological determinants of prognosis. I have suggested that the Gleason score be embellished with what I call the Gleason differential: a quantification of the amount (in percent) of Gleason grade 4 or 5 in the pathology specimen. Therefore, a patient with a Gleason score of 7 that

is (4,3) might have 95% Gleason grade 4 and only 5% Gleason grade 3 to give the following Gleason differential: GS(4,3)[95/5]. In contrast, he might only have 51% Gleason grade 4 or a Gleason differential of GS (4,3)[51/49]. Evaluations of the diagnostic biopsy material that quantitate the amount of Gleason grade 4 or 5 disease may allow for a further enhancement in the prognosis of PC.

These variables are part of the equation to determine extent and amount of PC as well as the ability to deliver specific kinds of therapy with greater or lesser probability of disease progression after completion of such therapy. Pending this kind of input, the astute physician, empowered patient, and partner can determine what other tests should be considered or discarded. Additionally, with this foundational information at hand, the health care team can use history to develop a risk assessment for the patient that relates to outcome: What is the probability that your treatment will be successful? Again, the latter presumes that the therapist delivering the treatment is as talented as the physicians involved in the studies that were the basis for the risk assessment.

## Cross One Bridge at a Time

A common path that patients and partners as well as physicians take after a diagnosis of PC is to immediately make the choice of a treatment option the main focus. Too often, a patient goes from a diagnosis to a bone scan, often a CT scan, and then to the discussion of treatment options. The medical detective work of assessing the patient's risk for organ-confined disease versus nonorgan-confined disease is just not done routinely.

The risk assessments involved with PC take the form of multiple inputs into a statistical evaluation in which the output has more statistical significance than any single input. In such a scenario, the whole is greater than the sum of its parts. These assessments are termed algorithms, nomograms, neural nets, and so on.[157,161-163] They look at data in terms of searching for meaningful variables and then combine these variables to provide a closer sense of the truth about a particular patient based on how other patients with the same variables fared in a large series of patients. This is the essence of what we call the Partin Tables.

Partin et al. looked at the findings of RP and noted whether or not the pathologic findings showed the PC to reflect OCD, and whether there was evidence of capsular penetration (CP), seminal vesicle (SV) or lymph node (LN) involvement.[107,160,164]

Statistical analysis was done to determine which presurgical findings would equate with a high probability of these RP findings upon pathologic review of the surgical specimens. This is the essence of many of the tools we use to assess risk for the hypothetical patient. Everyone is unique in his or her biology, but a general statement of risk can still be presented to the patient.

Unfortunately, despite the availability of this tool and many others similar to it, perhaps only 5–10% of physicians go through the discipline of doing the Partin Table and/or other algorithmic calculations. Sitting down and inputting medical variables of known significance and doing the homework involved in the risk assessment of the PC patient is a very crucial step in a logical, rational approach to this disease. Not only the patient but also the physician should be crossing one bridge at a time. When this is done, the PPP team reaches a superior understanding of the disease process and attains a greater sense of what is likely to be the reality for a particular patient.

Appendix F in *The Primer* goes into great depth about these diagnostic and staging variables. The reader is referred to Appendix F for further information. In addition, the May 2001 issue of the PCRI Insights newsletter contains a comprehensive review of risk assessment algorithms by Glenn Tisman, M.D. This issue can be obtained online at www.pcri.org or by calling the PCRI at (310) 743-2110. The software section on the PCRI website also has risk assessment computer programs that can be downloaded without charge.

What does all this lead to? It leads to a more accurate assessment of the patient's true status. Knowing where the PC may have spread gives direction to the PPP team to perform certain tests to exclude disease at those site(s). For example, if the algorithms show a high risk for lymph node disease, the staging process should include the monoclonal antibody scan called ProstaScint. However, if the risk is negligible for lymph node involvement, this study could be excluded. The same approach is used to evaluate disease at the different stations of involvement. Is there disease in the capsule of the prostate, the seminal vesicles, the lymph nodes, or the bones? If one finds a high probability of disease confined to the prostate, then local therapies such as RP, RT (3D conformal radiation, IMRT, seed implantation, HDR, or a combination of these radiation approaches), or cryosurgery can be used with a greater probability of success. However, there are caveats that relate to the successful use of these therapies as well.

## What Does This Mean for Patients?

Algorithms involve experiences of men who have gone before you. Take advantage of the information that others have provided you. Obtaining data from the algorithms is critical homework that must involve you and your medical coaches. Assessing your risk for PC spread to particular sites and evaluating those sites with special testing is an essential part of the successful management of the man with PC. Remember, if man does not learn from history, he is forced to repeat it.

## 6. KNOWING PROS AND CONS OF WEAPONRY: UNDERSTANDING PROS AND CONS OF TREATMENT OPTIONS

In winning a military battle, an understanding of the appropriate strategy for the situation at hand is critical for success. Military tactics, including the weapons used, must be matched intelligently to the circumstances that are present. The same is true for the management of PC and other illnesses. The most important aspect of this match is the realization that a local treatment will have its greatest chance of being curative if the biological expressions of disease suggest that it is likely that only local disease is present. Therefore, obtaining as many insights as possible into what constitutes a high probability of OCD is warranted.

The preceding sections have laid the groundwork, the reconnaissance so to speak, for the gathering of that information. The medical strategist takes these variables into account and builds a case for or against local therapy. The major algorithms such as the Partin 2001 Tables[160] and the nomograms from Kattan et al.,[165–167] D'Amico et al.,[79,161] Narayan et al.,[76] Bluestein et al.,[168] Gilliland et al.,[169] Lerner et al.,[170] Pisansky et al.,[171] and others[75,112,157,162,163,172–183] should be used. These only take minutes to do and there is little to lose in seeing if a consensus is present for organ-confined disease.

If an assumption is made that a patient has a high probability of organ-confined disease and that there are no medical issues or financial issues that preclude any particular choice of local procedure to cure PC, the $64000 question is this: "What procedure has the best track record?" Certainly, given the many publications on this subject over the last few years, one would have to state that overall there is no striking difference in success rates between any of the local therapies for PC–RP, RT of any type, or cryosurgery.[184–186] The longest follow-up period after definitive local therapy relates to RP. However, it appears unlikely that the 10- and 11-year data following RT are going to suddenly deteriorate or that the 15-year data after RP are going to change. The follow-up data after cryosurgery are at most 10 years old with most of the modern-day approaches to this technique beginning in 1992 with the work of Onik and Cohen et al.[187,188] The cryosurgery literature is more difficult to evaluate because there have been major technological advances in the last 10 years. These include the following:

- The use of temperature monitoring using thermocouples[146,189,190]
- The use of double and triple freezing techniques[146,189]
- The use of argon gas[191–193] instead of liquid nitrogen to induce the freezing necessary for creation of the iceball
- The recent use of templates to guide the placement of the cryosurgery probes, similar to those used in brachytherapy[194]

The fine points of RP, RT, and cryosurgery are extensively dealt with in *The Primer* (now available through amazon.com, Barnes & Noble, and Life Extension at (800) 544-4440).

The issue then is which of these local therapies, if any, does the patient choose. Assuming that the patient at risk is not a candidate for watchful waiting, any of these therapies might be a perfectly reasonable strategy to eradicate organ-confined or regionally confined PC. My recommendations to patients on this matter are based on the following differential factors:

- Age
- Overall medical status after a detailed examination
- Patient priorities
- Patient access to experts in the selected modality of therapy
- Financial and insurance issues
- Lower urinary tract symptoms (LUTS) at the time of diagnosis
- Prostate gland volume
- History of scar formation (keloids) after any prior surgery
- Baseline PAP
- Baseline plasma TGF-b1, IL-6, and IL-6 soluble receptor levels
- PSA response to ADT (androgen deprivation therapy) after 3 months of therapy

In essence, a combined modality analysis of sorts is being employed. This involves variables that have not been interactively evaluated as part of an effort to define the best local therapy for an individual patient. Hopefully, a true nomogram or artificial neural net (ANN) looking at such additional variables can validate their significance for such an analysis.

Some of these issues have been discussed in prior sections. A short review of each of these topics is justifiable for this section.

## Age

Traditionally, patients beyond age 70 are excluded as being candidates for RP. I believe that this decision should be individualized based on the patient's health, youthfulness for his age, and the other listed factors rather than using age as an arbitrary reason for excluding a patient. I have evaluated some men in their 50s who are much older in appearance and in biological status than their stated age. I have seen others in their late 70s who appear to be in their early 60s and who are healthier on examination than men in their 60s.

## Overall Medical Status after Detailed Examination

This has been alluded to in the section on medical record keeping and the use of summary and/or surveillance forms. Patients being considered for any invasive procedure should have a thorough physical examination. Factors that place them at much higher risk for morbidity after RP, RT, or cryosurgery should be candidly discussed with the patient and his partner.[195] Cardiovascular disease, type 2 diabetes, kidney disease, hypertension, and neurodegenerative diseases should be red flags that an invasive procedure may be associated with greater adverse effects.[195,196] The evaluation of the patient's cardiac status with triglyceride/HDL ratios[197,198] as well as the conventional LDL and total cholesterol levels, the use of hypersensitive C-reactive protein,[199–201] and homocysteine levels are reasonable to do in this setting (discussions of these topics can be found in several other protocols in this edition).

The use of fasting insulin levels and the ratio of AA to EPA may be an excellent screening tool to evaluate the overall health of a patient considering any of these procedures.[202–205] In addition to a very thorough internal medicine history and physical examination, the studies that I have found particularly revealing include a stress echocardiogram with calculation of the ejection fraction and electron beam tomography with coronary artery calcium scoring.[199]

A significant factor in patients having problems with RP, RT, or cryosurgery is small vessel disease due to diabetes or hypertension. Diabetic patients represent a great challenge because of the prolonged delay in return of urinary function after any local therapy. Tissue healing is not optimal in such a setting.

## Patient Priorities

The patient's inclinations toward a particular therapy are often a product of decades of programming that will not be undone in the course of weeks or even months. Some men are adamant about having surgery, while others are exactly the opposite. Some feel that RT is the choice for them, while others are more comfortable with freezing. The poet Robert Frost may have encountered this same problem and reflected upon it in "Fire and Ice"[206]:

> Some say the world will end in fire,
> Some say in ice.
> From what I've tasted of desire
> I hold with those who favor fire.
> But if I had to perish twice,
> I think I know enough of hate
> To say that for destruction ice
> Is also great
> And would suffice.

There are those patients who cannot decide between fire (RT), ice (cryosurgery), or surgery and who instead pursue objectified ongoing observation. But as my father used to tell me, "That's what makes horse racing."

## Patient Access to Experts in the Selected Modality of Therapy

I have no issues with any decision that a patient and his partner make if it has reasonable backing with biological data and the ability to involve physicians with gifted technical skills. Patients should interact with their fellow patients at support groups, asking about the details of experiences with local physicians in these fields. Patients and their partners should explore the Internet, looking for any listings of physicians considered to be outstanding in their skills.

Moreover, patients and their partners should have a formal consultation with the physician(s) that they are considering to see if there is rapport between all 3 parties and to witness the interaction of the physician with other patients in his or her medical office. The physician should be asked for names of patients who are willing to be telephoned by you and/or your partner. These should be patients who have undergone the procedure within the last 1–2 years. Obtaining 3 such names would be appropriate—perhaps one that had the procedure 6 months ago, another who had the procedure 12 months ago, and a third who had it 1 1/2–2 years ago. You should not be embarrassed to ask the physician about his success rate or about the incidence rates of complications his patients have experienced. These should be his figures and not those cited in someone else's series of patients.

## Financial and Insurance Issues

The choices being made are quality-of-life decisions that also can affect quantity of life. Some patients may elect to stay within their medical insurance plans and feel that this is adequate for them.

## Lower Urinary Tract Symptoms (LUTS) at the Time of Diagnosis

LUTS will often adversely affect the quality of life of a patient undergoing RT of any kind or cryosurgery. The physiological interaction is likely related to radiation urethritis due to RT or thermal (cold) injury to the urethra from cryosurgery.

LUTS can be quantified with the AUA symptom index score.[87,207] Patients should consider scores of 10 and higher as a relative negative risk factor in choosing RT or cryosurgery as a local therapy. A more powerful argument can be made for baseline AUA scores of 15–20 and higher. A study used a combined modality assessment to determine what findings are most significant for predicting bladder outflow obstruction. A combination of an AUA symptom index of greater than 20, a prostate gland volume of 40 g or more, and a urine flow of 10 mL or less per second, when present, predicted for obstruction 100% of the time.[89] Urine flow rate was determined using uroflowmetry.

The prophylactic and long-term use of alpha blockers (Flomax®, Cardura®, or Hytrin®) to reduce LUTS prior to, during, and after brachytherapy has been reported to reduce the time to return to baseline urinary function.[87]

## Prostate Gland Volume

Often, but not invariably, men with LUTS will have prostate gland enlargement due to BPH. The large gland volume is another confounding factor affecting potential radiation or cryotherapy-related injury to the urethra, rectum, and bladder. Options for the patient in such a situation include the use of ADT to reduce the gland size prior to local therapy. Usually, within 3 months of starting ADT, the gland volume will be reduced by as much as 40%. After 6 months of ADT, the gland volume may be reduced 60% or more from baseline. The proper use of ADT with monitoring of serum testosterone using the goal of less than 20 ng/dL may be a factor in why some men have dramatic reductions in gland size with ADT and others do not. The use of three-drug ADT involving an antiandrogen plus Proscar® or possibly another 5-alpha reductase inhibitor Avodart® (dutasteride) in conjunction with an LHRH-agonist like Lupron, Zoladex®, or Trelstar® LA has provided me with excellent results in both PC reduction and prostate gland volume reduction.

In men who are reluctant to receive ADT and/or do not have a dramatic response to alpha-1 blockers, choosing RP is an excellent way to eliminate LUTS and restore urinary function to a high level. The urologist is essentially providing the patient with a new urethra, without the adverse effect of compression of the urethra by an enlarged prostate. Urinary flow in such patients is restored to that of a young man. This presumes that the operating urologist is skilled in the RP procedure and has an impeccable track record with a complication rate for gross incontinence at less than 2%, but total continence rates in the order of 92–95% with no need for protective pads of any kind, and anastomotic stricture rates that are less than 5%.

## History of Scar Formation (Keloids) after Any Prior Surgery

If we could identify patients most likely to develop complications, we could direct them to other therapeutic strategies. An investigation that comes close to this was done by Park et al.[208] This study correlates the probability of developing a narrowing or stricture after RP to a patient history of excessive scar formation from the actual RP or evidence of such scarring in prior surgical procedures. This study spanned a 5-year period and involved 753 radical retropubic prostatectomies performed by a single surgeon. The overall incidence of stricture at the anastomosis or connection of the bladder neck and distal urethra (anastomotic stricture) was 4.8%. The only significant finding that predicted the development of such a stricture was the maximal width of the abdominal scar resulting from the skin incision made at the time of RP.

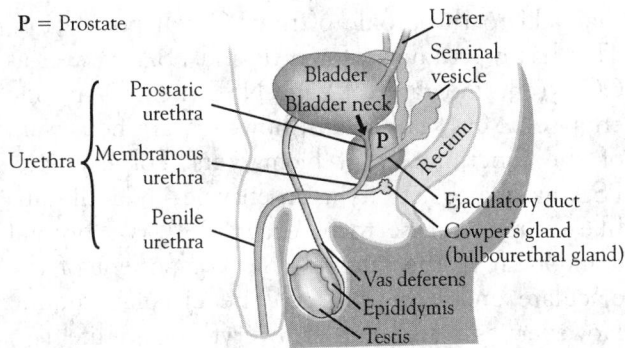

Figure 5. **The Anatomy of the Prostate in Relation to the Bladder Neck and Components of the Urethra.** During a radical prostatectomy (RP), the prostate and its prostatic urethra are excised and an anastomosis is made between the bladder neck tissue and the membranous urethra. (Modified from Figure 8 in *A Primer on Prostate Cancer, The Empowered Patient's Guide* by Strum, S.B. and Pogliano, D., Life Extension Media, 2002).

In other words, the patient's reaction to surgery at a skin level was reflected in the tissue healing at the site of union (anastomosis) between the bladder neck and membranous urethra joined together after the excision of the prostate and prostatic urethra (see Figure 5). Men with a maximal scar of greater than 10 mm were 8 times more likely to develop strictures than men with smaller scars. The percentage of men who required protective pads 1 year following radical retropubic prostatectomy in the stricture group was 46.2%, while the figure for those without a stricture was 12.5%.

The authors of this study speculated that prior history of excessive scar formation may have implications in the adverse outcomes of other surgical procedures such as coronary bypass grafts, angioplasties, bile duct operations, and so on. This is highly provocative, and the potential implication is that a history of excessive scar formation after any of the latter procedures may be a warning for those men considering RP as a possible choice of local therapy.

## Baseline PAP

The importance of the baseline PAP blood level has been published in at least 3 major papers.[77,78,209] These papers are referenced in detail in *The Primer*. The routine use of the PAP as part of our understanding of the biology of PC, its relation to the tumor cell population, and the probability of disease progression after RP or RT (with or without seed implantation) appears to be justified.

## Baseline Plasma TGF-b1, IL-6, and IL-6 Soluble Receptor Levels

Molecular biomarkers relate the mechanisms of biologic behavior, function, and cell–cell interaction that add to the profile of the PC cell population. This has been known for PAP and PSA as well as CGA (chromogranin A) and NSE (neuron-specific enolase). Many physicians, however, are not aware of the functionality of biomarkers. For example, PSA has major activity as an enzyme—a kallikrein-like serine protease to be exact. PSA is a normal component of the seminal fluid component of the ejaculate and helps to keep the ejaculate liquid. However, as stated earlier, everything in life is a two-edged sword.

PSA produced from malignant prostate cells functions to break down specific proteins. These glyco-proteins are found within the basement membrane of the microscopic glandular architecture. Simply, they are the ground substance to which the basal cells of the prostate glands are anchored. PSA degrades these proteins (fibronectin and laminin) and facilitates invasion by the PC cells. Thus, PSA made by the PC cell population is not only a biomarker of disease activity, but also a functional protein that is important to the survival of the cancer cell. Reducing PSA is therefore not only a good sign that a therapy is working, but also that one is reducing a substance that facilitates spread of the disease.[210] In another publication, PSA was shown to suppress T-cell mediated immunity.[211] This functional activity of PSA may be mediated by TGF-b1 production from the prostate cell.[212]

That cell products that we identify as biomarkers may have function appears to be the case for virtually every cell product identified. They have function as well as form. Another enzyme produced by both benign and malignant prostate cells is uPA. uPA was discussed earlier in this review (see the section titled General Preventive Measures). uPA is stimulated by IGF-1 and inhibited by GLA and EPA. uPA is believed to play a key mechanistic role in PC invasion and metastasis.[213]

TGF-b1 is a growth factor produced by the prostate cell as well as by cells of the bone matrix. Interleukin-6 (IL-6) is a cell product, or cytokine, that is made essentially by the primary tumor as well as by osteoblasts. IL-6 facilitates bone resorption by acting on IL-6 receptors located on the osteoclast and osteoclast precursor cells. This incredible cascade was illustrated in Figure 1 of this chapter. Studies published by Shariat et al. show a very strong positive correlation between higher plasma levels of pre-RP TGF-b1 and findings at RP of ECE (extracapsular extension), seminal vesicle involvement, and lymph node involvement.[214] In this

study, preoperative plasma TGF-b1 median levels of approximately 15 ng/mL was significantly associated with lymph node and bone metastases. Healthy noncancer controls and men with RP findings not indicating extra-prostatic involvement had median levels of TGF-b1 of 4.7–4.8 ng/mL.

In a subsequent study involving 302 men with clinically localized PC, the same investigators evaluated preoperative and postoperative plasma TGF-b1 levels, and also IL-6 and its soluble receptor (IL-6sR), to determine correlations with disease progression. Of the study participants, 88.8% of the men had PSA progression-free survival at 3 years and 85.1% remained progression-free at 5 years post-RP. Cancer progression occurred in 43 of the 302 men (14%), with average postoperative follow-up of 50.7 months. Of the 43 men with PC progression, 19 were categorized as having nonaggressive progression postoperatively because they had complete responses to salvage RT or because their PSA doubling times postoperatively were equal to or greater than 10 months.

The remaining 24 men had aggressive progression because of positive lymph nodes found at RP (n = 6), positive metastatic workup on bone or ProstaScint scan (n = 6), because their PSA doubling times were less than 10 months (n = 23), or they failed to respond to salvage RT (n = 14). What Shariat and colleagues found were significantly higher pre- and post-operative TGF-b1 levels and higher preoperative IL-6 and IL-6sR levels in men with "aggressive progression" versus those with "nonaggressive progression." These findings are summarized in Table 12.

This laboratory testing is allowing us to use the biology of the patient's tumor cell and host interaction to declare the probabilities of organ-confined disease versus nonorgan-confined disease. These findings are nicely in keeping with the Lerner algorithm from the Mayo Clinic in Rochester, Minnesota. In that large-scale study, 904 men with apparently pathologically organ-confined PC were found to have PSA recurrences within 5 years based on the RP Gleason score, baseline PSA, and whether or not the PC at surgery had a normal DNA amount (diploidy) or abnormal amount (aneuploidy). Even in the best of circumstances, with baseline PSA values of less than 10 ng/mL, a Gleason score at RP of 6, and diploidy, the data still show a biochemical failure rate of 15% within the first 5 years. If the RP specimen was aneuploid, this increases the failure probability to 30%. It would be of interest to see whether the TGF-b1

**Table 12: Plasma TGF-b1, IL-6, and IL-6 Soluble Receptor Pre-RP and Post-RP**

This battery of laboratory tests done on plasma can predict the findings at RP and also the patient's postoperative course. Modified from Shariat, S.F., Shalev, M., Menesses-Diaz, A. et al., *J. Clin. Oncol.* 19: 2856–64, 2001.[214]

| Preoperative Test Findings | | | Positive (+) or Negative (–) Correlations at RP | | | | |
| --- | --- | --- | --- | --- | --- | --- | --- |
| TGF-b1 | IL-6 | IL-6sR | ECE | SV | GS | LTvol | LN |
| –> | (++) | (++) | – | – | + | + | – |
| (++) | <–> | <–> | + | + | – | – | – |
| (++) | (++) | (++) | + | + | + | + | + |
| Postoperative Test Findings | | | Correlations with Clinical Course Postoperatively | | | | |
| (—) | (—) | (—) | Nonprogression of PC post-RP | | | | |
| <–> | (—) | (—) | Progression of PC post-RP | | | | |

Key: –> *not significantly elevated;* (++) *significantly elevated;* (—) *significantly decreased;* <–> *no significant change;* ECE, *extracapsular extension;* SV, *seminal vesicle involvement;* LN, *lymph node involvement;* GS, *Gleason score at RP* (+ = higher, – = lower); LTvol, *local tumor volume (cancer within prostate gland).*

status of the patient is independent of the ploidy status. Evolving algorithms using these kinds of inputs will clarify our recommendations to patients and their partners.

## PSA Response to ADT after 3 Months of Therapy

Michael Zelefsky of Memorial Sloan Kettering (New York City), a radiation oncologist, published a paper about the predictive value of the PSA after 3 months of ADT.[215] The purpose of his study was to identify prognostic variables that predict for improved biochemical and local control outcomes in patients with localized PC who had been treated upfront with ADT, which was then followed by three-dimensional conformal radiotherapy (3D-CRT).

Between 1969 and 1995, a total of 213 patients with apparently localized PC were treated with 3 months of ADT before 3D-CRT. The ADT consisted of leuprolide acetate and flutamide (ADT2). The purpose of ADT was to reduce the preradiotherapy target volume in order to decrease the dose delivered to adjacent normal tissues and minimize the risk of morbidity from high dose RT. The median pretreatment PSA level was 13.3 ng/mL (range of 1–360 ng/mL). The median 3D-CRT dose was 73.6 Gy (range of 64.8–81 Gy), and the median follow-up time was 3 years (range of 1–7 years).

The significant predictors for improved outcome identified by multivariate analysis included a pretreatment PSA level less than or equal to 10.0 ng/mL ($p < 0.001$), an ADT-induced preradiotherapy PSA nadir of less than

or equal to 0.5 ng/mL ($p < 0.001$), and a clinical stage less than or equal to T2c ($p < 0.04$). The 5-year PSA relapse-free survival rates were 93%, 60%, and 40% for patients with pretreatment PSA levels less than or equal to 10 ng/mL, 10–20 ng/mL, and greater than 20 ng/mL, respectively ($p < 0.001$). Patients with preradiotherapy nadir levels after 3 months of ADT2 that were less than or equal to 0.5 ng/mL experienced a 5-year PSA relapse-free survival rate of 74%, as compared with 40% for patients with higher nadir levels ($p < 0.001$). The incidence of a positive biopsy among 34 patients pretreated with ADT was 12%, as compared with 39% for 117 patients treated with 3D-CRT alone who underwent a biopsy ($p < 0.001$).

Zelefsky and colleagues concluded that, in settings of PC treated with ADT2 and high dose 3D-CRT, pretreatment PSA, preradiotherapy PSA nadir response, and clinical stage are important predictors of biochemical outcome. Patients with PSA nadir levels greater than 0.5 ng/mL after 3 months of ADT2 are more likely to develop biochemical failure after radiotherapy and may benefit from more aggressive therapies. A summary of these findings is shown in Table 13.

What Zelefsky et al. have done is to use the biological response of the tumor to indirectly gain insight into the tumor biology in order to help assess the probability of successful outcomes with radiation therapy. A low probability of success should prompt the PPP team to discuss different treatment strategies.

The reduction of PSA to a lowest point or nadir is the same principle used in our study on intermittent

**Table 13:** **Relationship of Pretreatment PSA Levels and 5-Year Relapse-Free Survival in PC Patients Treated with ADT2 and High-Dose 3D-CRT**[215]

| Prognostic Finding | Five-Year Relapse-Free Survival |
|---|---|
| PSA = 10 | 93% |
| PSA > 10 = 20 | 60% |
| PSA > 20 | 40% |
| PSA nadir = 0.5 after 3 m* | 74% |
| PSA nadir >0.5 after 3 m* | 40% |

*After 3 months of neoadjuvant androgen deprivation with flutamide, 250 mg every 8 hours, plus Lupron, 7.5 mg i.m. monthly. This is the PSA value after a full 3 months of ADT, that is, the PSA taken just prior to starting the fourth injection of Lupron.*

androgen deprivation (IAD) to identify men with a high probability of PC that most likely reflects a homogeneous tumor cell population of androgen-dependent cancer cells.[216] In our study, we used an ultrasensitive PSA and required a threshold of less than 0.05, 10 times more than the threshold of acceptability in the Zelefsky study. It is quite conceivable that the use of the PSA nadir is identifying a number of biological events that would equate with a better prognosis or response to therapy in general.

For example, the ability to drop the PSA to very low levels suggests that androgen-independent PC (AIPC) is not present. If it were, the efficacy of androgen deprivation would not decrease the PSA to the very low levels determined with an ultrasensitive PSA assay such as the Tosoh or DPC Immulite Third Generation assay. AIPC represents PC that has undergone mutation. It is associated with more aggressive PC that is also more likely to have left the prostate. If so, then RT would be less effective in preventing biochemical recurrence manifested by a persistently rising PSA after RT is completed. This may be one of the operative factors in the Zelefsky study.

Additionally, resistance factors to RT may have also developed in a setting of mutated tumor. This might be related to an increased amount of the antiapoptosis protein bcl-2, which confers radiation resistance. It could also be attributed to elevated levels of mutated p53.[217–219] Lastly, in a study on the use of upfront (neoadjuvant) androgen deprivation with RT, it was shown that levels of mutated p53 in PC tissue biopsied from patients failing RT were significantly increased in patients who had not received neoadjuvant ADT compared to those who did receive ADT (82% versus 38%, respectively).[220] bcl-2 and mutated p53 are adverse biochemical findings because they protect the cancer cell from undergoing apoptosis.

PSA also reflects tumor volume. RT is a volume-dependent modality. It is also reasonable to consider that the PSA threshold of 0.5 or less after 3 months of ADT2 required in the study reflects a significantly diminished tumor cell volume. This would enhance the efficacy of any form of RT because the target volume is smaller. ADT also decreases angiogenesis by reducing VEGF.[221] A major stimulus to increase VEGF and angiogenesis occurs in the centers of large tumors where oxygen tensions are low and cells cannot extract as much oxygen. This is called tumor hypoxia, and its occurrence is associated with resistance to radiation. If ADT is decreasing the size of the tumor, the probability of tumor hypoxia is less and also the ability of the tumor to nourish itself or spread via new blood vessel growth (angiogenesis) is less, again due to the effect of ADT.[221] Therefore, the Zelefsky publication is a landmark paper because it stimulates much thinking as to what explanation exists for its findings. It should also prompt others to test the many hypotheses that are implicit in this study.

All of the biological events above are pertinent to translating the findings of the patient's clinical situation into a real-time medical strategy. They should direct the team to select a particular tactic(s) pending the biological feedback obtained because, in biological reality, all of these tests are reflections of the tumor-host interaction. Therefore, in all 6 steps discussed so far, we are investigating biological indicators—medical gauges or LEDs—to help us obtain true information about the enemy and how our soldiers will likely fare in a particular medical-military tactic. This is the essence of Lewis Thomas's *The Lives of a Cell*, the foundation of Eastern philosophy that the microcosm reflects the macrocosm (and vice versa) and the truth behind optimizing outcomes for any issue vital to life.

## Hormone Therapy in Advanced PC

Hormone therapy may be used in advanced PC (stage 3) or cancer that spreads beyond the prostate (stage 4; metastasis often to the bones). Hormone therapies such as antiandrogens and estrogens (eg, ethinylestradiol) are used to reduce testosterone levels (androgen ablation therapy). Hormone analogues are also used as antiandrogens, that is, to interfere with the action of androgen.

A number of selective somatostatin analogues have been developed for clinical use in the treatment of PC. Somatostatin was first found in hypothalamic extracts and identified as a hormone that inhibited secretion of growth hormone. Somatostatins are regulatory hormones produced by neuroendocrine, inflammatory, and immune cells in the central nervous system and in most major peripheral organs. Somatostatin can act as an endocrine hormone, a neurotransmitter, or participate in paracrine/autocrine regulation; and when activated, many tumor cells produce somatostatin.[222–224]

Changes in PSA levels are commonly used to monitor response to PC therapy. A PSA value that declines by more than 50% is considered to indicate an objective clinical response to therapy in hormone-refractory disease. Often, measurement of another marker, chromogranin A (CgA), is required to accurately monitor response to treatment and identify some patients with advanced disease who do not have elevated serum PSA.[225]

A study reported in the *Journal of Urology* evaluated whether a combination therapy of ethinylestradiol and somatostatin analogue can reintroduce objective clinical responses in patients with metastatic androgen ablation refractory prostate cancer. The test subjects (10 patients with stage-D3 PC disease and bone metastases) had disease progression despite an initial response to combined androgen blockade and subsequent failure to antiandrogen withdrawal. The combined androgen blockade was discontinued and the patients were given 1 mg of oral ethinylestradiol daily and 73.9 mg of intramuscular lanreotide acetate (a somatostatin analogue) every 4 weeks. Serum PSA, CgA, the Eastern Cooperative Oncology Group (ECOG) Performance Status, and bone pain scores were monitored (median, 18 months; range, 10–24 months).

Although the number of patients in the study group was small, results were encouraging when combination therapy was used: 90% of the patients experienced an objective clinical response and an improvement in symptoms. In 9 of 10 subjects, PSA declined more than 50%, and in 3 subjects PSA normalized (<4 ng/mL). All subjects had significant improvement in bone pain (median duration 17.5 months) and ECOG Performance Status (median duration 18 months) without major treatment-related side effects. There was also a statistically significant decrease in serum CgA during administration and at the response to therapy (median 38.4%, range 28.6–64.9%) that was not increased at relapse. Although 2 patients died secondary to PC, all of the other patients were without disease progression.[226]

**Note:** *The ECOG Performance Status is used to assess disease progression, how the disease affects the patient's daily activities, and determine appropriate treatment and prognosis. The Status has grades 0 to 5: 0, fully active, no physical restrictions; 1, physical restrictions, but ambulatory and able to do light work; 2, ambulatory, can care for self, active more than 50% of waking hours, but unable to perform any work activity; 3, self-care is limited, in bed or chair more than 50% of waking hours; 4, completely disabled, no self-care, confined to bed or chair; 5, deceased.*

# 7. UNDERSTANDING ENEMY VULNERABILITY: LEARNING PRINCIPLES UNDERLYING TUMOR GROWTH

To understand the weakness and vulnerability of an enemy in military battle, one must first try to understand his apparent strengths. The analogy of the tumor or cancer cell being the societal equivalent to a terrorist is a strong one. What we learned and are still learning from September 11, 2001, is that we did not understand the strengths of the enemy. Hence, we were not successful in deterring a successful incursion by the terrorists on September 11. If we do not learn from this historical event, we will see history repeated. The same remarks about cancer are true.

What are the characteristics of malignancy that justify a metaphor with terrorists? First of all, both arenas often share common terminology. Some comparable words include "disorderly," "inflammatory," "primitive," "network," "radical," "invasive," "instability," "hits," "cells," "resistance," "surveillance," "eradication," "preemptive," "checkpoints," and "survival."

Every cancer, including PC, is a disordered and abnormal cell growth. Cancer cells have lost the ability to network and communicate in the way that normal cells do, and they no longer function as intended in the overall framework of body chemistry. Such cells take on a demeanor of juvenile delinquents, with no respect for parental direction. Attempts to restrict disruptive or nonproductive behavior are ignored. Such disruptive cells are usually censored and expelled by regulatory monitors—guardians of the genome, proteins such as p53, p21, and p27, which normally identify and biologically excise such maladapted cells. In malignant conditions, these regulatory proteins lose control for largely unknown reasons.

In one study involving the development of malignancy of the esophagus, antibodies to p53 were found in 4 of 36 (11%) premalignant lesions of the esophagus and in 10 of 33 (30%) of those with cancer of the esophagus. In 2 of the esophageal cancer patients, the p53 antibodies were detected prior to a clinical

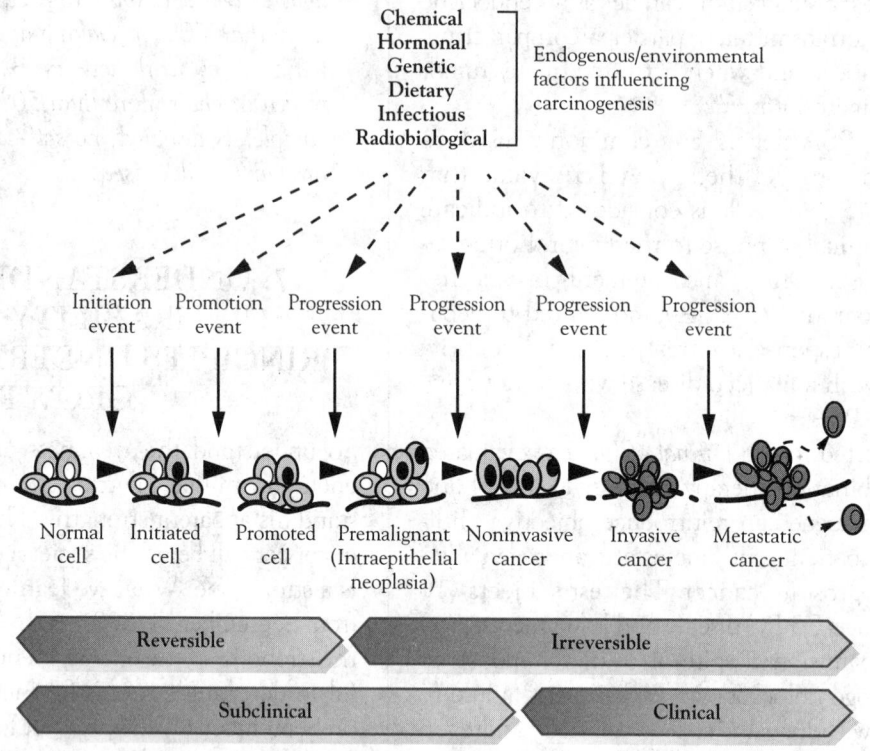

Figure 6. **The Evolution of Malignancy.** Initiation events, promotion events, and progression events are considered "hits" on the cells in question. As a cell goes through the evolution from normal to malignant, the cell's appearance (its phenotype) changes. Terms such as "metaplasia," "dysplasia," and finally "neoplasia" are used. Studies that will identify biochemical or molecular changes that occur prior to these changes, which are seen under the microscope, are needed. These will provide clues relating to what needs to be done to prevent or stop the evolution of malignancy. (Modified from Figure 10 in *A Primer on Prostate Cancer, The Empowered Patient's Guide.*)

diagnosis of cancer.[227] Therefore, the cellular counterparts of terrorists are finding a way past one of the surveillance mechanisms (p53) that usually stand guard to detect DNA damage and halt the machinery of the cell cycle in G1 or G2 when DNA defects are found (see Figure 3). In a later section, another mechanism that tumor cells and viruses use to get past the surveillance system will be discussed.

The development of malignancy results from a combination of hits on the cell—repeated insults. Initial factors that lead to cancer production (carcinogenesis) are shown in Figure 6. Ongoing promotional and progression events eventually lead to premalignant changes such as prostatic intraepithelial neoplasia (PIN), then to noninvasive cancer, and finally to invasive cancer. If not diagnosed early and eradicated, metastatic cancer may eventually develop.

Malignant tumors develop multiple genetic abnormalities that accumulate progressively in individual cells during the course of tumor evolution. For example, abnormalities involving p53 generally occur early in the development of invasive BCs.[228] What biological situation(s) or conditions allow p53 or other DNA

repair proteins, the guardians at the gate, to become mutated enough to allow such expressions? If we know what steps are involved in this process(es), we can avoid or reduce them and prevent initiation or promotional events.

The conditions favoring the above appear to include inflammatory situations that are associated with metabolic products that favor the development of dysplasia and neoplasia. These biologically inflamed situations are characterized by the production of reactive oxygen species (ROS) that damage cell membranes, that is, free radicals. For example, we know that ROS, or free radicals, cause oxidative damage to LDL cholesterol to eventuate in atheromatous plaques that are major factors in coronary artery disease. ROS damage the lipid membranes of the cell by means of an oxidative reaction called lipid peroxidation. The cell membrane is critical to the cell's integrity; it is involved in the selective entry and exit of substances (ligands) that interact at the membrane border by means of a chemical reaction with docking sites called receptors.

Damage to structures like the cell membrane allows the tumor cell access to vital cell functions. Tumor

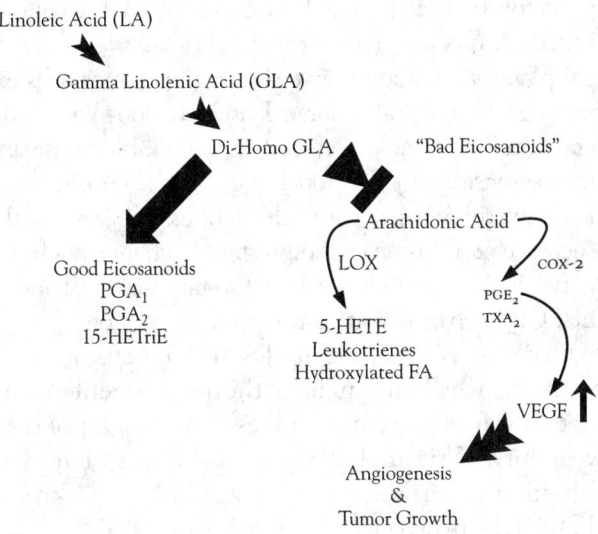

Linoleic Acid (LA)

Gamma Linolenic Acid (GLA)

Di-Homo GLA      "Bad Eicosanoids"

Arachidonic Acid

Good Eicosanoids
$PGA_1$
$PGA_2$
15-HETriE

LOX     COX-2

$PGE_2$
$TXA_2$

5-HETE
Leukotrienes
Hydroxylated FA

VEGF

Angiogenesis
&
Tumor Growth

**Figure 7. Arachidonic Acid Induces COX-2 Production.** Since AA is known to induce COX-2 synthesis by stimulating the early COX-2 gene, a major approach to preventing this occurrence is to decrease AA production. The pathway from DGLA to AA can be blocked by changes in the diet that involve (1) avoidance of insulin surges and (2) addition of EPA and DHA to the diet.

cells, or what causes them, along with viruses, inactivate other parts of the surveillance mechanisms of the healthy organism. The interferon-signaling pathway (ISP) is often knocked out by tumor cells because interferons are molecules that actively patrol against viruses and cancer cells. In situations where cancer has developed, the ISP is often damaged or inactivated. Therefore, tumor-promoting situations are ones in which there is vulnerability of the organism due to inflammatory conditions incited by events that lead to damage of the surveillance mechanisms and result in access to vital cell functions.

What is all this leading to? In earlier sections, the importance of the eicosanoids was discussed. These are the oldest hormonal substances known to scientists. Every cell membrane in every cell in the human body generates eicosanoids. This occurs via pathways that lead to a major metabolic crossroad—di-homo GLA (DGLA), a 20-carbon omega-6 fatty acid. DGLA is further metabolized to AA and its illness-producing metabolites (bad eicosanoids) or away from AA production and metabolized to good eicosanoids (see General Preventive Measures, Eicosanoid Balance). This balance is crucial to the maintenance of health and prevention of illness (see Figure 7).

Since eicosanoids are the oldest hormones, with origins that can be traced back to 500 million years ago, perhaps they are also the ones most likely to be vital keys in the initiation of malignancy and the perpetuation of cancer growth. Studies have shown that

the essential fatty acids, linoleic acid (LA) and AA, and the AA metabolite PGE2 stimulate tumor growth. In contrast, oleic acid (OA) and the omega-3 fatty acid, EPA, inhibit growth.[229,230] In cell cultures of the human PC cell line PC-3, expression of the c-fos gene and the early COX-2 gene is increased within minutes of adding AA. This expression is dependent upon the amount of AA present, that is, it is dose-dependent.[229] We also know that PGE2 is associated with the stimulation of VEGF and thus with angiogenesis and tumor growth (see Figure 7). These findings have huge implications for medical strategies.

Further insight into this strategy to decrease AA production comes from studies showing that aspirin and nonsteroidal anti-inflammatory drugs (NSAIDs) have been shown to reduce the incidence of malignancy. Both of these agents have in common the ability to antagonize the enzyme COX-2, which converts AA to PGE2. High doses of Celebrex® (celecoxib), a more selective COX-2 enzyme inhibitor, have been shown to prevent precancerous adenomatous polyps from progressing to overt colon cancer.[231] More drugs are being identified that act selectively on the COX-2 pathway. Agents such as silymarin (milk thistle), a known protector of liver cells (hepatocytes) against oxidative damage, have been shown to selectively inhibit the enzymes COX-2 and lipoxygenase (LOX) and also to downregulate interleukin-1 (IL-1). All of these are implicated in cancer initiation and growth.[232]

Another study of PC showed a significant degree of 15-LOX in PC biopsy specimens and correlated this with mutated p53 immunostaining in the same specimens. The findings of 15-LOX and mutated p53 were highly correlated with each other and with the Gleason score. In only 5 of 48 patients did normal tissue adjacent to cancerous foci display staining for 15-LOX-1. No staining for mutated p53 was observed in any of the normal tissues. In contrast, in PC foci, robust staining was observed for both 15-LOX-1 (36 of 48; 75%) and mutated p53 (19 of 48; 39%). Furthermore, the intensities of expression of 15-LOX-1 and p53 correlated positively with each other ($p < 0.001$) and with the degree of malignancy as assessed by Gleason grading ($p < 0.01$).[233]

Therefore, with an understanding that the AA-COX-2-PGE2 pathway is a major sequence associated with inducing and perpetuating malignancy and inflammation, we now have some additional means to undo proinflammatory and promalignant situations. Understanding how the tumor cell is initiated and perpetuated provides methods for us to prevent or lessen the events that result in tumor growth. The Sears approach emphasizes the importance of carbohydrate restriction to prevent insulin surges (hyperinsulinemia), along with the incorporation of healthy fats into the diet and the use of highly purified fish oil to supply EPA and DHA. These are all directed to push the eicosanoid imbalance that is so characteristic of illness back toward the direction of health. In Figure 7, the pathway between di-homo gamma-linolenic acid (DGLA) and AA is shown with an arrow and bar blocking the pathway. This pathway is stimulated by insulin, but inhibited by EPA and DHA. With dietary measures, we can implement the concepts of COX-2 and LOX inhibition.[40]

The interferon-signaling pathway (ISP) was mentioned earlier as one of the defensive pathways that healthy cells use against the development of malignancy and against invasion by viruses. In response to a cancer cell or a virus, the body produces interferon. Interferon communicates with the cell through interactions at the surface membrane (a lipid membrane) via interferon receptors. This interaction initiates a chain of communications involving a number of intracellular pathways whose end functions involve the following:

- Immune modulation
- Cell differentiation or maturity
- Apoptosis
- Changes in the cell cycle

All of these functions (and others) represent some of the security systems within the cell that are intended to prevent or to halt tumor growth. The very same processes also serve to protect normal cells from viral invasion. However, as part of tumor evolution, the selective pressure of mutations results in faults in this security system—the ISP. The paradox is that the defects in the ISP that may lead to the development of cancer cells may at the same time leave the very same cancer cells vulnerable to viral invasion. In this manner, biology represents a two-edged sword, not just for the normal cell, but also for the cancer cell. What has allowed the normal cell to become a cancer cell due to disruptions in the ISP at the same time leaves the cancer cell vulnerable to lethal attack by viruses.

A new arena of anticancer activity involves the use of viruses that kill tumor cells (oncolytic viruses). Vesicular stomatitis virus (VSV) is an RNA virus that may infect cattle to cause a temporary lip blister similar to cold sores in humans. In studies of human tumor cells, VSV destroys an impressive array of tumor types while leaving normal cells unharmed.[241,235]

Intravenously administered VSV has shown evidence of anticancer activity in tumor cells that have lost their interferon-induced antiviral response.[236] VSV has demonstrated oncolytic activity against tumor cells lacking normal p53. Other studies have shown that tumor cells expressing a protein called large T antigen along with PKR, a protein kinase molecule, lack an antiviral response and may be sensitive to VSV oncolysis.[234,237,238] (A discussion of oncolytic viruses with illustrations appears in the December 2002 issue of the Prostate Exchange published by the Educational Council for Prostate Cancer Patients [ECPCP]). Their website is http://www.ecpcp.org.

Other activities that disclose the modus operandi of the cancer cells include the recruitment of raw materials from native resources to use as part of their weaponry. This includes the utilization of iron to initiate and further tumor cell growth. It is known that ferric iron ($Fe^{+++}$) is reduced by a vital cell guardian—superoxide dismutase (SOD)—to ferrous iron ($Fe^{++}$). In the process of this reaction, a hydroxyl free radical ($OH^-$) is produced that causes DNA damage by DNA strand breaks, cross-linking, and point mutations.[239] These mutations are often clustered at apparent hot spots, many of which are similar to sites seen using iron to generate oxygen radicals.

These results suggest that human cells are able to produce oxygen radicals in response to tumor promoters and that this might play a significant role in the generation of tumors.[239] There are many publications on the decline of SOD with age. There is also much written about the association of malignancy and other degenerative processes with SOD deficiency states.[240] What appears critically important in this and all discussions throughout this volume is the balance of free radicals and free radical scavengers and the defense measures to combat the imbalance resulting in oxidative stress. In fact, in established malignancies, we are using chemotherapies and other approaches that employ the generation of free radicals to kill the very cancer cells that may have arisen from an imbalance of ROS. As stated earlier, biology is a two-edged sword. All of biology relates to balance and communication.

Table 14 lists characteristics of societal terrorism and compares these with cellular terrorism. Possible antidotes for the latter are suggested. Perhaps in solving one problem, we solve multiple problems.

# 8. ANTIANGIOGENESIS TREATMENTS, DIETARY CHANGES

Much of this has already been discussed in previous pages. The survival of the tumor cell population

## Table 14: Characteristics Common to Social and Cellular Terrorism

This table is intended to show the parallels between events that occur on a cellular level and on a societal level. Possible solutions to the cellular crises faced in PC are shown in the third column. Perhaps they will stimulate more thoughts on how we should be dealing with terrorism, which affects all humankind.

| Characteristics Common to Societal Terrorism | Characteristics Common to Biological (Cell) Terrorism | Solutions, Strategies, and Considerations |
|---|---|---|
| Unhealthy parenting; inadequate disciplinary measures during childhood and adolescence | Damage to p53, GST, and other guardians of the genome and cell cycle; demethylation and/or hypermethylation of DNA leading to DNA adducts, cross-linking, and/or point mutations | Genetic manipulations introducing native p53; use of ONYX-15 oncolytic virus that kills cells lacking native p53; glutathione supplements |
| Resistance to discipline, high rate of repeat offenses (recidivism) | Increased resistance to apoptosis; increase in bcl-2, bcl XL | Use of antisense oligonucleotides against bcl-2 and other antiapoptotic agents; use of Taxane chemotherapies that cause phosphorylation of bcl-2 |
| Creation of internal instability | DNA mutation; generation of arachidonic metabolites | Minimize genetic hits by reducing carcinogens in external and internal environments, such as excessive alcohol, cigarettes, automobile and airplane exhaust; dietary measures to prevent demethylation or hypermethylation, such as use of folate, B12, methionine |
| Incitement of population via inflammatory rhetoric | Production of proinflammatory chemicals, such as bad eicosanoids | Dietary lifestyle changes to avoid AA metabolite excesses; reduction of meat and egg yolk rich in AA; use of refined fish oil rich in EPA (Sears approach) |
| Hyperreactive to demands of society | Generation of excessive ROS | Decrease environmental exposure to ROS (UV light, ozone); stress avoidance; exercise in moderation; use free radical scavengers, such as selenium, vitamin E, SOD, DMSO, melatonin, fermented papaya, and so on |
| Illegal border crossings | Damage to cell membranes via lipid peroxidation (LPO) | Dietary changes to avoid AA metabolite excesses; use of CoQ10 to protect lipid membranes |
| Destruction and corruption of surveillance operations | Disruption of ISP; Ras gene activation that downregulates PKR signal transduction pathway | Oncolytic viruses, such as VSV and NVD to destroy tumor cells that have defects in the ISP; reolysin (oncolytic virus) that destroys tumors with Ras gene activation |
| Illegal appropriation of natural resources to create weapons of destruction | Utilization of bone-derived growth factors, such as TGF-b1, IGF-1, and IL-1, to promote tumor growth; use of iron to create OH radicals which damage DNA and lead to mutations | Stabilize bone microenvironment with bisphosphonates plus bone supplements and moderate resistive exercise; avoid dietary excess of iron; avoid blood transfusions (if possible); possible use of antimalarial compounds that kill tumor cells at iron-bearing sites |
| Ability to thrive in a low-level environment and resist elimination | Tumor growth in areas of tissue hypoxia (low levels of oxygen); radiation resistance of center of tumors where hypoxia exists | Diagnose tumors before they are bulky; cytoreduce tumors with androgen deprivation prior to RT; use of surgical debulking; use of hypoxic cell sensitizers with RT, such as 5-FU, cisplatin low-dose infusion |
| Recruitment of new terrorists as old ones die out | Increase in angiogenesis in areas of tissue hypoxia | Antiangiogenesis strategies such as doxycycline, androgen deprivation, reduction of PGE2 via zone approach; anti-VEGF monoclonal antibody therapy |
| Difficulty in eradication in general | Increase in telomerase | Use of telomerase inhibitors, such as use of histone deacetylase inhibitors, nerve growth factor,[241] and telomerase ASO |

*(Continued)*

**Table 14: Characteristics Common to Social and Cellular Terrorism—cont'd**

| Characteristics Common to Societal Terrorism | Characteristics Common to Biological (Cell) Terrorism | Solutions, Strategies, and Considerations |
|---|---|---|
| Difficulty in eradication of established terrorist cells | Low response rates to therapy in late diagnosed PC; higher probability of mutated disease in late diagnosed PC | Screening with earlier diagnosis; debulking of tumor surgically and with ADT |
| Spread of malignant credo to other parts of population | Invasion and metastasis | Antisense oligonucleotides (ASO) to uPA; early diagnosis and treatment; stabilize bone microenvironment |
| Suicide missions are common practice | Death of tumor cell population with death of host (patient) | Preventive medicine that invokes many of above approaches; learning early warning signals of cancer, routine use of effective screening, recognizing importance of trends and use of profiles in cancer behavior |

requires that the nutritional needs of the tumor cell be met. This may relate to the supply lines to the tumor—the vascular pathways that carry oxygen and amino acids, sugars, and fats required by the tumor for growth and function—or to the supplies themselves. Vascular pathways or blood vessels specifically arise through the process of angiogenesis, or new blood vessel growth. The major stimulant for that growth is hypoxia, or low levels of oxygen in the tissue. Hypoxia, which stimulates new blood vessel growth is also identified as a major factor relating to failure of radiation and chemotherapy protocols.

Tumor hypoxia has been shown to be an independent prognostic indicator of poor outcome in prostate, head and neck, and cervical cancers. Laboratory and clinical data have shown that hypoxia is also associated with a more malignant phenotype (observable physical or biochemical characteristics of an organism) as well as increased instability of the genome, resistance to apoptosis, increased angiogenesis and a greater propensity to metastasis.[242] In a study of the effect of hypoxia on radiation dose needed for tumor cell killing, the dose of radiation had to be increased by a factor of 2.6–2.8 if the tumor cell population contained an average of 20% hypoxic cells.[243]

Because tissue hypoxia or lower partial pressures of oxygen are found more frequently in tumor cells compared to normal cells,[244] consideration of therapies to reduce hypoxia and angiogenesis are reasonable strategies for clinical trials. The use of a Zone approach to calorie input (eating), according to the writings of Sears, has the potential to profoundly affect angiogenesis. This is because PGE2, a major metabolite of AA, is known to stimulate VEGF and hence angiogenesis.[44,245] A carbohydrate-restricted diet focused on preventing hyperinsulinemia and the use of highly refined fish oil supplementation containing EPA to shift the pathway from AA to favorable eicosanoids has been mentioned previously, but must be strongly reinforced as a simple, inexpensive foundation to lowering VEGF levels. This certainly should be studied in a clinical trial.

In a study by Fosslien et al., the induction of the COX-2 enzyme was associated with an increase in TGF-b1 and VEGF. Of interest is that these 3 agents favoring the growth of the cancer cells were co-localized.[245]

Measures to reduce angiogenesis could involve not only reduction in PGE2 production, but also the use of antiangiogenesis agents such as ADT, which decreases androgen levels and reduces VEGF.[221] Other therapies to reduce angiogenesis are shown in Table 15.

## Docetaxel and Management of Androgen-Independent Prostate Cancer

Androgen hormones are produced in the adrenal glands and testis. These hormones facilitate the growth of PC cells (testosterone in particular). Hormone therapy targeted at lowering testosterone levels can be an option when PC spreads beyond the prostate gland to other parts of the body, or if it comes back after being treated before, or if it is advanced and surgery and radiation are not good treatment options for a patient. Effective hormone therapy lowers PSA levels, an indicator of the amount of cancer in a patient's body.

Although hormone therapy (ADT) can lower androgen levels, it does not cure PC. It is a management strategy which can shrink the cancer or cause it to grow more slowly. Over time, PC can become androgen independent. Androgen-independent prostate cancer

**Table 15: Tactics to Reduce Angiogenesis**

Although the various tactics to reduce angiogenesis shown in this table are based on the peer-reviewed literature, only one treatment is commonly being used to reduce angiogenesis—androgen deprivation therapy, or ADT.

| Antiangiogenesis Tactics | Mechanism(s) | References |
|---|---|---|
| Reduction in VEGF | Reduction in PGE2 via COX-2; inhibition by dietary measures | 41, 44, 46, |
| Reduction in VEGF | Reduction in COX-2 with inhibitors such as Celebrex® | 245, 250 |
| | Reduction in testosterone via ADT | 221, 251, 252, |
| | Reduction in caloric intake (possibly) Use of vitamin E (possibly) | 33, 65 |
| Decrease in microvessel density (MVD) | Apoptosis of the endothelial cells using Hytrin® | 26 |
| Decrease in tumor-associated macrophage (TAM) activity | Reduction in TNF-alpha, such as Linomide, pentoxifylline (Trental®), thalidomide, and genistein, leads to decreased VEFG | 253, 254 |
| Increased production of GM-CSF | GM-CSF increases production of plasminogen activator inhibitor type 2 (PAI-2), such as Linomide | 253, 254 |
| Decrease TGF-b1 | Use of Losartan, Cozaar, Hyzaar; use of pentoxifylline | 212, 255 |
| Reduction of MMPs | Doxycycline (Periostat®) Other tetracyclines. | 256, 257 |

(AIPC; also hormone-refractory prostate cancer) does not require androgen hormones to grow. If PC becomes androgen-independent or hormone-refractory, effective treatment options are very limited.[246] However, use of docetaxel, a chemotherapy drug, has shown promise in AIPC patients.[247]

Docetaxel (Taxotere®) is a drug from the taxane family of medicines that is used in chemotherapy for some types of advanced cancers. It is synthesized from an extract of European yew needles (*Taxus baccata*).[248] Taxotere® was approved by the Food and Drug Administration (FDA) on June 22, 1998 for locally advanced or metastatic BC that had progressed during anthracycline-based treatment or had relapsed during anthracycline-based adjuvant therapy. On December 23, 1999, Taxotere® received FDA approval for locally advanced or metastatic nonsmall-cell lung cancer after prior platinum-based chemotherapy failed.

Docetaxel has shown promising results in the management of AIPC.[247–249] Used as a single agent, docetaxel had an overall PSA response rate (reduction) of 42% in four phase 2 studies.[248] Even more impressive were the results of docetaxel in combination with other chemotherapy drugs.[247,249] A review of clinical trials investigating docetaxel used alone or in combination with other agents found that when docetaxel was combined with other agents, it consistently demonstrated a palliative response.

The docetaxel-based regimens were moderately well tolerated and PSA decreased by 50% or more in over 60% of patients, indicating a decrease in measurable disease and suggesting improved survival.[247] Close patient monitoring is required because Taxotere® can cause allergic reactions, decreased red and white blood cells, and liver damage.

# 9. STABILIZING KEY ARENAS OF CONFLICT: FOCUS ON BONE INTEGRITY, BIOMARKERS, AND MORE

The old expression of "cross one bridge at a time" is valuable in approaching life's problems. In the various arenas encountered by the PPP in dealing with PC, this philosophical approach is sound advice. The crux of integrative or holistic medicine is the realization that fixing one aspect of health affects multiple areas—everything is interconnected. This is especially true for PC-related issues.

## Bone Integrity Affects the Natural History of Prostate Cancer

Bone integrity in a man with PC is often ignored until the patient is symptomatic. Not until recently have the issues of osteoporosis and its relationship to PC come to the medical forefront. Not only is bone integrity of vital consequence in the matter of PC spreading to the bone, but also in the realization that bone loss through resorption can lead to bone pain, compression of the bones of the vertebral column, and fracture of a weight-bearing bone in the hip or other bones affecting function. Such complications demand immediate attention and the need for surgical and/or radiation treatment. Frequently, the patient requires strong

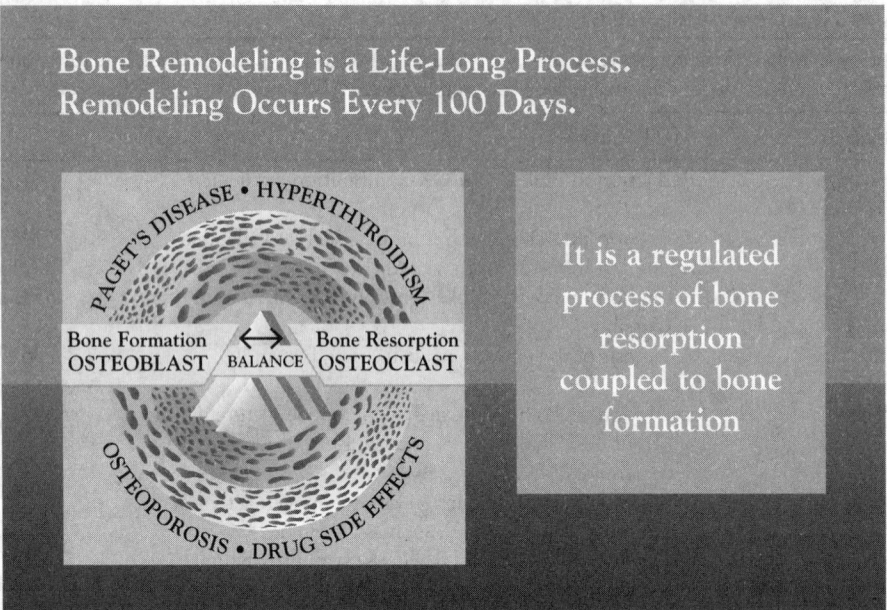

Figure 8. **The Dynamic Nature of Bone.** Think of bone dynamics as a mathematical equation. One side of the equation represents bone formation and the other represents bone loss or resorption. When bone resorption is decreased, the net result is that bone formation is favored, and vice-versa.

pain-killing medications. Such adverse occurrences clearly detract from the quality of life of the PC survivor, his family, and friends. Putting out this new fire also diverts attention away from the primary issues of control and eradication of the PC.

We know that the main danger in PC is its ability to metastasize to the bone. The bone is a favored place when PC cells metastasize. Stephen Paget discussed this in 1889 in his essays on *The Seed and the Soil*[258]:

> When a plant goes to seed, its seeds are carried in all directions; but they can grow only if they fall on congenial soil.

Paget recognized this inclination for cancer of the breast to spread to the bone. The same proclivity is found in PC. PC and BC are brother/sister diseases, strikingly alike in a multitude of ways. Most physicians consider the bone a static tissue, but it is exactly the opposite. The bone is constantly undergoing change in a process called remodeling. Bone tissue is formed and lost in the processes of bone formation and bone resorption (see Figure 8). This remodeling of bone tissue occurs every 100 days.

The dynamic nature of the bone tissue has been described in medical literature in thousands of peer-reviewed publications. Many patients and physicians are surprised to learn that the bone is extremely rich in growth factors. These growth factors have been implicated in PC growth and metastasis. Therefore, it should come as no surprise that PC cells consider

the bone a haven or sanctuary—congenial soil, to use the words of Paget. The rationale of current therapies in prostate, breast, and other cancers is to stabilize the bone microenvironment so that these bone-derived growth factors (BDGF) are not made readily available to nurture PC growth, invasion, and metastasis.

**The difference between evaluation of bone status using QCT versus DEXA.** Emphasizing the importance of the bone microenvironment in PC appears justified because there is a strong correlation with osteoporosis and osteopenia, as determined by bone mineral density examinations, at the time of diagnosis of PC.

In a report, osteoporosis was present in 63% of men at the time of diagnosis of PC, prior to any therapy. An additional 32% of men, in this same study population, had osteopenia.[259] In this landmark paper, the investigators evaluated DEXA bone mineral density testing and compared it to quantitative computerized tomography (QCT) bone mineral density testing in the same patients. A significantly greater percentage of men were found to have osteoporosis using the QCT methodology than the DEXA approach. DEXA bone mineral density evaluation picked up osteoporosis in only 5% of men. Therefore, using QCT technology, abnormalities in bone density were found in 95% of men compared to 34% of men with DEXA.

Studies done by Strum and Scholz have confirmed the results of Smith et al. (see Table 16). We found either osteoporosis (50%) or osteopenia (50%) in 100% of the men we studied with QCT. In the same

**Table 16:** **DEXA Scanning Underestimates the Occurrence of Osteoporosis in Men with PC**

The data from 2 separate groups evaluating DEXA versus QCT bone mineral density (done at the same time in men with PC) are strikingly alike. The evaluation of bone density with QCT should be a routine tactic in our goal to achieve and maintain bone integrity.

| Clinical Study | Osteopenia | Osteoporosis | Totals |
|---|---|---|---|
| Smith et al.[259] | | | |
| DEXA | 29% | 5% | 34% |
| QCT | 32% | 63% | 95% |
| Strum et al.[260] | | | |
| DEXA | 50% | 5% | 55% |
| QCT | 50% | 50% | 100% |

men, using DEXA, we found only 5% with osteoporosis and 50% with osteopenia.[260] A reasonable question is: Why are there such differences between the 2 techniques? The DEXA scan may read degenerative changes involving bone and joint tissues and calcium deposits within blood vessels as bone density.[261–265]

**The T score determines your status and risk of fracture.** The definitions used in the bone mineral density reports that are valid for men or women relate to the T scores. These reports are confusing even to radiologists who are experts in this field. The Z score is often relayed to patients and physicians in the radiology report as the final diagnosis or impression. The Z score compares the findings of the bone density exam, be it QCT or DEXA, with an age-matched population. This is of little actual value because what we are doing is comparing possible pathologic findings in a patient with known problems with osteoporosis or osteopenia in a general population of similar age. If I were 70 years old, I would not feel reassured that I am like most other 70-year-olds (who may also have osteoporosis or osteopenia) and therefore I am considered to be normal. I want my bone density to be compared to that of someone with healthy bone tissue that is not likely to fracture, or to release BDGF (bone-derived growth factors), which may initiate PC, stimulate its growth, or have a permissive action on bone metastases.

Therefore, it is the T score that is, or should be, the benchmark in bone mineral density (BMD) evaluations. The T score is based on World Health Organization (WHO) population studies that indicate how your bone density compares to that of a healthy 30- to 35-year-old (woman). There have been no T-score determinations set up for men. If the BMD is exactly 1 standard deviation below that which is considered to be normal bone density for a 30- to 35-year-old woman, the patient's T score is –1.0. If the BMD is one half of a standard deviation above what is considered normal for a 30- to 35-year-old, the T score is +0.5. More than 1 standard deviation below normal is considered to be the cut-off level to define abnormality. Therefore, if you have a T score of –1.1 or less, you have at least osteopenia. If the T score falls between –1.1 and –2.5, you are still in the range of osteopenia. Once below –2.5, the patient falls into the category of osteoporosis. The fracture risk doubles for each standard deviation below the normal T score.[266] Therefore, a person with a T score of –2.0 has twice the chance of fracturing a bone compared to a person with a T score of –1.0.

Osteoporosis is rampant in men newly diagnosed with PC. That is clear from previously cited studies. In light of the knowledge that bone loss occurs during treatment with any therapy that lowers male hormone, the PC patient undergoing almost all forms of ADT is in jeopardy of having abnormal bone density and a serious risk of osteoporosis. Add to this knowledge the fact that bone loss through the process of resorption may be stimulating the PC, and the issue of bone integrity becomes paramount.

In the context of PC, the bone tissue has to be regarded as a strategic area and must be stabilized, fortified, and brought to the status of a stronghold if we are to optimize our care of the PC patient.

**Resources for QCT testing.** Improving bone integrity mandates that we first assess bone integrity status to obtain a baseline. BMD evaluation and the value of the QCT technique has been emphasized in the preceding paragraphs. Since QCT technology is not readily known to most physicians, it is important that patients and partners share these new findings and seek out radiology facilities that have QCT bone densitometry equipment. Two references for sources of QCT testing are Mindways, Inc. and Image Analysis. Telephone numbers and websites for these nationally based organizations are Mindways, (877) 646-3929 (www.qct.com), or Image Analysis, (800) 548-4849 (www.image-analysis.com). For further information on maintaining bone integrity, refer to the protocol Cancer Treatment: The Critical Factors.

**Importance of bone integrity extends to cardiovascular risk and possibly Alzheimer's disease.** Studies have shown a relationship of abnormal bone density with an increased risk of cardiovascular disease.[267,268] It has been the observation of many that the loss of bone matrix detected by measurements of bone mineral density appears to relate to the deposition of calcium in arteries such as the coronaries, aorta, and femoral arteries. The loss of calcium from the bone matrix is a characteristic finding during excessive bone resorption. Hypothetically, it is reasonable to consider that calcium lost from the bone matrix may be pathologically deposited in blood vessels as well as associated with calcifications elsewhere, such as kidney stones, gall stones, and prostatic calculi. In fact, correlations between osteoporosis and an increased risk for kidney stone development have been reported.

An improvement in bone density with treatments that are designed to prevent kidney stones have likewise been reported.[269,270] Studies have shown that bisphosphonate compounds (such as alendronate [Fosamax®]) not only improve bone mineral density but also decrease a substance known as osteopontin, which has been implicated in kidney stone development.[271] Other studies have presented this unifying concept and have even linked bone loss and kidney stones with hypertension (high blood pressure).[272]

A biological marker involved in PC, especially androgen-independent PC, is IL-6.[273–275] IL-6 is a cell product that stimulates the maturation of osteoclasts, the cells that are major players in the breakdown (resorption) of bone. IL-6 is produced by osteoblasts[276] and stimulates the mature osteoclasts to break down bone. IL-6 has been identified as an inflammatory cytokine that is likely to play a major role in Alzheimer's disease (AD). Therefore, the emphasis on bone integrity is of potentially great magnitude. Maintaining bone integrity can now be seen to play a role in the following:

• Prevention and treatment of osteopenia or osteoporosis

• Decrease in cardiovascular disease

• Reduction in kidney stone formation

• Minimization of release of bone-derived growth factors that can stimulate prostate or BC

• Prevention of Alzheimer's disease

This again points out that a holistic approach to medicine is vital to our understanding of unifying concepts involved in both health and disease. The hip bone is connected not only to the thigh bone, but also to the heart, kidneys, prostate, breast, and brain.

AD is considered to be an inflammatory disease of the brain associated with the deposition of beta amyloid material. In prior discussions, the importance of the eicosanoid pathways was detailed and the role of the inhibition of AA formation and the prevention of metabolites of AA such as PGE2 and 5-HETE by dietary changes and by the use of EPA and DHA were stressed. COX-2 inhibitors that prevent AA metabolism to PGE2 have been shown to

be associated with a decreased incidence of AD. Even nonselective COX-2 inhibitors such as Motrin® are now shown to have a protective effect against the development of AD.

There are studies that show that all of these pathways are integrated in PC. COX-2 expression and PGE2 secretion are increased in prostatic intraepithelial neoplasia (PIN) and PC. An upregulation of PGE2 by IL-6 in a human cell line of PIN has been demonstrated. PGE2 further stimulates IL-6 soluble receptor release and other complex intracellular functions (gp130 dimerization, Stat-3 protein phosphorylation, and DNA binding activity).[277] These events, induced by PGE2, lead to increased PIN growth. Conversely, the use of a selective COX-2 inhibitor (eg, Celebrex®) decreases cell growth. Moreover, PIN cell growth stimulated by PGE2 was nullified by adding antibodies to IL-6. The authors concluded that increased expression of COX-2/PGE2 contributes to PC development and progression via activation of the IL-6 signaling pathway.

It should therefore come as no surprise to find that a study of animals fed diets varying in the ratio of AA to EPA reported that (1) higher AA-EPA-ratio diets led to findings of increased PGE2 production in the bone; (2) higher PGE2 in the bone was associated with increased bone resorption; and (3) lower AA-EPA ratios (reflecting higher intake of EPA) were associated with bone formation and decreased PGE2 concentrations.[204]

There is no doubt that the signaling pathways of communication between a PC tumor cell and bone (with osteoblasts and osteoclasts) are multidimensional. A conceptualized graphic of some of these interactions was shown in Figure 1.

**Clinical aspects of bone integrity in the treatment of PC patients.** Many of the salient points relating to the evaluation and treatment of bone integrity can be found in the protocol titled Osteoporosis. In addition to numerous articles written by me in the PCRI newsletter Insights, there is also a PowerPoint presentation on this subject that can be downloaded without charge. An update on this topic also appears in *The Primer* (available at www.lefprostate.org). In general, the main issues that still need a greater focus of attention include the following:

• Every man with PC and most likely every apparently healthy man aged 45 or over should be evaluated for osteoporosis and osteopenia. (Refer to the Osteoporosis protocol.)

• Significant bone loss in PC patients is underestimated by the use of DEXA scanning and should be evaluated with QCT bone density study instead.

- Bone resorption, and its correction, are easily evaluated by using a sensitive biomarker, as a biological endpoint (BEP), and the Pyrilinks-D (free deoxypyridinoline or free Dpd).

Dpd levels can be obtained from the second urine sample of the patient's day. This test is inexpensive and is an excellent tool to monitor the biological endpoint of bone resorption activity. In men, a normal value for Dpd is less than or equal to 5.4 (nanomoles Dpd/nanomoles creatinine) using the Metra Biosystems assay and up to 6.6 using the assay from Quest Laboratories.

In men, if the free Dpd exceeds the upper limit of normal, it is indicative of excessive bone resorption. This finding may be secondary to underlying PC in the bone or secondary to increased bone resorption due to ADT or illnesses such as diabetes, hyperthyroidism, Paget's disease of the bone, or hyperparathyroidism.

If the Pyrilinks-D level is abnormal, it should be corrected with the use of combination therapy employing a bisphosphonate compound, a calcium-containing bone supplement, and Rocaltrol® (synthetic vitamin D). The most active oral bisphosphonates are Fosamax® and Actonel®. The bone supplement is best taken in the evening between dinner and bedtime. Studies have shown that the administration of calcium in a bone supplement will reduce bone resorption by up to 20%, but only if it is administered in the evening.[278] This is apparently due to a circadian rhythm involving bone formation and bone loss.

The use of Rocaltrol® (calcitriol or 1,25-dihydroxy vitamin D3) requires a prescription. It is not to be confused with ordinary vitamin D3. There are an increasing number of articles relating to the use of standard dose[279] or high dose calcitriol,[280] used either alone or with chemotherapy such as Taxotere®[281] in combination with bisphosphonates to slow the doubling time of PSA and dramatically reduce PSA levels. This holds great promise for the PC survivor.

When bone resorption is halted, and the net effect favors bone formation, it is critical that not only sufficient calcium be available to restore bone density, but also other ingredients necessary for healthy bone formation. These include magnesium, boron, and silica, as well as vitamin K. The nature of the calcium salt used in these preparations is also of major significance, because calcium carbonate is not well absorbed in older patients when gastric HCL production is decreased. Calcium citrate, bisglycinate, and microfine calcium hydroxyapatite should be used preferentially. It is important for the PPP team to understand the importance of these substances in bone physiology and their interactions

with other cellular processes. A detailed description of these issues can be found in *The Primer*.

# 10. SUPPORTIVE CARE OF THE PATIENT

A military campaign is never successful unless the troops are supported in their efforts. Great military strategists win their battles because they realize the value of generous support for their soldiers. This is true in all endeavors; it is critical to invoke this principle in the support of the patient as he faces challenging crossroads in pursuit of quality and quantity of life. This is the essence of outstanding medical care and goes hand-in-hand with the physician-scientist whose prime directive is a strategy of success for the patient with whose life he is entrusted. This is an incredible opportunity for physicians, given the immediate intimacy with patients and their partners facing life-threatening illnesses. But what does supportive care mean?

Supportive care of the patient involves the fine-tuning needed to maximize efficacy while minimizing adverse effects. This is the basis for the concept of Therapeutic Index.

Therapeutic Index (TI) = Benefits of Therapy ÷ Adverse Effects of Therapy

Supportive care of the patient must be a conscious upfront concern with every aspect of the physician/patient encounter. The following list details some of the main supportive care issues that the PC patient may encounter. This is not an exhaustive list because an itemization of every supportive care measure (SCM) would involve numerous pages of text.

## Supportive Care Measures Involved in the Diagnosis, Evaluation, and Treatment of Men with Prostate Cancer

**Diagnosis.** *(1) DRE (digital rectal examination): This must be done gently, and with ample lubricant. The patient's rectal sphincter should be given time to adjust to the initial palpation of the gloved finger. This should not be a "ram job" that is too often described by traumatized patients. No patient should be reaching for the chandelier during a DRE. There may be an uncomfortable sense of fullness, an awkward feeling that there may be some leakage of seminal fluid, but if the physician is adept at doing a DRE, the patient should not be fearful of another such examination.[282] I have found that if I describe to the patient what I am doing, and feeling, during the entire procedure, the patient is more focused on listening to what I am saying than on any minor discomfort he may be experiencing.*

The physician's notes concerning the DRE should be detailed. An estimate of the gland volume, a notation of any areas suspicious for PC, and if present, their extent regarding size, should be clearly entered in the medical record. The use of descriptors such as moderately enlarged or 1+ enlarged is worthless. The physician should commit to an estimate of the gland volume in cubic centimeters. A T-stage designation, essentially equivalent to the clinical stage of the disease, should also be routinely recorded.

After the DRE is complete, the physician should have tissues available for the patient to wipe himself and allow him to use the restroom to clean himself up further and wash his hands. The patient should not spend the rest of the day sliding around on lubricant left over from the DRE. This may seem to be an excessive amount of words to spend on this subject, but this is one of the first physically intimate interactions the physician has with the patient. It should create a sense of trust that the physician is sensitive to this embarrassing and awkward situation.

*(2) Venipuncture (blood drawing): This is something that the physician's staff does, but it is also so potentially traumatizing that some discussion is necessary. Assuming a good-sized vein is found and the R.N. or laboratory technician has had no problem in obtaining blood, a gauze pad should be placed over the vein as the needle is withdrawn. The patient should be told to apply firm pressure with his fingers over this gauze pad and hold it for a few minutes.*

What I have seen too often is that the needle is withdrawn and almost immediately a bandage is applied to cover the venipuncture site. No mention is made for the patient to apply pressure for at least 3–4 minutes. It is as if the covering of the needle exit site with a bandage will eliminate the chance of bleeding after venipuncture. Too often, the patient is left with blood on his clothing, a hematoma at the site of the venipuncture, possible loss of use of that vein, and emotional stress the next time he has blood drawn. These 2 interactions are very simple, yet often poorly done.

*(3) TRUSP (transrectal ultrasound of the prostate) with biopsies: The procedure should be discussed in advance with the patient and his partner. The importance of avoiding drugs such as aspirin and NSAIDs for at least 10 days prior to prostate biopsies should be mentioned. Given the commonality of bleeding into the prostate and blood in the urine or semen after TRUSP with biopsies,[283,284] I believe it would be reasonable for physicians to do an in-office template bleeding time (TBT). This is a cheap and easy test to rule out a drug effect on the platelets that would be associated with an increased risk for prolonged bleeding after multiple biopsies.*

The Surgicutt TBT normal range is less than 9 minutes. Surgicutt is available through ITC, Inc. at www.itcmed.com. The U.S. customer service number is (800) 631-5945. Secondly, a urologist or other physician planning to do the biopsies should, as a matter of routine, check the patient's CBC (complete blood count), absolute platelet count, PT (prothrombin time), and the APTT (activated partial thromboplastin time). If the platelet count is normal (over 150 000) and the PT, PTT, and TBT are all within normal limits, then any potential risk for significant hemorrhage from TRUSP with biopsies as a result of a blood-related problem(s) would be excluded.

If bleeding is persistent after TRUSP with biopsies, Proscar® at a dose of 5 mg daily should be considered. Even in the face of coagulation abnormalities, as mentioned above, a report by Kearney et al. showed a marked decrease in gross bleeding (hematuria) with the use of Proscar®. Note that this study involved men with BPH and the bleeding that occurred was unrelated to prostate biopsies.[285] Critical to the results of this study are additional reports indicating the key role that androgens such as testosterone and dihydrotestosterone (DHT) play in increasing VEGF.[218,249,286] It should come as no surprise that Proscar® and/or other inhibitors of DHT formation would have the ability to decrease bleeding due to the hypervascularity of tissue known to occur in BPH and in PC.[287]

As part of the supportive care of the patient, physicians should employ such pharmacologic strategies in patients with persistent bleeding after TRUSP with biopsies. This intervention would take into account that the use of drugs such as Proscar® or other 5-alpha-reductase inhibitors such as Avodart® are effective at reducing angiogenesis by virtue of decreasing VEGF within prostatic tissue.

Additionally, other studies in BC patients have shown that the COX-2 enzyme is upregulated in BC tissue and that this is associated with an increase in tumor blood vessels (microvessel density) and VEGF.[288] We know that many PC patients will also have overexpression of COX-2 and this should suggest treatment by COX-2 inhibition, be it via dietary manipulation or by drugs. Therefore, in the management of persistent bleeding from prostate tissue or any tissue that may have an increase in blood vessels due to the activation of the COX-2/VEGF angiogenesis pathway, these measures are reasonable options to discuss with your physicians.

Not only is the bleeding complication of biopsy traumatic for the patient, but it also interferes with the interpretation of other investigational studies due to the effects of hemorrhage within the prostate. For example, if PC is diagnosed and an endorectal MRI is suggested for evaluation, the occurrence of any significant intraprostatic bleeding will complicate the interpretation of the MRI because cancer and hemorrhages both demonstrate the same low signal intensity.[289] It will take a minimum of 8 weeks for the postbiopsy hemorrhage to clear sufficiently to allow the endorectal MRI to be done under optimal conditions.

The patient's preparation for the TRUSP with biopsies should include a 1-day course of prophylactic antibiotics (Cipro, Floxin, or Levaquin) and a Fleet's enema to clear the rectal chamber.[290–292]

The patient should receive some type of pain medication prior to the actual biopsies.[293,294] It is amazing that a dentist will routinely give Novocain to fix dental cavities, but men going through 6–13 biopsies of their prostate gland have been offered local analgesia only for the last 5–6 years. Studies showing efficacy in reducing pain from the biopsy procedure have utilized injections of lidocaine (1%) into the tissue surrounding the prostate[294–297] or have used lidocaine gel (2%) as a lubricant for the insertion of the transrectal probe in order to provide analgesia during the biopsy procedure.[298,299] It is sad testimony that such studies were not done 10–15 years ago and that currently less than 50% of patients undergoing biopsy are offered periprostatic analgesia or some other approach to lessen their pain.[290,300,301]

Although not as distressing to the patient as a TRUSP with biopsies, the use of an endorectal probe during an endorectal MRI study can cause discomfort and pain. All along the road of diagnosis, evaluation, and management, the caring physician should be sensitive to any emotional or physical misery the man with PC may encounter. The road should be smoothed and the journey thus made easier. Insertion of an endorectal probe and inflation of the balloon surrounding the probe can be an unpleasant surprise. I have heard this from many men caught unaware. It is very simple to inform a patient who is planning this procedure about the possible discomfort and to propose workarounds.

Perhaps a complete liquid diet the day before and a Fleet's enema until clear on the morning of the endorectal MRI will lessen the discomfort because the rectal vault will be empty. The patient's primary physician may also prescribe Valium® 5 mg and Vicodin ES®, with 1 tablet of each medication to be taken about 30 minutes prior to the procedure. If the patient has not had prior experience with these drugs, his physician could prescribe a few extra tablets of each so that the patient can experience how he feels after taking this

combination. Of course, the patient should not consume alcoholic beverages or drive when these drugs are taken. This kind of approach can change the patient's experience from one characterized by anxiety and pain to one of assuredness and acceptable discomfort.

*(4) LUTS (lower urinary tract symptoms): In the course of the above evaluations leading to a diagnosis of PC, it is not uncommon for the physician to encounter men having problems with LUTS. Symptoms relating to slowness of urinary stream, difficulty in initiating urination, intermittent flow of the stream, dribbling of urine near the end of urination, getting up at night to urinate (nocturia), and other symptoms are cataloged objectively by the AUA symptom index score. This is described in detail in Appendix F (Forms) of The Primer.*

Out of these problems come opportunities for the physician focused on supportive care. He can not only lessen the problems caused by LUTS, but also implement a pharmacological strategy that has an anti-PC effect. The efficacy of multitasking relates to the fact that, more often than not, our therapies, if chosen carefully, can elicit multiple benefits. Clearly, if LUTS is treated with finasteride (Proscar®), we also are initiating the following biochemical effects:

- Inhibition of 5-alpha-reductase type 2, blocking conversion of testosterone to DHT
- Reduction in epidermal growth factor (EGF), especially in the periurethral zone[302]
- Reduction in both glandular and stromal elements within the prostate gland[303]
- Decrease in VEGF
- Decrease in microvessel density
- Decreased expression of basic fibroblast growth factor (bFGF)[304]
- Downregulation of androgen receptor (AR) expression[305]
- Decrease in IGF-1 gene expression in BPH patients[35]
- Increased programmed cell death of PC epithelial cells[306]

To add compliment to benefit, agents (alpha-1 blockers) that improve urine flow by affecting periurethral smooth muscle have been shown to be synergistic with Proscar® in causing prostate cell apoptosis.[306] These effects are not restricted to the benign prostate cell population of BPH, but are also operative in PC. In the study by Glassman et al.,[306] terazosin (Hytrin®), an alpha-1 blocker used in treating LUTS, was shown to cause apoptosis of prostate cells and to be synergistic with Proscar®. In our supportive care of PC patients, we can choose drugs that have multiple modes of biological action and by doing so improve the outcome for our patients. In other words, we can treat LUTS and improve the quality of life for men with these symptoms, while at the same time having a beneficial effect against PC.

Table 17 lists some of the literature citing activity of alpha-1-adrenoreceptor blocking agents in causing programmed cell death to prostate cells, both benign and malignant. Of the alpha-1 blockers used in the United States today to treat LUTS, 2 are in the piperazinyl quinazoline class; these are Hytrin® and Cardura® (doxazosin). These agents cause apoptosis of PC cells. The third agent, Flomax® (tamsulosin), an alpha-1 blocker in the sulphonamide class, does not have the apoptotic effects of either Hytrin® or Cardura®.

LUTS also has another potential role in the supportive care interactions between PC patients and their physicians—the choice of the primary PC treatment. The currently accepted choices of primary therapy include:

- RP
- RT of any kind, such as
  - **3D-conformal RT,**
    - Conventional brachytherapy,
    - High-dose rate brachytherapy,
    - Proton beam RT,
  - **Neutron beam RT**

- Cryosurgery
- ADT
- Watchful waiting

In the setting of significant lower urinary tract symptoms that are not responsive to available therapies, RP, done by a surgeon, will resolve the issue of LUTS. In contrast, RT will usually aggravate LUTS and not occasionally cause problems with urinary retention necessitating TURP (transurethral resection of the prostate). What an RP accomplishes in this respect is the removal of the prostatic urethra—the site of compression by tissue of the transition zone of the prostate. The transition zone is the portion of the zonal anatomy of the prostate gland that is significantly increased in men with BPH, a problem that commonly occurs in association with PC (see Figure 4).

It is reasonable to consider, in this respect, the use of ADT3, which combines an LHRH-agonist agent such as Lupron, Zoladex®, Trelstar® LA, or Viadur® with an antiandrogen such as Eulexin®, Casodex®, or Nilandron® and a 5-alpha reductase inhibitor such as Proscar® or Avodart®, as well as an alpha-1 blocker in light of the data presented in Table 17. If the ADT3 plus alpha-1 blocker is given with other supportive care measures, the patient has numerous ways to use this therapy with both therapeutic and prognostic strategies. This is especially true in men not physically fit enough to undergo an RP or in those with risk factors

**Table 17: Drugs Normally Used to Treat LUTS May Cause Apoptosis and Have Other Effects against Androgen Independent PC (AIPC)**

This table highlights how a physician utilizing the multitasking effects of drugs currently in use can enhance the supportive care of men with PC. These findings also suggest a possible role for these agents in the prevention of PC.

| Study Drug(s) | Cell Population | Biologic Effect(s) | Author | Reference |
|---|---|---|---|---|
| Hytrin® | BPH | Apoptosis increased | Glassman | 306 |
| Hytrin® | BPH with PC | Apoptosis increased; microvessel density (MVD) decreased; PSA expression in tissue decreased; VEGF unchanged | Kaledjian | 307 |
| Cardura® | PC (AIPC) | Apoptosis increased via bcl-2 downregulation | Ng | 308 |
| Both drugs | BPH | Apoptosis in epithelial and stromal cells; smooth muscle alpha-actin expression decreased | Chon | 309 |
| Both drugs | PC (AIPC) | Apoptosis of PC cells increased independently of alpha-1 blockade | Benning | 310 |
| Both drugs | BPH and PC | Apoptosis increased in dose-dependent manner | Kyprioanou | 311 |
| Both drugs | PC (AIPC) | Apoptosis synergistic with radiation therapy (RT) when Hytrin® or Cardura® given prior to or after RT; BAX or caspase-3 not increased | Cuellar | 312 |

that would suggest that RP is not likely to be curative. This will be discussed in a later section.

**Evaluation.** *(5) Choice of Diagnostic Studies to Evaluate Stage in Newly Diagnosed Men with PC:* Supportive care of the patient also involves a physician knowledgeable enough about PC to know when not to use health care dollars in ordering tests of negligible yield in the workup of a PC patient. This decreases the costs to patients, minimizes exposure to ionizing radiation, and reduces the workload on health care personnel when tests inappropriate to the patient's biological status are not needed.

This is especially true for CT scans of the pelvis and abdomen. Such studies done shortly after diagnosis are rarely abnormal. Eliminating such expensive procedures could better direct medical funds to more productive testing or treatment. In newly diagnosed PC patients with Gleason scores of less than (4,3)—validated by an expert laboratory or pathologist—a CT scan is not indicated unless the PSA exceeds 20 ng/mL. In a study of 425 PC patients, the authors concluded that in asymptomatic patients with newly diagnosed, untreated PC and serum PSA levels of less than 20 ng/mL, the likelihood of positive findings on abdominal/pelvic CT is extremely low (<1.0%).[313]

The same is also true of the bone scan in newly diagnosed patients with a baseline PSA of 10 ng/mL or less—assuming that the Gleason score is less than 7.[314] A study by Chybowski et al. concluded that the negative predictive value for a positive bone scan given a serum PSA of less than or equal to 20 ng/mL was 99.7%. Only 1 patient out of 306 with a PSA of less than or equal to 20 (PSA = 18.2) had a positive bone scan. Of the 207 patients with PSAs of less than or equal to 10 ng/mL, none had a positive bone

scan and only 1 of the 99 patients with a PSA of greater than 10 and less than or equal to 20 had a positive bone scan. It therefore appears reasonable to forego bone scanning in newly diagnosed, untreated PC patients who have PSAs of less than or equal to 10 ng/mL.[315] In another study, Oesterling et al. reported that only one abnormal bone scan out of a total of 200 bone scans (0.5%) would be missed if the requirement for performing a bone scan was a PSA greater than 10 ng/mL.[316]

In light of the fact that more and more men are being diagnosed with PSA levels of < 10, the impact on the health care economy when physicians order these tests in a reflex fashion is disastrous. Assuming that 180 000 men are newly diagnosed with PC each year in the United States and that at least 70% of them will have PSA levels at diagnosis below 10 ng/mL, and a negligible number will have PSA levels greater than 20 ng/mL, the health care financial waste is staggering (see Table 18).

Given that the average cost of a bone scan, CT scan of the pelvis, and CT scan of the abdomen is $600 per test, the waste in health care dollars is approximately $300 million each year! If we add to this a pelvic MRI study (not to be confused with an endorectal MRI), the cost could total $400 million per year. These sums represent flagrantly wasted economic resources, misused technician time, and unnecessary radiation exposure as well as inconvenience to patients. Most importantly, think of what some of this money could do in areas truly needing economic support, be it from private insurance carriers or in the United States to the taxpayer.

The major exception to the above is in the case of a patient with a Gleason score of (4,3) or higher at diagnosis. In such a setting of a high Gleason score, characterized by significant amounts of grade-4 and/or

**Table 18:** Implications of Misuse of Staging Studies in Newly Diagnosed PC Patients with a PSA of ≤ 10 ng/mL or ≤ 20 ng/mL.

Most newly diagnosed patients with PC are subjected to a bone scan as well as CT scans of the pelvis and abdomen and some patients are also advised to have a conventional pelvic MRI. The health care waste in the setting of a newly diagnosed patient having a validated Gleason score of less than (4,3), and a PSA of ≤ 10 ng/mL (bone scanning) or ≤ 20 ng/mL (CT pelvis, abdomen, MRI pelvis), misdirects money and effort away from a rational strategy that could offer far more guidance to the PC survivor, his partner, and his physician.

| Diagnostic Test | Setting | Yield | Suggestions/Ramifications |
|---|---|---|---|
| Bone scan | PSA = 10 ng/mL | 0.3–0.5% abnormal (1 in 200-333) | Forego bone scan; savings of $76 million/year in the United States |
| CT scan of pelvis | PSA = 20 ng/mL | <1% (<1 in 100) | Forego CT pelvis exam; savings of $108 million/year in the United States |
| CT scan of abdomen | PSA = 20 ng/mL | <1% (<1 in 100) | Forego CT abdominal exam; savings of $108 million/year in the United States |
| MRI pelvis | PSA = 20 ng/mL | 0.6% (1 in 150) | Forego MRI pelvis; savings of $160 million/year in the United States |
| Total | | | Savings of $300–400 million/year! |

grade-5 disease, for example, (4,3), (4,4), (4,5), (5,4), and (5,5), the PSA leak phenomenon must be taken into account.[130] Such patients may have low PSA levels, not uncommonly less than 5, yet have metastatic disease to bone. However, it must be emphasized that such patients have Gleason scores of 8–10 at the time of diagnosis or on the occasion that they are rebiopsied due to findings suggesting active PC.

**Treatment.** (6) *Testosterone Deprivation Therapy and Its Far-Reaching Implications: If there is any area of PC management that necessitates a comprehensive understanding by the physician, it is in knowing the spectrum of effects of ADT on male physiology. A lack of such understanding deprives the patient of available supportive care that can mean the difference between success and failure in the patient's life. This not only relates to preventing or minimizing side effects due to treatment, but also to the patient's compliance with therapy—whether he will remain on the medications used in ADT or stop them due to adverse effects.*

In the early 1980s, I began treating PC patients using antiandrogen therapy in combination with an LHRH agonist as one of the first American collaborators working with Fernand Labrie. My observation of patients taught me a great deal about the effects of an accelerated and intensified male menopause. The lowering of serum testosterone to castrate levels, defined as less than 20 ng/dL (<0.68 nmol/L), resulted in a spectrum of possible signs and symptoms that varied from man to man.

Some of these symptoms occurred acutely, while others developed over time. However, all were potentially troublesome, if not aggravating, for the patient.

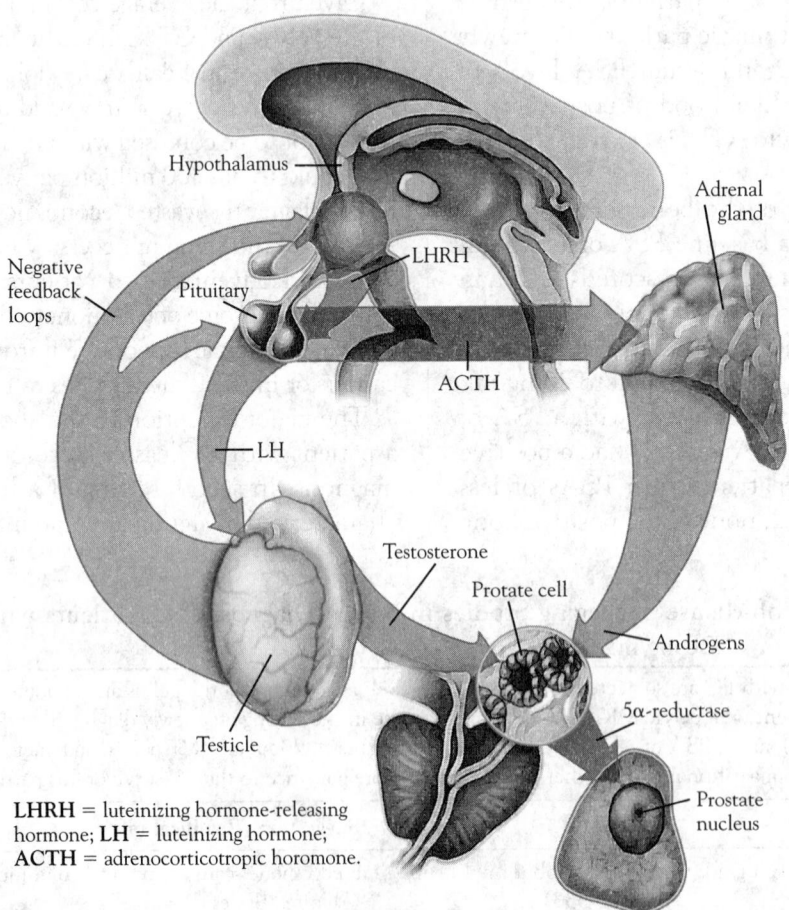

Figure 9. **The Hormonal Access Involved in PC Treatment.** LH-RH agonist therapy with drugs such as Lupron, Zoladex, and Trelstar LA block LH production from the pituitary. This results in a major decrease in the production of testosterone from the testicles. When this happens, a reflex pathway involving the hypothalamus sends messages to the pituitary to compensate for lack of testosterone. After orchiectomy, LH production increases (and FSH also). With LHRH-A therapy, these LH/FSH increases are blocked. The overall stimulation of the pituitary also results in increased ACTH levels that stimulate the adrenals to make adrenal androgen precursors. Anti-androgens are helpful to further block the effects of any uninhibited androgen. (Artwork reproduced with kind permission of graphic artist Kevin Somerville [ksomrvl@cox.net] and the editors of *Contemporary Urology* from Cain, M. and Fisher, H.A.: Androgen deprivation therapy: on methods, timing, and cost. *Contemp Urol* 4 : 79–86, 1992.)

If not treated in a preventive manner, such signs and symptoms can have a negative impact upon the patient's overall health.

Except for hot flashes and impotency, many symptoms resulting from androgen deprivation have been discounted by physicians as being due to old age or medical problems such as arthritis or heart disease. However, this constellation of clinical and laboratory abnormalities quickly develops in younger men or older men in otherwise good health after the initiation of ADT. This clearly suggests that these symptoms are not due to "old age" but are characteristics of the androgen deprivation syndrome (ADS).

ADS symptoms are directly or indirectly due to the drop in testosterone level that occurs following orchiectomy or use of an LHRH agonist (LHRH-A) such as Lupron, Zoladex®, Trelstar® LA, or Viadur®. In essence, men who are medically or surgically castrated undergo an accelerated and intensified form of male menopause that leads to many of the same symptoms that are seen in women going through female menopause. Patients treated with combined ADT (LHRH agonists or orchiectomy plus an antiandrogen such as Eulexin®, Casodex®, or Nilandron®) may have more severe ADS symptoms than those treated with an LHRH agonist or orchiectomy alone. This is because the additional use of an antiandrogen also helps to block residual testosterone from interacting at androgen receptor sites located throughout the body. LHRH agonists or orchiectomy suppress testicular androgen and not androgen synthesis from the adrenal glands. In fact, orchiectomy will result in increased production of adrenal androgen precursors due to a reflex stimulation of the hypothalamic-pituitary tract. This causes an increased production of LH along with an overflow stimulation of ACTH, which increases production of adrenal androgen precursors (see Figure 9).[317]

As mentioned in the section on LUTS, the addition of Proscar® will result in a further lowering of androgen effect. This is due to the ability of Proscar® to block the enzyme 5-alpha-reductase (type 2), which converts testosterone to DHT. DHT is therefore a metabolite of testosterone and is 5 times more potent than testosterone in stimulating cell growth. In addition to this, Proscar® also downregulates the expression of the androgen receptor. Therefore, it should not be surprising that ADT3, as described previously, would have the greatest potential for side effects due to androgen deprivation, but would also have a higher probability to have a greater antitumor effect on the PC cell population for the very same reason. If we were to routinely add the use of an alpha-1 blocker such as Hytrin® or Cardura®, we should have even greater effects against the PC population due to a decrease in microvessel density, downregulation of bcl-2, and enhanced apoptosis (as discussed in the section on LUTS and shown in Table 17).

In fact, the designation ADT4 could indicate the addition of a piperazinyl quinazoline compound of the alpha-1 blocker class to the standard ADT3 regimen of LHRH-A, antiandrogen, and 5-alpha-reductase inhibitor.

Androgen deprivation with 4 agents or ADT4 would involve the routine use of an agent of the quinazoline class of alpha-1 blockers such as Hytrin® or Cardura®. These agents will not only improve urinary flow, but also act to enhance the effects of ADT3. Therefore, the typical ADT4 regimen would include:

- LHRH-agonist: Lupron, Zoladex®, Trelstar® LA, or Viadur®
- Antiandrogen: Eulexin®, Casodex®, or Nilandron®
- 5-alpha-reductase inhibitor: Proscar® or Avodart®
- Alpha-1 blocker: Hytrin® or Cardura®

As emphasized earlier, there is a spectrum of side effects that may be seen with the use of ADT. These untoward effects are highly variable from man to man. Some men have no significant clinical symptomatology associated with the use of ADT, while others state they cannot function with a reasonable quality of life. The supportive care of the patient by the physician in using ADT is vital to the acceptability of this very important modality used in the treatment of PC. We can improve the therapeutic index of ADT by finding solutions to the problems that may occur as part of the androgen deprivation syndrome, or ADS.

Signs and symptoms that are part of the spectrum of ADS are shown in Table 19. These are divided into systems or tissues affected and the nature and onset of the symptoms, that is, acute and chronic. Again, it is of vital importance to understand that there is significant variability from patient to patient regarding frequency of occurrence and timing of all such findings.

To assess the significance of common ADS symptoms, we evaluated 177 hormone-naïve PC patients consecutively treated with an LHRH-agonist and an antiandrogen between 1994 and 1997. We asked patients to grade the frequency and severity of ADS as absent (grade 0), occasional (grade 1), frequent or bothersome (grade 2), or requiring drug therapy (grade 3). Other than loss of libido and impotence, Figures 10 and 11 depict the most commonly reported acute and chronic symptoms. Only grades 1, 2, or 3 findings are shown.

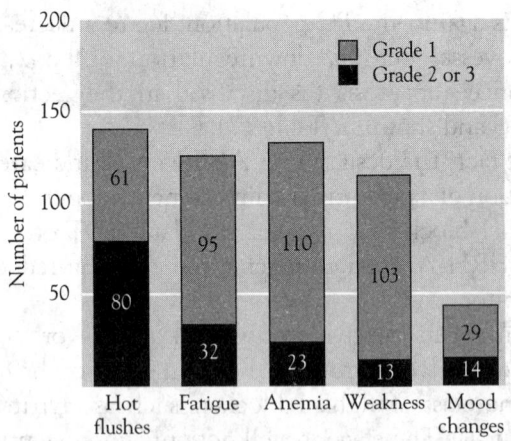

Figure 10. **Signs or Symptoms Relating to Most Common *Acute* Symptoms that May Be Seen in ADS.** Of the common side effects seen with ADT involving Grade 2 or 3 symptom intensity, hot flushes were most common at 45.1% (80/177) and fatigue was next at 18% (32/177). Although anemia occurred in 75% of the patients evaluated, it was found to be of Grade 2 to 3 intensity in only 23/177 or 12.9% of patients.

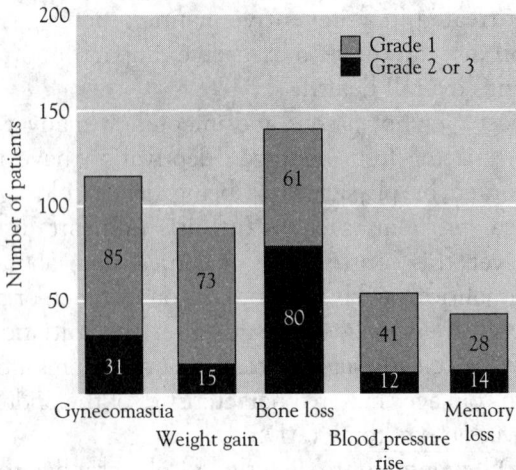

Figure 11. **Signs or Symptoms Relating to Most Common *Chronic* Symptoms that May Be Seen in ADS.** Of all findings that may occur in the chronic setting of androgen deprivation therapy, bone loss was most significant occurring in 45.1% of the patients studied.

Several patient-related and treatment-related factors were found to influence the incidence and severity of ADS symptoms (see Figures 12–14). Figure 12 depicts hot flashes with respect to age, Figure 13 relates to the intensity of anemia to the specific drugs used in ADT, and Figure 14 shows the effect of ADT duration on incidence of bone loss.

Finally, the incidence and intensity of bone loss are affected by the duration of ADT. This assumes that the patient on ADT is not receiving concomitant therapies

to prevent bone resorption, such as a bisphosphonate plus a bone supplement in conjunction with an exercise program. The mechanism of progressive bone loss during ADT relates to the fact that androgens are known inhibitors of osteoclast function. During ADT, this inhibition is lost and osteoclasts are activated, allowing for promotion of bone loss (resorption). Testosterone, therefore, is an anabolic steroid for bone, muscle and other tissues. The deprivation of androgens pushes the balance towards catabolism or breakdown.

## Table 19: Commonly Reported Acute and Chronic ADS Symptoms

These are possible findings that may occur in men receiving ADT. Many of these issues can be prevented, lessened, or resolved as part of the supportive care directed to the PC patient. This improves the therapeutic index of ADT. The PC patient and his partner, as a result, have an improved quality and quantity of life.

| System or Tissue Affected | Symptom Onset and Details | |
|---|---|---|
| | Acute (Symptoms in <2 Months) | Chronic (Symptoms in >6 Months) |
| Sexual | Decrease in libido; decrease in erectile ability | Penile shrinkage; testicular atrophy |
| Psychosocial | Mood "swings"; easy crying | Depression; hostility |
| Endocrine | Hot flashes; poor blood sugar control in patients with diabetes | Gynecomastia (breast enlargement) |
| Musculoskeletal | Loss of energy, feeling weak; aches and pains in joints and muscles | Decrease in strength and endurance; muscle atrophy; chronic fatigue-like symptoms; osteoporosis |
| Skin and nails | Increased dryness | Thinning of skin; nails brittle and break easily |
| Body mass | | Weight increase due to increased body fat; blood pressure control more difficult |
| Central nervous system | Decrease in short-term memory | Alzheimer's-like symptoms (severe short-term memory difficulties, inability to concentrate, and so on) |
| Hematologic | Anemia unrelated to blood loss, iron deficiency or bone marrow involvement | Chronic anemia |
| Urinary | Decrease or increase in urinary symptoms | |
| Lipids | | Increase in LDL cholesterol and/or triglyceride levels |

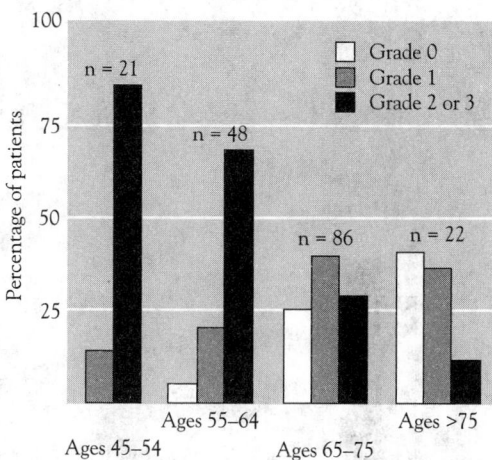

**Figure 12. Incidence and Severity of Hot Flushes Occurring in Younger Men on ADT.** Hot flushes were of significantly greater incidence and severity in patients less than 65 years of age. This most likely relates to the stronger stimulation by the hypothalamus on the pituitary to make LH in the absence of testosterone. The LH surges are believed to cause the severe hot flushes (flashes).

Clearly, a comprehensive care plan that takes the overall health of the PC patient into account must look at the impact of each and every ADS-related finding. Prevention of the undesirable consequences of ADT equates with a higher therapeutic index, which in turn means a higher quality of life for the PC survivor. Therefore, the intelligent use of ADT, as with any therapy, should take into account the following:

- Therapeutic purpose of ADT
- Nature of ADT (neoadjuvant, intermittent, or continuous treatment)
- Age and overall general health of the patient

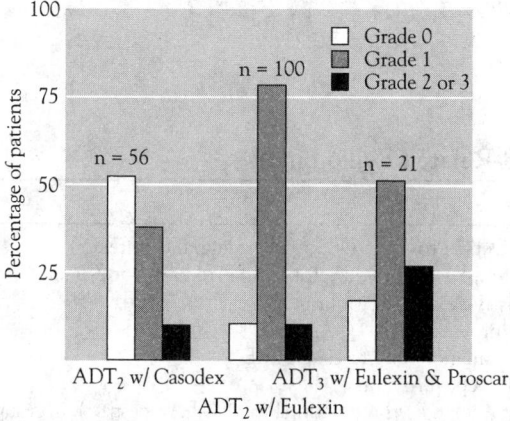

**Figure 13. Incidence and Intensity of Anemia Resulting from Androgen Deprivation May Relate to Intensity of ADT.** More intense anemia was observed with ADT$_2$ using Eulexin or in ADT$_3$ with the addition of Proscar. This strongly suggests that the degree of anemia may relate to the depth of androgen deprivation on a tissue level. Androgen receptors have been detected in the bone marrow. It therefore appears that three-drug ADT more profoundly affects androgen deprivation in this respect than two-drug ADT and that Eulexin has stronger anti-androgen effects than Casodex when using ADT$_2$.

- Degree of tolerance by the patient of the various ADT side effects
- Prevention or resolution of any signs and symptoms of ADS
- Net picture of pros versus cons

For example, the duration of neoadjuvant ADT rarely exceeds 1 year in patients who are candidates for potentially curative local therapies with RT or cryosurgery. Therefore, such patients have the potential risk for the typical acute ADS symptoms, but they will not experience chronic ADS symptoms to any significant extent. Patients who may be involved in this scenario include those with large-volume PC within the prostate with extracapsular extension (ECE). Such patients fare better when ADT is used upfront (neoadjuvant therapy), prior to the RT or cryosurgery, to decrease both the cancer volume as well as the gland volume. In *The Primer*, Physician's Note #5 relays such a story in the case of patient GB. The patient completed IMRT over 3 years ago and his PSA remains flat at 0.4 ng/mL.

Even with a highly responsive physician who is knowledgeable about ADS, acute ADS-related symptoms invariably compromise the lifestyles of healthy and active PC patients. This mandates that certain changes be made in the patient's diet, exercise, and work habits during ADT.

Chronic ADS symptoms are much more prevalent in PC patients treated with ADT than are currently recognized, and some are nearly inevitable in patients treated for longer than 1 year. For such patients, specific treatment strategies must be implemented to minimize or prevent the development of chronic ADS. Left untreated, chronic ADS is progressive with ongoing ADT and often leads to other medical complications. Useful preventive or active strategies against acute ADS-related symptoms are shown in Table 20, and chronic ADS-related symptoms in Table 21.

In the past, patients who were not candidates for local therapy were typically treated with continuous androgen blockade. Armed with our current knowledge about the signs and symptoms of acute and chronic ADS, we prevent or correct these findings with one or more of the therapies listed in Tables 20 and 21.

Another approach that avoids symptomatology attributable to chronic ADT is through the use of intermittent androgen deprivation (IAD). Depending on the required duration of ADT, individually determined for patients, IAD may be a reasonable alternative approach. This is an example of how therapy should be individualized to the patient's biological constitution. (A discussion of IAD with

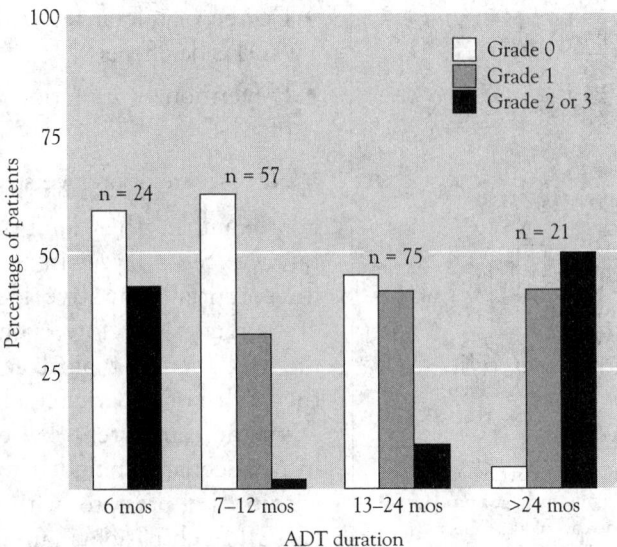

Figure 14. **ADT Duration Affects the Incidence and Severity of Bone Loss.** Symptoms and/or signs of bone loss invariably occur with the chronic administration of ADT. Of interest is that clinically significant bone loss is found also within the first 6 months of ADT and can affect the patient's quality of life. This often requires therapeutic intervention. It is suggested that all patients with PC, including those not receiving ADT, should understand the importance of bone integrity and the need to evaluate the bone mineral density and resorption status of the bones. PC patients should be actively treated with a combination of a bisphosphonate compound plus bone supplement and exercises. (Read the *Primer* for detailed information about bone integrity.)

graphs indicating outcomes using ADT2 versus ADT3 can be found in *The Primer*.)

Supporting the patient through measures such as some of those discussed relates to the fine-tuning that is characteristic of outstanding medical care. This is the essence of holistic medicine. There are other issues of supportive care that relate to the settings of pre- and post-operative care for a patient undergoing RP, cryosurgery, RT, and even watchful waiting. Some of these issues and possible

resolution therapies worthy of your review and subsequent discussion with your physician are outlined in Table 22.

*(7) Supportive Care for PC Patients Undergoing Chemotherapy: A comprehensive review of this topic is a book in itself and such a treatise is being considered. Due to limitations of space and time, this topic is not discussed at this time. The reader is advised to log on to the Prostate Chemotherapy protocol that can be accessed at www.lefprostate.org*

## Table 20:   Preventive and Active Treatments for Acute ADS-Related Symptoms

| Acute ADS-Related Symptom | Treatment Strategy |
| --- | --- |
| Hot flashes | Soy, genistein, Megace, Depo-Provera,[1] DES,[2] or venlafaxine (Effexor)[1] |
| Aches and pains in joints and muscles | Acetaminophen, ibuprofen, Fosamax®,[1] Actonel®,[1] Aredia®,[1] or Zometa®,[1] plus bone supplement, resistive exercise, walking |
| Fatigue and feeling weak | Walking, muscle stretching |
| Memory difficulties | Ginkgo biloba,[3] Eldepryl, memory exercises, DMAE[3] |
| Mood and emotional swings | Patience (may improve), Depo-Provera[1] |
| Symptomatic anemia (shortness of breath, chest pain, dizziness, severe weakness) | Injections of recombinant human erythropoietin (Procrit®,[1] Aranesp®[1]); iron supplementation only if documented iron deficiency via low ferritin or elevated serum transferrin receptor (>28)[3] |
| Increased urinary frequency | Hytrin®,[1] Cardura®,[1] Flomax®,[1] patience |
| Impotence and loss of libido | Viagra®,[1] Muse®[1] (alprostadil intraurethral pellet), or Caverject®,[1] or combinations of these. |

[1] *Physician's prescription is required to obtain medication.*
[2] *Not recommended in this setting due to toxicity.*
[3] *Available from health food suppliers, such as Life Extension.*

## Table 21:   Preventive and Active Treatments for Chronic ADS-Related Symptoms

| Chronic ADS-Related Symptom(s) | Treatment Strategy |
|---|---|
| Loss of muscle bulk and strength; worse in pectoral, biceps, and quadriceps | Exercise with light weights |
| Weight gain and fat redistribution | Sears's Omega Rx Zone approach; regular exercise |
| Chronic fatigue syndrome | Walking, regular exercise, avoid inactivity |
| Penile atrophy | Viagra®[1] and other similar agents |
| Gynecomastia | Breast radiation to prevent; liposuction or surgery to treat severe established cases |
| Osteoporosis | Fosamax®,[1] Actonel®,[1] Aredia®,[1] or Zometa®[1] plus bone supplement; synthetic vitamin D (Rocaltrol®[1]); aerobics, walking, resistive exercises |
| Alzheimer's-like symptoms | Ginkgo biloba,[3] DMAE[3]; see Life Extension's Alzheimer's disease protocol in this book; reading and other mind-stimulating activities |
| Increased serum cholesterol and triglyceride levels | Sears's Omega Rx Zone approach; if no help, Lipitor®,[1] Pravacol®,[1] Zocor®,[1] Mevacor®[1] (may require supplemental CoQ10[3]) |

[1] *Physician's prescription is required to obtain medication.*
[2] *Not recommended in this setting due to toxicity.*
[3] *Available from health food suppliers, such as Life Extension.*

## Table 22:   Some Considerations for Supportive Care Involved in Radical Prostatectomy, Radiation Therapy, Cryosurgery, and Watchful Waiting

Suggestions that can be discussed with your physician(s) to prevent adverse effects of any of the major therapies for PC (note that ADT and its supportive care were discussed in earlier sections).

| PC-Related Complication | Strategy for Resolution of Adverse Effects |
|---|---|
| | **Radical Prostatectomy** |
| Need for blood transfusions | Pre- or peri-operative use of Procrit®[1] or Aranesp®[1] and iron (only if biochemically indicated) |
| Incontinence | Kegel exercises (National Association for Continence at www.nafc.org); penile clamp, artificial urinary sphincter, urinary sling procedure |
| Impotence | Use of Viagra®,[1] Muse®,[1] combination therapy, injections of PGE1,[1] visual aids |
| Penile atrophy | Viagra®[1] and other similar new agents; PGE1[1] |
| Anastomotic stricture | Avoidance of surgery if history of exuberant scar formation (keloids); use of Pentoxifyllene[1] and vitamin E[2] |
| | **Radiation Therapy (Any Kind)** |
| Urinary obstructive symptoms | Pre-RT use of ADT to reduce gland volume plus use of Cardura®[1] or Hytrin®[1]; for post-RT problems, use of Hytrin®[1] or Cardura®[1] and, if severe, suprapubic tube; possibly transurethral laser surgery if scar tissue |
| Radiation injury to rectum (proctitis) | Rowasa[1] suppositories, Orgotein[1] or superoxide dismutase,[2] vitamin E,[2] Pentoxifyllene,[1] Sears' Omega Rx Zone approach[2] |
| Radiation injury to bladder (cystitis) | Rowasa[1] suppositories, Orgotein[1] or superoxide dismutase,[2] vitamin E,[2] Pentoxifyllene,[1] Sears' Omega Rx Zone approach[2]; avoid spicy foods, alcohol, coffee; use of calcium glycerophosphate[2]; trial of Elmiron®[1] |
| Impotence | Use of Viagra®,[1] Muse®,[1] combination therapy, injections of PGE1,[1] visual aids |
| Incontinence | Kegel exercises (National Association for Continence at www.nafc.org); penile clamp |
| | **Cryosurgery** |
| Urinary obstructive symptoms | ADT prior to cryosurgery to reduce gland volume; postcryosurgery use of suprapubic tube; Cardura®,[1] Hytrin®[1] |
| Incontinence | Kegel exercises (National Association for Continence at www.nafc.org); penile clamp, suprapubic tube |
| Impotence | Use of Viagra®,[1] Muse®,[1] combination therapy, injections of PGE1,[1] visual aids |
| | **Watchful Waiting (Objectified Ongoing Observations)** |
| Progressive disease that is clinically out of control | Interval testing and physical examination (DRE); graphing trends in PSA dynamics (velocity, doubling time); Sears' Omega Rx Zone approach[2]; modified citrus pectin[2]; dietary supplements[2] |

[1] *Doctors prescription is required to obtain medication*
[2] *Available from health food suppliers, such as Life Extension.*

# 11. BOOSTING MORALE OF THE TROOPS: FOSTERING A WILL TO LIVE, EMPOWERING THE PATIENT

The previous 10 sections have presented strategic issues that need to be addressed in our battle with PC. And, make no mistake, it is a battle—but one that can be won. There is much to be gained by many people in viewing this medical confrontation using a military metaphor. Such tactical thinking undoubtedly plays a pivotal role in achieving an optimal outcome for any life-endangering encounters.

However, all the good science and all the outstanding medicine in the world will not achieve its true goal of healing without the presence of spirit. This may not seem relevant to the man feeling the immediate threat of PC because of its philosophical orientation. But, I assure you, over the course of your journey, at some important crossroad in your life, it will be seen as the take-home lesson for all that has been written here. Your spirit, your will to live fully, is the crust of the holistic pie of life. Without this esprit, it is unlikely that you would have accepted the challenge of reading this chapter.

> Out of the night that covers me, black as the Pit from pole to pole,
> I thank whatever gods may be for my unconquerable soul.
> —Invictus, by William Ernest Henley

The basis for any victory must therefore involve morale—a state of spirit of a person or group as exhibited by confidence, cheerfulness, discipline, and willingness to perform assigned tasks. Morale, as defined in this fashion, and in the context of a war against PC, is embodied in acts reflecting empowerment of the patient and his partner.

Empowerment in this context becomes a process by which people assert control over factors that affect their health. This comes as a result of sharing resources and collaboration, which in turn lead to a more complete understanding of all aspects of a health issue.[318] My perspective developed through thousands of patient encounters each year with PC is that the empowered patient is better able to decide on treatments and choose physicians to guide him on his medical journey. The empowered patient is less anxious and more secure about his clinical course.[319] Empowerment, by its very nature, links people with resources.[320]

The empowered patient will explore options, look for new trials, participate in adjunctive or complementary therapies to enhance treatment outcomes, and be interactive in support groups. The empowered patient will take a politically active stance to increase funding, research, and awareness of the disease. The empowered patient is the purveyor of his medical records. The empowered patient views the physician as co-navigator, companion, and friend on his medical journey. An empowered patient expects bidirectional communication with his medical team to be the rule and not the exception.

In the process of opening channels of learning to the patient, we foster his empowerment and that of his partner, and that in turn encourages further learning. This extension of the physician as educator to the patient at a time of need is a manifestation of love. From this love comes wisdom in many walks of life.

> How do you choose to learn love?
> How do you choose to learn authentic empowerment—
> through doubt and fear, or through wisdom?
> —Gary Zukav

Those of you with PC are focused on your lives—your life is in jeopardy and what you took for granted before is no longer guaranteed to be there in the years to come. But

> Out of crisis comes opportunity.
> —Old Chinese saying

or

> A smooth sea never made a skilled mariner.
> —English proverb

During this crisis of PC, you will be provided multiple opportunities to overcome many obstacles. This is part of the lesson of life, of living, and of evolving. Remember that there are many out there without PC who will live their lives, day after day, without the appreciation to see the beauty of a tree or a sunrise; to say I love you; to smell the flowers; to marvel at the innocence of children; and to appreciate the uniqueness of your humanity. But this journey you are on should not be just an appreciation of life at a time of crisis, which is conveniently forgotten once the crisis is over. There are lessons here, crucial to your well-being and to that of your family, friends, community, and to all life forms.

> Life is the ultimate prize and it takes on ultimate value when suddenly we discover how tentative and fragile it can be.

*The essential art of living is to recognize and savor its preciousness when it is free of imminent threat or jeopardy.*
—Norman Cousins

Louis Armstrong said: "It's a wonderful world." The creation is wonder-full. We are part of that creation. We are also the caretakers of this wonderful world. PC should change your life; it should make you aware of this creation—not just the natural wonders, but the wonder of you and your fellow human-kind—all are linked together in a system longing for balance and communication. This is the essence of health for all biological systems. This is the heart of all that has been discussed in this chapter and throughout this book.

*Our humanity lies in our human unity.*
—Strum

This statement is not a political one. It is a socio-biological expression of what should be the underlying theme of virtually all life forms. On a biological level we are multicelled organisms that seek to achieve and maintain high levels of communication to remain in balance. It is a restatement of yin and yang. On every level of existence, from that of cellular interactions to the complexity of the individual human being to societies and governments, the call is the same: communication and balance. Without this, our health declines. Without this, our world dies.

My vision is for an empowered patient, who has an ability to use technological enhancements that provide the patient/physician team with far-reaching insights into the natural history and treatment of disease. At the same time, this empowerment embraces human unity—humanity—a realization that we are all in this together. The empowered patient shares his newfound understanding with others. He leaves the world of "I" and enters the world of "we."

The objective of this chapter on PC has been to provide specific and critical data that are an integral part of the comprehensive care of a patient with PC. The use of military metaphor has not been used simply as a literary tool, but more as a unique perspective—a different way of looking at things—that may yield new approaches in thinking about what tactics we could employ in our war against cancer. What may surprise the reader is the enormity of published information that is not routinely incorporated into the prevention and active treatment of

PC. Much of this involves an understanding of what encourages tumor growth and what enhances its rate of growth and ability to metastasize. The reader is encouraged not to look for a paragraph or two that summarizes all of what has been presented here; this is not realistic. Instead, read one section at a time and ask yourself: "Is this applicable to my situation?" If so, then take this information to your physician(s) and provide him with the appropriate references. Providing information in this manner improves your situation and that of all patients under the care of such physicians.

The first part of this chapter dealt with prevention. This is of importance not only to family members (and others) concerned about contracting PC, but also to patients seeking to slow disease progression and enhance the odds of a successful long-term outcome. As was discussed, many of the lifestyle changes that reduce PC risk also interfere with existing cancer cell proliferation.

Understanding the biological principles of the disease is crucial to understanding why such meticulous attention should be paid to keeping an accurate medical record of all test results, lifestyle changes, and therapeutic interventions. The medical record provides a basis for determining the status of the disease and what therapeutic modalities should be considered if adequate control of the disease has not been achieved.

By precisely assessing all of the measurable individual risk factors, a PC patient can better decide on the treatment options that offer the greatest opportunity for long-term control or cure, while minimizing potential side effects.

The knowledge base of how PC cells propagate and what can be done to interfere with these processes is colossal. This is good news for a PC patient who seeks a comprehensive scientific approach to eradicating his disease. Contrast this with a pancreatic cancer patient, who has little hope of survival beyond 12 months.

PC can easily be diagnosed at an early curable stage. Recurrence of existing disease can also be readily monitored. This is different from other cancers, in which a patient often waits for a dreaded physical symptom before learning the cancer has occurred or recurred. The bottom line is that a PC patient can exert a tremendous amount of control over his disease. What has been written here provides a systematic guide to taking advantage of the many technologies available today.

Life Extension has identified an extensive array of integrated PC therapies based on published scientific findings and the clinical experience of practicing oncologists. While this protocol provides information in a practical format, the cooperation of the attending physician is crucial.

## WHERE TO GO FROM HERE

While this chapter on PC provides an abundant quantity of life-saving guidance, many patients will need additional information to address their particular type and stage of disease.

For specific information about implementing some of the adjuvant drug therapies discussed in this chapter, refer to the protocol titled Cancer Treatment: The Critical Factors. Please remember that everything you read should be done so with the conscious thought of how this could apply to the current situation.

Those who have PC are urged to log on to www.lefprostate.org to read in-depth discussions that pertain to their stage of the disease and the different therapeutic modalities to consider.

## GLOSSARY OF TERMS

**3DCRT (3-DIMENSIONAL CONFORMAL RADIATION THERAPY):** An approach to radiation treatment planning that focuses on directing the radiation energy to the tumor target while sparing surrounding normal tissues.

**5-ALPHA REDUCTASE (5-AR):** The enzyme that converts testosterone to dihydrotestosterone (DHT).

**ADENOCARCINOMA:** A form of cancer that develops from a malignant abnormality in the cells comprising a glandular organ, such as the prostate. Almost all prostate cancers are adenocarcinomas.

**ADVANCED PROSTATE CANCER:** PC that is no longer organ-confined; systemic PC, sometimes with metastases to lymph nodes, seminal vesicles, bone, or vital organs of the body such as liver and/or lungs. Advanced PC is treated with systemic therapies currently in use such as androgen deprivation and chemotherapy.

**AGONIST:** A chemical substance, such as a drug, capable of combining with a receptor on a cell and initiating a reaction or activity. In PC, the LHRH agonist is also called LHRH-A. The most commonly used LHRH-As are Lupron and Zoladex®. Either of these agents interacts with the LHRH receptor and forms a complex that results in a decrease in the release of LH over a period of 2 weeks and hence a lowering in serum testosterone.

**ALGORITHM:** In PC, one of a group of systems whereby the human experiences of a number of patients are statistically or numerically analyzed to produce data that can be generalized to predict the probable disease status of patients who have not yet been treated and therefore have no empirical data of their own on which to base judgments regarding their disease status. Examples include the Partin Tables, Narayan Stage, and Kattan Nomograms.

**ALPHA-1 BLOCKERS:** Oral medications prescribed to improve urine flow by relaxing periurethral smooth muscle tissue; those of the quinazoline class (Hytrin® and Cardura®) have been shown to be synergistic with Proscar® in causing programmed cell death in prostate cells, both benign and malignant.

**ALPHA-TOCOPHEROL ISOMER:** A component of vitamin E.

**AMERICAN UROLOGICAL ASSOCIATION (AUA) SYMPTOM INDEX SCORE:** A series of subjective questions used by physicians to evaluate the extent of existing lower urinary tract symptoms.

**ANASTOMOSIS:** In PC, the surgical connection made between the bladder neck and the remaining urethra after the prostate is removed.

**ANASTOMOTIC STRICTURE:** In PC, a narrowing at the site of the anastomosis between the bladder neck and urethra after RP.

**ANDROGEN:** A hormone produced primarily by the testicles, but also in the cortex of the adrenal glands, that is responsible for male characteristics and the development and function of the male sexual organs and also affects muscle and bone mass, emotional stability, cognitive function, skin and hair, and so forth.

**ANDROGEN-DEPENDENT PC (ADPC):** Prostate cancer cells that depend on androgens for continued growth and vitality.

**ANDROGEN DEPRIVATION SYNDROME (ADS):** A constellation of symptoms directly or indirectly due to the drop in testosterone that occurs following surgical castration or the suppression of testicular and adrenal androgens by the use of medications.

**ANDROGEN DEPRIVATION THERAPY (ADT):** A PC treatment that is based on blocking the amount of available androgen to the PC cell.

**ANDROGEN-INDEPENDENT PC (AIPC):** PC cells that do not depend on androgen for growth.

**ANDROGEN RECEPTOR:** A structural entity that is essentially a docking site for androgen to communicate with the cell and affect cell function. The substance interacting with the receptor is called a ligand. The interaction of ligand and receptor is a major mode of biochemical communication in all life forms.

**ANEUPLOID:** Cells that have an abnormal number of sets of chromosomes. Aneuploid cancer cells tend not to respond as well to androgen deprivation therapy.

**ANGIOGENESIS:** Relating to the formation of blood vessels.

**ANTAGONIST:** A chemical that acts within the body to reduce the physiological activity of another chemical substance.

**ANTIGEN:** A substance that elicits a cellular-level immune response or causes the formation of an antibody.

**APOPTOSIS:** Programmed cell death due to an alteration in a critical substance or chemical necessary for cell viability. For example, the lack of male hormones causes apoptosis of androgen-dependent PC cells.

**ARACHIDONIC ACID (AA):** An omega-6 fatty acid that is known to generate free radicals and is considered an unfavorable eicosanoid. AA is metabolized via enzymes of the COX and LOX family to generate prostaglandins, thromboxanes, leukotrienes, hydroxylated fatty acids, lipoxins, and 5-HETE compounds that are implicated in cancer, inflammatory disease, immune dysfunction, and degenerative disorders. Organ meats and egg yolk are rich in AA.

**ARTIFICIAL NEURAL NET (ANN):** An approach to analyzing data that uses statistical analysis of historical data to produce systems that can predict probabilities of future outcomes based on inputted variables.

**BASELINE PSA:** The PSA level before a new treatment has begun; used to establish the efficacy of a therapy based on response of the PSA to treatment.

**BENIGN:** Not malignant; noncancerous.

**BENIGN PROSTATE HYPERPLASIA OR HYPERTROPHY (BPH):** A noncancerous condition of the prostate that results in the growth of both glandular and stromal (supporting connective) tissue, enlarging the prostate and potentially leading to obstructive symptoms relating to urine flow (see American Urological Association Symptom Index Score).

**BILATERAL:** Both sides; for example, a bilateral nerve-sparing RP is one in which the nerves on both sides of the prostate are left intact.

**BIOMARKER:** An indicator of biological activity of cells or tissues that can be used as a means to monitor a state of health or disease. PSA is one of the most useful biomarkers in medicine.

**BIOPSY:** Sampling of tissue from a specific part of the body in order to check for abnormalities such as cancer.

**BISPHOSPHONATES:** A class of compounds that stops bone loss (resorption) by actions directed against the osteoclast.

**BONE SCAN:** An imaging technique using a radioactive isotope that is selectively taken up by bone tissue to identify abnormal or cancerous growths within bone such as metastases.

**BRACHYTHERAPY:** A form of radiation therapy in which radioactive seeds or wires are used to deliver the radiation dose close to the site of a tumor. Seeds can be permanently implanted or radioactive wires can be temporarily introduced and then withdrawn after the radiation dose is delivered.

**CANCER:** The growth of abnormal cells in the body in an uncontrolled and disordered manner, invading surrounding tissues and sometimes spreading to distant sites within the body via the bloodstream and/or lymphatic system.

**CARCINOEMBRYONIC ANTIGEN (CEA):** A biomarker of PC that may be expressed in PC variants associated with higher Gleason scores, for example, Gleason scores 8–10 may indicate that androgen-independent cells are present.

**CASODEX®:** Brand name of an antiandrogen medication that functions by occupying and therefore blocking the androgen receptor, thus preventing natural androgens from stimulating cell growth.

**CAT or CT SCAN (COMPUTERIZED AXIAL TOMOGRAPHY):** An imaging method used to identify abnormalities by combining images from multiple X-rays under the control of a computer to produce cross-sectional or three-dimensional pictures of internal structures.

**CBC (COMPLETE BLOOD COUNT):** Complete blood workup including white blood count, hematocrit, and platelet count.

**cc (CUBIC CENTIMETERS):** Used as a measurement of prostate gland volume or amount of PC; cubic centimeters are equivalent to grams in determinations of prostate gland volume.

**cGy (centiGray):** A unit of measurement of radiation dose; 1 cGy equals the energy absorbed from ionizing radiation equal to 1 joule (a unit of energy) per kilogram.

**CHEMOTHERAPY:** The use of pharmaceuticals or other chemicals to kill cancer cells. In many cases these agents may also damage normal cells in the process of killing cancer cells, resulting in various adverse side effects.

**CHROMOGRANIN A (CGA):** A biomarker of PC that may be expressed in PC variants associated with higher Gleason scores, that is, Gleason scores 8–10. Progressive increases of CGA in the blood indicate an aggressive clone of PC is present that exhibits an increased tendency to metastasize to lymph nodes, liver, and lungs. CGA is produced by the neuroendocrine cells associated with androgen independent PC.

**CLINICAL STAGE:** The TNM (tumor, nodes, metastases) system of classification for communicating extent of disease in a specific patient based on all available information. This system has largely replaced the older Whitmore-Jewett staging classification system.

**CORE INVOLVEMENT:** Expressed as a percentage; indicates the amount of biopsy cores involved by PC divided by the total number of cores that have been sampled. If 12 cores of tissue were obtained and 6 showed PC, then the percentage core involvement would be 50%.

**COX-2 (CYCLOOXYGENASE 2):** The enzyme that converts arachidonic acid to prostaglandin E2. Inhibition of COX-2 is now an important approach to reducing the production of unfavorable eicosanoids implicated in the cause and progression of malignancy and inflammatory disorders.

**CRYOPROBES:** The hollow probes used to freeze tissue during a cryosurgery procedure.

**CRYOSURGERY:** The use of liquid nitrogen or argon gas circulated through cryoprobes to freeze and kill tissue, including any cancerous tissue.

**DEDIFFERENTIATION:** Relatively more primitive in appearance and function than well-differentiated cells that, by contrast, are mature and able to function properly. As the disease progresses, cancer cells become more dedifferentiated (ie, primitive) than normal cells, losing the characteristics that normal cells possess.

**DEXA SCAN:** An imaging procedure used to evaluate bone mineral density and evaluate the status of bone integrity as regards a diagnosis of osteopenia or osteoporosis. The DEXA may understate the true extent of abnormality by attributing unrelated conditions such as arthritis and vascular calcifications to normal bone density.

**DIAGNOSIS:** The evaluation of signs, symptoms, and tests to determine physical and biological causes of these signs and symptoms and evaluate whether a specific disease or disorder is involved.

**DIGITAL RECTAL EXAMINATION (DRE):** The use by a physician of a lubricated and gloved finger inserted into the rectum to feel for abnormalities of the prostate and rectum.

**DIHYDROTESTOSTERONE (DHT):** A male hormone 5 times more potent than testosterone; DHT is converted from testosterone within the prostate and in other tissues by the enzyme 5-alpha-reductase.

**DIPLOID:** Cells having one complete set of 46 normally paired chromosomes, that is, a normal amount of DNA. Diploid cancer cells grow relatively slowly and usually respond well to androgen deprivation therapy.

**DNA (DEOXYRIBONUCLEIC ACID):** The basic biologically active chemical that defines the physical development and growth of nearly all living organisms; a complex protein that is the carrier of genetic information.

**DOWNREGULATING (DOWNREGULATION):** Turning off a mechanism of action in the body at the biochemical level.

**DUTASTERIDE (AVODART®):** A 5-alpha-reductase inhibitor that prevents the conversion of testosterone to the 5 times more potent dihydrotestosterone (DHT). Unlike Proscar®, which blocks only 5-alpha reductase type 2, dutasteride also blocks 5-alpha reductase type 1.

**EICOSANOIDS:** Hormones made within the cell membrane of every living cell in the body controlling every physiological function. Eicosanoids have opposing actions operating as a check-and-balance system. Therefore, a balance of these opposing actions is essential for optimal health.

**EICOSAPENTENOIC ACID (EPA):** An omega-3 fatty acid that has been shown to inhibit the formation of AA by inhibiting the enzyme delta-5 desaturase, which converts DGLA to AA.

**EJACULATION:** The release of semen through the penis during orgasm.

**ENDOCRINE GLAND:** Any of various glands producing hormonal secretions that pass directly into the bloodstream. Examples of endocrine glands include the thyroid, parathyroids, anterior and posterior pituitary, pancreas, adrenals, pineal, and gonads.

**ENDORECTAL MRI:** Magnetic resonance imaging of the prostate using a probe inserted into the rectum.

**ENZYME:** Any of a group of chemical substances that are produced by living cells and cause particular chemical reactions to happen while not being changed themselves.

**EPITHELIAL CELL:** A cell type in the prostate gland that lines the ducts and functionally secretes substances such as PSA into the bloodstream or into the duct openings or lumens.

**EULEXIN®:** The brand name of an antiandrogen that blocks the androgen receptor and prevents testosterone and/or DHT from stimulating cell growth.

**EXTERNAL BEAM RADIATION THERAPY (EBRT):** A form of radiation therapy in which the radiation is delivered by a machine directed at the area to be radiated as opposed to radiation given within the target tissue, such as brachytherapy.

**EXTRACAPSULAR EXTENSION:** A disease status in PC in which the cancer has penetrated the outer shell or capsule of the prostate and extends into the periprostatic tissue.

**FINASTERIDE (PROSCAR®):** An inhibitor of the 5-alpha-reductase type 2 enzyme, which converts testosterone to the 5 times more potent dihydrotestosterone (DHT); used to treat BPH and PC.

**FOLLICLE STIMULATING HORMONE (FSH):** A hormone produced in the pituitary gland that, in males, stimulates cells (Sertoli cells) in the testicles to make sperm; may be a factor in PC growth because FSH receptors have been identified on PC cells.

**FREE PSA:** PSA unbound to any major protein; free PSA relates to benign prostate growth. The percentage of free PSA is one indicator of whether or not PC is likely present.

**FREE RADICALS:** Substances that damage cell membranes and disrupt the integrity of the cell; reactive oxygen species (ROS).

**GAMMA-LINOLENIC ACID (GLA):** One of the building blocks of eicosanoids that is metabolized to DGLA. The pathway that is taken after metabolism to DGLA is either toward AA and the unfavorable eicosanoids or toward the production of good eicosanoids such as PGA1 and PGA2.

**GAMMA-TOCOPHEROL ISOMER:** A component of vitamin E.

**GLAND:** A structure or organ that produces a substance that may be used in another part of the body.

**GLAND VOLUME:** The volume of the prostate gland in cubic centimeters or grams. (Both units of measurement, cubic centimeters and grams, yield the same result.)

**GLEASON GRADE:** After Donald Gleason, M.D., who developed the Gleason grading system as a tool to profile the aggressiveness of PC. A number from 1 to 5 that describes one of the 2 most predominant tissue patterns seen in the microscopic analysis of glandular architecture. The primary grade is the most predominant pattern, comprising 51–95% of the specimen, while the secondary grade comprises 5–49%.

**GLEASON SCORE (GS):** The two Gleason grades (represented as primary grade, secondary grade). An example of a high Gleason score would be (4,4) or (5,4) compared to a Gleason score of (3,3), the most common Gleason score at the time of diagnosis of PC.

**GLYCEMIC INDEX (GI):** A measurement of the rate of carbohydrate entry into the bloodstream.

**GLYCEMIC LOAD (GL):** The amount of insulin-stimulating carbohydrate multiplied by the glycemic index of the carbohydrate.

**HDR:** See High-Dose Rate Brachytherapy

**HEREDITARY:** Traits inherited from one's parents and from earlier generations via their DNA.

**HIGH-DOSE RATE (HDR) BRACHYTHERAPY:** Involves inserting iridium wires into the prostate gland through hollow plastic needles that are placed under transrectal ultrasound guidance. Once the radiation dose is delivered, the wires are withdrawn from the prostate.

**HORMONE:** Substances that are produced in the body that act as messengers, communicating information between cells. Usually peptides or steroids, they are produced by one tissue and delivered via the bloodstream to another tissue to affect physiological activity such as growth or metabolism.

**HYPERINSULINEMIA:** A state of high insulin levels in the blood that can be caused by disproportionate consumption of simple or complex carbohydrates in the diet in proportion to dietary proteins and fats.

**HYPOXIC CENTER:** The center of a PC tumor in which a state of lower oxygen tension exists. This stimulates VEGF, a substance that stimulates the blood vessel growth necessary for the nourishment of the tumor.

**IMAGING:** A radiology technique or method allowing a physician to see something that would not ordinarily be visible. Imaging studies include X-ray examinations, CT scans, bone or other nuclear medicine scans, and MRI and ProstaScint studies.

**INTENSITY MODULATED RADIATION THERAPY (IMRT):** An approach to external beam radiation therapy delivery using sophisticated computer planning to specify the tumor target dose and the amount of radiation allowable to nearby tissues and to modulate the intensity of the radiation as the delivery system rotates around the patient, thus minimizing damage to normal tissues.

**INTERFERON:** A molecule that is active against viruses and cancer cells.

**INTERLEUKIN-6 (IL-6):** A cell product made by the primary tumor as well as osteoblasts that facilitates bone resorption and promotes osteopenia and osteoporosis by stimulating mature osteoclasts to break down bone.

**INTERFERON-SIGNALING PATHWAY (ISP):** One of the defensive pathways that healthy cells use against the development of malignancy and invasion by viruses involving the interaction of interferon, which is produced in response to an invader.

**KATTAN NOMOGRAMS:** Various algorithms named after Michael Kattan that present probabilities of response to therapies, such as RP, external beam RT, and seed implantation based on a combination of biological inputs such as PSA, Gleason score, and clinical stage.

**KELOID:** Excessive scar tissue at the site of a surgery or an internal procedure. A history of this type of scar tissue formation may indicate the probability of the development of anastomotic stricture after RP.

**LACTIC DEHYDROGENASE (LDH):** Elevated levels of this substance are associated with high Gleason score PC. LDH used to be routinely included in the standard chemistry panel and was considered an excellent overall tumor marker. For reasons unclear, LDH has been omitted from the standard panel.

**LHRH ANTAGONIST:** An agent that blocks the LHRH receptor by pure antagonism without the initial release of LH, which is responsible for causing a testosterone surge seen with LHRH agonists; Abarelix (Plenaxis) is an example of an LHRH antagonist.

**LIGAND:** A protein or an enzyme that combines with its appropriate binding site or receptor. The interaction of a ligand and its receptor initiates a biochemical reaction leading to the synthesis of other substances, often proteins, hormones, or enzymes. Almost all reactions in the human body involve ligands interacting with their appropriate receptors.

**LNCaP:** One of the many PC cell lines. LNCaP is an androgen-dependent cell line.

**LOWER URINARY TRACT SYMPTOMS (LUTS):** Urinary difficulties including slow stream, urinary urgency, difficulty in starting urination, and incomplete emptying of the bladder. These symptoms are quantified in the AUA Symptom Index or Score.

**LUPRON:** Brand name of one of the drugs acting as an LHRH agonist.

**LUTEINIZING HORMONE (LH):** A pituitary hormone that stimulates the Leydig cells within the testicles to produce testosterone.

**LUTEINIZING HORMONE-RELEASING HORMONE (LHRH):** Hormone from the hypothalamus that interacts with the LHRH receptor in the pituitary to release LH which in turn stimulates Leydig cells in the testicles to make testosterone.

**LYMPH NODES:** Small glands occurring throughout the body that filter out bacteria and other toxins, including cancer cells. During the process of metastasis, they are one of the first sites of involvement when the cancer leaves the primary site of origin.

**MAGNETIC RESONANCE:** Absorption of specific frequencies of radio and microwave radiation by atoms placed in a strong magnetic field.

**MAGNETIC RESONANCE IMAGING (MRI):** Use of magnetic resonance with atoms in the body tissues to produce distinct cross-sectional or three-dimensional images of internal structures.

**MALIGNANCY:** A growth or tumor composed of cancerous cells.

**MALIGNANT:** Cancerous; tending to become progressively worse and to result in death; having the invasive and metastatic (spreading) properties of cancer.

**METASTASIS (pl. METASTASES):** Secondary tumor formed as a result of a cancer cell or cells from the primary tumor site traveling to a new site and growing there.

**MICROVESSEL DENSITY:** An objectified measurement of angiogenesis.

**mL (MILLILITER):** Unit of volume equal to one-thousandth of a liter.

**NARAYAN STAGE:** Part of the algorithm developed by Perry Narayan that assesses if the microscopic findings of PC were limited to one side of the prostate (Narayan B1) or both sides (Narayan B2).

**NERVE-SPARING:** A technique used in RP in which the erectile nerves are left intact by the surgeon.

**NEURON-SPECIFIC ENOLASE (NSE):** A biomarker of PC that may be expressed in PC variants associated with higher Gleason scores, that is, Gleason scores 8–10.

**ng (NANOGRAM):** Unit of measurement that is one-billionth of a gram.

**NOMOGRAM:** A graphic representation, often used in analyzing data, consisting of several lines marked off to scale. Specific variables such as PSA, Gleason score, clinical stage, and so on are given point values. The sum of all the points equates with the prognostic outcome.

**OBJECTIFIED ONGOING OBSERVATION:** A more appropriate term than watchful waiting that indicates that a patient not undergoing a definitive procedure using surgery or radiation or other treatments will be objectively monitoring his biological status in a consistent ongoing fashion.

**ONCOGENES:** Genes relating to tumor growth.

**ONCOLOGY:** The branch of medical science dealing with tumors. Oncologists study cancer and treat patients who are afflicted with cancer.

**ONCOLYTIC VIRUS:** A virus that can kill tumor cells having defects in the interferon-signaling pathway or by other mechanisms.

**ORGAN:** A group of tissues that work in concert to carry out a specific set of functions in the body.

**ORGAN-CONFINED DISEASE:** PC that is apparently confined to the prostate as determined either by clinical findings or, in the case of RP, by pathologic findings; PC that has not penetrated the prostate capsule.

**OSTEOBLAST:** A cell type within bone that promotes bone formation.

**OSTEOCLAST:** A cell type within bone that promotes breakdown of bone or bone resorption.

**OSTEOPENIA:** A condition of bone that indicates that an imbalance between bone formation and resorption is compromising bone integrity. Osteopenia indicates that the degree of bone loss is more than 1 standard deviation from the WHO definition of normal, but not more than 2.5 standard deviation below that level.

**OSTEOPOROSIS:** A reduction in bone mineral density that is more that 2.5 standard deviation below the normal level defined by the WHO.

**PARTIN TABLES:** Tables constructed based on results of the PSA, clinical stage, and Gleason score and associating those values with the findings at RP. Data involving thousands of men with PC used to predict the probability that the PC has penetrated the capsule, spread to the seminal vesicles or lymph nodes, or remained confined to the prostate. The tables were developed by a group of scientists at the Brady Institute for Urology at Johns Hopkins Medical Center.

**PATHOLOGIC STAGE:** The extent of disease as determined by a pathologist's microscopic analysis of tissue removed at the time of surgery.

**PERIPROSTATIC:** Pertaining to the soft tissues immediately adjacent to the prostate gland.

**PLOIDY:** DNA analysis to establish whether normal or abnormal numbers of pairs of chromosomes are present in a cell.

**PROCTITIS:** Inflammation of the rectum; may be an adverse effect of radiation therapy used to treat PC.

**PROSCAR®:** Brand name of finasteride, a 5-alpha-reductase inhibitor that blocks the conversion of testosterone to DHT.

**PROSTAGLANDIN:** An eicosanoid isolated from the prostate gland that acts locally, metabolizes rapidly, and has a hormone-like effect, stimulating target cells into action.

**PROSTAGLANDIN E2 (PGE2):** A major metabolite of arachidonic acid, known to stimulate VEGF and hence, angiogenesis.

**PROSTASCINT:** A monoclonal antibody (mAb) tagged with a radioactive isotope that is used to detect PC, particularly within lymph nodes. The ProstaScint mAb is directed against the prostate-specific membrane antigen (PSMA). PSMA is associated with androgen-independent PC. A few centers are using the ProstaScint scan to identify PC in the prostate gland.

**PROSTATE:** The gland surrounding the urethra and immediately below the bladder in males.

**PROSTATE CANCER (PC):** Adenocarcinoma of the prostate gland.

**PROSTATECTOMY:** Surgical removal of part or all of the prostate gland. If the entire gland is removed, a RP has been performed. Transurethral resection of the prostate (TURP), performed to improve urinary difficulties, is an example of removal of part of the gland.

**PROSTATE-SPECIFIC ANTIGEN (PSA):** A protein secreted by the normal epithelial cells of the prostate gland as well as by PC cells if they are present. Elevated PSA levels in the blood can be due to benign or malignant causes. After diagnosis of PC, this biomarker is typically used to monitor disease progression and/or response to therapy.

**PROSTATIC ACID PHOSPHATASE (PAP):** An enzyme or biomarker secreted by prostate cells that is associated with a higher probability of disease outside the prostate when pretreatment levels are 3.0 or higher. PAP elevations connote that the disease is not organ-confined disease.

**PROSTATIC INTRAEPITHELIAL NEOPLASIA (PIN):** A pathologically identifiable condition believed to be a possible precursor of PC; broken down into high-grade PIN or PIN 2 and PIN 3 versus low-grade PIN or PIN 1. High grade PIN is associated with having PC.

**PROSTATITIS:** Infection or inflammation of the prostate gland that can be treated with medication and/or prostate massage.

**PSA ASSAY:** The means by which a blood sample is analyzed to determine its PSA content. Various assays can result in different readings from the same sample; therefore, it is wise to use the same assay for each subsequent PSA test. Very sensitive assays that measure PSA down to 2 or 3 decimal points are called hypersensitive or

ultrasensitive PSA assays. These assays play a major role in early detection of relapse after RP or in the assessment of the tumor cell population in response to ADT.

**PSA DENSITY (PSAD):** The amount of PSA (expressed in nanograms) for each cubic centimeter of prostate volume; the serum PSA value divided by an accurate gland volume determination.

**PSA DOUBLING TIME (PSADT):** The length of time in months that it takes for the PSA to double in amount.

**PSA LEAK:** The secretion of PSA from the cells into the blood. Low levels of serum PSA are often associated with higher Gleason scores, as an expression of less PSA leak because more aggressive prostate cancers lose the ability to secrete PSA. Thus, PSA is an unreliable marker of disease progression in high-Gleason-score PC, such as Gleason scores 8–10.

**PSA RECURRENCE (PSAR):** Elevated PSA following treatment of PC, signaling that cancer cells are still present and that monitoring for disease progression is indicated.

**PSA RELAPSE-FREE SURVIVAL:** Survival of the patient that relates to no evidence of a progressively rising PSA.

**PSA TREND:** The slope that a series of PSA readings over time would exhibit on a graph.

**PSA VELOCITY (PSAV):** A statement of how fast the PSA is accelerating; the rate of change in PSA calculated per year of time.

**PYRILINKS-D (Dpd):** Deoxypyridinoline, or Dpd, is a laboratory test to monitor the biologic endpoint of bone resorption activity obtained by analysis of the second-voided urine of the day.

**QCT SCAN:** Quantitative CT bone densitometry; a superior way to evaluate bone density compared to the DEXA scan because it is uninfluenced by unrelated conditions such as arthritic changes and/or vascular calcifications. (Telephone numbers that may be helpful in finding QCT sites near you: Mindways, (877) 646-3929 (www.qct.com), or Image Analysis, (800) 548-4849 (www.image-analysis.com).)

**RADIATION THERAPY (RT):** The use of X-rays and other forms of radiation to destroy malignant cells and tissue.

**RADICAL PROSTATECTOMY (RP):** Surgical removal of the entire prostate gland and seminal vesicles.

**RECEPTOR:** A docking site on the cell membrane in the cell cytoplasm or in the nucleus that interacts with a ligand. All cells have multiple receptors.

**RECURRENCE:** The reappearance of disease manifested by clinically based findings, either upon physical examination or by the results of laboratory findings such as a rising PSA.

**RESORPTION:** Loss of bone caused by an imbalance in the dynamics of bone formation by osteoblasts or bone loss due to breakdown of the bone by osteoclasts.

**RISK ASSESSMENT:** An analysis of probabilities related to a specific patient's case, obtained by analyzing medical variables of known significance and used to derive an overall impression of how different disease management options would impact an optimal or suboptimal outcome for the patient.

**SCREENING:** Evaluation of populations of people who have no symptoms of the disease for which they are being evaluated in an effort to diagnose disease in its early stages.

**SEED IMPLANTATION (SI):** A treatment for PC in which radioactive seeds encased in titanium shells are permanently implanted into the prostate gland.

**SELENOMETHIONINE:** A substance that shows an inhibitory effect on certain PC cell lines that appear to be independent of androgen receptor or PSA pathways.

**SEMINAL VESICLES:** Glandular structures located above and behind the prostate that secrete and store seminal fluid. Seminal fluid is one component of ejaculate.

**STAGE:** See CLINICAL STAGE, PATHOLOGIC STAGE.

**SYSTEMIC:** Throughout the whole body; in PC, cancer that is no longer organ-confined.

**TESTOSTERONE (T):** The male hormone or androgen that comprises most of the androgens in a man's body. Chiefly produced by the testicles, testosterone is essential to virtually every male function from the brain to toenails.

**THERAPEUTIC INDEX (TI):** Treatment benefit divided by treatment side effects.

**THERMOCOUPLES:** In relation to PC, devices used during cryosurgery to monitor the temperature achieved by cryoprobes, thus helping to improve the therapeutic index of the procedure.

**TRANSFORMING GROWTH FACTOR BETA-1 (TGF-b1):** A growth factor produced by prostate cells as well as cells of the bone matrix. Elevated plasma levels of TGF-b1 obtained at baseline are associated with distant disease involving bone and/or lymph nodes.

**TRANSRECTAL:** Through the rectum (as in transrectal ultrasound of the prostate).

**TRANSRECTAL ULTRASOUND OF THE PROSTATE (TRUSP OR TRUS):** A method that uses the echoes of ultrasound waves to image the prostate by inserting an ultrasound probe into the rectum.

**TRANSURETHRAL:** Through the urethra. See Transurethral Resection of the Prostate.

**TRANSURETHRAL RESECTION OF THE PROSTATE (TURP):** A surgical procedure to remove prostate tissue obstructing the urethra.

**T SCORE:** A designation used in evaluation of bone mineral density that relates the patient's bone density to that found in a population of healthy women of approximately 30 years of age. The T score is in contrast to the Z score, which relates the patient's bone density to a pooled population of an age similar to the patient. The T score is the desired test result.

**TUMOR:** An excessive growth of cells caused by uncontrolled and disorderly cell replacement that can be either benign or malignant.

**TUMOR VOLUME:** The amount of tumor measured in cubic centimeters.

**ULTRASENSITIVE PSA ASSAY:** PSA assays that are able to measure very small amounts of PSA in the blood sample, reliable to the hundredth or even the thousandth of a nanogram per milliliter of blood. Tosoh and DPC Immulite Third Generation assays are examples of ultrasensitive PSA assays.

**UPREGULATING (UPREGULATION):** Turning on or increasing a mechanism of action at the biochemical level in the body.

**UROKINASE-TYPE PLASMINOGEN ACTIVATOR (uPA):** A substance believed to play a role in PC invasion and metastasis that is stimulated by IGF-1 and inhibited by GLA and EPA.

**UROLOGIST:** A surgically trained physician who specializes in disorders of the genitourinary system.

**VASCULAR ENDOTHELIAL GROWTH FACTOR (VEGF):** A substance known to stimulate blood vessel growth or angiogenesis and hence stimulate PC growth.

**VIADUR®:** Brand name of an LHRH agonist that is implanted under the skin and releases medication over the course of 1 year.

**VITAMIN E SUCCINATE:** Substance that inhibits the growth of PC cells of certain cell lines by suppressing androgen receptor expression and PSA expression.

**WATCHFUL WAITING (WW):** Objective ongoing observation and regular monitoring of a patient with PC without actual treatment or invasive therapies.

**ZOLADEX®:** Brand name of one of the LHRH-agonists.

**Z SCORE:** A designation of bone mineral density that relates the patient's bone density to that of a pooled population of similar age. See T Score.

## SUGGESTED READING

Those seeking additional information may order a copy of *A Primer on Prostate Cancer: the Empowered Patient's Guide*. *The Primer* reflects the synergistic efforts of Stephen B. Strum, a medical oncologist involved with PC since 1983, and Donna Pogliano, a partner of a PC warrior. *The Primer* is in full color with many graphic images, clinical vignettes, and a comprehensive appendix replete with material that is the essence of top-of-the-line health care as it relates to PC. *The Primer* is a working manual and companion tool to this protocol. *The Primer* is to be regarded as required reading for those serious at winning the war against PC. It is your basic field guide—but much more so. *The Primer* is available through Life Extension at (800) 544-4440 or on the Life Extension website at www.lefprostate.org. *The Primer* is also available through amazon.com, the Prostate Cancer Research Institute, the Educational Council for the Prostate Cancer Patient, and Barnes & Noble.

## ADDITIONAL READING

### Books about PC

- Patrick Walsh, M.D., Janet Farrar Worthington. *Dr. Patrick Walsh's Guide to Surviving Prostate Cancer*
- Sheldon Marks, M.D. *Prostate & Cancer: A Family Guide to Diagnosis, Treatment & Survival*

### Medical Journals Focused on PC

- *Urology*
- *Journal of Urology*
- *Prostate*
- *Prostate Cancer and Prostatic Diseases*

### PC Newsletters

- Prostate Cancer Research Institute's *PCRI Insights*
- Dr. Snuffy Myers's *Prostate Forum*
- ECPCP's (Education Center for Prostate Cancer Patients) *Prostate Exchange*
- PAACT's (Patient Advocates for Advanced Cancer Treatments) *Cancer Communication*

### Internet Websites

- PCRI (www.pcri.org)

## Internet-Based Tools (Software)

- PC Tools I and II (www.pcri.org)
- Kattan Nomograms (http://www.mskcc.org/mskcc/html/10088.cfm)

## Life Extension Suggestions

- **Modified citrus pectin:** 14–30 g daily without food
- **Lycopene:** 15–30 mg daily with food
- **Vitamin D:** 5000–8000 IU daily with food (depending on blood test results; optimal blood levels are 50–80 ng/mL)
- **Soy isoflavones** (including genistein): 100–200 mg daily with food
- **Green tea extract,** standardized to 98% polyphenols: 725–1450 mg daily
- **Omega 3 fatty acids:** 1400 mg EPA and 1000 mg DHA daily with food
- **Curcumin,** as highly absorbed BCM-95®: 400–1600 mg daily with food
- **Coenzyme Q10** (as ubiquinol): 200–400 mg daily with food
- **Melatonin:** 10–50 mg at bedtime
- **Selenium:** 200–400 mcg daily with food
- **Gamma E tocopherols:** 359–718 mg of gamma E–mixed tocopherols daily with food
- **Boron:** 3–9 mg daily with food
- **Zinc:** 15–50 mg daily with food
- **Milk thistle** (standardized extract): 750 mg daily
- **Gamma linolenic acid (GLA):** 300–600 mg daily with food

## STAYING INFORMED

The information published in these protocols is only as current as the day the book was sent to the printer. This protocol raises many issues that are subject to change as new data emerge. Furthermore, cancer is still a disease with unacceptably high mortality rates, and none of our suggested treatment regimens can guarantee a cure.

Life Extension is constantly uncovering information to provide cancer patients with more ammunition to battle their disease. A special website has been established for the purpose of updating patients on new findings that directly pertain to the cancer protocols published in this book. Whenever Life Extension discovers information that points to a better way of treating cancer, it will be posted on the website www.lefcancer.org.

Before utilizing the cancer protocols in this book, we suggest that you log on to www.lefcancer.org to see if any substantive changes have been made to the therapeutic recommendations described in this protocol. Based on the sheer number of newly published findings, there may be significant alterations to the information you have just read.

## REFERENCES

References available at: www.lef.org/dpt5/ch113

# 114

# *Raynaud's Phenomenon*

Raynaud's phenomenon (RP) can be a debilitating condition that causes periods of severely restricted blood flow to the fingers and toes (and sometimes to other parts of the body such as the nose or ears). In the worst-case scenario, this can result in amputation of the damaged digits.

The cause(s) of RP remain a mystery in many cases. The disease results in significant free-radical nerve damage in the affected tissues. This damage leads to local endothelial dysfunction, thickening of arterial walls, and formation of scar tissue, or fibrosis.[1] RP is closely associated with more serious diseases (especially scleroderma, a connective tissue disorder). Many scientists believe that RP may be the initial diagnosis, before the actual diagnosis of scleroderma is recognized. Other diseases associated with RP include systemic lupus erythematosus and arthritis. In each case, RP may contribute to the more serious disease by encouraging formation of scar tissue in the connective tissue and through arterial damage. Therefore, it is crucial that RP patients pursue aggressive antioxidant therapy to lower their risk of developing a more serious condition.

RP typically affects small blood vessels in the fingers and toes, but can affect the ears, nose, and tip of the tongue.[2-5] During episodes of RP, the affected area may become painful and turn blue.[5]

RP that occurs in the absence of another disease is referred to as primary RP. It is thought to involve a localized defect in the arteries and arterioles that deliver blood to the extremities. Because RP is associated with conditions (eg, migraine headaches and angina) caused by spasms of blood vessels (vasospasm), it may have a similar vasospastic mechanism.

RP that occurs in the presence of other diseases is called secondary RP. Occupational RP is a common form of secondary RP resulting from use of vibrating tools (eg, jackhammers).[5] Drugs or treatments used to treat high blood pressure (beta blockers), migraine headaches (ergotamine-containing drugs), and cancer (chemotherapy) have been known to cause RP.[5,6]

## OXIDATIVE DAMAGE: THE LASTING EFFECT OF RP

In normal healthy tissue, blood flow to the skin is regulated by a complex system that includes neural signals, hormones, and mediators released from circulating cells and blood vessels. When a person is either exposed to cold or experiencing emotional stress under normal conditions, arterioles constrict to return blood flow to the core of the body for warmth and protection.[5] This reaction is regulated by vasoconstrictive agents such as endothelin 1 and factors that impair production of nitric oxide, a potent vasodilator.[7-9]

In individuals with RP, the normal reaction is exaggerated (ie, blood circulation in the arterioles is greatly restricted, resulting in a visible progression of symptoms as blood flow to the affected areas drops). Skin turns white as it is deprived of blood, and then blue (cyanosis) due to the lack of blood and oxygen. Finally, skin has localized red flushing as the blood returns to the affected area.[10] This progression may be accompanied at first by a loss of sensation in the affected extremities, followed by a prickling, throbbing, or tingling sensation as circulation returns.[5]

Skin changes may migrate, moving from one finger to the next, sometimes even involving the thumb.[11] The tip of the nose, the earlobes, and (rarely) the cheeks or chin can also be affected.[2] Characteristic skin changes can occur in as little as 3 minutes. An episode can last from a few minutes to several hours[5]; however, episodes may last longer in people with connective tissue disorders such as scleroderma.[12]

Researchers working to discover the underlying mechanism of the condition have found that certain receptors, called alpha-2–adrenergic receptors, are hypersensitive in people with RP. Alpha-receptors are located on the membranes of vascular smooth muscle cells and help regulate vasoconstriction and smooth muscle contraction in blood vessel walls.[13] Studies found that blocking certain alpha-2 receptors reduced the number of vasospastic attacks in the fingers.[13,14]

No matter what the underlying cause, it is known that episodes of RP trigger significant free-radical nerve damage in affected tissues. During RP, blood flow is restricted and then restored, which causes ischemic reperfusion injury (ie, the same type of injury that can occur after a stroke, when returning blood flow to the brain causes additional damage). In RP, the ischemic reperfusion injury (which generates high levels of free radicals that attack the endothelium in arteries and surrounding tissue) causes scar tissue to form in connective tissue.[1]

This may help explain why RP is frequently associated with autoimmune connective tissue disorders such as scleroderma, lupus, and arthritis.[15] In about 20% of cases, RP is the first indicator of a more serious connective tissue disorder such as scleroderma, lupus, or arthritis, which means they should be closely monitored for these conditions.[15–17]

Episodes of RP are unpredictable and difficult to reproduce accurately in a clinical setting.[18] RP can remain dormant for years, only to resurface suddenly in response to infection, fatigue, or stress. If RP progresses, permanently decreased blood flow to the affected area can cause fingers to become thin and tapered, with smooth shiny skin and slow-growing nails. Often the most serious consequence is loss of sensitivity in the affected extremity. However, more severe cases of secondary RP can result in tissue death, finger deformity, skin ulceration, or gangrene.[19] RP can also affect the lungs. When the lungs are affected, breathing cold air triggers a coughing attack.[20] Vasospasm may also affect the heart, lungs, and kidneys.[17]

RP is also infrequently associated with hypothyroidism, alone or associated with scleroderma.[16] Treatment with supplemental thyroid hormones (such as those used to treat hypothyroidism) has been shown to resolve RP in extremely rare cases.[21]

## DIAGNOSING RP

Diagnosing RP is complicated because it can be mistaken for other conditions such as carpal tunnel syndrome, vascular disease, or thoracic outlet syndrome.[19] Therefore, physicians diagnose RP based on the presence of some of the following factors[5]:

- Periodic attacks of cyanosis
- Negative antinuclear antibody test result, which demonstrates the absence of lupus
- Normal erythrocyte sedimentation rate, which demonstrates the absence of major systemic inflammation

Although it is difficult to cause an attack of RP in a doctor's office,[18] submerging the patient's hands in ice, recording how long it takes for normal color to return to the hands, and performing a vascular assessment may determine severity of RP.

Because RP may be an important marker of more serious disease conditions, a full blood laboratory panel should be performed to rule out underlying autoimmune disorders, malignancies, kidney or liver dysfunction, and syndromes that affect blood or circulation.[19] In particular, an antinuclear antibody test and erythrocyte sedimentation rate should be performed to assess potential autoimmune conditions. Diagnosis of secondary RP includes periodic episodes of cyanosis, a positive antinuclear antibody test result, and an abnormal erythrocyte sedimentation rate.[5]

## CONVENTIONAL TREATMENT OF RP

Conventional treatment of RP is determined by type. In primary RP, treatment is often conservative, using self-help strategies such as preventing attacks and reducing symptoms. Pharmacologic treatment is rarely required and, unfortunately, antioxidant therapy is rarely recommended. When necessary, calcium channel blockers are considered the safest and most effective drugs. They relax smooth muscle and dilate small blood vessels, reducing the frequency and severity of attacks in primary and secondary RP.[5]

Treatment of secondary RP focuses on the underlying condition, such as scleroderma or lupus.[5] In addition to treatment of the underlying condition, the following drugs may be prescribed to control episodes of RP.[20]

### Calcium Channel Blockers

Calcium channel blockers are traditionally first-choice prescription medications to treat RP. These drugs block calcium channels in the smooth muscle of vessel walls, thereby preventing contraction. Nifedipine is considered the standard for treatment. Adverse effects of calcium channel blockers are frequent and include abnormal heart rhythm, flushing, swelling, and headache. These effects may subside over time, and long-acting preparations may minimize them. Diltiazem has fewer side effects but may be less effective. Calcium channel–blocking drugs improve symptoms only moderately in the treatment of secondary RP.[22]

### Vasodilators

Cilostazol, a relatively new vasodilator, has shown promise in the treatment of RP.[23] Sildenafil has also been used with some effectiveness.

### Prostaglandin E1

Transdermal patches containing prostaglandin E1 improved blood flow to skin capillaries and reduced the number of RP episodes in subjects with RP secondary to scleroderma.[24]

In addition to pharmaceutical treatments, the following therapies are used in treating RP.

## Paraffin

Regular paraffin (hot wax) treatment may be helpful, although it must be used with caution. Use only physician-prescribed hot wax units because wax that is too hot may damage fragile blood vessels. Never heat wax on a stove or in an electric cooking pot (such as a Crock-Pot). A physical or occupational hand therapist can provide training in the proper procedure.[20]

## LASER Irradiation

Low-level LASER treatment has been shown to reduce the frequency and severity of RP attacks. The conditions of people who had primary and secondary RP improved with LASER irradiation.[3,25] Patients with RP who received low-level LASER treatment experienced less response to cold.[3] Those with a decreased threshold for vasospasm experienced the greatest benefit.[25]

## Surgery

In selective cases of severe RP, doctors may recommend surgery to reestablish blood flow to an affected area by interrupting nerve pathways. In cervical sympathectomy, nerve pathways that may contribute to the symptoms of RP are interrupted. Early studies of this procedure show mixed results. There is little evidence that the benefits of surgery are longstanding. In localized digital sympathectomy, nerve pathways to specific digits or an area affected by RP (usually the fingers) are interrupted. The surgeon makes small incisions in the affected area and cuts nerves around blood vessels. This type of surgery is usually performed only on individuals who have failed to benefit from conservative medical treatment and continue to experience poor blood flow to affected areas, or individuals with severe or tissue-threatening RP (more common in secondary RP).[26]

# STRATEGIES TO REDUCE ATTACKS OF RP

A first line of defense against RP, whether primary or secondary, is to protect the extremities from common triggers of attacks such as cold or emotional and physical stress.

## Protect Your Body

Extreme changes in temperature are worse than cold alone. If you have RP:

- Keep your head and torso warm to enable blood to flow more freely to your hands and feet.[27]
- Wear socks to bed.

- Use an electric blanket to warm the sheets before getting into bed.
- Dress in loose layers of blended fabrics, including a sweater.
- Wear long underwear made of silk to protect against chills without overheating the body.
- Wear a warm hat and earmuffs to prevent heat loss through the head when outside.
- Use chemical-pack heaters inside socks and mittens.
- Warm body parts by using tubes of fabric filled with grain that can be warmed in a microwave and then applied to affected areas.
- Cover exposed skin (including nose and cheeks) in cold, windy weather.
- Avoid getting the skin wet or perspiring in cold weather. Moisture cools the skin as it evaporates.
- Wear an under layer of clothing in a material that wicks away moisture.
- Be prepared for temperature changes by having extra clothing available in the car or at work.
- Drink warm beverages.
- Carry an insulated hot water bottle on car trips.

## Protect Your Hands

Damp cold is more likely to precipitate an attack. Take the following steps to protect hands from cold temperatures.

- Wear mittens and wristlets outside in cold weather. Mittens warm hands more effectively than gloves because they pool heat from the entire hand. Wristlets keep cold air out of the gap between sleeves and mittens.
- Wear mittens to bed.
- Wear mittens when handling cold or frozen foods.[5]
- Use warm running water to clean vegetables; never cool water. An alternative is to use prewashed vegetables from the produce department.
- Run bath or shower water ahead of time to avoid touching cold water.
- Avoid touching cold water from garden hoses.
- Do not hang wet clothes outside.
- Do not shovel snow.
- Do not hold cold beverages. Use insulated cup holders and straws.

## Protect Your Skin

People with RP should take the following precautions with skin care because minor cuts and scrapes take longer to heal and are more susceptible to infection.

- Avoid skin injuries, particularly areas affected by RP.
- Wear gloves when using detergents or harsh chemicals.
- Wear gloves when gardening.
- Treat injuries without delay.
- Consult a healthcare provider if infection or skin ulcers develop.
- Use creams to keep skin soft. Rough, dry skin is more likely to tear.[28]

## Rewarm Affected Areas

A prolonged attack of RP can lead to tissue death, gangrene, and possibly amputation. Consider each attack an emergency and respond immediately. Try to remain calm when an attack begins. Gently rewarm fingers and toes as soon as possible. The sooner rewarming is started, the easier it will be to restore circulation and lessen the chance of damage. Try moving the affected part right away, which may avert the need for further measures. If moving the affected body part does not result in the alleviation of RP symptoms, try applying moist heat. Become familiar with the following rewarming strategies.[27]

- Do not clap hands together or rub them vigorously. Doing so can damage blood vessels.
- Place hands under armpits or between legs.
- Cup hands to the mouth and breathe on fingers.
- Have another person hold (but not rub) your hands.
- Wiggle fingers and toes.
- Walk (or otherwise move) around.
- Twirl arms around in the air in large circles until circulation returns. Avoid twirling arms, however, if scleroderma has damaged blood vessels.
- Run warm (but not hot) water over the affected body parts until normal color returns.
- Do not overheat hands to avoid constricting blood vessels and prolonging an attack.

## Avoid Vasoconstrictive Substances

Try not to consume food, medication(s), or be around substances that can constrict blood vessels.

- Do not smoke. Smoking constricts peripheral blood vessels[29] and reduces blood concentration of antioxidants such as ascorbic acid.[30,31]
- Avoid breathing second-hand smoke.

- Cut down on intake of caffeine-containing foods, beverages, and drugs. Caffeine, a vasoconstrictor, can be found in chocolate and some aspirin preparations, teas, and medications.[20]
- Do not use birth-control pills.[31]
- Avoid taking most over-the-counter decongestants, cold remedies, and diet pills.[5]
- Have a doctor monitor your condition closely if you take medications for migraines, high blood pressure, or heart problems. Some migraine headache, blood pressure, and heart medications can cause symptoms of RP.[5]

## Avoid Precipitating Activities

Attacks of RP may be initiated by operating vibrating equipment (eg, chain saws, jackhammers, or drills).[5] When using a vacuum cleaner, try wearing oven mitts to reduce the effect of the vibrations. Symptoms of RP can also be brought on by repetitive hand motions (such as typing, playing the piano or guitar, sewing, and chopping or dicing food). Do not carry heavy shopping bags with handles that restrict blood flow to fingers.

## Use Biofeedback

Blood vessels can be trained to relax using biofeedback.[5] In one form of biofeedback, "think" hands are warm. In another form of biofeedback, place hands in a bowl of warm water (in a warm room) for 5 minutes, then move to a cold room or cold environment. Then place hands in warm water again, this time for 10 minutes. Repeat the procedure several times a day for as many days as necessary to produce a conditioned reflex that is the opposite of the normal one; that is, when exposed to cold, blood vessels in fingers will dilate rather than constrict (without the aid of warm water). Success of biofeedback has been documented by studies. Biofeedback subjects showed significant elevations in blood flow to, and temperature of, the fingers and in skin conductance level beyond what could be explained by other differences in the study groups.[32] Improvement in symptoms was maintained for 9 weeks, 1 year, and 2 years in RP as well as 8 years in RP secondary to systemic lupus erythematosus.[33-35] Biofeedback is generally not as effective in treating secondary as primary RP. It may also not work as well for warming the feet.

# NUTRITIONAL APPROACHES TO RP

Although the causes of RP have remained mysterious, researchers understand the damage cascade that RP can touch off. During episodes of RP, high levels of free radicals are generated that damage the inner lining of arteries (endothelium) and surrounding tissue. The use of antioxidants in treating RP is based on research showing that levels of important antioxidants (such as vitamin E, vitamin C, and selenium) are depleted in RP patients.

## Vitamin E

Vitamin E, a key antioxidant that protects polyunsaturated fatty acids from oxidation,[36] has been found to have therapeutic effects in certain forms of RP. A clinical trial has shown that the alpha-tocopherol form of vitamin E was beneficial in treating occupational RP.[37]

## Vitamin C

Vitamin C is important for the synthesis of collagen, a key component of blood vessel walls. Studies have demonstrated that administering vitamin C improves blood flow. For example, in patients with atherosclerosis of the coronary arteries, the ascorbic acid form of vitamin C improved blood vessel vasoconstriction, thus improving blood flow through the arteries.[38] A deficiency of ascorbic acid and selenium has been found to raise the risk of scleroderma in people with RP.[30]

## Niacin

An experimental evaluation of the usefulness of no-flush niacin in treating RP concluded that it produced beneficial therapeutic effects on microcirculation, not only through vasodilation, but also through mechanisms such as an enhanced ability to break up clots (fibrinolysis) and lower lipids (fats) in the blood. Compared to standard drug treatment, few adverse effects were noted.[39] Another study found that long-term supplementation with nicotinate acid derivatives may improve peripheral circulation through a different effect than the one detected by short-term studies.[40] Niacin has also resulted in a significant improvement in the symptoms of RP and a reduction in the frequency of RP attacks.[41]

## Magnesium

Magnesium is essential to maintain relaxation of smooth muscle of the small arteries affected by RP.[42] Magnesium requirements increase with physical stress, which is a trigger associated with initiating RP episodes.[43] Red blood cell levels of magnesium were found to vary seasonally in women with primary RP. Magnesium levels were significantly lower in winter than summer.[44]

## Essential Fatty Acids

Omega-3 and gamma-linoleic acid (an omega-6 fatty acid found in evening primrose oil and borage oil) are anti-inflammatories shown to help relieve symptoms of RP. One study found that taking evening primrose oil dramatically decreased the number of RP attacks with the onset of cold weather, although there was no change in blood flow to the hands.[45] A clinical study found that ingesting fish oil increased the median time before onset of RP after exposure to cold (especially in people with primary RP). Fish oil also improved tolerance to cold exposure, as evidenced by significantly increased blood pressure in the fingers. Almost half the people who ingested fish oil did not exhibit RP symptoms in response to a cold water bath.[46]

## L-Arginine

L-arginine has been shown to reverse tissue damage caused by RP and improve symptoms in subsequent attacks. It stimulates production of nitric oxide, thus helping keep arteries open and relaxed.[47] Study results on L-arginine are mixed, with some showing efficacy and others showing none.

## Ginkgo Biloba

Ginkgo biloba is a well-tolerated plant extract. In one study, Ginkgo biloba reduced the frequency of weekly RP attacks by 56%.[48]

## Estrogens

Estrogen and related compounds increase nitric oxide synthesis, which in turn relaxes vascular smooth muscle and dilates arteries. Estrogen has been shown to reduce endothelial dysfunction in secondary RP.[9] Genistein (a phytoestrogen) has been shown to inhibit cold-induced vasoconstriction in the arterioles of RP patients.[14]

## N-Acetylcysteine

N-acetylcysteine (NAC), a powerful antioxidant, replenishes natural antioxidant molecules such as glutathione, which is active in preventing or reducing endothelial dysfunction in people with RP. In two studies, intravenous NAC reduced the frequency and severity of RP attacks in patients who had scleroderma[49] and enhanced global perfusion of the hands.[50]

## 7-Keto® DHEA (3-Acetyl-7-Oxo-Dehydroepiandrosterone)

Medical researchers believe that RP represents an abnormal response to cold by blood vessels. An article suggested that 7-Keto® may be helpful in preventing primary RP attacks by increasing the basal metabolic rate.[51]

## Life Extension Suggestions

- **Vitamin E (alpha-tocopherol):** 400 IU daily
- **Gamma E tocopherols:** at least 359 mg of gamma E–mixed tocopherols daily
- **Vitamin C:** 2500 mg daily
- **Niacin:** 750 mg or less daily. Use the lowest dose of niacin that relieves symptoms of RP. If you cannot tolerate the niacin flush, take 1500–4000 mg of inositol hexanicotinate (which does not typically cause flushing) in three divided doses.
- **Magnesium:** 1000 mg daily along with 1000 mg of elemental calcium
- **Gamma linolenic acid:** 1300–2600 mg daily
- **L-arginine:** 700–2250 mg daily
- **Fish oil:** 1400 mg of EPA and 1000 mg of DHA daily
- **Ginkgo biloba extract:** 120 mg daily
- **Selenium:** 200 mcg daily
- **N-acetyl-cysteine (NAC):** 600 mg daily
- **7-Keto® DHEA:** 25–100 mg daily

In addition to these supplements, hormone replacement therapy (with estrogen or phytoestrogen compounds) may be considered. Estrogen therapy should only be undertaken after blood tests have been performed and under the guidance of a qualified physician. Studies have shown that unopposed estrogen therapy can raise the risk of certain cancers. For more information on bioidentical hormonal therapy and on hormonal testing, call 1-800-226-2370 or visit Life Extension's *Blood Testing and Laboratory Services* online.

The following *blood tests* may be helpful:

- ESR (Sedimentation Rate)
- ANA (Antinuclear Antibody)
- Female Panel or Male Panel

## REFERENCES

References available at: www.lef.org/dpt5/ch114

# 115

# *Restless Legs Syndrome*

Restless legs syndrome (RLS) is a neurologic disorder associated with impaired sleep and characterized by throbbing, pulling, creeping, or other unpleasant sensations in the legs. Patients with RLS often complain of an almost irresistible urge to move their legs. The relentless and tormenting course of RLS symptoms often significantly diminishes quality of life for many of those affected and leads to significant emotional distress.[1]

*Sleepless nights* and *mental anguish* contribute to a considerable physical and psychological burden for those afflicted with RLS. Unfortunately, drugs used to treat psychological effects associated with RLS, such as tricyclic antidepressants (TCAs) and selective serotonin uptake inhibitors (SSRIs), may trigger or worsen RLS symptoms.[2–5]

Pharmaceutical treatment strategies, such as dopaminergic medications, can offer relief for those with RLS. However, a pitfall of dopaminergic drugs used at high doses is that quite often they may *exacerbate* RLS symptoms via a phenomenon known as *augmentation* or *rebound*. Fortunately, the 2012 approval of sustained release, transdermal *rotigotine* may overcome this roadblock.[6–9]

Many people do not realize that RLS can be classified as *primary* or *secondary*. Primary RLS has no known cause, whereas secondary RLS is related to another medical ailment. For example, secondary RLS is often associated with *high blood sugar*–related nerve damage or *chronic vascular disease*, such as deep vein thrombosis and arterial claudication.[10,11]

In this protocol, you will learn about possible causes of RLS and discover that treatment strategies vary based on the origins of the condition. You will also learn about convenient blood tests that might help uncover unexpected secondary causes of RLS symptoms.

## CAUSES OF RLS

### Primary RLS

The exact cause of primary RLS is unknown. However, there does appear to be a genetic component as approximately 40–50% of patients with primary RLS have a family history of the disorder and certain genetic variations are associated with the condition.[12–14]

Although many think of primary RLS as a disease of the peripheral nervous system, studies suggest that the central nervous system may also be involved. Because RLS is akin to some other movement disorders the neurotransmitter *dopamine*, which helps facilitate uniform, controlled movements, has been theorized to be a possible causative factor. Indeed, altered dopamine signaling within the brain has been observed in several RLS studies, but results have been insufficient to draw firm conclusions.[15–19] Additionally, alterations in dopamine signaling in the spinal cord have been observed, which lends further support to the hypothesis that dopamine is involved in RLS.[15,20]

### Secondary RLS

Over 20 medical conditions are connected to secondary RLS.[14]

Secondary RLS is a common complication of end-stage *kidney disease*. Estimates indicate that up to 60% of patients on dialysis have RLS.[21–23] People with *diabetes* or *impaired glucose tolerance* are more likely to have RLS, and RLS is a prominent part of diabetic peripheral neuropathy.[24–27] RLS may also be associated with *Parkinson's disease*, another disorder associated with dopaminergic dysfunction in the nervous system. However, the link has not yet been clearly established.[28,29] People with RLS also have an increased risk of developing *high blood pressure*, possibly due to overactivity of certain parts of the nervous system.[30,31]

*Chronic venous disorders* are a major contributor to secondary RLS. In a 2007 study, researchers found that *36% of patients suffering from chronic venous disease also had RLS. In comparison, the control group only had a 19% occurrence of RLS. However, when the control participants who showed positive for RLS were studied more closely, it was noted that 91% of them had mild indications of venous problems.*[11] In another study, participants with RLS who received medical treatment for chronic venous disease reported a *36% increase in quality of sleep and a 67% decrease in severity of symptoms.*[32]

## ROLE OF IRON IN RLS

One of the more commonly accepted hypotheses about the origins of RLS is that *iron metabolism* within the central nervous system plays a role.[14,33] As many as 25% of RLS patients have an iron deficiency,[34] and iron supplementation was shown to relieve RLS symptoms in iron-deficient subjects.[35]

Another study found that regular blood donors were more likely to develop RLS, particularly if they had reduced serum iron levels. Intravenous iron relieved RLS symptoms in this population.[36] Levels of ferritin (an iron storage protein) in the cerebrospinal fluid (CSF) may also be reduced in patients with RLS.[37] Iron levels in the substantia nigra (a brain region in which dopamine is produced) may be particularly important as a study using MRI imaging found reduced iron concentrations in the substantia nigra of RLS patients.[38,39] Other studies have further confirmed iron insufficiency in the substantia nigra as important for RLS. Also, people suffering from RLS often have abnormal levels of other proteins involved in iron handling (eg, ferroportin and transferrin).[40,41]

# CONVENTIONAL PHARMACOLOGIC TREATMENT

The main pharmacologic agents used to treat primary RLS are dopamine agonists, levodopa (L-DOPA), benzodiazepines, gabapentin, and opioids. However, treatment of primary RLS should not be considered until possible causes of secondary RLS are ruled out, especially venous disorders.[14]

## Dopamine Agonists

Dopamine agonists are drugs that directly activate dopamine receptors in the nervous system. They are currently considered the first-line therapy for severe RLS and are typically less associated with augmentation or rebound than high doses of L-DOPA. The following dopamine agonists, among others, are used to treat RLS.

**Ropinirole.** The efficacy of ropinirole has been demonstrated in 2 large, randomized, double-blind, placebo-controlled trials. In both studies, standardized assessment showed that (1) symptoms were significantly less, and (2) both quality and quantity of sleep were significantly improved in the ropinirole-treated groups compared with controls.[42,43]

**Pramipexole.** Pramipexole is highly effective in the reduction of periodic limb movements as well as improving subjective severity of RLS and sleep quality.[44,45] Compared to ropinirole, pramipexole is equally effective but with significantly lower incidence of nausea, vomiting, and dizziness.[46]

**Rotigotine.** On April 3, 2012, the Food and Drug Administration (FDA) approved topical delivery of rotigotine for the treatment of RLS.[6] Branded Neupro®, the topical delivery system represents a paradigm shift in the delivery of a dopamine agonist in the treatment of RLS. By delivering the drug in a sustained manner, Neupro® may lessen side effects common with orally administered dopamine agonists, which bombard dopamine receptors with a single, quickly absorbed dose.[7,8,47]

## Levodopa (L-DOPA)

L-DOPA serves as a precursor for dopamine in the human body. L-DOPA crosses the protective blood-brain barrier, whereas dopamine itself cannot. Once L-DOPA has entered the central nervous system, it is converted into dopamine with the aid of pyridoxal 5'-phosphate (the active form of vitamin B6).[48] In studies, L-DOPA reduced the number of periodic limb movements during sleep and improved sleep quality compared to placebo.[49–51] L-DOPA can provide relief within 20 minutes; however, it does not provide sustained relief for those with persistent symptoms. Levodopa/carbidopa is generally reserved for patients with infrequent symptoms, because of problems with augmentation and rebound.[52] Therefore, L-DOPA is recommended for intermittent treatment (less than 3 times a week) of bedtime symptoms or as prophylaxis during infrequent sedentary activities such as long plane trips, car rides, or theater events.[53] L-DOPA has a relatively benign side-effect profile, although there is some concern that it can cause symptoms to occur earlier in the day and more quickly at rest, and spread to the upper limbs.[54]

## DOPAMINERGIC DRUGS AND AUGMENTATION

A pitfall of dopaminergic drugs is that, paradoxically, they may cause or exacerbate RLS symptoms—a phenomenon known as *augmentation*. As many as 20–60% of patients treated with L-DOPA or dopamine agonists develop augmentation. Consequently, "it is important for physicians to carefully screen patients for changes in RLS symptoms for as long as they are on dopamine agents, with particular attention paid to those patients who present with the most severe RLS symptoms prior to treatment initiation."[55,56]

## Benzodiazepines

Benzodiazepines (eg, clonazepam and lorazepam) enhance the effect of the inhibitory neurotransmitter gamma-aminobutyric acid (GABA), giving them sedative, sleep-inducing, antianxiety, anticonvulsant, and amnesic qualities.[57] These drugs are often useful for treating insomnia associated with RLS.[58] A small placebo-controlled study measured the acute effects of 1 mg clonazepam on sleep and awakening quality in 10 RLS and 16 periodic limb movement disorder

(PLMD) patients. Insomnia associated with both RLS and PLMD was improved by clonazepam.[59] Benzodiazepines are sometimes combined with dopamine agonists in patients with refractory RLS.[52] These drugs can adversely impact cognitive ability and coordination and may rarely exacerbate anxiety and irritability.

## Gabapentin

Gabapentin is a medication often used to treat epilepsy and peripheral neuropathy; and some studies have also found that it may be useful in treating painful variants of RLS.[58,60–62] Gabapentin may be effective in individuals with RLS-associated neuropathic pain that has not responded to dopaminergic drugs.[52] The FDA approved Horizant® (gabapentin enacarbil) for the treatment of moderate-to-severe RLS in April 2011.

## Opioids

Low-dose opioids have been used successfully in some cases of RLS.[63,64] However, the mechanism by which they provide relief is not clear and the role of the endogenous opioids system in RLS is complex.[65] Opioids are typically reserved as a last-resort treatment for refractory RLS.

# LIFESTYLE CONSIDERATIONS AND NONPHARMACOLOGIC TREATMENTS

## Stimulant Avoidance

Certain chemicals (eg, nicotine and caffeine) stimulate both the central and peripheral nervous system, and can affect the body long after being ingested. As a result, many experts recommend that patients with RLS eliminate nicotine and avoid excess caffeine consumption throughout the day.[52,66] There is some controversy, however, regarding nicotine: There is a case report of nicotine actually helping alleviate symptoms in a patient,[67] and another case report of exacerbation of RLS symptoms following smoking cessation.[68] However, the evidence for nicotine as treatment for RLS is otherwise undocumented. In addition, excessive caffeine intake and nicotine use can also contribute to insomnia, which may exacerbate already existing RLS and increase daytime drowsiness.

## Exercise

Increased physical activity may be one way for RLS patients to reduce their symptoms. Risk factors for RLS can include a lack of regular physical activity,[69]

higher BMI, and obesity.[70] A randomized controlled trial found that aerobic exercise and lower-body resistance training 3 days per week significantly reduced symptoms of RLS.[71] Regular physical activity improved sleep patterns and reduced periodic limb movements (PLMs), and thus may be a useful nonpharmacologic treatment for PLMs.[72] However, it is important to not engage in physical activity shortly before going to bed, as this can exacerbate RLS symptoms.[70]

## Massage and Acupuncture

Both massage and acupuncture may produce some benefit for people with RLS.[73–75] A comprehensive review found that more research is needed to determine the benefit of acupuncture in RLS, as only 2 studies were deemed suitable for inclusion in the analysis.[76] However, one study did find that combining dermal needle therapy with medications and massage was more effective than medications and massage alone.[77] Similarly, massage of the affected regions of the leg may provide counterstimuli that can alleviate RLS symptoms.[78] Other massage techniques (eg, myofascial release, trigger point therapy, deep tissue massage), and enhanced external counter pulsation may also relieve RLS symptoms.[74,75]

# TARGETED NUTRITIONAL INTERVENTIONS

## Iron

Due to the presumed link between iron deficiency or altered iron metabolism in the brain and RLS,[79] one of the more common alternative treatments for RLS is iron supplementation.[80]

Various routes for iron supplementation have been studied as a treatment for RLS. Oral iron supplementation has been found to significantly ameliorate RLS in patients with low-normal levels of iron in their blood.[81] However, it is unclear whether oral iron supplements are as effective for patients with no signs of iron deficiency.[82] Oral iron supplementation is also beneficial for treating RLS in the elderly, particularly those with low iron levels.[35] Intravenous iron supplementation in the form of iron dextran has also been found to significantly reduce RLS symptoms.[83,84] Although intravenous iron may be more effective than oral iron supplementation, it can cause severe complications including anaphylaxis.[85] It is important to note that only those with a blood test-verified iron deficiency should take supplemental iron. Ingestion of excess iron has been linked to cancer, atherosclerosis, and other degenerative diseases.

## Folate

Folate deficiencies may also play a role in the development of RLS. Pregnancy often precipitates signs of RLS,[86] and folate levels are of paramount importance during pregnancy for healthy fetal development. Researchers have also found that pregnant women with low folate levels are more likely to develop RLS,[87] whereas women who take vitamins during pregnancy are less likely to develop RLS.[88] Low levels of folate may also play a role in nonpregnant RLS patients.[89] Older studies have found that folic acid supplementation can help treat certain paresthesias and other disorders of the peripheral nervous system as well.[90,91]

## Magnesium

Low levels of magnesium can cause neurons to become more easily excited, thus affecting a person's mental status. As a result, magnesium supplements are often used to stabilize neuronal membranes and prevent abnormal activity in the nervous system.[92] Magnesium supplementation has been studied as a treatment for RLS. One case study found that magnesium supplements were able to relieve symptoms of RLS and improve sleep.[93] A novel form of magnesium—*magnesium-l-threonate*—may be even more effective for RLS because it is better able to gain access to the central nervous system.[94] However, the impact of magnesium-L-threonate on RLS has yet to be clinically validated.

## Diosmin

The link between chronic venous disease and secondary RLS is well established.[11] Although it can be difficult to treat chronic venous issues, one therapy that has gained support is diosmin.

Diosmin is a natural venotonic that supports venous function, thereby preventing or reversing some of the changes of chronic venous disease. Used and researched extensively in Europe, micronized diosmin has been introduced to the United States and proven to be an effective treatment for chronic venous disease.[95,96] Although the effectiveness of diosmin for treating RLS has not been tested, it remains a promising possible treatment.

## Green Coffee Extract

Diabetes is a well-known risk factor for secondary RLS. However, less appreciated is that *prediabetes—subclinical* elevations in blood sugar—may also cause RLS while remaining under the diagnostic radar of most physicians.[10,24]

A study examining subjects with impaired glucose metabolism unearthed a significantly increased risk of RLS in this population. RLS affected *41%* of those with prediabetes, while only *18%* of those with healthy glucose tolerance experienced the condition.[24]

Maintaining healthy glucose metabolism, even for those not diagnosed with diabetes, may be helpful in RLS. Even slightly elevated blood sugar can damage delicate nerve cells and contribute to unpleasant sensations called *paresthesias*.[97] Evidence suggests that an extract from green coffee beans, which contains a powerful antioxidant called *chlorogenic acid*, may support healthy glucose metabolism.[98]

Life Extension suggests that all aging individuals should strive to maintain blood glucose levels at *70–85 mg/dL* for optimal health. Green coffee extract, with minimal caffeine content, represents a powerful tool for those aiming to maintain healthy blood sugar levels. It may also help control glucose elevations, which have been associated with RLS. However, this theory has yet to be tested in clinical trials.

## Valerian Root

Often used as an herbal sedative, valerian root has shown promise at reducing symptom severity of RLS. In an 8-week clinical trial, supplementation with 800 mg of valerian root daily resulted in improvements in daytime sleepiness and RLS symptoms.[99] Additional data also support the effectiveness of valerian root in treating insomnia in postmenopausal women.[100]

## EXPERIMENTAL ALTERNATIVE THERAPIES

Other less established interventions are also being explored for the treatment of RLS, including:

- **D-ribose.** D-ribose is a naturally occurring carbohydrate that is essential for the body. It may decrease the symptoms of RLS when taken daily.[101]
- **Vitamins C and E.** In a clinical trial among dialysis patients with RLS, supplementation with vitamins C and E significantly improved RLS symptoms.[102]
- **Near-infrared light.** Another RLS treatment that has shown promise is exposing the legs to near-infrared light for several sessions over a period of a week. This treatment may affect leg blood vessels in a way that relieves RLS symptoms.[103,104]

## Life Extension Suggestions

- **Iron:** 15 mg daily if blood testing reveals a deficiency
- **Vitamin C:** 1000–2000 mg daily
- **Folate** (preferably as L-methylfolate): 400–1000 mcg daily

- **Magnesium** (as magnesium-L-threonate): 140 mg daily
- **Diosmin:** 600 mg daily
- **Green coffee extract:** 200–400 mg before each heavy meal, up to 3 times daily
- **Valerian root:** 600–800 mg daily, 30 minutes–1 hour before bedtime
- **Natural vitamin E:** 100–400 IU alpha-tocopherol and 200 mg gamma-tocopherol daily
- **D-ribose:** 5–10 g daily in divided doses with food

In addition, the following *blood tests* may provide helpful information:

- Ferritin
- Fasting glucose
- Vitamin B12 and folate

## REFERENCES

References available at: www.lef.org/dpt5/ch115

# 116

# *Retinopathy*

Diabetic retinopathy (DR), the leading cause of visual disability and blindness among adults in the developed world, may affect as many as 20 million people. Early detection and treatment are keys to preventing vision loss and blindness associated with the disease. Unfortunately, only about half of those with diabetes have proper eye examinations on a yearly basis. It is very important that diabetics have a dilated eye exam each year.

Retinopathy damages the retina by destroying the capillaries (minuscule blood vessels connecting arteries and veins) that provide blood to the retina, the light-sensitive nerve tissue that sends visual images to the brain. With the onset of retinopathy, these vessels weaken or bulge with microaneurysms that may hemorrhage, leaking blood or fluid into surrounding tissue. New blood vessels that grow on the retina (and into the vitreous) can cause blurred vision and even temporary blindness. Ultimately, scar tissue forms, detaching the retina from the back of the eye and often causing permanent vision loss.

Chronically elevated blood insulin and glucose levels induce retinopathy. However, research shows that even after having long-term diabetes, lowering glucose has a positive effect on slowing the progression of retinopathy. A glycohemoglobin (also known as hemoglobin A1C or HbA1c) test is the best measurement of long-term glucose control. A high HbA1c number correlates with uncontrolled diabetes.

A study took place involving 834 people who were over the age of 30 years when they developed diabetes, and approximately 65 years at the start of the study. A HbA1c test, physical exam, and eye exam were performed at baseline, 4- and 10-year follow-up visits. In non–insulin-treated participants, those that had the highest HbA1c levels at baseline had nearly a 3-fold greater risk of developing retinopathy after 10 years than those with the lowest levels. In participants already showing proof of retinopathy at baseline, the presence of elevated HbA1c resulted in a 4-fold greater risk of retinopathy progression and a 14-fold greater risk of proliferative retinopathy.

In those people using insulin treatments and having the highest HbA1c levels, there was a 90%

greater risk of developing retinopathy than those with the lowest levels. Researchers concluded that controlling hyperglycemia, even later on in the course of diabetes, will result in a significant decrease in the incidence and progression of retinopathy as well as the development of visual loss.[1] Studies show that controlling excess serum insulin is also important in preventing retinopathy.[2-4]

There are additional precautions that can be taken to guard against the development of retinopathies. Vitamin B6 deficiency, for instance, is a proven cause of the disease. In order to rule out a nutritional deficiency as the cause of retinopathy, a 10-week program is suggested that incorporates a high-potency B-complex vitamin formula along with other supplements described in this protocol.

## RETINOPATHY OF PREMATURITY

Retinopathy of prematurity (ROP) is abnormal blood vessel development in the retina of the eye in a premature infant.[5] A study assessed retinopathy in 60 oxygen-treated, premature infants and their mothers. All 60 infants showed signs of acute oxidative stress. Concentrations of methionine-cysteine in plasma and selenium in blood were significantly lower in premature infants with moderate retinopathy than oxygen-treated premature infants without retinopathy. Mothers of premature infants with retinopathy showed the same pattern of deficiencies as their babies. Vitamin E treatment of premature infants seemed to have a positive effect against the development of ROP.[6]

The close correlation between antioxidant capacity of mothers and babies suggests that supplementation with sulfur-containing amino acids (methionine, cysteine) and folic acid during pregnancy might improve the antioxidant capacity of premature infants. An antioxidant cocktail of selenium plus vitamin E given to high-risk mothers (high risk factors include advanced age, smoking, and pregnancy-induced hypertension) before delivery might be useful in the prevention of retinopathy in premature infants.[6]

## PROTEIN GLYCATION

Glycation of proteins has been shown to play a prominent role in the development of many diseases related to diabetes, including atherosclerosis, cataract formation, and retinopathy. Oxidation induced by glycation can wreak havoc on the eye. Protein glycation occurs when sugar molecules inappropriately bind to protein molecules, forming cross-links that distort proteins and consequently render them useless. High blood sugar also increases glycation activity, which may also explain the various kinds of tissue damage that characterize advanced diabetes. Controlling blood sugar is a major means of preventing or at least slowing the onset and progression of DR. Glycation appears to increase oxidative processes, which may explain why both glycation and oxidation simultaneously increase with age.

Strategies for preventing diabetic complications should therefore aim to prevent the effects of both glycation and oxidative stress.

Aminoguanidine has been used successfully to protect against glycation.[7] Compounds produced through metabolism of sugars bind preferentially to aminoguanidine rather than lysine proteins. Thus, aminoguanidine is able to inhibit advanced glycation end-product (AGE) formation and help prevent the harmful development of collagen cross-links and changes in proliferation of mesangial cells.

Aminoguanidine used in the dose of 300 mg daily can specifically inhibit glycation, as can the nutrients keto-glutarate and pyruvate. Studies have shown aminoguanidine to be useful in slowing complications of diabetes, such as retinopathy. Aminoguanidine can also inhibit the formation of atherosclerotic plaques.

*Carnosine* is a naturally occurring antiglycation agent found in red meat. In the lens of the eye, protein cross-linking is part of cataract formation. Carnosine eye drops have been shown to delay vision impairment in humans; they are effective in 100% of cases of primary senile cataract and 80% of cases of mature senile cataract.[8] The most widely used antiglycating therapy is 1000 mg daily of oral supplemental carnosine.

*Benfotiamine*, a relative of vitamin B1 (thiamin), protects cells by preventing glycation and accelerated aging triggered by elevated sugar levels. The body has several natural mechanisms to cope with chemical toxins produced by excess glucose, and these defense systems all require vitamin B1 as a cofactor.[9] When the system is awash with excess glucose, thiamine supplies become depleted. Because thiamine is water-soluble and the body cannot retain thiamine at levels high enough to prevent cumulative damage, additional supplemental thiamine does not significantly protect against glucose-induced tissue damage.[10,11] Benfotiamine, however, is fat-soluble and can significantly increase thiamine levels within tissues as well as sustain them throughout the day.[9,11,12]

*Pyridoxal-5'-phosphate* (P5P), the biologically active form of vitamin B6, is a powerful inhibitor of both protein and fat glycation.[13,14] Glycation reductions by P5P are credited with reducing sugar-induced blood vessel damage from diabetes.[15,16]

## ANTIOXIDANTS AND RETINOPATHY

### Superoxide Dismutase and Retinal Damage

A newborn rat model of retinopathy was used to test the hypothesis that a lack of the antioxidant superoxide dismutase (SOD) contributes to retinal damage. The study concluded that delivery of SOD to the retina via long-circulating liposomes was beneficial, and suggested the potential value of restoration or supplementation of antioxidants in retinal tissue as a therapeutic strategy.[17] It is difficult to provide SOD directly to the retina, but adequate supplementation with nutrients (eg, zinc, copper, and manganese) provide the minerals needed for the formation of SOD in the cells.

### Decreased Retinal Antioxidant Activity in Diabetics

Enzymatic activities that protect the retina from reactive oxygen species were investigated in diabetic rats known to have retinopathy. Diabetes significantly decreased the activities of glutathione reductase and glutathione peroxidase in the retina. Activities of 2 other important antioxidant defense enzymes—superoxide dismutase (SOD) and catalase—were also decreased by >25% in the retinas of diabetic rats.[18]

The study showed that diabetes is associated with significant impairment of the antioxidant defense system and antioxidant supplementation can help alleviate the subnormal activities of antioxidant defense enzymes. Administration of supplemental vitamins C and E for 2 months prevented diabetes-induced impairment of the antioxidant defense system in the retina.[18] Another study found no protective effect from antioxidant nutrients for diabetic retinopathy. Authors concluded that further research is necessary to confirm associations between nutrient antioxidant intake and the disease.[19]

## CAROTENOIDS AND THE RETINA

Countless studies demonstrate an association between consumption of carotenoids and lowered risk of cancer and cardiovascular disease. *Carotenoids*, especially lutein and zeaxanthin, have also been found to help preserve eye health. Lutein is a pigment found in dark, green, leafy vegetables (eg, spinach, kale, broccoli, and collard greens). Zeaxanthin is found in fruits and vegetables with yellow hues (eg, corn, peaches, persimmons, and mangoes). Because lutein and zeaxanthin are structurally very similar, found in many of the same foods, and both present in the retina, they are often lumped together when discussed or studied. Lutein and zeaxanthin have been found to positively affect macular pigment density and help prevent age-related macular degeneration (AMD).

Although there are several hundred carotenoids in fruits and vegetables, only lutein and zeaxanthin are found in the retina.[20,21] Compared to other antioxidant concentrations found in the eye, German researchers found that lutein and zeaxanthin did not break down nearly as fast as lycopene and beta-carotene when exposed to free radical or UV light induced oxidative stress.[22] Authors suggested that perhaps the slow degradation of lutein and zeaxanthin may explain the strong presence of these carotenoids in the retina. Also, the quick breakdown of lycopene and beta-carotene may suggest why these carotenoids are lacking in the same retinal tissues.

Researchers have also found that lutein and zeaxanthin are more highly concentrated in the center of the macula. There, the amounts of lutein and zeaxanthin are much greater than their concentrations in the peripheral region. Using retinas from human donor eyes, investigators demonstrated that the concentration of lutein and zeaxanthin was 70% higher in rod outer segment (ROS) membranes (where the concentration of long-chain polyunsaturated fatty acids and susceptibility to oxidation is highest) than in residual membranes.[23] The fact that lutein and zeaxanthin are particularly concentrated in these parts of the eye suggests they may act as a shield or filter to help absorb harmful UVB light and dangerous free-radical molecules, both of which threaten retinal tissue.[24,25]

## TARGETED NUTRITIONAL THERAPIES

### Vitamin C

Another study investigated antioxidant activity in the lens and vitreous of diabetic and nondiabetic subjects. Researchers found significantly decreased glutathione peroxidase activity and lower vitamin C (ascorbic acid) levels in the lenses of diabetic patients, especially in the presence of retinal damage. Ascorbic acid is known to exert important antioxidant functions in the eye compartment. This study indicated that oxidative damage is involved in the onset of diabetic eye complications, in which the decrease in free radical scavengers was shown to be associated with oxidation of vitreous and lens proteins.[26]

### Vitamin B12

Vitamin B12 (cyanocobalamin, methylcobalamin, or hydroxycobalamin [a naturally occurring form]), is critical for several functions, such as folate metabolism, myelin synthesis, and normal development of red blood cells. A lack of this vitamin may leave the optic nerve more susceptible to damage. Studies have suggested that marginal vitamin deficiency plays an indirect, but important role in the development of diabetic complications.[27]

### Vitamin E

One study showed that reducing lipid peroxidation stress of the erythrocyte membrane using vitamin E (alpha-tocopherol nicotinate) therapy may be useful in slowing deterioration of microangiopathy in type 2 diabetes mellitus. The dose used was 300 mg, 3 times daily (after meals) for 3 months.[28] Researchers reported that vitamin E supplements normalized blood flow to the retina and kidneys. Following a 4-month clinical trial in which subjects were given doses of vitamin E that were 60 times the recommended daily allowance, kidney function improved and blood flow to the retina was increased almost to the normal rate. A large follow-up clinical trial was recommended.[29]

Another study evaluated the use of antioxidants as a prophylactic for eye disorders, such as macular degeneration, cataracts, ROP, and cystic macular edema. The study points to the positive role of antioxidants in both experimental research and clinical observations.[30]

### Green Tea

Green tea is another potent antioxidant that could be of use in the treatment of retinopathy. The active compound in green tea is catechins. Powerful polyphenolic antioxidants, catechins are astringent, water-soluble compounds that can be easily oxidized. They are a subgroup of flavonoids, weak phytoestrogenic compounds widely available in vegetables, fruit, tea, coffee, chocolate, and wine. The antioxidant potential of both green and black teas, as measured by the Phenol Antioxidant Index, was found to be significantly higher than that of grape juice and red wine. Green tea also has antiangiogenic properties, indicating it could be used for prevention and possibly treatment of degenerative eye disorders (eg, diabetic retinopathy) that also depend on the development of new blood vessels.[31,32]

### Silibinin

An in vitro study showed that silibinin (milk thistle extract) can normalize the degree of ribosylation and sodium pump activity, even in the presence of abnormally high glucose levels.[33] A similar protective effect of silibinin against ribosylation was found in the retina.[34] Thus, silibinin may be able to decrease the extent of diabetic neuropathy and retinopathy, 2 extremely serious complications of diabetes. Considering that silibinin has also been shown to protect the kidneys, another organ seriously damaged by glycation (kidney failure is a frequent cause of death in diabetics), silibinin should be seriously explored as an adjunct treatment in diabetes.

## Propionyl-L-Carnitine

Research examined the effect of propionyl-L-carnitine (an analogue of L-carnitine) on retinopathy in rats with laboratory-induced diabetes. Findings pointed to a potential therapeutic value of propionyl-L-carnitine for diabetic retinopathy.[35] L-carnitine, a natural substance found in meat, is related to B vitamins.

## Life Extension Suggestions

- **Comprehensive multinutrient formula:** per label instructions
- **Vitamin B12:** 1000 mcg of the methylcobalamin form, 1–4 times daily
- **Vitamin E:** 400 IU daily (containing approximately 200 mg gamma tocopherol)
- **Vitamin C:** 1000–4000 mg daily
- **Green tea:** 725 mg daily (standardized to contain 98% polyphenols and 45% EGCG)
- **Milk thistle:** 750 mg daily (standardized to contain 80% silymarin and 30% silibinins)
- **Carotenoid blend:** containing 3.75 of zeaxanthin/meso-zeaxanthin blend and 38 mg of lutein
- **Carnitine:** 1400 mg once or twice daily (containing 300 mg of propionyl L-carnitine per serving)
- **Carnosine:** 500 mg, 2–3 times daily
- **Benfotiamine:** 250 mg, 1–4 times daily
- **Pyridoxal 5'-phosphate:** 100 mg daily

In addition, the following *blood tests* may provide helpful information:

- Chemistry panel and complete blood count (CBC)
- Hemoglobin A1C

## REFERENCES

References available at: www.lef.org/dpt5/ch116

# 117

# Scleroderma

Scleroderma is a progressive autoimmune disorder that can disable its victims. In people with scleroderma, the body's immune system is activated, which results in inflammation and overproduction of thick layers of collagen. This resulting scar tissue can form anywhere in the body, especially in the skin. Other organ systems affected by scleroderma include the kidneys, lungs, heart, and eyes.

The cause of scleroderma is unknown. It affects women 4 times more frequently than men. Symptoms of scleroderma usually occur in people aged 35–65 years. While scleroderma is usually encountered in adults, it does occur (although rarely) in children.[1-3]

Managing scleroderma presents a challenge for physicians, and a multidisciplinary approach is usually best. Because it can affect such a variety of organ systems, people with systemic scleroderma often need to rely on the guidance of physicians from several specialties. It is very important that people with scleroderma work with physicians who are familiar with their disease, including dermatologists and rheumatologists, among others.

Because of the challenges associated with conventional treatment of scleroderma, many people with the condition turn to nutrient therapy to reduce inflammation, interfere with the creation of scar tissue, and reduce symptoms. It is imperative that your physician know all the therapies you are using and that you be an active self-advocate, asking for specific information, educating yourself about the disease, and seeking support.

## WHAT IS SCLERODERMA?

Scleroderma is a chronic disease characterized by 3 main features:

1. Formation of scar tissue in the tissue (fibrosis)
2. Changes in small blood vessels
3. An autoimmune response

Scleroderma primarily affects the skin. However, in more involved cases, it also affects internal organ systems including the lungs, kidneys, and heart. Scleroderma-like symptoms may also be part of a phenomenon called "mixed connective tissue disease." This diagnosis is reserved for patients who exhibit symptoms from several connective tissue diseases. These patients may have symptoms in common with systemic lupus erythematosus, polymyositis, and rheumatoid arthritis.

## TYPES OF SCLERODERMA

Scleroderma is often broken down into 2 subtypes, localized and systemic.

### Localized Scleroderma

Localized scleroderma is considered a mild form of scleroderma that affects the skin. Although it may affect muscles and joints, it does not affect organs. In a limited number of people, localized scleroderma may contribute to pulmonary hypertension after a decade or more, along with biliary cirrhosis. There are 2 common forms of localized scleroderma:

**Linear scleroderma.** Linear scleroderma is characterized by hardened skin affecting the underlying tissues (muscles, bones). It usually occurs on the arms, legs, and forehead on one side of the body and is more common in children.

**Morphea.** Morphea is characterized by patches of yellowish or ivory-colored rigid, dry skin that become hard, slightly depressed oval plaques. Morphea usually occurs on the trunk, although it may be widespread (generalized morphea).

### Systemic Scleroderma

Systemic scleroderma occurs throughout the body, affecting internal organs. Treatment for these individual complications is usually specific to each organ system. Systemic scleroderma can affect the connective tissue of the lung, kidney, heart, and other organs, as well as blood vessels, muscles, and joints. The skin thickening is symmetrical on both sides of the body, usually beginning on the fingertips and moving up the arms. Legs and thighs also are affected. Systemic scleroderma has several complications[4]:

- About 90% of patients experience problems in the esophagus and digestive tract. The lower two-thirds of the esophagus sometimes develops a tough inflexibility. The associated dysfunction of the lower esophageal sphincter may lead to gastroesophageal reflux.

- About 66% of patients experience kidney abnormalities. The kidneys may thicken as a result of fibrous collagen deposits forming in them.

- More than 50% of patients experience lung problems, including pulmonary hypertension and scarring within the lungs (interstitial fibrosis).

- About one-third of patients experience pericarditis (inflammation of the covering of the heart) or the deposition of scar tissue in the heart muscle (myocardial fibrosis), as well as thickening of the intramyocardial arterioles (small arteries within the middle portion of the heart).

In addition, a lesser form of scleroderma known by the acronym CREST may exist. CREST may occur alone or in combination with any autoimmune disease. There is no way to predict whether or when it will progress to diffuse scleroderma.[4] CREST stands for the following conditions occurring together:

- **C**alcinosis (the buildup of calcium deposits in the tissues). It may occur under the skin of the fingers, arms, feet, and knees, causing pain and infection if the calcium deposits pierce the surface of the skin.
- **R**aynaud's phenomenon, characterized by localized episodes of vasoconstriction in the fingers and extremities.
- **E**sophageal dysmotility, a malfunction in the ability to move the esophagus spontaneously.
- **S**clerodactyly, hardening of skin on the fingers.
- **T**elangiectasia, an abnormal dilatation of capillaries and small arteries that often forms an angioma (a swelling or tumor).

## SYMPTOMS AND DIAGNOSIS OF SCLERODERMA

Scleroderma is characterized by the overproduction and accumulation of collagen, the most abundant form of protein in the skin. The disease process involves activation of the immune system, along with vascular endothelial cell activation. Because of the vascular injury, scleroderma is often preceded by Raynaud's phenomenon (in about 95% of cases). During Raynaud's, small arteries in the fingers constrict, causing abnormal blood flow. As a result, the fingers turn white and become numb and cold. The majority of patients eventually diagnosed with scleroderma will report first suffering from Raynaud's. In most cases, the presence of Raynaud's and skin changes is enough to diagnose scleroderma.

There is no single test that can diagnose scleroderma. Rather, the diagnosis is based on symptoms and trademark characteristics of the disease. The following symptoms (with approximate percentages, when available, of patients in whom those organ systems are affected) may constitute scleroderma:

- Thickening of the skin (90%)
- Swelling of the hands and feet

- Pain and stiffness of the joints (30–50%)
- Joint contractures (fingers curling up, difficulty of movement)
- Raynaud's phenomenon (70–90%)
- Gastrointestinal tract problems (90%)
- Sjögren's syndrome (dry mucus membranes)
- Facial problems (tightening of skin, limiting mobility of mouth and eyelids; temporomandibular joint syndrome, or pain in the joint of the jaw)
- Dental problems (change in bite; loosening of teeth due to collagen deposition, increasing the size of the ligaments around the teeth; tooth sensitivity)
- Fatigue attributable to fibrosis in the heart muscle
- Generalized aching and weakness caused by fibrosis in the muscles (20%)
- Kidney, heart, and lung involvement

In addition, a variety of laboratory studies may help physicians pinpoint their diagnosis. People with scleroderma may have an elevated erythrocyte sedimentation rate (ESR) and suffer from anemia. Additional blood tests may reveal abnormalities in the gastrointestinal tract or kidneys. In addition, certain antibodies (eg, antitopoisomerase 1, antinucleolar, and anticentromere) may be present in the blood. Testing for these antibodies often helps physicians differentiate between localized and systemic scleroderma as well as help diagnose CREST.

Many patients describe the path toward diagnosis as one of the most difficult periods of the illness, in part because the difficulty of the diagnosis can lead both physicians and patients to label the symptoms as psychosomatic (ie, caused by the mind).

## CONVENTIONAL TREATMENT OF SCLERODERMA

Scleroderma therapy is guided by the specific needs of the patient; not all patients have the same symptoms. In general, conditions that may have been caused by scleroderma, such as heart or kidney failure, will be managed in much the same way as in any other patient. Conventional treatments, organized according to symptoms, are described in the following.

### Treatments for General Symptoms

D-penicillamine, because it was thought to interfere with the deposition of collagen, has been the treatment of choice for many years. However, studies found it ineffective in softening skin or preventing organ involvement.[5–7] High-dose D-penicillamine, up to 1000 mg daily, is associated with significant side effects. Research has found that low-dose penicillamine (125 mg every other day) is as effective as previously used high doses of penicillamine, with less toxicity.[8,9]

Gamma-interferon may inhibit the proliferation of fibroblasts, the cells that produce collagen. Steroids such as prednisone are frequently used for their anti-inflammatory action, which includes alteration of white blood cell function. However, steroids have significant side effects, including loss of bone density and weight gain. Steroids also suppress the body's natural ability to handle stress and are typically for short-term use.

Other treatments, including some with significant side effects, are being investigated for more serious forms of the disease. Immunosuppressive drugs that have been used for cancer chemotherapy and organ transplants may reduce the autoimmune response. These drugs kill cells that rapidly proliferate, which includes immune cells. High-dose cyclophosphamide is the drug of choice; azathioprine has fewer side effects but is less potent. Bone marrow transplants can be used in conjunction with these drugs. Some physicians, however, argue that this is unnecessary since the stem cells that produce white blood cells will not be affected by cytotoxic drugs.

Cyclosporin, which blocks the activation and stimulation of immune T cells, may also limit skin damage. However, cyclosporin causes kidney toxicity and does not affect pulmonary or cardiac complications; thus, it has a limited place in the treatment of systemic scleroderma.

Photopheresis, a procedure similar to dialysis, may help relieve some symptoms. During photopheresis, the patient's blood is removed, white blood cells are treated to quell autoimmune activity, and the blood is returned to the body. Research has been done using this treatment method for a variety of diseases, with encouraging results for scleroderma patients.[10] It is also believed that photopheresis, if used as a long-term treatment, is efficacious if started within the first 2 years following the onset of the disease, as long as there is no visceral involvement.[11]

Biomechanical stimulation has been shown in one small study to improve joint mobility and reduce edema.[12]

A new, experimental drug, halofuginone, is a collagen synthesis inhibitor that has shown promise in animal models of scleroderma. It was granted orphan drug status by the Food and Drug Administration (FDA) in 2000; orphan drug status is designed to encourage clinical research into a particular drug even though it has not been formally approved by the FDA.

## Treatments for Skin Disease and Musculoskeletal/Joint Pain

Swelling during the early stage of skin thickening may be controlled with steroids, but side effects must be considered. Some physicians feel that colchicine can reduce skin thickening if used early. Calcinosis can be treated with low-dose warfarin, colchicine, or probenecid, but may not be treated at all because it causes no clinical problems. Musculoskeletal and joint pain is commonly treated with nonsteroidal anti-inflammatory drugs or steroids. Topical pain relievers such as salicylate or capsaicin creams may be used.

Some centers specializing in dermatology offer PUVA therapy, in which repeated sessions of exposure to ultraviolet light are coupled with psoralen, a drug that makes the skin more sensitive to light. This technique has been found to soften skin and reduce the diameter of plaques, or even cure them. It is considered effective for localized disease.

Xerosis (ie, severe dry skin) is a common problem and can be treated with creams such as Lubriderm®, Eucerin®, Bag Balm®, histamine 2 blockers, or trazodone,[13] which has antiseptic properties. Skin should be kept moist and protected from cold, injury, or infection by clothing, especially gloves. Avoid strong detergents and soaps and use a humidifier.

## Treatments for Gastrointestinal Symptoms

Metoclopramide and cisapride can aid esophageal contraction and stomach emptying. Acid reflux (heartburn) can be managed by diet, sleeping on the left side, antacids, and proton pump inhibitors, including Prilosec® (omeprazole), Prevacid® (lansoprazole), Nexium® (esomeprazole), and others.

A balanced diet that includes nutritional supplements is considered vital to maintain body weight and health. Some literature advises avoiding caffeine, refined sugars, and food additives that have been implicated as carcinogens (eg, sodium nitrite) or have side effects (eg, caffeine, olestra, and monosodium glutamate [MSG]).

## Treatments for Pulmonary Symptoms

Fibrosis, or interstitial disease of the lungs, can be treated with steroids or immunosuppressants (eg, cyclophosphamide). Pulmonary hypertension will be treated with drugs that dilate the vessels, such as calcium channel blockers or epoprostenol.

## Treatments for Renal Symptoms

Kidney problems are thought to result from fibrosis and overall hypertension or high blood pressure. Therefore, it is critical to control blood pressure using angiotensin-converting enzyme (ACE) inhibitors.

---

### FOR MORE INFORMATION

The following protocols may also be of interest:

- Gastroesophageal Reflux Disease (GERD)
- Kidney Health
- Inflammation (Chronic)
- Pain (Chronic)
- Raynaud's Phenomenon

---

## NUTRITIONAL THERAPY

### Dimethylsulfoxide

Dimethylsulfoxide (DMSO), a solvent that readily penetrates the skin, is typically used to "carry" another substance. In scleroderma, it is used to soften the skin. Clinical studies with DMSO have yielded cautiously optimistic results. Cutaneous manifestations of scleroderma appear to resolve (albeit equivocally) following topical application of high concentrations of DMSO.[14] However, a significant number of patients (up to 25%) cannot withstand the skin toxicity sometimes associated with high-concentration DMSO; they must discontinue treatment.[15] Due to this risk, DMSO treatment should be highly individualized for maximum benefits.[16]

### Gamma-Linolenic Acid

Gamma-linolenic acid (GLA) is an essential fatty acid that is converted to the precursor for prostaglandin E1, a potent anti-inflammatory hormone-like fatty acid. Raising prostaglandin formation in scleroderma patients could be useful.[17,18] GLA has also been shown to reduce autoimmune dysfunction in rheumatoid arthritis patients. GLA can be obtained from evening primrose oil, borage oil, or black currant seed oil.

### Docosahexaenoic Acid and Eicosapentaenoic Acid

Docosahexaenoic acid (DHA) and eicosapentaenoic acid (EPA) are essential long-chain fatty acids with anti-inflammatory effects and are found in flaxseed oil and fish oil. Fish oils have been shown to help relieve Raynaud's, which is closely related to scleroderma.[19] Together, EPA and DHA suppress arachidonic acid, reducing inflammation and supporting healthy cell membranes.

### Antioxidants

Free-radical damage (oxidation) has long been suspected as a major mechanism of autoimmune disease. Low-density lipoproteins (LDLs) from patients with scleroderma are more susceptible to oxidation than those from healthy people[20] and patients with primary Raynaud's. Micronutrient antioxidant status in patients with primary Raynaud's and scleroderma revealed reduced vitamin C and selenium, especially in those patients with diffuse scleroderma.[21]

One study argued that autoimmune diseases are caused by a relative deficiency of vitamin E. This deficiency damages the membranes of lysosomes (cellular organelles that digest waste), allowing the escape of hydrolytic enzymes that denature (destroy) proteins to the point that they are no longer recognizable by the immune system and are attacked as if they were foreign particles. This process resembles the enhanced lipid peroxidation seen in patients with scleroderma, which is 4 times higher than a healthy person's. In one study, after supplementation with *vitamin E*, there was a decrease in the indicator of lipid peroxidation by two-thirds.[22] In a case study, vitamin E was administered to a 33-year-old woman with scleroderma who had several miscarriages. After 5 months of tocopherol nicotinate treatment, she conceived and later delivered a healthy baby.[23]

The antioxidant *N-acetylcysteine (NAC)* has shown promise in reducing the frequency of Raynaud's phenomenon in people with scleroderma. In one study, patients received NAC for 2 years through intravenous infusion. Imaging studies revealed that patients who underwent treatment with NAC had increased blood flow to their hands. The therapy also found negligible side effects, leading researchers to suggest that NAC was a successful vasodilator.[24] Another study examined the role of NAC in reducing pulmonary complications of scleroderma. In this study, macrophages taken from the lungs of patients with scleroderma were studied for their expression of inducible nitric oxide synthase (which causes vasoconstriction) and peroxynitrite (a pro-oxidant by-product of nitric oxide). Researchers found that concentrations of both chemicals were higher in the lungs of people with scleroderma and that NAC therapy reduced the expression of peroxynitrite, which may help reduce oxidant damage and thus fibrosis in the lungs.[25]

### Melatonin

Melatonin is a pineal hormone that is usually associated with sleep. Studies have revealed, however, that melatonin plays a varied role in the body. A study looked at the effect of concurrent melatonin and vitamin E treatment to reduce vascular damage among people with scleroderma. Researchers found that none of their test participants with stable or responding disease (all of them) experienced disease progression after 5 months of treatment.[26]

## Centella Asiatica

*Centella asiatica* is an herb found in Madagascar and East Africa. An extract of *Centella asiatica* has been used for wound healing and venous insufficiency. Various studies have shown active components in centella to be effective in scar management by aiding in the production of collagen type I.[27-29] Centella, under the name madecassol, has been used on localized and systemic scleroderma with positive results. A 6-month trial was carried out with 54 patients aged 15–70 years. A tablet, powder, or ointment combination was used on the patients. In 31 of the systemic scleroderma patients using 30 mg daily, indurative lesions, hyperpigmentation, or vascular trophic disorder decreased, and their general condition improved. Lack of disease progression corresponded with a subjective improvement in 10 patients. The researchers concluded that Madecassol works for oral and topical use in combined treatment of systemic scleroderma.[30] Centella, under the name gotu kola, is available in capsule or liquid form from several manufacturers.

## Vitamin D3

Vitamin D deficiency in scleroderma may be related to several factors including insufficient sun exposure due to disability and skin fibrosis and insufficient intake due to gut involvement and malabsorption.[31] Patients with vitamin D deficiency showed longer disease duration, lower diffusing lung capacity for carbon monoxide, higher estimated pulmonary artery pressure, and higher values of ESR and C-reactive protein (CRP) in comparison to patients with vitamin D insufficiency. Patients with vitamin D deficiency showed more severe disease in comparison to patients with vitamin D insufficiency, above all concerning lung involvement.[32]

## Life Extension Suggestions

- **DMSO:** concentrations as tolerated, applied to affected areas for 30 minutes daily, or 50% DMSO bath for hand immersion, with gradually increased duration and frequency, depending on tolerance
- **GLA:** 900–1800 mg daily
- **EPA/DHA:** 1400 mg EPA and 1000 mg DHA daily
- **NAC:** 600 mg daily
- **Melatonin:** 300 mcg–3 mg at bedtime (discontinue if symptoms or signs worsen)
- **Centella asiatica (gotu kola):** 300 mg daily, or topical centella ointment twice daily
- **Vitamin E:** 400 IU daily (with at least 200 mg gamma tocopherol)
- **Vitamin C:** 2500 mg daily
- **Beta-carotene:** 4500 IU daily
- **Selenium:** 200 mcg daily
- **Vitamin D3:** 5000–8000 IU daily

In addition, the following *blood tests* can provide helpful information:

- Erythrocyte Sedimentation Rate (ESR)
- Antinuclear Antibody (ANA)

## REFERENCES

References available at: www.lef.org/dpt5/ch117

# 118

# *Seasonal Affective Disorder*

Many people may feel sad or down during the winter months, when the days are shorter and temperatures drop. For some people, this condition goes beyond the winter "blahs" and develops into a subtype of clinical depression that lasts throughout the late fall and winter months. This condition is known as seasonal affective disorder, or SAD. The term SAD was introduced in 1984 and has since been included in the American Psychiatric Association's Diagnostic and Statistical Manual of Mental Disorders.

SAD is characterized by recurring, cyclic bouts of depression, increased appetite, and an increased need for sleep.[1,2] It contrasts with most depressive disorders, which are characterized by sleep disturbances and diminished appetite.[3] Besides mild depression, typical symptoms of SAD include anxiety, decreased activity, social withdrawal, increased sleep duration, increased appetite, weight gain, and carbohydrate craving.[4,5]

SAD occurs in about 10% of the general population, although it is about twice as common among people treated for depression.[6] It tends to be more common in the higher latitudes, where winter days are comparatively shorter than at latitudes nearer the equator, and it occurs more often in women than in men.[2,6,7] Studies have also shown that the tendency to develop SAD may run in families, which suggests a genetic component.[8] Family studies have shown that approximately 13–17% of people who have first-degree relatives with SAD will suffer from the condition themselves.[9–12] The occurrence of SAD seems to lessen after the age of 55 years.[6]

## WHAT CAUSES SAD?

The 24-hour sleep-wake cycle, known as the circadian rhythm, is governed in part by the regular rise and fall of hormones, especially melatonin. Melatonin, the master sleep hormone, is produced in the pineal gland. Researchers have identified a regular ebb and flow to human physiology and behavior throughout a normal 24-hour cycle.[13] Our overall pattern of sleep-wake depends on the proper functioning of an internal circadian clock, which lies deep in the brain. This circadian clock works with photosensors in the eyes to sense darkness. When darkness falls, the body begins to secrete melatonin, which is one of the factors that cause sleep. Melatonin continues to be secreted throughout the night, although levels alter, and toward dawn, melatonin secretion gradually diminishes, allowing for wakefulness in the morning.

When there is a problem with this system, sleep disorders and other psychological problems can occur. Research has identified a number of possible abnormalities that may help explain and offer therapeutic targets for SAD.

## The Melatonin Theory

Early research focused on the shorter photoperiod in winter, hypothesizing that shorter days led directly to SAD. Researchers initially attempted, with some success, to lengthen the photoperiod by exposing individuals to bright light in the morning and evening.[4,14] Next, researchers focused on the secretion of melatonin, which controls the sleep-wake cycle.

Although the 24-hour rhythm of melatonin secretion is generally the same in SAD patients and controls during winter months, researchers hypothesized that people with SAD had increased duration of melatonin secretion in the early morning hours.[15,16] This would explain why people with SAD have difficulty waking up and do not feel alert in the morning. Experiments with drugs to block melatonin secretion in the morning, thus decreasing the duration of its secretion, found the symptoms of SAD were relieved.[17]

## The Phase-Shift Theory

According to the phase-shift theory, developed in the late 1980s, people with SAD suffered from circadian rhythms that had fallen out of sync with the normal circadian cycle, which is not quite 24 hours long. Some people may be "phase-advanced" (ie, their bodies release melatonin too early in the evening) while others may be "phase-delayed" (ie, they continue to release melatonin for too long into the day). According to the phase-shift theory, this abnormality occurs because the seasonal changes in light exposure somehow disrupt normal functioning of the circadian clock.

## Retinal Hypersensitivity

One study found that the retinas of people with SAD are significantly less sensitive to light than those of controls, possibly because of neurotransmitter dysfunction.[18] However, other studies found that people with SAD are hypersensitive to light.[19]

## Neuroimmune Dysfunction

Significant wintertime elevations of interleukin-6, a proinflammatory cytokine, have been noted in patients with SAD.[20] Proinflammatory cytokines like interleukin-6 cause greater production of enzymes that deplete tryptophan from the blood. The result is serotonin deficiency in the brain (and the onset of depression).

Other studies have noted elevated neopterin (a marker of immune function) in response to reduced tryptophan in SAD patients.[21] These findings suggest that decreased tryptophan levels might lead to an overactive immune system.[22]

## Low Levels of Neurotransmitters

Research suggests that people with SAD, like those with most other depressive disorders, may have low or abnormal levels of important neurotransmitters, including serotonin (a precursor to melatonin), acetylcholine, and dopamine.[23-26]

Among people with SAD, serotonin levels vary from season to season, with some of the lowest levels observed during December and January.[27] This may explain why patients with SAD crave carbohydrates during the winter season: serotonin is involved in regulating feeding and satiety.[28] Studies have also shown the rate of production of serotonin in the brain is dependent on the length of exposure to bright sunlight and turnover of serotonin in the brain is much lower during the winter season.[29] Administration of m-chlorophenylpiperazine (a serotonin-like drug) produced increased activation and euphoria in depressed patients with SAD, but not in controls or in SAD patients during summer.[24] Some research suggests the change in serotonin levels may result from reduced levels of *vitamin D3*, which are often observed in cases of SAD. Administration of 400 or 800 IU of vitamin D3 to people with SAD during late winter appeared to improve mood.[30]

Untreated patients with SAD also have lower concentrations of norepinephrine compared to their normal counterparts.[24] Research suggests that reduced norepinephrine activity is linked to hypersomnia (ie, increased need for sleep), which is common among people with SAD.[31] Finally, low dopamine activity has been observed in SAD patients.[25,26]

# CONVENTIONAL TREATMENT OF SAD

First-line treatment for SAD is light therapy. During light therapy, patients are exposed to bright light early in the morning in an attempt to reduce the secretion of melatonin and stimulate a more natural waking cycle. Studies of patients with SAD indicate that bright light therapy in the morning produces greater therapeutic effect than evening light.[32,33]

Although bright light therapy is an effective method for treating SAD, some people do not respond due to side effects or lack of adherence to its use.[34] Lack of adherence may result from inconveniences associated with bright light therapy. First, bright light therapy is most effective if used early in the morning, but patients with SAD may have difficulty waking up.[34-37] Second, the devices used can be expensive and may not be covered by insurance.[34] Finally, light therapy is time consuming, with most studies recommending 30–45 minutes of direct exposure to the light source.

In addition to light therapy, a number of drugs may be prescribed, including the following.

## Selective Serotonin Reuptake Inhibitors

The selective serotonin reuptake inhibitors (SSRIs) fluoxetine and sertraline are the two antidepressants most commonly studied in the treatment of SAD.[38,39] SSRIs inhibit serotonin reuptake within synapses,[40] thus making more serotonin available to interact with serotonin receptors. Studies have also been conducted to determine the effects of SSRIs on melatonin levels in patients with SAD. Results have shown that fluoxetine significantly reduces melatonin levels in these patients, while other antidepressant agents (eg, tricyclics) elevate melatonin levels.[41] Because of the natural fluctuation in melatonin levels throughout the day, timing of SSRI administration may be an important consideration to ensure levels of melatonin are reduced at the appropriate time (ie, in the morning).

## Selective Noradrenaline Reuptake Inhibitor

Reboxetine is a novel selective noradrenaline reuptake inhibitor available in European countries; its application for approval in the United States has been denied by the Food and Drug Administration (FDA). It has been shown to be effective in treating depression.[42] A dose of 8 mg reboxetine daily has been shown to relieve both depressive and atypical symptoms associated with SAD within 2 weeks. Side effects included dry mouth and constipation, but they were generally transient and mild in intensity.[43]

## Modafinil

Modafinil, a drug known to promote wakefulness, has been studied in the treatment of SAD.[44] Modafinil is thought to selectively promote wakefulness by influencing the sleep-wake centers of the brain.[45] Studies using modafinil in the treatment of narcolepsy and major depressive disorder have indicated that modafinil can improve wakefulness and reduce fatigue.[46,47] In a study of treatment with 100 mg modafinil during week 1, followed by 100 mg or 200 mg for weeks 2–8, modafinil significantly improved SAD symptoms, reduced fatigue, and was well tolerated.[44]

# TARGETED NUTRITIONAL INTERVENTIONS FOR SAD

## Melatonin

Melatonin, a hormone produced in the pineal gland, is responsible for regulating sleep and core body temperature at night.[48] The role of melatonin in SAD is complicated and the subject of some controversy. Under normal circumstances, melatonin levels increase in the evening, prior to bedtime, peak in the middle of the night, and decrease gradually as morning approaches.[49] Among people with SAD, excessive duration of melatonin secretion has been implicated, but researchers are far from settled on this theory as the main cause of SAD. Nevertheless, low-dose melatonin taken at night has been shown to be effective in improving mood in patients with SAD.[50,51]

## Additional Support for SAD

Nutrient therapy for SAD operates along principles similar to those of pharmacologic therapy: increased serotonin levels may relieve symptoms. To understand how these nutrients work, it is necessary to understand how serotonin is synthesized. In the body, tryptophan is converted to 5-hydroxytryptophan (5-HTP) by the enzyme tryptophan hydroxylase; this conversion can be inhibited by a deficiency in vitamin B6 or insufficient magnesium.[52] In turn, 5-HTP is converted to serotonin, which is subsequently converted to melatonin, with S-adenosyl-L-methionine (SAMe) serving as the methylating agent.[49,53] Thus, any nutrients that support healthy levels of tryptophan or promote healthy methylation would theoretically help improve levels of serotonin and relieve the symptoms of SAD.

**Tryptophan.** Light therapy is usually considered the first-line treatment for SAD, but about 40% of patients treated with light therapy do not respond.[54] This may be due in part to a deficiency of tryptophan, which is necessary for the synthesis of serotonin and sometimes recommended as a natural antidepressant. Some data suggest that light stimulates the conversion of tryptophan to serotonin.[55] Some studies indicate that tryptophan may be used to enhance light therapy,[56] while others show that tryptophan can produce

benefits equal to those of light therapy in patients with SAD and may lengthen the time to relapse.[54] One study in patients with SAD who had been treated with light therapy noted rapid depletion of tryptophan resulted in a reversal of the therapeutic effects of bright light treatment.[55]

Tryptophan depletion in an experimental setting in patients with SAD has also been associated with an increase in plasma neopterin.[21] Neopterin is a marker of immune function; high levels are associated with increased immune system activity. This suggests low levels of tryptophan may cause elevated neopterin levels, which, in conjunction with reduced serotonin, may worsen depression associated with SAD.[21] These findings have important implications in patients with autoimmune disorders (eg, rheumatoid arthritis, multiple sclerosis, and Alzheimer's disease), in which levels of immune system cytokines (such as interleukin-6) may already be elevated.[57–59]

Tryptophan was a popular dietary supplement until 1989, when an epidemic outbreak of eosinophilia-myalgia syndrome (EMS) was associated with the use of tryptophan in the United States. About 95% of cases were traced to a single overseas supplier, although many people who took tryptophan from this supplier did not develop EMS. In 1989, the FDA issued a nationwide recall for all products containing tryptophan, and subsequently banned importation of tryptophan from overseas sources.[60]

**5-hydroxytryptophan.** 5-hydroxytryptophan (5-HTP) is the immediate precursor in the biosynthesis of serotonin from tryptophan. Oral 5-HTP crosses the blood-brain barrier easily and can be as effective as tryptophan in increasing levels of serotonin.[52] Administration of 200–600 mg 5-HTP has been shown to be effective in treating insomnia and improving quality of sleep.[61–63] 5-HTP has been found safe in treating SAD when used alone but has been shown to increase cortisol levels.[64] It is important to note that concomitant use of 5-HTP and SSRIs or monoamine oxidase inhibitors (MAOIs) can result in serotonin syndrome, a condition characterized by agitation, confusion, delirium, tachycardia, diaphoresis, and fluctuations in blood pressure.[65] However, no definitive cases of toxicity have emerged worldwide in the past 20 years in patients using 5-HTP alone as a dietary supplement.[60]

**Vitamin B6 and S-adenosyl-L-methionine (SAMe).** The conversion of tryptophan to 5-HTP can be inhibited by a deficiency of vitamin B6 or insufficient magnesium.[52] Also, the conversion of 5-HTP to serotonin, and serotonin's subsequent conversion into melatonin, rely on SAMe as a methylating agent.[49,53] Vitamin B6 is an important cofactor involved in the production of serotonin. Vitamin B6 deficiency should be considered in SAD; particularly in the elderly, who may suffer from vitamin deficiencies.[66]

**Magnesium.**   Studies indicate that a healthy circadian rhythm is associated with normally fluctuating magnesium levels, which peak in the evening, with fluctuations noted in the morning.[67,68] Insufficient magnesium levels can inhibit the conversion of tryptophan to 5-HTP, which can affect the production of serotonin and melatonin.[52] Research suggests that magnesium depletion may be associated with dysregulation of the biological clock, resulting from either an increase or decrease in melatonin, as is evident in SAD.[69]

**St. John's wort.**   St. John's wort has been shown to be effective against severe depression and depressive symptoms of SAD.[70,71] In one study, 900 mg of hypericum, an extract of St. John's wort, was found to be as effective as light therapy in SAD.[71] Another study found that 900 mg of hypericum in combination with bright light (3000 lux) or dim light (<300 lux) therapy reduced depressive symptoms in patients with SAD.[72] Its exact mechanism of action has not been clearly established; however, researchers propose that St. John's wort affects the uptake and reuptake of MAOIs like serotonin and norepinephrine.[73]

**Omega-3 fatty acids.**   Omega-3 fatty acids have a role in the synthesis of serotonin, and there is encouraging data about their use in depressive disorders. Also, because the incidence of SAD is associated with higher latitudes, it seems logical that people who live in the Arctic would suffer from very high rates of a winter depressive disorder. Researchers, however, have found that SAD is very rare among Icelandic peoples, who eat a lot of omega-3 fatty acids in cold water fish. When fish consumption goes down, the incidence of SAD begins to increase.[74–76]

As mentioned previously, proinflammatory cytokines cause greater production of enzymes that deplete tryptophan in the blood, which can result in serotonin deficiency in the brain. These new findings about cytokine-induced degradation of tryptophan explain why nutrients like fish oil (which suppress inflammatory cytokines) alleviate depression.

Although studies have not been conducted examining the role of omega-3 fatty acid supplementation in SAD, these essential oils have multiple health benefits, and considering the suggestive data in Arctic people who consume a lot of fish oil, it is probably prudent to add omega-3 fatty acids to a supplementation program.

## Life Extension Suggestions

- **Melatonin:** 2 mg, 15–30 minutes before bedtime
- **Tryptophan:** 500–2000 mg at night on an empty stomach or with a protein-free snack (carbohydrates may increase absorption)
- **5-HTP:** 50–200 mg at night on an empty stomach or with a protein-free snack (carbohydrates may increase absorption)
- **Vitamin B6:** 75–250 mg daily taken early in the day
- **S-adenosylmethionine** (SAMe): 200 mg daily
- **Magnesium:** 160–500 mg at bedtime
- **St. John's wort** (standardized to 0.3% hypericin): 300–900 mg daily on an empty stomach
- **Omega-3 fatty acids from fish oil:** 1400 mg EPA and 1000 mg DHA daily
- **Vitamin D:** 5000–8000 IU daily (depending on blood levels of 25-OH-vitamin D)

In addition, the following *blood tests* may provide helpful information:

- Vitamin D, 25-Hydroxy
- RBC magnesium
- Vitamin B6
- Omega Score®

## REFERENCES

References available at: www.lef.org/dpt5/ch118

# 119

# *Sinusitis*

Sinusitis is inflammation of the sinuses, which are small air-filled cavities within the bones of the face surrounding the nose.[1–4] Sinusitis symptoms include congestion, mucus discharge, and facial pain. The condition affects an estimated 16% of the U.S. adult population, resulting in millions of primary care office visits each year.[5,6]

*Sinusitis* should not be confused with *rhinitis,* which is characterized by inflammation associated with the mucosal surface of the nasal cavity.[7] However, since most cases of sinusitis also include symptoms of rhinitis, the term *rhinosinusitis* is often used.[1,8]

Sinusitis can be *acute, subacute, chronic,* or *recurrent acute*; categorization is dependent on duration and frequency of symptoms.[5,9] Acute sinusitis typically causes mild symptoms that resolve on their own, but very rarely may progress into severe or even life-threatening complications, such as a brain abscess.[10–13] Chronic sinusitis causes persistent symptoms and is often difficult to treat.[5]

Conventional pharmaceutical options to reduce inflammation in the sinuses and nasal passages include corticosteroids and decongestants, although some people receive limited, or minimal symptom relief.[14] Moreover, antibiotics are often needlessly overprescribed since most cases of acute sinusitis are caused by viruses, which do not respond to antibiotics, and chronic sinusitis can be caused by chronic inflammation or anatomic irregularities.[5,15,16] The inappropriate use of antibiotics can lead to antibiotic-resistant organisms and an unnecessary increase in antibiotic-related adverse events such as diarrhea.[6,17]

This protocol will describe the human sinuses as well as the causes, risk factors, and symptoms of sinusitis. Conventional treatment options will be examined along with an underutilized drug-free method for relieving sinusitis symptoms. Also, a variety of scientifically studied natural sinusitis therapies will be reviewed.

## The Human Sinuses

The paranasal sinuses comprise 4 pairs of interconnected, mucous membrane-lined cavities that drain into the nasal cavity and are formed within the skull

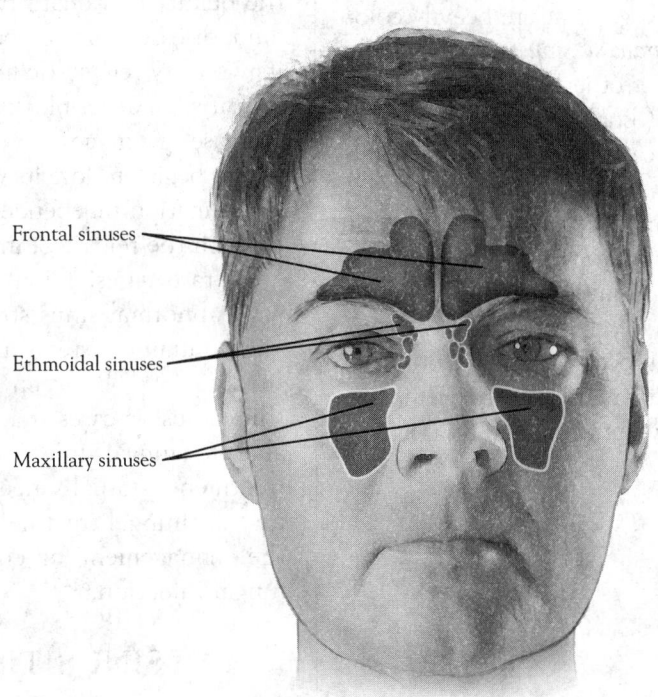

Frontal sinuses

Ethmoidal sinuses

Maxillary sinuses

Anatomy of the sinuses

| Name | Location |
|------|----------|
| Frontal sinuses | Above the eyes in the brow area |
| Maxillary sinuses | Inside each cheekbone |
| Ethmoid sinuses | Behind the bridge of the nose and between the eyes |
| Sphenoid sinuses | Deeper behind the ethmoids, above the nose, and behind the eyes |

bones that surround the nose.[2,18,19] Each of the sinus cavities are named after the particular facial bone(s) that shape(s) them, including[2]:

The sinuses circulate air and are lined with specialized cells that produce mucus and cells that possess tiny hairs called cilia.[20] The sinuses contain a thin layer of watery mucus that traps and filters out pathogens and other harmful particles from inhaled air, while the cilia rhythmically pulsate or "beat," sweeping the stagnant mucus out of the sinuses and into the nasal cavity.[2,21] In addition to catching unwanted material before it reaches the lungs, mucus and cilia also work together to warm and humidify the sinuses and nasal cavities so they remain moist and do not dry out during breathing.[2,22] The sinuses also generate high concentrations of nitric oxide, a free radical and immune mediator, which may serve to maintain sterility, strengthen immune defense against viruses and bacteria, and enhance the efficiency of cilia in clearing excess mucus.[20,23]

## CAUSES AND RISK FACTORS

In contrast to the *nasal passages* that are heavily colonized with bacteria, the *paranasal sinuses* are generally free from harmful bacteria or other pathogens.[20] However, the drainage openings (ostia) that allow the sinuses to empty into the nasal cavity are relatively small, and thus vulnerable to becoming easily blocked.[24,25] When this drainage system is blocked, the stagnant mucus begins to accumulate, allowing bacteria and other pathogens to colonize in the sinus cavity, resulting in inflammation and infection (ie, sinusitis).[1,24]

Blockage of the ostia can occur as a result of direct mechanical obstruction or injury that causes swelling in the nose.[2,20] The following represents potential causes of ostia blockage[1,5,20]:

### Swelling Factors

- Viral upper respiratory tract infection (ie, common cold)
- Allergies (eg, hay fever)
- Cystic fibrosis
- Chemical inhalation (eg, tobacco smoke)
- Immune disorders

- Facial injury
- Changes in atmospheric pressure (eg, flying, scuba diving)
- Overusing nasal decongestant sprays

### Mechanical and Anatomical Obstructions

- Deviated septum
- Nasal polyps
- Foreign body
- Congenital deformity
- Tumor
- Nasal bone spur

Although there are multiple risk factors that can contribute to ostia obstruction, allergic inflammation and viral upper respiratory infections (URIs) are the most significant.[20] Infection with a common cold virus is the most frequent cause of viral sinusitis.[26,27] Bacterial sinusitis is much less common, arising as a complication of viral sinusitis in about 0.5–2% of cases.[5,28]

Other conditions that reduce the clearance of mucus from the sinuses can also contribute to sinusitis.[20] For instance, the common cold virus appears to impair mucus clearance from the sinuses by disrupting the structure and function of the cilia.[20,21] This increases the chances of developing sinusitis, particularly in the maxillary sinuses where the direction of drainage is against gravity.[5,21]

Since the function of cilia is largely dependent on the quality and quantity of the surrounding mucosal fluid, diseases that dry out the mucosal layer or affect its viscosity (eg, cystic fibrosis) may also contribute to sinusitis.[1,20] Ostia blockage is also associated with an increase in mucosal viscosity because the trapped mucus begins to lose its water content. Likewise, sinus inflammation independently thickens sinus secretions through the release of inflammatory debris.[2,20]

In rare cases, fungi can cause sinusitis.[2] People with abnormal sinus structures or those with weakened immune systems are more vulnerable to fungal sinusitis.[2,26,29] Between 6% and 9% of all resistant rhinosinusitis cases that require surgery are attributable to fungal infection.[30] Unfortunately, surgical treatment is usually needed, since evidence suggests that antifungal treatment is of little to no benefit in the management of chronic rhinosinusitis due to fungal infection.[31-33]

## SINUSITIS SYMPTOMS

Distinguishing between sinusitis and other nasal conditions such as allergic rhinitis and the common cold can be difficult since the symptoms are often similar.[27] *Viral sinusitis* is the most common form of sinus infection, and typically produces symptoms similar to those of the common cold that last approximately 10 days.[5,6,27] However, symptoms of acute *bacterial* sinusitis typically last 10–30 days and are more severe than those of the common cold or viral sinusitis.[2,5,27]

Throbbing facial pain or pressure is a prominent feature in many cases of sinusitis. This symptom typically originates in the same location as the affected sinus (eg, in the forehead, cheeks, nose, or between the eyes). The pain associated with sinusitis is a result of increased pressure caused by trapped air and mucus, which pushes on the sinus mucous membrane and bony wall behind it. Sinus pain can also be caused by negative pressure within the sinuses, which occurs due to blocked sinus openings that do not allow air to enter, thus creating a vacuum space.[2]

Sinusitis is also often marked by a change in the characteristics of nasal secretions, which progress from clear and watery to thick and opaque (eg, white, yellowish, greenish, or blood-tinged).[2,20] The mucus becomes thick because it loses its water content while trapped in the sinus cavity. It also becomes saturated with inflammatory mediators,[2] and appears discolored as it mixes with neutrophils, a type of white blood cell.[34]

Other symptoms linked to sinusitis include[1,21,22,26]:

- Headache
- Postnasal drip
- Sore throat
- Reduced sense of smell and taste
- Halitosis (ie, bad breath)
- Ear pain/pressure
- Nasal congestion and runny nose
- Cough (may be worse at night)
- Fever
- Fatigue
- Aching teeth

When symptoms of the common cold or viral sinusitis do not improve after 10 days or worsen after 5 days, bacterial sinusitis may be suspected.[20,27]
Sinusitis can be classified as follows[9]:

- *Acute*—Symptoms last <4 weeks
- *Subacute*—Symptoms last 4–8 weeks
- *Chronic*—Symptoms last >8 weeks
- *Recurrent acute*—Symptoms occur 3 or more times per year and last <2 weeks

# DIAGNOSIS AND CONVENTIONAL TREATMENT

Sinusitis is usually diagnosed based on a physician's assessment of a patient's symptoms and medical history. In some cases, when a patient presents with a history of upper respiratory infection and symptoms lasting 7–10 days, a bacterial culture may be obtained. Some other procedures can help aid diagnosis, but are typically not required in uncomplicated cases; these include radiography, computed tomography, endoscopic visualization of ostia secretions, and sinus puncture in cases that have failed other treatments.[35]

Conventional treatment recommendations for acute sinusitis are largely dependent upon the underlying cause of infection.[26] The majority of sinusitis cases are caused by viral infection, and antibiotics are generally not needed in these cases.[6,19,26] Since the symptoms of viral sinusitis are mild-to-moderate and typically resolve on their own within 10 days or less, they can often be managed via self-care techniques and/or home remedies.[5,6,26,36]

## Self-Care Strategies

The following self-care strategies may provide relief from sinusitis symptoms:

- Get adequate rest to help the body fight infection and speed up recovery.[21,26]
- Elevate the head while sleeping by using an extra pillow to reduce congestion and keep the sinuses draining properly.[21,26]
- Stay hydrated with water, as this helps to thin out mucus secretions and promote drainage.[1,26] Sipping hot beverages may also help, since they can dilate blood vessels and promote drainage.[21,37]
- Avoid alcohol and caffeine consumption, since they can cause dehydration and contribute to nasal and sinus swelling.[21,26]
- Eat a healthy, well-balanced diet, which includes plenty of fruits and vegetables; a diet rich in antioxidants may boost immune function and help fight infection.[1]
- Try steam inhalation 3–4 times daily to open sinus passages, which can reduce pain and help clear mucus.[19] This can be done by draping a towel over the head and inhaling rising steam from a bowl of hot water.[26] Breathing in the warm, moist air of a hot shower or use of a humidifier may also be beneficial.[1,19,26]
- Apply a warm, damp towel to painful sinus areas several times per day.[1,21,26]
- Rinse out nasal passages with a saline nasal spray several times per day. This helps reduce congestion

by loosening mucus and cleaning out sinuses and nasal passages.[1,21,22,26,27] This technique may also have a moisturizing effect, which can reduce the crusting of nasal secretions.[27] Nasal irrigation with a sea salt solution appears to be as effective as saline nasal wash and topical nasal steroids for the management of chronic rhinosinusitis.[38,39]

## Medications

Treatment with one or more of the following medications may also help.

**Decongestants.** Also known as α-adrenergic agonists, decongestants cause blood vessel constriction, thereby reducing airway resistance by increasing the size of the airway lumen.[20,27,40] Oral decongestants such as pseudoephedrine (eg, Sudafed®) are less potent than topical nasal decongestant sprays such as oxymetazoline (eg, Afrin®) and phenylephrine (eg, Neo-Synephrine®).[27] Unlike topical nasal decongestants, oral decongestants are associated with systemic side effects, including increased blood pressure, restlessness, insomnia, and urinary retention.[20,27] Although topical nasal decongestants are preferred for these reasons, their use should be limited to no more than 3–5 consecutive days. This is because they quickly induce tolerance, which means that higher and higher doses will be needed to achieve the same effect.[27] Furthermore, if a nasal decongestant spray is overused and then abruptly stopped, an extreme increase in nasal congestion (ie, rebound congestion) may be experienced.[26,27] Similarly, continued overuse of nasal decongestant sprays can cause a phenomenon known as rhinitis medicamentosa, in which congestion worsens despite continued or even increased medication use.[41]

**Mild analgesics.** Over-the-counter pain relievers such as aspirin, acetaminophen (Tylenol®), or ibuprofen (Advil® or Motrin®) may be helpful for temporarily relieving sinus pain and headache.[21,26] Refer to the Acetaminophen and NSAID Toxicity protocol especially when using acetaminophen over an extended period.

**Intranasal corticosteroids.** Although nasal steroids may decrease the inflammatory response associated with sinusitis, clinical trials have shown conflicting results.[20] The Food and Drug Administration (FDA) has not approved their use for the treatment of acute sinusitis.[5] However, nasal steroids may still be of benefit, since they are able to decrease swelling of the sinus passages associated with allergies and allow the sinuses to drain.[2] As a result, nasal steroids may be of benefit to individuals whose nasal allergies (eg, hay fever) predispose them to developing sinusitis.[20]

**Antibiotics.** Although bacterial sinusitis is less common and more severe than viral sinusitis, it may resolve without the need for antibiotics.[26] As a result, sinusitis treatment guidelines do not recommend taking antibiotics within the first week of illness, unless the symptoms are particularly severe (eg, high fever or extreme pain). The cautious use of antibiotics for the treatment of sinusitis is warranted because they are not usually helpful, and are also associated with negative side effects, antibiotic resistance, and increased medical costs.[6] If deemed necessary, antibiotics that may be prescribed include amoxicillin, doxycycline, and trimethoprim-sulfamethoxazole.[26] A typical course of antibiotic treatment for severe bacterial sinusitis will last 10–14 days, and should not be discontinued early just because symptoms have resolved.[27]

## Surgical Intervention

Surgical intervention is usually a last resort, and thus reserved for cases of chronic sinusitis that have not responded to drug therapy.[2,20] For example, allergic fungal sinusitis represents up to 9% of all sinusitis cases requiring surgery.[30] The goal of surgery is to improve drainage by removing or reducing sinus obstruction.[2] Most surgical procedures for sinusitis are aided by endoscopic visualization.[20] Surgery can be performed to enlarge sinus openings, remove nasal polyps, and correct anatomical abnormalities (eg, deviated septum).[1,2,20] For most patients, surgery results in lasting symptom improvement and an increased quality of life[2,20]; however, symptoms may reoccur.[2]

---

### DRUG-FREE SINUSITIS RELIEF WITH THERAPEUTIC ULTRASOUND

Chronic sinusitis is notoriously difficult to treat and causes significant suffering for those it afflicts. Antibiotics and/or corticosteroid therapies may fail to provide relief in some cases, leaving surgery as a last resort.[5]

*Therapeutic ultrasound*, in which low-frequency ultrasound waves are applied to the sinuses, appears to be an effective drug-free treatment for chronic, as well as acute sinusitis, with little potential for side effects.[42]

In a 2010 study on 22 subjects with a history of chronic rhinosinusitis that had failed aggressive medical management, therapeutic ultrasound 3 days per week for 6 sessions led to a 34% improvement on a standardized assessment of sinusitis symptoms.[43] A 2012 study on 30 chronic rhinosinusitis patients who received therapeutic ultrasound 3 days per week for 10 sessions revealed a reduction of sinusitis symptoms of up to 65%.[44] A 2010 case report showed that this same treatment regimen resolved sinusitis symptoms in a patient who had been suffering from chronic sinusitis for a year. After the treatment, the patient only experienced mild nasal obstruction.[45] In a larger 2010 trial involving 42 subjects with acute sinusitis, therapeutic ultrasound administered for 4 consecutive days provided as much relief from symptoms as the antibiotic amoxicillin.[46]

Therapeutic ultrasound has been shown to disrupt *biofilms*.[47] A biofilm is a layer of mucus-like film secreted by some pathogens that helps infectious organisms colonize a surface. Organisms embedded in a biofilm are very difficult to eradicate. In the sinus cavities, biofilms appear to contribute to persistent infection and are associated with sinusitis.[48,49] Therapeutic ultrasound appears to disrupt biofilm, which may contribute to its efficacy in relieving sinusitis symptoms.[42,43,47]

# TARGETED NATURAL INTERVENTIONS

In addition to the natural therapies listed below, which have been studied in the context of sinusitis, those with acute sinusitis should refer to the Common Cold protocol, since a majority of sinusitis cases arise from complications of the common cold.[1,36,50]

## Lactoferrin

Lactoferrin and its active metabolite, lactoferricin, are multifunctional proteins known to possess antibacterial, antifungal, and antiviral activities, as well as immune regulatory and anti-inflammatory actions.[51] Lactoferrin is a component of whey protein that can also be found in high concentrations within mucosal secretions, such as airway mucus, tears, and breast milk.[52,53] Lactoferrin is produced and stored within the cells of the nasal mucosa and is presumed important as a first line of defense against invading pathogens.[53]

Research suggests that lactoferrin may be beneficial for alleviating the symptoms and complications of the common cold for at least two reasons. First, it can kill bacteria through the binding of iron molecules that would otherwise be needed for essential bacterial functions.[52,53] Second, lactoferrin exerts an antioxidant effect by preventing the formation of free radicals, thus decreasing nasal tissue oxidative damage.[53]

Studies suggest that decreased levels of lactoferrin may play a role in the development of chronic sinusitis, especially when nasal polyps, asthma, and/or allergies are involved.[51,54] Lactoferrin production is reduced in people with sinus conditions compared to healthy subjects. Moreover, lactoferrin levels are particularly low in sinusitis patients with nasal polyps. The low levels of lactoferrin associated with sinusitis are due to both its decreased expression/down-regulation as well as its increased utilization to fight infection.[53]

## Vitamin C

Since the human body cannot synthesize vitamin C, it must be acquired from the diet.[55] Research shows a sufficient daily intake of ascorbic acid is required for the immune system to defend the body against infections (especially viral infections).[56]

Evidence suggests that supplementation with 1000 mg daily of vitamin C can decrease the risk of catching a cold.[57] When given in doses greater than 200 mg daily, vitamin C has been shown to reduce the duration of cold symptoms by 1–4 days.[58] Vitamin C markedly improves immune function by enhancing natural killer cell activity, interferons (signaling proteins that boost immune response), macrophages, T-lymphocyte production, cell movement (ie, chemotaxis), and cell-mediated immunity.[58,59]

Individuals with sinusitis typically exhibit decreased serum levels of vitamin C.[60,61] Topical vitamin C may be associated with enhanced mucociliary clearance of the paranasal sinuses through the loosening of thick mucus secretions and an increase in ciliary beat frequency.[60,62] Oral vitamin C supplementation also reliably decreases plasma levels of histamine, a known contributor to inflammation and nasal congestion, especially among people with allergy-induced sinusitis.[63,64]

## Zinc

Zinc is an essential trace element required for a variety of metabolic processes,[65] including the maintenance of a healthy immune function.[52] Unfortunately, zinc deficiency is prevalent throughout developed Western countries.[66] Zinc deficiency, which is common among the elderly and the young, is linked to the impairment of many components of immune response, including T- and B-lymphocyte function, natural killer cell activity, macrophage phagocytosis, and antibody formation.[66-68] As a result, zinc deficiency is associated with an increased risk of infection.[66,67] In one study, children with chronic rhinosinusitis exhibited lower levels of antioxidants, including zinc, than healthy control subjects.[61] Correcting zinc deficiency through supplementation is efficacious for a variety of viral infections.[67,68] This may be partly attributable to zinc's positive effect on the expression of interleukin-2 and interferon-γ, as well as on natural killer and cytotoxic T cells, which help the immune system kill viruses.[69]

Zinc supplementation has long been considered an effective therapy for reducing the duration of the common cold.[52,68] A 2011 study concluded that zinc supplementation significantly reduced both duration and severity of the common cold when administered within 24 hours of the onset of symptoms. This study also revealed that zinc supplementation over 5 months was helpful for preventing infection by common cold viruses.[70] Likewise, a clinical study involving zinc nasal gel (given within 1–2 days of illness onset) found that zinc was able to reduce the severity and duration of common cold symptoms among healthy adults.[71] In a 2012 study, researchers found that the combination of zinc plus vitamin C was more efficacious than placebo at reducing runny nose, and it also appeared to accelerate recovery in common cold patients.[66]

## N-Acetyl Cysteine

N-acetyl cysteine (NAC) may reduce the viscosity and improve the clearance of mucus. NAC has antioxidant properties, which can help protect against free radical damage. It may also help restore healthy sinus conditions that have deteriorated due to sinusitis.[72]

A 2010 study found that NAC is capable of fighting infections, such as those that cause sinusitis, through its ability to break down biofilms. Biofilms are essentially a community of bacteria that adhere to surfaces, including moist mucus membranes. These biofilms are known to produce resistant communities of bacteria and are estimated to be involved in at least 60% of all chronic and/or recurrent infections. NAC has been shown to reduce the adhesion of biofilms to mucus membranes (eg, antibiotics or nasal steroids).[73]

## Vitamin E

Numerous studies have demonstrated that vitamin E may have a positive effect on the human immune system. For instance, elderly patients who took 200 IU of vitamin E daily for 1 year were 20% less likely to catch a cold.[74] In one study, children with chronic rhinosinusitis were found to have lower serum levels of several antioxidants, including vitamin E, than healthy children.[61] A 2011 study found that topical vitamin E (in combination with other antioxidant oils) was able to persistently reverse oxidative stress and nasal inflammation, similar to that by viral infections, chronic sinusitis, and allergic disease.[75] Furthermore, animal studies show that vitamin E may affect the risk and severity of viral respiratory infections.[76]

## Rosmarinic Acid

Rosmarinic acid is an antioxidant compound found in rosemary.[77] In experimental animal models, rosmarinic acid has been shown to reduce allergic inflammatory reactions by decreasing histamine release and inhibiting the expression of interleukin (IL)-1β, IL-6, and tumor necrosis factor-alpha (TNF-α).[78] This mechanism of action may be significant for individuals suffering from chronic sinusitis caused by allergies.

## Bromelain

Bromelain, which is a proteolytic enzyme complex found in pineapple, is frequently used to treat sinusitis because it reduces inflammation and loosens mucus. Specifically, bromelain may inhibit pro-inflammatory prostaglandin biosynthesis and prostaglandin E1 accumulation. This in turn inhibits the release of leukocyte enzymes. Among sinusitis patients, bromelain has been shown to hasten symptom recovery and resolve inflammation better than standard treatment or placebo. Typical oral doses of bromelain are 500–2000 mg daily.[63]

## Eucalyptus

Cineole is the main ingredient of eucalyptus oil. It has anti-inflammatory and antimicrobial properties, and it also affects ciliary beat frequency.[79] Studies have confirmed that cineole can thin, drain, and reduce mucus secretions. In a clinical study involving 152 patients with acute rhinosinusitis, cineole was associated with significant symptom improvement at 4 and 7 days when compared to placebo. The authors concluded that cineole is safe and effective for the treatment of acute rhinosinusitis, and suggested that it be utilized prior to the initiation of antibiotics.[80] In 2008, a similar study was conducted among 150 patients with acute and viral rhinosinusitis. These authors also found that treatment with cineole resulted in reduced symptoms at 4 and 7 days, and concluded that this treatment effect was clinically relevant.[79]

## Herbal Combination Formula

A combination of gentian root, primula flower, elder flower, sorrel herb, and verbena herb is frequently used in the treatment of acute and chronic rhinosinusitis.[81,82] Results from a 2011 laboratory study demonstrated that this formula shows a broad spectrum of antiviral activity against viruses commonly known to cause respiratory infections.[81] A more concentrated version of the formula (ie, dry extract) reduced exudate volume and leukocyte numbers in an animal study. It also reduced the expression of cyclooxygenase-2 protein and lowered prostaglandin E2 levels. Therefore, the rationality for using the combination formula to manage sinusitis is partly based on its significant anti-inflammatory effects.[82] Since inflammation of the mucosa can often lead to a loss of smell, researchers theorize that this combination of herbs may be useful for this indication as well.[83]

## Xylitol Nasal Irrigation

Xylitol is a sugar alcohol that appears to enhance the body's natural defense against bacterial pathogens. An animal model showed that administering xylitol solution simultaneously with a bacterial pathogen reduced the amount of bacteria detectable upon a later examination of the sinuses.[84] In one trial, 20 subjects with chronic rhinosinusitis were randomized and instructed to rinse their sinuses daily with either a xylitol or saline solution. Fifteen subjects completed the study. Nasal irrigation with the xylitol solution was associated with a significant improvement on a standardized assessment of sinusitis symptoms.[85] Another trial designed to assess the effects of xylitol nasal irrigation compared to placebo in the treatment of chronic sinusitis is recruiting participants as of November 2012.[86]

## Black Cumin Seed Oil

*Nigella sativa*, also known as black cumin, is a flowering plant that grows in Eastern Europe, the Middle East, and Western Asia. The small black seeds of nigella sativa have a rich history of medical use in the Middle East and Asian countries. Modern scientific inquiry has examined the potential benefit of black cumin seeds and the oil derived from them in a variety of contexts ranging from cardiovascular disease to cancer.[87–90] Several lines of evidence suggest that black cumin seed oil and some of its active constituents are powerful anti-inflammatory agents and also combat oxidative stress.[91–93] In an animal model of rhinosinusitis, an active constituent derived from black cumin seed was found to be as effective as antibiotic therapy in reducing manifestations of sinusitis such as vascular congestion, inflammation, and epithelial injury in sinus tissue.[94]

## Life Extension Suggestions

- **Lactoferrin** (providing 95% of apolactoferrin [285 mg]): 300 mg daily
- **Vitamin C:** 1000–5000 mg or more daily
- **Zinc:** 30 mg daily
- **N-acetyl cysteine (NAC):** 600–1800 mg daily
- **Vitamin E:** 400 IU daily with at least 200 mg gamma tocopherol
- **Rosmarinic acid:** 100–200 mg daily
- **Bromelain:** 500–2000 mg daily
- **Black cumin seed oil:** 1000 mg daily
- **Herbal combination formula (gentian root, primula flower, elder flower, sorrel herb, and verbena herb):** per label instructions
- **Nasal wash containing xylitol:** per label instructions

## REFERENCES

References available at: www.lef.org/dpt5/ch119

# 120

# Sjögren's Syndrome

Approximately 4 million Americans suffer from Sjögren's syndrome, which was first identified in 1933 by the Swedish ophthalmologist Henrik Sjögren. About 90% of victims are women with a mean age of 50 years, although Sjögren's can strike any age group, including children.[1]

The main symptoms of Sjögren's are chronic dryness of the eyes and mouth; however, it is also associated with dryness in external genitalia as well as the ear, nose, and throat area. There may also be decreased secretions in the gastrointestinal tract.

Sjögren's is an autoimmune disorder. Symptoms associated with Sjögren's are caused by the infiltration of immune-system cells (usually B and T lymphocytes) into glands responsible for secreting fluid. The disease can occur alone (primary Sjögren's) or in conjunction with other autoimmune diseases (secondary Sjögren's). Sjögren's has been associated with rheumatoid arthritis, systemic lupus erythematosus, scleroderma, and other connective tissue diseases.[1] It has also been associated with autoimmune disorders in the thymus gland; studies have shown that patients with Sjögren's may also suffer from thyroid disorders.[2]

Traditional treatment relies on cholinergics (ie, drugs that stimulate the parasympathetic nervous system); however, they can have significant side effects. Nutritional therapy focuses on essential fatty acids, which have been shown to modulate the immune system. Lifestyle changes are also a valuable therapeutic tool.

Although the disease rarely shortens a patient's life span, Sjögren's can have devastating effects. Ocular (eye) dryness can lead to chronic keratoconjunctivitis and corneal ulcers; oral dryness can result in severe and chronic dental decay, fissures, infections, as well as difficulty speaking and swallowing. The disease is often accompanied by depression, fatigue, and fever. Elevated liver enzymes occur in 25% of patients, liver enlargement in 33%, Raynaud's syndrome in 20%, fibromyalgia in 55%, and lymphoma in less than 5%.[3]

Oral symptoms of Sjögren's syndrome include reduced saliva; a dry, sticky mouth; and difficulty chewing and swallowing. Decreased saliva makes the oral cavity more acidic; the lowered pH, along with the reduction in the number of antibacterial enzymes normally present in human saliva, makes tooth decay a significant problem. Dental caries is considered a potential marker for the disease.[4] Dry mouth can also affect speech, taste, and tolerance to dental prostheses.

Chronic dryness of the eye causes inflammatory reactions,[5] leaving a feeling of grittiness in the eye and intolerance to light. The roughened surface of the eye caused by the dryness causes light to scatter, resulting in blurred vision. Dry eye also renders eyes more sensitive to irritants and susceptible to infections, which can result in corneal ulcerations if left untreated. Eyelid dermatitis may be another manifestation of primary Sjögren's syndrome.

Other symptoms associated with Sjögren's include the following:

- Nasal dryness, nosebleeds, congestion, impaired taste and smell, as well as more serious conditions (eg, bronchitis and pneumonia) caused by damage to mucous glands in the nose

- Dryness in eustachian tubes, which can lead to a clogged feeling in the ear and impaired hearing

- Itchy, dry skin

- Vaginal dryness

- Nutritional malabsorption, caused by affected mucous lining of the stomach

- Pancreatitis

Individuals with Sjögren's may develop neurologic problems, such as impaired memory and reduced concentration.[6] A French study linked the onset of facial palsy involving cranial nerves to Sjögren's.[7]

Because it progresses slowly, Sjögren's syndrome is frequently misdiagnosed and left untreated.[8] Symptoms of primary Sjögren's syndrome—dryness, fatigue, pain, head and neck complaints, hoarseness, or hearing loss—can also occur as a result of medication use, anxiety and depression, or normal aging.[9,10] In a Chinese study, the average time between onset of symptoms and establishment of diagnosis was 7.8 years, indicating that most cases were either improperly diagnosed or neglected.[11]

Sjögren's is diagnosed on the basis of the presence of symptoms and specific autoantibodies. During diagnosis, the physician will ask questions to determine if a patient is suffering from dry eyes or mouth and will test the functioning of salivary and ocular glands. In addition, tests could be conducted to detect antibodies to Ro/SS-A or La/SS-B antigens. Researchers have also discovered increased levels of the antibody interleukin-18, an immunoregulatory and proinflammatory cytokine in patients with Sjögren's.[12] This cytokine interferes with acetylcholine, the messenger chemical that triggers saliva production.

# SJÖGREN'S: AN AUTOIMMUNE DISEASE

Like other autoimmune diseases, Sjögren's syndrome results from the immune system mistakenly attacking healthy tissue. The autoimmune response is not fully understood and may have multiple causes, including mimicry molecules, immature T cells, and leaky gut syndrome. Mimicry molecules excite the immune system to attack molecules they resemble. Immature T cells are those that have not been "trained" long enough in the thymus and cannot properly differentiate between harmful antigens and healthy tissues. Finally, leaky gut syndrome, characterized by an overly permeable intestinal wall, can arouse an allergic response by releasing large molecules into the bloodstream. In general, allergic reactions were found to be more common in people with Sjögren's syndrome.[13]

When healthy tissues such as excretion glands are attacked because of an autoimmune response, they become clogged with circulating immune complexes.[14] These large molecules are formed by the combination of an antibody and an antigen. When lodged in the salivary and lachrymal glands (produce tears), they block these glands from supplying their watery and mucosal secretions.

Some researchers think that the underlying cause of autoimmune disorders (like Sjögren's) may be a flawed T cell response. T cells are lymphocytes that are "trained" in the thymus gland for their role in the immune system. However, if T cells are not "schooled" long enough in the thymus before being released, they tend to behave erratically, attacking healthy tissue.

Patients with Sjögren's show significant defects in T cell immunity.[15] Japanese researchers found that estrogen deficiency contributes to this dysfunctional T-cell response.[16]

Depression, which is associated with Sjögren's,[17] can trigger the production of cytokines that interfere with salivary and lachrymal gland production.

# PHARMACEUTICAL TREATMENT OF SJÖGREN'S

Few pharmaceutical treatments have shown efficacy for Sjögren's syndrome. The most common regimen includes drugs known as cholinergics as well as interferon-alpha.[18]

## Cholinergics

Cholinergics activate the parasympathetic system by mimicking acetylcholine, a neurotransmitter that stimulates the lachrymal and salivary glands. The two cholinergics prescribed most frequently follow.

**Pilocarpine.** Pilocarpine has been shown to reduce symptoms of xerostomia (dry eye). It can cause gastrointestinal upset.[19]

**Cevimeline.** Cevimeline (30 mg) taken 3 times daily seems to be well tolerated and provide substantive relief of dry eye. Twice that dose was associated with an increase in the occurrence of adverse events, particularly gastrointestinal tract disorders. Cevimeline taken over prolonged periods or in too high doses can cause drowsiness, excessive sweating, interference with night vision, as well as more serious side effects.[20]

## Interferon

Interferon has also been used in the treatment of Sjögren's. Among patients with primary Sjögren's syndrome, interferon has been shown to improve salivary output and decrease complaints of xerostomia without causing significant adverse medical events.[21]

# SJÖGREN'S AND HORMONE DEFICIENCIES

## Dehydroepiandrosterone

Restoring dehydroepiandrosterone (DHEA) levels modulates immune and inflammatory responses. Women with primary Sjögren's show decreased serum concentration of DHEA and an increased cortisol/DHEA ratio.[22] Because most people over age 35 years are deficient in DHEA, Life Extension believes that patients with Sjögren's should have their DHEA levels tested and if necessary, supplement with this vital hormone. Retesting is recommended 3–6 weeks after therapy is initiated to ascertain whether optimal DHEA levels have been obtained.

## Estrogen

Sjögren's syndrome has also been linked to estrogen deficiencies in menopausal women.[23] While no human studies have been conducted on the value of estrogen restoration therapy among Sjögren's patients, Life Extension believes that women >35 years should have a complete hormone profile performed and correct any hormonal deficiencies. Women with hormone-dependent cancers, however, are generally advised against hormone restoration with estrogen. Hormone restoration might be especially important among Sjögren's patients who suffer from a disease associated with hormonal deficiencies, even if the mechanism is incompletely understood.

# LIFESTYLE MANAGEMENT STRATEGIES

## Exercise

Exercise has also been shown to be anti-inflammatory, stimulating the production of anti-inflammatory cytokines and inhibiting proinflammatory cytokines.[24] Psychological stress disrupts the network of signals linking the nervous, endocrine, and immune systems. In addition, stress reduction can significantly affect cellular immune response.[25] A variety of exercise methods will supply symptomatic relief.

## Avoid Dry Eye

- Tear substitutes are efficient in mild to moderate cases of dry eye, although some may increase patients' complaints due to the preservatives they contain. Preservatives can be avoided by using monodose disposable packaging or brands that are preservative-free.[26] Research suggests that topical cyclosporine is a promising possibility in treating dry eye.[27]

- Studies have demonstrated that calcium carbonate in a petroleum base relieved dry eye when applied to the lower eyelid.[28]

- For mild to moderate dry eye, slow-melting lubricating pellets, available by prescription and inserted into the lower pocket of the eyelid twice daily, will bring relief. Lubricating ointments are best used at night as they tend to blur vision during the day.

- Moisture-chamber eyeglasses will help preserve tear volume by minimizing airflow over the surface of the eye.

- Closing tear ducts by using collagen or silicone plugs can increase tear volume by reducing drainage. Collagen plugs are absorbed; silicone plugs are easily removed. Lower tear ducts (punta) are sealed first; a determination is then made about sealing the upper punta. If permanent closure seems warranted, electrocautery or an argon laser can permanently close the punta.[3]

- Avoiding dust, fumes, and excessive makeup (especially around the margin of the eyelid) may also help.

## Protect Your Teeth Against Dental Caries

- Brush frequently, both before and after meals, using an electric toothbrush. Floss and irrigate the teeth

(using a Waterpik® or other tool) frequently. Among Sjögren's patients, oral hygiene is crucial in combating tooth decay. See a dentist regularly to monitor tooth decay and loss of enamel.

- Use a pH-balanced mouthwash to lower acidity. Try 1/4 teaspoon of baking soda dissolved in 1/4 cup of warm water. Alcohol-free *goldenseal* (*H. canadensis*) can be used as an antibacterial mouthwash. Goldenseal can help compensate for lower levels of antibacterial enzymes in the saliva. Dissolve 30 drops in 2 oz of water and swish the solution in the mouth.

- Avoid sugary foods. Bacteria produce acid for 20 minutes whenever sugar is ingested. Avoid acidic foods, including citrus fruits.

- Drink nonacidic bottled water.[29]

- Use a straw to protect the mouth when drinking soft drinks and other acidic beverages.

- Avoid abrasive toothpastes that can harm already compromised tooth enamel. Certain toothpastes (eg, Biotene®) have been specially formulated for individuals with dry mouth.

## Fight Oral Dryness

- Drink plenty of water to replace lost moisture in the oral cavity. Remember to avoid acidic beverages like tomato and orange juice.

- Sugarless candy or sugar-free chewing gum kept in the mouth can stimulate saliva flow. Xylitol, a sugar substitute used in candy and gum, is thought by some to inhibit dental caries. Never sleep with anything in the mouth. Many health food stores carry rice- or barley-sweetened candies.

- Avoid caffeine, which is a diuretic.

- Oral interferon-alpha in lozenge form, available by prescription, will significantly increase saliva flow.[30]

## Protect Your Nose and Throat

- Use a humidifier to keep the air moist.

- Breathe through the nose rather than the mouth; a soft cervical collar will inhibit open-mouth breathing at night by supporting the jaw. Keep your bedroom cool.[3]

- A mixture of saline and aloe, which can relieve dry nasal membranes and nosebleeds, is gentle enough for repeated use.

## Avoid Skin and Vaginal Dryness

- Avoid antibacterial and abrasive soaps; use soaps with added oils or moisturizers and moisturize the skin after bathing.

## TARGETED NUTRITIONAL STRATEGIES

### Essential Fatty Acids: Supporting Healthy Glands

Traditional drugs offer considerable potency in dealing with Sjögren's syndrome, but side effects make them a mixed blessing. In addition, pharmacologic approaches target symptoms without addressing underlying causes or related health issues. Nutritional support may be successful, not only in mitigating the side effects of drugs, but in lowering doses as well.

Essential fatty acids (EFAs) and eicosanoids, short-lived "messenger" hormones derived from EFAs, have been implicated in the abnormal function of salivary and lachrymal glands. Measurements in Sjögren's syndrome patients have shown that EFA deficiencies are present,[31] and controlled clinical trials of supplementation with EFAs, including gamma-linolenic acid (GLA), have yielded positive results.[32]

**Omega-3 and omega-6 fatty acids.** Omega-3 and omega-6 essential fatty acids (EFAs) have been shown to alleviate symptoms of autoimmune disease by supporting the immune system and reducing inflammation.[32–35] EFAs accomplish this in several ways:

- Determining whether genes are expressed
- Producing eicosanoids and cytokines
- Activating antioxidant enzymes

Cytokines are intercellular messenger chemicals that can be pro- or anti-inflammatory. Essential fatty acids support production of anti-inflammatory cytokines.[33]

GLA is important to the production of the anti-inflammatory prostaglandin E1 (PGE1). Evening primrose oil, which is rich in GLA, may correct immunologic defects, halt atrophy of salivary and lachrymal glands, and increase PGE1. Direct supplementation with GLA has resulted in clinical improvement in Sjögren's syndrome, scleroderma, and other conditions (eg, high blood pressure and high cholesterol).[36]

### Green Tea Extract

Green tea's antioxidant and anti-inflammatory effects have led scientists to propose that it may have a role in fighting autoimmune diseases such as Sjögren's syndrome. In the laboratory, green tea catechins stimulated changes in human cells that make them less susceptible to autoimmune attack by the immune system. Additionally, green tea dramatically decreased inflammation in healthy tissues, another change indicative of decreased autoimmune activity.[37]

### Thymus Extract

There is evidence that thymus extracts can improve the functioning and numbers of T cells and stimulate conversion of immature T6 cells (thymocytes) into nondedicated T3 cells.[38,39] Thymomimetic drugs, such as levamisole and isoprinosine, stimulate the thymus and may be beneficial to T cell development.[40] Because immature T cells have been implicated in Sjögren's syndrome, Life Extension believes that thymus extract may help reduce the severity of symptoms associated with the disease.

### Digestive Support

The amino acid *L-glutamine* heals the intestinal lining and improves its mucosal structure.[41] Beneficial intestinal bacteria, such as *Lactobacillus acidophilus* and *Bifidobacterium bifidus*, and fructooligosaccharides (ie, a form of sugar that can enhance beneficial bacteria) provide gastrointestinal tract support by increasing the gut population of healthy microflora.

### Life Extension Suggestions

- **Fish oil** (with olive polyphenols): 1400 mg EPA and 1000 mg DHA daily.
- **Gamma linolenic acid (GLA):** 300–600 mg daily
- **Probiotics:** per label instructions
- **Freeze-dried gland extract** (from thymus, lymph, and spleen): 580 mg daily
- **L-glutamine:** 500–1000 mg daily
- **DHEA:** 15–25 mg daily for women, and 25–75 mg daily for men (depending on blood test results)
- **Green tea extract** (standardized to 98% polyphenols): 725–1450 mg daily
- **Goldenseal** (*H. canadensis*): per label instructions

In addition, the following *blood tests* may be helpful:

- Female Panel or Male Panel (includes DHEA-S, free and total testosterone, estradiol, progesterone [female panel only], TSH and vitamin D)

## REFERENCES

References available at: www.lef.org/dpt5/ch120

# 121

# *Skin Aging*

With a surface area of about 16–22 square feet, skin is far more than merely a protective barrier. Skin is an *organ*, and it serves to regulate excretion of metabolic waste products, regulates temperature, and includes receptors for pain, tactile sensation, and pressure. Accordingly, the health and appearance of your skin, like the health of your other organs, correlates with the *lifestyle* and *dietary habits* that you choose, as well as with critical age-related factors such as *hormonal imbalance.*

Skin is central in the social and visual experience, as it clearly reflects the consequences of aging. Skin aging is influenced by many factors including *ultraviolet radiation, excess alcohol consumption, tobacco abuse,* and *environmental pollution.*[1] In addition, few people realize that as their *body weight* increases and their *blood sugar* levels rise, biochemical reactions *disrupt* the very structural framework of their skin. Combined, these factors lead to cumulative deterioration in skin appearance and function.

Within the skin, aging is associated with a loss of fibrous tissue, slower rate of cellular renewal, and a reduced vascular and glandular network. Barrier function that maintains cellular hydration also becomes impaired. The subcutaneous tissue (hypodermis) flattens, particularly in the face, hands, and feet.

Depending on genetic makeup and lifestyle, normal physiologic functions within the skin may decline by 50% by middle age.[2,3]

Unless you take action to support the skin's *intrinsic* defense systems, the youthful qualities of your skin will rapidly deteriorate. Fortunately, by harnessing insights garnered through the latest scientific innovations, you can dramatically *slow,* and potentially *reverse,* the signs and symptoms of accelerated skin aging.

Throughout this Life Extension protocol, you will learn about internal *and* external strategies to combat accelerated skin aging, including *topical interventions* containing scientifically advanced ingredients that help support youthful skin structure and function, and targeted *nutritional supplements* that fortify your skin form the inside out.

## SKIN ANATOMY AND FUNCTION

In its entirety, the skin is comprised of three distinctive layers: *epidermis, dermis,* and *hypodermis.* Each layer exhibits unique cellular makeup and physiologic function.

The *epidermis* (outermost layer) is comprised of *keratin,* which strengthens the skin, and *melanin,* found in the basal layer of the epidermis, responsible for depth of skin color. Important cellular components in immune recognition of pathogens, called Langerhans cells, also reside in the epidermis. The epidermis provides protection against the environment; the *stratum corneum* is the primary barrier.

The *dermis* is directly below the epidermis and provides a kind of scaffold for strength and support. Unlike the epidermis, the dermis contains nerves, blood vessels, and fibroblasts that provide sensory receptors, deliver nutrients, and maintain the structural foundation of the skin. The most abundant connective material within the dermis is *collagen,* a fibrous protein whose primary function is to maintain skin firmness. *Elastin* protein fibers combine with collagen to give the skin elasticity. The base of the dermis is composed of substances such as complex sugars (*glycosaminoglycans*), *glycoproteins, hyaluronic acid,* and *chondroitin sulfate.* These substances combined form a "cementing and gelling" base that binds to water molecules, allows nutrients and oxygen into the tissue and protects the dermal structural layer. It is within the dermis that new cells are produced and eventually migrate toward the outer layers (the epidermis).

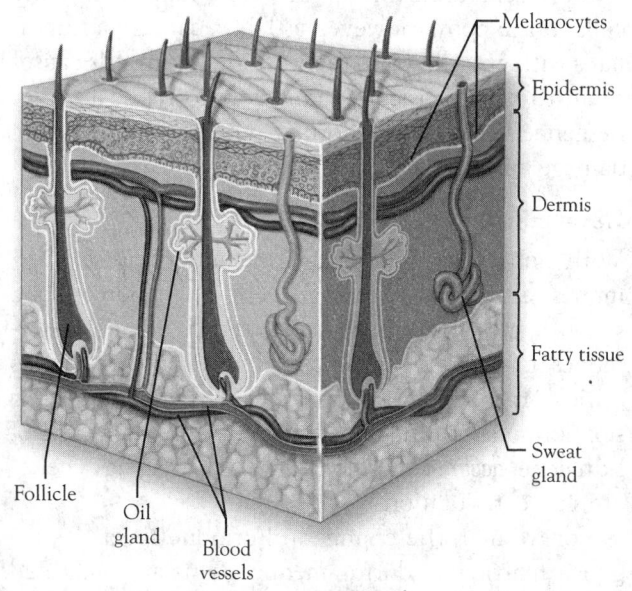

**Skin Anatomy**

The bottom layer of the skin is the *hypodermis*. It contains adipocytes (fat cells) that insulate the body and help to preserve heat, as well as other connective tissues.

Skin contains the *sebaceous glands* and *sweat glands* (eccrine and apocrine), which help to prevent dryness, protect skin against bacteria, and maintain core body temperature (thermoregulation).

## FACTORS CONTRIBUTING TO SKIN AGING

Premature skin aging is the result of several factors such as intense physical and psychological stress, alcohol intake, poor nutrition, overeating, environmental pollution, and UV exposure.

### Intrinsic Factors in Skin Aging

Intrinsic skin aging is determined primarily by genetic factors, hormonal status, and metabolic reactions, such as *oxidative stress*. Skin is at risk for similar degenerative effects seen in other organs, yet due to its visibility, skin outwardly discloses many aspects of inner health.

### Genetics

Cellular aging is the process by which a cell becomes old and can no longer replicate. Known as "replicative senescence," this phenomenon can be the result of DNA damage induced by factors such as UV radiation, toxins, or age-related deterioration. A hallmark of replicative senescence is the shortening of *telomeres*, the "caps" at the ends of DNA strands that help ensure chromosomal stability.[4-6]

Skin cells are some of the most rapidly dividing cells in the body. However, as DNA damage accumulates with age, the rapid replication of skin cells causes them to be intrinsically vulnerable to replicative senescence, especially if efforts to protect skin cells from damage are not taken.[4,7,8]

### Hormones

With aging, there is a decline in the level of sex hormones (estrogen, testosterone, dehydroepiandrosterone sulfate), and growth hormone.[9,10] These particular hormones have great influence on the skin. *Balance* is critical in the realm of hormones, and while *escalating* sex hormones during puberty increase the incidence of skin acne, *declining* hormonal levels with aging accelerate skin deterioration.[11]

For women, the change in hormone levels, estrogen in particular, during menopause is accompanied by significant changes within the skin.[12] Estrogens influence skin thickness, wrinkling, and moisture.[13-15] Estrogen binds to receptors on skin cells, activating gene expression that modulates skin cell renewal.[12,16] With declining estrogen levels, skin cellular renewal becomes sluggish, resulting in thinning of the epidermal and dermal layers. Capillary blood circulation velocity decreases significantly[17] and the ability for the skin to maintain hydration, strength and elasticity suffers as a result.[12]

### Oxidative Stress

As the outermost barrier separating internal tissue from the environment, the skin is regularly exposed to UV radiation and air pollution. These exposures induce the production of highly volatile molecules called *free radicals*, which go on to wreak havoc in the cellular environment of the skin. Chronic free radical assault leads to the appearance of uneven, blotchy pigmentation, and subverts the structural framework of the skin, giving rise to wrinkles and sagging skin.[18] Free radicals also arise from internal, metabolic reactions like *glycation* from elevated blood sugar, so simply avoiding exposure to UV light is not adequate for optimal protection.

Oxidative stress plays a central role in initiating and driving events that cause skin aging at the cellular level.[19] Oxidative stress breaks down protein (collagen), alters cellular renewal cycles, damages DNA, and promotes the release of proinflammatory mediators (cytokines), which trigger the generation of inflammatory skin diseases. It is also established that free radicals participate in the pathogenesis of allergic reactions in the skin.[18-22]

In addition to the skin's antioxidant defense, epidermal immune cells called *Langerhans* cells help protect the skin by recognizing antigens (foreign substances) and inducing antibody defense responses. As observed in aging skin there is a reduced number of immune Langerhans cells, thereby affecting skin's ability to ward off stressors or infection that may impact its health.[2,23] This is critical, because with advancing age, skin immunity declines, increasing the incidence of infection, malignancies and structural deterioration (skin aging).[2,23]

### Elevated Blood Sugar Levels and Glycation

While external factors such as sun exposure can accelerate extrinsic skin aging, scientific evidence points to another culprit: *glucose-driven* intrinsic aging. Glucose is a vital cellular fuel. However, based on the accelerated rate of aging seen in diabetics, chronic glucose exposure has long been known to affect how the body ages by a process called *glycation*.[24]

The same browning reaction that occurs when meat is cooked at high heat takes place at a slower rate to long-lived tissue proteins such as collagen in the body.[25] When the proteins in meat are exposed to heat and carbohydrates in the absence of moisture, they cause it to turn brown in a chemical process called the Maillard reaction. Similarly, in the human body, once sugars enter the circulation, they attach themselves to the amino groups of tissue proteins such as collagen to slowly rearrange their youthful structure into the main culprits of damage, called *advanced glycation end products* (AGEs). AGE molecules are particularly destructive since they can undergo extensive cross-linking with other proteins to form strong chemical bridges. As a result, once healthy collagen fibers lose their elasticity, becoming rigid, more brittle, and prone to breakage.[26] Strong scientific evidence also indicates that glycation reactions are promoted by oxidative stress and lead to the production of reactive oxygen species in the skin.[27]

This assault on the skin's structural support system contributes to the aging of tissues and, when accelerated by hyperglycemia, to the gradual development of diabetic complications. Not surprisingly, collagen abnormalities with aging and in diabetes share similar roots and have widespread consequences for the skin, such as thinning, discoloration, loss of elasticity, and tendency to rashes and infections.

Laboratory research shows that once formed, AGEs can be self-perpetuating—directly inducing the cross-linking of collagen even in the absence of glucose.[28] Glycation also induces fibroblast apoptosis (cell death), which creates a state of cellular senescence that has been shown to switch fibroblasts from a matrix-producing to a matrix-degrading state.[29] In this state, the secretion of collagen-degrading enzymes, called matrix metalloproteinases (MMPs), increases and levels of their inhibitors decline.[30]

In fact, glycation directly increases the release of MMP-1, which preferentially breaks down collagen.[31] While these assaults on the skin occur internally, external sources of oxidative stress can also aggravate skin aging. In particular, sun exposure increases levels of MMP-1 in the skin.[32]

## Extrinsic Factors in Premature Skin Aging
### UV Radiation and "Photoaging"

The intrinsic ageing of the skin is exacerbated by environmental (extrinsic) factors. One of the most important extrinsic factors in accelerated skin ageing is *solar ultraviolet radiation* (UVR). Epidemiological and clinical studies have identified excessive sun exposure

as a primary causal factor in various skin diseases including, premature aging, inflammatory conditions, melanoma and non-melanoma skin cancers.[33,34]

A series of deleterious biochemical reactions occur within the skin when it is exposed to excess UV radiation; this process is referred to as *photoaging*.

Chronic sun exposure damages the dermal connective tissue and alters normal skin metabolism. In addition to depressing immunity, and stimulating oxidative stress and inflammation, UV radiation increases the production of *matrix metalloproteinases* (MMPS), enzymes that *degrade collagen*.[35] The destruction of collagen is a major contributor to the loss of skin suppleness and structure that occurs with advancing age.

The major targets of UV irradiation in the skin are the surface epidermal layers; this results in the depletion of antioxidants such as *alpha-tocopherol* (vitamin E) and *ascorbic acid* (vitamin C), which decreases the overall antioxidant capacity within the skin.[19] Secondarily to the depletion of vital antioxidant molecules in the epidermis, intrinsic antioxidant defense systems begin to fail; these include *superoxide dismutase*, *catalase*, and *glutathione-S-transferase*.[36]

---

## UV WAVELENGTHS AND THEIR EFFECTS ON THE SKIN

**UV-A radiation (long wave)** accounts for a large percentage of total UVR (90–95%) and penetrates deeper into the epidermis and dermis of the skin. UV-A radiation induces oxidative stress that stimulates post-UV inflammation and hyperpigmentation (melanin production). Ironically, it is oxidative stress that creates the "tanned" skin so often mistakenly associated with health and vitality. A suntan is evidence of *skin damage*, and represents the skin's attempt to protect itself from further damage.

**UV-B radiation (mid wave)**, although it comprises only about 5% of the total UVR, is highly damaging to DNA and epidermal keratinocytes. UVB radiation is mainly responsible for nonmelanoma skin cancer.

UV-B radiation also stimulates the synthesis of vitamin D within the skin. However, obtaining optimal 25-hydroxyvitamin D levels of 50–80 ng/mL through sun exposure only is not ideal, as the damaging consequences of excess sun exposure will override the beneficial effects of vitamin D. Therefore, supplementation with about 5000–8000 IU of vitamin D daily is a more favorable method for ensuring optimal vitamin D status for most individuals.

---

### Environmental Toxins

Tobacco use is a major factor that contributes to many chronic diseases and reduced life expectancy.[37,38] Studies have confirmed that smoking tobacco damages the skin via multiple mechanisms as well.[39]

On the molecular level, tobacco smoke produces oxidative stress, impairs circulation, and triggers DNA damaging reactions, making the skin more vulnerable to disease and aging.[39,40] Visually, "smoker's skin" is characterized by increased lines and wrinkles, uneven tone, dehydration, and dull and frail skin. Interestingly, smokers who quit have noted dramatic improvements in the visual appeal of their skin, and a more youthful skin appearance has been observed within 9 months after smoking cessation.[39]

In addition to UV radiation and smoking, pollution is a factor in premature skin aging.[41] Epidemiologic studies have correlated pollution levels with poor health status. Specifically, recent studies relate particle pollution to advanced skin aging. Most notably, skin hyperpigmentation and sluggish skin cell renewal has been observed in both human and animal studies.[41,42] For information to help reduce the consequences of environmental toxin exposure, see Life Extension's Metabolic Detoxification protocol.

# COMBATTING SKIN AGING

## Dietary Strategies to Promote Youthful Skin Appearance

As skin is the "visual" organ, the beauty industry's primary objective is to improve the appearance of skin with sophisticated topical treatments and interventions. However, often overlooked is the need support the health and beauty of skin from within through proper nutrition.[4]

In addition to the well-documented role of a wholesome, plant-based diet in maintaining the youthful vivacity of the skin, modern nutritional science is elucidating the relationship between *specific nutrients* and optimal skin health.

Sadly, the typical North American diet falls considerably short of providing the nutritional composition needed to keep skin healthy and vibrant.

- **Macronutrient Composition and Glycemic Load.** The North American diet contains excessive amounts of simple carbohydrates and saturated fats. Not surprisingly, this dietary pattern correlates with an increased appearance of skin wrinkles.[43-46]

  The *glycemic index* measures how rapidly and significantly foods cause blood sugar elevations following consumption. Epidemiology data suggest that a high glycemic diet may contribute to inflammatory skin conditions such as acne, rosacea, psoriasis, and eczema as well.[43,47,48]

  Insulin resistance and inflammation disrupt sebum production, cause collagen malformation, and excite the *epidermal growth factor receptor*, which is involved in tissue renewal, but can also stimulate inflammatory reactions in the skin cells.[43-46]

  When sugar comes in contact with collagen (a protein), a devastating reaction, called *glycation*, occurs resulting in the formation of tissue-destroying advanced glycation end products (AGES).[49] Glycation occurs in all tissues of the body, but is accelerated by a high sugar diet and, within the skin, excessive sun exposure.[49-51]

  Protein glycation and AGE formation are accompanied by increased free radical activity in skin collagen, which accelerates skin aging.[52] All of these changes create an environment within the skin that favors degradation of collagen, thus compromising the integrity and regeneration of skin tissue.

- **Fatty Acid Composition.** Within the skin, fatty acids make up an integral component of cell walls (membranes) that help maintain cell structure and function. Clinical studies show that the healthy balance of fatty acids in skin dramatically decreases with aging and increased oxidative stress, such as that caused by chronic sun exposure.[53,54] Therefore, obtaining the right amount (and type) of fats through diet or supplementation is critical to maintain healthy skin as we age.[53-56] Traditional and non-Westernized diets offer a more balanced intake of omega-6 to omega-3 fatty acids (typically at a ratio of about 4:1).[55,57] Today, the North American diet provides a ratio of about 15:1 or more of omega-6s to omega-3s.[57,58] Excessive amounts of the omega-6 fat arachidonic acid, found in relatively high quantities in egg yolks, poultry skin, and organ meats from animals fed corn-based diets have a proinflammatory effect in the body (including the skin). Conversely, fish oil rich in the omega-3 oils eicosapentaenoic and docosahexaenoic acids (EPA and DHA) inhibit the production of inflammatory metabolites. Due to their ability to modulate inflammation, long-chain omega-3 fatty acids are effective in the management of inflammatory skin conditions, such as acne, psoriasis, eczema, and rosacea.[55,56]

- **Micronutrient and Antioxidant Density.** For some time, nutrition experts have recommended choosing whole foods that are micronutrient- and antioxidant-dense over commercially manufactured, overly processed foods negligible in micronutrients, yet rich in fat and carbohydrate calories. This is a critical consideration for skin health as well.

Clinical studies have shown that *catechins* from green tea, *anthocyanins* from dark berries and red cabbage, *bioflavonoids* from citrus, *carotenoids* such as lycopene and lutein from tomatoes, *resveratrol* from red wine and *genistein* from soy offer potent secondary antioxidant protection in the skin.[59,60] By including these types of foods more often in the diet, the antioxidant defenses in the skin can be optimized.

- **Sodium and Hypertension.** The North American diet relies heavily on over-processed, salty foods and some studies suggest that high sodium intake increases the risk of developing hypertension.[61,62] Studies have shown that those with borderline and established hypertension have significantly lower skin capillary densities than non-hypertensive subjects.[63] A recent trial proved that by reducing sodium intake in hypertensive subjects, even modestly, microcirculation and capillary densities in the skin can be improved.[64]

- **Caloric Intake.** Data indicate that calorie restriction (CR) promotes longevity through improving body composition and optimizing metabolic function.[65] Caloric restriction may promote healthier skin aging due to improved skin cell renewal and repair mechanisms as well.[66] To learn more about the numerous benefits associated with caloric restriction, see Life Extension's Caloric Restriction protocol.

## OPTIMAL DIET FOR SKIN HEALTH

Studies indicate that the *Mediterranean diet* is linked with improved health and longevity. The Mediterranean dietary pattern centers upon fruits, vegetables, whole grains, legumes, monounsaturated fats (MUFA, such as those found in *olive oil*), and a healthy ratio of omega-3 to omega-6 polyunsaturated fatty acids (PUFAs).

An impressive amount of epidemiological data link the Mediterranean diet with improved cardiovascular, cognitive, and metabolic health.[67–70]

The unique properties of this diet are also of particular interest for the skin. The Mediterranean diet may exert an anti-inflammatory effect due in part to its emphasis on extra virgin olive oil, which is high in compounds that modulate oxidative stress and quell inflammatory reactions. A particularly interesting olive oil compound is *oleocanthal*. This compound has been recently been shown to possess anti-inflammatory actions similar to ibuprofen.[68,71] In one hospital-based study in Italy, researchers gathered and compared medical and lifestyle history, as well as sun exposure habits and dietary patterns from over 300 controls to over 300 cases of cutaneous melanoma patients. Upon analysis and careful control for sun exposure and pigmentary characteristics, shellfish, fish rich in omega-3 fatty acids, regular tea drinking, and greater consumption of fruits and vegetables were associated with improved skin health.[59]

## SKIN HEALTH AND GUT HEALTH—IS THERE A CONNECTION?

Human skin harbors a variety of microorganisms, collectively known as the skin microbiota. Within the skin, there is a complex network of interactions between the microbes and cells of the epidermis. Friendly bacteria, such as *Lactobacillus* and *Bifidobacteria* are well documented for effectively treating certain infections, promoting healthy immunity, and reducing skin inflammation.[72–74]

Orally administered pre- and probiotics have been shown *in vivo* to rebalance the skin microbiota and optimize skin barrier function.[75,76] Additionally, oral probiotics boost cellular antioxidant capacity and combat inflammation as well.[72]

Moreover, probiotics help to neutralize toxic byproducts, defend the lining of the intestine, increase the bioavailability of some nutrients and reinforce the intestinal barrier against infectious microbes that may harm healthy skin.[75–77]

## MEDICAL PROCEDURES AND MODALITIES TO COMBAT SKIN AGING

As the quest for youth and beauty continues to evolve, research advancements within the cosmetic and medical aesthetics industry have seen exponential growth over the last 20 years.[78] Within corrective dermatology, the most sought after treatments include those with the least amount of down time and minimal risk. These include lasers, intense pulsed light, hyaluronic acid based fillers, botulinum toxin (BOTOX®), chemical peeling, radiofrequency, and dermabrasion procedures.[79]

Medically supervised treatments such as exfoliation-type (microdermabrasion) or chemical peels have been performed for years to rejuvenate the skin. Glycolic acid chemical peels offer a non-invasive treatment to help renew skin surface. After application, the peel lifts off the surface layer of the skin to bring out a radiant glow and minimize visibility of fine lines and wrinkles. Although chemical peels are used mostly on the face, they can also be used to improve the skin on the neck and hands.[80]

With advanced technology there are now a multitude of devices and mechanisms available to thermally treat the skin. These include laser or intense pulsed light (IPL) skin resurfacing and may require a mild anesthetic and short recovery period. To date, fractional laser resurfacing have become popular in medical aesthetic practices as they have exhibited favorable outcomes with minimal recovery time. In general, this type of treatment involves the application of a focused laser light to the skin. With the heat generated by the light, upper and middle layers of skin are removed. After skin healing, general results show a visible improvement in skin coloration and softening of fines lines and wrinkles.[79,81]

To help restore volume, smooth skin appearance and minimize fine lines and wrinkles, semi-permanent (BOTOX®, Juvederm®), and more permanent dermal fillers (Restylane®) are treated to the eye area, forehead and nasolabial folds (smile lines). The procedure occurs with a local injection to the treated area of the face. Depending on the type of filler used, results generally last 3–4 months (BOTOX®), 6 months to a year (Juvederm®), or up to 3 years (Restylane®).[82]

In the last few years, skin cell regenerating creams have been brought to market in the hope to combat the signs of skin aging. Of particular interest is stem cell therapy. Adult stem cells are found in different tissues, such as the brain, bone marrow, blood vessels, muscle and skin. They generally will remain inactive until they are activated by injury or for example, chronic photodamage to the skin. Once activated, stem cells can regenerate a range of cell types from the originating organ. In skin, stem cells that lie just beneath the surface have been used to engineer new skin tissue that can be grafted on to burn victims.[83]

One of the most recent treatments in stem therapy include the use of adipose-derived stem cells (ADSC), which have been shown to in animal studies to combat free radical damage and age spots, and promote wound healing in the skin upon injection.[84,85] Experiments suggest that ADSCs, when injected subcutaneously, stimulate collagen synthesis and the formation of new blood vessels (angiogenesis).[84] These findings indicate that ADSCs may be an effective anti-aging strategy for maintaining skin vitality.

## HORMONE THERAPY AND SKIN AGING

As outlined earlier in this protocol, age-related changes in hormone levels, especially those that occur during menopause for women, have dramatic effects on skin health. Therefore, utilizing natural *bioidentical hormone replacement therapy* as a means to maintain hormones in a youthful range is a provocative strategy for combatting skin aging. Indeed, several trials have shown that hormone replacement therapy improves skin quality.

To assess the effects of *estrogen replacement therapy* on skin aging, 40 postmenopausal women received systemic estrogen replacement therapy for seven 28-day cycles. By the end of the trial, skin elasticity and hydration improved significantly, with no adverse effects reported.[86]

In another trial, researchers aimed to assess the effects of systemic estrogen therapy on skin collagen in postmenopausal women. Researchers found that by 16 weeks of treatment, collagen content had significantly *increased* in facial skin, resulting in improved texture and firmness.[88] There are also some studies that have noted visual improvements in skin dispigmentation (age spots) and wrinkle reduction in peri- and post-menopausal women treated with systemic transdermal estradiol-based creams.[86,88,89]

### DHEA and Melatonin

The sleep hormone (melatonin) and the anti-stress hormone (DHEA) are both found in human skin. Both are converted into entities with biological roles within the skin. DHEA is converted into estrogen- and androgen-type metabolites unique to the skin.[90] Melatonin is synthesized in skin. In low concentrations it can stimulate cell growth. This type of on-site, organ-specific production of hormones is called intracrine biosynthesis. Intracrine biosynthesis allows different organs to manufacture the substances they need without flooding the entire body with growth factors.

Although the exact roles of DHEA and melatonin in human skin are still under scrutiny, researchers have identified several mechanisms through which these hormones protect against aging, maintain the health of skin, and affect how sunlight reacts with skin cells.

*DHEA* has beneficial effects beyond its conversion to skin-friendly hormones. DHEA itself has powerful skin protective effects. A study in the Journal of Surgical Research demonstrates the extraordinary ability of topically applied DHEA to protect skin's delicate blood vessels. Researchers found that if DHEA was applied after a serious burn, the blood vessels underlying the burned area are protected.[91] DHEA also has antioxidant action against peroxyl and superoxide free radicals, and also limits the bioactivation of some toxins.[92–94] DHEA blunts chemical carcinogen-induced DNA damage as well.[95,96]

A 2008 clinical trial found that topical DHEA improved skin brightness and texture in postmenopausal women after 4 months of treatment.[97]

*Melatonin* is an antioxidant hormone that protects against UV radiation.[98] A group at the University of Zurich has shown that topical melatonin gives excellent protection against sunburn if applied before sun exposure.[99] Melatonin may be involved in repairing burned skin as well.[100] Moreover, melatonin appears to play a role in regulating blood circulation within the skin as well.[101]

An animal model of pressure-ulceration revealed that melatonin, both topically and systemically, ameliorated disruption in antioxidant defense system within the skin.[102]

# NUTRITIONAL SUPPLEMENTATION TO COMBAT SKIN AGING

Already a well-established strategy for women in Asian and European cultures, targeted oral nutritional supplementation to support skin health and beauty is a more recent introduction in North America. Unlike topical products, which are applied to targeted areas, these nutritional formulations are taken orally then metabolized and distributed throughout the body. Additionally, the bloodstream continuously supplies these bioactive compounds to all skin compartments (ie, epidermis, dermis, subcutaneous fat). Therefore, by working systemically, nutricosmetics are able to further protect and support the health of the skin.[103]

### Nutritional Support for General Skin Health

Minerals such as selenium, copper, and molybdenum are required cofactors for the maintenance of antioxidant defense systems in the skin.

Recently, certain natural ingredients such as *curcumin*, resveratrol, *coenzyme Q10*, and *superoxidase dismutase (SOD)*-enriched melon extract, have been shown to stimulate the production of these primary defense antioxidants.[104–106]

There is some clinical research showing that *selenium*-dependent glutathione peroxidase enzyme activity is low in participants with acne vulgaris. One study examined the effect of selenium and *vitamin E*, in which acne patients took 200 mcg of selenium with 10 mg of vitamin E twice per day for 12 weeks. At the end of the trial, a reduced number of lesions and visual skin improvements were observed, especially in

participants with low baseline glutathione peroxidase activity.[107,108]

*Carotenoids* are a group of fat soluble compounds found in orange and red fruits and vegetables that confer antioxidant protection within the skin.[109] *Lycopene*, found predominantly in tomatoes and tomato-based products, is well-supported in the scientific literature for skin photoprotection. When skin is subjected to UV light stress, more skin lycopene is destroyed compared with beta-carotene, suggesting a role of lycopene in photoprotection against UV damage in tissues. In one trial, 20 women ingested 16 mg of lycopene daily for 12 weeks. After being exposed to UV radiation and in comparison to the control group, the lycopene-supplemented group had a significant reduction in post-UV exposure reddening and inflammation. The researchers concluded that lycopene effectively protected the skin from acute and potentially long-term photodamage.[110]

In another study, researchers investigated the effect of a tomato-based drink on markers of inflammation, immunity and oxidative stress within the skin. Subjects were given either a drink containing 5.7 mg of lycopene, along with several other tomato-derived antioxidants, or placebo for 26 days. At the end of the trial, inflammatory intermediates were more than 34% lower in the group that consumed the tomato-based drink.[111]

Trials (in animals and in humans) have shown that *coenzyme Q10* suppresses the UV radiation–induced inflammatory response in skin cells. In an 8-year prospective study of 117 patients with melanoma, CoQ10 plasma levels predicted the risk of metastasis. CoQ10 levels were significantly lower in patients than in control subjects and in patients who developed recurring melanoma than those who did not.[112]

Another nutrient of interest for skin health is *vitamin D*, which is synthesized in the skin upon exposure to UV-B radiation.[113] Insufficient vitamin D levels have been linked in epidemiology studies to decreased physical performance, poor cardiac health, autoimmune disease, neurologic disorders, several cancers, and increased overall mortality.[114] In its active form as *calcitriol*, vitamin D contributes to healthy skin cell renewal and repair. It also supports the skin's immune system and can neutralize free radicals within the epidermal layers.[113–115]

However, with the notable dangers associated with excess sun exposure, vitamin D deficiency is an epidemic in North America and throughout the world.[115,116] With more frequent sunscreen use (although required), less sun exposure, and natural aging, the skin's ability to manufacture vitamin D is compromised, emphasizing the need for dietary and supplemental intake.[113–116]

## Photoprotective Nutrients

### Plant Polyphenols

Polyphenols are a large family of naturally occurring compounds that are widely distributed in plant-based foods. Dietary sources of polyphenols include onions (*flavonols*), cacao beans, grape seeds (*proanthocyanidins*), tea (*catechins*), apples and red wine (*flavonols and catechins*), citrus fruits (*flavanones*), berries and cherries (*anthocyanidins*), and soy (*isoflavones*).

A variety of polyphenols possess substantial skin photoprotective effects.[60] Once ingested, this type of antioxidant is rapidly utilized in the body, therefore *daily* consumption of polyphenols is recommended to provide efficient skin protection.

The role of dietary components, such as, catechins from green tea and proanthocyanidins from grape seeds, have been assessed in prevention of UV-induced skin carcinogenesis *in vitro* and *in vivo* in animal models.[117–120] A recent trial published in the *Journal of Nutrition* found that when women consumed a beverage containing 1402 mg of catechins daily, skin was better protected against harmful UV radiation; the intervention also improved overall skin quality (elasticity, roughness, hydration) over 12 weeks.[121]

### Fern Extract (Polypodium Leucotomos)

Extracts from the leaves of a certain species of fern, *Polypodium leucotomos* (PL) have been shown in clinical studies to effectively block ultraviolet (UV)-induced skin phototoxicity.[122–125]

In one study, 53 patients with sun allergy condition (Idiopathic photodermatoses), consumed 480 mg PL extract daily while exposing themselves to sunlight. Over 73% of the patients had a benefit from the administered PL, with significant reduction of skin reaction or irritation and subjective symptoms. With no side effects observed, the study authors concluded that oral supplementation with PL effectively and safely provides photoprotection.[122]

Another clinical trial found that oral PL effectively reduced skin reddening induced by artificial UVR. Moreover, upon histological examination of skin biopsies taken from the subjects who consumed PL extract, decreased skin cell DNA damage and immune activation was noted.[125] The authors of this study concluded that "*oral administration of PL is an effective systemic chemophotoprotective agent leading to significant protection of skin against UV radiation.*"

PL extract appears to be especially effective in those whose skin is particularly sensitive to the sun.

Several studies have found that oral PL blunts dermal allergic responses to sun exposure in those prone to such reactions.[126]

A comprehensive review by Gonzalez[123] of the mechanisms by which PL combats photoaging states the following:

*"PL is a natural mixture of phytochemicals endowed with powerful antioxidant properties. Its short-term effects include inhibition of reactive oxygen species production induced by UV radiation, DNA damage, isomerization and decomposition of trans-urocanic acid [an endogenous sunscreen-like agent], prevention of UV-mediated apoptosis and necrosis, as well as degradative matrix remodeling, which is the main cause of photoaging. These short-term effects translate into long-term prevention of photoaging and photocarcinogenesis. A striking property is that PL can exert its effect when administered orally. Together, these effects postulate PL as a natural photoprotective agent and a potential adjuvant to phototherapy for various skin diseases."*

In addition, a recent animal model elucidated further mechanisms by which PL guards against photodamage.[127] This experiment found that PL dramatically *reduced* the sun-induced expression of COX-2, which drives inflammation and contributes to skin cancer growth, while it simultaneously *increased* the expression of a major DNA repair protein, P53. In animals fed PL, UVR exposure induced *25% fewer* DNA mutations than in animals receiving a control diet.

## Natural Ingredients to Restore Skin

### Plant-Based Ceramides

*Ceramides* make up the lipid-rich protective layer within the epidermis. Although present in other tissues, their highest concentration is found in the skin. We can obtain ceramides through foods, mainly rice bran, wheat flour, and wheat germ oil. Ceramide concentrations decrease naturally with age and since they play an important role in preventing dehydration in the skin, oral supplemented plant-based ceramides may help to combat breakdown associated with aging.[128–130]

In a randomized trial, 51 women (aged 20–63 years) with dry skin were given either 350 mg of a non-GMO wheat extract containing ceramides or placebo for 3 months. After evaluating skin hydration in the legs, arms, and face at the beginning and end of trial, a significant increase in skin hydration and an improvement in the clinical signs of dryness were observed at the end of 3 months.[131] When combined with antioxidants in oral formulations, it has been shown that ceramides further optimize systemic absorption and utilization of water-soluble antioxidants, such as ascorbic acid (vitamin C).[129–131]

### Soy Compounds

Recent research has confirmed the antioxidant and DNA protective effects of *soy isoflavones* in skin. It is the protective effect of *genistein* that is believed to block UV-induced cellular damage.[132] In addition to the photoprotective benefits, active components of soy have demonstrated other beneficial effects for the skin. For instance, soy protein peptides have favorably stimulated collagen and hyaluronic acid production within the dermis *in vitro*.[133]

Since they exert weak estrogenic activity, soy isoflavones may assist in delaying accelerated skin aging due to hormonal decline in postmenopausal women.[132,134] For example, to assess the effect of soy isoflavones on skin aging, 30 postmenopausal women were administered 100 mg/day of isoflavone-rich soy extract for 6 months. At the end of the study, researchers observed that over 86% of the women experienced significant increases in skin thickness, collagen and elastin fibers, and microcapillary density.[132] In another trial, skin benefits were observed when 40-mg soy isoflavones were taken daily for 12 weeks.[134]

## Topical Interventions in Skin Aging

Since their introduction in the 1980s, "*cosmeceuticals*" (a topical product that exerts both *cosmetic* and *therapeutic* benefits), have continued to evolve to ward off the signs of skin aging.[135] *Sunscreens* are the most important cosmeceutical, and *retinoids* have proven their safety and effectiveness in reducing photodamaged skin and are now a mainstream treatment for skin anti-aging.[136] However, emerging categories of cosmeceuticals are proving effective in maintaining vibrant skin.

Generally, there are three categories of cosmeceuticals on the market. These include exfoliating and whitening agents, antioxidants and regenerating products, such as peptides, and stem cell-based skincare.[137–139]

The use of alpha-hydroxy acids (AHAs) has been shown to improve skin texture and reduce the signs of aging by promoting cell shedding in the outer layers of the epidermis and by restoring hydration. They are used often to improve skin texture and for treating mild to moderate photodamage.[140,141]

The most common ingredients used in formulations and peels include:

- Citric acid
- Glycolic acid
- Lactic acid
- Malic acid
- Pyruvic acid
- Tartaric acid

### Cutting-Edge Topical Ingredients

*Peptide-based creams* represent a breakthrough in skin-care technology. Within the skin, collagen deterioration results in the formation of protein fragments, called *peptides*. These fragments are then recognized by collagen-producing cells, which respond by increasing collagen production in order to repair the damaged skin. However, with advancing age, this positive feedback between skin breakdown and the initiation of new collagen formation becomes inefficient.

Researchers have discovered that application of these protein fragments directly to the skin *circumvents* the natural deterioration in collagen turnover. Therefore, by applying specialized peptides to your skin, you can effectively "trick" collagen-producing cells into ramping up collagen production.[138,142]

One such peptide is *palmitoyl tetrapeptide-3*. This synthetic amino-peptide complex effectively stimulates collagen synthesis by interacting with receptors that turn on genes responsible for cell proliferation and renewal. This patented pentapeptide significantly enhances the production of collagen and elastin within the extracellular matrix of the skin. This increased production complements the volumizing action of *hyaluronic acid*, thereby resulting in visibly reduced wrinkle depth, density, and number. Studies show that this patented ingredient is as effective as the vitamin A derivative retinol in reducing the signs of photoaging, yet it does not cause the skin irritation associated with retinol.[143]

*Argireline* (acetyl hexapeptide-3) is a relatively new topical antiwrinkle ingredient that reduces pre-existing wrinkle depth through a novel mechanism. This active peptide works by significantly downregulating muscle contraction, interfering with the neurotransmitters that make your muscles contract, thereby preventing the formation of unwanted lines and wrinkles. This natural ingredient appears to be especially beneficial for visibly reducing wrinkle depth around the eyes and forehead.[138,144,145]

### Matrixyl® Synthe'6™

The breakdown of skin scaffolding is a major cause of wrinkles. A compound known as Matrixyl® Synthe'6™ has been found to complete the maturation and stabilization of fibers, thereby *stimulating* the scaffolding of skin molecules.

In a controlled clinical study, 25 women aged 42–70 were assigned to one of two groups. Cream was applied *2 times daily*.[146] One group applied a placebo cream, while the other group applied a 2% solution of Matrixyl® synthe'6™. Scientists later measured the participants' wrinkles and crow's feet.

The researchers found that frown lines among the Matrixyl® synthe'6™ group were *lifted* by *28%*, and the volume of wrinkles was diminished by *31%*. And this anti-wrinkling effect was observed in just *2 months*.

Also, scientists observed that, in the test group, crow's feet were *lifted* by *12.6%*, and their volume was reduced *21.1%*.

Matrixyl® Synthe'6™ actively *promotes* the synthesis of *six* skin matrix constituents—*collagen I, III,* and *IV, hyaluronic acid, fibronectin,* and *laminin*. These skin matrix constituents are found in the lower epidermis, where cells communicate with each other and with the cells in the dermal layer.

### Hylasome® EG10

Excessive dryness of the skin promotes fine lines and weakens cells. It can cause lipids in the skin's fatty layer to crystallize, causing dull and flaking skin.

*Hyaluronic acid*, a natural skin constituent, is a good moisturizer owing to its ability to capture water molecules, which reduces the visibility of lines. It is also a volumizing agent. For these reasons, hyaluronic acid is an ingredient in several skincare applications.[147]

However, scientists have now developed a potent new generation of this compound—an aqueous gel of cross-linked hyaluronic acid, called *Hylasome® EG10*. This gel forms a thin film on the skin and continuously delivers the *larger* amount of water bound by this new compound.

When Rutgers University scientists tested this unique gel on human skin, they found that skin cells treated with Hylasome® EG10 held *6 times more* moisture in total, and *5 times more* moisture in the *stratum corneum* (extreme outer) layer, than cells treated with hyaluronic acid. This greater moisturizing effect was observed even *24 hours* after application.[148]

Hylasome® EG10 also exhibited ability to *combat* oxidation and free radical attack, which can damage skin structure and cause wrinkles.

### Vegetal Filling Spheres

Deterioration of skin matrix, combined with moisture loss, results in indentations and wrinkles. But a new compound attacks this problem from deep inside the indentations.

*Vegetal filling spheres* are derived from wheat protein, which is a *biopolymer* known for its hydrating capacities.

Scientists applied either vegetal filling spheres, or placebo, to the crow's feet of 30 volunteers. They observed a *31% decrease* in the total wrinkle surface, and a *27% decrease* in wrinkle length. And this effect was seen in just *1 hour*.[149]

Researchers found the spheres had settled inside the wrinkle indentations deep within the lower epidermis. There, they acted like microscopic sponges, trapping moisture that would normally be lost through the skin surface.

The observed result was a *physicochemical effect*: the spheres expanded with moisture and physically *plumped* wrinkles—transforming the skin surface from wrinkled to smooth.

Remarkably, the plumping effect occurs immediately after application—and is long-lasting. There is also a durable *increase* in hydration of the middle and upper layers of the epidermis.

### Poly P

Skin cell proliferation and collagen synthesis both slow down as we age, producing visible lines.

However, *inorganic phosphates*, found in almost all cells, were found to inhibit this deterioration. Called *Poly P*, these phosphates *promote tissue remodeling*.[150]

Poly P communicates with skin cells at the dermal layer where *fibroblasts*—responsible for cell renewal—are produced. Scientists believe this interaction *increases* production of skin cells, which surface to replace old cells. Also, Poly P is believed to *increase* the production of collagen.

Boosting production of both collagen and dermal cells *improves* skin volume and tone, making Poly P a key compound in any modern skincare product.

Studies have confirmed the efficacy of topical formulations containing multiple bioactives, such as a combination of stem cell growth factors, peptides and antioxidant based formulations to combat skin damage and aging.

In a 3-month trial, 37 females with mild to severe signs of photodamage were treated with a facial serum containing naturally occurring stem cell growth factors, peptides and antioxidants, applied twice daily. As early as 1 month, significant visual reductions in wrinkles and improvements in skin texture and radiance were noted; progress continued into months 2 and 3.[151]

## Natural and Complementary Topical Therapies

Due to the increasing demand for natural ingredients in topical skin care products, antioxidants are being increasingly used in anti-aging skincare. Targeting similar cellular mechanisms as nutritional approaches, topical antioxidants are effective in warding off damaging free radicals and reducing inflammation within the epidermal layers.

Among the most commonly used are ascorbic acid (Vitamin C), tocopherols (Vitamin E), alpha lipoic acid, and coenzyme Q10. Emerging natural antioxidants proving effective include EGCG (from green tea), resveratrol, Centella asiatica (Gotu Kola), proanthocyanidins (grapeseed), curcumin, pomegranate, silymarin/silibinin (milk thistle), coffee berry, melatonin, and marine-based ingredients.[152-154]

When applied topically, antioxidants have been shown to provide powerful anti-inflammatory, photoprotective, and antiaging skin benefits.[152-160]

In one trial, two different antioxidants were used to stimulate collagen production and improve chronically sun damaged skin. Over 6 months, a cream consisting of 5% Vitamin C and 0.1% madecassoside (Centella asiatica) was applied daily to 20 females with photodamaged skin. At the end of trial, a significant improvement in wrinkles, firmness, roughness, and skin hydration was observed.[156]

In another trial, researchers assessed the effects of an antioxidant rich cream on the aging face in over 30 women (mean age of 54 years). For 12 weeks, the women were treated with a 5% alpha lipoic acid (ALA) cream (twice daily) or placebo cream. In addition to visible skin improvements, the researchers used laser profilometry to measure skin variables and found there was a 50% average reduction in skin roughness in the ALA-treated skin over the placebo-treated skin. Researchers concluded the ALA antioxidant cream was effective in improving clinical characteristics of aging and photodamaged skin.[161]

Another ingredient used for its powerful skin anti-aging properties is hyaluronic acid, a sugar-like molecule found in the tissues throughout the body. Originally recognized for its antioxidant effects and wound healing properties,[162] hyaluronic acid is used in topical formulations and non-permanent dermal fillers to combat skin aging.[163] Within the skin hyaluronic acid is an important component of the structural foundation in the dermis. Its primary function is to attract and bind to water to moisturize and give skin cells volume, while visually smoothing the appearance of skin.[163,164]

### Botanimoist® AMS

Keratinocytes produce keratin, the material comprising fibrous proteins responsible for strengthening skin membranes. So loss of hydration in keratinocytes causes a weakening of skin cells, resulting in a sagging, wrinkling effect. Also, a depletion of cellular moisture causes lines to be more visible.

Scientists tested hydrating capability of a dried extract of apple fruit, called Botanimoist® AMS (apple moisturizing saccharide) in a placebo-controlled human study. A single topical application of this extract resulted in an 88.9% increase in skin hydration—after just 30 minutes (Botanigenics).

Even after 6 hours, skin hydration of participants treated with Botanimoist® AMS remained 30.6% higher than the hydration level of untreated skin.

### Pichia-Fermented Resveratrol

Skin often suffers from insufficient hydration, oxidative stress, or slow collagen turnover. These factors cause weakened cellular structure and result in wrinkles. Also, inflammation of the skin promotes aging.

Resveratrol has long been known as an antioxidant and anti-inflammatory, as well as a mimetic of some of the benefits of calorie restriction. It appears to work partly by activating the sirtuin 1 gene and enhancing the functioning of mitochondria, cellular energy factories.[165]

The application of resveratrol to the skin is linked to antiaging and anti-inflammatory effects. When one study showed that topical application of resveratrol prevented skin cancer in mice treated with a carcinogen, this further suggested a role for resveratrol as a topical skincare agent.[166]

Scientists then investigated ways to utilize resveratrol to generate a more direct and potent effect on skin appearance. They developed a special resveratrol, which is fermented by Pichia pastoris yeast, and tested it on the skin of humans.[167]

In a double-blind, placebo-controlled, 22-person study, participants applied Pichia resveratrol to one side of their faces twice a day. Skin hydration was measured by a special technique known as corneometric reading, and high-resolution photos were taken.

The resveratrol-treated sides of the volunteers' faces showed a 36% greater degree of hydration over the control sides. Wrinkles were dramatically lifted, and expression lines were noticeably smoothed. These effects were observed after just 28 days.[167]

## Life Extension Suggestions

Youthful looking, vibrant skin is within reach—if you dedicate yourself to comprehensive skin care.

Any truly effective skin care regimen begins with a nutrient-dense, plant-based diet like the Mediterranean diet. Plenty of physical activity and adequate water intake ensure healthy circulation within the skin.

Supplementation with clinically tested natural ingredients complements the use of conventional and natural topical interventions to dualistically promote skin vibrance.

## Topical Interventions

- *Sunscreen* (with dual protection against UVA and UVB, in a photostable complex; premium products also contain added active ingredients that offer support for skin structure and function): Follow label directions.
- *Light daily moisturizer*: A comprehensive daily moisturizer should include a combination of *moisturizing agents*, *antioxidants*, and *bioactive peptides*.
- *Intensive nighttime moisturizer*: A heavier nighttime cream containing hydrating moisturizers as well as the natural hormones DHEA and melatonin will support structural regeneration within facial skin while you sleep.
- *Targeted topical support*.

Look for specially formulated blends of functional ingredients specifically designed for your skin concerns, such as:

- Those with troublesome *dark circles* and "*bags*" under their eyes should consider an under-eye serum containing *oxidoreductase* enzymes to support microcirculation;
- Those with uneven skin tone should consider a serum containing a high-potency concentration of *vitamin C*.

## Supplemental Nutrients to Support Skin Health

- **Curcumin** (as highly absorbed BCM-95®): 400–800 mg daily
- ***trans*-Resveratrol**: 250–500 mg daily
- **Coenzyme Q10** (CoQ10): 100–200 mg daily

- **Melon and wheat sprout extracts** (containing super oxide dismutase): 2100 mg daily
- **Selenium**: 200–400 mcg daily
- **Vitamin E** (as high gamma tocopherol mix): 350 mg daily
- **Vitamin A** (as *beta*-carotene): 5000 IU daily
- **Omega-3s from fish oil**: 1400 EPA and 1000 mg daily
- **Lycopene**: 15 mg daily
- **Vitamin D**: 5000–8000 IU daily (Dosing should always be based on blood test results with a goal of achieving a 25-hydroxyvitamin D blood level of 50–80 ng/mL.)
- **Green tea,** standardized extract: 725–1450 mg daily
- **Grape extract** (from whole grape): 150 mg daily
- **Blend of dark berry extracts**: 700–1400 mg daily
- **Fern (*Polypodium leucotomos*) extract**: 240–480 mg daily, 30 minutes prior to sun exposure
- **Non-GMO wheat oil extract** (providing ceramides): 350 mg daily
- **Soy isoflavone blend**: 135–270 mg daily

In addition, the following *blood testing* resources may be helpful:

- Omega Score®
- Vitamin D, 25-Hydroxy
- Female Comprehensive Hormone panel or Male Comprehensive Hormone panel; or Female panel or Male panel

## REFERENCES

References available at: www.lef.org/dpt5/ch121

# 122

# *Stress Management*

Although the human body is relatively adept at managing *acute* physical and/or psychological stressors, *chronic* psychological stress can produce a variety of adverse effects.

Chronic unremitting stress can increase our risk of suffering from a barrage of anxiety- and pressure-related diseases ranging from *high blood pressure* and *dementia* to *depression*. Chronic stress also increases our risk for some types of *cancer*.[1-6] According to reports by the American Academy of Family Practice and the Russian Department of Family Care, nearly *two-thirds* of doctor's office visits are related to stress.[7-9]

Regrettably, while chronic stress produces significant adverse health effects, conventional medicine often relies on psychoactive drugs to *mask* stressed patients' symptoms. At the same time, mainstream stress management strategies often fail to address biochemical abnormalities, such as imbalanced *adrenal hormone levels*, that contribute to the detrimental health effects of chronic stress.[10-12]

At the core of chronic stress is deregulation of the *hypothalamic-pituitary-adrenal (HPA) axis*, an interconnected network of physiologic command terminals that governs the production of stress hormones such as *cortisol* and catecholamines (like *epinephrine* and *norepinephrine*). Chronic stress leads to *desynchronization* of the HPA axis and subsequent imbalances in stress hormone levels, a critical feature of stress-related illness.

Upon reading this Life Extension protocol, you will appreciate the dangers of chronic stress, understand how it contributes to various diseases, and know how you can optimize your stress response by combining healthy lifestyle habits with scientifically studied natural therapies.

## THE DEADLY CONSEQUENCES OF CHRONIC STRESS

The consequences of chronic stress can be devastating. A chilling example is *stress cardiomyopathy*, a spontaneous weakening of the heart that predisposes victims to arrhythmia and even *sudden cardiac death*. While the mechanism is not clearly understood, it is thought that chronic stress-induced elevations in epinephrine (adrenaline) overstimulate the cardiac muscle, altering its function and causing atrial remodeling.[13,14]

Another striking example is a condition the Japanese refer to as *karoshi* (death from overworking); this condition was recognized in post–World War II Japan. Overworked and severely emotionally and physically stressed Japanese high-level executives suffered strokes and heart attacks at alarming rates at relatively young ages. Researchers discovered that the death of these otherwise healthy men was due to chronic, unremitting stress. Government estimates in 1990 put the number of men dying each year from karoshi at over 10 000.[9,15]

Prolonged stress has been linked with elevated circulating markers of *inflammation* and increased *intima media thickness*, a measure of *atherosclerosis* progression.[16,17] Chronic stress considerably increases the risk of *anxiety* and *depression* by causing structural and functional changes in the brain as well.[5,18] Moreover, those who do not properly manage and adapt to chronic stress are more likely to be *overweight* and develop *sexual dysfunction*.[19]

## Health Risks Associated with Chronic Stress

| Stressor | Health Outcome | Increased Risk |
|---|---|---|
| Sleep disturbances[20] | Early death from all causes | 170% |
| | Occupational injuries | 38% (Men) |
| | Early death from all causes | 32% |
| | Death from respiratory disease | 79% |
| Perceived stress[21] | Death from heart attacks | 159% |
| | Death from external causes | 207% |
| | Suicide | 491% |
| Adverse childhood experiences[22] | Death by age 65 | 140% |
| | Risk of type 2 diabetes in women | 100% |
| Stress at work[23-25] | Death from heart attack | 181% |
| | Early death from all causes | 65% |
| Not enough reward for effort at work[26] | Poor self-rated health | Up to 280% |
| Divorce[27] | Total and cardiovascular death | 37% (Men) |
| Major negative life events[28] | Breast cancer | 533% |

# HOW THE BODY RESPONDS TO STRESS

When an individual experiences a stressor, physical or emotional, internal or environmental, the body initiates a complex system of adaptive reactions to help cope with the stress. This reactive response results in the release of *glucocorticoids*, also known as stress hormones, and *catecholamines*, which stimulate adaptive changes in a variety of bodily systems.

## The "Fight or Flight" Response

Under short-term circumstances, stress-induced changes prioritize functions involved in escaping danger; for example—redirection of blood flow to the muscles from most other body parts, increased blood pressure and blood sugar levels, dilation of pupils, and inhibition of digestion for energy conservation. During this time, fatty acids and glucose (blood sugar) are liberated from storage sites into the bloodstream where they become readily available for utilization by the muscles. This is known as the *fight-or-flight response*. This reactive and adaptive protection system originates in the brain.

Upon perception of stress, specialized neurons in the paraventricular nucleus of the *hypothalamus* (a major endocrine-regulating brain region) respond by releasing, among other compounds, *corticotrophin releasing hormone* (CRH) and *vasopressin* (VP). Subsequently, these hormones stimulate the release of *adrenocorticotropic hormone* (ACTH) from the *pituitary* gland.

After entering circulation and reaching the *adrenal* glands, ACTH stimulates the production of *glucocorticoids* and *catecholamines*, which then act throughout the body to induce the adaptive changes mentioned in the opening paragraph of this section. Cumulatively, this brain-endocrine coordination comprises the *hypothalamic-pituitary-adrenal* (HPA) axis.

While the fight-or-flight response is undoubtedly necessary to initiate an autonomous response to impending danger in an acute situation (the "rush" you feel when you hear an unexpected loud noise, for example, is the fight-or-flight response in action), it can become devastating when active, even at a low-level, for a protracted period of time.[29]

We modern humans live in an environment filled with emotional stressors, such as financial worries, and deadline pressures at work or school. All of these modern worries *chronically activate* the HPA axis in an evolutionarily unnatural way, leading to elevated stress hormone levels and accompanying physiologic changes throughout the day.

A few components of the fight-or-flight response are especially damaging to health when the stress response is active over a prolonged timeframe—*insulin resistance* and *high blood pressure*.[30]

The elevation in blood pressure and deteriorating insulin sensitivity contribute, along with several other stress-related physiologic irregularities, to a compromised health state that predisposes chronically stressed individuals to an onslaught of age-related diseases.

Eventually, chronic elevations in glucocorticoid levels damage and destroy neurons in the region of the hypothalamus responsible for regulating CRH release.[31] This gives rise to erratic or insufficient HPA axis activation and may lead to the mood disorders (eg, depression, anxiety, and fatigue) commonly observed in individuals who have been under great stress for a long time.

## A Closer Look at Cortisol

Cortisol is, in many ways, a paradoxical hormone. A certain amount of cortisol is necessary for optimal health, but too much or too little can be unhealthy. As mentioned above, during acute episodes of stress, more cortisol is released to help the body cope with physical or psychological stressors.[32] Its primary functions in the body follow:

- Regulation of blood glucose levels by a process called *gluconeogenesis* in the liver
- Regulation of the immune system
- Regulation of carbohydrate, protein, and lipid metabolism

Essentially, cortisol is regarded as an anti-inflammatory hormone, blood glucose modulator, immune-modifier, and adaptation hormone.[33] Depending on diet, exercise, stress, and time of day, serum levels of cortisol can vary.

During healthy conditions, cortisol levels peak in the early morning hours (usually around 8AM) and dip to their lowest between midnight and 4AM. The complex process of cortisol biosynthesis and release is sensitive to disruption by both internal and external factors.[32,34,35] In the face of chronic psychological stress, for example, the adrenal glands excrete an abnormal amount of cortisol in an abnormal rhythm.

Cortisol, being a catabolic hormone (a hormone that breaks down tissues), when out of balance and unregulated can have detrimental effects on body composition. Moreover, *too much* cortisol can suppress the immune system, while *too little* can lead to autoimmunity and rheumatologic disorders.[33,36–39]

Cortisol receptors are expressed throughout the body, including in the brain; therefore, derangement of the biosynthesis, metabolism, and release of cortisol can disrupt many physiologic systems.[32,34,35]

## THE ISSUE OF "ADRENAL FATIGUE"

An alternative medical term that often finds its way into discussions about stress is "*adrenal fatigue*." Although "adrenal fatigue" is not a recognized diagnosis in conventional medicine, Life Extension believes that symptoms often attributed to "adrenal fatigue" arise from *multifactorial pathologic processes* involving, among other systems, the HPA axis, and that these conditions must be treated as such.

On the other hand, *Addison's disease*, sometimes referred to as "*adrenal insufficiency*," is a medical condition that can be life threatening. Addison's disease is typically the result of an autoimmune disorder, but can arise due to genetic abnormalities as well. Consequences of Addison's disease are much more severe and acute than those induced by stress; the condition should be closely monitored by a qualified healthcare professional. For those who would like more information, Addison's disease is discussed in our Adrenal Disorders (Addison's Disease and Cushing's Syndrome) protocol.

## RECOGNIZING WHEN STRESS IS GETTING THE BEST OF YOU

Everyone has an inborn ability to handle stress. However, tolerance is variable as some people can handle only low levels and short durations of stress, while others adapt and can accommodate higher levels stress for more prolonged periods. Hans Selye, in 1935, devised the term *stress* as a factor that induced behavioral changes in mammals. He then furthered this notion to include higher level organisms (humans) as being effected by stress in a harmful way.[40]

According to Selye, there are 3 states the body faces when dealing with stress. The first being the *alarm state* early on in the process, followed by the *resistance state* where the body attempts to adapt to the added stress (release of cortisol), and finally, after stress overwhelms and weakens the system, the *exhaustion state*.[39,41] These 3 "states" can be analogously detailed as physiologic mechanisms:

1. Alarm state: adaptation to acute stress; "fight-or-flight" response

2. Resistance state: emergence of consequences of prolonged stress response activation (ie, insulin resistance)

3. Exhaustion state: decline in responsiveness and sensitivity of primary relays of the HPA axis (ie, hypothalamic deterioration/dysfunction leading to

erratic/insufficient stress hormone and catecholamine production and subsequent mood disorders and fatigue)

The same imbalances in the HPA axis and stress response mechanisms that contribute to these signs and symptoms also contribute to the deadly sequelae of more serious stress-related illness. Therefore, recognizing that you are experiencing some or all of the following symptoms is an important initial step towards achieving better overall health and mitigating your risk for various diseases.

Signs that you are suffering the effects of chronic stress may include the following:

1. Excessive fatigue after minimal exertion; feeling "overwhelmed" by relatively trivial problems

2. Trouble waking in the morning, even after adequate sleep

3. Relying on coffee (caffeine) and other "energy" drinks for a pick me up

4. Perceived energy burst after 6:00 PM

5. Chronic low blood pressure

6. Hypersensitivity to cold temperatures

7. Increased premenstrual symptoms (PMS) symptoms

8. Depression and/or labile mood swings

9. Mental "fog" and poor memory

10. Decreased sex drive

11. Anxiety

12. Craving sugar and salty foods

13. Decreased appetite

14. Imbalanced immune system

15. Chronic allergies

16. Generalized weakness and dizziness upon standing

Some of these symptoms may mimic, or overlap, with dysfunction of the thyroid gland, gonadal (sex) hormones, malnutrition, depression, chronic fatigue states, chronic illness, infection, alcohol and drug abuse, and heavy metal toxicity.[42,43] Therefore, it is very important to rule out other possible causes before attributing symptoms to chronic stress alone.

## IMPAIRED STRESS RESPONSE: A MAJOR CAUSE OF ANXIETY AND DEPRESSION

Often, chronic stress is accompanied by mood disorders, particularly anxiety and depression. In fact, depression and anxiety can both be viewed as manifestations of an impaired stress response; the underlying physiology of both is similar.

In fact, the chronic elevation in glucocorticoids caused by chronic stressors in modern society can lead to physical changes in brain structure.

For example, dendrites, the branches of neurons that receive signals from other neurons, are shifted into less functional patterns upon chronic exposure to glucocorticoids. This has been documented in key brain regions associated with mood, short-term memory, and behavioral flexibility.[44] Furthermore, glucocorticoids cause receptors for the mood-regulating neurotransmitter *serotonin* to become less sensitive to activation.[45,46] Other detrimental effects of chronic stress include both increased susceptibility to neuronal damage and impaired neurogenesis, the process by which new neurons are "born."[44]

Interestingly, emerging research suggests that certain psychoactive drugs, like those used to treat anxiety and depression, may stabilize mood not only by acting upon neurotransmitter levels, but by modulating the action of glucocorticoids receptors within the brain.[47] These new findings strongly support the idea that in order to alleviate mood disorders, controlling stress response is an important aspect of treatment. Several genetic and epidemiologic studies have linked excessive stress as well as the inability to efficiently adapt to stress to increased rates of anxiety and depression.[48,49]

# CHRONIC STRESS AND NUTRITION

Deficiencies, toxicities, and lifestyle habits impact the adrenal gland. Deficiencies in vitamin C and vitamin B5, which are essential co-factors in cortisol production and adrenal health, are 2 examples.[50,51] Copper is a mineral that is essential in some bodily enzymatic reactions, but may disrupt adrenal function if levels are too high.[52]

Even relative imbalances between minerals can affect cortisol levels. It has been documented that abnormal ratios of copper to zinc cause adrenal cortex disruption.[42,43] A well-balanced multivitamin can complement a healthy diet to help ensure that vitamin and mineral intake is sufficient to support optimal adrenal function.

The fatty acid content of the diet also contributes considerably to stress response physiology. Relative imbalances of omega-6 fatty acids to omega-3 fatty acids create conditions that favor heightened inflammation and impaired stress response.[53]

For example, a clinical trial examined the effects of parenteral fish oil infusions on the stress response induced by injections of an endotoxin called lipopolysaccharide. The group who received fish oil exhibited a much less severe stress response, with plasma norepinephrine levels remaining 7-fold lower and ACTH levels 4-fold lower than the control group.[54] Upon examination, it was found that the platelet phospholipid omega-3 content had increased substantially in fish oil group, reflecting a lowered omega-6 to omega-3 ratio, a state less conducive of inflammation.

It is believed that a diet high in omega-3 fatty acids may attenuate the effects of chronic stress by limiting the influence of inflammation on stress physiology.[53]

Since cholesterol is a building block of the cortisol hormone, ingestion in the diet of *some* saturated fat is important. However, the liver will synthesize cholesterol, if poor dietary ingestion occurs, from acetate.[55] Of course, too much cholesterol has its drawbacks as well, so a happy medium must be reached. Both extremes of dietary fat ingestion have ill effects on the human body. Life Extension suggests an optimal total cholesterol level of 160–180 mg/dL.

# LIFESTYLE STRATEGIES FOR OVERCOMING CHRONIC STRESS

Thierry Hertoghe, an internationally noted endocrinologist, recommends a few lifestyle modifications that one should adhere to before consideration of natural or pharmacologic therapies. Lifestyle modifications alone for some with mild to moderate forms of impaired stress response may ease symptoms.[41,56,57] Dietary supplements and/or hormone therapy can complement lifestyle modification to resolve adrenal dysfunction.[58]

The obvious recommendation of *avoiding stressful situations and occurrences* goes without saying. If commuter stress, for example, is affecting your body, moving to a home closer to your workplace or finding a job closer to home is an obvious solution. If working third shift causes disruption in your cortisol levels or circadian rhythm resulting in disease, then change your work schedule to eliminate this stressor.[59] Smoking, and *extremely* vigorous or protracted bouts of exhaustive exercise impact the adrenals in a negative way as well.[36,60,61]

With regard to the diurnal biorhythms of cortisol release, a few things increase cortisol at the inappropriate time. The consumption of alcohol and caffeinated beverages such as tea and coffee before bedtime is not recommended as caffeine can increase serum cortisol levels, which is counterproductive during the evening hours when the normal trough is expected.[62] Additionally, caffeine and alcohol affect the release of *melatonin* (melatonin counters some of the negative effects of cortisol), causing a relative reduction in melatonin secretion during the night when a spike is usually seen.[63]

Other therapies such as *acupuncture, traditional Chinese medicine (TCM), ayurvedic medicine, massage therapy, relaxation, yoga,* and even *music therapy* have shown success in stress management.[64–66]

Several published studies suggest that *owning a pet* is associated with improved physical and psychological health.[67,68] For chronically stressed individuals, adopting a dog or cat may help ameliorate some of the symptoms and effects of chronic stress.[69]

# ALTERNATIVE STRESS MANAGEMENT STRATEGIES

## Hormonal Therapy

**Dehydroepiandrosterone.** Dehydroepiandrosterone (DHEA), also an adrenal hormone, counters the action of cortisol in many tissues.[70] The balance between cortisol and DHEA is generally maintained in youth. However, as we age, DHEA levels decline sharply.[71] The unabated action of cortisol in the presence of declining DHEA levels can contribute to stress-related diseases.

Furthermore, DHEA replacement therapy can restore balance between cortisol and DHEA.[72] DHEA has been shown to reduce the negative impact of elevated levels of cortisol on the brain of dementia and Alzheimer's disease study subjects.[73] The heart benefits as well, with a decline in the incidence of coronary artery disease with DHEA supplementation.[74-76] In the context of metabolic syndrome, which is characterized by abdominal obesity, lipid disorders, insulin resistance, and hypertension, DHEA reduces lipid levels, lowers adipose tissue formation, and reduces cardiovascular risk.[77,78]

DHEA also has a positive effect on cognitive function and mood.[79-81] DHEA appears to be beneficial in those with glucose intolerance and diabetes, lowering average serum glucose levels and averting the destructive effects of diabetes.[82,83] There have been reports of cancer risk reduction with DHEA supplementation as well.[84] With regards to age related bone mineral loss, DHEA supplementation has been shown to combat osteoporosis.[85]

A great deal of insight into the function of the adrenal glands can be gained through testing blood levels of DHEA and cortisol. Deviations from the natural rhythm of adrenal function can be detected by an *AM/PM cortisol test*, in which levels of the adrenal hormone are tested early in the morning and early in the evening the same day. A *DHEA sulfate (DHEA-S) blood test* can determine if DHEA levels are sufficient.

Supplemental doses of DHEA typically range from 10–25 mg daily for women and 25–75 mg daily for men, but should always be determined based on DHEA-S blood tests. Life Extension suggests that in order to counter the negative effects of aberrant cortisol production, DHEA-S blood levels should remain between 350–490 μg/dL for men and 275–400 μg/dL for women.

**Melatonin.** The hormone melatonin, which is released from the small gland at the base of the brain called the pineal gland, is known for its relationship with the sleep cycle. Melatonin has an antagonistic effect on cortisol, and the circadian rise in melatonin levels at night correlates with a drop in cortisol.[86] Low levels of melatonin can mean inappropriate and undesirable glucocorticoid signaling during the night when it should be at the lowest.

Chronic, late-night stress, whether physical or psychological, can result in an inappropriately elevated nighttime cortisol level; shift work is an example of such a stressor.[87] This chronic disruption and inappropriate release of cortisol at night may impair the normal circadian corticosteroid output in the morning.[58,88–90]

Melatonin is also a hormone with great penetration into the nucleus of the cells and is one of the most important *antioxidant* hormones as it protects cellular (mitochondrial and nuclear) DNA from damage.[91] Melatonin has been found to affect the levels of cortisol and the balance between DHEA and cortisol in circulation.[88–90] Doses differ in individuals but can start as low as 0.3 mg; some may require up to 10 mg daily.

**Maintaining sex hormone balance.** Imbalances in sex hormones (testosterone for men; estrogen and progesterone for women) may exacerbate the detrimental effects of chronic stress. Some experimental data indicates that having low levels of sex hormones impairs the response to cortisol in the brain.[92] Over time, this may lead to an overcompensatory increase in stress hormone production by the adrenal glands, which could become damaging.

Likewise, human trials have confirmed that steroid hormones exert considerable influence over the stress response. In a small trial of women who were overcoming cocaine addiction, higher progesterone levels were associated with a blunted stress response to a drug cue.[93]

In another clinical trial, menopausal women treated long-term with hormone replacement therapy (HRT) coped with stress better than non-HRT users in an experimental setting.[94]

The biological actions of the sex hormone progesterone within the brain are calming; therefore, age-related declines in progesterone levels may predispose women to anxiety. Specifically, some metabolites of progesterone have been shown to function as ligands at the GABA-α receptor subunit, which is inhibitory upon activation.[95]

Stressed men and women should review Life Extension's Male Hormone Restoration and Female Hormone Restoration protocols.

# NUTRIENTS TO COUNTERACT THE EFFECTS OF STRESS

## B-Complex Vitamins

Several members of the B-vitamin family impact varying aspects of stress response physiology. For example, pantothenic acid is necessary for the synthesis of coenzyme A (CoA), which is integral in the production of cholesterol and in steroid hormone biosynthesis.[96,97] Pantothenic deficiency is rather rare, but can result in adrenal insufficiency.[98–101]

Another correlation between B vitamins was revealed in a clinical trial that found that injecting either ACTH (adrenocorticotropic hormone) or cortisol into healthy subjects for 4 days significantly decreased levels of folic acid and B12.[102] These findings suggest that not only are B vitamins important to promote healthy stress response, but stress itself may lower B-vitamin blood levels. Therefore, B-vitamin supplementation may ameliorate the effects of stress from multiple angles.

## Vitamin C (Ascorbic Acid)

Another crucial vitamin in adrenal function and maintenance of healthy levels of cortisol and DHEA is vitamin C.[103,104] Deficiencies of this vitamin can have profound effects on adrenal function.[105,106] The benefits of vitamin C are multiple, acting as an anti-inflammatory and co-factor in soft tissue synthesis and repair.[107–109]

Ultra-marathon runners who were given 1500 mg vitamin C after a race displayed less dramatic elevations in cortisol and epinephrine levels than is typical after such extreme stress.[60] This same study found that vitamin C was able to suppress inflammation in the runners.

## Minerals

*Calcium*, *magnesium*, *sodium*, and *potassium* are all macro elements. A macro element means that they are found in our bodies in greater quantities than other elements or minerals. These 4 macro elements are important in supporting and maintaining balanced adrenal function[106,110] as well as in the formation and release of adrenal hormones.

*Manganese*, *zinc*, *chromium*, and *selenium* are some of the trace elements that have an impact on the function of the adrenal glands. Research shows that deficiencies in these trace elements can have a negative effect on adrenal function.[111–113]

## L-Theanine

L-theanine, an amino acid found exclusively in *green tea*, has traditionally been used to enhance relaxation and improve concentration and learning ability.[114–117]

L-theanine is chemically related to the neurotransmitter *glutamate* and binds to glutamate receptors in the brain.[118] Unlike glutamate, however, which can cause a state called *excitotoxicity* that can destroy nerve cells, L-theanine *protects* brain cells against excitotoxicity, calming the nerve networks in the brain.[119–121]

Animal studies verify the behavioral benefits of these biochemical effects. In vitro studies show that L-theanine reduces electrical activity associated with anxiety.[122] L-theanine reduces evidence of anxiety and depression in several different animal models of stress.[123,124] In one animal model, L-theanine led to decreases in nearly all frequencies of brainwave activity, indicating a state of calmness and relaxation.[122] Moreover, L-theanine has been shown to act synergistically with the GABAergic drug midazolam, a relative of *Valium*®.[124]

Brainwave studies have shed some light on the mechanism by which L-theanine may appease anxiety. In one study, healthy subjects took a soft drink containing green tea enriched with L-theanine while their brainwave power was measured.[125] Power was initially reduced in all frequencies and areas during the first hour, indicating relaxation. Later changes indicated both an increase in mental performance and a higher degree of relaxation. In this case, L-theanine seemed to produce desirable increases in attention accompanied by durable relaxation—meaning subjects could concentrate better without being distracted by anxiety.

Another brainwave study demonstrated that L-theanine significantly increased activity in the frequency band associated with relaxation without inducing drowsiness.[126] A third trial concluded that L-theanine plays a general role in sustaining attention during a long-term difficult task.[127]

Another way to assess stress and anxiety is by measuring vital signs such as heart rate and salivary content of certain proteins that are increased during stress. Japanese researchers did just that with 12 subjects during a mental arithmetic test given as an acute stressor.[128] Results showed that the supplement reduced heart rate response to the acute stress task compared with placebo. In addition, heart rate variability was improved, a sign that L-theanine was modulating the sympathetic nervous system, or "fight-or-flight" response.

## Omega-3 Fatty Acids (Fish Oil)

Research indicates that intake of fish oil or omega-3 essential fatty acids (n-3 EFA) can act in an *adaptogenic* fashion to help ameliorate the effects of stress.[129,130]

Omega-3 fatty acids balance the effects of omega-6 metabolism.[131–133] Fatty acid balance is also critical for glucocorticoid hormone receptor function.[134–136] Omega-3 fatty acids have been documented to be successful in treating those suffering from depression and anxiety disorders, which themselves can be a consequence or inducer of stress.[137–139]

## Phosphatidylserine

The phospholipid phosphatidylserine (PS), which is found in cell membranes, is a critical component for healthy cellular communication. Several studies have shown that a diet rich in PS is able to balance the HPA axis and limit the negative consequences of overactivation of the adrenal cortex.[140–144] PS also helps attenuate the increase in cortisol levels during periods of intense, acute stress.[145]

## Herbal Therapies

**Sedative herbs.** Sedative herbs such as hops, passionflower, poppy, and valerian can provide calming effects to reduce stress. Herbal *lemon balm* (*Melissa officinalis*) has been shown in a number of studies to reduce stress. This is yet another herb that has shown benefit in reducing negative effects of stress on the body.[146–148]

In a recent small clinical trial including 20 stressed volunteers, a standardized lemon balm extract (Cyracos®) was shown to significantly combat anxiety symptoms and insomnia.[149] The extract *"reduced anxiety manifestations by 18%, ameliorated anxiety-associated symptoms by 15% and lowered insomnia by 42%."*

**Adaptogenic herbs.** A class of herbs known as *adaptogens* are helpful in regulation of the HPA axis. Nikolai Lazarev, a noted Russian pharmacologist during the cold war era, coined the term "adaptogenic herb" to describe about 25 of the hundreds of medicinal herbs having particular properties.[150] These properties are unique to this class of herbs making them important for human health.

To be classified as an adaptogen, herbs must have the following 3 properties: no toxicity associated with them; have a normalizing ability (ie, the same dose can raise or lower physiologic properties), and the mechanisms by which the herbs carry out their effects must be due to more than one physiologic or pharmacologic mechanism.[9,151–153] Unlike any other compound, adaptogens *condition* the body to respond favorably to stress.

Adaptogenic herbs can become an important supplement to support a healthy HPA axis stress response. The list of adaptogenic herbs includes about 25 known, and

of these several have been studied for their effects on the HPA system, including ginseng (*Panax ginseng*), Eleuthero (*Eleutherococcus senticosus*), Rhodiola (*Rhodiola rosea*), Cordyceps (*Cordyceps sinensis*), and Ashwaghanda (*Withania somnifera*), to name a few.[9,150,154–156]

**Rhodiola.** The adaptogenic herb Rhodiola (*Rhodiola rosea*) has demonstrated improvements in both physical endurance and cognitive performance in many studies.[156–158] Its ability to reduce fatigue associated with stress is documented in well-designed research papers.[156,159,160] The apparent mechanism of action of Rhodiola is related to its ability to assist neurotransmitter transport in the brain and blunt catecholamine release.[161,162]

In a large, phase 3, placebo-controlled clinical trial conducted in Sweden in 2009, studying participants aged 20–55 years with a diagnosis of stress-related fatigue[159] received either Rhodiola extract or placebo. Subjects taking the Rhodiola extract had significantly lower cortisol responses to chronic stress than the placebo recipients—as a result, they had lower scores on scales of burnout and improved performance on cognitive tests.

**Ashwagandha.** Ashwagandha, also known as *Withania somnifera*, is an important ayurvedic medicinal herb. It has many uses in traditional Indian medicine such as treatments for stress, fatigue, pain, diabetes, GI and rheumatologic disorders.[163] Ashwagandha has shown promise in neuroprotection as scientists have discovered that this adaptogenic herb prevents damage to neurons and improves neurologic function in the face of stress.[164–166] Additionally, data suggest that Ashwagandha may reduce the harmful effects of stress on male reproductive capacity.[167]

A double-blind, randomized, placebo-controlled clinical trial assessed the effects of ashwagandha in 130 chronically stressed subjects.[168] Over a 60-day period, doses ranging from 125–500 mg daily of a patented ashwagandha extract (Sensoril®) significantly improved scores on a standardized measurement of stress intensity and favorably modulated several biomarkers associated with cardiovascular health, including C-reactive protein and blood pressure. Moreover, at the end of the study period, subjects that received 500 mg of ashwagandha daily had cortisol levels nearly 30% lower than subjects who took a placebo, and their DHEA-S levels were significantly higher as well.

**Ginseng.** Probably the most recognized of the adaptogen herbs in the West is ginseng (*Panax ginseng* [*P. ginseng*]). There are 11 species of this medicinal herb, *P. ginseng* being among the most widely studied.[169,170] American ginseng (*Panax quinquefolius*) is another species within the Panax genus that shares medicinal properties.[171] Siberian ginseng (*Eleutherococcus senticosus*), while not technically a true ginseng botanical, has similar beneficial properties and is closely related to the Panax family of plants.[172]

A wealth of studies show stress-reducing properties of true ginseng and the other ginseng-related herbals.[173,174] For example, the isolated polysaccharides from *P. ginseng* have demonstrated antifatigue properties in one study.[175]

American ginseng extract shows a reduction in oxidative endothelial damage due to diabetes.[176,177] Antidepressive effects and the positive modulation that benefits the HPA axis is outlined in a research paper on protective ginsenosides in Panax and other ginseng plants showing usefulness in the management of chronic stress.[178,179]

**Licorice (*Glycyrrhiza glabra* and *G. uralensis*).** A mainstay in TCM, licorice extracts may be of benefit for those who have reached the exhaustion stage and are no longer producing sufficient cortisol.

Licorice has the ability to decrease the breakdown or metabolism of hydrocortisone by the liver, thus increasing the amount of cortisol in circulation and reducing the strain on the adrenal glands to produce it.[180] The combination of low doses of licorice with supplemental DHEA may help balance the HPA axis.[181]

It is important to understand that licorice may not be ideal for everyone dealing with day-to-day stress. In high doses over prolonged periods, licorice may cause electrolyte imbalance (hypokalemia) and elevations in blood pressure, a syndrome called hypermineralocorticoidism.[182] Due to its ability to increase cortisol levels, licorice is best reserved for those individuals who are experiencing fatigue due to chronic stress and also have low cortisol levels.

**Holy basil.** Increased cortisol and blood glucose levels are common in people with disorders of the adrenal gland.[183] Increased blood glucose is also seen in people receiving chronic glucocorticoid treatment.[184] *Ocimum sanctum*, or holy basil, is an herb widely grown in India that is known for its ability to control blood sugar.[185] A study in mice showed that extracts of *Ocimum sanctum* decreased serum concentrations of both cortisol and glucose. This study suggested that *Ocimum sanctum* extract could potentially regulate diabetes mellitus that has developed secondary to corticosteroid treatment.[186] Ocimumosides A and B, which are novel compounds isolated from an extract of holy basil leaves, were shown to normalize

hyperglycemia, plasma cortisol levels, and adrenal hypertrophy in rats.[187]

Furthermore, clinical trials in humans have also shown the benefits of holy basil extract for improving immune function as well as decreasing stress and depression associated with anxiety. Studies in healthy human subjects showed that treatment with 300 mg of holy basil extract for 4 weeks increased antibody levels and cells in the immune system.[188] In a clinical trial, 35 subjects with generalized anxiety disorder were treated with 500 mg of holy basil extract twice daily for 60 days. At the end of the study, these subjects showed decreased stress and depression, improved attention, and an increased ability to adapt to changes.[189]

***Bacopa monnieri.*** The herb *Bacopa monnieri* is used in the classical Indian medicinal system of ayurveda as a tonic for the nervous system and is known to promote mental health.[190] It has also been shown to possess antianxiety properties. Experiments have shown that rats fed with extracts of *Bacopa* showed decreased anxiety, which was comparable to that in rats fed lorazepam, a common antianxiety drug. The *Bacopa*-fed rats did not show any adverse effects on physical activity.[190] *Bacopa* possesses adaptogenic properties and evidence shows that it can normalize levels of corticosterone and noradrenaline in rodents exposed to stressful conditions.[191] In a clinical trial on the mental and emotional effects of *Bacopa* in the elderly, 54 subjects aged 65 years or older were given 300 mg *Bacopa* or placebo for 12 weeks. Subjects receiving *Bacopa* showed significantly reduced anxiety and improved cognitive performance.[57] At the time of this writing, a clinical trial is currently underway in Australia to test the effects of *Bacopa* and another herb, pycnogenol, in reducing cognitive decline with aging. The trial will evaluate the effects of *Bacopa* supplementation for up to a year on mood, cognition, blood pressure, inflammation, and oxidative stress, among other tests.[192]

***Schisandra chinensis.*** Exposure to chronic stress leads to sustained increases in cortisol levels and deleterious effects on various body systems.[193] *Schisandra chinensis* is traditionally used in East Asia for its antistress properties. It was found that *Schisandra* reduced the levels of corticosterone and glucose and preserved the structure of the adrenal cortex in rats exposed to stress.[194] Athletes exposed to acute exercise show increased levels of cortisol and nitric oxide (which helps in conducting signals between cells) in the blood and saliva. However, extremely well-trained athletes who are exposed to chronic exercise-related stress do not show such increases. When such subjects are given *Schisandra*, they start showing increased cortisol and nitric oxide levels, meaning they further adapted to heavy physical loading. Thus, adaptogens such as *Schisandra* may increase the body's ability to respond to stress stimuli.[195]

*Cordyceps sinensis.*   Oxidative stress damages cells and is associated with various health disorders. *Cordyceps sinensis* is a type of mushroom used in Chinese medicine that has been found to boost the immune system and possesses antitumor and antioxidant properties.[196] An experimental study showed that *Cordyceps* extract stimulated corticosterone production in mice.[197] Another study found that orally administered *Cordyceps* extract increased swimming capacity and reduced fatigue in mice.[198] Also, the weight changes in adrenal glands, which are considered a stress index, were suppressed in rats following a 48-hour stress period.[198] Furthermore, a polysaccharide isolated from *Cordyceps* was found to reduce plasma glucose levels in diabetic and hyperglycemic mice.[199]

In a clinical trial, *Cordyceps* powder was provided for 2 weeks to sedentary male subjects who then underwent exhaustive exercise. Exercise tolerance and catecholamine and cortisol levels were compared before and after *Cordyceps* treatment. Subjects receiving *Cordyceps* showed improved exercise tolerance, increased levels of epinephrine and norepinephrine, and a slight decrease in cortisol levels. Overall, *Cordyceps* supplementation appeared to improve energy generation and reduce fatigue.[200]

## Life Extension Suggestions

Maintaining balance in today's stressful world requires a multimodal approach that encompasses healthy eating habits, getting plenty of exercise, and using innovative natural ingredients to support the body's natural adaptive abilities. Regular blood testing of DHEA-S as well as morning and evening cortisol levels help ensure that stress hormones remain in balance.

### Hormonal Therapies
- **DHEA:** 15–25 mg daily for women (depending on blood test results); 25–75 mg daily for men (depending on blood test results)
- **Melatonin:** 0.3–5 mg before bed (sometimes up to 10 mg)

- **Bioidentical hormone replacement therapy:** Refer to Life Extension's Male Hormone Restoration or Female Hormone Restoration protocols

### Nutritional Therapies
- **B-complex vitamin**
  - **Thiamine (B1):** 75–125 mg daily
  - **Riboflavin (B2):** 50 mg daily
  - **Niacin (B3):** 50–190 mg daily
  - **Folate** (preferably as L-methylfolate): 400–1000 mcg daily
  - **Vitamin B12:** 300–600 mcg daily
  - **Biotin:** 300–3000 mcg daily
  - **Pantothenic acid:** 100–600 mg daily
- **Vitamin C:** 1000–2000 mg daily
- **Fish oil** (with olive polyphenols): 2000–4000 mg daily
- **Phosphatidylserine:** 100–600 mg daily
- **L-theanine:** 200–400 mg daily
- **Calcium:** 200–1200 mg daily
- **Magnesium:** 140–500 elemental mg of highly-absorbable magnesium
- **Zinc:** 30 mg daily
- **Chromium (Crominex™):** 500 mcg daily
- **Selenium:** 200 mcg daily
- **Manganese:** 1 mg daily
- **Comprehensive multivitamin formula:** per label instructions (*Note*: some of the nutrients mentioned in the protocol [ie, zinc, selenium, manganese, and vitamin C] can be obtained by taking a high-quality multivitamin/mineral supplement).

### Herbal Therapies
- **Lemon balm extract:** 300–600 mg daily
- **Valerian root:** 400–1000 mg daily
- **Licorice root:** 450–900 mg daily (for those with low cortisol levels)

### Adaptogens
- *Rhodiola rosea*, standardized extract: 250–500 mg daily
- **Ashwagandha**, standardized extract (Sensoril®): 125–250 mg daily
- **Panax ginseng**, standardized extract: varying doses
- **Holy basil** (standardized to 2.5% triterpene acids): 600 mg daily
- *Schisandra chinensis* extract (standardized to 9% total schisandrins): 250 mg daily
- **Standardized blend of bacopa, ashwagandha, and cordyceps extracts:** 516 mg daily

In addition, the following *blood testing* resources may be helpful:

- Cortisol AM/PM
- Cortisol, 24 hour (urine test)
- Female Comprehensive Hormone panel or Male Comprehensive Hormone panel; or Female panel or Male panel; or Dehydroepiandrosterone sulfate (DHEA-S)
- Omega Score®

## REFERENCES

References available at: www.lef.org/dpt5/ch122

# 123

---

# *Stroke*

---

Stroke is a major killer of Americans, claiming a life every 4 minutes, and is a leading cause of disability.[1,2] According to a 2012 report from the American Heart Association, about half of stroke survivors 65 or older had some difficulty with movement on one side of their body and over a quarter were institutionalized or in a nursing home 6 months following their stroke.[1]

A stroke is the result of loss of blood flow, and subsequently oxygen, to part of the brain. Stroke can be caused by either blockage, or rupture and subsequent hemorrhage (bleeding), of a blood vessel in the brain.[3]

About 54% of stroke deaths happen outside of the hospital. This is partly because many stroke victims do not get to the hospital in time to receive potentially life-saving treatment.[1,4]

Receiving *emergency treatment within 4.5 hours* of stroke onset can mean the difference between life and death.[5,6] Unfortunately, one study showed that the median time to emergency department admission was *16 hours* after onset of stroke symptoms. Only about half of the patients in this study were able to identify one stroke symptom.[7] Knowledge of signs and symptoms of stroke can help victims and their caregivers obtain emergency treatment in a timely manner.[1,2]

In addition to knowing how to react if stroke symptoms occur, Life Extension emphasizes the need for *all* aging individuals to take *proactive stroke prevention* measures. Also, recognition of an epidemic of "silent" strokes is critical. Silent strokes, or mini-strokes, do not cause outright stroke symptoms, but are associated with cognitive dysfunction and increase risk for overt stroke. Estimates indicate that over a quarter of the elderly population has experienced a silent stroke.[8–10] Being aware of and taking steps to modify factors that increase stroke risk is paramount in reducing the likelihood of having a stroke or silent stroke.[10,11] In one study, over 40% of possible stroke patients were unable to identify one stroke risk factor.[12]

Maintaining optimal *blood pressure* levels is one of the most important ways to minimize stroke risk. For example, research suggests that people with blood pressure lower than 120/80 mmHg are about half as likely to suffer a stroke as those with higher blood pressure. It has also been reported that each 20/10 mmHg increase over

115/75 mmHg *doubles the risk* of several vascular complications, including heart attack, heart failure, stroke, and kidney disease.[13] Similarly, having *impaired glucose tolerance* nearly doubles stroke risk. *Low levels of HDL-cholesterol* ("good cholesterol") and *heart rhythm irregularities* also significantly increase chances of having a stroke, and people with *sleep apnea* have twice the risk.[1]

The good news is that dietary and lifestyle management strategies coupled with natural compounds and certain drugs can target stroke risk factors. Also, comprehensive *blood testing* can help identify correctable factors involved in stroke and thus help guide prevention strategies.

This protocol will review the different types of stroke and their causes, risk factors, signs, and symptoms. Conventional treatments will be discussed, and strategies to mitigate stroke risk using integrative and scientifically studied natural modalities will be examined.

## TYPES OF STROKE

There are 2 main kinds of stroke, *ischemic stroke*, which makes up about 87% of all strokes, and *hemorrhagic stroke*.[1] *Transient ischemic attacks (TIAs)* and *silent strokes* are less severe types of stroke, but both can have long-term consequences such as memory impairment.[14–18]

### Ischemic Stroke

An ischemic stroke arises from blockage of blood supply to part of the brain. There are two kinds of ischemic stroke: *thrombotic* and *embolic*.

**Thrombotic stroke.** A thrombotic stroke is caused by a blood clot forming in a blood vessel leading to or in the brain and disrupting blood flow to part of the brain.[19]

**Embolic stroke.** Embolic stroke occurs when a blood vessel supplying the brain is blocked by circulating debris (ie, an embolus) that originated elsewhere in the body, such as when clots form on artificial heart valves or in the upper chamber of the heart. Embolic strokes are typically caused by blood clots.[19]

### Hemorrhagic Stroke

Strokes caused by blood vessel(s) breaking and leaking blood into the brain are called hemorrhagic strokes. Hemorrhagic strokes account for about 13% of all strokes, but are responsible for more than 30% of all stroke deaths. There are two types of hemorrhagic stroke: *intracerebral and subarachnoid*.[1,19]

**Intracerebral hemorrhage.** Intracerebral hemorrhage is the most common form of hemorrhagic stroke. It occurs when a blood vessel within the brain ruptures and leaks blood into the surrounding tissue. High blood pressure is the primary cause of this type of hemorrhage. Most intracerebral hemorrhages are accompanied by a sudden onset of symptoms, such as loss of consciousness, nausea or vomiting, numbness of the face, or severe headache with no known cause.[20]

**Subarachnoid hemorrhage.** Subarachnoid hemorrhage is usually caused by an *aneurysm*, a bulge in a blood vessel wall, bursting in a large artery on or near the delicate membrane surrounding the brain. Blood spills into the area around the brain, which is filled with protective *cerebrospinal fluid (CSF)*. This causes the brain to be surrounded by blood-contaminated CSF. While there are no warning signs for a subarachnoid hemorrhage, symptoms could include a sudden severe headache often described by patients as the "worst headache of my life." At least 30% of subarachnoid hemorrhages lead to a condition called *vasospasm*, which occurs when blood vessels irritated by excess blood begin to spasm and narrow in size. This makes it difficult to supply the brain with enough blood to survive.

## Transient Ischemic Attack

A transient ischemic attack (TIA), or "mini stroke," can cause symptoms similar to a stroke, but they usually last only a few hours and are resolved within 24 hours. An example of a symptom shared by both stroke and TIA is visual abnormalities such as sudden vision loss. Since TIAs are short (ie, transient), they do not result in significant permanent brain damage.[16,21] However, history of TIA increases future stroke risk.[22,23]

## Silent Stroke

Silent strokes lack overt stroke-like symptoms and commonly go unnoticed.[24] However, silent strokes typically cause lesions in the brain, which can be detected using imaging such as magnetic resonance imaging (MRI). These lesions, known as *brain infarcts*, are associated with age-dependent memory loss and reduced brain volume.[14] Studies suggest that silent stroke is a *hidden epidemic* among Americans, with up to 40% of people over age 70 exhibiting signs.[10] It is estimated that silent strokes are 5 times more common than symptomatic strokes.[15]

A silent stroke differs from a TIA in that TIA symptoms are detectable but usually only last a short time.[16] Silent strokes can be the result of minor hemorrhages, or they could be lacunar infarcts, in which a penetrating artery becomes occluded, resulting in lesions in the brain's white matter.[25,26] In a study of 2040 stroke-free subjects with an average age of 62, over 10% showed signs of silent stroke when examined by MRI, even though they were not aware of any symptoms.[18]

## COMPLICATIONS OF STROKE

Cognitive abilities, perception, coordination, speech, and balance can be impaired by a stroke. Paralysis is also possible. The specific effects depend on the location and extent of brain damage. For example, since the right hemisphere of the brain controls movement of the left side of the body, a stroke in the right hemisphere can cause paralysis on the left side of the body. A stroke in the cerebellum can cause problems with balance and coordination, and a brainstem stroke can damage involuntary "life-support" functions such as breathing, heart rate, and could lead to death. The 5 most common complications of stroke that render many patients disabled are aphasia, pain, pseudobulbar affect, vascular dementia, and paralysis/spasticity.[28–30]

### Aphasia

About 25% of all stroke survivors experience aphasia, or impairment of the ability to speak and understand spoken or written language. Aphasia is the result of stroke-induced damage to brain regions involved in speech and language processing. Many patients with aphasia benefit from speech/language therapy.[29,31]

### Pain

Stroke victims may experience pain immediately following a stroke or weeks to months later. Some stroke victims experience local or mechanical pain that may be isolated to joints. This type of pain is caused by damaged muscle or other soft tissue. Other victims may experience a chronic central pain caused by damage to the brain. Central pain occurs because the damaged brain does not interpret pain messages properly and may register even the slightest touch as painful.[30]

Brain Regions and Their Corresponding Functions

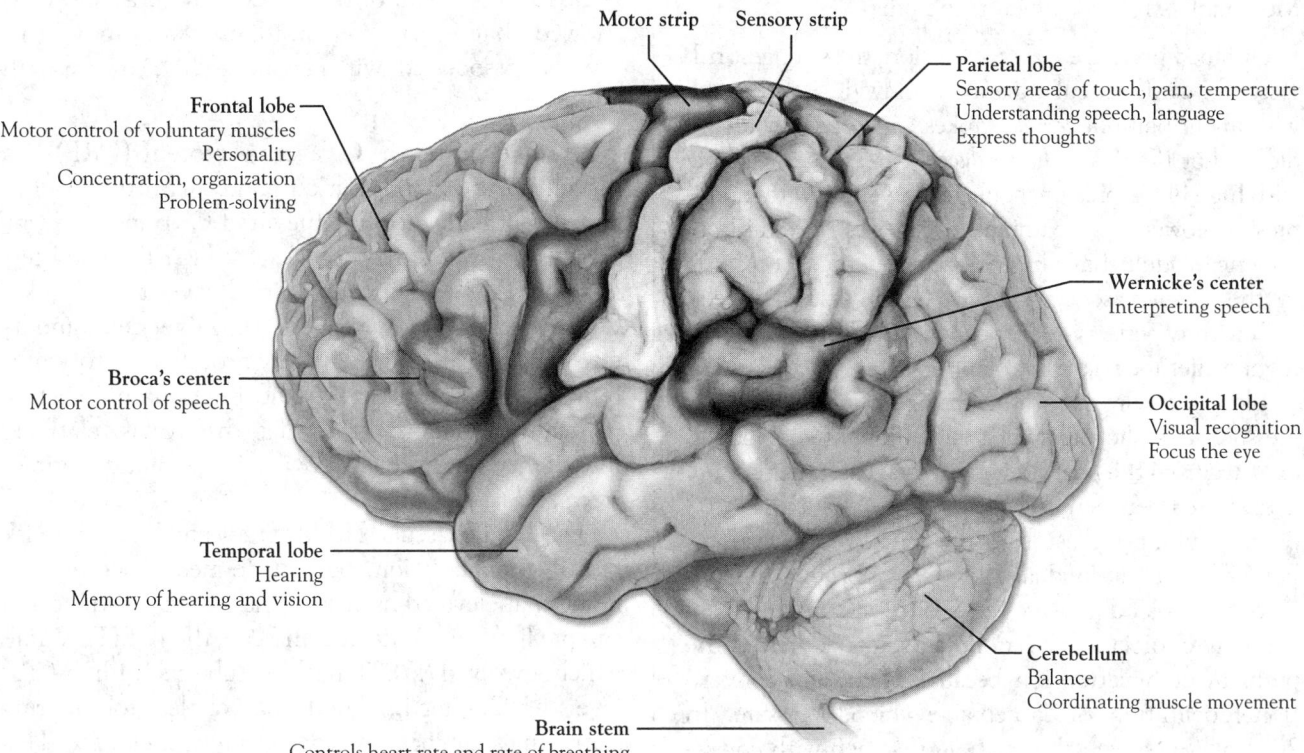

Motor strip    Sensory strip

**Parietal lobe**
Sensory areas of touch, pain, temperature
Understanding speech, language
Express thoughts

**Frontal lobe**
Motor control of voluntary muscles
Personality
Concentration, organization
Problem-solving

**Wernicke's center**
Interpreting speech

**Broca's center**
Motor control of speech

**Occipital lobe**
Visual recognition
Focus the eye

**Temporal lobe**
Hearing
Memory of hearing and vision

**Cerebellum**
Balance
Coordinating muscle movement

**Brain stem**
Controls heart rate and rate of breathing

## Pseudobulbar Affect

A stroke that damages areas in the brainstem and cerebral cortex can cause a condition called pseudobulbar affect, which results in uncontrollable episodes of laughing or crying that often disrupt normal social interaction. Up to 52% of stroke victims report at least some symptoms of pseudobulbar affect.[32,33]

## Vascular Dementia

It is estimated that almost one-fifth of stroke victims will develop problems with their mental and cognitive abilities.[28] This loss of intellectual ability is called vascular dementia and results from tissue damage caused by reduced blood flow to the brain. Evidence suggests that stroke doubles the risk of dementia.[34] Common symptoms of vascular dementia include memory loss, confusion, and decreased attention span.[35]

## Paralysis and Spasticity

Some stroke victims experience complete paralysis (ie, the inability to voluntarily move muscles). In other cases, patients may experience a tightening or stiffness of muscles that impairs movement of the arms and/or legs. This condition, called spasticity, occurs because messages from parts of the brain to

muscles are not properly conveyed.[36] In some cases, the damaged brain sends signals to muscles to contract for long periods of time, causing painful muscle spasms similar to severe cramping.[37]

## RISK FACTORS FOR STROKE

### Nonmodifiable Risk Factors

Age, gender, race, ethnicity, and genetics have all been identified as nonmodifiable risk factors for stroke, with age being the most important.[38–40]

**Age.** The stroke rate more than doubles in men and women for each 10 years over age 65.

**Gender.** Stroke rates are higher in men than women, but more women die of stroke each year.

**Race and ethnicity.** Stroke rates vary extensively among different racial groups. For example, African Americans are statistically twice as likely to die from strokes as whites. Stroke incidence has risen sharply in Chinese and Japanese populations. Specifically, stroke leads heart disease as a cause of death in Japan.

**Genetics/hereditary factors.** The Framingham Offspring Study demonstrated that family history of stroke is a strong predictor of future stroke risk.

## Modifiable Risk Factors

Modifiable stroke risk factors include:

**High blood pressure.** Hypertension, the strongest risk factor for cardiovascular disease worldwide, is associated with about half of *ischemic* strokes.[41] Also, estimates indicate that 17–28% of *hemorrhagic* strokes among people with high blood pressure could be prevented with blood-pressure-lowering treatment.[42] About one-third of American adults have high blood pressure.[43] According to the Cardiovascular Lifetime Risk Pooling Project, men with hypertension throughout middle age have the highest lifetime risk for stroke.[44]

Blood pressure is measured as systolic and diastolic pressure. Systolic pressure is measured when blood is expelled from the heart as it contracts. Diastolic pressure is measured between contractions. Systolic is the "top" or "first" number, diastolic is the "bottom" or "second." For most aging individuals, Life Extension recommends an optimal blood pressure target of 115/75 mmHg.

Many clinicians have not adequately addressed the problem of hypertension because of the lax conventional definition of "acceptable" blood pressure. In 2012, it was shown that men and women with consistent blood pressure below 120/80 mmHg had the lowest lifetime risk of stroke and cerebrovascular disease.[44] It has also been reported that each 20/10 mmHg increase over 115/75 mmHg *doubles the risk* of several vascular complications, including heart attack, heart failure, stroke, and kidney disease.[13] Unfortunately, studies have shown that some medical professionals are unlikely to aggressively treat hypertension until blood pressure levels reach 160/90 mmHg.[45]

Elevated blood pressure can contribute significantly to *endothelial dysfunction*, which is impairment of normal function of the *endothelium*, the delicate cellular lining of the inside of blood vessels.[46,47] High blood pressure can alter the endothelium and decrease the motility of the arteries and stiffen the arterial wall.[48] When arteries become stiff, they no longer contract and dilate normally, placing stress on the heart.[49] High blood pressure also contributes to atherosclerosis and blood clot formation. Refer to the High Blood Pressure protocol for more information.

**Elevated homocysteine.** Homocysteine is an amino acid derivative that can damage blood vessels. High homocysteine levels have been associated with an increased risk of stroke recurrence (1.74-fold) and all-cause death (1.75-fold).[50] Homocysteine disrupts endothelial tissue and inhibits the growth of new endothelial cells, which contributes to atherosclerotic plaque formation. Homocysteine can also disrupt the function of brain cells and compromise their survival.[51]

Life Extension recommends an optimal homocysteine level of <8 µmol/L. One comprehensive review showed that every 2.5 µmol/L increase above this level is associated with about a 20% increase in stroke risk.[52]

**C-reactive protein.** C-reactive protein (CRP) is a protein in the blood that correlates with the level of systemic inflammation.[53] Elevated CRP measured by a *high-sensitivity C-reactive protein (hsCRP)* blood test is associated with incidence and severity of stroke. C-reactive protein is synthesized by liver cells, and its rate of synthesis is regulated by proinflammatory proteins such as interleukin-6 and interleukin-1. While in healthy humans the level of hsCRP is relatively low, it becomes elevated with inflammation, infection, and tissue damage.[54]

The Cardiovascular Health Study and Emerging Risk Factors Collaboration, both performed a decade ago, found that elevated hsCRP is a risk factor for stroke and can predict stroke outcome. In 2008, the JUPITER trial, which involved 17802 healthy subjects with hsCRP levels ≥ 2.0 mg/L, found that cholesterol-lowering statin drugs significantly reduced stroke incidence. This may be due in part to an anti-inflammatory effect of statins.[55,56] In a group of Chinese patients, high levels of CRP (>3 mg/L) 15 days before ischemic stroke onset independently predicted death within 3 months.[53] Another study involving 467 subjects found that elevated (highest versus lowest quartile) hsCRP was associated with a more than 4-fold increase in risk of death over 4 years of follow-up after first ischemic stroke.[56]

The plasma level of hsCRP is a powerful predictor of endothelial dysfunction, stroke, and vascular death in individuals without known cardiovascular disease. Levels of hsCRP higher than 1.5 mg/L are associated with an increased risk of death after ischemic stroke.[57] Elevated levels of hsCRP may also be a predictor of secondary cerebrovascular events after an initial stroke.[58] Life Extension recommends an optimal blood level for hsCRP of <0.55 mg/L in men and <1.50 mg/L in women.

**Excess fibrinogen.** Fibrinogen is a component of blood involved in the clotting/coagulation process. It is converted through enzymatic reactions into the protein fibrin, which binds with other proteins to form a clot. High levels of fibrinogen are associated with cerebrovascular disease, even when other known risk factors such as cholesterol are normal.[59] A study in a Taiwanese population indicated that excess fibrinogen is a major independent predictor of future stroke risk.[60] Life Extension recommends an optimal fibrinogen blood level of 295–369 mg/dL.

**High LDL cholesterol.** Cholesterol, found in all the body's cells, is important for normal cellular function. Cholesterol is carried to and from cells by lipoproteins (high-density lipoprotein [HDL] and low-density lipoprotein [LDL]). LDL ("bad cholesterol") can contribute to buildup of plaque in arterial walls.[61] Studies indicate that high levels of LDL and triglycerides are associated with increased risk of stroke and TIA. Statins, drugs that lower LDL cholesterol, reduce stroke risk by as much as 18% and reduce stroke-related deaths by 13%.[62] High levels of HDL ("good cholesterol") are associated with reduced risk of stroke or cerebrovascular disease.[63]

Cholesterol-lowering statin drugs not only reduce the incidence of first stroke, but also reduce chances of having a second, often more debilitating stroke. Statin use is recommended in those who have already experienced a stroke or TIA and have an LDL cholesterol level of ≥100 mg/dL, with the aim of reaching an optimal level of 70 mg/dL.[64] Life Extension recommends optimal HDL levels ≥50 mg/dL. Refer to the Cholesterol Management protocol for more information.

**Insulin resistance/glucose intolerance.** Insulin resistance is a metabolic disorder characterized by reduced sensitivity to the hormone insulin, which regulates blood sugar levels. Insulin signals cells to uptake glucose from the blood. In conditions where insulin levels are low or insulin does not function properly, such as diabetes, blood sugar levels are abnormal. Insulin resistance occurs when insulin levels are normal but its ability to regulate blood sugar is impaired. This results in elevated blood sugar. The insulin-resistant state is associated with hypertension, endothelial dysfunction, abnormal fibrinogen levels, and increased concentrations of LDL particles in the bloodstream.[65]

In a multiethnic, population-based study of nondiabetic individuals, insulin resistance was associated with a 2.8-fold increased occurrence of a first ischemic stroke.[66] This result corroborates previous observational findings that insulin resistance is an independent risk factor for stroke. In the Helsinki Policeman Study, which involved 970 healthy men aged 34–64, the rate of stroke incidence was 2-fold higher in diabetes-free patients with higher insulin concentrations (top tertile) compared to those with lower insulin concentrations over a 22-year follow-up.[65,67] Refer to the Diabetes protocol for more information.

**Sleep apnea.** Many aging individuals suffer from episodic breathing lapses during sleep. This is called sleep apnea. The most common form of sleep apnea occurs when the upper airway collapses (partially or completely) for intermittent periods. This results in characteristic gasping or choking during nighttime breathing.[68]

Sleep apnea deprives its victims of oxygen during sleep. Lack of oxygen due to sleep apnea is associated with inflammation, endothelial dysfunction, and oxidative stress. All of these factors compromise the integrity of blood vessels, increasing the likelihood a stroke-causing blood clot will form. Sleep apnea is independently associated with significantly increased stroke risk, ranging from about 1.5-fold to over 4-fold across several studies, but also may aggravate stroke risk factors such as high blood pressure, atrial fibrillation, and diabetes.[68] One study showed that people with sleep apnea are more likely to die within the first month following stroke than those who breathe normally during sleep.[69]

Many people with sleep apnea may not know they have it. Participating in a clinical sleep study is the most accurate way to assess sleep quality. Identification and correction of sleep apnea can significantly reduce overall cardiovascular risk.[70]

## STROKE DIAGNOSIS AND TREATMENT

Ischemic stroke damage is time dependent. Following initial arterial occlusion, cell death cascades to greater areas of the brain until blood flow is reestablished.[71] Hemorrhagic stroke damage is also time dependent. As blood continues to leak from the original rupture site, the area of the brain damaged by the hematoma increases.[72] It is therefore critical to treat stroke victims as fast as possible to avoid widespread brain damage.

Once a stroke victim has arrived at the hospital, physicians use imaging tests to determine the type of stroke (ischemic or hemorrhagic) that occurred.[73] Determining the type of stroke is critical because the medications used to treat ischemic stroke will not work for hemorrhagic stroke, and vice versa.[74]

### Brain Imaging

Brain imaging can help detect strokes and determine their nature.

**Computerized tomography angiography (CTA).** CTA is utilized to look for aneurysms, arterial and venous malformations, as well as narrowing of arteries in the neck and brain.

**Computerized tomography (CT).** CT is a medical imaging tool that can be used to identify cerebral hemorrhaging.

**Magnetic resonance imaging (MRI).** MRI techniques can aid in the diagnosis of stroke.[75]

**Magnetic resonance angiography (MRA).** MRA uses a magnetic field, radio waves, and a dye injected into the veins to evaluate arteries in the neck and brain.

## Emergency Treatment of Ischemic Stroke

Treatment of ischemic stroke *within 4.5 hours of symptom onset* is critical. Studies show that rapid dissolution of the blood clot within 4.5 hours of symptom onset can dramatically reduce brain damage.[74] Unfortunately, many ischemic stroke patients do not get to the hospital and receive the appropriate thrombolytic agent until significant brain damage has already occurred.[7]

**Intravenous injection of tissue plasminogen activator (tPA).** tPA is approved by the Food and Drug Administration to treat acute ischemic stroke.[76] tPA is an enzyme that converts plasminogen to plasmin—the major enzyme that stimulates clot breakdown. It helps decrease ischemic injury and salvage brain tissue. tPA administration within 4.5 hours of symptom onset is a first choice therapy among patients with no contraindications.[5,6] Unfortunately, studies indicate that only 2–8% of ischemic stroke patients receive this potentially life-saving treatment.[77] One study found that 18% of these treatment omissions are avoidable.[78] In fact, in many instances, even eligible patients may be denied tPA treatment.[77] Sadly, bureaucratic barriers, such as legal liability concerns and insufficient insurance reimbursement, contribute to these deadly denials.[79] Another reason often cited for tPA avoidance during acute ischemic stroke treatment is bleeding risk. Physicians often hesitate to treat ischemic stroke victims with tPA if the patient has been taking warfarin for fear of brain hemorrhage. However, evidence suggests that warfarin-treated stroke victims whose INR is ≤1.7 can be treated with tPA without excess risk of intracranial hemorrhage.[80] Part of the burden of ensuring timely treatment lies with the patient and/or their caregivers as well. Doctors cannot deliver tPA within the critical 4.5-hour window if a stroke victim arrives at the hospital long after this period has expired. Unfortunately, one study showed that the median time to emergency department admission was *16 hours* after onset of stroke symptoms.[7] Calling 911 immediately upon experiencing stroke symptoms is the patient's and his/her caregivers' role in ensuring optimal stroke treatment.

**Aspirin and antiplatelet agents.** Aspirin is established as an important treatment for ischemic stroke. Studies have shown that 160- or 300-mg doses of aspirin given within 48 hours of ischemic stroke onset can reduce the death rate over time (at hospital discharge or at 6 months).[71]

**Surgical procedures.** If necessary, emergency procedures must be performed as soon as possible. For example, if a burst aneurysm (a weakness in a blood vessel) causes associated subarachnoid hemorrhage in the brain, a surgeon can clip the aneurysm and stop the bleeding. Another procedure, called balloon angioplasty, can be used to improve blood flow in occluded arteries.[81]

**Secondary ischemic stroke prevention.** After stroke, there is a significant risk of a repeat stroke or secondary stroke.[82] To help prevent secondary stroke, patients may be prescribed antiplatelet therapy, including low-dose aspirin or Plavix®, or anticoagulant therapy such as long-term warfarin (Coumadin®).[83–85]

## Emergency Treatment of Hemorrhagic Stroke

Emergency treatment of hemorrhagic stroke focuses on controlling bleeding and reducing pressure in the brain. Surgical procedures are often used to drain the blood that collects outside the blood vessels during a hemorrhage (hematoma).[86] If older types of anticoagulant medication (eg, Coumadin®) had been taken to prevent blood clots, intervention with vitamin K may be used to counteract the effects of warfarin. Anticlotting agents (eg, aspirin and tPA) may increase bleeding and cannot be used.[81]

The medication nimodipine, a calcium channel blocker, is often used to help control vasospasm and may improve outcome among patients with subarachnoid hemorrhage. Nimodipine lowers central blood pressure, and its ability to control vasospasm is thought to be due to inhibition of vasoconstriction.[20,87–89] An experimental drug called clazosentan, an endothelin receptor antagonist, has been reported in some human and animal studies to reduce the risk of blood vessel spasm and constriction after hemorrhagic stroke and greatly improve chances of survival.[90–92] However, other studies have failed to corroborate these findings, so more investigation is needed.[93]

**Secondary hemorrhagic stroke prevention.** Following acute treatment, medications may be prescribed to control blood pressure, which is a major risk factor for a second stroke.[94] Prescription medications for lowering blood pressure include diuretics, calcium channel blockers, beta blockers, ACE inhibitors, and others.[95]

# APPROACHES TO STROKE RISK REDUCTION

Stroke risk reduction hinges upon targeting a variety of known risk factors such as high blood pressure, elevated cholesterol, and insulin resistance, as well as improving dietary and lifestyle habits. However, one of conventional medicine's most powerful ischemic stroke risk-reduction strategies is to mitigate the likelihood of blood clots using anticoagulants and antiplatelet medications. It is critical to understand that these medications reduce ischemic stroke risk but *increase* hemorrhagic stroke risk. Hemorrhagic stroke risk reduction strategies primarily focus on reducing blood pressure rather than avoiding clotting.[64,71,96–98]

## Anticoagulant Medications

**Warfarin.** Warfarin (Coumadin®), an anticoagulant, has been associated with a 64% reduction in ischemic stroke risk.[99] Warfarin reduces blood clotting by antagonizing the effects of vitamin K.[100] However, warfarin can interact with other drugs, and people taking warfarin require constant monitoring to protect against excessive bleeding.

**Dabigatran and rivaroxaban.** Recently approved oral anticoagulant drugs are now available to treat blood clots after orthopedic surgeries and may reduce stroke risk is some populations.[101–103] Dabigatran (Pradaxa®), which is a direct thrombin inhibitor, and rivaroxaban (Xarelto™), which inhibits an enzyme involved in coagulation called factor Xa, are examples of anticoagulants that have recently been approved for human use.

These newer therapies may have significant benefits over warfarin, which interferes with vitamin K metabolism. First, they both inhibit clotting factors that do not depend on vitamin K, so they are less sensitive to fluctuations of dietary vitamin K intake. Dabigatran does not exhibit major interactions with foods or other medications.[104] Unlike warfarin, people taking these medications do not need regular blood testing to monitor coagulation.[105] In clinical trials, both treatments were at least as effective as warfarin for reducing stroke risk in patients with atrial fibrillation, and preventing/treating deep vein thrombosis, with a reduced risk of bleeding.[106–108] For more information see the Blood Clot Prevention protocol.

*Advantages* of Pradaxa® versus Warfarin include:

- Rapid onset of action.
- Predictable, consistent anticoagulant effects.
- Low potential for drug–drug interaction.

- No requirement for anticoagulant blood test monitoring.
- Preliminary efficacy and safety advantages versus warfarin based on initial head-to-head, hard-endpoint data.
- No need to maintain low vitamin K levels. Insufficient vitamin K promotes arterial calcification.

*Disadvantages* of Pradaxa® versus Warfarin include:

- No antidote for reversal of over anticoagulation effect. When too much warfarin is given and the patient's INR indicates that they are at risk for a major bleed (or are pathologically bleeding), vitamin K can be injected to immediately reverse warfarin's anticoagulant effect. If too much Pradaxa® is taken, there is no immediate antidote.
- No long-term safety data on Pradaxa® (the case with virtually all newly approved drugs).
- More expensive than warfarin.

## Antiplatelet Medications

Platelets are cell fragments in the blood involved in clot formation. Antiplatelet drugs make these cell fragments less sticky and less likely to clot. The most frequently used antiplatelet medication is aspirin. Aggrenox®, a combination of low-dose aspirin and the antiplatelet drug dipyridamole, may be prescribed instead.[109] Other alternatives include clopidogrel (Plavix®) or ticlopidine (Ticlid®).[110–113]

## Left-Atrial-Appendage Occlusion

For some patients with atrial fibrillation and who cannot take anticoagulants or other blood-thinners, a surgical procedure called left-atrial-appendage occlusion has been shown to inhibit clot formation and decrease stroke risk.[114,115] The left atrial appendage is a muscular pouch that serves as a reservoir for one of the chambers of the heart (left atrium). In the presence of arrhythmia, blood in the appendage is prone to clotting.[116]

# NATURAL STRATEGIES TO REDUCE STROKE RISK

Conventional medications and surgeries used to prevent stoke and cerebrovascular disease are often associated with side effects and are limited in their ability to target the multiple factors that contribute to stroke. Life Extension emphasizes a global stroke prevention strategy. This strategy includes a series of preventive measures such as reducing chronic inflammation, maintaining healthy body weight, reducing cholesterol, suppressing homocysteine and fibrinogen levels, and lowering blood pressure.[117]

## Diet

**Mediterranean diet.** The traditional Mediterranean diet is rich in fruits, vegetables, whole grains, and fish, and low in red meat and sweets.[118] Adherence to a Mediterranean diet is associated with reduced all-cause mortality and lower incidence of several age-related diseases, including stroke.[118,119] A 2011 study found that strict adherence to a Mediterranean diet decreased the likelihood of ischemic stroke irrespective of cholesterol levels, age, and gender.[120] In a separate population study, adherence to a Mediterranean diet significantly decreased the risk of ischemic stroke, heart attack, and vascular death.[121] In a study surveying over 70000 American women, a "prudent" diet of fruits, vegetables, fish, and whole grains was associated with a lower risk of total and ischemic stroke compared to a "Western" diet high in processed meats, refined grains, and sweets.[122] Consuming a Mediterranean diet low in red meat and rich in fresh fruits and vegetables can also curtail excess homocysteine levels in people genetically prone to high homocysteine.[123]

## Targeted Nutritional Interventions

**Olive leaf and olive oil.** The *Olea Europaea* plant is an important constituent of the diet of Mediterranean cultures, and has antihypertensive and antiatherosclerotic effects.[124] The leaves of the olive tree contain the active compounds oleuropein and oleacein. In a human trial, 1000 mg daily of *olive leaf extract* reduced blood pressure.[125] Pretreatment with 100 mg/kg of olive leaf extract has also been shown to reduce brain damage in a rat model of ischemic stroke.[126] Olive oil also contains heart-healthy compounds. A French study showed that older subjects who consume olive oil in both cooking and in dressing have a 41% lower ischemic stroke risk compared with people who never use olive oil.[127]

**Nattokinase.** A 2008 study demonstrated that nattokinase, an enzyme extracted from fermented soybeans, is helpful in reducing blood pressure in patients with hypertension.[128] The participants that received 2000 fibrinolytic units (FU) of nattokinase daily for 8 weeks had a reduction in systolic and diastolic pressure of almost 6 mmHg and 3 mmHg, respectively. Nattokinase breaks apart the protein fibrinogen, which contributes to blood viscosity and clotting. This reduction in blood viscosity may be one of the ways that nattokinase affects blood pressure. Nattokinase also inhibits the elevation of angiotensin II in the bloodstream.[129]

**L-carnitine, acetyl-L-carnitine, and propionyl-L-carnitine.** L-carnitine is an essential co-factor in the metabolism of lipid molecules into cellular energy. L-carnitine has been shown to be neuroprotective in rat models of ischemic stroke.[130] Laboratory studies on human tissue specimens demonstrate that L-carnitine causes vasodilation. In one laboratory study, L-carnitine selectively inhibited a platelet-activating factor, demonstrating that L-carnitine has a protective effect against thrombosis in ischemic stroke. In a sample of nine ischemic muscle specimens from five patients with vascular disease, L-carnitine levels were low, but were restored 2 days after a single injection followed by a 30-minute infusion of propionyl-L-carnitine.[131] In an animal model of ischemic stroke, pretreatment with acetyl-L-carnitine decreased brain damage.[132]

**Vinpocetine.** Vinpocetine is derived from the chemical vincamine, which is an extract from the leaves of the lesser periwinkle plant. Since its synthesis in the 1960s, vinpocetine has shown both neuroprotective and cerebral blood flow-enhancing properties. It is widely used in cerebrovascular disease in Japan, Hungary, Poland, Russia, and Germany.[133]

Vinpocetine has neuroprotective effects due to its ability to block sodium channels and calcium channels in brain cells, preventing excitotoxicity and death of brain tissue.[134] Animal models reveal a role for vinpocetine in blocking inflammatory processes. This is significant because chronic inflammation leads to endothelial dysfunction and atherosclerosis, increasing the risk for stroke. In an animal model of ischemic stroke, damage to a brain area known as the hippocampus was reduced from 77% in untreated animals to 37% in animals treated with vinpocetine.[133]

**Vitamin D.** Evidence from clinical trials suggests that vitamin D plays a modest role in blood pressure control.[135] Vitamin D regulates blood pressure by modulating calcium–phosphate metabolism, controlling endocrine glands, and improving endothelial function. Vitamin D deficiency appears to be an independent risk factor for stroke incidence in Japanese–American men[136] and Korean men.[137] A recent study also showed that individuals whose vitamin D levels were >30 ng/mL had the lowest incidence of heart attack and stroke.[137] Vitamin D may also promote normal insulin metabolism.[117]

**Vitamin B6, B12, and folic acid.** B-vitamin therapy has been shown to lower homocysteine levels and independently reduce stroke risk.[138] Homocysteine levels can become elevated when serum B12 level are below 400 pmol/L.[139] Analysis of data on 5522 participants in a large trial to assess the role of B vitamins in stroke risk reduction (the HOPE-2 trial) demonstrated that treatment with folic acid and vitamins B6 and B12 lowered plasma homocysteine levels and overall stroke incidence. In this study, the incidence of both ischemic and hemorrhagic stroke was lower in the vitamin group compared to the placebo group.[138] A 2012 review of 19 different studies found that B-vitamin supplementation reduces stroke risk by approximately 12%.[140] Another 2012 study supported those findings by demonstrating that supplementation with folic acid can reduce stroke incidence by 8%.[141]

**Omega-3 fatty acids.** Omega-3 fatty acids are found in certain fat sources such as coldwater fish and flaxseed oil.[117] Studies have demonstrated that omega-3 fatty acids help regulate blood pressure and reduce platelet aggregation, inflammation, LDL-cholesterol, and other atherosclerosis risk factors.[142] A 2006 review article indicated that omega-3 fatty acids have a significant protective effect against cerebrovascular disease.[143] In a mouse model of ischemia, 3 months of treatment with docosahexaenoic acid (DHA) blunted inflammatory responses after an ischemic stroke and decreased brain damage.[144]

Omega-3 intake may slow the progression of atherosclerosis by reducing plasma triglyceride levels.[145] In short-term clinical trials, consumption of omega-3 fatty acids stimulated nitric oxide production, which enhances the dilation of arteries and improves blood flow throughout the body. Omega-3 fatty acids have also been shown to improve endothelial function and prevent abnormal heart rhythms (arrhythmias).[145–147] The American Heart Association suggests that some people may not get enough omega-3 fatty acids through diet alone and that these individuals should consider taking a dietary supplement.[142]

**Garlic.** Some clinical trials have found that increased consumption of garlic can lower blood pressure in hypertensive patients. Consumption of approximately 10 000 mcg of the active ingredient *allicin*, the amount contained in about 4 cloves of garlic, per day appears to be necessary to lower blood pressure.[117] A review of studies demonstrated that garlic consumption appears to lower systolic and diastolic blood pressure by an average of 16 and 9 mmHg, respectively.[148]

**Dehydroepiandrosterone.** Dehydroepiandrosterone (DHEA), an endogenous steroid hormone derived from cholesterol, is the most abundant circulating steroid in humans. DHEA improves arterial dilation and protects against endothelial dysfunction, a risk factor for stroke.[149] In a study of over 300 postmenopausal women, higher levels of DHEA-S, a major metabolic derivative of DHEA, were associated with less severe stroke.[150]

**Vitamin C.** Vitamin C, also known as ascorbic acid, is a water-soluble antioxidant that improves endothelial function. Numerous observational and clinical studies have documented that dietary intake of vitamin C can lower blood pressure and heart rate. Evaluation of published clinical trials has shown that intake of 250 mg vitamin C twice daily lowered systolic and diastolic blood pressure by about 7 mmHg and 4 mmHg, respectively. Vitamin C may lower blood pressure by reducing binding of angiotensin II to its receptor. Vitamin C also appears to enhance antihypertensive effects of some blood pressure medications.[117]

**Flavonoids.** Flavonoids are naturally occurring antioxidants found in fruits, vegetables, red wine, and tea.[117] A 2012 study showed that increased intake of flavonoids is associated with reduced risk of ischemic stroke in women, and consumption of citrus fruits can reduce overall stroke risk.[151] An animal model showed that a single intravenous dose of the flavonoid *resveratrol* improved cerebral blood flow by 30% and protected against ischemia-induced brain damage.[152]

**Rutin.** Rutin is a flavonoid that occurs naturally in buckwheat and some fruits (eg, apples).[153,154] Rutin inhibits *protein disulfide isomerase (PDI)*, an enzyme that participates in blood clot formation. Among nearly 5000 agents screened as potential PDI inhibitors in one study, rutin was one of the most potent.[155] An animal model showed that rutin inhibits the formation of blood clots.[155]

## Life Extension Suggestions

- **Olive leaf extract** (standardized to 16% oleuropein, or 80 mg): 1000 mg daily
- **Garlic extract** (standardized to 10000 ppm allicin potential [12 mg]): 1200–4800 mg daily
- **Vitamin D:** 5000–8000 IU daily; depending upon blood levels of 25-OH-vitamin D
- **Nattokinase:** 2000–4000 FU daily
- **Vinpocetine:** 10–30 mg daily
- **Fish oil** (with olive polyphenols): providing 1400 mg EPA and 1000 mg DHA daily
- **Vitamin B6:** 250 mg daily
- **Vitamin B12:** 1000–5000 mcg daily
- **Folic acid:** 800–1000 mcg daily
- **Resveratrol:** 250 mg daily

- **Green tea extract** (standardized to 98% polyphenols): 725–1450 mg daily
- **Vitamin C:** 1000–2000 mg daily
- **Rutin:** 500 mg daily
- **L-carnitine:** 500–2000 mg daily
- **Acetyl-L-carnitine:** 1000–2000 mg daily
- **Propionyl-L-carnitine:** 300–600 mg daily
- **DHEA:** 25–50 mg daily (depending on blood test results)

In addition, the following *blood tests* may be helpful:

- Male or Female Panel (includes homocysteine, C-reactive protein, vitamin D, glucose, cholesterol, and triglyceride tests)

- Fibrinogen
- Fasting Insulin
- Vitamin D, 25-Hydroxy
- Omega Score®

## REFERENCES

References available at: www.lef.org/dpt5/ch123

# 124

# Surgical Preparation

Surgery has been referred to as "benign violence"[1]— an appropriate term for the calculated and deliberate wounding of a human body, even when the goal is curing disease.

Indeed, from a biological standpoint, surgery causes many of the same kinds of tissue damage that occur during a traumatic injury. While this injury may be necessary and beneficial, the body does not discriminate between a surgeon's scalpel and any other kind of trauma. In fact, studies have shown that patients are under great physical stress both during and after surgery. However, few conventional physicians recommend proven ways to speed recovery and produce better patient outcomes.

In general, surgery can be divided into 3 main phases: the preoperative period, period during surgery, and postoperative (or recovery) period. At each of these stages, patients can take an active role in their own well-being by following documented steps to support their body's antioxidant stores, reduce inflammation, and modulate immune responses that accompany surgery. By paying careful attention to nutritional status, patients can speed their recovery and experience more successful results.[2,3]

## PHASES OF SURGERY

### The Preoperative Period

In an ideal situation, patients undergoing surgery will have adequate time before the operation to prepare themselves emotionally and physically. This preparation will likely include dietary supplementation as well as mental and emotional preparation. The healthier patients are when they go into surgery, the healthier they are likely to be during the postoperative phase.

Each of the 3 phases of a surgical procedure poses different threats to the patient's well-being, although there may be considerable overlap. The most variable phase is the preoperative, or preparatory phase. In the case of emergency surgery, this period may be limited to a few hours (and in the case of trauma a few minutes). In most cases, however, both the patient and surgical team have longer to prepare, and it is during this period that many nutritional interventions can be made. One overlooked statistic is that up to 50% of patients admitted to hospitals are malnourished.[4] This startling statistic underscores the critical importance of proper nutritional intervention.

Two significant threats to the patient's well-being during the preoperative period are continued progression of the disease that has made the operation necessary (for instance, a growing cancer) and the patient's degree of apprehension and anxiety. Certain preoperative procedures, such as prolonged fasting, may also exert negative effects.

**Disease progression.** Virtually all disease processes that require surgery, including traumatic injury, impose substantial oxidative threats to tissue.[5] For instance, initial oxidative (free radical) damage can be caused by impaired blood supply as a tumor presses on major vessels or diverts blood from healthy tissues. Toxins may be released from infected or malignant tissue or by release of intracellular contents, including protein-damaging enzymes, from dying cells.[6]

Blood released from normal circulation into various body compartments, such as the abdomen, can itself produce oxidative damage.[7] An early response to oxidative damage is inflammation, which is aimed at destroying unhealthy tissue or invading infectious agents. As inflammation grows, however, additional oxidant damage is produced by white blood cells that are attracted to the area by signaling chemicals called cytokines and chemokines.[8] Many of these cells, particularly white blood cells called neutrophils, release toxic reactive oxygen species, which cause further tissue damage.[9]

Similarly, in the case of infection, the body's powerful immune response calls inflammatory cells to the infected tissue, where they release agents that oxidize lipids in cell membranes, causing the membranes to leak and cells to die.[10] Inflammation also changes blood vessel walls, making them "leaky" and allowing blood components to seep into tissues, causing swelling and loss of plasma proteins.[11] These oxidative and inflammatory reactions impair local tissue function and sap the body of proteins, minerals, and other substances necessary for maintaining normal blood pressure and overall tissue health.[12]

A healthy diet and appropriate nutritional supplements can help prepare a patient for surgery by maximizing reserves of proteins, essential fatty acids, vitamins, and minerals. Specific nutrient and supplements can also help bolster the immune system, minimize oxidative damage, and keep inflammation under control.

**Psychological stress.** Psychological and emotional stress reduces the body's immune function and renders people more vulnerable to disease. Scientists today understand that much of this effect is mediated by brain structures that influence production of stress-induced hormones (eg, corticosteroids).[13,14] Every person who will be undergoing a surgical procedure, no matter how minor, has some degree of anxiety about the procedure, its outcomes, and potential complications. Outcomes of surgical procedures are almost always improved by a reasonably long preoperative planning period, which gives the surgical team and patient a maximum opportunity for physical and technical preparation. Excessively long preoperative periods, however, may be associated with increased amounts of worry, anxiety, and stress; these factors can have a negative impact on surgical outcomes.[15]

The oft-repeated phrase "just relax" is not only entirely ineffective, but there is even evidence that patients "ordered" to relax actually experience increased stress levels. Instead, one of the most effective interventions to reduce patient stress levels is communication; patients with a high degree of so-called health literacy are known to have shorter hospital stays, fewer complications, and better overall outcomes.[16,17] Health literacy is easy to attain; the Partnership for Clear Health Communication promotes a program called "Ask Me 3," which recommends that patients get the following three questions answered by a physician regarding any disease or treatment:

1. What is my main problem?
2. What do I need to do?
3. Why is it important for me to do this?

Getting these questions answered is a major step in improving health literacy and reducing stress levels. Also, many physicians appreciate being asked to present information to patients in this format.

Other nonmedical strategies for reducing preoperative anxiety and stress have shown to be helpful in varying degrees. Hypnosis has been found to be effective in reducing both preoperative anxiety and postoperative complications.[18,19] A related technique called guided imagery, in which a skilled therapist works with the patient to envision low-stress and positive concepts, has also been documented to reduce anxiety, safely lower pulse and blood pressure, and shorten hospital stays.[20,21] In other studies, patients using guided imagery required 50% less pain medication than controls.[22,23]

**Preoperative fasting.** Practically since the inception of general anesthesia for surgery, doctors have worried about the effects of a full stomach on an unconscious patient. The chief risk is aspiration of stomach contents into the lungs, which can cause severe inflammation,

infection, and death. Modern anesthesia practices, however, such as careful control of the patient's airway, close monitoring, and selective use of appropriate anesthetic drugs has dramatically reduced this risk.[24] Periods of fasting, such as the traditional "nothing by mouth (or NPO) after midnight" on the night before surgery can produce dehydration, low blood sugar, and a variety of other complications. Increasingly, anesthesiologists are recognizing both the biological and psychological value of permitting patients a reasonable oral intake, at least of liquids, until about 4 hours before the surgical procedure. Patients are encouraged to discuss this practice with their physicians well in advance of surgery.

**Glucose control.** Life Extension also suggests that patients with poor glucose control discuss intensive insulin therapy with the surgeon before surgery. Studies indicate that surgery-induced insulin resistance, leading to elevated glucose levels during surgery, raises the risk of complications and death. Intensive insulin therapy, a procedure in which glucose levels are closely monitored during surgery, can help reduce complications and lower the risk of death.[25] The recommended glucose range is 80–120 mg/dL. However, this practice is not standard in hospitals and requires intensive monitoring from nurses and other members of the surgical team. Nevertheless, because of the benefits, patients may want to discuss intensive insulin therapy with their surgical team to see if it is warranted.

**Aspirin therapy.** Patients may also want to discuss aspirin therapy before surgery. Aspirin is a well-known antiplatelet used for prevention of heart attack and to mitigate damage of ongoing heart attacks. Some studies suggested that aspirin therapy may benefit certain patients before surgery, especially heart patients and those undergoing carotid endarterectomy.[26] However, because aspirin affects the blood's ability to clot, no surgery patients should begin aspirin therapy unless under the direct supervision of their surgical team.

## The Operation Itself

The surgical procedure itself is the phase over which patients have the least control. From the moment the patient enters the operating room, virtually all vital functions are taken over by members of the surgical team. The "ABCs," or airway, breathing, and circulation, are typically managed by the anesthesiologist. While many anesthetic agents are aimed at attaining unconsciousness and managing pain, many other medications are given to support pulse and blood pressure, prevent infection and blood loss, and counter the side effects of other medications. It is not unusual for a patient to experience the effects of more than 10 medications during a major surgical procedure. Blood transfusions can also have untoward effects, especially with regard to calcium status.[27]

While each medication has its purpose, they also have inevitable unwanted effects, with many medications being potent oxidants and others stimulating immune or inflammatory responses, particularly in the lungs, which are directly exposed to inhaled anesthetic gasses.[28,29] Most medications have effects on the liver's ability to detoxify other drugs and toxins. Anesthesiologists typically plan the array of medications carefully to minimize these effects. It has been shown that certain of the most commonly used anesthetic gasses actually provide some protection against oxidative damage.[30,31]

The oxygen provided during the procedure is itself a mixed blessing. Critical for maintaining normal cellular processes and proper wound healing, supplemental oxygen also produces increased levels of reactive oxygen species that can damage tissues. Surgical procedures themselves are known to reduce circulating levels of vitamins A, E, and other naturally occurring antioxidants.[32,33] Good pre- and post-operative nutrition, with special attention to maintaining adequate antioxidant status, can help minimize these effects; studies of administration of antioxidants during surgery are showing some promise.[34,35]

The majority of physiologic stress produced by an operation is the result of direct tissue damage from cutting, clamping, suturing, and otherwise manipulating organs and other structures. Reduced blood flow produces ischemia (lack of oxygen), resulting in cell death and release of intracellular components that produce an acidic environment. Enzymes released from injured cells can further damage adjacent tissue.

When blood flow is restored to an ischemic area, reperfusion injury occurs, with suddenly elevated oxygen levels causing transient oxidative damage and the restored blood flow sweeping tissue toxins into general circulation.[6] Oxidant molecules produce the same sort of damage to cell membranes (lipid peroxidation) as the disease process itself.[10] Similarly, oxidant damage results in stimulation of inflammatory processes and release of cytokines, with further oxidant injury caused by inflammatory cells attacking injured tissue.[6,7,9] While this inflammatory response represents the first stages of healing, it can often become exaggerated and contribute to both local and systemic stressors that impede, rather than improve recovery.[36]

Finally, although not a major factor during the operation, bacterial and fungal organisms may gain access to normally sterile body areas, especially during so-called dirty cases, in which the bowel or other naturally contaminated organs must be opened. Drainage of abscesses and other infected tissue can also allow infectious organisms to enter into otherwise sterile tissue, setting the stage for a postoperative infection, with its attendant oxidative and inflammatory consequences.[36]

Oxidant and inflammatory stresses are not limited to the surgical region. Surgery itself is now widely recognized as a systemic inflammatory stress that can cause injury in areas far removed from the surgical site.[37,38] For example, surgery can impact the function of blood vessels during the procedure, causing blood pressure instability.[39]

Some of the most profound effects of surgical procedures may impact the gastrointestinal tract. There is now good evidence that surgery (and anesthesia) may produce "leaky gut" effects, permitting entry of toxins and microorganisms into circulation and affecting long-term outcomes.[40] Many surgeons and anesthesiologists are now interested in the use of antioxidant and immune-modulating nutrients during surgery to ameliorate these effects.[36,41]

## The Postoperative (Recovery) Period

During the postoperative phase, the patient and surgical team have many opportunities to collaborate in maximizing nutrient contributions to the healing and recovery process. As in the preoperative period, considerable benefit has been demonstrated from nonmedical interventions such as hypnosis and guided imagery. The latter, in particular, has been shown to reduce pain, anxiety, and length of hospital stay in patients undergoing diverse surgical procedures.[18,20,42]

The greatest biological threats to the postoperative patient arise from intricate relationships between regrowth of healing tissue, inflammation, and infection. A certain amount of inflammation is necessary for proper wound healing—cytokines and other inflammatory mediators are required for the production of vascular endothelial growth factor, which is vital for assuring a strong blood supply to new tissue.[43,44] Inflammatory cells and their chemical products are also required to fight the ever present threat of infection; however, excessive inflammation can also impair the healing process.

Supplemental oxygen is a very frequent part of the postoperative treatment regimen; surgeons are naturally anxious to provide adequate oxygen to meet the increased metabolic demands of rapidly healing tissue.[45,46] Wound healing is known to be accelerated by moderately elevated tissue oxygen levels. In fact, hyperbaric oxygen therapy (oxygen treatment at higher-than-normal pressures) is now used for treatment of slow-healing wounds and many burns,[47] where it has been shown to increase vascular endothelial growth factor levels.[48]

As with intraoperative oxygen therapy, however, this benefit is not without its costs in terms of increased tissue levels of reactive oxygen species. A judicious mix of increased oxygen supply with antioxidant supplementation seems to provide maximum wound healing benefits with minimum systemic exposure to free oxygen radicals.[45,48–50]

In addition to wounds and tissue damage inflicted by surgery itself, postoperative patients are at risk for a number of complications caused by decreased mobility. Early complications include partial lung collapse that results from shallow, painful breathing,[51] bladder infections from indwelling catheters,[52] local inflammation of the healing wound,[53] and inflammation caused by blood clots developing in nonmoving lower extremities.[54] These complications are so common, in fact, that surgical interns are taught the mnemonic "wind, water, wound, walk" when considering likely sources of a fever in the first few postoperative days.[55] All of these complications are the result of inflammatory processes amplified by surgery. Nutritional modulation of the inflammatory response may help blunt these complications.[41]

Perhaps the most severe postoperative complication is development of pressure ulcers, or bedsores. These ulcers develop at pressure points in patients who are unable or unwilling (because of pain) to shift their positions in bed; early signs of their development can be present within 2 hours of pressure being applied.[56] Constant pressure reduces local blood flow, producing ischemia (reduced oxygen levels) and lack of nutrients. This situation rapidly produces increased tissue levels of metabolic waste products (eg, lactic acid) and eventually results in cell death, with release of toxins and enzymes into adjacent tissue. Once again, inflammation is triggered in previously healthy tissue, attracting inflammatory cells that cause further tissue damage. Necrosis (cell death) can occur very rapidly in these ulcers, resulting in the development of potentially large masses of dead and dying tissue, which are a breeding ground for bacteria.

For these reasons, bedsores can be life-threatening. Their prevention is one of the chief priorities of the surgical team in the postoperative period. Poor nutritional status is a major risk factor for their development,[57] and many nutritional interventions are known to be helpful.[58,59]

Proper wound healing also requires both energy and an adequate supply of the chemical building materials of new tissue. Requirements for calories, protein, and vitamins in the postoperative period are higher than practically any other period in the lifetime of an adult.[60] Formerly, surgeons sharply limited the amount and pace of postoperative feedings, believing the gut needed a lengthy recovery period from anesthesia and surgery. Today, most surgeons recognize the critical nature of early restoration of feedings, preferably via the gastrointestinal route.[61,62] This practice has been shown not only to maximize nutritional intake, but also reduce "leaky gut" effects produced by systemic inflammation in response to surgery.[40]

Finally, surgery suppresses immune response.[36] For this reason, the risk of infection, already elevated by the operation itself, rises still higher in the postoperative period as all branches of the immune system slowly emerge from their depressed state. Many nutrients contribute to the postoperative recovery of the immune system, and the new field of immunonutrition has developed around a growing understanding of the effects of certain nutrients on immune and inflammatory responses.[63]

# TARGETED NUTRITIONAL STRATEGIES

## Immunonutrition

Most surgeons now recognize that good attention to nutrition, including its effects on antioxidant and inflammatory status, can have a major positive impact on the outcome of a surgical procedure.[41] A comprehensive nutritional program begun in the weeks prior to surgery and continued at the earliest possible postoperative moment is known to increase survival, reduce complications, minimize length of hospital stay, keep costs down, and significantly enhance quality of life.[60]

Immunonutrition aims to provide the proper nutrient mix to boost healthy immune function while suppressing the exaggerated inflammatory response.[61,64] A variety of nutrient formulas and routes of delivery have been tested. The most promising results come from nutrient formulas provided by mouth or feeding tube (enteral route) rather than intravenous feedings. Such feedings reduce atrophy of the intestinal lining and prevent the increase in gut permeability that is a consequence of the inflammatory response.[40]

Patients given enteral (orally administered) supplements have been shown to have fewer infections,[65] shorter stays in intensive care, and fewer overall hospital days.[61] They have improved wound healing compared with patients receiving standard nutrition.[66] Starting immunonutrition supplements up to 5 days before surgery may provide even greater benefits,[67] including beneficial immune system effects,[68] fewer postoperative infections,[69] and reduced costs.[70]

**Omega-3 fatty acids.** While many different mixtures of nutrients have been used in immunonutrition, several main components appear to provide maximum benefit. The goal of reducing exaggerated inflammatory response to surgery is met through the inclusion of omega-3 fatty acids, largely derived from fish oils.[61] These fatty acids can shift the production of cytokines away from those that stimulate inflammation.[71] They also make cell and mitochondrial membranes more resistant to oxidant stress,[72] which reduces tissue damage and prevents amplification of the inflammatory response. Most effective immunonutrient supplements contain substantial quantities of omega-3 fatty acids.

**Amino acids.** The amino acids arginine, glutamine, and taurine are conditionally essential amino acids, which means that under certain stressful conditions (including trauma and surgery), the body cannot synthesize them in normal amounts; it must therefore rely on external supplemental sources.[73,74]

- *Arginine.* Arginine provides a substrate for nitric oxide production, which enhances blood flow by relaxing blood vessels.[61] It also stimulates and activates immune system cells.[65] Trauma and surgery increase levels of the enzyme arginase, which reduces arginine levels.[75] Arginine supplementation, alone or in combination, has been observed to enhance wound healing[69] and prevent pressure ulcers.[76]

- *Glutamine.* Glutamine is a major component of proteins produced during clotting.[77] Supplementation with glutamine also speeds wound healing.[78]

- *Taurine.* Taurine is required for mitochondrial energy production and efficient utilization of other nutrients.[79] It has been documented to improve cardiac surgery outcomes by protecting heart muscle against ischemic damage.[80]

**Ribonucleic acids.** Ribonucleic acids (RNA) are crucial to protein synthesis in wound healing, as well as the expression of gene products of immune system cells. While the precise mechanism is unknown, immunonutritional supplements containing RNA appear to improve immune responses and more rapidly overcome immune depression induced by surgery.[81] Like other nutrient combinations, these supplements are effective when given both preoperatively[68] and in the early postoperative period.[66]

More than 170 studies have been published on various immunonutrient combinations that have shown positive results.[61] Patients given a preoperative formula containing omega-3 fatty acids and arginine had significantly improved systemic immune responses, gut oxygen levels, and gut perfusion compared with control patients.[82] In a different study, patients supplemented with arginine, glutamine, and omega-3 fatty acids had higher postoperative total protein and immunoglobulin levels, higher levels of infection-fighting white blood cells, and lower levels of pro-inflammatory cytokines and tumor necrosis factor than unsupplemented controls, demonstrating that these supplements enhanced host defenses while modulating the exaggerated inflammatory response.[64]

Wound healing is also improved by immunonutritional mixtures. A 2005 study demonstrated that a postoperative formula containing arginine, omega-3 fatty acids, and RNA increased protein synthesis in surgical wounds, and supplemented patients experienced fewer wound healing complications than unsupplemented control patients.[66] Enhancement of host defenses by immunonutritional supplements[72] results in fewer postoperative complications, such as pneumonia[83] and pressure ulcers.[76]

## Other Nutrients that Enhance Surgical Outcomes

In addition to immunonutrients, supplementation with many other biologically active materials can help prepare a person for surgery. Ensuring that the body is replete with antioxidants is one easy and powerful way to avoid antioxidant depletion during surgery.[84] Maximizing anti-inflammatory status and boosting immune function to achieve proper balance of host defense against infection while minimizing exaggerated inflammatory response to surgery is another. Also, ensuring adequate protein intake prior to surgery is an important way of providing the soon-to-be-healing body with building blocks of new tissue. All of these effects can be achieved with a reasonable program of supplementation in the weeks prior to surgery.

**Amino acids.** In addition to being a good source of immunonutrition, amino acids are the building blocks of proteins, which are the chief components of structural tissue. Enzymes that catalyze all biological processes are also proteins. Surgery dramatically increases the daily requirement of protein, particularly if there is substantial blood loss. Supplements containing amino acids or whole proteins have been shown in animal models and human trials to enhance surgical outcomes.[85–87] Supplements may improve wound healing,[85] reduce the rate and severity of pressure ulcers,[59,88,89] and improve fat mass (a good thing following surgery).[90]

Almost all known vitamins are essential in each of the phases of surgery, either as vital cofactors in protein or nucleic acid synthesis for rapidly healing tissue or as potent antioxidants that can minimize tissue damage and the heightened inflammatory response caused by surgery. Blood levels of many of the vitamins are markedly reduced during surgery, and there is good evidence for both pre- and post-operative supplementation.

**Vitamin C.** Vitamin C is an antioxidant required for protein synthesis, making it indispensable in wound and fracture healing; fractures in animal models heal faster when they receive vitamin C supplementation.[91,92] In humans, vitamin C contributes to the strength of healing wounds and reduces the degree and severity of postoperative pressure ulcers.[58,86,88]

**Vitamin E.** Vitamin E is a potent antioxidant and fat-soluble vitamin found in large amounts in skin, where it may improve wound healing and scar appearance.[86,93] By scavenging reactive oxygen species, vitamin E can reduce tissue damage caused by free radicals, thereby reducing surgically induced inflammation. Like vitamin A, vitamin E levels are depleted during surgical procedures, especially those that require use of a heart–lung machine.[33] In animal models, supplements containing vitamin E promote fracture healing[91,94] and mitigate the deleterious effects of hyperbaric (high pressure) oxygen.[4] In humans, vitamin E also assists in the healing of bone necrosis following radiation treatment.[95] Vitamin E, administered directly into coronary blood vessels during open-heart surgery, has been shown to reduce reperfusion oxidative injury to cardiac muscle cells.[34]

Because vitamin E can inhibit platelet aggregation, vitamin E supplementation should be considered on a case-by-case basis (well in advance of surgery) to determine whether the benefit exceeds the risk. Another way to enhance vitamin E function without direct vitamin E supplementation is to consider alpha-lipoic acid, which has been shown to support vitamin E's antioxidant function in patients undergoing hyperbaric oxygen treatment.[45]

**Lipoic acid.** Lipoic acid is an effective antioxidant that may have a role in preoperative care. In a rat model of skin injury, pretreatment with lipoic acid sped the healing of skin wounds by protecting skin cells from oxidant damage.[96] In humans, lipoic acid helped combat free radical damage caused by high tissue concentrations of oxygen.[45]

**Vitamin A.** Vitamin A is essential for surgical patients; it stimulates the production of transforming growth factor beta-1, which accelerates skin and intestinal wound healing.[97] Supplements containing vitamin A have been especially useful in the prevention of pressure ulcers[76] and treatment of burn patients.[98] Vitamin A has also been shown to mitigate the effects of inflammation caused by radiation treatments that often accompany cancer surgery.[99]

In addition to vitamins, a number of other micronutrients and conditionally essential nutrients, many with antioxidant or anti-inflammatory effects, have been found to improve surgical outcomes and prevent complications.

**Omega-3 fatty acids.** Omega-3 fatty acids have already been mentioned as key components of immunonutrient formulas. Fish oil supplements have independently been documented to reduce the exaggerated inflammatory response caused by surgery, producing decreased cytokine levels.[75,100,101] Supplementation with fish oil rich in omega-3 fatty acids reduced infection rates and showed promise for shortening length of hospital stay.[71] The same group of investigators also demonstrated postoperative improvements (in liver and pancreatic function) in cancer patients supplemented with fish oil.[102] Cancer patients given 5 days of omega-3 supplementation before their surgery had dramatically reduced blood levels of inflammatory mediators in the postoperative days.[103] In a 2004 study, preoperative supplementation with fish oil demonstrated a decrease in deaths following surgery.[104] This study also showed a lower requirement for mechanical ventilation postoperatively and shorter length of hospital stay in the group supplemented preoperatively.

**Coenzyme Q10.** Coenzyme Q10 (CoQ10) is an antioxidant molecule intimately involved in intracellular energy management. Like other antioxidants, its levels plummet sharply during surgery, presumably because of rapid consumption by oxidant species.[84] Diminished levels of CoQ10 and other conditionally essential antioxidants may also worsen cardiac output, especially in people with preexisting heart disease.[74] Poor cardiac output results in poor perfusion of other organs, can delay healing, and set the stage for other complications. Preoperative treatment with CoQ10 can restore cardiac muscle function and protect against hypoxic (low oxygen) damage.[80,105] One study of a supplement containing CoQ10, taurine, and carnitine demonstrated improved cardiac blood volumes in cardiac surgery patients.[79]

**Zinc.** Zinc is a mineral that functions as an important coenzyme in the production of collagen (chief protein in healing wound tissue); in addition, it has an important antioxidant function in skin.[106] The earliest sign of zinc deficiency in humans is often the development of skin breakdown, and topical zinc treatments have been used for centuries with good effect.[107] Animals made zinc deficient have slower rates of collagen accumulation in wounds and diminished wound strength, while zinc supplementation prior to creation of the wound (preoperatively) increased the strength of the healing wound.[108,109] Quantitative studies of the effects of zinc supplementation in mice demonstrate that adequate zinc has an antioxidant function and hastens wound healing, while deficiency or very high doses delay healing.[110,111] Zinc may help in the healing, not only of skin wounds, but also bone; a study demonstrated that zinc supplementation hastened the healing of leg fractures in rats.[112]

In studies of patients with pressure ulcers, supplementation with a combination of zinc, arginine, and vitamin C produced significant improvement in treated patients compared with controls given placebo.[58,88] A similar supplement was shown to delay the onset of pressure ulcers in a group of patients recovering from hip surgery.[113] This combination is now widely recognized for patients undergoing surgery of any kind.[76]

**Melatonin.** Melatonin is a pineal gland hormone with antioxidant functions.[114] It appears to fundamentally affect a variety of brain functions related to relaxation, sleep, and anxiety; also, its natural secretion is perturbed by surgery[115] and anesthesia.[116] These disturbances may contribute to the well-known phenomena of postoperative delirium[117] and "ICU psychosis," in which patients become agitated, confused, and combative while in intensive care. Melatonin supplementation has been suggested in this setting.[118]

Melatonin has been demonstrated to be as effective at reducing anxiety before a procedure as the commonly used benzodiazepine drug midazolam.[119] As a premedication, melatonin has the added advantage of not producing postoperative impairments in mental function, as do the benzodiazepines.[120] There is emerging clinical evidence that melatonin may positively modify surgically induced general inflammation. In a study of newborns, melatonin given postoperatively significantly reduced inflammatory cytokine levels.[121]

**Curcumin.** Curcumin is a major component of turmeric. It is an antioxidant and potent inhibitor of nuclear factor-kappa B, which plays a central role in "translating" inflammatory stimuli into activation of the inflammatory response. There has been tremendous interest in the role of nuclear factor-kappa B inhibition as a means of reining in overactive inflammatory reactions in sepsis, cancer, and autoimmune diseases.[122]

A study of topical curcumin delivered in a collagen-based film demonstrated enhanced wound healing and tissue proliferation in wounds covered with the film, as well as more-efficient free radical scavenging than in wounds covered with a non-curcumin-containing film.[123] In an animal model of radiation-induced impaired wound healing, pretreatment with curcumin

enhanced wound closure compared with controls.[124] This study has profound implications for human cancer surgeries often complicated by the effects of radiation treatment.

Curcumin has also demonstrated powerful antioxidant effects on skin cells in culture, protecting cells against damage caused by hydrogen peroxide.[125] These mechanisms together may explain the more rapid healing of experimentally-induced surgical wounds in animals treated with curcumin.[126,127] There is limited research on the effect of curcumin in the context of surgery, but it has been observed to be safe and well-tolerated in human trials as an anti-inflammatory and chemoprotective agent.[128,129]

## Life Extension Suggestions

Nutrients that might be helpful before and after surgery include:

- **Fish oil** (with olive polyphenols and sesame lignans): 1400 mg EPA and 1000 mg DHA daily
- **L-arginine:** 2250–9000 mg daily (in divided doses)
- **Glutamine:** 1000–3000 mg daily
- **Vitamin C:** 2000–3000 mg daily
- **Vitamin E:** 400 IU daily (with at least 200 mg gamma tocopherol)
- **Vitamin A:** 25 000 IU daily
- **Lipoic acid:** 300–600 mg daily
- **CoQ10:** 300 mg daily
- **Zinc:** 30 mg daily
- **Melatonin:** 300 mcg–10 mg, usually taken before bedtime; begin with the smallest possible dose
- **Curcumin** (as highly absorbed BCM-95®): 400–800 mg daily
- **Whey or plant protein:** 17 g or more daily
- **RNA (ribonucleic acid):** 500–2000 mg daily

Importantly, the surgeon should be aware of any dietary supplements consumed. Some supplements, such as vitamin E and Ginkgo biloba, increase the risk of bleeding during surgery. Many physicians will recommend that patients discontinue these supplements up to 14 days before surgery.

## REFERENCES

References available at: www.lef.org/dpt5/ch124

# 125

# *Thyroid Regulation*

Millions of Americans suffer from fatigue, weight gain, depression, and cognitive impairment. Many believe that they have no choice but to accept these seemingly "age-related" declines in quality of life.

*Underactive* thyroid (hypothyroidism) is often overlooked or misdiagnosed and can be the underlying cause of these symptoms. Patients and their doctors often disregard these common signs of thyroid hormone deficiency, mistaking them for normal aging.[1]

*Overactive* thyroid (hyperthyroidism) afflicts fewer people than hypothyroidism, yet the symptoms can be equally devastating. Subclinical hyperthyroidism, characterized by suppressed thyroid-stimulating hormone (TSH) levels accompanied by normal thyroid hormones (T4 and T3) levels,[2] has been associated with increased rates of cardiovascular disease; arrhythmia in particular.[3] Overt hyperthyroidism compromises bone health,[4] elevates blood glucose levels,[5] and often causes anxiety.[2]

Fortunately, a simple blood test for TSH, T3, and T4 can reveal an underlying thyroid condition and help direct treatment to improve the symptoms.[1,2]

In this protocol we will discuss the function and regulation of the thyroid gland, and the systemic implications of both hypothyroidism and hyperthyroidism. We will examine the importance of proper testing and interpretation of thyroid hormone levels and reveal natural approaches for maintaining optimal thyroid hormone levels.

## ROLE OF THE THYROID

The thyroid is a butterfly-shaped organ located just below the Adam's apple in the neck. Made up of small sacs, this gland is filled with an iodine-rich protein called thyroglobulin along with the thyroid hormones thyroxine (T4) and small amounts of triiodothyronine (T3).

The primary function of these two hormones is to regulate metabolism by controlling the rate at which the body converts oxygen and calories to energy. In fact, the metabolic rate of every cell in the body is regulated by thyroid hormones, primarily T3.[6]

In healthy individuals the gland is imperceptible to the touch. A visibly enlarged thyroid gland is referred to

as a goiter. Historically, goiter was most frequently caused by a lack of dietary iodine.[7] However, in countries where salt is iodized, goiter of iodine deficiency is rare.

## THYROID REGULATION

The production of T4 and T3 in the thyroid gland is regulated by the hypothalamus and pituitary gland. To ensure stable levels of thyroid hormones, the hypothalamus monitors circulating thyroid hormone levels and responds to low levels by releasing thyrotropin-releasing hormone (TRH). This TRH then stimulates the pituitary to release thyroid stimulating hormone (TSH).[8,9] When thyroid hormone levels increase, production of TSH decreases, which in turn slows the release of new hormone from the thyroid gland.

Cold temperatures can also increase TRH levels. This is thought to be an intrinsic mechanism that helps keep us warm in cold weather.[10]

Elevated levels of cortisol, as seen during stress and in conditions such as Cushing's syndrome, lowers TRH, TSH, and thyroid hormone levels as well.[11,12]

The thyroid gland needs iodine and the amino acid L-tyrosine to make T4 and T3. A diet deficient

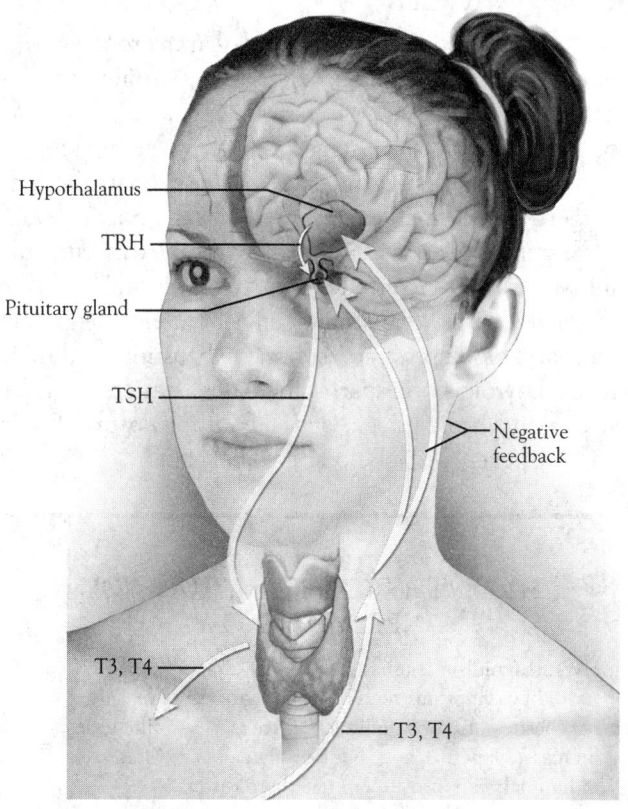

Thyroid hormone regulation

in iodine can limit how much T4 the thyroid gland can produce and lead to hypothyroidism.[13]

T3 is the biologically active form of thyroid hormone. The majority of T3 is produced in the peripheral tissues by conversion of T4 to T3 by a selenium-dependent enzyme. Various factors including nutrient deficiencies, drugs, and chemical toxicity may interfere with conversion of T4 to T3.[14]

Another related enzyme converts T4 to an inactive form of T3 called reverse T3 (rT3). rT3 does not have thyroid hormone activity; instead it blocks the thyroid hormone receptors in the cell hindering action of regular T3.[15]

Ninety-nine percent of circulating thyroid hormones are bound to carrier proteins, rendering them metabolically inactive. The remaining "free" thyroid hormone, the majority of which is T3, binds to and activates thyroid hormone receptors, thereby exerting biological activity.[16] Very small changes in the amount of carrier proteins will affect the percentage of unbound hormones. Oral contraceptives, pregnancy, and conventional female hormone replacement therapy may increase thyroid carrier protein levels, thereby lowering the amount of free thyroid hormone available.[17]

# THYROID DYSFUNCTION

## Hyperthyroidism

In hyperthyroidism, the thyroid gland produces too much thyroid hormone, which can significantly accelerate the body's metabolism. Typical symptoms of hyperthyroidism include sudden weight loss, a rapid heartbeat, sweating, nervousness, or irritability. Hyperthyroidism affects about 1% of the population.[3]

Extreme hyperthyroidism, or thyrotoxicosis, can culminate in what's referred to as "thyroid storm."[18] In this medical emergency, patients suffer from elevated heart rates and blood pressure, extreme exhaustion, and high fever. Thyroid storm sharply increases a patient's risk for stroke and heart attack, and is fatal for up to 50% of patients, even with the best medical care.[19]

---

### HYPERTHYROIDISM: WHAT YOU NEED TO KNOW

Hyperthyroidism is usually caused by Graves disease characterized by symptoms such as rapid heartbeat, sweating, nervousness, tremors, muscle weakness, sleep difficulties, increased appetite, and sudden weight loss.[20] Affected individuals can also experience thyroid storm—a potentially deadly medical emergency.[18]

---

### Medical Treatment of Graves Disease[21]

- Antithyroid drugs, such as *methimazole* or *propylthiouracil*, inhibit the production of T3
- Radioactive iodine, which causes destruction of the overactive thyroid gland
- Surgical removal of the thyroid gland (thyroidectomy)
- Beta-blockers may be used to control the high blood pressure and increased heart rate associated with hyperthyroidism

### Nutritional Support for Hyperthyroidism

- Increased thyroid activity increases loss of L-carnitine through the urine. Individuals suffering from hyperthyroidism may, therefore, require supplemental L-carnitine.[22]
- L-carnitine supplementation helped prevent or reverse muscle weakness and other symptoms in individuals suffering from hyperthyroidism. Clinical trials have shown that doses of 2000–4000 mg/day of L-carnitine are helpful in individuals who suffer from hyperthyroidism.[23]
- Passion flower (*Passifloraincarnata*) and valerian (*Valerianaofficinalis*) are botanicals that have a calming effect on the nervous system[24,25] and thus may help control the symptoms of an overactive thyroid.

---

## Hypothyroidism

Hypothyroidism is a condition in which the thyroid gland does not make enough thyroid hormones, characterized by a reduction in metabolic rate. The main symptoms of hypothyroidism are fatigue, weakness, increased sensitivity to cold, constipation, unexplained weight gain, dry skin, hair loss or coarse dry hair, muscle cramps, and depression. However, most symptoms take years to develop. The slower the metabolism gets, the more obvious the signs and symptoms will become. If hypothyroidism goes untreated, the signs and symptoms could become severe, such as a swollen thyroid gland (goiter), slow thought processes, or dementia.[26]

Subclinical hypothyroidism, an often underdiagnosed thyroid disorder, manifests as elevated TSH, normal T4 and normal T3 levels.[27] Individuals with subclinical hypothyroidism are at greater risk for developing overt hypothyroidism.[28] An August 2010 study reported that 8.3% of women with no history of thyroid disease suffer from subclinical hypothyroidism.[27] An article in the American Family Physician in 2005 estimated that about 20% of women over the age of 60 suffer from subclinical hypothyroidism.[29]

There is evidence that the standard reference range for TSH (blood) may cause many cases of hypothyroidism to be missed. Most physicians accept a reference range for TSH between 0.45 and 4.5 µIU/mL to indicate normal thyroid function. In reality, however, a TSH reading of more than 2.0 may indicate lower-than-optimal thyroid hormone levels.[30]

According to a study reported in *Lancet*, various TSH levels that fall within normal range are associated with adverse health outcomes [23]:

- TSH>2.0: Increased 20-year risk of hypothyroidism and increased risk of thyroid autoimmune disease

- TSH at 2.0–4.0: Hypercholesterolemia and cholesterol levels decline in response to T4 therapy

- TSH>4.0: Greater risk of heart disease

There is another and separate problem brought on by these overly broad normal ranges for TSH. People already diagnosed and being treated for hypothyroidism are often not taking correct doses of thyroid replacement hormone. A November 2010 study reported that about 37% of people being treated for hypothyroidism were taking incorrect doses, about half too much and another half too little.[31]

Consequences of hypothyroidism include:

**Gastrointestinal problems.** Hypothyroidism is a common cause of constipation. Constipation in hypothyroidism may result from diminished motility of the intestines. In some cases, this can lead to intestinal obstruction or abnormal enlargement of the colon.[32] Hypothyroidism is also associated with decreased motility in the esophagus, which causes difficulty swallowing, heartburn, indigestion, nausea, or vomiting. Abdominal discomfort, flatulence, and bloating occur in those with small intestinal bacterial growth secondary to poor digestion.[28]

**Depression and psychiatric disorders.** Panic disorders, depression, and changes in cognition are frequently associated with thyroid disorders.[33] Hypothyroidism is often misdiagnosed as depression.[34] A study published in 2002 suggests that thyroid function is especially important for bipolar patients: "Our results suggest that nearly three-quarters of patients with bipolar disorder have a thyroid profile that may be suboptimal for antidepressant response."[35]

**Cognitive decline.** Patients with low thyroid function can suffer from slowed thinking, delayed processing of information, difficulty recalling names, and so on.[36] Patients with subclinical hypothyroidism show signs of decreased working memory[37] as well as decreased speed of sensory and cognitive processing.[38] An evaluation of thyroid hormones along with TSH may help avoid misdiagnosis as being depressed.[39]

**Cardiovascular disease.** Hypothyroidism and subclinical hypothyroidism are associated with increased levels of blood cholesterol, increased blood pressure, and increased risk of cardiovascular disease.[40] Even those with subclinical hypothyroidism were almost 3.4 times as likely to develop cardiovascular disease than those with healthy thyroid function.[41]

- **High blood pressure.** Hypertension is relatively common among patients with hypothyroidism. In a 1983 study, 14.8% of patients with hypothyroidism had high blood pressure compared with 5.5% of patients with normal thyroid function.[42] "*Hypothyroidism has been recognized as a cause of secondary hypertension. Previous studies … have demonstrated elevated blood pressure values. Increased peripheral vascular resistance and low cardiac output has been suggested to be the possible link between hypothyroidism and diastolic hypertension.*"[43]

- **High cholesterol and atherosclerosis.** "*Overt hypothyroidism is characterized by hypercholesterolemia and a marked increase in low-density lipoproteins (LDL) and apolipoproteinB.*"[44] These changes accelerate atherosclerosis, which causes coronary artery disease.[39] The risk of heart disease increases proportionally with increasing TSH, even in subclinical hypothyroidism.[45] Hypothyroidism caused by autoimmune reactions is associated with stiffening of the blood vessels.[46] Thyroid hormone replacement may slow the progression of coronary heart disease by inhibiting the progression of plaques.[47,48]

- **Homocysteine.** Treating hypothyroid patients with thyroid hormone replacement might attenuate homocysteine levels, an independent risk factor for cardiovascular disease: "*A strong inverse relationship between homocysteine and free thyroid hormones confirms the effect of thyroid hormones on homocysteinemetabolism.*"[49]

- **Elevated C-reactive protein.** Both overt and subclinical hypothyroidism are associated with increased levels of low-grade inflammation, as indicated by elevated C-reactive protein (CRP). A 2003 clinic study observed that CRP values increased with progressive thyroid failure and suggested it may count as an additional risk factor for the development of coronary heart disease in hypothyroid patients.[50]

**Metabolic syndrome.** In a study of more than 1500 subjects, researchers found that those with metabolic syndrome had statistically significantly higher TSH levels (meaning lower thyroid hormone output) than healthy control subjects. Subclinical hypothyroidism was also correlated with elevated triglyceride levels and increased blood pressure. Slight increases in

TSH may put people at higher risk for metabolic syndrome.[51]

**Reproductive system problems.** In women, hypothyroidism is associated with menstrual irregularities and infertility.[52] Proper treatment can restore a normal menstrual cycle and improve fertility.[53]

**Fatigue and weakness.** The well known and common symptoms of hypothyroidism, such as chilliness, weight gain, paresthesia (tingling or crawling sensation in the skin) and cramps are often absent in elderly patients compared with younger patients; fatigue and weakness are common in hypothyroid patients.[54]

# TESTING THYROID FUNCTION

## Thyroid Stimulating Hormone

Thyroid stimulating hormone (TSH) level is the most common test for screening for thyroid dysfunction. In the last decade, the diagnostic strategy for using TSH measurements has changed as a result of the sensitivity improvements in these assays. It is now recognized that the TSH measurement is a more sensitive test than T4 for detecting both hypo- and hyperthyroidism.[55] As a result, some countries now promote a TSH-first strategy for diagnosing thyroid dysfunction in patients.[56]

In 2008 many labs adopted the reference range for TSH, 0.45–4.50 µIU/mL, recommended by both the Endocrine Society and the American Medical Association. Although this range is an improvement over the previous 0.45–5.5 mIU/L, it is still considered too broad by many clinicians.[55,56,57]

The American Association of Clinical Endocrinologists now recommends an upper limit of 3.0 mIU/L.[57] The guidelines for diagnosing thyroid disease from the National Academy of Clinical Biochemistry point out that *"more than 95% of normal individuals have TSH levels below 2.5 µIU/mL."*[58] This panel suggests that the upper limit of TSH should be reduced to 2.5 µIU/mL.[59]

On the other hand, current studies also suggest that TSH values below the normal range may represent thyroid hormone excess and, in elderly patients, might be associated with an increased risk of death due to cardiovascular disease.[60,61]

Life Extension suggests an optimal level of TSH between 1.0 and 2.0 µIU/mL, as some studies have noted that a TSH above 2.0 may be associated with adverse cardiovascular risk factors.[23] In addition, a TSH between 1.0 and 2.0 µIU/mL has been associated with the lowest subsequent incidence of abnormal thyroid function.[62]

However, while a measure of TSH alone is a useful screening tool in assessing thyroid function, Life Extension advocates additional testing, including free T3 and T4 levels, to provide a more complete evaluation of the thyroid.

Note: TSH values do fluctuate with time of day, infection, and various other factors. In a 2007 survey published in the Archives of Internal Medicine, values spontaneously returned to normal in more than 50% of patients with abnormal TSH levels when the test was repeated at a later date.[63] No single measurement of TSH should be considered diagnostic.

## Basal Body Temperature

An alternative method for assessing thyroid status that was widely used in the past, before the development of accurate thyroid function blood tests, is the basal body temperature test. The temperature is taken when the body is at complete rest, immediately after waking, and before beginning any activity. The normal basal temperature is 97.6–98.2 °F, and some alternative practitioners believe that a 5-day consecutive temperature reading below 97.6 °F is indicative of hypothyroidism. One study showed a significant correlation between basal body temperature and low thyroid function in whiplash patients. The authors of this study conclude that basal body temperature "seems to be a sensitive screening test, in combination with laboratory analysis, for the hypothyroidism seen after whiplash trauma."[64] However, there are many reasons for alteration of basal body temperature; a thyroid panel blood test should be taken to accurately evaluate the thyroid function.

## Tests for T4 and T3

Thyroid hormones can be tested in both their free and protein-bound forms. Tests for the protein-bound forms and unbound form of T4 or T3 are generally referred to as total T4 or total T3, respectively; unbound forms are called free T4 and free T3. Each of these tests gives information about how the body is making, activating, and responding to thyroid hormone. Levels of free T3 and T4 will be below normal in clinical hypothyroidism. In subclinical hypothyroidism, the TSH will be elevated while the thyroid hormone levels are still in the normal reference range.

## Reverse T3

Certain individuals with apparently normal T4 and T3 hormone levels still display the classic symptoms of hypothyroidism. This may be due to an excessive production of rT3. rT3 is inactive and may interfere with the action of T3 in the body. Stress and extreme exercise may play a role in lowering thyroid hormone action by suppressing production of TSH and T3 and elevating rT3 levels.[11,65]

## Autoimmune Antibodies

When evaluating the thyroid, it is also important to consider that the most common cause of overt hypothyroidism in the United States is an autoimmune disorder known as Hashimoto's thyroiditis.[66] In this condition, the body produces antibodies to the thyroid gland and damage the gland. Hashimoto's thyroiditis is diagnosed by standard thyroid testing in conjunction with testing for the presence of these antibodies called antithyroglobulin antibodies (AgAb) and thyroperoxidase antibodies (TPOAb). Some people with celiac disease or sensitivity to gluten are at increased risk for developing autoimmune thyroid disease and should be evaluated.[67]

Elevated thyroid antibodies are often associated with chronic urticaria, also called hives. Studies report that as many as 57.4% of patients with hives have antithyroidantibodies.[68,69] A 2010 paper[70] suggested that treatment with T4 improved the itching associated with urticaria, but did not advise treatment with T4 unless the patient was hypothyroid.

## Additional Testing

Sometimes *biopsy* or *enzymatic studies* are required to establish a definite diagnosis for thyroid dysfunction. Major abnormalities of the thyroid gland detected in a physical exam can be further assessed by *ultrasound* or a procedure known as *scintigraphy*.

## Hypothalamic Pituitary Axis (HPA)

There is an intimate relationship between the thyroid, adrenal glands, and sex hormones.[71] If hypothyroidism is suspected, evaluation of adrenal glands as well as sex hormones is suggested.

---

## HYPOTHYROIDISM: WHAT YOU NEED TO KNOW

- Thyroid diseases occur about five times more frequently in women than in men. As many as 20% of women over 60 years old have subclinical hypothyroidism.[29]
- If untreated, chronic hypothyroidism can result in myxedema coma, a rare, life-threatening condition. Mental dysfunction, stupor, cardiovascular collapse, and coma can develop after worsening of chronic hypothyroidism as well.[72]
- An autoimmune disease called Hashimoto's thyroiditis is the most common cause of low thyroid function in the United States. The body's immune system mistakenly attacks the thyroid tissue, impairing the ability to make hormones.[73] Hypothyroidism caused by Hashimoto's disease is treated with thyroid hormone replacement agents.

- Hashimoto's disease usually causes hypothyroidism, but may also trigger hyperthyroid symptoms.[66]
- Hyperthyroidism is usually caused by Graves disease, in which antibodies are produced that bind to TSH receptors in the thyroid gland, stimulating excess thyroid hormone production.[18]
- The distinction between Hashimoto's thyroiditis and Graves disease may not be as important as once thought. In 2009 researchers wrote: *"Hashimoto's and Graves' disease are different expressions of a basically similar autoimmune process, and the clinical appearance reflects the spectrum of the immune response in a particular patient."*[74] The two diseases can overlap causing both thyroid gland stimulation and destruction simultaneously or in sequence.[75] Some clinicians consider the two conditions different presentations of the same disease.[76] About 4% of patients with Graves disease displayed some symptoms of Hashimoto's thyroiditis during childhood.[77]
- Pregnant women are especially at risk for hypothyroidism. During pregnancy, the thyroid gland produces more thyroid hormone than when a woman is not pregnant,[78] and the gland may increase slightly in size.
- Uncontrolled thyroid dysfunction during pregnancy can lead to preterm birth, mental retardation, and hemorrhage in the postpartum period.[79] It is important to work closely with a physician to monitor thyroid function during pregnancy.
- Tests to diagnose and monitor hypothyroidism include thyroid stimulating hormone (TSH), total T4, total T3, free T4 (fT4), free T3 (fT3), rT3, thyroid peroxidase antibody (TPOAb), and thyroglobulin antibody (TgAb)

---

# THYROID HORMONE REPLACEMENT

The most common treatment for low thyroid hormone levels consists of thyroid hormone replacement therapy. The goal of thyroid hormone replacement is to relieve symptoms and provide sufficient thyroid hormone to decrease elevated TSH levels to within the normal range.[80]

Conventional treatment almost always begins with synthetic T4 (levothyroxine) preparations such as Synthroid® or Levoxyl®. Low doses are usually used at first because a rapid increase in thyroid hormone may result in cardiac damage.[81]

Sometimes hypothyroid symptoms persist despite T4 treatment. In a 2001 study, T4 therapy was no more effective than placebo in improving cognitive function and psychological well-being in patients with symptoms of hypothyroidism, despite improvement in free T3 levels.[82] A December 2010 study compared the T3 and T4 levels of hypothyroid patients treated with T4 alone against the levels found in healthy people; researchers reported that T4 supplementation alone did not increase T3 to the same level as found in healthy people.[83] Deficiencies in nutrients like selenium can disable the body from converting T4 to biologically active T3.

In an animal study, rats with their thyroid gland removed were treated with T4 alone. Researchers found that no single dose restored normal concentrations of TSH, T4, and T3 in the blood, tissues, and organs.[84] The following year the same authors reported that a combination of T4 and T3 was able to normalize hormone levels in both blood and tissues.[85] Other studies have failed to demonstrate any advantage of combination therapy, although the results do suggest the possibility of a subset of hypothyroid patients who would benefit from combination therapy.[86,87]

One combination option is a drug called Thyrolar®, which combines synthetic T3 and T4 in a fixed 1:4 ratio. Caution should be used, however, in administering T3 to older individuals because excess T3 may cause adverse cardiac events in this population.[88]

Another T3 option is a drug called Cytomel®, which is a synthetic form of T3. This can be used in combination with T4.

## Desiccated Thyroid

Armour Thyroid, Nature-Throid, and Westhroid are prescription medications that contain desiccated porcine thyroid gland. Natural thyroid extracts have been used since 1892 and were approved by the Food and Drug Administration in 1939. Armour Thyroid and most other natural glandular preparations are made to standards approved by the United States Pharmacopoeia.

Armour Thyroid is preferred by some clinicians because it may achieve results in patients that fail to respond to levothyroxine alone. Patients with hypothyroidism show greater improvements in mood and brain function if they receive treatment with Armour Thyroid rather than Synthroid®.[89] One argument favoring natural hormones is that other naturally occurring hormones and chemicals found in these preparations may buffer or enhance the effect of the active hormones.[80,85]

Ultimately, there may not be a single correct approach to low thyroid hormone levels. Instead, the best option may be to monitor thyroid levels through regular blood testing and systematically try various protocols to see what yields the best resolution of symptoms. Some people may prefer to begin with desiccated thyroid, while others may find it preferable to begin with T4 supplementation then move to a combination T3–T4 therapy if they experience no improvement from T4 alone.

## Absorption of Thyroid Hormone Medications

Coffee,[90] aluminum antacids,[91] ferrous sulfate (iron),[92] calcium carbonate,[93] soy,[94] and possibly grapefruit juice[95] can all decrease the absorption of thyroid hormone prescriptions. Most doctors simply advise patients to take thyroid away from any food or medication.

While most people take thyroid hormone in the morning, a December 2010 paper suggests that it is more effective to take thyroid just before bed.[96]

# NUTRIENTS TO SUPPORT THYROID FUNCTION

## Iodine

The body needs iodine to make thyroid hormone. As of the late 1990s, 32 European countries were still affected by iodine deficiency.[97] In 2007, the World Health Organization estimated that over 30% of the world's population (2 billion) has insufficient iodine intake as measured by urinary iodine excretion below 100 µg/L.[98] Iodized salt has proven to be effective at preventing iodine deficiency. The Morton Salt Company began selling iodized salt in the United States in 1924.[99]

Hypothyroidism in the unborn child, congenital hypothyroidism, or cretinism is frequently caused by iodine deficiency. In industrialized countries, the incidence is about 1 case in 4500 live births. Yet, the incidence of cretinism can increase to as much as 1 case in 20 live births in areas that have iodine deficiency.[100] Because of this, iodine deficiency remains one of the leading causes of mental retardation.[101]

During pregnancy T4 production doubles, causing increases in daily iodine requirements.[102] Iodine deficient pregnant women cannot produce the thyroid hormones needed for proper neurologic development of their growing babies, and are at high risk of giving birth to infants with cognitive impairment and learning delay. Even moderate iodine deficiency in a pregnant woman can lower her infant's IQ 8–16 points.[103,104]

People who avoid iodized salt or adhere to a salt-restricted diet may become iodine deficient.[105] Vegetarians are also at risk of developing iodine deficiency, especially if they eat food grown in low iodine soil.[106] Vegans who avoid sea vegetables are also at higher risk.[107]

Diets both low and high in iodine are associated with hypothyroidism. This is supported by studies showing that both low and high urinary iodine excretion are associated with hypothyroidism.[108] High intake of iodine also increases the risk of Hashimoto's thyroiditis.[109]

Iodine or foods high in iodine, such as seaweed, are thought useful in treating hypothyroidism, but this is probably only true for people who are iodine deficient.[106,107] In 2007, Teas and colleagues[110] reported a slight increase in TSH levels in healthy postmenopausal women who consumed 5 g/day of seaweed (*Alariaesculenta*). A 2008 trial measuring the effect of eating kombu

(*Laminaria japonica*) seaweed in Japanese adults found that eating 15 and 30 g of kombu (containing 35 and 70 mg of iodine, respectively) daily for 7–10 days significantly increased TSH (which reflects lower thyroid hormone output).[111]

The upper intake level (UL) of iodine for adults is 1.1 mg per day. The safety of therapeutic doses of iodine above the established UL is evident in the lack of toxicity in people living in the northern coastal regions of Japan, whose diets contain large amounts of seaweed with a daily iodine intake of 50 000–80 000 mcg (50–80 mg).[112] Studies using 3.0–6.0 mg iodine per day to effectively treat fibrocystic breast disease may reveal an important role for iodine in maintaining normal breast tissue architecture and function.[113] Iodine may also have important antioxidant functions in breast tissue and other tissues that concentrate iodine.[114]

Life Extension's review of the scientific literature suggests an iodine intake up to 1150 mcg daily is reasonable. However, the amount of supplemental iodine needed for an individual varies widely based on the factors listed above. It is important to test thyroid function when supplementing with iodine since both low and excessively high intake can contribute to hypothyroidism.

## Selenium

After iodine, selenium is probably the next most important mineral affecting thyroid function. The thyroid contains more selenium by weight than any other organ.[115] Selenium is a necessary component of the enzymes that remove iodine molecules from T4 converting it into T3; without selenium, activation of thyroid hormone is not possible. When patients suffering from various forms of thyroid disease were tested for selenium levels, all were found to be lower than in normal healthy people.[116] Some researchers suggest that selenium supplementation improves conversion of T4 to T3.[117] Selenium also plays a role in protecting the thyroid gland itself. The cells of the thyroid generate hydrogen peroxide and use it to make thyroid hormone. Selenium protects the thyroid gland from the oxidative damage caused by these reactions. Without adequate selenium, high iodine levels lead to destruction of the thyroid gland cells.[115,118]

People living in areas with low selenium content in the soil are more likely to develop Hashimoto's disease.[119] This may be because a selenium deficiency makes the enzyme glutathione peroxidase less effective.[120] Therefore, selenium supplementation has been suggested for treating Hashimoto's disease.[121]

In a placebo-controlled study published in 2002, researchers in Germany reported on an experiment in which they gave 200 mcg of sodium selenite daily to patients with Hashimoto's disease and high levels of thyroid peroxidase antibodies. After 3 months, the thyroid peroxidase antibody levels of the patients taking selenium declined by 66.4% compared to their pretreatment values, and antibody levels returned to normal in nine of the selenium treated patients.[122] Austrian researchers reported in 2008 that they were unable to duplicate the results of the earlier study when they did not limit the study population to those with high levels of thyroid peroxidase antibodies. They suggest that selenium supplementation might be of greater benefit to patients with higher disease activity.[123]

Selenium deficiency is also common in celiac disease, which may be the tie-in to increased frequency of thyroid problems with celiac disease.[124]

During severe or prolonged infection, blood levels of selenium, T4, T3, and TSH decrease, and the conversion of T4 to T3 slows, inducing a hypothyroid state.[125] Because the enzymes that moderate this conversion require selenium, it has been hypothesized that supplementing extra selenium might prevent this decrease in T3 during illness. Supplying extra selenium may decrease mortality from infection, but it does not normalize thyroid hormone levels.[126] It seems that the suppression of T3 during sickness is mediated by cytokines, in particular interleukin-6 (IL-6).[127] It may be that IL-6 and other cytokines generated by infection limit production of selenium enzymes and interfere with hormone production.

## Zinc

Zinc may be helpful in patients with low T3 and may contribute to conversion of T4 to T3. In animal studies, zinc deficiency lowered T3 and free T4 concentrations by approximately 30%. Levels of total T4 were not affected by zinc deficiency.[128] In a group of patients with low levels of free T3, normal T4, elevated rT3, and mild to moderate zinc deficiency, oral zinc supplementation for 12 months normalized the serum levels of free T3 and total T3, decreased rT3, and normalized TSH levels.[129]

Like iodine, too much zinc may suppress thyroid function.[130] Very high doses of zinc interfere with copper absorption and can lead to a serious and potentially fatal copper deficiency.[131–133] Therefore, taking copper when supplementing with zinc is advised.

## Iron

Iron deficiency hinders manufacture of thyroid hormone by reducing activity of the enzyme thyroid peroxidase. In one study, 15.7% of women with subclinical hypothyroidism were iron deficient compared to only 9.8% of the control group.[134] Iron-deficiency anemia decreases and iron supplementation improves the beneficial effects of iodine supplementation.[118] Treating iron-deficient hypothyroid patients with levothyroxine (T4) along with iron improves their iron deficiency anemia more than treatment with iron alone.[135]

## Copper

An August 2010 study revealed that copper is important for normal brain development; its deficiency leaves the hypothalamus unable to regulate thyroid hormone effectively. Copper-deficient pregnant rats give birth to infant rats that produce 48% less T3 than those born from healthy mothers.[136]

## Vitamin E

Vitamin E may reduce the oxidative stress caused by hypothyroidism. In one animal study, vitamin E was shown to protect animals from increased oxidation and thyroid cell damage.[137] In another study, vitamin E reduced the amount of thyroid cell replication in animals with induced hypothyroidism.[138]

## Vitamin D

Deficiency of vitamin D may increase risk of autoimmune thyroid disease. When adjusted for age, presence of thyroid antibodies was inversely correlated with vitamin D levels in a group of 642 participants (244 males and 398 females) in New Delhi, India.[139] Moreover, other evidence suggests that compared to the general population, vitamin D deficiency is more common among individuals with thyroid cancer or thyroid nodules.[140] Given the many benefits of adequate vitamin D, it makes sense to supplement if needed.

## Vitamin B12

Hypothyroid patients are often vitamin B12 deficient. In a 2008 paper, Pakistani doctors reported that of 116 hypothyroid patients tested for vitamin B12, approximately 40% were deficient.[141] The link between B12 deficiency and low thyroid function is not clear, nor is it clear whether thyroid function will improve with B12 supplementation.[142] However, since low B12 causes serious neurologic damage, all hypothyroid patients should be tested.

## DHEA and Pregnenolone

Japanese researchers reported that concentrations of DHEA, DHEA sulfate, and pregnenolone sulfate are significantly lower in hypothyroid patients compared to age- and sex-matched healthy controls.[143]

## Turmeric (*Curcuma longa*) Extract

A 2002 study found that treatment with turmeric extract in rats reduced the impact of chemically induced hypothyroidism in terms of thyroid weight, T4, T3, and cholesterol levels.[144] Results of a similar trial on rats treated with vitamin E and curcumin, a component found in turmeric, showed that treatment prevented a decline in basal body temperature and protected the liver.[145]

## Rhodiola Rosea

Given the fact that stress can influence thyroid status, it may be beneficial for some individuals with hypothyroidism to consider adaptogenic herbs such as *Rhodiola*.[146,147] Adaptogenic herbs support the adrenal glands and can improve the body's response to stress.[148]

# DIETARY RECOMMENDATIONS

Some foods contain goitrogenic substances that reduce the utilization of iodine. These foods include canola oil, vegetables from the Brassica family (eg, cabbage[149] and Brussels sprouts[150]), cassava,[151] and millet.[152] The actual content of goitrogens in these foods is relatively low, however, and cooking significantly reduces the impact of these goitrogens on thyroid function.[153]

Studies show conflicting information concerning the impact of soy on the thyroid. Isoflavone molecules in soy do inhibit an enzyme involved in thyroid hormone synthesis,[154,155] but that has not translated into poor thyroid function in otherwise healthy individuals with adequate iodine intake.[156–158]

For those with hypothyroidism, raw goitrogenic foods and soy foods that have not undergone fermentation and/or food processing should be consumed in moderation and discontinued if symptoms appear.

## Life Extension Suggestions

**Thyroid hormone supplementation:** If hormones are necessary, work with an experienced medical provider to find a hormone supplement that works best for you.

**TSH target:** An ideal TSH level is between 1 and 2 μIU/mL. TSH levels lower than this may increase risks and symptoms associated with hyperthyroidism. TSH levels higher than this may increase risks and symptoms associated with hypothyroidism.

- **Iodine**: Up to 1150 mcg daily
- **Selenium**: 200–400 mcg daily
- **Zinc**: 30–80 mg daily
- **Copper**: 1–2 mg daily
- **Natural Vitamin E**: 400 IU alpha-tocopherol and 200 mg gamma-tocopherol
- **Vitamin C**: 1000–2000 mg daily
- **Iron**: Check for deficiency and correct if low
- **Vitamin B12** (as methylcobalamin): 1000–2000 mcg daily
- **DHEA**: The exact dosage to be taken should be determined by blood testing and the advice of a physician. Typical dosages range from 15–75 mg daily taken in the morning. DHEA serum blood tests are suggested 3–6 weeks after initiating DHEA replacement therapy to optimize individual dosing.
- **Pregnenolone**: Check for deficiencies and correct if low. Typical dosages are 50–100 mg daily. A complete hormone profile is suggested when supplementing with pregnenolone as it may affect levels of other hormones, such as progesterone, estrogen, testosterone, and/or DHEA.
- **Rhodiola**, standardized extract: 250–500 mg daily
- **L-tyrosine**: 500–1000 mg daily

In addition, the following blood testing resources may be helpful:

- Thyroid Panel (TSH, T4, Free T4, Free T3)
- Reverse T3
- Thyroid Antibody Panel
- Female Comprehensive Hormone Panel or Male Comprehensive Hormone Panel; or Female Panel or Male Panel
- Vitamin D, 25-Hydroxy

**Caution:** Cancer patients should avoid taking L-phenylalanine and L-tyrosine. Certain cancers, such as melanoma, depend on these amino acids to fuel their growth. Supplemental use of L-phenylalanine and L-tyrosine may raise or normalize blood pressure. Insomnia may occur from overstimulation if taken too close to bedtime. Individuals with the rare metabolic disorder phenylketonuria should avoid phenylalanine. Those suffering from migraine headaches should also avoid L-phenylalanine and L-tyrosine because they form tyramine, a substance that may trigger migraines.

## REFERENCES

References available at: www.lef.org/dpt5/ch125

# 126

# Trauma and Wound Healing

Trauma is a stressful event caused by either a mechanical or chemical injury. Depending on its level, trauma can have serious short-term and long-term consequences. The role of healthy nutrition, both in promoting healing and avoiding complications associated with trauma, has long been acknowledged in trauma recovery.

Trauma varies in intensity, ranging from serious burns or traffic accidents to the gradual, cumulative trauma that occurs with repetitive overuse of muscles and joints (such as strenuous weight lifting). Minor injuries, often no more than minor irritants, are relatively frequent. However, any traumatic event, even a minor one, affects the body's natural metabolic balance and initiates a cascade of reactions aimed at repair and restoration of function.

Over the past few decades, trauma has become increasingly common.[1] This may be due in part to newer, more dangerous pastimes and sports. People have also learned a great deal about recovering from trauma, including nutritional approaches to maximize healing.

## TISSUE RESPONSE TO TRAUMA

Trauma (or any injury) results in tissue damage. Immediately after traumatic injury, a pattern of local reactions and systemic changes is launched. This reparative process involves almost all organ systems.

The local response to trauma serves three goals: stop blood loss, clear tissue debris, and restore normal biological function to affected area with use of scar tissue.

### Limitation of Blood Loss

This begins with a brief constriction of blood vessels to reduce blood flow to the affected area. Meanwhile, platelets are activated to form a clot or mesh of fibrin to block the bleeding blood vessels. Platelets then release substances such as histamine, serotonin, and cytokines, which activate the next stage of healing, inflammation.

### Clearing of Tissue Debris

Once the bleeding is under control, the body begins to remove damaged and dysfunctional tissue through inflammatory response. Only after the debris is completely reabsorbed can the body lay down a new tissue framework. Inflammation requires the activation of certain enzyme systems and pro-inflammatory cells that dissolve damaged tissue.

During this inflammatory period, blood flow to the wound is increased. This vasodilation, which follows intense vasoconstriction seen immediately after the wound is created, is mediated by chemicals such as histamine, prostaglandins, and those found in the complement cascade, which is part of the immune system response to injury. Under their influence, blood vessel walls in the area of the wound become leaky, allowing repair cells and protein-rich plasma to gather in damaged tissues. This process results in swelling.

Plasma spilling into the wound serves multiple functions. It dilutes any irritants in the injured area and brings protein molecules called fibrinogen, which link with each other and form a fibrin mesh big enough to occupy the entire wound. This clot helps trap foreign particles, enhances immune cell effectiveness, and forms scaffolding over which new tissues are laid down.

Neutrophils are among the first white blood cells to arrive at the injury site. They remove dead and dying cells, blood clots, and the fibrin mesh to clean up the wound. Other immune cells including monocytes, lymphocytes, eosinophils, and basophils follow neutrophils. Together these immune cells engulf and digest any bacteria.

## Scar Tissue and Long-Term Healing

Once bleeding has stopped and the body's immediate inflammatory response has been activated, long-term healing and tissue regeneration can begin. The growth of new tissue consists of 3 different processes:

- Angiogenesis, or creation of new blood vessels
- Formation of granulation tissue
- Remodeling of the scar to suit changing functional requirements

**Angiogenesis.** The cells lining damaged capillaries start multiplying to form fresh blood vessels, a process known as angiogenesis. New capillaries not only help clear dead tissue, but also support growing cells by supplying oxygen and nutrients.

**Granulation and remodeling.** Once the wound is free of debris and new blood vessels have begun to form, repair cells called fibroblasts lay down a scaffolding of collagen. This collagen network matures into granulation tissue, which forms the foundation of scars. Granulation tissue matures as collagen fibers become increasingly interlinked. Externally, the scar can be seen to contract and close the wound; this process of collagen maturation and remodeling continues for a lifetime.

## SYSTEMIC RESPONSE TO INJURY

Four major organ systems are involved in wound healing: the sympathetic nervous system, endocrine organs, cardiovascular system, and an acute phase reaction involving the liver. During the immediate systemic response, the wounded person becomes alert, opium-like substances are released to decrease pain, heart and respiratory rates quicken, blood glucose levels rise, and the basal metabolic rate speeds up. This is a stress reaction, with organ systems functioning at supraphysiologic levels. Unless supported by appropriate nutritional therapy, a sustained level of stress takes a toll on the body's physiology.

The systemic response is produced as local chemical mediators spill into blood vessels from the wound. They activate circulating monocytes (a kind of immune cell) to release chemical messengers called cytokines, which cause the various metabolic changes seen after trauma. In cases of major trauma, there may be generalized fever, increased oxygen consumption, and increased metabolism of fats, glucose, and proteins.

As the reaction is prolonged over days or weeks, local lymph nodes and the spleen enlarge to supply immune cells.

## MALNUTRITION IN TRAUMA PATIENTS

The body needs a certain amount of nutrients to maintain a constant, healthy state. This need is determined by the basal metabolic rate. Any external or internal trauma raises the metabolic rate, and greater amounts of oxygen and nutrients are required to supply enough fuel and amino acids for repair and recovery.

Energy expenditure may rise by 10–50% to support the intense metabolic workload.[2] Protein and amino acid requirements increase to support formation of new tissues and proliferation of immune cells, maintain lean body mass (or muscle protein), and replace protein lost to perspiration, bleeding, and excretion.

A positive nutritional balance is reflected in rapid healing of wounds, an efficient immune response, the absence of infections or sepsis (shock), and maintenance of a lean body mass.

Population studies indicate that 9–44% of people with wound and surgical trauma are malnourished.[3] The condition often goes unrecognized and untreated in hospitals, and some studies have explored the increased risk of malnutrition during hospital stays, based on the common occurrence of clinically significant weight loss observed in hospitalized surgical patients.[4]

Biologically, it is difficult to achieve usual levels of nutrition after major trauma because many important nutrients are channeled into the healing effort. In addition, many trauma patients suffer from altered levels of consciousness, poor appetite, reduced digestive function, compromised blood circulation, and a radical alteration of normal daily routines.

There are also pronounced changes in the way the body metabolizes nutrients and food. Under normal circumstances, carbohydrates and fat are used to produce or store energy, and protein is used for developing and maintaining lean body mass. In this nonstressed condition, 90% of energy is supplied by carbohydrates or fat, and proteins contribute only 5–8% of total calories.

By contrast, during trauma, proteins (including muscle mass) are broken down to yield as much as 30% of caloric needs. Even when nutrients are supplemented, proteins will be utilized to provide 20–25% of caloric needs.

Compared to fat, protein yields less energy per gram. The patient becomes hypermetabolic, requiring higher-than-normal levels of calories and protein. Abnormal metabolism is caused by the release of stress hormones such as cortisol and catecholamines. This hypermetabolic state contributes to rapid loss of lean body mass, even when the patient is well fed. It is critical that trauma patients maintain an adequate supply of protein and calories to protect their lean muscle mass and supply their healing body with necessary nutrients.

## COMPLICATIONS OF TRAUMA

Besides the danger posed by trauma and the risk of malnutrition, patients are also at risk for complications resulting from their injury. Wound repair may be impeded by the following complications:

- **Infection.** Wound infection can occur in cases of extensive wound area, poor host defenses, and improper wound care.

- **Keloid.** Keloid is a bulky protrusion of scar tissue formed as a result of abnormal collagen synthesis. It can spread to the adjoining skin.

- **Gangrene.** Gangrene is dead wound tissue formed by the decay of body tissues. It can be caused by infection, blood clots, or lack of blood flow. This condition is most common in the extremities.

- **Rapid weight loss.** This results from protein–calorie malnutrition.

- **Compromised immune system.** The malnourished patient can quickly exhibit symptoms of decreased immune function, such as infection.

Extreme injuries can also provoke an uncontrollable inflammatory response, overwhelming vital organ systems like the heart and lungs. This life-threatening condition, known as systemic inflammatory response syndrome, is a major problem in the management of multiple traumas. While optimal levels of inflammation can clear debris and initiate healing, these reactions need to be regulated vigilantly. Enzymes and chemicals that dissolve dead tissue can also damage living tissue. If inflammation overwhelms the control mechanism, it can reach life-threatening proportions.

---

## WHAT YOU HAVE LEARNED SO FAR

- Trauma is a generic term for physical or chemical injury. The intensity of trauma ranges from an acute, life-threatening event to gradual, cumulative injuries.
- The body's response to trauma involves both a local and systemic reaction. Inflammation, blood clotting, and immune system activation are all necessary elements of healing after trauma.
- During trauma, the body functions at an enhanced physiologic rate. The body's requirement for calories, protein, and nutrients is greatly enhanced, leading to a risk of malnourishment among trauma patients.
- Nutritional supplementation is critical to helping the healing process.

---

# TARGETED NUTRITIONAL STRATEGIES

## Essential Nutrients for Wound Healing

Based on extensive biological and metabolic changes that occur after trauma, nutritional supplementation is often required. The following nutritional factors have been shown to support the body's enhanced metabolic demands.

**Calories.** Wound healing consumes energy. Ordinarily, carbohydrates and fats are the main sources of energy. During the stress response, proteins are also broken down to provide energy. To prevent loss of lean body mass, sufficient energy supply has to be maintained. After trauma, caloric requirements may be increased up to 25–30 calories per kilogram of body weight daily.[5]

**Carbohydrates.** Carbohydrates are a rich source of cellular energy during wound healing. After a wound, carbohydrates:

- Help meet the body's heightened energy requirements

- Aid in fibroblast movement, which is vital in wound healing
- Enhance white blood cell activity to strengthen immune response

**Protein.** Proteins are a vital component of collagen synthesis. Therefore, insufficient protein can affect the rate and quality of wound healing. Trauma increases the demand for protein. This requirement is further increased in the event of sepsis or stress. Wound healing requires 1.5–3 g per kilogram (of body weight) per day of protein; this requirement may vary depending on the type of wound.[5]

**Fats.** Fats are a concentrated source of calories. Supplementation with certain fatty acids is essential. They play the chief role in cell membrane structure and function, as well as help wound healing. It is recommended that 20% of calories be obtained from fat, especially monounsaturated fat. Fats are also implicated in the synthesis of new cells; therefore, low fat levels would delay wound healing.

**Vitamin A.** Vitamin A is indispensable for normal growth and differentiation of skin, making it significant in wound healing. Vitamin A increases the strength of scar tissue. It is required for an adequate inflammatory response and has been used to counteract the catabolic effect glucocorticosteroids exert on wound healing.[6] The improvement in wound healing from vitamin A supplementation is also attributed to an increase in collagen cross-linking, which results in higher tensile strength.[7]

**Vitamin C.** Wound healing requires more vitamin C than diet alone can provide.[8] As vitamin C is water soluble, it has to be taken daily. Vitamin C is important for proper function of the enzyme protocollagen hydroxylase, which generates collagen. Vitamin C forms bonds between strands of collagen fibers and helps provide extra strength and stability. It is also essential for synthesis of the intracellular matrix of tissues such as bone, skin, blood vessel walls, and connective tissue. Finally, vitamin C is a potent antioxidant; studies have shown elevated levels of reactive oxygen species (a kind of free radical) in wounds.[9,10]

**Zinc.** Zinc is a trace mineral present in the body in only a small quantity. However, it is found in many tissues, including bone, skin, muscle, and organs, and is required in as many as 300 enzymatic reactions. Zinc is used in DNA synthesis, cell division, and protein synthesis; also, it mediates the maturation of T-lymphocytes.[11] The body's need for zinc increases during cell proliferation and protein secretion.

**Water.** Meeting hypermetabolic needs may leave the body dehydrated. Not only is it essential to maintain hydration, but the need for hydration increases if a wound is draining or a person is on an air-fluidized therapy bed. Trauma patients' daily requirement of water may range from 1500–2000 mL.[5]

## The Therapeutic Role of Nutrition

Hypermetabolic effects of stress may require special or high-dose nutrients for enhanced wound healing and uneventful recovery.

**Arginine.** Arginine fuels the cellular immune response and fights against bacterial challenges. It is an essential precursor to protein synthesis at the wound site and increases local wound immune function. Researchers have found that in the case of trauma and surgery, arginine requirements increase to 17–25 g of oral arginine daily, in contrast to the normal daily requirement of 5 g.[12,13] Enhanced wound healing has been observed with large doses of arginine.[14]

**Glutamine.** Glutamine is a key substrate for fast-growing and multiplying cells, including white blood cells. Glutamine stimulates the proliferation of fibroblasts, thereby helping in wound closure. It is the major amino acid lost during any tissue injury, implying a significant role in the preservation of lean body mass. According to researchers, glutamine possesses anabolic properties, which are effective in wound healing only when present in amounts 2–7 times greater than required in healthy persons.[15]

**Bromelain.** Bromelain is a proteolytic enzyme derived from pineapple stem. This anti-inflammatory enzyme possesses the ability to break down or dissolve proteins. This property can be utilized to reduce muscle and tissue swelling, especially following injuries or surgery.[8] Use of oral bromelain over the postoperative period results in faster resolution of swelling and decreased dependence on analgesics in fracture patients.[16] Similar results have been recorded after dental surgery[17] and musculoskeletal trauma.[18]

**Glucosamine.** Glucosamine provides the raw material needed to repair connective tissue found in skin, tendons, ligaments, and joints.[19,20] Animal studies show that levels of glucosamine increase in injured tissue during healing.[21] Reviews of perioperative nutrition in humans recommend glucosamine 1500 mg daily until healing is complete.[8]

**Aloe vera.** The healing properties of aloe vera have been known for centuries. Used as a topical application, aloe stimulates collagen synthesis and has been shown to promote wound healing.[22] Animal studies have demonstrated beneficial effects of aloe vera in healing frostbite, electrical injuries, and diabetes.[23–26] Aloe vera improves the permeability of cell walls, boosts nutrient influx into cells, and removes toxins from cells.[27]

**Curcumin.** Curcumin, an extract of the spice turmeric, is used to reduce inflammation as well as treat wounds and skin ulcers. Research shows that it has antioxidant properties and other health benefits.[28] It also improves formation of new skin and the migration of immune cells necessary for wound healing.[29] Specifically, it has been shown to enhance muscle regeneration in muscle injury.[30]

**Omega-3 fatty acids.** Omega-3 fatty acids, including eicosapentaenoic acid (EPA) and docosahexaenoic acid (DHA), are anti-inflammatory and have wide-ranging effects. They stimulate the immune system by enhancing T-cell and natural killer cell activity. Because the body's need for fats increases under conditions of stress, omega-3 fatty acids play an important role in the healing process.

## Boosting Growth Factors

Growth factors are small proteins that enable cells to communicate. There are seven major growth factor families: epidermal growth factor, transforming growth factor-beta, insulin-like growth factor 1, interleukins, platelet-derived growth factor, fibroblast growth factor, and colony-stimulating factors.

Growth factors have a number of functions in wound healing[31]:

- Forming granulation tissue
- Increasing connective tissue by creating new blood supply
- Promoting remodeling and growth of new skin
- Attracting proteins and immune cells to fight infection

Studies have shown that various growth factors are diminished after trauma. For instance, serum levels of insulin-like growth factors are decreased during critical illness.[32] Nutrients that stimulate secretion of growth factors may assist recovery from trauma. Various supplements have been studied for the ability to boost growth factors, including the amino acid arginine, omega-3 fatty acids, and nucleotides.[33]

Arginine, a semi-essential amino acid, helps in wound healing and recovery from stress. In addition, arginine enhances immune response of trauma patients. In a study of healthy people and surgical and intensive care unit patients, arginine was shown to increase lymphocyte and monocyte proliferation and enhance helper T cell formation.[34] Arginine also increases intestinal calcium absorption and collagen synthesis.

Ornithine alpha-ketoglutarate (OKG), a salt formed of 2 molecules of ornithine and one molecule of alpha-ketoglutaric acid, is a promising anticatabolic agent that promotes wound healing and protein synthesis. Researchers have hypothesized that OKG works by upregulating glutamine and arginine production.[35]

Glutamine supplementation in critically ill patients has been shown to improve gut-associated lymphoid tissue function and enhance immune defense against infection.[36]

## Life Extension Suggestions

After an injury, it is very important to maintain an adequate supply of calories to support the increased metabolic state. The following guidelines are suggested:

- Fifty-five percent of calories should come from carbohydrates, mainly complex carbohydrates found in whole-grain foods.
- Twenty percent of calories should come from fats. The addition of EPA/DHA omega-3 fatty acids can help supply these essential fatty acids.
- Twenty-five percent of calories should come from protein. The addition of whey protein to the diet can help guarantee that adequate protein is ingested.

It is also very important that trauma patients stay properly hydrated. They should drink plenty of water throughout the day.

In severe wound conditions, physicians sometimes use hyperbaric oxygen therapy.

In addition, the following vitamins and nutrients may aid the healing process:

- **Vitamin A:** 25 000 IU daily as beta carotene
- **Vitamin C:** 1000–4000 mg daily
- **Zinc:** 30–90 mg daily
- **L-arginine:** 2250–9000 mg daily
- **L-ornithine:** 750–3000 mg daily
- **Glutamine:** 1000–3000 mg daily
- **Bromelain:** 500 mg twice daily in an enteric-coated form
- **Glucosamine:** 1500 mg daily
- **Aloe:** per label instructions
- **Curcumin** (as highly absorbed BCM-95®): 400–800 mg daily
- **Omega-3 fatty acids:** 1400 mg EPA and 1000 mg DHA daily
- **Whey or plant protein blend:** 17 g or more daily

## REFERENCES

References available at: www.lef.org/dpt5/ch126

# 127

# *Urinary Tract Infection (UTI)*

A urinary tract infection (UTI) is a common infection that occurs along the urinary tract, which includes the bladder, kidneys, ureters, and urethra; they are usually caused by bacteria.[1-5] Infections of the *lower* urinary tract (ie, bladder and urethra) commonly cause urinary urgency, pain during urination, or cloudy, pink, or red-colored urine.[2,6] Less common and potentially more severe are infections of the *upper* urinary tract, which comprises the kidneys and ureters; kidney infection (pyelonephritis) is associated with fever, vomiting, and flank pain.[3,7,8]

In 2007, UTIs accounted for *8.6 million doctor's office visits*, making them one of the most common bacterial infections encountered by outpatient caregivers; costs associated with UTI management have been estimated to be *$1.6 billion annually*.[2,9] UTIs are considerably more common among women, nearly half of whom will experience a UTI during their lifetime.[2,3,7,10]

Doctors routinely prescribe *powerful antibiotics* to treat UTIs, and individuals with recurrent UTI may be prescribed a longer course of treatment.[2,11] This may lead to the emergence of *antibiotic-resistant bacterial strains*, which can cause UTIs that are more serious and difficult to treat.[2,12,13]

Scientific studies suggest that *natural compounds* such as those found in extracts of *Hibiscus sabdariffa* and *cranberry* may reduce adherence of bacteria to the urinary tract, thereby reducing UTI recurrence.[14-17] In addition, *probiotics* represent a potential treatment option, as these "good bacteria" may be able to displace pathogenic bacteria and modulate the immune system to help fight infections.[18-20]

This protocol will outline the biology and development of UTIs, and explain how they are conventionally treated; some novel and emerging treatment strategies will also be examined. Dietary and lifestyle considerations that may reduce UTI risk will be discussed, as will a number of scientifically-studied natural interventions that may support the health of the urinary tract.

## BIOLOGY AND DEVELOPMENT OF URINARY TRACT INFECTIONS

A UTI typically arises when microorganisms like bacteria or fungi enter the urinary tract through the urethra.[2] UTIs can also occur in association with use of urinary catheters, which are medical devices that drain the bladder.[21,22]

There are many different bacteria that can cause UTIs, with *Escherichia coli* (*E. coli*) being the most common.[23,24] Less commonly, fungi (esp. *Candida* species) may cause UTIs; this is more frequent in hospital settings or individuals with predisposing diseases and/or structural abnormalities of the urinary tract.[23,25,26]

The bacteria that cause UTIs are similar to those naturally found in the colon and other areas of the body, but they have some characteristics that allow them to cause UTIs.[2] One of the most important, especially in the case of *E. coli*, is the ability of these bacteria to adhere to the mucous membranes in the urinary tract.[11,27,28] The mucous membranes of the lower urinary tract contain a variety of molecules, including mannose, a sugar. Strains of *E. coli* can adhere (or attach to) these mannose molecules using small projections, called fimbriae.[28-32] This binding prevents bacteria from being cleared from the urinary tract by the flow of urine, which is normally a deterrent to bacterial colonization.[33] Once the bacteria bind to the cells that line the urinary tract, they may then invade these cells. This process also helps the bacteria avoid being killed by antibiotics or the immune system.[32-35]

Although most research has focused on *E. coli* infections of the urinary tract in otherwise healthy individuals, the general process is similar for other forms of UTI.[36] In the case of catheter-associated UTIs, which account for up to 40% of hospital-acquired infections, bacteria can gain access to the urinary tract via the catheter itself.[21]

## CAUSES AND RISK FACTORS

In women, symptomatic UTIs are typically caused by the spread of potentially pathogenic bacteria from the bowel to the urinary tract.[2,37] Although UTIs can occur in anyone, certain factors increase risk, including female gender, sexual intercourse, family and personal history of UTIs, pregnancy, allergies, diabetes, abnormalities in the flow of urine, sustained urinary catheterization, incontinence, low estrogen levels, and antibiotic use.

### Female Gender

UTIs are more common in women than men; the majority of females report having had a UTI by 32 years of age.[2,11] This may be because (1) women have shorter urethras than men, which makes it easier for bacteria to access their bladders, and (2) the urethral opening is closer to the external genitalia and anus, thus increasing the risk of bacterial cross-contamination.[4,11,38,39]

## Sexual Intercourse

Sexual intercourse is a risk factor for UTIs.[2,4,40] This is particularly true for women who have sexual intercourse more than once per week.[41] Women who use diaphragms for contraception also have an increased risk of developing UTIs.[40] A new sexual partner in the past year is another sexually related risk factor for UTI in women.[42]

## Family History

Having one or more first-degree female relatives (mother or sister) with a history of UTIs increases personal risk.[2]

## Personal History

Having a personal history of UTIs, either recurrent or otherwise, is another major risk factor for the development of a subsequent UTI.[40–42]

## Pregnancy

Pregnancy appears to increase the risk that a UTI will spread and cause *pyelonephritis*, a serious infection of the kidneys associated with fever, chills, and flank pain. This is because pregnancy can cause hormonal changes, as well as shifts in the position of the urinary tract, which make it easier for bacteria to spread to the kidneys.[11,38]

## Allergies

Women who are allergic to compounds that may come in contact with the genital area, such as bubble baths, vaginal creams, and soaps may be at greater risk of developing UTIs because irritation of this sensitive region may allow bacteria access to the urinary tract.[38]

## Diabetes

Patients being treated for diabetes have an increased risk of developing *asymptomatic bacteriuria* (bacteria in the urine that does not cause symptoms), UTIs, and pyelonephritis.[1,41] Diabetes impairs the immune system and makes it harder for the body to fight off infection.[4] In addition to the more common UTIs caused by *E. coli*, people with diabetes are also more likely to acquire UTIs caused by other bacteria, including *Klebsiella* and group B *Streptococcus*.[23]

## Urinary Flow Abnormalities

Disruptions in urinary flow can also predispose people to UTIs. Anatomical abnormalities that affect the urinary tract can lead to recurring UTIs in children. Anything else that blocks the flow of urine, such as kidney stones, a narrow urethra, or an enlarged prostate also increases the risk of UTI.[1,4,43]

## Urinary Catheters

People who require a urinary catheter have a higher incidence of UTI.[23] Use of a urinary catheter disrupts the body's natural defense against bacterial infections and provides an easier route by which bacteria can travel to the bladder. As a result, it is recommended that urinary catheters be used for the shortest possible time to reduce the risk of UTIs.[1,11,21,43]

## Incontinence

Incontinence is associated with an increase in UTIs[41] as well as acute pyelonephritis.[42]

## Low Estrogen Levels

The risk of UTI increases after menopause as estrogen levels in the body drop. Estrogen is responsible for maintaining the health of vaginal walls; when estrogen levels are low, either due to menopause, surgery, or congenital problems, vaginal walls become thin, which increases susceptibility to invading bacteria.[38,43] Some studies have found that estrogen prescriptions, such as creams and vaginal rings, may help prevent UTIs.[44]

## Antibiotic Use

Patients who have taken antibiotics recently may have an increased risk of developing a UTI. Antibiotics deplete the urinary tract of the beneficial bacteria *Lactobacilli*, which are protective against *E. coli* and other infectious bacteria.[38]

# SIGNS AND SYMPTOMS

A variety of signs and symptoms may suggest lower and/or upper UTI.

*Cystitis* involves the lower urinary tract, and typical signs/symptoms include the following[4,38,43]:

- Painful stinging or burning sensation during urination
- The need to urinate more frequently
- Cloudy, red, pink, or dark-colored urine
- Discomfort or pressure in the lower abdomen
- Urine with a strong odor

- Pain in the pelvic area (women) or rectum (men)
- Fever

Pyelonephritis is a serious infection involving the upper urinary tract (kidneys). Signs/symptoms of pyelonephritis include the following[2,11,45]:

- High fever
- Flank/abdominal pain
- Chills
- Vomiting
- Frequent/painful urination

## INTERSTITIAL CYSTITIS/PAINFUL BLADDER SYNDROME

While pelvic pain, urinary urgency, and nighttime urination are associated with UTI, these symptoms may be the result of a different, somewhat more obscure condition called *interstitial cystitis* or, sometimes, *painful bladder syndrome*.[46–50]

As with UTIs, interstitial cystitis affects women more often than men and can considerably decrease quality of life. Unfortunately, opinions about interstitial cystitis, and the techniques used to diagnose and treat it, are somewhat inconsistent within conventional medicine; this leads to delayed diagnosis in many cases. One reason for this is that a specific cause has not been identified; upon examination, bacteria are not present in the urine of those with interstitial cystitis. Inflammatory damage to the bladder lining (urothelial cell barrier) and some level of immune system derangement are thought to be involved, but the origins of these phenomena are unclear.[46–49]

Since little is understood about the development of interstitial cystitis, protocols for its treatment lack a robust evidence base and often depend upon physicians' clinical experience or data from relatively small clinical trials. After diagnosing a patient with interstitial cystitis, which can only be accomplished by ruling out other causes of symptoms since no laboratory test can identify the condition, physicians may prescribe a number of therapies, including, among others, the following[46–49]:

- Some antidepressants (eg, amitriptyline)
- Dimethyl sulfoxide (DMSO) (injected into the bladder)
- Antihistamines
- Behavioral therapy (eg, retraining voiding patterns)[51]
- Pentosan polysulfate sodium (Elmiron®)
- Transcutaneous electrical nerve stimulation (TENS)
- Intravesical lidocaine (ie, injection of the local anesthetic lidocaine into the bladder)
- Corticosteroids

Despite the fact that an estimated 180 different strategies have been tried as potential treatments for interstitial cystitis, very few have shown to be effective. One such drug is pentosan, which is approved by the Food and Drug Administration (FDA) to treat interstitial cystitis and marketed under the brand name Elmiron®.[47] Pentosan is thought to work by supporting the integrity of the urothelial layer in the bladder.[52]

## DIAGNOSIS AND CONVENTIONAL TREATMENT

### Diagnosis

UTIs may be difficult to diagnose in some cases, since patients may not always have typical symptoms.[53] Also, other conditions have symptoms in common with UTI (eg, gonorrhea, chlamydia, interstitial cystitis, and diabetes).

The presence of red or white blood cells, bacteria or certain chemicals in the urine usually indicates a UTI.[1,54] Most frequently, a urine dipstick test is used to confirm the diagnosis of UTI in individuals with suggestive symptoms. This test evaluates a urine sample to detect *nitrites*, which are chemicals produced by *E. coli*, a bacteria that can cause UTIs; it also measures levels of proteins produced by immune cells responding to the infection. In some complicated cases, a urine culture may be used to help guide treatment.[53]

### Conventional Treatment

**Antibiotics.** The standard treatment for a UTI is a course of one or more antibiotics. No single antibiotic is recommended for treating every UTI, but nitrofurantoin (Furadantin®), trimethoprim-sulfamethoxazole (Bactrim™), pivmecillinam (Selexid®), fosfomycin trometamol (Monurol®), fluoroquinolone (eg, Cipro®), and beta-lactam (eg, Augmentin®) may all be used.[7,55]

Although many antibiotics can be used to treat UTIs, one of the main factors that determines which antibiotics are chosen is the bacterial resistance pattern. There are strains of *E. coli* that are resistant to antibiotics and are found throughout the world.[2,56,57] Other strains of bacteria that cause UTIs, including species of *Proteus* and *Klebsiella*, have also developed resistance to specific antibiotics.[56] As a result, the choice of antibiotic is usually governed by susceptibility of the pathogenic organism responsible for an individual's case and/or community history of microbial antibiotic resistance.[2] This is typically determined by regional rates reported by local hospitals, although this information can overestimate the prevalence of resistance among bacteria in a region.[2,13] Some guidelines recommend avoiding a particular antibiotic if local resistance rates to that antibiotic are greater than 20%.[58]

## NOVEL AND EMERGING TREATMENTS

### Topical Estrogen for Recurring UTI

Low estrogen levels thin the walls of the vagina, increasing a woman's risk of developing UTIs.[38] As a result, topical estrogen may represent a treatment option in some cases of UTI among women.

Two different methods of administering topical estrogen have been effective at reducing the frequency of recurring UTIs in postmenopausal women. These include an estradiol-releasing ring and intravaginal estriol cream.[59-61] Estradiol-releasing rings may also acidify the urine, which may help combat intravaginal bacterial growth. As of late 2012, a phase 4 clinical trial is examining the efficacy of intravaginal estrogen and lactobacilli for preventing recurrent UTIs.[62]

## FimH Inhibitors

One of the most important early steps for bacteria to infect the urinary tract is their adhesion to the outside of the cells that line the urinary tract. Bacteria use small finger-like projections, called fimbriae, to bind to the urinary tract lining. Fimbriae are coated with proteins, called lectins, which mediate this process.[29] Researchers have discovered that one of these lectins, known as *FimH*, is crucial for this process; they have therefore developed medications that inhibit the activity of FimH.[63,64]

To make even better therapies, scientists have developed many different compounds that can inhibit FimH and are continuously tweaking the molecules to improve their effectiveness. The most promising compounds have a similar core structure and are called alpha-D-mannosides. Although these drugs have not yet been tested in humans, studies have found that these chemicals can significantly reduce the amount of bacteria that colonize the bladder in animal models of UTI.[63,64] In some studies, the FimH blockers drastically reduce the amount of bacteria in the bladder by approximately as much as standard antibiotic treatments.[63] These FimH blockers have also been effective in animal models of catheter-associated UTIs.[65]

## Hyaluronic Acid and Chondroitin Sulfate Injections

Another emerging treatment focuses on the bladder wall. The cells that line the inside of the bladder, known as urothelial cells, are an important part of the body's defense against UTIs.[66,67] These cells help keep undesirable substances (eg, bacteria) from penetrating into the deeper layers of the bladder and also make substances, known as *proteoglycans*, which form a layer of *glycosaminoglycans (GAGs)* on the inner surface of the bladder. Any damage to the GAG layer facilitates the adhesion of bacteria to the bladder wall and may play a role in recurrent UTIs.[66,68]

New treatments that focus on restoring the integrity of the GAG wall are being developed for preventing recurrent UTIs. These treatments involve injecting some of the substances used to construct GAG, such as *hyaluronic acid* and *chondroitin sulfate*, directly into the bladder. This process is also known as intravesical administration. Intravesical administration of hyaluronic acid and chondroitin sulfate has been shown to reduce the number of UTIs in women with recurrent UTIs.[66,68-70] Mild bladder irritation has been reported as a side effect of this treatment in some patients.[66,69] Although this treatment is available in Canada and Europe, it has not been FDA-approved for use in patients because of limited clinical trial data.

# DIETARY AND LIFESTYLE CONSIDERATIONS

## Fluid Intake

Physicians often recommend that patients with UTIs increase their fluid intake. The theory behind this recommendation is that increasing fluid intake will increase the amount of urine produced, which will help flush out bacteria.[71] Although this is a common physician suggestion, it is not clear how effective it is at treating or preventing UTIs. Some early studies found that more frequent urination reduces the amount of bacteria in the urine. However, studies examining whether increased urination reduces the incidence of UTI have not yielded conclusive results.[71,72] Regardless, poor fluid intake is a risk factor for recurrent UTI in female children,[73,74] and increased fluid intake does appear to be protective against more serious upper UTIs that can affect the kidneys.[72]

## Behavioral Measures

Some behavioral changes may also help prevent UTIs, particularly in children. Recurrent UTIs in female children are associated with infrequent urination, delaying urination after the urge to urinate manifests, and delaying of defecation, but not poor bathroom hygiene.[73,74] Similarly, women who delay urination for more than 1 hour post-urge have an increased risk of developing UTIs, which suggests that urinating shortly after feeling the need to urinate could help prevent UTIs. Avoiding diaphragms and spermicide as contraception methods may also prevent UTIs.[75] Although some sources suggest that urinating shortly before and after intercourse also helps to reduce a female's risk of developing UTIs,[38,76] there is no conclusive evidence that frequent voiding or voiding after intercourse significantly reduces UTI risk.[2,75] Other behavioral interventions that may reduce the risk of developing a UTI include wearing cotton underwear, avoiding tight-fitting clothing, and wiping from front-to-back to prevent transportation of bacteria from the anus to the urethra.[43]

# TARGETED NATURAL INTERVENTIONS

## Cranberry

Cranberries contain substances that may be able to treat or prevent UTIs. Cranberry juice and powders made from cranberry extract have been used for decades to prevent or treat UTIs. Originally, it was hypothesized that one of the components in cranberry—quinic acid—increased the levels of a natural antibacterial agent in the urine, known as hippuric acid. However, it is not clear if there is a significant increase in hippuric acid levels in the urine after cranberry consumption.[77,78]

Evidence suggests that substances known as proanthocyanidins, which are found in cranberries, may interfere with the adhesion of bacteria (particularly *E. coli*) to the walls of the urinary tract.[77–79] By preventing *E. coli* from binding to urinary tract cells, proanthocyanidins can keep bacteria from fully colonizing and invading the urinary tract. One of the advantages of using cranberry juice or related products is that cranberries are relatively inexpensive, natural, and should not contribute to the growing problem of antibiotic resistance.[79]

One study found that both cranberry juice and cranberry tablets were effective at reducing UTIs (compared to placebo) in women who developed at least one UTI per year. This study also found that cranberry tablets were a more cost-effective option compared to cranberry juice.[80] Another study found that consuming cranberry juice 3 times per day produced a trend towards reducing the incidence of UTIs during pregnancy.[81] Yet another study compared cranberry extract to low-dose trimethoprim (a commonly used antibiotic) for prevention of recurrent UTIs in older women. This study found that regular use of trimethoprim was only slightly better than 500 mg of cranberry extract daily for preventing the recurrence of UTIs. It also found that women taking trimethoprim were more likely to withdraw from the study due to side effects.[82]

Although there are many studies that have examined the potential benefits of cranberry for UTIs, a recent comprehensive review concluded that the benefits of consuming cranberry juice for UTIs were minimal. However, many of the studies included in this review used sugar-laden cranberry juice cocktails; the high sugar content and the fact that many of these beverages are blends of different juices (reducing the proanthocyanidin content) may also obscure the benefits of cranberries.[78]

## D-mannose

D-mannose is a sugar that can be found in, among other things, cranberries. One of the interesting aspects of D-mannose is that it is able to bind to the cells that line the urinary tract[76] and prevent bacteria, such as *E. coli*, from adhering to the lining of the urinary tract.[76,83]

## Blueberry

Much like cranberries, blueberries contain compounds that can inhibit the adhesion of *E. coli* to the cells that line the urinary tract.[84] In addition, both blueberries and cranberries contain compounds that are able to help prevent large aggregates of bacteria from forming.[85] The clinical effect of blueberries on UTIs has yet to be thoroughly investigated.

## Probiotics

Probiotics—beneficial bacteria that reside in the gut and positively impact the health of their host—are a promising natural treatment for UTIs. There are many possible ways that probiotics may prevent UTIs: they may compete with other bacteria for resources, secrete natural antibacterial chemicals (called bacteriocin), and prevent pathogenic bacteria from adhering to the urinary tract.[18]

Bacteria in the *Lactobacillus* family, normally found in the female vagina, are thought to prevent UTIs.[18] Taking antibiotics or using spermicidal agents can kill off these *Lactobacilli*, which can then increase the risk of UTI.[86] In addition, recurrent UTIs are often associated with decreased levels of *Lactobacillus* bacteria and increased colonization with *E. coli*.[19] As a result, supplementing the vaginal flora with probiotic *Lactobacilli* may represent a viable technique for preventing UTIs.[19,86,87] In particular, there is evidence that the *Lactobacillus rhamnosus* GR-1 and *Lactobacillus reuterii* RC-14 strains are clinically effective.[88]

*Lactobacillus* bacteria also may prevent UTIs by stimulating the immune system and producing substances that kill infectious bacteria, such as hydrogen peroxide and lactic acid.[18] A study comparing *Lactobacillus* bacteria to regular doses of trimethoprim-sulfamethoxazole (an antibiotic combination) found that the antibiotics were only slightly more effective than the probiotic treatment for uncomplicated UTI; however, probiotics were more effective in complicated cases, which was likely due to the presence of baseline antibiotic resistance rates in these cases. The authors also point out that probiotics had the advantage of not increasing the risk of antibiotic-resistant microorganisms.[20]

## Berberine

Berberine, a chemical known as a plant alkaloid, has historically been used in Chinese and ayurvedic medicine. It can be found in many plants, including goldenseal, Oregon grape, coptis, barberry, and turmeric.[89] Berberine has natural antibacterial properties and is effective at inhibiting the growth of many opportunistic pathogens, including *E. coli*.[90] Some studies have found that berberine prevents *E. coli* from adhering to cells that line the urinary tract, thus providing a possible mechanism of action for its UTI-preventative properties.[91] One study suggested that berberine may represent a new target for the development of pharmaceuticals.[92] Berberine may not be safe for pregnant women, however, because it can induce uterine contractions and may cause jaundice in newborns.[89]

## Hibiscus

Hibiscus is a family of plants that has traditionally been used to treat many different infections, including UTIs. Hibiscus plants contain many compounds that have antibacterial, antifungal, and antioxidant properties.[93] One compound in particular, gossypetin, has been shown to have antibacterial activity against common UTI-causing bacteria, including *E. coli* and *Pseudomonas aeurginosa*.[14] In a double-blind, placebo-controlled clinical trial, 61 women with a history of frequent UTIs were randomly assigned to one of three groups receiving a daily dose of 200 mg of hibiscus extract standardized to 90% polyphenols, 200 mg of hibiscus extract standardized to 60% polyphenols, or placebo. Compared to the control group, women taking the hibiscus concentrations experienced 77% fewer incidence of UTIs, as well as overall improvement in urinary comfort.[17]

## Vitamin C

Vitamin C, also known as ascorbic acid, is one of the most commonly used vitamin supplements and has a variety of effects on the human body. One potential benefit is that it may acidify the urine, which helps inhibit the growth of infectious bacteria in the urinary tract.[94] This acidification may also convert bacterial nitrites into nitric oxide, which is toxic to bacteria.[76] In addition, vitamin C is important for the function of the immune system.[76] Studies have found that taking 100 mg of vitamin C daily during pregnancy can reduce the incidence of UTIs.[95]

## General Support for Healthy Bladder Function

**Pumpkin seed extract.** Urinary urgency and/or frequency are often associated with UTI. To this end, for those afflicted by UTIs, especially chronic UTI sufferers, taking steps to improve bladder tone and support healthy voiding patterns may be beneficial.

Although not studied specifically in the context of UTI, *pumpkin seed extract* has been shown to support bladder function and combat the symptoms associated with an overactive bladder. In an animal study, rats supplemented with pumpkin seed extract exhibited significantly improved bladder function and decreased urinary frequency.[96] In a human study involving 39 postmenopausal women, 6 weeks of supplementation with pumpkin seed extract plus soybean germ extract led to significant decreases in daytime and nighttime urination.[97] In a similar study among 45 men, this same combination extract led to reduced nighttime urination and improved sleep satisfaction after 6 weeks of supplementation.[98]

## Life Extension Suggestions

- **Cranberry extract:** 500 mg daily
- **Hibiscus,** standardized extract: 200 mg daily
- **D-mannose:** 1000–2000 mg daily
- **Vitamin C:** 1000–2000 mg daily
- **Blueberry extract:** 500–2000 mg daily
- **Probiotics** (eg, *Lactobacillus rhamnosus* and *Lactobacillus reuteri*): 5 billion cfu
- **Goldenseal extract** (providing berberine): 250 mg daily
- **Pumpkin seed extract and soy isoflavones:** 624–936 mg daily

In addition, the following *blood testing* resource may be helpful:

- **Female panel**

## REFERENCES

References available at: www.lef.org/dpt5/ch127

# 128

# *Uterine (Endometrial) Cancer*

Cancer of the uterus is the most common cancer of the female reproductive tract, with an annual rate of 21 per 100 000 women.[1] The majority of uterine (endometrial) cancer cases occur around or after menopause between the ages of 60 and 75 years. In the United States, 2–3% of women will develop cancer of the uterus during their lifetimes.[2]

The primary symptom of uterine cancer is abnormal vaginal bleeding. Obesity and a diet high in animal fats and low in fruits and vegetables are associated with the development of uterine cancer.[3,4] The relationship between unopposed estrogen exposure and uterine cancer is well established.[5–7] The incidence of uterine cancer has increased in the past 50 years because of longer female life expectancy and an increase in the use of unopposed estrogen therapy. However, enhanced methods of diagnosis have improved detection rates.[8]

Fortunately, most uterine cancers are detected at an early stage, leading to successful cure rates. The usual treatment for uterine cancer is a complete hysterectomy (removal of the uterus).[9] Depending on the severity and spread of the cancer, radiation therapy is sometimes recommended.[10] A healthy diet and lifestyle together with hormonal and dietary supplements may impede the development of uterine cancer and stop its spread in those who already have it.[11,12]

## WHAT IS UTERINE CANCER?

The uterus (or womb) is a thick-walled, hollow, muscular organ, shaped like an inverted pear in the female pelvis.[13] The uterus is where a fetus grows. The innermost layer of the uterus (the endometrium) is shed during menstruation. Cancer of the uterus is a disease in which malignant (cancer) cells form in the tissues of the endometrium (*metra* is Greek for womb). Therefore, uterine cancer is often also referred to as endometrial cancer.[14]

Uterine cancer can spread outward through the layers of the uterus.[15] Cancerous cells may invade nearby structures such as the cervix, fallopian tubes, and vagina.[9,16] Untreated uterine cancer cells can spread via the lymphatic system to nearby lymph nodes.[17] If left untreated and allowed to progress, uterine cancer can spread via the bloodstream, which may result in the spread of cancer to the lungs, liver, bone, and brain.[10]

## SYMPTOMS OF UTERINE CANCER

The primary symptoms of uterine cancer are abnormal vaginal bleeding and pelvic pain.[18] This commonly occurs in postmenopausal women but may also occur in menstruating women who experience irregular bouts of bleeding. It is imperative that any abnormal bleeding or discharge from the vagina be evaluated by a physician.[9]

## UNMODIFIABLE RISK FACTORS FOR UTERINE CANCER

### Age

In 95% of cases, uterine cancer occurs around or after menopause, usually between the ages of 60 and 75 years.[19] It also occurs more often in obese, postmenopausal women[20] who have had no or very few pregnancies.[21]

### Ethnicity

Caucasian women have a 2.88% lifetime risk of developing uterine cancer compared with the 1.69% risk for African-American women.[1] However, mortality rates are nearly twice as high in the latter group,[22] who have more aggressive tumors and more accompanying illnesses and complications.[23]

### Genetics

Most cases of uterine cancer appear sporadically. However, approximately 10% of cases are thought to be hereditary.[24] There may be 2 forms of inherited uterine cancer—the first involving a genetic tendency for inheriting uterine cancer alone and the second involving a family cancer syndrome called Lynch syndrome type 2, or hereditary nonpolyposis colorectal cancer.[25] There is a 40–60% lifetime risk of developing uterine cancer in an individual with Lynch syndrome type 2.[25] Genetic blood testing is available to identify individuals who carry this syndrome.[26]

## CAUSES OF UTERINE CANCER

### Unopposed Estrogen

When estrogen is taken without the counterbalancing effects of progesterone, it is referred to as unopposed estrogen.[7] Increased exposure to unopposed estrogen from supplemental hormone replacement therapy (HRT) or through excessive estrogen generated in the body[5,9,27] is the most common risk factor for uterine cancer. Women who take unopposed estrogen replacement therapy (ERT) may be at risk of uterine cancer,[28] even after discontinuing ERT.[29]

Women using unopposed estrogen for more than 2 years have a 2- to 3-fold increased risk of uterine cancer,[8] whereas women receiving progestin in conjunction with estrogen have no increased risk.[29] The addition of progestin to HRT reduces the risk of uterine cancer by lowering the exposure of the endometrium to unopposed estrogen.[30] For further information on hormone supplementation, see the Female Hormone Restoration protocol.

Endometrial cell growth is finely sensitive to the effects of estrogen that are unopposed by progesterone.[27] A possible precursor lesion for uterine cancer may be endometrial hyperplasia (abnormal growth).[31] Endometrial hyperplasia occurs when uterine lining cells become overstimulated, dense, and thickened. In most cases, endometrial hyperplasia is caused by estrogen stimulation.[14,32,33] This tissue may consist of normal cells or abnormal cells, and only 2% of cases of hyperplasia of normal cells will develop into uterine cancer. In contrast, 25–100% of abnormal cell hyperplasia will progress into uterine cancer, indicating that abnormal cell hyperplasia is probably a precursor to uterine cancer.[34,35]

## Obesity

Obesity is associated with a significantly increased risk of endometrial cancer in both premenopausal[36,37] and postmenopausal women.[38] Fat cells produce 10–15% of estrogens. Estrogens are formed when androgens (male hormones) are converted to estrogens via aromatization (conversion) outside of the ovaries.[3,39] In obese females, elevated levels of estrogens from fat can stimulate the endometrial lining of the uterus and increase the risk of uterine cancer.[21,40] See the protocol on Obesity and Weight Loss, which outlines an integrative approach to counteracting obesity.

## Ovulation Problems

Ovulation problems and hormone imbalances in which excess androgens are produced, such as polycystic ovary syndrome (ovaries with many abnormal cysts), may result in excessive production of estrogens.[41] This hormonal imbalance places women at increased risk of uterine cancer.[42,43]

## No Pregnancies

During pregnancy, the hormonal balance shifts toward more progesterone and less estrogen.[44] If a woman does not go through a pregnancy, she does not benefit from this hormonal shift (more progesterone and a lower estradiol level), which provides protection against uterine cancer.[42] Women who have never been pregnant or have gone through only one pregnancy are more likely to develop uterine cancer than women who have had multiple pregnancies.[45]

## Late Menopause

The average age for a woman to stop menstruating is 51 years old.[46] Women who experience menopause at a much later age will produce hormones (including estrogen) for a longer time.[19] This increased exposure to estrogen is associated with uterine cancer.[42]

## Tamoxifen

Tamoxifen is a medication that is often prescribed to breast cancer survivors. Unfortunately, tamoxifen users have a 2- to 3-fold increased risk of uterine cancer.[47] Women taking tamoxifen should be monitored closely by their physician.[48] See the protocol on Breast Cancer for more information.

## Western Diet

The rates of uterine cancer increase in first and second generation Japanese women born in the United States,[49] suggesting that the Western diet, high in animal fat, may be a risk factor for uterine cancer.[50] The intake of animal protein and fat increases the risk of myoma, a benign (noncancerous) fibroid.[51] It also increases the risk of uterine cancer. Conversely, eating fresh fruits and vegetables[52] and more fiber decreases the risk.[21] The protocol on Uterine Fibroids describes nutritional supplements that support healthy uterine structure and function.

### WHAT YOU HAVE LEARNED SO FAR

- Uterine cancer is a disease in which malignant (cancer) cells form, typically in the lining of the uterus (endometrium).
- Uterine cancer is highly curable by removal of the uterus (hysterectomy) if surgery is performed before the spread of the cancer.
- Taking tamoxifen and increased exposure to estrogens, whether from unopposed estrogen therapy or excess body fat, are the most common risk factors for developing uterine cancer.[53,54]
- Possible signs of uterine cancer include unusual vaginal discharge or bleeding.

- The risk of uterine cancer can be reduced by lowering and balancing levels of estrogens in the body,[55-57] for example, by correcting obesity or adding progestin.[3,39]
- It is important to make lifestyle and dietary changes, and to balance hormones, if you are at increased risk of uterine cancer.

## DIAGNOSING UTERINE CANCER

The following are some of the tools used to diagnose uterine cancer.

### Biopsy

Although somewhat uncomfortable, a biopsy of the endometrial lining is a useful tool for the diagnosis of uterine cancer.[58,59] Physicians do not usually recommend a biopsy as a general screening tool but it is the procedure of choice for high-risk individuals.[59] If the biopsy test result is positive for uterine cancer, the physician will discuss all treatment options.

### Dilation and Curettage (D&C)

If the biopsy test result is negative but the patient is at high risk of uterine cancer, the patient may need to have a D&C.[60] In this procedure, the physician dilates the woman's cervix and removes a sample of uterine tissue. The physician or a technician examines the tissue sample under a microscope for the presence of cancerous cells. A D&C is more accurate than an endometrial biopsy for diagnosing uterine cancer.[61]

### Pap Test

The Pap (short for Papanicolaou) test detects cervical cancer but is not a good test for detecting uterine cancer. A Pap test will fail to diagnose uterine cancer about 87% of the time.[62] Occasionally, uterine cells shed and appear on a Pap test. When this occurs in a postmenopausal woman, further evaluation is required. About 25% of postmenopausal women with *abnormal* uterine cells on their Pap tests will have uterine cancer.[60] However, about 6% of postmenopausal women whose Pap test results show *normal* uterine cells actually have uterine cancer.[63]

## PREDICTING THE PROGNOSIS

Once uterine cancer has been diagnosed, magnetic resonance imaging (MRI) is often performed to evaluate the extent of disease. MRI is particularly useful in determining the depth of cancer invasion within the uterus.[64] Patients thought to have more advanced disease may be referred to a gynecologic cancer center for extensive surgery and treatment.[19,60]

## UNDERSTANDING THE STAGING SYSTEM

Approximately 75% of women with uterine cancer have stage 1 (mild) disease. Of these women, almost 90% have no sign of cancer 5 years after surgery.[18] The possibility of curing the disease decreases as the cancer becomes more advanced.[18] Advanced disease has a poor prognosis; the 5-year survival rate for stage 3 is 29% and declines to 10% for stage 4.[65]

**International Federation of Gynecologists and Obstetricians (FIGO) Uterine Cancer Staging System**[60]

| | |
|---|---|
| Stage 1 (mild) | Cancer found only in uterus |
| Stage 2 | Cancer in uterus and cervix, but not outside uterus |
| Stage 3 | Cancer in uterus and beyond, but not outside pelvis |
| Stage 4 (most advanced stage) | Cancer beyond pelvis, in bladder, bowel, or other areas of the body |

## DECODING THE PATHOLOGY REPORT

After the surgeon removes the uterine cancer tissue, it is sent to the pathology laboratory for analysis. A technician examines the tissue for the absence or presence of hormone receptors (places where hormones can attach) within the tumor.[66] Most uterine cancer cells possess receptors for estrogen or progesterone, or both.[67,68] This is why uterine cancer is often classified as a hormonally responsive cancer.

Patients who have tumors that test positive for progesterone and/or estrogen receptors typically have longer survival rates than patients whose tumors lack these hormone receptors.[69,70] However, progesterone receptors appear to be a stronger predictor of long-term survival than estrogen receptors.[71] Tumors with progesterone receptors have a much greater response to progestin therapy than do tumors without progesterone receptors.[30,72]

If the cancerous tissue contains estrogen and/or progesterone receptors, it may be responsive to hormonal therapy, particularly if the cancer recurs.[66,73-75] Therefore, it is recommended that the cancerous tissue be analyzed for the presence of estrogen and/or progesterone receptors at the time of surgery.[66,73,74,76]

## MEDICAL TREATMENT

The following surgeries and therapies are used to treat uterine cancer.

## Surgery

Removing the cancer in an operation is the most common treatment of uterine cancer. During surgery, the physician evaluates the extent of the cancer and uses a staging guide to assess each patient's cancer stage. The following surgical procedures may be used.

**Radical hysterectomy.** The primary treatment of uterine cancer is a hysterectomy in which the uterus, fallopian tubes, cervix, ovaries, surrounding tissue, and lymph glands are removed. A radical hysterectomy is usually done through the abdomen.

**Total hysterectomy.** This type of hysterectomy involves removal of just the uterus and cervix. It can be done through the abdomen or vagina. Sometimes a total vaginal hysterectomy can be done with the aid of a laparoscope (a viewing instrument passed through a small incision in the abdomen).

**Bilateral salpingo-oophorectomy.** A bilateral salpingo-oophorectomy is the removal of both ovaries and both fallopian tubes via surgery. It is done in conjunction with a hysterectomy.

## Radiation

If the cancer is confined to the uterine lining, usually no additional treatment after surgery is needed. However, if the cancer has spread further, then radiation treatment after surgery may be indicated.[10]

Depending on the results of the surgical staging and the existence of high-risk factors, radiation may be recommended immediately after surgery (postoperative) to minimize the possibility of the cancer returning.[77] Radiation has been shown to decrease the incidence of both pelvic and vaginal cancer recurrences.[60] Radiation appears to benefit women who have cancer in their para-aortic lymph nodes[16,77] and improves the 5-year survival rate by nearly 40%.[78] Brachytherapy is a one-time intravaginal radiation treatment that produces a high dose of radiation close to the cancer and a lesser dose in healthy tissues, thus producing fewer adverse effects.

## Hormonal Therapy

Endometrial cancer is a hormone-dependent disease. Therefore, hormonal therapy added to standard treatments may improve the outcome in the early stages of the disease.[79-82] Hormonal therapy is not usually recommended as standard treatment when uterine cancer is diagnosed; however, it has been used after hysterectomy with some success.[74,79] Hormonal therapy has also been demonstrated to be useful in treating selected patients who have widespread uterine cancer

that has returned after treatment; it is used primarily to relieve symptoms.[77,83]

Uterine cancer with progesterone receptors is more responsive to progestin therapy than if progesterone receptors are lacking.[72] Therefore, future therapeutic regimens targeted at enhancing progesterone receptor expression have the potential to improve outcomes in women with uterine cancer.[30,67] Progestin therapy is most commonly prescribed in pill form, but intramuscular injection of medroxyprogesterone acetate (MPA; a synthetic progestin) and intravaginal forms are also available.[76,79] Adverse effects of progestins are usually minor and include weight gain, edema (swelling), and headache; however, blood clots can occur.[84-86] Unlike synthetic progestins (such as MPA), micronized progesterone has been reported to cause only fatigue and sleepiness.

**Heading toward hormones.** Therapy with one of a number of progestational agents has been the conventional approach to the management of endometrial carcinoma in cases where surgery or radiation therapy is not recommended, particularly in obese women. Progestins such as MPA in particular are considered useful in treating uterine cancer.[82] MPA has been widely used both intramuscularly and orally in a variety of doses and schedules.

While the role of MPA in the palliative treatment of advanced disease is well accepted, opinion is divided on its role in the adjuvant setting (treatment given after surgery to increase the chances of a cure). The commonly used progestational agents megestrol acetate, hydroxyprogesterone, and MPA all produce similar response rates, and the antiestrogen tamoxifen produces responses in 10–25% of patients in the final phase of medical treatment.

Natural progesterone is obtained primarily from plant sources and is currently available in oral and injectable forms as well as topical gels. An oral micronized progesterone preparation is also available. It has improved bioavailability and fewer reported adverse effects when compared with synthetic progestins.[87] Natural progesterone is used to prevent uterine cancer. However, there is little evidence that progesterone can be used to treat uterine cancer once it has been diagnosed.[87]

## Treatment of Recurrent Cancer

The likelihood that uterine cancer may recur depends on the extent of the disease and success of the initial treatment.[77] Approximately 34% of all recurrences are detected within 1 year and 76% within 3 years of primary treatment. The cancer usually recurs in the pelvis (ie, locally), not in distant parts of the body.[88]

Chemotherapy and hormonal therapy are not recommended as standard treatment when uterine cancer is initially diagnosed.[88–90] However, they are sometimes recommended if the cancer recurs after surgery and radiation.[77,90]

# DIETARY MANAGEMENT STRATEGIES

Nutritional factors have been estimated to contribute to 20–60% of cancers and almost one-third of deaths from cancer in Western countries.

## Low-Fat Diet

A diet high in animal fat, particularly red meat, may be associated with a small to moderately increased risk of uterine cancer.[50,91] This is probably because high-fat (and sugar) diets cause increased body fat content, which in turn results in high levels of estrogens. Estrogens are known for their proliferative effects on estrogen-sensitive tissues, resulting in tumor development. There is a stronger association between dietary fat and uterine cancer in women who have high circulating levels of estrogen, such as those with a higher body mass index (BMI) and users of unopposed estrogens.[92] A low-fat diet may be linked to lower estrogen levels and thereby protect against uterine cancer.[11]

## Fish and Flaxseed

Oily fish such as salmon, herring, mackerel, bluefin tuna, and sardines contain high levels of essential omega-3 polyunsaturated fatty acids. Omega-3 fatty acids reduce the risk of certain hormone-dependent cancers by exerting favorable effects on estrogen metabolism, such as decreasing estrogen stimulation of these tumors and competitive inhibition of omega-6 fatty acids, which are associated with cancer development.[93]

The American Heart Association recommends 2 servings of fatty fish per week to obtain cardiovascular benefits from omega-3 fatty acids.[94] Two to three servings of fatty fish per week are also suggested to prevent uterine cancer.[20,93]

Other primary sources of dietary alpha-linolenic acid (which can be converted into omega-3 fatty acids) are ground flaxseed, soybeans, pumpkin seeds, and walnuts.[94] Ground flaxseed is a good source of omega-3 fatty acids[95,96] and is "as effective as oral estrogen–progesterone to improve mild menopausal symptoms" and lower glucose and insulin levels.[97]

## Fruits and Vegetables

Significant protection against uterine cancer (a 40–60% reduction) was found to be conferred by elevated intake of most fresh fruits and vegetables and whole-grain foods.[52] Therefore, a diet rich in fruits, vegetables, whole grains, and fiber most likely will help protect against uterine cancer.[83,98–100]

Various nutrients found in fruits and vegetables seem to have the ability to detoxify certain carcinogens (cancer-causing agents).[101] For example, the risk of uterine cancer is inversely related to intake of beta-carotene and fiber.[83] Fruits and vegetables that contain high amounts of vitamin A,[4] beta-carotene,[52] and vitamin C[5] may decrease the risk of uterine cancer.

In addition, cruciferous vegetables may have favorable effects on estrogen metabolism,[91] and thus reduce the risk of developing uterine cancer.[102] Examples of cruciferous vegetables include cabbage, Brussels sprouts, bok choy, kale, kohlrabi, broccoli, and watercress.

Vegetables from the allium group (*allium* is Latin for garlic) also may reduce the risk of uterine cancer by interrupting cancer cells' reproductive cycle.[103,104] Examples of allium vegetables include garlic, onions, scallions, leeks, chives, and shallots.

## Whole Grains and High-Fiber Foods

A diet rich in whole grains and high-fiber foods has been closely correlated with reduced uterine cancer risk.[4,83,105] These foods are rich in antioxidants, which are important in cancer prevention.[50,106] Low levels of antioxidants within the uterus and surrounding pelvic organs may allow proliferating free radicals to cause damage and prevent optimal functioning.[107] Many of these types of foods also contain plant estrogens (phytoestrogens), which exert protective hormonal effects against hormone-related cancers such as zuterine, breast, and prostate cancer.[108,109] Examples of whole grains include brown rice, oatmeal, pearl barley, whole wheat, and whole rye. High-fiber foods include legumes, beans, seeds, and nuts.

## Soy

Nutritional studies indicate that people in Asian countries consume approximately 10 times the amount of fermented soy as the average American. A diet rich in fermented soy reduces the risk of uterine cancer.[110,111] The consumption of soy foods also provides high amounts of fiber, which is protective against uterine cancer.[108,109]

Fermented soy foods include miso, tempeh, and natto. Soy milk, soy flour, and textured soy protein are used to make a variety of soy-based products including soy burgers (veggie burgers), soy cheese, and soy ice cream and yogurts.

# TARGETED NATURAL INTERVENTIONS

The following are some of the dietary supplements that have been found to prevent and, in some cases, treat uterine cancer.

## Coffee

Coffee, especially brews enriched with chlorogenic acid, protect cells against the DNA damage that leads to aging and cancer development.[112–114] Growing tumors develop the ability to invade local and regional tissue by increasing their production of "protein-melting" enzymes called matrix metalloproteinases. Chlorogenic acid—present in coffee—strongly inhibited matrix metalloproteinase activity.[115,116] Women with the highest coffee intake were 30% less likely to develop endometrial cancer than those who consumed none.[117]

## Vitamin A and Carotenoids

Carotenoids such as alpha-carotene, beta-carotene, lutein, and lycopene have been shown to be protective against uterine cancer.[11,52,83,118,119] Vitamin A inhibits uterine tumor growth.[4,118,120]

Vitamin A can be obtained from liver and yellow or orange vegetables. The Council for Responsible Nutrition (CRN) suggests taking 10 000 IU of vitamin A if you have a low dietary retinol intake or 5000 IU of vitamin A if you already have a high dietary retinol intake. The dosage for optimum health and for cancer prevention is not defined, but several cancer studies have shown benefits of 25 000 IU per day.[121–124]

## Vitamin C

Vitamin C is an important antioxidant and has been linked to reduced risk of uterine cancer.[2,5,21,52] It is believed that vitamin C works against cancer by enhancing the immune system and suppressing cancer cell growth.[125,126] In addition, vitamin C causes the formation of collagen,[127] which can wall off tumors[125,128,129] and help block the spread of cancer.[130,131] Vitamin C can be obtained by eating citrus fruits and dark green, leafy vegetables.[132,133] Many people prefer to take vitamin C in the form of a dietary supplement. Clinical studies have used up to 10 g (10 000 mg) daily.[132,133]

## Lignans

Lignans are found in high concentrations in flaxseed and sesame. Once consumed, lignans are converted in the intestines into enterolactone. Enterolactone has been shown to inhibit angiogenesis and promote cancer cell apoptosis.[134,135]

When researchers assessed lignan intake and cancer status among nearly 1000 women, they concluded that postmenopausal women with the highest dietary lignan intake experienced a 43% lower risk of developing uterine cancer.[110] Also, lignans have reduced the incidence of uterine cancer in rats.[136]

## Melatonin

Melatonin is a hormone secreted by the pineal gland. It is responsible for sleep patterns and can enhance immunologic activity.[137] Melatonin may help prevent cancer, especially cancers related to hormonal activity such as breast, prostate, and uterine cancers.[138–142]

The melatonin dose for insomnia is normally 3–6 mg at bedtime.[143,144] However, the majority of clinical cancer studies have used much higher doses, up to 20 mg of melatonin at bedtime.[138–140,142]

## Ginseng

Ginseng is an herb that has been used in Asian medicine for thousands of years. In experimental conditions, ginseng destroys cancerous tumors by attacking them at the cellular level[145] and preventing cancer spread.[146] Moreover, Siberian ginseng but not Asian ginseng (*Panax ginseng*) or North American ginseng (*Panax quinquefolius*) has been shown to bind to estrogen receptors.[147,148]

Preliminary clinical trials with 2 drugs made with Panax ginseng (panaxel and bioginseng) were carried out in patients with precancerous lesions of the endometrium. Bioginseng caused regression of these precancerous lesions (adenomatous cystic hyperplasia) of the endometrium in some patients. Thus, bioginseng appears to hold considerable promise for uterine cancer prevention.[145]

A multicenter cancer-prevention study of hepatocellular carcinoma (a type of liver cancer) was conducted in Korea where participants took 1 g of red ginseng powder per day for 5 years in an attempt to prevent this type of liver cancer.[149,150]

In a randomized, multicenter, double-blind study of symptomatic postmenopausal women, a standardized ginseng extract was found to improve quality of life and overall relief of symptoms without increasing thickening of the endometrium or raising estradiol levels.[151]

Adverse effects of ginseng are rare, but may include nervousness, insomnia, blood-clotting problems, high blood pressure, diarrhea, and rarely, breast tenderness and irregular menstruation in women.[152]

## Allicin

Allicin is the major ingredient in fresh crushed garlic. Allicin is also found in onions, scallions, leeks, chives, and shallots. These vegetables have been shown to reduce the risk of uterine cancer by interrupting the reproductive cycle of the cancer cells.[103,104,153]

## Polysaccharide K

Polysaccharide K (PSK), which is a specially prepared polysaccharide extract from the mushroom *Coriolus versicolor*, has been studied extensively in Japan where it is used as a nonspecific biological response modifier to enhance the immune system in cancer patients.[154–156] PSK suppresses tumor cell invasiveness by down-regulating several invasion-related factors.[157] PSK has been shown to enhance natural killer (NK) cell activity in multiple studies.[158–161]

In a clinical trial evaluated the effects of PSK in individuals with uterine or cervical cancer, study participants received postradiation therapy PSK (3 g daily) for 2 weeks per month. The 5-year survival in those with stage 3B cancer who received PSK was 65% compared to 49% in those not receiving PSK.[162]

## Selenium

Because selenium is a trace mineral found in soil, the amount of selenium in plant foods relates to the quality of the soil the plants are grown in. Therefore, diet is not the best method of obtaining reliable amounts of selenium.[163]

A low concentration of selenium in the body may be a contributing factor in uterine carcinogenesis.[164,165] Selenium works against cancer cells through antioxidant activity,[166] preventing or slowing tumor growth.[167] Selenium is linked to a decreased risk of developing various types of gynecologic cancers.[164,168–170]

A dosage of 400 mcg has been proposed as a safe daily dietary selenium intake.[171] High doses (more than 910 mcg/day) can result in a rare condition called selenosis, characterized by gastrointestinal upset, hair loss, white blotchy nails, fatigue, and irritability.[163,172]

## Calcium

Daily use of calcium supplements appears to lower endometrial cancer risk,[173] especially in women whose calcium intake is low because they do not eat dairy products.[83,91]

The amount of calcium supplementation varies, depending on how much calcium is consumed in the diet.[174] However, the American College of Obstetricians and Gynecologists recommends that women take 1000 mg/day of calcium if they are younger than age 50 and 1200 mg/day of calcium if they are age 50 and above.[175,176]

## SUMMARY

The complications of uterine cancer are related to the natural progression of the disease or the adverse effects of surgery, chemotherapy, or radiation. Thromboembolic disease (a tendency toward blood clots) has long been associated with uterine cancer.

Most of the adverse effects of chemotherapeutic agents are predictable and can be lessened with adjuvant medications or by taking nutritional supplements because poor nutrition is a risk factor.

The complications related to radiation can be acute (such as low blood cell counts) and chronic (gastrointestinal, genitourinary, and pulmonary). Gastrointestinal symptoms are controlled with supportive therapy such as eating a glutamine-rich diet, drinking enough water, and avoiding high-fiber foods while symptoms persist. For further information on some of the topics outlined in this protocol, read the following protocols:

- Cancer Surgery
- Cancer Radiation Therapy
- Chemotherapy
- Obesity and Weight Loss
- Female Hormone Restoration
- Breast Cancer

### Life Extension Suggestions

Women who have uterine cancer should consult their physician before taking any nutritional supplements, especially if they are receiving conventional medical treatment.

- **Apple pectin:** 2.8 g daily, with water
- **Calcium:** 1000–1200 mg daily
- **Green coffee bean extract:** 400 mg, 3 times daily
- **Essential fatty acid:** 4.8 g eicosapentaenoic acid (EPA) and 2.4 g docosahexaenoic acid (DHA) daily
- **Ground flaxseed:** 3 tablespoons (25–40 g) daily, with water
- **Garlic:** 1200 mg daily
- **Lignans:** 75–125 mg daily

- **Melatonin:** 6–20 mg, 1–2 hours before sleeping (nighttime)
- **PSK** (from the mushroom *Coriolus versicolor*): 3 g daily
- **Siberian ginseng:** 200–1000 mg daily
- **Cruciferous vegetable extract:** per label instructions
- **Vitamin A:** 25 000 IU daily
- **Vitamin C:** 2.5–5 g daily

- **Multivitamin/multimineral supplement (without copper):** containing 20 mg beta-carotene, 15 mg lycopene, and 200 mcg selenium daily

## REFERENCES

References available at: www.lef.org/dpt5/ch128

# 129

---

# Uterine Fibroids

---

The uterus is one organ in a complex system that composes the structures common to the internal genitalia of a woman. The uterus is a hollow, pear-shaped organ of reproduction in which the fertilized egg is implanted and the fetus develops. However, the uterus, which is composed of the cervix, body, and fundus, can experience stress beyond its role in pregnancy.

One such uterine anomaly is the formation of fibrous or fully developed connective tissue, resulting in abnormal muscle cells, referred to as a uterine fibroid or myoma. A myoma is a benign neoplasm, affecting 20–30% of all women by the age of 40 and more than 50% of women overall. Uterine fibroids are much more common among African Americans than Caucasians, although the reason for this is not clearly understood.

A fibroid can form on the interior muscular wall, as well as the exterior of the uterus. Fibroids are spherical, firm lumps that most often occur in groups. Symptoms of uterine fibroids (and their impact on general health) include abnormally heavy menstrual periods (with the likelihood of anemia), shortened menstrual cycles (less than 28 days), metrorrhagia (unexplained uterine bleeding), fatigue, increased vaginal discharge, painful sexual intercourse, and pain or pressure in the bowel or bladder. Some women, however, judge their condition to be asymptomatic, with the diagnosis of uterine fibroids being made only after a routine pelvic examination.

## HORMONAL INFLUENCE

Since fibroids tend to increase during pregnancy and decrease during menopause, presumably due to fluctuating levels of estrogen, uterine fibroids are considered to be estrogen-dependent.[1] To further substantiate this finding, in leiomyomas (leio meaning smooth; myomas meaning a common benign fibroid tumor on the uterine muscle), estrogen levels were persistently elevated whereas progesterone showed contradictory levels from test results, some showing low concentrations and others showing elevations.[2] Thus, the recommendation of progesterone is clouded.

As late as 1995, various researchers stated that estrogen did not directly stimulate myoma growth, but it is actually progesterone and progestins that promote fibroids. Various practitioners have, however, reported excellent results regarding uterine fibroids and progesterone usage. Because progesterone research is confounding, women using progesterone should be closely monitored. The consensus is more unified, however, that women with uterine fibroids should attempt to lessen the entry of exogenous estrogen substances into their systems.

Practitioners report that fibroids the size of a 13-week fetus (the size at which Western medicine begins discussing the need for a hysterectomy) have been successfully treated using the reduced-estrogen method. The accompanying heavy uterine bleeding has also been controlled with this conservative treatment.

Various researchers believe that women with fibroids, due to the estrogen load that a contraceptive delivers, should avoid oral contraception. Other practitioners, who believe the only notable association with oral contraception is a significantly increased risk among women who used oral contraceptives at age 13–16 years, question this theory.[3] The risk of developing a uterus that is not strong physically appears to increase with early menarche, parity, or history of infertility. It seems prudent to select an alternative form of birth control other than oral contraceptives if health of the reproductive system is questioned.

Controlling estrogen levels is difficult in our estrogen-laden environment. Estrogen has become a significant problem because the hormone has ways of entering our food and water supply. Various agricultural chemicals mimic the activity and structural description of estrogen, provoking heightened estrogen receptivity on estrogen receptor sites. Pesticides initially invade our airspace and then later appear as residual by-products in the food chain. Urine, contaminated with high levels of residual estrogen from birth control pills, can seep back into water supplies through inadequate sewage treatment procedures. Obviously, estrogen replacement therapy at menopause can worsen uterine fibroids due to increased levels of circulating estrogen.

## DETOXIFICATION OF HORMONES

Three types of estrogen make up the total estrogen load in a female. These include estradiol, estrone, and estriol. Both estradiol and estrone have been implicated as being carcinogenic under certain circumstances. There is some evidence that estriol is not only noncarcinogenic, but also anticarcinogenic.

Mother Nature did not leave females without a defense in regard to downgrading the carcinogenic status of various female hormones. One adaptation is intricately provided by way of the hard-working liver. In fact, the liver is the most active metabolic processing center in the body. Among the many vital metabolic functions assigned to the liver is detoxification or excretion of hormones such as estrogen. The liver metabolizes estrogen (so it can be eliminated from the body) by converting it to estrone and eventually to estriol, which has very little ability to stimulate the uterus. If the liver is not effectively metabolizing estradiol, the uterus may become "overestrogenized" and respond with fibroids.

The implications of good liver function are manifold. Most individuals can benefit from nutritional support applied to improve liver performance. Herbs such as silibinin (milk thistle), dandelion, goldenseal, barberry, and artichoke have moved from folklore to accepted herbal pharmacology as agents for improving liver function. Choline, inositol, and methionine are also often included in a hepatic protocol.

Liver health is not always easy to assess because satisfactory liver results can sometimes be obtained even when the liver is being severely challenged. This can occur through the principle of homeostasis: the body constantly strives for correction in the face of perilous internal mayhem. Because of toxins constantly bombarding the liver, women with fibroids in particular should consider additional liver support. Once the liver has been assisted, conversion of estradiol to estriol is much easier.

## DRUG THERAPY TO REDUCE EXCESS ESTROGEN

Estrogen is a growth-stimulating hormone. As stated earlier, fibroids typically shrink after menopause because of the reduction in endogenous (self-produced) estrogen that accompanies menopause. Women with uterine fibroids should have their blood estrogen level checked. If blood testing reveals too much estrogen, consider asking your doctor to prescribe a low dose (1 mg every few days) aromatase-inhibiting drug such as anastrozole (Arimidex®). By having a physician adjust the dose of Arimidex®, women may be able to lower excess estrogen, thereby helping to shrink fibroids and possibly reducing breast cancer risk. When Arimidex® was compared to tamoxifen in a breast cancer prevention trial, Arimidex®

was slightly more effective and virtually free of side effects.[4]

## THE ROLE OF THE THYROID GLAND

The health of the thyroid gland should be considered in any debility in the reproductive organs. Hypothyroidism can be the primary causative agent in abnormal Pap smears (Papanicolaou test), menorrhagia (abnormally heavy or long menstrual periods), ovarian cysts, metrorrhagia (bleeding other than that caused by menstruation), infertility, and unsuccessful pregnancies. Fibroid tumors are rare in women with hypothyroidism who have been maintained on adequate thyroid therapy. It is possible to produce fibroids in experimental animals by injections of estrogen, and there is evidence of excess estrogens in women with hypothyroidism.

In hypothyroidism, there is increased activity of the pituitary gland aimed at trying to stimulate the thyroid to produce more hormone secretions, and increased pituitary activity may cause the ovaries to increase their estrogen output. Unless the health of the thyroid is considered in assessing any "female" complaint, the individual may be at risk for unnecessary physical suffering and emotional debility. A few grains of thyroid extract can often reverse impending disaster in the reproductive tract. The importance of a thyroid evaluation by a competent endocrinologist cannot be overemphasized.

Interestingly, women with endometriosis and antithyroidal antibodies have significantly higher values of polychlorinated biphenyls (PCBs).[5] PCBs represent a family of more than 200 structurally related chemicals that were once used as industrial coolants in power transformers. Because PCBs were found to cause cancer in laboratory animals, their use has been banned for more than 20 years in the United States. However, PCBs still persist in the environment and mimic the action of thyroxin, a hormone produced by the thyroid gland. It is thought that PCBs affect not only the thyroid gland, but also the reproductive system in animals.

The luteinizing hormone (LH), responsible for ovulation, and the follicle-stimulating hormone (FSH), responsible for follicle maturation, respond to stimuli from gonadotropin-releasing hormone (GnRH) released from the hypothalamus. When a GnRH analogue (GnRHa) was given as leuprolide acetate, significant tumor reduction was achieved.[6] In another study, nonmenopausal women (110, with mean age of 42.1 years) with symptomatic uterine leiomyomata (smooth benign fibroid tumors) were studied to determine the efficacy of leuprolide, administered intramuscularly at a dose of 3.75 mg every 4 weeks for 16 weeks. Initial results revealed that the uterine size decreased to 50% of its original volume in 33 (37.5%) of 88 women who entered the study with a hypertrophic uterus. Eighty fibromas, measured separately, decreased by greater than 50% of the initial size in 47 (52.8%) of the women tested.[7] Amenorrhea (or absent menstrual periods) and an attendant increase in hemoglobin levels were produced by way of the GnRH inhibitor.

Because of cost and side effects (hot flashes being the major complaint followed by isolated incidences of hypertension and headache), continued use of GnRH inhibitors is often considered prohibitive. However, important correlations may be taken from GnRHa research that relate to the thyroid gland. What leuprolide is accomplishing by way of inhibition of LH and FSH, hypothyroidism may be undoing by stimulating these hormones into greater activity.

In a condition of hypothyroidism, the thyrotropin-releasing factor, elaborated in the hypothalamus, is continually being secreted to arouse greater thyroid activity from the anterior pituitary. The body may not allow for thyroid hormone stimulation without stimulation of LH and FSH as well. The thyrotropin-releasing factor may arouse other areas in the anterior pituitary in its effort to goad the production of increased thyroid hormone release.

GnRH is capable of inciting additional production from both LH and FSH, which in sequence stimulate the uterus. A reduction in GnRH can actually diminish fibroid size and symptoms. It is likely that the thyrotropin-releasing factor can elicit a similar stimulatory effect on LH and FSH. The anterior pituitary secretes the growth hormone, thyrotropin, adrenocorticotropic hormone, melanocyte-stimulating hormone, FSH, LH, prolactin, and endorphins. This cascade likely best describes why hypothyroidism is the purveyor of so many reproductive tract anomalies and why it must be considered in any treatment protocol.

Obtaining satisfactory laboratory results regarding thyroid performance is sometimes difficult. This unfortunate situation has led alternative practitioners to resort to temperature analysis to demonstrate thyroid function. This is a noninvasive, reliable test that can highlight the need for thyroid support. Sometimes a glass-bulb thermometer is used under the arm. At other times, physicians monitor the readings via the traditional sublingual method. Consistent readings below 97.6 °F are suggestive of an underactive thyroid gland.

# THE ROLE OF HEAVY METAL CONTAMINATION

Women with hormonal disorders often present with high levels of mercury and cadmium excretion.[5] Cadmium excretion was pronounced for the following groups of women: those with technical professions, thyroid dysfunctions, and habitual abortions and uterine fibroids. Evaluation of heavy metal and pesticide contamination should be included in a woman's test panel if she has hormonal irregularities or specific fertility disorders. The effects of these pollutants could affect the thyroid gland, with the consequence being a disordered uterus. They could also stimulate the uterus by mimicking the activity of estrogen.

Chelation with ethylenediaminetetraacetic acid (EDTA) is sometimes used to extract toxic mineral accumulations from the body. Most toxic minerals are divalent, that is, they carry 2 positive charges ready to link up with 2 negative ions. Divalent minerals include divalent mercury, aluminum, and cadmium, along with some essential minerals such as calcium, magnesium, zinc, copper, and manganese, as well as other trace minerals. EDTA, in the presence of divalent minerals, binds or attracts these hazardous minerals by drawing the positive charge into itself. An EDTA/mineral complex is then formed and remains in solution and is capable of passing through the blood vessels to the kidney and out of the body. EDTA is best described as a pharmacologically neutral "escort" molecule that transports divalent ions out of the body. The beneficial minerals are then either replaced by way of nutritional supplementation or through direct administration of the minerals in an intravenous solution. (See the Heavy Metal Detoxification protocol for additional information about chelation.)

Kelp, in a general nutritive tonic, can also extract cadmium by preventing its absorption in the gastrointestinal (GI) tract. When consumed daily, seaweed has advantages beyond ridding the body of heavy metal stores. It is regarded by some as a powerful ally in healing and lessening the severity of fibroids. Mercury can also be mobilized and transported from the body by way of vitamin C, cysteine, glutathione, and selenium. Concern about heavy metal and pesticide contamination has been expressed in more than 68 reports, with the consensus being that women who experience hormonal irregularities or specific fertility disorders should be examined for heavy metal poisoning. (See the

Heavy Metal Detoxification protocol for additional information about potential sources of heavy metal contamination.)

## DIETARY SUGGESTIONS

If organic fruits and vegetables are available and affordable to the consumer, their consideration is likely indicated. Health practitioners recommend a diet centered on whole foods, with fresh fruits and vegetables, nuts, seeds, and whole grains being emphasized. Lignins, found in all whole grains, are antiestrogenic. Lignins are present in decreasing order in flaxseed, rye, buckwheat, millet, oats, barley, corn, rice, and wheat.

Fiber-rich diets can assist in extracting excessive estrogen stores from the body. The positive effects of a high-fiber compared to a low-fiber diet (28 g daily compared to 12 g) were illustrated when fecal weight and fecal excretion of estrogens in the vegetarian's diet were contrasted to that of nonvegetarian (eating both animal and vegetable substances).[8] Foods thought best to be avoided, either because of their low-fiber content or history of promoting fibroid growth, include dairy products, red meat, fried fatty foods, sugar, salt, caffeine, and alcohol.

Much debate has focused on whether soy products should be included in the diet of women with estrogen excess. Genistein and daidzein, both regarded as isoflavones, appear in soy and have estrogen activity. Researchers, representing the "pro" and "con" of the estrogen debate, present their views with conviction. In countries where soy is a main part of the diet, there are claims that reproductive tract disease is less frequent than in regions or cultures where soy is not included in the diet. The premise is that the weaker estrogen constituents of soy bind to the estrogen receptor, making less available to the binding site for the stronger, more ominous estrogen. Conversely, it appears that menarche (the onset of the menses or the menstrual period) may actually be hastened in the precocious child who uses soy products. Because of the dichotomies regarding soy usage, it is considered wise to avoid large amounts of genistein in conditions that are estrogen receptor-positive.

A more slender frame may benefit women with fibroids as well. Judicious undereating may be beneficial to the uterus, providing less quantities of estrogen by way of lessening the overconsumption of hormone-rich foodstuffs.

### Additional Suggestions

Nutritional supplementation for uterine fibroids should include antiestrogenic substances such as flavonoids which have 1/400–1/50 000 the estrogenic effect that synthetic estrogen has. Flavonoids contribute very little to the total body supply of estrogen. Various herbs (saw palmetto, historically used for benign prostatic hyperplasia), lady's mantle, chaste tree berries, and yarrow flowers have been cited for their antiestrogenic values. Other supplements recommended for uterine fibroids include immune-enhancing nutrients such as coenzyme Q10 (CoQ10), vitamin C, zinc, arginine/lysine combination, maitake mushrooms, and vitamin A. The antioxidant activity of beta-carotene, vitamin C, vitamin E, and selenium is also recommended.

As a possible addition to a nutritional protocol, a woman with fibroids should consider pancreatic enzymes. Pancreatic enzymes have many uses, but when used to reduce unusual cell, tissue, or muscle mass (such as in cancer and fibroids), pancreatic enzymes should be consumed between meals. Although not universally accepted, the logic behind using pancreatic enzymes is that the enzymes will digest fibrous/smooth muscle tissue and dissolve fibroids. When taken with food, pancreatic enzymes assist in digestion and do not resolve tissue.

## SURGICAL INTERVENTION

Some women prefer an abdominal/pelvic surgical intervention (a myomectomy) that removes the fibroids and muscle tissue, but spares the uterus. However, 15–30% of women who have a myomectomy eventually require further surgery because fibroids can recur. A myomectomy requires a search for a very competent surgeon because greater skill is required in the procedure. Even if a woman is not concerned about protecting her fertility, a myomectomy should still be considered as an alternative to a hysterectomy. A hysterectomy appears to be too great a sacrifice for a condition that is considered to be benign 99.9% of the time. However, 30% of hysterectomies performed are to remove fibroids.

It is thought that much of an individual's sexual response is psychic in origin. Therefore, if a woman considers that her internal feminization is a part of her sexual mystique, then the absence of her uterus could prove to be her undoing: 25% of women who have a hysterectomy report increased difficulty becoming sexually aroused and then having a disappointing orgasm, if it occurs. The uterus contracts on the impulses of the orgasm, making the sensation deeper and more satisfying. The uterus also responds pleasurably to breast stimulation. Without a uterus, no such response occurs. When the uterus is removed because of fibroids, the ovaries are usually left intact. This lessens the degradation.

Research indicates that a retained sexual nature retards aging. Some women recount the removal of their uterus as entering the operating room young and emerging old. Chronic dysthymia (despondency) is frequently observed. Many women are also disappointed in their lack of bladder control after surgery. Others are plagued by intestinal adhesions which are not considered to be rare following abdominal surgery and can actually be life-threatening. Alternatives to radical surgery should first be carefully explored before any decision to operate is made.

## Life Extension Suggestions

Women experiencing poor uterine health should consider the following suggestions, acting on those most appropriate for each individual:

- **Evaluate the thyroid gland**
- **Restrict exogenous estrogen**
- **Detoxification of hormones/liver support**
  - **Milk thistle:** 750 mg standardized extract (containing 80% silymarin and 30% silibinins)
  - **Artichoke leaf:** 500 mg standardized extract, 1–3 times daily
  - **Dandelion tincture:** 5–10 mL, 3 times daily (or dandelion root, 200–500 mg capsules twice daily)
  - **Goldenseal:** 400 mg daily
  - **Choline, inositol, and methionine** (complexed in a formulary to yield 1000 mg of choline and inositol daily): These nutrients may also be purchased separately as choline bitartrate, 0.5 tsp, twice daily; inositol, two 500-mg capsules daily; methionine powder, 500 mg daily
  - **Calcium-d-glucarate:** 137.5–400 mg daily
- **Antiestrogenic substances/uterine support**
  - **Vitex (chaste tree berry),** standardized extract: 20–40 mg daily
  - **Soy isoflavones:** 135 mg (including 28 mg genistein) daily

- **Cruciferous vegetable extract:** containing at least 80–160 mg of indole-3-carbinol (I3C) and 14–28 mg di-indolyl-methane (DIM) daily
- **Comprehensive multinutrient formula:** per label instructions
- **Zinc:** 30–90 mg daily
- **Vitamin A:** 5000 IU (as 90% beta-carotene and 10% acetate) daily in divided doses
- **Beta-carotene:** 4500 IU daily
- **Vitamin D:** 5000–8000 IU daily, depending on blood levels of 25-OH-vitamin D
- **Arginine/lysine:** 500 mg of each daily, with vitamins C and B6 to assist absorption
- **Saw palmetto:** 320 mg daily
- **Coenzyme Q10**, as ubiquinol: 50–200 mg daily
- **Iodine:** 1–3 mg daily
- **Progesterone cream:** per label instructions; depending on blood levels
- **Detoxification of heavy metals**
  - **EDTA:** per label instructions
  - **L-glutathione:** 50–150 mg daily
  - **L-cysteine:** 200–600 mg daily
  - **Selenium:** 200–400 mcg daily
- **Additional suggestion**
  - **Pancreatin 8x blend:** 400–1200 mg daily between meals

In addition, the following *blood tests* may provide helpful information:

- Female Comprehensive Hormone panel
- Thyroid Antibody panel
- Heavy Metals panel
- 24-hour Urinary Hormone profile

## REFERENCES

References available at: www.lef.org/dpt5/ch129

# 130

# Vertigo

Vertigo is the feeling of spinning or falling through space when there is no motion. Sensations associated with vertigo include a sense of spinning, tumbling, falling forward or backward, or the ground rolling beneath one's feet. It may be difficult to focus visually; many people find it uncomfortable to keep their eyes open during vertigo spells. Sweating, nausea, and vomiting are also common. Depending on the cause, vertigo can last from a few minutes to days.

Vertigo is not a disease, but a symptom of a broad range of disorders, diseases, and conditions, including the following:

- Diseases or disorders of the inner ear (such as motion sickness; the formation of "sludge" in the inner ear, which causes the inner ear to send a confusing motion signal to the brain; or tumors in the inner ear)

- Injuries or other damage to the inner ear (eg, from drugs [including aspirin and some diuretics, chemotherapeutics, and antibiotics])

- Diseases or disorders of the brain (such as tumors, migraine, transient ischemic attack or stroke, or a psychiatric disease or disorder)

- Disorders affecting the acoustic nerve, which connects the inner ear to the brain

- Ménière's disease or Ménière's syndrome

- Viral and bacterial infections

- Allergies

- Multiple sclerosis

- Damage to the nerves in the neck that help the brain monitor the relative position of the neck and trunk (this form of vertigo, called cervical vertigo, often occurs after an injury such as a whiplash injury but may be associated with arthritis in the neck or degenerative cervical spine disease)

- Low blood pressure

Under normal circumstances, the brain relies on three sensory systems to maintain spatial orientation: the vestibular system (inner ear), visual system (eyes), and somatosensory system (conveys information from the skin, joint, and muscle receptors). These 3 systems overlap, allowing the brain to assemble an accurate sense of spatial orientation. However, a compromised system or conflicting signals can cause vertigo.

The vestibular system is most often involved with vertigo. The sensory organs for the vestibular system are located in the bony labyrinths of the inner ear. They include 3 semicircular canals and an otolithic apparatus on each side. The otolithic apparatus consists of tiny particles of calcium carbonate suspended in a gelatinous matrix in two structures called the utricle and saccule. These particles shift in response to movement in a straight line, stimulating cilia (hairlike fibers) that are embedded in the gel. Movement at an angle is detected by the semicircular canals. These components work together to provide a sense of spatial orientation.

Broadly classified, vertigo is usually either physiologic or pathologic. Physiologic vertigo is normal and occurs when there is a conflict between the signals sent to the brain by the vestibular system and the other balance-sensing systems of the body. It can also occur when the head is subjected to unfamiliar movements, such as the rolling motion associated with seasickness, spinning for an extended period, or when the head is held in an unusual position (eg, head and neck are tilted back for an extended period). Physiologic vertigo is usually easily corrected, either by moving the head and neck into a more normal position or focusing on an external reference point to give the vestibular system an opportunity to stabilize. This is why a person with motion sickness is advised to look into the distance and focus on some faraway point, such as the horizon.

Pathologic vertigo occurs because of lesions or disorders in any of the three sensory systems (usually the vestibular system). Pathologic vertigo is further broken down into the following:

- **Labyrinthine dysfunction.** Labyrinthine dysfunction can occur as a result of any disease or condition that affects the ability of the vestibular organs (the labyrinths) to communicate with the brain.

- **Vertigo of the vestibular nerve.** Diseases of the eighth (vestibular) cranial nerve cause vertigo of the vestibular nerve.

- **Central vertigo.** Lesions on the brainstem or cerebellum (parts of the nervous system in which information from the vestibular system is integrated with information from the eyes and musculoskeletal position sensors, or proprioceptors) can cause central vertigo.

- **Psychogenic vertigo.** Psychogenic vertigo usually occurs with panic attacks or agoraphobia (fear of open spaces).

No matter what the cause, vertigo is common, affecting millions of people annually. Episodes of vertigo increase with age, accounting for more than 61% of all cases of dizziness by age 65 years.[1] The overall incidence of dizziness, vertigo, and imbalance is 5–10% of the overall population and 40% in patients older than 40 years.

## TYPES OF VERTIGO

### Benign Paroxysmal Positional Vertigo

Benign paroxysmal positional vertigo (BPPV) occurs after a sudden movement of the head. It is one of the most common types of vertigo.[2] Women are affected twice as often as men, and the average age of onset is the mid-50s.[3]

BPPV is usually harmless and often no cause is detected (ie, idiopathic). In some cases, however, BPPV is caused by age-related degeneration or head trauma.[4] Patients with BPPV have short-lived episodes of temporary dizziness, lightheadedness, imbalance, and nausea. Symptoms of BPPV, which usually develop suddenly after a change in head position, may be severe enough to cause vomiting.[5] Typical motions that cause episodes of BPPV include getting out of bed, rolling over, bending down, and looking up while standing.[6] One of the characteristic symptoms of BPPV is rapid movement of the eye in one direction followed by a slow drift back to its original position. This involuntary movement of the eyes is a type of nystagmus. Doctors can sometimes tell what kind of vertigo is present by the nature of the nystagmus.

BPPV occurs when debris from the otoliths settles into the posterior semicircular canal. This renders the canal oversensitive to the pull of gravity, producing a constant sense of motion or falling.[7]

### Ménière's Syndrome and Ménière's Disease

The terms Ménière's disease and Ménière's syndrome are sometimes used interchangeably. However, even though both involve the inner ear apparatus, they are not the same disorder. Ménière's disease develops due to idiopathic (or unknown) causes, while Ménière's syndrome is secondary to other diseases such as inner ear inflammation caused by syphilis, thyroid disease, or head trauma. Of the two, the most common is idiopathic Ménière's disease.

Ménière's of either variety is recognized by a classic triad of symptoms: vertigo; low-frequency, fluctuating hearing loss; and tinnitus (ringing in the ears).[8] Also, the condition is characterized by a condition known as endolymphatic hydrops, or increased hydraulic pressure in the inner ear's endolymphatic system. Although researchers have long suspected that endolymphatic hydrops was the underlying cause of the symptoms of Ménière's disease, newer studies have called into question an even deeper cause. The endolymphatic hydrops in Ménière's disease may be caused by neurotoxicity and progressive damage to the cochlear nerve in the ear; the increased pressure is a result rather than a cause.[9,10] Some early research has suggested that nerve cell toxicity is mediated by nitric oxide, which is an important mediator in the inflammatory process. This suggests that agents that block nitric oxide may someday be important in the treatment of Ménière's.[9,11]

In the meantime, while researchers are still pursuing these findings, other treatments may come to the forefront. For instance, because people with Ménière's disease have been shown to have characteristic abnormalities in their inner ear and an elevated level of free radicals,[12] free radical scavengers may be of benefit in treating Ménière's.

People who have Ménière's may experience attacks of vertigo that last 1–8 hours. These attacks (and the accompanying tinnitus) can be severe. There may also be an aura (such as a sensation of seeing lights or smelling odors). These symptoms may last an indefinite period. In the worst cases, hearing loss is permanent.[13]

### Vestibular Neuronitis

Vestibular neuronitis involves an attack of vertigo that occurs without accompanying disruption of hearing. Its symptoms may persist for up to several weeks before clearing, but usually abate within a matter of days. It is sometimes referred to as vestibular neuropathy.[14]

### Labyrinthitis

Labyrinthitis is an acute inflammation of the labyrinths, often caused by viral infections, although it can also be caused by reactions to medications or toxins. People with labyrinthitis experience an acute onset of severe vertigo that lasts several days to a week. It is typically accompanied by hearing loss and tinnitus.

### Phobic Postural Vertigo

Phobic postural vertigo is the second most common diagnosis in people with dizziness or vertigo, although there is some debate about whether this is a single disorder or represents a group of different conditions with possible different causes.[15] Phobic postural vertigo, which is characterized by nonrotational vertigo with postural and gait instability, mainly occurs in people with an obsessive-compulsive personality.[16]

## Migraine-Associated Vertigo

Migraine-associated vertigo is a disorder that can accompany a migraine headache. In medical practices focused on treating migraine, 27–42% of patients report episodic vertigo. A large number (about 36%) of these patients also experienced vertigo during headache-free periods.[17]

## Posttraumatic Vertigo

Posttraumatic vertigo immediately follows head trauma. In most cases, it causes damage to the inner ear mechanisms in the absence of other central nervous system signs. The interval between injury and onset of symptoms can be days or even weeks. The mechanism for the delay of symptoms is uncertain but includes hemorrhage into the labyrinth, with later development of labyrinthitis in the fluids of the inner ear.[18]

## Central Nervous System Dysfunction

Central nervous system dysfunction causes of vertigo are varied and include brainstem vascular disease, arteriovenous malformation, tumor of the brainstem and cerebellum, multiple sclerosis, and vertebrobasilar migraine.[19]

# CONVENTIONAL TREATMENT OF VERTIGO

Although BPPV and some other common causes of vertigo are relatively harmless and disappear over time, there are other forms whose appearance might signify the beginning of a more serious condition. Because of this, it is always recommended that any case of vertigo be evaluated by an experienced physician.

The conventional treatment of vertigo depends on its underlying cause. In the case of BPPV, the most common therapy is repositioning exercises that redistribute the calcium carbonate back throughout the inner ear. There are various forms of repositioning exercises, including the Epley maneuver. In the Epley maneuver, the person lies down and the head is moved from side to side, with each position being held about 20 seconds. This has been shown to redistribute the calcium deposits in the inner ear, thus reestablishing normal function.[20] Nonsurgical, nonpharmaceutical

exercises such as the Epley maneuver have an excellent record of reversing vertigo caused by BPPV.

Treatment of Ménière's is aimed at controlling the vertigo, usually through salt restriction or diuretics to relieve the elevated pressure in the endolymphatic sac. Similarly, glucocorticoids may be prescribed. For severe cases, surgery is sometimes recommended to decompress the endolymphatic sac. Unfortunately, no effective therapy for tinnitus or hearing loss has been identified.

Other pharmaceuticals used to suppress vestibular abnormalities include anticholinergics, benzodiazepines, and antihistamines. Some patients with nausea use antiemetics.

# NUTRITIONAL APPROACHES TO VERTIGO

As a symptom, vertigo is always a reason to see a physician. At the same time, however, for conditions in which vertigo persists (eg, Ménière's disease), a number of nutrients might be considered to counteract the effects.

## Antioxidants

Antioxidants mitigate the damaging effects of free radicals on tissues, cell membranes, and DNA. Vitamin C, vitamin E, lipoic acid, and glutathione are among the most important antioxidants. Vitamin C has been shown to have a beneficial effect on patients with Ménière's disease when given in combination with glutathione.[21] Glutathione, which is a powerful antioxidant, has been demonstrated to be effective in treating vertigo induced by Ménière's disease.[12] Because glutathione is poorly absorbed by the body, Life Extension recommends taking precursors to glutathione, including N-acetylcysteine and lipoic acid. It is worth noting, however, that the role of L-glutamate has been studied in vertigo with somewhat conflicting results. There is some evidence that the neurotoxicity associated with some forms of vertigo is mediated by glutamate.[11] Glutamate-blocking drugs have also been proposed as treatment for vertigo.[22]

## Vitamin B6

Studies have reported positive effects using vitamin B6 on drug-induced vertigo and nausea, suggesting that vitamin B6 appears to offer protection against this form of vertigo.[23]

## Ginkgo Biloba

Researchers in Poland have found that vertigo induced by vestibular receptor impairment can be reduced by Ginkgo biloba extract. According to their study, almost all of the 45 patients who received 120 mg twice daily of Ginkgo biloba extract for 30 days showed a significantly increased ability to compensate for vestibular lesions and subsequently experienced fewer episodes of vertigo.[24] These results confirmed the earlier work performed by researchers who found that patients who received Ginkgo biloba extract at 80 mg twice daily had their vertigo and dizziness reduced by as much as 65%.[25] Positive results have also been found in trials of people with vertigo of various causes.[26–28]

## Coenzyme Q10

During a multicenter clinical trial of 2664 patients with congestive heart failure, 73% reported a decrease in the incidence of vertigo after only 3 months of treatment with 50–150 mg of coenzyme Q10 (CoQ10) daily.[29]

## Ginger

Volunteers who took ginger and were then subjected to induced motion sickness (which includes vertigo as a symptom) experienced delayed onset of motion sickness and reported a shorter recovery time.[30]

These results have been confirmed by other studies that showed that ginger reduced motion sickness and its associated vertigo.[31,32] One researcher hypothesized that the positive effects of ginger were likely the result of its effect on the gastric system.[33]

## Life Extension Suggestions

- **Vitamin C:** 1000–6000 mg daily with food with 600–1800 mg of **N-acetylcysteine** daily
- **Vitamin B6:** 150 mg with food, while vertigo persists
- **Ginkgo biloba:** 120 mg daily
- **CoQ10:** 50–200 mg daily with food
- **Ginger:** per label instructions (especially for motion sickness)
- **Vitamin E:** 400 IU daily with at least 200 mg gamma tocopherol
- **R-lipoic acid:** 240–480 mg daily

---

## REFERENCES

References available at: www.lef.org/dpt5/ch130

# Appendix A

# Selected References: Aspirin, Metformin, and Cimetidine in the Treatment and/or Prevention of Cancer

## ASPIRIN

Routine aspirin or nonsteroidal anti-inflammatory drugs for the primary prevention of colorectal cancer: U.S. Preventive Services Task Force recommendation statement. *Annals of internal medicine*. Mar 6 2007;146(5):361-364.

Alfonso LF, Srivenugopal KS, Arumugam TV, Abbruscato TJ, Weidanz JA, Bhat GJ. Aspirin inhibits camptothecin-induced p21CIP1 levels and potentiates apoptosis in human breast cancer cells. *International journal of oncology*. Mar 2009;34(3):597-608.

Algra AM, Rothwell PM. Effects of regular aspirin on long-term cancer incidence and metastasis: a systematic comparison of evidence from observational studies versus randomised trials. *The lancet oncology*. May 2012;13(5):518-527.

Asano TK, McLeod RS. Nonsteroidal anti-inflammatory drugs and aspirin for the prevention of colorectal adenomas and cancer: a systematic review. *Diseases of the colon and rectum*. May 2004;47(5):665-673.

Avivi D, Moshkowitz M, Detering E, Arber N. The role of low-dose aspirin in the prevention of colorectal cancer. *Expert opinion on therapeutic targets*. Mar 2012;16 Suppl 1:S51-62.

Bardia A, Ebbert JO, Vierkant RA, Limburg PJ, Anderson K, Wang AH, . . . Cerhan JR. Association of aspirin and nonaspirin nonsteroidal anti-inflammatory drugs with cancer incidence and mortality. *Journal of the National Cancer Institute*. Jun 6 2007;99(11):881-889.

Bastiaannet E, Sampieri K, Dekkers OM, de Craen AJ, van Herk-Sukel MP, Lemmens V, . . . Liefers GJ. Use of aspirin postdiagnosis improves survival for colon cancer patients. *British journal of cancer*. Apr 24 2012;106(9):1564-1570.

Benamouzig R, Uzzan B, Little J, Chaussade S. Low dose aspirin, COX-inhibition and chemoprevention of colorectal cancer. *Current topics in medicinal chemistry*. 2005;5(5):493-503.

Bosco JL, Palmer JR, Boggs DA, Hatch EE, Rosenberg L. Regular aspirin use and breast cancer risk in US Black women. *Cancer causes & control : CCC*. Nov 2011;22(11):1553-1561.

Bosetti C, Gallus S, La Vecchia C. Aspirin and cancer risk: a summary review to 2007. *Recent results in cancer research. Fortschritte der Krebsforschung. Progres dans les recherches sur le cancer*. 2009;181:231-251.

Bosetti C, Gallus S, La Vecchia C. Aspirin and cancer risk: an update to 2001. *European journal of cancer prevention : the official journal of the European Cancer Prevention Organisation (ECP)*. Dec 2002;11(6):535-542.

Bosetti C, Rosato V, Gallus S, Cuzick J, La Vecchia C. Aspirin and cancer risk: a quantitative review to 2011. *Annals of oncology : official journal of the European Society for Medical Oncology / ESMO*. Jun 2012;23(6):1403-1415.

Burn J, Gerdes AM, Macrae F, Mecklin JP, Moeslein G, Olschwang S, . . . Bishop DT. Long-term effect of aspirin on cancer risk in carriers of hereditary colorectal cancer: an analysis from the CAPP2 randomised controlled trial. *Lancet*. Dec 17 2011;378(9809):2081-2087.

Chan AT. Aspirin and chemoprevention of cancer: reaching beyond the colon. *Gastroenterology*. Oct 2012;143(4):1110-1112.

Chan AT, Giovannucci EL, Meyerhardt JA, Schernhammer ES, Curhan GC, Fuchs CS. Long-term use of aspirin and nonsteroidal anti-inflammatory drugs and risk of colorectal cancer. *JAMA : the journal of the American Medical Association*. Aug 24 2005;294(8):914-923.

Chan AT, Giovannucci EL, Meyerhardt JA, Schernhammer ES, Wu K, Fuchs CS. Aspirin dose and duration of use and risk of colorectal cancer in men. *Gastroenterology*. Jan 2008;134(1):21-28.

Chan AT, Ogino S, Fuchs CS. Aspirin use and survival after diagnosis of colorectal cancer. *JAMA : the journal of the American Medical Association*. Aug 12 2009;302(6):649-658.

Chen W, Zhu H, Jia Z, Li J, Misra HP, Zhou K, Li Y. Inhibition of peroxynitrite-mediated DNA strand cleavage and hydroxyl radical formation by aspirin at pharmacologically relevant concentrations: implications for cancer intervention. *Biochemical and biophysical research communications*. Dec 4 2009;390(1):142-147.

Choe KS, Cowan JE, Chan JM, Carroll PR, D'Amico AV, Liauw SL. Aspirin use and the risk of prostate cancer mortality in men treated with prostatectomy or radiotherapy. *Journal of clinical oncology: official journal of the American Society of Clinical Oncology.* Oct 1 2012;30(28):3540-3544.

Corley DA, Kerlikowske K, Verma R, Buffler P. Protective association of aspirin/NSAIDs and esophageal cancer: a systematic review and meta-analysis. *Gastroenterology.* Jan 2003;124(1):47-56.

Cuzick J, Otto F, Baron JA, Brown PH, Burn J, Greenwald P, . . . Thun M. Aspirin and non-steroidal anti-inflammatory drugs for cancer prevention: an international consensus statement. *The lancet oncology.* May 2009;10(5):501-507.

Dhillon PK, Kenfield SA, Stampfer MJ, Giovannucci EL. Long-term aspirin use and the risk of total, high-grade, regionally advanced and lethal prostate cancer in a prospective cohort of health professionals, 1988-2006. *International journal of cancer. Journal international du cancer.* May 15 2011;128(10):2444-2452.

Din FV, Theodoratou E, Farrington SM, Tenesa A, Barnetson RA, Cetnarskyj R, . . . Dunlop MG. Effect of aspirin and NSAIDs on risk and survival from colorectal cancer. *Gut.* Dec 2010;59(12):1670-1679.

Dube C, Rostom A, Lewin G, Tsertsvadze A, Barrowman N, Code C, . . . Moher D. The use of aspirin for primary prevention of colorectal cancer: a systematic review prepared for the U.S. Preventive Services Task Force. *Annals of internal medicine.* Mar 6 2007;146(5):365-375.

DuPont AW, Arguedas MR, Wilcox CM. Aspirin chemoprevention in patients with increased risk for colorectal cancer: a cost-effectiveness analysis. *Alimentary pharmacology & therapeutics.* Aug 1 2007;26(3):431-441.

Fernandez Calderon M, Betes Ibanez MT. [Aspirin in the primary prevention of colorectal cancer]. *Anales del sistema sanitario de Navarra.* May-Aug 2012;35(2):261-267.

Flossmann E, Rothwell PM. Effect of aspirin on long-term risk of colorectal cancer: consistent evidence from randomised and observational studies. *Lancet.* May 12 2007;369(9573):1603-1613.

Fontaine E, McShane J, Page R, Shackcloth M, Mediratta N, Carr M, . . . Poullis M. Aspirin and non-small cell lung cancer resections: effect on long-term survival. *European journal of cardio-thoracic surgery : official journal of the European Association for Cardio-thoracic Surgery.* Jul 2010;38(1):21-26.

Garcia-Albeniz X, Chan AT. Aspirin for the prevention of colorectal cancer. *Best practice & research. Clinical gastroenterology.* Aug 2011;25(4-5):461-472.

Garcia-Rodriguez LA, Huerta-Alvarez C. Reduced risk of colorectal cancer among long-term users of aspirin and nonaspirin nonsteroidal antiinflammatory drugs. *Epidemiology (Cambridge, Mass.).* Jan 2001;12(1):88-93.

Garcia Rodriguez LA, Gonzalez-Perez A. Risk of breast cancer among users of aspirin and other anti-inflammatory drugs. *British journal of cancer.* Aug 2 2004;91(3):525-529.

Gee JR, Jarrard DF, Bruskewitz RC, Moon TD, Hedican SP, Leverson GE, . . . Messing EM. Reduced bladder cancer recurrence rate with cardioprotective aspirin after intravesical bacille Calmette-Guerin. *BJU international.* Mar 2009;103(6):736-739.

Giovannucci E, Rimm EB, Stampfer MJ, Colditz GA, Ascherio A, Willett WC. Aspirin use and the risk for colorectal cancer and adenoma in male health professionals. *Annals of internal medicine.* Aug 15 1994;121(4):241-246.

Habel LA, Zhao W, Stanford JL. Daily aspirin use and prostate cancer risk in a large, multiracial cohort in the US. *Cancer causes & control : CCC.* Jun 2002;13(5):427-434.

Hassan C, Rex DK, Cooper GS, Zullo A, Launois R, Benamouzig R. Primary prevention of colorectal cancer with low-dose aspirin in combination with endoscopy: a cost-effectiveness analysis. *Gut.* Aug 2012;61(8):1172-1179.

Henschke UK, Luande GJ, Choppala JD. Aspirin for reducing cancer metastases? *Journal of the National Medical Association.* Aug 1977;69(8):581-584.

Hoffmeister M, Chang-Claude J, Brenner H. Individual and joint use of statins and low-dose aspirin and risk of colorectal cancer: a population-based case-control study. *International journal of cancer. Journal international du cancer.* Sep 15 2007;121(6):1325-1330.

Holmes MD, Chen WY, Li L, Hertzmark E, Spiegelman D, Hankinson SE. Aspirin intake and survival after breast cancer. *Journal of clinical oncology : official journal of the American Society of Clinical Oncology.* Mar 20 2010;28(9):1467-1472.

Jacobs EJ, Newton CC, Gapstur SM, Thun MJ. Daily aspirin use and cancer mortality in a large US cohort. *Journal of the National Cancer Institute.* Aug 22 2012;104(16):1208-1217.

Jacobs EJ, Rodriguez C, Mondul AM, Connell CJ, Henley SJ, Calle EE, Thun MJ. A large cohort study of aspirin and other nonsteroidal anti-inflammatory drugs and prostate cancer incidence.

*Journal of the National Cancer Institute.* Jul 6 2005; 97(13):975-980.

Jacobs EJ, Thun MJ, Bain EB, Rodriguez C, Henley SJ, Calle EE. A large cohort study of long-term daily use of adult-strength aspirin and cancer incidence. *Journal of the National Cancer Institute.* Apr 18 2007;99(8):608-615.

Jankowska H, Hooper P, Jankowski JA. Aspirin chemoprevention of gastrointestinal cancer in the next decade. A review of the evidence. *Polskie Archiwum Medycyny Wewnetrznej.* Oct 2010;120(10):407-412.

Jayaprakash V, Menezes RJ, Javle MM, McCann SE, Baker JA, Reid ME, . . . Moysich KB. Regular aspirin use and esophageal cancer risk. *International journal of cancer. Journal international du cancer.* Jul 1 2006;119(1):202-207.

Jayaprakash V, Rigual NR, Moysich KB, Loree TR, Nasca MA, Menezes RJ, Reid ME. Chemoprevention of head and neck cancer with aspirin: a case-control study. *Archives of otolaryngology—head & neck surgery.* Nov 2006;132(11):1231-1236.

Langley RE, Burdett S, Tierney JF, Cafferty F, Parmar MK, Venning G. Aspirin and cancer: has aspirin been overlooked as an adjuvant therapy? *British journal of cancer.* Oct 11 2011;105(8):1107-1113.

Larsson SC, Giovannucci E, Wolk A. Long-term aspirin use and colorectal cancer risk: a cohort study in Sweden. *British journal of cancer.* Nov 6 2006;95(9):1277-1279.

Lee CS, McNamara D, O'Morain CA. Aspirin as a chemoprevention agent for colorectal cancer. *Current drug metabolism.* Nov 2012;13(9):1313-1322.

Lim WY, Chuah KL, Eng P, Leong SS, Lim E, Lim TK, . . . Seow A. Aspirin and non-aspirin nonsteroidal anti-inflammatory drug use and risk of lung cancer. *Lung cancer (Amsterdam, Netherlands).* Aug 2012;77(2):246-251.

Liu E, Sakoda LC, Gao YT, Rashid A, Shen MC, Wang BS, . . . Hsing AW. Aspirin use and risk of biliary tract cancer: a population-based study in Shanghai, China. *Cancer epidemiology, biomarkers & prevention : a publication of the American Association for Cancer Research, cosponsored by the American Society of Preventive Oncology.* May 2005;14(5): 1315-1318.

Lloyd FP, Jr., Slivova V, Valachovicova T, Sliva D. Aspirin inhibits highly invasive prostate cancer cells. *International journal of oncology.* Nov 2003;23(5):1277-1283.

Luo T, Yan HM, He P, Luo Y, Yang YF, Zheng H. Aspirin use and breast cancer risk: a meta-analysis. *Breast cancer research and treatment.* Jan 2012;131(2):581-587.

Mangiapane S, Blettner M, Schlattmann P. Aspirin use and breast cancer risk: a meta-analysis and meta-regression of observational studies from 2001 to 2005. *Pharmacoepidemiology and drug safety.* Feb 2008;17(2):115-124.

McCaffrey P. Aspirin use reduces skin-cancer risk. *The lancet oncology.* Jan 2006;7(1):16.

Mills EJ, Wu P, Alberton M, Kanters S, Lanas A, Lester R. Low-dose aspirin and cancer mortality: a meta-analysis of randomized trials. *The American journal of medicine.* Jun 2012;125(6):560-567.

Mione M, Zon LI. Cancer and inflammation: an aspirin a day keeps the cancer at bay. *Current biology : CB.* Jul 10 2012;22(13):R522-525.

Morgan G. Potential contribution of aspirin to cancer control programmes. *Ecancermedicalscience.* 2008;2:100.

Moyad MA. An introduction to aspirin, NSAIDs, and COX-2 inhibitors for the primary prevention of cardiovascular events and cancer and their potential preventive role in bladder carcinogenesis: part I. *Seminars in urologic oncology.* Nov 2001;19(4):294-305.

Moyad MA. An introduction to aspirin, NSAids, and COX-2 inhibitors for the primary prevention of cardiovascular events and cancer and their potential preventive role in bladder carcinogenesis: part II. *Seminars in urologic oncology.* Nov 2001;19(4):306-316.

Neill AS, Nagle CM, Protani MM, Obermair A, Spurdle AB, Webb PM. Aspirin, nonsteroidal anti-inflammatory drugs, paracetamol and risk of endometrial cancer: a case-control study, systematic review and meta-analysis. *International journal of cancer. Journal international du cancer.* Mar 1 2013;132(5):1146-1155.

Ou YQ, Zhu W, Li Y, Qiu PX, Huang YJ, Xie J, . . . Yan GM. Aspirin inhibits proliferation of gemcitabine-resistant human pancreatic cancer cells and augments gemcitabine-induced cytotoxicity. *Acta pharmacologica Sinica.* Jan 2010;31(1):73-80.

Paterson JR, Lawrence JR. Salicylic acid: a link between aspirin, diet and the prevention of colorectal cancer. *QJM : monthly journal of the Association of Physicians.* Aug 2001;94(8):445-448.

Pennarun B, Kleibeuker JH, van Ek WB, Kruyt FA, Hollema H, de Vries EG, de Jong S. Targeting FLIP and Mcl-1 using a combination of aspirin and sorafenib sensitizes colon cancer cells to TRAIL. *The Journal of pathology.* Feb 2013; 229(3):410-421.

Ratnasinghe LD, Graubard BI, Kahle L, Tangrea JA, Taylor PR, Hawk E. Aspirin use and mortality from cancer in a prospective cohort study. *Anticancer research*. Sep-Oct 2004;24(5B):3177-3184.

Reimers MS, Bastiaannet E, van Herk-Sukel MP, Lemmens VE, van den Broek CB, van de Velde CJ, . . . Liefers GJ. Aspirin use after diagnosis improves survival in older adults with colon cancer: a retrospective cohort study. *Journal of the American Geriatrics Society*. Dec 2012;60(12):2232-2236.

Rothwell PM. Aspirin in prevention of sporadic colorectal cancer: current clinical evidence and overall balance of risks and benefits. *Recent results in cancer research. Fortschritte der Krebsforschung. Progres dans les recherches sur le cancer*. 2013;191:121-142.

Rothwell PM, Fowkes FG, Belch JF, Ogawa H, Warlow CP, Meade TW. Effect of daily aspirin on long-term risk of death due to cancer: analysis of individual patient data from randomised trials. *Lancet*. Jan 1 2011;377(9759):31-41.

Rothwell PM, Price JF, Fowkes FG, Zanchetti A, Roncaglioni MC, Tognoni G, . . . Meade TW. Short-term effects of daily aspirin on cancer incidence, mortality, and non-vascular death: analysis of the time course of risks and benefits in 51 randomised controlled trials. *Lancet*. Apr 28 2012;379(9826):1602-1612.

Rothwell PM, Wilson M, Elwin CE, Norrving B, Algra A, Warlow CP, Meade TW. Long-term effect of aspirin on colorectal cancer incidence and mortality: 20-year follow-up of five randomised trials. *Lancet*. Nov 20 2010;376(9754):1741-1750.

Rothwell PM, Wilson M, Price JF, Belch JF, Meade TW, Mehta Z. Effect of daily aspirin on risk of cancer metastasis: a study of incident cancers during randomised controlled trials. *Lancet*. Apr 28 2012;379(9826):1591-1601.

Salinas CA, Kwon EM, FitzGerald LM, Feng Z, Nelson PS, Ostrander EA, . . . Stanford JL. Use of aspirin and other nonsteroidal antiinflammatory medications in relation to prostate cancer risk. *American journal of epidemiology*. Sep 1 2010; 172(5):578-590.

Sandler RS, Halabi S, Baron JA, Budinger S, Paskett E, Keresztes R, . . . Schilsky R. A randomized trial of aspirin to prevent colorectal adenomas in patients with previous colorectal cancer. *The New England journal of medicine*. Mar 6 2003;348(10):883-890.

Schror K. Pharmacology and cellular/molecular mechanisms of action of aspirin and non-aspirin NSAIDs in colorectal cancer. *Best practice & research. Clinical gastroenterology*. Aug 2011;25(4-5):473-484.

Shebl FM, Sakoda LC, Black A, Koshiol J, Andriole GL, Grubb R, . . . Hsing AW. Aspirin but not

ibuprofen use is associated with reduced risk of prostate cancer: a PLCO study. *British journal of cancer*. Jun 26 2012;107(1):207-214.

Suh O, Mettlin C, Petrelli NJ. Aspirin use, cancer, and polyps of the large bowel. *Cancer*. Aug 15 1993;72(4):1171-1177.

Swede H, Mirand AL, Menezes RJ, Moysich KB. Association of regular aspirin use and breast cancer risk. *Oncology*. 2005;68(1):40-47.

Tan XL, Reid Lombardo KM, Bamlet WR, Oberg AL, Robinson DP, Anderson KE, Petersen GM. Aspirin, nonsteroidal anti-inflammatory drugs, acetaminophen, and pancreatic cancer risk: a clinic-based case-control study. *Cancer prevention research*. Nov 2011;4(11):1835-1841.

Thun MJ, Blackard B. Pharmacologic effects of NSAIDs and implications for the risks and benefits of long-term prophylactic use of aspirin to prevent cancer. *Recent results in cancer research. Fortschritte der Krebsforschung. Progres dans les recherches sur le cancer*. 2009;181:215-221.

Thun MJ, Jacobs EJ, Patrono C. The role of aspirin in cancer prevention. *Nature reviews. Clinical oncology*. May 2012;9(5):259-267.

Thun MJ, Namboodiri MM, Heath CW, Jr. Aspirin use and reduced risk of fatal colon cancer. *The New England journal of medicine*. Dec 5 1991;325(23):1593-1596.

Tian Y, Ye Y, Gao W, Chen H, Song T, Wang D, . . . Ren C. Aspirin promotes apoptosis in a murine model of colorectal cancer by mechanisms involving downregulation of IL-6-STAT3 signaling pathway. *International journal of colorectal disease*. Jan 2011;26(1):13-22.

Urick ME, Giles JR, Johnson PA. Dietary aspirin decreases the stage of ovarian cancer in the hen. *Gynecologic oncology*. Jan 2009;112(1):166-170.

Van Dyke AL, Cote ML, Prysak G, Claeys GB, Wenzlaff AS, Schwartz AG. Regular adult aspirin use decreases the risk of non-small cell lung cancer among women. *Cancer epidemiology, biomarkers & prevention : a publication of the American Association for Cancer Research, cosponsored by the American Society of Preventive Oncology*. Jan 2008;17(1):148-157.

Walker AJ, Grainge MJ, Card TR. Aspirin and other non-steroidal anti-inflammatory drug use and colorectal cancer survival: a cohort study. *British journal of cancer*. Oct 23 2012;107(9):1602-1607.

Yang P, Zhou Y, Chen B, Wan HW, Jia GQ, Bai HL, Wu XT. Aspirin use and the risk of gastric cancer: a meta-analysis. *Digestive diseases and sciences*. Jun 2010;55(6):1533-1539.

Zaridze D, Borisova E, Maximovitch D, Chkhikvadze V. Aspirin protects against gastric cancer: results of a case-control study from Moscow, Russia. International journal of cancer. Journal international du cancer. Aug 12 1999;82(4):473-476.

## METFORMIN

Alimova IN, Liu B, Fan Z, Edgerton SM, Dillon T, Lind SE, Thor AD. Metformin inhibits breast cancer cell growth, colony formation and induces cell cycle arrest in vitro. *Cell cycle (Georgetown, Tex.)*. Mar 15 2009;8(6):909-915.

Anisimov VN. Metformin for aging and cancer prevention. *Aging (Albany NY)*. Nov 2010;2(11): 760-774.

Antonoff MB, D'Cunha J. Teaching an old drug new tricks: metformin as a targeted therapy for lung cancer. *Seminars in thoracic and cardiovascular surgery*. Autumn 2010;22(3):195-196.

Ashinuma H, Takiguchi Y, Kitazono S, Kitazono-Saitoh M, Kitamura A, Chiba T, . . . Tatsumi K. Antiproliferative action of metformin in human lung cancer cell lines. *Oncology reports*. Jul 2012;28(1):8-14.

Beck E, Scheen AJ. [Anti-cancer activity of metformin: new perspectives for an old drug]. *Revue medicale suisse*. Sep 1 2010;6(260):1601-1607.

Belda-Iniesta C, Pernia O, Simo R. Metformin: a new option in cancer treatment. *Clinical & translational oncology : official publication of the Federation of Spanish Oncology Societies and of the National Cancer Institute of Mexico*. Jun 2011;13(6):363-367.

Ben Sahra I, Le Marchand-Brustel Y, Tanti JF, Bost F. Metformin in cancer therapy: a new perspective for an old antidiabetic drug? *Molecular cancer therapeutics*. May 2010;9(5):1092-1099.

Bodmer M, Becker C, Meier C, Jick SS, Meier CR. Use of metformin and the risk of ovarian cancer: a case-control analysis. *Gynecologic oncology*. Nov 2011;123(2):200-204.

Bodmer M, Meier C, Krahenbuhl S, Jick SS, Meier CR. Long-term metformin use is associated with decreased risk of breast cancer. *Diabetes care*. Jun 2010;33(6):1304-1308.

Bonanni B, Puntoni M, Cazzaniga M, Pruneri G, Serrano D, Guerrieri-Gonzaga A, . . . Decensi A. Dual effect of metformin on breast cancer proliferation in a randomized presurgical trial. *Journal of clinical oncology : official journal of the American Society of Clinical Oncology*. Jul 20 2012;30(21): 2593-2600.

Bosco JL, Antonsen S, Sorensen HT, Pedersen L, Lash TL. Metformin and incident breast cancer among diabetic women: a population-based case-control study in Denmark. *Cancer epidemiology, biomarkers & prevention : a publication of the American Association for Cancer Research, cosponsored by the American Society of Preventive Oncology*. Jan 2011;20(1):101-111.

Bost F, Sahra IB, Le Marchand-Brustel Y, Tanti JF. Metformin and cancer therapy. *Current opinion in oncology*. Jan 2012;24(1):103-108.

Cantrell LA, Zhou C, Mendivil A, Malloy KM, Gehrig PA, Bae-Jump VL. Metformin is a potent inhibitor of endometrial cancer cell proliferation—implications for a novel treatment strategy. *Gynecologic oncology*. Jan 2010;116(1):92-98.

Chaiteerakij R, Yang JD, Harmsen WS, Slettedahl SW, Mettler TA, Fredericksen ZS, . . . Roberts LR. Risk factors for intrahepatic cholangiocarcinoma: Association between metformin use and reduced cancer risk. *Hepatology*. Feb 2013;57(2):648-655.

Col NF, Ochs L, Springmann V, Aragaki AK, Chlebowski RT. Metformin and breast cancer risk: a meta-analysis and critical literature review. *Breast cancer research and treatment*. Oct 2012;135(3):639-646.

Decensi A, Puntoni M, Goodwin P, Cazzaniga M, Gennari A, Bonanni B, Gandini S. Metformin and cancer risk in diabetic patients: a systematic review and meta-analysis. *Cancer prevention research*. Nov 2010;3(11):1451-1461.

Del Barco S, Vazquez-Martin A, Cufi S, Oliveras-Ferraros C, Bosch-Barrera J, Joven J, . . . Menendez JA. Metformin: multi-faceted protection against cancer. *Oncotarget*. Dec 2011;2(12):896-917.

Dowling RJ, Goodwin PJ, Stambolic V. Understanding the benefit of metformin use in cancer treatment. *BMC medicine*. 2011;9:33.

Garcia A, Tisman G. Metformin, B(12), and enhanced breast cancer response to chemotherapy. *Journal of clinical oncology : official journal of the American Society of Clinical Oncology*. Jan 10 2010;28(2):e19; author reply e20.

Gonzalez-Angulo AM, Meric-Bernstam F. Metformin: a therapeutic opportunity in breast cancer. *Clinical cancer research : an official journal of the American Association for Cancer Research*. Mar 15 2010; 16(6):1695-1700.

Goodwin PJ, Stambolic V. Obesity and insulin resistance in breast cancer—chemoprevention strategies with a focus on metformin. *Breast (Edinburgh, Scotland)*. Oct 2011;20 Suppl 3: S31-35.

Goodwin PJ, Stambolic V, Lemieux J, Chen BE, Parulekar WR, Gelmon KA, . . . Shepherd LE.

Evaluation of metformin in early breast cancer: a modification of the traditional paradigm for clinical testing of anti-cancer agents. *Breast cancer research and treatment.* Feb 2011;126(1):215-220.

Grenader T, Goldberg A, Shavit L. Metformin as an addition to conventional chemotherapy in breast cancer. *Journal of clinical oncology : official journal of the American Society of Clinical Oncology.* Dec 10 2009;27(35):e259; author reply e260.

Guppy A, Jamal-Hanjani M, Pickering L. Anticancer effects of metformin and its potential use as a therapeutic agent for breast cancer. *Future oncology (London, England).* Jun 2011;7(6):727-736.

Hadad S, Iwamoto T, Jordan L, Purdie C, Bray S, Baker L, . . . Thompson AM. Evidence for biological effects of metformin in operable breast cancer: a pre-operative, window-of-opportunity, randomized trial. *Breast cancer research and treatment.* Aug 2011;128(3):783-794.

Hirsch HA, Iliopoulos D, Tsichlis PN, Struhl K. Metformin selectively targets cancer stem cells, and acts together with chemotherapy to block tumor growth and prolong remission. *Cancer research.* Oct 1 2009;69(19):7507-7511.

Iliopoulos D, Hirsch HA, Struhl K. Metformin decreases the dose of chemotherapy for prolonging tumor remission in mouse xenografts involving multiple cancer cell types. *Cancer research.* May 1 2011;71(9):3196-3201.

Jalving M, Gietema JA, Lefrandt JD, de Jong S, Reyners AK, Gans RO, de Vries EG. Metformin: taking away the candy for cancer? *European journal of cancer.* Sep 2010;46(13):2369-2380.

Jiralerspong S, Gonzalez-Angulo AM, Hung MC. Expanding the arsenal: metformin for the treatment of triple-negative breast cancer? *Cell cycle (Georgetown, Tex.).* Sep 1 2009;8(17):2681.

Kobayashi M, Kato K, Iwama H, Fujihara S, Nishiyama N, Mimura S, . . . Masaki T. Antitumor effect of metformin in esophageal cancer: In vitro study. *International journal of oncology.* Feb 2013;42(2):517-524.

Koch L. Cancer: Long-term use of metformin could protect against breast cancer. *Nature reviews. Endocrinology.* Jul 2010;6(7):356.

Kumar S, Meuter A, Thapa P, Langstraat C, Giri S, Chien J, . . . Shridhar V. Metformin intake is associated with better survival in ovarian cancer: A case-control study. *Cancer.* Feb 1 2013;119(3):555-562.

Landman GW, Kleefstra N, van Hateren KJ, Groenier KH, Gans RO, Bilo HJ. Metformin associated with lower cancer mortality in type 2 diabetes: ZODIAC-16. *Diabetes care.* Feb 2010;33(2):322-326.

Lee DJ, Kim B, Lee JH, Park SJ, Hong SP, Cheon JH, . . . Kim WH. [The effect of metformin on responses to chemotherapy and survival in stage IV colorectal cancer with diabetes]. *The Korean journal of gastroenterology = Taehan Sohwagi Hakhoe chi.* Dec 2012;60(6):355-361.

Lee JH, Jeon SM, Hong SP, Cheon JH, Kim TI, Kim WH. Metformin use is associated with a decreased incidence of colorectal adenomas in diabetic patients with previous colorectal cancer. *Digestive and liver disease : official journal of the Italian Society of Gastroenterology and the Italian Association for the Study of the Liver.* Dec 2012;44(12):1042-1047.

Lee MS, Hsu CC, Wahlqvist ML, Tsai HN, Chang YH, Huang YC. Type 2 diabetes increases and metformin reduces total, colorectal, liver and pancreatic cancer incidences in Taiwanese: a representative population prospective cohort study of 800,000 individuals. *BMC cancer.* 2011;11:20.

Libby G, Donnelly LA, Donnan PT, Alessi DR, Morris AD, Evans JM. New users of metformin are at low risk of incident cancer: a cohort study among people with type 2 diabetes. *Diabetes care.* Sep 2009;32(9):1620-1625.

Liu B, Fan Z, Edgerton SM, Yang X, Lind SE, Thor AD. Potent anti-proliferative effects of metformin on trastuzumab-resistant breast cancer cells via inhibition of erbB2/IGF-1 receptor interactions. *Cell cycle (Georgetown, Tex.).* Sep 1 2011;10(17):2959-2966.

Malki A, Youssef A. Antidiabetic drug metformin induces apoptosis in human MCF breast cancer via targeting ERK signaling. *Oncology research.* 2011;19(6):275-285.

Martin-Castillo B, Vazquez-Martin A, Oliveras-Ferraros C, Menendez JA. Metformin and cancer: doses, mechanisms and the dandelion and hormetic phenomena. *Cell cycle (Georgetown, Tex.).* Mar 15 2010;9(6):1057-1064.

McCarty MF. mTORC1 activity as a determinant of cancer risk—rationalizing the cancer-preventive effects of adiponectin, metformin, rapamycin, and low-protein vegan diets. *Medical hypotheses.* Oct 2011;77(4):642-648.

Nobes JP, Langley SE, Klopper T, Russell-Jones D, Laing RW. A prospective, randomized pilot study evaluating the effects of metformin and lifestyle intervention on patients with prostate cancer receiving androgen deprivation therapy. *BJU international.* May 2012;109(10):1495-1502.

Oleksyszyn J. The complete control of glucose level utilizing the composition of ketogenic diet with the gluconeogenesis inhibitor, the anti-diabetic drug metformin, as a potential anti-cancer therapy. Medical hypotheses. Aug 2011;77(2):171-173.

Papanas N, Maltezos E, Mikhailidis DP. Metformin and cancer: licence to heal? Expert opinion on investigational drugs. Aug 2010;19(8):913-917.

Pollak MN. Investigating metformin for cancer prevention and treatment: the end of the beginning. Cancer discovery. Sep 2012;2(9):778-790.

Rattan R, Ali Fehmi R, Munkarah A. Metformin: an emerging new therapeutic option for targeting cancer stem cells and metastasis. Journal of oncology. 2012; 2012:928127.

Rattan R, Giri S, Hartmann LC, Shridhar V. Metformin attenuates ovarian cancer cell growth in an AMP-kinase dispensable manner. Journal of cellular and molecular medicine. Jan 2011;15(1):166-178.

Rattan R, Graham RP, Maguire JL, Giri S, Shridhar V. Metformin suppresses ovarian cancer growth and metastasis with enhancement of cisplatin cytotoxicity in vivo. Neoplasia (New York, N.Y.). May 2011;13(5):483-491.

Rozengurt E, Sinnett-Smith J, Kisfalvi K. Crosstalk between insulin/insulin-like growth factor-1 receptors and G protein-coupled receptor signaling systems: a novel target for the antidiabetic drug metformin in pancreatic cancer. Clinical cancer research : an official journal of the American Association for Cancer Research. May 1 2010;16(9):2505-2511.

Schneider MB, Matsuzaki H, Haorah J, Ulrich A, Standop J, Ding XZ, . . . Pour PM. Prevention of pancreatic cancer induction in hamsters by metformin. Gastroenterology. Apr 2001;120(5):1263-1270.

Schott S, Bierhaus A, Schuetz F, Beckhove P, Schneeweiss A, Sohn C, Domschke C. Therapeutic effects of metformin in breast cancer: involvement of the immune system? Cancer immunology, immunotherapy : CII. Sep 2011;60(9):1221-1225.

Soranna D, Scotti L, Zambon A, Bosetti C, Grassi G, Catapano A, . . . Corrao G. Cancer risk associated with use of metformin and sulfonylurea in type 2 diabetes: a meta-analysis. The oncologist. 2012;17(6):813-822.

Tseng CH. Diabetes, metformin use, and colon cancer: a population-based cohort study in Taiwan. European journal of endocrinology / European Federation of Endocrine Societies. Sep 2012;167(3):409-416.

Vazquez-Martin A, Oliveras-Ferraros C, Cufi S, Del Barco S, Martin-Castillo B, Lopez-Bonet E, Menendez JA. The anti-diabetic drug metformin suppresses the metastasis-associated protein CD24 in MDA-MB-468 triple-negative breast cancer cells. Oncology reports. Jan 2011;25(1):135-140.

Vazquez-Martin A, Oliveras-Ferraros C, Del Barco S, Martin-Castillo B, Menendez JA. The anti-diabetic drug metformin suppresses self-renewal and proliferation of trastuzumab-resistant tumor-initiating breast cancer stem cells. Breast cancer research and treatment. Apr 2011;126(2):355-364.

Vazquez-Martin A, Oliveras-Ferraros C, del Barco S, Martin-Castillo B, Menendez JA. The antidiabetic drug metformin: a pharmaceutical AMPK activator to overcome breast cancer resistance to HER2 inhibitors while decreasing risk of cardiomyopathy. Annals of oncology : official journal of the European Society for Medical Oncology / ESMO. Mar 2009;20(3):592-595.

Wang LW, Li ZS, Zou DW, Jin ZD, Gao J, Xu GM. Metformin induces apoptosis of pancreatic cancer cells. World journal of gastroenterology : WJG. Dec 21 2008;14(47):7192-7198.

Wright JL, Stanford JL. Metformin use and prostate cancer in Caucasian men: results from a population-based case-control study. Cancer causes & control : CCC. Nov 2009;20(9):1617-1622.

Wu B, Li S, Sheng L, Zhu J, Gu L, Shen H, . . . Di W. Metformin inhibits the development and metastasis of ovarian cancer. Oncology reports. Sep 2012;28(3):903-908.

Wu N, Gu C, Gu H, Hu H, Han Y, Li Q. Metformin induces apoptosis of lung cancer cells through activating JNK/p38 MAPK pathway and GADD153. Neoplasma. 2011;58(6):482-490.

Wysocki PJ, Wierusz-Wysocka B. Obesity, hyperinsulinemia and breast cancer: novel targets and a novel role for metformin. Expert review of molecular diagnostics. May 2010;10(4):509-519.

Yang Y. Metformin for cancer prevention. Frontiers of medicine. Jun 2011;5(2):115-117.

Yasmeen A, Beauchamp MC, Piura E, Segal E, Pollak M, Gotlieb WH. Induction of apoptosis by metformin in epithelial ovarian cancer: involvement of the Bcl-2 family proteins. Gynecologic oncology. Jun 1 2011;121(3):492-498.

Yurekli BS, Karaca B, Cetinkalp S, Uslu R. Is it the time for metformin to take place in adjuvant treatment of Her-2 positive breast cancer? Teaching new tricks to old dogs. Medical hypotheses. Oct 2009;73(4):606-607.

Zakikhani M, Blouin MJ, Piura E, Pollak MN. Metformin and rapamycin have distinct effects on the AKT pathway and proliferation in breast cancer cells. Breast cancer research and treatment. Aug 2010;123(1):271-279.

Zhang Z, Dong L, Sui L, Yang Y, Liu X, Yu Y, . . . Feng Y. Metformin reverses progestin resistance in endometrial cancer cells by downregulating GloI expression. International journal of gynecological cancer : official journal of the International Gynecological Cancer Society. Feb 2011;21(2):213-221.

Zhang ZJ, Zheng ZJ, Kan H, Song Y, Cui W, Zhao G, Kip KE. Reduced risk of colorectal cancer with metformin therapy in patients with type 2 diabetes: a meta-analysis. Diabetes care. Oct 2011;34(10):2323-2328.

Zhang ZJ, Zheng ZJ, Shi R, Su Q, Jiang Q, Kip KE. Metformin for liver cancer prevention in patients with type 2 diabetes: a systematic review and meta-analysis. The Journal of clinical endocrinology and metabolism. Jul 2012;97(7):2347-2353.

Zhu Z, Jiang W, Thompson MD, McGinley JN, Thompson HJ. Metformin as an energy restriction mimetic agent for breast cancer prevention. Journal of carcinogenesis. 2011;10:17.

Zhuang Y, Miskimins WK. Metformin induces both caspase-dependent and poly(ADP-ribose) polymerase-dependent cell death in breast cancer cells. Molecular cancer research : MCR. May 2011;9(5):603-615.

# CIMETIDINE

Adams WJ, Lawson JA, Morris DL. Cimetidine inhibits in vivo growth of human colon cancer and reverses histamine stimulated in vitro and in vivo growth. Gut. Nov 1994;35(11):1632-1636.

Adams WJ, Lawson JA, Nicholson SE, Cook TA, Morris DL. The growth of carcinogen-induced colon cancer in rats is inhibited by cimetidine. European journal of surgical oncology : the journal of the European Society of Surgical Oncology and the British Association of Surgical Oncology. Aug 1993;19(4):332-335.

Adams WJ, Morris DL. Short-course cimetidine and survival with colorectal cancer. Lancet. Dec 24-31 1994;344(8939-8940):1768-1769.

Adams WJ, Morris DL, Ross WB, Lubowski DZ, King DW, Peters L. Cimetidine preserves non-specific immune function after colonic resection for cancer. The Australian and New Zealand journal of surgery. Dec 1994;64(12):847-852.

Bai D, Yang G, Yuan H, Li Y, Wang K, Shao H. Perioperative cimetidine application modulates natural killer cells in patients with colorectal cancer: a randomized clinical study. Journal of Tongji Medical University = Tong ji yi ke da xue xue bao. 1999;19(4):300-303.

Bobek V, Boubelik M, Kovarik J, Taltynov O. Inhibition of adhesion breast cancer cells by

anticoagulant drugs and cimetidine. Neoplasma. 2003;50(2):148-151.

Burtin C, Noirot C, Scheinmann P, Galoppin L, Sabolovic D, Bernard P. Clinical improvement in advanced cancer disease after treatment combining histamine and H2-antihistaminics (ranitidine or cimetidine). European journal of cancer & clinical oncology. Feb 1988;24(2):161-167.

Deva S, Jameson M. Histamine type 2 receptor antagonists as adjuvant treatment for resected colorectal cancer. Cochrane database of systematic reviews. 2012;8:CD007814.

Dillman RO, Soori G, DePriest C, Nayak SK, Beutel LD, Schiltz PM, . . . O'Connor AA. Treatment of human solid malignancies with autologous activated lymphocytes and cimetidine: a phase II trial of the cancer biotherapy research group. Cancer biotherapy & radiopharmaceuticals. Oct 2003;18(5):727-733.

Eaton D, Hawkins RE. Cimetidine in colorectal cancer—are the effects immunological or adhesion-mediated? British journal of cancer. Jan 21 2002; 86(2):159-160.

Fujiwara S, Noguchi T, Suehiro S, Kikuchi R, Noguchi T, Uchida Y. [A case of multiple lung metastases of colon cancer with long-term survival following 5'-DFUR and cimetidine therapy]. Gan to kagaku ryoho. Cancer & chemotherapy. Aug 2003;30(8):1177-1181.

Hayashi A, Kobayashi K, Imaeda Y, Matsumoto S. [Cimetidine inhibits the adhesion of cancer cells with sialyl Lewis epitope onto the vascular endothelium]. Gan to kagaku ryoho. Cancer & chemotherapy. Oct 2003;30(11):1788-1790.

Inhorn L, Williams SD, Nattam S, Stephens D. High-dose cimetidine for the treatment of metastatic renal cell carcinoma. A Hoosier Oncology Group study. American journal of clinical oncology. Apr 1992;15(2):157-159.

Jiang CG, Liu FR, Xu HM, Wu T, Gao J. [Effects of cimetidine on the biological behaviors of human gastric cancer cells]. Zhonghua yi xue za zhi. Jul 11 2006;86(26):1813-1816.

Jiang CG, Liu FR, Yu M, Li JB, Xu HM. Cimetidine induces apoptosis in gastric cancer cells in vitro and inhibits tumor growth in vivo. Oncology reports. Mar 2010;23(3):693-700.

Kawase J, Kobayashi K, Imaeda Y, Umemoto S, Matsumoto S. [An interesting change of E-selectin in cimetidine administration during anticancer drug use]. Gan to kagaku ryoho. Cancer & chemotherapy. Oct 2005;32(11):1578-1579.

Kawase J, Kobayashi K, Imaeda Y, Umemoto S, Ozawa S, Matsumoto S. [Effect of cimetidine on E-selectin expression on the vascular endothelium stimulated by anti-cancer drug]. Gan to kagaku ryoho. Cancer & chemotherapy. Nov 2007;34(12):1902-1904.

Kikuchi Y, Oomori K, Kizawa I, Kato K. Augmented natural killer activity in ovarian cancer patients treated with cimetidine. European journal of cancer & clinical oncology. Sep 1986;22(9):1037-1043.

Kobayashi K, Matsumoto S, Morishima T, Kawabe T, Okamoto T. Cimetidine inhibits cancer cell adhesion to endothelial cells and prevents metastasis by blocking E-selectin expression. Cancer research. Jul 15 2000;60(14):3978-3984.

Kubecova M, Kolostova K, Pinterova D, Kacprzak G, Bobek V. Cimetidine: an anticancer drug? European journal of pharmaceutical sciences : official journal of the European Federation for Pharmaceutical Sciences. Apr 18 2011;42(5):439-444.

Kubota T, Fujiwara H, Ueda Y, Itoh T, Yamashita T, Yoshimura T, . . . Yamagishi H. Cimetidine modulates the antigen presenting capacity of dendritic cells from colorectal cancer patients. British journal of cancer. Apr 22 2002;86(8):1257-1261.

Langman MJ, Dunn JA, Whiting JL, Burton A, Hallissey MT, Fielding JW, Kerr DJ. Prospective, double-blind, placebo-controlled randomized trial of cimetidine in gastric cancer. British Stomach Cancer Group. British journal of cancer. Dec 1999;81(8):1356-1362.

Li B, Cao F, Zhu Q, Li B, Gan M, Wang D. Perioperative Cimetidine Administration Improves Systematic Immune Response and Tumor Infiltrating Lymphocytes in Patients with Colorectal Cancer. Hepato-gastroenterology. Aug 22 2012;60(122).

Li Y, Yang GL, Yuan HY, Bai DJ, Wang K, Lin CR, . . . Feng MH. Effects of perioperative cimetidine administration on peripheral blood lymphocytes and tumor infiltrating lymphocytes in patients with gastrointestinal cancer: results of a randomized controlled clinical trial. Hepato-gastroenterology. Mar-Apr 2005;52(62):504-508.

Lin CY, Bai DJ, Yuan HY, Wang K, Yang GL, Hu MB, . . . Li Y. Perioperative cimetidine administration promotes peripheral blood lymphocytes and tumor infiltrating lymphocytes in patients with gastrointestinal cancer: Results of a randomized controlled clinical trial. World journal of gastroenterology : WJG. Jan 2004;10(1):136-142.

Links M, Clingan PR, Phadke K, O'Baugh J, Legge J, Adams WJ, . . . Morris DL. A randomized trial of cimetidine with 5-fluorouracil and folinic acid in metastatic colorectal cancer. European journal of surgical oncology : the journal of the European Society of Surgical Oncology and the British Association of Surgical Oncology. Oct 1995;21(5):523-525.

Liu FR, Jiang CG, Li YS, Li JB, Li F. Cimetidine inhibits the adhesion of gastric cancer cells expressing high levels of sialyl Lewis x in human vascular endothelial cells by blocking E-selectin expression. International journal of molecular medicine. Apr 2011;27(4):537-544.

Marshall ME, Mendelsohn L, Butler K, Cantrell J, Harvey J, Macdonald J. Treatment of non-small cell lung cancer with coumarin and cimetidine. Cancer treatment reports. Jan 1987;71(1):91-92.

Matsumoto S, Imaeda Y, Umemoto S, Kobayashi K, Suzuki H, Okamoto T. Cimetidine increases survival of colorectal cancer patients with high levels of sialyl Lewis-X and sialyl Lewis-A epitope expression on tumour cells. British journal of cancer. Jan 21 2002;86(2):161-167.

Mavligit GM. Immunologic effects of cimetidine: potential uses. Pharmacotherapy. 1987;7(6 Pt 2):120S-124S.

McCarty MF. Cimetidine as an adjuvant for allogeneic lymphocyte immunotherapy of cancer. Medical hypotheses. Jun 1985;17(2):155-156.

Nagano T, Matsuda H, Park YC, Kurita T. [Successful treatment of metastatic renal cell carcinoma with cimetidine—report of two cases]. Nihon Hinyokika Gakkai zasshi. The japanese journal of urology. Oct 1996;87(10):1201-1204.

Siegers CP, Andresen S, Keogh JP. Does cimetidine improve prospects for cancer patients?. A reappraisal of the evidence to date. Digestion. Sep-Oct 1999;60(5):415-421.

Surucu O, Middeke M, Hoschele I, Kalder J, Hennig S, Dietz C, Celik I. Tumour growth inhibition of human pancreatic cancer xenografts in SCID mice by cimetidine. Inflammation research : official journal of the European Histamine Research Society ... [et al.]. Mar 2004;53 Suppl 1:S39-40.

Svendsen LB, Ross C, Knigge U, Frederiksen HJ, Graversen P, Kjaergard J, . . . Sparso BH. Cimetidine as an adjuvant treatment in colorectal cancer. A double-blind, randomized pilot study. Diseases of the colon and rectum. May 1995;38(5):514-518.

Tang NH, Chen YL, Wang XQ, Li XJ, Yin FZ, Wang XZ. Cooperative inhibitory effects of antisense oligonucleotide of cell adhesion molecules and cimetidine on cancer cell adhesion. World journal of gastroenterology : WJG. Jan 2004;10(1):62-66.

Tatokoro M, Fujii Y, Kawakami S, Fukui N, Komai Y, Saito K, . . . Kihara K. Favorable response to combination treatment of cimetidine, cyclooxygenase-2

inhibitor and renin-angiotensin system inhibitor
in metastatic renal cell carcinoma: Report of three
cases. International journal of urology : official
journal of the Japanese Urological Association.
Sep 2008;15(9):848-850.

Tatokoro M, Fujii Y, Kawakami S, Saito K, Koga F,
Matsuoka Y, . . . Kihara K. Phase-II trial of combination treatment of interferon-alpha, cimetidine, cyclooxygenase-2 inhibitor and renin-
angiotensin-system inhibitor (I-CCA therapy)
for advanced renal cell carcinoma. Cancer
science. Jan 2011;102(1):137-143.

Tomita K, Izumi K, Okabe S. Roxatidine- and
cimetidine-induced angiogenesis inhibition
suppresses growth of colon cancer implants in
syngeneic mice. Journal of pharmacological
sciences. Nov 2003;93(3):321-330.

Tonnesen H, Knigge U, Bulow S, Damm P, Fischerman
K, Hesselfeldt P, . . . et al. Effect of cimetidine on
survival after gastric cancer. Lancet. Oct 29 1988;
2(8618):990-992.

Tonnesen H, Knigge UP, Bulow S, Damm P, Fischerman
K, Hesselfeldt P, . . . et al. [Cimetidine treatment of
stomach cancer]. Ugeskrift for laeger. Jun 12 1989;
151(24):1549-1551.

Uotila P. Inhibition of prostaglandin E2 formation
and histamine action in cancer immunotherapy.
Cancer immunology, immunotherapy : CII.
Sep 1993;37(4):251-254.

Wen QS, Zhang GZ, Kong XT. [Modulation effect of
cimetidine on the production of IL-2 and interferon-
gamma in patients with gastric cancer]. Zhonghua
zhong liu za zhi [Chinese journal of oncology].
Jul 1994;16(4):299-301.

Yoshimatsu K, Ishibashi K, Hashimoto M, Umehara A,
Yokomizo H, Yoshida K, . . . Ogawa K. [Effect of
cimetidine with chemotherapy on stage IV
colorectal cancer]. Gan to kagaku ryoho. Cancer
& chemotherapy. Oct 2003;30(11):1794-1797.

Yoshimatsu K, Ishibashi K, Yokomizo H, Umehara A,
Yoshida K, Fujimoto T, . . . Ogawa K. [Can the survival of patients with recurrent disease after curative
resection of colorectal cancer be prolonged by the
administration of cimetidine?]. Gan to kagaku ryoho.
Cancer & chemotherapy. Nov 2006;33(12):
1730-1732.

Zeng P, Xiao J, Lei Y. [Cell-mediated immune
function in NPC patients treated with cimeti-
dine]. Zhonghua zhong liu za zhi [Chinese
journal of oncology]. May 1995;17(3):223-225.

# Index